MOVEMENT DISORDERS

MOVEMENT DISORDERS
Neurologic Principles and Practice

Editors

Ray L. Watts, M.D.

Associate Professor of Neurology
Director, Division of Movement Disorders
Department of Neurology
Emory University School of Medicine
Atlanta, Georgia

William C. Koller, M.D., Ph.D.

Professor and Chairman
Department of Neurology
University of Kansas Medical Center
Kansas City, Kansas

McGraw-Hill
Health Professions Division

New York   St. Louis   San Francisco   Auckland   Bogotá   Caracas   Lisbon   London   Madrid
Mexico City   Milan   Montreal   New Delhi   San Juan   Singapore   Sydney   Tokyo   Toronto

McGraw-Hill

A Division of The McGraw·Hill Companies

34567890 QPK QPK 90432109

ISBN 0-07-035203-8

This book was set in Palatino by Monotype Composition Co., Inc. The editors were Joseph A. Hefta and Lester A. Sheinis; the production supervisor was Clare Stanley. The cover was designed by Edward Schultheis. The project was managed by Barbara Karni for Monotype Editorial Services. Quebecor Printing/Kingsport was printer and binder.

This book is printed on acid-free paper.

About the cover: The large encompassing sphere represents normal movement. The four overlapping spheres are subsets of normal movement. The sphere at 12 o'clock with the smaller sphere represents akinetic/bradykinetic movement disorders. The sphere at 3 o'clock represents altered movement paths, such as in cerebellar disorders. The sphere at 6 o'clock represents hyperkinetic disorders. The sphere at 9 o'clock represents interrupted movement. (Graphic provided by Allen S. Mandir, M.D., Ph.D.)

Library of Congress Cataloging-in-Publication Data
Movement disorders: neurologic principles and practice / editors,
  Ray L. Watts, William C. Koller.
      p.   cm.
    Includes bibliographical references and index.
    ISBN 0-07-035203-8
    1. Movement disorders.   I. Watts, Ray L. (Ray Lannom).   date.
  II. Koller. Willam C.   date.
    [DNLM: 1. Movement Disorders.   WL 390 M9356 1996]
  RC376.5.M69   1996
  616.8′3—dc20
  DNLM/DLC
  for Library of Congress   96-35518

To our families, whose love, support, and forbearance were critical to the success of the project, and to our patients, whose courage and perseverance in the face of adversity are inspirational for us all

CONTENTS

CONTRIBUTORS *xi*
PREFACE *xv*
COLOR PLATES *Fall between pages 368 and 369*

PART I
INTRODUCTION TO MOVEMENT DISORDERS

1. Approach to the Patient with a Movement Disorder and Overview of Movement Disorders *3*
   Asha Kishore and Donald B. Calne

2. Neurobehavioral Aspects of Movement Disorders *15*
   Dean J. Foti and Jeffrey L. Cummings

3. Neuroimaging of Movement Disorders *31*
   David J. Brooks

PART II
NEUROSCIENTIFIC FOUNDATIONS

4. Oxidative Phosphorylation Diseases and Movement Disorders *51*
   John M. Shoffner

5. Anatomy of the Basal Ganglia and Related Motor Structures *73*
   Garrett E. Alexander

6. Physiology of the Basal Ganglia and Pathophysiology of Movement Disorders of Basal Ganglia Origin *87*
   Thomas Wichmann and Mahlon R. DeLong

7. Functional Biochemistry and Molecular Neuropharmacology of the Basal Ganglia and Motor Systems *99*
   Brian J. Ciliax, J. Timothy Greenamyre, and Allan I. Levey

8. Neurotrophic Factors *117*
   Clifford W. Shults

9. Neuropathology of Movement Disorders: An Overview *125*
   Suzanne S. Mirra, Julie A. Schneider, and Marla Gearing

PART III
CLINICAL DISORDERS

SECTION I
Parkinsonian States

PARKINSON'S DISEASE

10. Epidemiology and Genetics of Parkinson's Disease *137*
    Caroline M. Tanner, Jean P. Hubble, and Piu Chan

11. Neurochemistry and Neuropharmacology of Parkinson's Disease *153*
    G. Frederick Wooten

12. Etiology of Parkinson's Disease *161*
    Yoshikuni Mizuno, Shin-ichirou Ikebe, Nobutaka Hattori, Hideki Mochizuki, Yuko Nakagawa-Hattori, and Tomoyoshi Kondo

13. Clinical Manifestations of Parkinson's Disease *183*
    Henry L. Paulson and Matthew B. Stern

14. Pharmacological Treatment of Parkinson's Disease *201*
    Werner Poewe and R. Granata

15. Transplantation Strategies for Parkinson's Disease *221*
    C. Warren Olanow, Thomas B. Freeman, and Jeffrey H. Kordower

16. Stereotaxic Surgery and Deep Brain Stimulation for Parkinson's Disease and Movement Disorders *237*
    Jerrold L. Vitek

17. Neurobehavioral Abnormalities in Parkinson's Disease *257*
    Eldad Melamed

18. Parkinson's Disease: Neuropathology *263*
    Julian Fearnley and Andrew J. Lees

AKINETIC-RIGID SYNDROMES

19. Progressive Supranuclear Palsy *279*
    Lawrence I. Golbe

vii

20. Multiple-System Atrophy 297
   Lisa M. Shulman and William J. Weiner

OTHER PARKINSONIAN SYNDROMES

21. Infectious and Postinfectious Parkinsonism 307
   Puiu Nisipeanu, Diana Paleacu, and Amos D. Korczyn

22. Toxin-Induced Parkinsonian Syndromes 315
   Rajesh Pahwa

23. Drug-Induced Parkinsonism 325
   Jean P. Hubble

24. Other Degenerative Syndromes That Cause
   Parkinsonism 331
   Wolfgang H. Oertel and J.C. Möller

25. Other Central Nervous System Conditions That
   May Cause or Mimic Parkinsonism 345
   Jacob I. Sage

26. Heredofamilial Parkinsonian Syndromes 351
   Zbigniew K. Wszolek and Ronald F. Pfeiffer

SECTION II

Tremor Disorders

27. Essential Tremor 365
   William C. Koller and Karen L. Busenbark

28. Uncommon Forms of Tremor 387
   Bala V. Manyam

29. The Pathophysiology of Tremor 405
   Rodger J. Elble

SECTION III

Dystonic Disorders

30. Childhood Dystonia 419
   Susan B. Bressman and Stanley Fahn

31. Adult-Onset Idiopathic Torsion Dystonia 429
   Eduardo S. Tolosa and Masso J.F. Martí

32. Treatment of Dystonia 443
   Joseph Jankovic

33. Symptomatic Dystonias 455
   *Justo Garcia de Yébenes, Rosario Sánchez Pernaute,
   and Cesar Tabernero*

SECTION IV

Choreatic Disorders

34. Genetics and Molecular Biology of Huntington's
   Disease 477
   James F. Gusella and Marcy E. MacDonald

35. Clinical Features and Treatment of Huntington's
   Disease 491
   Frederick J. Marshall and Ira Shoulson

36. Neuropathology and Pathophysiology of
   Huntington's Disease 503
   Steven M. Hersch and Robert J. Ferrante

37. Tardive Dyskinesia 519
   Christopher G. Goetz

38. Other Choreatic Disorders 527
   Margery H. Mark

SECTION V

Myoclonic Disorders

39. Classification, Clinical Features, and Treatment
   of Myoclonus 541
   José A. Obeso

40. Pathophysiology of Myoclonic Disorders 551
   Camilo Toro and Mark Hallett

SECTION VI

Tic Disorders

41. Pathophysiology and Differential Diagnosis of
   Tics 561
   Jorge L. Juncos and Alan Freeman

42. Tourette's Syndrome 569
   Roger M. Kurlan

SECTION VII

Cerebellar Disorders

43. Clinical Features and Treatment of Cerebellar
   Disorders 577
   Sid Gilman

44. Pathophysiology of Cerebellar Disorders 587
   Darry S. Johnson and Erwin B. Montgomery, Jr.

SECTION VIII

Other Movement Disorders

45. Corticobasal Degeneration 611
   *Ray L. Watts, Randall P. Brewer, Julie A. Schneider,
   and Suzanne S. Mirra*

46. Wilson's Disease 623
   Ronald F. Pfeiffer

47. Stiff-Person Syndrome 639
   Oscar S. Gershanik

48. Gait and Balance Disorders 649
   John G. Nutt and Fay B. Horak

SECTION IX

Special Considerations

49. Movement Disorders in Childhood   *661*
George W. Paulson and Carson R. Reider

50. Movement Disorders and Aging   *673*
Ali H. Rajput

51. Movement Disorders Specific to Sleep and the Nocturnal Manifestations of Waking Movement Disorders   *687*
David B. Rye and Donald L. Bliwise

52. Psychogenic Movement Disorders   *715*
Néstor Gálvez-Jiménez and Anthony E. Lang

53. Systemic Illnesses That Cause Movement Disorders   *733*
Amy Colcher and Howard I. Hurtig

APPENDIX   Support Organizations for Patients and Educational Organizations for Physicians   *743*

INDEX   *751*

CONTRIBUTORS

Garrett E. Alexander, M.D., Ph.D.* [5]
Department of Neurology, Emory University School of
Medicine, Atlanta, Georgia

Donald L. Bliwise, Ph.D. [51]
Department of Neurology and Emory University Sleep
Disorders Center, Emory University School of Medicine,
Atlanta, Georgia

Susan B. Bressman, M.D.* [30]
Neurological Institute, Columbia-Presbyterian Medical
Center, New York, New York

Randall P. Brewer, M.D. [45]
Department of Neurology, Emory University School of
Medicine, Atlanta, Georgia

David J. Brooks, M.D.* [3]
MRC Cyclotron Unit, Hammersmith Hospital, London,
United Kingdom

Karen L. Busenbark, R.N. [27]
Department of Neurology, University of Kansas Medical
Center, Kansas City, Kansas

Donald B. Calne, M.D.* [1]
Neurodegenerative Disorders Center, University of British
Columbia, Vancouver, British Columbia, Canada

Piu Chan, M.D., Ph.D. [10]
The Parkinson's Institute, Sunnyvale, California

Brian J. Ciliax, Ph.D. [7]
Department of Neurology, Emory University School of
Medicine, Atlanta, Georgia

Amy Colcher, M.D. [52]
Movement Disorders Center, Department of Neurology,
Graduate Hospital, Philadelphia, Pennsylvania

Jeffrey L. Cummings, M.D.* [2]
Department of Neurology, Department of Psychiatry and
Behavioral Sciences, University of California at Los
Angeles School of Medicine; Behavioral Neuroscience
Section, West Lost Angeles Veterans Affairs Medical
Center, Los Angeles, California

Mahlon R. DeLong, M.D.* [6]
Department of Neurology, Emory University School of
Medicine, Atlanta, Georgia

Rodger J. Elble, M.D.* [29]
Department of Neurology and the Center for Alzheimer
Disease and Related Disorders, Southern Illinois
University School of Medicine, Springfield, Illinois

Stanley Fahn, M.D. [30]
Department of Neurology, Columbia-Presbyterian Medical
Center, New York, New York

Julian Fearnley, M.D., M.R.C.P. [18]
National Hospital for Neurology and Neurosurgery,
London, United Kingdom

Robert J. Ferrante, Ph.D. [36]
Geriatric Research and Education Clinical Center, Bedford
Veterans Administration Medical Center, Bedford,
Massachusetts; Departments of Neurology and Pathology,
Boston University School of Medicine, Boston,
Massachusetts

Dean J. Foti, M.D., FRCPC [2]
Division of Neurology, Vancouver Hospital and Health
Sciences Center, University of British Columbia,
Vancouver, British Columbia, Canada

Alan Freeman, M.D. [41]
Division of Movement Disorders, Department of
Neurology, Emory University School of Medicine, Atlanta,
Georgia

Thomas B. Freeman, M.D., [15]
Departments of Neurosurgery and Pharmacology,
University of South Florida, Tampa, Florida

Nestor Gálvez-Jiménez, M.D. [52]
Morton and Gloria Shulman Movement Disorders Centre,
Toronto Hospital Western Division; Department of
Medicine (Neurology), University of Toronto, Toronto,
Ontario, Canada

Marla Gearing, Ph.D. [9]
Department of Pathology and Laboratory Medicine
(Neuropathology), Veterans Medical Center
Administration, Emory University School of Medicine,
Atlanta, Georgia

The number in brackets following the contributor's name refers to the chapter written or cowritten by the contributor. Asterisks
indicate corresponding authors.

Oscar S. Gershanik, M.D.* [47]
Extrapyramidal Disease Section, Centro Neurologico,
Hospital Frances, Buenos Aires, Argentina

Sid Gilman, M.D.* [43]
Department of Neurology, University of Michigan Medical
Center, Ann Arbor, Michigan

Christopher G. Goetz, M.D.* [37]
Department of Neurological Sciences, Rush-Presbyterian-
St. Luke's Medical Center, Chicago, Illinois

Lawerence I. Golbe, M.D.* [19]
Department of Neurology, Robert Wood Johnson Medical
School, University of Medicine and Dentistry of New
Jersey, New Brunswick, New Jersey

R. Granata, M.D. [14]
Department of Neurology, University of Innsbruck,
Innsbruck, Austria

J. Timothy Greenamyre, M.D., Ph.D. [7]
Division of Movement Disorders, Department of
Neurology, Emory University School of Medicine, Atlanta,
Georgia

James F. Gusella, Ph.D.* [34]
Molecular Neurogenetics Unit, Neuroscience Center,
Massachusetts General Hospital, Boston, Massachusetts

Mark Hallett, M.D.* [40]
National Institute of Neurological Disorders and Stroke,
National Institutes of Health, Bethesda, Maryland

Nobutaka Hattori, M.D. [12]
Department of Neurology, Juntendo University School of
Medicine, Tokyo, Japan

Steven M. Hersch, M.D., Ph.D.* [36]
Department of Neurology, Emory University School of
Medicine, Atlanta, Georgia

Fay B. Horak, Ph.D. [48]
R.S. Dow Neurological Sciences Institute, Legacy Good
Samaritan Hospital, Portland, Oregon

Jean P. Hubble, M.D.* [23]
Department of Neurology, The Ohio State University
Medical Center, Columbus, Ohio

Howard I. Hurtig, M.D.* [53]
Movement Disorders Center, Department of Neurology,
Graduate Hospital, Philadelphia, Pennsylvania

Shin-ichirou Ikebe, M.D. [12]
Division of Movement Disorders, Department of
Neurology, Juntendo University School of Medicine,
Tokyo, Japan

Joseph Jankovic, M.D.* [32]
Department of Neurology, Baylor College of Medicine,
Houston, Texas

Darry S. Johnson, M.D. [44]
Department of Neurology, University of Arizona College
of Medicine, Tucson, Arizona

Jorge L. Juncos, M.D. [41]
Division of Movement Disorders, Department of
Neurology, Emory University School of Medicine, Atlanta,
Georgia

Asha Kishore, M.D. [1]
Neurodegenerative Disorders Center, University of British
Columbia, Vancouver, British Columbia, Canada

Wiliam C. Koller, M.D., Ph.D.* [27]
Department of Neurology, University of Kansas Medical
Center, Kansas City, Kansas

Tomoyoshi Kondo, M.D. [12]
Department of Neurology, Juntendo University School of
Medicine, Tokyo, Japan

Amos D. Korczyn, M.D.* [21]
Department of Neurology, Ichilov Hospital; Sackler School
of Medicine, Tel Aviv Medical Center, Tel Aviv, Israel

Jeffrey H. Kordower, Ph.D. [15]
Department of Neurological Sciences, Rush-Presbyterian-
St. Luke's Medical Center, Chicago, Illinois

Roger M. Kurlan, M.D.* [42]
Department of Neurology, University of Rochester
Medical Center, Rochester, New York

Anthony E. Lang, M.D.* [52]
Morton and Gloria Shulman Movement Disorders Centre,
Toronto Hospital Western Division; Department of
Medicine (Neurology), University of Toronto, Toronto,
Ontario, Canada

Andrew J. Lees, M.D.* [18]
National Hospital for Neurology and Neurosurgery,
London, United Kingdom

Allan I. Levey, M.D., Ph.D.* [7]
Department of Neurology, Emory University School of
Medicine, Atlanta, Georgia

Marcy E. MacDonald, Ph.D. [34]
Molecular Neurogenetics Unit, Neuroscience Center,
Massachusetts General Hospital, Boston, Massachusetts

Bala V. Manyam, M.D.* [28]
Department of Neurology, Southern Illinois University
School of Medicine, Springfield, Illinois

Margery H. Mark, M.D.* [38]
Department of Neurology, Robert Wood Johnson Medical
School, University of Medicine and Dentistry of New
Jersey, New Brunswick, New Jersey

Frederick J. Marshall [35]
Department of Neurology, University of Rochester
Medical Center, Rochester, New York

Masso J.F. Martí, M.D. [31]
Neurology Service, Hospital Clínic i Provincial de
Barcelona; University of Barcelona, Barcelona, Spain

Eldad Melamed, M.D.* [17]
Department of Neurology and National Parkinson's
Disease Foundation Research Center, Beilinson Medical
Center, Petah Tiqwa; Sackler School of Medicine, Tel Aviv
Medical Center, Tel Aviv, Israel

Suzanne S. Mirra, M.D. [9*, 45]
Department of Pathology and Laboratory Medicine
(Neuropathology), Emory University School of Medicine;
Veterans Administration Medical Center, Atlanta, Georgia

Yoshikuni Mizuno, M.D.* [12]
Department of Neurology, Juntendo University School of
Medicine, Tokyo, Japan

Hideki Mochizuki, M.D. [12]
Department of Neurology, Juntendo University School of
Medicine, Tokyo, Japan

J.C. Möller, M.D. [24]
Department of Neurology, Philipps-Universität Marburg,
Marburg, Germany

Erwin B. Montgomery, Jr., M.D.* [44]
Department of Neurology, University of Arizona College
of Medicine, Tucson, Arizona

Yuko Nakagawa-Hattori, M.D. [12]
Department of Neurology, Juntendo University School of
Medicine, Tokyo, Japan

Puiu Nisipeanu, M.D. [21]
Department of Neurology, Sackler School of Medicine, Tel
Aviv Medical Center, Tel Aviv, Israel

John G. Nutt, M.D.* [48]
Department of Neurology, Oregon Health Sciences
University, Portland, Oregon

José A. Obeso, M.D.* [39]
Functional Neurology and Neurosurgery Center, Clínica
Quirón, San Sebastian; Centro de Enfermedades del
Sistema Nervioso, Hospiten, Tenerife, Spain

Wolfgang H. Oertel, M.D.* [24]
Department of Neurology, Philipps-Universität Marburg,
Marburg, Germany

C. Warren Olanow, M.D.* [15]
Department of Neurology, Mt. Sinai Medical Center, New
York, New York

Rajesh Pahwa, M.D.* [22]
Department of Neurology, University of Kansas Medical
Center, Kansas City, Kansas

Diana Paleacu, M.D. [21]
Department of Neurology, Sackler School of Medicine, Tel
Aviv Medical Center, Tel Aviv, Israel

George W. Paulson, M.D.* [49]
Department of Neurology, The Ohio State University
Medical Center, Columbus, Ohio

Henry L. Paulson, M.D., Ph.D. [13]
Department of Pharmacology, University of Pennsylvania
and Movement Disorders Center, Graduate Hospital,
Philadelphia, Pennsylvania

Rosario Sánchez Pernaute [33]
Servicio de Neurología, Fundación Jímenez Diaz, Madrid,
Spain

Ronald F. Pfeiffer, M.D.* [46]
Department of Neurology, University of Tennessee School
of Medicine, Memphis, Tennessee

Werner Poewe, M.D.* [14]
Department of Neurology, University of Innsbruck,
Innsbruck, Austria

Ali H. Rajput, M.D.* [50]
Department of Neurology, University of Saskatchewan;
Royal University Hospital, Saskatoon, Saskatchewan,
Canada

Carson R. Reider, M.S. [49]
Department of Neurology, The Ohio State University
Medical Center, Columbus, Ohio

David B. Rye, M.D., Ph.D.* [51]
Department of Neurology and the Emory University Sleep
Disorders Center, Emory University School of Medicine,
Atlanta, Georgia

Jacob I. Sage, M.D.* [25]
Department of Neurology, Robert Wood Johnson Medical
School, University of Medicine and Dentistry of New
Jersey, New Brunswick, New Jersey

Julie A. Schneider, M.D. [45]
Department of Neurological Sciences, Rush-Presbyterian-
St. Luke's Medical Center, Chicago, Illinois

John M. Shoffner, M.D.* [4]
Department of Genetics and Molecular Medicine,
Department of Neurology, Emory University School of
Medicine, Atlanta, Georgia

Ira Shoulson, M.D.* [35]
Department of Neurology, University of Rochester
Medical Center, Rochester, New York

Lisa M. Shulman, M.D. [20]
Department of Neurology, University of Miami School of
Medicine, Miami, Florida

Clifford W. Shults, M.D.* [8]
Department of Neurosciences, University of California at
San Diego, La Jolla, California; Neurology Service,
Veterans Administration Medical Center, San Diego,
California

Matthew B. Stern, M.D.* [13]
Movement Disorders Center, Department of Neurology,
Graduate Hospital, Philadelphia, Pennsylvania

Cesar Tabernero, M.D. [33]
Servicio de Neurología, Fundación Jímenez Diaz, Madrid,
Spain

Caroline M. Tanner, M.D.* [10]
The Parkinson's Institute, Sunnyvale, California

Eduardo S. Tolosa, M.D.* [31]
Neurology Service, Hospital Clínic i Provincial de
Barcelona; University of Barcelona, Barcelona, Spain

Camilo Toro, M.D. [40]
Human Motor Control Section, National Institute of
Neurological Disorders and Stroke, National Institutes of
Health, Bethesda, Maryland

Jerrold L. Vitek, M.D., Ph.D.* [16]
Division of Movement Disorders, Department of
Neurology, Emory University School of Medicine, Atlanta,
Georgia

Ray L. Watts, M.D.* [45]
Division of Movement Disorders, Department of
Neurology, Emory University School of Medicine, Atlanta,
Georgia

William J. Weiner, M.D.* [20]
Department of Neurology, University of Miami Medical
School, Miami, Florida

Thomas Wichmann, M.D. [6]
Division of Movement Disorders, Department of
Neurology, Emory University School of Medicine, Atlanta,
Georgia

G. Frederick Wooten, M.D.* [11]
Department of Neurology, University of Virginia Health
Sciences Center, Charlottesville, Virginia

Zbigniew K. Wszolek, M.D.* [26]
Section of Neurology, University of Nebraska Medical
Center, Omaha, Nebraska

Justo Garcia de Yébenes, M.D.* [33]
Servicio de Neurología, Fundación Jímenez Díaz, Madrid,
Spain

PREFACE

When we were first approached by McGraw-Hill to consider editing this book, we were impressed by their desire to produce an authoritative and comprehensive text on the neurologic basis of movement disorders with emphasis on pathophysiology and treatment, in the vein of their landmark publications Adams and Victor's *Principles of Neurology* and Harrison's *Principles of Internal Medicine*. Given the rapid development of neuroscience research and the fact that movement disorders is one of the most rapidly expanding fields in clinical neuroscience, we felt that a comprehensive new text based on neuroscientific principles that addressed the full spectrum of movement disorders would represent an important contribution. We enlisted the support of internationally renowned colleagues from around the world, and have been gratified by their response. Their outstanding contributions make up the 53 chapters that follow.

The book is organized into three major parts: (I) Introduction to Movement Disorders, (II) Neuroscientific Foundations, and (III) Clinical Disorders. In Part I, Chapter 1 provides an overview of the spectrum of movement disorders, describes how they are identified and differentiated phenomenologically, and examines how a given patient is approached systematically. Chapter 2 covers the very important neurobehavioral aspects of movement disordes based upon neuroanatomical links between regions of the brain that control movement, cognition, and limbic functions. Chapter 3 addresses how functional neuroimaging of movement disorders provides important pathophysiologic and diagnostic information, especially when structure appears intact on routine studies employing computed tomography or magnetic resonance imaging. Part II covers the neuroscientific principles that underpin our current understanding of the pathological anatomy, pathophysiology, biochemistry, and molecular neuropharmacology of movement disorders. Also covered are the normal anatomy, physiology, and biochemistry of brain regions that are involved in movement control. The potentially critical role of neurotrophic factors in health and motor system disease, as well as the possible therapeutic implications, is also discussed. Part III addresses the broad spectrum of neurological disorders that constitute the field of movement disorders as we currently understand it. Sections within Part III cover parkinsonian states (Chapters 10 to 26), tremor disorders (Chapters 27 to 29), dystonic disorders (Chapters 30 to 33), choreatic disorders (Chapters 34 to 38), myoclonic disorders (Chapters 39 and 40), tic disorders (Chapters 41 and 42), cerebellar disorders (Chapters 43 and 44), other movement disorders (Chapters 45 to 48), and special considerations, such as movement disorders in childhood (Chapter 49), movement disorders and aging (Chapter 50), movement disorders and sleep (Chapter 51), psychogenic movement disorders (Chapter 52), and systemic illnesses that cause movement disorders (Chapter 53). All of the chapters on specific movement disorders focus on genetics, epidemiology, biochemical pathology, anatomical localization, pathophysiology, and neuroimaging and how this knowledge affects accurate clinical diagnosis and therapeutics. Most movement disorders are very treatable for the most part, but successful therapy is predicated upon a timely and accurate diagnosis and an understanding of the biochemistry of the system(s) involved.

In every chapter, the latest neuroscientific discoveries are examined in the context of clinical and therapeutic relevance to individual patients with movement disorders. Given this emphasis, the audience for this book will be broad, encompassing medical students, house staff in training, clinicians in practice and academics, neuroscientists with an interest in research related to movement disorders, and other health care professionals involved in the care of patients with movement disorders.

We have strived for accuracy of all information presented, but in such a rapidly changing field new knowledge may emerge between the time the manuscript is written and the book is published. Such is the nature of medical science in the modern era.

We owe special thanks to several individuals who were instrumental in bringing the work to fruition. Our deepest appreciation is extended to our wives, Nancy and Vicki, and our children, Justin, Alexander, Evan, Emily, and Olivia and Todd, Chad, and Kyle, for their encouragement, support, and sacrifices, which made the work possible and enjoyable. Joseph Hefta, medical editor in the Health Professions Division at McGraw-Hill, was tireless and persistent as a facilitator, and his gentlemanly demeanor under all circumstances was very much appreciated. The editorial assistance of Lisa Taylor, administrative assistant in the Department of Neurology at Emory University, was crucial in all aspects of the editorial process, and the book could not have been completed without her tireless effort and long hours of hard work. Her kind and gentle manner, even in periods of intense activity, was appreciated by everyone. We are grateful for the secretarial assistance of Selena Nelson, Claire Guest, and Pat Melching; the many hours of library work checking references by Robert Redden and Walt Hubert; the editorial and production work done by Neil Saunders and the staff of Monotype Composition Company, Inc.; and the administrative support of the Department of Neurology at Emory University and the University of Kansas. We are especially indebted to our colleagues at Emory University, the University of Kansas, and other institutions who contributed chapters, reviewed the scope and contents of the book, and critiqued various aspects. This has been a collaborative process that has yielded a unique product that we hope will serve as a helpful information source for all who are involved in the care and study of patients with neurological disorders that affect movement.

PART I

INTRODUCTION TO MOVEMENT DISORDERS

APPROACH TO THE PATIENT WITH A MOVEMENT DISORDER AND OVERVIEW OF MOVEMENT DISORDERS

ASHA KISHORE and DONALD B. CALNE

HYPERKINETIC DISORDERS
    Dystonia
    Tremor
    Myoclonus
    Chorea
    Pseudoathetosis
    Paroxysmal Dyskinesias (PDS)
    Painful Legs and Moving Toes (PLMT)
    Periodic Leg Movement of Sleep (PLMS)
    Restless Leg Syndrome (RLS)
    Alien Limb
    Tics
    Stereotypy
    Akathisia
    Phantom Dyskinesia
    Hemifacial Spasm (HS)
    Startle Disease or Hyperekplexia
    Stiff-Person Syndrome
HYPOKINETIC DISORDERS
APPROACH TO A PATIENT WITH A MOVEMENT
    DISORDER

The term "movement disorder" is used in two contexts: (1) as a physical sign of involuntary movement or abnormal movement and (2) to describe the syndrome that causes the involuntary movement. Movement disorders occur in a heterogenous group of conditions in which abnormalities in the form and velocity of movements of the body predominate. The abnormal movements in these disorders occur in a conscious patient. Many diseases are associated with more than one type of movement disorder (e.g., chorea, dystonia, and parkinsonism may be seen in Huntington's disease (HD) and Wilson's disease). Abnormalities of movement may be the only manifestation of a disease (e.g., essential tremor (ET), hemifacial spasm, or hemiballismus), or they can be part of a constellation of neurological manifestations of a disease (e.g., HD, progressive supranuclear palsy (PSP), Creutzfeldt-Jakob disease).

Diagnosis of a patient with a movement disorder includes: (1) identifying the type and pattern of the movement disorder; (2) determining whether it is an isolated movement disorder or is associated with other neurological signs; and (3) delineating of the probable etiology (hereditary, sporadic, primary or secondary to a known neurological disease). A carefully taken history with inquiries into the specific characteristics of the movement, presence of heredity, inciting events, exposure to drugs or toxins, and time course of the disease will help to narrow the differential diagnosis and allow one to determine which investigations should be undertaken (see Table 1-1).

Some movement disorders are known to be associated with pathological changes in the basal ganglia (e.g., Parkinson disease (PD), HD), whereas the pathology in many others is still unclear (e.g., idiopathic torsion dystonia (ITD), tardive dyskinesia (TD), Tourette's syndrome, and ET). Abnormal movements are classified according to their clinical phenomenology. This approach broadly categorizes movement disorders as those in which (1) there is excess movement (*hyperkinesias*) or (2) there is a paucity of voluntary and automatic movement that is unaccounted for by weakness or spasticity (*hypokinesias*). The term dyskinesia is used to describe any involuntary or unwanted movement. ET is the commonest movement disorder, followed by idiopathic PD, dystonia, and drug-induced movement disorders.

Hyperkinetic Disorders

An understanding of the clinical patterns of abnormal involuntary movements is necessary to subcategorize these disorders as chorea, dystonia, myoclonus, ballism, tics, tremor, etc. Identification of the type of involuntary movement may be difficult, especially when a combination of different types of movements occurs in the same individual. Repeated examinations and analysis of video records are helpful in such instances. The characteristics that enable these differentiations to be made are: distribution, velocity, amplitude, stereotypy, rhythmicity, suppressibility, relation to posture, activity, sleep, precipitating and relieving factors, diurnal variation, and associated or related sensory and emotional components.

1. Specific distribution, for example, restless-leg syndrome (RLS) and painful legs and moving toes (PLMT);
2. Specific actions, for example, task-specific tremor and dystonia;
3. Speed: slow—for example, dystonia, athetosis, and dystonic tics; quick—for example, myoclonus and myoclonic tics; intermediate: for example, chorea, tremor, and asterixis;
4. Rhythm: continuous—for example, tremor, PLMT; intermittent: for example, asterixis.
5. Relation to posture: RLS only in lying position, tremor at rest, postural, and action and orthostatic tremors;
6. Relation to sleep: sleep-induced, for example, paroxysmal nocturnal dystonia or hypnogenic myoclonus; persistent in sleep: for example, palatal myoclonus.
7. Relation to voluntary movement: for example, action tremor, and action dystonia.
8. Associated sensory symptoms: PLMT, RLS, and phantom dyskinesias.
9. Suppressibilty: volitional in tics, by sensory tricks in dystonia, and by activity in rest tremor.

TABLE 1-1 Approach to a Patient with a Movement Disorder

1. Careful history: With special attention to history of present illness; past medical history; current medications; prior history of medications, toxin exposure, and infections; review of systems; family history (pedigree analysis, if indicated); social history.
2. Thorough physical examination: With special attention to the neurological and mental status examination. Of particular importance: Presence of involuntary movements, facial expression, eye movements and speech, motor examination of the limbs (strength, muscle tone, and coordination), posture and gait, and reflexes.
3. Ancillary studies
   a. Laboratory
      (1) *Routine:* electrolytes (including calcium and phosphorus), BUN/creatinine, liver function tests (including bilirubin total/direct, transaminase levels, alkaline phosphatase), LDH, CPK, globulin and albumin levels, uric acid, complete blood count (including WBC and RBC indices), platelet count, prothrombin time and partial thromboplastin time, thyroid function tests (thyroxine, T3 resin uptake (free T4 index), TSH), serum test for syphilis (FTA)
      (2) *When indicated by history, examination, and/or differential diagnosis:*
         (a) Urine and/or serum toxin and/or heavy metal screen
         (b) Urine collection (24-hour) for copper (along with creatinine and total protein)
         (c) Serum ceruloplasmin (+/− copper) level
         (d) Arterial blood gases
         (e) Peripheral blood smear examination for acanthocytes
         (f) Parathyroid hormone
         (g) Collagen vascular disease/antiphospholipid antibody workup, including antinuclear antibodies, rheumatoid factor, lupus anticoagulant, and antiphospholipid antibodies
         (h) Antistreptolysin O titers (acute and convalescent)
         (i) Viral titers (acute and convalescent)
         (j) Lumbar puncture for pressure measurements and CSF examination (with analyses for glucose, protein, and cell counts with differential, infectious agents, and inflammatory conditions—IgG index, oligoclonal bands . . .)
         (k) Serum folate, vitamin B_{12}, biopterin levels
         (l) Serum lactate and pyruvate
         (m) Serum and urine organic acids and amino acids
         (n) Antineuronal antibodies (serum and/or CSF)
   b. Lumbar puncture (see 3.a(2).(j).)
   c. Ophthalmologic slit-lamp examination
      (for Kayser-Fleischer rings)
   d. Genetic testing (also Table 1-4)
   e. Electrophysiological
      (1) EEG
      (2) EMG/nerve conditions studies
      (3) Evoked responses (VER, BAER, SSER, P300)
      (4) Electronystagmography
      (5) Accelerometric/electromyographic tremor and involuntary movement analysis
      (6) Cortical potentials/Bereitschaftpotential analysis
      (7) Electrical or magnetic transcranial stimulation for central motor pathway conduction studies
      (8) Movement time/reaction time analysis
      (9) Balance platform and gait laboratory assessment
      (10) Jerked locked EEG backaveraging for myoclonus
      (11) Polysomnography/sleep analysis
   f. Neuroimaging (see also Tables 1-4 to 1-7 and Chapter 3)
      (1) Computed tomographic scan(s): head, spine
      (2) Magnetic resonance imaging: head, spine
      (3) Positron emission tomography (PET) and single-photon emission computed tomography (SPECT)
   g. Neuropsychological Testing[65]
   h. Tissue biopsy
      (1) Muscle, nerve, skin, rectal mucosa, bone marrow—for storage/metabolic and inflammatory disorders
      (2) Muscle platelets—oxidative phosphorylation disorders
      (3) Brain—degenerative, infectious, and inflammatory disorders

BUN, blood urea nitrogen; LDH, lactate dehydrogenase; CPK, creatine phosphokinase; WBC, white blood cell; RBC, red blool cell; TSH, thyroid-stimulating hormone; FTA, free treponemal antibody; CSF, cerebrospinal fluid.

10. Aggravating factors: stress and anxiety make all involuntary movements worse, whereas rest and sleep relieve most of them.
11. Precipitating factors: alcohol, caffeine, stress, fatigue, and cold in paroxysmal nonkinesigenic dystonia; quick movements in paroxysmal kinesigenic dyskinesia; and prolonged exercise in paroxysmal exercise-induced dystonia.

DYSTONIA

Dystonia is an abnormal movement characterized by sustained muscle contractions, frequently causing twisting and repetitive movements or abnormal postures.[1] There are often quick components superimposed on the slow movements. Dystonia as a disease can be classified based on its etiology as idiopathic (primary) and symptomatic (secondary). Both primary and secondary dystonias can be familial or sporadic[2] (see Chaps. 30, 31, and 33).

Dystonia can involve any part of the body. According to the site of involvement, dystonia is classified as (1) focal, for example, blepharospasm and torticollis; (2) segmental (when two or more contiguous parts are affected, e.g., Meige's syndrome), (3) multifocal (when two or more noncontiguous parts are involved; (4) hemidystonia; and (5) generalized (crural with involvement of other parts). Hemidystonia calls for investigation of secondary causes, especially stroke, tumor, vascular malformation, and multiple sclerosis[3,4] (see Chap. 33).

RELATION TO ACTIVITY

Dystonia may occur when a body part is at rest (dystonia at rest) or only when a limb is used to perform a voluntary activity (action dystonia). Action dystonia appears only with action whereas a dystonia at rest may be aggravated during action. It is useful to differentiate this relation to activity. ITD generally begins as specific action dystonia, most commonly, dystonia in a foot only when walking. As the disease advances dystonia occurs with nonspecific movements of the involved limb, later with movements of other parts of the body (overflow dystonia) and, ultimately, at rest. Thus any dystonia at rest usually represents a more severe form of dystonia than pure action dystonia. Action dystonia may be task-specific and occur only with specific actions such as occupational cramps (writer's, typist's, and musicians' cramp). Later in the course, less specific actions may induce it.

Dystonic movements are generally slow and arrhythmic; however, they can also be rapid, resembling myoclonus, and these dystonic movements are called myoclonic dystonia. Unless the accompanying dystonia is recognized, the quick movement may be incorrectly diagnosed as myoclonus. EMG in these patients shows prolonged EMG bursts typical of dystonia, rather than the characteristic short-duration bursts seen in myoclonus.[5] A subgroup of patients with idiopathic dystonia has been identified who have shock-like arrhythmic myoclonic spasms and postures. This has been identified to be a genetic variant of ITD, which has an autosomal-dominant pattern of inheritance and responds to alcohol.[6,7] Dystonia can also be associated with fast rhythmic tremulous movements (dystonic tremor).[8]

Dystonia tends to increase with stress, fatigue, and emotional upset. It is relieved by sleep and rest. An interesting feature of dystonia is the patient's frequent ability to suppress a spasm or movement by "sensory tricks" that are usually tactile or proprioceptive stimuli, for example, spasmodic torticollis can sometimes be relieved by placing a hand on the chin or the side of the face (patients may develop pressure palsy of the ulnar nerve if they use this "trick" excessively). Patients with blepharospasm may get relief from touching the skin around the eye. This phenomenon is unique to dystonia, and a positive history can be useful for diagnosis.

Most dystonia is sustained throughout the day. However, it may have a diurnal pattern, with appearance or worsening toward the end of the day, as in the work described by Segawa and colleagues.[9] This condition, with onset in childhood, begins with dystonia in the legs and is dominantly inherited. There may be associated features of parkinsonism, and it can present with an unusual gait, leading to frequent falls; it is commonly mistaken for cerebral palsy. It is extremely sensitive to small doses of L-dopa and, because of this, early diagnosis is essential. This disorder is also termed "L-dopa-responsive dystonia" (DRD)[10] (see Chaps. 30 and 32).

The age of onset of dystonia is important for prognosis as young-onset dystonia tends to evolve into a generalized condition where as adult onset disease is more likely to remain focal.

In primary dystonias the only abnormal finding is dystonia. However, not all isolated dystonias are primary. Approximately 30 percent of dystonias are symptomatic. Onset with dystonia at rest, early occurrence of sustained postures, early affectation of speech (except spasmodic dysphonia), oculogyric crises, sudden onset, rapid course, and hemidystonia should prompt a search for an identifiable cause. Few of the symptomatic dystonias are amenable to treatment, with the notable exception being Wilson's disease. The presence of additional neurological signs, such as spasticity, dementia, cerebellar signs, oculomotor deficits, retinal changes, amyotrophy, or sensory changes, is suggestive of secondary dystonia. Dystonia in association with parkinsonism can occur in idiopathic parkinsonism (IP) as a part of the disease, in patients on chronic L-dopa therapy, in the juvenile dystonia-parkinsonism syndrome, in progressive supranuclear palsy (PSP), corticobasal degeneration (CBD), and the dystonia-parkinsonism syndrome of the Philippines (lubag)[11] (see Chaps. 13, 14, 19, 20, 24, 26, 33, 45, 46, and 49).

Exposure to drugs (D2 dopamine receptor antagonists, L-dopa, anticonvulsants), anoxia, birth injury, toxic exposure (Mn, CO, carbon disulfide, methanol), head injury, stroke, and encephalitis all can cause dystonia (see Chap. 33). Refer to Chaps. 30, 31, and 33 for detailed discussions on the inherited causes of primary and secondary dystonia. There are no diagnostic laboratory tests for primary dystonia.

Acute dystonic reactions consist of sustained painful muscular spasms producing twisting and pulling movements occurring within minutes to hours of exposure to a neuroleptic drug. Torticollis, retrocollis, trismus, blepharospasm, and ocular deviations are the usual manifestations. This represents an idiosyncratic reaction to a dopamine receptor (D2) blocker, and it occurs most commonly in juveniles or young adults.

PSYCHOGENIC DYSTONIA

It is important to rule out a conversion reaction or malingering. False give-way weakness, sensory complaints in the involved limb, multiple somatizations, incongruous and inconsistent postures and limb movements, deliberate slowness of movement, presence of an overt psychiatric disorder, and relief with psychiatric treatment are signs suggestive of nonorganic illness.[12] However, it should be remembered that some organic dystonia, for example, spasmodic torticollis, can undergo spontaneous remission[13] (see Chap. 52).

TREMOR

Tremor comprises involuntary oscillations of a body part produced by alternating or synchronous contractions of reciprocally innervated muscles.[14] It may be fine or coarse, fast or slow, present at rest or when maintaining a posture, or during movement (kinetic tremor).

PHYSIOLOGICAL TREMOR

Muscle fibers whose motor units are being recruited at subtetanic rates produce vibrations. These tremors are of very small amplitude and are demonstrable only by means of an accelerometer or other amplifier systems. When muscle contractions are maintained, the amplitude of this tremor increases, and movement becomes visible to the naked eye.[15] When the tremor becomes noticeable when the arms are held outstretched against gravity or when a person tries to drink from a cup or write, it is called *enhanced physiological tremor.* Anxiety and fear are precipitants. Medical conditions, such as thyrotoxicosis, hypoglycemia, and alcohol withdrawal, and drugs, such as beta 2 agonists (bronchodilators), amphetamines, L-dopa, sodium valproate, lithium, and xanthines, for example, caffeine, can enhance physiological tremor and should be excluded before considering a diagnosis of ET (see Chaps. 27–29).

ET

Tremor is the major clinical manifestation of ET and other neurological signs are typically absent, although one may find mild abnormalities of tone, posture, and balance[16] (see Chap. 27). There is often cogwheeling caused by coarse tremor interrupting the passive movement. ET is typically a postural tremor but may be accentuated by goal-directed movements. Occasionally, it may be present at rest.[16,17] In some patients the tremor becomes manifest only on assuming certain postures, and it may change with alteration in posture. The site of involvement in most cases is the hands, and it is frequently asymmetric initially. Flexion-extension movements of the hand and adduction-abduction movements of the fingers are the commonest types of movement. Occasionally, pronation-supination movements may be seen. The next most common sites of involvement are the cervical and cranial musculature. Tremor may involve the tongue, voice, head, lips, or chin, alone or in combination. Legs and trunk can also be involved.[18] ET can begin at any age. Senile tremor has all the features of ET.[19] Fatigue, emotional upset, and central nervous system (CNS) stimulants can all worsen the tremor. Alcohol can ameliorate ET in many patients even in small quantities. Although this therapeutic effect of alcohol is characteristic of ET, other forms of tremor may also respond, to some extent.[20]

PARKINSONIAN TREMOR

Tremor at rest, at a frequency of 4–5 Hz, is the most characteristic and the most prominent type of tremor in PD, but postural and kinetic tremor are also frequently seen. Onset of tremor is usually in one of the hands[21]; rarely, it may begin in the legs. Rest tremor (RT) is uncommon in other parkinsonian syndromes.[22] Rest tremor is intermittent in the early stages and obvious only under emotional or physical stress. In such instances it can be precipitated by simultaneous mental exercise (serial seven subtractions) and contralateral tight hand gripping. Some patients with ET may develop RT in the late stages. Pathological studies have shown that appearance of RT in ET does not indicate an additional diagnosis of PD.[23] The risk of PD is not increased in ET[22] (see Chaps. 13, 29, and 50).

INTENTION TREMOR

These are rhythmic involuntary oscillations that undergo exacerbation as the hand or foot approaches the target of a voluntary movement. It indicates involvement of the cerebellum or its connections (see Chaps. 28, 43, and 44).

ORTHOSTATIC TREMOR

This is probably a variant of ET. It begins within seconds of assuming a standing posture and involves the trunk and legs. Sitting, standing, or lying can alleviate the tremor. The majority of patients have a postural tremor of the hands and a family history of ET[24] (see Chap. 28).

"WING BEATING" TREMOR

This large-amplitude tremor is brought out when the arms are extended and after a short latency. The tremor results in the arm being thrown up and down. It can increase in severity and even result in imbalance and falls. Changes of posture of the extended arm may alter the severity of the tremor. It is typically seen in Wilson's disease (see Chap. 46).

PSYCHOGENIC TREMOR

This should be suspected when the movements do not have the features of other recognized forms of tremor. Sudden onset, fluctuations in the frequency and direction, influence of distraction, presence of secondary gains, and dramatic response to placebo strengthen the suspicion (see Chap. 52).

Spontaneous clonus can present as rhythmic involuntary oscillations at a joint resembling a tremor, but the context in which it occurs (pyramidal signs, hyperreflexia) helps to differentiate it from tremor.

MYOCLONUS

Myoclonus describes sudden shock-like muscle contractions. They can be focal, multifocal, or generalized. Myoclonus may be regular and rhythmic like tremor, but it is usually random and irregular like chorea. It differs from tremor in that there are visible pauses in between the jerks. It differs from chorea, which is flowing and resembles fragments of normal movements. Tics can resemble myoclonus but are voluntarily suppressible for short periods; furthermore, an inner buildup of tension occurs during the suppression of tics.

Myoclonus is a sign of CNS dysfunction and has been classified as cortical or subcortical in origin (see Chaps. 39 and 40). Cortical myoclonus is an epileptic phenomenon and the technique of back-averaging the electroencephalogram (EEG), using the electromyogram (EMG) activity as a trigger, will demonstrate the transient time-locked cortical event preceding the myoclonic jerk.

As an epileptic phenomenon, myoclonus is almost always associated with other forms of seizures and is more common in children and adolescents. Chronic prolonged focal myoclonic jerking in a child should arouse suspicion of a focal chronic progressive encephalitis. Repetitive, focal, regular myoclonic jerking without loss of consciousness (epilepsia partialis continua) is a focal motor seizure and is of cortical origin.

The combination of myoclonic and generalized seizures with ataxia and dementia signifies a progressive myoclonic epilepsy (PME) syndrome. Detailed investigations, including tissue studies, are required for a definitive diagnosis. The common causes of PME are neuronal ceroid lipofuscinosis, mitochondrial encephalomyopathy, sialidosis, Lafora body disease, Unverricht-Lundborg disease (Baltic myoclonus), GM2 gangliosidosis, and dentatorubropallidoluysian atrophy (DRPLP).

Some specific categories or types of myoclonus are: (a) *Action myoclonus* describes arrhythmic muscular jerking induced by voluntary movement. It can be accentuated by attempts to perform a precise movement (intention myoclonus). Myoclonus also may be provoked by certain sensory stimuli. (b) *Dyssynergia cerebellaris myoclonica* (Ramsay-Hunt syndrome) includes action myoclonus, cerebellar ataxia and, in late stages, dementia and seizures. (c) *Lance-Adams syndrome* comprises chronic action myoclonus in a patient who has sustained an episode of cerebral anoxia; it is often accompanied by cerebellar ataxia.[25] Dramatic response to 5-hydroxytryptophan (5-HTP) is another feature of this condition. (d) *Segmental myoclonus (spinal myoclonus)* involves repetitive myoclonic jerking of an arm or leg and activity in the flexors usually predominates. Spinal cord trauma, tumor, or inflammatory lesions may be responsible.[26] (e) *Palatal myoclonus* involves rhythmic jerking of the soft palate, often in conjunction with the pharynx, larynx, extraocular muscles, and diaphragm. These can persist in sleep and occur at a frequency of around 120 per minute (i.e., 2/s). The site of the lesion is often the inferior olive, central tegmental tract, or dentate nucleus, and the etiologic workup should include: vascular, neoplastic, inflammatory, degenerative, or metabolic causes, such as dialysis encephalopathy.[27] A response to 5-HTP can be diagnostic. (f) *Asterixis* (negative myoclonus) results in brief lapses of posture manifesting as flaps of the dorsiflexed hand. However, it is less rhythmic than tremor. EMG reveals irregular silent periods during these flaps. It is commonly seen in the setting of metabolic encephalopathies, as a reaction to general anesthesia, and during anticonvulsant therapy.

CHOREA

Chorea and *ballism* can be defined separately as clinically distinct signs but they often merge together and resemble each other. In addition, they may also have a common anatomic and physiological basis (see Chaps. 34–38). Chorea consists of arrhythmic, rapid, often jerky movements that may be simple or complex and are usually distal and of low amplitude. Choreic movements are purposeless, but patients may incorporate them into a deliberate movement as if to make them less noticeable. The movements may be very discrete or resemble fidgetiness, which may be considered normal, especially in children. Facial grimacing and abnormal respiratory sounds are other manifestations of chorea. Chorea is often associated with hypotonia of the limbs. The knee jerk may be pendular. Large-amplitude, proximal choreic movements are called *ballism*. The movements are often violent and flinging in nature. The causative lesion is usually vascular. Ballism is usually limited to one side of the body (hemiballism), but it may occur bilaterally (biballism). Monoballism is confined to one limb. Metabolic disturbances, such as nonketotic hyperglycemia or hypoglycemia, are also known to produce choreoballism.

Chorea may be the only neurological sign of disease (e.g., rheumatic chorea, thyrotoxicosis, vascular disease) or it may be present as part of the neurological spectrum of a disease (HD, neuroacanthocytosis) (see Table 1-2).

Tardive dyskinesia (TD) or tardive chorea is defined as abnormal involuntary movement appearing after treatment with a neuroleptic drug for 3 months or more in patients with no other identifiable cause for a movement disorder[28] (see Chap. 37). TD can persist after withdrawal of the offending drug and, in most instances, is unmasked only when the dose of drug is reduced or stopped. Although chorea in other diseases is typically nonstereotyped, tardive chorea may be stereotyped.[29] Rhythmical and complex chewing movements (oral-buccal-lingual dyskinesia) represent the classic presentation of TD. The oral movements of TD are more complex than those seen in other choreatic disorders. Irregular and frequent tongue protrusion is called flycatcher

TABLE 1-2 Causes of Chorea

Hereditary-dominant	HD, PDS, DPRLA, neuroacanthocytosis, benign hereditary chorea
Hereditary-recessive	Wilson's disease, Niemann-Pick disease, Pelizaeus-Merzbacher disease, Hallervorden-Spatz disease, ataxia telengiectasia, Lesch-Nyhan disease
Maternal inheritance	Mitochondrial encephalopathies
Autoimmune	Rheumatic chorea, chorea gravidarum, systemic lupus erythematosis (SLE), periarteritis nodosa, Behçet's disease
Vascular	Infarcts
Metabolic	Hypo- or hypernatremia, hypocalcemia, hypo- or hyperglycemia, hyperthyroidism, renal failure, hypoparathyroidism.
Toxins	Mercury, carbon monoxide
Inflammatory	Encephalitis, AIDS
Drugs	Neuroleptics, metoclopramide, L-dopa, anticonvulsants, steriods, oral contraceptives

AIDS, acquired immune deficiency syndrome; DRPLA, L-dopa-responsine dystonia; PDS, paroxysmal dyskinesias.

tongue. Tardive chorea, when confined to the trunk or distal extremities and unaccompanied by orofacial dyskinesia, may not be recognized as drug-induced. TD may involve the abdominal and pelvic muscles producing truncal or pelvic rocking or thrusting movements.

Respiratory dyskinesias can result in involuntary chest and diaphragmatic movements that resemble hyperventilation related to anxiety.[30] The typical chorea in TD is brief but frequently may be associated with more sustained movements (tardive dystonia). In drug-induced tardive syndromes, it is common to see choreatic/dyskinetic movements and dystonic movements in the same patient, and these may be accompanied by tardive akathisia (motor restlessness) as well.

PSEUDOATHETOSIS

Athetosis is a term that formerly was used for writhing movements. It has now largely been replaced by the term dystonia, but the term pseudoathetosis persists. Proprioceptive sensory loss can lead to abnormal slow movements resembling athetosis or dystonia. These can occur with lesions anywhere along the proprioceptive sensory pathways from parietal cortex, thalamus, spinal cord, dorsal root ganglia, and peripheral nerves.[31] The involuntary movements may be suppressed by supporting the limb, unlike the dystonia seen in other conditions.

PAROXYSMAL DYSKINESIAS (PDS)

PDSs are a heterogeneous group of disorders characterized by involuntary movements in bursts with return to normality within variable periods. The movements are sometimes bizarre and may be mistaken for a hysterical disease. Attacks are generally painless and stereotyped. There is no alteration of consciousness, incontinence of urine, postictal confusion, or amnesia. The most widely used classification, put forth by Lance, divides PDSs into prolonged attacks lasting for more than 5 minutes (paroxysmal dystonia) and brief attacks precipitated by movement lasting less than 5 minutes (paroxysmal kinesigenic choreoathetosis [PKC]).[32] Both can be familial or sporadic, and the latter may be primary or secondary.

PKC is precipitated by such movements as a sudden change of posture after a period of resting, rising from a chair, turning in bed, or running. It can last for seconds to a few minutes. Emotional upset and excitement can trigger an attack. Hyperventilation may also induce an episode. Sensory symptoms can precede the attack, and they usually take the form of numbness, pins and needles, or stiffness.[32–34] Most of the brief attacks are dystonic in nature with extension of the leg with equinovarus posturing, arm abduction, wrist extension, and elbow flexion. There may be facial grimacing or torsion of the trunk. In some patients the movements are choreatic or ballistic.[35] The attacks may be suppressed by rest or pressure on the affected limb. Attacks may be unilateral or bilateral. Seizures are the most common neurological disorder associated with PKCs. The familial and primary sporadic PKCs are benign nonprogressive conditions responsive to anticonvulsant treatment (see Chaps. 32, 33, and 38).

Paroxysmal dystonia is often familial but may also be sporadic and is frequently triggered by stress, fatigue, caffeine, or alcohol. It can last for minutes to hours. Several sensory phenomena or an aura can precede the attack, and they usually involve the limb in which the abnormal movement appears. The patient may describe the symptoms as tightening, stiffness, pins and needles, or vague indescribable sensations. The dystonic posturing begins in one limb and may progress to involve all four limbs with facial grimacing and arching of the back. When bilateral, it can affect postural stability and result in a fall. Orofacial dystonia can lead to dysarthria. Chorea may be superimposed on dystonia in varying proportions.[32] Most patients are able to suppress their attacks partially or completely with rest. Others gain reported benefit from physical or mental activity or rubbing the affected limb.[36,37] The attacks usually respond to clonazepam or other benzodiazepines. Both normal and abnormal EEGs have been reported with PDSs.[33,34] Secondary causes should be sought in nonfamilial, nonkinesigenic PDSs. Potential etiologies include multiple sclerosis, myelopathy, encephalitis, head injury, cerebral ischemia, cerebral palsy, focal seizures, radiculopathy, thyrotoxicosis, hypoglycemia, hemiparesis, psychogenic, and reflex sympathetic dystrophy.[38]

Familial paroxysmal dystonia can be induced by exercise. The attacks are usually provoked by prolonged exertion, rather than sudden movements. In a report of one family, dystonia could be induced focally in any limb by exercise or sensory stimulation restricted to that limb.[39]

Paroxysmal nocturnal dystonia occurs during nonrapid eye movement (non-REM) sleep (see Chap. 51). Attacks are restricted to the night during sleep or on awakening in the morning. They may occur several times during the night and are sometimes associated with epileptic seizures.[40,41] Some patients have both daytime and nocturnal attacks. The ictal EEG is usually normal. The pathogenesis of this condition has remained controversial, and it is considered to be a variant of frontal lobe seizures by some.[42,43] Both familial and sporadic paroxysmal nocturnal dystonia cases occur.

PAINFUL LEGS AND MOVING TOES (PLMT)

The motor component of this syndrome is usually confined to the toes but may involve proximal parts of the legs. The movements are generally continuous, stereotyped, and flexion-extension or adduction-abduction movements of the toes.[44] Rarely, the upper limbs can be affected.[45] The movements tend to disappear during sleep although, rarely, they can persist. Immersing the body in hot or cold water will sometimes relieve the symptoms and rest can be helpful. The sensory symptoms may range in severity from mild to excruciating pain, which has a deep, boring quality. The pain is not distributed in any dermatomal, myotomal, or peripheral nerve distribution. It differs from akathisia in that there is no subjective desire to move the limbs, and patients strive to stop the movements. The movements give no relief from the sensory phenomena. The neurological examination is normal, except in cases associated with peripheral neuropathy or radiculopathy (see Chap. 51).

PERIODIC LEG MOVEMENT OF SLEEP (PLMS)

Nocturnal myoclonus or PLMS is distinct from the hypnic jerks experienced by normal individuals on falling asleep (see Chap. 51). The movements of PLMS consist of repetitive stereotyped extension of the big toe. The ankle, knee, and the hip may flex after the toe has extended.[46] The myoclonic jerks are generally bilateral but may involve either leg alone. The events occur in clusters lasting from 10 minutes to several hours and in some people throughout nocturnal sleep. PLMS can be associated with RLS.[47] The movements are characteristically periodic and recur on a regular basis every 30 seconds for prolonged periods during stages 1 and 2 of non-REM sleep.

RESTLESS LEG SYDROME (RLS)

RLS (Ekbom's syndrome) is a symptom complex of discomfort in the legs that is characteristically relieved by movement (see Chap. 51). The abnormal sensations are deep seated and usually localized to the lower limbs although, rarely, similar symptoms also occur in the upper extremities. The abnormal sensations are described as crawling, pulling, stretching, itching, or creeping, all typically felt in the bone, muscles, or tendons. The symptoms are maximal when the patient is in bed at night, usually within 15–20 minutes of assuming the recumbent posture. In milder cases patients get relief by massaging their legs or kicking their legs in the air. In severe cases patients need to pace the floor for temporary relief. RLS differs from akathisia, which also causes discomfort and the desire to move but occurs during the day. RLS is not accompanied by other neurological symptoms or signs. An association has been reported with several medical conditions such as diabetes, vitamin deficiencies, pregnancy, uremia, malabsorption, carcinoma, chronic pulmonary disease, amyloidosis, etc.[48] Many of these conditions are associated with sensory neuropathy, and thus, some of these cases are likely to represent secondary RLS.

ALIEN LIMB

To diagnose alien limb, there should be either a feeling of "foreignness" about movements of the affected limb or a lack of recognition of movement in the affected limb(s).[49] The movements in alien limb are complex and look purposeful, although they are involuntary. Patients try to restrain the limb, punish it, or personify it and talk to it. The movements may be groping, pushing aside, striking, or prehension of body parts or clothing. Alien hand occurs in a nonparalyzed limb and in the absence of any sensory loss; thus, it is different from anosognosia.

An alien hand can occur after surgical transection of the corpus callosum, tumors of the medial portion of the hemisphere invading the corpus callosum, or infarction of the medial frontal cortex.[50–52]

Alien limb phenomenon occurs in a significant proportion of patients with corticobasal degeneration (CBD). It may take the form of simple hand or leg levitation, involuntary groping of the hands to the face or other body parts, or complex movements, such as exploring a purse, removing eye glasses, or touching the examiner.[53] Often there are associated features such as apraxia, dystonia, and cortical sensory loss (see Chap. 45).

TICS

A tic is an involuntary, rapid, nonrhythmic movement (motor tic) or sound (vocal tic) (see Chaps. 41 and 42) Tic occurs on a background of normal activity. Motor and vocal tics can be either simple or complex. A simple motor tic is an abrupt, brief, isolated movement, such as an eye blink, shoulder shrug, facial grimace, contraction of abdominal muscle, or head jerk (clonic tic). Slower sustained movements can also occur and are called dystonic tics, for example, neck turning, blepharospasm, etc. Complex motor tics include stereotyped facial expressions or patterned coordinated repetitive movements, such as touching or grooming behavior, smelling objects or body parts, shaking hands, scratching, kicking, squatting, or obscene gesturing. The coordinated nature of the tics makes it difficult to differentiate them from voluntary movements. Many of these overlap with compulsive behavior. Simple vocal tics usually consist of throat clearing, grunting, coughing, clicking, snorting, or animal sounds, such as hissing, barking, growling, hooting, or quacking. Complex vocal tics include words and phrases but, more often, obscene utterances or religious profanities. Tics are exacerbated by stress, anxiety, and fatigue and are relieved by concentration on a task or absorbing activities, such as reading or playing a musical instrument. They are usually first reported by parents, friends, and teachers. Tics are variable in frequency, duration, amplitude, and location. Tics are usually multifocal and can migrate from one location to the other, but the most common sites of occurrence are the face, head, neck, and shoulders.

Tics are seen in normal people (mannerisms). Transient tic disorder occurs in up to 15 percent of children and adolescents and usually takes the form of a simple motor or vocal tic. It may last only a brief period, occurring for periods of 2 weeks to a year. There may be transient periods of recurrence in adult life during periods of stress (see Chaps. 41 and 42).

Dopamine-blocking drugs can cause tics as a tardive syndrome,[54] but such agents can also be used to treat tics. Chronic tic disorder typically begins before the 21 years of age and persists for more than a year. In Tourette's syndrome (TS) the tics are chronic, multifocal, motor, and vocal. TS is associated with attention deficit disorder with hyperactivity, sleep disorders, obsessive-compulsive behavior, echolalia (repeating sounds and words from an external source, usually, the last sound), echopraxia (repeating movements of another person), palilalia (repeating one's own words or sounds with increasing speed and decreasing clarity), coprolalia (obscene utterances), and copropraxia (obscene gesturing) (see Chap. 42).

Characteristic features of tics include:[55]

1. Occurrence of an unusual sensation and an irresistible urge to move before the tic. Execution of the tic relieves the tension that mounts before the movement. The association of sensory phenomena before an involuntary move-

ment can also occur in akathisia, phantom dyskinesia, RLS, and PLMTs. In akathisia the restlessness is constant without a buildup before the movement. In akathisia the movements are stereotyped, repetitive, continuous, and the usual patterns are pacing, crossing and uncrossing of legs, or stamping of the feet.

2. Ability to voluntarily suppress the tic for a short time. Voluntary suppression usually leads to a buildup and rebound exacerbation of tics. However, patients with tremor, dystonia, chorea, and ballism may also be able to suppress their movements temporarily by change of position, autohypnosis, or biofeedback.

3. Occurrence during all stages of sleep.

STEREOTYPY

These movements occur continuously. Stereotypy is seen in Rett syndrome (RS), autism, mental retardation, schizophrenia, TD, and Lesch-Nyhan syndrome. In RS these movements consist of stereotypic hand washing, hand wringing, squeezing, clapping, and mouthing. The movements seen in classical tardive dyskinesia are often rhythmical and may be classified as stereotypic movements (see Chaps. 24, 33, 37, and 49).

AKATHISIA

The motor activity in akathisia is described by patients as a voluntary effort to relieve uncomfortable sensations. Akathisia is usually expressed as changes in body position, standing, or pacing. In milder forms this can be voluntarily suppressed. In severe cases the need for motor activity is beyond control.[56]

Acute akathisia can occur after the administration of an antipsychotic drug. It is dose-related, and the onset of symptoms may coincide with an increase in dose. Acute akathisia can occur within minutes of administration of the offending drug. Patients are usually young, with short periods of exposure to antipsychotics, and they have no manifestations of TD.[56] Tardive akathisia implies that the symptoms appear long after the start of neuroleptic treatment (more than 3 months) and persist despite the reduction or discontinuation of the drug. The condition has a high incidence of orofacial and limb dyskinesia in association with subjective restlessness.

The characteristic syndrome entails the inability to remain seated, repetitive shifting of weight, rocking of the trunk while standing, pacing or, in severe cases, marching. Continuous shuffling and feet tapping are difficult to differentiate from choreoathetotic dyskinesia. The subjective distress with the need to move is crucial in differentiating akathisia from TD.

PHANTOM DYSKINESIA

Amputees can experience paresthesiae and other sensory phenomena with associated involuntary movements of the stump (spontaneously or in the presence of exposure to dopamine-blocking drugs).[57,58]

HEMIFACIAL SPASM (HS)

In HS unilateral contraction of the facial muscles involving the eyelids, cheek, and the corner of the mouth occurs (see Chaps. 31 and 32). It usually involves both upper and lower parts of the face and may be continuous or intermittent. The attacks can be provoked by voluntary forced contraction of the facial muscles, followed by relaxation. The cause may consist of any irritative lesion of the ipsilateral facial nerve. In the absence of an obvious lesion it is sometimes thought to be caused by facial nerve compression by a blood vessel in its intracranial course. In HS, the EMG may reveal some degree of denervation in the facial muscles. Hemifacial spasm can be distinguished from early blepharospasm, because the latter is seldom unilateral.

STARTLE DISEASE OR HYPEREKPLEXIA

Abnormal excessive startle in response to a sudden unexpected stimulus can occur in three distinct conditions: Startle disease or hyperekplexia, startle epilepsy, and a condition called the Jumping Frenchmen of Maine (see Chaps. 39 and 40).

Startle disease is a rare and poorly understood condition that can be both familial and sporadic. In a mild form it results in an exaggeration of the normal startle response. When patients with severe symptoms are startled, they experience generalized muscle stiffness with loss of postural control and falling. As soon as they hit the ground there is recovery of normal muscle tone and control of voluntary muscles.[59] The attacks are precipitated by emotional tension and fatigue. Alcohol, phenobarbital, and chlordiazepoxide can lessen the intensity to some extent.

STIFF-PERSON SYNDROME

This is a rare condition with continuous isometric contractions of somatic muscles, frequently involving the trunk and, occasionally, the limbs. The contractions are painful and may result in opisthotonos. Chap. 47 discusses the disorder in detail.

Hypokinetic Disorders

BRADYKINESIA

Bradykinesia is slowness of movement execution with progressive reduction in the speed and amplitude of repetitive movements. It is usually associated with rigidity. Bradykinesia is evident in the typical appearance of a patient with PD, and examples are slowness of limb and body movements, reduced facial expression, low voice volume, monotonous speech, and reduced blinking. Bradykinesia can be demonstrated by asking the patient to perform hand and foot movements. A sample of the handwriting may reveal micrographia, and arm swing is reduced when walking.

RIGIDITY

Rigidity is an increase in muscle tone during passive movement. Asymmetric rigidity is an important diagnostic clue for PD. Rigidity may be smooth (lead pipe) or ratchety (cogwheel in the presence of tremor). Rigidity is usually more evident in the distal joints of the limb. To properly assess rigidity the patient being examined must be able to relax. Voluntary activation of the contralateral muscles (e.g., drawing circles in the air) increases tone in the side being examined and may bring out an asymmetry that was undetected in the resting state (augmentation).

POSTURAL INSTABILITY

In the majority of patients with PD, postural and gait abnormalities occur within 5 years of the onset of symptoms.[60] Righting reflexes are impaired, and this can be tested by instructing the patient to maintain balance with the feet separated after the examiner's sudden pull from behind.

PARKINSONIAN SYNDROMES

The constellation of tremor, rigidity, bradykinesia, and loss of postural reflexes constitute parkinsonism. Although classically seen in PD (Chap. 13), parkinsonism may have other causes. In the elderly these include dopamine-blocking drugs (Chap. 23), PSP (Chap. 19), multiple system atrophy (MSA) (Chap. 20), striatonigral degeneration (SND) (Chap. 20), Shy-Drager syndrome (SDS) (Chap. 20), cortico basal degeneration (CBD) (Chap. 45), Alzheimer's disease (AD) with parkinsonism (Chap. 2), and diffuse Lewy body disease (DLD) (Chap. 24). Parkinsonism in a young person may be caused by juvenile-onset dystonia/parkinsonism (Chap. 24), Westphal variant of HD (Chaps. 35 and 49), Wilson's disease (Chap. 46), L-dopa-responsive dystonia (Chap. 30), Hallervorden-Spatz disease (Chap. 24), and progressive pallidal degeneration (Chap. 24).

IDIOPATHIC PARKINSONISM (IP)/PARKINSON'S DISEASE (PD)

The typical patient is between 50 and 70 years old. In some cases symptoms can start before the age of 40 years. The diagnosis is generally made when two of three cardinal features of parkinsonism are present, that is, tremor, rigidity, or bradykinesia. Some patients may have postural instability and gait abnormality as early manifestations of the disease.[61] However, postural instability and slowness may be seen in normal healthy elderly individuals.[62,63] Hence, postural instability is better used as an adjunct to the diagnosis (see Chap. 13). Some slowing of movement and stooped posture is common in old age and should not lead to a diagnosis of IP (see Chap. 50). Depression is another common condition that may mimic IP when psychomotor retardation is present (because of the reduced facial animation and slowness of movements), although both conditions frequently coexist.

In the early stages of the disease oligosymptomatic patients may not satisfy all inclusion criteria. Calne et al. have proposed stratifying patients into three groups of increasing diagnostic certainty—possible, probable, and definite.[64] Exclusion criteria are summarized in Table 1-3.

TABLE 1-3 Exclusion Criteria for Idiopathic Parkinsonism

1. Neuroleptics, calcium channel-blocking drugs
2. Exposure to toxins; MPTP, CO inhalation, manganese, methanol, *n*-hexane
3. Definite encephalitis
4. Strokes and stepwise deterioration
5. Repeated head injury
6. Early and severe dementia or autonomic dysfunction
7. Cerebellar signs, supranuclear gaze palsy, and negative response to high doses of L-dopa.

MPTP, 1-methyl-4-phenyl-1,2,3,6-tetrahydropyridine.

PSP

PSP should be suspected in the presence of symmetrical onset of parkinsonian symptoms, frequent falls as an early manifestation, prominent axial rigidity, early dysarthria, lack of tremor, frontal lobe dementia, lack of significant L-dopa responsiveness, and impaired vertical gaze (see Chap. 19).

MSA

MSA is a single term that encompasses three of the commonest forms of "atypical" parkinsonism, namely, SND, SDS, and sporadic olivopontocerebellar atrophy (OPCA) (Chap. 20).

SDS presents as akinetic-rigid parkinsonism with early and prominent autonomic dysfunction in the form of urinary incontinence, postural hypotension, upper airway obstruction, cardiac arrhythmia, and pupillary changes (see Chap. 20).

SND is suspected in the presence of an akinetic-rigid parkinsonism unresponsive to L-dopa. A confirmed diagnosis requires autopsy (see Chap. 20).

OPCA has parkinsonism and cerebellar ataxia as major features. It can occur as a familial condition with autosomal-dominant inheritance and phenotypic heterogeneity. Some of the common associated signs are disorders of eye movement, dementia, retinal degeneration, and pyramidal tract signs. Sporadic cases are included under MSA (see Chap. 20).

CBD

The clinical manifestations of CBD are rigid-bradykinetic parkinsonism with cortical signs such as apraxia, cortical sensory loss, and the alien hand phenomenon. Asymmetric onset, dystonic limb postures, myoclonus, lack of L-dopa responsiveness, and gradual progression are other characteristic features (see Chap. 45).

ALZHEIMER'S DISEASE (AD) WITH PARKINSONISM

Many patients with AD have mild parkinsonism. When these signs are present early in the course of AD, they may be mistaken for IP. It can also be difficult to exclude the possibility of diffuse Lewy body disease when dementia and parkinsonism are initial manifestations (see Chaps. 2, 24, and 45).

Approach to a Patient with a Movement Disorder

Much of this book is dedicated to how patients with specific movement disorders present to the clinician and how they

TABLE 1-4 Molecular Genetics in Movement Disorders

Name of Disease	Type of Inheritance
Huntington's disease (HD)	AD
ET	AD
ITD	AD
Neuroacanthocytosis	AD/AR/X-linked
Lubag	X-linked
Paroxysmal dyskinesias	AD
Spinocerebellar ataxia (SCA 1 and 2)	AD
Machado-Joseph disease (familial OPCA)	AD
DRD	AD
Tourette's syndrome	AD
Startle disease	AD
Benign hereditary chorea	AD
Familial parkinsonism	AD
DRPLA	AD

DRD, L-dopa-responsive dystonia; DRPLA, dentatorubropallidoluysian atrophy.

are treated. Although each disorder may be approached somewhat differently, a systematic approach to the patient with a movement disorder will lead to a correct differential diagnosis and the ultimately correct diagnosis. Then a specific treatment plan for the individual patient with his or her unique attributes can be delineated. Table 1-1 provides a general framework for how to approach a patient with a movement disorder.

Table 1-4 provides information regarding modes of inheritance in specific movement disorders known to be genetically determined. Gene testing is available for HD, DRPLA, DRD, ITD, autosomal-dominant spinocerebellar ataxias SCA 1 and 2, Machado-Joseph disease, and some types of familial parkinsonism. These disorders are addressed in detail in subsequent chapters throughout the book.

Tables 1-5 to 1-8 provide information regarding different approaches to the *neuroimaging of movement disorders* and patterns of abnormality encountered using the various neuroimaging techniques in different movement disorders. Chapter 3 covers neuroimaging in detail, and chapters throughout the book deal with neuroimaging in individual disorders in greater detail.

TABLE 1-5 Causes of Basal Ganglia Calcification

Hypo- and pseudohypoparathyroidism
Fahrs syndrome
CO intoxication
Birth anoxia
Tuberous sclerosis
Mitochondrial encephalopathies
Radiation and methotrexate therapy
AIDS
Congenital folate deficiency, dihydropteridine reductase deficiency.
Japanese B encephalitis, herpes simplex encephalitis
Down syndrome
Cockayne's syndrome

AIDS, acquired immune deficiency syndrome.

TABLE 1-6 MRI Hyperintense Signal in Basal Ganglia

Wilson's disease
Creutzfeldt-Jakob disease
Manganese toxicity
Hepatic encephalopathy
Calcified basal ganglia
AIDS
Normal aging

MRI, magnetic resonance imaging; AIDS, acquired immune deficiency syndrome

TABLE 1-7 MRI Hypointense Signal in Basal Ganglia

Wilson's disease
Leigh's disease
CO intoxication
Anoxia
Hallervorden-Spatz disease
Cyanide poisoning
Methanol intoxication
GM2-gangliosidosis
Hemolytic uremic disease
Wasp sting encephalopathy

MRI, magnetic resonance imaging.

TABLE 1-8 PET Neuroimaging in Specific Movement Disorders

Movement Disorder	MRI	PET-FDG/FD
HD	Caudate atrophy	Hypometabolism in caudate and frontal lobes[66,67]
ITD	Normal	FD and FDG scans normal[68,69]
Wilson's disease	Hypo- or hyperintensities in basal ganglia, thalamus, midbrain and frontal lobes	Hypometabolism in striatum, frontal-parietal cortices and white matter; reduced FD uptake[70]
IP	Normal	Reduced FD uptake in striatum, especially putamen[71]; hypermetabolism in palladium in FDG scan[22]
PSP	Midbrain atrophy	Reduced FD uptake in striatum[73]
MSA/SDS	Cerebellar and brain stem atrophy; hyperintensity in dorsolateral putamen	Reduced FD uptake in caudate and putamen; frontal and striatal hypometabolism in FDG scan[74,75]
CBD	Contralateral and later bilateral frontoparietal atrophy	Asymmetric parietal and frontal hypometabolism in FDG scan; asymmetric reduction of striatal FD uptake[76]

FD, L-(18F) fluorodopa; FDG, L-(18F) fluorodeoxyglucose; PET, position emission tomography; MRI, magnetic resonance imaging.

Acknowledgment

We thank Susan Calne for editorial assistance.

References

1. Ad Hoc Committee (1984): Ad Hoc Committee of the Dystonia Medical Research Foundation met in February, 1984. Its members included Drs. A. Barbeau, D. B. Calne, S. Fahn, C.D. Marsden, J. Menkes and G.F. Wooten.

2. Fahn S: Concept and classification of dystonia. *Adv Neurol* 50:1–8, 1988.

3. Pettigrew LC, Jankovic J: Hemidystonia: A report of 22 patients and a review of the literature. *J Neurol Neurosurg Psychiatry* 48:650–657, 1985.

4. Marsden CD, Obeso JA, Zarranz JJ, Lang AE: The anatomical basis of symptomatic hemidystonia. *Brain* 108:463–484, 1985.

5. Obeso JA, Rothwell JC, Lang AE, Marsden CD: Myoclonic dystonia. *Neurology* 33:825–830, 1983.

6. Kurlan R, Behr J, Medved L, Shoulson I: Myoclonus and dystonia: A family study. *Adv Neurol* 50:385–389, 1988.

7. Quinn NP, Rothwell JC, Thompson PD, Marsden CD: Hereditary myoclonic dystonia, hereditary torsion dystonia, and hereditary essential myoclonus: An area of confusion. *Adv Neurol* 50:391–401, 1988.

8. Jedynak CP, Bonnet AM, Agid Y: Tremor and idiopathic dystonia. *Mov Disord* 6:230–236, 1991.

9. Segawa M, Hosaka A, Miyagawa F, et al: Hereditary progressive dystonia with marked diurnal variation. *Adv Neurol* 14:215–233, 1976.

10. Nygaard TG, Marsden CD, Duvoisin RC: Dopa responsive dystonia. *Adv Neurol* 50:377–384, 1988.

11. Lee LV, Kupke KG, Caballar-Onazaga F, et al: The phenotype of the X-linked dystonia-parkinsonism syndrome—an assessment of 42 cases in the Philippines. *Medicine* 70:179–187, 1991.

12. Fahn S, Williams DT: Psychogenic dystonia. *Adv Neurol* 50:431–455, 1988.

13. Friedman A, Fahn S: Spontaneous remissions in spasmodic torticollis. *Neurology* 36:398–400, 1986.

14. Jankovic J, Fahn S: Physiological and pathological tremors: Diagnosis, mechanism and management. *Ann Intern Med* 93:460–465, 1980.

15. Young RR, Weigner AW: Tremor, in Swash M, Kennard C (eds): *Scientific Basis of Clinical Neurology*. Edinburgh: Churchill Livingstone, 1985, pp 116–132.

16. Larsen TA, Calne DB: Essential tremor. *Clin Neuropharmacol* 6:185–206, 1983.

17. Critchley M: Observations on essential (heredofamilial) tremor. *Brain* 72:113–139, 1949.

18. Koller WC, Biary N: Metoprolol compared to propranolol in the treatment of essential tremor. *Arch Neurol* 41:171–172, 1984.

19. Sutherland JM, Edwards VE, Eadie MJ: Essential (hereditary or senile) tremor. *Med J Aust* 2:244–247, 1975.

20. Rajput AH, Jamieson H, Hirsh S, Quraishi A: Relative efficacy of alcohol and propranolol in action tremor. *Can J Neurol Sci* 2:31–35, 1975.

21. Findley LJ, Gresty MA: Tremor. *Br J Hosp Med* 26:16–32, 1981.

22. Rajput AH, Rozdilsky B, Ang L, Rajput A: Clinicopathological observations in essential tremor: Report of six cases. *Neurology* 41:1422–1424, 1991.

23. Rajput AH, Rozdilsky B, Ang L: Occurrence of resting tremor in Parkinson's disease. *Neurology* 41:1298–1299, 1991b.

24. Fitzgerald PM, Jankovic J: Orthostatic tremor: An association with essential tremor. *Mov Disord* 1:60–64, 1991.

25. Lance JW, Adams RD: The syndrome of intention or action myoclonus as a sequel to hypoxic encephalopathy. *Brain* 86:111–136, 1963.

26. Frenken CWGM, Notermans SLH, Korten JJ, Horstink MWIM: Myoclonic disorders of spinal origin. *Clin Neurol Neurosurg* 79:107–118, 1978.

27. Lapresle J: Palatal myoclonus. *Adv Neurol* 43:265–273, 1986.

28. Baldessarini RJ, Cole JO, Davis JM, et al: Tardive dyskinesia: Summary of a task force report of the American Psychiatric Association. *Am J Psychiatry* 137:1163–1172, 1980.

29. Shoulson I. On chorea. *Clin Neuropharmacol* 9(suppl 2):S85–S99, 1986.

30. Faheem AD, Brightwell DR, Burton GC, Struss A: Respiratory dyskinesia and dysarthria from prolonged neuroleptic use: Tardive dyskinesia? *Am J Psychiatry* 139:517–518, 1982.

31. Sharp FR, Rando TA, Greenberg SA, et al: Pseudochoreoathetosis: Movements associated with loss of proprioception. *Arch Neurol* 51(11):1103–1109, 1994.

32. Lance JW: Familial paroxysmal dystonic choreoathetosis and its differentiation from related syndromes. *Ann Neurol* 2:285–293, 1977.

33. Stevens H: Paroxysmal choreoathetosis—a form of reflex epilepsy. *Arch Neurol* 14:415–420, 1966.

34. Jung S, Chen KM, Brody JA: Paroxysmal choreoathetosis. *Neurology* 23:749–755, 1973.

35. Pryles CV, Livingston S, Ford FR: Familial paroxysmal choreoathetosis of Mount and Rebaback. *Pediatrics* 9:44–47, 1952.

36. Weber MB: Familial paroxysmal dystonia. *J Nerv Ment Dis* 145:221–226, 1967.

37. Walker ES: Familial paroxysmal dystonic choreoathetosis: A neurologic disorder simulating psychiatric illness. *Johns Hopkins Med J* 148:108–113, 1981.

38. Bennett DA, Goetz CG: Acquired paroxysmal dyskinesias, in Joseph AB, Young RR (eds): *Movement Disorders in Neurology and Neuropsychiatry*. Boston: Blackwell Scientific Publications, 1992, pp 540–556.

39. Plant GT, Williams AC, Earl CJ, Marsden CD: Familial paroxysmal dystonia induced by exercise. *J Neurol Neurosurg Psychiatry* 47(3):275–9, 1984.

40. Lugaresi E, Cirignotta F, Montagna P: Nocturnal paroxysmal dystonia. *J Neurol Neurosurg Psychiatry* 49(4):375–380, 1986.

41. Veggiotti P, Zambrino CA, Balottin U, Lanzi G: Concurrent nocturnal and diurnal paroxysmal dystonia. *Child Nerv Syst* 9(8):458–461, 1993.

42. Oguni M, Oguni H, Kozasa M, Fukuyama Y: A case with nocturnal paroxysmal unilateral dystonia and interictal right frontal epileptic EEG focus: A lateralized variant of nocturnal paroxysmal dystonia. *Brain Dev* 14(60):412–416,1992.

43. Meierkord H, Fish DR, Smith SJ, et al: Is nocturnal paroxysmal dystonia a form of frontal lobe epilepsy? *Mov Disord* 7(1):38–41, 1992.

44. Spillaine JD, Nathan PW, Kelly RE, Marsden CD: Painful legs and moving toes. *Brain* 94:541–556, 1971.

45. Montagna P, Cirignotta F, Sacqugna T, et al: "Painful legs and moving toes" associated with polyneuropathy. *J Neurol Neurosurg Psychiatry* 46:399–403, 1983.

46. Coleman RM: Periodic movements in sleep (nocturnal myoclonus) and restless leg syndrome, in Guilleminault C (ed): *Sleeping and Waking Disorders: Indications and Techniques*. Menlo Park, CA: Addison Wesley, 1982, pp 265–296.

47. Lugaresi E, Cirignotta F, Coccagna G, Montagna P: Nocturnal myoclonus and restless leg syndrome. *Adv Neurol* 43:295–307, 1986.

48. Ekbom KA: Restless legs, in Vinken PJ, Bruyn GW (eds): *Handbook of Clinical Neurology: Diseases of Nerves*. Amsterdam: Elsevier Science Publishers, 1970, part 2, pp 311–320.

49. Levine DN: The alien hand, in Joseph AB, Young RR (eds): *Movement Disorders in Neurology and Neuropsychiatry*. Boston: Blackwell Scientific Publications, 1992, chap 88, pp 691–695.

50. Bogen JE: The callosal syndrome, in Heilman KM, Valenstein E (eds): *Clinical Neuropsychology*. New York: Oxford University Press, 1979, pp 308–359.

51. Goldenberg G, Mayer NH, Toglia JV: Medial frontal cortex infarction and the alien hand sign. *Arch Neurol* 36:683–686, 1981.

52. Levine DN, Rinn WE: Opticosensory ataxia and alien hand syndrome after posterior cerebral artery infarction. *Neurology* 36:1094–1097, 1986.

53. Riley DE, Lang AE, Lewis A, et al: Cortico-basal ganglionic degeneration. *Neurology* 1203–1212, 1990.

54. Klawans HL, Falk DK, Nausieda PA, Weiner WJ: Guilles de la Touretteås syndrome after long-term chlorpromazine therapy. *Neurology* 28:1064–68, 1978.

55. Jankovic J: The neurology of tics, in Marsden CD, Fahn S (eds): *Movement Disorders 2*. London: Butterworth, 1987, chap 19, pp 383–405.

56. Gibb WRG, Lees Aj: The clinical phenomenon of akathisia. *J Neurol Neurosurg Psychiatry* 49:881–886, 1986.

57. Barnes TRE, Braude WM: Akathisia variants and tardive dyskinesia. *Arch Gen Psychiatry* 42:874–878, 1985.

58. Jankovic J, Glass JP: Metoclopramide-induced phantom dyskinesia. *Neurology* 35:432–435, 1985.

59. Andermann F, Andermann E: Startle disease or hyperekplexia (letter). *Ann Neurol* 16:367–368, 1984.

60. Martilla RJ, Rinne UK: Disability and progression of Parkinsonås disease. *Acta Neurol Scand* 56:159–169, 1977.

61. Jankovic J, McDermott M, Carter J, et al: Variable expression of Parkinsonås disease: A base line assessment of the DATATOP cohort. *Neurology* 40:1529–1534, 1990.

62. Duncan G, Wilson JA: Normal elderly have some signs of PS (letter). *Lancet* 2:1392, 1989.

63. Weiner WJ, Nora LM, Glantz RH: Elderly inpatients: Postural reflex impairment. *Neurology* 34:945–947, 1984.

64. Calne DB, Snow BJ, Lee CS: Criteria for diagnosing Parkinsonås disease. *Ann Neurol* 32:S125–S127, 1992.

65. Pillon B, Dubois B, Agid Y: Testing cognition may contribute to the diagnosis of movement disorders. *Neurology* 1996; 46:329–334.

66. Hayden MR, Martin WRW, Stoessl AJ, et al: Positron emission tomography in the early diagnosis of Huntingtonås disease. *Neurology* 36:888–894, 1986.

67. Martin WRW, Clark CM, Ammann W, et al: Cortical glucose metabolism in Huntingtonås disease. *Neurology* 42:223–229, 1992.

68. Leenders KL, Quinn N, Frackowiak RSJ, Marsden CD: Brain dopaminergic system studied in patients with dystonia using positron emission tomography. *Adv Neurol* 50:243–247, 1988.

69. Stoessl AJ, Martin WRW, Clark CM, et al: PET studies in cerebral glucose metabolism in idiopathic torticollis. *Neurology* 36:653–657, 1986.

70. Snow BJ, Bhatt MH, Martin WRW, Calne DB: Dopaminergic metabolism in Wilsonås disease studied with positron emission tomography. *J Neurol Neurosurg Psychiatry* 53:12–17, 1990.

71. Leenders KL, Salmon EP, Tyrell P, et al: The nigrostiatal dopaminergic system assessed in-vivo by positron emission tomography in healthy volunteer subjects and patients with Parkinsonås disease. *Arch Neurol* 47:1290–1298, 1990.

72. Martin WRW, Stoessl AJ, Adam MJ, et al: Parkinsonås disease. *Adv Neurol* 45:95–98, 1986.

73. Bhatt MH, Snow BJ, Martin WRW, Peppard RF, et al: Positron emission tomography in progressive supra nuclear palsy. *Arch Neurol* 48:389–391, 1991.

74. Bhatt MH, Snow BJ, Martin WRW, Calne DB: Positron emission tomography in Shy-Drager syndrome. *Ann Neurol* 28:101–103, 1990.

75. Eidelberg D, Takikawa S, Moeller JR, et al: Striatal hypometabolism distinguishes striatonigral degeneration from Parkinsonås disease. *Ann Neurol* 33:518–527, 1993.

76. Sawle GV, Brooks DJ, Marsden CD, Frackowiak RSJ: Corticobasal degeneration. *Brain* 114:541–556, 1991.

Chapter 2

NEUROBEHAVIORAL ASPECTS OF MOVEMENT DISORDERS

DEAN J. FOTI and JEFFREY L. CUMMINGS

NEUROBEHAVIORAL ASPECTS OF MOVEMENT
 DISORDERS
FRONTAL SUBCORTICAL CIRCUITS
NEUROPSYCHIATRIC DISTURBANCES
 Depression
 Mania
 Psychosis
 Personality Alterations
 Obsessive-Compulsive Disorder
 Anxiety
 Sleep and Sexual Disturbances
COGNITIVE DISTURBANCES
 Executive Function
 Memory
 Speech and Language
 Visuospatial Function
 Praxis
DEMENTIA
 Huntington's Disease
 Progressive Supranuclear Palsy
 Parkinson's Disease
 Multiple-System Atrophies
 Wilson's Disease
 Rarer Movement Disorders with Prominent Dementia
COMMENT

Neurobehavioral Aspects of Movement Disorders

Behavioral changes accompany most movement disorders and were frequently acknowledged in the initial reports of basal ganglia diseases. Kinnier Wilson used the term "psychical" in reference to the behavior of eight of the twelve patients he reported with "Wilson's disease" in 1912.[1] Similarly, George Huntington referred to "insanity with a tendency to suicide" as an essential feature of the disease that bears his name.[2] James Parkinson's essay on the shaking palsy refers to the "unhappy sufferer," but his comment "the senses and intellect remain uninjured" was considerably less accurate.[3] However, an appreciation of the shared substrate of behavior and movement disorders was not fully understood for many years, and a multitude of psychodynamic and "reactive" theories were proposed,[4-6] or cognitive and emotional disorders were simply ignored and left unstudied. A compelling argument for common neurophysiological processes under-

lying motion and emotion is the high frequency of intellectual impairment, depression and personality changes in diseases of the basal ganglia as well as the common occurrence of motor disorders seen in schizophrenia, affective disorders, and obsessive-compulsive disorder.[7] The psychosocial aspects of movement disorders do play a role in behavioral and affective changes of basal ganglia diseases, but animal experiments,[8] progress in understanding of frontal-subcortical circuits,[9-13] and evidence from focal lesions of the basal ganglia[14,15] have clarified the anatomic substrate of behavior changes in conditions with basal ganglia dysfunction.

The principal theme developed in this chapter is that behavioral changes are common to a number of movement disorders and are an expression of the interruption of specific components of frontal-subcortical circuits. An initial summary of the relevant frontal-subcortical circuits as they apply to behavior is presented, followed by an overview of neurobehavioral aspects of movement disorders, divided into the various behavioral "domains" of the basal ganglia: neuropsychiatric, mild cognitive, and dementia.

Frontal Subcortical Circuits

There are five circuits linking the frontal lobes and subcortical structures: motor, oculomotor, dorsolateral prefrontal, lateral orbitofrontal, and anterior cingulate.[9-12] The latter three originate in the prefrontal cortex and are responsible for distinct neurobehavioral syndromes involving cognition and emotion.[9] All circuits share common structures and organization, originating in the frontal lobe with sequential projections to the striatum, globus pallidus (GP)/substantia nigra (SN), and thalamus, ultimately linking back to the frontal lobe (Fig. 2-1). Each circuit has a direct and indirect (via GP externa and subthalamic nucleus) pathway from the striatum to the GP interna/SN. The circuits are adjacent to each other but remain anatomically segregated. In general, the inputs to the circuits are broad and may involve functionally related structures outside of the circuit, whereas the output is more specific to localized cortical areas.

The dorsolateral prefrontal circuit (Fig. 2-1) originates in the frontal lobe convexity and projects to the dorsolateral head of the caudate, with subsequent projections to the more lateral dorsomedial GP and rostral SN.[11,12] These neurons then project to the ventral anterior (VA) and medial dorsal (MD) thalamic nuclei, which connect back to the dorsolateral prefrontal cortex. Disruption of this circuit results in a dorsolateral prefrontal syndrome with deficits in executive function and motor programming.[9,13] These patients exhibit difficulties in maintaining or shifting set, generating organizational strategies and retrieving memories, and they have reduced verbal and nonverbal fluency.[16,17] Functional aspects of this area are assessed by the Wisconsin Card Sort Test (WCST) and are impaired in Huntington's disease (HD),[18,19] which affects primarily the caudate nucleus, and in Parkinson's disease (PD), especially when the medial SN projections to the caudate are involved.[20-23]

The lateral orbitofrontal circuit (Fig. 2-1) originates in the inferolateral prefrontal cortex and projects to the ventromedial caudate nucleus, which then projects to the dorsomedial

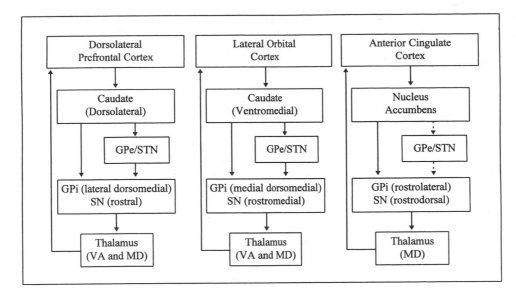

FIGURE 2-1 Three behaviorally relevant frontal-subcortical circuits. *Dotted arrows* are postulated connections. GPe/STN, indirect pathway via globus pallidus externa/subthalamic nucleus; GPi, globus pallidus interna; SN, substantia nigra; VA, ventral anterior; MD, medial dorsal.

GP and rostromedial SN.[11,12] These projections are areas similar to the dorsolateral frontal circuit, but more medial in all the structures. The return path is via the VA and DM thalamic nuclei, which project back to the orbitofrontal cortex. The integrity of this circuit is important in the inhibition of interference from external cues and in self-monitoring.[9] Disturbance of the orbitofrontal circuit results in significant personality alterations consisting primarily of disinhibition and irritability.[9] These personality alterations are well known in the early stages of HD,[24,25] where the medial caudate neurons are preferentially affected.[26,27] A study of Mendez and coworkers[15] in patients with focal caudate lesions highlights the separation of the ventral and dorsal caudate into distinct circuits. Patients with ventral lesions were significantly more disinhibited, euphoric, and inappropriate. Similar behavioral changes are prominent in other disorders primarily affecting the caudate, such as idiopathic calcification of the basal ganglia (ICBG)[28,29] and neuroacanthocytosis.[30]

The third "behavioral" circuit is the anterior cingulate circuit (Fig. 2-1), originating in the anterior cingulate gyrus and projecting to the ventral (or limbic) striatum. The latter includes the nucleus accumbens, olfactory tubercle, and parts of the ventromedial caudate and putamen.[11,12] There are multiple additional limbic inputs to the ventral striatum. The ventral striatum then connects to the ventral and rostrolateral GP and rostrodorsal SN, which in turn project to the paramedian part of the MD nucleus of the thalamus, which ultimately projects back to the anterior cingulate cortex. Dysfunction in this circuit results in the medial frontal-anterior cingulate syndrome with apathy and reduced initiative.[9] Akinetic mutism with profound apathy is reported in bilateral anterior cingulate lesions.[31] The integrity of this circuit is critical for drive and motivation. Disruption of anterior cingulate and orbitofrontal circuits is implicated in obsessive-compulsive disorder and apathy associated with a number of movement disorders.[9]

Disruption of multiple frontal-subcortical circuits in patients with basal ganglia disease results in the frequent occurrence of personality and mood disorders, as well as cognitive dysfunction. Thus, movement disorders can be considered markers of disease affecting structural and neurochemical components of frontal-subcortical circuits. Movement abnormalities occur primarily with diseases affecting caudate, putamen, and subthalamic nucleus, whereas disorder of prefrontal cortex and thalamus have less effect on motility.

Neuropsychiatric Disturbances

Degenerative diseases of the basal ganglia are associated with movement disorders and neuropsychiatric syndromes.[7] Behavioral changes are also noted in focal disease of the basal ganglia.[14,15] The nature of neuropsychiatric symptoms found in movement disorders is often very similar to that seen in primary psychiatric disease, and there is support from neuroimaging studies indicating that identical regions may be involved. The neuropsychiatric symptoms include depression, mania, personality change, psychosis, obsessive-compulsive disorder, anxiety, apathy, sexual behavior changes, and sleep disturbance.

DEPRESSION

Depression refers to an alteration in mood with significant sadness, hopelessness, and anhedonia, often associated with changes in appetite, loss of sexual drive, sleep disturbance, psychomotor retardation, and fatigue.[7] Depression occurs in a number of movement disorders (Table 2-1). Difficulties in assessing the prevalence of depression in movement disorders arise primarily from variability in assessment. Only more recent studies have used standardized questionnaires.[32,33] There is also the variability of selection criteria and referral biases. Finally, depression in hypokinetic movement disorders such as PD can be more complicated to assess, as psychomotor slowing is an integral aspect of the motor disorder of depression.

Dysfunction in either the orbitofrontal or dorsolateral frontal circuit is associated with depression.[9] In particular, the caudate appears to have a key role in mediating mood, as disorders of the caudate nucleus have a high rate of depres-

TABLE 2-1 Movement Disorders with Depression

Parkinson's disease
Huntington's disease
Idiopathic calcification of the basal ganglia
Wilson's disease
Vascular parkinsonism
Progressive supranuclear palsy
Neuroacanthocytosis
Dystonia
  Idiopathic torsion dystonia
  Meige's syndrome
Spinocerebellar degenerations
Gilles de la Tourette's disorder

sion.[33] Depression has been associated with orbital and caudate hypometabolism on positron emission tomography (PET) in both PD and HD.[34,35] Other studies have shown dorsolateral frontal hypometabolism in idiopathic depression.[36]

PARKINSON'S DISEASE

Depression is common in patients with PD. The frequency of depression overall is approximately 40 percent, with variability in reported rates from 4 to 70 percent, depending on methodology and threshold for diagnosis.[32,33] A confounding aspect in the use of depression inventories in PD is the overlap of motor manifestations, but cluster analysis has shown that depressed and nondepressed PD patients can be distinguished, using rating scale scores.[37,38] The severity of the depression is sufficient to meet criteria for a major depressive episode in slightly more than half of those with mood disorders, with the others manifesting dysthymia or minor depression.[33] Postencephalitic parkinsonism has approximately the same frequency of depression as idiopathic PD but more prominent personality and behavioral changes.[39]

The nature of the depression of PD is not identical to that seen in idiopathic depression; there is more sadness without significant guilt or self-blame and a high rate of anxiety.[33,40–43] Psychotic depression is rare. However, anxiety is seen more often among elderly depressed than younger depressed patients[44] and may not be specific to PD. There is a low suicide rate in PD despite a high frequency of suicidal ideation.[33] A few studies have reported more depression among those with right hemiparkinsonism.[45] Brown and coworkers[40] studied the longitudinal course of depression in 152 PD patients and found that it showed little variability, with major depression persisting over 2 years and only a small proportion of the nondepressed group developing depression. Depression is associated with greater cognitive dysfunction in PD.[46–48] Those with depression perform more poorly on executive function tasks, such as the WCST, verbal fluency, and trail making. Longitudinal follow-up of depressed versus nondepressed PD patients over a 4-year period by Starkstein and coworkers[45] showed a significantly greater decline in cognitive function in depressed patients.

The etiology of depression in PD is not fully determined. The contributions of reactive[49,50] versus endogenous[46] factors remains to be identified. Depression often predates motor disabilities.[47] In one study, 43% of depressed PD patients were depressed before the onset of motor deficits.[51] PD patients are more depressed than other disabled patients matched for severity of functional impairment.[52] These findings argue against a predominant psychosocial model. There is a serotonergic deficit in PD, which may be important in mediating depression.[53,54] Studies of nondepressed versus depressed PD patients showed lower cerebrospinal fluid (CSF) 5-hydroxyindoleacetic acid (5-HIAA) in the depressed group, but severity of depression did not correlate with the level, nor did all depressed patients have low CSF 5-HIAA.[55] The role of dopamine in PD with depression is not clear. The relationship to motor disabilities has been assessed in a number of studies, and the majority have found little correlation with mood, although there is some suggestion that depression is more common in patients with dopamine-responsive deficits such as rigidity and bradykinesia and less common with tremor.[33] The role for dopamine in mood is supported by the reported increased severity of depressive symptomatology during the "off" state.[56,57] Differences in neurotransmitter changes because of variable cell loss in subcortical nuclei in PD[58] may explain why only a subgroup of patients become depressed.

Functional imaging has shown selective differences between depressed and nondepressed PD patients. Using PET Ring and colleagues[34] have recently shown a selective decrease in medial frontal metabolism in both depressed PD patients as well as in those with idiopathic depression, whereas these changes were not present in nondepressed PD patients. Mayberg et al.[35] also showed selective hypometabolism in the inferior frontal lobe in depressed, as opposed to nondepressed, PD patients.

A model has been proposed by Cummings[33] for the pathogenesis of depression in PD that hinges on biochemical abnormalities in the cortex and basal ganglia, resulting in the behaviors of decreased reward mediation, environmental dependency, and inadequate stress response. These behavioral deficiencies result in symptoms of apathy, worthlessness, helplessness, hopelessness, and dysphoria.

HUNTINGTON'S DISEASE

Depression is also particularly common in HD, with approximately half of the patients affected and 30 percent meeting criteria for a major depressive episode.[24,25,27,59] It is the second most common neuropsychiatric disorder in HD (after dementia)[25] and may precede the neurological symptoms by 2 to 20 years.[24] Suicide is four to six times more common in HD than in other depressed patients and up to 20 times higher in the age group from 50 to 69 years.[25,60] Increased impulsivity because of associated dysfunction of the orbitofrontal circuit may result in the higher rate of suicide. Interruption of the anterior cingulate circuit by dysfunction in the ventral striatum may result in diminished motivation in combination with reduced reinforcement of reward-oriented behavior, behavioral changes that manifest in the symptoms of worthlessness, hopelessness, and apathy.

OTHER MOVEMENT DISORDERS

Depression is the second most common psychiatric manifestation in Wilson's disease, occurring in 20–30 percent.[61,62,63] Only personality alterations are more common. Depression is unlikely to be purely reactive, as it frequently presents before diagnosis or disability. However, it is generally poorly responsive to treatment of the copper disorder.[63]

Other movement disorders in which depression occurs include progressive supranuclear palsy (PSP), neuroacanthocytosis, idiopathic calcification of the basal ganglia (ICBG), and in Gilles de la Tourette's disorder (GTD).[28,30,64–67]

MANIA

Mania seen in the course of primary bipolar disorder frequently has an associated movement disorder of hyperkinesis.[68] Similarly, classic movement disorders have been associated with mania (Table 2-2). Secondary mania is characterized by elated and/or irritable mood for at least 1 week, with three of the associated features of hyperactivity, pressured speech, flight of ideas, grandiosity, decreased sleep, distractibility, and lack of judgment in the absence of delirium or dementia.[7,69] Hypomania has similar diagnostic criteria but shorter duration of at least 4 days with milder symptoms producing less interference with functioning.[69] Secondary mania has been associated with a wide variety of neurological, metabolic, and toxic etiologies.[7,68]

The most important movement disorder associated with mania is HD.[25,27,70] Approximately 10 percent of HD patients develop hypomania with increased energy, elevated mood, decreased sleep, pressured speech, and, sometimes, associated hypersexuality. Dewhurst et al.[70] reported grandiose delusions in 5 of 102 HD patients hospitalized in a psychiatric facility. There are reports of hypomania and mania in Wilson's disease,[62] postencephalitic parkinsonism,[71] and Gerstmann-Straussler-Scheinker disease,[72] a familial prion disease with cerebellar symptoms and dementia. Although mania does not occur in untreated PD, drug-induced mania, hypomania, and euphoria occurs in 1.5–12 percent of patients treated with L-dopa or bromocriptine.[73–75] Mania has been reported with selegiline.[76] The risk of these drug-induced behaviors is higher in PD patients with a past history of hypomania or mania.[75]

The pathogenesis of secondary mania is not yet determined, but evidence from focal lesions suggests that the region abutting the third ventricle near the hypothalamus in the midline is of importance in the mediation of manic symptoms.[77] Mania and hemiballismus have been described following right thalamic infarction,[78] and the majority of focal lesions producing mania occur on the right side of the brain.[77]

PSYCHOSIS

Psychosis is a loss of reality testing resulting from the inability to accurately evaluate perceptions or thoughts, leading the patient to make incorrect inferences about external reality.[7,69]

TABLE 2-2 Movement Disorders with Hypomania/Mania

Huntington's disease
Wilson's disease
Parkinson's disease (related to treatment with dopaminergic medications)
Postencephalitic parkinsonism
Sydenham's chorea
Gerstmann-Straussler-Scheinker disease

Like mania, there are a number of secondary causes of psychosis. The anatomic correlates of secondary psychosis involve subcortical structures, as well as cortex, particularly temporoparietal cortex.[79] However, the relationship of a schizophreniform psychosis to the basal ganglia is specifically linked to diseases that affect primarily the caudate nucleus. Mendez et al.[15] reported a woman with paranoia, fear of germs, and auditory hallucinations on the basis of a caudate lesion. No other focal lesions of the basal ganglia are known to produce psychosis.[14] The etiologies of the degenerative basal ganglia disorders with psychosis also support involvement of the caudate. Schizophreniform psychosis (with disordered thought content and form) is more common in HD and ICBG, which structurally affect predominantly the caudate.[24,26,28,29,80] In contrast, Wilson's disease, Hallervorden-Spatz's disease, and idiopathic PD are associated less commonly with psychosis and have minimal structural effects on the caudate.[61,63,80,81] The psychosis in the caudate disorders tends to be refractory to management.[25,59]

Psychosis occurs in 6–25 percent of HD patients, although the number presenting with psychosis is less clear.[24,27] The early occurrence of behavioral changes in the absence-of-movement disorder may relate to the preferential early loss of spiny neurons in the medial caudate.[25,26] There is no significant correlation between psychosis severity and duration of symptoms or between cognitive impairment and psychosis,[59] but the number of studies addressing these issues is limited.

Psychosis may be seen in ICBG at an early age before the emergence of the movement disorder[28,29] and in a variety of other disorders (Table 2-3). Wilson's disease is associated with many behavioral changes, but a recent retrospective review found that schizophreniform psychosis was uncommon (1 percent).[61] Schizophreniform states with delusions, hallucinations, and catatonia were often seen in postencephalitic parkinsonism, and patients were susceptible to recurrence of psychosis when treated with L-dopa.[39,82,83] Psychosis in idiopathic PD is primarily drug-related (L-dopa, dopamine agonists, selegiline, anticholinergics, amantadine), occurring in 10–50 percent.[73,84] Dementia and age are important risk factors for drug-induced psychosis in PD.[75,84] It occurs most often in the setting of a clear sensorium, with primarily visual hallucinations, but a confusional psychosis can occur with dementia or anticholinergic use.[84] Finally, delusions and hal-

TABLE 2-3 Movement Disorders with Psychosis

Huntington's disease
Idiopathic calcification of the basal ganglia
Sydenham's chorea
Postencephalitic parkinsonism
Parkinson's disease (related to treatment with dopaminergic medications)
Vascular parkinsonism
Diffuse Lewy body disease
Wilson's disease
Thalamic degenerations
Spinocerebellar degenerations
Prion diseases
    Creutzfeldt-Jakob disease
    Gerstmann-Straussler-Scheinker disease

lucinations are common in the Lewy body dementias, which present with an extrapyramidal disorder and dementia.[85]

The relationship between movement disorders and psychosis is founded in the disruption of structures of the limbic striatum. The structures are either affected directly, as in HD, or disturbed functionally, as in the thalamic degenerations. Dopamine also plays a role, as psychosis is rarely seen in dopamine-deficient disorders such as idiopathic PD but is prominent in HD, in which there is relative preservation of dopamine.[86] The variety of motor abnormalities that occurs in schizophrenia[7] may reflect similar dysfunction in frontal-subcortical circuits. The cognitively impaired schizophrenic with preexisting dysfunction in these circuits appears to be more susceptible to developing tardive dyskinesia, lending support to an association between psychosis and frontal-subcortical circuit dysfunction.[87,88]

PERSONALITY ALTERATIONS

Personality refers to a behavioral style: one's feelings, attitudes, mood, and pattern of behavior.[7,69] The disturbances noted in movement disorders include apathy, irritability, lability, impulsivity, aggression, agitation and, sometimes, even violence. The presentation of personality changes before the appearance of the movement disorder argues for a neuroanatomic substrate for the behavioral alterations. Similar behaviors occur in the setting of frontal lobe injuries,[16] and disruption of prefrontal projections is essential in the production of personality change in movement disorders.

Apathy is frequently reported in globus pallidus lesions resulting from carbon monoxide poisoning, with concomitant "psychic akinesia."[89] This can often be reversed by external stimuli, an observation also made with postencephalitic parkinsonism.[71] Similarly, patients with HD have early loss of spontaneity but will engage in tasks when external stimuli are supplied.[90,91] Once the stimulation is removed, inertia returns. These deficits are likely mediated by disruption of the medial frontal-anterior cingulate subcortical circuit.[9]

Early personality change with irritability, indifference, and lability of mood is described in PSP.[92] One third of patients with the parkinsonism-dementia complex of Guam develop early disturbances in personality and mood, with apathy, irritability, depression, restlessness, agitation, and even violent behavior.[82,93] Wilson's disease presents with personality changes in 20–46 percent; patients are described as irritable, emotional, reckless, disinhibited, bizarre, and sometimes aggressive.[61,62,80] Personality changes in HD are ubiquitous, with apathy, irritability, lability, and impulsivity frequently described.[24,25,27,59,70] Aggression in HD can occur in the setting of personality disorders, psychosis, or depression, with a frequency of approximately 60 percent.[25] Folstein[27] found that 30.6 percent of 182 HD patients met criteria for intermittent explosive disorder and 5.9 percent for antisocial personality disorder. Irritability and lability occur early in HD when the ventromedial caudate is preferentially affected, disrupting connections to the orbitofrontal cortex.

Aggressive behavior, hyperactivity, and temper outbursts are described in 60–70 percent of patients with GTD and, in one large study, 49 percent met criteria for attention deficit disorder with hyperactivity.[66,67,94] There is no clear relationship between the severity of the tics and behavioral difficul-

ties, and the extent of the genetic connection between GTD and attention deficit disorder continues to be debated.[67,94]

PARKINSON'S DISEASE PERSONALITY

The issue of personality in PD has been much discussed, and still no definitive conclusions have been reached. Fifty years ago, PD was considered by some to be a consequence of disordered personality.[5,6] Sands believed that the suppression of emotions ultimately resulted in the symptoms of PD.[6] Although our current understanding of neuropharmacology and neuropathology may dismiss such considerations, the "premorbid personality" of PD remains contentious.[95–98] PD patients are reported to have reduced risk-taking behavior with decreased novelty-seeking.[13,95,99] They are often described as rigid, frugal, and contemplative, and these characteristics may result in difficulties in novel situations. These interpretations of "personality" may reflect their decreased mental flexibility from underlying cognitive impairment.

Previous studies by Riklan et al.[100] and Smythies[96] found no evidence for a PD personality using standardized personality questionnaires. However, more recent studies, also retrospectively biased, showed that PD patients were morally rigid, cautious, and less flexible and exhibit less novelty-seeking, compared to others with similar disability produced by rheumatoid arthritis[97] or orthopedic conditions.[98] Hubble and coworkers[101] found PD patients to be quieter, less flexible, and more cautious than controls in a retrospective survey of current and premorbid personality. The assessment of current status did not correlate with degree of motor disability but did correlate with depression scores. Twin studies also support a distinctive premorbid personality style, with the affected twin being more introverted.[102] The inverse association between smoking and PD[103–105] may be a reflection of premorbid personality traits.

Hubble and Koller[95] have summarized four potential interpretations of a PD personality: personality contributes to the development of PD; PD causes the personality (the change represents a preclinical phase of disease); personality type and PD may develop in the same at-risk population and, finally, the personality may reflect the early expression of a depressed mood in patients who are at risk for both depression and PD. Until means of detecting PD at a very early presymptomatic stage are developed, this issue will remain unresolved.

OBSESSIVE-COMPULSIVE DISORDER

Obsessive-compulsive disorder (OCD) is characterized by recurrent obsessions and/or compulsions that interfere significantly with normal routine and are experienced as distressing (ego-dystonic).[7,69] Obsessions may be thoughts, images, or impulses and frequently include ideas of dirt, disease, or aggressive or sexual acts. Compulsions are repetitive behaviors or mental acts and typically involve hand-washing, checking, counting, touching, and avoiding. The compulsive behaviors are aimed at reducing stress or preventing a dreaded situation. However, they are often excessive or not connected in a realistic fashion with what they were designed to neutralize or prevent.

The relationship between movement disorders and OCD is most strongly exemplified in consideration of the high association between GTD and OCD.[106,107] The frequency of obsessive-compulsive behavior in GTD varies from 30–90 percent, depending on biases in referral population, diagnostic criteria, and method of data acquisition.[108] Larger studies, which used standardized evaluation techniques, found an overall frequency of obsessive-compulsive behavior in 50 percent of GTD patients.[108–110] Similarly, one sees a higher rate of tics in primary OCD, with 15 percent of children meeting criteria for GTD after 2–7 years of follow-up in a study of primary OCD (GTD excluded).[111] Family pedigrees are suggestive of gender-specific phenotypic expression within GTD families, with females predominantly developing OCD and males GTD.[112] The severity of OCD in GTD is generally milder and may be more suitably considered as obsessive-compulsive behavior.[108] The nature of the behaviors differs somewhat from primary OCD, with more touching and aligning rituals in GTD, as opposed to a higher number of germ-related cleaning rituals in primary OCD.[108]

The relationship between OCD and the basal ganglia has been developing from a number of viewpoints, both clinical and neurobiological.[113–116] Focal lesions of the basal ganglia have produced symptoms typical of OCD, although the anxiety or distress from withholding compulsions is frequently lacking.[14,115] OCD has been reported in many movement disorders (Table 2-4). Postencephalitic parkinsonism produces some of the most striking examples, with attacks of compulsive counting and forced thinking frequently associated with oculogyric crises.[39,117,118] Sometimes, forced grunting or shouting similar to tics of GTD occurred at the same time.[7] OCD has been reported in PSP[119] and in PD, particularly when the right hemisphere is preferentially involved.[98,120] OCD also occurs in choreiform disorders, such as Sydenham's chorea and HD.[7,25,114,121] OCD has been infrequently reported in HD, perhaps because repetitive behaviors were misinterpreted as perseverative rather than recognized as obsessional features associated with the behaviors.[25]

The neurobiological mechanisms of OCD appear to involve a disturbance in the ventral striatum or pallidum with disruption of the orbitofrontal subcortical circuit. Volumetric magnetic resonance imaging studies in GTD have shown reduced size of the left caudate, putamen, and pallidum.[122,123] PET studies in primary OCD demonstrate increased metabolism in orbitofrontal cortex bilaterally, and response to treatment is associated with a reduction in metabolism in the left caudate.[113,116] The failure of the basal ganglia to suppress or inhibit overlapping motor, cognitive, and limbic circuits may result in recurrent excitation, producing these stereotyped behaviors or movement disorder.[106,116,124,125] Baxter et al. proposed that the loss of gating function of the basal ganglia is responsible for the release of ritualistic behavior.[113] The eventual identification of the GTD gene will contribute significantly to the understanding of OCD.

ANXIETY

Anxiety is a feeling of worry, uneasiness, dread, or foreboding in the absence of an appropriately threatening stimulus.[7] Anxiety occurs in the setting of a number of psychiatric

TABLE 2-4 Movement Disorders with Obsessive-Compulsive Disorder

Gilles de la Tourette's disorder
Postencephalitic parkinsonism
Parkinson's disease
Manganese-induced parkinsonism
Vascular parkinsonism
Progressive supranuclear palsy
Huntington's disease
Sydenham's chorea
Meige's syndrome

disorders, including depression, mania, OCD, and schizophrenia. Thus, anxiety may occur in a number of disorders discussed earlier in the chapter. Movement disorders that may initially present with prominent anxiety include Wilson's disease and HD.[25,61,62,70] Dewhurst et al. reported that anxiety was present at admission in 12 of 102 patients with HD,[70] but the exact prevalence is not known accurately. As discussed previously in this chapter, depression in PD is often associated with significant anxiety. Anxiety is a common side effect of medication, occurring in 20 percent of advanced PD patients treated with selegiline.[126] Falling dopamine levels during "off" periods are usually associated with significant anxiety, as well as mood changes,[43,56,57] and should prompt readjustment of medications.

Just as anxiety occurs commonly in the setting of movement disorders and psychiatric disease, disorders of motor activity are usually associated with the autonomic arousal of anxiety.[7] There is often pacing, increased respirations, widening of palpebral fissures, raising of eyebrows, and rigid posturing of the body. It is likely that parallel circuits are activated via the limbic striatal circuits, and multiple neurotransmitters, including gamma-aminobutyric acid, norepinephrine, dopamine, and serotonin, are involved.

SLEEP AND SEXUAL DISTURBANCES

Movement disorders can be associated with prominent alterations in sleep and sexual behavior. This relationship is based on the high frequency of neurochemical alterations occurring in the subcortical or brain stem nuclei and their projections. The projections between the ventral striatum and hypothalamus are also essential in these basic life functions. A few pertinent relationships will be highlighted; complete discussion is beyond the scope of this chapter. (See also Chap. 51.)

Sleep disorders can be divided into hypersomnias, insomnias, and parasomnias (sleep-related conditions that do not affect the total amount of sleep).[7] Hypersomnias with increased total sleep time and excessive daytime sleepiness have been reported in patients with focal basal ganglia lesions.[14] Postencephalitic parkinsonism is associated with persisting disturbances in sleep, including sleep-wake reversal and drowsiness alternating with insomnia.[82] Early somnolence was also noted in 14 percent of patients with Parkinsonism-dementia/ALS of Guam.[127] Whipple's disease, a disorder with hypersomnolence, diarrhea, cognitive deficits, and supranuclear gaze palsy, is associated with a unique movement disorder of oculomasticatory myorhythmia.[128] Excessive daytime sleepiness may be associated with neurogenic sleep apnea that can occur in the multiple system atrophies because of autonomic dysfunction.[7] Insomnia and, sometimes, excessive daytime sleepiness occur with nocturnal myoclonus and restless legs syndrome.[7]

Parasomnias are commonly related to the side effects of dopaminergic agents, with sleep fragmentation, vivid dreams, nightmares, and night terrors.[129,130] Increasing parasomnias often precede a dopaminergic psychosis and may be an early warning of the need for intervention. Machado-Joseph disease, an autosomal dominant degenerative disorder that presents with a mixture of cerebellar and extrapyramidal signs, has sleep disturbance in 50 percent of patients with nocturnal cries, nightmares, and disrupted REM sleep.[82,131]

Sexual behavior may be similarly divided into hypersexuality, hyposexuality, and sexual deviations.[7] Hypersexuality and hyposexuality are commonly seen in primary psychiatric disease and are frequently a consequence of drugs used in their treatment.[7] Hypersexuality occurs as a side effect of dopaminergic medication in 0.9–3 percent of PD patients and may occur either with or without mania or psychosis.[75,84,132] Reduced sexual inhibitions, including inappropriately disrobing and masturbating in public, have been reported in Wilson's disease.[62,63] Increased fecundity and alteration in libido occur in 25 percent of patients with HD and, again, may occur independently of mania or psychosis.[25,27,70] Paraphilias are also seen in HD with sexual aggression, exhibitionism, and voyeurism.[25] Compulsive sexual touching and exhibitionism may occur in the spectrum of behavioral changes associated with GTD.[7,67] Paraphilias occurred in patients with postencephalitic parkinsonism, including pedophilia, exhibitionism, and sadism.[71]

Disturbances in sexual behavior have been linked to pathological involvement of structures in the brain stem and diencephalon. Gorman and Cummings[133] suggest that the inferior frontal cortex, hypothalamus, amygdaloid nuclei, and medial striatal/septal region are relevant areas in the production of sexual dysfunction. The medial striate region in HD is affected early and may underlie the changes in sexual behavior.[25] The similarity of these abnormal sexual behaviors to those seen in frontal lobe injury suggests that the disruption of the orbitofrontal-ventral striatal circuit may be mediating the behavioral change.

Cognitive Disturbances

There has been extensive investigation of the cognitive disturbances associated with movement disorders, particularly PD and HD. Many studies have been hampered by the comorbid motor deficits that interfere with neuropsychological evaluation, but great strides have been made in isolating individual cognitive domains. Other confounding aspects have been the inclusion of heterogeneous populations with both early cognitive decline and advanced dementia, variable severity of motor deficits among subjects, and lack of control for the effects of medication and mood disorders.[134] Cognitive disturbance can occur because of the isolated effects of sub-

cortical pathology, but many movement disorders have additional cortical pathology, which further confounds the characterization of the cognitive deficits. The extent of research in this area is vast. This part of the chapter will summarize pertinent aspects of cognitive dysfunction in the absence of overt dementia. A discussion of dementia follows in the final segment of this chapter.

EXECUTIVE FUNCTION

Executive function can be broadly defined as the ability to plan, organize, and regulate goal-directed behavior. The frontal lobes are critical for executive function.[16] Many cognitive domains are affected by disturbances of executive function. Impaired executive function is the core early deficit in disorders of the basal ganglia and results in difficulties in the generation, maintenance, shifting, and blending of set.[135–139] The interruption of the striatal-pallidothalamic-dorsolateral frontal circuit is likely the underlying basis for the disturbance in executive function.

Executive dysfunction can be shown in focal lesions of the basal ganglia in the absence of any other coexisting pathology.[14] However, these disturbances are generally milder than those seen in the degenerative subcortical diseases, such as PD, HD, or PSP. Patients with focal caudate lesions showed impairment on the WCST; fewer concepts were found than by controls.[15]

PARKINSON'S DISEASE

Deficits of executive function in early PD have been consistently demonstrated, although the nature of the deficit is somewhat controversial. Nondemented PD patients showed decreased generation and maintenance of set and slowness in shifting set in new learning situations but no impairments in overlearned tasks.[21,134] In general, PD patients benefit from external cues and structure, and the deficit tends not to be perseverative but rather difficulty shifting attention to a novel stimulus.[138] Deficits in maintaining set, partially by disengaging from infrequent cues more easily and an inability to ignore irrelevant stimuli, may contribute to apparent bradyphrenia when attempting to solve problems.[20,140,141] Canavan[22] demonstrated a significant effect of age on cognition with a worsening performance on the WCST only in a subset of PD patients who were older. Deficits have been noted in the temporal ordering of events within a procedural task.[135] Overall, executive function is impaired early in PD but may differ from cortical dysexecutive syndromes with fewer perseverative errors.

HUNTINGTON'S DISEASE

HD patients often complain early in their course of organizational difficulties, such as scheduling daily activities, organizing their work, and following recipes.[90,142] They have particular difficulties in changing mental set, making multiple perseverative errors on tests such as the WCST.[136,143] These deficits tend to be more severe than in PD and interfere substantially with evaluation of other domains of cognitive function.

OTHER MOVEMENT DISORDERS

Executive dysfunction can be seen in many other movement disorders, usually in the setting of a subcortical dementia[144] (see later in chapter). Few studies have investigated executive tasks in the early course of basal ganglia disease in patients without dementia. However, a study by Pillon and coworkers[145] showed that PSP patients in the early stages of cognitive decline were more impaired than HD and PD patients on frontal lobe testing. Most of the multiple-system atrophies produce only mild intellectual impairment.[82] Robbins and coworkers[146] found executive deficits in striatonigral degeneration in the absence of significant intellectual impairment. Deficits in set shifting and working memory were qualitatively different from those of PSP and PD patients, more closely resembling errors made by patients with frontal lobe dysfunction.[147]

MEMORY

Memory can be divided into the domains of declarative and procedural.[148] Declarative memory involves items or episodes that are accessible to conscious recollection, whereas procedural memory involves perceptual or motor skills not readily accessible to conscious recall. The hippocampal memory system is essential in the storage of new information, whereas frontal-subcortical circuits are strategic in the organized recall of information. The basal ganglia are important in procedural memory. Thus, it is not surprising that the memory deficits encountered in movement disorders consist of a retrieval deficit for declarative memory and abnormalities in procedural memory.

Impaired declarative memory has been demonstrated in focal lesions of the caudate, with poor retrieval rather than a storage deficit.[14,15] Memory defects in HD and PD are similar in character, but they are more severe in HD. The deficits parallel those seen in focal caudate lesions, with impaired retrieval of declarative memories.[142,143,149,150] Disordered executive function may contribute to the memory retrieval deficit, as both HD and PD patients show poor learning strategies and impaired temporal sequencing of memories.[136,149] In newly diagnosed PD patients, Taylor and coworkers[151] showed poor strategy for recall of semantically related words, whereas patients were no different from controls in recalling unrelated words or in tests of spatial memory. Similar poor strategies for recalling recent and remote memories have been demonstrated in PSP.[152]

Procedural memory has been studied extensively in early HD. Impairment in motor learning with sparing of declarative memory has been shown reliably in some HD patients.[136,142,153,154] However, variations occur in early HD, with deficits in declarative memory in some and in procedural memory in others.[19,136,150] Impaired procedural learning has been demonstrated in a serial reaction time paradigm in PSP.[139]

Examination of remote memory in HD has shown defective recall with a flat temporal gradient. Beatty et al.[155] showed a deficit of equal severity in recalling information from sequentially more remote decades, which differs significantly from the patterns seen in early Alzheimer's disease or Korsakoff patients. This pattern supports the role of the basal ganglia in "accessing" stored declarative information.

SPEECH AND LANGUAGE

Aphasia is not commonly seen in disorders restricted to the basal ganglia, but speech disorders with altered verbal output are common. Disorders of verbal output include aphasia, reiterative speech disorders, and dysarthria.

Aphasia from focal subcortical lesions is usually associated with damage to the white matter pathways[156,157] and, thus, generally is not seen in degenerative diseases of the basal ganglia. Aphasia occurs in movement disorders when there is concomitant cortical pathology. Aphasia is reported in corticobasal-ganglionic degeneration in 21 percent of cases.[82,158] The nature of the aphasia has not been well characterized; it has mostly nonfluent features and is usually mild. One case presented as a primary progressive aphasia with characteristics of a transcortical motor aphasia.[159] Creutzfeldt-Jakob disease frequently has associated aphasia during its course,[39] and it may present with a mixed transcortical aphasia and echolalia.[160]

More subtle language deficits in sentence comprehension, especially with syntactically embedded questions, have been described in early PD.[161] In demented PD patients, deficits were noted in phrase length, speech melody, information content of spontaneous speech, and comprehension of verbal and written commands when compared with nondemented PD.[162] Verbal fluency is reduced in both PD and HD, in addition to reduced word retrieval on confrontational naming.[162,163] Reduction in the expression and comprehension of prosody have also been noted in HD, hypothesized to reflect decreased emotional cognition.[164]

Reiterative speech disorders occur in movement disorders. Echolalia, the tendency to repeat words and phrases just addressed to the patient, has been reported in HD, neuroacanthocytosis, catatonia, postencephalitic parkinsonism, GTD, and startle diseases (hyperekplexia, latah, miryachit).[160,165] Macpherson and coworkers[160] have postulated that echolalia may be a result of involvement of frontal-subcortical circuits, with interruption of "inhibiting" responses and the presence of environmental dependency. Palilalia, the involuntary repetition of words or phrases usually at the end of a phrase, also occurs in movement disorders such as postencephalitic parkinsonism, ICBG, and PD.[166]

Disturbed rate, volume, and initiation of speech are commonly seen with focal lesions of the basal ganglia.[156,157] Degenerative diseases of the basal ganglia show similar speech abnormalities. Dysarthric speech, sometimes to the point of unintelligibility, occurs frequently in HD.[143,166] Perseverative features, decreased initiation, and respiratory dyskinesias may further impair articulation. Hypokinetic movement disorders often produce dysarthria, hypophonia, and occasionally mutism.[166]

VISUOSPATIAL FUNCTION

Visuospatial function encompasses a number of aspects: sensory perception, motor, attention, cognition, and body-spatial orientation.[167] Tests for these different categories have been devised in an attempt to understand visuospatial function in health and disease. There have been extensive studies on the integrity of visuospatial function in movement disorders. As in other areas of cognition, methodological issues have hampered definitive conclusions. These include the interference of motor disability, inconsistent assessment of organizational (executive) dysfunction, and inadequate attention to the presence of dementia or depression. However, clever paradigms with minimal motor components have been devised to try to account for some of these issues.

PARKINSON'S DISEASE

Visuospatial dysfunction is frequently reported in PD, but conclusions as to whether it is an integral part of the disorder are mixed.[137,167–171] Cummings and Huber[167] reviewed the reported abnormalities in the subcategories of visuospatial function, identifying abnormalities in PD in all areas except visual sensory abilities and visual recognition (right-left orientation, recognition of familiar faces and places). A progressive pattern of increasing deficit with advancing disease has been noted: early impairment on rod orientation tests, followed by difficulties with line orientation, block design, and picture arrangement and, finally, deficits in nonfamiliar-face discrimination. Some deficits, such as copying complex figures, recognition of embedded figures, and performance of a task requiring spatial updating, can be accounted for by confounding impairment in executive or motor function.[137,171] However, the consistency of results across many studies, lack of correlation within tests to severity of motor disability, and lack of improvement with L-dopa argue in favor of visuospatial deficit in PD.[167]

OTHER MOVEMENT DISORDERS

Visuospatial function has been less extensively evaluated in HD. HD patients with only mild intellectual decline performed poorly on tests of egocentric orientation, such as determining direction or position based on an internal representation of space (i.e., one's own position)[143,172,173] Deficits of visuospatial function have been described in olivopontocerebellar atrophy, perhaps implicating cerebellocortical loops in visuospatial organization.[174] In striatonigral degeneration, mixed results have been reported, with most investigations yielding deficits similar to those of PD.[82,146] Finally, severe visuospatial and constructional disturbances secondary to parietal lobe involvement are common in corticobasal-ganglionic degeneration.[159,175]

PRAXIS

Apraxia is the inability to perform a motor act despite intact comprehension, motor and sensory skills, and cooperation.[176] Ideomotor apraxia is the inability to carry out an action to command despite retained spontaneous ability to perform the action. Ideational apraxia is the inability to carry out a sequence of actions, especially when handling actual objects. The main movement disorder with disordered praxis is corticobasal-ganglionic degeneration, which frequently presents with asymmetric ideomotor limb apraxia.[82,158,177] Apraxia was reported in 71 percent of cases in one series and may lead to complete loss of limb function.[158] Apraxia of gaze, eyelid opening, and speech can occur. The disorder is attributed primarily to neuronal loss and achromasia in the frontoparietal cortex, although a role for the basal ganglia cannot be excluded.[177]

The only other movement disorder with frequent apraxia is Creutzfeldt-Jakob disease, where it forms a component of the dementia and may appear early in the course in association with extrapyramidal or cerebellar signs.[39,178] PD was reported to have increased apraxia by Grossman et al.[161] but others have not confirmed this in early, nondemented PD patients.[179]

Dementia

Dementia is an acquired syndrome of intellectual impairment as a consequence of brain dysfunction.[39] The clinical criteria for dementia are varied, accounting for differing reported rates of dementia in movement disorders. Many studies have used criteria from the *Diagnostic and Statistical Manual of Mental Disorders* (DSM) III-R for defining dementia, which requires a decline in intellectual function of sufficient severity to interfere with social and occupational function.[69] The degree to which functioning is impaired because of intellectual, as opposed to motor disability, is sometimes difficult to determine in movement disorders. DSM-IV includes "executive function" as an additional area of cognitive impairment, reflecting the increased recognition of subcortical dementia and executive abnormalities within movement disorders.

Dementia in disorders of the basal ganglia is predominantly of the subcortical type. The cardinal features include psychomotor slowing, memory retrieval deficits, abnormal cognition with an impaired ability to manipulate knowledge, alterations in mood or personality, and abnormalities in speech.[64,144] Aphasia, apraxia, agnosia, and amnesia are usually absent. *Dilapidation in cognition* has been used to describe the intellectual impairment, referring to the executive function deficits.[180] Patients may perform individual aspects of a task properly but fail at integrating all necessary sequences and components. The mood and personality disturbances most frequently consist of depression and a lack of motivation or initiative. Although the division of dementias into cortical and subcortical types has been challenged frequently,[181,182] based on a lack of anatomic specificity, it remains a useful clinical phenomenological distinction. Perhaps more accurate terminology would use frontal-subcortical systems dementia, as it is the disruption of the three behavioral circuits described earlier that produces the cardinal manifestations. Table 2-5 lists movement disorders with a predominant subcortical pattern of dementia.

In addition to the subcortical dementia, one may observe a mixed cortical-subcortical dementia in association with movement disorders (Table 2-5). PD, for example, is associated with three types of dementia: a typical subcortical dementia, a cortical dementia clinically and neuropathologically indistinguishable from Alzheimer's disease (AD), and a disorder variably termed diffuse Lewy body disease (DLBD), cortical Lewy body dementia, or senile dementia of the Lewy body type.[85,183–188] The dementias of PD are discussed in more detail below.

The remainder of this chapter will review the common movement disorders with prominent dementia.

HUNTINGTON'S DISEASE

Dementia in HD is considered one of the cardinal features of the disease, although the reported cross-sectional prevalence

TABLE 2-5 Movement Disorders with Dementia

Subcortical Pattern	Cortical Pattern
Parkinsonism	Corticobasal-ganglionic degeneration
Parkinson's disease	
Progressive supranuclear palsy	Cortical Lewy body disease
	Creutzfeldt-Jakob disease
Hallervorden-Spatz disease	Gerstmann-Straussler-Scheinker disease
Idiopathic calcification of the basal ganglia	
Postencephalitic parkinsonism	Parkinson's disease + Alzheimer's disease
Parkinsonism-dementia/ALS of Guam	
Olivopontocerebellar atrophy	
Dentatorubropallido-luysian atrophy	
Spinocerebellar degenerations	
Vascular	
Lacunar state	
Binswanger disease	
Manganese toxicity	
Thalamic degenerations	
Hydrocephalus	
Dementia syndrome of depression	
Whipple disease	
Dementia pugilistica	
Hyperkinetic	
Huntington's disease	
Wilson's disease	
Neuroacanthocytosis	

has varied widely from 15–95 percent, depending on diagnostic criteria.[143] The characteristics of the dementia conform to a subcortical type, with early changes in personality and mood with or without psychosis, followed by cognitive deficits primarily in the realms of memory retrieval deficits, executive dysfunction, and slowing of cognition.[18,19,70,90,91,142,143] Higher cortical deficits, such as aphasia, agnosia, and apraxia, are typically lacking. There appears to be little relationship between the extent of psychopathology and the severity of cognitive deficits.[25,29] The intellectual impairment progresses as the disease advances and has been correlated with duration of illness,[90] as well as with extent of atrophy of subcortical structures, particularly the head of the caudate, on both computed tomography and magnetic resonance imaging.[189,190] Striatal glucose metabolic rate, measured by PET, has also been correlated with extent of neuropsychological deficit.[191]

The nature of the behavioral and neuropsychological deficits in HD is similar to that seen in patients with frontal lobe lesions.[39] The dementia in HD is attributed to striatal degeneration and interruption of frontal subcortical circuits, although some authors feel that the inconsistent neuropathological changes reported in the cerebral cortex may be relevant.[26]

PROGRESSIVE SUPRANUCLEAR PALSY

PSP is an example of a disorder with pure subcortical neuropathological changes manifesting with dementia. Personality

change with apathy may occur early along with mild cognitive deficits; the cognitive impairment usually progresses to moderate intellectual impairment with deficits in memory retrieval and slowing of information processing and manipulation.[64,82,139,145] Dementia has been found in the later stages by the majority of authors.[82] Hypometabolic changes in the dorsal frontal lobe on PET support a relationship between dementia and interruption of frontal-subcortical circuits.[192,193]

PARKINSON'S DISEASE

The frequency of dementia in PD is variably reported, ranging from 4 to 93 percent, with an overall frequency of 39.9 percent based on a review of 27 studies.[186] The variability arises from differing methods of cognitive assessment, definition of dementia, and study populations. The best current prevalence data from the general population suggests that dementia in PD occurs in 41 percent,[194] higher than previously estimated at 29 percent.[195] The rate of dementia in PD is higher than in the general population matched for age and sex. The risk for dementia developing in PD over a 3- to 5-year period is approximately four times greater than that in the general population matched for age and sex.[195,196] Risks for dementia include older age of onset and the types with predominant rigidity.[186,194,197] Progression of disability and mortality is also higher in demented PD patients, compared with that of nondemented PD.[45,194,195]

There are clinical subtypes of dementia within PD, and these may correlate with different underlying pathologies.[186,198] Mild cognitive deficits in PD are almost ubiquitous, and the pattern of cognitive change was discussed previously in this chapter under the section entitled Cognitive Disturbances. The dementia in PD is most commonly mild to moderate in severity, with bradyphrenia, memory retrieval deficits, impaired set shifting and maintenance, impaired problem solving, poor visuospatial function, decreased word list generation, and prominent mood disorder.[20,73,134,186] However, more severe dementia in PD does occur and is usually but not invariably associated with AD-type pathology; advanced dementia can occur in the absence of AD-type changes, either in the nucleus basalis or cerebral cortex.[183–185,198,199] The frequency of AD-type pathology is debated (10–60 percent), depending on neuropathological criteria and methods, but may be greater than in an age-matched population. Dementia with combined pathology tends to have mixed cortical and subcortical features.[198,200] The implications of a possible overlap between AD and PD is uncertain and may reflect either a neuropathological spectrum of two diseases or a unique disorder that resembles AD and PD superficially.[183]

Neurochemical changes may also contribute to dementia in PD. Cholinergic function is most deficient in PD patients with dementia but does not always correlate with the extent of AD-type pathology.[200,201] Dementia in PD also correlates with extent of cell loss in the medial substantia nigra.[23] A combination of dopaminergic and cholinergic deficits is likely of relevance neurochemically, although other neurotransmitters may also be involved.

A final type of dementia associated with PD is a dementia occurring with cortical Lewy bodies. Since the use of antiubiquitin stains to identify Lewy bodies in the cortex became customary, the "Lewy body dementias" have become the second most common type of dementia after AD, occurring in 7–30 percent of referral populations.[85,202] However, Lewy bodies using this technique have been found in essentially 100 percent of PD patients, even those without dementia.[203,204] In the patients meeting dementia criteria, AD and Lewy body pathology may both occur, either independently or together. Although consensus pathological or clinical criteria is lacking for the Lewy body dementias (LBD), clinical characterization suggest two basic forms of LBD[205]: (1) "pure" LBD with no AD changes on pathology, clinically presenting with prominent rigidity early in the course and dementia only in the later stages, and (2) "common" LBD with concomitant AD pathology (plaques more than tangles), presenting with cognitive and neuropsychiatric disturbances and milder but definite extrapyramidal features.

Clinical criteria attempting to distinguish LBD from AD have been proposed and include fluctuating cognitive impairment, psychotic features with complex visual hallucinations and paranoid delusions, spontaneous extrapyramidal features or marked neuroleptic sensitivity, and repeated unexplained falls.[206] However, these features do not occur in all LBD patients, and the criteria have yet to be validated in a prospective fashion.[205] The exact relationship to AD and PD remains to be determined, as does the role of the Lewy body in cognitive dysfunction.

MULTIPLE-SYSTEM ATROPHIES

The multiple-system atrophies include olivopontocerebellar atrophy (OPCA), striatonigral degeneration (SND), and Shy-Drager syndrome (SDS). These disorders have both familial and sporadic forms. Dementia has been found frequently in certain subgroups of the OPCAs, but dementia is not present until the very late stages in some families.[82] Classification of these disorders continues to be problematic, and it is difficult to establish any clear profiles of dementia across all subgroups.

Patients with sporadic versus familial OPCA were compared by Berciano,[207] who found dementia in 35 percent of the former and 57 percent of the latter, mostly in the middle-to-late stages of the disease. Dementia may occur early and was a dominant feature in 11 to 22 percent of cases, respectively. For the most part, the dementias have the subcortical pattern of cognitive impairment, with gradually progressive cognitive decline involving slowness of information processing, apathy, frontal/executive dysfunction, and impaired visuoconstructional skills.[39,82,174] Deficits of cortical function, such as aphasia, apraxia, and agnosia, have generally been absent, although two members of one family reported with OPCA type V (as classified by Konigsmark and Weiner) were described with aphasia.[208] The occurrence of aphasia may relate to cortical neuronal loss described in this subgroup.

Cognitive impairment in SND and SDS is usually mild, with impairments predominantly involving executive function.[82,146] Patients generally do not meet criteria for dementia. The deficits are milder than in PSP and similar to those observed in the early stages of PD, although the limited number of studies have produced conflicting results.

WILSON'S DISEASE

Intellectual impairment has been reported in Wilson's disease, but the deficits are mild in severity, compared with those seen in PSP and HD.[63,209] As noted earlier in the chapter, personality alterations may occur early in the disease and often predate cognitive or neurological decline.[210] Failure to progress in school may be an early sign in juvenile onset cases. Neuropsychological changes include retrieval deficits on the Wechsler Memory Scale, decline in Full Scale IQ, and poor concentration.[63,209] Dening and Berrios[61] classified only 11 of 45 patients suspected of cognitive deficits as being intellectually impaired in a retrospective review. The cognitive deficits may respond to a reduction in copper.[63,211] The relationship between cognitive, neuropathological, and radiological changes in Wilson's disease has not been systematically assessed.

RARER MOVEMENT DISORDERS WITH PROMINENT DEMENTIA

Dementia is a prominent feature of some less common basal ganglia disorders. ICBG is a familial disorder with extensive calcification of the basal ganglia, despite normal serum calcium and phosphate. It presents with chorea or a parkinsonian-type extrapyramidal disorder. The younger onset form of ICBG presents primarily with psychosis, whereas the later-onset variety (mean age, 49.4 years) presents with dementia and movement disorder.[28,29] Dementia typical of a subcortical process, with memory retrieval deficits and poor concentration, is characteristic.[39]

Hallervorden-Spatz disease is a rare familial disorder with deposition of iron-containing pigment in the GP and ventral substantia nigra.[39] The dementia syndrome includes psychomotor slowing, poor memory, impaired attention and concentration, and diminished intellectual function.[212] The movement disorder is heterogeneous, with rigidity, dystonic posturing, and chorea predominating.

Parkinsonism-dementia/ALS complex of Guam presents with early, often severe dementia, which may be the most prominent disability.[82,93,127] The mental status changes are inexorably progressive, with personality changes, mental slowing, poor memory, and frequent mood disorders.

Finally, thalamic degenerations are a heterogeneous group of rare disorders in which there are cognitive and behavioral changes consisting of amnesia, confusion, apathy, and labile affect in association with a variety of motor disorders such as involuntary movements, chorea, ataxia, and myoclonus.[39,213] Akinetic mutism may occur. The amnestic quality of the memory defects is in contrast to the more typical retrieval deficit seen in subcortical dementias, and reflects involvement of the hippocampal-thalamic memory storage system.

Comment

The interruption of the three frontal-subcortical circuits mediating behavior results in neuropsychiatric and cognitive disturbances in most movement disorders. These neurobehavioral changes can occur with both focal basal ganglia lesions and degenerative diseases involving subcortical structures. Early behavioral changes are common, and awareness of the association with movement disorders may allow earlier diagnosis and potentially more efficacious therapy.

Acknowledgments

This work was supported by the Department of Veterans Affairs and National Institute of Aging Alzheimer's Disease Center Grant AG10123.

References

1. Wilson SAK: Progressive lenticular degeneration: A familial nervous disease associated with cirrhosis of the liver. *Brain* 34:295–507, 1912.
2. Huntington G: On chorea. *Med Surg Rep* 26:317–321, 1872.
3. Parkinson J: *An Essay on the Shaking Palsy.* London: Sherwood, Neely and Jones, 1817.
4. Booth G: Psychodynamics in parkinsonism. *Psychosom Med* 10:1–4, 1948.
5. Lit AC: Man behind a mask: An analysis of the psychomotor phenomena of Parkinson's disease. *Acta Neurol Belg* 68:863–874, 1968.
6. Sands I: The type of personality susceptible to Parkinson's disease. *Mt Sinai J Med* 9:792–794, 1942.
7. Cummings JL: *Clinical Neuropsychiatry.* New York: Grune & Stratton, 1985.
8. Denny-Brown D: *The Basal Ganglia and Their Relation to Disorders of Movement.* Oxford: Oxford University Press, 1962.
9. Cummings JL: Frontal-subcortical circuits and human behavior. *Arch Neurol* 50:873–880, 1993.
10. Alexander GE, Crutcher MD: Functional architecture of basal ganglia circuits: Neural substrates of parallel processing. *Trends Neurosci* 13:266–271, 1990.
11. Alexander GE, DeLong MR, Strick PL: Parallel organization of functionally segregated circuits linking basal ganglia and cortex. *Annu Rev Neurosci* 9:357–381, 1986.
12. Alexander GE, Crutcher MD, DeLong MR: Basal ganglia-thalamocortical circuits: Parallel substrates for motor, oculomotor, prefrontal and limbic functions. *Prog Brain Res* 85:119–146, 1990.
13. Saint-Cyr JA, Taylor AE, Nicholson K: Behavior and the basal ganglia. *Adv Neurol* 65:1–128, 1995.
14. Dubois B, Defontaines B, Deweer B, et al: Cognitive and behavioral changes in patients with focal lesions of the basal ganglia. *Adv Neurol* 65:29–41, 1995.
15. Mendez MF, Adams NL, Lewandowski KS: Neurobehavioral changes associated with caudate lesions. *Neurology* 39:349–354, 1989.
16. Stuss DT, Benson DF: *The Frontal Lobes.* New York: Raven Press, 1986.
17. Benton AL: Differential behavioral effects in frontal lobe disease. *Neuropsychologia* 6:53–60, 1968.
18. Butters N, Sax D, Montgomery K, Tarlow S: Comparison of the neuropsychological deficits associated with early and advanced Huntington's disease. *Arch Neurol* 35:585–589, 1978.
19. Brandt J: Cognitive impairments in Huntington's disease: Insights into the neuropsychology of the striatum, in Boller F, Grafman J (eds): *Handbook of Neuropsychology.* Amsterdam: Elsevier, 1991, vol 5, pp 241–264.
20. Levin BE, Tomer R, Rey GF: Cognitive impairments in Parkinson's disease. *Neurol Clin* 10:471–485, 1992.
21. Rashkin SA, Borod JC, Tweedy J: Neuropsychological aspects of Parkinson's disease. *Neuropsychol Rev* 1:185–219, 1990.
22. Canavan AGM: The performance on learning tasks of patients in the early stages of Parkinson's disease. *Neuropsychologia* 27:141–156, 1989.
23. Rinne JO, Rummukainen J, Paljarvi L, Rinne VK: Dementia in Parkinson's disease is related to neuronal loss in the medial substantia nigra. *Ann Neurol* 26:47–50, 1989.
24. Morris M: Psychiatric aspects of Huntington's disease, in Harper PS (ed): *Huntington's Disease.* Philadelphia: WB Saunders, 1991, pp 81–126.
25. Cummings JL: Behavioral and psychiatric symptoms associated with Huntington's disease. *Adv Neurol* 65:179–186, 1995.
26. Vonsattel J-P, Myers RH, Stevens TJ, et al: Neuropathological classification of Huntington's disease. *J Neuropathol Exp Neurol* 44:559–577, 1985.
27. Folstein SE: *Huntington's Disease: A Disorder of Families.* Baltimore: John Hopkins University Press, 1989, pp 49–64.
28. Cummings JL, Gosenfeld LF, Houlihan JP, McCaffrey T: Neuropsychiatric disturbances associated with idiopathic calcification of the basal ganglia. *Biol Psychiatry* 18:591–601, 1983.
29. Francis AF: Familial basal ganglia calcification and schizophreniform psychosis. *Br J Psychiatry* 135:360–362, 1979.
30. Wyszynski B, Merriam A, Medalia A, et al: Choreoacanthocytosis: Report of a case with psychiatric features. *Neuropsychiatr Neuropsychol Behav Neurol* 2:137–144, 1989.
31. Barris RW, Schuman HR: Bilateral anterior cingulate gyrus lesions. *Neurology* 3:44–52, 1953.
32. Santamaria J, Tolosa E: Clinical subtypes of Parkinson's disease and depression, in Huber SJ, Cummings JL (eds): *Parkinson's Disease: Behavioral and Neuropsychological Aspects.* New York: Oxford University Press, 1992, pp 217–228.
33. Cummings JL: Depression and Parkinson's disease: A review. *Am J Psychiatry* 149:443–454, 1992.
34. Ring HA, Bench CJ, Trimble MR, et al: Depression in Parkinson's disease: A positron emission study. *Br J Psychiatry* 165:333–339, 1994.
35. Mayberg HS, Starkstein SE, Sadzot B, et al: Selective hypometabolism in the inferior frontal lobe in depressed patients with Parkinson's disease. *Ann Neurol* 28:57–64, 1990.
36. Baxter LR Jr, Schwartz JM, Phelps ME, et al: Reduction of prefrontal cortex glucose metabolism common to three types of depression. *Arch Gen Psychiatry* 46:243–250, 1989.
37. Levin BE, Llabre MM, Weiner WJ: Parkinson's disease and depression: Psychometric properties of the Beck Depression Inventory. *J Neurol Neurosurg Psychiatry* 51:1401–1404, 1988.
38. Starkstein SE, Preziosi TJ, Forrester AW, Robinson RG: Specificity of affective and autonomic symptoms of depression in Parkinson's disease. *J Neurol Neurosurg Psychiatry* 53:869–873, 1990.
39. Cummings JL, Benson DF: *Dementia: A Clinical Approach,* 2d ed. Boston: Butterworth-Heinemann, 1992.
40. Brown RG, MacCarthy B, Gotham AM, et al: Depression and disability in Parkinson's disease: A follow-up study of 132 cases. *Psychol Med* 18:49–55, 1988.
41. Taylor AE, Saint-Cyr JA, Lang AE, Kenny FT: Parkinson's disease and depression: A critical re-evaluation. *Brain* 109:279–292, 1986.
42. Gotham AM, Brown RG, Marsden CD: Depression in Parkinson's disease: A quantitative and qualitative analysis. *J Neurol Neurosurg Psychiatry* 49:381–389, 1986.
43. Schiffer RB, Kurlan R, Rubin A, et al: Evidence for atypical depression in Parkinson's disease. *Am J Psychiatry* 145:1020–1022, 1988.
44. Alexopoulos GS, Young RC, Meyer BS, et al: Late onset depression. *Psychiatr Clin North Am* 11:101–115, 1988.

45. Starkstein SE, Bolduc PL, Mayberg HS, et al: Cognitive impairments and depression in Parkinson's disease: A follow-up study. *J Neurol Neurosurg Psychiatry* 53:597–602, 1990.

46. Mayberg HS, Solomon DH: Depression in Parkinson's disease: A biochemical and organic viewpoint. *Adv Neurol* 65:49–60, 1995.

47. Mayeux R, Stern Y, Rosen J, Leventhal J: Depression, intellectual impairment, and Parkinson's disease. *Neurology* 31:645–650, 1981.

48. Starkstein SE, Preziosi TJ, Bolduc PL, Robinson RG: Depression in Parkinson's disease. *J Nerv Ment Dis* 178:27–31, 1990.

49. Dakof GA, Mendelsohn GA: Parkinson's disease: The psychological aspects of a chronic illness. *Psychol Bull* 99:375–387, 1986.

50. MacCarthy B, Brown R: Psychosocial factors in Parkinson's disease. *Br J Clin Psychol* 28:41–52, 1989.

51. Santamaria J, Tolosa E, Valles A: Parkinson's disease with depression: a possible subgroup of idiopathic parkinsonism. *Neurology* 36:1130–1133, 1986.

52. Ehmann TS, Beninger RJ, Gawel MJ, Riopelle RJ: Depressive symptoms in Parkinson's disease: A comparison with disabled control subjects. *J Geriatr Psychiatry Neurol* 2:3–9, 1990.

53. Sano M, Stern Y, Cote L, et al: Depression in Parkinson's disease: A biochemical model. *J Neuropsychiatr Clin Neurosci* 2:88–92, 1990.

54. Mayeux R, Stern Y, Sano M, et al: The relationship of serotonin to depression in Parkinson's disease. *Mov Disord* 3:237–244, 1988.

55. Mayeux R, Stern Y, Williams JBW, et al: Clinical and biochemical features of depression in Parkinson's disease. *Am J Psychiatry* 143:756–759, 1986.

56. Brown RG, Marsden CD, Quinn N, Wyke MA: Alterations in cognitive performance and affect-arousal during fluctuations in motor function in Parkinson's disease. *J Neurol Neurosurg Psychiatry* 57:454–465, 1984.

57. Menza MA, Sage J, Marshall E, et al: Mood changes and "on-off" phenomena in Parkinson's disease. *Mov Disord* 5:148–151, 1990.

58. Jellinger K: Overview of morphological changes in Parkinson's disease. *Adv Neurol* 45:1–18, 1986.

59. Caine ED, Shoulson I: Psychiatric syndromes in Huntington's disease. *Am J Psychiatry* 140:728–733, 1983.

60. Schoenfeld M, Myers RH, Cupples LA, et al: Increased rate of suicide among patients with Huntington's disease. *J Neurol Neurosurg Psychiatry* 47:1283–1287, 1984.

61. Dening TR, Berrios GE: Wilson's disease: Psychiatric symptoms in 195 cases. *Arch Gen Psychiatry* 46:1126–34, 1989.

62. Akil M, Schwartz JA, Dutchak D, et al: The psychiatric presentations of Wilson's disease. *J Neuropsychiatr Clin Neurosci* 3:377–382, 1991.

63. Akil M, Brewer GJ: Psychiatric and behavioral abnormalities in Wilson's disease. *Adv Neurol* 65:171–178, 1995.

64. Albert ML, Feldman RG, Willis AL: The subcortical dementia of progressive supranuclear palsy. *J Neurol Neurosurg Psychiatry* 37:121–130, 1974.

65. Kurlan R: Tourette's syndrome: Current concepts. *Neurology* 39:1625–1630, 1989.

66. Robertson MM, Trimble MR, Lees AJ: The psychopathology of the Gilles de la Tourette's syndrome. *Br J Psychiatry* 152:383–390, 1988.

67. Comings DE, Comings BG: Comorbid behavioral disorder, in Kurlan R (ed): *Handbook of Tourette's Syndrome and Related Tic and Behavioral Disorders*. New York: Marcel Dekker, 1993, pp 111–147.

68. Stasiek C, Zetin M: Organic manic disorders. *Psychosomatic* 26:394–402, 1985.

69. American Psychiatric Association: *Diagnostic and Statistical Manual and Mental Disorders* (DSM-IV), 4th ed. Washington, DC: American Psychiatric Press, 1994.

70. Dewhurst K, Oliver J, Trick KLK, McKnight AL: Neuro-psychiatric aspects of Huntington's disease. *Confin Neurol* 31:258–268, 1969.

71. Fairweather DS: Psychiatric aspects of the post-encephalitic syndrome. *J Ment Sci* 93:201–254, 1947.

72. Farlow MR, Yee RD, Dlouhy SR, et al: Gerstmann-Straussler-Scheinker disease. I. Extending the clinical spectrum. *Neurology* 39:1446–1452, 1989.

73. Mayeux R: Parkinson's disease: A review of cognitive and psychiatric disorders. *Neuropsychiatr Neuropsychol Behav Neurol* 3:3–14, 1990.

74. Goodwin FK: Psychiatric side effects of L-dopa in man. *JAMA* 218:1915–1920, 1971.

75. Factor SA, Molho ES, Podskalny GD, Brown D: Parkinson's disease: Drug-induced psychiatric states. *Adv Neurol* 65:115–138, 1995.

76. Kurlan R, Dimitsopulos T: Selegiline and manic behavior in Parkinson's disease. *Arch Neurol* 49:1231, 1992.

77. Cummings JL, Mendez MF: Secondary mania with focal cerebrovascular lesions. *Am J Psychiatry* 141:1084–1087, 1984.

78. Kulisevsky J, Berthier ML, Pujol J: Hemiballismus and secondary mania following a right thalamic infarction. *Neurology* 43:1422–1424, 1993.

79. Cummings JL: Psychosis in neurologic disease: Neurobiology and Pathogenesis. *Neuropsychiatr Neuropsychol Behav Neurol* 5:144–150, 1992.

80. Beckson M, Cummings JL: Psychosis in basal ganglia disorders. *Neuropsychiatr Neuropsychol Behav Neurol* 5:126–131, 1992.

81. Jackson JA, Free GBM, Pike HV: The psychic manifestations in paralysis agitans. *Arch Neurol Psychiatry* 10:680–684, 1923.

82. Cohen S, Freedman M: Cognitive and behavioral changes in the parkinson-plus syndromes, in Weiner WJ, Lang AE (eds): *Adv Neurol* 65:139–157, 1995.

83. Calne DB, Stern GM, Laurence DR, et al: L-dopa in post-encephalitic parkinsonism. *Lancet* 1:744–746, 1969.

84. Cummings JL: Behavioral complications of drug treatment of Parkinson's disease. *J Am Geriatr Soc* 33:708–716, 1991.

85. Perry RH, Irving D, Blessed G, et al: Senile dementia of Lewy body type: A clinically and neuropathologically distinct type of Lewy body dementia in the elderly. *J Neurol Sci* 95:119–139, 1990.

86. Spokes EGS: Dopamine in Huntington's disease: A study of postmortem brain tissue. *Adv Neurol* 23:481–493, 1979.

87. Wegner JT, Kane JM, Weinhold P, et al: Cognitive impairment in tardive dyskinesia. *Psychiatry Res* 16:331–337, 1985.

88. Waddington JL: Psychopathological and cognitive correlates of tardive dyskinesia in schizophrenia and other disorders treated with neuroleptic drugs. *Adv Neurol* 65:211–229, 1995.

89. Laplane D, Baulac M, Wildocher D, Dubois B: Pure psychic akinesia with bilateral lesion of the basal ganglia. *J Neurol Neurosurg Psychiatr* 47:377–385, 1984.

90. Caine ED, Hunt RD, Weingartner H, Eber MH: Huntington's dementia: Clinical and neuropsychological features. *Arch Gen Psychiatry* 35:377–384, 1978.

91. Folstein SE, Brandt J, Folstein MF: The subcortical dementia of Huntington's disease, in Cummings JL (ed): *Subcortical Dementia*. Oxford: Oxford University Press, 1990, pp 87–107.

92. Steele JC, Richardson JC, Olszewski J: Progressive supranuclear palsy. *Arch Neurol* 10:333–358, 1964.

93. Elizan TS, Hirano A, Abrams BM, et al: Amyotrophic lateral sclerosis and parkinsonism dementia of Guam. *Arch Neurol* 14:356–368, 1966.

94. Walkup JT, Scahill LD, Riddle MA: Disruptive behavior, hyperactivity, and learning disabilities in children with Tourette's syndrome. *Adv Neurol* 65:259–272, 1995.

95. Hubble JP, Koller WC: The Parkinsonian personality. *Adv Neurol* 65:43–48, 1995.

96. Smythies JR: The previous personality in parkinsonism. *J Psychosom Res* 11:169–171, 1967.

97. Eatough VM, Kempster PA, Stern GM, Lees AJ: Premorbid personality and idiopathic Parkinson's disease, *Adv Neurol* 53:335–337, 1990.

98. Menza MA, Forman NE, Goldstein HS, Golbe LI: Parkinson's disease, personality, and dopamine. *J Neuropsychiatr Clin Neurosci* 2:282–287, 1990.

99. Menza MA, Golbe LI, Cody RA, et al: Dopamine-related personality traits in Parkinson's disease. *Neurology* 43:505–508, 1993.

100. Riklan M, Weiner H, Diller L: Somato-psychologic studies in Parkinson's disease. I. An investigation into the relationship of certain disease factors to psychological functions. *J Nerv Ment Dis* 129:263–272, 1959.

101. Hubble JP, Venkatesch R, Hassanein RES, et al: Personality and depression in Parkinson's disease. *J Nerv Ment Dis* 181:657–662, 1993.

102. Ward CD, Duvoisin RC, Ince SE, et al: Parkinson's disease in 65 pairs of twins and in a set of quadruplets. *Neurology* 33:815–825, 1983.

103. Rajput AD, Offord KP, Beard M, Kurland LT: A case-control study of smoking habits, dementia and other illnesses in idiopathic Parkinson's disease. *Neurology* 37:226–232, 1987

104. Bauman RJ, Jameson HD, McKean HE, et al: Cigarette smoking and Parkinson's disease. I. A comparison of cases with matched neighbors. *Neurology* 20:839–843, 1980.

105. Morens DM, Grandinetti, Reed D, et al: Cigarette smoking and protection from Parkinson's disease: False association of etiologic clue? *Neurology* 45:1041–1051, 1995.

106. Cummings JL, Frankel M: Gilles de la Tourette syndrome and the neurological basis of obsession and compulsion. *Biol Psychiatry* 20:1117–1126, 1985.

107. Pauls D, Towbin K, Leckman J, et al: Gilles de la Tourette's syndrome and obsessive-compulsive disorder: Evidence supporting a genetic relationship. *Arch Gen Psychiatry* 43:1180–1182, 1986.

108. Como PG: Obsessive-compulsive disorder in Tourette's syndrome. *Adv Neurol* 65:281–291, 1995.

109. Caine ED, McBride MC, Chiverton P, et al: Tourette's syndrome in Monroe County school children. *Neurology* 38:472–475, 1988.

110. Singer HS, Rosenberg LA: The development of behavioral and emotional problems in Tourette's syndrome. *Pediatr Neurol* 5:41–44, 1989.

111. Leonard HL, Swedo SE, Rapoport JL, et al: Tourette syndrome and obsessive-compulsive disorder, *Adv Neurol* 58:83–93, 1992.

112. Pauls DL, Pakstis AJ, Kurlan R, et al: Segregation and linkage analysis of Gilles de la Tourette's syndrome and related disorders. *J Am Acad Child Adolesc Psychiatry* 29:195–203, 1990.

113. Baxter LR, Schwartz JM, Bergmann KS, et al: Caudate glucose metabolic rate changes with drug and behavior therapy for obsessive-compulsive disorder. *Arch Gen Psychiatry* 49:681–690, 1992.

114. Rapoport JL, Wise SP: Obsessive-compulsive disorder: Evidence for basal ganglia dysfunction. *Psychopharmacol Bull* 24:380–384, 1988.

115. Laplane D, Levasseur M, Pillon B, et al: Obsessive-compulsive and other behavioural changes with bilateral basal ganglia lesions. *Brain* 112:699–725, 1989.

116. Baxter LR, Schwartz JM, Guze BH, et al: Neuroimaging in obsessive-compulsive disorder: seeking the mediating neuroanatomy, in Jenike MA, Baer L, Minichiello WE (eds): *Obsessive-compulsive Disorders: Theory and Management.* Chicago: Year Book Medical, 1990, pp 167–188.

117. Claude H, Baruk H, Lamache A: Obsessions-impulsions consecutives a l'encephalite epidemique. *Encephale* 22:716–720, 1922.

118. Jenike MA: Obsessive-compulsive disorder: A question of a neurologic lesion. *Compr Psychiatry* 25:298–304, 1984.

119. Destee A, Gray F, Parent M, et al: Comportement compulsif d'allure obsessionnelle et paralysie supranucleaire progressive. *Rev Neurol (Paris)* 146:12–18, 1990.

120. Tomer R, Levin BE, Weiner WJ: Obsessive-compulsive symptoms and motor asymmetries in Parkinson's disease. *Neuropsychiatr Neuropsychol Behav Neurol* 6:26–30, 1993.

121. Cummings JL, Cunningham K: Obsessive-compulsive disorder in Huntington's disease. *Biol Psychiatry* 31:263–270, 1992.

122. Peterson B, Riddle MA, Cohen DJ, et al: Reduced basal ganglia volumes in Tourette's syndrome using three-dimensional reconstruction techniques from magnetic resonance images. *Neurology* 43:941–949, 1993.

123. Singer HS, Reiss AL, Brown JE, et al: Volumetric MRI changes in basal ganglia of children with Tourette's syndrome. *Neurology* 43:950–956, 1993.

124. Leckman JF, Pauls DL, Peterson BS, et al: Pathogenesis of Tourette's syndrome: Clues from the clinical phenotype. *Adv Neurol* 58:15–24, 1992.

125. Instel TR: Toward a neuroanatomy of obsessive-compulsive disorder. *Arch Gen Psychiatry* 49:739–744, 1992.

126. Yahr MD, Mendoza MR, Moros D, Bergmann KJ: Treatment of Parkinson's disease in early and late phases: Use of pharmacological agents with special reference to deprenyl (selegiline). *Acta Neurol Scand Suppl* 95:95–102, 1983.

127. Roger-Johnson P, Garruto P, Yanagihara R, et al: Amyotrophic lateral sclerosis and parkinsonism dementia on Guam: A thirty year evaluation of clinical and neuropathological trends. *Neurology* 36:7–13, 1986.

128. Schwartz MA, Selhorst JB, Ochs AL, et al: Oculomasticatory myorhythmia: A unique movement disorder occurring in Whipple's disease. *Ann Neurol* 20:677–683, 1986.

129. Nausieda PA, Wiener WJ, Kaplan LR, et al: Sleep disruption in the course of chronic L-dopa therapy: An early feature of the L-dopa psychosis. *Clin Neuropharmacol* 5:183–194, 1982.

130. Sharf B, Moskovitz C, Lupton MD, Klawans HL: Dream phenomena induced by chronic L-dopa therapy. *J Neural Transm* 43:143–151, 1978.

131. Spinella GM, Sheridan PH: Research initiative on Machado-Joseph disease: National Institute of Neurological Disorders and Stroke Workshop summary. *Neurology* 42:2048–2051, 1992.

132. Uitti RJ, Tanner CM, Rajput AH, et al: Hypersexuality with antiparkinsonian therapy. *Clin Neuropharmacol* 12:375–383, 1989.

133. Gorman DG, Cummings JL: Hypersexuality following septal injury. *Arch Neurol* 49:308–310, 1992.

134. Levin BE, Tomer R, Rey G: Clinical correlates of cognitive impairments in Parkinson's disease, in Huber SJ, Cummings JL (eds): *Parkinson's Disease: Behavioral and Neuropsychological Aspects.* New York: Oxford University Press, 1992, pp 97–106.

135. Taylor AE, Saint-Cyr JA: Executive function, in Huber SJ, Cummings JL (eds): *Parkinson's Disease: Behavioral and Neuropsychological Aspects.* New York: Oxford University Press, 1992, pp 74–85.

136. Saint-Cyr JA, Taylor AE, Lang AE: Procedural learning and neostriatal dysfunction in man. *Brain* 111:941–959, 1988.

137. Levin BE, Katzen HL: Early cognitive changes and nondementing behavioral abnormalities in Parkinson's disease. *Adv Neurol* 65:85–95, 1995.

138. Owen AM, Roberts AC, Hodges JR, et al: Contrasting mechanisms of impaired attentional set-shifting in patients with frontal lobe damage or Parkinson's disease. *Brain* 116:1159–1175, 1993.

139. Grafman N: Frontal lobe function in progressive supranuclear palsy. *Arch Neurol* 47:533–558, 1990.

140. Wright MJ, Burns RJ, Geffen GM, et al: Covert orientation of visual attention in Parkinson's disease. *Neuropsychologia* 28:151–159, 1990.

141. Downes JJ, Roberts AC, Sahakian BJ, et al: Impaired extradimensional shift performance in medicated and unmedicated Parkinson's disease: Evidence for a specific attentional dysfunction. *Neuropsychologia* 27:1329–1343, 1989.

142. Shoulson I: Huntington's disease: Cognitive and psychiatric features. *Neuropsychiatr Neuropsychol Behav Neurol* 3:15–22, 1990.

143. Morris M: Dementia and cognitive changes in Huntington's disease. *Adv Neurol* 65:187–200, 1995.

144. Cummings JL: Introduction, in Cummings JL (ed): *Subcortical Dementia.* New York: Oxford University Press, 1990, pp 3–16.

145. Pillon B, Dubois B, Ploska A, Agid Y: Severity and specificity of cognitive impairment in Alzheimer's, Huntington's, and Parkinson's diseases and progressive supranuclear palsy. *Neurology* 41:634–643, 1991.

146. Robbins TW, James M, Lange KW, et al: Cognitive performance in multiple system atrophy. *Brain* 114:271–291, 1992.

147. Robbins TW, James M, Owen AM, et al: Cognitive deficits in progressive supranuclear palsy, Parkinson's disease, and multiple system atrophy in tests sensitive to frontal lobe dysfunction. *J Neurol Neurosurg Psychiatry* 57:79–88, 1994.

148. Cohen NJ, Eichenbaum H, DeAcedo H, Corkin S: Different memory systems underlying acquisition of procedural and declarative knowledge. *Ann N Y Acad Sci* 444:54–71, 1985.

149. Butters N, Wolfe J, Marone M, et al: Memory disorders associated with Huntington's disease: verbal recall, verbal recognition, and procedural memory. *Neuropsychologia* 23:729–743, 1985.

150. Butters N, Sax D, Montgomery K, Tarlow S: Comparison of the neuropsychological deficits associated with early and advanced Huntington's disease. *Arch Neurol* 35:585–589, 1978.

151. Taylor AE, Saint-Cyr JA, Lang AE: Memory and learning in early Parkinson's disease. *Brain Cogn* 2:211–232, 1990.

152. Litvan I, Grafman J, Gomez C, Chase TN: Memory impairment in patients with progressive supranuclear palsy. *Arch Neurol* 46:765–767, 1989.

153. Heindel WC, Butters N, Salmon DP: Impaired learning of a motor skill in patients with Huntington's disease. *Behav Neurosci* 102:141–147, 1988.

154. Bylsma FW, Brandt J, Strauss ME: Aspects of procedural memory are differentially impaired in Huntington's disease. *Arch Clin Neuropsychiatry* 5:287–297, 1990.

155. Beatty WW, Salmon DP, Butters N, et al: Retrograde amnesia in patients with Alzheimer's disease or Huntington's disease. *Neurobiol Aging* 9:181–186, 1988.

156. Alexander M, Naeser MA, Palumbo CL: Correlations of subcortical CT lesions sites and aphasia profiles. *Brain* 110:961–991, 1987.

157. Alexander M: Clinical-anatomical correlations of aphasia following predominantly subcortical lesions, in Boller F, Grafman J (eds): *Handbook of Neuropsychology.* New York: Elsevier, 1989.

158. Riley DE, Lang AE, Lewis A, et al: Cortical-basal ganglionic degeneration. *Neurology* 40:1203–1212, 1990.

159. Lippa CF, Cohen R, Smith TW, Drachman DA: Primary progressive aphasia with focal neuronal achromasia. *Neurology* 41:882–886, 1991.

160. McPherson SE, Kuratani JD, Cummings JL, et al: Creutzfeldt-Jakob disease with mixed transcortical aphasia: Insights into echolalia. *Behav Neurol* 7:197–203, 1994.

161. Grossman M, Carvel S, Goloomp S, et al: Sentence comprehension and praxis deficits in Parkinson's disease. *Neurology* 41:1620–1626, 1991.

162. Cummings JL, Darkins A, Mendez M, et al: Alzheimer's disease and Parkinson's disease: Comparison of Speech and Language alterations. *Neurology* 38:680–684, 1988.

163. Podoll K, Caspary P, Lange HW, Noth J: Language functions in Huntington's disease. *Brain* 111:1475–1503, 1988.

164. Speedie LJ, Brake N, Folstein SE, et al: Comprehension of prosody in Huntington's disease. *J Neurol Neurosurg Psychiatry* 53:607–610, 1990.

165. Ford RA: Neurobehavioural correlates of abnormal repetitive behaviour. *Behav Neurol* 4:113–119, 1991.

166. Benson DF, Ardila A: *Aphasia: A clinical perspective.* New York: Oxford University Press, 1996.

167. Cummings JL, Huber SJ: Visuospatial abnormalities in Parkinson's disease, in Huber SJ, Cummings JL (eds): *Parkinson's Disease: Behavioral and Neuropsychological Aspects.* New York: Oxford University Press, 1992, pp 59–73.

168. Levin BE, Llabre MM, Reisman S, et al: Visuospatial impairment in Parkinson's disease. *Neurology* 41:365–369, 1991.

169. Mohr E, Litvan I, Williams J, et al: Selective deficits in Alzheimer and parkinsonian dementia: Visuospatial function. *Can J Neurol Sci* 17:292–297, 1990.

170. Stelmach GE, Phillips JG, Chau AW: Visuo-perceptual processing in parkinsonians. *Neuropsychologia* 27:485–493, 1989.

171. Brown RG, Marsden CD: Visuospatial function in Parkinson's disease. *Brain* 109:987–1002, 1986.

172. Potegal M: A note on spatial-motor deficits in patients with Huntington's disease: A test of a hypothesis. *Neuropsychologia* 9:233–235, 1971.

173. Brouwers P, Cox C, Martin A, et al: Differential perceptual spatial impairment in Huntington's and Alzheimer's dementia. *Arch Neurol* 41:1073–1076, 1984.

174. Botez MI, Botez T, Eli R, Attig E: Role of the cerebellum in complex human behavior. *Ital J Neurol Sci* 10:291–300, 1989.

175. Gibb WRG, Luthert PJ, Marsden CD: Corticobasalganglionic degeneration. *Brain* 112:1171–1192, 1989.

176. Benson DF, Geschwind N: Aphasia and related disorders: A clinical approach, in Mesulam MM (ed): *Principles of Behavioral Neurology.* Philadelphia: FA Davis, 1985, pp 193–238.

177. Rebeiz JJ, Kolodny EH, Richardson EP: Corticodentatonigral degeneration with neuronal achromasia. *Arch Neurol* 18:20–33, 1968.

178. Brown P, Cahtala F, Castaigne P, Gajdusek DC: Creutzfeldt-Jakob disease: Clinical analysis of a consecutive series of 230 neuropathologically verified cases. *Ann Neurol* 20:597–602, 1986.

179. Lees AJ, Smith E: Cognitive deficits in the early stages of Parkinson's disease. *Brain* 106:257–270, 1983.

180. McHugh PR, Folstein MF: Psychiatric syndromes of Huntington's chorea: A clinical and phenomenologic study, in Benson DF, Blumer D (eds): *Psychiatric Aspects of Neurologic Disease.* New York: Grune & Stratton, 1975, pp 267–285.

181. Mayeux R, Stern Y, Rosen J, Benson DF: Is "subcortical dementia" a recognizable clinical entity? *Arch Neurol* 14:278–283, 1983.

182. Whitehouse PJ: The concept of subcortical and cortical dementia: Another look. *Ann Neurol* 19:1–6, 1986.

183. Grossman M: Alzheimer's disease and parkinsonism, in Stern MB, Kolley WC (eds): *Parkinsonian Syndromes.* New York: Marcel Dekker, 1993, pp 249–277.

184. Xuereb JH, Tomlinson BE, Irving D, et al: Cortical and subcortical pathology in Parkinson's disease: Relationship to parkinsonian dementia. *Adv Neurol* 53:35–40, 1990.

185. Boller F, Mizutani T, Roessmann U, Pierluigi G: Parkinson's disease, dementia, and Alzheimer disease: Clinicopathological correlations. *Ann Neurol* 7:329–335, 1980.

186. Cummings JL: Intellectual impairment in Parkinson's disease: Clinical, pathologic, and biochemical correlates. *J Geriatr Psychiatry Neurol* 1:24–36, 1988.

187. Yoshimura M: Cortical changes in the parkinsonian brain: A contribution to the delineation of diffuse Lewy body disease. *J Neurol* 229(1):17–32, 1983.

188. Okazaki H, Lipkin LE, Aronson SM: Diffuse intracytoplasmic ganglionic inclusion (Lewy type) associated with progressive dementia and quadriparesis in flexion. *Exp Neurol* 20:237–244, 1961.

189. Starkstein SE, Brandt J, Bylsma F, et al: Neuropsychological correlates of brain atrophy in Huntington's disease: A magnetic resonance imaging study. *Neuroadiology* 34:487–489, 1992.

190. Bamford KA, Caine ED, Kido DK, et al: Clinical-pathologic correlation in Huntington's disease: A neuropsychological and computed tomography study. *Neurology* 39:796–801, 1989.

191. Berent S, Giordani B, Lehtinen S, et al: Positron emission tomographic scan investigations of Huntington's disease: Cerebral metabolic correlates of cognitive function. *Ann Neurol* 23:541–546, 1988.

192. D'Antona R, Baron JC, Samson Y, et al: Subcortical dementia: Frontal cortex hypometabolism detected by positron tomography in patients with progressive supranuclear palsy. *Brain* 108:785–799, 1985.

193. Foster NL, Gilman S, Berent S, et al: Cerebral hypometabolism in progressive supranuclear palsy studied with positron emission tomography. *Ann Neurol* 24:399–406, 1988.

194. Mayeux R, Denaro J, Hemenegildo N, et al: A population-based investigation of Parkinson's disease with and without dementia: Relationship to age and gender. *Arch Neurol* 49:492–497, 1992.

195. Rajput AH: Prevalence of dementia in Parkinson's disease, in Huber SJ, Cummings JL (eds): *Parkinson's Disease: Behavioral and Neuropsychological Aspects.* New York: Oxford University Press, 1992, pp 119–131.

196. Mindham RHS, Ahmed SWA, Clough CG: A controlled study of dementia in Parkinson's disease. *J Neurol Neurosurg Psychiatry* 45:969–974, 1982.

197. Huber S, Paulson G, Shuttleworth E: Relationship of motor symptoms, intellectual impairment, and depression in Parkinson's disease. *J Neurol Neurosurg Psychiatry* 51:855–858, 1988.

198. Ross GW, Mahler ME, Cummings JL: The dementia syndromes of Parkinson's disease: Cortical and subcortical features, in Huber SJ, Cummings JL (eds): *Parkinson's Disease: Behavioral and Neuropsychological Aspects.* New York: Oxford University Press, 1992, pp 132–148.

199. Whitehouse PJ, Hedreen JC, White CL, et al: Basal forebrain in the dementia of Parkinson's disease. *Ann Neurol* 13:243–248, 1983.

200. Gaspar P, Gray F: Dementia in idiopathic Parkinson's disease. A neuropathological study of 32 cases. *Acta Neuropathol* 64:43–52, 1984.

201. Perry EK, Curtis M, Dick DJ, et al: Cholinergic correlates of cognitive impairment in Parkinson's disease: Comparison with Alzheimer's disease. *J Neurol Neurosurg Psychiatry* 48:413–421, 1985.

202. Lennos G, Lowe J, Morrell K, et al: Anti-ubiquitin immunocytochemistry is more sensitive than conventional techniques in the detection of diffuse Lewy body disease. *J Neurol Neurosurg Psychiatry* 52:67–71, 1989.

203. Perry E, McKeith I, Thompson P, et al: Topography, extent, and clinical relevance of neurochemical deficits in dementia of Lewy body type, Parkinson's disease, and Alzheimer's disease. *Ann N Y Acad Sci* 640:197–202, 1991.

204. Hughes A, Daniel S, Blankson S, Lees A: A clinicopathologic study of 100 cases of Parkinson's disease. *Arch Neurol* 50:140–148, 1993.

205. Olichney JM, Galasko D, Corey-Bloom J, Thal LJ: The spectrum of diseases with diffuse Lewy bodies. *Adv Neurol* 65:159–170, 1995.

206. McKeith IG, Perry RH, Fairbairn AF, et al: Operational criteria for senile dementia of Lewy body type (SDLT). *Psychol Med* 22:911–922, 1992.

207. Berciano J: Olivopontocerebellar atrophy: A review of 117 cases. *J Neurol Sci* 53:253–272, 1982.

208. Konigsmark BW, Weiner LP: The olivopontocerebellar atrophies: A review. *Medicine* 49:227–241, 1970.

209. Medalia A, Isaacs-Glabermann K, Scheinberg H: Neuropsychological impairment in Wilson's disease. *Arch Neurol* 45:502–504, 1988.

210. Martin JP: Wilson's disease, in Vinken PJ, Bruyn GW (eds): *Diseases of the Basal Ganglia. Handbook of Clinical Neurology.* New York: American Elsevier, 1968, vol 6, pp 267–278.

211. Rosselli M, Lorenzana P, Rosselli A, Vergara I: Wilson's disease, a reversible dementia: Case report. *J Clin Exp Neuropsychol* 9:399–406, 1987.

212. Dooling EC, Schoene WC, Richardson EP Jr: Hallervorden-Spatz syndrome. *Arch Neurol* 30:70–83, 1974.

213. Martin JJ: Thalamic degenerations, in Vinken PJ, Bruyn GW (eds): *System Disorders and Atrophies. Handbook of Clinical Neurology.* Amsterdam: North Holland Publishing Co., 1975, vol 21/1, pp 587–604.

Chapter 3

NEUROIMAGING OF MOVEMENT DISORDERS

DAVID J. BROOKS

ROLE OF THE BASAL GANGLIA
AKINETIC-RIGID SYNDROMES
    Parkinson's Disease
    Detection of Preclinical Disease
    Atypical Parkinsonian Syndromes
INVOLUNTARY MOVEMENT DISORDERS
CONCLUSION

The role of structural imaging in the understanding and diagnosis of movement disorders is a limited one. Computed tomography/magnetic resonance imaging (CT/MRI) findings in nondegenerative disorders, such as idiopathic dystonia and Tourette's syndrome, tend to be normal, although cases of acquired dystonia may show structural lesions in the lentiform nucleus or posterior thalamus.[1-3] Idiopathic Parkinson's disease (PD) patients may show increased signal from the substantia nigra on T_2-weighted MRI, but this is not a consistent finding.[4,5] Multisystem degenerations with associated parkinsonism, such as striatonigral degeneration and progressive supranuclear palsy, may on occasion be distinguishable from idiopathic PD if reduced T_2-weighted lentiform nucleus signal or evidence of brain stem and/or cerebellar atrophy is present.[5,6] These differential MRI findings, however, are unreliable. Although MRI signal changes, generally manifested as raised T_2-weighted signal, can be found in the lentiform nucleus and other areas of gray matter in established neurological Wilson's disease,[7] this modality is insensitive for detecting subclinical cerebral involvement in the hepatic form. Altered MRI signal in striatum and later caudate atrophy are evident in established cases of Huntington's disease,[8,9] but asymptomatic gene carriers generally have normal findings.

Functional imaging provides a sensitive means of detecting and characterizing regional changes in brain metabolism and receptor binding in movement disorders. There are three main approaches to functional imaging: Positron emission tomography (PET) allows quantitative examination of regional cerebral blood flow (rCBF), glucose and oxygen metabolism (rCMRGlc, $rCMRO_2$), and brain pharmacology. Single-photon emission tomography (SPECT) gives semiquantitative estimates of rCBF and receptor binding. The third approach involves the use of magnetic resonance to measure changes in brain activation and metabolite levels. The bulk of reports concerning in vivo brain function in movement disorders have, to date, concerned PET, so this chapter will concentrate on this technique but compares SPECT findings where relevant. There are two basic approaches to examining the changes in cerebral function that are associated with movement disorders: First, abnormalities in resting levels of regional cerebral metabolism, blood flow, and neuroreceptor binding can be examined. Second, abnormal cortical and subcortical activity associated with either involuntary movements per se can be studied, or patients with movement disorders can be asked to perform motor tasks in order to reveal abnormalities in patterns of cerebral activation.

Role of the Basal Ganglia

When a movement is made, it is first necessary to decide its nature; select basic parameters such as direction, force, velocity, and acceleration; and then to prepare and execute the action. It is also essential that inappropriate muscular contraction (i.e., contraction of antagonists and unrelated muscles) is inhibited and that sequential patterns of movement are performed in the correct order. When the movement is novel, skill acquisition may also be required. The exact role that the basal ganglia play in controlling motor function is still uncertain, but it has been suggested that they may play a primary role in all these aspects of motor control.

Animal studies have revealed that the basal ganglia are components of segregated parallel anatomic "loops" involving frontal cortex.[10] A dorsolateral prefrontal loop links this prefrontal area via dorsal head of caudate nucleus and anterior globus pallidus to the ventral anterior and dorsomedial thalamic nuclei which, in turn, project back to prefrontal cortex. A motor loop links posterior lateral and mesial premotor areas and sensorimotor cortex via dorsal posterior putamen and posterior inferior globus pallidus to the ventrolateral thalamus which, in turn, projects back to the posterior lateral premotor and supplementary motor areas. As a consequence, the most likely function of the basal ganglia would seem to be to modulate the higher functions performed by the frontal areas from which they receive and to which they send projections.

Functional imaging allows us to examine patterns of basal ganglia activation, as evidenced by blood flow changes, associated with performance of different motor tasks and so helps us draw conclusions over their possible role. Using $H_2^{15}O$ PET, it has been reported that performance of paced joystick movements leads to a similar level of lentiform nucleus activation, whether the directions of the movements are freely chosen, instructed by the pitch of a tone, or fixed in the same forward direction.[11,12] There is a suggestion, however, that the focus of putamen activation may become more anteriorly sited when motor decisions are being made (M Jueptner, unpublished observations). Extension of the index finger has also been shown to be associated with equivalent lentiform nucleus activation irrespective of whether movements are self-paced or cued.[13] Taken together, these observations suggest that, although they are involved, the basal ganglia do not play a primary role in making decisions over direction and timing of volitional movements.

The role of the basal ganglia in skill acquisition has also been studied with PET. In an initial study, subjects were asked to keep the tip of a metal stylus against a 2-cm metal target on a 20-cm disk diameter that rotated at 60 rpm (a pursuit rotor task), and then serial blood flow measurements were performed over 60 minutes as proficiency was gained.[14] The contralateral lentiform nucleus was activated by this pursuit, but levels of activated putamen rCBF stayed constant, although subjects acquired greater skill, as evidenced by an increased time on target. This finding suggests that the basal ganglia are not primarily involved in the process of procedural learning.

A lack of involvement of the putamen in procedural learning can also be drawn from two other studies.[15,16] In the first, subjects were asked to perform paced sequential thumb oppositions against each finger of the right hand and underwent repetitive measurements of rCBF. Familiarity with the paradigm led to no change in levels of basal ganglia activity. In the second, regional cerebral activation associated with performance of repetitive opposition of all fingers simultaneously to the thumb was compared with that associated with performance of a complex sequence of finger opposition movements. Again, similar activation increases in contralateral putamen rCBF were found. These PET studies, therefore, argue against the basal ganglia playing a primary role in either acquisition of skilled movement.

The role of the basal ganglia in acquiring a correct sequence of finger movements has also been explored.[17] Levels of basal ganglia rCBF obtained while subjects learned a new eight-move sequence of keypresses by trial and error were compared with levels when the subjects performed a prelearned sequence of finger movements. The lentiform nucleus was equally activated whether sequences of movements were being acquired or performed automatically. The authors concluded that the lentiform nucleus was not involved in the process by which complex sequential movements become familiar. A follow-up of this study with a higher-sensitivity camera has confirmed this finding but suggested that the location of the lentiform activation focus moves more anteriorly during active learning (M Jueptner, unpublished observations). It was also possible to demonstrate head-of-caudate activation during learning on this occasion, though as the caudate activation occurred in association with dorsal prefrontal activation, it may, however, have simply reflected increased afferent input from that structure.

Levels of basal ganglia activation have also been examined when paced joystick movements in freely chosen directions were performed at increasing frequencies and when a Morse key was pressed with increasing force by the index finger.[18,19] Both joystick and finger movements activated the putamen, but levels of blood flow remained constant as frequency and force of movement increased. These findings are, therefore, against the basal ganglia playing a primary role in determining basic movement parameters.

So what is the role of the basal ganglia? It has recently been shown that, whether limb movements are simply imagined or actually performed, there is a similar level of activation of the lentiform nucleus.[20] This would be compatible with the basal ganglia having a role in both movement preparation and execution. One possible role, compatible with all of the above published PET findings, is that when a motor decision is made by higher centers, the lentiform nuclei facilitate the required movement by continuously focusing and filtering

mizing the pattern of muscular activity in the light of sensory feedback, so that the goal state is reached efficiently. In other words they act to optimize motor programs. As the motor program is optimized it is relayed to the primary motor cortex for execution at the appropriate force and velocity and to the cerebellum if automaticity is required. At the same time the basal ganglia may act to filter out unwanted muscular contractions. This suggested role for the basal ganglia would explain their activation during imaginary actions and also their lack of primary involvement in making motor decisions and determining the basic parameters of movement. It is also compatible with the observation that pallidotomy in PD results in improvement rather than disability. If, once optimized by the basal ganglia, a program is dumped in the cerebellum, its future automatic running would not require pallidal output. This would also explain why basal ganglia degeneration can lead to slow hypometric movements or involuntary movements in the various subcortical degenerations.

Akinetic-Rigid Syndromes

PARKINSON'S DISEASE

Currently, there is no in vivo biological marker for PD. As a consequence, clinical or pathological criteria have to be applied to make a diagnosis. Clinically, it is conventional to regard PD as a condition characterized by the presence of extrapyramidal rigidity, a 3- to 5-Hz rest tremor with or without a 4- to 8-Hz postural component, and bradykinesia.[21] A good response to L-dopa and asymmetrical onset of limb involvement are supporting diagnostic features. Atypical features include supranuclear gaze difficulties, cerebellar or pyramidal signs, and early onset of autonomic, gait, or bulbar problems. Although these are reasonable diagnostic guidelines, a significant minority of patients with atypical parkinsonian syndromes (striatonigral degeneration, Steele-Richardson-Olszewski syndrome) can retain a reasonable L-dopa response throughout their illness, and a few never show atypical features.[22]

The pathological hallmark of PD is generally agreed to be degeneration of pigmented and other brain stem nuclei (substantia nigra compacta, locus ceruleus, dorsal nuclei of the vagus, nucleus accumbens, and nucleus basalis of Meynert) associated with neuronal Lewy inclusion bodies.[23] The Lewy body is an eosinophilic inclusion with a characteristic halo, is made up of neurofilaments, and has ubiquitin immunoreactivity. Loss of cells from the substantia nigra in PD results in profound dopamine depletion in the striatum, ventral projections to putamen being more affected than dorsal projections to head of caudate.[24–27]

In a recent pathological series, all PD patients examined were found to have occasional cortical, as well as brain stem, Lewy bodies.[21] When cortical involvement becomes extensive, the condition is usually termed diffuse Lewy body disease (DLBD), rather than PD, but currently it remains unclear whether DLBD and PD are opposite ends of a spectrum. Cases of DLBD can present as L-dopa-responsive akinetic-rigid syndromes, but this condition may also manifest as isolated dementia indistinguishable from Alzheimer's disease.[28] To confuse the issue further, cases of LBD have been reported that had poorly L-dopa-responsive parkinsonism,[21] supranuclear gaze problems,[29,30] isolated dystonia,[31] and isolated autonomic failure.[32] As a consequence, if one is trying to determine the etiology of Parkinson's disease, defined as brain stem LBD, it may be necessary to include these other syndromes within the spectrum if they occur in at-risk subjects such as relatives of patients with typical disease.

STUDIES ON RESTING METABOLISM

PET measurements of rCMRGlc with [18]FDG primarily reflect the metabolism of nerve terminal synaptic vesicles whereas rCMRO$_2$ studies with [15]O$_2$ are also influenced by somatic metabolism. Levels of metabolism in the basal ganglia, therefore, reflect the synaptic activity of interneurons and, to a lesser extent, afferent projections to those nuclei, rather than that of basal ganglia efferent projections. Monkeys made hemiparkinsonian by administering the nigral toxin 1-methyl-4-phenyltetrahydropyridine (MPTP) show an increase in external, but not internal, pallidal glucose utilization.[33] Striatal output projections are GABAergic and inhibitory in action. Increased lateral pallidal metabolism after nigral destruction suggests that the nigrostriatal dopaminergic system normally has an inhibitory action on striatoexternal pallidal projections.

Using PET, increased rCMRO$_2$ and rCMRGlc can be demonstrated in the lentiform nucleus contralateral to the affected limbs in hemiparkinsonian patients with early disease.[34,35] Unfortunately, the current resolution of PET is not sufficient to separately resolve external pallidal activity. When treated subjects with bilateral PD are studied, metabolism of the lentiform nuclei tends to be normal or mildly reduced; however, covariance analysis can sensitively demonstrate an abnormal inverse relationship between lentiform nucleus and frontal metabolism in these patients which correlates with disease severity.[36] L-dopa therapy appears to have little effect on resting striatal metabolism.[37] This is not entirely surprising, as nigrostriatal projections account for only a small percentage of the total striatal synaptic activity and, therefore, large changes in activity of the dopaminergic system after administration of exogenous dopa may lead to only small overall changes in total resting striatal activity.

Nondemented hemiparkinsonian patients, early into their disease, show small but significant decreases in frontal blood flow and metabolism contralateral to their affected limbs.[35,38] Bilaterally affected PD patients show more diffuse cortical hypometabolism, levels of glucose use correlating with psychometric performance.[39,40] [18]FDG scans of frankly demented PD patients generally show an Alzheimer's disease pattern of impaired brain glucose use, posterior parietal and temporal association areas being most affected.[35,41–43] Only one demented PD patient has had pathological findings correlated with [18]FDG PET, and no cortical changes of either Alzheimer's disease or DLBD involvement were evident.[44] As a consequence, it remains unclear whether the pattern of glucose hypometabolism in demented PD patients reflects coincidental Alzheimer's disease, cortical LBD, loss of cholinergic projections, or another degenerative process. As lesions of

the nucleus basalis of Meynert in primates result in transient diffuse cortical hypometabolism,[45] it would seem that loss of cholinergic projections is an unlikely explanation of the pattern of reduced [18]FDG uptake found in demented PD patients.

Recently, clinical criteria have been suggested that may help to distinguish cortical LBD dementia from Alzheimer's disease.[46] Distinguishing features are said to include more prominent rigidity and a greater prevalence of hallucinations and fluctuating confusion in the former. We have studied patients who had clinically probable DLBD, based on the above criteria. Their [18]FDG PET scans have, to date, been indistinguishable from those seen in patients with Alzheimer's disease (N Turjanski and DJ Brooks, unpublished observations).

CEREBRAL ACTIVATION STUDIES

When normal subjects perform paced movements of a joystick in freely selected directions with their right hand, there are associated rCBF increases in the contralateral lentiform nucleus and sensorimotor cortex (SMC) and bilaterally in anterior cingulate, supplementary motor area (SMA), lateral premotor cortex (PMC), and dorsolateral prefrontal cortex (DLPFC).[11] Self-paced extension of the index finger results in a pattern of activation similar to that associated with moving a joystick in freely chosen directions.[13] When PD patients, scanned after cessation of treatment for 12 hours, perform the same motor tasks, normal activation of SMC, PMC, and lateral parietal association areas occurs, but there is selectively impaired activation of the contralateral lentiform nucleus, the anterior cingulate, SMA, and DLPFC, that is, those cortical areas that receive their main input from the basal ganglia.

It is thought that the SMA and DLPFC play a crucial role in preparing and generating volitional motor programs whereas PMC may play a greater role in facilitating motor responses to external cues.[47–50] An inability to activate SMA and DLPFC in PD during movements that are self-paced or in freely selected directions could explain the difficulty patients with this disease experience in initiating volitional movements. Jenkins et al.[51] have demonstrated that when apomorphine, a combined D$_1$ and D$_2$ agonist, is given subcutaneously to PD patients, resolution of their akinesia is associated with a significant increase in SMA and DLPFC blood flow, providing further evidence for the role of these structures in the generation of motor programs (see Fig. 3-1). Normal levels of SMA activation in PD after apomorphine and L-dopa administration have also been reported, using ^{133}Xe SPECT.[52,53]

Pallidotomy has recently come back into fashion as a surgical therapy for PD. The rationale underlying this approach is that the loss of striatal dopamine in PD is associated with reduced inhibition of the internal globus pallidus (GP$_i$), resulting in excessive output to the ventral thalamus. As this output is inhibitory, it results in impaired activation of SMA and prefrontal cortex. By lesioning the motor GP$_i$ it is argued that this excessive inhibition will be removed and, therefore, that volitional movements will be facilitated in PD patients. Rigidity and bradykinesia are improved by 30–40 percent on semiquantitative scoring in most series, but the main effect

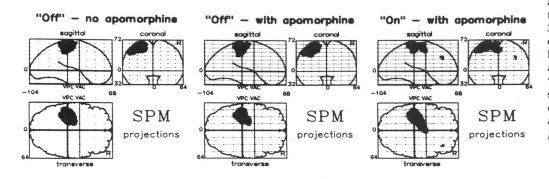

Parkinson's disease — 7 subjects
(joystick activation)

"Off" — no apomorphine   "Off" — with apomorphine   "On" — with apomorphine

SPM projections   SPM projections   SPM projections

p<0.05 corrected   MRC CU

FIGURE 3-1 A PET activation study in PD before and after apomorphine. Patients were asked to move a joystick in freely chosen directions every 3 seconds. Before treatment, only the primary motor and lateral premotor cortex is activated, but after switching "on" after apomorphine, the supplementary motor area and dorsal prefrontal cortex also activate. (*Courtesy of Dr. IH Jenkins.*)

of pallidotomy appears to be to raise the threshold for L-dopa-induced dyskinesias considerably benefiting end-stage PD patients with this problem.[54-56] Two PET activation studies on the functional effects of pallidotomy in PD have now been reported. The first demonstrated significantly increased activation of SMA, lateral premotor cortex, and dorsal prefrontal cortex in a single PD case during arm movements after pallidotomy while off medication.[57] The patient was asked to perform paced joystick movements in freely selected directions and showed an improvement in both his response times and the number of completed movements after surgery. The second study concerned six PD patients who were scanned at rest and while reaching out to grasp lighted targets every 3 seconds while off medication.[58] There was no change in patient performance after pallidotomy, but the patient group again showed significantly increased SMA activation. This externally cued motor task failed to activate prefrontal areas. These two activation studies, therefore, lend support to the hypothesis that pallidotomy results in removal of excess pallidal inhibitory drive to frontal association areas in PD.

THE PRESYNAPTIC DOPAMINERGIC SYSTEM

After its intravenous administration, ^{18}F-dopa is taken up by the terminals of the nigrostriatal dopaminergic projections and converted to ^{18}F-dopamine and, subsequently, dopamine metabolites.[59] The rate of striatal ^{18}F accumulation reflects both transport of ^{18}F-dopa into striatal vesicles and its subsequent decarboxylation by dopa decarboxylase. ^{11}C-Nomifensine and cocaine analogues such as ^{123}I-β-CIT and ^{11}C-CFT bind to dopamine reuptake sites on nigrostriatal terminals and also provide a measure of integrity of nigrostriatal projections.[60-63] The tracer ^{11}C-dihydrotetrabenazine is a marker of vesicle monoamine transporters.[64]

Garnett and Nahmias[65] published the first reports on striatal ^{18}F-dopa uptake in PD. Their subjects were early cases with hemiparkinsonism, and PET showed normal caudate but bilaterally reduced putamen tracer uptake, with activity being most depressed in the putamen contralateral to the

affected limbs. These studies were the first demonstration that subclinical involvement of dopaminergic projections to the putamen contralateral to clinically unaffected limbs in PD could be detected. These observations have been reproduced with ^{18}F-dopa PET[66-69] and also with the cocaine PET tracer ^{11}C-CFT[62] (see Fig. 3-2). The tracers ^{123}I-β-CIT and ^{11}C-dihydrotetrabenazine also provide a sensitive means of discriminating PD patients from normal subjects, although ^{11}C-β-CIT has proved disappointing in this respect.[63,70,71] Striatal uptake of ^{18}F-dopa, ^{11}C-nomifensine, and ^{123}I-β-CIT have all shown an inverse correlation with degree of locomotor disability in PD.[63,66,67,72-74] Patients with a sustained response to L-dopa show greater striatal ^{18}F-dopa accumulation than those with fluctuating responses.[68]

On average, PD patients show a 50 percent loss of specific putamen ^{18}F-dopa and ^{11}C-nomifensine uptake,[67,72,73] compared to a 60–80 percent loss of ventrolateral nigra compacta cells at post mortem.[26,75] As putamen dopamine levels are reduced by over 90 percent in PD,[27,76] striatal uptake of ^{18}F-dopa is more likely to reflect the terminal density of the nigrostriatal projections, rather than levels of endogenous dopamine. At onset of symptoms, PD patients show approximately a 30 percent loss of ^{18}F-dopa uptake in the putamen contralateral to the affected limbs.[77] ^{18}F-dopa PET, therefore, provides a potential means of detecting subclinical nigral dysfunction in subjects at risk for parkinsonism. It may well be that cocaine-based PET and SPECT tracers will prove even more sensitive for this purpose in the future; a direct comparison of these tracers with ^{18}F-dopa PET is yet to come.

DETECTION OF PRECLINICAL DISEASE

Using ^{18}F-dopa PET, Calne et al.[78] studied four asymptomatic subjects who had been exposed to the nigral toxin MPTP. These workers were able to demonstrate subnormal striatal tracer uptake in two of these four subjects. We have used ^{18}F-dopa PET to study 28 asymptomatic relatives in 5 kindreds with familial PD. Each of these kindreds contained at least two affected individuals with L-dopa-responsive par-

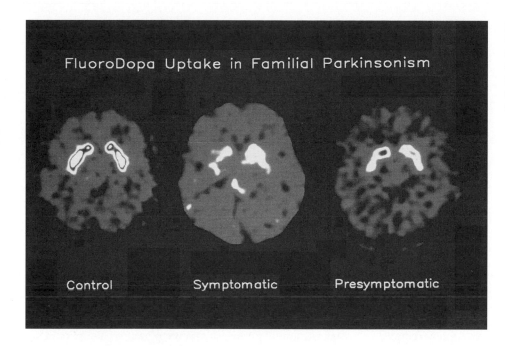

FluoroDopa Uptake in Familial Parkinsonism

Control   Symptomatic   Presymptomatic

FIGURE 3-2 PET images of striatal ^{18}F-dopa uptake in a normal subject, a parkinsonian patient, and his presymptomatic relative. It can be seen that the relative has abnormal dopaminergic function. See Color Plate 1. (*Courtesy of Dr. GV Sawle.*)

kinsonism indistinguishable from sporadic PD. Four of these kindreds had unknown pathology; in three, the index case had disease onset in the sixth or seventh decades, typical of the sporadic disease, while in the fourth kindred disease onset was in the fourth decade.[79] The fifth kindred is known to have DLBD.[80] The index patient developed parkinsonism at age 18, along with panic attacks, and he later became demented. He died at age 33. Panic attacks, along with parkinsonism, were a presenting feature in other affected members of this kindred.

Affected individuals from each of these five kindreds all showed a pattern of striatal ^{18}F-dopa uptake compatible with the presence of sporadic PD, that is, putamen tracer uptake was more reduced than caudate. Of the 28 asymptomatic at-risk relatives from these five kindreds that have been scanned to date, 5 had an isolated postural tremor on examination. Of these 28 asymptomatic relatives, studied, 11 have shown levels of putamen ^{18}F-dopa uptake reduced more than 2 SD below the normal mean, including 4 of the 5 relatives with isolated postural tremor. The other 7 of these 11 had no clinical signs but, 2 years after PET, 3 have subsequently developed parkinsonism.

Our ^{18}F-dopa PET findings in these kindreds have, to date, found a 39 percent prevalence of dopaminergic dysfunction in asymptomatic relatives of index patients with familial parkinsonism (see Fig. 3-2). This is significantly higher than the 15 percent prevalence normally quoted for the presence of a positive family history in PD, and our PET findings also suggest that isolated postural tremor is a feature of familial parkinsonism. Our results are most compatible with a dominant inheritance of disease in the five kindreds that we have studied but are also compatible with nigral dysfunction arising from exposure to a common environmental toxin, assuming that individual members had variable susceptibility to this agent.

We have also now studied 24 asymptomatic co-twins of affected PD patients with ^{18}F-dopa PET.[81] Sixteen were mono-zygotic (MZ) co-twins, ages 54–81 years, and five of these showed putamen ^{18}F-dopa uptake reduced 2 SDs below the normal mean. Of these five, three had isolated postural tremor on examination, and in one of these an orthostatic component was evident. This co-twin has now become brad-ykinetic. A fourth exhibited an occasional tremor of the left arm while lying on the PET scanner while the fifth had borderline bradykinesia of finger movements. None of these co-twins were aware of any problem at the time of PET. A sixth MZ co-twin with an isolated postural tremor had low normal putamen ^{18}F-dopa uptake.

Eight dizygotic (DZ) asymptomatic co-twins, ages 23–67 years, also underwent ^{18}F-dopa PET. Two of them have shown reduced putamen ^{18}F-dopa uptake in the absence of any clinical signs. A third DZ co-twin with a postural tremor on examination had low normal putamen ^{18}F-dopa uptake. In summary, our ^{18}F-dopa PET findings suggest concordances of 31 and 25 percent for nigral dysfunction in MZ and DZ co-twins, respectively. These are higher than the clinical concordances (2–12 percent) reported in previous clinical surveys. We were unable to demonstrate a significant difference in prevalence of nigral dysfunction between the MZ and DZ co-twin cohorts. This was also the case in a recent German ^{18}F-dopa PET study, in which five DZ and two MZ PD co-twins all showed abnormal findings.[82] Three of our five co-twins with isolated postural tremor had reduced putamen ^{18}F-dopa uptake, and the uptake in the other two was at the low end of normal. This provides further evidence that postural tremor may be a phenotype of familial parkinsonism. After 2 years of follow-up, two of seven of our asymptomatic co-twins with reduced levels of putamen ^{18}F-dopa uptake have now developed clear signs of parkinsonism.

The finding of similar concordances for reduced putamen ^{18}F-dopa uptake in MZ and DZ co-twins could be interpreted as being more in favor of an environmental than a genetic etiology for PD. One of the MZ co-twins with reduced puta-men ^{18}F-dopa uptake separated from his family in Massachusetts and moved to North Carolina at the age of 15 and, therefore, if this twin pair were exposed to a common environmental insult it must have occurred before that time. Our ^{18}F-dopa PET data, however, do not have the power to rule out an autosomal dominant mode of transmission with low penetrance and are also compatible with a mitochondrial mode of inheritance in PD.

Tremor and PD

Our ^{18}F-dopa PET studies on the role of inheritance in PD showed a strong correlation between the presence of isolated postural tremor in relatives of PD patients and the presence of nigral dysfunction. We have further addressed the relationship between tremor and PD by performing ^{18}F-dopa PET studies patients with isolated 4- to 8-Hz postural tremor or isolated predominant 3- to 5-Hz rest tremor.[83] All of our patients with familial essential tremor had putamen ^{18}F-dopa uptake within the normal range. Having said that, mean putamen ^{18}F-dopa uptake for the cohort was reduced by 13 percent, and we cannot exclude the presence of minor degrees of dopaminergic dysfunction. Two of the 12 patients in the sporadic ET group had putamen ^{18}F-dopa uptake reduced below the normal range, with one lying within the PD range. This last patient has subsequently developed bradykinesia and a rest tremor. Overall, our findings confirm that isolated postural tremor can be associated with nigral dysfunction and can be a presenting feature of PD but do not indicate a direct relationship between familial ET and PD. A more recent study with ^{123}I-β-CIT SPECT has also failed to find any evidence of nigrostriatal dysfunction in essential tremor.[84] The presence of putative clinical predictors of possible PD proved to be unhelpful: 9 of our 12 sporadic ET patients had a low-amplitude breakthrough rest tremor; 6 had reduced arm swing; and 5 had cogwheel rigidity on synkinesis, but only 2 of these patients showed reduced putamen ^{18}F-dopa uptake.

All of our 11 rest tremor patients had reduced ^{18}F-dopa uptake in the putamen contralateral to the affected limbs, with 9 values falling within the PD range. Caudate tracer uptake was relatively preserved, which is typical of the pattern seen in sporadic PD. Although none of these 11 patients had associated bradykinesia and only 4 showed cogwheel rigidity on synkinesis, our ^{18}F-dopa PET findings suggest that all of these patients had "tremulous PD." Despite the mean 50 percent loss of putamen dopamine terminal function in our rest tremor patients, only 44 percent of them showed a response to L-dopa. This would suggest that the presence of rest tremor is not determined by damage to the nigrostriatal dopaminergic system alone.

In summary, ^{18}F-dopa PET findings suggest that isolated rest tremor is a forme fruste of PD and confirm that isolated postural tremor can, on occasion, be associated with nigral dysfunction. ^{18}F-dopa PET and ^{123}I-β-CIT SPECT findings are currently against, however, an association between familial essential tremor and PD.

The Role of Aging in Progression of Parkinson's Disease

There is still debate over whether PD is initiated by a subclinical toxic or infective insult in early life but only becomes clinically apparent when additional nigral loss from natural attrition causes the cell population to fall below a critical threshold or whether it represents an ongoing active degenerative process.[85] In order to try to distinguish between these possibilities, several groups have studied the relationship between age and striatal ^{18}F-dopa uptake cross-sectionally in normal subjects over an age range of 20–80 years. Results have been conflicting, with two groups reporting no age effect on striatal tracer uptake[86,87] but another group consistently reporting a small but significant decline of ^{18}F-dopa uptake with age.[88,89]

In order to overcome the drawbacks of cross-sectionally acquired data, two groups have carried out longitudinal ^{18}F-dopa PET studies on PD progression. Bhatt et al.[90] measured striatal ^{18}F-dopa uptake on two occasions over 3 years in groups of nine PD and seven normal subjects. PD patients had had clinical symptoms on average for 4 years before PET. Both the PD and normal groups showed a similar 5 percent fall in mean striatal-cerebellar ^{18}F-dopa uptake ratios. These workers concluded that the decline in nigral function in PD was slow and similar to that associated with natural aging. In contrast, Morrish et al.[91] have reported a mean 14 percent annual decline in specific putamen ^{18}F-dopa uptake in a group of 10 PD patients with clinical symptoms present for an average of 18 months, whereas controls showed no significant change in uptake. This latter finding is more suggestive of an ongoing degenerative rather than an aging process. More recently, Vingerhoets et al.[92] have also demonstrated a more rapid decline in striatal ^{18}F-dopa uptake in PD than in controls. Currently, the exact contribution of aging to PD progression remains uncertain. Recent pathological studies suggest that the pattern of nigral cell and striatal dopamine loss from natural aging and PD are different.[26,93] As there is evidence of reactive microglia in the nigra in PD patients at autopsy, which is indicative of an ongoing inflammatory process, it seems unlikely that aging alone is responsible for the onset of symptoms and disease progression in PD.[94]

Fetal Graft Function in Parkinson's Disease

PD has now been treated with striatal implants of fetal mesencephalic tissue with varying degrees of success in a number of centers. ^{18}F-dopa PET provides a means of examining graft function post-transplantation. Sawle et al.[95] reported ^{18}F-dopa PET findings on two PD patients before, and serially for 13 months after, fetal engraftment into the putamen contralateral to the more affected limbs. Patency of the blood-graft barrier was established at 6 months in one of these subjects using gadolinium (Gd)-enhanced MRI. Both of these patients maintained a sustained clinical improvement of the limbs contralateral to the putamen engrafted. In a follow-up study these workers were able to demonstrate continuing graft function in the two patients both clinically and with PET 3 years after surgery[96] and, indeed, positive 5-year follow-up data are now available. Since then, these workers have transplanted another four PD patients, all of whom are showing PET evidence of graft function 1 year after surgery. Clinically successful fetal transplantation with corroborative ^{18}F-dopa PET findings has also been reported for two PD patients in a French study[97] and for four PD patients in a series from Tampa, Florida[98] with 6-month–1-year follow-up data. One of the transplanted PD patients in the Florida series subsequently died from an unrelated cause, and at post mortem viable tyrosine hydroxylase (TH) staining graft tissue forming connections with host neurons was seen.[99] This finding confirms that ^{18}F-dopa PET is measuring graft function, rather than simply reflecting a host reaction to foreign tissue or the presence of blood-brain barrier breakdown. As a consequence of these pilot data, two major studies on the efficacy of implantation of fetal cells in PD are now being organized by the NIH in the United States.

THE POSTSYNAPTIC STRIATAL DOPAMINE SYSTEM

At least five different subtypes of dopamine receptors have now been described, but broadly they fall into D1 type (D1, D5), which are adenyl cyclase-dependent, and D2 type (D2, D3, D4), which are not. Striatal D1 and D2 receptors are primarily involved in modulating locomotor function. In untreated hemiparkinsonian patients, later shown to be L-dopa responsive, ^{11}C-SCH23390 PET has shown no side-to-side difference in striatal uptake, suggesting that D1 binding is normal.[100] In contrast, PD patients who have been exposed to L-dopa for several years show a reduction in striatal D1 binding.[101] This reduction is found in both patients with sustained and fluctuating responses to treatment, but a trend was seen for a greater reduction in the latter.

A number of PET and SPECT ligands have been used to study striatal D2 receptor binding in PD. Leenders et al.[102] first reported normal striatal uptake of ^{11}C-methylspiperone (MSP) in four untreated PD patients. Brücke et al.[103] and Schwarz et al.[104] also noted normal striatum-frontal uptake ratios of ^{123}I-iodobenzamide (IBZM) in de novo PD patients who were later shown to be responsive to dopaminergic agents. Subsequently, ^{11}C-raclopride PET studies have demonstrated mean 10–20 percent increases in putamen D2 binding in de novo PD contralateral to the more affected limbs.[105-108] Overall, PET and SPECT findings suggest that in untreated PD putamen, D2 binding is normal or mildly upregulated whereas caudate D2 binding is normal. Where putamen ^{18}F-dopa and ^{11}C-raclopride uptake have both been measured in de novo PD patients, an inverse correlation between the binding of the two tracers has been found.[109] It has been suggested that the presence of normal striatal ^{123}I-IBZM uptake in de novo PD correlates well with subsequent response to apomorphine.[104] Around 20 percent of the PD cases with normal striatal D2 binding, however, have a poor apomorphine response, so the presence of normal striatal D2 binding does not reliably exclude atypical disease.

Striatal D2 binding in treated PD cases appears to be either normal or decreased. Initial studies using ^{11}C-MSP PET reported normal[110,111] and reduced[102] tracer uptake. Brücke et al.[103] reported a 17 percent decrease of striatal ^{123}I-IBZM uptake in medicated PD patients. More recent ^{11}C-raclopride PET studies have helped to clarify the situation. De novo PD patients with initially increased putamen ^{11}C-raclopride binding show a tendency for this to normalize after some months of exposure to L-dopa.[108,112] Chronically treated PD cases retain normal putamen D2 binding but developed reduced caudate D2 binding, irrespective of whether their response to treatment is sustained or fluctuating.[101,105]

In summary, functional imaging suggests that untreated PD patients have mildly raised putamen D2 but normal D1 binding. Chronic exposure to L-dopa results in normalization of putamen D2 binding while caudate D2 and both caudate and putamen D1 binding become reduced. PD cases who develop a fluctuating response to therapy with dyskinesias do not differ significantly from those with a sustained L-dopa response in terms of striatal D1 and D2 binding.

ATYPICAL PARKINSONIAN SYNDROMES

MULTIPLE-SYSTEM ATROPHY

This condition, also known as Shy-Drager syndrome, includes striatonigral degeneration (SND), olivopontocerebellar atrophy (OPCA), and progressive autonomic failure (PAF) in its spectrum. About 10 percent of cases initially diagnosed as PD are found to have multiple system atrophy (MSA) at autopsy.[113] The pathology of MSA is distinct from PD and consists of neuronal loss from the nigra and striatum, brain stem and cerebellar nuclei, and intermediolateral columns of the cord with argyrophilic neuronal and glial inclusions.[114] In its early stages MSA may present as an akinetic-rigid syndrome or as progressive ataxia. Around 50 percent of patients with the akinetic-rigid variant show an initial response to L-dopa, making it difficult to distinguish them from PD on clinical criteria.[22]

Metabolic Studies

There have been three [18]FDG PET studies on regional cerebral glucose utilization in clinically probable striatonigral degeneration.[115] De Volder et al.[115] studied seven cases, two of which had additional autonomic failure and cerebellar ataxia and, therefore, had the full syndrome of MSA. They found a 46 and 36 percent reduction in the level of putamen and caudate glucose metabolism, respectively, with a lesser reduction in frontal function. Cerebellar metabolism was reduced in the two patients with ataxia. Otsuka et al.[43] have also reported significantly reduced striatal glucose metabolism in eight patients with probable SND, whereas striatal glucose metabolism was preserved in eight PD patients. More recently, Eidelberg et al.[116] demonstrated that reduced levels of striatal glucose metabolism discriminated eight out of ten L-dopa nonresponsive SND patients from L-dopa-responsive PD patients in whom metabolism was either normal or raised. Proton magnetic resonance spectroscopy (PMRS) has also been used to discriminate SND from PD. Davie et al.[117] were able to demonstrate reduced N-acetylaspartate (NAA) to creatine ratios in the signal from the lentiform nucleus in six out of seven clinically probable SND cases whereas eight of their nine PD patients had normal ratios.

Fulham et al.[118] examined [18]FDG uptake in seven OPCA patients with autonomic failure and in eight PAF patients. They found significantly reduced cerebellar and frontal glucose use in the OPCA patients and normal levels of rCMRGlc in PAF. These findings suggest that PET may provide a potential means of determining whether patients presenting with isolated autonomic failure have PAF or MSA. Glucose use has also been examined in cases of sporadic and familial

OPCA without autonomic failure or rigidity.[119,120] These patients have shown reduced cerebellar and brain stem rCMRGlc, with individual levels correlating inversely with the level of ataxia present.

Neuropharmacology

As in PD, specific putamen ^{18}F-dopa and ^{11}C-nomifensine uptake is reduced to around 50 percent of normal levels in SND and individual levels of putamen ^{18}F-dopa uptake correlate with locomotor function.[67,72,121] In patients with the full syndrome of MSA, caudate ^{18}F-dopa and ^{11}C-nomifensine uptake are significantly more depressed compared with PD, but reduced caudate ^{18}F-dopa uptake only discriminates SND from PD with 70 percent specificity.[43,121,122] The lateral nigra sends dopamine projections to the putamen whereas the medial nigra projects to caudate. The above PET findings suggest that medial nigra is more severely involved in MSA than PD, and pathological studies corroborate this conclusion.[22,25,123]

Striatal dopamine D2 binding has been studied with ^{11}C-raclopride PET in SND.[105] A mild but significant reduction in mean caudate (10 percent) and putamen (11 percent) tracer uptake was found, equivalent to a mean 14 and 15 percent loss of caudate and putamen D2 binding. Only 2 of the 10 SND patients, however, had individually significantly reduced caudate and putamen ^{11}C-raclopride uptake. A reduction in mean striatal ^{11}C-MSP binding in four SND cases has also been reported,[110] but again the SND and normal ranges of tracer uptake overlapped. Schwarz et al.[104] have shown reduced striatal ^{123}I-IBZM uptake in 8 of 12 de novo parkinsonian patients who had a negative apomorphine response. Overall, functional imaging suggests that loss of striatal D2 sites occurs in SND but that a significant number of parkinsonian patients who respond poorly to L-dopa retain normal levels of striatal D2 binding. It is likely, therefore, that degeneration of brain stem and pallidal, rather than striatal, projections is responsible for their poor L-dopa-responsive rigidity.

Striatal opioid binding has also been compared in SND and PD.[124] ^{11}C-diprenorphine is a nonspecific opioid antagonist binding with equal affinity to μ, κ, and δ sites. In PD all individual values of caudate and putamen tracer uptake lay within 2.5 SD of the normal mean, whereas mean putamen uptake was reduced in SND, and three of the seven patients individually had significantly reduced binding.

[18]F-dopa uptake has also been studied in patients with pure autonomic failure.[121] Those few PAF patients who have come to pathology have shown degeneration of the intermediolateral columns of the spinal cord similar to that seen in MSA but also LBDs in the nigra and sympathetic ganglia similar to those seen in PD patients.[32] In contrast to PD patients, however, the PAF patients showed little nigral cell loss. Striatal ^{18}F-dopa uptake was found to be normal in five of seven PAF patients, suggesting that their dysautonomia was not associated with underlying nigral dysfunction. Two patients, however, showed reduced putamen ^{18}F-dopa uptake, and one of these subsequently developed a pseudobulbar palsy, suggestive of MSA.

It has been suggested that SND, OPCA, and PAF all represent extremes of an MSA spectrum. Argyrophilic neuronal and glial inclusions characteristic of MSA have been reported in both isolated SND and OPCA.[114] Functional imaging provides an opportunity to detect the presence of subclinical multisystem dysfunction in vivo in patients with apparently isolated neurological syndromes. Four studies have examined striatal function in OPCA: Rinne et al.[125] studied 10 sporadic OPCA patients who had autonomic failure with ^{18}F-dopa and ^{11}C-diprenorphine PET. Of these 10, 7 had no signs of parkinsonism whereas soft signs were present in the other 3. Of the 10, 7, including 2 of 3 with soft signs of parkinsonism, had reduced putamen ^{18}F-dopa uptake whereas four had reduced putamen ^{11}C-diprenorphine binding. Otsuka et al.[126] have also reported reduced levels of mean caudate and striatal ^{18}F-dopa uptake in a group of five patients with sporadic OPCA whereas Gilman and coworkers have demonstrated striatal glucose hypometabolism in sporadic OPCA.[120] Davie et al.[117] studied five sporadic OPCA patients with PMRS and found a reduction in the lentiform NAA:creatine signal ratio. It would seem, therefore, that a majority of sporadic OPCA cases with autonomic failure show subclinical evidence of striatonigral dysfunction when studied with functional imaging.

PROGRESSIVE SUPRANUCLEAR PALSY

This condition is generally taken to refer to Steele-Richardson-Olszewski syndrome and is characterized pathologically by neurofibrillary tangle formation and neuronal loss in the basal ganglia, superior colliculi, brain stem nuclei, and periaqueductal gray matter.[127] There are, however, a number of other degenerative causes of supranuclear-gaze palsy. The full PSP syndrome comprises a L-dopa-resistant akinetic-rigid syndrome with supranuclear down-gaze palsy, bulbar palsy, and dementia of frontal type. In the early stages of the disease, however, the patient may present as an isolated akinetic-rigid syndrome, making a distinction from other parkinsonian disorders difficult.[128,129]

Metabolic Studies

There have been a number of studies of rCBF and rCMRGlc in patients with probable PSP, several of whom have later had the diagnosis confirmed at autopsy.[130–135] Cortical metabolism tends to be globally depressed in this condition. Frontal areas are particularly affected, and levels of metabolism correlate with both performance on psychometric tests of frontal function and disease duration.[131] Hypofrontality is not specific for PSP, however, and can be seen in SND, Pick's disease, and Huntington's disease. Recently, a patient with clinically probable PSP with appropriate [18]FDG PET findings was found to have progressive subcortical gliosis at post mortem.[136] Additionally, as basal ganglia, cerebellar, and thalamic metabolism may all be depressed in PSP, [18]FDG PET scans cannot be used to reliably distinguish PSP from SND. Preservation of striatal metabolism in PD distinguishes this condition from PSP.

Neuropharmacology

Three studies[67,133,137] have reported that striatal ^{18}F-dopa uptake in PSP is significantly reduced, with individual levels of uptake correlating inversely with disease duration. Unlike PD, putamen and caudate ^{18}F-dopa uptake appear to be equally affected in PSP, suggesting that the nigra is uniformly involved, which is in agreement with pathological reports.[138,139] In practice, 90 percent of PSP patients can be discriminated from PD patients on the basis of caudate involvement.[122] There appears to be no correlation between putamen or caudate ^{18}F-dopa uptake in the PSP and locomotor function. Unlike PD and SND, in which locomotor disability appears to result primarily from loss of dopaminergic fibers, loss of mobility in PSP is probably a consequence of degeneration of pallidal and brain stem projections.

Striatal dopamine D2 receptor density in PSP has been studied with both PET and SPECT in a number of centers.[103,105,140,141] It is generally agreed that mean caudate and putamen D2 binding is reduced in PSP, although not all individuals show significant dopamine receptor loss. It is likely that in some cases of PSP, as in SND, degeneration of pallidal and brain stem projections is responsible for the poor L-dopa responsiveness of this akinetic-rigid syndrome, rather than a primary loss of dopamine receptors. One study has examined opioid binding in PSP.[124] Striatal ^{11}C-diprenorphine was reduced in all six patients studied and, unlike SND, where caudate function was spared, caudate and putamen appeared to be equally affected in PSP.

CORTICOBASAL DEGENERATION
This syndrome, also known as corticobasal ganglionic degeneration, corticodentatonigral degeneration, and neuronal achromasia, has characteristic clinical features.[142] Patients present with an akinetic-rigid, apraxic limb that may exhibit alien behavior. Cortical sensory loss, dysphasia, myoclonus, supranuclear-gaze problems, and bulbar dysfunction may also be evident. Intellect is spared until the late stage of the disease. Eventually, all four limbs become involved, and the patient's condition is invariably poorly L-dopa-responsive. The pathology consists of collections of swollen, achromatic, tau-positive-staining Pick's cells, but no argyrophilic Pick bodies are present.[143] The posterior frontal, inferior parietal, and superior temporal lobes, as well as the dentate nuclei and substantia nigra, are targeted.

There have been three PET and one SPECT series published on patients with the clinical syndrome of CBD. Sawle et al.[144] studied six patients with ^{18}F-dopa and [15]O₂. Striatal ^{18}F-dopa uptake was strikingly asymmetrical, being most depressed contralateral to the more affected limbs. Caudate and putamen tracer uptake were similarly depressed in patients with CBD, in contrast to those with PD. As might be predicted from the distribution of the pathology, cortical rCMRO₂ was most significantly reduced in posterior frontal, inferior parietal, and superior temporal regions. Again, these rCMRO₂ reductions were strikingly asymmetrical, being most severe contralateral to the more affected limbs.

Eidelberg et al.[145] have studied five CBD patients with PET. They found relatively reduced inferior parietal, hippocampal, and thalamic glucose utilization contralateral to the more affected limbs, as compared with ipsilateral values. This contrasted with PD patients, who showed symmetrical levels of glucose utilization. Striatal ^{18}F-dopa uptake was also reduced. Blin et al.[146] have also reported asymmetric reductions in inferior parietal and thalamic FDG uptake in CBD. A single case studied with IBZM SPECT was recently reported as showing a severe asymmetrical reduction of striatal D2 binding.[147] The above PET findings can help to distinguish CBD from Pick's disease, in which inferior frontal hypometabolism predominates; from PD, in which cortex glucose metabolism is preserved or symmetrically involved and caudate ^{18}F-dopa uptake is spared; and from PSP, in which frontal and striatal metabolism are more symmetrically reduced.

SUMMARY
Table 3-1 summarizes the functional imaging characteristics of parkinsonian syndromes.

Involuntary Movement Disorders

DYSTONIA
Idiopathic torsion dystonia (ITD) is a dominantly inherited condition with 40 percent penetrance and variable phenotype.[148] It has been linked to a locus on chromosome 9 in some caucasian and jewish kindreds.[149,150] Pathological studies have failed to identify consistent structural or neurotransmitter abnormalities in ITD, although depressed levels of brain stem and basal ganglia monoamines have been reported in one patient.[151,152] Patients with acquired hemidystonia often have structural lesions of the lentiform nucleus or posterior thalamus,[1,3] and it has been suggested that ITD arises because of dysfunction of projections from these structures to frontal association areas.

A problem with a number of PET studies concerning dystonia has been the heterogeneity of the patient groups recruited. Familial, sporadic, and acquired dystonia have been

TABLE 3-1 PET Findings in Akinetic-Rigid Syndromes

	PD	PD-Dementia	SND	PSP	CBD
Metabolism	Normal	Low parietal/temporal	Low striatal/frontal	Low striatal/frontal	Low thalamic/ inferior parietal
[18]F-dopa CFT/CIT	Putamen <caudate	Putamen <caudate	Putamen <caudate	Low putamen & caudate	Low putamen & caudate
Striatal D2 sites	Raised if untreated, normal/low if treated	—	Low	Low	Low
Opioid sites	Normal		Low putamen	Low putamen & caudate	—

considered together, and patients with focal or hemidystonia have been favored in order to provide side-to-side comparisons of basal ganglia function. As a consequence, the relevance of some of these PET findings to familial ITD is uncertain.

Studies on Resting Metabolism and Cerebral Activation

Two studies have reported increased resting lentiform nucleus metabolism in dystonia. Chase et al.[153] studied six patients with sporadic cases of idiopathic dystonia with [18]FDG, all of whom had normal CT or MRI. Three of the six dystonics had increased lenticular glucose use contralateral to the more affected limbs, and after thalamotomy one of these three patients showed partial resolution of their lentiform nucleus hypermetabolism. Eidelberg et al.[154] showed increased lentiform nucleus rCMRGlc contralateral to the affected limbs in two patients with idiopathic hemidystonia, one familial and the other sporadic, both of whom had normal MRI.

In contrast to the above two studies, Gilman et al.,[155] Otsuka et al.,[156] and Stoessl et al.[157] were all unable to find any consistent pattern of altered rCMRGlc in either patients with sporadic asymmetrical ITD or torticollis. Stoessl et al., however, noted a reduced covarience between striatal and thalamic rCMRGlc in his torticollis patients and postulated that dysfunction of striatal-thalamic projections were present. More recently, Karbe et al.[158] have reported a reduction in striatal and frontal rCMRGlc in ITD.

Cerebral activation studies appear to give a more consistent picture. Tempel and Perlmutter[159] examined the integrity of central sensory connections in a group of 11 subjects with idiopathic hemi- or focal dystonia. They used vibrotactile stimulation to activate the SMC and measured the resultant increase in blood flow. The dystonic subjects had a 20 percent attenuation of their SMC blood flow response to tactile stimulation, compared with that of normal controls. This was true whether the affected or "normal" hand was stimulated, Tempel and Perlmutter and suggested that this reduced SMC activation was a consequence of abnormal function of basal ganglia-thalamic-SMC projections. There were, however, some difficulties with the above study: The first was that some subjects developed dystonic spasms in response to the vibrotactile stimulus, which could possibly have influenced the rCBF response. Tempel and Perlmutter controlled for this by having some controls imitate dystonic spasms during stimulation and showed that their SMC activation was increased, rather than diminished, by voluntary posturing. A second problem was that their dystonic patients were on average 25 years older than their controls. More recently, the same group compared the cerebral activation associated with vibrotactile stimulation in six unilateral cases of writer's cramp and eight age-matched normal controls.[160] In this study attenuated activation of caudal SMA, as well as sensorimotor cortex, was demonstrated in their dystonic patients.

We have performed PET activation studies on ITD patients while they were off of medication, measuring the associated rCBF changes while they performed paced joystick movements with their right hands. Two motor paradigms were used: In a "fixed" paradigm the joystick was always moved in a forward direction whereas in a "free" paradigm the joystick was moved in freely selected directions, avoiding repetition. Then rCBF levels associated with the motor tasks were compared with those for resting blood flow, which was normal for these patients when compared with that of age-matched controls.

The first study involved six familial ITD patients who were all able to perform the motor paradigms but took about 20 percent longer than controls to respond to the buzzer and complete joystick movements in both stereotyped and freely chosen directions.[161] Although bradykinetic compared to age-matched controls, the ITD patients showed significantly increased contralateral putamen, supplementary motor, lateral premotor, and dorsolateral prefrontal area activation. Activation of contralateral sensorimotor cortex was reduced to 40 percent, of normal despite the presence of cocontraction during right arm movements. The authors concluded that dystonic limb movements are associated with inappropriate overactivity of the lentiform nucleus and frontal association area projections.

We then repeated this study using a fresh group of eight familial ITD cases and a higher-resolution PET camera.[162] The observation of increased contralateral lentiform nucleus, premotor cortex, and dorsolateral prefrontal cortex activation in dystonia on arm movement was confirmed and, additionally, were now able to show that it is specifically the rostral lateral and mesial premotor areas that are overactive in dystonia whereas the caudal lateral premotor and supplementary motor areas and the primary sensorimotor cortex all have significantly attenuated activation. This finding, therefore, lends support to the observations of Perlmutter and Tempel and suggests that sensorimotor cortex and caudal SMA activation is impaired in ITD. This pattern of activation in dystonia is, therefore, very different from the pattern associated with PD, in which striatal, SMA, and prefrontal areas are underfunctioning while primary motor cortex activates normally.[11]

The cortical regions with attenuated activation in ITD (primary sensorimotor and caudal premotor) are executive areas that send direct pyramidal tract projections to the spinal cord; rostral premotor and dorsal prefrontal areas send no such projections. It would seem, therefore, that dystonic limb movements are associated with inappropriate overactivity of basal ganglia-frontal association area projections whereas the associated bradykinesia may arise from underfunctioning motor executive cortical areas. Such a phenomenon could be explained if the pathology of ITD were to directly affect both the basal ganglia and the executive motor areas, disinhibiting the former but inhibiting the latter.

If this hypothesis is correct, one might predict that patients with acquired dystonia because of focal basal ganglia or thalamic lesions would show normal activation of executive cortical areas, as these should be free of pathology. Inappropriate overactivity of basal ganglia projections to rostral premotor and dorsal prefrontal cortex, however, would persist. We have scanned five such patients with acquired hemi- or focal dystonia while performing paced joystick movements in freely chosen directions.[163] In contrast to the ITD patients, the secondary dystonia group showed reduced rather than raised contralateral lentiform nucleus activation in association with joystick movements, reflecting the presence of their structural lesions, and raised rather than reduced primary motor cortex activation. In common with ITD, premotor and dorsolateral prefrontal cortex activation was increased. These findings, therefore, support overactivity of basal ganglia projection areas (rostral premotor and dorsal prefrontal cortex) on limb movement as being the unifying mechanism of dystonia and lend credence to the idea that the pathology of ITD has a direct inhibitory effect on primary motor cortex function.

The question then arises: What is the significance of the frontal association area overactivity that is evident in both idiopathic and acquired dystonia? Three possibilities can be envisaged: First, the overactivity represents a primary dysfunction of motor planning circuitary. Second, the functional deficit in dystonia is at an executive level, and the prefrontal cortex becomes overactive in a conscious attempt to try to suppress the unwanted movents. Third, the frontal overactivity simply represents a secondary phenomenon reflecting primary basal ganglia overactivity.

In order to examine the function of planning circuitry in ITD, we next studied the cerebral activation associated with imagination of joystick movements in freely chosen directions.[20] Rate of imagined movement was paced at 3-s intervals by a tone. In both ITD patients and age-matched controls, imagination of movement led to significant activation of dorsolateral prefrontal and rostral supplementary motor areas and lentiform nucleus but not sensorimotor cortex. No significant differences in activated rCBF changes were found between the normal and dystonic cohorts. We, therefore, concluded that the primary deficit in idiopathic dystonia must lie at an executive rather than at a planning level.

In summary, PET activation findings in idiopathic and acquired dystonia are compatible with inappropriate overactivity of the basal ganglia and their frontal projections on limb movement underlying this condition. Whether the frontal association area overactivity is simply secondary to primary basal ganglia overactivity or represents an adaptive phenomenon in a conscious attempt to suppress the syndrome is unclear. In idiopathic dystonia significant underfunctioning of primary sensorimotor and caudal premotor executive areas is also evident, suggesting that the pathology of ITD may also directly affect these circuits.

The Dopaminergic System

Initial reports on dopaminergic function in dystonia did not tend to involve patients with familial ITD. Leenders et al.[164] reported striatal ^{18}F-dopa uptake in four patients with hemidystonia, three of whom had dystonia-parkinsonism rather than ITD, and two other patients with torticollis. One of the hemidystonic cases had a calcified lesion in the midbrain tegmentum. The six subjects all had low striatal ^{18}F-dopa uptake, and in the four hemidystonics this was most depressed in the striatum contralateral to the affected limbs. The four hemidystonic patients also had striatal D2 binding, measured with ^{11}C-methylspiperone. In three this was normal, but the patient with the midbrain lesion showed increased striatal D2 binding, possibly reflecting upregulation secondary to nigrostriatal dopaminergic dysfunction. Martin et al.[165] measured striatal ^{18}F-dopa uptake in four dystonic subjects. One of these had dopa-responsive dystonia, and his striatal ^{18}F-dopa uptake was normal. The other three had

sporadic ITD, and two of these showed reduced tracer uptake. More recently, Otsuka et al.[156] have reported mildly raised striatal ^{18}F-dopa uptake in eight patients with ITD.

The only study to entirely involve familial ITD cases was from Playford et al.,[166] who scanned 11 such cases with ^{18}F-dopa PET. Eight of these patients had normal striatal tracer uptake, but three showed mild impairment of putamen ^{18}F-dopa uptake. These three had the most severe disease and were on high doses of anticholinergics. It was concluded that nigral dysfunction had low penetrance in ITD and was either an epiphenomenon or medication related. Two asymptomatic obligate gene carriers that were studied both had normal striatal ^{18}F-dopa uptake.

Dopa-responsive dystonia (DRD) is a familial disorder and, in the majority of cases, is linked to GTP-cyclohydrolase 1 deficiency, with the genetic defect located on chromosome 14.[167] This enzyme constitutes part of the tetrahydrobiopterin synthetic pathway, the cofactor for tyrosine hydroxylase; therefore, sufferers are unable to manufacture dopa and, hence, dopamine from endogenous tyrosine but can still convert exogenous L-dopa to dopamine. DRD cases generally present in childhood with diurnally fluctuating dystonia, and they later develop background parkinsonism.[168] Occasionally, the condition presents as pure parkinsonism in adulthood. Two centers have reported ^{18}F-dopa PET findings in DRD. Sawle et al.[169] studied six subjects with clinically typical disease and found normal striatal tracer uptake in four of the six and mildly reduced uptake in both caudate and putamen of the other two. Snow et al.[170] have studied 10 DRD patients and found normal striatal ^{18}F-dopa uptake in all of their cases. The finding of normal striatal ^{18}F-dopa uptake in DRD helps to distinguish this condition from sporadic dystonia-parkinsonism, in which severely reduced putamen ^{18}F-dopa uptake is found.[171]

In summary, PET studies on resting metabolism in dystonia have produced inconsistent findings, possibly because of the heterogeneity of the patient groups studied. Activation studies on ITD patients suggest that the lentiform nucleus, supplementary motor area, and prefrontal cortex are overactive when these patients perform motor tasks while sensorimotor cortex activation is impaired. The majority of ITD patients have normal striatal ^{18}F-dopa uptake, as do the majority of patients with dopa-responsive dystonia.

CHOREA

Huntington's disease (HD) is an autosomal dominantly transmitted disorder because of an excess of CAG repeats (>38) in the IT15 gene on chromosome 4.[172] The function of this gene is uncertain, but its mRNA is expressed in all tissues. The pathology of HD targets the striatum and involves a loss of medium spiny projection neurones. Those patients with predominant chorea show a selective loss of striatolateral pallidal projections, containing GABA and enkephalin, whereas those with a predominant akinetic-rigid syndromes show additional severe loss of striatomedial pallidal fibers containing GABA and dynorphine.[173] Other degenerative disorders associated with chorea are neuroacanthocytosis (NA) and dentatorubropallidoluysian atrophy (DRPLA), as is benign familial chorea (BFC). NA is a familial disorder of unknown etiology also associated with seizures, dementia, self-injurious behavior, and an axonal neuropathy.[174] DRPLA is a dominantly inherited disorder that arises because of an excess of CAG repeats in a gene on chromosome 12.[175] In addition, the inflammatory diseases systemic lupus erythematosus (SLE) and Sydenham's chorea (SC) can also be associated with chorea. Patients with tardive dyskinesia (TD) may exhibit chorea, although orolingual stereotypes are more characteristic. The pathology of TD is uncertain; neurochemical studies on a primate TD model have reported severe depletion of subthalamic levels of GABA,[176] while postmortem studies on human TD cases have found low subthalamic glutamate decarboxylase activity.[177]

Metabolic Studies

A number of studies have established that affected HD patients have severely reduced rCMRGlc and $rCMRO_2$ of the caudate and lentiform nuclei and that this can be seen in early disease when CT and MRI tend to be normal.[178-180] Levels of resting putamen and caudate rCMRGlc correlate with locomotor function and cognition, respectively, of these patients.[181,182] In early HD cortical metabolism is preserved, but it subsequently declines as dementia becomes prominent, the frontal cortex being targeted.[39,183] Caudate hypometabolism is also found in NA and DRPLA and may be reduced in BFC, so its presence does not distinguish these degenerative choreiform disorders.[184-187] In contrast to the degenerative causes of chorea, striatal rCMRGlc has been reported to be elevated in chorea secondary to SLE,[188] Sydenham's chorea,[189] and tardive dyskinesia.[190]

The future role for functional imaging in degenerative choreas is likely to lie in providing an objective means of following disease progression and the functional effects of neuroprotective agents or cell implants, rather than being used as a diagnostic tool. The sensitivity of [18]FDG PET for the detection of subclinical striatal hypometabolism in subjects at risk for HD and its subsequent rate of decline is, therefore, of relevance and is still being established. Grafton et al.[191]

studied 54 subjects at risk for HD and found low caudate metabolism in 12 cases. Nine of 12 patients identified as high risk from either DNA linkage studies or their subsequent clinical course had low caudate metabolism—a concordance of 75 percent. Results from other centers have been less striking. Young et al.[192] found no abnormalities of caudate metabolism in 29 at-risk subjects while Hayden et al.[193] reported reduced caudate glucose use in 3 of 8 high-risk subjects. Grafton has since followed the progression of decline in caudate rCMRGlc in his cohort of HD patients and found a mean annual reduction of 3.1 percent.[9]

Neuropharmacology

The medium spiny striatal neurons that degenerate in HD bear D1, D2, opioid, and benzodiazepine receptors. A number of PET and SPECT studies, using tracers such as ^{11}C-MSP,[111,180,194] ^{18}F-FESP,[141] and ^{123}I-IBZM,[103] have established that striatal D2 binding is severely reduced in affected HD patients. Turjanski et al.[195] have used ^{11}C-SCH23390 and ^{11}C-raclopride PET to study both D1 and D2 binding in HD. They found a parallel reduction in striatal binding to these receptor subtypes irrespective of whether patients had predominant chorea or rigidity, although rigid cases were most severely affected (see Fig. 3-3). Mild cases showed at least a 40 percent loss of dopamine receptor binding, suggesting that ^{11}C-SCH23390 and ^{11}C-raclopride PET should be capable of detecting subclinical dysfunction in asymptomatic HD gene carriers. Weeks et al.[196] have recently tested this and were able to show a significant parallel loss of striatal D1 and D2 binding in 50 percent of asymptomatic adults with the HD mutation. These findings suggest that levels of striatal dopamine receptor binding will provide a sensitive objective means of following HD progression. If one wants, in the future, to follow the function of implants of fetal striatal cells in HD, then monitoring striatal dopamine receptor binding has an obvious advantage over monitoring rCMRGlc. Regeneration of dopamine receptors would be a clear indication

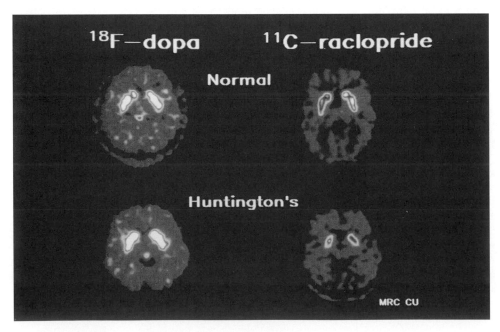

FIGURE 3-3 PET images of ^{18}F-dopa and ^{11}C-raclopride uptake in Huntington's disease. It can be seen that the presynaptic dopaminergic system is intact, but a profound loss of dopamine D2 receptors has occurred in HD. See Color Plate 2. (*Courtesy of Dr. N Turjanski.*)

of graft function, whereas improved rCMRGlc could also reflect active graft rejection. The former has been demonstrated with PET using a rodent model of HD.[197]

Weeks et al.[198] also examined opioid binding in affected HD patients. Conventional region-of-interest analysis showed that mean caudate and putamen ^{11}C-diprenorphine uptake were reduced by 23 and 16 percent in a group of five cases, so this tracer does not provide as sensitive a measure of striatal dysfunction as dopaminergic markers. Using statistical parametric analysis, these workers were able to detect additional reductions in ^{11}C-diprenorphine binding in cingulate areas, whereas increased binding was found in thalamus and prefrontal areas. This increased binding may well reflect increased occupancy of these opioid sites by endogenous endorphins secondary to loss of striatal projections. Striatal benzodiazepine (BDZ) binding has also been examined in HD with ^{11}C-flumazenil.[199] The density of BDZ sites is low in this region, but it proved possible to demonstrate a 26 percent reduction in the caudate ^{11}C-flumazenil volume of distribution.

The finding of reduced striatal D2 binding is, again, not specific for HD. A mean 70 percent reduction of striatal ^{11}C-raclopride binding has been reported in three neuroacanthocytosis patients.[200] While striatal D2 binding is severely reduced in degenerative causes of chorea, normal binding has been reported in a case of SLE chorea.[195] Additionally, two PET studies have established, using the tracers [76]Br-BSP and ^{11}C-MSP, that striatal D2 binding is preserved in tardive dyskinesia.[201,202] This finding argues against the hypothesis that TD results from striatal D2 receptor supersensitivity after prolonged exposure to neuroleptic and suggests that down stream changes in GABA transmission may be of greater relevance.

Conclusion

This chapter has reviewed the way in which functional imaging can demonstrate and distinguish the characteristic patterns of derangement of regional cerebral metabolism and neuropharmacology in the different causes of parkinsonian syndromes, dystonia, and chorea. PET is able to detect subclinical functional abnormalities in at-risk subjects for PD and HD and has provided strong support for a role of inheritance in the former. Both PET and SPECT provide an objective means of monitoring the therapeutic effects of implants of fetal cells in movement disorders. In the future they are also likely to play a role in establishing the role of nerve growth factors and neuroprotective agents in the treatment of subcortical degenerative diseases.

The use of PET for studying patterns of cerebral activation in normal subjects, PD patients, and dystonia patients performing motor tasks has also been reviewed. These studies have provided insight into the role of the basal ganglia in motor control and are compatible with their acting to focus and filter motor programs. They have also identified the system (supplementary motor area and dorsal prefrontal cortex) whose reduced activation appears to underlie akinesia and whose inappropriate overactivity may be responsible for dystonia. In the future, functional imaging is likely to help in the identification of the anatomic substrates of other involuntary movements, such as tics, chorea, and myoclonus.

References

1. Marsden CD, Obeso JA, Zarranz JJ, Lang AE: The anatomical basis of the symptomatic hemidystonias. *Brain* 108:463–483, 1985.
2. Calne DB, Lang AE: Secondary dystonia. *Adv Neurol* 50:9–33, 1988.
3. Bhatia KP, Marsden CD: The behavioural and motor consequences of focal lesions of the basal ganglia in man. *Brain* 117:859–876, 1994.
4. Duguid JR, De La Paz R, DeGroot J: Magnetic resonance imaging of the midbrain in Parkinson's disease. *Ann Neurol* 20:744–747, 1986.
5. Rutledge JN, Hilal SK, Silver AJ, et al: Study of movement disorders and brain iron by MR. *AJR* 149:365–379, 1987.
6. Drayer BP, Olanow W, Burger P, et al: Parkinson Plus syndrome: Diagnosis using high field MR imaging of brain iron. *Radiology* 159:493–498, 1986.
7. Starosta-Rubinstein S, Young AB, Kluin K, et al: Clinical assessment of 31 patients with Wilson's disease: Correlations with structural changes on magnetic resonance imaging. *Arch Neurol* 44:365–370, 1987.
8. Savoiardo M, Strada L, Oliva D, et al: Abnormal MRI signal in the rigid form of Huntington's disease. *J Neurol Neurosurg Psychiatry* 54:888–891, 1991.
9. Grafton ST, Mazziotta JC, Pahl JJ, et al: Serial changes of cerebral glucose metabolism and caudate size in persons at risk for Huntington's disease. *Arch Neurol* 49:1161–1167, 1992.
10. Alexander GE, Crutcher MD, Delong MR: Basal ganglia thalamo-cortical circuits: Parallel substrates for motor, oculomotor, "prefrontal" and "limbic" functions. *Prog Brain Res* 85:119–146, 1990.
11. Playford ED, Jenkins IH, Passingham RE, et al: Impaired mesial frontal and putamen activation in Parkinson's disease: A PET study. *Ann Neurol* 32:151–161, 1992.
12. Deiber M-P, Passingham RE, Colebatch JG, et al: Cortical areas and the selection of movement: A study with positron emission tomography. *Exp Brain Res* 84:393–402, 1991.
13. Jahanshahi M, Jenkins IH, Brown RG, et al: Self-initiated versus externally triggered movements: I. Measurements of regional cerebral blood flow and movement related potentials in normals and Parkinson's disease. *Brain* 118:913–934, 1995.
14. Grafton ST, Mazziotta JC, Presty S, et al: Functional anatomy of human procedural learning determined with regional cerebral blood flow and PET. *J Neurosci* 12:2542–2548, 1992.
15. Friston KJ, Frith CD, Passingham RE, et al: Motor practice and neurophysiological adaptation in the cerebellum: A positron tomography study. *Proc R Soc Long B* 248:223–228, 1992.
16. Shibasaki H, Sadato N, Lyshkow H, et al: Both primary motor cortex and supplementary motor area play an important role in complex finger movement. *Brain* 116:1387–1398, 1993.
17. Jenkins IH, Brooks DJ, Nixon PD, et al: Motor sequence learning: A study with positron emission tomography. *J Neurosci* 14:3775–3790, 1994.
18. Jenkins IH, Passingham RE, Frackowiak RSJ, Brooks DJ: The effect of movement rate on cerebral activation: A study with positron emission tomography. *Mov Disord* 9 (suppl 1):118, 1994.
19. Dettmers C, Fink G, Lemon RN, et al: Relationship between force and cerebral blood flow in primary and cingular motor area. *Neurology* 44 (suppl 2):A232, 1994.

20. Ceballos-Baumann AO, Marsden CD, Passingham RE, et al: Cerebral activation with performing and imagining movement in idiopathic torsion dystonia (ITD): A PET study. *Neurology* 44 (suppl 2):A338, 1994.

21. Hughes AJ, Daniel SE, Kilford L, Lees AJ: The accuracy of the clinical diagnosis of Parkinson's disease: A clinicopathological study of 100 cases. *J Neurol Neurosurg Psychiatry* 55:181–184, 1992.

22. Fearnley JM, Lees AJ: Striatonigral degeneration: A clinicopathological study. *Brain* 113:1823–1842, 1990.

23. Jellinger K: The pathology of parkinsonism, in Marsden CD, Fahn S (eds): *Movement Disorders 2*. London: Butterworth, 1987, pp 124–165.

24. German DC, Manaye K, Smith WK, et al: Midbrain dopaminergic cell loss in Parkinsons disease: Computer visualization. *Ann Neurol* 26:507–514, 1989.

25. Spokes EGS, Bannister R, Oppenheimer DR: Multiple system atrophy with autonomic failure: Clinical, histological, and neurochemical observations on four cases. *J Neurol Sci* 43:59–62, 1979.

26. Fearnley JM, Lees AJ: Ageing and Parkinson's disease: Substantia nigra regional selectivity. *Brain* 114:2283–2301, 1991.

27. Kish SJ, Shannak K, Hornykiewicz O: Uneven pattern of dopamine loss in the striatum of patients with idiopathic Parkinson's disease. *N Engl J Med* 318:876–880, 1988.

28. Byrne E, Lennox G, Lowe J, Godwin-Austin RB: Diffuse Lewy body disease: Clinical features in 15 cases. *J Neurol Neurosurg Psychiatry* 52:709–717, 1989.

29. Lewis AJ, Gawell MJ: Diffuse Lewy Body disease with dementia and oculomotor dysfunction. *Mov Disord* 5:143–147, 1990.

30. Fearnley JM, Revesz T, Brooks DJ, et al: Diffuse Lewy body disease presenting with a supranuclear downgaze palsy. *J Neurol Neurosurg Psychiatry* 54:159–161, 1991.

31. Sage JI, Miller DC, Golbe LI, et al: Clinically atypical expression of pathologically typical Lewy-body parkinsonism. *Clin Neuropharmacol* 13:36–47, 1990.

32. Vanderhaegen JJ, Perier O, Sternon JE: Pathological findings in idiopathic orthostatic hypotension: Its relationship with Parkinson's disease. *Arch Neurol* 22:207–214, 1970.

33. Crossman AR: A hypothesis on the pathophysiological mechanisms that underlie L-dopa- or dopamine agonist-induced dyskinesia in Parkinson's disease: Implications for future strategies in treatment. *Mov Disord* 5:100–108, 1990.

34. Miletich RS, Chan T, Gillespie M, et al: Contralateral basal ganglia metabolism is abnormal in hemiparkinsonian patients: An FDG-PET study. *Neurology* 38:S260, 1988.

35. Wolfson LI, Leenders KL, Brown LL, Jones T: Alterations of regional cerebral blood flow and oxygen metabolism in Parkinson's disease. *Neurology* 35:1399–1405, 1985.

36. Eidelberg D, Moeller JR, Dhawan V, et al: The metabolic topography of parkinsonism. *J Cereb Blood Flow Metab* 14:783–801, 1994.

37. Leenders KL, Wolfson L, Gibbs JM, et al: The effects of L-dopa on regional cerebral blood flow and oxygen metabolism in patients with Parkinson's disease. *Brain* 108:171–191, 1985.

38. Perlmutter JS, Raichle ME: Regional blood flow in hemiparkinsonism. *Neurology* 35:1127–1134, 1985.

39. Kuhl DE, Metter EJ, Riege WH, Markham CH: Patterns of cerebral glucose utilisation in Parkinson's disease and Huntington's disease. *Ann Neurol* 15 (Suppl):S119–S125, 1984.

40. Peppard RF, Martin WRW, Guttman M, et al: The relationship of cerebral glucose metabolism to cognitive deficits in Parkinson's disease. *Neurology* 38 (Suppl 1):364, 1988.

41. Kuhl DE, Metter EJ, Benson DF, et al: Similarities of cerebral glucose metabolism in Alzheimer's and Parkinsonian dementia. *J Cereb Blood Flow Metab* 5:S169–S170, 1985 (abstr.).

42. Kuhl DE, Metter EJ, Riege WH: Patterns of local cerebral glucose utilisation determined in Parkinson's disease by the 18F-fluorodeoxyglucose method. *Ann Neurol* 15:419–424, 1984.

43. Otsuka M, Ichiya Y, Hosokawa S, et al: Striatal blood flow, glucose metabolism, and ^{18}F-dopa uptake: Difference in Parkinson's disease and atypical parkinsonism. *J Neurol Neurosurg Psychiatry* 54:898–904, 1991.

44. Schapiro MB, Grady C, Ball MJ, et al: Reductions in parietal/temporal cerebral glucose metabolism are not specific for Alzheimer's disease. *Neurology* 40 (suppl 1):152, 1990.

45. Kiyosawa M, Baron JC, Hamel E, et al: Time course of effects of unilateral lesions of the nucleus basalis of Meynert on glucose utilisation by the cerebral cortex: Positron emission tomography in baboons. *Brain* 112:435–455, 1989.

46. McKeith I, Fairbairn A, Perry R, et al: Neuroleptic sensitivity in patients with senile dementia of Lewy body type. *BMJ* 305:673–678, 1992.

47. Thaler DE, Passingham RE: The supplementary motor cortex and internally directed movement, in Crossman AR, Sambrook M (eds): *Neural Mechanisms in Disorders of Movement*. London: Libby, 1989, pp 175–181.

48. Goldberg G: Supplementary motor area structure and function: Review and hypotheses. *Behav Brain Sci* 8:567–616, 1985.

49. Mushiake H, Inase M, Tanji J: Selective coding of motor sequence in the supplementary motor area of the monkey cerebral cortex. *Exp Brain Res* 82:208–210, 1990.

50. Goldman-Rakic PS: Circuitry of primate prefrontal cortex and regulation of behaviour by representational memory, in Plum F (ed): *The Nervous System: Higher Functions of the Brain*. Bethesda, MD: American Physiology Society, 1987, pp 373–417.

51. Jenkins IH, Fernandez W, Playford ED, et al: Impaired activation of the supplementary motor areain Parkinson's disease is reversed when akinesia is treated with apomorphine. *Ann Neurol* 32:749–757, 1992.

52. Rascol O, Sabatini U, Chollet F, et al: Supplementary and primary sensory motor area activity in Parkinson's disease: Regional cerebral blood flow changes during finger movements and effects of apomorphine. *Arch Neurol* 49:144–148, 1992.

53. Rascol O, Sabatini U, Chollet F, et al: Normal activation of the supplementary motor area in patients with Parkinson's disease undergoing long-term treatment with L-dopa. *J Neurol Neurosurg Psychiatry* 57:567–571, 1994.

54. Laitinen LV, Bergenheim AT, Hariz MI: Leksell's posteroventral pallidotomy in the treatment of Parkinson's disease. *J Neurosurg* 76:53–61, 1992.

55. Dogali M, Fazzini E, Kolodny E, et al: Stereotaxic ventral pallidotomy for Parkinson's disease. *Neurology* 45:753–761, 1995.

56. Vitek JL, Baron M, Kaneoke Y, et al: Microelectrode-guided pallidotomy is an effective treatment for medically intractable Parkinson's disease. *Neurology* 44 (suppl 2):A304, 1994.

57. Ceballos-Baumann AO, Obeso JA, Delong MR, et al: Functional reafferentation of striatal-frontal connections after posteroventral pallidotomy in Parkinson's disease. *Lancet* 344:814, 1994.

58. Grafton ST, Waters C, Sutton J, et al: Pallidotomy increases activity of motor association cortex in Parkinson's disease— A positron emission tomographic study. *Ann Neurol* 37:776–783, 1995.

59. Firnau G, Sood S, Chirakal R, et al: Cerebral metabolism of 6-[18F]fluoro-L-3,4-dihydroxyphenylalanine in the primate. *J Neurochem* 48:1077–1082, 1987.

60. Tedroff J, Aquilonius S-M, Laihinen A, et al: Striatal kinetics of [11C]-(+)-nomifensine and 6-[18F]fluoro-L-dopa in Parkinson's disease measured with positron emission tomography. *Acta Neurol Scand* 81:24–30, 1990.

61. Tedroff J, Aquilonius S-M, Hartvig P, et al: Monoamine re-uptake sites in the human brain evaluated in vivo by means of 11C-nomifensine and positron emission tomography: The effects of age and Parkinson's disease. *Acta Neurol Scand* 77:192–201, 1988.

62. Frost JJ, Rosier AJ, Reich SG, et al: Positron emission tomographic imaging of the dopamine transporter with ¹¹C-WIN 35,428 reveals marked declines in mild Parkinson's disease. *Ann Neurol* 34:423–431, 1993.

63. Marek KL, Seibyl JP, Sandridge B, et al: SPECT imaging with [I-123]b-CIT demonstrates striatal dopamine transporter loss in parkinsonism. *Neurology* 44 (suppl 2):A352, 1994 (abstr.).

64. Kilbourn MR, Lee LC, Jewett DM, et al: In vitro and in vivo binding of a dihydrotetrabenazine to the vesicular monoamine transporter is stereospecific. *J Cereb Blood Flow Metab* 15 (suppl 1):S650, 1995.

65. Nahmias C, Garnett ES, Firnau G, Lang A: Striatal dopamine distribution in Parkinsonian patients during life. *J Neurol Sci* 69:223–230, 1985.

66. Leenders KL, Palmer A, Turton D, et al: Dopa uptake and dopamine receptor binding visualized in the human brain in vivo, in Fahn S, Marsden CD, Jenner P, Teychenne P (eds): *Recent Developments in Parkinson's Disease*. New York: Raven Press, 1986, pp 103–113.

67. Brooks DJ, Ibaez V, Sawle GV, et al: Differing patterns of striatal ¹⁸F-dopa uptake in Parkinson's disease, multiple system atrophy and progressive supranuclear palsy. *Ann Neurol* 28:547–555, 1990.

68. Leenders KL, Palmer AJ, Quinn N, et al: Brain dopamine metabolism in patients with Parkinson's disease measured with positron emission tomography. *J Neurol Neurosurg Psychiatry* 49:853–860, 1986.

69. Martin WRW, Stoessl AJ, Adam MJ, et al: Positron emission tomography in Parkinson's disease: Glucose and dopa metabolism. *Adv Neurol* 45:95–98, 1986.

70. Koeppe RA, Frey KA, Vander Borght TM, et al: Kinetic evaluation of [C-11]dihydrotetrabenazine (DTBZ) by dynamic PET: A marker for the vesicular dopamine transporter. *J Cereb Blood Flow Metab* 15 (suppl 1):S651, 1995.

71. Laihinen AO, Rinne JO, Nagren KA, et al: PET studies on brain monoamine transporters with carbon-11-beta-CIT in Parkinson's disease. *J Nucl Med* 36:1263–1267, 1995.

72. Salmon EP, Brooks DJ, Leenders KL, et al: A two-compartment description and kinetic procedure for measuring regional cerebral [11C]nomifensine uptake using positron emission tomography. *J Cereb Blood Flow Metab* 10:307–316, 1990.

73. Leenders KL, Salmon EP, Tyrrell P, et al: The nigrostriatal dopaminergic system assessed in vivo by positron emission tomography in healthy volunteer subjects and patients with Parkinson's disease. *Arch Neurol* 47:1290–1298, 1990.

74. Brcke T, Asenbaum S, Pirker W, et al: Quantification of dopaminergic nerve cell loss in Parkinson's disease with [I-123]-b-CIT. *J Cereb Blood Flow Metab* 15 (suppl 1):S37, 1995.

75. Rinne JO, Rummukainen J, Lic M, et al: Dementia in Parkinson's disease is related to neuronal loss in the medial substantia nigra. *Ann Neurol* 26:47–50, 1989.

76. Bernheimer H, Birkmayer W, Hornykiewicz O, et al: Brain dopamine and the syndromes of Parkinson and Huntington: Clinical, morphological, and neurochemical correlations. *J Neurol Sci* 20:415–455, 1973.

77. Morrish PK, Sawle GV, Brooks DJ: Clinical and [¹⁸F]dopa PET findings in early Parkinsons disease. *J Neurol Neurosurg Psychiatry* 59:597–600, 1995.

78. Calne DB, Langston JW, Martin WR, et al: Positron emission tomography after MPTP: Observations relating to the cause of Parkinson's disease. *Nature* 317:246–248, 1985.

79. Sawle GV, Wroe SJ, Lees AJ, et al: The identification of presymptomatic parkinsonism: Clinical and [¹⁸F]dopa PET studies in an Irish kindred. *Ann Neurol* 32:609–617, 1992.

80. Mark MH, Burn DJ, Bergen M, et al: Familial diffuse Lewy body disease: An ¹⁸F-dopa PET study. *Mov Disord* 7 (suppl 1):142, 1992.

81. Burn DJ, Mark MH, Playford ED, et al: Parkinson's disease in twins studied with ¹⁸F-dopa and positron emission tomography. *Neurology* 42:1894–1900, 1992.

82. Holthoff VA, Vieregge P, Kessler J, et al: Discordant twins with Parkinson's disease-positron emission tomography and early signs of impaired cognitive circuits. *Ann Neurol* 36:176–182, 1994.

83. Brooks DJ, Playford ED, Ibanez V, et al: Isolated tremor and disruption of the nigrostriatal dopaminergic system: An ¹⁸F-dopa PET study. *Neurology* 42:1554–1560, 1992.

84. Asenbaum S, Brucke T, Pirker W, et al: Imaging of striatal dopamine reuptake sites with [¹²³I]b-CIT and SPECT assists successfully in the diagnosis of movement disorders. *J Cereb Blood Flow Metab* 15 (suppl 1):S754, 1995.

85. Calne DB, Eisen A, McGeer EG, Spencer P: Alzheimer's disease, Parkinson's disease and motoneurone disease: abiotrophic interaction between aging and environment. *Lancet* 1:1067–1070, 1986.

86. Sawle GV, Colebatch JG, Shah A, et al: Striatal function in normal aging: Implications for Parkinsons disease. *Ann Neurol* 28:799–804, 1990.

87. Eidelberg D, Takikawa S, Dhawan V, et al: Striatal F-18 dopa uptake—Absence of an aging effect. *J Cereb Blood Flow Metabol* 13:881–888, 1993.

88. Martin WRW, Palmer MR, Patlak CS, Calne DB: Nigrostriatal function in humans studied with positron emission tomography. *Ann Neurol* 26:535–542, 1989.

89. Cordes M, Snow BJ, Cooper S, et al: Age-dependent decline of nigrostriatal dopaminergic function—A positron emission tomographic study of grandparents and their grandchildren. *Ann Neurol* 36:667–670, 1994.

90. Bhatt MH, Snow BJ, Martin WRW, et al: Positron emission tomography suggests that the rate of progression of idiopathic parkinsonism is slow. *Ann Neurol* 29:673–677, 1991.

91. Morrish PK, Sawle GV, Brooks DJ: An [¹⁸F]dopa PET and clinical study of the rate of progression of Parkinson's disease. *Brain* 119:585–591, 1996.

92. Vingerhoets FJG, Snow BJ, Lee CS, et al: Longitudinal fluoro-dopa positron emission tomographic studies of the evolution of idiopathic parkinsonism. *Ann Neurol* 36:759–764, 1994.

93. Kish SJ, Shannak K, Rajput A, et al: Aging produces a specific pattern of striatal dopamine loss: Implications for the etiology of idiopathic Parkinson's disease. *J Neurochem* 58:642–648, 1992.

94. McGeer PL, Itagaki S, Akiyama H, McGeer EG: Rate of cell death in Parkinsonism indicates active neuropathological process. *Ann Neurol* 24:574–576, 1988.

95. Sawle GV, Bloomfield PM, Bjorklund A, et al: Transplantation of fetal dopamine neurons in Parkinson's disease: PET [¹⁸F]-6-L-fluorodopa studies in two patients with putaminal implants. *Ann Neurol* 31:166–173, 1992.

96. Linvall O, Sawle G, Widner H, et al: Evidence for long term survival and function of dopaminergic grafts in progressive Parkinsons disease. *Ann Neurol* 35:172–180, 1994.

97. Peschanski M, Defer G, Nguyen JP, et al: Bilateral motor improvement and alteration of L-dopa effect in two patients with Parkinson's disease following intrastriatal transplantation of fetal ventral mesencephalon. *Brain* 117:487–499, 1994.

98. Freeman TB, Olanow CW, Hauser RA, et al: Bilateral fetal nigral transplantation into the post-commisural putamen as a treat-

ment for Parkinson's disease: Six months follow-up. *Ann Neurol* 38:379–388, 1995.

99. Kordower JH, Freeman TB, Snow BJ, et al: Neuropathological evidence of graft survival and striatal reinnervation after the transplantation of fetal mesencephalic tissue in a patient with Parkinson's disease. *N Engl J Med* 332:1118–1124, 1995.

100. Rinne JO, Laihinen A, Nagren K, et al: PET demonstrates different behaviour of striatal dopamine D1 and D2 receptors in early Parkinson's disease. *J Neurosci Res* 27:494–499, 1990.

101. Turjanski N, Lees AJ, Brooks DJ: Striatal D_1 and D_2 receptor status in L-dopa treated Parkinson's disease patients with and without dyskinesia: A PET study. *Mov Disord* 9 (suppl 1):151, 1994.

102. Leenders KL, Herold S, Palmer AJ, et al: Human cerebral dopamine system measured in vivo using PET. *J Cereb Blood Flow Metabol* 5 (suppl 1):S157–S158, 1985.

103. Brcke T, Podreka I, Angelberger P, et al: Dopamine D_2 receptor imaging with SPECT: Studies in different neuropsychiatric disorders. *J Cereb Blood Flow Metab* 11:220–228, 1991.

104. Schwarz J, Tatsch K, Arnold G, et al: ^{123}I-iodobenzamide-SPECT predicts dopaminergic responsiveness in patients with de-novo parkinsonism. *Neurology* 42:556–561, 1992.

105. Brooks DJ, Ibanez V, Sawle GV, et al: Striatal D_2 receptor status in Parkinson's disease, striatonigral degeneration, and progressive supranuclear palsy, measured with ^{11}C-raclopride and PET. *Ann Neurol* 31:184–192, 1992.

106. Leenders KL, Antonini A, Schwarz J, et al: Brain dopamine D_2 receptors in "de novo" drug-naive parkinsonian patients measured using PET and ^{11}C-raclopride. *Mov Disord* 7 (suppl 1):141, 1992.

107. Rinne UK, Leihinen A, Rinne JO, et al: Positron emission tomography demonstrates dopamine D2 receptor supersensitivity in the striatum of patients with early Parkinson's disease. *Mov Disord* 5:55–59, 1990.

108. Antonini A, Schwarz J, Oertel WH, et al: [^{11}C]raclopride and positron emission tomography in previously untreated patients with Parkinson's disease: Influence of L-dopa and lisuride therapy on striatal dopamine D_2-receptors. *Neurology* 44:1325–1329, 1994.

109. Sawle GV, Playford ED, Brooks DJ, et al: Asymmetrical presynaptic and postsynaptic changes in the striatal dopamine projection in dopa-naive parkinsonism: Diagnostic implications of the D_2 receptor status. *Brain* 116:853–867, 1993.

110. Shinotoh H, Aotsuka A, Yonezawa H, et al: Striatal dopamine D_2 receptors in Parkinson's disease and striato-nigral degeneration determined by positron emission tomography, in Nagatsu T, et al: (eds): *Basic, Clinical, and Therapeutic Advances of Alzheimer's and Parkinson's diseases*. New York: Plenum Press, 1990, vol 2, pp 107–110.

111. Hagglund J, Aquilonius SM, Eckernas SA, et al: Dopamine receptor properties in Parkinson's disease and Huntington's chorea evaluated by positron emission tomography using 11C-N-methyl-spiperone. *Acta Neurol Scand* 75:87–94, 1987.

112. Rinne JO, Laihinen A, Rinne UK, et al: PET study on striatal dopamine D2 receptor changes during the progression of early Parkinson's disease. *Mov Disord* 8:134–138, 1993.

113. Quinn N: Multiple system atrophy—The nature of the beast. *J Neurol Neurosurg Psychiatry* 52:78–89, 1989.

114. Papp MI, Lantos PL: The distribution of oligodendroglial inclusions in multiple system atrophy and its relevance to clinical symptomatology. *Brain* 117:235–243, 1994.

115. De Volder AG, Francard J, Laterre C, et al: Decreased glucose utilisation in the striatum and frontal lobe in probable striatonigral degeneration. *Ann Neurol* 26:239–247, 1989.

116. Eidelberg D, Takikawa S, Moeller JR, et al: Striatal hypometabolism distinguishes striatonigral degeneration from Parkinson's disease. *Ann Neurol* 33:518–527, 1993.

117. Davie CA, Wenning GK, Barker GJ, et al: Differentiation of multiple system atrophy from idiopathic Parkinson's disease using proton magnetic resonance spectroscopy. *Ann Neurol* 37:204–210, 1995.

118. Fulham MJ, Dubinsky RM, Polinsky RJ, et al: Computed tomography, magnetic resonance imaging, and positron emission tomography with [^{18}F]fluorodeoxyglucose in multiple system atrophy and pure autonomic failure. *Clin Autonomic Res* 1:27–36, 1991.

119. Rosenthal G, Gilman S, Koeppe RA, et al: Motor dysfunction in olivopontocerebellar atrophy is related to cerebral metabolic rate studied with positron emission tomography. *Ann Neurol* 24:414–419, 1988.

120. Gilman S, Koeppe RA, Junck L, et al: Patterns of cerebral glucose metabolism detected with positron emission tomography differ in multiple system atrophy and olivopontocerebellar atrophy. *Ann Neurol* 36:166–175, 1994.

121. Brooks DJ, Salmon EP, Mathias CJ, et al: The relationship between locomotor disability, autonomic dysfunction, and the integrity of the striatal dopaminergic system, in patients with multiple system atrophy, pure autonomic failure, and Parkinson's disease, studied with PET. *Brain* 113:1539–1552, 1990.

122. Burn DJ, Sawle GV, Brooks DJ: The differential diagnosis of Parkinsons disease, multiple system atrophy, and Steele-Richardson-Olszewski syndrome: Discriminant analysis of striatal 18F-dopa PET data. *J Neurol Neurosurg Psychiatry* 57:278–284, 1994.

123. Goto S, Hirano A, Matsumoto S: Subdivisional involvement of nigrostriatal loop in idiopathic Parkinsons disease and striatonigral degeneration. *Ann Neurol* 26:766–770, 1989.

124. Burn DJ, Rinne JO, Quinn NP, et al: Striatal opioid receptor binding in Parkinsons disease, striatonigral degeneration, and Steele-Richardson-Olszewski syndrome: An ^{11}C-diprenorphine PET study. *Brain.* In press.

125. Rinne JO, Burn DJ, Mathias CJ, et al: PET studies on the dopaminergic system and striatal opioid binding in the olivopontocerebellar atrophy variant of multiple system atrophy. *Ann Neurol* 37:568–573, 1995.

126. Otsuka M, Ichiya Y, Kuwabara Y, et al: Striatal ^{18}F-dopa uptake and brain glucose metabolism by PET in patients with syndrome of progressive ataxia. *J Neurol Sci* 124:198–203, 1994.

127. Steele JC, Richardson JC, Olszewski J: Progressive supranuclear palsy: A heterogeneous degeneration involving the brain stem, basal ganglia, and cerebellum, with vertical gaze and pseudobulbar palsy. *Arch Neurol* 10:333–359, 1964.

128. Maher ER, Lees AJ: The clinical features and natural history of the Steele-Richardson-Olszewski syndrome (progressive supranuclear palsy). *Neurology* 36:1005–1008, 1986.

129. Jackson JA, Jankovic J, Ford J: Progressive supranuclear palsy: Clinical features and response to treatment in 16 patients. *Ann Neurol* 13:273–278, 1983.

130. D'Antona R, Baron JC, Samson Y, et al: Subcortical dementia: Frontal cortex hypometabolism detected by positron tomography in patients with progressive supranuclear palsy. *Brain* 108:785–800, 1985.

131. Blin J, Baron JC, Dubois P, et al: Positron emission tomography study in progressive supranuclear palsy. *Arch Neurol* 47:747–752, 1990.

132. Foster NL, Gilman S, Berent S, et al: Cerebral hypometabolism in progressive supranuclear palsy studied with positron emission tomography. *Ann Neurol* 24:399–406, 1988.

133. Leenders KL, Frackowiak RS, Lees AJ: Steele-Richardson-Olszewski syndrome: Brain energy metabolism, blood flow and fluorodopa uptake measured by positron emission tomography. *Brain* 111:615–630, 1988.

134. Goffinet AM, De Volder AG, Gillain C, et al: Positron tomography demonstrates frontal lobe hypometabolism in progressive supranuclear palsy. *Ann Neurol* 25:131–139, 1989.

135. Otsuka M, Ichiya Y, Kuwabara Y, et al: Cerebral blood flow, oxygen and glucose metabolism with PET in progressive supranuclear palsy. *Ann Nucl Med* 3:111–118, 1989.

136. Foster NL, Gilman S, Berent S, et al: Progressive subcortical gliosis and progressive supranuclear palsy can have similar clinical and PET abnormalities. *J Neurol Neurosurg Psychiatry* 55:707–713, 1992.

137. Bhatt MH, Snow BJ, Martin WRW, et al: Positron emission tomography in progressive supranuclear palsy. *Arch Neurol* 48:389–391, 1991.

138. Jellinger K, Riederer P, Tomananga M: Progressive supranuclear palsy: Clinico-pathological and biochemical studies. *J Neural Transm* (suppl 16):111–128, 1980.

139. Kish SJ, Chang LJ, Mirchandani LJ, et al: Progressive supranuclear palsy: Relationship between extrapyramidal disturbances, dementia, and brain neurotransmitter markers. *Ann Neurol* 18:530–536, 1985.

140. Baron JC, Maziere B, Loc'h C, et al: Loss of striatal ([76Br])bromospiperone binding sites demonstrated by positron tomography in progressive supranuclear palsy. *J Cereb Blood Flow Metabol* 6:131–136, 1986.

141. Wienhard K, Coenen HH, Pawlik G, et al: PET studies of dopamine receptor distribution using [18F]fluoroethylspiperone: Findings in disorders related to the dopaminergic system. *J Neural Transm* 81:195–213, 1990.

142. Riley DE, Lang AE, Lewis A, et al: Cortical-basal ganglionic degeneration. *Neurology* 40:1203–1212, 1990.

143. Feaney MB, Ksiezakreding H, Liu WK, et al: Epitope expression and hyperphosphorylation of tau protein in corticobasal degeneration—differentiation from progressive supranuclear palsy. *Acta Neuropatholog* 90:37–43, 1995.

144. Sawle GV, Brooks DJ, Marsden CD, Frackowiak RSJ: Corticobasal degeneration: A unique pattern of regional cortical oxygen metabolism and striatal fluorodopa uptake demonstrated by positron emission tomography. *Brain* 114:541–556, 1991.

145. Eidelberg D, Dhawan V, Moeller JR, et al: The metabolic landscape of cortico-basal ganglionic degeneration: Regional asymmetries studied with positron emission tomography. *J Neurol Neurosurg Psychiatry* 54:856–862, 1991.

146. Blin J, Vidhailhet M-J, Pillon B, et al: Corticobasal degeneration: Decreased and asymmetrical glucose consumption as studied by PET. *Mov Disord* 7:348–354, 1992.

147. Frisoni GB, Pizzolato G, Zanetti O, Bianchetti A, et al: Corticobasal degeneration—Neuropsychological assessment and dopamine D-2 receptor SPECT analysis. *Eur Neurol* 35:50–54, 1995.

148. Fletcher NA, Harding AE, Marsden CD: A genetic study of idiopathic torsion dystonia in the United Kingdom. *Brain* 113:379–395, 1990.

149. Ozelius L, Kramer PL, Moskowitz CB, et al: Human gene for torsion dystonia located on chromosome 9q32-34. *Neuron* 2:1427–1434, 1989.

150. Kramer PL, De Leon D, Ozelius L, et al: Dystonia gene in Ashkenazi Jewish population is located on chromosome 9q32-34. *Ann Neurol* 27:114–120, 1990.

151. Hornykiewicz O, Kish SJ, Becker LE, et al: Brain neurotransmitters in dystonia musculorum deformans. *N Engl J Med* 315:347–352, 1986.

152. Jankovic J, Svendsen CN: Brain neurotransmitters in dystonia. *N Engl J Med* 316:278–279, 1987.

153. Chase T, Tamminga CA, Burrows H: Positron emission studies of regional cerebral glucose metabolism in idiopathic dystonia. *Adv Neurol* 50:237–241, 1988.

154. Eidelberg D, Dhawan V, Cedarbaum J, et al: Contralateral basal ganglia hypermetabolism in primary unilateral limb dystonia. *Neurology* 40 (suppl 1):399, 1990.

155. Gilman S, Junck L, Young AB, et al: Cerebral metabolic activity in idiopathic dystonia studied with positron emission tomography. *Adv Neurol* 50:231–236, 1988.

156. Otsuka M, Ichiya Y, Shima F, et al: Increased striatal 18F-dopa uptake and normal glucose metabolism in idiopathic dystonia syndrome. *J Neurol Sci* 111:195–199, 1992.

157. Stoessl AJ, Martin WRW, Clark C, et al: PET studies of cerebral glucose metabolism in idiopathic torticollis. *Neurology* 36:653–657, 1986.

158. Karbe H, Volthoff VA, Rudolf J, et al: Positron emission tomography demonstrates frontal cortex and basal ganglia hypometabolism in dystonia. *Neurology* 42:1540–1544, 1992.

159. Tempel LW, Perlmutter JS: Abnormal vibration-induced cerebral blood flow responses in idiopathic dystonia. *Brain* 113:691–707, 1990.

160. Tempel LW, Perlmutter JS: Abnormal cortical responses in patients with writer's cramp. *Neurology* 43:2252–2257, 1993.

161. Playford ED, Passingham RE, Marsden CD, Brooks DJ: Increased activation of frontal areas during arm movement in idiopathic torsion dystonia. *Mov Disord.* In press.

162. Ceballos-Baumann AO, Pasingham RE, Warner T, et al: Overactivity of rostral and underactivity of caudal frontal areas in idiopathic torsion dystonia: A PET activation study. *Ann Neurol* 37:363–372, 1995.

163. Ceballos-Baumann AO, Passingham RE, Marsden CD, Brooks DJ: Overactivity of primary and accessory motor areas after motor reorganisation in acquired hemi-dystonia: A PET activation study. *Ann Neurol* 37:746–757, 1995.

164. Leenders KL, Quinn N, Frackowiak RSJ, Marsden CD: Brain dopaminergic system studied in patients with dystonia using positron emission tomography. *Adv Neurol* 50:243–247, 1988.

165. Martin WRW, Stoessl AJ, Palmer M, et al: PET scanning in dystonia. *Adv Neurol* 50:223–229, 1988.

166. Playford ED, Fletcher NA, Sawle GV, et al: Integrity of the nigro-striatal dopaminergic system in familial dystonia: An 18F-dopa PET study. *Brain* 116:1191–1199, 1993.

167. Ichinose H, Ohye T, Takahashi E, et al: Hereditary progressive dystonia with marked diurnal fluctuation caused by mutations in the GTP-cyclohydrolase-1 gene. *Nature Genet* 8:236–242, 1994.

168. Nygaard TG, Trugman JM, de Yebenes JG, Fahn S: Dopa-responsive dystonia: The spectrum of clinical manifestations in a large North American family. *Neurology* 40:66–69, 1990.

169. Sawle GV, Leenders KL, Brooks DJ, et al: Dopa-responsive dystonia: [18F]dopa positron emission tomography. *Ann Neurol* 30:24–30, 1991.

170. Snow BJ, Nygaard TG, Takahashi H, Calne DB: Positron emission tomography studies of dopa-responsive dystonia and early-onset idiopathic parkinsonism. *Ann Neurol* 34:733–738, 1993.

171. Turjanski N, Bhatia K, Burn DJ, et al: Comparison of striatal 18F-dopa uptake in adult-onset dystonia-parkinsonism, Parkinson's disease, and dopa-responsive dystonia. *Neurology* 43:1563–1568, 1993.

172. The Huntington's Disease Collaborative Research Group: A novel gene containing a trinucleotide repeat that is expanded and unstable on Huntington's disease chromosomes. *Cell* 72:971–983, 1993.

173. Albin RL, Reiner A, Anderson KD, et al: Striatal and nigral neuron subpopulations in rigid Huntington's disease: Implications for the functional anatomy of chorea and rigidity-akinesia. *Ann Neurol* 27:357–365, 1990.

174. Hardie RJ, Pullon HWH, Harding AE, et al: Neuroacanthocytosis: A clinical, haematological, and pathological study of 19 cases. *Brain* 114:13–50, 1991.

175. Yazawa T, Nukina N, Hashida H, et al: Abnormal gene product identified in hereditary dentatorubralpallidoluysian atrophy (DRPLA) brain. *Nature Genet* 10:99–103, 1995.

176. Gunne LM, Haggstrom J-E, Sjoquist B: Association with persistent neuroleptic-induced dyskinesia of regional changes in brain GABA synthesis. *Nature* 309:347–349, 1984.

177. Andersson U, Haggstrom J-E, Levin ED, et al: Reduced glutamate decarboxylase activity in the subthalamic nucleus of patients with tardive dyskinesia. *Mov Disord* 4:37–46, 1989.

178. Kuhl DE, Phelps ME, Markham CH, et al: Cerebral metabolism and atrophy in Huntington's disease determined by 18FDG and computed tomographic scans. *Ann Neurol* 12:425–434, 1982.

179. Hayden MR, Martin WRW, Stoessl AJ, et al: Positron emission tomography in the early diagnosis of Huntington's disease. *Neurology* 36:888–894, 1986.

180. Leenders KL, Frackowiak RSJ, Quinn N, Marsden CD: Brain energy metabolism and dopaminergic function in Huntington's disease measured in vivo using positron emission tomography. *Mov Disord* 1:69–77, 1986.

181. Young AB, Penney JB, Starosta-Rubinstein S, et al: PET scan investigations of Huntington's disease: Cerebral metabolic correlates of neurological features and functional decline. *Ann Neurol* 20:296–303, 1986.

182. Berent S, Giordani B, Lehtinen S, et al: Positron emission tomographic scan investigations of Huntington's disease—Cerebral metabolic correlates of cognitive function. *Ann Neurol* 23:541–546, 1988.

183. Kuwert T, Lange HW, Langen KJ, et al: Cortical and subcortical glucose consumption measured by PET in patients with Huntington's disease. *Brain* 113:1405–1423, 1990.

184. Dubinsky RM, Hallett M, Levey R, Di Chiro G: Regional brain glucose metabolism in neuroacanthocytosis. *Neurology* 39:1253–1255, 1989.

185. Hosokawa S, Ichiya Y, Kuwabara Y, et al: Positron emission tomography in cases of chorea with different underlying diseases. *J Neurol Neurosurg Psychiatry* 50:1284–1287, 1987.

186. Kuwert T, Lange HW, Langen KJ, et al: Normal striatal glucose consumption in two patients with benign hereditary chorea as measured by positron emission tomography. *J Neurol* 237:80–84, 1990.

187. Suchowersky O, Hayden MR, Martin WRW, et al: Cerebral metabolism of glucose in benign hereditary chorea. *Mov Disord* 1:33–45, 1986.

188. Guttman M, Lang AE, Garnett ES, et al: Regional cerebral glucose metabolism in SLE chorea: Further evidence that striatal hypometabolism is not a correlate of chorea. *Mov Disord* 2:201–210, 1987.

189. Weindl A, Kuwert T, Leenders KL, et al: Increased striatal glucose consumption in Sydenham chorea. *Mov Disord* 8:437–444, 1993.

190. Pahl JJ, Mazziotta JC, Cummings J, et al: Positron emission tomography in tardive dyskinesia and Huntington's disease. *J Cereb Blood Flow Metab* 7:1253–1255, 1987.

191. Grafton ST, Mazziotta JC, Pahl JJ, et al: A comparison of neurological, metabolic, structural, and genetic evaluations in persons at risk for Huntington's disease. *Ann Neurol* 28:614–621, 1990.

192. Young AB, Penney JB, Starosta-Rubinstein S, et al: Normal caudate glucose metabolism in persons at-risk for Huntington's disease. *Arch Neurol* 44:254–257, 1987.

193. Hayden MR, Hewitt J, Martin WRW, et al: Studies in persons at risk for Huntington's disease. *N Engl J Med* 317:382–383, 1987.

194. Wong DF, Links JM, Wagner HN Jr, et al: Dopamine and serotonin receptors measured in-vivo in Huntington's disease with C-11 N-methylspiperone PET imaging. *J Nucl Med* 26:P107, 1985.

195. Turjanski N, Weeks R, Dolan R, et al: Striatal D_1 and D_2 receptor binding in patients with Huntington's disease and other choreas: A PET study. *Brain* 118:689–696, 1995.

196. Weeks RA, Harding AE, Brooks DJ: PET demonstrates a parallel loss of D_1 and D_2 dopamine receptors in asymptomatic mutation carriers of Huntingtons disease. *Ann Neurol* 40:49–54, 1996.

197. Torres EM, Fricker RA, Hume SP, et al: Assessment of striatal graft viability in the rat in vivo using a small diameter PET scanner. *Neuroreport* 6:2017–2021, 1995.

198. Weeks RA, Cunningham V, Waters S, et al: A comparison of region of interest and statistical parametric mapping analysis in PET ligand work: ^{11}C-diprenorphine in Huntington's disease and Tourette's syndrome. *J Cereb Blood Flow Metab* 15 (Suppl 1): S41, 1995.

199. Holthoff VA, Koeppe RA, Frey KA, et al: Positron emission tomography measures of benzodiazepine receptors in Huntington's disease. *Ann Neurol* 34:76–81, 1993.

200. Brooks DJ, Ibanez V, Playford ED, et al: Presynaptic and postsynaptic striatal dopaminergic function in neuroacanthocytosis: A positron emission tomographic study. *Ann Neurol* 30:166–171, 1991.

201. Andersson U, Eckernas SA, Hartvig P, Ulin J, et al: Striatal binding of ^{11}C-NMSP studied with positron emission tomography in patients with persistent tardive dyskinesia: No evidence for altered dopamine receptor binding. *J Neural Transm* 79:215–226, 1990.

202. Blin J, Baron JC, Cambon H, et al: Striatal dopamine D_2 receptors in tardive dyskinesia: PET study. *J Neurol Neurosurg Psychiatry* 52:1248–1252, 1989.

PART II

NEUROSCIENTIFIC FOUNDATIONS

Chapter 4 _____

OXIDATIVE PHOSPHORYLATION DISEASES AND MOVEMENT DISORDERS

JOHN M. SHOFFNER

OXPHOS: BIOCHEMISTRY AND GENETICS
AGE-RELATED ABNORMALITIES IN OXPHOS AND
    mtDNA
SOMATIC mtDNA MUTATIONS IN THE CENTRAL
    NERVOUS SYSTEM
INHERITED AND SOMATIC MUTATIONS: POSSIBLE
    INTERACTIONS IN NEURODEGENERATIVE
    DISEASES
    Myoclonic Epilepsy and Ragged-Red Fiber Disease
        (MERRF)
    Leber's Hereditary Optic Neuropathy (LHON) and
        Dystonia
    Leigh's Disease (Subacute Necrotizing
        Encephalopathy)
    Parkinson's Disease
    Ataxias and Other Movement Disorders
OXPHOS DISEASE ASSESSMENT IN PATIENTS WITH
    MOVEMENT DISORDERS
OXPHOS DISEASE THERAPY

For almost 3 decades, laboratory criteria used in the diagnosis of an oxidative phosphorylation (OXPHOS) disease depended on searching for elevations of lactate, pyruvate, and alanine in blood, urine, or cerebrospinal fluid (CSF) and on performing a muscle biopsy to look for the presence of ragged-red muscle fibers (RRF), abnormal cytochrome c oxidase histochemistry, abnormal mitochondrial ultrastructure, and OXPHOS enzyme abnormalities. Once genetic mutations in the mitochondrial DNA (mtDNA) were discovered in 1988,[1,2] it became clear that these observations were present in only a subset of patients with OXPHOS diseases. The term *OXPHOS disease* now encompasses an enormous array of clinical disorders whose onset can occur at any time from birth to old age. Clinical diseases are no longer confined to rare neuromuscular disorders with RRFs and structurally abnormal mitochondria. In fact, as more is learned about the relationships among mtDNA mutations, nuclear DNA mutations, and OXPHOS disease expression, the catalogue of patient phenotypes suggests that OXPHOS diseases may be one of the most commonly encountered classes of degenerative diseases.

Basal ganglia structures appear to be particularly vulnerable to OXPHOS dysfunction. Consequently, movement disorders are an important manifestation of OXPHOS diseases in both pediatric and adult patients. In children, high levels of certain mtDNA mutations are associated with a form of rapid degeneration in basal ganglia and brain stem structures that is often referred to as Leigh's disease or subacute necrotizing encephalopathy.[3,4] In 1995, a novel mtDNA mutation was discovered that produces generalized dystonias in children.[5,6] Abnormalities in OXPHOS as well as candidate mutations in the mtDNA are being investigated for their role in producing adult-onset movement disorders such as Parkinson's disease.[7,8] This chapter reviews basic aspects of OXPHOS biochemistry, OXPHOS genetics, mtDNA mutations that can cause movement disorders, and modern approaches to patient diagnosis.

OXPHOS: Biochemistry and Genetics

OXPHOS consists of five protein-lipid enzyme complexes, which are located in the mitochondrial inner membrane. These enzymes contain flavins (FMN, FAD), quinoid compounds (coenzyme Q_{10}), and transition metal compounds (iron-sulfur clusters, hemes, protein-bound copper)[9,10] and are designated complex I (nicotinamide adenine dinucleotide (NADH) ubiquinone oxidoreductase), complex II (succinate: ubiquinone oxidoreductase), complex III (ubiquinol:ferrocytochrome c oxidoreductase), complex IV (cytochrome C oxidase), and complex V (adenosine triphosphate (ATP) synthase) (Fig. 4-1). Complexes I and II collect electrons from the catabolism of fats, proteins, and carbohydrates and transfer them to ubiquinone (coenzyme Q_{10}). The electrons then move sequentially through complex III, cytochrome c, complex IV, and, finally, they react with oxygen, the terminal electron acceptor. Complexes I, III, and IV use the energy in electron transfer to pump protons across the inner mitochondrial membrane, producing a proton gradient. Complex V uses the potential energy stored in the proton gradient to condense adenosine diphosphate (ADP) and inorganic phosphate (P_i) into ATP. The resulting ATP is exchanged across the inner membrane with ADP by the adenine nucleotide translocase. Genetic regulation of OXPHOS depends on developmental stage-specific and tissue-specific control of nuclear OXPHOS gene expression. The highly variable energy demands for each tissue are regulated by tissue-specific mechanisms that modulate ATP production. Tissue-specific OXPHOS isoforms and transcriptional control of OXPHOS are two methods that tissues use to regulate OXPHOS activity.

The human mtDNA is a 16,569 nucleotide pair, double-stranded, circular molecule that codes for two ribosomal RNAs (rRNA) and 22 transfer RNAs (tRNA) required for mitochondrial protein synthesis and 13 polypeptides that, together with polypeptides coded by the nuclear DNA, are essential to the assembly and function of OXPHOS enzyme complexes I, III, IV, and V (Fig. 4-2).[11] The high mtDNA copy number and cytoplasmic location of mitochondria produce genetic characteristics that are unique to the mtDNA. Current concepts in mitochondrial genetics embody four main features: (1) maternal inheritance, (2) replicative segregation, (3) threshold expression of phenotype, and (4) an accumulation of somatic mtDNA mutations with aging and in degenerative diseases.

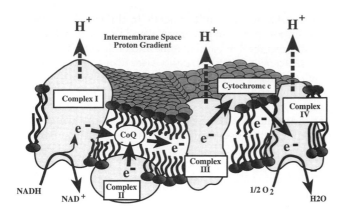

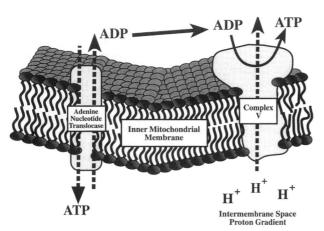

FIGURE 4-1 Oxidative phosphorylation. Dashed arrows indicate proton (H⁺) translocation into the space between the inner and outer membrane (intermembrane space). e⁻, electron flow through OXPHOS; CoQ, ubiquinone (coenzyme Q) *(From Shoffner et al.[10] Used with permission.)*

FIGURE 4-2 Mitochondrial DNA gene arrangement (* = mtDNA genes coded on the L-strand). The mtDNA map positions are according to the Human Gene Mapping conventions. The mitochondrial genome is composed of 16,569 np which contains the following features: *D-Loop:* This is a 1122-np stretch of mtDNA, extending from np 16,024 to 576, which is responsible for directing replication and transcription. It consists of the termination associated sequence (TAS, np 16,157–16,172), the origin of H-strand replication (O_H, np 110–441), the 7S-like DNA region (O_L, 16,104–16,106), conserved sequence block (CSB) I (CSBI, np 213–235), II (CSBII, np 299–315), and III (CSBIII, np 346–363), mtTF binding sites (np 233–260, 276–303, 418–445, and 523–550), the mitochondrial replication primer (np 317–321), the L-strand promoter (P_L, np 392–445), the major H-strand promotor (P_{H1}, np 545–567), and the minor H-strand promotor (P_{H2}, np~ 645). The membrane attachment site is located at approximately np 15,925–499. Other regulatory sequences are located outside the D-loop and include the origin of light strand replication (O_L, np 5721–5798) and a transcription terminator that regulates the rRNA and mRNA ratio (np 3237–3249). *Ribosomal RNAs (rRNA):* 12S rRNA (np 648–1601), 16S rRNA (np 1671–3229). *Transfer RNAs (tRNAs):* alanine (A, Ala, np 5587–5655), arginine (R, Arg, np 10405–10469), asparagine (N, Asn, np 5657–5729), aspartate (D, Asp, np 7518–7585), cysteine (C, Cys, np 5761–5826), glutamate (E, Glu, np 14674–14742), glutamine (Q, Gln, np 4329–4400), glycine (G, Gly, np 9991–10058), histadine (H, His, np 12138–12206), isoleucine (I, Ile, np 4263–4331), leucine (L(UUR), Leu, np 3230–3304 and L(CUN), np 12266–12336), lysine (K, Lys, np 8295–8364), methionine (M, Met, np 4402–4469), phenylalanine (F, Phe, np 577–647), proline (P, Pro, np 15955–16023), serine (S(UCN), Ser, np 7445–7516, and S(AGY), np 12207–12265), threonine (T, Thr, np 15888–15953), tryptophan (W, Trp, np 5512–5576), tyrosine (Y, Tyr, np 5826–5891), valine (V, Val, np 1602–1670). *OXPHOS subunits:* (A) Complex I: NADH dehydrogenase (ND) 1 (ND1, np 3307–4262), ND2 (np 4470–5511), ND3 (np 10059–10404), ND4 (np 10760–12137), ND4L (np 10470–10766), ND5 (np 12337–14148), ND6 (np 14149–14673). (B) Complex III: cytochrome b (Cytb, np 14747–15887). (C) Complex IV: cytochrome c oxidase I (COI, np 5904–7444), COII (np 7586–8262), COIII (np 9207–9990). (D) Complex V: ATPase 6 (ATP-6, np 8527–9207), ATPase 8 (ATP-8, np 8366–8572). *(From Shoffner et al.[10] Used with permission.)*

Maternal transmission of mtDNA defines the inheritance pattern of this genome in all vertebrates. Although low levels of paternally transmitted mtDNA have been identified in mice that represent about 0.01 percent of the total mtDNA,[12] paternal transmission of mtDNA has not been observed in human pedigrees. The mtDNA is normally homoplasmic, meaning that the same mtDNA sequence exists in all cells. However, pathogenic mtDNA mutations are frequently heteroplasmic, which means that mtDNAs with both normal and mutant sequences coexist. An important factor in determining the relative proportions of normal and mutant mtDNAs is the replicative potential of the cell line. For example, skeletal muscle, cardiac muscle, and neurons have a low replicative potential accounting for their ability to maintain high proportions of mutant mtDNAs. In contrast, hematopoietic cells replicate throughout an individual's life, resulting in highly variable concentrations of mutant and normal mtDNAs. Hence, replicative segregation accounts for a significant proportion of the variation in cellular genotypes observed in patients with OXPHOS diseases that are caused by heteroplasmic mtDNA mutations.

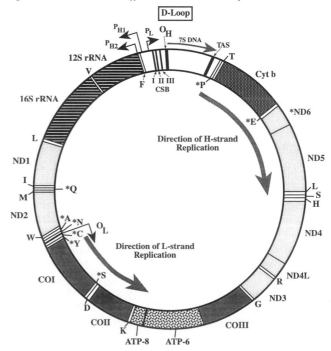

Age-Related Abnormalities in OXPHOS and mtDNA

Aging is associated with a wide variety of degenerative changes in cells, including a progressive decline in mitochondrial respiratory function. Although numerous mechanisms have been proposed to account for the variable rates of cellular senescence among tissues, the mitochondrial theory of aging[13,14] is gaining significant experimental support. This hypothesis has three main assumptions.

The first assumption is that free radicals are continuously produced in the mitochondria by OXPHOS as well as by other reactions. Although approximately 90–95 percent of the oxygen delivered to the cell is reduced to H_2O by complex IV, up to 1–2 percent of the oxygen may be converted to oxygen radicals by direct transfer of electrons from reduced mitochondrial flavins, coenzyme Q_{10}, and cytochrome b,[15,16] thus generating superoxide radicals at a rate of about 10^7 molecules of O_2/mitochondrion/day.[17,18]

The second assumption is that free radical production is stimulated by inhibition of the electron transport chain and, thus, is a self-perpetuating process. Inhibition of the electron transport chain may stimulate oxygen radical generation by increasing the electronegativity of the early stages of OXPHOS.[19] Subsequent oxidative degradation of mitochondrial lipids, proteins, and mtDNAs would impair OXPHOS efficiency and stimulate more free radical accumulation. Single-electron transfer reactions produce a variety of free radicals that are cytotoxic, including the superoxide radical, the hydroxyl radical, lipid radicals, and possibly even reactive polypeptide compounds.[20] Once formed, the destructive potential of the mitochondrial oxygen radicals may be propagated by the autocatalytic formation of lipid radicals.[21-23] The polyenoic fatty acyl chains, such as phosphatidylcholine and phosphatidylethanolamine, which compose about 80 percent of the mitochondrial membrane phospholipids, are highly susceptible to oxygen radical modification.[24,25]

The third assumption is that the accumulation of mtDNA damage blocks mitochondrial biogenesis, resulting in permanent organelle dysfunction and, ultimately, in cell death. Damage to the mtDNA can be caused by oxygen radicals. The mtDNA is susceptible to oxygen radical damage because of its proximity to the site of oxygen radical production (OXPHOS), a lack of protective histones, and minimal mtDNA repair mechanisms. Oxygen radicals react with DNA at the sugar-phosphate backbone, producing a break in the DNA or at a single nucleotide, which results in an alteration in DNA coding.[18,26-28] Free radical-mediated DNA damage can be assessed by measuring levels of a guanine oxidation product called 8-hydroxydeoxyguanosine. This altered nucleotide can cause base substitutions by pairing with adenine rather than cytosine, thus causing G:C to T:A transversion mutations.[29] Consistent with these concepts, human mtDNA accumulates 16 times more oxidized bases than the nuclear DNA,[18,28,30] shows an age-related increase in 8-hydroxydeoxyguanosine in diaphragm[31] and brain,[32] and is more susceptible to alkylating agents and polycyclic aromatic hydrocarbons than nuclear DNA.[33,34] Pathogenic mtDNA point mutations also increase with age. The MTTL1*MELAS3243G mutation was identified in brain, extraocular muscle, skeletal

muscle, and heart,[35,36] and the MTTK*MERRF8344G mutation increased with age in extraocular muscle and skeletal muscle of aging subjects.[37] In addition to single-nucleotide changes, pathogenic mtDNA rearrangements in which essential mtDNA genes are deleted increase with age in brain,[38-40] heart,[41-47] skeletal muscle,[48] liver,[49,50] kidney,[50] and various other tissues.[50] MtDNA deletions impair OXPHOS by removing large segments of mtDNA that code for OXPHOS polypeptides and mitochondrial tRNAs.[9] The smaller size of the deleted mtDNAs may impart a replicative advantage over the larger, normal mtDNAs, thus favoring their accumulation within the cell. Alternatively, the local reduction in OXPHOS production of ATP resulting from the deleted molecules may signal the nucleus to stimulate mtDNA replication, thus expanding populations of mutant mtDNAs.

Consistent with the age-related increases in damaged mtDNA, OXPHOS function declines, and morphological alterations in mitochondria occur with advancing age. Measurements of the maximal oxygen uptake during exercise demonstrated that the oxidative work capacity for individuals declined by about 1 percent per year.[33] When various biochemical approaches were used to assess OXPHOS function in human skeletal muscle,[51,52] cardiac muscle,[53] liver,[49] and lymphocyte mitochondria,[54-56] a significant decline in respiratory function was observed. Histochemical techniques demonstrated that complex IV-deficient muscle fibers accumulated in essentially all muscle groups with advancing age and reached their highest number in levator palpebrae and extraocular eye muscles.[57-59] Immunohistochemical analysis of eye muscles, using subunit-specific antisera raised against human heart complex IV, demonstrated complete loss of the mtDNA-encoded subunits and variable reductions in the nuclear-encoded subunits.[59] Mitochondria of old organisms and cultured cells show decreased numbers, increased size, and various morphological abnormalities.[60] For example, one study found that exercise training in young men increased the total mitochondrial volume by 100 percent by increasing the mitochondrial number. In contrast, aged men show about a 20 percent increase in total mitochondrial volume by increasing the size of existing mitochondria.[61] One possible interpretation of this data is that aging may be associated with a diminished capacity to replace damaged mitochondria, thus allowing somatic mtDNA mutations to be maintained within certain cell types.

Somatic mtDNA Mutations in the Central Nervous System

Somatic mtDNA mutations appear to be distributed randomly throughout the mtDNA, thus resulting in a heterogenous mixture of mutations that include mtDNA rearrangements, mtDNA point mutations, and oxidized mtDNA nucleotides. Although this heterogeneity complicates the accurate measurement of the total quantity of damaged mtDNAs within a tissue, important insights into age-related accumulations of damaged mtDNAs emerged when mtDNA rearrangements were used as a marker for the extent of cellular mtDNA damage. Because over 100 different breakpoints for mtDNA deletions are known,[62] the markers used for mtDNA damage assessment represent only a small fraction of the total mtDNA damage. Although essentially any mtDNA rearrangement can be used to assess the extent of age-related damage to the mtDNA, a commonly used marker for mtDNA damage is a 4977 nucleotide pair deletion that extends from the ND5 gene to ATPase 8 gene (mtDNA[4977] deletion), removing genes that encode polypeptide subunits for complexes I, IV, and V, as well as for numerous tRNAs.[42]

Recent experiments with neuropathologically normal brain indicated that the susceptibility of the central nervous system to somatic mtDNA mutations is high and that a preferential accumulation of these mutations occurs with age in specific brain regions. Of the various brain regions examined, somatic mtDNA deletion accumulation was highest in the substantia nigra, caudate, and putamen of the basal ganglia.[39,40] When the mtDNA[4977] deletion was used as a marker for age-related mtDNA damage, this single mtDNA rearrangement accounted for approximately 10 percent of the the total mtDNA in the putamen of individuals over 75 years of age.[39] In this study, lower levels of the mtDNA[4977] deletion were observed and ranged from approximately 2 to 4 percent of the total mtDNA in different cortical regions, the globus pallidus, and the hippocampus. The lowest levels of the mtDNA[4977] deletion were observed in the cerebellum and myelinated axons. These regions had essentially no detectable accumulations of the mtDNA[4977] deletion with age. Although the basis for this regional variability in somatic mtDNA mutations within the brain is unknown, differences in regional metabolic rates among basal ganglia, cortical, and cerebellar structures,[63] as well as regional differences in free radical generation, may contribute to the variability in neuronal susceptibility to somatic mtDNA mutations. For example, dopaminergic neurons generate H_2O_2 in conjunction with oxidative deamination of dopamine by monoamine oxidase B (MAO-B) at the outer mitochondrial membrane and by the autooxidation of dopamine during the formation of neuromelanin. Dopaminergic neurons which arise from the pars compacta of the substantia nigra innervate the corpus striatum (caudate and putamen) and send projections to the cerebral cortex.[64] In contrast, the cerebellum is devoid of dopaminergic innervation. Free radical production could also be enhanced by the interaction between neuromelanin, a dopamine and lipofuscin polymer, and iron, which is present at higher levels in substantia nigra and corpus striatum than in cerebral cortex or cerebellum. Hence, mtDNA mutations might accumulate in dopaminergic neurons because of their high endogenous generation of oxygen radicals.

The unique susceptibility of specific brain regions to mtDNA damage is further emphasized by quantitating the percentage of mtDNA[4977] deletions in other highly oxidative tissues, such as cardiac muscle. The mtDNA[4977] deletion is essentially absent in normal hearts from individuals less than 40 years of age.[41,42,45] However, hearts from individuals over 40 years of age show an age-related increase in the mtDNA[4977] deletion, ranging from 0.00022 to 0.007 percent.[41,42] The levels of mtDNA damage observed in the cortex and putamen from individuals of advanced age[39] were much higher than the levels found in hearts. The maximum heart mtDNA[4977] deletion level was 0.007 percent, which was comparable to that of aged cerebellum but was 220-fold less than the deletion levels of aged cortex and 1667-fold less than the deletion levels of aged putamen.

Inherited and Somatic Mutations: Possible Interactions in Neurodegenerative Diseases

When organs are rank ordered according to oxygen consumption per gram of tissue, the heart has the highest rate of consumption, followed by kidney, brain, liver, and skeletal muscle.[65] However, OXPHOS diseases generally produce central nervous system dysfunction, myopathies, and cardiomyopathies early during the course of the disease. In contrast, liver and kidney generally have minor clinical manifestations. Hence, the differential sensitivity of these organs to OXPHOS dysfunction appears to be from the interaction of complex variables that include the pathogenicity of the mtDNA mutation (i.e., the severity of the mutation's effect on OXPHOS function), replicative segregation of mutant and normal mtDNAs, the different energetic requirements of human organs and tissues, the different abilities of human organs and tissues to compensate for cellular injury, interactions with nuclear genes, interactions with environmental factors, and the accumulation of somatic mtDNA mutations. When the inherited mtDNA mutation has a highly pathogenic effect, ATP generation rapidly falls early in life below critical energetic thresholds, resulting in pediatric diseases. When the effect of the mtDNA mutation on OXPHOS function is milder, individuals may not exhibit clinical symptoms until later in life, thus permitting additional factors such as environmental toxins or possibly even the accumulation of somatic mtDNA mutations to hasten the appearance of disease manifestations.

Evidence is accumulating that brains of patients with various types of neurodegenerative diseases such as Huntington's disease[66] and Alzheimer's disease (AD)[67] can harbor increased levels of somatic mtDNA mutations, relative to those of age-matched controls. Huntington's disease is a neurodegenerative disease that is characterized by dementia and choreoathetoid movements, inherited in an autosomal-dominant fashion with complete penetrance, and is caused by the expansion of a trinucleotide $(CAG)_n$ repeat within the coding region of the Huntington gene on chromosome 4.[68] Oxidative phosphorylation dysfunction in patients with Huntington's disease has been implicated by metabolic and biochemical studies of patient brains and may contribute to the degenerative process. Cerebral cortex and basal ganglia structures showed significant increases in lactate, as detected by $_1$H-NMR measurements.[69] Defects in oxidative phosphorylation were observed in brains[70,71] and platelets[72] from patients with Huntington's disease. One possible mechanism for these OXPHOS abnormalities is a gradual decline in cellular energetics because of the accumulation of somatic mtDNA mutations. In support of this hypothesis, the mtDNA[4977] mutation was 11-fold higher in temporal cortex and 5-fold higher in frontal cortex in the brains of 22 patients with Huntington's disease than in age-matched control brains.[66]

Alzheimer's disease (AD) is characterized by a dementia that usually begins after 60 years of age. The major neuropathological features include senile plaques, neurofibrillary tangles within neuronal perikarya, and amyloid angiopathy. Several neurotransmitter systems are perturbed in AD, with cholinergic deficiency being most prominent and associated with neuron loss in the nucleus basalis of Meynert.[73] Evidence for OXPHOS dysfunction in AD has been controversial, and data interpretation is complex. Complex IV (cytochrome c oxidase) abnormalities were identified in platelets[74] in one study but not in a second study in which platelet OXPHOS measurements in patients with AD were compared to measurements in patients with multi-infarct dementia and in age-matched controls.[75] Regional abnormalities in brain OXPHOS enzymology were identified by two groups,[76,77] but an analysis of complex IV (cytochrome c oxidase) activity by a third group was normal in temporal cortex.[78] The identification of an OXPHOS defect in tissue homogenates is dependent on how widely the abnormality is expressed in the tissue that is being analyzed. Hence, abnormalities that are confined to discrete populations of neurons can be missed. This explanation for the variation observed in the brain OXPHOS measurements is supported by experiments using the complex IV histochemical reaction or in situ hybridization of complex IV mRNA to assess OXPHOS in tissue sections from AD brain. An abnormal complex IV histochemical reaction was observed in the dentate gyrus and hippocampus in brain sections from patients with AD but not in occipital cortex from patients or controls.[79] In a separate study, a reduction in the mRNA for the mtDNA-encoded subunit II of complex IV was also observed in the dentate gyrus and hippocampus of AD brain.[80]

Although the precise cause of the biochemical defects observed in AD is unclear, inherited and somatic mtDNA mutations may be an important part of the neurodegenerative process. Maternally inherited mutations in the mtDNA were identified in patients with AD that may increase an individual's susceptibility to developing this disease[8] (see Parkinson's Disease section for a discussion of these mtDNA mutations). In addition, the mtDNA[4977] deletion was also observed to accumulate in the brains of patients with AD.[67,81] Corral-Debrinski et al.[67] identified a 15-fold increase in the mtDNA[4977] deletion level in the frontal cortex of AD patients who were below 75 years of age, relative to that of age-matched controls. In individuals who were above 75 years of age, the mtDNA[4977] deletion level in frontal cortex was four-fold lower than that of age-matched controls. Because control brains from individuals who are above 75 years of age showed a dramatic increase in the mtDNA[4977] deletion level, the reason for this age-related difference in the AD brains was unclear. The apolipoprotein E4 allele on chromosome 19, which is associated with an increased risk of developing AD, was similar in the two age groups (29 percent in the <75 year old group and 33 percent in the >75 year old group). Hence, more extensive neuronal loss in individuals who are >75 years of age is a possible explanation for these results. The assessment of OXPHOS by histochemical investigations of complex IV or in situ molecular genetic approaches may provide more insight into this phenomenon and its relationship to the pathogenesis of AD.

MYOCLONIC EPILEPSY AND RAGGED-RED FIBER DISEASE (MERRF)

MERRF is a chronic neurodegenerative disease that can begin at any age, ranging from late childhood to adulthood. The clinical features that are most predictive for a diagnosis of MERRF are epilepsy (myoclonic epilepsy, generalized seizures, or focal seizures), cerebellar ataxia, and a RRF myopathy. The probability that a patient has MERRF is further increased when multifocal neurological manifestations such as dementia, corticospinal tract degeneration, peripheral neuropathy, optic atrophy, and deafness are identified in conjunction with multisystem involvement that includes myopathy, proximal renal tubule dysfunction, cardiomyopathy, and lactate, pyruvate, and alanine elevations in blood, urine, and CSF. The myoclonus in MERRF patients is best categorized as cortical reflex myoclonus and can be associated with epileptiform discharges and photic sensitivity with large-amplitude occipital wave forms on electroencephalogram, as well as giant cortical somatosensory evoked responses.[82-84] Fig. 4-3 demonstrates the features of the myoclonus and ataxia detected by accelerometers placed on the arm of a MERRF patient. Myoclonic jerks occur at rest (Fig. 4-3, Panel A) and increase in frequency and amplitude with movement. Although the cerebellar ataxia can be difficult to appreciate during a routine neurological examination in patients with severe myoclonus, accelerometer recordings (Fig. 4-3, Panel B) give a clear representation of the cerebellar ataxia. While at rest the patient has no detectable tremor, but with movement a low-frequency action tremor appears. Patients with MERRF often demonstrate characteristic accumulations of lipomas in the anterior and posterior cervical region[85-87] (Fig. 4-4). Neuropathological analyses of the brains from patients with MERRF revealed multifocal degeneration involving the dentatorubral and pallidoluysian systems, substantia nigra, cerebellar cortex, inferior olivary nucleus, locus ceruleus, gracile and cuneate nuclei, and the pontine tegmentum.[88-92] The pathology in the spinal cord resembled that found in Friedriech's ataxia.[88,92]

The majority of MERRF cases are caused by an A-to-G mutation that alters a conserved nucleotide in the TΨC loop of the tRNA[Lysine] at position 8344 of the mtDNA (MTTK*MERRF8344G).[93] This mutation was the first mitochondrial tRNA mutation discovered, as well as the first gene mutation discovered to cause a type of epilepsy. When greater than 90 percent mutant mtDNAs are present in multiple-organ systems, the risk for developing MERRF is high.[83,93] A small percentage of MERRF patients harbor a T-to-C mutation at position 8356 of the mtDNA (MTTK*MERRF8356C).[94,95] The MTTK*MERRF8356C mutation alters a moderately conserved nucleotide that is predicted to disrupt base pairing in the stem of the TΨC loop. Both the dihydrouridine loop and the TΨC loop appear to be involved in interactions with the ribosome.[96] OXPHOS enzymological analysis of individuals from the same pedigree revealed that complex I- and complex IV-specific activities were severely reduced.[83] This is consistent with the protein synthesis defects observed in MERRF patient cells, since complexes I and IV have the greatest number of mtDNA encoded subunits and thus would be most sensitive to a protein synthesis defect.[97-99]

The inhibitory effect of the MTTK*MERRF8344G mutation on mitochondrial protein synthesis has been confirmed in cybrid cell lines.[98] Cybrid cell lines are made by separating the cytoplasm from the nucleus of donor cell line and fusing the cytoplasm with a specially constructed recipient cell line

A. Right arm at rest

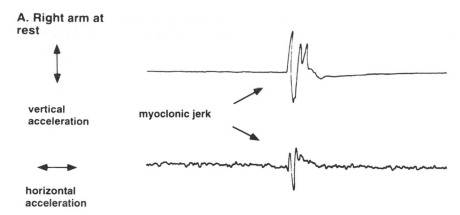

vertical acceleration

myoclonic jerk

horizontal acceleration

B. Outstretched right arm

cerebellar ataxia

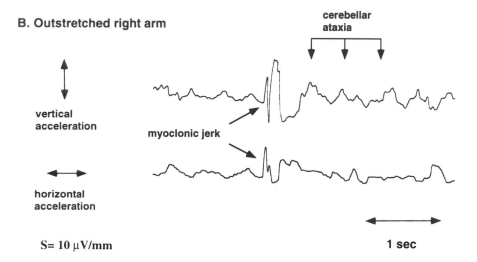

vertical acceleration

myoclonic jerk

horizontal acceleration

S= 10 μV/mm

1 sec

FIGURE 4-3 Myoclonus and ataxia, as detected by hand accelerometers in a patient with MERRF. Horizontal and vertical movements were detected by accelerometers placed on the hand of a patient with MERRF and the MTTK*MERRF8344G mutation. Accelerometer measurements were performed by Dr. Alan Freeman, Dr. Jorge Juncos, and Dr. Ray Watts in the Movement Disorders Clinic, Emory University Department of Neurology. *(From Shoffner et al.[108] Used with permission.)*

that lacks mtDNA referred to as ρ^0 cells. This approach is important for establishing the pathogenicity of a mtDNA mutation. If the OXPHOS defect is transferred from the donor cell line to the recipient cell line (ρ^0 cells) along with the mtDNA, then the mutation is coded in the mtDNA. If it is not, the mutation is presumed to be nuclear.[100–102] This approach is described in greater detail in the Fig. 4-5 legend. This experiment was important in proving that the MTTK*MERRF8344G mutation is solely responsible for the mitochondrial translation defect.[98]

Heteroplasmic myotubes with varying percentages of the MTTK*MERRF8344G mutation demonstrated a sharp decline in mitochondrial protein synthesis levels when the intracellular percentage of mutant mtDNAs exceeded 85 percent.[97] At this point, the translation efficiency of COI, an mtDNA-encoded polypeptide of cytochrome c oxidaze (complex IV), and the cytochrome c oxidase enzyme activity dramatically declined, indicating that the MTTK*MERRF8334G mutation is functionally recessive. When the mutant mtDNAs exceeded 85 percent, severe clinical manifestations developed with only small decreases in the percentage of normal mtDNAs.[93] This implied that patients born with high percentages of mutant mtDNAs would be acutely sensitive to further inhibition of OXPHOS function. It is possible that the relatively small reductions in OXPHOS function[49,51,57–59] associated with the age-related accumulation of somatic mtDNA mutations[41–43,45] could accelerate the appearance of or worsen disease manifestations.

FIGURE 4-4 Cervical lipomas are often identified in patients with myoclonic epilepsy and RRF disease (MERRF). A patient with the MTTK*MERRF8344G mutation and a prominent cervical lipoma is shown here (arrow).

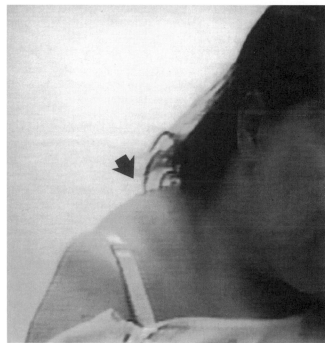

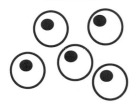

**ρ° Cell Line
HPRT Deficient**

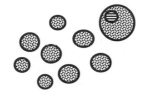

**Enriched cytoplasmic fragments
purified from patient lymphoblasts.**

Although the cell line has mitochondria,
no mtDNAs are present. Due to the absence
of a functional OXPHOS, cell growth is
dependent on uridine.

These fragments contain mitochondria
with a pathogenic mtDNA mutation. Intact
lymphoblasts contaminate the mixture.

Electrofusion is used to fuse the ρ° cells with
the cytoplasmic fragments from the patient.
Based on the resistance of the cybrids to
6-thioguanine and the ability of the cybrids
to grow in the absence of uridine, the cybrid
cell line is selectively grown from the mixture.

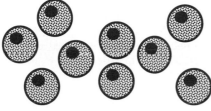

Cybrid cell line with ρ° cell line nuclear DNA (HPRT deficient) and
mitochondria containing mutant mtDNAs from the patient's lymphoblast
cell line.

= nuclear DNA that has normal HPRT activity and is sensitive to the
effects of 6-thioguanine

= nuclear DNA that has no HPRT activity and is resistant to the
effects of 6-thioguanine

FIGURE 4-5 Construction of cybrid cell lines for assessing the
pathogenicity of a mtDNA mutation. In order to investigate
whether an OXPHOS defect or a specific mtDNA point
mutation segregates with a patients's mtDNA, rather than the
nuclear DNA, cultured cells from a patient who harbors a
candidate mtDNA mutation are enucleated, and the cytoplasmic
fragments containing the patient's mitochondria and mtDNAs
are fused to a recipient ρ° cell line. This procedure is complex
in that the technique used for separating the nucleus and
cytoplasm yields a complex mixture that is enriched for these
cellular components but also contains whole cells. Hence, when
fusions between donor and recipient cell lines are performed,
the final mixture contains the newly formed cybrids plus
unfused nuclei and cytoplasmic fragments, patient donor cells,
and intact recipient (ρ°) cells. Selection of the cybrids takes
advantage of several unique properties of these cell lines. The
ρ° cells are formed by depleting the mtDNA by means of long-
term culture in ethidium bromide.[205] Once the mtDNAs are
depleted, the ρ° cells become dependent on uridine for survival,
because their OXPHOS deficiency inhibits the dihydrouridine
dehydrogenase activity necessary for de novo uridine
monophosphate synthesis.[206,207] Although the patient mtDNA
may harbor a mutation that impairs OXPHOS, acquisition of
patient mtDNAs that result in even mild increases in ATP
production relieves the pyrimidine auxotrophy and permits the
cytoplasmic hybrids (cybrids) to grow in media lacking uridine,
thus permitting selective growth of the cybrids over any
recipient ρ° cells. In order to separate the cybrids from intact
patient donor cells, the culture conditions are manipulated to
take advantage of the fact that the nuclear DNA of the cybrid is
derived from the ρ° cells, which is a cell line (WAL-2A) that is
deficient in hypoxanthine-guanine phophoribosyltransferase
(HPRT), thus making these cells resistant to the effects of 6-
thioguanine. 6-Thioguanine is a purine analogue that is toxic to
cells once a phophoribosyl moiety is transferred to the base by

Some patients with MERRF are easily recognized, and
genetic testing for the MTTK*MERRF8344G or the
MTTK*MERRF8356C mutations in leukocyte, platelet, or
muscle mtDNA will establish the diagnosis, whereas patients
with less severe disease manifestations may require more
extensive investigations to assess whether an OXPHOS disease is present. Replicative segregation of mutant and normal
mtDNAs between tissues can result in highly variable percentages of the MTTK*MERRF8344G mutation among an
individual's organs. Skeletal muscle frequently has high percentages of the MTTK*MERRF8344G mutation in severely
affected individuals ranging from 80 to almost 100 percent.[93,97,103] Less severely affected family members harbor
lower percentages of the MTTK*MERRF8344G mutation.[93,103]
Relative to skeletal muscle, fibroblasts and lymphocytes have
lower levels of the MTTK*MERRF8344G mutation.[103] Hence,
genetic testing for this mutation can facilitate the patient
diagnosis, but accurate prognosis in a single patient is difficult.

When patients have less severe clinical manifestations and
the diagnosis of MERRF is not apparent, a variety of approaches that assess OXPHOS can be helpful. Abnormalities
in CNS energy metabolism of MERRF patients can be detected by imaging techniques such as positron emission tomography (PET) and ^{31}P NMR analyses of brain,[86,104] as well
as ^{31}P NMR analysis of skeletal muscle.[83] Quantitative organic
acid and amino acid analyses can show elevations in lactate,
pyruvate, and alanine. Defects in the highly energy dependent proximal renal tubules manifest as generalized amino-
acidurias and can be an important clue to the presence of
an OXPHOS disease.[105] Normal results of 31P NMR investigations or metabolic testing do not exclude the possibility that a
patient has MERRF. Abnormalities observed in type I muscle
fibers include RRFs with Gomori-trichrome staining, reduced
activity with cytochrome c oxidase staining, and increased
activity with succinate dehydrogenase staining. Small blood
vessels within the skeletal muscle can show evidence of a
mild vasculopathy with increased complex II (succinate dehydrogenase) activity, a reduced complex IV (cytochrome c
oxidase) activity, and abnormal mitochondrial ultrastructure
within the vascular smooth muscle cells.[106] Although myopathic changes are frequently observed in muscle biopsies
from patients with MERRF, neuropathic changes are uncommon. Ultrastructural examination of muscle often demonstrates structurally abnormal mitochondria with paracrystalline inclusions, which are condensations of mitochondrial
creatine kinase that are located in the space between the
inner and outer mitochondrial membrane.[107] Biochemical investigations of OXPHOS function can also be either normal
or abnormal, depending on the extent of skeletal muscle
involvement. The most common abnormality that is observed
in mitochondria isolated from the skeletal muscle biopsy
before freezing is a combined defect in complexes I and
IV.[10,108,109] This is a frequently observed biochemical abnormal-

HPRT. Hence, the addition of 6-thioguanine to the culture
media is toxic to intact donor cells that have HPRT activity but
not to the HPRT-deficient ρ° cells. By taking advantage of these
properties, a cybrid cell line can be selectively cultured for
additional analyses.

ity in patients with OXPHOS diseases that is caused by defects in mitochondrial protein synthesis.

LEBER'S HEREDITARY OPTIC NEUROPATHY (LHON) AND DYSTONIA

Adult and pediatric onset dystonias represent a complex group of disorders in which patients experience involuntary sustained muscle contractions in a focal, segmental, or generalized distribution. Although basal ganglia dysfunction is the most likely cause of these muscle spasms, precise neuroanatomic or biochemical localization of the defect has not been possible.[110] Pathological analyses of brains from patients with idiopathic dystonias are generally normal.[111] Although the clinical features are highly variable, the most severe variant of the disease, generalized dystonia, generally has its onset in childhood, whereas the less severe focal and segmental dystonias generally become symptomatic during adult life. The inheritance of idiopathic dystonia is complex. Cases can be sporadic within a family, show autosomal-dominant inheritance,[110,112-117] or display maternal inheritance of a mtDNA mutation.[5,6,118-125]

Recent biochemical and mtDNA studies provided evidence that OXPHOS defects are an important cause for dystonias. Biochemical evidence for an impairment of OXPHOS was first demonstrated in platelets from a cohort of patients with focal, segmental, and generalized dystonias.[126] Complex I specific activity as determined by the nicotinamide adenine dinucleotide (NADH)-ubiquinone assay was significantly reduced in all patients with dystonia relative to controls. Moreover, the patients with segmental or generalized dystonias had greater reductions in this enzyme activity relative to controls than did patients with focal dystonias. The biochemical assessment of OXPHOS in other tissues, such as skeletal muscle and mtDNA sequencing, will be important in exploring this association further.

The first genetic mutation found to cause a maternally inherited form of dystonia was a G-to-A transition in the ND6 gene at position 14459 of the mtDNA (MTND6*LDYT14459A).[5,6] This mutation can be either heteroplasmic or homoplasmic in patients and has been recognized in three unrelated families. The MTND6*LDYT14459A mutation was first identified in a large Hispanic family in which individuals manifested a pattern of vision loss consistent with LHON or a generalized dystonia with basal ganglia degeneration that was referred to as bilateral striatal necrosis.[125] The vision loss presented with acute or subacute, painless loss of central visual acuity in both eyes. Additional disease manifestations included early-onset dementia with asymmetric dystonia, bulbar dysfunction, corticospinal tract abnormalities, and short stature. The onset of the striatal necrosis was between 1.5 and 9 years of age. Significant variability in the severity of disease penetrance among family members occurred with the mildest clinical cases presenting as adolescent onset LHON and the most severe clinical cases presenting with infantile bilateral striatal necrosis. In an African-American family, a 42-year-old mother and her 19-year-old daughter experienced a subacute vision loss.[5] The ophthalmological evaluation was consistent with LHON from the presence of bilateral central scotomas, nerve fiber layer degeneration, optic atrophy, and the transient appearance of peripapillary telangiectasias. Fig. 4-6 illustrates the nerve fiber layer degeneration observed in these individuals. Although the daughter had a normal neurological examination except for the vision loss, her head magnetic resonance imaging (MRI) demonstrated a unilateral lesion in the right putamen and bilateral lesions in the caudate nucleus, features that are not generally seen in most patients with LHON (Fig. 4-7). No other individuals in the family were known to be affected. In the Caucasian family, a single individual was affected with a generalized dystonia and basal ganglia degeneration. Her symptoms began at about 3 years of age with a mild right hemidystonia, which progressed gradually to a generalized dystonia. As in the other two families with the MTND6*LDYT14459A mutation, bilateral basal ganglia lesions were evident on head MRI and CT. These three families had distinct mtDNA haplotypes, indicating that the MTND6*LDYT14459A mutation occurred independently in Hispanic, Caucasian, and African-American mtDNA lineages.

Histochemistry and electron microscopy of skeletal muscle and quantitative organic acid and amino acid analyses in blood and urine were essentially normal. Measurement of skeletal muscle OXPHOS activity in the 19-year-old daughter from the African-American family revealed a prominent abnormality in the specific activity of complex I.[5] To investigate whether the impaired complex I activity was specific to this mutation, the complex I activity was determined in lymphoblast mitochondria from patients and controls and in cybrid cell lines. Analysis of OXPHOS in Epstein-Barr virus-transformed lymphoblasts confirmed the complex I defect noted in patient skeletal muscle.[127] In addition, this complex I defect

FIGURE 4-6 Fundus photograph of the left eye of a 42-year-old mother with LHON who harbors the MTND6*LDYT14459A mutation and is from an African-American family. The fundus had similar appearances in both eyes. Abnormal disk pallor is associated with absence of nerve fiber layer striations temporal to the disk. The nerve fiber layer striations that are visible above and below each disk appear coarsened and whitish. Note the abrupt transition between atrophic sectors and zones of nerve fiber preservation (arrow). Dr. Stephen Pollok, Department of Ophthalmology, Duke University performed the ophthalmological examination and also provided the fundus photograph.

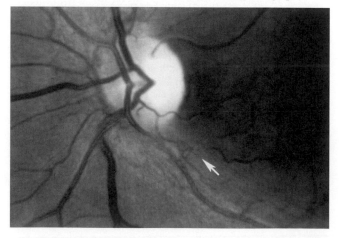

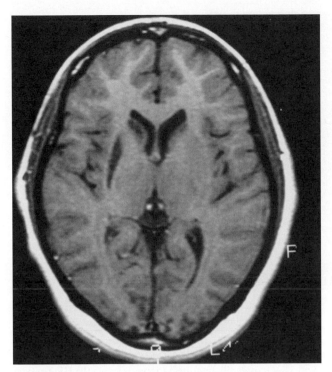

FIGURE 4-7 T_1-weighted MR image from a 19-year-old female with LHON who harbors the MTND6*LDYT14459A mutation and is from an African-American family. Lesions are present in the right putamen and bilaterally in the caudate nuclei.

transferred to a recipient ρ^0 cell line along with the MTND6*LDYT14459A mutation, thus confirming that the MTND6*LDYT14459A mutation is the cause for this unique form of LHON and dystonia.

Dystonia with basal ganglia lesions and complex neurodegeneration has also been observed in conjunction with another mtDNA mutation that causes LHON. LHON was the first human disease to be associated with a mtDNA point mutation.[2] The most common cause for LHON is an A-to-G mutation in the ND4 subunit gene of complex I at position 11,778 of the mtDNA (MTND4*LHON11778G).[2] This mutation accounts for approximately 50 to 70 percent of cases in Europe and over 90 percent of the cases in Japan.[128] Although most individuals with the MTND4*LHON11778G mutation generally have an uncomplicated optic atrophy, atypical presentations do occur. A Swedish LHON family that was homoplasmic for the MTND4*LHON11778G mutation had complex neurological manifestations in addition to the classic ophthalmological findings.[129] These included bilateral lesions in the putamen on MRI, tremor, ataxia, posterior column dysfunction, dystonia, corticospinal tract dysfunction, and extrapyramidal rigidity. Muscle biopsy revealed a subsarcolemmal increase in mitochondria, as well as a few fibers with paracrystalline inclusions. To determine whether this unique phenotype is a part of the spectrum of MTND4*LHON11778G expression or whether the pathogenicity of this mutation was augmented by other mtDNA mutations within this patient's mtDNA, it will be necessary to sequence the patient's mtDNA to exclude the possibility that this family harbors additional deleterious mtDNA muta-

tions. To date, the mtDNA sequence for this family has not been reported.

The biochemical results obtained in platelets,[126] skeletal muscle,[5] and lymphoblast cell lines[127] and the confirmed pathogenicity of the MTND6*LDYT14459A mutation in the ND6 gene[5,6,127] suggest that complex I defects are important considerations in patients with dystonia. Interestingly, the basal ganglia structures, as well as the lateral geniculate body, appear particularly susceptible to missense mutations involving complex I genes. Further biochemical and genetic investigations of OXPHOS will be important in defining the contribution of mtDNA mutations to the dystonias.

LEIGH'S DISEASE (SUBACUTE NECROTIZING ENCEPHALOPATHY)

Leigh's disease or subacute necrotizing encephalopathy is a severe neurodegenerative disorder in which OXPHOS defects are an important cause of the prominent neuropathological changes observed in basal ganglia structures. This disease is suspected when cranial nerve abnormalities, respiratory dysfunction, ataxia, dystonias, and developmental abnormalities are observed in conjunction with bilateral, symmetrical, hyperintense signals on T_2-weighted MRI images in the basal ganglia, cerebellum, or brain stem (Fig. 4-8). The age of onset for disease manifestations is usually during infancy or early childhood. Less commonly, disease manifestations begin in adolescence or adulthood. The neuropathological changes in Leigh's disease are characterized by demyelination, gliosis, areas of necrosis, and capillary proliferation that is most severe in basal ganglia structures, the cerebellum, and the brain stem (Fig. 4-9).

OXPHOS defects may be the most commonly encountered abnormalities in patients with Leigh's disease. Most patients with Leigh's disease and OXPHOS defects can be classified into one of the following categories: a maternally inherited complex V defect, a maternally inherited mitochondrial protein synthesis defect, or an autosomal-recessive complex IV defect. The complex V defects associated with Leigh's disease can be caused by either a heteroplasmic T-to-G mutation in the ATPase 6 gene at position 8993 of the mtDNA (MTATP6*NARP8993G)[3,4] or a heteroplasmic T-to-C mutation at the same nucleotide position (MTATP6*NARP8993C).[130] The MTATP6*NARP8993G mutation changes an evolutionarily conserved leucine at amino acid position 156 of the ATPase 6 polypeptide to an arginine. This amino acid change is highly significant in that a neutral or uncharged amino acid (leucine) is replaced by a basic or charged amino acid (arginine) within the proton channel of complex V. This amino acid alteration impairs proton translocation, thus reducing the rate of ATP synthesis.[131,132] The MTATP6*NARP8993G mutation is the most frequently encountered of the two mutations and was originally identified in patients with cerebellar ataxia plus pigmentary retinopathy syndromes.[133] Individuals with Leigh's disease who harbor this mutation are normal at birth and frequently develop disease manifestation during the first year of life. In 50 patients with Leigh's disease in whom PDH complex defects were excluded, 20 percent of the patients harbored the MTATP6*NARP8993G mutation.[134] In patients with clinical presentations that are consistent with

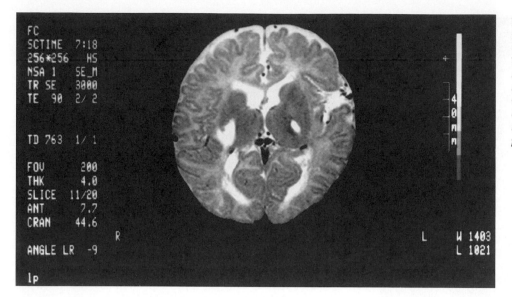

FIGURE 4-8 T₂-weighted brain MR image of a patient with Leigh's disease. Bilateral lesions of the basal ganglia, thalamus, and associated structures are evident and are characteristic MRI findings that are important in the clinical diagnosis of this disorder. *(From Shoffner et al.[10] Used with permission.)*

Leigh's disease who were evaluated in our clinic and diagnostic laboratory, approximately 7 percent of the cases harbored a mutation at position 8993 of the mtDNA.

As with mitochondrial tRNA mutations (i.e., MTTK*MERRF8344G and MTTL1*MELAS3243G mutations), the MTATP6*NARP8993G mutation acts in a recessive manner. Patients generally are asymptomatic when the levels of the MTATP6*NARP8993G mutation in organs is less than approximately 60 to 70 percent of the total mtDNA. Patients that harbor between approximately 70 and 90 percent mutant mtDNAs in their organs have highly variable disease manifestations. The most severe phenotype, Leigh's disease, occurs when systemic levels of the MTATP6*NARP8993G mutation exceed 90 percent of the total mtDNA.[3,4,131,134] In mildly affected individuals, a pigmentary retinopathy can be the only clinical manifestation. In more severely affected individuals, cerebellar ataxia and pigmentary retinopathy are commonly observed together. Brain imaging of these patients can show cerebellar atrophy or olivopontocerebellar atrophy (Fig. 4-10). Additional manifestations that can be observed are hypertrophic cardiomyopathy, sensory and motor neuropathies, muscle weakness, and elevated lactate or alanine levels in blood or urine. Hence, a careful family history is important in patients with cerebellar ataxia plus pigmentary retinal degeneration to differentiate those families with maternally inherited disorders from those families with autosomal-dominant, cerebellar ataxia variants.

Other causes for Leigh's disease include mitochondrial protein synthesis defects produced by mtDNA rearrangements, the MTTL1*MELAS3243G mutation, the MTTL1*MELAS3271C mutation, or the MTTK*MERRF8344G mutation. An autosomal-recessive mutation in a nuclear DNA-encoded subunit of complex IV was proposed as a cause for Leigh's disease; however, the precise nuclear DNA mutation was not identified.[135] Many Leigh's disease patients have OXPHOS defects but do not harbor one of the known mtDNA mutations and, in our experience, OXPHOS defects are much more common than pyruvate dehydrogenase complex abnormalities. Hence, these patients could harbor either

FIGURE 4-9 (A) Hematoxylin-eosin stain of medulla from patient III-4 shows bilateral necrotizing lesions. (B) High-power view (×250) of this section demonstrates capillary proliferation and gliosis. Adjacent sections were used for analysis of the MTATP6*NARP8993G mutation. *(From Shoffner et al.[4] Used with permission.)*

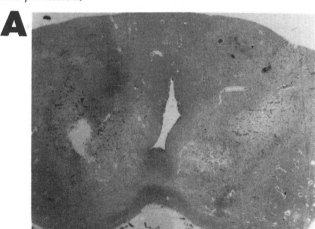

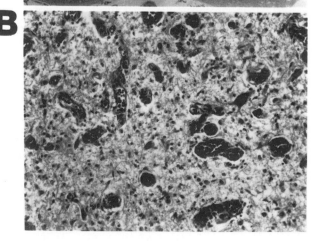

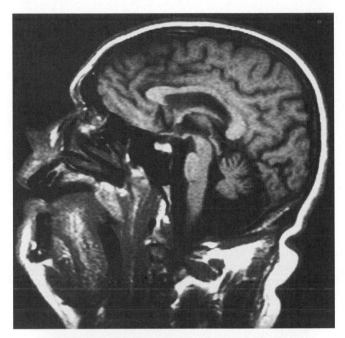

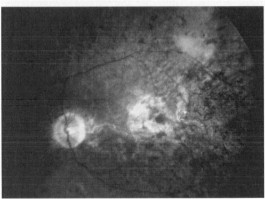

FIGURE 4-10 A head MR image from a patient who harbors the MTATP6*NARP8993G mutation demonstrates the features of olivopontocerebellar atrophy *(top).* This individual also had a severe pigmentary retinopathy with bone spicule formation *(bottom).* The neurological and ophthalmological examinations of this patient were performed by Dr. Nancy Newman, Department of Ophthalmology, Emory University. *(From Shoffner and Wallace.[10] Used with permission.)*

a nuclear DNA or mtDNA mutation, requiring careful evaluation of these patients before genetic counseling.

PARKINSON'S DISEASE

Parkinson's disease (PD) is characterized clinically by akinesia, tremor, rigidity, and gait disturbance and neuropathologically by Lewy body formation in the pigmented nuclei and nucleus basalis with the loss of dopaminergic neurons from the substantia nigra, from which neurons project into the striatum, particularly the dorsal putamen.[136,137] The clinical symptoms are responsive to dopamine supplementation. Patients with PD show substantial clinical, pathological, bio-

chemical, and genetic heterogeneity. An interesting area of clinical and neuropathological overlap occurs with individuals who have Alzheimer's disease (AD). Frequently, AD patients exhibit extrapyramidal signs of PD,[138] and 20 to 40 percent have coexisting neuropathological features of PD, including substantia nigra degeneration and Lewy body accumulation (AD + PD).[139,140] Cases displaying cortical Lewy bodies have been called "diffuse Lewy body disease"[141–143] and are increasingly recognized with and without concomitant AD pathology. Thus, the clinical and neuropathological features of AD and PD overlap extensively, suggesting that they may represent a spectrum of diseases with related causal mechanisms.

Recent toxicological, biochemical, and genetic investigations suggest that OXPHOS defects may play a role in the pathogenesis of AD and PD.[144] The neurotoxin 1-methyl-4-phenyl-1,2,3,6-tetrahydropyridine (MPTP) provided the first biochemical evidence that OXPHOS defects may be linked to PD. MAO B, which is localized in glia cells, converts MPTP to 1-methyl-4-phenylpyridinium (MPP+).[145] MPP+ is actively transported into dopaminergic neurons[146] and concentrated in the mitochondria,[147] where it inhibits complex I.[148,149] The impairment of ATP generation and the associated increase of free radical production may be important factors contributing to the death of the dopaminergic neurons in individuals exposed to this toxin. The neuroleptic medications represent additional classes of compounds that may exert a toxic effect on the basal ganglia by inhibiting complex I activity.[150] Haloperidol, chlorpromazine, thiothixene, and clozapine were observed to inhibit complex I activity in a dose-dependent manner in rat brain mitochondria. Patients treated with haloperidol, loxapine, fluphenazine, or thiothixene had reduced complex I activities in platelet mitochondria. These results suggest that complex I inhibition may be important in producing the extrapyramidal side effects associated with the use of neuroleptic medications.

Further evidence for a role of OXPHOS in PD was obtained by biochemical, immunohistochemical, immunoblot, and genetic approaches. When patients with idiopathic PD were tested for OXPHOS defects, abnormalities in complex I were detected in PD brains,[151–154] blood platelets,[151,155–160] and skeletal muscle.[144,151,161,162] For the OXPHOS analyses performed in platelet mitochondria, 24 percent (32/131) of the individuals tested were untreated PD patients.[151,155–160] However, extensive overlap in the enzyme levels of patients and controls exists in these data sets. When the 5 percent confidence level of the control OXPHOS activities is used as the lower limits of normal, only a subset of PD patients can be definitively identified as abnormal.[144,162] Despite this variance in the data, a subset of PD patients do appear to harbor OXPHOS defects. Hence, the occurrence of OXPHOS defects in various tissue types suggests that some PD patients harbor systemic OXPHOS defects. Although a reduction in complex I activity is the most frequently observed abnormality in PD patients, reductions in the specific activities of other OXPHOS complexes can also be present.[157,160,162,163] Patients in whom the complex I defects were localized to the substantia nigra had normal OXPHOS enzyme activities in cerebral cortex, cerebellum, caudate, globus pallidus, and tegmentum.[151,154] By contrast, patients with multiple-systems atrophy who had severe substantia nigra neuronal degeneration, received similar doses of L-dopa, and experienced similar agonal states before death were found to have normal OXPHOS activity in substantia nigra,[154] thus supporting the specificity of the finding in patients with PD. To date, an inhibitory effect of L-dopa on complex I activity has not been confirmed in human platelet mitochondria[155] or rat skeletal muscle.[164] However, the results of one study indicated that chronic L-dopa administration was associated with a reversible decrease in complex I activity in rat striatum and substantia nigra.[165] The results of immunohistochemical and immunoblot investigations of OXPHOS subunits in PD brain are complex. One group showed a reduction of complex I subunits by immunohistochemical methods,[166] whereas a second group observed no abnormalities in their PD patients.[154] Immunoblot analysis of complex I subunits isolated from PD patient striatum revealed decreased antibody cross-reactivity of complex I subunits,[152] but these changes did not correlate with OXPHOS activities in these regions, which showed only a decrease in complex III specific activity.[163] The complexities inherent in interpreting these techniques were recently reviewed.[167]

The OXPHOS defects identified in AD and PD patients suggested that inherited mutations in cytoplasmic or nuclear OXPHOS genes may be important in the pathogenesis of these diseases. Evaluating this possibility has been difficult because of the highly variable penetrance of late-onset AD and PD cases, the complexity of OXPHOS genetics, and potential interactions between genetics and environmental factors. To screen for candidate mtDNA mutations, the mtDNAs from 92 patients were surveyed with 14 restriction endonucleases to identify novel site variants. Four candidate mtDNA mutations were identified: an A-to-G mutation in the tRNA^{Glutamine} gene at position 4,336 of the mtDNA (MTTQ*ADPD4336G), an A-to-G mutation in the ND1 gene at position 3397 (MTND1*ADPD3397G), a nine-base pair insertion in the 12S rRNA gene at positions 956–965 (MT12S*ADPD956-965ins), and a G-to-A mutation in the 16S rRNA gene at position 3196 (MT16S*AD3196A).[8] All of these mutations were homoplasmic, except for the MT16S*AD3196A mutation, which was heteroplamic. Three candidate mutations, MTND1*ADPD3397G, MT12S*ADPD956-965ins, and MT16S*AD3196A mutations, were observed at low frequency in the patient groups, making an assessment of their significance difficult. The MTTQ*ADPD4336G mutation has the strongest correlation with AD, AD + PD, and PD. The frequencies of the MTTQ*ADPD4336G mutation have been updated since our original investigations,[8] with data obtained from brain samples from neuropathologically characterized patients with AD or AD + PD contributed by Dr. Flint Beal (Massachusettes General Hospital, Boston, MA) and leukocyte samples from clinically characterized patients with PD contributed by Dr. Stephen Fink and colleagues (The Movement Disorders Clinic, Massachusettes General Hospital, Boston, MA). This mutation was present in 1.9 percent (2/104) of brains with AD pathology, 6.2 percent (5/81) of brains with AD + PD pathology, and 2.6 percent (2/114) of clinically defined PD cases, giving an overall total of 3.3 percent (10/299). Hence, the overall frequency of the MTTQ*ADPD4336G site variant was present at a significantly higher frequency in the total

patient population than in the general caucasian population (0.7 percent; 12/1691). This mutation was not identified in other ethnic groups (0 percent; 0/1345) and appeared to characterize caucasian mtDNA lineages. We hypothesized that the presence of this site variant in the general caucasian population could simply reflect the prevalence of AD and PD, since 10 to 20 percent of the general population who live past 85 years of age develop AD or PD. With 1691 individuals from the caucasian population tested, approximately 169–338 would be at risk for these diseases. Of the individuals at risk for AD and PD, 3.3 percent or between 6 and 11 individuals would be predicted to harbor the MTTQ*ADPD4336 site variant, a range that approximates the observed 12 caucasians found with population screening. This site variant was also equally distributed among AD, AD + PD, and PD patients from various regions of the United States. Hence, it appeared unlikely that sampling bias caused the increased frequency in AD and PD patients. Dr. Gino Cortopassi's group at University of Southern California, Los Angeles analyzed 137 AD cases and 266 age-matched controls for the MTTQ*ADPD4336G mutation.[168] In the AD group, 6 percent of individuals had the MTTQ*ADPD4336G mutation, whereas only 0.3 percent of age-matched controls had this mutation. Hence, the frequency for the MTTQ*ADPD4336G mutation was significantly increased in patients relative to that of controls. This analysis indicated that the mean risk for individuals with this mutation for developing AD or AD + PD may be about 16-fold higher than that for individuals who do not harbor this mutation.

Although these various observations are suggestive that mtDNA mutations may contribute to the risk of manifesting AD and PD, substantially more data will be required before an association between these or any mtDNA mutations and AD or PD can be established. Obtaining definitive data to prove causality is particularly problematic, because all of the identified mtDNA mutations occurred in the late-onset cases of AD and PD. Therefore, when the mtDNA mutations are pathological, the mutations must be mild, and their penetrance may be dependent on additional genetic and environmental factors. Such factors could include abnormally metabolized environmental neurotoxins,[169,170] direct respiratory inhibitors such as MPTP, nuclear mutants that either affect OXPHOS or cell structure and physiology, and complex interactions between cellular energetics, calcium regulation, and excitotoxic neuronal damage.[171,172] Hence, an array of mtDNA genotypes may exist in the general population that confers susceptibility to neuronal losses and, hence, neurodegenerative diseases.

ATAXIAS AND OTHER MOVEMENT DISORDERS

Cerebellar ataxia is a commonly observed movement disorder in patients with OXPHOS diseases that can be caused by a variety of mtDNA mutations that include complex mtDNA rearrangements in which large segments of mtDNA are duplicated or deleted, point mutations in which single-nucleotide substitutions occur within transfer RNA (tRNA) genes, or missense mutations in mitochondrial genes encoding OXPHOS polypeptides. Although more than 30 pathogenic mtDNA point mutations and more than 60 different types of mtDNA deletions are known,[10,173] cerebellar ataxia may be observed in conjunction with the MTATP6*NARP8993G, MTATP6*NARP8993C, MTTK*MERRF8344G, and MTTL1*MELAS3243G mutations and mtDNA rearrangements. The importance of cerebellar ataxia in the patients who harbor the MTTK*MERRF8344G, MTATP6*NARP8993G, or the MTATP6*NARP8993C mutations has already been reviewed.

The most commonly encountered mtDNA mutation that can cause ataxia is an A-to-G mutation in the tRNA[Leucine(UUR)] gene at position 3243 of the mtDNA (MTTL1*MELAS3243G).[174] The MTTL1*MELAS3243G mutation was originally recognized as a cause for a type of "stroke in the young" called mitochondrial encephalomyopathy, lactic acidosis, and stroke-like episodes (MELAS).[174] This mutation accounts for approximately 80 percent of the MELAS cases.[175] Patients are generally below 45 years of age and present with a large- or small-vessel stroke that can be associated with a migraine headache and/or seizures. Delineating this presentation from the long list of other causes of stroke in the young can be difficult and is assisted by recognizing myopathy, ataxia, cardiomyopathy, diabetes mellitus, retinitis pigmentosa, proximal renal tubule defects, or lactic acidosis and hyperalaninemia. Because these systemic manifestations are not present in all patients, biochemical and genetic studies of OXPHOS can be essential in establishing the diagnosis. Cerebellar ataxia is often observed in patients with MELAS and may precede the development of stroke by many years. However, careful patient evaluation usually reveals manifestations in other organs, thus distinguishing these patients from other classes of cerebellar ataxia. An additional phenotype that is easily recognized clinically and can be caused by the MTTL1*MELAS3243G mutation is the Kearns-Sayre syndrome, which is a disorder characterized by early-onset (<20 years of age) ptosis, ophthalmoplegia, and variable manifestations of multiorgan degeneration or a chronic progressive external ophthalmoplegia (CPEO) syndrome, which is characterized by similar, though usually less severe, and later-onset (>20 years of age) of disease manifestations.[176] The MTTL1*MELAS3243G mutation is an important cause for Kearns-Sayre and CPEO syndromes and should be considered in the differential diagnosis of these disorders. The identification of this mutation is important in these patients, because it is maternally inherited and is associated with a greater risk of stroke than the mtDNA rearrangements.

Recent investigations suggest that diabetes mellitus is the most common disease manifestation produced by this mutation.[177] In three large screening studies performed on Japanese patients with noninsulin-dependent diabetes mellitus (NIDDM) and insulin-dependent diabetes mellitus (IDDM) and two studies of Caucasians with NIDDM, 1.6 percent (17/1095) of the Japanese individuals[178–180] and 1.1 percent (3/283) of the Caucasian individuals[181,182] harbored the MTTL1*MELAS3243G mutation. Because diabetes mellitus is a common disease affecting as many as 5–10 percent of Japanese and Western populations,[183] and because approximately 1 percent of randomly selected patients with adult-onset diabetes mellitus may harbor the MTTL1*MELAS3243G mutation,[180] as many as 2.5 million individuals in the United States are predicted to harbor this mutation.

Additional mtDNA mutations that can cause MELAS are all mutations involving the tRNA[Leucine(UUR)] gene and include a T-to-C mutation at position 3271, which accounts for about 7 percent of the MELAS cases,[174,175] rare mutations at positions 3256[184] and 3291[185] in patients with MELAS and possibly at position 3252, in which a single individual had a stroke-like episode at 58 years of age and her daughter had a mitochondrial encephalomyopathy.[186] Severe basal ganglia degeneration with extensive cerebral calcifications or Fahr's syndrome was observed in a patient with a single nucleotide deletion that removed one of the T:A nucleotide pairs between positions 3271 and 3273 of the mtDNA.[187] Fahr's syndrome is a nonspecific clinical classification in which patients have nonarteriosclerotic bilateral calcification of the cortex, pallidum, striatum, centrum semiovale, and dentate nucleus (Fig. 4-11).[188–191] Presenting symptoms are highly heterogeneous and include seizures, dementia, parkinsonism, retinitis pigmentosa, and a variety of endocrine disturbances.

Ptosis, ophthalmoplegia or ophthalmoparesis, and a RRF myopathy represent a clinical triad that is highly predictive for the presence of a mtDNA mutation. Patients with these manifestations can be classified into one of three groups, according to their age of onset and the severity of their clinical symptoms. The most severe variant is the Kearns-Sayre (KS) syndrome, which is characterized by infantile, childhood, or adolescent onset of disease manifestations and significant multisystem involvement that includes cardiac abnormalities (cardiomyopathies and cardiac conduction defects), diabetes mellitus, cerebellar ataxia, deafness, and evidence of multifocal neurodegeneration. "CPEO plus" refers to a disorder of intermediate severity that has an adolescent or adult onset and variable involvement of tissues other than the eyelids and eye muscles. The mildest variant is isolated CPEO, in which clinical signs and symptoms develop during adulthood and are limited to the eyelids and eye muscles. In each of these classification groups, patients worsen with age. Individuals who are initially classified as isolated CPEO can progress to CPEO plus, and patients with KS syndrome often develop more severe multisystem involvement. The highly variable clinical course experienced by patients with these phenotypes reflects the combined effects of the quantity and pathogenicity of the inherited mtDNA mutation and may also reflect the accumulation of somatic mtDNA mutations.

The most common cause for KS and CPEO syndromes is mtDNA rearrangements, which are characterized as mtDNA deletion mutations and mtDNA duplication mutations. The mtDNA deletion mutation has the simplest structure and consists of a mtDNA molecule that is missing contiguous tRNA and OXPHOS polypeptide genes, thus yielding a mtDNA molecule that is smaller than the normal 16.6-kb mtDNA.[192] The mtDNA deletions are heteroplasmic, remove 9 to 50 percent of the mitochondrial genome, commonly remove mitochondrial genes encoding subunits of OXPHOS enzymes and tRNA genes and, rarely, remove the rRNA genes.[173] The smallest known mtDNA deletion is a single nucleotide deletion in the tRNA[Leucine(UUR)] gene at position 3271 of the mtDNA that caused extensive cerebral calcifications and neurodegeneration or Fahr's disease.[187] The structurally more complex mtDNA duplication mutation produces a mtDNA molecule that is larger than the normal mtDNA and

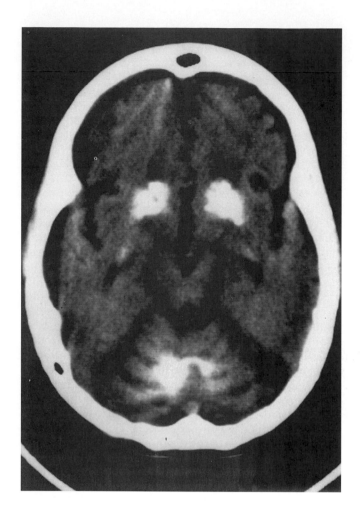
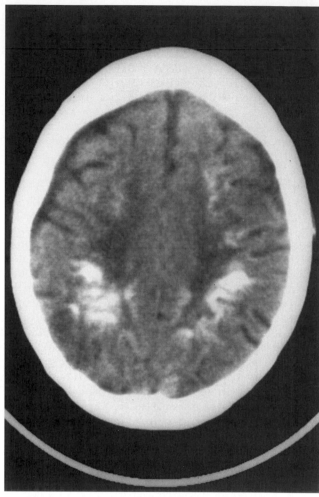

FIGURE 4-11 CT scan of the brain from a patient with Fahr's disease, caused by a single base pair deletion between positions 3271 and 3271 of the mtDNA. Marked bilateral calcification of the basal ganglia, thalamus, cerebellum, and white matter is shown. The head CT was provided by Dr. Martin G. Bialer, Department of Pediatrics, North Shore University Hospital-Cornell University Medical College, Manhasset, NY. (*From Shoffner et al.*[187] *Used with permission.*)

contains two tandemly arranged mtDNA molecules consisting of a full-length 16.6-kb mtDNA coupled to a mtDNA deletion mutation.[193,194] The mtDNA duplication mutation appears to be stable in tissues with a high replicative capacity, such as hematopoietic cells, and is easily detected by Southern blot analysis.[195] In contrast, the mtDNA deletion mutation is absent or present at low concentrations in highly replicative tissues and is difficult to detect by means of standard diagnostic approaches. Cells with predominantly normal mtDNAs may have a replicative advantage over cells with predominantly mutant mtDNAs, thus acounting for the difficulty in detecting mtDNA deletion mutations in the blood cells of patients with KS and CPEO syndromes.[196] This is supported by the observation that the mtDNA deletion mutation level can decrease rapidly in cultured myoblast cell lines, suggesting that myoblasts with predominantly normal mtDNAs have a survival advantage.[197] In contrast, tissues with a low replicative capacity, such as skeletal muscle and brain, can contain all three types of mtDNAs: the mtDNA duplication mutation, the mtDNA deletion mutation, and normal mtDNA. Hence, skeletal muscle is the optimal tissue for detection of mtDNA rearrangements because of its low replicative capacity, ability to retain mtDNA mutations, and easy accessibility.

Approximately 80 percent of patients with KS syndrome, 70 percent with CPEO plus, and 40 percent with CPEO harbor mtDNA rearrangements.[198,199] In most patients with mtDNA rearrangements, the mutation was not inherited but appears to be a spontaneous event that occurred after fertilization of the oocyte. Because of replicative segregation of mutant and normal mtDNAs, the identification of maternal inheritance of a mtDNA rearrangement by clinical criteria can be difficult and can require analysis of skeletal muscle mtDNA from a maternal lineage relative of the proband. Of the two classes of mtDNA rearrangements, the mtDNA duplication mutation has the greatest probability of being maternally transmitted. Hence, characterization of the mtDNA rearrangement is important for genetic counseling of the patient and family members.

Patients with cerebellar ataxia who are not easily categorized into one of the conventional OXPHOS disease categories and who do not harbor one of the common mtDNA mutations can have OXPHOS defects.[108] In two unrelated patients with spinocerebellar ataxia, no evidence of other systemic manifestations, and no identifiable family history of the disease, OXPHOS biochemistry indicated that a complex IV defect was present in one individual and that defects of multiple OXPHOS complexes were present in the second patient. Other identifiable causes for their spinocerebellar ataxia, such as mtDNA rearrangements, MTTL1*MELAS3243G, MTTK*MERRF8344G, MTATP6*NARP8993G, MTATP6*NARP8993C mutations, and $(CAG)_n$ trinucleotide repeat expansion in the ataxin-1 gene on chromosome 6 (spinocerebellar ataxia, type I)[200] were not found. Although the identification of a pathogenic mutation in a nuclear OXPHOS gene or in a mtDNA gene is essential to validating the relationship between the skeletal muscle OXPHOS defects and their clinical manifestations, these results suggested that various types of spinocerebellar degeneration may be caused by OXPHOS defects. Biochemical and genetic investigations of additional patients with spinocerebellar ataxia will be important in assessing this possibility.

OXPHOS Disease Assessment in Patients with Movement Disorders

The identification of patients with OXPHOS diseases requires application of the principles of both mitochondrial and Mendelian genetics. OXPHOS defects can result from mutations in any of the vast array of nuclear and mitochondrial OXPHOS genes. Hence, all forms of Mendelian inheritance, including autosomal-dominant, recessive, and X-linked inheritance patterns, are possible. Maternal inheritance of homoplasmic or heteroplasmic mutations, abnormalities of the interactions between nuclear DNA and mtDNA genes, and spontaneous mutations must be considered.

The basic elements of an OXPHOS evaluation are metabolic studies of blood, urine and, sometimes, CSF and a muscle biopsy that is processed immediately for histochemistry, electron microscopy, OXPHOS enzymology, and a mtDNA mutation screen. The most commonly observed metabolic abnormalities are elevations in lactate, pyruvate, and alanine in blood, urine, or CSF. A defect in the highly energy-dependent proximal renal tubules manifests as a generalized aminoaciduria and can be an important clue to the presence of an OXPHOS disease.[105] Because metabolic tests can be normal in patients with OXPHOS diseases, most patients require a muscle biopsy for diagnosis. Pathological analysis of the muscle biopsy, using various histochemical techniques and electron microscopy, can be helpful in supporting the diagnosis of an OXPHOS disease. The modified Gomori-trichrome stain and the more sensitive succinate dehydrogenase and cytochrome c oxidase reactions are useful in the diagnosis of mitochondrial myopathies. Muscle fibers develop abnormal segments of fiber degeneration and mitochondrial proliferation that alternate with normal segments. The mitochondria stain red with the modified Gomori-tri-

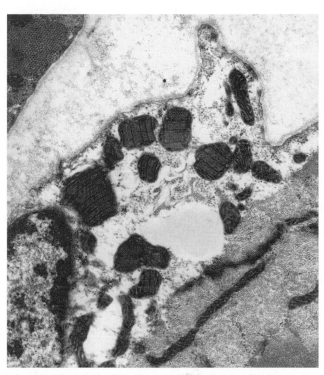

FIGURE 4-12 Skeletal muscle ultrastructure in a patient with a mitochondrial myopathy. Paracrystalline inclusions represent aggregations of mitochondrial creatine kinase. This ultrastructural observation is characteristic of OXPHOS diseases that are caused by defects in mitochondrial protein synthesis, such as mtDNA rearrangements and tRNA point mutations. OXPHOS diseases caused by missense mutations in mtDNA genes coding for polypeptide subunits are not associated with paracrystalline inclusions.

chrome stain, show an increase in the intensity of the succinate dehydrogenase reaction, or show a decreased cytochrome c oxidase reaction. A mitochondrial myopathy can be particularly difficult to diagnose in older patients because of significant overlap between the frequency of RRFs in patients and controls. RRFs normally accumulate with advancing age in conjunction with a decline in OXPHOS function. When the succinate dehydrogenase histochemical reaction is used to detect RRFs, 1–4 abnormal fiber segments can be evident in transverse sections of muscle per low-powered field.[201] Ultrastructural analysis of the muscle often reveals structurally abnormal mitochondria with paracrystalline inclusions, which are intermembranous condensations of mitochondrial creatine kinase (Fig. 4-12),[107] but this analysis can show normal mitochondrial ultrastructure in some individuals. These pathological findings are most commonly found in patients with mtDNA mutations that cause defects in mitochondrial protein synthesis, such as mtDNA rearrangements, the MTTK*MERRF8344G mutation, and the MTTL1*MELAS3243G mutation. Diseases associated with mtDNA missense mutations in OXPHOS polypeptide genes such as the MTATP6*NARP8993G mutation rarely show diagnostic abnormalities on electron microscopy or histochemical analyses. In patients under approximately 5 years of age, histochemical or ultrastructural abnormalities are unusual.

The presence of an OXPHOS disease can be confirmed by biochemical and/or genetic testing. When specific mutations are not implicated, OXPHOS enzyme analysis in skeletal muscle mitochondria is essential to OXPHOS disease diagnosis. Although it is now possible to achieve a precise diagnosis of certain OXPHOS diseases by means of DNA analysis alone, OXPHOS enzymology is the only means of diagnosing many cases. To perform accurate assessments of this delicate enzyme system, mitochondria should be immediately isolated from fresh muscle biopsies. This approach avoids artifacts in OXPHOS enzyme analysis that can be associated with freezing the biopsy before mitochondrial isolation.[202] A small portion of the biopsy is frozen in liquid nitrogen for DNA or RNA extraction. Finally, lymphoblast and/or myoblast cell lines can be established for cellular respiration studies, for somatic cell genetic studies, and as a source of total genomic DNA for future analyses. This integrated clinical, metabolic, and biochemical approach increases the probability of reaching a correct genetic diagnosis which is essential for accurate genetic counseling and effective patient management. The mtDNA mutations that cause defects in mitochondrial protein synthesis have their most pronounced effects on complexes I and IV, which are the OXPHOS enzymes with the greatest number of polypeptide subunits encoded by the mtDNA. When defects in these OXPHOS complexes are observed in conjunction with a RRF myopathy, patients have a high probability of harboring a mtDNA mutation that impairs mitochondrial protein synthesis.[83,93]

Patients with very high concentrations of a mtDNA mutation in a stable tissue such as skeletal muscle generally have the most severe disease manifestations. However, formulating an accurate prognosis based on mtDNA quantitation from a single tissue is difficult. Replicative segregation of normal and mutant mtDNAs accounts for a significant amount of this variability in disease expression, because different tissues within the same individual can have large differences in the amounts of mutant mtDNAs. In addition, some of the techniques used for quantitation of normal and mutant mtDNAs have limitations. Mutation quantitation is most accurate for mtDNA point mutations that can be assessed by Southern blot using restriction endonucleases that permit the unambiguous recognition of the mtDNA mutation.

OXPHOS Disease Therapy

Although rapid advancements in the diagnosis and genetic counseling of patients with OXPHOS diseases developed over the past several years, little change in the approaches used to treat patients has occurred. An important limitation of therapeutic trials is that the large number of pathogenic mtDNA mutations, the replicative segregation of mutant and normal mtDNAs, tissue-specific thresholds for phenotype expression, and the accumulation of somatic mtDNA mutations make the formation of a homogeneous treatment group difficult. To date, most attempts to improve OXPHOS function have used vitamins, coenzymes, and metabolic interme-

diates (reviewed in Refs 10 and 109). Of these treatments, coenzyme Q10 (CoQ10) received the greatest attention. Numerous case reports suggested that CoQ10 can produce a mild-to-moderate improvement in cellular energetics. The most dramatic clinical responses included improvements in cardiac conduction defects and in respiratory failure in patients with KS and CPEO syndromes and in the frequency of stroke-like episodes in MELAS patients. Although some investigators found CoQ10 treatment ineffective when heterogeneous patient populations were studied,[203] a multicenter, double-blind study of CoQ10 at doses of 2 mg/kg/day in patients with KS and CPEO syndromes demonstrated a decrease in postexercise blood lactate levels in approximately 30 percent of individuals and an improvement of intention tremor in approximately 10 percent of individuals with cerebellar ataxia.[204] Further studies using genetically homogeneous groups of patients are needed to clarify the efficacy of CoQ10 therapy. Based on our clinical experience with CoQ10 dosing and based on the doses reported in patients who experienced positive therapeutic responses, we administer CoQ10 at a dose of 4.3 mg/kg/day to both pediatric and adult patients and adjust the dose to maintain blood levels between 3 and 4 mg/ml. If a positive clinical or metabolic response has not been identified after 10–12 months of treatment, the CoQ10 is discontinued. Although considerable experience has developed with the administration of CoQ10 to a variety of patients with OXPHOS diseases, the effects of CoQ10 on the progression of movement disorders has not been investigated. Although little is known about the effects of CoQ10 on disease progression, we have not observed significant improvements in motor control in patients with ataxias or extrapyramidal disease manifestations.

Acknowledgments

This work was supported by NIH Grants NS33999, M01RR-00039, M01RR-00827, and 1P30AG10130-01.

References

1. Holt IJ, Harding AE, Morgan HJA: Deletions of muscle mitochondrial DNA in patients with mitochondrial myopathies. *Nature* 331:717–719, 1988.
2. Wallace DC, Singh G, Lott MT, et al: Mitochondrial DNA mutation associated with Leber's hereditary optic neuropathy. *Science* 242:1427–1430, 1988.
3. Tatuch Y, Christodoulou J, Feigenbaum A, et al: Heteroplasmic mitochondrial DNA mutation (T to G) at 8993 can cause Leigh disease when the percentage of abnormal mtDNA is high. *Am J Hum Genet* 50:852–858, 1992.
4. Shoffner JM, Fernhoff PM, Krawiecki NS, et al: Subacute necrotizing encephalopathy: Oxidative phosphorylation defects and the ATPase 6 point mutation. *Neurology* 42:2168–2174, 1992.
5. Shoffner JM, Brown MB, Stugard C, Jun AS, Pollok S, Haas RH, Kaufman A, Koontz D, Kim Y, Graham JR, Smith E, Dixon J, Wallace DC: Leber's hereditary optic neuropathy plus dystonia is caused by a mitochondrial DNA point mutation. *Ann Neurol* 38:163–169, 1995.

6. Jun AS, Brown MD, Wallace DC: A mitochondrial DNA mutation at np 14459 of the ND6 gene associated with maternally inherited Leber's hereditary optic neuropathy and dystonia. *Proc Natl Acad Sci USA* 91:6206–6210, 1994.

7. O'Brien TW, Denslow ND, Anders JC, Courtney BC: The translation system of mammalian mitochondria. *Biochim Biophys Acta* 1050:174–178, 1990.

8. Shoffner JM, Brown MD, Torroni A, et al: Mitochondrial DNA mutations associated with Alzheimer's and Parkinson's disease. *Genomics* 17:171–184, 1993.

9. Shoffner JM, Wallace DC: Oxidative phosphorylation diseases: Disorders of two genomes. *Adv Hum Genet* 19:267–330, 1990.

10. Shoffner JM, Wallace DC: *Oxidative phosphorylation diseases*, in Scriver CR, Beaudet AL, Sly WS, Valle D (eds): *The Metabolic and Molecular Bases of Inherited Disease.* New York: McGraw-Hill, 1995, pp 1535–1610.

11. Anderson S, Bankier AT, Barrell BG, et al: Sequence and organization of the human mitochondrial DNA genome. *Nature* 290:457–465, 1981.

12. Gyllensten U, Wharton D, Josefsson A, Wilson AC: Paternal inheritance of mitochondrial DNA in mice. *Nature* 352:255–257, 1991.

13. Linnane AW, Marzuki S, Ozawa T, Tanaka M: Mitochondrial DNA mutations as an important contributor to aging and degenerative diseases. *Lancet* i:642–645, 1989.

14. Miquel J, Economos AC, Fleming J, Johnson JEJ: Mitochondrial role in cell aging. *Exp Gerontol* 15:575–591, 1980.

15. Chance B, Sies H, Boveris A: Hydroperoxide metabolism in mammalian organs. *Physiol Rev* 59:527–605, 1979.

16. Boveris A, Oshino N, Chance B: The cellular production of hydrogen peroxide. *Biochem J* 128:617–630, 1972.

17. Forman HJ, Boveris A: Superoxide radical and hydrogen peroxide in mitochondria, in Pryor WA (ed): *Free Radicals in Biology.* New York: Academic Press, 1982, pp 65–90.

18. Richter C, Park JW, Ames BN: Normal oxidative damage to mitochondrial and nuclear DNA is extensive. *Proc Natl Acad Sci U S A* 85:6465–6467, 1988.

19. Bandy B, Davison AJ: Mitochondrial mutations may increase oxidative stress: Implications for carcinogenesis and aging? *Free Radic Biol Med* 8:523–539, 1990.

20. Dean RT, Gebicki J, Gieseg S, et al: Hypothesis: A damaging role in aging for reactive protein oxidation products? *Mutat Res* 275:387–393, 1992.

21. Horton AA, Fairhurst S: Lipid peroxidation and mechanisms of toxicity. *CRC Crit Rev Toxicol* 18:27–79, 1987.

22. Recknagel RO, Glende EAJ, Britton RS: Free radical damage and lipid peroxidation, in Meeks RG, Harrison SD, Bull RJ (eds): *Hepatotoxicology.* Boca Raton, FL: CRC Press, 1991, pp 401–436.

23. Esterbauer H, Eckl P, Ortner A: Possible mutagens derived from lipids and lipid precursors. *Mutat Res* 238:223–233, 1990.

24. Daum G: Lipids of mitochondria. *Biochim Biophys Acta* 822:1–42, 1985.

25. Bindoli A: Lipid peroxidation in mitochondria. *Free Radic Biol Med* 5:247–261, 1988.

26. Imlay JA, Linn S: DNA damage and oxygen radical toxicity. *Science* 240:1302–1309, 1988.

27. Halliwell B, Aruoma OI: DNA damage by oxygen-derived species. Its mechanism and measurement in mammalian systems. *FEBS Lett* 281:9–19, 1991.

28. Richter C: Do mitochondrial DNA fragments promote ageing and cancer? *FEBS Lett* 241:1–5, 1988.

29. Kouchakdijan M, Bodepudi V, Shibutani S, et al: NMR structural studies of the ionizing radiation adduct 7-hydro-8-oxodeoxyguanosine (8-oxo-7H-dG) opposite deoxyadenosine in a DNA duplex. 8-Oxo-7H-dG(syn)-dA(anti) alignment at lesion site. *Biochemistry* 30:1403–1412, 1991.

30. Hruszkewycz AM, Bergtold DS: The 8-hydroxyguanine content of isolated mitochondria increases with lipid peroxidation. *Mutat Res* 244:123–128, 1990.

31. Hayakawa M, Torii K, Sugiyama S, et al: Age-associated accumulation of 8-hydroxydeoxyguanosine in mitochondrial DNA of human diaphragm. *Biochem Biophys Res Commun* 179:1023–1029, 1991.

32. Mecocci P, MacGarvey U, Kaufman AE, et al: Oxidative damage to mitochondrial DNA shows marked age-dependent increases in human brain. *Ann Neurol* 34:609–616, 1993.

33. Backer JM, Weinstein IB: Mitochondrial DNA is a major cellular target for a dihydrodiol-epoxide derivative of benzo[alpha]pyrene. *Science* 209:297–299, 1980.

34. Wunderlich V, Schutt M, Bottger M, Graffi A: Preferential alkylation of mitochondrial deoxyribonucleic acid by N-methyl-N-nitrosourea. *Biochem J* 118:99–109, 1970.

35. Munscher C, Muller-Hocker J, Kadenbach B: Human aging is associated with various point mutations in tRNA genes of mitochondrial DNA. *Biol Chem Hoppe Seyler* 374:1099–1104, 1993.

36. Zhang C, Linnane AW, Nagley P: Occurrence of a particular base substitution (3243 A to G) in mitochondrial DNA of tissues of ageing humans. *Biochem Biophys Res Commun* 195:1104–1110, 1993.

37. Munscher C, Muller-Hocker J, Kadenbach B: The point mutation of mitochondrial DNA characteristic for MERRF disease is found also in healthy people of different ages. *FEBS Lett* 317:27–30, 1993.

38. Ikebe S, Tanaka M, Ohno K, et al: Increase of deleted mitochondrial DNA in the striatum in Parkinson's disease and senescence. *Biochem Biophys Res Commun* 170:1044–1048, 1990.

39. Corral-Debrinski M, Horton T, Lott MT, et al: Mitochondrial DNA deletions in human brain: Regional variability and increase with advanced age. *Nature Genet* 2:324–329, 1992.

40. Soong NW, Hinton DR, Cortopassi G, Arnheim N: Mosaicism for a specific somatic mitochondrial DNA mutation in adult human brain. *Nature Genet* 2:318–323, 1992.

41. Corral-Debrinski M, Shoffner JM, Lott MT, Wallace DC: Association of mitochondrial DNA damage with aging and coronary atherosclerotic heart disease. *Mutat Res* 275:169–80, 1992.

42. Corral-Debrinski M, Stepien G, Shoffner JM, et al: Hypoxemia is associated with mitochondrial DNA damage and gene induction. Implications for cardiac disease. *JAMA* 266:1812–1816, 1991.

43. Hattori K, Tanaka M, Sugiyama S, et al: Age-dependent increase in deleted mitochondrial DNA in the human heart: Possible contributory factor to presbycardia. *Am Heart J* 121:1735–1742, 1991.

44. Sugiyama S, Hattori K, Hayakawa M, Ozawa T: Quantitative analysis of age associated accumulation of mitochondrial DNA with deletion in human hearts. *Biochem Biophys Res Commun* 180:894–899, 1991.

45. Cortopassi GA, Arnheim N: Detection of a specific mitochondrial deletion in tissues of older individuals. *Nucleic Acids Res* 18:6927–6933, 1990.

46. Arnheim N, Cortopassi G: Deleterious mitochondrial DNA mutations accumulate in aging human tissues. *Mutat Res* 275:157–167, 1992.

47. Ozawa T, Tanaka M, Sugiyama S, et al: Multiple mitochondrial DNA deletions exist in cardiomyocytes of patients with hypertrophic or dilated cardiomyopathy. *Biochem Biophys Res Commun* 170:830–836, 1990.

48. Katayama M, Tanaka M, Yamamoto H, et al: Deleted mitochondrial DNA in the skeletal muscle of aged individuals. *Biochem Int* 25:47–56, 1991.

49. Yen T-C, Su J-H, King K-L, Wei Y-H: Ageing-associated 5 kb deletion in human liver mitochondrial DNA. *Biochim Biophys Res Commun* 178:124–131, 1991.

50. Cortopassi GA, Shibata D, Soong N-W, Arnheim N: A pattern of accumulation of a somatic deletion of mitochondrial DNA in aging tissues. *Proc Natl Acad Sci USA* 89:7370–7374, 1992.

51. Trounce I, Byrne E, Marzuki S: Decline in skeletal muscle mitochondrial respiratory chain function: Possible factor in ageing. *Lancet* i:637–639, 1989.

52. Cardellach F, Galofre J, Cusso R, Urbano-Marquez A: Decline in skeletal muscle mitochondrial respiration chain function with ageing. *Lancet* 2:44–45, 1989.

53. Abu-Erreish GM, Sanadi DR: Age-related changes in cytochrome concentration of myocardial mitochondria. *Mech Ageing Dev* 7:425–432, 1978.

54. Beregi E, Regius O: Relationship of mitochondrial damage in human lymphocytes and age. *Aktull Gerontol* 13:226–228, 1983.

55. Beregi E: Relationship between ageing of the immune system and ageing of the whole organism, in Bergener M, Ermini M, Stahelin HB (eds): *Dimensions in Ageing*. London: Academic Press, 1986, pp 35–50.

56. Tauchi H, Sato T: Cellular changes in senescence: Possible factors influencing the process of cellular ageing, in Bergener M, Ermini M, Stahelin HB (eds): Thresholds in Ageing. London: Academic Press, 1985, pp 91–113.

57. Muller-Hocker J: Cytochrome c oxidase deficient cardiomyocytes in the human heart: An age-related phenomenon. *Am J Pathol* 134:1167–1171, 1989.

58. Muller-Hocker J: Cytochrome c oxidase deficient fibers in the limb muscle and diaphragm of man without muscular disease: An age-related alteration. *J Neurol Sci* 100:14–21, 1990.

59. Muller-Hocker J, Schneiderbanger K, Stefani FH, Kadenbach B: Progressive loss of cytochrome c oxidase in the human extraocular muscles in ageing—a cytochemical-immunohistochemical study. *Mutat Res* 275:115–124, 1992.

60. Bittles AH: The role of mitochondria in cellular ageing, in Warnes AM (ed): Human, Ageing and Later Life. London: Edward Arnold, 1989, pp 29–37.

61. Kiessling KH, Pilstrom I, Karlsson J, Piehl K: Mitochondrial volume in skeletal muscle from young and old physically untrained and trained healthy men and from alcoholics. *Clin Sci* 44:547–554, 1973.

62. Wallace DC, Lott MT, Torroni A, Brown MD: Report of the committee on human mitochondrial DNA. *Cytogenet Cell Genet* 59:727–757, 1992.

63. Phelps ME, Mazziotta JC, Huang SC: Study of cerebral function with positron computed tomography. *J Cereb Blood Flow Metab* 2:113–162, 1982.

64. Gerfen CR: The neostriatal mosaic: Multiple levels of compartmental organization in the basal ganglia. *Annu Rev Neurosci* 15:285–320, 1992.

65. Schoolwerth AC, Drewnowska K: *Renal metabolism*, in Schrier RW, Gottschalk CW (eds): *Diseases of the Kidney*. Boston: Little, Brown, 1993, pp 233–260.

66. Horton TM, Graham BH, Corral-Debrinski M, Shoffner JM, Beal MF, Wallace DC: Marked increase in mitochondrial DNA deletion levels in the cerebral cortex of Huntington's disease patients. Neurology 45:1879–1883, 1995.

67. Corral-Debrinski M, Horton T, Lott MT, et al: Marked changes in mitochondrial DNA deletion levels in Alzheimer brains. *Genomics* 23:471–476, 1994.

68. Huntington's Disease Collaborative Research Group: A novel gene containing a trinucleotide repeat that is expanded and unstable on Huntington's disease chromosomes. *Cell* 72:971–983, 1993.

69. Jenkins BG, Koroshetz WJ, Beal MF, Rosen BR: Evidence for impairment of energy metabolism in vivo in Huntington's disease using localized 1H-NMR spectroscopy. *Neurology* 43:2689–2695, 1993.

70. Mann VM, Cooper JM, Javoy-Agid F, et al: Mitochondrial function and parental sex effect in Huntington's disease. *Lancet* 336:749, 1990.

71. Brennan WA, Bird ED, Aprille JR: Regional mitochondrial respiratory activity in Huntington's disease brain. *J Neurochem* 44:1948–1950, 1985.

72. Parker WD, Boyson SJ, Luder AS, Parks JK: Evidence for a defect in NADH:ubiquinone oxidoreductase (complex I) in Huntington's disease. *Neurology* 40:1231–1234, 1990.

73. Whitehouse PJ, Price DL, Struble RG, et al: Alzheimer's disease and senile dementia: Loss of neurons in the basal forebrain. *Science* 215:1237–1239, 1982.

74. Parker WD, Filley CM, Parks JK: Cytochrome oxidase deficiency in Alzheimer's disease. *Neurology* 40:1302–1303, 1990.

75. Van Zuylen AJ, Bosman GJCGM, Ruitenbeek W, et al: No evidence for reduced thrombocyte cytochrome oxidase activity in Alzheimer's disease. *Neurology* 42:1246–1247, 1992.

76. Kish S, Bergeron C, Rajput A, et al: Brain cytochrome c oxidase in Alzheimer's disease. *J Neurochem* 59:776–779, 1992.

77. Reichmann H, Florke S, Hebenstreit G, et al: Analyses of energy metabolism and mitochondrial genome in post-mortem brain from patients with Alzheimer's disease. *J Neurol* 240:377–380, 1993.

78. Cooper JM, Wischik C, Schapira AHV: Mitochondrial function in Alzheimer's disease. *Lancet* 341:969–970, 1993.

79. Simonian NA, Hyman BT: Functional alterations in Alzheimer's disease: Diminution of cytochrome oxidase in the hippocampal formation. *J Neuropath Exp Neurol* 52:580–585, 1993.

80. Chandrasekaran K, Stoll J, Brady DR, Rapoport SI: Distribution of cytochrome oxidase (COX) activity and mRNA in monkey and human brain: COX mRNA distribution correlates with neurons vulnerable to Alzheimer pathology. *Soc Neurosci Abstr* 18:557, 1992.

81. Blanchard BJ, Park T, Fripp WJ, et al: A mitochondrial DNA deletion in normally aging and in Alzheimer brain tissue. *Neuroreport* 4:799–802, 1993.

82. Rosing HS, Hopkins LC, Wallace DC, et al: Maternally inherited mitochondrial myopathy and myoclonic epilepsy. *Ann Neurol* 17:228–237, 1985.

83. Wallace DC, Zheng XX, Lott MT, et al: Familial mitochondrial encephalomyopathy (MERRF): Genetic, pathophysiological, and biochemical characterization of a mitochondrial DNA disease. *Cell* 55:601–610, 1988.

84. Thompson PD, Hammans SR, Harding AE: Cortical reflex myoclonus in patients with the mitochondrial DNA transfer RNA-Lys(8344) (MERRF) mutation. *J Neurol* 241:335–340, 1994.

85. Calabresi PA, Silvestri G, DiMauro S, Griggs RC: Ekbom's syndrome: Lipomas, ataxia, and neuropathy with MERRF. *Muscle Nerve* 17:943–945, 1994.

86. Berkovic SF, Carpenter S, Evans A, et al: Myoclonus epilepsy and ragged-red fibres (MERRF). I. A clinical, pathological, biochemical, magnetic resonance spectrographic and positron emission tomographic study. *Brain* 112:1231–1260, 1989.

87. Holme E, Larsson N-G, Oldfors A, et al: Multiple symmetric lipomas with high levels of mtDNA wi the tRNA-Lys A to G (8344) mutation as the only manifestation of disease in a carrier of myoclonus epilepsy and ragged-red fibers (MERRF) syndrome. *Am J Hum Genet* 52:551–556, 1993.

88. Sasaki H, Kuzuhara S, Kanazawa I, et al: Myoclonus, cerebellar disorder, neuropathy, mitochondrial myopathy, and ACTH deficiency. *Neurology* 33:1288–1293, 1983.

89. Nakano T, Sakai H, Amano N, et al: An autopsy case of degenerative type myoclonus epilepsy associated with Friedreich's ataxia and mitochondrial myopathy. *Brain Nerve* 34:321–332, 1982.

90. Fukuhara N: MERRF: A clinicopathological study. Relationships between myoclonus epilepsies and mitochondrial myopathies. *Rev Neurol (Paris)* 147:476–479, 1991.

91. Fukuhara N: Myoclonus epilepsy and mitochondrial myopathy, in Scarlato G, Cerri C (eds): *Mitochondrial Pathology in Muscle Diseases*. Padua, Italy: Piccin Medical Books, 1983, pp 88–110.

92. Takeda S, Wakabayashi K, Ohama E, Ikuta F: Neuropathology of myoclonus epilepsy associated with ragged-red fibers (Fukuhara's disease). *Acta Neuropathol (Berl)* 75:433–440, 1988.

93. Shoffner JM, Lott MT, Lezza AM, et al: Myoclonic epilepsy and ragged-red fiber disease (MERRF) is associated with a mitochondrial DNA tRNA(Lys) mutation. *Cell* 61:931–937, 1990.

94. Silvestri G, Moraes CT, Shanske S, et al: A new mutation in the tRNA-Lys gene associated with myoclonic epilepsy and ragged-red fibers (MERRF). *Am J Hum Genet* 51:1213–1217, 1992.

95. Zeviani ML, Muntoni F, Savarese N, et al: A MERRF/MELAS overlap syndrome associated with a new point mutation of mitochondrial DNA tRNA-Lys gene. *Eur J Hum Genet* 1:80–87, 1993.

96. Rich A, RajBhandary UL: Transfer RNA: Molecular structure, sequence, and properties. *Annu Rev Biochem* 45:805–860, 1976.

97. Boulet L, Karpati G, Shoubridge E: Distribution and threshold expression of the tRNA-Lys mutation in skeletal muscle of patients with myoclonic epilepsy and ragged-red fibers (MERRF). *Am J Hum Genet* 51:1187–1200, 1992.

98. Chomyn A, Meola G, Bresolin N, et al: In vitro genetic transfer of protein synthesis and respiration defects to mitochondrial DNA-less cells with myopathy-patient mitochondria. *Mol Cell Biol* 11:2236–44, 1991.

99. Wallace DC, Yang J, Ye J, et al: Computer prediction of peptide maps: Assignment of polypeptides to human and mouse mitochondrial DNA genes by analysis of two-dimensional-proteolytic digest gels. *Am J Hum Genet* 38:461–481, 1986.

100. King MP, Attardi G: Human cells lacking mtDNA: Repopulation with exogenous mitochondria by complementation. *Science* 246:500–503, 1989.

101. Bunn CL, Wallace DC, Eisenstadt JM: Cytoplasmic inheritance of chloramphenicol resistance in mouse tissue culture cells. *Proc Natl Acad Sci USA* 71:1681–1685, 1974.

102. Wallace DC, Bunn CL, Eisenstadt JM: Cytoplasmic transfer of chloramphenicol resistance in human tissue culture cells. *J Cell Biol* 67:174–188, 1975.

103. Larsson N-G, Tulinius MH, Holme E, et al: Segregation and manifestations of the mtDNA tRNA-lys A to G (8344) mutation of myoclonus epilepsy and ragged-red fibers (MERRF) syndrome. *Am J Hum Genet* 51:1201–1212, 1992.

104. Eleff SM, Barker PB, Blackband SJ, et al: Phosphorus magnetic resonance spectroscopy of patients with mitochondrial cytopathies demonstrates decreased levels of brain phosphocreatine. *Ann Neurol* 27:626–630, 1990.

105. Shoffner JM, Voljavec AS, Dixon J, et al: Renal amino acid transport in adults with oxidative phosphorylation diseases. *Kidney Int* 47:1101–1107, 1995.

106. Hasagawa H, Matsuoka T, Goto Y, Nonaka I: Cytochrome c oxidase activity is deficient in blood vessels of patients with myoclonus epilepsy with ragged-red fibers. *Acta Neuropathol* 85:280–284, 1993.

107. Stadhouders A, Jap P, Walliman TH: Biochemical nature of mitochondrial crystals. *J Neurol Sci* 98(suppl):304–305, 1990.

108. Shoffner JM, Kaufman A, Koontz D, et al: Oxidative phosphorylation diseases in cerebellar ataxia. *Clin Neurosci* 2:43–53, 1995.

109. Shoffner JM, Wallace DC: Oxidative phosphorylation diseases and mitochondrial DNA mutations: Diagnosis and treatment. *Annu Rev Nutr* 14:535–568, 1994.

110. Hornykiewicz O, Kish SJ, Becker LE, et al: Brain neurotransmitters in dystonia musculorum deformans. *N Engl J Med* 315:347–353, 1986.

111. Zweig RM, Hedreen JC, Jankel WR, et al: Pathology in brainstem regions of individuals with primary dystonia. *Neurology* 38:702, 1988.

112. Bressman SB, De Leon D, Brin M, et al: Idiopathic dystonia among Ashkenazi Jews: Evidence for autosomal recessive dominant inheritance. *Ann Neurol* 26:612–620, 1989.

113. Fletcher NA, Harding AE, Marsden CD: A genetic study of idiopathic torsion dystonia in the United Kingdom. *Brain* 113:379–395, 1990.

114. Waddy HM, Fletcher NA, Harding AE, Marsden CD: A genetic study of idiopathic focal dystonias. *Ann Neurol* 29:320–324, 1991.

115. Zilber N, Korczyn AD, Kahana E, et al: Inheritance of idiopathic torsion dystonia among Jews. *J Med Genet* 21:13–20, 1984.

116. Bundey S, Harrison MJG, Marsden CD: A genetic study of torsion dystonia. *J Med Genet* 12:12–19, 1975.

117. Eldridge R: The torsion dystonias: Literature review and genetic and clinical studies. *Neurology* 20(suppl 1):1–78, 1970.

118. Parker WDJ, Oley CA, Parks JK: A defect in mitochondrial electron-transport activity (NADH-coenzyme Q oxidoreductase) in Leber's hereditary optic neuropathy. *N Eng J Med* 320:1331–1333, 1989.

119. Wallace DC: A new manifestation of Leber's disease and a new explanation for the agency responsible for its unusual pattern of inheritance. *Brain* 93:121–132, 1970.

120. Wallace DC: Leber's optic atrophy: A possible example of vertical transmission of a slow virus in man. *Aust Ann Med* 19:259–262, 1970.

121. Mackey D, Howell N: A variant of Leber hereditary optic neuropathy characterized by recovery of vision and by an unusual mitochondrial genetic etiology. *Am J Hum Genet* 51:1218–1228, 1992.

122. Howell N, Kubacka I, Xu M, McCullough DA: Leber hereditary optic neuropathy: Involvement of the mitochondrial ND1 gene and evidence for an intragenic suppressor mutation. *Am J Hum Genet* 48:935–942, 1991.

123. Johns DR, Neufeld MJ, Park RD: An ND-6 mitochondrial DNA mutation associated with Leber hereditary optic neuropathy. *Biochem Biophys Res Commun* 187:1551–1557, 1992.

124. Johns DR, Hehrer KL, Miller NR, Smith KH: Leber's hereditary optic neuropathy: Clinical manifestations of the 14484 mutation. *Arch Ophthalmol* 111:495–498, 1993.

125. Novotny EJJ, Singh G, Wallace DC, et al: Leber's disease and dystonia: A mitochondrial disease. *Neurology* 36:1053–1060, 1986.

126. Benecke R, Strumper P, Weiss H: Electron transfer complex I defect in idiopathic dystonia. *Ann Neurol* 32:683–686, 1992.

127. Jun AS, Trounce IA, Brown MD, et al: Use of transmitochondrial cybrids to assign a complex I defect to the mitochondrial DNA, NADH dehydrogenase subunit 6, nucleotide pair 14459 mutation that causes Leber hereditary optic neuropathy and dystonia. *Mol Cell Biol.*

128. Nakamura M, Ara F, Yamada M, et al: High frequency of mitochondrial ND4 gene mutation in Japanese pedigrees with Leber hereditary optic neuropathy. *Jpn J Ophthalmol* 36:56–61, 1992.

129. Larsson NG, Andersen O, Holme E, et al: Leber's hereditary optic neuropathy and complex I deficiency in muscle. *Ann Neurol* 30:701–708, 1991.

130. Santorelli FM, Shanske S, Jain KD, et al: A T to C mutation at nt 8993 of mitochondrial DNA in a child with Leigh syndrome. *Neurology* 44:972–974, 1994.

131. Trounce I, Neill S, Wallace D: Cytoplasmic transfer of the mtDNA nt 8993 T to G (ATP 6) point mutation associated with Leigh syndrome into mtDNA-less cells demonstrates cosegregation with a decrease in state II respiration and ADP/O ratio. *Proc Natl Acad Sci USA* 91:8334–8338, 1994.

132. Tatuch Y, Pagon RA, Vlcek B, et al: The 8993 mtDNA mutation: Heteroplasmy and clinical presentation in three families. *Eur J Hum Genet* 2:35–43, 1994.

133. Holt IJ, Harding AE, Petty RK, Morgan HJA: A new mitochondrial disease associated with mitochondrial DNA heteroplasmy. *Am J Hum Genet* 46:428–33, 1990.

134. Santorelli FM, Shanske S, Macaya A, et al: The mutation at nt 8993 of mitochondrial DNA is a common cause of Leigh's syndrome. *Ann Neurol* 34:827–834, 1993.

135. Miranda DF, Ishii S, DiMauro S, Shay JW: Cytochrome c oxidase (COX) deficiency in Leigh's syndrome: Genetic evidence for a nuclear DNA-encoded mutation. *Neurology* 39:697–702, 1989.

136. Alexander GE, DeLong MR, Strick PL: Parallel organization of functionally segregated circuits linking basal ganglia and cortex. *Annu Rev Neurosci* 9:357–381, 1986.

137. Brooks DJ, Ibanez V, Sawle GV, et al: Differing patterns of striatal 18F-dopa uptake in Parkinson's disease, multiple system atrophy, and progressive supranuclear palsy. *Ann Neurol* 28:547–555, 1990.

138. Chui HC, Teng EL, Henderson VW, Moy AC: Clinical subtypes of dementia of the Alzheimer type. *Neurology* 35:1544–1550, 1985.

139. Mirra SS, Heyman A, McKeel D, et al: The Consortium to Establish a Registry for Alzheimer's Disease (CERAD). Part II: Standardization of the neuropathologic assessment of Alzheimer's disease. *Neurology* 41:479–486, 1991.

140. Ditter SM, Mirra SS: Neuropathologic and clinical features of Parkinson's disease in Alzheimer's disease patients. *Neurology* 37:754–760, 1987.

141. Dickson DW, Crystal H, Mattiace LA, et al: Diffuse Lewy body disease: Light and electron microscopic immunocytochemistry of senile plaques. *Acta Neuropathol (Berl)* 78:572–584, 1989.

142. Perry RH, Irving D, Blessed G, et al: Senile dementia of Lewy body type: A clinically and neuropathologically distinct form of Lewy body dementia in the elderly. *J Neurol Sci* 95:119–139, 1990.

143. Hansen L, Salmon D, Galasko D, et al: The Lewy body variant of Alzheimer's disease: A clinical and pathologic entity. *Neurology* 40:1–8, 1990.

144. Wallace DC: Mitochondrial genetics: A paradigm for aging and degenerative diseases? *Science* 256:628–32, 1992.

145. Salach JI, Singer TP, Castagnoli NJ, Trevor A: Oxidation of the neurotoxic amine 1-methyl-4-phenyl-1,2,3,6-tetrahydropyridine (MPTP) by monoamine oxidases A and B and suicide inactivation of the enzymes by MPTP. *Biochem Biophys Res Commun* 125:831–835, 1984.

146. Javitch JA, D'Amato RJ, Strittmatter SM, Snyder SH: Parkinsonism-inducing neurotoxin, N-methyl-4-phenyl-1,2,3,6-tetrahydropyridine: Uptake of the metabolite N-methyl-4-phenylpyridine by dopamine neurons explains selective toxicity. *Proc Natl Acad Sci USA* 82:2173–2177, 1985.

147. Ramsay RR, Dadgar J, Trevor A, Singer TP: Energy-driven uptake of N-methyl-4-phenylpyridine by brain mitochondria mediates the neurotoxicity of MPTP. *Life Sci* 39:581–588, 1986.

148. Ramsay RR, Salach JI, Dadgar J, Singer TP: Inhibition of mitochondrial NADH dehydrogenase by pyridine derivatives and its possible relation to experimental and idiopathic parkinsonism. *Biochem Biophys Res Commun* 135:269–75, 1986.

149. Nicklas WJ, Vyas I, Heikkila RE: Inhibition of NADH-linked oxidation in brain mitochondria by 1-methyl-4-phenyl-pyridine, a metabolite of the neurotoxin, 1-methyl-4-phenyl-1,2,5,6-tetrahydropyridine. *Life Sci* 36:2503–2508, 1985.

150. Burkhardt C, Kelly JP, Lim Y-H, et al: Neuroleptic medications inhibit complex I of the electron transport chain. *Ann Neurol* 33:512–517, 1993.

151. Mann VM, Cooper JM, Krige D, Daniel SE, Schapira AH, Marsden CD: Brian, skeletal muscle and platelet homogenate mitochondrial function in Parkinson's disease. *Brain* 115:333–342, 1992.

152. Mizuno Y, Ohta S, Tanaka M, et al: Deficiencies in complex I subunits of the respiratory chain in Parkinson's disease. *Biochem Biophys Res Commun* 163:1450–1455, 1989.

153. Schapira AH, Cooper JM, Dexter D, et al: Mitochondrial complex I deficiency in Parkinson's disease. *Lancet* 1:1269, 1989.

154. Schapira AH, Cooper JM, Dexter D, et al: Mitochondrial complex I deficiency in Parkinson's disease. *J Neurochem* 54:823–827, 1990.

155. Benecke R, Strumper P, Weiss H: Electron transfer complexes I and IV of platelets are abnormal in Parkinson's disease but normal in Parkinson-plus syndromes. *Brain* 116:1451–1463, 1993.

156. Krige D, Carroll MT, Cooper JM, et al: Platelet mitochondrial function in Parkinson's disease: The Royal Kings and Queens Parkinson Disease Research Group. *Ann Neurol* 32:782–788, 1992.

157. Yoshino H, Nakagawa-Hattori Y, Kondo T, Mizuno Y: Mitochondrial complex I and II activities of lymphocytes and platelets in Parkinson's disease. *J Neural Transm* 4:27–34, 1992.

158. Bravi, D., Anderson JJ, Dagani F, et al: Effect of aging and dopaminergic therapy on mitochondrial respiratory function in Parkinson's disease. *Mov Disord* 7:228–231, 1992.

159. Parker WD, Boyson SJ, Parks JK: Abnormalities of the electron transport chain in idiopathic Parkinson's disease. *Ann Neurol* 26:719–23, 1989.

160. Haas RH, Nasirian F, Nakano K, et al: Low platelet mitochondrial complex I and complex II/III activity in early untreated Parkinson's disease. *Ann Neurol* 37:714–722, 1995.

161. Bindoff LA, Birch Machin M, Cartlidge NE, et al: Mitochondrial function in Parkinson's disease. *Lancet* 2:49, 1989.

162. Shoffner JM, Watts RL, Juncos JL, et al: Mitochondrial oxidative phosphorylation defects in Parkinson's disease. *Ann Neurol* 30:332–339, 1991.

163. Mizuno Y, Suzuki K, Ohta S: Postmortem changes in mitochondrial respiratory enzymes in brain and a preliminary observation in Parkinson's disease. *J Neurol Sci* 96:49–57, 1990.

164. Dagani F, Ferrari R, Anderson JJ, Chase TN: L-DOPA does not affect electron transfer chain enzyme and respiration of rat muscle mitochondria. *Mov Disord* 6:315–319, 1991.

165. Przedborski S, Jackson-Lewis V, Muthane U, et al: Chronic L-dopa administration alters cerebral mitochondrial respiratory chain activity. *Ann Neurol* 34:715–723, 1993.

166. Hattori NB, Tanaka M, Ozawa T, Mizuno Y: Immunohistochemical studies on complexes I, II, III, and IV of mitochondria in Parkinson's disease. *Ann Neurol* 30:563–571, 1991.

167. Schapira AHV: Evidence for mitochondrial dysfunction in Parkinson's disease—a critical appraisal. *Mov Disord* 9:125–138, 1994.

168. Cortopassi GA, Hutchin TP: Germline inheritance of a rare mtDNA variant leads to greatly increased risk for Alzheimer's disease. *Am J Hum Genet* 55:A149, 1994.

169. Armstrong M, Daly AK, Cholerton S, et al: Mutant debrisoquine hydroxylation genes in Parkinson's disease. *Lancet* 339:1017–1018, 1992.

170. Smith CA, Gough AC, Leigh PN, et al: Debrisoquine hydroxylase gene polymorphism and susceptibility to Parkinson's disease. *Lancet* 339:1375–1377, 1992.

171. Dugan LL, Choi DW: Excitotoxicity, free radicals, and cell membrane changes. *Ann Neurol* 35:S17–S21, 1994.

172. Beal MF: Does impairment of energy metabolism result in excitotoxic neuronal death in neurodegenerative illnesses? *Ann Neurol* 31:119–130, 1992.

173. Wallace DC, Lott MT, Torroni A, et al: Report of the committee on human mitochondrial DNA, in Cuticchia AJ, Pearson PL (eds): *Human Gene Mapping*. Baltimore: Johns Hopkins University Press, 1994, pp 813–845.

174. Goto Y-I, Nonaka I, Horai S: A new mutation in the tRNA-Leu(UUR) gene associated with mitochondrial myopathy, lactic acidosis, and stroke-like episodes. *Biochim Biophys Acta* 1097:238–240, 1991.

175. Goto Y, Horai S, Matsuoka T, et al: Mitochondrial myopathy, encephalopathy, lactic acidosis, and stroke-like episodes (MELAS). *Neurology* 42:545–550, 1992.

176. Rowland LP: Molecular genetics, pseudogenetics, and clinical neurology. *Neurology* 33:1179–1195, 1983.

177. Van den Ouweland JMW, Lemkes HHPJ, Ruitenbeek W, et al: Mutation in mitochondrial tRNALeu(UUR) gene in a large pedigree with maternally transmitted type II diabetes mellitus and deafness. *Nature Genet* 1:368–371, 1992.

178. Kadowaki T, Kadowaki H, Mori Y, et al: A subtype of diabetes mellitus associated with a mutation of mitochondrial DNA. *N Engl J Med* 330:962–968, 1994.

179. Katagiri H, Asano T, Ishihara H, et al: Mitochondrial diabetes mellitus: Prevalence and clinical characterization of diabetes due to mitochondrial tRNA-Leu(UUR) gene mutation in Japanese patients. *Diabetologia* 37:504–510, 1994.

180. Otabe S, Sakura H, Shimokawa K, et al: The high prevalence of the diabetic patients with a mutation in the mitochondrial gene in Japan. *J Clin Endocrinol Metab* 79:768–771, 1994.

181. Alcolado JC, Majid A, Brockington M, et al: Mitochondrial gene defects in patients with NIDDM. *Diabetologia* 37:372–376, 1994.

182. Van den Ouweland JMW, Lemkes HHPJ, Trembath RC, et al: Maternally inherited diabetes and deafness is a distinct subtype of diabetes and associates with a single point mutation in the mitochondrial tRNA-Leu(UUR) gene. *Diabetes* 43:746–751, 1994.

183. WHO Study Groups: Diabetes mellitus: Report of a WHO Study Group. *World Health Organ Tech Rep Ser* 727:1–113, 1985.

184. Sato W, Hayasaka K, Shoji Y, et al: A mitochondrial tRNA-Leu(UUR) mutation at 3256 associated with mitochondrial myopathy, encephalopathy, lactic acidosis, and stroke-like symptoms. *Biochem Mol Biol Int* 33:1055–1061, 1994.

185. Goto Y-I, Tsugane K, Tanabe Y, et al: A new point mutation at nucleotide pair 3291 of the mitochondrial tRNA-Leu(UUR) gene in a patient with mitochondrial myopathy, encephalopathy, lactic acidosis, and stroke-like episodes (MELAS). *Biochem Biophys Res Commun* 202:1624–1630, 1994.

186. Morten KJ, Cooper JM, Brown GK, et al: A new point mutation associated with mitochondrial encephalomyopathy. *Hum Molec Genet* 2:2081–2087, 1993.

187. Shoffner JM, Bialer MG, Pavlakis SG, et al: Mitochondrial encephalomyopathy caused by a single nucleotide deletion in the mitochondrial tRNA-leucine(UUR) gene. *Neurology* 45:286–292, 1995.

188. Lowenthal A: Striopallidodentate calcifications, in Vinken PJ, Bruyn GW, Klawans HL (eds): *Handbook of Clinical Neurology: Extrapyramidal Disorders*. New York: Elsevier Science Publishers, 1986, pp 417–436.

189. Babbitt DP, Tang TT, Dobbs J, Berk R: Idiopathic familial cerebrovascular ferrocalcinosis (Fahr's disease) and review of differential diagnosis of intracranial calcification in children. *Am J Roentgenol* 105:352–358, 1969.

190. Bonneman CG, Meinecke P, Reich H: Encephalopathy with intracerebral calcification, white matter lesions, growth hormone deficiency, microcephaly, and retinal degeneration: Two sibs confirming a probable district entity. *J Med Genet* 28:708–711, 1991.

191. Kousseff BG: Fahr disease: Report of a family and a review. *Acta Paediat Berg* 33:57–61, 1980.

192. Holt IJ, Cooper JM, Morgan-Hughes JA, Harding AE: Deletions of muscle mitochondrial DNA. *Lancet* 1:1462, 1988.

193. Poulton J, Deadman ME, Gardiner RM: Tandem direct duplications of mitochondrial DNA in mitochondrial myopathy: Analysis of nucleotide sequence and tissue distribution. *Nucleic Acids Res* 17:10223–10229, 1989.

194. Poulton J, Deadman ME, Bindoff L, et al: Families of mtDNA rearrangements can be detected in patients with mtDNA deletions: Duplications may be a transient intermediate form. *Hum Mol Genet* 2:23–30, 1993.

195. Ballinger SW, Shoffner JM, Gebhart S, et al: Mitochondrial diabetes revisited. *Nature Genet* 7:458–459, 1994.

196. Shoffner JM, Lott MT, Voljavec AS, et al: Spontaneous Kearns-Sayre/chronic external ophthalmoplegia plus syndrome associated with a mitochondrial DNA deletion: A slip-replication model and metabolic therapy. *Proc Natl Acad Sci USA* 86:7952–7956, 1989.

197. Moraes CT, Schon EA, DiMauro S, Miranda AF: Heteroplasmy of mitochondrial genomes in clonal cultures from patients with Kearns-Sayre syndrome. *Biochem Biophys Res Commun* 160:765–71, 1989.

198. Holt IJ, Harding AE, Cooper JM, et al: Mitochondrial myopathies: Clinical and biochemical features of 30 patients with major deletions of muscle mitochondrial DNA. *Ann Neurol* 26:699–708, 1989.

199. Moraes CT, DiMauro S, Zeviani M, et al: Mitochondrial DNA deletions in progressive external ophthalmoplegia and Kearns-Sayre syndrome. *N Engl J Med* 320:1293–1299, 1989.

200. Orr HT, Chung M-Y, Banfi S, et al: Expansion of an unstable trinucleotide CAG repeat in spinocerebellar ataxia type 1. *Nat Genet* 4:221–226, 1993.

201. Rifai Z, Welle S, Kamp C, Thornton CA: Ragged red fibers in normal aging and inflammatory myopathy. *Ann Neurol* 37:24–29, 1995.

202. Zheng XX, Shoffner JM, Voljavec AS, Wallace DC: Evaluation of procedures for assaying oxidative phosphorylation enzyme activities in mitochondrial myopathy muscle biopsies. *Biochim Biophys Acta* 1019:1–10, 1990.

203. Matthews PM, Ford B, Dandurand RJ, et al: Coenzyme Q10 with multiple vitamins is generally ineffective in treatment of mitochondrial disease. *Neurology* 43:884–890, 1993.

204. Bresolin N, Doriguzzi C, Ponzetto C, et al: Ubidecarenone in the treatment of mitochondrial myopathies: A multi-center double-blind trial. *J Neurol Sci* 100:70–78, 1990.

205. Trounce IA, Kim YL, Jun AS, Wallace DC: Assessment of mitochondrial oxidative phosphorylation in patient muscle biopsies, lymphoblasts, and transmitochondrial cell lines, in Attardi GM, Chomyn A (eds): *Mitochondrial Biogenesis and Genetics*. San Diego, Academic Press, 1996.

206. Gregoire M, Morais R, Quilliam MA, Gravel D: On auxotrophy for pyrimidines of respiration-deficient chick embryo cells. *Eur J Biochem* 142:49–55, 1984.

207. Chen JJ, Jones ME: The cellular location of dihydroorotate dehydrogenase: Relation to de novo biosynthesis of pyrimidines. *Arch Biochem Biophys* 176:82–90, 1976.

Chapter 5

ANATOMY OF THE BASAL GANGLIA AND RELATED MOTOR STRUCTURES

GARRETT E. ALEXANDER

OVERVIEW OF MOTOR SYSTEM
    Descending and Reentrant Pathways
    Parallel Organization
CORTICAL MOTOR AREAS
    Corticospinal System
    Motor Cortex
    Lateral Premotor Areas
    Supplementary Motor Area
    Cingulate Motor Areas
BASAL GANGLIA ORGANIZATION
    Functional Segregation of Basal Ganglia Circuitry
    Basal Ganglia Skeletomotor Circuit

The basal ganglia have been implicated in a variety of movement disorders, and as such their structure and organization are of interest to those wishing to understand the pathophysiology of these same conditions. However, the basal ganglia cannot be understood in isolation. They are part of a complex, reentrant system that processes information received from widespread parts of cerebral cortex and returns the processed results, by way of the thalamus, to discrete portions of the frontal lobe. The basal ganglia also have some limited downstream projections to brainstem structures, some of which project in turn to spinal levels. Thus, to understand the roles of the basal ganglia in normal motor control and in various types of movement disorders, it is necessary to understand not only the internal organization of these structures but also their relationships with the various cortical and subcortical systems with which they interact.

Overview of Motor System

To place the basal ganglia in perspective, we briefly consider a large-scale overview of how the motor system is organized. The neuronal substrates for many reflexes and basic movement synergies are present at spinal levels, but it is the elaborate system of cortical and subcortical motor circuitry that provides the flexible control over segmental mechanisms necessary for adaptive and skilled motor acts.

DESCENDING AND REENTRANT PATHWAYS

As indicated schematically in Fig. 5-1, the segmental circuitry associated with the motor nuclei of the spinal cord is influenced by two principal categories of descending pathways: those originating from the cerebral cortex and those arising from various brainstem nuclei, many of which are themselves recipients of descending cortical influences. The cortical motor fields, whose descending projections serve, both directly and indirectly, to modulate the output of the segmental motor apparatus, are influenced in turn by other cortical areas (sensory and associative) and by outputs from the basal ganglia and the cerebellum.

These last two stuctures can each be viewed as parallel, *reentrant* processing stations that receive separate, but largely similar, inputs from widespread cortical areas (including motor, premotor, and somatosensory cortex) and return their own respective influences to specific, and largely separate, portions of the precentral motor fields via basal ganglia- and cerebellar-specific connections within the ventrolateral ("motor") thalamus. As indicated in Fig. 5-1, both the basal ganglia and the cerebellum also direct some of their outflow to brain stem descending systems.

PARALLEL ORGANIZATION

The parallel organization of the motor system is noteworthy. As discussed in more detail below, we now know that there are at least six separate cortical motor fields in the primate brain, all of which contribute both to the descending and to the reentrant pathways depicted in Fig. 5-1. The basal ganglia are clearly organized for parallel processing, with multiple functionally segregated channels passing through each of the constituent nuclei. And it has long been known that the cerebellum is organized along parallel lines. Although we will not consider the cerebellar circuits any further in the present chapter, it is worth emphasizing that the parallel features of cerebellar architecture are at least as impressive as those of the basal ganglia.[1,2] For example, the "vestibular/oculomotor," "spinal," and "cerebral" subdivisions of cerebellar cortex (so designated because of their characteristic inputs) each project their separate outputs through corresponding functional channels via the cerebellar output nuclei. And these functional subdivisions are maintained along the reentrant, cerebellothalamic pathways as well (see Chap. 44).

Cortical Motor Areas

All of the known motor fields are contained within the frontal lobes. In nonhuman primates, at least six discrete motor areas have been identified thus far. In addition to primary motor cortex (Brodmann's area 4), there are five nonprimary motor fields or "premotor" areas, two on the lateral convexity and three within the medial wall of the hemisphere. In man, it is still common to distinguish only two premotor areas, the lateral premotor cortex lying immediately rostral to the primary motor cortex and the supplementary motor area on the medial surface of the hemisphere. There is now evidence, however, that a third (and possibly a fourth) premotor area can also be distinguished within human cingulate cortex. From the available evidence, it would seem likely that the functional organization of the premotor fields will prove to

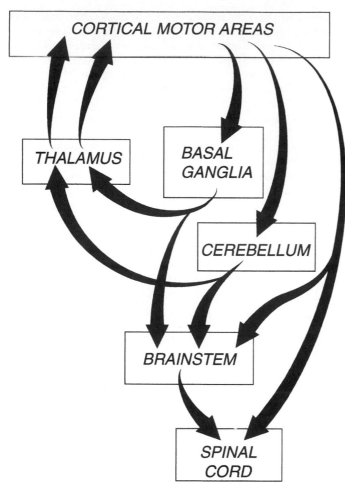

FIGURE 5-1 Schematic illustration of the principal relationships among the major components of the motor system. Note that the basal ganglia and cerebellum may be viewed as key elements in two parallel reentrant systems that return their influences to cortex through discrete and separate portions of the ventrolateral thalamus. This figure also emphasizes the parallel projections of the cerebral cortex to multiple levels of the motor system.

be similar in humans and nonhuman primates, although there are obvious limitations on the precision with which such questions can be addressed directly in human subjects.

The locations of the known motor fields in the monkey are indicated in Fig. 5-2. On the lateral surface of the hemisphere are the primary motor cortex (MC) and the dorsal (PMd) and ventral (PMv) premotor areas. Within the medial wall of the hemisphere are the supplementary motor area (SMA) and the rostral (CMAr) and caudal (CMAc) cingulate motor areas. Each of the five nonprimary motor areas is connected reciprocally to MC, and like MC they each contain complete somatotopic maps.[3-9] All six precentral motor fields also share other important characteristics. Each is reciprocally connected with a portion of the motor thalamus, each receives a characteristic set of inputs from the parietal lobe, and each sends substantial projections both to the basal ganglia and to the cerebellum.[10-13] And though tradition has led

us to think of MC as being "primary" among motor areas, there is abundant evidence that this cortical area is not alone in having direct, descending projections to the segmental motor apparatus.

CORTICOSPINAL SYSTEM

All six of the cortical motor fields send direct projections to the ventral horn of the spinal cord at both cervical and lumbar levels.[3,5,8,14,15] These projections are glutamatergic[16] and excitatory, although they facilitate both inhibitory and excitatory circuitry at spinal levels.

In the human, approximately one million corticospinal fibers pass through each medullary pyramid, compared with about 250,000 in the monkey.[17] Comparative studies indicate that the corticospinal projections have emerged and been selectively strengthened in various species (especially primates) roughly in accordance with an increasing capacity for the execution of movements that are highly fractionated (that is, in which closely approximated structures, such as

FIGURE 5-2 Locations of the six known precentral motor fields in the monkey. Also indicated is the pre-SMA, which has recently been differentiated from the SMA proper. MC, primary motor cortex; CMAc, caudal cingulate motor area; CMAr, rostral cingulate motor area; PMd, dorsal premotor area; PMv, ventral premotor area; pre-SMA, presupplementary motor area; SMA, supplementary motor area. The arcuate, central, and cingulate sucli have been opened, with their respective boundaries indicated by broken lines and their fundi shown as solid lines.

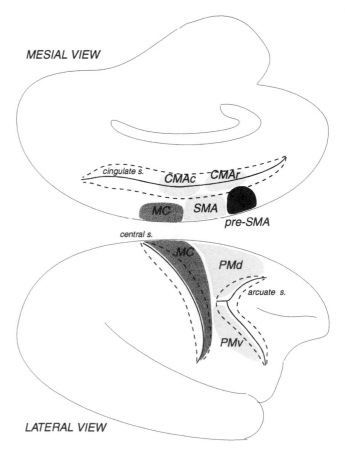

fingers, are moved in relative independence).[18,19] Selective lesions of the corticospinal pathway lead to the specific loss of ability to perform movements of this type. But the capacity for making fractionated movements is not based on simple point-to-point mappings of corticomotoneurons onto spinal motoneurons in the fashion of a telephone switchboard. Instead, there is substantial convergence and divergence of connections between these two sets of neurons.

Thus, for example, injections of individual corticospinal axons with anatomic tracers have shown that each axon can give rise to a surprisingly large number of terminal branches that diverge to innervate multiple separate spinal motor nuclei.[20] And, conversely, the ventral horn at a given level of the spinal cord receives somatotopically specific corticospinal inputs from several different cortical motor fields.[12,21] Studies using spike-triggered averaging (in which the action potentials of individual corticomotoneurons are correlated with rectified EMG activity recorded from a number of different muscles) have shown that most corticospinal neurons appear to have direct, presumably monosynaptic connections with more than one motoneuron.[22,23] In most cases, the "muscle field" of a given cortical neuron is restricted to a relatively small number of functionally related muscles (generally two to three), and the amount of facilitation (or suppression) provided to each muscle is usually different.[24] In some cases, individual corticospinal neurons have been shown to exert reciprocal effects on muscles that are functional antagonists (e.g., flexors versus extensors of a finger),[25] and thus far there have been no reports of neurons that provide postspike facilitation to both agonists and antagonists of the same joint. The relative weakness of the postspike EMG facilitation that is associated with the activity of any single corticospinal neuron suggests that convergent input from many such cells is necessary in order for EMG activity to be initiated in a given motor unit.[23,24] In fact, anatomic studies suggest that while each spinal motoneuron may receive up to several thousand synapses in all, it is unlikely to receive more than one synaptic contact from any single corticospinal axon. Corticospinal neurons that influence a particular muscle are often clustered together, but their individual motor fields may differ significantly from one another (i.e., although all of the cells within a cluster may influence a single muscle in common, they may each provide additional facilitation to differing sets of functionally related muscles).[24]

How, then, can somatotopic specificity and the capacity for fractionated movements be explained in the face of the striking convergence and divergence of descending corticospinal projections from the various cortical motor fields? The answer to this question is not yet known with any certainty. However, evidence from other systems would suggest that much of the gross topography/somatotopy within the motor system may be genetically determined, while the fine-tuning (e.g., in terms of the response properties of individual neurons) may depend significantly upon experience and associated activity-dependent changes in local synaptic strengths. Convergent corticospinal inputs to a given motor unit might be differentially strengthened (or weakened) by experience according to activity-dependent synaptic learning rules. As discussed below in connection with the basal ganglia, such processes could lead to the coordination of functionally related but spatially distributed corticospinal neurons, or clusters of such neurons, and thereby account for movement fractionation despite the absence of one-to-one mapping between cortical and spinal motoneurons.

MOTOR CORTEX

Primary motor cortex, MC, is coextensive with Brodmann's area 4, the agranular cortex within and immediately rostral to the anterior bank of the central sulcus that contains giant layer V pyramidal neurons. Given the massive contribution of MC to the corticospinal tract, it is not surprising that the functions of this area are often viewed in terms of its contribution to this pathway, especially as reflected by the motor deficits that result from corticospinal lesions. A more direct and positive indication of the functions of the MC has been obtained in studies of the activity of MC pyramidal tract neurons (PTNs) in the behaving primate.[26] MC PTNs have been shown to discharge prior to the onset of muscular activity and to have properties similar in many respects to those of spinal alpha-motoneurons, with patterns of discharge that are highly correlated with force and with the length/tension properties of muscles. The PTNs also exhibit rate modulation in relation to increasing force and are recruited in an orderly manner in relation to size. A direct action of PTNs on alpha-motoneurons has been demonstrated by spike-triggered averaging techniques.[27]

Although the functions of the MC are partially reflected by the actions of its PTNs and the deficits resulting from lesions of the corticospinal tract, the role of the MC in motor control is clearly not limited to its corticospinal output. The MC also contributes substantial projections to each of the premotor areas and to several somatosensory areas (including areas 3a, 1, 2, and 5), as well as to the ventrolateral thalamus (VPLo, VLo, VLc), basal ganglia (putamen), and cerebellum (via the various precerebellar nuclei). These additional outputs presumably serve to inform the target areas of the "intended" movement ("corollary discharge") and to exert some influence over the outputs from these areas. Evidence in monkeys suggests that these noncorticospinal projections from the MC are derived largely from separate populations of non-PTNs, rather than from PTN collaterals.[28]

Functional analyses of the cortical motor fields in humans have been facilitated by imaging techniques that permit assessments of regional cerebral blood flow (rCBF) and regional oxidative metabolism and by electrical recordings of event-related cerebral potentials. During voluntary movements of a limb, focal increases in cerebral blood flow are seen within the contralateral MC and within the SMA, usually on both sides.[29-34] During the planning or preparation for a movement that is merely rehearsed but not executed, increases in blood flow are seen within the SMA and within premotor cortex on the lateral surface of the hemisphere but not within MC.[35]

Studies of event-related potentials in humans[36,37] suggest that early during the preparation for a voluntary movement (several hundred milliseconds before EMG onset) both MC and the SMA become active bilaterally, giving rise to the slow negative potential referred to as the "readiness potential" or Bereitschaftspotential (BP). In scalp recordings the BP is centered over the vertex,[36,38] but in subdural recordings it has been shown to arise from discrete foci within MC and the SMA.[37] The BP appears to be associated only with self-initiated movements and reportedly is not observed in movements that are triggered by external stimuli.[39] Following the BP, and approximately 250–400 ms before EMG onset, a second potential can be discerned, the so-called "negative slope" (NS). In scalp recordings the NS is centered over the contralateral centroparietal region,[38] but in subdural recordings it has been found to arise from separate foci within the SMA and contralateral MC.[37] Both the BP and the NS are reduced in amplitude in patients with unilateral lesions of prefrontal cortex.[40] The NS also appears to depend on input from the lateral parietal cortex (Brodmann's areas 7, 39, and 40).[41]

Following the NS is another, steeper, negative potential, the motor potential (MP), which begins shortly (50–100 ms) before EMG onset and continues (in the form of several subsets of potentials) throughout the movement. In both scalp and subdural recordings the various components of the MP appear to arise exclusively from the contralateral MC and somatosensory cortices.[36–38]

Although the techniques available for functional studies in humans do not have the spatial or temporal resolution of the single cell recording techniques that have been used to study motor physiology in behaving monkeys, the two approaches have yielded results that are largely congruent. Thus, for example, during the preparation for movement, much higher proportions of neurons become active in the lateral premotor areas and the SMA than in the MC, while the reverse is seen during movement execution.[42–44]

LATERAL PREMOTOR AREAS

The concept of a premotor cortex that could be structurally and functionally differentiated from primary MC was first articulated in a systematic way by Fulton more than half a century ago. Until relatively recently, the premotor cortex was thought to consist of a single, homogeneous region that was more or less coextensive with the expanse of agranular cortex (Brodmann's area 6) lying immediately rostral to the MC on the lateral surface of the hemisphere. Based on studies in the monkey, we now recognize at least two subdivisions of this region, the dorsal premotor area, PMd, and the ventral premotor area, PMv. Each contains a complete somatotopic map, and each projects strongly to spinal levels.[4,21,45,46]

Single cell recording studies in monkeys have shown that the PMd contains large numbers of neurons that discharge selectively during the preparation of goal-directed limb movements.[47–52] Neurons in PMv show preferential activation in association with visually guided limb movements, and lesions of this region have consistently resulted in impairments in visually guided reaching.[6,53,54]

Clinical and experimental studies in humans have suggested several roles for the premotor cortex of the lateral convexity, without distinguishing between dorsal and ventral subfields. One such role is the control of proximal limb musculature and interlimb coordination.[55–58] This is consistent with the anatomic evidence indicating heavy projections from this region to the medial pontomedullary reticular formation, whose spinal projections constitute the bulk of the ventromedial descending brain stem system that is associated with control of the proximal musculature.[59] Not only do patients with premotor lesions manifest proximal weakness (of shoulder and/or hip musculature), their apraxic deficits also seem confined mainly to movements involving proximal musculature. Thus, such patients may have difficulty making coordinated rotatory movements of both shoulders (though independent movements of either shoulder are performed with ease, within the limits of any associated proximal weakness).[58] Such proximal limb-kinetic apraxia contrasts sharply with the bimanual—i.e., distal—apraxic deficits associated with lesions of the SMA.

Studies in humans have shown maximal increases in rCBF in lateral premotor areas during voluntary movements that require sensory guidance.[35] Patients with premotor lesions have been shown to have specific impairments in using sensory cues (visual, auditory, or tactile) to recall previously learned movements, although they have no difficulty in retrieving the same movements on the basis of spatial cues.[60] Such observations have led to suggestions that the lateral premotor cortex may function as a higher motor association area. This is consistent with studies of the preparatory discharges of monkey PMd neurons, which appear to encode salient task contingencies that the subject must take into account in planning an appropriate motor response.[49,50] Premotor lesions of the dominant hemisphere are associated with motor dysgraphia and/or motor dysphasia.[61] In a recent study it was found that lateral as well as medial premotor areas show preferential increases in rCBF during motor tasks that require the subject to select among several possible arm movements.[62] These and other findings have prompted the suggestion that human lateral premotor cortex must play an important role in the preparation for movement,[63] a suggestion that is strongly supported by chronic neurophysiological studies in awake, behaving monkeys.

SUPPLEMENTARY MOTOR AREA

Penfield and Welch coined the term "supplementary motor area" for the agranular cortex of area 6 that lies within the medial wall of the hemisphere, from which complex movements could be evoked by electrical stimulation both in humans and in subhuman primates. Since those initial studies, the SMA had been considered until recently to be coextensive with the entire expanse of mesial area 6. However, there is now general agreement that the most rostral portion, the newly designated pre-SMA, should be distinguished from the SMA proper because the former lacks direct connections with the MC, lacks direct projections to spinal levels, and (unlike the SMA) receives direct input from the dorsolateral prefrontal cortex.[64,65] Thus, although neurons in the pre-SMA show clear involvement in the preparation and execution of limb movements,[44,65,66] this portion of area 6 should no longer be considered a premotor area in the strictest sense of having direct connections with the MC and with the segmental motor apparatus.[4] Nevertheless, the SMA and the pre-SMA do share strong, reciprocal connections with each other, indicating that the pre-SMA is likely to play a significant role in high level motor control.

The SMA receives inputs from widely distributed areas of the cerebral cortex, particularly from frontal and parietal regions (areas 2, 5, and 7b). The latter regions are likely to be involved in the tactile guidance of exploratory limb movements. Some of these corticocortical connections may also play a role in the modulation of transcortical reflexes by the SMA. Studies in the monkey suggest that projections from SMA to MC may have an inhibitory effect on MC neuronal responses to spinal inputs[55] (but see also the negative results of Ref. 67). The release of this inhibitory control over MC output in response to somatosensory input may explain why lesions of the SMA are frequently associated with involuntary grasping of objects which come into contact with the hand.[55,68]

A further perspective on the role of the SMA in controlling voluntary movements has been suggested by reports that SMA lesions in humans may lead to a severe poverty of movement (akinesia) and mutism.[69–71] It is noteworthy in this regard that a major output of the basal ganglia is directed (via the thalamus) to the SMA. It remains uncertain, however, whether the akinesia and mutism reported after lesions involving the SMA can be explained simply in terms of the loss of basal ganglia influences on the cerebral cortex. A role of the SMA in speech production, suggested by the lesion reports, is also supported by data from functional imaging studies[72] and from reports of vocalization and speech arrest induced by electrical stimulation of this region in humans.[73,74]

Participation of the SMA in complex motor functions is supported by single-cell recordings in the SMA of monkeys, which have revealed changes in neuronal activity related not only to movement execution but also to the preparation for movement and motor set.[43,44,75,76] Many SMA neurons show selective, sustained activation following an instruction that permits the subject to prepare for an upcoming movement and then cease firing as the movement begins. Such findings are consistent with the results of human studies of event-related potentials (BP, see above)[36 38] and local cerebral blood flow[62,77] that have implicated the SMA in neural processes underlying the preparation for movement. What has yet to be determined is precisely how the lateral and medial premotor areas differ in respect to their respective contributions to the processes underlying movement preparation.

Lesions of the SMA are associated with impaired control of bimanual movements both in humans and monkeys.[78,79] This may be related to the fact that even unilateral limb movements tend to result in bilateral activation of the SMA. Nevertheless, in single-cell recording studies in monkeys the large majority of SMA neurons show restricted, contralateral sensorimotor fields, and microstimulation of the SMA results in focal movements of contralateral body parts (in accordance with a clearly evident somatotopy).[15,44,80–83] However, a recent study has shown that the SMA—but not MC—also contains a select population of neurons that discharge exclusively during coordinated, bilateral movements of the digits and not during movements of either hand by itself.[84] Taken together, these findings suggest that the SMA may play a special role in the coordination of movements involving both sides of the body.

The SMA has also been implicated recently in the control of sequential movements. Lesions of this area in monkeys appear to interfere with the capacity to learn or reproduce remembered sequences of movements.[54] Single-cell recordings have shown that neurons in the SMA, but not in MC, discharge selectively during or in anticipation of a particular sequence of movements (and not in relation to the same components executed in a different sequence).[85] And functional imaging studies in humans have shown changes in rCBF in the region of the SMA associated with the learning of motor sequences.[86]

CINGULATE MOTOR AREAS

The cingulate motor areas have come to be recognized as such only relatively recently. In monkeys, at least two can be identified within the cingulate sulcus, CMAr in Brodmann's area 23c and CMAc in area 24c.[5,8,87] Both of these premotor fields project directly to the spinal cord and to the basal ganglia.[3,5] CMAr receives strong connections from the dorsolateral prefrontal cortex and from the pre-SMA.[64,88–90]

A recent study of neuronal activity in the cingulate motor areas of the monkey demonstrated movement-related neurons in CMAr and in CMAc, with the caudal area containing a higher proportion of neurons discharging selectively in relation to self-initiated rather than stimulus-triggered movements.[87] One or both of these areas may correspond to the gigantopyramidal field within the depths of the cingulate sulcus of humans.[91] Electrical stimulation of this region has been shown to evoke complex motor responses in man.[92] Studies of regional cerebral blood flow in human subjects show that cortex within the cingulate sulcus is activated in association with various complex motor tasks.[62,93]

Basal Ganglia Organization

The basal ganglia consist of the striatum (comprising the putamen and caudate nucleus, which together constitute the neostriatum, and the ventral striatum—also known as the limbic striatum), the globus pallidus, the substantia nigra, and the subthalamic nucleus. Each of these nuclei has distinct functional subdivisions that may include skeletomotor, oculomotor, associative, and/or limbic territories. The functional subdivisions are differentiated on the basis of their respective physiological properties and their interconnections with cortical and thalamic territories of the same functionalities.[94] As a consequence of this organization, the basal ganglia can be viewed as components among a family of reentrant loops that are organized in parallel, each taking its origin from a particular set of functionally related cortical fields (skeletomotor, oculomotor, etc.), passing through the functionally corresponding portions of the basal ganglia and returning to parts of those same cortical fields by way of specific basal ganglia-recipient zones in the dorsal thalamus. This scheme is depicted schematically in Fig. 5-3.

FUNCTIONAL SEGREGATION OF BASAL GANGLIA CIRCUITRY

The skeletomotor circuit, which we shall consider in more detail below, takes its origin from the cortical motor and premotor fields of the frontal lobe and from various somatosensory fields within the parietal lobe. The striatal portion of the circuit lies mainly within the putamen. The oculomotor circuit originates within the frontal and supplementary eye fields, with the striatal component lying within the body of

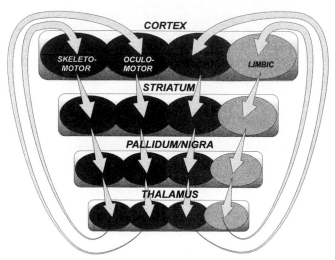

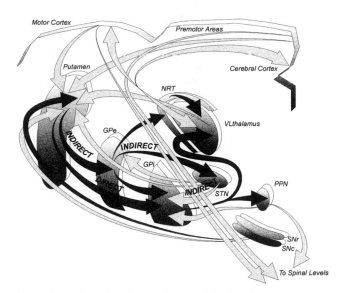

FIGURE 5-3 Parallel, functionally segregated basal ganglia-thalamocortical loops. Each of these partially closed reentrant pathways engages a separate portion of cortex, basal ganglia, and thalamus. See text for details.

the caudate nucleus. The associative circuits take their origin from the dorsolateral prefrontal cortex and from the orbitofrontal cortex, and their striatal components lie principally within the head of the caudate nucleus. The limbic circuit arises from the anterior cingulate cortex (rostral to the cingulate motor areas), with the striatal and pallidal components lying uniquely within the ventral striatum and the ventral pallidum. The basis for these functional demarcations is reviewed in more detail in Ref. 94.

Due to maintained segregation along each of these corticobasal ganglia-thalamocortical circuits, there is little direct communication among the separate functional domains, except by way of corticocortical interactions. Although virtually the entire cortical mantle is mapped topographically onto the striatum, often considered the "input" portion of the basal ganglia, the cortically directed signals from the basal ganglia output nuclei (internal pallidum and substantia nigra pars reticulata) are returned exclusively to foci within the frontal lobe (after first passing through the corresponding portions of the thalamus). Because of their parallel organization, it is generally suspected that the operations performed at corresponding stations along each of these loops are quite similar.

BASAL GANGLIA SKELETOMOTOR CIRCUIT

The skeletomotor and oculomotor circuits have been studied in most detail, both anatomically and physiologically. Because of its special relevance for movement disorders, the skeletomotor circuit will be the principal focus of the remaining discussion. The major components of this circuit are depicted in Fig. 5-4.

PUTAMEN

Like the cerebellum, the basal ganglia receive prominent input from most of the sensorimotor territories of the cerebral cortex, including primary and secondary somatosensory areas, MC, and each of the five premotor areas.[4,95–103] As noted, the striatum serves as the input nucleus for the basal ganglia.

FIGURE 5-4 Functional organizaton of the basal ganglia skeletomotor circuit. The direct and indirect pathways through the basal ganglia are indicated. Excitatory pathways are indicated by light shading, inhibitory by dark shading. Connections between thalamus and cortex are reciprocal. Connections to and from SNr (which parallel those of GPi) are not shown. A further simplification shows the thalamostriate projection arising from VL thalamus rather than from the centromedian nucleus. GPe, external segment of globus pallidus; GPi, internal segment; NRT, thalamic reticular nucleus; PPN, pedunculopontine nucleus; SNc, substantia nigra pars compacta; SNr, pars reticulata; STN, subthalamic nucleus; VL thalamus, ventrolateral thalamus.

The coordinated topography of corticostriatal input imposes a well-defined somatotopic organization on the target nucleus for sensorimotor inputs, which for primates coincides roughly with the putamen.[75,104,105] The majority of the putamen-projecting sensorimotor areas also sends topographic projections to the subthalamic nucleus.[106] Both the corticostriatal and the corticosubthalamic projections are excitatory and, probably, glutamatergic.[107–110]

In the putamen, as in the rest of the striatum, the large majority of neurons (>75 percent in primates, up to 95 percent in rodents) are of the medium spiny type (MSN).[111] MSNs are GABA (gamma-aminobutyric acid)-ergic projection neurons,[112] and in primates they comprise two distinct populations, one projecting to the external segment of the globus pallidus (GPe) and the other projecting either to the internal segment of the globus pallidus (GPi) or to the substantia nigra pars reticulata (SNr).[113,114] At rest, putamen projection neurons are nearly silent,[115,116] but most have well-defined sensorimotor fields and discharge selectively in relation to specific parameters of movement or specific aspects of the preparation for movement.[44,66,75,117,118]

The other type of putamen neuron that has been well studied is the large, aspiny interneuron.[119,120] Unlike MSNs, the large interneurons are spontaneously active (with discharge rates of 3–7 Hz), and they do not discharge in relation to specific parameters of movement preparation or execution. Rather, they discharge briefly (only one or two spikes) and synchronously after the presentation of a conditioned sensory stimulus that signifies the imminent delivery of a reward.[121] In this respect, their behavior is similar to that of dopamine neurons (see below). The spontaneously active interneurons appear to be cholinergic,[122] but their synaptic influence on neighboring MSNs has not been directly determined. Electron microscopic studies have shown that cholinergic synapses on the somata and dendritic shafts and spines of MSNs are of the symmetrical type,[123] which suggests that the aspiny interneurons may have an inhibitory effect on MSNs.

INTERNAL PALLIDUM AND SUBSTANTIA NIGRA PARS RETICULATA

Those portions of GPi and SNr that receive input from the putamen constitute the sensorimotor output nuclei of the basal ganglia, sending GABAergic projections to their respective targets in both the ventrolateral thalamus (n. ventralis lateralis and n. ventralis anterior) and the centromedian nucleus of the thalamus.[124–130] Anatomically, GPi and SNr share many common features, and from a functional standpoint they can be viewed as two subdivisions of a single basal ganglia output nucleus.[131,132] Neurons in the sensorimotor territories of GPi/SNr have movement-related receptive fields that are similar to those of the putamen's MSNs, but GPi/SNr neurons differ from MSNs in that they have relatively high spontaneous discharge rates (60–80 Hz) that are modulated both upward and downward, depending on their particular sensorimotor response fields.[133–135] Neurons in the sensorimotor territory of GPe have discharge properties and sensorimotor fields that are comparable to those in GPi/SNr.[133]

EXTERNAL PALLIDUM AND SUBTHALAMIC NUCLEUS

The basal ganglia output nuclei (GPi/SNr) receive not only *direct* input from the striatum via the GPi- and SNr-projecting MSNs but also an important converging source of information via what has come to be termed the *indirect* pathway through the basal ganglia.[136] The direct and indirect pathways are illustrated in Fig. 5-4. The indirect pathway takes its origin from the GPe-projecting MSNs. In turn, the GABAergic neurons of GPe project mainly to the subthalamic nucleus,[137] whose excitatory glutamatergic neurons send feedforward connections to GPi/SNr, completing one arm of the indirect pathway.[138–140] Subthalamic neurons also send glutamatergic feedback connections to GPe and to the putamen.[139,141,142]

Recently, a second arm of the indirect pathway has been revealed: GPe projects not only to the subthalamic nucleus but also to the output nuclei, GPi/SNr.[143,144] A remarkable consequence of this is that activation of MSNs associated with either arm of the *indirect pathway* should *increase* basal ganglia output by increasing neuronal activity at the level of GPi/SNr: in one case, by disinhibiting the subthalamic nucleus with its excitatory projections to GPi/SNr; in the other, by directly disinhibiting GPi/SNr. In contrast, activation of MSNs associated with the *direct pathway* should *decrease* basal ganglia output by directly suppressing activity at the level of GPi/SNr. Given the reentrant nature of basal ganglia-thalamocortical connections, cortically initiated activation of the direct pathway might therefore be expected to result in positive feedback at cortical levels, with corresponding activation of the indirect pathway giving rise, conversely, to negative feedback.

GPe sends an inhibitory, feedforward projection to the nucleus reticularis of the thalamus (NRT),[145] which in turn imposes a robust, GABAergic modulation on the basal ganglia-recipient nuclei of the ventrolateral thalamus.[146] There appears to be a functional consistency among the various GPe projections, in that cortically induced activations of GPe-projecting MSNs should have the net effect of producing negative feedback at cortical levels, based on the functional effects of each of the known GPe projections—including both arms of the indirect pathway and the GPe projections to the NRT.

On the other hand, the role of the NRT in basal ganglia operations may be much more complicated. It is generally accepted that the NRT plays an important role in gating thalamocortical transmission from the dorsal thalamus, and that it does so in a roughly topographic manner that links specific portions of the NRT with specific thalamic nuclei and their cortical target zones.[146] The NRT receives collateral excitatory inputs from corticothalamic as well as thalamocortical fibers that must pass through this nucleus en route to their respective termination zones in cortex and thalamus. In addition, the NRT may also receive collateral input[147] from both the inhibitory pallidothalamic pathway[124,148] and the excitatory thalamostriate projections.[149]

PEDUNCULOPONTINE NUCLEUS

While the pedunculopontine nucleus (PPN) is not generally considered to be part of the basal ganglia, this structure has strong, reciprocal connections with the basal ganglia output nuclei and with the subthalamic nucleus, and it also sends unreciprocated projections to the dopaminergic neurons of the substantia nigra pars compacta (SNc; see below), as well as to the putamen and caudate nucleus.[128,129,137,142,150–153] In primates, the majority of pallidal inputs to the PPN are apparently collaterals of pallidothalamic projections.[141,151,152] The PPN contains two populations of neurons, one cholinergic and the other noncholinergic.[154] It is mainly the noncholinergic neurons that project back to GPi/SNr and the subthalamic nucleus,[154,155] whereas the cholinergic neurons project primarily to the thalamus.[156,157] The noncholinergic neurons have excitatory effects on their basal ganglia targets,[158–160] and there is some evidence that they may use glutamate as their transmitter.[161]

As with GPi/SNr, there is a convergence of inputs from both the direct and indirect pathways at the level of the PPN. In this case, however, activation of either pathway at the level of the MSNs leads to the same polarity of response within the PPN (that is, activation of PPN by disinhibited subthalamic inputs, or direct disinhibition of PPN by inputs from GPe or from GPi/SNr).

Until recently, descending projections of the basal ganglia output nuclei have received relatively little attention, it having been generally assumed that directly descending basal ganglia influences on the skeletomotor system extended no further caudally than the PPN. Studies in rats, however, have also revealed substantial PPN outflow to the reticulospinal system.[162,163] These findings have not yet been extended to primates.

FUNCTIONAL SEGREGATION OF PATHWAYS

One of the remarkable features of basal ganglia circuitry is that functionally discrete channels of information processing are maintained throughout the various corticobasal ganglia-thalamocortical pathways[164-166] in the face of layer-to-layer connectivity that is highly convergent.[111,167] In the case of the skeletomotor pathways, for example, basal ganglia neurons have been shown to have highly refined sensorimotor fields that are comparable in their somatotopic and behavioral specificity to the sensorimotor fields of neurons at cortical levels.[44,168-170]

Recent anatomic studies using transneuronal tracers have revealed at least three separate channels of arm representation that extend continuously throughout the basal ganglia-thalamocortical pathways.[95] Each channel originates in a separate cortical motor area (MC, PMv, or SMA) and remains segregated from the others throughout the entire corticobasal ganglia-thalamocortical loop.

On the other hand, at the cellular level there is considerable convergence of inputs along these same pathways. Based on electron microscopic analyses, it has been estimated that the convergence ratio along the corticostriatal pathways, which provide approximately half of the excitatory input to the neostriatum, may be on the order of 5000:1. Cell counts in the human striatum and globus pallidus[171,172] suggest minimum convergence ratios on the order of 300:1 and 100:1, respectively, for the striatal projections to GPe and GPi.

The mechanisms that underlie the development and maintenance of functional specificity in basal ganglia networks (despite the abundant anatomic convergence) have yet to be identified. Much of this organization may be genetically determined, but experience-dependent synaptic modification may also play a role. If synaptic plasticity in basal ganglia networks operates according to principles of Hebbian learning,[173] and there is some evidence that this may be the case (see below), the correlative nature of this type of learning might well be expected to strengthen preferentially those connections that link neurons with similar functional properties.[174]

DOPAMINE AND THE SUBSTANTIA NIGRA PARS COMPACTA

Another important feature of basal ganglia organization is the pervasive role of dopamine. The functionality of dopamine in basal ganglia operations appears to be very complex. Dopaminergic input to the putamen consists of nigrostriatal projections that originate in the substantia nigra pars compacta (SNc),[141] and the cortical motor and premotor areas receive separate dopaminergic projections from the ventral tegmental area.[175-177] At the network level, dopamine appears to have differential effects on the direct and indirect pathways, tending to activate striatal MSNs that project directly to GPi while suppressing those that project to GPe.[136] Given the fact that there appear to be reciprocal reentrant effects associated with differential activation of the direct versus indirect pathways (i.e., positive feedback to cortex via the direct pathway and negative feedback via the indirect: see above), the differential effects of dopamine on these two pathways suggest that its overall impact on basal ganglia operations may include the enhancement of positive feed-

back, and suppression of negative feedback, returned to the various cortical areas that receive basal ganglia influences.

Dopamine has also been shown to have a role in synaptic plasticity within the striatum, being implicated in both long-term potentiation (LTP) and long-term depression (LTD).[178-180] The nigrostriatal pathway provides an extraordinarily dense dopaminergic input to each MSN, which is comparable in magnitude to the 5,000 or so corticostriatal synapses that individual MSNs receive.[181] The behavioral correlates of dopamine neurons have been studied in considerable depth.[182,183] Unlike nearly all the other basal ganglia motor circuit neurons, except perhaps the large, aspiny interneurons of the striatum,[115,121] dopamine neurons do not show activity changes in relation to movement per se but discharge instead in relation to conditions involving the probability and imminence of behavioral reinforcement.[182,183]

The newly discovered facts that dopamine may play a crucial role in the cellular mechanisms of LTD and LTP within the striatum and that dopamine neurons discharge selectively in relation to specific reward contingencies combine to suggest the intriguing hypothesis that dopamine neurons may play an important role in determining when striatal synapses should be strengthened or weakened. In this respect, dopamine neurons might be seen as playing a role in striatal information processing analogous to that played by an "adaptive critic" in certain types of connectionist networks that are capable of autonomous learning.[184]

It is noteworthy, however, that the striatum is not the only basal ganglia structure for which there is evidence of adaptive synapses. With their combined voltage dependency and ligand specificity, N-methyl-D-aspartate (NMDA) receptors are widely assumed to play a role in at least one form of activity-dependent synaptic plasticity, namely LTP.[185] Evidence for the existence of NMDA receptors has been found in a number of basal ganglia nuclei that are believed to receive significant glutamatergic input, including the striatum (putamen and caudate nucleus),[108,119,186] the subthalamic nucleus,[107,186] and the SNc.[187] NMDA receptors have also been demonstrated at cortical levels,[186,188,189] where the phenomenon of LTP has been documented in many regions including some of the sensorimotor fields.[190-193] Taken together, these findings indicate that adaptive synapses may be distributed at multiple junctures along the basal ganglia-thalamocortical pathways.

Acknowledgments

This chapter was made possible by support from the National Institutes of Health (NS-17678 and NS-31937) and from the Office of Naval Research (N00014-92-J-1132).

References

1. Brooks VB, Thach WT: Cerebellar control of posture and movement, in Brookhart JM, Mountcastle VB, Brooks VB (eds): *Handbook of Physiology. The Nervous System:* Motor Control. Bethesda, MD: American Physiological Society, 1981, sect 1, vol 2, part 1, pp 877–946.
2. Ito M: *The Cerebellum and Neural Control.* New York: Raven Press, 1984.

3. Hutchins KD, Martino AM, Strick PL: Corticospinal projections from the medial wall of the hemisphere. *Exp Brain Res* 715:667–672, 1988.

4. Dum RP, Strick PL: The origin of corticospinal projections from premotor areas in the frontal lobe. *J Neurosci* 11:667–689, 1991.

5. He S-Q, Dum RP, Strick PS: Topographic organization of corticospinal projections from the frontal lobe: Motor areas on the medial surface of the hemisphere. *J Neurosci.* 15:3284–3306, 1995.

6. Gentilucci M, Fogassi L, Luppino G, et al: Functional organization of inferior area 6 in the macaque monkey I. Somatotopy and the control of proximal movements. *Exp Brain Res* 71:475–490, 1988.

7. Rizzolatti G, Camarda R, Fogassi L, et al: Functional organization of inferior area 6 in the macaque monkey II. Area F5 and the control of distal movements. *Exp Brain Res* 71:491–507, 1988.

8. Luppino G, Matelli M, Camarda R, et al: Corticospinal projections from mesial frontal and cingulate areas in the monkey. *Neuroreport* 5:2545–2548, 1994.

9. Matelli M, Camarda R, Glickstein M, et al: Afferent and efferent projections of the inferior area 6 in the macaque monkey. *J Comp Neurol* 251:281–298, 1986.

10. Matelli M, Luppino G, Fogassi L, et al: Thalamic input to inferior area 6 and area 4 in the macaque monkey. *J Comp Neurol* 280:468–488, 1989.

11. Schell GR, Strick PL: The origin of thalamic inputs to the arcuate premotor and supplementary motor areas. *J Neurosci* 4:539–560, 1984.

12. Dum RP, Strick PL: Premotor areas: Nodal points for parallel efferent systems involved in the central control of movement, in Humphrey DR, Freund H-J (eds): *Motor Control: Concepts and Issues.* New York: John Wiley & Sons, 1991, pp 383–397.

13. Holsapple JW, Preston JB, Strick PL: The origin of thalamic inputs to the 'hand' representation in the primary motor cortex. *J Neurosci* 11:2644–2654, 1991

14. He S-Q, Dum RP, Strick PS: Topographic organization of corticospinal projections from the frontal lobe: Motor areas on the lateral surface of the hemisphere. *J Neurosci* 13:952–980, 1993.

15. Hummelsheim H, Wiesendanger M, Bianchetti M, et al: Further investigations of the efferent linkage of the supplementary motor area (SMA) with the spinal cord of the monkey. *Exp Brain Res* 65:75–82, 1986.

16. Valtschanoff JG, Weinberg RJ, Rustioni A: Amino acid immunoreactivity in corticospinal terminals. *Exp Brain Res* 93:95–103, 1993.

17. DeMyer W: Number of axons and myelin sheaths in adult human medullary pyramids. *Neurology* 9:42–47, 1959.

18. Kuypers HGJM: Anatomy of the descending pathways, in Brookhart JM, Mountcastle VB, Brooks VB, et al (eds): *Handbook of Physiology. The Nervous System: Motor Control.* Bethesda, MD: American Physiological Society, 1981, sect 1, vol 2, part 1, pp 597–666.

19. Bortoff GA, Strick PS: Corticospinal terminations in two New-World primates: Further evidence that corticomotoneuronal connections provide part of the neural substrate for manual dexterity. *J Neurosci* 13:5105–5118, 1993.

20. Shinoda Y, Yokota J, Futami T: Divergent projection of individual corticospinal axons to motorneurons of multiple muscles in the monkey. *Neurosci Lett* 23:7–12, 1981.

21. Murray EA, Coulter JD: Organization of corticospinal neurons in the monkey. *J Comp Neurol* 195:339–365, 1981.

22. Fetz EE, Cheney PD: Postspike facilitation of forelimb muscle activity by primate corticomotoneuronal cells. *J Neurophysiol* 44:751–772, 1980.

23. Fetz EE, Cheney PD, Mewes K, et al: Control of forelimb muscle activity by populations of corticomotoneuronal and rubromotoneuronal cells. *Prog Brain Res* 80:437–449, 1989.

24. Lemon R: The output map of the primate motor cortex. *Trends Neurosci* 11:501–506, 1988.

25. Buys EJ, Lemon RN, Mantel GWH, et al: Selective facilitation of different hand muscles by single corticospinal neurones in the conscious monkey. *J Physiol (Lond)* 381:529–549, 1986.

26. Evarts EV: Role of motor cortex in voluntary movements in primates, in Brookhart JM, Mountcastle VB, Brooks VB, et al (eds): *Handbook of Physiology. The Nervous System: Motor Control.* Bethesda, MD: American Physiological Society, 1981, sect 1, vol 2, part 2, pp 1083–1120.

27. Cheney PD, Fetz EE: Functional classes of primate corticomotoneuronal cells and their relation to active force. *J Neurophysiol* 44:773–791, 1980.

28. Jones EG, Wise SP: Size, laminar and columnar distribution of efferent cells in the sensory-motor cortex of monkeys. *J Comp Neurol* 175:391–437, 1977.

29. Colebatch JG, Deiber M-P, Passingham RE, et al: Regional cerebral blood flow during voluntary arm and hand movements in human subjects. *J Neurophysiol* 65:1392–1401, 1991.

30. Rao SM, Binder JR, Hammeke TA, et al: Somatotopic mapping of the human primary motor cortex with functional magnetic resonance imaging. *Neurology* 45:919–924, 1995.

31. Grafton ST, Woods RP, Mazziotta JC: Within-arm somatotopy in human motor areas determined by positron emission tomography imaging of cerebral blood flow. *Exp Brain Res* 95:172–176, 1993.

32. Kawashima R, Itoh H, Ono S, et al: Activity in the human primary motor cortex related to arm and finger movements. *Neuroreport* 6:238–240, 1995.

33. Boecker H, Kleinschmidt A, Requardt M, et al: Functional cooperativity of human cortical motor areas during self-paced simple finger movements. A high-resolution MRI study. *Brain* 117:1231–1239, 1994.

34. Remy P, Zilbovicius M, Leroy-Willig A, et al: Movement- and task-related activations of motor cortical areas: A positron emission tomographic study. *Ann Neurol* 36:19–26, 1994.

35. Roland PE, Larsen B, Lassen NA, et al: Supplementary motor area and other cortical areas in organization of voluntary movements in man. *J Neurophysiol* 43:118–136, 1980.

36. Deecke L, Grozinger B, Kornhuber HH: Voluntary finger movement in man: Cerebral potentials and theory. *Biol Cybern* 23:99–119, 1976.

37. Neshige R, Lüders H, Shibasaki H: Recording of movement-related potentials from scalp and cortex in man. *Brain* 111:719–736, 1988.

38. Barrett G, Shibasaki H, Neshige R: Cortical potentials preceding voluntary movement: Evidence for three periods of preparation in man. *Electroencephalogr Clin Neurophysiol* 63:327–339, 1986.

39. Papa SM, Artieda J, Obeso JA: Cortical activity preceding self-initiated and externally triggered voluntary movement. *Mov Disord* 6:217–224, 1991.

40. Singh J, Knight RT: Frontal lobe contribution to voluntary movements in humans. *Brain Res* 531:45–54, 1990.

41. Knight RT, Singh J, Woods DL: Pre-movement parietal lobe input to human sensorimotor cortex. *Brain Res* 498:190–194, 1989.

42. Wise SP: The primate premotor cortex: Past, present, and preparatory. *Ann Rev Neurosci* 8:1–19, 1985.

43. Tanji J, Kurata K: Contrasting neuronal activity in supplementary and precentral motor cortex of monkeys. I. Responses to instructions determining motor responses to forthcoming modalities. *J Neurophysiol* 53:129–141, 1985.

44. Alexander GE, Crutcher MD: Preparation for movement: Neural representations of intended direction in three motor areas of the monkey. *J Neurophysiol* 64:133–150, 1990.

45. Biber MP, Kneisley LW, LaVail JH: Cortical neurons projecting to the cervical and lumbar enlargements of the spinal cord in young and adult rhesus monkeys. *Exp Neurol* 59:492–508, 1978.

46. Martino AM, Strick PL: Corticospinal projections originate from the arcuate premotor area. *Brain Res* 404:307–312, 1987.

47. Godschalk M, Lemon RN, Nijs HGT, et al: Behaviour of neurons in monkey peri-arcuate and precentral cortex before and during visually guided arm and hand movements. *Exp Brain Res* 44:113–116, 1981.

48. Godschalk M, Lemon RN, Kuypers HGJM, et al: The involvment of monkey premotor cortex neurones in preparation of visually cued arm movements. *Behav Brain Res* 18:143–157, 1985.

49. Kurata K, Wise SP: Premotor cortex of rhesus monkeys: Set-related activity during two conditional motor tasks. *Exp Brain Res* 69:327–343, 1988.

50. Mauritz K-H, Wise SP: Premotor cortex of the rhesus monkey: Neuronal activity in anticipation of predictable environmental events. *Exp Brain Res* 61:229–244, 1986.

51. Wise SP, Mauritz K-H: Set-related neuronal activity in the premotor cortex of rhesus monkeys: Effects of changes in motor set. *Proc R Soc Lond [Biol]* 223:331–354, 1985.

52. Weinrich M, Wise SP, Mauritz K-H: A neurophysiological study of the premotor cortex in the rhesus monkey. *Brain* 107:385–414, 1984.

53. Rizzolatti G, Matelli M, Pavesi G: Deficits in attention and movement following the removal of postarcuate (area 6) and prearcuate (area 8) cortex in macaque monkeys. *Brain* 106:655–673, 1983.

54. Passingham RE: Two cortical systems for directing movement, in Bock G, O'Connor M, Marsh J (eds): *Motor Areas of the Cerebral Cortex. Ciba Foundation Symposium 132.* New York: John Wiley & Sons, 1987, pp 151–161.

55. Wiesendanger M: Organization of secondary motor area of cerebral cortex, in Brookhart JM, Mountcastle VB, Brooks VB (eds): *Handbook of Physiology. The Nervous System: Motor Control.* Bethesda, MD: American Physiological Society, 1981, sect 1, vol 2, part 2, pp 1121–1147.

56. Freund H-J: Premotor areas in man. *Trends Neurosci* 7:481–483, 1984.

57. Freund H-J, Hummelsheim H: Premotor cortex in man: Evidence for innervation of proximal limb muscles. *Exp Brain Res* 53:479–482, 1984.

58. Freund H-J, Hummelsheim H: Lesions of premotor cortex in man. *Brain* 108:697–773, 1985.

59. Lawrence DG, Kuypers HG: The functional organization of the motor system in the monkey. II. The effects of lesions of the descending brain stem pathways. *Brain* 91:15–26, 1968.

60. Halsband U, Freund H-J: Premotor cortex and conditional motor learning in man. *Brain* 113:207–222, 1990.

61. Freund H-J: Motor dysfunction in Parkinson's disease and premotor lesions. *Europ Neurol* 29(suppl 1):33–37, 1989.

62. Deiber M-P, Passingham RE, Colebatch JG, et al: Cortical areas and the selection of movement: A study with positron emission tomography. *Exp Brain Res* 84:393–402, 1991.

63. Freund H-J: Premotor area and preparation of movement. *Rev Neurol (Paris)* 146:543–547, 1990.

64. Lu M-T, Preston JB, Strick PL: Interconnections between the prefrontal cortex and the premotor areas in the frontal lobe. *J Comp Neurol* 341:375–392, 1994.

65. Matsuzaka Y, Aizawa H, Tanji J: A motor area rostral to the supplementary motor area (presupplementary motor area) in the monkey: Neuronal activity during a learned motor task. *J Neurophysiol* 68:653–662, 1992

66. Alexander GE, Crutcher MD: Neural representations of the target (goal) of visually guided arm movements in three motor areas of the monkey. *J Neurophysiol* 64:164–178, 1990.

67. Schmidt EM, Porter R, Mcintosh JS: The effects of cooling supplementary motor area and midline cerebral cortex on neuronal responses in area-4 of monkeys. *Electroencephalogr Clin Neurophysiol* 85:61–71, 1992.

68. Smith AM, Bourbonnais D, Blanchette G: Interactions between forced grasping and a learned precision grip after ablation of the supplementary motor area. *Brain Res* 222:395–400, 1981.

69. LaPlane D, Talairach J, Meininger V, et al: Clinical consequences of corticectomies involving the supplementary motor area in man. *J Neurol Sci* 34:301–314, 1977.

70. Masdeu JC, Schoene WC, Funkenstein H: Aphasia following infarction of the left supplementary motor area. *Neurology* 28:1220–1223, 1978.

71. Damasio AR, VanHoesen GW: Structure and function of the supplementary motor area. *Neurology* 30:3591980.

72. Larsen B, Skinhoj E, Lassen NA: Regional cortical blood flow variations in the right and left hemisphere during automatic speech. *Brain* 101:193–209, 1978.

73. Penfield W, Welch K: The supplementary motor area of the cerebral cortex. *Arch Neurol Psychiatry* 66:289–317, 1951.

74. Talairach J, Bancaud J: The supplementary motor area in man. *Int J Neurol* 5:330–347, 1966.

75. Crutcher MD, Alexander GE: Movement-related neuronal activity selectively coding either direction or muscle pattern in three motor areas of the monkey. *J Neurophysiol* 64:151–163, 1990.

76. Kurata K, Tanji J: Contrasting neuronal activity in supplementary and precentral motor cortex of monkeys. II. Responses to movement triggering vs. nontriggering sensory signals. *J Neurophysiol* 53:142–152, 1985.

77. Fox PT, Fox JM, Raichle ME, et al: The role of cerebral cortex in the generation of voluntary saccades: A positron emission tomographic study. *J Neurophysiol* 54:348–369, 1985.

78. Brinkman C: Supplementary motor area of the monkey's cerebral cortex: Short- and long-term deficits after unilateral ablation and the effects of subsequent callosal section. *J Neurosci* 4:918–929, 1984.

79. Schell G, Hodge CJ, Cacayosin E: Transient neurological deficit after therapeutic embolization of the arteries supplying the medial wall of the hemisphere including the supplementary motor area. *Neurosurgery* 18:353–356, 1986.

80. Macpherson JM, Marangoz C, Miles TS, et al: Microstimulation of the supplementary motor area (SMA) in the awake monkey. *Exp Brain Res* 45:410–416, 1982.

81. Mitz AR, Wise SP: The somatotopic organization of the supplementary motor area: Intracortical microstimulation mapping. *J Neurosci* 7:1010–1021, 1987.

82. Tanji J: Comparison of neuronal activities in the monkey supplementary and precentral motor areas. *Behav Brain Res* 18:137–142, 1985.

83. Wise SP, Tanji J: Supplementary and precentral motor cortex: Contrast in responsiveness to peripheral input in the hindlimb area of the unanesthetized monkey. *J Comp Neurol* 195:433–451, 1981.

84. Tanji J, Okano K, Sato KC: Neuronal activity in cortical motor areas related to ipsilateral, contralateral and bilateral digit movements of the monkey. *J Neurophysiol* 60:325–343, 1988.

85. Mushiake H, Inase M, Tanji J: Selective coding of motor sequence in the supplementary motor area of the monkey cerebral cortex. *Exp Brain Res* 82:208–210, 1990.

86. Jenkins IH, Brooks DJ, Nixon PD, et al: Motor sequence learning: A study with positron emission tomography. *J Neurosci* 14:3775–3790, 1994.

87. Shima K, Aya K, Mushiake H, et al: Two movement-related foci in the primate cingulate cortex observed in signal-triggered and self-paced forelimb movements. *J Neurophysiol* 65:188–202, 1991.

88. Bates JF, Goldman-Rakic PS: Prefrontal connections of medial motor areas in the rhesus monkey. *J Comp Neurol* 336:211–228, 1993.

89. Morecraft RJ, VanHoesen GW: Frontal granular cortex input to the cingulate (M3), supplementary (M2) and primary (M1) motor cortices in the rhesus monkey. *J Comp Neurol* 337:669–689, 1993.

90. Luppino G, Matelli M, Camarda R, et al: Corticocortical connections of area F3 (SMA-proper) and area F6 (pre-SMA) in the macaque monkey. *J Comp Neurol* 338:114–140, 1993.

91. Braak H: A primitive gigantopyramidal field buried in the depth of the cingulate sulcus of the human brain. *Brain Res* 109:219–233, 1976.

92. VanBuren JM, Fedio P: Functional representation on the medial aspect of the frontal lobes in man. *J Neurosurg* 44:275–289, 1976.

93. Paus T, Petrides M, Evans AC, et al: Role of the human anterior cingulate cortex in the control of oculomotor, manual and speech responses: A positron emission tomography study. *J Neurophysiol* 70:453–469, 1993.

94. Alexander GE, Crutcher MD, DeLong MR: Basal ganglia-thalamocortical circuits: Parallel substrates for motor, oculomotor, 'prefrontal' and 'limbic' functions. *Prog Brain Res* 85:119–146, 1990.

95. Hoover JE, Strick PL: Multiple output channels in the basal ganglia. *Science* 259:819–821, 1993.

96. Flaherty AW, Graybiel AM: Two input systems for body representations in the primate striatal matrix: Experimental evidence in the squirrel monkey. *J Neurosci* 13:1120–1137, 1993.

97. Flaherty AW, Graybiel AM: Corticostriatal transformations in the primate somatosensory system. Projections from physiologically mapped body-part representations. *J Neurophysiol* 66.1249–1263, 1991.

98. Künzle H: Bilateral projections from precentral motor cortex to the putamen and other parts of the basal ganglia. An autoradiographic study in Macaca fascicularis. *Brain Res* 88:195–209, 1975.

99. Künzle H: Projections from the primary somatosensory cortex to basal ganglia and thalamus in the monkey. *Exp Brain Res* 30:481–492, 1977.

100. Künzle H: An autoradiographic analysis of the efferent connections from premotor and adjacent prefrontal regions (areas 6 and 9) in macaca fascicularis. *Brain Behav Evol* 15:185–234, 1978.

101. Cavada C, Goldman-Rakic PS: Topographic segregation of corticostriatal projections from posterior parietal subdivisions in the macaque monkey. *Neuroscience* 42:683–696, 1991.

102. Selemon LD, Goldman-Rakic PS: Longitudinal topography and interdigitation of cortico-striatal projections in the rhesus monkey. *J Neurosci* 5:776–794, 1985.

103. Yeterian EH, Pandya DN: Striatal connections of the parietal association cortices in rhesus monkeys. *J Comp Neurol* 332:175–197, 1993.

104. Alexander GE, DeLong MR: Microstimulation of the primate neostriatum. II. Somatotopic organization of striatal microexcitable zones and their relation to neuronal response properties. *J Neurophysiol* 53:1417–1430, 1985.

105. Crutcher MD, DeLong MR: Single cell studies of the primate putamen. I. Functional organization. *Exp Brain Res* 53:233–243, 1984.

106. Hartmann-von Monakow K, Akert K, Künzle H: Projections of the precentral motor cortex and other cortical areas of the frontal lobe to the subthalamic nucleus in the monkey. *Exp Brain Res* 33:395–403, 1978.

107. Nakanishi H, Kita H, Kitai ST: An N-methyl-D-aspartate receptor mediated excitatory postsynaptic potential evoked in subthalamic neurons in an in vitro slice preparation of the rat. *Neurosci Lett* 95:130–134, 1988.

108. Cherubini E, Herrling PL, Lanfumey L, et al: Excitatory amino acids in synaptic excitation of rat striatal neurones in vitro. *J Physiol (Lond)* 400:677–690, 1988.

109. Kawaguchi Y, Wilson CJ, Emson PC: Intracellular recording of identified neostriatal patch and matrix spiny cells in a slice preparation preserving cortical inputs. *J Neurophysiol* 62:1052–1068, 1989.

110. Wilson CJ: Postsynaptic potentials evoked in spiny neostriatal projection neurons by stimulation of ipsilateral and contralateral neocortex. *Brain Res* 367:201–213, 1986.

111. Wilson CJ, Groves PM: Fine structure and synaptic connections of the common spiny neuron of the rat neostriatum: A study employing intracellular injection of horseradish peroxidase. *J Comp Neurol* 194:599–615, 1980.

112. Kita H, Kitai ST: Glutamate decarboxylase immunoreactive neurons in rat neostriatum: Their morphological types and populations. *Brain Res* 447:346–352, 1988.

113. Selemon LD, Goldman-Rakic PS: Topographical intermingling of striatonigral and striatopallidal neurons in the rhesus monkey. *J Comp Neurol* 297:359–376, 1990.

114. Flaherty AW, Graybiel AM: Output architecture of the primate putamen. *J Neurosci* 13:3222–3237, 1993.

115. Kimura M, Kato M, Shimazaki H: Physiological properties of projection neurons in the monkey striatum to the globus pallidus. *Exp Brain Res* 82:672–676, 1990.

116. Alexander GE, DeLong MR: Microstimulation of the primate neostriatum. I. Physiological properties of striatal microexcitable zones. *J Neurophysiol* 53:1401–1416, 1985.

117. Liles SL: Activity of neurons in putamen during active and passive movements of wrist. *J Neurophysiol* 53:217–236, 1985.

118. Kimura M, Aosaki T, Hu Y, et al: Activity of primate putamen neurons is selective to the mode of voluntary movement: Visually guided, self initiated or memory guided. *Exp Brain Res* 89:473–477, 1992.

119. Kawaguchi Y: Large aspiny cells in the matrix of the rat neostriatum in vitro: Physiological identification, relation to the compartments and excitatory postsynaptic currents. *J Neurophysiol* 67:1669–1682, 1992.

120. Wilson CJ, Chang HT, Kitai ST: Firing patterns and synaptic potentials of identified giant aspiny in the rat neostriatum. *J Neurosci* 10:508–519, 1990.

121. Kimura M: The role of primate putamen neurons in the association of sensory stimuli with movement. *Neurosci Res* 3:436–443, 1986.

122. Bolam JP, Wainer BH, Smith AD: Characterization of cholinergic neurons in rat striatum. A combination of choline acetyltransferace immunocytochemistry, Golgi-impregnation and electron microscopy. *Neuroscience* 12:711–718, 1984.

123. Phelps PE, Houser CR, Vaughn JE: Immunocytochemical localization of choline acetyltransferase within the rat neostriatum: A correlated light and electron microscopic study of cholinergic neurons and synapses. *J Comp Neurol* 238:286–307, 1985.

124. Uno M, Ozawa N, Yoshida M: The mode of pallido-thalamic transmission investigated with intracellular recording from cat thalamus. *Exp Brain Res* 33:483–507, 1978.

125. Yamamoto T, Samejima A, Oka H: An intracellular analysis of the entopeduncular inputs on the centrum medianum-parafascicular nuclear complex in cats. *Brain Res* 348:343–347, 1985.

126. Penney JB Jr, Young AB: GABA as the pallidothalamic neurotransmitter: Implications for basal ganglia function. *Brain Res* 207:195–199, 1981.

127. Carpenter MB, Nakano K, Kim R: Nigrothalamic projections in the monkey demonstrated by autoradiographic technics. *J Comp Neurol* 165:401–416, 1976.

128. Kim R, Nakano K, Jayaraman A, et al: Projections of the globus pallidus and adjacent structures: An autoradiographic study in the monkey. *J Comp Neurol* 169:263–290, 1976.

129. DeVito JL, Anderson ME: An autoradiographic study of efferent connections of the globus pallidus. *Exp Brain Res* 46:107–117, 1982.

130. Ueki A, Uno M, Anderson A, et al: Monosynaptic inhibition of thalamic neurons produced by stimulation of the substantia nigra. *Experientia* 33:1480–1482, 1977.

131. Nauta HJW: A proposed conceptual reorganization of the basal ganglia and telencephalon. *Neuroscience* 4:1875–1881, 1979.

132. Parent A: *Comparative Neurobiology of the Basal Ganglia*. New York: John Wiley & Sons, 1986.

133. Mitchell SJ, Richardson RT, Baker FH, et al: The primate globus pallidus: Neuronal activity related to direction of movement. *Exp Brain Res* 68:491–505, 1987.

134. DeLong MR, Crutcher MD, Georgopoulos AP: Relations between movement and single cell discharge in the substantia nigra of the behaving monkey. *J Neurosci* 3:1599–1606, 1983.

135. Hamada I, DeLong MR, Mano N-I: Activity of identified wrist-related pallidal neurons during step and ramp wrist movements in the monkey. *J Neurophysiol* 64:1892–1906, 1990.

136. Alexander GE, Crutcher MD: Functional architecture of basal ganglia circuits: Neural substrates of parallel processing. *Trends Neurosci* 13:266–271, 1990.

137. Carpenter MB, Jayaraman A: Subthalamic nucleus of the monkey: Connections and immunocytochemical features of afferents. *J Hirnforsch* 31:653–668, 1990.

138. Smith Y, Parent A: Neurons of the subthalamic nucleus in primates display glutamate but not GABA immunoreactivity. *Brain Res* 453:353–356, 1988.

139. Robledo P, Feger J: Excitatory influence of rat subthalamic nucleus to the substantia nigra pars reticulata and the pallidal complex: Electrophysiological data. *Brain Res* 518:47–54, 1990.

140. Kita H, Kitai ST: Efferent projections of the subthalamic nucleus in the rat: Light and electron microscopic analysis with the PHA-L method. *J Comp Neurol* 260:435–452, 1987.

141. Parent A: Extrinsic connections of the basal ganglia. *Trends Neurosci* 13:254–258, 1990.

142. Nakano K, Hasegawa Y, Tokushige A, et al: Topographical projections from the thalamus, subthalamic nucleus and pedunculopontine tegmental nucleus to the striatum in the Japanese monkey, Macaca fuscata. *Brain Res* 537:54–68, 1990.

143. Hazrati L-N, Parent A, Mitchell S, et al: Evidence for interconnections between the two segments of the globus pallidus in primates: A PHA-L anterograde tracing study. *Brain Res* 533:171–175, 1990.

144. Bolam JP, Smith Y: The striatum and the globus pallidus send convergent synaptic inputs onto single cells in the entopeduncular nucleus of the rat: A double anterograde labelling study combined with postembedding immunocytochemistry for GABA. *J Comp Neurol* 321:456–476, 1992.

145. Hazrati L-N, Parent A: Projection from the external pallidum to the reticular thalamic nucleus in the squirrel monkey. *Brain Res* 550:142–146, 1991.

146. Jones EG: *The Thalamus*. New York: Plenum Press, 1985.

147. Jones EG: some aspects of the organization of the thalamic reticular complex. *J Comp Neurol* 162:285–308, 1975.

148. Uno M, Yoshida M: Monosynaptic inhibition of thalamic neurons produced by stimulation of the pallidal nucleus in cats. *Brain Res* 99:377–380, 1975.

149. Wilson CJ, Chang HT, Kitai ST: Disfacilitation and long-lasting inhibition of neostriatal neurons in the rat. *Exp Brain Res* 51:227–235, 1983.

150. DeVito JL, Anderson ME, Walsh KE: A horseradish peroxidase study of afferent connections of the globus pallidus in Macaca mulatta. *Exp Brain Res* 38:65–73, 1980.

151. Harnois C, Filion M: Pallidofugal projections to thalamus and midbrain: A quantitative antidromic activation study in monkeys and cats. *Exp Brain Res* 47:277–285, 1982.

152. Hazrati L-N, Parent A: Contralateral pallidothalamic and pallidotegmental projections in primates: An anterograde and retrograde labeling study. *Brain Res* 567:212–223, 1991.

153. Smith Y, Hazrati L-N, Parent A: Efferent projections of the subthalamic nucleus in the squirrel monkey as studied by PHA-L anterograde tracing method. *J Comp Neurol* 294:306–323, 1990.

154. Lee HJ, Rye DB, Hallanger AE, et al: Cholinergic vs. noncholinergic efferents from the mesopontine tegmentum to the extrapyramidal motor system nuclei. *J Comp Neurol* 275:469–492, 1988.

155. Rye DB, Saper CB, Lee HJ, et al: Pedunculopontine tegmental nucleus of the rat: Cytoarchitecture, cytochemistry and some extrapyramidal connections of the mesopontine tegmentum. *J Comp Neurol* 259:483–528, 1987.

156. Hallanger AE, Levey AI, Lee HJ, et al: The origins of cholinergic and other "nonspecific" afferents to the thalamus in the rat. *J Comp Neurol* 262:105–124, 1987.

157. Hallanger AE, Wainer BH: Ascending projections from the pedunculopontine tegmental nucleus and the adjacent mesopontine tegmentum in the rat. *J Comp Neurol* 274:483–518, 1988.

158. Gonya-Magee T, Anderson ME: An electrophysiological characterization of projections from the pedunculopontine area to entopeduncular nucleus and globus pallidus in the cat. *Exp Brain Res* 49:269–279, 1983.

159. Hammond C, Rouzaire-Dubois B, Feger J, et al: Anatomical and electrophysiological studies on the reciprocal projections between the subthalamic nucleus and nucleus tegmenti pedunculopontinus in the rat. *Neuroscience* 9:41–52, 1983.

160. Scarnati E, Prioa A, DeLoreto S, et al: The reciprocal electrophysiological influence between the nucleus tegmenti pedunculopontinus and the substantia nigra in normal and decorticated rats. *Brain Res* 423:116–124, 1987.

161. Scarnati E, Prioa A, Campana E, et al: A microiontophoretic study on the nature of the putative synaptic neurotransmitter in the pedunculopontine-substantia nigra pars compacta excitatory pathway in the rat. *Exp Brain Res* 62:470–478, 1986.

162. Nakamura Y, Kudo M, Tokuno H: Monosynaptic projection from the pedunculopontine tegmental region to the reticulospinal neurons of the medulla oblongata: An electron microscopic study in the cat. *Brain Res* 524:353–356, 1990.

163. Nakamura Y, Tokuno H, Moriizumi T, et al: Monosynaptic nigral inputs to the pedunculopontine tegmental nucleus neurons which send their axons to the medial reticular formation in the medulla oblongata. An electron microscopic study in the cat. *Neurosci Lett* 103:145–150, 1989.

164. Nambu A, Yoshida S, Jinnai K: Projection on the motor cortex of thalamic neurons with pallidal input in the monkey. *Exp Brain Res* 71:658–662, 1988.

165. Nambu A, Yoshida S, Jinnai K: Discharge patterns of pallidal neurons with input from various cortical areas during movement in the monkey. *Brain Res* 519:183–191, 1990.

166. Nambu A, Yoshida S, Jinnai K: Movement-related activity of thalamic neurons with input from the globus pallidus and projection to the motor cortex of the monkey. *Exp Brain Res* 84:279–284, 1991.

167. Yelnick J, Percheron G, Francois C: A golgi analysis of the primate globus pallidus. II. Quantitative morphology and spatial orientation of dendritic aborizations. *J Comp Neurol* 227:200–213, 1984.

168. Crutcher MD, DeLong MR: Single cell studies of the primate putamen. II. Relations to direction of movement and pattern of muscular activity. *Exp Brain Res* 53:244–258, 1984.

169. Georgopoulos AP, DeLong MR, Crutcher MD: Relations between parameters of step-tracking movements and single cell discharge in the globus pallidus and subthalamic nucleus of the behaving monkey. *J Neurosci* 3:1586–1598, 1983.

170. DeLong MR, Crutcher MD, Georgopoulos AP: Primate globus pallidus and subthalamic nucleus: Functional organization. *J Neurophysiol* 53:530–543, 1985.

171. Schroder KE, Hopf A, Lange H, et al: Morphemetrisch-statistche Strukturanalysen des Striatum, Pallidum und Nucleus Subthalamicus beim Menschen. I. Striatum.. *J Hirnforsch* 16:333–350, 1975.

172. Thorner G, Lange H, Hopf A: Morphometrisch-statische Strukturanalysen des Striatum, Pallidum und Nucleus Subthalamicus beim Menschen. II. Pallidum. *J Hirnforsch* 16:401–413, 1975.

173. Brown TH, Kairiss EW, Keenan CL: Hebbian synapses: Biophysical mechanisms and algorithms. *Annu Rev Neurosci* 13:475–511, 1990.

174. Linsker R: Perceptual neural organization: Some approaches based on network models and information theory. *Annu Rev Neurosci* 13:257–281, 1990.

175. Smiley JF, Williams SM, Szigeti K, et al: Light and electron microscopic characterization of dopamine-immunoreactive axons in human cerebral cortex. *J Comp Neurol* 321:325–335, 1992.

176. DeKeyser J, Herregodts P, Ebinger G: The mesoneocortical dopamine neuron system. *Neurology* 40:1660–1662, 1990.

177. Gaspar P, Berger B, Febvret A, et al: Catecholamine innervation of the human cerebral cortex as revealed by comparative immunohistochemistry of tyrosine hydroxylase and dopamine-beta-hydroxylase. *J Comp Neurol* 279:249–271, 1989.

178. Calabresi P, Maj R, Pisani A, et al: Long-term synaptic depression in the striatum: Physiological and pharmacological characterization. *J Neurosci* 12:4224–4233, 1992.

179. Calabresi P, Pisani A, Mercuri NB, et al: Long-term potentiation in the striatum is unmasked by removing the voltage-dependent magnesium block of NMDA receptor channels. *Eur J Neurosci* 4:929–935, 1992.

180. Walsh JP: Depression of excitatory synaptic input in rat striatal neurons. *Brain Res* 608:123–128, 1993.

181. Doucet G, Descarries L, Garcia S: Quantification of the dopamine innervation in adult rat neostriatum. *Neuroscience* 19:427–445, 1986.

182. Schultz W, Romo R: Dopamine neurons of the monkey midbrain: Contingencies of responses to stimuli eliciting immediate behavioral reactions. *J Neurophysiol* 63:607–624, 1990.

183. Romo R, Schultz W: Dopamine neurons of the monkey midbrain: Contingencies of responses to active touch during self-initiated arm movements. *J Neurophysiol* 63:592–606, 1990.

184. Barto AG: Reinforcement learning and adaptive critic methods, in White DA, Sofge DA (eds): *Handbook of Intelligent Control: Neural, Fuzzy, and Adaptive Approaches.* New York: Van Nostrand Reinhold, 1992, pp 469–491.

185. Rauschecker JP: Mechanisms of visual plasticity: Hebb synapses, NMDA receptors, and beyond. *Physiol Rev* 71:587–615, 1991.

186. Young AB, Dauth GW, Hollingsworth Z, et al: Quisqualate- and NMDA-sensitive [3H]glutamate binding in primate brain. *J Neurosci Res* 27:512–521, 1990.

187. Mercuri NB, Stratta F, Calabresi P, et al: A voltage-clamp analysis of NMDA-induced respnses on dopaminergic neurons of the rat substantia nigra zona compacta and ventral tegmental area. *Brain Res* 593:51–56, 1992.

188. Kobayashi T, Nagao T, Fukuda H, et al: NMDA receptors mediate neuronal burst firing in rat somatosensory cortex in vivo. *Neuroreport* 4:735–738, 1993.

189. Armstrong JM, Welker E, Callahan CA: The contribution of NMDA and non-NMDA receptors to fast and slow transmission of sensory information in the rat SI barrel cortex. *J Neurosci* 13:2149–2160, 1993.

190. Iriki A, Pavlides C, Keller A, et al: Long-term potentiation in the motor cortex. *Science* 245:1385–1387, 1989.

191. Iriki A, Pavlides C, Keller A, et al: Long-term potentiation of thalamic input to the motor cortex induced by coactivation of thalamocortical and corticocortical afferents. *J Neurophysiol* 65:1435–1441, 1991.

192. Bindman LJ, Murphy KPSJ, Pockett S: Postsynaptic control of the induction of long-term changes in efficacy of transmission at neocortical synapses in slices of rat brain. *J Neurophysiol* 60:1053–1065, 1988.

193. Baranyi A, Szente MB: Long-lasting potentiation of synaptic transmission requires postsynaptic modifications in the neocortex. *Brain Res* 423:378–384, 1987.

Chapter 6

PHYSIOLOGY OF THE BASAL GANGLIA AND PATHOPHYSIOLOGY OF MOVEMENT DISORDERS OF BASAL GANGLIA ORIGIN

THOMAS WICHMANN and MAHLON R. DELONG

ANATOMY OF THE BASAL GANGLIA
FUNCTIONAL CONSIDERATIONS
    Motor Functions of the Basal Ganglia
    Segregation versus Convergence
    "Scaling" versus "Focusing"
    Motor Subcircuits
MOVEMENT DISORDERS
    Hypokinetic Movement Disorders
    Hyperkinetic Movement Disorders
CONCLUSION

The basal ganglia are implicated in a wide spectrum of movement disorders. In recent years, significant advances have led to major insights into the anatomy and function of the basal ganglia and into the pathophysiology of disorders that involve these structures. In the following, the anatomy and physiology of the basal ganglia and the pathophysiological mechanisms underlying both hypo- and hyperkinetic movement disorders are considered.

Anatomy of the Basal Ganglia

Anatomic and physiological studies indicate that the basal ganglia are components of larger segregated circuits, which also involve parts of the cortex and thalamus.[1-3] (see also chapter 5). These circuits appear to be similarly organized in anatomic terms and have been named according to the presumed functions of their cortical areas of origin. In the monkey, functionally segregated "motor," "oculomotor," "associative," and "limbic" circuits have been identified. Each of these circuits originates in a specific cortical area, passes through separate portions of the basal ganglia and thalamus, and then projects back onto the original cortical area. In each of these circuits, the striatum functions as the "input" stage of the basal ganglia, whereas the internal segment of the globus pallidus (GPi) and the pars reticulata of the substantia nigra (SNr) serve as output stations. GPi and SNr may be viewed as components of a single output structure divided by the internal capsule in a manner similar to

that of the division of the striatum into the caudate nucleus and putamen.

Movement disorders appear to result from disturbances in the motor circuit. This circuit is comprised of pre- and postcentral sensorimotor fields, as well as the motor territories of the basal ganglia and the ventral anterior and ventrolateral thalamus (VA/VL). Cortical projections from the sensorimotor fields terminate largely in the postcommissural putamen, the motor portion of the striatum (Fig. 6-1). Putamenal output is in turn directed toward motor portions of GPi/SNr via two pathways, a "direct" monosynaptic pathway from the putamen to motor portions of GPi/SNr and an "indirect" pathway passing through the motor areas of the external pallidal segment (GPe) and the subthalamic nucleus (STN). Although it appears that different populations of neurons in STN innervate GPi and SNr (e.g., see Ref. 4), these connections are generally considered functionally similar. There are also direct reciprocal connections between GPe and GPi/SNr that circumvent the STN (e.g., see Ref. 5). GPi/SNr motor output is directed not only to VA/VL, where it influences the activity of thalamocortical projection neurons, but also to the pedunculopontine nucleus (PPN) in the midbrain. The role of this projection remains uncertain, but it may offer direct access of basal ganglia output to bulbar and spinal cord centers, circumventing the cortex. With the exception of the excitatory (glutamatergic) projection between STN and GPi/SNr, the intrinsic connections of the basal ganglia, as well as their outputs to thalamus, superior colliculus and midbrain, are all inhibitory and GABAergic.

Release of dopamine from terminals of the nigrostriatal projection, which arises from the substantia nigra pars compacta (SNc), appears to facilitate transmission over the direct pathway via activation of D1 receptors and to inhibit transmission over the indirect pathway via activation of D2 receptors (e.g., see Refs. 6 and 7). Both D1 and D2 receptors are located on dendritic spines of striatal output neurons, which receive cortical input. This location enables dopamine released in the striatum to modulate corticostriatal transmission. The overall effect of dopamine released in the striatum appears to be a reduction of basal ganglia output, leading, by disinhibition, to increased activity of thalamocortical projection neurons and a facilitation of movement. Conversely, reduction of striatal dopamine, as occurs in parkinsonism, should increase basal ganglia outflow and inhibit movement. In addition, basal ganglia output may be modulated by extrastriatal release of dopamine. For example, SNc sends dopaminergic projections to STN and GPi, and dopamine may reach the SNr via dendritic release (e.g., see Refs. 8–10). In these nuclei, dopamine may act presynaptically on striatal efferents or postsynaptically on output neurons.

Functional Considerations

By virtue of their anatomic connections, the basal ganglia are likely involved in the modulation and fine tuning of the activity of large portions of the frontal cortex, having a role in the control of movements, and in limbic and associative functions. The anatomic similarities between the different cortical-basal ganglia-thalamocortical circuits suggest that

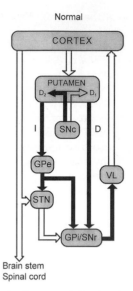

FIGURE 6-1 Schematic diagram of the basal ganglia-thalamocortical circuitry under normal conditions. Inhibitory connections are shown as filled arrows, excitatory connections as open arrows. D, direct pathway; I, indirect pathway; GPe, external segment of the globus pallidus; GPi, internal segment of the globus pallidus; SNr, substantia nigra, pars reticulata; SNc, substantia nigra, pars compacta; STN, subthalamic nucleus; VL, ventrolateral thalamus.

the function of the basal ganglia in the different circuits is also similar, and that conclusions drawn from the study of one circuit are, at least to some extent, also applicable to the others. Among the circuits passing through the basal ganglia, the motor circuit is certainly most studied and best understood, particularly because it is hoped that a better understanding of the physiology and pathophysiology of this circuit may aid in the development of new therapeutic strategies to treat movement disorders more effectively.

MOTOR FUNCTIONS OF THE BASAL GANGLIA

Although the basal ganglia have been implicated in a wide variety of motor functions, including the planning, initiation, and execution of movements, the evidence from behavioral studies in animals and humans for a specific role of the basal ganglia in the control of movement is not entirely conclusive. Many speculations regarding the role of the basal ganglia in the control of normal behavior have been based on the study of deficits arising from functional or structural abnormalities affecting the basal ganglia. For instance, a role of the basal ganglia in initiation of movement is suggested by the severe disturbance of this in Parkinson's disease (i.e., akinesia), although support for this from animal experiments is lacking. Similarly, a role of the basal ganglia in movement execution, as suggested by the development of bradykinesia in parkinsonian subjects, is not firmly established, because data from lesions in animals and man are inconsistent regarding this point (e.g., see Refs. 11–18). A role of the basal ganglia in the control of sequential or simultaneous movements has been inferred from the fact that parkinsonian patients do poorly in motor tasks that involve such movements.[19–24] More

recently, it was shown that such patients appear to rely more on external cues when performing these movements than do normal controls. This led to the hypothesis that the basal ganglia-thalamocortical circuitry may have a role in the generation or use of internally cued sequential or simultaneous movements.[20–22] Similarly, observations of deficits in parkinsonian patients have also been used to argue for a role of the basal ganglia in the execution of learned movements (e.g., see Refs. 25 and 26).

Although these findings clearly establish a role for the basal ganglia in the development of movement disorders, they do not by themselves constitute evidence for a role of these structures in the control of normal movement, because abnormal basal ganglia output may simply disrupt cortical activity nonspecifically. For instance, it has always been puzzling that lesions of the basal ganglia outflow nuclei have relatively minor long-term effects on motor performance.[11,12,18,27,28] Although this finding may be explainable by the action of compensatory mechanisms "downstream" from the basal ganglia, and thus may not negate a "motor function" of the basal ganglia, it indicates that these structures are not essential in motor control.

More direct evidence for involvement of these structures in the control of normal movement comes from electrophysiological studies recording the discharge of single basal ganglia neurons. Such studies have indeed shown that many neurons in the basal ganglia exhibit discharge correlated with certain aspects of limb or eye movements. Although mostly correlative and thus inadequate to establish a *causal* relationship between basal ganglia discharge and aspects of behavior, these studies still provide the best available insights into basal ganglia function, and the considerations outlined below, therefore, largely focus on results from these experiments.

SEGREGATION VERSUS CONVERGENCE

The apparent parallel organization of basal ganglia-thalamocortical pathways and the paucity of interneurons or axon collaterals in the basal ganglia nuclei (e.g., see Refs. 29–32) suggests that the flux of information in the different circuits remains largely segregated. Indeed, electrophysiological recording studies have shown that the discharge of individual neurons in the basal ganglia in a wide variety of behavioral paradigms does not appear to contain new information or extract features that were not already apparent in the discharge of the respective cortical source regions. On the other hand, it is almost certain that some degree of convergence of information does take place within the basal ganglia, because the number of striatal neurons receiving cortical afferents is much smaller than the number of cortical neurons sending these projections, and the number of output neurons in the striatum in turn is larger than the number of target neurons in GP/SN. Pallidal neurons have large dendritic fields that are traversed by a multitude of striatal efferent fibers,[33–35] an arrangement that may form the anatomic basis for convergence. This "funneling" of information may permit recombination of cortical inputs, which may serve as an important mechanism of modulation of cortical activity. Convergence takes place probably within, rather than between circuits, because convergence of information across the boundaries of the major basal ganglia circuits has never been demonstrated convincingly.

Under physiological conditions, most neurons in the basal ganglia output nuclei appear to respond to a narrow range of input stimuli, which suggests that convergence may not play an important role in normal basal ganglia function. This view is further supported by cross-correlation studies that show that the discharge of neighboring pallidal neurons is not correlated.[36,37] Recording in monkeys depleted of dopamine supply to the basal ganglia, however, has shown that, compared to the normal state, motor-related neurons in both segments of the globus pallidus and in STN lose part of their specificity for individual movements, and that the degree of synchrony between neighboring neurons is increased.[36,38–41] This suggests that dopamine may help to maintain segregation between the different circuits passing through the basal ganglia. Segregation of basal ganglia circuits, as well as channels within individual circuits, may thus be a dynamic, rather than static phenomenon, with dopamine playing a gate-keeper role in maintaining specificity. It is unknown whether this role is restricted to striatal dopamine, or may extend to extrastriatal dopamine or even to other neuromodulators in the basal ganglia (such as serotonin).

"SCALING" VERSUS "FOCUSING"

Tonic high-frequency inhibitory output of motor areas of the basal ganglia to the thalamus probably restrains the overall amount of movements to the appropriate amount. Facilitation of a particular desired movement is likely the result of phasic reduction of basal ganglia output, leading to a (brief) disinhibition of thalamocortical neurons (e.g., see Ref. 42). Given the polarities of connections in the motor circuit, this disinhibition should primarily be the result of the transmission of phasic cortical inputs to striatal neurons that give rise to the direct pathway (e.g, see Ref. 43). In contrast, phasic activity over the indirect pathway should lead to increased GPi/SNr discharge,[43] and to further suppression of thalamocortical neurons and movement.

The temporal interplay between the activity of direct and indirect inputs to the basal ganglia output nuclei may give the basal ganglia a role in influencing characteristics of movements as they are carried out. The basal ganglia may thus act to scale certain movement parameters, such as amplitude or velocity ("scaling" hypothesis). The motor circuit may also act to compare phasic neuronal responses, that reflect processed efferent copies of motor commands from precentral motor areas, with proprioceptive feedback. A signal from this comparator would then be projected back to the precentral motor areas via the thalamus. In this case the motor circuit would scale movements by constraining motor commands issued to the periphery to lie within desired limits.

In addition, basal ganglia output may act to focus the cortical selection of movements ("focusing" hypothesis, e.g., see Refs. 18, 44, and 45) by facilitation of intended movements, and inhibition of related but unwanted ones involving the same or nearby joints. A potential anatomic substrate for such a "center-surround" mechanism has been proposed,[46] based on the finding that STN efferents to GPi may terminate broadly, whereas the direct putamen-GPi projection may terminate more specifically on individual pallidal cells. More

recent data, however, argue in favor of a more specific manner of arborization of subthalamopallidal efferents.[47,48] By amplifying phasic activity both in the direct and in the indirect pathway (i.e., by providing a "gain" higher than 1), the contribution of the basal ganglia in the "focusing" model would be to sharpen the contrast in activity between cortical areas that govern wanted and unwanted movements and, thereby, to stabilize and select individual movements. It is clear, however, that during initiation and execution of individual movements most neurons in the basal ganglia do *not* alter their firing. For instance, with intended elbow flexion, neurons related to orofacial or leg movements are not likely to discharge. This implies that selection may take place only for selected movements that warrant the particular inhibition provided by transmission via the indirect pathway. The mechanisms by which this selection would be achieved are entirely unclear but would likely be located at the cortical level.

MOTOR SUBCIRCUITS

Combined single-cell and behavioral studies in primates have shown that discharge of basal ganglia neurons in the motor territory of the basal ganglia in relation to movement is heterogeneous, primarily with regard to the timing of discharge in relation to behavioral events. This may not only be because of technical or species differences but may also be explainable by the observation from recent anatomic and physiological studies[49–52] that the motor circuit encompasses several segregated subcircuits, which emanate from different cortical areas (e.g., supplementary motor area [SMA], and arcuate premotor area [APA]). The function of these cortical areas and, thus, the function of the associated motor subcircuits, may differ, and such differences may determine discharge characteristics of individual associated basal ganglia neurons, such as the timing of neuronal discharge in relation to movement. Neuronal activity related to execution or termination of movement may be more commonly found in neurons belonging to a subcircuit originating in the primary motor cortex.[52] In contrast, discharge of basal ganglia neurons that discharge long before onset of movement and electromyogram (EMG) activity ("preparatory discharge,"[53–57]) may predominate in basal ganglia neurons that belong to a subcircuit that originates in SMA or other mesial motor areas. Such preparatory or "set"-related activity may encode certain characteristics of the upcoming movement, for instance, the direction, amplitude, or target location, or may be related to spatial memory, attention, or other factors.

It should be clear from these considerations that a role of the basal ganglia in motor control is likely, but that most evidence for specific functions is indirect, allowing no firm conclusions regarding the precise role of these structures in planning, execution, or termination of movement.

Movement Disorders

More progress has recently been made in understanding the pathophysiological mechanisms underlying the major movement disorders of basal ganglia origin than in the elucidation of the role of the basal ganglia in the control of normal movement. This group of disorders involves disruption of the delicate balance between the activity of the direct and the indirect pathways which appears to characterize the normal state. *Hypo*kinetic movement disorders are thought to arise from a relative preponderance of activity of the indirect pathway, leading to an increase of (inhibitory) basal ganglia output to the thalamus. Conversely, *hyper*kinetic disorders are likely the result of a shift of the balance towards the direct pathway, leading to reduced basal ganglia output.

HYPOKINETIC MOVEMENT DISORDERS

GENERAL PATHOPHYSIOLOGICAL MODEL

Parkinson's disease is the prototypic hypokinetic movement disorder. Clinically, parkinsonism is characterized by the tetrad of akinesia, bradykinesia, rigidity, and tremor. The term "akinesia" is defined as poverty of movement, secondary to impaired movement initiation. "Bradykinesia" refers to slowness of movement and "rigidity" to increased resistance to passive stretch. Parkinsonian tremor consists of low-frequency oscillations, mainly occurring at rest. Pathologically, it is characterized by degeneration of the dopaminergic nigrostriatal projection. The study of the pathophysiological mechanisms resulting from degeneration of nigrostriatal fibers has been greatly facilitated by the introduction of an animal model that reproduces many of the pathological and behavioral abnormalities of human parkinsonism, i.e., the primate treated with 1-methyl-4-phenyl-1,2,3,6-tetrahydropyridine (MPTP).[2,39,58,59]

Recent electrophysiological experiments and studies of the metabolic activity in the basal ganglia of such monkeys suggest that loss of dopaminergic input to the striatum leads to overall increased activation of the indirect pathway and decreased activity in the direct pathway (Fig. 6-2). Both changes result in increased basal ganglia output to the thalamus, leading to increased inhibition of thalamocortical neurons. In accordance with this, microelectrode recording has shown that the tonic activity in GPe is decreased, whereas the neuronal activity in STN and GPi is increased relative to pre-MPTP levels.[38–40,60] In support of the concept that increased output from the basal ganglia motor circuit is important in parkinsonian pathophysiology, inactivation of motor portions of STN or GPi markedly ameliorates parkinsonian motor signs.[58,61–64]

In addition to the above-mentioned changes in overall basal ganglia activity, phasic neuronal responses to joint manipulation in STN, GPi, and thalamus[38–41] occur more often, are more pronounced, and show widened receptive fields after treatment with MPTP. There is also a marked change in the synchrony of discharge in the basal ganglia. Cross-correlation studies have revealed that a substantial proportion of neighboring neurons in GPi and STN discharge in unison in MPTP-treated primates.[40] This is in contrast to the virtual absence of synchronized discharge of such neurons in normal monkeys (e.g., see Ref. 37).

Following the encouraging results of lesions of the basal ganglia output structures on parkinsonian signs in MPTP-treated primates, stereotactic lesioning of these nuclei has recently been reintroduced as a treatment for Parkinson's disease.[65–70] This has offered an opportunity to directly study

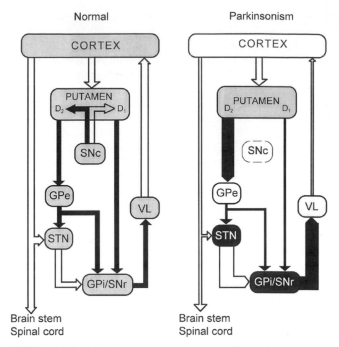

FIGURE 6-2 Activity changes in the basal ganglia-thalamocortical circuitry in Parkinson's disease. Degeneration of the nigrostriatal pathway leads to differential changes in the two striato-pallidal projections, indicated by the thickness of the connecting arrows. Basal ganglia output to the thalamus is increased. For abbreviations see legend to Fig. 6-1.

some of the abnormalities as they occur in the human disorder. Thus, electrophysiological recording during these procedures has revealed that neuronal discharge rates in GPi are increased relative to GPe and are characterized by frequent burst discharges and a high degree of synchronous discharge of neighboring neurons (although studies in normal controls are not feasible, of course).[71]

The clinical results of these new lesioning strategies also support the concept that Parkinson's disease is characterized by increased basal ganglia output. For instance, both GPi lesions[65–70] and high-frequency stimulation of the subthalamic nucleus (presumably leading to inactivation of the nucleus) have been shown to be remarkably effective in the amelioration of parkinsonian signs, as well as drug-induced dyskinesias and motor fluctuations.[72] Positron emission tomography (PET) studies have demonstrated that the decreased cortical activation seen in parkinsonian patients is at least partially resolved after stereotactic pallidotomy, concomitant with recovery of motor function.[68,73,74]

AKINESIA, BRADYKINESIA, RIGIDITY

Akinesia, usually the earliest sign of parkinsonism in MPTP-treated primates, is seen after doses of the neurotoxin small enough to damage almost exclusively the dopamine supply to the striatum, making it very likely that most parkinsonian abnormalities result from dopamine loss in the basal ganglia. In all stages of parkinsonism, most importantly in the earliest, dopamine depletion is consistently greatest in the sensorimotor territory of the striatum, the putamen, which implicates abnormalities in the motor circuit in the development of parkinsonism. This is further supported by recent PET studies[75] of preclinical and clinical parkinsonian patients, in which reduced putaminal [18F]dopa uptake has consistently been the earliest sign of striatal dopamine deficiency, with relative sparing of the dopaminergic innervation to other striatal areas (e.g., the caudate). The involvement of the motor circuit is also supported by the finding that lesions of the motor territory within the GPi and the STN have striking effects on parkinsonian signs, including akinesia, bradykinesia, and rigidity.[58,61,66–69,74,76–80]

The changes in tonic and phasic activity of basal ganglia output (see above) are probably transmitted via cortical motor areas, resulting in akinesia, bradykinesia, and rigidity. Increased tonic inhibition of thalamocortical neurons by excessive output from GPi/SNr may reduce the responsiveness of cortical mechanisms involved in motor control and may prevent the faithful transmission to the cortex of superimposed phasic reductions in activity that occur during movement execution, which may interfere with the normal scaling of movement. Increased *tonic* inhibition of thalamocortical neurons by increased basal ganglia output in parkinsonism may also render precentral motor areas less responsive to other inputs normally involved in initiating movements, or may interfere with "set" functions that have been shown to be highly dependent on the integrity of basal ganglia pathways.[81] Increased gain in the feedback from proprioceptors, reflected by increased *phasic* activity in the basal ganglia, may signal excessive movement or velocity to precentral motor areas, leading to a slowing or premature arrest of ongoing movements, as well as to greater reliance upon external cues during movement.

Some evidence for the involvement of abnormal activity in cortical areas that belong to the motor circuit and are presumably related to motor planning comes from studies of the Bereitschaftspotential (readiness potential), a slow negative cortical potential that precedes self-paced movements and is thought to reflect the neural activity in SMA.[82] The early portion of the Bereitschaftspotential is smaller in parkinsonian patients than in age-matched controls,[74,83] suggesting a deficit in the normal function of the SMA in the early stages of preparation for self-initiated movements. PET studies of cerebral blood flow in human patients have revealed that dopamine loss in the striatum leads to decreased blood flow (thus, by inference, reduced synaptic activity) in the SMA, motor cortex, and dorsolateral prefrontal cortex (e.g., see Refs. 68, 74, 75, 84–87).

Although the pathophysiological changes in basal ganglia discharge underlying akinesia, bradykinesia and rigidity are thought to be the same in general terms, that is, changes of tonic or phasic basal ganglia output, the expression of these signs may depend on abnormalities in different motor subcircuits. Conceivably, akinesia, a defect in movement preparation and initiation, may be related to abnormal discharge in the subcircuit whose activity is mostly "preparatory," that is, the subcircuit emanating from SMA and mesial cortical motor areas. In contrast, bradykinesia and rigidity may result from abnormalities in the subcircuit arising from primary motor cortex (see, e.g., discussion in Ref. 49).

The concept that increased inhibition of thalamocortical neurons by increased output from GPi/SNr will ultimately result in akinesia is probably too simplistic, because lesions of the areas of the thalamus that receive basal ganglia input (VL/VA) do not result in akinesia (e.g., see Refs. 88–91). Abnormal basal ganglia output to targets other than the thalamus (for instance, the PPN) may, therefore, also play a role in the development of akinesia.

Abnormalities of neuronal activity in the basal ganglia and cortex will eventually lead to abnormal activity in the spinal cord. One of the main consequences of these "downstream" effects appears to be increased alpha-motoneuron excitability.[92] Although the precise mechanism for this is elusive, abnormal processing of information transmitted to the spinal cord by Ia afferents has been implicated. In support of this concept, dorsal root section abolishes parkinsonian rigidity,[93] although Ia fiber activity appears to be normal in parkinsonian subjects.[94] As a possible explanation, altered basal ganglia output, mediated via the pontine nucleus gigantocellularis and the dorsal longitudinal fasciculus of the reticulospinal projection, may lead to increased inhibition of Ib interneurons which, in turn, may disinhibit alpha-motoneurons.[95] Abnormalities of long-latency reflexes (LLRs) may also play a role in abnormal alpha-motoneuron excitability. In parkinsonian subjects, the reflex gain in LLRs seems to be relatively fixed and abnormally high.[96] The abnormal phasic responses generated within the basal ganglia of MPTP-treated primates[38–40] could be responsible for increased LLR production (acting through the motor circuit projection to the supplementary motor area) or may reflect abnormally large inputs to the striatum from the motor or somatosensory cortices that are engaged in the LLR production and whose altered responsiveness may result from increased tonic output from GPi and SNr.

TREMOR

Although tremor in Parkinson's disease has been largely considered as a result of thalamic oscillatory discharge, it has more recently been linked to abnormal discharge in the basal ganglia (e.g., see Ref. 97). This possibility is in large part based on the observation that surgical interruption of pallidal outflow, either by disruption of pallidal efferents or by lesions of GPi, can produce lasting relief of tremor in parkinsonian patients,[76,98,99] and lesions of the STN in MPTP-treated African green monkeys reduce tremor significantly.[58] This may be explainable by increased tonic basal ganglia output to the thalamus, which may promote oscillatory activity through increased hyperpolarization in that nucleus.[100,101] This tendency for rhythmic oscillations of thalamocortical neurons may be further enhanced by periodic bursting in reticular thalamus during moments of immobility. Alternatively, it has been speculated that loss of dopamine in the basal ganglia output nuclei (GPi/SNr), rather than the striatum, may be important in the generation of tremor (discussed in Refs. 62, and 102). In support of this, it appears that those primate species (African green monkeys) which, when treated with MPTP, lose the dopamine supply to GPi, tend to develop tremor, whereas those species (macaques) that appear to have preserved dopamine input to GPi do not develop tremor.[40,62,103] The local loss of dopamine may lead to unmasking of pacemaker-like properties[104] in the basal ganglia nuclei themselves, which have been demonstrated by intracellular recordings from GP in brain slices from adult guinea pigs when the recorded cells were abruptly depolarized from a hyperpolarized membrane potential.[104] Furthermore, bursts of spikes synchronous with visible tremor have also been recorded in the STN and GPi of MPTP-treated monkeys[38,40,97] and in parkinsonian patients undergoing pallidotomy (e.g., Refs. 40, 71, and 97). Oscillations generated in motor areas of the basal ganglia output nuclei or the thalamus will eventually lead to rhythmic activity in thalamocortical cells, which in turn may lead to oscillations in corticospinal projection neurons. In parkinsonian patients undergoing stereotactic thalamotomy, neurons discharging at the parkinsonian tremor frequency have indeed been detected in areas of the thalamus that receive basal ganglia input (discussed in Ref. 105).

NONMOTOR PHENOMENA

Parkinson's disease clearly encompasses more than motor phenomena. Although a detailed discussion of the pathogenesis of nonmotor signs of parkinsonism is beyond the scope of this chapter, it is likely that these abnormalities rely on abnormal discharge in nonmotor circuits of the basal ganglia, which may be affected by dopamine loss in much the same way as the motor circuit. For instance, oculomotor abnormalities appear to be the result of dopaminergic loss in the "oculomotor" basal ganglia-thalamocortical circuit.[106] Similarly, some of the cognitive and psychiatric disturbances seen in parkinsonian patients are reminiscent of syndromes seen after lesions of the dorsolateral prefrontal cortex (problems with executive functions) or of the anterior cingulate (apathy, personality changes). These symptoms may be the result of loss of dopamine in the dorsolateral or ventral caudate nucleus, respectively.[107] Finally, disturbance of the normal function of cortical-basal ganglia-thalamocortical circuits has also been implicated in the occurrence of obsessive-compulsive symptoms in some parkinsonian patients, as well as in patients with other diseases of presumed basal ganglia origin, such as Tourette's syndrome.[108,109]

HYPERKINETIC MOVEMENT DISORDERS

Just as Parkinson's disease and Huntington's disease represent opposite extremes clinically, so do the underlying pathophysiological mechanisms. The main hyperkinetic symptoms, chorea, ballismus, and dystonia, may all be characterized by reduced basal ganglia output to the thalamus, leading to disinhibition of thalamocortical neurons, which in turn leads to the development of involuntary movements. The term *chorea* refers to discrete involuntary arrhythmic jerky movements, whereas *ballismus* refers to more proximal involuntary movements, resembling throwing motions of larger amplitude. The term *dystonia* refers to slower, more sustained movements and abnormal postures with cocontraction of antagonist muscles.

HEMIBALLISM

Hemiballism; results in the majority of cases from lesions involving the STN.[110–115] In terms of the anatomic model outlined above, such lesions interrupt the indirect pathway, leaving activity along the direct pathway unopposed (Fig. 6-3).

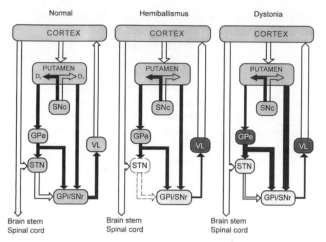

FIGURE 6-3 Activity changes in the basal ganglia-thalamocortical circuitry in hemiballism *(center panel)* and in dystonia *(right panel)*. The two conditions may differ in preferential involvement of the indirect pathway in hemiballism and involvement of the direct pathway in dystonia. As in all hyperkinetic movement disorders, the net result is reduced basal ganglia output to the thalamus in either case. For abbreviations see legend to Fig. 6-1.

This leads to the development of involuntary movements. Electrophysiological experiments have directly demonstrated that fiber-sparing STN lesions result in reduced activity in both GPi and GPe, concomitant with the development of chorea, and that the proportion of cells that responds to somatosensory examination with increases in discharge is dramatically reduced in both nuclei under these conditions.[116] Recently, it was also shown (in an MPTP-treated animal) that STN lesions lead to increases in discharge in thalamic areas that receive input from the basal ganglia, presumably because of reduced (inhibitory) GPi/SNr output to the thalamus, following the loss of excitatory drive from the STN on GPi/SNr neurons (Yoshi Kaneoke et al., unpublished observations).

HUNTINGTON'S DISEASE

This is the classic basal ganglia disorder characterized by chorea. Pathologically, striatal projection neurons degenerate in this disorder (see also Chap. 36). This process, however, is not random but follows a sequence in most patients, which allows chorea to develop. Thus, initially, striatal output neurons projecting to GPe are preferentially affected, leading to reduced inhibition of neurons in that nucleus and, subsequently, increased inhibition of STN neurons, resulting in decreased GPi output, the hallmark of hyperkinetic disorders. In later stages of the disease, inhibitory striatal output neurons to GPi also degenerate, which results in disinhibition of GPi neurons. Increased activity of GPi neurons will reduce the amount of chorea and may later even lead to the development of parkinsonian features.

DRUG-INDUCED DYSKINESIAS

Chronic administration of dopaminergic drugs to parkinsonian patients may lead to the development of dyskinesias by shifting the balance between direct and indirect pathway toward the direct pathway, resulting in decreased basal ganglia output. Dopamine receptor activation may result in activation of the direct pathway (via dopamine D1 receptors) and inhibition of the putamen-GPe connection (part of the indirect pathway, via D2 receptors). Both changes will again lead to reduced basal ganglia output and, presumably, to increased activity of thalamocortical neurons. It is unknown why this phenomenon occurs predominantly after previous damage to the nigrostriatal system (Parkinson's disease) and prolonged exposure to dopaminergic agonists. Compensatory changes in dopamine receptor number or binding characteristics in response to dopamine depletion may be essential for this phenomenon (for discussion see, e.g., see Ref. 117).

DYSTONIA

The pathophysiology of dystonia is less well understood than the pathophysiology of chorea. This is in part because the term dystonia describes a symptom that may arise from a variety of probably unrelated disease processes, for instance, basal ganglia diseases, but also cerebellar[118–120] or brain stem disorders.[120,121] Dystonia of basal ganglia origin often develops after focal striatal lesions, particularly of the putamen, weeks or months after the inciting basal ganglia lesion, suggesting that it results from secondary changes, rather than from the primary lesion. Thus, compensatory changes in the affinity or number of dopamine receptors in the remainder of the striatum, or a reorganization of striatal topography, may eventually lead to changes in the activity of the other basal ganglia structures. Dystonia is often seen in the context of parkinsonism, and a subgroup of patients with dystonia will respond to treatment with L-dopa (e.g., see Refs. 122 and 123). In most cases, however, damage to the nigrostriatal tract is probably not necessary for the development of dystonia (see, e.g., discussion in Ref. 124). Rather, dystonia appears to develop frequently in individuals who have been exposed to dopaminergic drugs. There is no consensus whether stimulation of D1 receptors, D2 receptors, or both are needed for dystonia to occur.

Mitchell et al.[125] have shown in 2-deoxyglucose studies that synaptic activity in GPi and STN is increased in MPTP-treated monkeys, which were rendered dystonic by injections of dopaminergic agonists. This result, in conjunction with studies in monkeys rendered dystonic by small ibotenic-acid lesions of the putamen in which the concentration of met-enkephalin in GPe (indicating the activity of the putamen-GPe pathway) was reduced,[126] suggests that reduction of activity of the putamen-GPe connection, resulting in increased inhibition of both STN and GPi, may be involved in the development of dystonia of striatal origin. In addition, overactivity in the direct pathway may also contribute significantly to decreased GPi output (Fig. 6-3).

Given these considerations, the pathophysiology of chorea and that of dystonia of basal ganglia origin are remarkably similar at the level of gross changes in the neuronal activity in the basal ganglia output nuclei. The reasons why these changes lead in some cases to chorea but in others to dystonia are unclear, but it may be an issue of timing or the extent of abnormal discharge in the basal ganglia, with reductions

in discharge being shorter and more focal in chorea and prolonged and widespread in dystonia, thus leading to jerky involuntary movement in the former and agonist/antagonist cocontraction in the latter. As pointed out above, decreased GPi output may result from decreased excitation of GPi via the indirect pathway or from increased inhibition in the direct pathway. As in the case of hemiballism, reduced excitatory input to GPi via the indirect pathway can clearly lead to chorea. Conceivably, increased inhibition via the direct pathway may be more important in dystonia (see Fig. 6-3). Furthermore, compensatory mechanisms, particularly involving the striatal or extrastriatal dopamine system, may also differ. For instance, the differences in the affinity or distribution of striatal dopamine receptors, or the intactness of dopamine supply to extrastriatal sites, may play a role in this regard. We have seen significant dystonia in MPTP-treated macaques (a species that maintains a relatively intact extrastriatal dopamine supply after MPTP-treatment), whereas MPTP-treated African green monkeys (in whom extrastriatal dopamine is destroyed) have not shown this sign.

Conclusion

Although the evidence from animal experiments and ablative procedures in man have lent support to a model of normal function and the pathophysiological considerations outlined above, the models clearly fall short of "explaining" the role of the basal ganglia in voluntary movement and movement disorders. The reason for this lies in the unavailability of feasible methods to clearly establish the physiological function of the basal ganglia in motor control. As mentioned above, the most powerful tool for studies of this kind, single-cell recording studies in behaving primates, help to support anatomic concepts of the basal ganglia circuitry but cannot establish a clear motor function because they are correlative. The study of deficits that result from basal ganglia abnormalities also fails in this regard, because studies on individuals with such disorders demonstrate merely that altered basal ganglia output disturbs motor performance but not that these structures are important for normal movement. Furthermore, movement disorders such as Parkinson's disease affect not only the basal ganglia but also cortical and other subcortical regions (e.g., see Refs. 127–130), rendering the reduction of the pathophysiology of movement disorders to abnormalities in the basal ganglia alone too simplistic.

In fact, lesions of these structures often lead to results that are difficult to understand, given the current models of basal ganglia function. For instance, the models predict that reduced basal ganglia output should always lead to excess movement, as it is seen, for instance, after lesions of the STN (e.g., see Ref. 116). Pallidal lesions in normal or parkinsonian monkeys or in parkinsonian patients, however, have not been associated with involuntary movement other than occasional transient dyskinesias[28,76,131] (but see Ref. 18). Furthermore, if the basal ganglia play an important role in motor control, as generally believed, it is expected that reduction of basal ganglia output should lead to disturbances of normal movement. As mentioned above, however, neither GPi nor STN lesions in man or experimental animals lead to significant long-term abnormalities of voluntary movement.[28,58,62,131] It appears that voluntary movement can be controlled with reduced or absent GPi/SNr activity. Basal ganglia output may, therefore, be either relatively unimportant for movement initiation or execution, or its loss can be rapidly and readily compensated for by other parts of the motor system. In contrast, increased basal ganglia output, as seen in Parkinson's disease, appears to severely disrupt motor performance on a more permanent basis.

Overall, our understanding of the contribution of the basal ganglia to movement and behavior lags far behind our understanding of the pathophysiology of Parkinson's disease and other movement disorders. Although impressive advances in the understanding and treatment of these disorders have been made in recent years, more comprehensive knowledge of normal basal ganglia functioning will ultimately be necessary to maximize therapeutic outcome for patients affected by basal ganglia disorders.

References

1. Alexander GE, DeLong MR, Strick PL: Parallel organization of functionally segregated circuits linking basal ganglia and cortex. *Annu Rev Neurosci* 9:357–381, 1986.
2. Albin RL, Young AB, Penney JB: The functional anatomy of basal ganglia disorders. *Trends Neurosci* 12:366–375, 1989.
3. Alexander GE, Crutcher MD, DeLong MR: Basal ganglia-thalamocortical circuits: Parallel substrates for motor, oculomotor, 'prefrontal' and 'limbic' functions. *Prog Brain Res* 85:119–146, 1990.
4. Parent A, Smith Y: Organization of efferent projections of the subthalamic nucleus in the squirrel monkey as revealed by retrograde labeling methods. *Brain Res* 436:296–310, 1987.
5. Hazrati LN, Parent A, Mitchell S, Haber SN: Evidence for interconnections between the two segments of the globus pallidus in primates: A PHA-L anterograde tracing study. *Brain Res* 533:171–175, 1990.
6. Gerfen CR, Engber TM, Mahan LC, et al: D1 and D2 dopamine receptor-regulated gene expression of striatonigral and striatopallidal neurons. *Science* 250:1429–1432, 1990.
7. Gerfen CR, Engber TM, Mahan LC, et al: D1 and D2 dopamine receptor-regulated gene expression of striatonigral and striatopallidal neurons. Glutamate and Parkinson's disease. *Ann Neurol* 35:639–645, 1994.
8. Lavoie B, Smith Y, Parent A: Dopaminergic innervation of the basal ganglia in the squirrel monkey as revealed by tyrosine hydroxylase immunohistochemistry. *J Comp Neurol* 289:36–52, 1989.
9. Cheramy A, Leviel V, Glowinski J: Dendritic release of dopamine in the substantia nigra. *Nature* 289:537–542, 1981.
10. Gauchy C, Desban M, Glowinski J, Kemel ML: NMDA regulation of dopamine release from proximal and distal dendrites in the cat substantia nigra. *Brain Res* 635:249–256, 1994.
11. DeLong MR, Coyle JT: Globus pallidus lesions in the monkey produced by kainic acid: Histologic and behavioral effects. *Appl Neurophysiol* 42:95–97, 1979.
12. Horak FB, Anderson ME: Influence of globus pallidus on arm movements in monkeys. I. Effects of kainic-induced lesions. *J Neurophysiol* 52:290–304, 1984.
13. Hore J, Villis T: Arm movement performance during reversible basal ganglia lesions in the monkey. *Exp Brain Res* 39:217–228, 1980.
14. MacLean PD: Effects of lesions of globus pallidus on species-typical display behavior of squirrel monkeys. *Brain Res* 149:175–196, 1978.
15. Ranson SW, Berry C: Observations on monkeys with bilateral lesions of the globus pallidus. *Arch Neurol Psychiatry* 46:504–508, 1941.
16. Strub RL: Frontal lobe syndrome in a patient with bilateral globus pallidus lesions. *Arch Neurol* 46:1024–1027, 1986.
17. Kato M, Kimura M: Effects of reversible blockade of basal ganglia on a voluntary arm movement. *J Neurophysiol* 68:1516–1534, 1992.
18. Mink JW, Thach WT: Basal ganglia motor control. III. Pallidal ablation: Normal reaction time, muscle cocontraction, and slow movement. *J Neurophysiol* 65:330–351, 1991.
19. Bennett KM, Marchetti M, Iovine R, Castiello U: The drinking action of Parkinson's disease subjects. *Brain* 118:959–970, 1995.
20. Cunnington R, Iansek R, Bradshaw JL, Phillips JG: Movement-related potentials in Parkinson's disease. Presence and predictability of temporal and spatial cues. *Brain* 118:935–950, 1995.
21. Martin KE, Phillips JG, Iansek R, Bradshaw JL: Inaccuracy and instability of sequential movements in Parkinson's disease. *Exp Brain Res* 102:131–140, 1994.
22. Georgiou N, Bradshaw JL, Iansek R, et al: Reduction in external cues and movement sequencing in Parkinson's disease. *J Neurol Neurosurg Psychiatry* 57:368–370, 1994.
23. Benecke R, Rothwell JC, Dick JP, et al: Disturbance of sequential movements in patients with Parkinson's disease. *Brain* 110:361–379, 1987.
24. Benecke R, Rothwell JC, Dick JP, et al: Simple and complex movements off and on treatment in patients with Parkinson's diesease. *J Neurol Neurosurg Psychiatry* 50:296–303, 1987.
25. Rolls ET: Neurophysiology and cognitive functions of the striatum. *Rev Neurol* 150:648–660, 1994.
26. Marsden CD: Which motor disorder in Parkinson's disease indicates the true motor function of the basal ganglia? *Ciba Found Symp* 107:225–241, 1984.
27. Trouche E, Beaubaton D, Amato G, et al: Changes in reaction time after pallidal or nigral lesion in the monkey. *Adv Neurol* 40:29–38, 1984.
28. DeLong MR, Georgopoulos AP: Motor functions of the basal ganglia, in Brookhart JM, Mountcastle VB, Brooks VB, Geiger SR (eds): *Handbook of Physiology. The Nervous System: Motor Control.* Bethesda, MD: American Physiological Society, 1981, sect 1, vol 2, part 2, pp 1017–1061.
29. Francois C, Percheron G , Yelnik J, Heyner S: A golgi analysis of the primate globus pallidus. I. Inconstant processes of large neurons, other neuronal types, and afferent axons. *J Comp Neurol* 227:182–199, 1984.
30. Yelnik J, Percheron G, Francois C: A golgi analysis of the primate globus pallidus. II. Quantitative morphology and spatial orientation of dendritic arborizations. *J Comp Neurol* 227:200–213, 1984.
31. Yelnik J, Francois C, Percheron G, Heyner S: Golgi study of the primate substantia nigra. I. Quantitative morphology and typology of nigral neurons. *J Comp Neurol* 265:455–472, 1987.
32. Francois C, Yelnik J, Percheron G: Golgi study of the primate substantia nigra. II. Spatial organization of dendritic arborizations in relation to the cytoarchitectonic boundaries and to the striatonigral bundle. *J Comp Neurol* 265:473–493, 1987.
33. Percheron G, Yelnick J, Francois C: A golgi analysis of the primate globus pallidus. III. Spatial organization of the striatopallidal complex. *J Comp Neurol* 227:214–227, 1984.
34. Francois C, Percheron G, Yelnick J, Heyner S: A golgi analysis of the primate globus pallidus. I. Inconstant processes of large neurons, other neuronal types, and afferent axons. *J Comp Neurol* 227:182–199, 1984.

35. Yelnick J, Percheron G, Francois C: A golgi analysis of the primate globus pallidus. II. Quantitative morphology and spatial orientation of dendritic arborizations. *J Comp Neurol* 227:200–213, 1984.

36. Nini A, Feingold A, Slovin H, Bergman H: Neurons in the globus pallidus do not show correlated activity in the normal monkey, but phase-locked oscillations appear in the MPTP model of parkinsonism. *J Neurophysiol.* 74:1800–1805, 1995.

37. Wichmann T, Bergman H, DeLong MR: The primate subthalamic nucleus. I. Functional properties in intact animals. *J Neurophysiol* 72:494–506, 1994.

38. Filion M, Tremblay L, Bedard PJ: Abnormal influences of passive limb movement on the activity of globus pallidus neurons in parkinsonian monkeys. *Brain Res* 444:165–176, 1988.

39. Miller WC, DeLong MR: Altered tonic activity of neurons in the globus pallidus and subthalamic nucleus in the primate MPTP model of parkinsonism, in Carpenter MB, Jayaraman A (eds): *The Basal Ganglia II.* New York: Plenum Press, 1987, pp 415–427.

40. Bergman H, Wichmann T, Karmon B, DeLong MR: The primate subthalamic nucleus. II. Neuronal activity in the MPTP model of parkinsonism. *J Neurophysiol* 72:507–520, 1994.

41. Vitek JL, Ashe J, DeLong MR, Alexander GE: Altered somatosensory response properties of neurons in the 'motor' thalamus of MPTP treated parkinsonian monkeys. *Soc Neurosci Abstr* 16:425, 1990.

42. Chevalier G, Deniau JM: Disinhibition as a basic process in the expression of striatal functions. *Trends Neurosci* 13:277–280, 1990.

43. Kita II: Physiology of two disynaptic pathways from the sensorimotor cortex to the basal ganglia output nuclei, in Percheron G, McKenzie JS, Feger J (eds): *The Basal Ganglia IV. New Ideas and Data on Structure and Function.* New York: Plenum Press, 1994, pp 263–276.

44. Mink JW, Thach WT: Basal ganglia motor control. I. Nonexclusive relation of pallidal discharge to five movement modes. *J Neurophysiol* 65:273–300, 1991.

45. Mink JW, Thach WT: Basal ganglia motor control. II. Late pallidal timing relative to movement onset and inconsistent pallidal coding of movement parameters. *J Neurophysiol* 65:301–329, 1991.

46. Hazrati LN, Parent A: Convergence of subthalamic and striatal efferents at pallidal level in primates: An anterograde double-labeling study with biocytin and PHA-L. *Brain Res* 569:336–340, 1992.

47. Smith Y, Sidibe M, Shink E: A light and electron microscopic analysis of the interconnections between the two pallidal segments and the subthalamic nucleus in the squirrel monkey. *Soc Neurosci Abstr* 20:332, 1994 (abstr.).

48. Shink E, Bevan MD, Bolam JP, Smith Y: The subthalamic nucleus and the external pallidum: Two tightly interconnected structures that control the output of the basal ganglia in the monkey. *Neuroscience.* 73:335–357, 1996.

49. Hoover JE, Strick PL: Multiple output channels in the basal ganglia. *Science* 259:819–821, 1993.

50. Nambu A, Yoshida S-I, Jinnai K: Discharge patterns of pallidal neurons with input from various cortical areas during movement in the monkey. *Brain Res* 519:183–191, 1990.

51. Yoshida S, Nambu A, Jinnai K: The distribution of the globus pallidus neurons with input from various cortical areas in the monkeys. *Brain Res* 611:170–174, 1993.

52. Jinnai K, Nambu A, Yoshida S, Tanibuchi I: The two separate neuron circuits through the basal ganglia concerning the preparatory or execution processes of the motor control, in Mano N, Hamada I, DeLong MR (eds): *Role of the Cerebellum and Basal Ganglia in Voluntary Movement.* Amsterdam: Elsevier, 1993, pp 153–163.

53. Romo R, Schultz W: Role of primate basal ganglia and frontal cortex in the internal generation of movement. III. Neuronal activity in the supplementary motor area. *Exp Brain Res* 91:396–407, 1992.

54. Schultz W, Romo R: Role of primate basal ganglia and frontal cortex in the internal generation of movement. I. Preparatory activity in the anterior striatum. *Exp Brain Res* 91:363–384, 1992.

55. Alexander GE, Crutcher MD: Preparation for movement: Neural representations of intended direction in three motor areas of the monkey. *J Neurophysiol* 64:133–150, 1990.

56. Alexander GE, Crutcher MD: Neural representations of the target (goal) of visually guided arm movements in three motor areas of the monkey. *J Neurophysiol* 64:164–178, 1990.

57. Jaeger D, Gilman S, Aldridge JW: Primate basal ganglia activity in a precued reaching task: Preparation for movement. *Exp Brain Res* 95:51–64, 1993.

58. Bergman H, Wichmann T, DeLong MR: Reversal of experimental parkinsonism by lesions of the subthalamic nucleus. *Science* 249:1436–1438, 1990.

59. DeLong MR: Primate models of movement disorders of basal ganglia origin. *Trends Neurosci* 13:281–285, 1990.

60. Filion M, Tremblay L: Abnormal spontaneous activity of globus pallidus neurons in monkeys with MPTP-induced parkinsonism. *Brain Res* 547:142–151, 1991.

61. Aziz TZ, Peggs D, Sambrook MA, Crossman AR: Lesion of the subthalamic nucleus for the alleviation of 1-methyl-4-phenyl-1,2,3,6-tetrahydropyridine (MPTP)-induced parkinsonism in the primate. *Mov Disord* 6:288–292, 1991.

62. Wichmann T, Bergman H, DeLong MR: The primate subthalamic nucleus. III. Changes in motor behavior and neuronal activity in the internal pallidum induced by subthalamic inactivation in the MPTP model of parkinsonism. *J Neurophysiol* 72:521–530, 1994.

63. Wichmann T, Baron MS, DeLong MR: Local inactivation of the sensorimotor territories of the internal segment of the globus pallidus and the subthalamic nucleus alleviates parkinsonian motor signs in MPTP treated monkeys, in Percheron G, McKenzie JS, Feger J (eds): *The Basal Ganglia IV: New Ideas and Data on Structure and Function.* New York: Plenum Press, 1994, pp 357–363.

64. Guridi J, Herrero MT, Luquin R, et al: Subthalamotomy improves MPTP-induced parkinsonism in monkeys. *Stereotact Funct Neurosurg* 62:98–102, 1994.

65. Laitinen LV, Bergenheim AT, Hariz MI: Leksell's posteroventral pallidotomy in the treatment of Parkinson's disease. *J Neurosurg* 76:53, 1992.

66. Baron M, Vitek J, Turner R, et al: Lesions in the sensorimotor region of the internal segment of the globus pallidus (GPi) in parkinsonian patients are effective in alleviating the cardinal signs of Parkinson's disease. *Soc Neurosci* 19:1584, 1993.

67. Iacono RP, Lonser RR: Reversal of Parkinson's akinesia by pallidotomy. *Lancet* 343:418–419, 1994.

68. Dogali M, Fazzini E, Kolodny E, et al: Stereotactic ventral pallidotomy for Parkinson's disease. *Neurology* 45:753–761, 1995.

69. Laitinen LV: Pallidotomy for Parkinson's disease. *Neurosurg Clin N Am* 6:105–112, 1995.

70. Sutton JP, Couldwell W, Lew MF, et al: Ventroposterior medial pallidotomy in patients with advanced Parkinson's disease. *Neurosurgery* 36:1118–1125, 1995.

71. Vitek JL, Kaneoke Y, Turner R, et al: Neuronal activity in the internal (GPi) and external (GPe) segments of the globus pallidus (GP) of parkinsonian patients is similar to that in the MPTP-treated primate model of parkinsonism. *Soc Neurosci Abstr* 19:1584, 1993.

72. Pollak B, Benabid AL, Gross C, et al: Effects de la stimulation do noyan sous-thalamique dans la maladie de Parkinson. *Rev Neurol (Paris)* 149:175–176, 1994.

73. Ceballos-Bauman AO, Obeso JA, Vitek JL, et al: Restoration of thalamocortical activity after posteroventrolateral pallidotomy in Parkinson's disease. *Lancet* 344:814, 1994.

74. Obeso JA, Rothwell JC, Ceballos-Bauman A, et al: The mechanism of action of pallidotomy in Parkinson's disease (PD): Physiological and imaging studies. *Soc Neurosci Abstr* 21:1982, 1995(abstr.).

75. Brooks DJ: Detection of preclinical Parkinson's disease with PET. *Neurology* 41(suppl 2):24–27, 1991.

76. Svennilson E, Torvik A, Lowe R, Leksell L: Treatment of parkinsonism by stereotactic thermolesions in the pallidal region. A clinical evaluation of 81 cases. *Acta Psychiat Neurol Scand* 35:358–377, 1960.

77. Laitinen LV: Leksell's posteroventral pallidotomy in the treatment of Parkinson's disease. *J Neurosurg* 76:53–61, 1992.

78. Bakay RAE, DeLong MR, Vitek JL: Posteroventral pallidotomy for Parkinson's disease (letter). *J Neurosurg* 77:487–488, 1992.

79. Vitek JL, Baron M, Kaneoke Y, et al: Microelectrode-guided pallidotomy is an effective treatment for medically intractable Parkinson's disease. *Neurology* 44 (suppl. 2):A304 (Abstr. 703p), 1994.

80. Baron MS, Vitek JL, Turner RS, et al: Treatment of medically intractable Parkinson's disease with micro-electrode guided pallidotomy: One year follow-up. *Mov Disord* 44 (suppl. 2):A304 (Abstr. 702p), 1994.

81. Alexander GE, Crutcher MD: Functional architecture of basal ganglia circuits: Neural substrates of parallel processing. *Trends Neurosci* 13:266–271, 1990.

82. Deecke L: Cerebral potentials related to voluntary actions: Parkinsonism and normal subjects, in Delwaide PJ, Agnoli A (eds): *Clinical Neurophysiology in Parkinsonism.* Amsterdam: Elsevier, 1985, pp 91–105.

83. Dick JPR, Rothwell JC, Day BL, et al: The Bereitschaftspotential is abnormal in Parkinson's disease. *Brain* 112:233–244, 1989.

84. Calne D, Snow BJ: PET imaging in parkinsonism. *Adv Neurol* 60:484, 1993.

85. Eidelberg D: Positron emission tomography studies in parkinsonism. *Neurol Clin* 10:421, 1992.

86. Eidelberg D, Moeller JR, Dhawan V, et al: The metabolic topography of parkinsonism. *J Cereb Blood Flow Metab* 14:783–801, 1994.

87. Brooks DJ: Functional imaging in relation to parkinsonian syndromes. *J Neurol Sci* 115:1–17, 1993.

88. Narabayashi H: Surgical treatment in the L-dopa era, in Stern G (ed): *Parkinson's Disease.* London: Chapman & Hall, 1990, pp 597–646.

89. Narabayashi H, Maeda T, Yokochi F: Long-term follow up study of nucleus ventralis intermedius and ventrolateralis thalamotomy using a microelectrode technique in parkinsonism. *Appl Neurophysiol* 50:330–337, 1987.

90. Narabayashi H: Stereotaxic Vim thalamotomy for treatment of tremor. *Eur Neurol* 29:S29–S32, 1989.

91. Hassler R, Mundinger F, Riechert T: Stereotaxis in parkinsonian syndromes. Berlin: Springer-Verlag, 1979.

92. Marsden CD: The mysterious motor function of the basal ganglia: The Robert Wartenburg lecture. *Neurology* 32:514–539, 1982.

93. Pollack LT, Davis L: Muscle tone in parkinsonian states. *Arch Neurol Psychiatry* 23:303–319, 1930.

94. Burke D, Gandevia SC, McKeon B: Monosynaptic and oligosynaptic contributions to human ankle jerk and H reflex. *J Neurophys* 52:435–448, 1984.

95. Delwaide PJ, Pepin JL, Maertens de Noordhout A: Short-latency

96. Lee RG, Murphy JT, Tatton WG: Long-latency myotatic reflexes in man: Mechanisms, functional significance, and changes in patients with Parkinson's disease or hemiplegia, in Desmedt JE (ed): *Motor Control Mechanisms in Health and Disease.* New York: Raven Press, 1983, pp 489–507.

97. Vitek JL, Wichmann T, DeLong MR: Current concepts of basal ganglia neurophysiology with respect to tremorgenesis, in Findley LJ, Koller W (eds): *Handbook of Tremor Disorders.* New York: Marcel Dekker, 1994, pp 37–50.

98. Spiegel EA, Wycis HT: Ansotomy in paralysis agitans. *Arch Neurol Psychiatry* 71:598–614, 1954.

99. Hassler R, Reichert T, Mundinger F, et al: Physiological observations in stereotaxic operations in extrapyramidal motor disturbances. *Brain* 83:337–350, 1960.

100. Buzsaki G, Smith A, Berger S, et al: Petit mal epilepsy and parkinsonian tremor: Hypothesis of a common pacemaker. *Neuroscience* 36(1):1–14, 1990.

101. Llinas RR: The intrinsic electrophysiological properties of mammalian neurons: Insights into central nervous system function. *Science* 242:1654–1664, 1988.

102. Dacko S, Smith MG, Schneider JS: Immunohistochemical study of the pallidal complex in symptomatic and asymptomatic MPTP-treated monkeys, normal human, and Parkinson's disease patients. *Soc Neurosci Abstr* 16:428, 1990.

103. Bernheimer H, Birkmayer W, Hornykiewicz O, et al: Brain dopamine and the syndromes of Parkinson and Huntington. *J Neurol Sci* 20:415–455, 1973.

104. Nambu A, Llinas R: Electrophysiology of the globus pallidus neurons: An in vitro study in guinea pig brain slices. *Soc Neurosci Abstr* 16:428, 1990 (abstr.).

105. Pare D, Curro'Dossi R, Steriade M: Neuronal basis of the parkinsonian resting tremor: A hypothesis and its implications for treatment. *Neuroscience* 35:217–226, 1990.

106. Pifl C, Bertel O, Schingnitz G, Hornykiewicz O: Extrastriatal dopamine in symptomatic and asymptomatic rhesus monkeys treated with 1-methyl-4-phenyl-1,2,3,6-tetrahydropyridine (MPTP). *Neurochem Int* 17:263–270, 1990.

107. Cummings JL: Frontal-subcortical circuits and human behavior. *Arch Neurol* 50:873–880, 1993.

108. Hollander E, Cohen L, Richards M, et al: A pilot study of the neuropsychology of obsessive-compulsive disorder and Parkinson's disease: Basal ganglia disorders. *J Neuropsychiatry Clin Neusosci* 5:104–107, 1993.

109. Cummings JL, Cunningham K: Obsessive-compulsive disorder in Huntington's disease. *Biol Psychiatry* 31:263–270, 1992.

110. Carpenter MB, Whittier JR, Mettler FA: Analysis of choreoid hyperkinesia in the rhesus monkey: Surgical and pharmacological analysis of hyperkinesia resulting from lesions in the subthalamic nucleus of Luys. *J Comp Neurol* 92:293–332, 1950.

111. Whittier JR, Mettler FA: Studies of the subthalamus of the rhesus monkey. II. Hyperkinesia and other physiologic effects of subthalamic lesions with special references to the subthalamic nucleus of Luys. *J Comp Neurol* 90:319–372, 1949.

112. Crossman AR, Sambrook MA, Jackson A: Experimental hemichorea/hemiballismus in the monkey. Study on the intracerebral site of action in a drug-induced dyskinesia. *Brain* 107:579–596, 1984.

113. Hammond C, Feger J, Bioulac B, Souteyrand JP: Experimental hemiballism in the monkey produced by unilateral kainic acid lesion in corpus Luysii. *Brain Res* 171:577, 1979.

114. Kase CS, Maulsby GO, DeJuan E, Mohr JP: Hemi-chorea-hemiballism and lacunar infarction in the basal ganglia. *Neurology* 31:452–455, 1981.

115. Hamada I, DeLong MR: Excitotoxic acid lesions of the primate

subthalamic nucleus result in transient dyskinesias of the contralateral limbs. *J Neurophysiol* 68:1850–1858, 1992.

116. Hamada I, DeLong MR: Excitotoxic acid lesions of the primate subthalamic nucleus result in reduced pallidal neuronal activity during active holding. *J Neurophysiol* 68:1859–1866, 1992.

117. Gerfen CR: Dopamine receptor function in the basal ganglia. *Clin Neuropharmacol* 18:S162–S177, 1995.

118. Tranchant C, Maquet J, Eber AM, et al: Angiome caverneux cerebelleux, dystonie cervicale et diaschisis cortical croise. *Rev Neurol* 147:599–602, 1991.

119. Gille M, Jacquemin C, Kiame G, et al: Myelinolyse centropontine avec ataxie cerebelleuse et dystonie. *Rev Neurol* 149:344–346, 1993.

120. Janati A, Metzer WS, Archer RL, et al: Blepharospasm associated with olivopontocerebellar atrophy. *J Clin Neuroophthalmol* 9:281–284, 1989.

121. Krauss JK, Mohadjer M, Braus DF, et al: Dystonia following head trauma: A report of nine patients and review of the literature. *Mov Disord* 7:263–272, 1992.

122. Nygaard TG: Dopa-responsive dystonia. *Curr Opin Neurol* 8:310–313, 1995.

123. Patel K, Roskrow T, Davis JS, Heckmatt JZ: Dopa responsive dystonia. *Arch Dis Child* 73:256–257, 1995.

124. Playford ED, Fletcher NA, Sawle GV, et al: Striatal [18F]dopa uptake in familial idiopathic dystonia. *Brain* 116:1191–1199, 1993.

125. Mitchell IJ, Luquin R, Boyce S, et al: Neural mechanisms of dystonia: Evidence from a 2-deoxyglucose uptake study in a primate model of dopamine agonist-induced dystonia. *Mov Disord* 5:49–54, 1990.

126. Hantraye P, Riche D, Maziere M, Isacson O: A primate model of Huntington's disease: Behavioral and anatomical studies of unilateral excitotoxic lesions of the caudate-putamen in the baboon. *Exp Neurol* 108:91–104, 1990.

127. Forno LS, Langston JW, DeLanney LE, et al: Locus ceruleus lesions and eosinophilic inclusions in MPTP-treated monkeys. *Ann Neurol* 20:449–455, 1986.

128. Forno LS, DeLanney LE, Irwin I, Langston JW: Similarities and differences between MPTP-induced parkinsonism and Parkinson's disease. *Adv Neurol* 60:600–608, 1993.

129. Gibb WR: Neuropathology of Parkinson's disease and related syndromes. *Neurol Clin* 10:361–376, 1992.

130. Jellinger KA: Pathology of Parkinson's disease. Changes other than the nigrostriatal pathway. *Mol Chem Neuropathol* 14:153–197, 1991.

131. Laitinen LV, Bergenheim AT, Hariz MI: Ventroposterolateral pallidotomy can abolish all parkinsonian symptoms. *Stereotact Funct Neurosurg* 58:14–21, 1992.

_____

Chapter 7

FUNCTIONAL BIOCHEMISTRY AND MOLECULAR NEUROPHARMACOLOGY OF THE BASAL GANGLIA AND MOTOR SYSTEMS

BRIAN J. CILIAX, J. TIMOTHY GREENAMYRE, and ALLAN I. LEVEY

OVERVIEW OF THE NEUROCHEMISTRY OF MOTOR CIRCUITS
MOLECULAR PHARMACOLOGY OF DOPAMINE IN BASAL GANGLIA
    Anatomy of Dopaminergic Transmission in Basal Ganglia
    Dopamine Receptor Pharmacology in Basal Ganglia
    Molecular Diversity of Dopamine Receptors
MOLECULAR PHARMACOLOGY OF ACETYLCHOLINE IN BASAL GANGLIA
    Anatomy and Physiology of Cholinergic Transmission in Basal Ganglia
    Molecular Diversity of ACh Receptors
    Pharmacology and Signal Transduction Mechanisms of Muscarinic Receptors
    Selective Expression of Muscarinic Receptor Subtypes in Basal Ganglia
MOLECULAR PHARMACOLOGY OF GLUTAMATE IN BASAL GANGLIA
    Anatomy and Physiology of Glutamate in Basal Ganglia
    Altered Glutamatergic Neurotransmission in Parkinson's Disease
    Therapeutic Manipulation of Glutamatergic Neurotransmission

In recent years there has been an explosion of information about the molecular biology and neuropharmacology of motor pathways, including identification of many classical and nonclassical neurotransmitters and, more remarkably, an unanticipated diversity of genes encoding the receptors, transporters, and other proteins that mediate the effects of these transmitters. Although this complexity challenges attempts to understand the molecular and synaptic organization of motor circuits, the heterogeneity also provides new opportunities for therapeutic interventions. Because most hypokinetic and hyperkinetic disorders may ultimately be manifest because of perturbations in the neural activity of different

motor pathways (Chap. 6), knowledge of molecules that govern the activity of each synapse in motor circuits has tremendous implications for understanding the pathogenesis and treatment of movement disorders. Clinicians can expect to have available a new armamentarium of drugs aimed at these molecular targets in the near future that offer hope for more effective and selective therapies, both symptomatic and neuroprotective. The purpose of this chapter is to review some of the key advances in understanding the molecular pharmacology of dopamine, acetylcholine (ACh), and glutamate, three of the primary neurotransmitters regulating basal ganglia activity, and to integrate this information with current views of the anatomy, physiology and pathophysiology of motor pathways (Chaps. 5 and 6).

Overview of the Neurochemistry of Motor Circuits

The principal transmitters in basal ganglia and other motor regions have been the subject of several excellent reviews[1,2] and are summarized in Fig. 7-1. Glutamate and gamma-aminobutyric acid (GABA) mediate the main flow of information processing along excitatory and inhibitory pathways, respectively, in the basal ganglia and associated pathways. As explained in the previous chapter, motor circuitry is initiated in cortical regions that transmit parallel glutamatergic projections to striatum. The putamen is the region of striatum that processes the motor component of basal ganglia-thalamocortical circuits, whereas caudate and nucleus accumbens mediate cognitive, emotive, and limbic processes. In putamen, spiny neurons receive the excitatory synaptic inputs from neocortex, as well as thalamus.[3] Spiny neurons are the principal input and output cells, and they account for more than three-quarters of the total striatal neuronal population. Two distinct populations of spiny neurons in turn project downstream to the globus pallidus internal segment (GPi), although the information is processed via separate routes termed the direct and indirect pathways.[4-7] The GPi is the major output nucleus of the basal ganglia circuit, providing tonic GABAergic inhibitory output to motor nuclei in the thalamus and the mesopontine tegmentum.

The neurochemistry of the direct and indirect pathways through basal ganglia are key to understanding pharmacological approaches to treatment of movement disorders. The balance of activity in these pathways is believed to play an important role in the normal operations of basal ganglia[6,7] and also in the genesis of movement disorders,[8-10] as discussed in Chapters 5 and 6. The spiny neurons in striatum that give rise to these projections are neurochemically and anatomically distinct, although both subpopulations receive direct synaptic innervation from motor cortex.[11] The direct pathway originates from a subpopulation of GABA and substance P-containing neurons that project directly (hence, the direct pathway) to the GPi and substantia nigra pars reticulata (SNr), which are the basal ganglia output nuclei (GPi/SNr). The indirect pathway starts from a separate subpopulation of spiny neurons that coexpress GABA and enkephalin and

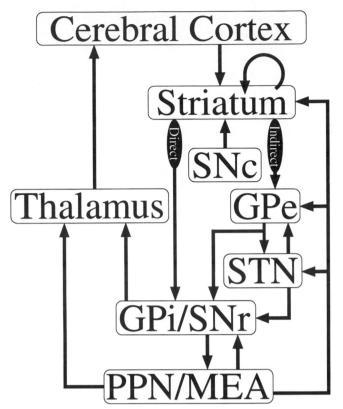

FIGURE 7-1 Schematic of basal ganglia circuitry model. Direct and indirect pathways originating from striatum are named according to the immediacy of their regulation of the basal ganglia output nuclei, GP1/SNr. The projections from each region are color coded by their major neurotransmitters in the Color Gallery. GPe, globus pallidus external segment; GPi/SNr, globus pallidus internal segment/substantia nigra pars reticulata; PPN/MEA, pedunculopontine nucleus/midbrain extrapyramidal area; SNc, substantial nigra pars compacta; STN, subthalamic nucleus. See Color Plate 3.

project to the external segment of globus pallidus (GPe). GPe sends a GABAergic projection to the subthalamus (STN), which in turn provides glutamatergic innervation of GPi/SNr. Thus, the basal ganglia output nuclei receive opposing inhibitory and excitatory signals from the direct and indirect pathways, respectively.

This model of basal ganglia circuits suggests that the basal activity of the pallidal neurons is kept in check by a balance of the direct and indirect pathways, with the direct pathway tending to reduce basal ganglia output and the indirect pathway tending to increase the output. Because GPi is GABAergic, the high basal discharge of these pallidal neurons results in tonic inhibitory control over the thalamus. During normal movement, changes in the balance of the direct and indirect pathways reduce GPi/SNr inhibition of thalamus, allowing engagement of thalamocortical circuits necessary for the speed and guidance of movements. An imbalance of activity, however, in the direct and indirect pathways can perturb the normal degree of GPi/SNr inhibition of thalamocortical activity, producing either hypokinetic or hyperkinetic move-

ment disorders.[2,9,10] For example, in Parkinson's disease (PD), models suggest that activity is reduced in the direct pathway and increased in the indirect pathway, both leading to enhanced GPi/SNr activity and excessive inhibition of thalamus.[2,9,10]

These pathways provide a diversity of sites for therapeutic drugs to influence basal ganglia output and restore function in movement disorders. The striatum is particularly enriched with a variety of neurochemicals, including extremely high levels of dopamine, ACh, and their receptors,[1,12,13] and is thus often suggested to be a principal site of action of the commonly used dopaminergic and anticholinergic therapies. Glutamate is also the major excitatory transmitter at the corticostriate synapse.[1,3] Each of these transmitters has the potential to differentially modulate the activity of the direct and indirect striatal output pathways. Moreover, the transmitters have known or potentially important roles at downstream sites, where they can alter subthalamic, pallidal, and thalamic activity. In addition to this anatomic complexity, there are often multiple physiological responses to a single transmitter within a given structure.

Recent advances in molecular biology have led to the discovery of large gene families encoding heterogeneous receptor subtypes for dopamine,[14–16] ACh,[17,18] glutamate,[19] and other transmitters. Indeed, for glutamate alone, there are now more than 100 types of genetically distinct receptors. Although the present level of understanding of the precise physiological roles of each of the receptors is extremely limited, it is nonetheless clear that the multiplicity of effects of each transmitter is in part governed by the differential expression of the genes. Somewhat surprisingly, it appears that almost all therapeutic drugs presently used for movement disorders bind to numerous receptor subtypes. Hence, drugs intended to augment or block a particular neurotransmitter produce complex effects at many sites, of which only some are therapeutic, whereas others lead to undesirable side effects. Thus, identification of the molecular sites of action of therapeutic drugs will facilitate development of new compounds that are targeted to the key receptor subtypes located in select basal ganglia pathways. Such "magic bullet" therapies offer the promise of increased efficacy for a variety of movement disorders and also reduced side effects, compared to that offered by drugs presently available. The remainder of the chapter focuses on the receptor gene families for dopamine, ACh, and glutamate and summarizes relevant information about the expression and function of the subtypes in basal ganglia.

Molecular Pharmacology of Dopamine in Basal Ganglia

ANATOMY OF DOPAMINERGIC TRANSMISSION IN BASAL GANGLIA

Dopaminergic innervation of motor striatum originates principally from the A9 cell group in substantia nigra pars compacta,[20] wherein neurons are arranged in interdigitated clusters that project to either caudate or putamen.[21] Dopaminergic terminals synapse predominantly on dendritic shafts and spines of striatal medium spiny neurons,[22,23] where they appear to regulate responsiveness to cortical and thalamic excitatory drive.[24,25] Distinct subpopulations of dopamine neurons project to the patch and matrix compartments (for a review, see Ref. 2). These compartments represent separate subchannels of afferent and efferent circuits through basal ganglia. Based on corticostriatal connections, the striatal patch compartment processes limbic information, whereas the striatal matrix processes sensorimotor information.[2] Substantia nigra pars compacta neurons also extend dendrites into pars reticulata, where they release dopamine, modulating GABA release, neuronal activity in pars reticulata and, subsequently, basal ganglia output to thalamus.[20,26] In primate, dopaminergic neurons are separated into dorsal and ventral groups, which project to ventral and dorsolateral striatum, respectively.[27] It is unclear whether these subgroups are equivalent to dorsal and ventral tiers described in lower species,[28–30] because a detailed analysis in primates is lacking; however, one report does indicate a similar type of organization.[31] Thus, ventrally located dopamine neurons in primates project to motor striatum and are the neurons most vulnerable in PD and 1-methyl-4-phenyl-1,2,3,6-tetrahydropyridine (MPTP) toxicity, whereas dorsally located neurons are relatively spared.[32–37] These subgroups of dopamine neurons differentially express calbindin[36] and neuromelanin;[33,35] however, any role these markers play in the fate of these cells is unclear.

DOPAMINE RECEPTOR PHARMACOLOGY IN BASAL GANGLIA

Dopamine has diverse effects mediated by two subfamilies of dopamine receptors, D1 and D2, which are defined by pharmacological, anatomic, and biochemical criteria.[38] Receptors from both families have been shown to be concentrated in striatum by functional and radioligand binding assays.[39–49] Receptors in the D1 subfamily are positively coupled to adenylate cyclase, whereas those of the D2 subfamily are either not coupled or negatively coupled.[16,38,50] Selective drugs have been used to demonstrate that D1 and D2 receptor subfamilies have a multitude of roles in behavior, electrophysiology, regulation of neurotransmitter release, and induction of gene expression.[51–53] Thus, the role of dopamine in basal ganglia function and movement disorders is complex.

Dopamine receptor stimulation causes stereotypy and increased locomotion, whereas pharmacological blockade causes catalepsy and parkinsonism, and both D1-like and D2-like receptors are important for these actions.[51,53,54] The role of D2-like receptors in motor function has long been established, largely because of the early availability of D2-specific drugs. Neuroleptics, which induce catalepsy and block stereotypy and locomotion induced by apomorphine or amphetamine, were found to be high-affinity antagonists of D2-like receptors. In addition, D2-specific agonists produced the same behavioral syndrome as the nonselective agonists and were effective treatments for animals with nigrostriatal lesions, as well as patients with PD. Thus, D2-like receptors are clearly involved in dopaminergic regulation of motor control.

Until recently, elucidation of the specific role of D1-like receptors in basal ganglia function has been limited by the lack of ideal D1-specific agonists. The most widely used D1 agonist, SKF 38393, was originally chosen because of its high specificity and its ability to traverse the blood-brain barrier. SKF 38393, however, is only a partial agonist at D1-like receptors, with approximately one-third the efficacy of dopamine.[55] Although studies reporting positive results with this compound demonstrate that submaximal stimulation of D1-like receptors is effective in certain assays, the numerous negative results must be interpreted with caution. Thus, previous views that D1-like receptor stimulation had no locomotor effects and that D1 agonists were ineffective therapies for akinesia induced by nigrostriatal denervation need to be reevaluated with full D1-specific agonists. In fact, recent studies using more efficacious D1 agonists demonstrate a clear role for D1-like receptors in motor performance and the potential to reverse parkinsonism in MPTP-treated monkeys.[56,57] Moreover, a full D1 agonist is able to stimulate c-*fos* (a putative marker of neuronal activation) expression in normosensitive striatum,[58] whereas SKF38393 is effective only in 6-hydroxydopamine (OHDA)-lesioned striatum. Thus, reevaluation of D1 receptor function using full, D1-specific agonists will shed new light on the respective roles of dopamine receptor subfamilies in basal ganglia circuitry.

D1 and D2 receptors mediate the locomotor effects of dopamine through an interdependent-synergistic mechanism,[51,53] which is corroborated by electrophysiology and immediate early gene-induction studies.[52,59–65] Locomotion elicited by either D1 or D2 receptor stimulation can be blocked by removing all endogenous stimulation of the other receptor subfamily via antagonists or dopamine depletion. Locomotion can be restored in the depleted animals with subthreshold doses of an agonist for the other receptor subfamily. Conversely, in normal animals, subthreshold doses of one agonist will potentiate the locomotor effects of the other. This could have important therapeutic implications, particularly when considering selective D1 and D2 agonists as primary or adjunctive treatments for PD and suggests that the output of both direct and indirect pathways must be altered (see below) for successful dopamine replacement therapy.

L-dopa therapy is very effective in reversing the akinesia, rigidity, and bradykinesia of PD; however, several complications may occur during the course of treatment, including the development of tolerance and dyskinesias. It has recently been shown that both D1 and D2 agonists can elicit dyskinesias in proportion to their therapeutic efficacy[66] and that the dosing regimen is critical for initiating both sensitization to locomotor responses and side effects.[67,68] Thus, dopamine elicits complex changes in basal ganglia, which occur at distinct cellular and subcellular levels, via pre- and postsynaptic mechanisms, and which now are known to be mediated by an increasingly large family of dopamine receptor subtypes.

MOLECULAR DIVERSITY OF DOPAMINE RECEPTORS

Molecular biology has led to a great increase in understanding dopamine receptor subtypes. In humans, at least five distinct genes encode functional dopamine receptor subtypes, some of which have multiple isoforms. Each subtype belongs to one of the two pharmacologically defined subfamilies. Excellent reviews of the gene family are available.[16,50] All dopamine receptors identified to date are members of the superfamily of G protein-coupled receptors and have seven transmembrane regions. Each receptor consists of a single protein that, when activated by dopamine, stimulates a guanosine triphosphate (GTP)-binding protein effector. Receptor subtypes of the D1 subfamily have long carboxy termini, whereas those of the D2 subfamily have long third intracellular loops. These domains are believed to specify which G protein subtype(s) are activated. The D1 subclass consists of D1, D1$_B$, and D5 gene products, the receptors are highly conserved (~80 percent homologous) in the transmembrane regions, and all bind D1-selective ligands with high affinity and activate adenylyl cyclase.[69–71] The D1$_B$ receptor, cloned from rats,[69] and the D5 receptor,[71] cloned from humans, may be species variants of the same gene. The D2 subclass consists of D2, D3, and D4 receptors; these clones also have marked sequence homology in transmembrane regions (~75 percent homologous), and all bind D2-selective ligands with high affinity.[72–74] D2, D3, and D4 inhibit adenylate cyclase (dependent upon the type of cell line transfected, suggesting that the subtypes couple to different G proteins expressed in the different cell lines).[75–77] Clozapine, an atypical antipsychotic free of extrapyramidal side effects, has a 10-fold higher affinity for D4 receptor than D2 or D3 receptors, suggesting that D4 may be the site of action for clozapine's antipsychotic properties and that D4 may have a role in limbic function.[74] Several polymorphisms of human D4 have been identified, each with a different number of a 16 amino acid repeat in the third intracellular loop, which subtly alters the receptor's affinity for neuroleptics.[78] The classification of the dopamine receptor gene family, including binding properties, selective agonists and antagonists, and general distributions in brain are summarized in Table 7-1.

The distribution of each dopamine receptor subtype is distinct, suggesting a specific role for each. In the striatum, D1 and D2 receptor mRNAs are the most abundant subtypes.[67,71,73,79–81] Furthermore, D1 and D2 receptor proteins are immunolocalized to striatum (Figs. 7-2 and 7-3) and each accounts for the vast majority of binding sites for the respective subfamilies.[82]

A critical question in models of basal ganglia circuits is whether D1 and D2 receptors are segregated or colocalized to the striatonigral and striatopallidal neurons. If the receptors are segregated, dopamine can differentially regulate the direct and indirect pathways by concomitant stimulation of D1 and D2 receptors in striatum. In the segregation model, dopamine binding to D1 receptors activates striatonigral neurons via stimulation of adenylyl cyclase, whereas dopamine binding to D2 receptors inhibits striatopallidal neurons via inhibition of adenylyl cyclase. Several lines of evidence support this segregation model. First, D1 and D2 selective drugs have been shown to selectively modulate the expression of the immediate early gene c-*fos* in different projection neurons.[52,58,83,84] D1 *agonists* increase expression in striatonigral neurons, suggesting D1 is excitatory and D2 *antagonists* increase expression in striatopallidal neurons, suggesting D2 is inhibitory. Second, nigrostriatal 6-hydroxydopamine lesions in rat result in elevated GABA and benzodiazepine binding sites in the entopeduncular nucleus (EPN, the rodent homolog of GPi) and SNr, but reduced binding sites in globus pallidus (GP, the rodent homolog of GPe), suggesting differential regulation by dopamine of striatonigral and striatopallidal GABAergic efflux.[85] Third, in primates with MPTP lesions, GPe activity is decreased, whereas GPi activity is increased,[86,87] consistent with reduced D2 inhibition of striatopallidal neurons and reduced D1 excitation of striatonigral neurons. Fourth, local injection of D1 agonists into striatum increases GABA and dynorphin release from striatonigral terminals in pars reticulata,[88] whereas local injection of D2 agonist into striatum decreases GABA release from striato-

FIGURE 7-2 Immunocytochemical localization of dopaminergic (D1 and D2) and muscarinic cholinergic (m4) receptor subtypes in monkey basal ganglia. Low-power darkfield micrograph of immunoperoxidase-stained brain tissue sections through neostriatum and globus pallidus. Note intense staining (white areas) of all three receptors in caudate (C) and putamen (Pu), and selective localization to either globus pallidus interna (GPi) for D1 and m4 or globus pallidus externa (GPe) for D2, suggesting selective expression of the subtypes in the striatofugal neurons and terminals of the direct or indirect pathways, respectively. Coronal sections; lateral portion positioned on the left and medial on the right; scale bars = 100 μm.

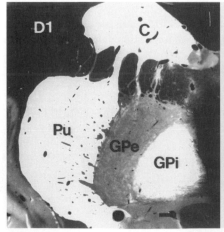
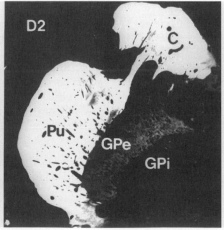
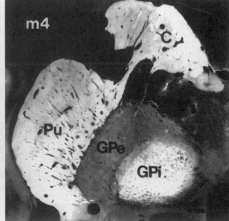

TABLE 7-1 Dopamine Receptor Subtypes

Receptor Subtype	Pharm. Class	Isoforms	Second Messenger	Selective Agonists	Selective Antagonists	Localization
D1 Subfamily			Increase cAMP	SKF 38393 CY 208-243 (partial agonists) A 77636 SKF 82958 (full agonists)	SCH 23390 (some 5-HT effects) SCH 39166 (no 5-HT effects)	
D1 (D1A)	D1					Striatal spiny neurons (direct pathway)
D5 (D1B)	D1	Pseudogenes on chrom. 1 and 2, polymorphisms				Cortex, thalamus cholinergic striatal neurons, SNc
D2 Subfamily			Decrease cAMP	Bromocriptine Quinpirole	Spiroperidol (some 5-HT effects) Raclopride	
D2 (D2A)	D2	Short/long splice variants, 6 introns				Striatal spiny neurons (indirect pathway) SNc (autoreceptor)
D3 (D2B)	D2	2 splice variants (truncated), 5 introns		7-OH-DPAT PD 128,907		Ventral striatum, limbic regions
D4 (D2C)	D2	Polymorphisms (2–10 repeats)			Clozapine (some muscarinic + 5-HT effects) L 745870 U 101958	Poorly understood

pallidal terminals in GP.[89] Fifth, blockade, by dopamine denervation or dopaminergic antagonists, produces different regulatory effects on precursor mRNAs and peptide levels of substance P and met-enkephalin in striatonigral and striatopallidal neurons, respectively.[67,90–95] Thus, in the dual-pathway model, the release of dopamine in striatum has opposite effects on the subpopulations of striatal output neurons. Do-

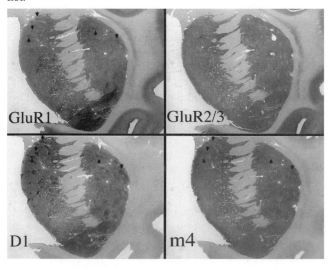

FIGURE 7-3 Comparison of the distributions of GluR1, GluR2/3, D1, and m4 proteins in human striatum. Note that GluR1, D1, and m4 are all enriched in patches (arrows), but GluR2/3 is not.

pamine, however, ultimately produces the same result through each pathway: inhibition of GPi/SNr and disinhibition of thalamus. Applying this model to nigrostriatal degeneration as it occurs in PD, loss of dopamine reduces the tonic stimulation by D1 receptors on striatonigral neurons and the tonic inhibition by D2 receptors on striatopallidal neurons. Both effects are predicted to lead to an excitation of GPi/SNr and a consequent excessive inhibition of the thalamocortical motor circuits, and they result in bradykinesia, rigidity, and other hallmarks of the disease.[2,9,10]

At least two critical issues complicate this simplified model of D1 and D2 receptor segregation in basal ganglia function. First, although the cellular effects of dopamine agonists are still poorly understood (for review, see Ref. 25), most electrophysiology studies indicate that dopamine and dopaminergic agonists (mixed and selective) all produce inhibition or decreased responsiveness to excitatory (corticostriatal) drive in striatal output neurons.[63,96–110] The actions of dopamine, however, may be complex in that they are dependent on the actions of other neurotransmitter systems. For example, when nigrostriatal and corticostriatal stimulation are paired, a subpopulation of striatal neurons is excited and another subpopulation is inhibited, consistent with segregation of D1 and D2 receptors.[111] Striatal afferent interactions are probably even more complex, because responses of striatal output neurons have been shown to be critically dependent on which dopamine receptor subfamilies and glutamate receptor subfamilies are coactivated; thus, D1 increases and D2 decreases NMDA responses in striatal slices,[112,113] which is also consistent with the prediction of opposing actions of dopamine through the different receptor subtypes. Therefore, electrophysiology studies analyzing passive membrane properties, using injections of electric current into striatal neurons, are unlikely to detect such dopaminergic regulation of specific ligand-gated ion channels. Pharmacological methodology, as used in these more recent studies, should provide a better approach for analyzing these electrophysiological effects. Interaction with other neurotransmitter/neuropeptide systems (GABA, enkephalin, substance P, dynorphin, ACh, and serotonin) could also influence the effects of dopamine, as could other dopamine receptor molecular subtypes expressed pre- and postsynaptically in basal ganglia circuitry. Thus, much research remains to be conducted before we have a complete understanding of the neurophysiology of dopamine in basal ganglia.

The second issue complicating the dual-pathway model is that the cellular localization of D1 and D2 gene products has been controversial, with different methods producing conflicting results. In situ hybridization has shown that D1 and D2 mRNAs are expressed in about 50 percent of the striatal neurons,[114,115] D1 mRNA is localized to substance P-containing striatonigral neurons and D2 mRNA is localized to enkephalinergic striatopallidal neurons.[67,80] In contrast, a study using polymerase chain reaction (PCR) to amplify mRNAs from individual cells indicated that D1, D2, and D3 receptor mRNAs are all expressed in retrogradely labeled striatonigral neurons.[116] More recent reports, however, indicate that this holds for only a fraction of neurons.[117] The discrepancy between in situ hybridization and PCR data may reflect sensitivity differences between the two methods. Because the level of receptor protein may differ from that of corresponding mRNA, subtype-specific antibodies were developed for direct detection of dopamine receptor proteins in striatum by immunocytochemistry. These studies found that D1 and D2 receptor proteins are each localized to 50 percent of striatal cells.[11,118,119] Furthermore, D1 receptor protein is enriched in retrogradely labeled striatonigral neurons, but D2 is not, as predicted by the D1/D2 segregation hypothesis.[120,121] Electron microscopic immunocytochemistry studies agree with these findings, in that postsynaptic D1 and D2 receptor proteins are enriched in subsets of dendrites and spines,[11,82,122] where they probably modulate cortical and thalamic inputs. Finally, ultrastructural double labeling of D1 and D2 with different chromogens demonstrated no colocalization.[11] Therefore, although physiological and molecular biology issues remain to be resolved, direct anatomic evidence supports the conclusion that D1 and D2 receptor proteins are differentially expressed in striatonigral and striatopallidal neurons, respectively.

Several other elements in the basal ganglia pathways selectively express different dopamine receptor subtypes and offer selective targets for manipulation of specific components of basal ganglia-thalamocortical circuitry. D1 receptors are relatively enriched in the patch compartment in striatum[11,122] (Fig. 7-3). D1 receptors are concentrated in GPi of primate, and D2 is concentrated in GPe (Fig. 7-2), suggestive of selective expression of these subtypes in the striatonigral and striatopallidal neurons, respectively, and subsequent transportation to the terminal fields. D1 and D2 receptors are expressed on local axon collaterals in striatum.[11,122] Interest-

ingly, D1 receptors increase GABA release and D2 receptors decrease GABA release in striatum.[123] In substantia nigra, D2 receptor mRNA is expressed in pars compacta neurons,[47,115] and D2 receptor protein is concentrated on nigrostriatal terminals and dendrites,[124] where they may act as autoreceptors in regulation of synthesis, release and re-uptake of dopamine, as well as of the firing rate of substantia nigra pars compacta neurons. D5 receptor mRNA and protein are expressed in cerebral cortex, striatum, thalamus, and brain stem, predominantly in perikarya and proximal dendrites (Ciliax and Levey, unpublished observations).[125–127] Giant Betz cells in motor cortex, magnocellular neurons in red nucleus and large putatively cholinergic interneurons in striatum are particularly enriched with D5. D1 and D5 receptors are both widely expressed in pyramidal neurons of cerebral cortex (Ciliax and Levey, unpublished observations).[128,129] Less is known about the cellular and subcellular distributions of D3 and D4 receptor proteins in brain, because highly specific probes for each remain to be developed and fully characterized. Radioligand binding with relatively selective ligands and in situ hybridization indicates that D3 receptors are present in cortex and striatum and could serve as novel targets for dopaminergic drugs; however, selective enrichment of D3 in ventral striatum suggests that such compounds could have significant psychiatric side effects.[73,130] D4 mRNA localization by Northern blot analysis indicates that this subtype is expressed in cortex and striatum.[74] Thus, much progress has been made in understanding the molecular neuropharmacology of the dopamine system in basal ganglia, whereas functional studies of each receptor subtype await the development of more specific drugs.

Molecular Pharmacology of Acetylcholine in Basal Ganglia

ANATOMY AND PHYSIOLOGY OF CHOLINERGIC TRANSMISSION IN BASAL GANGLIA

ACh's effects on basal ganglia are generally considered to reside in striatum, where there are exceptionally high levels of virtually all pre- and postsynaptic cholinergic markers. Striatal ACh is derived almost exclusively from large aspiny interneurons. Although these neurons are rare (e.g., ~3 percent of total striatal neurons), they are tonically active and play a key role in motor learning.[131] The cholinergic terminals derived from these neurons ramify extensively and synapse predominantly on spiny neurons,[3,132] where ACh is in an ideal position to modulate postsynaptically the responsiveness of the spiny neurons to the excitatory cortical and thalamic inputs located on the spine heads.[133] Physiological studies have shown that ACh elicits mixed excitatory and inhibitory responses to evoked activity.[134,135] The complex nature of the responses may result in part from the nonclassical manner in which this transmitter modulates excitatory transmission in striatum[3] and in part from stimulation of a diverse group of receptors localized on the same or different neurons. ACh also has well-described actions on presynaptic nerve terminals in striatum. For example, ACh regulates its own release via autoreceptors on cholinergic terminals,[136] as well as the release of dopamine, glutamate (from corticostriate terminals),[137] and GABA (from spiny neuron axon collaterals and interneurons).[138] Moreover, much evidence suggests that subclasses of muscarinic receptors differentially regulate release of these transmitters.[137,138]

Although the role of ACh in striatum has been most widely investigated, ACh could also strongly influence motor function via actions in GP, STN, substantia nigra (SN), and thalamus. Cholinergic fibers innervate each of these sites in human brain[139] and appear to be derived from the PPN.[140] The PPN resides in the mesopontine tegmentum and contains both cholinergic and glutamatergic components (see Chap. 51). The region of the PPN itself receives basal ganglia output, with direct projections from GPi and SNr, and projects caudally to motor structures in brain stem.[141] In PD, there is pathological involvement of the PPN.[142] Moreover, there is a dramatic increase (>200 percent) in muscarinic binding sites in GPi in this disease, possibly reflecting compensatory upregulation of the receptors in the face of reduced cholinergic activity.[143] Thus, in addition to the intrinsic cholinergic system in striatum, the PPN and other extrastriatal sites are also likely to be important mediators of cholinergic effects on basal ganglia and motor functions.

MOLECULAR DIVERSITY OF ACh RECEPTORS

The effects of ACh are mediated by two classes of receptors, the G protein-coupled muscarinic family and the ligand-gated ion channel nicotinic family. Both classes of receptor are abundant in the brain and basal ganglia structures. Nicotinic receptors have an unknown role in central motor functions. In contrast, muscarinic cholinergic transmission has been known to be crucial for basal ganglia function for many years. For instance, antimuscarinic drugs are effective treatments for PDs, tremor, and dystonia.[144] Although still widely used, particularly for the latter conditions, these drugs have side effects such as confusion and sedation that frequently limit their tolerability. The identification of five genes encoding closely related receptors[17] now offers the possibility that different subtypes are responsible for the effects on movement, cognition, and arousal.

The classification of the muscarinic ACh receptor (mAChR) gene family, including binding properties, signal transduction mechanisms, and distributions in brain, is summarized in Table 7-2.

PHARMACOLOGY AND SIGNAL TRANSDUCTION MECHANISMS OF MUSCARINIC RECEPTORS

The m1-m5 muscarinic ACh receptor subtypes identified by molecular cloning[17] cannot be subclassified as readily as the dopamine subtypes. The correspondence of the receptor proteins to pharmacologically defined binding sites (M1-M3) previously identified in tissues is uncertain, because even the most selective ligands bind to multiple receptor proteins with high affinity.[145] This is very different from the dopamine subclasses, which have ~100-fold differences in affinities for D1 and D2-selective ligands.[146] The m1, m3, and m5 receptors are functionally related; all preferentially couple to phosphatidylinositol metabolism. The m2 and m4 subtypes both inhibit adenyl cyclase activity, but m4 may also stimulate this enzyme in some cells. The cloned receptors also selectively modulate a variety of ion channels.[18] Thus, the cloned muscarinic receptors have important structural and functional differences when expressed in tissue culture, indicating that different subtypes are likely to mediate distinct responses in brain. The lack of highly selective compounds, however, for individual receptor subtypes continues to impede progress in understanding the roles of the mAChR in basal ganglia and other brain functions.

Nonetheless, comparisons of the clinical usefulness of anticholinergic drugs with the binding affinities for the cloned mAChR subtypes may provide clues to the identification of therapeutically relevant receptors. For instance, three of the most commonly used anticholinergic therapies, including benztropine (Cogentin), biperiden (Akineton), and trihexyphenidyl (Artane), each have the highest affinity for m1 and m4 receptors.[147] This suggests that both of these receptor

TABLE 7-2 Muscarinic Acetylcholine Receptor Subtypes

Molecular Subtype	Pharm. Subclass	Isoforms	Second Messenger	Basal Ganglia Localization
m1	M1	None	Increase PI hydrolysis	Striatal spiny neurons (direct and indirect pathways)
m2	M2	None	Decrease cAMP	Cholinergic striatal interneurons, PPN, cortex, thalamus
m3	M3 > M1 > M2	None	Increase PI hydrolysis	Subthalamus and widespread regions outside striatum
m4	M1 and M2	None	Decrease cAMP	Striatal spiny neurons (direct pathway)
m5	M1 > M2	None	Increase PI hydrolysis	SNc (nigrostriatal terminals?)

cAMP, cyclic AMP; PI, phosphatidylinositol; PPN, pedunculopontine nucleus; SNc, subtantia nigra pars compacta.

subtypes are good candidates for mediating the therapeutic effects. However, because these drugs, have only about two- to five-fold differences in affinity for m1 and m4, it is not possible to determine whether one or both of these receptors is clinically important. Moreover, other subtypes also bind with high affinities to some of these drugs. Therefore, these considerations do not minimize the potential relevance of other receptors for which selective compounds have yet to be developed. As described below, the patterns of expression of the genetically distinct receptors provide additional clues to the functions of these subtypes.

SELECTIVE EXPRESSION OF MUSCARINIC RECEPTOR SUBTYPES IN BASAL GANGLIA

Surprisingly, all mAChR mRNAs and proteins have been detected in basal ganglia[114,148–150] and are thus likely to play different roles in the circuits. Subtype-specific antibodies have been developed, enabling quantification and more precise immunocytochemical localization of the subtypes in brain.[149,150] The m1, m2, and m4 receptors account for the vast majority of striatal muscarinic binding sites in rat[149,150] and human[151] brain, as measured by immunoprecipitation. Importantly, the m4 subtype is the most abundant mAChR in neostriatum, accounting for 50 percent of total mAChR, which further suggests that it may be a key target for anticholinergic drugs for movement disorders.

The cellular and regional distributions of the receptors provide insight into the functional roles of the subtypes in striatum. Receptor autoradiography has been used to determine that subclasses of binding sites are heterogeneously distributed in patch or matrix compartments in the primate neostriatum.[1,12,13] As shown in Figs. 7-2 and 7-3, m4 receptor immunoreactivity is also very dense in monkey and human caudate, putamen, and nucleus accumbens, with increased levels in patches. The other muscarinic receptor proteins do not show such differential localization in patch and matrix divisions. The m4 patches correspond to those high in D1 and glutamate receptor subunit GluR1 (Fig. 7-3). Because patch and matrix compartments are well established as having different afferent and efferent connections,[1,2] this finding suggests that cholinergic stimulation of m4 receptors may selectively modulate particular basal ganglia channels.

Distinct direct and indirect pathway striatal projection neurons provide another level of striatal compartmentalization. Intermingled subpopulations of projection neurons[2] are located within the matrix, with evidence that they are regulated by different receptor subtypes. As described above, segregation of D1 and D2 receptors may explain the opposing effects of dopamine on the neurons, which give rise to the direct and indirect pathways, as well as the imbalance in the pathways in PD. By analogy, selective localization of muscarinic receptor subtypes in the striatal output pathways also might enable differential cholinergic modulation of the striatal outflow pathways. Indeed, the m4 mRNA and protein are present in about 40–50 percent of spiny neurons in rat striatum,[114,152] particularly those that express substance P,[153] and, thus, probably project via the direct pathway to basal ganglia output nuclei. There also appears to be selective localization of m4 in nonhuman primates, as shown in Fig. 7-2. This

immunocytochemical preparation shows intense m4 immunoreactivity in the caudate and putamen. In addition, m4 receptors are dense in the terminal zone of the direct pathway projection neurons in GPi, with comparatively little m4 in the indirect pathway projection site in GPe. **This finding suggests the possibility that m4, like D1, is localized specifically on the terminals of direct pathway projection neurons.** The other mAChR subtypes also appear to have selective localizations. For instance, m1 is expressed in all of the spiny projection neurons, whereas the m2 receptor is expressed in the cholinergic interneurons only.[114,152,153] An example of m2 immunoreactive cholinergic interneurons in the human neostriatum is shown in Fig. 7-4. Electron microscopic studies have also delineated differences in the subcellular distributions of the subtypes.[152] Whereas m1 is mostly postsynaptic on the dendrites and spines of all spiny neurons, m4 is postsynaptic in the spines of a subset of spiny neurons, as well as presynaptically localized in axon terminals, many of which appear to be GABAergic and are probably from the axon collaterals of the direct pathway projection neurons. In contrast, m2 is abundant in cholinergic nerve terminals, where the presynaptic receptor controls transmitter release. **Thus, differential expression and trafficking of the mAChR subtypes allows ACh to have different effects on direct and indirect pathway spiny neurons, as well as on interneurons.** Several other basal ganglia structures also express mAChR subtypes. As described above, the m4 receptor protein is highly enriched in GPi (Fig. 7-2). Because mAChR mRNAs are not detected in GPi,[114] the protein is probably synthesized in neurons that project to this site. One excellent possibility is that m4 is localized on the GABAergic terminals of the striatal projection neurons, which express m4 mRNA[114] and protein.[152] Another possibility, however, is that m4 is present on glutamatergic terminals derived from subthalamus, which also expresses the m4 mRNA.[114] Interestingly, there is substantial upregulation of mAChR binding sites in GPi in Parkinson's disease, perhaps secondary to reduced cholin-

FIGURE 7-4 Immunocytochemical localization of muscarinic cholinergic m2 receptor subtype in large striatal interneurons. Several examples of human striatal interneurons expressing m2. These neurons have the same frequency, size, and morphology as giant aspiny interneurons, and m2 colocalizes with choline acetyltransferase immunoreactivity, a marker for cholinergic neurons.

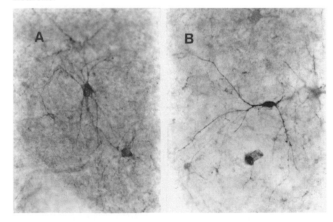

ergic transmission from PPN.[143] Given the crucial pathophysiological role of excessive pallidal drive in Parkinsonism, novel antagonists or agonists selectively acting on m4 receptors could potentially provide an excellent means of dampening pallidal discharge by altering the release of GABA and/or glutamate. Depending on the effect, a drug with the opposing action might be extremely useful for hyperkinetic disorders. The subthalamus also expresses relatively high levels of m3 mRNA[114] and protein,[150] making this receptor another potentially valuable target for new therapeutic agents. The PPN expresses high levels of m2 protein,[154] where it probably functions as an autoreceptor, as it does on other cholinergic neuronal populations. Finally, the dopaminergic neurons in SN are one of few sites in brain with m5 mRNA[114] and with no other reported receptor subtypes. Although there are only very low levels of m5 protein (e.g., where detectable accounting for less than 2 percent of total mAChR,[155]) this receptor might be localized on nigrostriatal terminals, because dopamine release in striatum is known to be regulated by a muscarinic receptor.[156]

Thus, the diversity of mAChR subtypes at critical basal ganglia sites provides an excellent opportunity for new magic bullet therapies. Together with the burgeoning knowledge of the pathophysiological changes in the circuits in various movement disorders, the next decade should bring a variety of selective muscarinic compounds to the clinic that can be rationally chosen to intervene at overactive or underactive synapses.

Molecular Pharmacology of Glutamate in Basal Ganglia

ANATOMY AND PHYSIOLOGY OF GLUTAMATE IN BASAL GANGLIA

Glutamate is the principal excitatory neurotransmitter in the brain. Within the basal ganglia circuitry, it plays a prominent role in the physiology of the cortex, striatum, GP, STN, SN, and thalamus. The striatum receives a massive, somatotopically organized, glutamatergic projection from virtually all areas of neocortex.[157,158] In addition, the centromedian and parafascicular thalamic nuclei send glutamatergic projections to striatum.[159] Terminals from cortex synapse almost exclusively on heads of dendritic spines, whereas those from thalamus synapse mostly with dendrites and, less frequently, with spines.[159] Individual dendritic spines of striatal neurons receive convergent input from cortical glutamatergic afferents and dopaminergic nigrostriatal cells. Cortical glutamatergic neurons also send projections to STN, SN, and thalamus. Other regions of the basal ganglia, the GPe, GPi, and SNc/SNr, receive excitatory glutamatergic input from the STN.[159] In short, all portions of these motor pathways receive and/or send glutamatergic projections. In movement disorders affecting the basal ganglia, there are alterations in glutamatergic neurotransmission and, as discussed below, the glutamate system may represent an important new target for therapeutic intervention.[160]

Glutamate is termed a "mixed agonist," because it activates several classes of receptors. Each class of receptor has a distinct pharmacology and physiology, and the receptors are named for the agonist compounds specific in eliciting a given physiological response. Thus, the receptors are called N-methyl-D-aspartate (NMDA), alpha-amino-3-hydroxy-5-methyl-4-isoxazole-propionic acid (AMPA), and kainate receptors. All of these receptors are ligand-gated ion channels ("ionotropic receptors"); in other words, the binding of glutamate to the receptors leads to rapid opening of an associated ion channel. In addition, other glutamate receptors, termed metabotropic receptors, are linked to G-proteins and are associated with slower changes in cyclic nucleotides or phosphoinositol metabolism.[161]

When glutamate is released from a nerve terminal and interacts with postsynaptic ionotropic receptors, it leads to opening of cation channels. This causes membrane depolarization and increases the probability that the postsynaptic cell will initiate an action potential. Glutamate receptors are located on virtually all neurons in the central nervous system, and glutamate is capable of exciting almost all cells of the central nervous system. Excitatory postsynaptic potentials are commonly composed of both AMPA and NMDA receptor-mediated components. The role of the third type of ionotropic receptor, the kainate receptor, is uncertain and will not be considered further. Metabotropic receptors are enriched in the basal ganglia, where recent studies indicate that they have important physiological functions.

NMDA RECEPTORS

The pharmacology of the NMDA receptor is exceedingly complex. In addition to a binding site for glutamate, there is also a binding site for glycine. Both the glutamate and glycine sites must be occupied for receptor activation to occur.[162] Thus, glutamate and glycine are referred to as "coagonists" of the NMDA receptor. It is important to note that the glycine binding site on the NMDA receptor is distinct from the glycine receptor found in spinal cord. Unlike the glycine receptor, the glycine binding site on the NMDA receptor is strychnine-insensitive. A variety of competitive antagonists acting at both the glutamate and the glycine site of the NMDA receptor are now available for experimental use.[163] Either class of competitive antagonist can completely block NMDA receptor activation.

NMDA receptor activation is also modulated by polyamines such as spermine and spermidine.[164] The NMDA receptor is also influenced to a large extent by extracellular pH (protons). As pH is reduced, there is progressively less activation of the NMDA receptor. This regulatory mechanism may be important under conditions of ischemia, where extracellular pH is reduced. Apparently, polyamines potentiate receptor function by reducing the tonic inhibition caused by protons at physiological pH.[165] It appears that certain drugs antagonize the NMDA receptor by acting at the polyamine site; they have therefore been termed "polyamine antagonists." Extracellular Zn^{2+} can also act as an antagonist of the NMDA receptor. The exact site at which it acts and its mechanism of action are not well defined. The NMDA receptor can also be antagonized by drugs that act within the ion channel to block current flow. Such drugs include phencyclidine (PCP), MK-801, and remacemide.[166]

One of the most important and defining features of the NMDA receptor is the voltage-dependent blockade of the receptor ion channel by Mg^{2+}.[167] At resting membrane potential (about -70 mV), ambient extracellular concentrations of Mg^{2+} block the NMDA receptor ion channel and prevent current flow, even when the glutamate and glycine sites are occupied. Because the Mg^{2+} blockade is voltage-dependent, however, the degree of Mg^{2+} block is reduced as a neuron becomes depolarized. Thus, with graded depolarization, the amount of Ca^{2+} current flowing inward through the NMDA receptor ion channel increases. Unlike the AMPA receptor, the NMDA receptor ion channel is highly permeable to Ca^{2+}; it also allows influx of Na^+. Calcium permeability of the NMDA receptor is important for its physiological function, as well as for the toxic events associated with NMDA receptor activation, as discussed below.

The NMDA receptors appear to be multimeric heteromers.[168–172] Two families of NMDA receptor subunits have been identified. The NMDAR 1 subunit is widely and rather uniformly distributed in the central nervous system, but it exists in at least eight alternatively spliced variants, which differ in their properties and distributions. Homomeric NMDAR 1 receptors contain each of the regulatory sites found on native NMDA receptors, but agonist-induced current flow is greatly reduced, compared to that of native NMDA receptors. The other family of NMDA receptor subunits, NMDAR 2A–D, shows a much more restricted anatomic distribution. Each of these subunits can combine with the NMDAR 1 subunit to form NMDA receptors, which have large current fluxes and distinctive pharmacological and physiological properties. It is believed that most NMDA receptors are heteromeric and that distinct receptor subtypes with characteristic pharmacological and physiological properties are found in different brain regions.

Receptor binding studies indicate that NMDA receptors are found throughout the basal ganglia but are most abundant in striatum.[173] Lower levels are seen in GP, STN, SN, and thalamus. Within the striatum, there is evidence from receptor binding studies that NMDA receptors are preferentially enriched in striatonigral projection neurons.[173] Recent studies have begun to delineate the regional and cellular distributions of NMDA receptor subunit mRNAs and proteins. An antibody that recognizes all isoforms of the NMDAR 1 gene product shows an extremely widespread distribution, with moderate to intense staining in striatum, and lower but detectable levels in GP, STN, SNc/SNr, and thalamus.[174] Similarly, an antibody directed against exon 5 of NMDAR 1 also shows extensive staining throughout the basal ganglia and other brain regions.[175] An example of this immunoreactivity in SNc/SNr is shown in Fig. 7-5; staining is particularly prominent in dendrites in SNr. The mRNAs for the NMDAR 2 family of subunits are differentially distributed in basal ganglia structures.[176] In the striatum, NMDAR 2B is the predominant species, but NMDAR 2A is also detectable. Elsewhere, in the GP, STN, and SN, NMDAR 2D is most abundant. Interestingly, NMDAR 2C, generally considered a cerebellar subunit, is relatively enriched in SNc. Within the striatum, differences in cellular expression of NMDA receptor subunit genes and isoforms have been described.[177] Enkephalin-positive projection neurons have higher levels of NMDAR 1 and NMDAR 2B message than intrinsic somatostatin and cholinergic neurons. In contrast, these interneurons express NMDAR 2D mRNA, but the enkephalin-positive neurons do not. Thus, there is evidence that different populations of striatal neurons express distinct heteromeric forms of the NMDA receptor. This likely results in different pharmacological profiles and heterogeneous physiological responses to receptor activation.

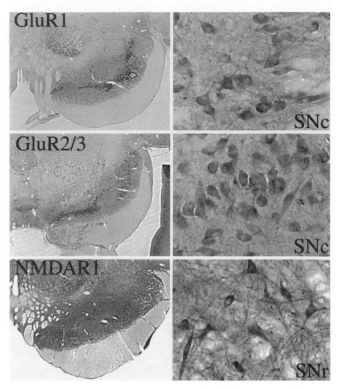

FIGURE 7-5 Immunocytochemistry of glutamate receptor subunits in monkey substantia nigra. GluR1 and GluR2/3 immunoreactive neurons are relatively concentrated in the SNc. In contrast, the NMDAR1 subunit is more abundant in SNr, where much of the immunoreactivity is found in dendrites.

AMPA RECEPTORS

Activation of AMPA receptors by glutamate appears to mediate most of the fast, excitatory neurotransmission in the central nervous system. This class of receptor was previously called the "quisqualate receptor," but the name was changed with the recognition that quisqualate can activate several receptor classes. The binding of glutamate or AMPA to the receptor is associated with influx of Na^+ from the extracellular space to the intracellular compartment. Although AMPA receptors are permeable primarily to Na^+, it has been reported that some native AMPA receptors are highly permeable to Ca^{2+}.[178] As discussed below, this is probably a result of the subunit composition of individual AMPA receptors. Several selective antagonists of the AMPA receptor have been developed in recent years.[163] The most specific of these competitive antagonists is 6-nitro-7-sulfamoylbenzo[f]quinoxaline-2,3-dione (NBQX). Another class of AMPA receptor antagonist appears to act noncompetitively, perhaps at the level of a modulatory protein associated with the receptor. The prototypical noncompetitive AMPA antagonist is GYKI 52466.

Like other ligand-gated ion channels, the AMPA receptors are believed to be multimeric heteromers composed of several distinct subunits. The AMPA receptor subunits were the first of the glutamate receptors to be cloned.[19,179] GluR1–GluR4 (also known as GluR A–GluR D) are AMPA receptor subunits, which can assemble in various combinations to form functional receptors. The specific subunit composition of a given AMPA receptor determines its precise physiological and pharmacological properties. The subunit composition of native AMPA receptors is unknown and is likely to vary regionally.

The permeability of AMPA receptors to Ca^{2+} is determined by receptor subunit composition. GluR1 and GluR3 can form homomeric or heteromeric receptor channels that are permeable to Ca^{2+}. The inclusion of a GluR2 subunit in the receptor assembly, however, prevents Ca^{2+} permeability.[180] The impermeability of GluR2 subunits to Ca^{2+} is based on the substitution of an arginine for a glutamine within a putative transmembrane domain of the subunit protein. Further complexity in the composition of AMPA receptors is achieved by alternative splicing. Thus, slightly different messenger RNA splice variants, termed "flip" and "flop," exist for each of the AMPA receptor subunits GluR1 through GluR4.[181] These splice variants give rise to receptors with distinct physiological and pharmacological profiles, different anatomic distributions, and characteristic developmental profiles.

Several laboratories have developed antibodies to GluR subunits.[182,183] Antibodies recognizing GluR1 label medium spiny, medium aspiny, and large aspiny, neurons of the striatum. Moreover, the GluR1 subunit appears to be enriched in striosomes corresponding to substance P-enriched and calbindin-poor regions. In addition, in the human striatum, GluR1 patches colocalize with dopamine D1 receptor patches (Fig. 7-3). In contrast, antibodies that recognize GluR2/3 and GluR 4 do not show differential striosomal versus matrix staining. GluR2/3 antibodies primarily label medium spiny neurons, and GluR4 antibodies do not label striatal neurons. In the rat striatum, GluR1 does not colocalize with striatopallidal or striatonigral projection neurons, but it does colocalize with parvalbumin-positive interneurons.[184] In contrast, GluR2/3 is localized to most projection neurons.

GluR1 is also found in GPe, GPi, STN, and SNc/SNr. Figure 7-6 shows GluR1 immunoreactivity in striatum and GPe/Gpi in human brain, and demonstrates stained neurons in the GPi. Fig. 7-7 shows the intense GluR1 immunoreactivity in monkey STN, and Fig. 7-5 shows labeled neurons in SN. Neurons enriched in GluR2/3 are found in GPi (Fig. 7-6) and in SNc/SNr (Fig. 7-5), and there are GluR4 immunoreactive neurons in SNr. Finally, it should be noted that GluR4 and, to a lesser extent, GluR1 may be located in glial cells in some brain regions.

METABOTROPIC RECEPTORS

Unlike NMDA, AMPA, and kainate receptors, the metabotropic receptors are not directly coupled to ion channels but

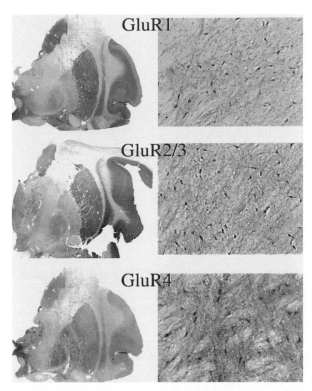

FIGURE 7-6 Distribution of GluR1, GluR2/3, and GluR4 in human basal ganglia; panels on right show higher magnification of cells in the GPi. Note that each of the subunits shows both cellular and neuropil staining in this nucleus.

are coupled, instead, to G proteins. Molecular cloning studies have demonstrated the existence of at least eight distinct metabotropic receptor genes (mGluR1-8), at least six of which (mGluR1-5 and mGluR7) are expressed in brain (for a review, see Ref. 185). Depending on the receptor subtype and the cell type, metabotropic receptors may mediate inositol phosphate metabolism, release of arachidonic acid, or changes in cyclic AMP levels. Additionally, some mGluRs are located on presynaptic nerve terminals and appear to modulate neurotransmitter release. Unfortunately, the exact functional roles of metabotropic receptors in the brain have not been well defined because of a lack of potent, subtype-selective antagonists. Nevertheless, clues to their importance in basal ganglia function are emerging. Activation of mGluRs in striatum or STN elicits dopamine-dependent rotational behavior in rats.[186,187] It has also been shown that activation of striatal mGluRs modulates NMDA receptor function,[188] an effect that may be mediated by phosphorylation. Also, activation of mGluRs presynapticaly inhibits corticostriatal transmission and appears to be crucial to the phenomenon of long-term depression of synaptic transmission in striatum.[64]

Analysis of the regional and cellular distributions of mGluR message in the basal ganglia reveals that these receptors have distinct localizations.[189] Nearly all striatal neurons express low but detectable levels of mRNA for mGluR1 and moderate levels of mGluR3. Expression of mGluR4 is low and heterogeneous, with both labeled and unlabeled neurons present. The mGluR5 signal is intense in about 75 percent

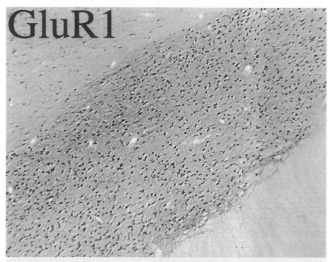

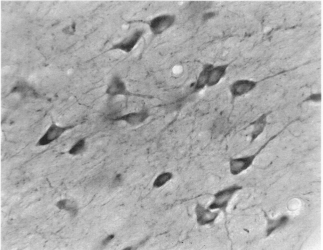

FIGURE 7-7 GluR1 immunoreactivity in the monkey subthalamic nucleus. Bottom panel shows a higher magnification (×40).

TABLE 7-3 Glutamate Receptor Subtypes in the Basal Ganglia

Receptor Type	Basal Ganglia Localization
NMDA	
NMDAR 1	Striatum: *projection neurons > intrinsic neurons*; GPE; GPi; STN; SNc; SNr
NMDAR 2A	Striatum
NMDAR 2B	Striatum: *projection neurons > intrinsic neurons*
NMDAR 2C	SNc
NMDAR 2D	Striatum: *intrinsic neurons >> projection neurons*; GPe; GPi; STN; SNc; SNr
AMPA	
GluR1	Striatum: *patch > matrix; intrinsic neurons >> projection neurons?; medium spiny, medium aspiny & large aspiny neurons*; GPe; GPi; STN; SNc; SNr
GluR2/3	Striatum: *medium spiny neurons*; GPi; SNc
GluR4	GPi; SNr; glia
Metabotropic	
mGluR1	Striatum < GPe < GPi < STN < SNc < SNr
mGluR2	STN
mGluR3	Striatum; glia
mGluR4	Striatum
mGluR5	Striatum: *projection neurons >> intrinsic neurons*; >> GPe; GPi; STN; SNc; SNr

of striatal neurons but is entirely absent in the remainder. Double-label studies indicate that mGluR5 mRNA is highly expressed in enkephalin-positive projection neurons but not in cholinergic or somatostatin interneurons.[190] It is also found in nonenkephalinergic, presumably, substance P-containing projection neurons. Lastly, the mRNA for mGluR2 was absent in all but one to two percent of striatal neurons. Similarly, other basal ganglia regions show differential expression of mGluRs that undoubtedly confer distinct physiological properties in those nuclei.

The distributions of glutamate receptors in the basal ganglia are summarized in Table 7-3.

ALTERED GLUTAMATERGIC NEUROTRANSMISSION IN PARKINSON'S DISEASE

Dopaminergic denervation of the striatum, reproduced in animal models of PD, causes complex changes in the functional circuitry of the basal ganglia (see Chap. 6). Striatal GABAergic neurons projecting directly to GPi/SNr become underactive, thus causing a disinhibition of these GABAergic nuclei. In addition, striatal GABAergic neurons projecting to GPe become overactive. Therefore, the firing rate of the GPe GABAergic projection to STN decreases, leading to overactivity of STN which, via its glutamatergic projections, overstimulates GPi/SNr. Thus, in the setting of nigrostriatal dopamine depletion, the activity of the GABAergic output nuclei is increased by two simultaneous but distinct mechanisms: reduced GABAergic inhibition from the striatum and increased excitatory input from the STN. As a result of the overactivity of the GABAergic projections from GPi/SNr, neurons of the ventrolateral thalamus that project to cortex become underactive. This reduction in the outflow from the motor thalamus to the motor cortex is believed to underlie many of the clinical manifestations of PD.

Based on this scheme, it can be anticipated that there might be regulatory changes in basal ganglia glutamate receptors. After striatal dopamine depletion there is electrophysiological evidence for increased spontaneous release of glutamate in striatum.[191] Further evidence for enhanced glutamatergic activity under conditions of reduced dopaminergic tone comes from studies by Yamamoto and others, which have shown that chronic D2 receptor blockade or dopaminergic denervation cause elevated extracellular levels of basal and potassium-releasable glutamate in striatum.[192,193] In a rodent model of unilateral DA denervation, there is a downregulation of striatal NMDA receptors but not of AMPA receptors.[194] These results complement the work of Klockgether and Turski, which showed that microinjection of NMDA, but not of AMPA, into the anterior striatum produces signs of parkinsonism in rats.[195]

Downstream from the striatum, overactivity of the excitatory glutamatergic projections from STN to the basal ganglia output nuclei appears to play a major role in the pathophysiology of parkinsonian motor signs (see Chap. 6). Using a rodent model, it has been shown that striatal dopaminergic denervation also leads to metabolic activation of the basal ganglia output nuclei, presumably because of increased excitatory input from STN.[194] Consistent with this interpretation, selective lesions of STN reduce metabolic activity in these nuclei.[196] Moreover, in dopamine-depleted rats, STN lesions normalize metabolic activity in the basal ganglia output nuclei.[197] In the rodent model of unilateral DA depletion, there is a selective downregulation of AMPA receptors but not of NMDA receptors in the basal ganglia output nuclei, consistent with the hypothesized importance of AMPA receptors in these regions.[194] These results are also consonant with the work of Klockgether and Turski, showing that micro injection of AMPA, but not of NMDA, into the basal ganglia output nuclei induces parkinsonism in rats.[195]

In conclusion, it appears that AMPA and NMDA receptor systems in the basal ganglia are regulated differently in response to dopaminergic denervation of the striatum. Whether there is the same relationship between striatal NMDA receptors and output nuclei AMPA receptors in the primate brain remains to be investigated. The molecular basis of this glutamate receptor regulation is currently being studied. Identification of the specific receptor subunits involved in these pathways, and elucidation of how they regulate, is expected to lead to improved therapies as the glutamatergic system becomes a target for antiparkinsonian pharmacological interventions.

THERAPEUTIC MANIPULATION OF GLUTAMATERGIC NEUROTRANSMISSION

Support for the hypothesis that excessive subthalamic activity plays an important role in regulating basal ganglia output—and parkinsonian signs—was provided by experiments in MPTP-treated parkinsonian monkeys. Bergman and colleagues showed that small, axon-sparing lesions of the subthalamic nucleus could ameliorate all signs of parkinsonism in the monkeys.[198] The apparent role of glutamatergic neurotransmission in the functional anatomy of the basal ganglia, in general, and in subthalamic output, in particular, raises the possibility that modulation of this neurotransmitter may be beneficial therapeutically in PD. Moreover, evidence suggests that AMPA and NMDA receptor antagonists might exert antiparkinsonian effects at anatomic sites that are, at least in part, distinct.[194,195] Specifically, NMDA antagonists may exert antiparkinsonian actions at the level of the striatum, whereas AMPA antagonists may act primarily in the basal ganglia output nuclei, GPi/SNr. There is considerable experimental evidence from animal models of PD, indicating the feasibility of this approach.[199,200] In rodent and primate models of PD, glutamate antagonists have been administered locally by stereotactic injection, and systemically as monotherapy and in combination with conventional antiparkinsonian agents.[201-203]

Finally, it is worth noting that at least three drugs used in current clinical practice for PD are NMDA receptor antagonists. Amantadine is a relatively weak blocker of the NMDA receptor ion channel;[204,205] it also appears to have effects on the GABAergic and cholinergic systems. Of its defined mech-

anisms of action, it is most potent as an NMDA antagonist. Memantine is a more potent analogue of amantadine that is available in Europe. At therapeutic doses, brain levels of memantine are sufficient to block NMDA receptors.[206] Budipine is a moderately effective antiparkinsonian drug, whose mechanism of action has been unknown. Recently, it was shown that it is also an NMDA antagonist.[205,207] It is anticipated that by the time this book is published, newer and more specific glutamate receptor antagonists will have been evaluated in controlled clinical trials in PD.

Acknowledgments

The authors wish to thank Michael Crutcher, Steven Hersch, Thomas Wichmann, Howard Rees, and David Rye for helpful discussions and other contributions. This work was supported in part by National Institute of Health Grants PO1 NS31937 and R29 NS34861, and by the American Parkinson Disease Association.

References

1. Graybiel A: Neurotransmitters and neuromodulators in the basal ganglia. *Trends Neurosci* 13:244–254, 1990.
2. Gerfen C: The neostriatal mosaic: Multiple levels of compartmental organization in the basal ganglia. *Annu Rev Neurosci* 15:285–320, 1992.
3. Wilson CJ: Basal ganglia, in Shepard, GM (ed): *The Synaptic Organization of the Brain* New York, Oxford University Press, 1990, pp 279–316.
4. Reiner A, Anderson KD: The patterns of neurotransmitter and neuropeptide co-occurrence among striatal projection neurons: Conclusions based on recent findings. *Brain Res Rev* 15:251–265, 1990.
5. Gerfen CR, Young WS, III: Distribution of striatonigral and striatopallidal peptidergic neurons in both patch and matrix compartments: An in situ hybridization histochemistry and fluorescent retrograde tracing study. *Brain Res* 460:161–167, 1988.
6. Alexander G, Delong M, Strick P: Parallel organization of functionally segregated circuits linking basal ganglia and cortex. *Annu Rev Neurosci* 9:357–381, 1986.
7. Alexander GE, Crutcher MD: Functional architecture of basal ganglia circuits: Neural substrates of parallel processing. *Trends Neurosci* 13:266–271, 1990.
8. Penney JBJ, Young AB: Striatal inhomogeneities and basal ganglia function. *Mov Disord* 1:3–15, 1986.
9. DeLong MR: Primate models of movement disorders of basal ganglia origin. *Trends Neurosci* 13:281–285, 1990.
10. Albin RL, Young AB, Penney JB: The functional anatomy of basal ganglia disorders. *Trends Neurosci* 12:366–375, 1989.
11. Hersch SM, Ciliax BJ, Gutekunst C-A, et al: Electron microscopic analysis of D1 and D2 dopamine receptor proteins in the dorsal striatum and their synaptic relationships with motor corticostriatal afferents. *J Neurosci* 15:5222–5237, 1995.
12. Richfield EK, Young AB, Penney JB: Comparative distribution of dopamine D1 and D2 receptors in the basal ganglia of turtles, pigeons, rats, cats, and monkeys. *J Comp Neurol* 262:446–463, 1987.
13. Nastuk MA, Graybiel AM: Autoradiographic localization and biochemical characteristics of M1 and M2 muscarinic binding sites in the striatum of the cat, monkey, and human. *J Neurosci* 8:1052–1062, 1988.

14. Niznik HB, Van Tol HHM: Dopamine receptor genes: New tools for molecular psychiatry. *J Psychiatr Neurosci* 17:158–180, 1992.

15. Sibley DR, Monsma FJ, Jr: Molecular biology of dopamine receptors. *Trends Pharmacol Sci* 13:61–69, 1992.

16. Gingrich JA, Caron MG: Recent advances in the molecular biology of dopamine receptors. *Annu Rev Neurosci* 16:299–322, 1993.

17. Hulme EC, Birdsall NJM., Buckley NJ: Muscarinic receptor subtypes. *Annu Rev Pharmacol Toxicol* 30:633–673, 1990.

18. Caulfield MP: Muscarinic receptors: Characterization, coupling and function. *Pharmacol Ther* 58:319–379, 1993.

19. Keinänen K, Wisden W, Sommer B, et al: A family of AMPA-selective glutamate receptors. *Science* 249:556–560, 1990.

20. Bjorklund A, Lindvall O: Dopamine-containing systems in the CNS, in Bjorklund A, Hokfelt T, (eds): *Classical Transmitters in the CNS: Handbook of Chemical Neuroanatomy*. New York: Elsevier, 1984, part 1, pp 55–122.

21. Parent A, Mackey A, De Bellefeuille L: The subcortical afferents to caudate nucleus and putamen in primate: A fluorescence retrograde double labeling study. *Neuroscience* 10(4):1137–1150, 1983.

22. Pickel VM, Beckley SC, Joh TH, Reis DJ: Ultrastructural immunocytochemical localization of tyrosine hydroxylase in the neostriatum. *Brain Res* 225(2):373–385, 1981.

23. Arluison M, Dietl M, Thibault J: Ultrastructural morphology of dopaminergic nerve terminals and synapses in the striatum of the rat using tyrosine hydroxylase immunocytochemistry: A topographical study. *Brain Res Bull* 13(2):269–285, 1984.

24. Bouyer JJ, Park DH, Joh TH, Pickel VM: Chemical and structural analysis of the relation between cortical inputs and tyrosine hydroxylase-containing terminals in rat neostriatum. *Brain Res* 302(2):267–275, 1984.

25. Wilson CJ: Basal ganglia, in GM Shepherd (ed): *The Synaptic Organization of the Brain,* 3d ed. New York: Oxford University Press, 1990, pp 279–316.

26. Gauchy C, Kemel ML, Desban M, et al: The role of dopamine released from distal and proximal dendrites of nigrostriatal dopaminergic neurons in the control of GABA transmission in the thalamic nucleus ventralis medialis in the cat. *Neuroscience* 22(3):935–946, 1987.

27. Lynd-Balta E, Haber SN: The organization of midbrain projections to the striatum in the primate: Sensorimotor-related striatum versus ventral striatum. *Neuroscience* 59(3):625–640, 1994.

28. Jimenez-Castellanos J, Graybiel AM: Subdivisions of the dopamine-containing A8-A9-A10 complex identified by their differential mesostriatal innervation of striosomes and extrastriosomal matrix. *Neuroscience* 23(1):223–242, 1987.

29. Gerfen CR, Herkenham M, Thibault J: The neostriatal mosaic: II. Patch- and matrix-directed mesostriatal dopaminergic and non-dopaminergic systems. *J Neurosci* 7(12):3915–3934, 1987.

30. Gerfen CR, Baimbridge KG, Thibault J: The neostriatal mosaic: III. Biochemical and developmental dissociation of patch-matrix mesostriatal systems. *J Neurosci* 7(12):3935–3944, 1987.

31. Langer LF, Graybiel AM: Distinct nigrostriatal projection systems innervate striosomes and matrix in the primate striatum. *Brain Res* 498:344–350, 1989.

32. German DC, Dubach M, Askari S, et al: 1-Methyl-4-phenyl-1,2,3,6-tetrahydropyridine-induced parkinsonian syndrome in Macaca fascicularis: Which midbrain dopaminergic neurons are lost? *Neuroscience* 24(1):161–174, 1988.

33. Hirsch E, Graybiel AM, Agid YA: Melanized dopaminergic neurons are differentially susceptible to degeneration in Parkinson's disease. *Nature* 334(6180):345–348, 1988.

34. German DC, Manaye K, Smith WK, et al: Midbrain dopaminergic cell loss in Parkinson's disease: Computer visualization. *Ann Neurol* 26(4):507–514, 1989.

35. Hirsch EC, Graybiel AM, Agid Y: Selective vulnerability of pigmented dopaminergic neurons in Parkinson's disease. *Acta Neurol Scand Suppl* 126:19–22, 1989.

36. German DC, Manaye KF, Sonsalla PK, Brooks BA: Midbrain dopaminergic cell loss in Parkinson's disease and MPTP-induced parkinsonism: Sparing of calbindin-D28k-containing cells. *Ann NY Acad Sci* 648:42–62, 1992.

37. Graybiel AM, Moratalla R, Quinn B, et al: Early-stage loss of dopamine uptake-site binding in MPTP-treated monkeys. *Adv Neurol* 60:34–39, 1993.

38. Andersen PH, Gingrich JA, Bates MD, et al: Dopamine receptor subtypes: Beyond the D1/D2 classification. *Trends Pharmacol Sci* 11(6):231–236, 1990.

39. Kebabian JW, Calne DB: Multiple receptors for dopamine. *Nature* 277(5692):93–96, 1979.

40. Stoof JC, Kebabian JW: Two dopamine receptors: Biochemistry, physiology and pharmacology. *Life Sci* 35(23):2281–2296, 1984.

41. Filloux FM, Wamsley JK, Dawson TM: Presynaptic and postsynaptic D1 dopamine receptors in the nigrostriatal system of the rat brain: A quantitative autoradiographic study using the selective D1 antagonist SCH 23390. *Brain Res* 408:205–209, 1987.

42. Dawson TM, Gehlert DR, McCabe RT, et al: D-1 dopamine receptors in the rat brain: A quantitative autoradiographic analysis. *J Neurosci* 6(8):2352–2365, 1986.

43. Dawson TM, Gehlert DR, Wamsley JK: Quantitative autoradiographic localization of central dopamine D-1 and D-2 receptors. *Adv Exp Med Biol* 204(93):93–118, 1986.

44. Wamsley JK, Gehlert DR, Filloux FM, Dawson TM: Comparison of the distribution of D-1 and D-2 dopamine receptors in the rat brain. *J Chem Neuroanat* 2(3):119–137, 1989.

45. Boyson SJ, McGonigle P, Molinoff PB: Quantitative autoradiographic localization of the D1 and D2 subtypes of dopamine receptors in rat brain. *J Neurosci* 6(11):3177–3188, 1986.

46. Dubois A, Savasta M, Curet O, Scatton B: Autoradiographic distribution of the D1 agonist [3H]SKF 38393, in the rat brain and spinal cord: Comparison with the distribution of D2 dopamine receptors. *Neuroscience* 19(1):125–137, 1986.

47. Mansour A, Meador WJ, Bunzow JR, et al: Localization of dopamine D2 receptor mRNA and D1 and D2 receptor binding in the rat brain and pituitary: An in situ hybridization-receptor autoradiographic analysis. *J Neurosci* 10(8):2587–2600, 1990.

48. Richfield EK, Young AB, Penney JB: Comparative distribution of dopamine D-1 and D-2 receptors in the basal ganglia of turtles, pigeons, rats, cats, and monkeys. *J Comp Neurol* 262(3):446–463, 1987.

49. Richfield EK, Debowey DL, Penney JB, Young AB: Basal ganglia and cerebral cortical distribution of dopamine D1- and D2-receptors in neonatal and adult cat brain. *Neurosci Lett* 73(3):203–208, 1987.

50. Sibley DR, Monsma FJJ, Shen Y: Molecular neurobiology of dopaminergic receptors. *Int Rev Neurobiol* 35:391–415, 1993.

51. Clark D, White FJ: D1 dopamine receptor—the search for a function: A critical evaluation of the D1/D2 dopamine receptor classification and its functional implications. *Synapse* 1(4):347–388, 1987.

52. Paul ML, Graybiel AM, David JC, Robertson HA: D1-like and D2-like dopamine receptors synergistically activate rotation and c-fos expression in the dopamine-depleted striatum in a rat model of Parkinson's disease. *J Neurosci* 12(10):3729–3742, 1992.

53. Waddington JL, Daly SA: Regulation of unconditioned motor behaviour by D1:D2 interactions, in Waddington JL (ed): *D1:D2 Dopamine Receptor Interactions* New York: Academic Press, 1993, pp 51–78.

54. Jenner P: The rationale for the use of dopamine agonists in Parkinson's disease. *Neurology* 45(suppl 3):S6–12, 1995.

55. Bryson SE, Drew GM, Hall AS, et al: Characterization of the dopamine receptor expressed by rat glomerular mesangial cells in culture. *Eur J Pharmacol* 225(1):1–5, 1992.

56. Taylor JR, Lawrence MS, Redmond DE Jr, et al: Dihydrexidine, a full dopamine D1 agonist, reduces MPTP-induced parkinsonism in monkeys. *Eur J Pharmacol* 199(3):389–391, 1991.

57. Kebabian JW, Britton DR, DeNinno MP, et al: A-77636: A potent and selective dopamine D1 receptor agonist with antiparkinsonian activity in marmosets. *Eur J Pharmacol* 229(2-3):203–209, 1992.

58. Wirtshafter D, Asin KE: Interactive effects of stimulation of D1 and D2 dopamine receptors on fos-like immunoreactivity in the normosensitive rat striatum. *Brain Res Bull* 35(1):85–91, 1994.

59. Robertson G, Vincent S, Fibiger H: D1 and D2 dopamine receptors differentially regulate c-fos expression in striatonigral and stratopallidal neurons. *Neuroscience* 49:285–296, 1992.

60. Keefe K, Gerfen C: D1-D2 dopamine receptor synergy in striatum: Effects of intrastriatal infusions of dopamine agonists and antagonists on immediate early gene expression. *Neuroscience* 66(4):903–913, 1995.

61. Carlson JH, Bergstrom DA, Walters JR: Stimulation of both D1 and D2 dopamine receptors appears necessary for full expression of postsynaptic effects of dopamine agonists: A neurophysiological study. *Brain Res* 400(2):205–218, 1987.

62. Walters JR, Bergstrom DA, Carlson JH, et al: D1 dopamine receptor activation required for postsynaptic expression of D2 agonist effects. *Science* 236(4802):719–722, 1987.

63. Wachtel SR, Hu XT, Galloway MP, White FJ: D1 dopamine receptor stimulation enables the postsynaptic, but not autoreceptor, effects of D2 dopamine agonists in nigrostriatal and mesoaccumbens dopamine systems. *Synapse* 4(4):327–346, 1989.

64. Calabresi P, Maj R, Pisani A, et al: Long-term synaptic depression in the striatum: Physiological and pharmacological characterization. *J Neurosci* 12(11):4224–4233, 1992.

65. White FJ, Hu X-T: Electrophysiological correlates of D1:D2 interactions, in Waddington JL (ed): *D1:D2 Dopamine Receptor Interactions.* New York: Academic Press, 1993, pp 79–114.

66. Gomez-Mancilla B, Bedard PJ: Effect of D1 and D2 agonists and antagonists on dyskinesia produced by L-dopa in 1-methyl-4-phenyl-1,2,3,6-tetrahydropyridine-treated monkeys. *J Pharmacol Exp Ther* 259(1):409–413, 1991.

67. Gerfen CR, Engber TM, Mahan LC, et al: D1 and D2 dopamine receptor-regulated gene expression of striatonigral and striatopallidal neurons. *Science* 250(4986):1429–1432, 1990.

68. Blanchet PJ, Calon F, Martel JC, et al: Continuous administration decreases and pulsatile administration increases behavioral sensitivity to a novel dopamine D2 agonist (U-91356A) in MPTP-exposed monkeys. *J Pharmacol Exp Ther* 272(2):854–859, 1995.

69. Tiberi M, Jarvie KR, Silvia C, et al: Cloning, molecular characterization, and chromosomal assignment of a gene encoding a second D1 dopamine receptor subtype: Differential expression pattern in rat brain compared with the D1A receptor. *Proc Natl Acad Sci U S A* 88:7491–7495, 1991.

70. Sunahara RK, Niznik HB, Weiner DM, et al: Human dopamine D1 receptor encoded by an intronless gene on chromosome 5. *Nature* 347:80–83, 1990.

71. Sunahara RK, Guan HC, O'Dowd BF, et al: Cloning of the gene for a human dopamine D5 receptor with higher affinity for dopamine than D1. *Nature* 350(6319):614–619, 1991.

72. Bunzow JR, Van Tol HH, Grandy DK, et al: Cloning and expression of a rat D2 dopamine receptor cDNA. *Nature* 336(6201):783–787, 1988.

73. Sokoloff P, Giros B, Martres MP, et al: Molecular cloning and characterization of a novel dopamine receptor (D3) as a target for neuroleptics. *Nature* 347(6289):146–151, 1990.

74. Van Tol HH, Bunzow JR, Guan HC, et al: Cloning of the gene for a human dopamine D4 receptor with high affinity for the antipsychotic clozapine. *Nature* 350(6319):610–614, 1991.

75. Tang L, Todd RD, Heller A, O'Malley KL: Pharmacological and functional characterization of D2, D3 and D4 dopamine receptors in fibroblast and dopaminergic cell lines. *J Pharmacol Exp Ther* 268(1):495–502, 1994.

76. Chio CL, Lajiness ME, Huff RM: Activation of heterologously expressed D3 dopamine receptors: Comparison with D2 dopamine receptors. *Mol Pharmacol* 45(1):51–60, 1994.

77. Potenza MN, Graminski GF, Schmauss C, Lerner MR: Functional expression and characterization of human D2 and D3 dopamine receptors. *J Neurosci* 14(3 Pt 2):1463–1476, 1994.

78. Van Tol HH, Wu CM, Guan HC, et al: Multiple dopamine D4 receptor variants in the human population [see comments]. *Nature* 358(6382):149–52, 1992.

79. Weiner DM, Levey AI, Sunahara RK, et al: D1 and D2 receptor messenger RNA in rat brain. *Proc Natl Acad Sci U S A* 88:1859–1863, 1991.

80. Le Moine C, Normand E, Bloch B: Phenotypical characterization of the rat striatal neurons expressing the D1 dopamine receptor gene. *Proc Natl Acad Sci USA* 88(10):4205–4209, 1991.

81. Van Tol HHM, Bunzow JR, Guan H-C, et al: Cloning of the gene for a human dopamine D4 receptor with high affinity for the antipsychotic clozapine. *Nature* 350:610–614, 1991.

82. Levey AI, Hersch SM, Rye DB, et al: Localization of D1 and D2 dopamine receptors in brain with subtype-specific antibodies. *Proc Natl Acad Sci U S A* 90(19):8861–8865, 1993.

83. Robertson GS, Fibiger HC: Neuroleptics increase c-fos expression in the forebrain: Contrasting effects of haloperidol and clozapine. *Neuroscience* 46(2):315–328, 1992.

84. Berretta S, Robertson HA, Graybiel AM: Dopamine and glutamate agonists stimulate neuron-specific expression of Fos like protein in the striatum. *J Neurophysiol* 68(3):767–777, 1992.

85. Pan H, Penney J, Young A: Gamma-aminobutyric acid and benzodiazepine receptor changes induced by unilateral 6-hydroxydopamine lesions of the medial forebrain bundle. *J Neurochem* 45:1396–1404, 1985.

86. Filion M, Tremblay L, Bedard PJ: Effects of dopamine agonists on the spontaneous activity of globus pallidus neurons in monkeys with MPTP-induced parkinsonism. *Brain Res* 547(1):152–161, 1991.

87. Wichmann T, DeLong MR: Pathophysiology of parkinsonian motor abnormalities. *Adv Neurol* 60:53–61, 1993.

88. You ZB, Herrera-Marschitz M, Nylander I, et al: The striatonigral dynorphin pathway of the rat studied with in vivo microdialysis—II. Effects of dopamine D1 and D2 receptor agonists. *Neuroscience* 63(2):427–434, 1994.

89. Ferre S, O'Connor W, Fuxe K, Ungerstedt U: The striopallidal neuron: A main locus for adenosine-dopamine interactions in the brain. *J Neurosci* 13(12):5402–5406, 1993.

90. Morris BJ, Hollt V, Herz A: Dopaminergic regulation of striatal proenkephalin mRNA and prodynorphin mRNA: Contrasting effects of D1 and D2 antagonists. *Neuroscience* 25(2):525–532, 1988.

91. Morris BJ, Hunt SP: Proenkephalin mRNA levels in rat striatum are increased and decreased, respectively, by selective D2 and D1 dopamine receptor antagonists. *Neurosci Lett* 125(2):201–204, 1991.

92. Young WSd, Bonner TI, Brann MR: Mesencephalic dopamine neurons regulate the expression of neuropeptide mRNAs in the rat forebrain. *Proc Natl Acad Sci USA* 83(24):9827–9831, 1986.

93. Pollack AE, Wooten GF: Differential regulation of striatal preproenkephalin mRNA by D1 and D2 dopamine receptors. *Brain Res* 12(1-3):111–119, 1992.

94. Hong JS, Yoshikawa K, Kanamatsu T, Sabol SL: Modulation of striatal enkephalinergic neurons by antipsychotic drugs. *Fed Proc* 44(9):2535–2539, 1985.

95. Cruz CJ, Beckstead RM: Quantitative radioimmunocytochemical evidence that haloperidol and SCH 23390 induce opposite changes in substance P levels of rat substantia nigra. *Brain Res* 457(1):29–43, 1988.

96. Bloom FE, Costa E, Salmoiraghi GC: Anesthesia and the responsiveness of individual neurons of the caudate nucleus of the cat to acetylcholine, norepinephrine and dopamine administered by microelectrophoresis. *J Pharmacol Exp Ther* 150(2):244–252, 1965.

97. Bernardi G, Marciani MG, Morocutti C, et al: The action of dopamine on rat caudate neurones intracellularly recorded. *Neurosci Lett* 8:235–240, 1978.

98. Herrling PL, Hull CD: Iontophoretically applied dopamine depolarizes and hyperpolarizes the membrane of cat caudate neurons. *Brain Res* 192(2):441–462, 1980.

99. Johnson SW, Palmer MR, Freedman R: Effects of dopamine on spontaneous and evoked activity of caudate neurons. *Neuropharmacology* 22(7):843–851, 1983.

100. Brown JR, Arbuthnott GW: The electrophysiology of dopamine (D2) receptors: A study of the actions of dopamine on corticostriatal transmission. *Neuroscience* 10(2):349–355, 1983.

101. Mercuri N, Bernardi G, Calabresi P, et al: Dopamine decreases cell excitability in rat striatal neurons by pre- and postsynaptic mechanisms. *Brain Res* 358(1-2):110–121, 1985.

102. Abercrombie ED, Jacobs BL: Dopaminergic modulation of sensory responses of striatal neurons: Single unit studies. *Brain Res* 358(1-2):27–33, 1985.

103. Calabresi P, Mercuri N, Stanzione P, et al: Intracellular studies on the dopamine-induced firing inhibition of neostriatal neurons in vitro: evidence for D1 receptor involvement. *Neuroscience* 20(3):757–771, 1987.

104. Hu XT, Wang RY: Comparison of effects of D-1 and D-2 dopamine receptor agonists on neurons in the rat caudate putamen: An electrophysiological study. *J Neurosci* 8(11):4340–4348, 1988.

105. Hu XT, Wang RY: Haloperidol and clozapine: Differential effects on the sensitivity of caudate-putamen neurons to dopamine agonists and cholecystokinin following one month continuous treatment. *Brain Res* 486(2):325–333, 1989.

106. Hu XT, Wachtel SR, Galloway MP, White FJ: Lesions of the nigrostriatal dopamine projection increase the inhibitory effects of D1 and D2 dopamine agonists on caudate-putamen neurons and relieve D2 receptors from the necessity of D1 receptor stimulation. *J Neurosci* 10(7):2318–2329, 1990.

107. Hu XT, White FJ: Repeated D1 dopamine receptor agonist administration prevents the development of both D1 and D2 striatal receptor supersensitivity following denervation. *Synapse* 10(3):206–216, 1992.

108. Hu XT, Brooderson RJ, White FJ: Repeated stimulation of D1 dopamine receptors causes time-dependent alterations in the sensitivity of both D1 and D2 dopamine receptors within the rat striatum. *Neuroscience* 50(1):137–147, 1992.

109. White FJ, Hu XT, Brooderson RJ: Repeated stimulation of dopamine D1 receptors enhances the effects of dopamine receptor agonists. *Eur J Pharmacol* 191(3):497–499, 1990.

110. Bickford-Wimer P, Kim M, Boyajian C, et al: Effects of pertussis toxin on caudate neuron electrophysiology: Studies with dopamine D1 and D2 agonists. *Brain Res* 533(2):263–267, 1990.

111. Hirata K, Yim CY, Mogenson GJ: Excitatory input from sensory motor cortex to neostriatum and its modification by conditioning stimulation of the substantia nigra. *Brain Res* 321(1):1–8, 1984.

112. Levine MS, Cepeda C, Day M, et al: Dopaminergic modulation of responses evoked by activation of excitatory amino acid receptors in the neostriatum is dependent upon specific receptor subtypes, in Ariano MA, Surmeier DJ (eds): *Molecular and Cellular Mechanisms of Neostriatal Function.* New York: Springer-Verlag, 1995, pp 217–228.

113. Cepeda C, Buchwald N, Levine M: Neuromodulatory actions of dopamine in the neostriatum are dependent upon the excitatory amino acid receptor subtypes activated. *Proc Natl Acad Sci U S A* 90:9576–9580, 1993.

114. Weiner DM, Levey AI, Brann MR: Expression of muscarinic acetylcholine and dopamine receptor mRNAs in rat basal ganglia. *Proc Natl Acad Sci U S A* 87:7050–7054, 1990.

115. Weiner DM, Levey AI, Sunahara RK, et al: D1 and D2 dopamine receptor mRNA in rat brain. *Proc Natl Acad Sci U S A* 88(5):1859–1863, 1991.

116. Surmeier DJ, Eberwine J, Wilson CJ, et al: Dopamine receptor subtypes colocalize in rat striatonigral neurons. *Proc Natl Acad Sci U S A* 89(21):10178–10182, 1992.

117. Surmeier DJ, Cantrell AR, Carter-Russell H: Dopaminergic and cholinergic modulation of calcium conductances in neostriatal neurons, in Ariano MA, Surmeier DJ (eds): *Molecular and Cellular Mechanisms of Neostriatal Function.* New York: Springer-Verlag, 1995, pp 193–215.

118. McVittie LD, Ariano MA, Sibley DR: Characterization of antipeptide antibodies for the localization of D2 dopamine receptors in rat striatum. *Proc Natl Acad Sci USA* 88(4):1441–1445, 1991.

119. Huang Q, Zhou D, Chase K, et al: Immunohistochemical localization of the D1 dopamine receptor in rat brain reveals its axonal transport, pre- and postsynaptic localization, and prevalence in the basal ganglia, limbic system, and thalamic reticular nucleus. *Proc Natl Acad Sci U S A* 89(24):11988–11992, 1992.

120. Ince ES, Ciliax BJ, Levey AI: Expression of dopamine receptor proteins in striatonigral projection neurons. *Soc Neurosci Abstr* 21(2):1424, 1995.

121. Ince E, Ciliax B, Levey A: Differential expression of D1 and D2 dopamine and m4 muscarinic acetylcholine receptors in identified striatonigral neurons. Unpublished.

122. Ciliax BJ, Hersch SM, Levey AI: Immunocytochemical localization of D1 and D2 receptors in rat brain, in Niznik HB (ed): *Dopamine Receptors and Transporters: Pharmacology, Structure, and Function.* New York: Marcel Dekker, 1994, pp 383–399.

123. Girault JA, Spampinato U, Glowinski J, Besson MJ: In vivo release of [3H]gamma-aminobutyric acid in the rat neostriatum—II. Opposing effects of D1 and D2 dopamine receptor stimulation in the dorsal caudate putamen. *Neuroscience* 19(4):1109–1117, 1986.

124. Hersch SM, Yi H, Ciliax BJ, Levey AI: Electron microscopic localization of the dopamine transporter in the striatum and substantia nigra. *Soc Neurosci Abstr* 21(1):781, 1995.

125. Beischlag TV, Marchese A, Meador-Woodruff JH, et al: The human dopamine D5 receptor gene: Cloning and characterization of the 5'-flanking and promoter region. *Biochemistry* 34:5960–5970, 1995.

126. Huntley GW, Morrison JH, Prikhozhan A, Sealfon SC: Localization of multiple dopamine receptor subtype mRNAs in human and monkey motor cortex and striatum. *Brain Res* 15(3-4):181–188, 1992.

127. Rappaport MS, Sealfon SC, Prikhozhan A, et al: Heterogeneous distribution of D1, D2 and D5 receptor mRNAs in monkey striatum. *Brain Res* 616(1-2):242–250, 1993.

128. Smiley JF, Levey AI, Ciliax BJ, Goldman-Rakic P: D1 dopamine receptor immunoreactivity in human and monkey cerebral cortex: predominant and extrasynaptic localization in dendritic spines. *Proc Natl Acad Sci USA* 91(12):5720–5724, 1994.

129. Bergson C, Mrzljak L, Smiley J, et al: Regional, cellular, and subcellular variations in the distribution of D_1 and D_5 dopamine receptors in primate brain. *J Neurosci* 15(12):7821–7836, 1995.

130. Sokoloff P, Giros B, Martres MP, et al: Localization and function of the D3 dopamine receptor. *Arzneimittelforschung* 42(2A):224–230, 1992.

131. Aosaki T, Tsubokawa H, Ishida A, et al: Responses of tonically active neurons in the primate's striatum undergo systematic changes during behavioral sensorimotor conditioning. *J Neurosci* 14:3969–3984, 1994.

132. Izzo PN, Bolam JP: Cholinergic synaptic input to different parts of spiny striatonigral neurons in the rat. *J Comp Neurol* 269:219–234, 1988.

133. Kemp JM, Powell TPS: The termination of fibres from the cerebral cortex and thalamus upon dendritic spines in the caudate nucleus: A study with the Golgi method. *Phil Trans Roy Soc Lond* B 262:429–439, 1971.

134. Kitai ST, Surmeier DJ: Cholinergic and dopaminergic modulation of potassium conductances in neostriatal neurons. *Adv Neurol* 60:40–52, 1993.

135. Calabresi P, Mercuri N, Bernardi G: Chemical modulation of synaptic transmission in the striatum. *Prog Brain Res* 99:299–308, 1993.

136. Weiler MH: Muscarinic modulation of endogenous acetylcholine release in rat neostriatal slices. *J Pharmacol Exp Ther* 250:617–623, 1989.

137. Sugita S, Uchimura N, Jiang Z-G, North RA: Distinct muscarinic receptors inhibit release of gamma-aminobutyric acid and excitatory amino acids in mammalian brain. *Proc Natl Acad Sci U S A* 88:2608–2611, 1991.

138. Marchi M, Sanguineti P, Raiteri M: Muscarinic receptors mediate direct inhibition of GABA release from rat striatal nerve terminals. *Neurosci Lett* 116:347–351, 1990.

139. Mesulam M-M, Mash D, Hersh L, et al: Cholinergic innervation of the human striatum, globus pallidus, subthalamic nucleus, substantia nigra, and red nucleus. *J Comp Neurol* 323:252–268, 1992.

140. Rye DB, Saper CB, Lee HJ, Wainer BH: Pedunculopontine tegmental nucleus of the rat: Cytoarchitecture, cytochemistry, and some extrapyramidal connections of the mesopontine tegmentum. *J Comp Neurol* 259:483–528, 1987.

141. Rye DB, Lee HJ, Saper CB, Wainer BH: Medullary and spinal efferents of the pedunculopontine tegmental nucleus and adjacent mesopontine tegmentum in the rat. *J Comp Neurol* 269:315–341, 1988.

142. Zweig RM, Jankel WR, Hedreen JC, et al: The pedunculopontine nucleus in Parkinson's disease. *Ann Neurol* 26:41–46, 1989.

143. Griffiths PD, Sambrook MA, Perry R, Crossman AR: Changes in benzodiazepine and acetylcholine receptors in the globus pallidus in Parkinson's disease. *J Neurol Sci* 100:131–136, 1990.

144. Jabbari B, Scherokman B, Gunderson C, et al: Treatment of movement disorders with trihexyphenidyl. *Mov Disord* 4:202–212, 1989.

145. Dorje F, Wess J, Lambrecht G, et al: Antagonist binding profiles of five cloned human muscarinic receptor subtypes. *J Pharmacol Exp Ther* 256:727–733, 1991.

146. Sibley D, Monsma F: Molecular biology of dopamine receptors. *Trends in Pharm Sci* 13:61–69, 1992.

147. Bolden C, Cusack B, Richelson E: Antagonism by antimuscarinic and neuroleptic compounds at the five cloned human muscarinic cholinergic receptors expressed in chinese hamster ovary cells. *J Pharmacol Exp Ther* 260:576–580, 1992.

148. Vilaro MT, Mengod G, Palacios JM: Advances and limitations of the molecular neuroanatomy of cholinergic receptors: The example of multiple muscarinic receptors. *Prog Brain Res* 98:95–101, 1993.

149. Levey A, Kitt C, Simonds W, et al: Identification and localization of muscarinic acetylcholine receptor proteins in brain with subtype-specific antibodies. *J Neurosci* 11:3218–3226, 1991.

150. Levey AI, Edmunds SM, Heilman CJ, et al: Localization of muscarinic m3 receptor protein and M3 receptor binding in rat brain. *Neuroscience* 63:207–221, 1994.

151. Flynn D, Ferrari-DiLeo G, Mash D, Levey A: Differential regulation of molecular subtypes of muscarinic receptors in Alzheimer's disease. *J Neurochem* 64:1888–1891, 1995.

152. Hersch SM, Gutekunst CA, Rees HD, et al: Distribution of m1-m4 muscarinic receptor proteins in the rat striatum: Light and electron microscopic immunocytochemistry using subtype-specific antibodies. *J Neurosci* 14:3351–3363, 1994.

153. Bernard V, Normand E, Bloch B: Phenotypical characterization of the rat striatal neurons expressing muscarinic receptor genes. *J Neurosci* 12:3591–3600, 1992.

154. Rye D, Thomas J, Levey A: Distribution of molecular muscarinic (m1-m4) receptor subtypes and choline acetyltransferase in the pontine reticular formation of man and non-human primates. *Sleep Res Abst* 24:59, 1995.

155. Yasuda RP, Ciesla W, Flores LR, et al: Development of antisera selective for m4 and m5 muscarinic cholinergic receptors: Distribution of m4 and m5 receptors in rat brain. *Mol Pharmacol* 43:149–157, 1993.

156. Marchi M, Paudice P, Gemignani A, Raiteri M: Is the muscarinic receptor that mediates potentiation of dopamine release negatively coupled to the cyclic GMP system? *J Neurosci Res* 17:142–145, 1987.

157. Divac I, Fonnum F, Storm-Mathisen J: High affinity uptake of glutamate in terminals of corticostriatal axons. *Nature* 266:377–378, 1977.

158. Young A, Bromberg M, Penney J: Decreased glutamate uptake in subcortical areas deafferented by sensorimotor cortical ablation in the cat. *J Neurosci* 1:241–249, 1981.

159. Parent A: Extrinsic connections of the basal ganglia. *Trends Neurosci* 13:254–258, 1990.

160. Blandini F, Porter R, Greenamyre J: Glutamate and Parkinson's disease. *Mol Neurobiol* 12:73–94, 1996.

161. Schoepp D, Conn P: Metabotropic glutamate receptors in brain function and pathology. *TIPS* 14:13–29, 1993.

162. Kleckner N, Dingledine R: Requirement for glycine in activation of NMDA receptors expressed in Xenopus oocytes. *Science* 241:835–837, 1988.

163. Greenamyre J, Porter R: Anatomy and physiology of glutamate in the CNS. *Neurol* 44(suppl 8):S7–S13, 1994.

164. Williams S, Johnston D: Muscarinic depression of synaptic transmission at the hippocampal mossy fiber synapse. *J Neurophysiol* 64:1089–1097, 1990.

165. Traynelis S, Hartley M, Heinemann S: Control of proton sensitivity of the NMDA receptor by RNA splicing and polyamines. *Science* 268:873–876, 1995.

166. Kemp J, Foster A, Wong E: Non-competitive antagonists of excitatory amino acid receptors. *Trends Neurosci* 10:294–299, 1987.

167. Nowak L, Bregestovski P, Ascher P: Magnesium gates glutamate-activated channels in mouse central neurons. *Nature* 307:462–465, 1984.

168. Ishii T, Moriyoshi K, Sugihara H, et al: Molecular characterization of the N-methyl-D-aspartate receptor subunits. *J Biol Chem* 268:2836–2843, 1993.

169. Kutsuwada T, Kashiwabuchi N, Mori H, et al: Molecular diversity of the NMDA receptor channel. *Nature* 358:36–41, 1992.

170. Meguro H, Mori H, Araki K, et al: Functional characterization of a heteromeric NMDA receptor channel expressed from cloned cDNAs. *Nature* 357:70–74, 1992.

171. Monyer H, Sprengel R, Schoepfer R, et al: Heteromeric NMDA receptors: Molecular and functional distinction of subtypes. *Science* 256:1217–1221, 1992.

172. Moriyoshi K, Masu M, Ishii T, et al: Molecular cloning and characterization of the rat NMDA receptor. *Nature* 354:31–37, 1991.

173. Albin RL, Makowiec RL, Hollingsworth ZR, et al: Excitatory amino acid binding sites in the basal ganglia of the rat: A quantitative autoradiographic study. *Neuroscience* 46:35–48, 1992.

174. Petralia R, Yokotani N, Wenthold R: Light and electron microscope distribution of the NMDA receptor subunit NMDAR1 in the rat nervous system using a selective antipeptide antibody. *J Neurosci* 14:667–696, 1994.

175. Nash N, Heilman C, Rees H, Levey A: Novel human NMDA receptor subunits: Cloning and immunological characterization of exon 5 containing isoforms. *Soc Neurosci Abstr* 21:1111, 1995.

176. Standaert D, Testa C, Young A, Penney J: Organization of N-methyl-D-aspartate glutamate receptor gene expression in the basal ganglia of the rat. *J Comp Neurol* 343:1–16, 1994.

177. Landwehrmeyer G, Standaert D, Testa C, et al: NMDA receptor subunit mRNA expression by projection neurons and interneurons in rat striatum. *J Neurosci* 15:5297–5307, 1995.

178. Brorson J, Bleakman D, Chard P, Miller R: Calcium directly permeates kainate/α-amino-3-hydroxy-5-methyl-4-isoxazolepropionic acid receptors in cultures of cerebellar Purkinje neurons. *Mol Pharmacol* 41:603–608, 1992.

179. Hollmann M, O'Shea-Greenfield A, Rogers S, Heinemann S: Cloning by functional expression of a member of the glutamate receptor family. *Nature* 342:643–648, 1989.

180. Hollmann M, Hartley M, Heineman S: Ca2+ permeability of KA-AMPA-gated glutamate receptor channels depends on subunit composition. *Science* 252:851–853, 1991.

181. Sommer B, Keinanen K, Verdoorn T, et al: Flip and flop: A cell specific functional switch in glutamate-operated channels. *Science* 249:1580–1585, 1990.

182. Martin LJ, Blackstone CD, Levey AI, et al: AMPA glutamate receptor subunits are differentially distributed in rat brain. *Neuroscience* 53:327–358, 1993.

183. Petralia RS, Wenthold RJ: Light and electron immunocytochemical localization of AMPA-selective glutamate receptors in the rat brain. *J Comp Neurol* 318:329–354, 1992.

184. Tallaksen-Greene S, Albin R: Localization of AMPA-selective excitatory amino acid receptor subunits in identified populations of striatal neurons. *Neuroscience* 61:509–519, 1994.

185. Pin J-P, Duvoisin R: The metabotropic glutamate receptors: Structure and functions. *Neuropharmacology* 34:1–26, 1995.

186. Kaatz K, Albin R: Intrastriatal and intrasubthalamic stimulation of metabotropic glutamate receptors: A behavioral and FOS immunohistochemical study. *Neuroscience* 66:55–65, 1995.

187. Sacaan A, Bymaster F, Schoepp D: Metabotrophic glutamate receptor activation produces extrapyramidal motor system activation that is mediated by striatal dopamine. *J Neurochem* 59:245–251, 1992.

188. Colwell C, Levine M: Metabotropic glutamate receptors modulate N-methyl-D-aspartate receptor function in neostriatal neurons. *Neuroscience* 61:497–507, 1994.

189. Testa C, Standaert D, Young A, Penney J: Metabotropic glutamate receptor mRNA expression in the basal ganglia of the rat. *J Neurosci* 14:3005–3018, 1994.

190. Testa C, Standaert D, Landwehrmeyer G, et al: Differential expression of mGluR5 metabotropic glutamate receptor mRNA by rat striatal neurons. *J Neurosci* 354:241–252, 1995.

191. Calabresi P, Mercuri N, Sancessario G, Bernardi G: Electrophysiology of dopamine-denervated striatal neurons. Implications for Parkinson's disease. *Brain* 116:433–452, 1993.

192. Yamamoto B, Cooperman M: Differential effects of chronic antipsychotic drug treatment on extracellular glutamate and dopamine concentrations. *J Neurosci* 14:4159–4166, 1994.

193. Abarca J, Gysling K, Roth R, Bustos G: Changes in extracellular levels of glutamate and aspartate in rat substantia nigra induced by dopamine receptor ligands: In vivo microdialysis studies. *Neurochem Res* 20:159–169, 1995.

194. Porter R, Greene J, Higgins D, Greenamyre J: Polysynaptic regulation of glutamate receptors and mitochondrial enzyme activity in the basal ganglia of rats with unilateral dopamine depletion. *J Neurosci* 14:7192–7199, 1994.

195. Klockgether T, Turski L: Toward an understanding of the role of glutamate in experimental parkinsonism: Agonist-sensitive sites in the basal ganglia. *Ann Neurol* 34:585–593, 1993.

196. Blandini F, Greenamyre J: Effects of subthalamic nucleus lesion on basal ganglia mitochondrial enzyme activities. *Brain Res* 669:59–66, 1995.

197. Blandini F, Garcia-Osuna M, Greenamyre J: Subthalamic ablation reverses changes in basal ganglia oxidative metabolism and motor response to apomorphine induced by nigrostriatal lesion. *Soc Neurosci Abstr* 21:913, 1995.

198. Bergman H, Wichmann T, DeLong M: Reversal of experimental parkinsonism by lesions of the subthalamic nucleus. *Science* 249:1436–1438, 1990.

199. Greenamyre J: Dopamine interactions in the basal ganglia: Implications for Parkinson's disease. *J Neural Transm Park Dis Dement Sect* 91:255–269, 1993.

200. Starr M: Glutamate/dopamine D_1/D_2 balance in the basal ganglia and its relevance to Parkinson's disease. *Synapse* 19:264–293, 1995.

201. Klockgether T, Turski L, Zhang Z, et al: The AMPA receptor antagonist NBQX has antiparkinsonian effects in monoamine-depleted rats and MPTP-treated monkeys. *Ann Neurol* 30:717–723, 1991.

202. Greenamyre J, Eller R, Zhang Z, et al: Antiparkinsonian effects of remacemide hydrochloride, a glutamate antagonist, in rodent and primate models of Parkinson's disease. *Ann Neurol* 35:655–661, 1994.

203. Steece-Collier K, Pazmino R, Greenamyre J: Antiparkinsonian effects of the novel NMDA antagonist CP-101, 606. *Soc Neurosci Abstr* 21:1256, 1995.

204. Kornhuber J, Bormann J, Hubers M, et al: Effects of the 1-amino-adamantines at the MK-801-binding site of the NMDA-receptor-gated ion channel: A human postmortem brain study. *Eur J Pharmacol* 206:297–300, 1991.

205. Porter R, Greenamyre J: Variations in the regional pharmacology of NMDA receptor channel blockers: Implications for therapeutic potential. *J Neurochem* 64:614–623, 1995.

206. Kornhuber J, Bormann J, Retz W, et al: Memantine displaces [³H]MK-801 at therapeutic concentrations in postmortem human frontal cortex. *Eur J Pharmacol* 166:589–590, 1989.

207. Klockgether T, Jacobsen P, Löschmann P, Turski L: The antiparkinsonian agent budipine is an N-methyl-D-aspartate antagonist. *J Neural Transm Park Dis Dement Sect* 5:101–106, 1993.

Chapter 8 _____

NEUROTROPHIC FACTORS

CLIFFORD W. SHULTS

TRANSFORMING GROWTH FACTOR-BETA (TGF-β)
   FAMILY
      Glial Cell Line–Derived Neurotrophic Factor
      TGF-β1,2 and 3
NEUROTROPHINS
      BDNF
      NT-3
      NT-4/5
FIBROBLAST GROWTH FACTORS
OTHER TROPHIC FACTORS
      Ciliary Neurotrophic Factor (CNTF)
      Epidermal Growth Factor (EGF)/Transforming
         Growth Factor-ALPHA (TGF-α)
      Insulin
SUMMARY

The initial concept of neurotrophic factors was shaped by the original studies of nerve growth factor (NGF), which was the first neurotrophic factor identified.[1] These early studies indicated that neurotrophic factors are produced in the target tissue and retrogradely transported to the neurons, which are dependent on exposure to the trophic factor for survival. For example, a trophic factor, which is supportive of the survival of the dopaminergic neurons in the substantia nigra pars compacta (SNpc), would be produced in the striatum and retrogradely transported to the neurons in the SNpc. Recent studies have expanded our understanding of modes of actions of neurotrophic factors.[2] Neurotrophic factors can be produced not only by targets of the neurons but also by adjacent cells, such as glia and ensheathing cells of peripheral nerves, and act on the nearby neurons. Neurotrophic factors can also be produced by neurons and act in a paracrine, autocrine and, perhaps, even an intracrine fashion.

A trophic factor could be important in a neurological disorder by virtue of a role in the pathogenesis or as a treatment of the disorder. Although there is, as yet, no example in which a deficiency of a specific neurotrophic factor is the unequivocal cause of a neurological disorder, it is plausible that a deficiency of a neurotrophic factor could be the cause or a contributing factor in the development of a disorder. In fact, there appears to be a relative deficiency in fibroblast growth factor-2 (FGF-2) in the nigral dopaminergic neurons in parkinsonian brains (see below).

Trophic factors hold great promise in the treatment of neurological disorders and could potentially act by a number of mechanisms. Because Parkinson's disease (PD) is the movement disorder in which neurotrophic factors have been studied most extensively, it is used here as a model for the ways in which neurotrophic factors could be used. First, a trophic factor could slow the progressive loss of dopaminergic neurons in the SNpc, which underlies PD. Second, a trophic factor could enhance the activity of remaining nigral dopaminergic neurons. Third, a trophic factor could stimulate remaining dopaminergic neurons in the SNpc and their axons projecting to the striatum to sprout collateral axons and reinnervate the striatum. Fourth, trophic factors could also be indirectly useful in the treatment of PD, when used in conjunction with transplantation of dopaminergic neurons, or other catecholaminergic cells, to the striatum in parkinsonian patients. Finally, investigators have recently discovered that certain trophic factors can cause proliferation of embryonic neuronal progenitor cells in vitro. This discovery raises the possibility that trophic factors could be used to grow relatively pure cultures of fetal dopaminergic neurons, which could later be transplanted in parkinsonian patients. Because most of the work directed toward a possible role for trophic factors in pathogenesis or treatment of movement disorders has been directed toward PD, most of the studies discussed will be related to PD. The reader may find a number of earlier reviews useful.[3–8]

Transforming Growth Factor-Beta (TGF-β) Family

The TGF-β superfamily is a large family of trophic factors that includes TGF-β1,2,3,4, and 5, glial cell line-derived neurotrophic factor (GDNF), and distantly related factors such as activins/inhibins and bone morphogenic proteins.[9]

GLIAL CELL LINE–DERIVED NEUROTROPHIC FACTOR

GDNF was purified from a rat glial cell line on the basis of its ability to promote dopamine uptake in cultures of embryonic mesencephalic cells.[10] In Lin's initial study,[10] GDNF was also demonstrated to increase the survival of dopaminergic neurons but not of serotonergic or gamma-aminobutyric acids (GABAergic) neurons, in the embryonic midbrain cultures, as well as to increase the neurite outgrowth and the average size of the dopaminergic neurons.

During development of the mesostriatal dopaminergic system in the rat, the message for GDNF is sequentially expressed in the midbrain, then in the striatum.[11] At embryonic day 15.5, a time at which nigral dopaminergic neurons have undergone their final division and the initial innervation of the striatum by nigral dopaminergic axons is occurring, abundant message for GDNF is found in the midbrain, but little message for GDNF is expressed in the developing striatum. At postnatal day 1, as connections between the nigral dopaminergic neurons and their targets in the striatum mature, message for GDNF is reduced in the midbrain but is conspicuously increased in the striatum. This pattern of expression of message for GDNF suggests that it acts first as a locally derived trophic factor and then as a target-derived trophic factor.

The message for GDNF is also expressed in many other regions of the nervous system and in nonneural tissue, including muscle.[12–17] For example, the message for GDNF has been found in the striatum, hippocampus, cortex and spinal cord in the adult rat and human brain.[14] The widespread distribution of GDNF suggests that it is also a trophic factor for nondopaminergic neurons, and a number of studies have shown this to be the case. Both in vitro and in vivo, GDNF has been shown to support the survival of motor neurons.[18–21] GDNF has also been reported to attenuate the convulsions and loss of hippocampal neurons in kainic acid-treated rats[22] and to promote the survival of cultured neurons from peripheral autonomic ganglia.[23]

The original study of Lin et al. directed the focus of the first in vivo studies of GDNF toward its effects on the mesostriatal dopaminergic system.[10] Studies have indicated that GDNF may be useful in the treatment of Parkinson's disease (PD) by a number of the mechanisms discussed in the introduction to this chapter. Recent studies have indicated that GDNF can support the survival of injured nigral dopaminergic neurons. Tomac et al. found that supranigral or intrastriatal injection of GDNF in mice before or after treatment with 1-methyl-4-phenyl-1,2,3,6-tetrahydropyridine (MPTP) exerted protective or reparative effects on the mesostriatal dopaminergic system.[24] Beck et al. found that daily supranigral injections of GDNF in rats with transection of the medial forebrain bundle increased the survival of the axotomized nigral dopaminergic neurons.[25] Kearns and Gash reported that intranigral administration of GDNF decreased the loss of tyrosine hydroxylase-immunoreactive neurons in the SNpc that occurred after intranigral or intrastriatal administration of 6-hydroxydopamine.[26]

Implicit in the studies mentioned above is the ability of GDNF to increase the activity of nigral dopaminergic neurons. This has been directly studied in intact rats and monkeys. Hudson et al. reported that a single unilateral intranigral injection of GDNF in intact rats induced an increase in motor activity, sprouting of tyrosine hydroxylase immunoreactive fibers toward the injection site, increased tyrosine hydroxylase-immunoreactivity in the ipsilateral striatum and increase in the level of dopamine in the SNpc.[27] Similarly, Shults et al. reported that a series of unilateral intrastriatal injections of GDNF increased contraversive amphetamine-induced rotation, the size of the nigral dopaminergic neurons ipsilateral to the injection, and the number of tyrosine hydroxylase-immunoreactive profiles reminiscent of growth cones in the injected striatum.[28] Gerhardt et al. reported an increase in the functional activity of the mesostriatal dopaminergic system after a single intrastriatal or intranigral injection of GDNF in normal monkeys.[29]

The report by Tomac et al.[24] suggests that GDNF can cause regeneration of the mesostriatal dopaminergic system. Hoffer et al. reported that in rats with nearly complete unilateral lesions of the nigrostriatal dopaminergic system, a single injection of GDNF into the lesioned SNpc resulted in attenuation of apomorphine-induced rotation and an increase in the levels of dopamine in the lesioned SNpc. Interestingly, despite the improvement in rotational behavior, the reinnervation of the striatum by dopaminergic axons from the SNpc did not occur.[30]

The early study by Strömberg et al. indicated that GDNF may be useful in transplantation of nigral dopaminergic neurons. They reported that repeated intraocular injections of GDNF increased the outgrowth of dopaminergic fibers and the number of dopaminergic neurons in animals with grafts of fetal mesencephalon in the anterior chamber of the eye.[12]

TGF-β1, 2, AND 3

Other members of the TGF-β superfamily have also been shown to be trophic for mesencephalic dopaminergic neurons in vitro. Krieglstein and Unsicker reported that TGF-β1, 2, and 3 promoted survival of dopaminergic neurons isolated from the embryonic rat midbrain.[31] TGF-β1, 2, and 3 also protected the dopaminergic neurons against toxicity of N-methyl-4-phenylpyridinium (MPP$^+$). Poulsen et al. demonstrated that TGF-β2 and 3, but not TGF-β1 supported the survival of dopaminergic neurons from the embryonic rat midbrain.[11] Poulsen et al. also studied the distribution of the message for TGF-β1, 2, and 3 and GDNF in the developing rat brain. At embryonic day 15.5, message for TGF-β2 and GDNF are present in close proximity to the dopaminergic neurons in the developing midbrain. At postnatal day 1, the message for GDNF is present in the striatum, the message for TGF-β2 is present in the frontal, entorhinal, perirhinal and piriform cortices; and the message for TGF-β3 is present in the olfactory bulb. The differences in the distributions of mRNA for TGF-β2 and 3 and GDNF suggests that members of the TGF-β superfamily may be associated with different parts of the mesencephalic dopaminergic system. GDNF appears be associated with the nigrostriatal system, and TGF-β2 appears be associated with the mesocortical system.

Neurotrophins

NGF was the first neurotrophic factor to be characterized.[1] In 1989, Liebrock et al. determined the structure of a second protein that is trophic for neurons, brain-derived neurotrophic factor (BDNF).[32] Recognition that BDNF and NGF share approximately 50 percent homology in amino acid sequence suggested that they might be members of a larger family of neurotrophic molecules. Soon after this homology was reported, five groups identified a third molecule that is similar in amino acid sequence to NGF and BDNF.[33–37] The family of trophic factors was named the neurotrophins, and the third member to be recognized was designated neurotrophin-3 (NT-3). Shortly thereafter, neurotrophin-4/5 (NT-4/5) was identified in vipers and humans.[38,39] The most recent member of the neurotrophin family to be discovered is neurotrophin-6 (NT-6).[40] Members of the neurotrophin family exist naturally as homodimers. They act through the Trk family of receptors, which are tyrosine kinases.[41] NGF binds to Trk-A; BDNF and NT-4/5 act through Trk-B; and NT-3 acts primarily through Trk-C. Trk-B and Trk-C exist both as full-length and truncated forms that lack the tyrosine kinase domain. The full-length forms of Trk-B are found in the central nervous system on neurons, and the truncated forms are found on nonneuronal cells such as astrocytes and ependyma. Trk-C appears to be exclusively found on neurons and blood vessels.[42]

There is, as yet, no evidence that a deficit of any of the neurotrophins is the cause of a specific movement disorder. One study of three families with autosomal-dominant inherited parkinsonism found no linkage with polymorphic markers linked to the BDNF gene.[43] Mutant mice lacking BDNF were found to have severe degeneration in several sensory ganglia, but midbrain dopaminergic did not appear affected.[44,45]

BDNF

Despite the finding that BDNF appears not to be necessary for the development of mesencephalic dopaminergic neurons,[44,45] anatomic studies of the distribution of the message of both BDNF and TrkB suggest that BDNF plays a role(s) in function of the basal ganglia. In vitro and in vivo studies have supported this notion. Hofer et al. found a small but detectable level of mRNA for BDNF in the striatum of the adult rat,[46] and Okazawa et al. reported that oral administration of L-dopa increased expression of BDNF mRNA in the striatum of mice.[47] The message for TrkB is present in the SNpc but also is present in the striatum.[42,48] BDNF injected into the striatum diffuses a short distance, and some is retrogradely transported to the SNpc.[49,50] Production of BDNF in the target, the striatum, and the retrograde transport of the trophic factor to the dependent cells, dopaminergic neurons in the SNpc, is consistent with established mechanisms for the effect of a trophic factor.[2]

There are alternative mechanisms by which BDNF might have an effect on the dopaminergic neurons of the SNpc. Recent studies have indicated that BDNF may serve autocrine or paracrine functions for the neurons.[51,52] Gall and coworkers reported that the message for BDNF is expressed in cells in the dopaminergic neurons in the medial SNpc and VTA, as well as in adjacent regions in the mesencephalon.[53] It is conceivable that BDNF, which is produced by dopaminergic neurons in the mesencephalon, may have an autocrine or paracrine effect on these neurons.

A role for BDNF in function of the mesostriatal dopaminergic system is further supported by in vitro studies. Hyman et al. and Knüsel et al. reported that BDNF supported the survival of dopaminergic neurons and promoted dopamine uptake in cultures of fetal mesencephalic cells.[54–56] Of considerable interest were the further observations that BDNF promoted survival in vitro of fetal dopaminergic neurons treated with MPP+ and 6-hydroxydopamine (6-OHDA), toxins relatively selective for dopaminergic neurons.[54,57,58]

A number of in vivo studies have indicated that BDNF may be useful in the treatment of PD by virtue of its ability to protect and enhance the activity of nigral dopaminergic neurons. Early studies, in rats with transection of the nigrostriatal dopaminergic axons, did not demonstrate ability of BDNF to protect the nigral dopaminergic neurons.[59] Frim et al. reported that implantation into the mesencephalic tegmentum of fibroblasts, which had been genetically engineered to produce BDNF, reduced the loss of nigral neurons caused by intrastriatal infusion of MPP+.[60] Recently, Shults et al. demonstrated in rats that intrastriatal injections of BDNF reduced the apomorphine-induced rotation and the loss of striatal dopaminergic axons and nigral neurons caused by intrastriatal injection of 6-OHDA.[61]

BDNF has also been shown to enhance the activity of nigral dopaminergic neurons in vivo. Altar and colleagues[62,63] reported that chronic supranigral infusion of BDNF in rats resulted in amphetamine-induced rotation contraversive to the side of BDNF infusion (the pattern of rotation is consistent with increased activity of the dopaminergic system on the side of infusion) and increased the ratio of homovanillic acid to dopamine, an index of dopamine turnover. Shults and colleagues have reported that a single, unilateral injection of BDNF into the mesencephalon of rats resulted in an increase in amphetamine-induced, contraversive rotation that persisted for a number of months after the single treatment.[64] Shen et al. reported that chronic supranigral infusions of BDNF increased the number of active dopaminergic neurons, the average firing rate, and the number of action potentials contained within bursts of the dopaminergic neurons.[65]

Investigators have yet to demonstrate that BDNF can support sprouting of collateral axons from residual dopaminergic neurons in animal models of PD. However, Lucidi-Phillipi et al. reported that fibroblasts genetically engineered to produce BDNF, when implanted in the SNpc in intact rats, induced sprouting of dopaminergic fibers into the grafted fibroblasts.[66] BDNF may be useful when used in conjunction with transplanted fetal nigral dopaminergic neurons. Sauer et al. reported that BDNF enhanced the function but not the survival of fetal nigral neurons grafted to the striatum in rats.[67]

NT-3

The role of NT-3 in the mesostriatal dopaminergic system has been less thoroughly studied than that of BDNF. The message for NT-3 is present in the dopaminergic neurons of the medial SNpc, ventral tegmental area (VTA), and retrorubral nucleus in the rat.[53] In fact, more of the dopaminergic neurons of the ventral mesencephalon appeared to contain message for NT-3 than contained message for BDNF. Hyman et al. reported that NT-3 supported survival of dopaminergic and GABAergic cells in cultures of mesencephalic cells from rat embryos.[55] However, Knüsel et al. reported that, unlike BDNF, NT-3 did not increase dopamine uptake in cultured mesencephalic cells.[56] Altar et al. reported that both BDNF and NT-3 reversed rotational behavior deficits and augmented striatal dopaminergic and serotonergic metabolism in a model of PD in which there is a partial lesion of the nigrostriatal dopaminergic system.[68]

NT-4/5

NT-4/5 has been studied less extensively than BDNF and NT-3. Because both it and BDNF act through Trk-B, it is not surprising that the effects of NT-4/5 in studies in the basal ganglia have been similar.[63,69]

In addition to their effects on the nigrostriatal dopaminergic system, BDNF and NT-4/5 have been shown to be protective of striatal neurons in vitro.[69–71] This effect may be a result of an increase in calcium binding proteins, such as calbindin and calretinin. However, implantation into the striatum of fibroblasts that had been genetically engineered to produce NGF, but not those engineered to produce BDNF, reduced the size of the lesion caused by excitotoxins.[77] These results suggest that neurotrophins may be useful in degenerative disorders of the striatum such as Huntington's disease.

In addition to its effects on the basal ganglia, BDNF has been shown to have a protective effect on a number of other neuronal types, including motor neurons.[73–77]

Fibroblast Growth Factors

During the past seven years, a number of pieces of data have accumulated to indicate that FGF-1 (acidic FGF, or aFGF) and FGF-2 (basic FGF, or bFGF) can have trophic effects on mesencephalic dopaminergic cells.[3–5,8,78] FGF-1 and FGF-2 were the first members of the FGF family of trophic factors to be isolated and are the most thoroughly characterized.[78] To date, seven other members of the FGF family have been identified.

A number of anatomic studies have demonstrated the presence of FGF-1 and FGF-2 message and protein in the dopaminergic neurons in the ventral mesencephalon.[79–82] Tooyama et al. extended the anatomic studies to parkinsonian brains.[83] This group reported that in brains from patients without neurological disease, approximately 94 percent of the pigmented neurons in the SNpc were immunoreactive for FGF-2. In parkinsonian brains, both the number of pigmented neurons and number of FGF-2-immunoreactive cells were severely depleted, but the reduction in FGF-2-immunoreactive neurons, 4.7 percent of that of control brains, was even greater than that of pigmented neurons, 30.3 percent that of control brains. In the parkinsonian brains only 8.2 percent of the remaining pigmented neurons contained FGF-2-immunoreactive material. This group also reported that in Huntington's disease there is an increase in FGF-1-immunoreactive material in the striatum, which appears to accompany the gliosis.[84]

Four high-affinity FGF receptors have been identified.[78] There appear to be overlapping recognition and specificity among the four known high-affinity FGF receptors; one high-affinity receptor may bind with similar affinity to several of the known FGFs, and one FGF may bind with similar affinity to several of the high-affinity receptors. Wanaka carried out in situ hybridization studies and found a wide distribution of the message for FGFR-1 in the rat brain.[85] The neurons of the SNpc and VTA showed moderate binding. Little signal for the bFGF receptor could be detected in the striatum.

A number of groups have demonstrated that FGF-2 increases dopamine uptake and/or survival of dopaminergic neurons in cultures of fetal mesencephalic cells.[86–90] A number of the studies have indicated that the effects of FGF-2 require the presence of glia. A number of studies have indicated that FGF-2 has a trophic effect on the nigrostriatal dopaminergic system in vivo. Otto and Unsicker reported that implantation of Gelfoam, which had been soaked in bFGF into one striatum in MPTP-treated mice, increased the levels of dopamine and tyrosine hydroxylase activity in the striatum bilaterally.[91] Implantation of the Gelfoam also increased the density of tyrosine hydroxylase immunoreactive axons in the striatum but only in the side of Gelfoam implantation. The effect of FGF-2 was noted if the FGF-2 was administered at the time of

MPTP administration or 8 days later. A subsequent study from this group indicated that treatment with FGF-2 did not induce greater gliosis than did treatment with cytochrome c, suggesting that increased gliosis was not the cause of the benefit from FGF-2 treatment.[92] Date and colleagues noted a similar phenomenon in young mice that received intrastriatal injections of FGF-1 at 2, 7, and 12 days after administration of MPTP.[93] However, administration of FGF-1 in aged mice treated with MPTP had no effect.

Matsuda and colleagues reported that addition of FGF-2 to grafts of fetal dopaminergic neurons transplanted into the striatum of hemiparkinsonian rats, at a dose of 5 ng but not 50 ng, enhanced the reduction in rotational asymmetry.[94] Gage's group reported that grafting of fibroblasts genetically engineered to produce FGF-2 with fetal nigral dopaminergic neurons in hemiparkinsonian rats substantially increased the number of dopaminergic neurons surviving in the grafted striatum.[95]

Ray et al. reported that treatment of embryonic neurons from the hippocampus could cause proliferation and perpetuation of the neurons.[96] This finding raises the possibility that dopaminergic neurons could be grown and purified in vitro and later transplanted to patients with PD.

Other Trophic Factors

CILIARY NEUROTROPHIC FACTOR (CNTF)

Hagg and Varon reported that in rats with transection of the nigrostriatal axons, infusion of ciliary neurotrophic factor CNTF into the rostral SNpc reduced the loss of neurons in the SNpc.[97] Although treatment with CNTF prevented death of the dopaminergic neurons, it did not prevent loss of tyrosine hydroxylase, the rate-limiting enzyme in synthesis of dopamine, from the neurons. These data suggest that CNTF has a general neuroprotective effect, but the ability to protect or induce recovery of function within the mesostriatal dopaminergic system remains to be established.

EPIDERMAL GROWTH FACTOR (EGF)/
TRANSFORMING GROWTH FACTOR-ALPHA (TGF-α)

Epidermal growth factor (EGF) and transforming growth factor-alpha (TGF-α) are structurally similar, and both bind with high affinity to and appear to mediate their effects through a common receptor, the EGF-receptor.[98] Mogi et al. reported that levels of EGF-like and TGF-α-like material, as well as interleukin-1β-like and interleukin-6-like material, were significantly higher in the striatum from parkinsonian brains than from controls brains.[99] They commented that the increase in these cytokines, which can be trophic for neurons, in the parkinsonian striatum could be a compensatory, neurotrophic response to degeneration in the nigrostriatal system. Although this hypothesis is quite plausible, the cytokines could also play a role in the degenerative process.

EGF has been reported to have trophic effects on mesencephalic dopaminergic neurons both in vitro and in vivo, but appears to exert its effect through stimulation of proliferation of glia.[4] Alexi and Hefti reported that TGF-α increased number of surviving dopaminergic neurons and dopamine up-take in cultures of embryonic dopaminergic neurons, but the effect may have been mediated by glia.[100]

INSULIN

Moroo et al. reported the loss of insulin receptor-immunore-active material in neurons of the SNpc, but not oculomotor nucleus, in parkinsonian brains. Such loss was not noted in brains from patients who had suffered from Alzheimer's disease or amyotrophic lateral sclerosis.[101] This observation provides support for the hypothesis that reduction in trophic support to the dopaminergic neurons in the SNpc may contribute to degeneration of the SNpc found in PD.

Summary

Only within the past decade, the number of neurotrophic factors identified, our understanding of the actions of neurotrophic factors, and our appreciation of the relevance of neurotrophic factors to movement disorders have all increased enormously. Studies have suggested that deficiencies in neurotrophic factors may be involved in the pathogenesis of certain movement disorders. For example, FGF-2-immunoreactive material has been reported by one group to be strikingly reduced in the SNpc in parkinsonian brains. Numerous in vitro and in vivo studies have indicated that neurotrophic factors may be useful in the treatment of PD through a number of mechanisms. GDNF and BDNF currently appear to be the most promising trophic factors to become useful in the treatment of PD. A limited number of studies have also indicated that neurotrophic factors may also be useful in the treatment of degenerative disorders of the striatum, such as Huntington's disease. If the pace of research into the possible use of neurotrophic factors as treatments in neurological disorders continues as it has during the past decade, one should expect that neurotrophic factors will surely be added to our treatments of PD and certain other movement disorders.

References

1. Levi-Montalcini R. The nerve growth factor 35 years later. *Science* 237:1154–1162, 1987.
2. Korsching S: The neurotrophic factor concept: A reexamination. *J Neurosci* 13:2739-2748, 1993.
3. Shults CW: Future perfect? Presymptomatic diagnosis, neural transplantation, and trophic factors, in Cedarbaum JM, Gancher ST (eds): *Parkinson's Disease–Neurologic Clinics.* Philadelphia: WB Saunders, 1992, pp 567–593.
4. Shults CW: Trophic factors—potential therapies, in Koller WC, Paulson G (eds): *Therapy of Parkinson's Disease,* 2d ed. New York: Marcel Dekker, 1994, pp 559–570.
5. Hefti F: Neurotrophic factor therapy for nervous system degenerative diseases. *J Neurobiol* 25:1418–1435, 1994.
6. Lindsay RM, Wiegand SJ, Altar CA, DiStefano PS. Neurotrophic factors: From molecule to man. *Trends Neurosci* 17:182–190, 1994.
7. Lindvall O, Odin P: Clinical application of cell transplantation and neurotrophic factors in CNS disorders. *Curr Opin Neurobiol* 4:752–757, 1994.
8. Unsicker K: Growth factors in Parkinson's disease. *Prog Growth Factor Res* 5:73–87, 1994.
9. Miyazono K, Ichijo H, Heldin C-H: Transforming growth factor-β: Latent forms, binding proteins and receptors. *Growth Factors* 8:11–22, 1993.
10. Lin L-F H, Doherty DH, Lile JD, et al: GDNF: A glial cell line-derived neurotrophic factor for midbrain dopaminergic neurons. *Science* 260:1130–1132, 1993.
11. Poulsen KT, Armanini MP, Klein RD, et al: TGFβ2 and TGFβ3 are potent survival factors for midbrain dopaminergic neurons. *Neuron* 13:1245–1252, 1994.
12. Strömberg, I, Björklund L, Johansson M, et al: Glial cell line-derived neurotrophic factor is expressed in the developing but not adult striatum and stimulates developing dopamine neurons *in vivo. Exp Neurol* 124:401–412, 1993.
13. Schaar DG, Sieber B-A, Dreyfus CF, Black IB: Regional and cell-specific expression of GDNF in rat brain. *Exp Neurol* 124:368–371, 1993.
14. Springer JE, Mu X, Bergmann LW, Trojanowski JQ: Expression of GDNF mRNA in rat and human nervous tissue. *Exp Neurol* 127:167–170, 1994.
15. Suter-Crazzolara C, Unsicker K: GDNF is expressed in two forms in many tissues outside the CNS. *Neuroreport* 5:2486–2488, 1994.
16. Springer JE, Seeburger JL, He J, et al: cDNA sequence and differential mRNA regulation of two forms of glial cell line-derived neurotrophic factor in Schwann cells and rat skeletal muscle. *Exp Neurol* 131:47–52, 1995.
17. Choi-Lundberg DL, Bohn MC: Ontogeny and distribution of glial cell line-derived neurotrophic factor (GDNF) mRNA in rat. *Dev Brain Res* 85:80–88, 1995.
18. Henderson CE, Phillips HS, Pollock RA, et al: GDNF: A potent survival factor for motoneurons present in peripheral nerve and muscle. *Science* 266:1062–1064, 1994.
19. Zurn AD, Baetge EE, Hammang JP, et al: Glial cell line-derived neurotrophic factor (GDNF), a new neurotrophic factor for motoneurones. *Neuroreport* 6:113–118, 1994.
20. Yan Q, Matheson C, Lopez O: *In vivo* neurotrophic effects of GDNF on neonatal and adult facial motor neurons. *Nature* 373:341–344, 1995.
21. Oppenheim RW, Houenou L, Johnson JE, et al: Developing motor neurons rescued from programmed and axotomy-induced cell death by GDNF. *Nature* 373:344–346, 1995.
22. Martin D, Miller G, Rosendahl M, Russell DA: Potent inhibitory effects of glial derived neurotrophic factor against kainic acid mediated seizures in the rat. *Brain Res* 683:172–178, 1995.
23. Ebendal T, Tomac A, Hoffer BJ, Olson L: Glial cell line-derived neurotrophic factor stimulates fiber formation and survival in cultured neurons from peripheral autonomic ganglia. *J Neurosci Res* 40:276–284, 1995.
24. Tomac A, Lindqvist E, Lin L-F H, et al: Protection and repair of the nigrostriatal dopaminergic system of GDNF *in vivo. Nature* 373:335–339, 1995.
25. Beck KD, Valverde J, Alexi R, et al: Mesencephalic dopaminergic neurons protected by GDNF from axotomy-induced degeneration in the adult brain. *Nature* 373:339–341, 1995.
26. Kearns CM, Gash DM: GDNF protects nigral dopamine neurons against 6-hydroxydopamine in vivo. *Brain Res* 672:104–111, 1995.
27. Hudson J, Granholm A-C, Gerhardt GA, et al: Glial cell line-derived neurotrophic factor augments midbrain dopaminergic circuits in vivo. *Brain Res Bull* 36:425–432, 1995.
28. Shults CW, Shin C, Ernesto C: Effects of intrastriatal injections of glial cell line-derived neurotrophic factor (GDNF) in rats. *Neurology* 45:A335, 1995.

29. Gerhardt G, Cass WA, Zhang Z, et al: Effects of glial cell line-derived neurotrophic factor (GDNF) on the nigrostriatal dopamine system in non-human primates. *Soc Neurosci Abst* 20:1102, 1994.

30. Hoffer BJ, Hoffman A, Bowenkamp K, et al: Glial cell line-derived neurotrophic factor reverses toxin-induced injury to midbrain dopaminergic neurons in vivo. *Neurosci Lett* 182:107–111, 1994.

31. Krieglstein K, Unsicker K: Transforming growth factor-β promotes survival of midbrain dopaminergic neurons and protects them against N-methyl-4-phenylpyridinium ion toxicity. *Neuroscience* 63:1189–1196, 1994.

32. Leibrock J, Lottspeich F, Hohn A, et al: Molecular cloning and expression of brain-derived neurotrophic factor. *Nature* 341:149–152, 1989.

33. Ernfors P, Ibáñez, Ebendal T, et al: Molecular cloning and neurotrophic activities of a protein with structural similarities to nerve growth factor: Developmental and topographical expression in the brain. *Proc Natl Acad Sci USA* 87:5454–5458, 1990.

34. Hohn A, Leibrock J, Bailey K, Barde Y-A: Identification and characterization of a novel member of the nerve growth factor/brain-derived neurotrophic factor family. *Nature* 344:339–341, 1990.

35. Kaisho Y, Yoshimura K, Nakahama K: Cloning and expression of a cDNA encoding a novel human neurotrophic factor. *FEBS Lett* 266:187–191, 1990.

36. Maisonpierre PC, Belluscio L, Squinto S, et al: Neurotrophin-3: A neurotrophic factor related to NGF and BDNF. *Science* 247:1446–1451, 1990.

37. Rosenthal A, Goeddel DV, Nguyen T, et al: Primary structure and biological activity of a novel human neurotrophic factor. *Neuron* 4:767–773, 1990.

38. Ip NY, Ibáñez CF, Nye SH, et al: Mammalian neurotrophin-4: Structure, chromosomal localization, tissue distribution, and receptor specificity. *Proc Natl Acad Sci U S A* 89:3060–3064, 1992.

39. Berkemeier LY, Winslow JW, Kaplan DR, et al: Neurotrophin-5: A novel neurotrophic factor that activates trk and trkB. *Neuron* 7:857–866, 1991.

40. Gotz R, Koster R, Winkler C, et al: Neurotrophin-6 is a new member of the nerve growth factor family. *Nature* 372:266–269, 1994.

41. Barbacid M: The Trk family of neurotrophin receptors. *J Biol* 25:1386–1403, 1994.

42. Altar CA, Siuciak JA, Wright P, et al: *In situ* hybridization of trkB and trkC receptor mRNA in rat forebrain and association with high-affinity binding of [¹²⁵I]BDNF, [¹²⁵I]NT-4/5 and [¹²⁵I]NT-3. *Eur J Neurosci* 6:1389–1405, 1994.

43. Gasser T, Wszolek ZK, Trofatter J, et al: Genetic linkage studies in autosomal dominant parkinsonism: Evaluation of seven candidate genes. *Ann Neurol* 36:387–396, 1994.

44. Ernfors P, Lee K-F, Jaenisch R: Mice lacking brain-derived neurotrophic factor develop with sensory deficits. *Nature* 368:147–149, 1994.

45. Jones KR, Fariñas I, Backus C, Reichardt LF: Targeted disruption of the BDNF gene perturbs brain and sensory neuron development but not motor neuron development. *Cell* 76:989–999, 1994.

46. Hofer M, Pagliusi SR, Hohn A, et al: Regional distribution of brain-derived neurotrophic factor mRNA in the adult mouse brain. *EMBO J* 9:2459–2464, 1990.

47. Okazawa H, Murata M, Wantanabe M, et al: Dopaminergic stimulation up-regulates the in vivo expression of brain derived neurotrophic factor (BDNF) in the striatum. *FEBS Lett* 3123:138–142, 1992.

48. Lindsay RM, Altar CA, Cedarbaum JM, et al: The therapeutic potential of neurotrophic factors in the treatment of Parkinson's disease. *Exp Neurol* 124:103–118, 1993.

49. Anderson KD, Alderson RF, Altar CA, et al: The differential distributions of exogenous BDNF, NGF and NT-3 in the brain corresponds to the relative abundance and distribution of high and low-affinity neurotrophin receptors. *J Comp Neurol* 357:1–22, 1995.

50. Mufson EJ, Kroin JS, Sobreviela T, et al: Intrastriatal infusions of brain-derived neurotrophic factor: Retrograde transport and colocalization with dopamine containing substantia nigra neurons in rat. *Exp Neurol* 129:15–26, 1994.

51. Schecterson LC, Bothwell M: Novel roles for neurotrophins are suggested by BDNF and NT-3 mRNA expression in developing neurons. *Neuron* 9:449–463, 1992.

52. Acheson A, Conover JC, Fandl JP, et al: A BDNF autocrine loop in adult sensory neurons prevents cell death. *Nature* 374:450–453, 1995.

53. Gall CM, Gold SJ, Isackson PJ, Seroogy KB: Brain-derived neurotrophic factor and neurotrophin-3 mRNAs are expressed in ventral midbrain regions containing dopaminergic neurons. *Mol Cell Neurosci* 3:56–63, 1992.

54. Hyman C, Hofer M, Barde Y-A, et al: BDNF is a neurotrophic factor for dopaminergic neurons of the substantia nigra. *Nature* 350:230–232, 1991.

55. Hyman C, Juhasz M, Jackson C, et al: Overlapping and distinct actions of the neurotrophins BDNF, NT-3, and NT-4/5 on cultured dopaminergic and GABAergic neurons of the ventral mesencephalon. *J Neurosci* 14:335–347, 1994.

56. Knüsel B, Winslow JW, Rosenthal A, et al: Promotion of central cholinergic and dopaminergic neuron differentiation by brain-derived neurotrophic factor but not neurotrophin 3. *Proc Natl Acad Sci USA* 88:961–965, 1991.

57. Spina MB, Squinto SP, Miller J, et al: Brain-derived neurotrophic factor protects dopamine neurons against 6-hydroxydopamine and N-methyl-4-phenylpyridinium ion toxicity: Involvement of the glutathione system. *J Neurochem* 59:99–106, 1992.

58. Beck KD, Knüsel B, Winslow JW, et al: Pretreatment of dopaminergic neurons in culture with brain-derived neurotrophic factor attenuates toxicity of 1-methyl-4-phenylpyridinium. *Neurodegeneration* 1:27–36, 1992.

59. Knüsel B, Beck KD, Winslow JW, et al: Brain-derived neurotrophic factor administration protects basal forebrain cholinergic but not nigral dopaminergic neurons from degenerative changes after axotomy in the adult rat brain. *J Neurosci* 12:4391–4402, 1992.

60. Frim DM, Uhler TA, Galpern WR, et al: Implanted fibroblasts genetically engineered to produce brain-derived neurotrophic factor prevent 1-methyl-4-phenylpyridinium toxicity to dopaminergic neurons in the rat. *Proc Natl Acad Sci USA* 91:5104–5108, 1994.

61. Shults C, Kimber T, Altar CA: BDNF attenuates the effects of intrastriatal injection of 6-hydroxydopamine. *Neuroreport* 6:1109–1112, 1995.

62. Altar CA, Boylan CB, Jackson C, et al: Brain-derived neurotrophic factor augments rotational behavior and nigrostriatal dopamine turnover *in vivo. Proc Natl Acad Sci USA* 89:11347–11351, 1992.

63. Altar CA, Boylan CB, Fritsche M, et al: The neurotrophins NT-4/5 and BDNF augment serotonin, dopamine, and GABAergic systems during behaviorally effective infusions to the substantia nigra. *Exp Neurol* 130:31–40, 1994.

64. Shults CW, Matthews RT, Altar CA, et al: A single intramesencephalic injection of brain-derived neurotrophic factor induces persistent rotational asymmetry in rats. *Exp Neurol* 125:183–194, 1994.

65. Shen R-Y, Altar CA, Chiodo LA: Brain-derived neurotrophic factor increases the electrical activity of pars compacta dopamine neurons *in vivo. Proc Natl Acad Sci USA* 91:8920–8924, 1994.

66. Lucidi-Phillipi CA, Gage FH, Shults CW, et al: Brain-derived neurotrophic factor-transduced fibroblasts: Production of BDNF and effects of grafting to the adult rat brain. *J Comp Neurol* 354:361–376, 1995.

67. Sauer H, Fischer W, Nikkhah G, et al: Brain-derived neurotrophic factor enhances function rather than survival of intrastriatal dopamine cell-rich grafts. *Brain Res* 626:37–44, 1993.

68. Altar CA, Boylan CB, Fritsche M, et al: Efficacy of brain-derived neurotrophic factor and neurotrophin-3 on neurochemical and behavioral deficits associated with partial nigrostriatal dopamine lesions. *J Neurochem* 63:1021–1032, 1994.

69. Widmer HR, Hefti F: Neurotrophin-4/5 promotes survival and differentiation of rat striatal neurons developing in culture. *Eur J Neurosci* 6:1669–1679, 1994.

70. Mizuno K, Carnahan J, Nawa H: Brain-derived neurotrophic factor promotes differentiation of striatal GABAergic neurons. *Dev Biol* 165:243–256, 1994.

71. Nakao N, Kokaia Z, Odin P, Lindvall O: Protective effects of BDNF and NT-3 but not PDGF against hypoglycemic injury to cultured striatal neurons. *Exp Neurol* 131:1–10, 1995.

72. Frim DM, Uhler TA, Short MP, et al: Effects of biologically delivered NGF, BDNF and bFGF on striatal excitotoxic lesions. *Neuroreport* 4:367–370, 1993.

73. Yan Q, Elliott J, Snider WD: Brain-derived neurotrophic factor rescues spinal motor neurons from axotomy-induced cell death. *Nature* 360:753–755, 1992.

74. Ip NY, Li Y, Yancopoulos GD, Lindsay RM: Cultured hippocampal neurons show responses to BDNF, NT-3, and NT-4, but not NGF. *J Neurosci* 13:3394–3405, 1993.

75. Yan Q, Matheson C, Lopez OT, Miller JA: The biological responses of axotomized adult motoneurons to brain-derived neurotrophic factor. *J Neurosci* 14:5281–5291, 1994.

76. Cheng B, Goodman Y, Begley JG, Mattson MP: Neurotrophin-4/5 protects hippocampal and cortical neurons against energy deprivation—and excitatory amino acid-induced injury. *Brain Res* 650:331–335, 1994.

77. Friedman B, Kleinfeld D, Ip NY, et al: BDNF and NT-4/5 exert neurotrophic influences on injured adult spinal motor neurons. *J Neurosci* 15:1044–1056, 1995.

78. Baird A: Fibroblast growth factors: Activities and significance of non-neurotrophin growth factors. *Curr Opin Neurobiol* 4:78–86, 1994.

79. Bean AJ, Elde R, Cao, et al: Expression of acidic and basic fibroblast growth factors in the substantia nigra of rat, monkey, and human. *Proc Natl Acad Sci USA* 88:10237–10241, 1991.

80. Stock A, Kuzis K, Woodward WR, et al: Localization of acidic fibroblast growth factor in specific subcortical neuronal populations. *J Neurosci* 12:4688–4700, 1992.

81. Cintra A, Cao Y, Oellig C, et al: Basic FGF is present in dopaminergic neurons of the ventral midbrain of the rat. *Neuroreport* 2:597–600, 1991.

82. Bean AJ, Oellig C, Pettersson RF, Hökfelt T: Differential expression of acid and basic FGF in the rat substantia nigra during development. *Neuroreport* 3:993–996, 1992.

83. Tooyama I, Kawamata T, Walker D, et al: Loss of basic fibroblast growth factor in substantia nigra neurons in Parkinson's disease. *Neurology* 43:372–376, 1993.

84. Tooyama I, Kremer HPH, Hayden MR, et al: Acidic and basic fibroblast growth factor-like immunoreactivity in the striatum and midbrain in Huntington's disease. *Brain Res* 610:1–7, 1993.

85. Wanaka A, Johnson EM, Milbrandt J: Localization of FGF receptor mRNA in the adult rat central nervous system by in situ hybridization. *Neuron* 5:267–281, 1990.

86. Ferrari G, Minozzi M-C, Toffano G, et al: Basic fibroblast growth factor promotes the survival and development of mesencephalic neurons in culture. *Dev Biol* 133:140–147, 1989.

87. Knüsel B, Michel PP, Schwaber JS, Hefti F: Selective and nonselective stimulation of central cholinergic and dopaminergic development in vitro by nerve growth factor, basic fibroblast growth factor, epidermal growth factor, insulin and the insulin-like growth factors I and II. *J Neurosci* 10:558–570, 1990.

88. Engele J, Bohn MC: The neurotrophic effects of fibroblast growth factors on dopaminergic neurons in vitro are mediated by mesencephalic glia. *J Neurosci* 11:3070–3078, 1991.

89. Hartikka J, Staufenbiel M, Lübbert H: Cyclic AMP, but not basic FGF, increases the in vitro survival of mesencephalic dopaminergic neurons and protects them from MPP+-induced degeneration. *J Neurosci Res* 32:190–201, 1992.

90. Park TH, Mytilineou C: Protection from 1-methyl-4-phenylpyridinium (MPP+) toxicity and stimulation of regrowth of MPP+-damaged dopaminergic fibers by treatment of mesencephalic cultures with EGF and basic FGF. *Brain Res* 599:83–97, 1992.

91. Otto D, Unsicker K: Basic FGF reverses chemical and morphological deficits in the nigrostriatal system of MPTP-treated mice. *J Neurosci* 10:1912–1921, 1990.

92. Otto D, Unsicker K: FGF-2 in the MPTP model of Parkinson's disease: Effects on astroglial cells. *Glia* 11:47–56, 1994.

93. Date I, Notter MFD, Felten SY, Felten DL: MPTP-treated mice but not aging mice show partial recovery of the nigrostriatal dopaminergic system by stereotaxic injection of acidic fibroblast growth factor (aFGF). *Brain Res* 526:156–160, 1990.

94. Matsuda S, Saito H, Nishiyama N: Basic fibroblast growth factor ameliorates rotational behavior of substantia nigral-transplanted rats with lesions of the dopaminergic nigrostriatal neurons. *Jpn J Pharmacol* 59:365–370, 1992.

95. Takayama H, Ray J, Raymon HK, et al: Basic fibroblast growth factor increases dopaminergic graft survival and function in a rat model of Parkinson's disease. *Nature Medicine* 1:53–58, 1995.

96. Ray J, Peterson D, Schinstine M, Gage FH: Proliferation, differentiation, and long-term culture of primary hippocampal neurons. *Proc Natl Acad Sci USA* 90:3602–3606, 1993.

97. Hagg T, Varon S: Ciliary neurotrophic factor prevents degeneration of adult rat substantia nigra dopaminergic neurons *in vivo*. *Proc Natl Acad Sci USA* 90:6315–6319, 1993.

98. Adamson ED: Developmental activities of the epidermal growth factor receptor. *Curr Top Dev Biol* 24:1–29, 1990.

99. Mogi M, Harada M, Kondo T, et al: Interleukin-1β, interleukin-6, epidermal growth factor and transforming growth factor-a are elevated in the brain from parkinsonian patients. *Neurosci Lett* 180:147–150, 1994.

100. Alexi T, Hefti F: Trophic actions of transforming growth factor a on mesencephalic dopaminergic neurons developing in culture. *Neuroscience* 55:903–918, 1993.

101. Moroo I, Yamada T, Makino H, et al: Loss of insulin receptor immunoreactivity from the substantia nigra pars compacta neurons in Parkinson's disease. *Acta Neuropathol* 87:343–348, 1994.

Chapter 9 _____

NEUROPATHOLOGY OF MOVEMENT DISORDERS: AN OVERVIEW

SUZANNE S. MIRRA, JULIE A. SCHNEIDER, and MARLA GEARING

GROSS NEUROPATHOLOGIC EXAMINATION IN MOVEMENT DISORDERS
MICROSCOPIC EXAMINATION OF THE BRAIN IN MOVEMENT DISORDERS
IDIOPATHIC PARKINSON'S DISEASE
DEMENTIA WITH LEWY BODIES
PROGRESSIVE SUPRANUCLEAR PALSY
    Gross Neuropathology
    Microscopic Changes
    Heterogeneity
CORTICOBASAL DEGENERATION
    Neuropathology
    Neuropathologic and Clinical Heterogeneity
MULTIPLE-SYSTEM ATROPHY
    Neuropathology
    Cytoplasmic Inclusions
SUMMARY

The neuropathologic diagnosis and assessment of movement disorders present special challenges to neuropathologists and clinicians alike. Clinical-pathological studies affirm diagnostic problems in assessing patients with parkinsonism[1,2] and the relatively low accuracy of conventional diagnostic criteria for the clinical diagnosis of Parkinson's disease (PD). Hughes and colleagues[3] found that only 76 of 100 patients clinically diagnosed as having idiopathic PD exhibited nigral Lewy bodies at autopsy. Neuropathologic diagnoses on the remaining 24 cases included progressive supranuclear palsy (PSP), multiple system atrophy (MSA) and Alzheimer's disease (AD); the diagnostic accuracy rate improved dramatically on retrospective application of recommended criteria. Larsen and coworkers[4] reviewed the literature and found that 20–30 percent of cases clinically diagnosed as having PD fail to exhibit Lewy bodies along with cell loss in the substantia nigra; these investigators proposed the establishment of levels of probability for the clinical diagnosis of PD, analogous to those widely adopted for the clinical diagnosis of Alzheimer's disease (AD).[5] In contrast, for AD, the accuracy of the clinical diagnosis was 87 percent for 106 subjects enrolled in the multicenter longitudinal study CERAD (Consortium to Establish a Registry for Alzheimer's Disease)[6] and assessed using standard clinical and neuropathologic batteries.[7,8] Efforts are already underway to establish standard criteria for the neuropathologic diagnosis of PSP and corticobasal degeneration (CBD);[9,10] additional work is warranted, however, to standardize the neuropathologic diagnosis of PD and other movement disorders. As difficulties associated with the clinical diagnosis of movement disorders may be problematic, neuropathologists examining autopsy brains derived from such individuals must evaluate the material in a manner sufficiently comprehensive so as to encompass a broad range of diagnostic possibilities. We believe that many neurodegenerative disorders or overlapping pathologies remain undetected at autopsy if a complete assessment is not carried out.

Gross Neuropathologic Examination in Movement Disorders

Gross examination of the brains of individuals with movement disorders is often informative and may guide additional microscopic studies. Many of the same principles governing the gross and even microscopic assessment of brains derived from individuals with AD and non-AD dementias pertain to movement disorders. The reader is referred to two publications in which guidelines with color illustrations are provided for nonspecialist pathologists.[11,12]

In all cases, the convexity should be carefully evaluated before cutting the brain for the presence and distribution of cortical atrophy, exemplified by narrowing of the gyri and widening of the sulci. Perirolandic atrophy, i.e., involvement of the precentral and postcentral gyri, often asymmetric, is characteristic, although not pathognomonic of CBD (as depicted in Chap. 45), and the pathologist may wish to sample cortex from both hemispheres for comparison of microscopic features. When feasible, it is advisable to have a pathologist examine the entire brain, before any dissection for research or other purposes. Otherwise, significant asymmetry may be overlooked.

Evaluation of the base of the brain includes assessment of the circle of Willis for atherosclerosis or other changes. In addition, degeneration of the brain stem and cerebellum, such as that seen in olivopontocerebellar atrophy (OPCA) or MSA, may be appreciated when the base of the pons, the cerebellar peduncles, the inferior olivary nuclei or the cerebellar hemispheres or vermis exhibit external evidence of atrophy (see Chap. 20).

Sections through the cerebral hemispheres, cut either in coronal or other planes for comparison with neuroimaging studies, may also be revealing. On these sections, cortical atrophy is exemplified by narrowing of the cortical ribbon, widening of sulci, enlarged Sylvian fissures, reduction in the volume of underlying white matter of the centrum semiovale or corpus callosum, and ventricular enlargement. Asymmetrical atrophy, such as that seen in the frontoparietal cortex in CBD or in the frontal, temporal or, rarely, the parietal lobe in Pick's disease, may be apparent. Enlargement of the temporal horn of the lateral ventricle often reflects narrowing of the entorhinal cortex, a very common feature in AD. The hippocampus is involved in a broad range of neurodegenerative disorders and other conditions and should always be examined; it is often atrophic in AD, a condition that frequently coexists with PD and other disorders. The amygdala, too, is virtually always involved in AD, and it is also a common site for detection of Lewy bodies in Lewy body dementia.

Gross examination of subcortical gray matter, especially the basal ganglia, also provides clues to the underlying pathology. For example, variable atrophy with flattening of the normally convex contour of the head of the caudate nucleus is seen in Huntington's disease[13] as discussed in Chap. 36. Brownish discoloration and atrophy of the putamen are characteristic features of striatonigral degeneration.[14] Atrophy of the bilateral globus pallidus may be appreciated in PSP when there is extensive neuronal loss and gliosis in this region (see Chap. 19). Rusty discoloration of the pallidum and nigra are seen in Hallervorden-Spatz disease, although the associated iron deposits and ovoids or swollen axons are observed to variable degrees in these regions in other more common neurodegenerative disorders. Necrosis and cystic degeneration of the globus pallidus may be seen in carbon monoxide poisoning, although bilateral and symmetrical lacunes caused by cerebrovascular disease occur in the pallidum as well. The subthalamic nucleus is often narrowed and, occasionally, is barely discernible in PSP.

The midbrain often displays aqueductal enlargement in PSP. Pallor of the substantia nigra occurs not only in idiopathic PD, where it may be asymmetric, but also in a number of movement disorders, including PSP, CBD, and MSA. Nigral pallor is also observed in about 25–30 percent of individuals with neuropathologically confirmed AD in whom there is concomitant PD pathology (defined by CERAD as nigral degeneration and Lewy bodies at any site). The cerebral peduncles may be reduced in size in CBD, and this change may be asymmetrical, reflecting Wallerian degeneration secondary to degeneration of motor cortex.

Sections through the brain stem and cerebellum may reveal grossly apparent loss of myelinated fibers or atrophy of the base of the pons, along with reduction in size of the middle cerebellar peduncles in MSA or olivopontocerebellar atrophy (OPCA). The fourth ventricle may be enlarged in long-standing or severe cases of PSP, as well as in OPCA or MSA. Pallor of the locus ceruleus is seen with idiopathic PD, PSP, and AD.[11] The inferior olivary nuclei may appear atrophic in OPCA; although these nuclei are often involved at a microscopic level in PSP, this change is rarely detected grossly. Cerebellar cortical atrophy, such as that associated with OPCA, may be appreciated if the cerebellar folia are widely separated from one another and firmer than normal. The dentate nucleus may appear discolored or have a distorted contour in several disorders including PSP, particularly when there is underlying grumose degeneration.

Microscopic Examination of the Brain in Movement Disorders

Adequate histopathologic assessment of movement disorder cases requires extensive sampling of potentially involved regions of the brain and spinal cord. In addition, because cognitive dysfunction, neurobehavioral problems, and speech abnormalities are frequently observed in patients with movement disorders, the neuropathologic workup should probably include an assessment of those changes associated with dementia. A reasonable workup, in our view, would involve sampling the following structures: Focal regions of cerebral cortical atrophy should be examined along with representative sections from frontal, temporal, parietal, occipital, ante-

rior cingulate, and insular cortex similar to those recommended for AD.[8,11] Perirolandic cortex, if possible bilateral, should be examined whenever corticobasal degeneration or atypical parkinsonism is considered, even if this cortex appears grossly normal. Hippocampus, entorhinal cortex and amygdala, sites which exhibit a spectrum of neurodegenerative changes including Lewy bodies, should also be examined in all cases. In addition, sections of basal ganglia, substantia innominata, thalamus, subthalamic nucleus, hypothalamus, midbrain, pons, medulla, and cerebellum including hemisphere, vermis, deep white matter and dentate nucleus should be taken. These subcortical sections may be crucial for making the diagnosis of such disorders as PSP, which can be easily overlooked if structures such as the subthalamic or inferior olivary nuclei are not examined. Spinal cord, when available, should be sampled at all levels, (e.g. cervical, thoracic, and lumbar).

Routine staining with hematoxylin-eosin preparation along with a battery of special stains is recommended. These include silver stains such as Bielschowsky and Sevier Munger preparations for detection of neurofibrillary tangles seen in PSP, AD, and other disorders, senile plaques, neuropil threads, and Pick bodies. The Gallyas silver stain is preferred by some for use in staging of neurofibrillary degeneration as proposed by Braak and Braak[16] and is considered the stain of choice for glial and neuronal inclusions in MSA, PSP, CBD, and Pick's disease (see ref. 17 for review).

Immunohistochemistry is an important adjunct for the neuropathological assessment of many neurodegenerative disorders, including those associated with parkinsonism and/or dementia. Use of tau antibodies will reveal tau-positive structures in CBD, PSP, AD, and Pick's disease (see ref. 18 for review). Ubiquitin immunohistochemistry enhances the detection of cortical Lewy bodies,[19] highlights the intriguing immunoreactive neurites within CA2-3 of the hippocampus in a spectrum of cases exhibiting cortical and nigral Lewy bodies[20–22] and labels the glial and neuronal cytoplasmic inclusions associated with MSA.[17] The ballooned achromatic neurons characteristic of CBD but seen in many other disorders[23] label intensely with antibodies to neurofilament protein. Antibodies to beta-amyloid peptide (Aβ) are useful in estimating the extent and distribution of amyloid deposition in senile plaques and blood vessels, not only in AD but also in all neurodegenerative disorders.

We believe that neuropathologists must balance their responsibility to provide diagnoses, thorough assessment, and correlation with clinical, neuropsychological, neuroimaging, and genetic and molecular data with the practical considerations of reducing costs in the laboratory. Evaluations similar to those described above are expensive and unless additional support for the autopsy becomes available, such neuropathology assessments will be increasingly difficult to implement outside of the scope of funded research investigations.

In the following pages of this chapter, we briefly highlight the neuropathological hallmarks of selected movement disorders and related conditions. As each of these disorders has been described in detail in the chapters that follow, we have not attempted to be totally comprehensive but rather have stressed key features. We have also emphasized the commonality, heterogeneity, and overlap among movement disorders and other neurodegenerative disorders.

Idiopathic Parkinson's Disease

A detailed description of the neuropathology and anatomic basis of PD is provided by Fearnley and Lees in Chapter 18. The reader is also referred to Forno's excellent review on the neuropathology of PD.[24]

The major gross finding in idiopathic PD is pallor of the substantia nigra (Fig. 9-1), the result of loss of pigmented dopaminergic neurons, most prominently within the ventral lateral cell groups.[25] Occasionally, the pallor and nigral degeneration are asymmetric. Microscopic examination of the nigra in idiopathic PD reveals variable neuronal loss and gliosis, along with evidence of "pigmentary incontinence" exemplified by the finding of neuromelanin within macrophages or, occasionally, free within the neuropil.

The presence of single or multiple Lewy bodies within pigmented neurons of the nigra, as depicted in Figure 9-2, is characteristic, although not pathognomonic, of idiopathic PD. Lewy bodies are concentric eosinophilic cytoplasmic inclusions with peripheral halos and dense cores (see ref. 26 for review). Ultrastructurally, they are composed of a dense osmiophilic core surrounded by radiating 8- to 10-nm filaments. Lewy bodies label with antibodies to neurofilament protein[27] and contain epitopes spanning the entire primary sequences of all three neurofilament subunits.[28,29] They are widely distributed within cortical and subcortical sites and, as reviewed by Forno,[24] may be found in the locus ceruleus, nucleus basalis of Meynert, dorsal motor nucleus of the vagus, hypothalamus, Edinger-Westphal nucleus, raphe nuclei, olfactory bulb, and autonomic ganglia. Lewy bodies are also found in the cerebral cortex in 100 percent of cases of idiopathic PD, according to Hughes et al.,[3] assume a more amorphous appearance than their subcortical counterparts (Fig. 9-3) and may be difficult to detect on standard stains. Their detection may be enhanced by ubiquitin immunohistochemistry.[19]

In her recent review, Forno[24] adopted the operational definition of PD as a "distinctive progressive disorder characterized by tremor, rigidity, and bradykinesia, and pathologically by nerve cell loss in the substantia nigra and the presence of Lewy's intraneuronal inclusion bodies." Yet, as Forno and others point out, the presence of similar neuropathologic features in primary dementia cases reinforces the notion that there is no absolute gold standard for the neuropathologic diagnosis of PD. As emphasized by Koller,[30] the

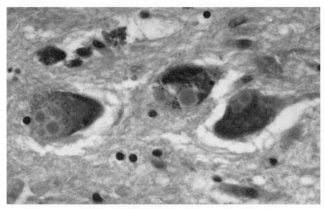

FIGURE 9-2 Three pigmented neurons from the substantia nigra contain multiple Lewy bodies within their cytoplasm. Macrophages filled with neuromelanin are seen at top left. Hematoxylin-eosin stain.

specificity and sensitivity of PD pathology is not clearly established, and the spectrum of pathology underlying dementia in PD is poorly understood. At least some cases of PD with dementia show concomitant AD neuropathology.[3,31,32] In addition, cell loss, gliosis, and Lewy body formation may be seen in the nucleus basalis of Meynert, but these changes apparently do not distinguish cases of PD with and without dementia. We agree that additional longitudinal clinical-pathological studies are needed to understand the underpinnings of dementia and other features of idiopathic PD.

Dementia with Lewy Bodies

The brains of individuals presenting with primary dementia may exhibit neuropathologic features virtually indistinguishable from those described above in idiopathic PD. Regardless of nosological considerations, given the differences in clinical presentation, it is amazing but true that making a distinction between idiopathic PD and DLB, based upon current neuropathologic approaches alone, is a difficult if not impossible task.

As reviewed by Hansen and Crain,[12] numerous names have been applied to the DLB. Some reflect the frequent

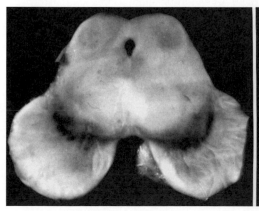
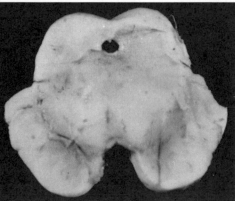

FIGURE 9-1 In contrast to the normally pigmented substantia nigra on the left, marked pallor is appreciated in the nigra of an individual with idiopathic Parkinson's disease.

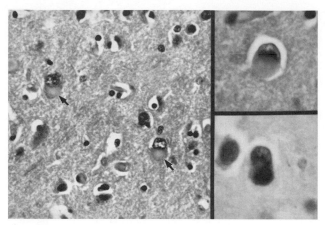

FIGURE 9-3 Cortical Lewy bodies, indicated by arrows, are seen in two neurons (*left*, hematoxylin-eosin stain). Single cortical Lewy bodies are depicted at higher magnification (*upper right*, hematoxylin-eosin stain; *lower right*, ubiquitin immunohisto-chemistry).

coexistence of AD neuropathology, e.g. "AD + PD"[33] or "Lewy body variant of AD."[34] In fact, in clinical-pathological studies of patients diagnosed as having AD, CERAD autopsy findings reveal PD changes in at least one-fifth of AD cases.[6,8] Although, extrapyramidal signs in AD are not invariably accompanied by PD pathology,[35] a prospective CERAD study revealed that extrapyramidal dysfunction occurs more frequently in AD patients with coexistent PD pathology than in those with "pure AD" pathology[36]; in agreement with Hansen et al.,[37,38] these AD + PD cases show fewer neurofibrillary tangles.

The term "diffuse Lewy body disease" is also widely used for DLB,[39] whereas some investigators reserve this term for dementia associated with Lewy bodies in the absence of significant AD changes (in our hands, such cases are quite rare). Indeed, clinical, neuropathologic, and neurobiological distinctions between diffuse Lewy body disease and AD have been suggested.[20,34,40–44]

Clinical diagnostic criteria of DLB have been proposed and evaluated by McKeith and coworkers[45,46] and, at a 1995 workshop of the Consortium on Dementia with Lewy bodies held at Newcastle on Tyne, criteria for the clinical and patho-

logical diagnosis of DLB were formulated by consensus.[47] In addition to progressive cognitive decline, the conferees agreed that features necessary for the diagnosis of probable DLB should include at least two of the following: fluctuating cognition with pronounced variations in attention and alertness, recurrent visual hallucinations that are typically well formed and detailed, and spontaneous motor features of parkinsonism (see Chap. 24). Supportive features included repeated falls, syncope, transient loss of consciousness, and neuroleptic sensitivity.

Not unexpectedly, the essential neuropathologic feature required by the Consortium for the diagnosis of DLB was the presence of Lewy bodies.[47] Associated but not essential histopathologic features included "Lewy-related neurites,"[20,22,40] and microvacuolization or spongiform change[48] described below, plaques, neurofibrillary tangles, and regional neuronal loss, especially in nigra, locus ceruleus, and nucleus basalis of Meynert.

Dickson and coworkers first reported ubiquitin-immunoreactive neurites in CA2-3 of Ammon's horn of the hippocampus (Fig. 9-4) in diffuse Lewy body disease[20,21] but not in patients with "pure AD." We sought to determine the specificity and sensitivity of this observation in a series of 120 cases of diverse neurodegenerative disease[22] and found that this change occurred not only in cases of AD with concomitant PD changes but also in two cases of idiopathic PD and two cases of PSP, all of which had concomitant cortical Lewy bodies. We concluded that this neuritic change coexists with cortical Lewy bodies but is independent of other pathologies, such as AD. Nor are these neurites observed in disorders with nigral degeneration without Lewy bodies, e.g., striatonigral degeneration. Although there is some evidence both in humans and in rodents that there are links between the CA2-3 region of hippocampus and the catecholaminergic system, the absence of tyrosine hydroxylase immunoreactivity militates against their catecholaminergic origin. Similar ubiquitin-immunoreactive neurites have been observed in the brain stem in idiopathic PD,[49] particularly in the region of the dorsal vagus nucleus. More investigation is needed to understand the significance of these changes.

Another intriguing feature prominent in some cases of AD with coexistent PD pathology (AD + PD) is that of spongiform change in the gray matter mimicking that of Creutz-

FIGURE 9-4 CA2-3 neurites in hippocampus in case of AD with concomitant PD pathology (nigral degeneration and Lewy bodies in cortical and subcortical sites). Ubiquitin-immunoreactive neurites (arrows) are seen at low power view of Ammon's horn of hippocampus (*left*) and at a higher magnification (*right*). Ubiquitin immuno-histochemistry.

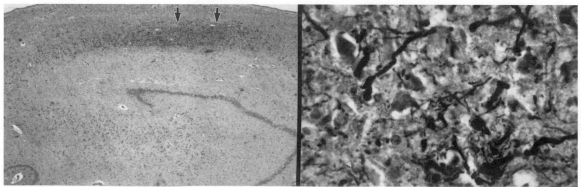

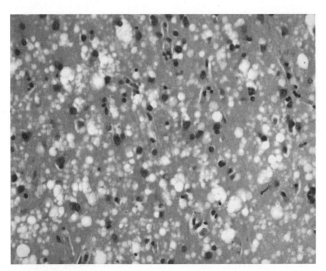

FIGURE 9-5 Florid spongy change mimicking that of Creutz-feldt-Jakob disease is appreciated in entorhinal cortex in case of AD with concomitant PD pathology (nigral degeneration and Lewy bodies in cortical and subcortical sites).

feldt-Jakob disease (CJD) (Fig. 9-5). Unlike CJD, however, this vacuolization change occurs in a stereotypical distribution, predominantly involving the entorhinal, superior temporal and insular cortex as well as the amygdala.[48] The spongy change in these regions is usually interspersed with typical AD changes and Lewy bodies. To our knowledge, similar spongiform changes have not been observed in idiopathic PD.

Progressive Supranuclear Palsy

GROSS NEUROPATHOLOGY

The gross changes in the brain of an individual with PSP, however subtle, may provide clues to the underlying pathology. The globus pallidus, a site of predilection, may be shrunken in cases with extensive neuronal loss and gliosis (Fig. 9-6). Atrophy of the subthalamic nucleus is more com-

monly observed. Examination of the midbrain usually reveals pallor of the substantia nigra which, of course, is not specific for PSP. However, when accompanied by enlargement of the aqueduct of Sylvius, PSP should be suspected. The aqueduct is variably enlarged secondary to involvement of the periaqueductal gray matter and superior colliculi. In long-standing cases, the third and fourth ventricles, too, may be dilated.

MICROSCOPIC CHANGES

The histopathology and the distribution of changes in PSP, as originally described by Steele et al.[50] are relatively stereotypical. Globose neurofibrillary tangles within neurons of subcortical nuclei are the major neuropathologic hallmark (Fig. 9-7), along with variable neuronal loss and gliosis. These changes are most commonly encountered in the globus pallidus, substantia nigra, subthalamic nucleus, colliculi, red nucleus, inferior olivary nucleus, and dentate nucleus. Sparse cortical tangles are also encountered (see ref. 51 for review). Braak et al.[52] found tangles largely confined to the allocortex in six PSP patients; transentorhinal tangles were found in all cases, whereas the brains derived from three moderately demented patients showed severe changes in the superficial entorhinal region as well. Hof et al.[53] observed tangles in the hippocampus and neocortex in six PSP patients; tangles were especially prominent in the primary motor cortex, where they occurred in moderate numbers.

As clearly summarized by Chin and Goldman,[17] there has been increasing recognition of glial tangle pathology in PSP. Several major morphological types have been described and are best appreciated on Gallyas silver and tau immunohistochemical preparations: tufted astrocytes, thorn-shaped astrocytes, coiled bodies, and interfascicular threads. Although none of these changes is absolutely specific for PSP, the tufted astrocytes are particularly characteristic. They consist of tufts of radiating fibers, often surrounding a central astrocytic nucleus.

Another interesting histopathologic feature strongly associated with but not pathognomonic for PSP is grumose degeneration, an eosinophilic granular change in the dentate nucleus attributed to clusters of distended axon terminals

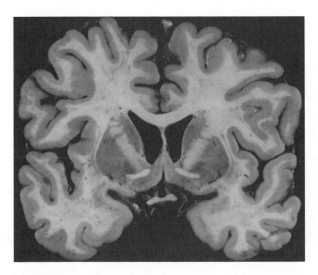

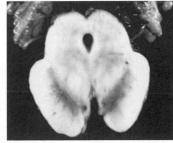

FIGURE 9-6 Progressive supranuclear palsy. Atrophy and slight discoloration of bilateral globus pallidus are appreciated on this coronal section (*left*). The midbrain exhibits characteristic enlargement of the aqueduct of Sylvius and pallor of the substantia nigra (*right*).

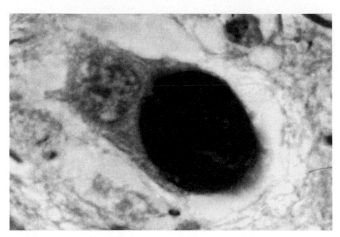

FIGURE 9-7 Progressive supranuclear palsy. A neuron in the globus pallidus contains a characteristic globose neurofibrillary tangle. Sevier-Munger silver preparation.

and preterminals with accumulations of organelles.[54] Grumose degeneration is associated most commonly with PSP[54] but has also been described in Ramsey Hunt syndrome,[55] dentatorubral-pallidoluysian atrophy,[56] Machado-Joseph's disease,[57,58] and early onset AD.[59] We have observed grumose degeneration in two cases of CBD,[60] one with combined PSP-CBD features and the second with typical clinical and neuropathological features of CBD.

HETEROGENEITY

In a study of 20 patients of neuropathologically diagnosed PSP,[61] we found that PSP exhibits remarkable neuropathologic and clinical heterogeneity. The clinical diagnosis of PSP was made in 10 of these individuals, whereas probable AD was the primary diagnosis in another 7. In addition to PSP neuropathology, 12 of the 20 patients (60 percent) showed concomitant pathological changes of AD, PD, or both disorders. Other coexisting pathologies included CBD (two patients) and hippocampal sclerosis. Our observations indicate that AD and PD changes coexist with PSP neuropathology in a substantive proportion of patients. Moreover, our results suggest that PSP may be underdiagnosed and deserves more prominence in the differential diagnosis of dementing illness.

Other investigators, too, have observed heterogeneity of neuropathologic features in PSP and overlap between PSP, CBD, and Pick's disease.[62–67] Indeed, this overlap has been a confounding factor as investigators have sought to formulate neuropathologic criteria for the diagnosis of PSP.[9,10] Both clinical markers and neuropathologic features are required for diagnosis; neither alone is considered sufficient to differentiate CBD, PSP, Pick's disease, and postencephalitic parkinsonism.[10]

AD and PD features have also been observed by others in PSP. Diffuse plaques have been observed in this disorder, as well as in other neurodegenerative diseases.[68,69] Lewy bodies have been noted in brain stem nuclei and cerebral cortex in PSP.[70,71]

Corticobasal Degeneration

NEUROPATHOLOGY

The neuropathological features of CBD are illustrated and described in Chap. 45. CBD is characterized by cortical atrophy involving the frontal parietal lobe, often asymmetrical and predominantly involving perirolandic cortex. In some cases, especially those with atypical clinical presentation, we find that the atrophy involves more rostral frontal cortex.[60] Loss of volume of the centrum semiovale and thinning of the corpus callosum reflect the loss of cortical neurons. Degeneration of motor cortex may lead to ipsilateral atrophy of the cerebral peduncle or other evidence of Wallerian degeneration.

Microscopic examination of regions of cortical degeneration reveal neuronal loss and gliosis and, often, striking loss of myelin and axons in underlying white matter. A characteristic histopathologic feature of CBD, seen on routine hematoxylin-eosin preparations or with neurofilament immunohistochemistry, is the ballooned or achromatic neuron. These abnormal neurons are prominent in areas of cortical degeneration, usually in the deeper layers, but they may be observed in subcortical regions as well. As discussed elsewhere in this chapter, they are not specific for CBD and occur in a variety of disorders. Degeneration of the substantia nigra is usually pronounced in CBD, although involvement of other subcortical structures, such as basal ganglia and dentate nucleus, is much more variable.

Neurofibrillary tangles (NFT) within neurons and glial cells and abundant tau pathology are increasingly recognized features of CBD, best seen with Gallyas silver stain and tau immunohistochemistry (see Ref. 17). Unlike the inclusions in MSA, those in CBD are generally ubiquitin-negative. The neuronal tangles occur in the basal ganglia and brain stem, and their ultrastructure has been variously reported as composed of 15-nm straight tubules versus that of twisted filaments with a long periodicity. Two major types of glial inclusions are described: coiled bodies similar to those seen in PSP and so-called, "astrocytic plaques," described by Feany and Dickson.[72] These "plaques" consist of loose aggregates of distended tau-positive distal astrocyte processes without central nuclei or amyloid. Although closely associated with CBD, they have also been observed in PSP.[60,73] The enormous extent of tau histopathology in both white and gray matter in CBD, as observed by Feany and coworkers,[67,74] is remarkable. These investigators found that large numbers of tau-positive neuropil threads distinguish CBD from PSP and Pick's disease. These threads are more numerous in CBD, particularly in the white matter, where the number of threads and oligodendroglial inclusions is very high, compared with that in other disorders.

NEUROPATHOLOGIC AND CLINICAL HETEROGENEITY

In a study of 11 cases of neuropathologically diagnosed CBD, we found considerable clinical and neuropathologic heterogeneity.[60] Of the 11 patients in our series, 7 presented with unilateral limb dysfunction, although the remaining 4 patients had less typical presentations, including memory loss, behavioral changes, and difficulties with speech or gait. All 11 patients eventually developed extrapyramidal signs, as well as cortical features, most commonly, apraxia. Neuropathologic study revealed predominant neuronal loss and gliosis of perirolandic cortex in 7 of 11 patients; degeneration of more rostral frontal cortex was observed in 3 of the 4 patients with atypical clinical presentations. All cases displayed ballooned neurons, tau-positive neuronal and glial inclusions, threads and grains, and nigral degeneration. Of the 11 patients, 6 manifested overlapping neuropathologic features of one or more disorders, including AD, PSP, PD, and hippocampal sclerosis. Interestingly, these six patients had all exhibited memory loss early in the course of their illness. Our findings suggest that CBD is a pathologically and clinically heterogeneous disorder with substantial overlap with other neurodegenerative disorders.

There are no universally accepted standard criteria for the diagnosis of CBD, and the clinical diagnosis may be difficult.[2] Hauw and coworkers[9,10] examined the validity and reliability of neuropathologic diagnoses of PSP and related disorders, and they proposed criteria for CBD. Exclusion criteria proposed by Litvan and colleagues,[10] however, would eliminate patients with coexisting PD, AD, or certain other pathologies. Our findings suggest that a substantial proportion of otherwise typical CBD patients would be excluded on the basis of these exclusion criteria.

In our view, it is the compendium of neuropathologic findings, often in concert with clinical features, that allows the diagnosis of CBD. Each of the neuropathologic features, in and of itself, is nonspecific. Ballooned neurons have been seen in a variety of central nervous system (CNS) disorders,[23] including Pick's disease, CJD,[75] PSP,[76] amyotrophic lateral sclerosis (ALS),[77] and AD.[23] Moreover, tau positive inclusions occur in AD, Pick's disease and PSP,[67] although there are distinctions as described above and reviewed by Chin and Goldman[17] and Feany et al.[67] We observed tau-positive "astrocytic plaques," considered to be a specific marker for CBD,[67,72] in 10 of 11 of our CBD patients but, as discussed above, they may also be seen in PSP.

Similarly, focal or asymmetric cortical degeneration occurs in other disorders, e.g., Pick's disease, frontal lobe dementia, and ALS with frontal lobe dementia. Some authors have suggested that all neurodegenerative disorders with focal cortical degeneration, including CBD, be classified as "asymmetric cortical degenerative syndromes" or "Pick's complex."[78]

Indeed, there is substantial pathological overlap between CBD and Pick's disease. In addition to focal and often asymmetric cortical degeneration, Pick's disease and CBD show ballooned neurons, variable degeneration of the substantia nigra and basal ganglia, and tau-positive inclusions. Yet, Pick's bodies, typically numerous in Pick's disease, are absent or infrequently noted in CBD. Moreover, the hippocampus, a principal site of pathology in Pick's disease, is typically spared in CBD. Neurofibrillary tangles, glial inclusions, and tau-related pathology are more prominent in Pick's disease than previously appreciated (see Ref. 17 for review). As reviewed by Schneider and coworkers,[60] CBD and Pick's disease also have overlapping clinical features. Extensive clinical-pathological overlap between CBD and PSP has also been observed, as discussed earlier. Patients with both disorders

present with an extrapyramidal syndrome that usually fails to respond to dopaminergic agents. Moreover, eye movement abnormalities, dystonic posturing, and gait imbalance occur in both PSP and CBD; the evolution and predominance of these signs differ in classic cases. This clinical overlap is not surprising, given the similar distribution of subcortical pathology in both conditions.

Multiple-System Atrophy

The nonfamilial forms of MSA include OPCA, striatonigral degeneration (SND), and Shy-Drager syndrome (see Chap. 20). This group of conditions is characterized by parkinsonism, autonomic dysfunction, and pyramidal and cerebellar symptoms or signs. Advances in our understanding of the neuropathology of MSA, supported by findings of functional neuroimaging and other studies, have affirmed the notion that the disorders included under the rubric of MSA have common pathogenetic links and represent a unified group of disorders.

NEUROPATHOLOGY

The neuropathologic features of OPCA include atrophy of the pons, middle cerebellar peduncles, and inferior olivary nuclei. The cerebellum exhibits variable loss of Purkinje cells in the cortex; the dentate nucleus displays gliosis, but its neurons are generally well preserved. The spinal cord may exhibit degeneration of the posterior columns and spinocerebellar tracts. This disorder may be associated with Shy-Drager syndrome with SND and loss of neurons in the intermediolateral cell column of the thoracic spinal cord and Onuf's nucleus in the sacral cord.

SND, which may coexist with OPCA and Shy-Drager syndrome, is generally characterized clinically by bradykinesia and rigidity unresponsive to L-dopa therapy. At autopsy, the brain exhibits bilateral brownish discoloration and atrophy (Fig. 9-8) of the putamen with extensive neuronal loss and, often, florid gliosis. The globus pallidus may also be involved to a lesser extent. The substantia nigra exhibits pallor with loss of neurons and generally mild-to-moderate gliosis but, with rare exceptions, Lewy bodies are not seen.

CYTOPLASMIC INCLUSIONS

A major advance in our understanding of MSA was the finding of glial cytoplasmic inclusions (GCI) by Papp and coworkers,[79,80] confirmed by many groups[81–83] (see Ref. 17 for review). Currently, cytoplasmic inclusions, found in neurons and glial cells, are well-recognized as a key feature of MSA pathology. Measuring about 2 to 25 μm, these inclusions are found in OPCA, SND, Shy-Drager syndrome and nonfamilial forms of MSA. The GCI preferentially involve small cells resembling oligodendroglia in the white matter, whereas the neuronal inclusions tend to involve cells in the pons, basal ganglia, and other sites. The inclusions are slightly eosinophilic, stain black on silver stains and label consistently with antibodies to ubiquitin and alpha-β-crystallin; they also label to varying degrees with antibodies to alpha- and beta-tubulin and microtubule-associated proteins (MAP), such as MAP5

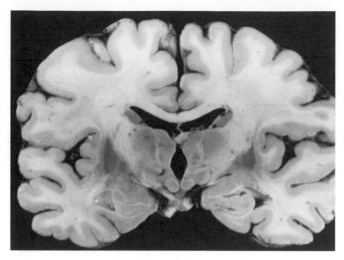

FIGURE 9-8 Striatonigral degeneration. Atrophy of the lenticular nuclei with marked discoloration of the bilateral putamen is appreciated on this coronal section.

and tau. Their ultrastructural appearance and immunohistochemical properties suggest a relationship to the microtubular system. In general, GCI seem to increase in parallel with the numbers of interfascicular oligodendroglia and parallel the degeneration seen in the gray and white matter, although they are also seen in areas that are minimally involved or uninvolved. As discussed by Chin and Goldman,[17] it is still unclear as to whether oligodendroglial cells are specifically targeted in MSA, or whether the inclusions represent a reactive change secondary to neuronal damage.

Papp and Lantos[84] mapped GCI in the brains of 14 patients with various combinations of OPCA, SND, and autonomic failure. The inclusions were common in primary and higher motor areas of cortex, as well as within the pyramidal, extrapyramidal, and corticocerebellar systems. They were rarely found in visual and auditory pathways. These investigators have adopted a "lumper's" approach and believe that GCIs signify a marker of MSA that unifies OPCA, SND, and Shy-Drager syndrome. This view is supported by a recent positron emission tomography (PET) study of patients with OPCA showing subclinical evidence of striatonigral dysfunction and emphasizing the unity of MSA-associated disorders.[85]

Summary

The extensive overlap observed among movement disorders and other neurodegenerative disorders suggests common pathophysiological mechanisms. The increasing recognition of widespread tau-associated and glial pathology in these disorders, discussed earlier in this chapter and in two excellent reviews by Feany and Dickson[18] and Chin and Goldman,[17] highlights the potential relationship of disorders such as CBD, Pick's disease, and PSP and provokes questions about their relationship to AD. Ultrastructural and molecular studies in these disorders have shown both similarities and differences regarding the morphology of the inclusions and biochemical properties of the tau polypeptides.[75,86]

Although the apolipoprotein E ϵ4 allele is recognized as a major risk factor for familial and sporadic AD,[87,88] we have

noted an increased frequency of the apoE ϵ4 allele in those disorders characterized by tau cytoskeletal pathology, that is, CBD, PSP, and Pick's disease.[89] Although others have not observed this trend in PSP,[90] another group has recently reported an increased ϵ4 allele frequency in Pick's disease.[91]

In summary, there is considerable overlap among the movement disorders and other neurodegenerative disorders. Common clinical features may lead to diagnostic problems, such as distinguishing the dementia of AD, PD, and PSP. Furthermore, for a patient in whom one disorder, for example, PSP, has been diagnosed, a physician might be reluctant to assign a second diagnosis, for example, AD. The commonality and overlap among the neurodegenerative diseases may be clarified by prospective clinical and neuropathologic studies of larger series of patients. Ideally, to facilitate sharing of information, such studies should use standardized evaluation batteries, such as those developed by CERAD for AD[7,8] to assess PSP, PD, and other movement disorders.

Acknowledgments

The authors thank Elizabeth Lakin, HT-ASCP, for assistance with histopathology and Linda McGuire for assistance with the manuscript. This work was supported by a Veterans Affairs Merit Award and by NIH Grants AG10130 and AG06790.

References

1. Rajput AH, Rozdilsky B, Rajput A: Accuracy of clinical diagnosis in parkinsonism—A prospective study. *Can J Neurol Sci* 18:275–278, 1991.
2. Litvan I, Agid Y, Goetz C, et al: Accuracy of the clinical diagnosis of corticobasal degeneration: A clinicopathological study. *Neurology.* In Press.
3. Hughes AJ, Daniel SE, Kilford L, Lees AJ: Accuracy of clinical diagnosis of idiopathic Parkinson's disease: A clinicopathological study of 100 cases. *J Neurol Neurosurg Psychiatry* 55:181–184, 1992.
4. Larsen JP, Dupont E, Tandberg E: Clinical diagnosis of Parkinson's disease: Proposal of diagnostic subgroups classified at different levels of confidence. *Acta Neurol Scand* 89:242–251, 1994.
5. McKhann G, Drachman D, Folstein M, et al: Clinical diagnosis of Alzheimer's disease: Report of the NINCDS-ADRDA workgroup under the auspices of the Department of Health and Human Services Task Force on Alzheimer's Disease. *Neurology* 34:939–944, 1984.
6. Gearing M, Mirra SS, Hedreen JC, Hansen LA, et al: Neuropathology confirmation of the clinical diagnosis of Alzheimer's disease: CERAD (Consortium to Establish a Registry for Alzheimer's Disease). Part X. *Neurology* 45:461–466, 1995.
7. Morris JC, Heyman A, Mohs RC: The Consortium to Establish a Registry for Alzheimer's Disease (CERAD). Part I. Clinical and neuropsychological assessment of Alzheimer's disease. *Neurology* 39:1159–1165, 1989.
8. Mirra SS, Heyman A, McKeel D, et al: The Consortium to Establish a Registry for Alzheimer's Disease (CERAD). Part II. Standardization of the neuropathologic assessment of Alzheimer's disease. *Neurology* 41:479–486, 1991.
9. Hauw JJ, Daniel SE, Dickson D, et al: Preliminary NINDS neuropathologic criteria for Steele-Richardson-Olszewski syndrome (progressive supranuclear palsy). *Neurology* 44:2015–2019, 1994.

10. Litvan I, Hauw JJ, Bartko, et al: Validity and reliability of the preliminary NINDS neuropathologic criteria for progressive supranuclear palsy and related disorders. *J Neuropathol Exp Neurol* 55:97–105, 1996.

11. Mirra SS, Hart MN, Terry RD: Making the diagnosis of Alzheimer's disease: A guide for practicing pathologists. *Arch Pathol Lab Med* 117:132–144, 1993.

12. Hansen LA, Crain BJ: Making the diagnosis of mixed and non-Alzheimer's dementias. *Arch Pathol Lab Med* 119:1023–1031, 1995.

13. Vonsattel JP, Myers RH, Stevens TJ, et al: Neuropathological classification of Huntington's disease. *J Neuropathol Exp Neurol* 44:559–577, 1985.

14. Takei Y, Mirra SS: Striatonigral degeneration: A form of multiple system atrophy with clinical Parkinsonism. *Prog Neuropathol* 2:60–77, 1973.

15. Mirra SS, Gearing M, Hughes J, et al: Interlaboratory comparison of neuropathology assessments in Alzheimer's disease: A study of the Consortium to Establish a Registry for Alzheimer's Disease (CERAD). *J Neuropathol Exp Neurol* 53:303–315, 1994.

16. Braak II, Braak E: Neuropathological staging of Alzheimer-related changes. *Acta Neuropathol* 82:239–259, 1991.

17. Chin SS-M, Goldman JE: Glial inclusions in CNS degenerative diseases. *J Neuropathol Exp Neurol* 55:499–508, 1996.

18. Feany MB, Dickson DW: Neurodegenerative disorders with extensive tau pathology: A comparative study and review. *Ann Neurol* 40:139–148, 1996.

19. Lennox G, Lowe J, Morrell K, et al: Anti-ubiquitin immunocytochemistry is more sensitive than conventional techniques in the detection of diffuse Lewy body disease. *J Neurol Neurosurg Psychiatry* 52:67–71, 1989.

20. Dickson DW, Ruan D, Crystal H, et al: Hiippocampal degeneration differentiates diffuse Lewy body disease (DLBD) from Alzheimer's disease: Light and electron microscopic immunocytochemistry of CA2-3 neurites specific to DLBD. *Neurology* 41:1402–1409, 1991.

21. Dickson DW, Schmidt ML, Lee VM-Y, et al: Immunoreactivity profile of hippocampal CA2-3 neurites in diffuse Lewy body disease. *Acta Neuropathol* 87:269–276, 1994.

22. Kim H, Gearing M, Mirra SS: Ubiquitin-positive CA2-3 neurites in hippocampus coexist with cortical Lewy bodies. *Neurology* 45:1768–1770, 1995.

23. Dickson DW, Yen S-H, Suzuki KI, et al: Ballooned neurons in select neurodegenerative diseases contain phosphorylated neurofilament epitopes. *Acta Neuropathol* 71:216–223, 1986.

24. Forno LS: Neuropathology of Parkinson's disease. *J Neuropathol Exp Neurol* 55:259–272, 1996.

25. Fearnley JM, Lees AJ: Aging and Parkinson's disease: Substantia nigra regional selectivity. *Brain* 114:2283–2301, 1991.

26. Pollanen MS, Dickson DW, Bergeron C: Pathology and biology of the Lewy body. *J Neuropathol Exp Neurol* 52:183–191, 1993.

27. Goldman JE, Yen S-H, Chiu F-C, Peress NS: Lewy bodies of Parkinson's disease contain neurofilament antigens. *Science* 221:1082–1084, 1983.

28. Hill WD, Lee VM-Y, Hurtig HI, et al: Epitopes located in spatially separate domains of each neurofilament subunit are present in Parkinson's disease Lewy bodies. *J Comp Neurol* 309:150–160, 1991.

29. Schmidt ML, Murray J, Lee VM-Y, et al: Epitope map of neurofilament protein domains in cortical and peripheral nervous system Lewy bodies. *Am J Pathol* 139:53–65, 1991.

30. Koller WC: How accurately can Parkinson's disease be diagnosed. *Neurology* 42(suppl 1):6–16, 1992.

31. Boller F, Mizutani T, Roessmann U, Gambetti P: Parkinson disease, dementia, and Alzheimer disease: Clinicopathologic correlations. *Ann Neurol* 7:329–335, 1980.

32. Hakim AM, Mathieson G: Basis of dementia in Parkinson's disease (letter). *Lancet* 1:729, 1978.

33. Ditter SM, Mirra SS: Neuropathologic and clinical features of Parkinson's disease in Alzheimer's disease patients. *Neurology* 37:754–760, 1987.

34. Hansen L, Salmon D, Galasko D, et al: The Lewy body variant of Alzheimer's disease: A clinical and pathologic entity. *Neurology* 40:1–8, 1990.

35. Morris JC, Drazner M, Fulling K, et al: Clinical and pathological aspects of parkinsonism in Alzheimer's disease: A role for extranigral factors? *Arch Neurol* 46:651–657, 1989.

36. Hulette C, Mirra S, Wilkinson, Heyman A, et al: The Consortium to Establish a Registry for Alzheimer's Disease (CERAD). Part IX. A prospective cliniconeuropathologic study of Parkinson's features in Alzheimer's disease. *Neurology* 45:1991–1995, 1995.

37. Hansen LA, Masliah E, Galasko D, Terry RD: Plaque-only Alzheimer disease is usually the Lewy body variant, and vice versa. *J Neuropathol Exp Neurol* 52:648–654, 1993.

38. Hansen LA, Galasko D, Samuel W, et al: Apolipoprotein E ∈-4 is associated with increased neurofibrillary pathology in the Lewy body variant of Alzheimer's disease. *Neurosci Lett* 182:63–65, 1994.

39. Dickson DW, Davies P, Mayeux R, et al: Diffuse Lewy body disease: Neuropathological and biochemical studies of six patients. *Acta Neuropathol (Berl)* 75:8–15, 1987.

40. Dickson DW, Crystal H, Mattace LA, et al: Diffuse Lewy body disease: Light and electron microscopic immunocytochemistry of senile plaques. *Acta Neuropathol* 78:572–584, 1989.

41. Bergeron C, Pollanen M: Lewy bodies in Alzheimer's disease—one or two diseases? *Alzheimer Dis Assoc Disord* 3:197–204, 1989.

42. Crystal HA, Dickson DW, Lizardi JE, et al: Antemortem diagnosis of diffuse Lewy body disease. *Neurology* 40:1523–1528, 1990.

43. Perry RH, Irving D, Blessed G, et al: Senile dementia of Lewy body type: A clinically and neuropathologically distinct form of Lewy body dementia in the elderly. *J Neurol Sci* 95:119–139, 1990.

44. Byrne EJ, Lennox G, Lowe J, Godwin-Austen RB: Diffuse Lewy body disease: Clinical features in 15 cases. *J Neurol Neurosurg Psychiatry* 52:709–717, 1989.

45. McKeith IG, Fairbairn AF, Perry RH, Thompson P: The clinical diagnosis and misdiagnosis of senile dementia of Lewy body type (SDLT). *Br J Psychiatry* 165:324–332, 1994.

46. McKeith IG, Fairbairn AF, Bothwell RA, et al: An evaluation of the predictive validity and inter-rater reliability of clinical diagnostic criteria for senile dementia of Lewy body type. *Neurology* 44:872–877, 1994.

47. McKeith IG, Galasko D, Kosaka K, et al: Consensus guidelines for the clinical and pathological diagnosis of dementia with Lewy bodies (DLB): Report of the Consortium on DLB International Workshop. *Neurology* 47, 1996.

48. Hansen L, Masliah E, Terry RD, Mirra SS: A neuropathological subset of Alzheimer's disease with concomitant Lewy body disease and spongiform change. *Acta Neuropathol* 78:194–201, 1989.

49. Gai WP, Blessing WS, Blumberger PC: Ubiquitin-positive degenerating neurites in the brainstem in Parkinson's disease. *Brain* 118:1447–1460, 1995.

50. Steele JC, Richardson JC, Olszewski J: Progressive supranuclear palsy: A heterogeneous degeneration involving the brain stem, basal ganglia and cerebellum with vertical gaze and pseudobulbar palsy, nuchal dystonia and dementia. *Arch Neurol* 10:333–359, 1964.

51. Jellinger KA, Bancher C: Neuropathology, in Litvan I, Agid Y (eds): *Progressive Supranuclear Palsy: Clinical and Research Approaches.* New York: Oxford University Press, 1992, pp 44–88.

52. Braak H, Jellinger K, Braak E, Bohl J: Allocortical neurofibrillary changes in progressive supranuclear palsy. *Acta Neuropathol* 84:478–483, 1992.

53. Hof PR, Delacourte A, Bouras C: Distribution of cortical neurofibrillary tangles in progressive supranuclear palsy: A quantitative analysis of six cases. *Acta Neuropathol* 84:45–51, 1992.

54. Mizusawa H, Yen S-H, Hirano A, Llena JF: Pathology of the dentate nucleus in progressive supranuclear palsy: A histological, immunohistochemical and ultrastructural study. *Acta Neuropathol (Berl)* 78:419–428, 1989.

55. Kobayashi K, Morikawa K, Fukutani Y, et al: Ramsey Hunt syndrome: Progressive mental deterioration in association with unusual cerebral white matter change. *Clin Neuropathol* 13:88–96, 1994.

56. Yamashita S, Iwamoto H, Hara M, et al: Sisters with early onset hereditary dentatorubral-pallidoluysian atrophy of childhood—DNA analysis and clinicopathological findings (title translated from Japanese). *No To Hattatsu* 27:473–479, 1995.

57. Kogure T, Oda T, Katoh Y: Autopsy cases of hereditary ataxia pathologically diagnosed as the Japanese type of Joseph disease-cliniconeuropathological findings (title translated from Japanese). *Seishin Shinkeigaku Zasshi* 92:161–183, 1990.

58. Iwabuchi K, Nagatomo H, Tanabe T, et al: An autopsied case of type 2 Machado-Joseph's disease or spino-pontine degeneration (title translated from Japanese). *No To Shinkei* 45:733–740, 1993.

59. Hattori H, Tanaka S, Kondoh H, et al: A case of juvenile Alzheimer's disease with various neurological features such as myoclonus, showing grumose degeneration in the dentate nucleus (title translated from Japanese). *Rinsho Shinkeigaku* 30:647–653, 1990.

60. Schneider JA, Watts RL, Gearing M, et al: Corticobasal degeneration: Neuropathological and clinical heterogeneity. *Neurology.* In Press.

61. Gearing M, Olson DA, Watts RL, Mirra SS: Progressive supranuclear palsy: Neuropathologic and clinical heterogeneity. *Neurology* 44:1015–1024, 1994.

62. Gibb WRG, Luthert PJ, Marsden CD: Corticobasal degeneration. *Brain* 112:1171–1192, 1989.

63. Arima K, Murayama S, Oyanagi S, et al: Presenile dementia with progressive supranuclear palsy tangles and Pick bodies: An unusual degenerative disorder involving the cerebral cortex, cerebral nuclei, and brain stem nuclei. *Acta Neuropathol* 84:128–134, 1992.

64. D'Amato CJ, Foster NL, Hicks SP, Sima AAF: Swollen cortical neurons and Lewy bodies accompanying progressive supranuclear palsy and Creutzfeldt-Jakob's disease. *J Neuropathol Exp Neurol* 51:324 (abs), 1992.

65. Ikeda K, Akiyama H, Haga C, et al: Argyrophilic thread-like structure in corticobasal degeneration and supranuclear palsy. *Neurosci Lett* 174:157–159, 1994.

66. Jendroska K, Rossor MN, Mathias CJ, Daniel SE: Morphological overlap between corticobasal degeneration and Pick's disease: A clinicopathological report. *Mov Disord* 10:111–114, 1995.

67. Feany MB, Mattiace LA, Dickson DW: Neuropathologic overlap of progressive supranuclear palsy, Pick's disease, and corticobasal degeneration. *J Neuropathol Exp Neurol* 55:53–67, 1996.

68. Mann DMA, Jones D: Deposition of amyloid (A4) protein within the brains of persons with dementing disorders other than Alzheimer's disease and Down's syndrome. *Neurosci Lett* 109:68–75, 1990.

69. Sasaki S, Maruyama S, Toyoda C: A case of progressive supranuclear palsy with widespread senile plaques. *J Neurol* 238:345–348, 1991.

70. D'Amato CJ, Sima AF, Foster NL, et al: Cerebral Lewy bodies with progressive supranuclear palsy. *J Neuropathol Exp Neurol* 50:308 (abs), 1991.

71. Mori H, Yoshimura M, Tomonaga M, Yamanouchi H: Progressive supranuclear palsy with Lewy bodies. *Acta Neuropathol (Berl)* 71:344–346, 1986.

72. Feany MB, Dickson DW: Widespread cytoskeletal pathology characterizes corticobasal degeneration. *Am J Pathol* 146:1388–1396, 1995.

73. Nishimura T, Ikeda K, Akiyama H, et al: Immunohistochemical investigation of tau-positive structures in the cerebral cortex of patients with progressive supranuclear palsy. *Neurosci Lett* 201:123–126, 1995.

74. Feany MB, Ksiezak-Reding H, Liu WK, et al: Epitope expression and hyperphosphorylation of tau protein in corticobasal degeneration: Differentiation from progressive supranuclear palsy. *Acta Neuropathol* 90:37–43, 1995.

75. Nakazato Y, Hirato J, Ishida Y, et al: Swollen cortical neurons in Creutzfeldt-Jakob disease contain a phosphorylated neurofilament epitope. *J Neuropathol Exp Neurol* 49:197–205, 1990.

76. Mackenzie IRA, Hudson LP: Achromatic neurons in the cortex of progressive supranuclear palsy. *Acta Neuropathol* 90:615–619, 1995.

77. Manetto V, Sternberger NH, Petty G, et al: Phosphorylation of neurofilaments is altered in amyotrophic lateral sclerosis. *J Neuropathol Exp Neurol* 47:642–653, 1986.

78. Kertesz A, Hudson L, Mackenzie IRA, Munoz DG: The pathology and nosology of primary progressive aphasia. *Neurology* 44:2065–2072, 1994.

79. Papp MI, Kahn JE, Lantos PL: Glial cytoplasmic inclusions in the CNS of patients with multiple system atrophy (striatonigral degeneration, olivopontocerebellar atrophy and Shy-Drager syndrome). *J Neurol Sci* 94:79–100, 1989.

80. Papp MI, Lantos PL: Accumulation of tubular structures in oligodendroglial and neuronal cells as the basic alteration in multiple system atrophy. *J Neurol Sci* 107:172–182, 1992.

81. Nakazato Y, Yamazaki H, Hirato J, et al: Oligodendroglial microtubular tangles in olivopontocerebellar atrophy. *J Neuropathol Exp Neurol* 49:521–530, 1990.

82. Abe H, Yagishita S., Amano N, et al: Argyrophilic glial introcytoplasmic inclusions in multiple system atrophy: Immunocytochemical and ultrastructural study. *Acta Neuropathol* 84:273–277, 1992.

83. Kobayashi K, Miyazu K, Katsukawa K, et al: Cytoskeletal protein abnormalities in patients with olivopontocerebellar atrophy—an immunocytochemical and Gallyas silver impregnation study. *Neuropathol Appl Neurobiol* 18:237–249, 1992.

84. Papp MI, Lantos PL: The distribution of oligodendroglial inclusions in multiple system atrophy and its relevance to clinical symptomatology. *Brain* 117:235–243, 1994.

85. Rinne JO, Burn DJ, Mathias CJ, et al: Positron emission tomography studies on the dopaminergic system and striatal opioid binding in the olivopontocerebellar atrophy variant of multiple system atrophy. *Ann Neurol* 37:568–573, 1995.

86. Ksiezak-Reding H, Morgan K, Mattiace LA, et al: Ultrastructural and biochemical composition of paired helical filaments in corticobasal degeneration. *Am J Pathol* 145:1496–1508, 1994.

87. Corder EH, Saunders AM, Strittmatter WJ, et al: Gene dose of apolipoprotein E type 4 allele and the risk of Alzheimer's disease in late onset families. *Science* 261:921–923, 1993.

88. Strittmatter WJ, Saunders AM, Schmechel D, et al: Apolipoprotein E: High-avidity binding to beta-amyloid and increased frequency of type 4 allele in late-onset familial Alzheimer disease. *Proc Natl Acad Sci U S A* 90:1977–1981, 1993.

89. Schneider JA, Gearing M, Robbins RS, et al: Apolipoprotein E genotype in diverse neurodegenerative disorders. *Ann Neurol* 38:131–135, 1995.

90. Tabaton M, Rolleri M, Masturzo P, et al: Apolipoprotein E epsilon 4 allele frequency is not increased in progressive supranuclear palsy. *Neurology* 45:1764–1765, 1995.

91. Farrer LA, Abraham CR, Volicer L, et al: Allele e4 of apolipoprotein E shows a dose effect on age at onset of Pick disease. *Exp Neurol* 136:162–170, 1995.

PART III
CLINICAL DISORDERS

Chapter 10

EPIDEMIOLOGY AND GENETICS OF PARKINSON'S DISEASE

CAROLINE M. TANNER, JEAN P. HUBBLE, and PIU CHAN

EPIDEMIOLOGY OF PARKINSON'S DISEASE
    Incidence and Prevalence Rates
    Mortality
    Risk Factors
GENETICS OF PARKINSON'S DISEASE
    Familial Parkinson's Disease
    Twin Studies
    Mitochondrial Inheritance
    Susceptibility Genes
CONCLUSIONS

Parkinson's disease was described in 1817,[1] yet its etiology remains unknown. In the 1950s, Kurland[2] in Rochester, Minnesota, and Gudmundsson[3] in Iceland provided the first community-based estimates of Parkinson's disease prevalence, finding it to be one of the most common neurodegenerative disorders of the elderly. Epidemiology has played an important role not only in health planning but also as a tool for the investigation of the cause of Parkinson's disease. One proposed cause, genetics, has risen and fallen in popularity several times since 1817. The flowering of modern molecular genetics has provided important new approaches for evaluating the contribution of genetic factors to Parkinson's disease. Because these technological advances are scientifically most useful when applied to well-characterized populations, both genetics and epidemiology will be considered in this chapter. First, however, we offer some definitions and sound a cautionary note.

In this chapter, the term Parkinson's disease will be used to refer to a specific entity. The proposed definition is a narrow one, reflecting almost exactly the syndrome originally described by Parkinson. Parkinson's disease is defined as a slowly progressive neurodegenerative disorder with no identifiable cause. Pathologically, Parkinson's disease is characterized by loss of pigmented neurons and gliosis, most prominently in the substantia nigra pars compacta and locus ceruleus, and by the presence of ubiquitin-positive eosinophilic cytoplasmic inclusions in degenerating neurons.[4] Because there is no antemortem biological marker for Parkinson's disease, in living subjects diagnosis is based entirely on the neurological examination. The cardinal signs of Parkinson's disease are bradykinesia, rest tremor, cogwheel rigidity, and postural reflex impairment. Neurological signs suggesting more extensive injury of the motor or sensory pathways extending beyond the pigmented brain stem nuclei are not included in this definition of Parkinson's disease. These signs are suggestive of other neurodegenerative disorders, often termed "atypical parkinsonism," including progressive supranuclear palsy, striatonigral degeneration, and other less common conditions.[5]

A particular diagnostic and nosological problem is presented by persons with the cardinal signs of Parkinson's disease but having also an associated dementia. Although, not surprisingly, at postmortem persons with these clinical signs show pathological changes in cortical areas, the nature of the cortical change may be parkinsonian (i.e., Lewy bodies) or Alzheimer-like (i.e., neurofibrillary tangles). A reliable method for making this distinction before death has not been developed. For simplicity, those persons in whom the motor changes of Parkinson's disease occur before or coincidentally with cognitive difficulties will be considered as having Parkinson's disease, whereas those with dementia preceding motor abnormalities will not be included.

Epidemiological and genetic investigations of Parkinson's disease are complicated by the very nature of Parkinson's disease. First, because the diagnosis of Parkinson's disease is dependent entirely on the neurological history and examination, some persons may be misclassified. In one series, 20 percent of patients diagnosed in life as having Parkinson's disease had some other diagnosis, usually, some form of atypical parkinsonism, at autopsy.[6] Because cases in which the clinical diagnosis is in question are more likely to be referred for autopsy, this rate is likely higher than that which would be found if all cases were evaluated pathologically. Nonetheless, these results highlight the possibility that some cases of atypical parkinsonism may be erroneously diagnosed as Parkinson's disease. Inclusion of these cases in risk factor studies would likely lessen the likelihood that a variable associated with Parkinson's disease can be clearly identified. Their inclusion in genetic studies may lead to erroneous conclusions about the contribution of heredity.

Second, although diagnostic criteria are not uniformly applied in contemporary studies of Parkinson's disease, differences in case ascertainment and diagnosis were even greater in the past. These differences may profoundly affect comparisons and study conclusions. So-called "meta-analyses" of Parkinson's disease epidemiological studies are nearly impossible. For example, a study using tremor as the only diagnostic criterion for Parkinson's disease will likely include many persons with other disorders. Potential erroneous outcomes include overestimation of disease frequency, loss of power in assessing risk factors, and overestimation of the role of genetics by inclusion of persons with other heritable movement disorders.

Third, the clinical manifestations of Parkinson's disease may be preceded by a long "latent" stage.[7] The existence of "presymptomatic" Parkinson's disease is suggested by the finding of Lewy bodies in the brains of persons not known to have clinical evidence of Parkinson's disease during life. "Incidental Lewy bodies" and clinical Parkinson's disease are both age-related phenomena.[8,9] If these incidental Lewy body cases represent subclinical Parkinson's disease, then many persons with the identical pathological process will be overlooked, using current diagnostic methods in which biological disease markers are lacking. The possibility of a long latent period makes identification of environmental risk factors difficult. Similarly, the identification of familial patterns of disease is made difficult when pathologically affected family members die before clinical signs are apparent.

Fourth, Parkinson's disease is a disorder of late life. This is particularly problematic in genetic investigations, because very few families will include living members from more than one or two generations. As a result, clinical information and diagnostic accuracy are limited for ancestral generations. Even more scarce are blood and tissue for thorough molecular genetic investigations. Finally, Parkinson's disease is a relatively rare disorder. As a result, even studies canvassing relatively large populations will identify relatively few cases, and the potential error in any single study may be significant.

Despite the challenges outlined in the preceding paragraphs, epidemiological and genetic investigations have added considerably to our understanding of Parkinson's disease and serve as an impetus for future study. These results will be summarized in the remainder of this chapter.

Epidemiology of Parkinson's Disease

INCIDENCE AND PREVALENCE RATES

Incidence is the most accurate estimate of disease frequency, as it is the measure of the number of new cases occurring in a given time period for a specific location. It is relatively unaffected by factors affecting disease survival. This is particularly true for a slowly progressive disorder such as Parkinson's disease. However, measurements of disease incidence are the most difficult, and only 10 such studies in Parkinson's disease have been reported (Table 10-1). The incidence rates in these studies ranged from 4.5–21/100,000 population/year, reflecting, at least in part, variations in study design such as ascertainment methods and case definition. For example, some researchers included both Parkinson's disease and

postencephalitic parkinsonism when calculating incidence rates, although today these disorders are thought to be quite distinct. Similarly, persons with parkinsonism in addition to cerebellar and pyramidal dysfunction were included in Gudmundsson's incidence rates as examples of "arteriosclerotic parkinsonism,"[3] although such cases would likely not be considered as Parkinson's disease by most present-day physicians. Others made the diagnosis of parkinsonism solely based on medical record[10] and may have included persons with other disorders, such as essential tremor. In fact, a study conducted in Finland found that 201 of 775 patients who carried the diagnosis of Parkinson's disease on the basis of medical records were considered to have essential tremor when examined.[13]

Prevalence measures the total number of current cases in a population at a given time. Three approaches have been used to estimate the prevalence of Parkinson's disease. The first method estimates prevalence based on clinical populations, most often at an academic referral center. This technique is inherently inaccurate, as social or economic factors may determine who seeks medical care at a given clinical site. In addition there may be an overrepresentation of midstage disease cases with mildly affected individuals not requiring or seeking care at a referral center and end-stage patients being unable to travel to the clinic. The second approach estimates prevalence from health service records, and it is subject to biases similar to those in the first method, although larger, more diverse clinical populations can be surveyed. In settings in which health care is universally available and uniformly delivered, good estimates can be obtained using this method. The third method estimates prevalence based on door-to-door screening of a target population, followed by a physician examination of screen-positive individuals. This method is the most accurate, but the time and expense involved limit its widespread application. Crude estimates

TABLE 10-1 Estimated Incidence and Crude Prevalence of Parkinson's Disease in Community-Based Studies

Reference	Location	Incidence per 100,000/yr	Prevalence per 100,000
Kurland[2]	Rochester, NY	20	187
Brewis[10]	Carlisle, UK	12	113
Jenkins[11]	Victoria, Australia		85
Gudmundsson[3]	Iceland	16	162
Kessler[12]	Baltimore, MD		128*
Marttila[13]	Turku, Finland	15	120
Rosati[14]	Sardinia, Italy	4.9	66
Harada[15]	Yonago, Japan	10	81
Rajput[16]	Rochester, NY	21	
Sutcliffe[17]	Northampton, UK		108
Ashok[18]	Benghazi, Libya	4.5	31
Mutch[19]	Aberdeen, Scotland		164
D'Alessandro[20]	San Marino		152
Shi[21]	Shanghai, China		18
Okada[22]	Izumo City, Japan		82
Granieri[23]	Ferrara, Italy	10	165
Mayeux[24]	New York, NY		100
Caradoc-Davies[25]	Dunedin, New Zealand		110
Svenson[26]	Alberta, Canada		110

*Males only.

of Parkinson's disease prevalence have been reported to vary from 18/100,000 persons in a Shanghai, China, population survey[21] to 328/100,000 in a door-to-door survey of the Parsi community in Bombay, India (a population in which 44 percent of persons are aged 50 or older)[30] (Tables 10-1 and 10-2). As might be predicted, the prevalence estimates derived by means of door-to-door methods are greater than those derived from other methods for comparable populations.

AGE-SPECIFIC DISTRIBUTION

Both the incidence and the prevalence of Parkinson's disease increase with increasing age of the population surveyed (Table 10-3). Parkinson's disease is rare before age 50, and incidence and prevalence increase steadily until around the 9th decade for incidence or the 10th decade for prevalence, when rates appear to decline. This apparent decline among the most elderly likely represents an artifact resulting from poor ascertainment and the very few people in these age groups.

GENDER-SPECIFIC DISTRIBUTION

Parkinson's disease appears to be slightly more common in men than in women in most studies (Table 10-4). Most dramatic is the finding of a more than threefold-increased prevalence in men, compared to women, in China.[27] More typically, rates in men are elevated but are less than twice the rates in women. The observed male preponderance is less robust than the association with increasing age, and there is considerable variability across studies. Moreover, because these observations are based on prevalence surveys, differences in survival, access to health care, and differences in the underlying composition of the population may contribute to this apparent increased risk of Parkinson's disease for men. The validity of this association must be validated in prospective studies of disease incidence.

RACE-SPECIFIC DISTRIBUTION

The prevalence of Parkinson's disease appears to vary internationally (Tables 10-1 and 10-2), possibly reflecting variations in risk determined by the racial composition of the populations surveyed. Caucasians in Europe and North America usually have a higher prevalence, whereas rates are intermediate for Asians in Japan and China and lowest for blacks in Africa. These data have been interpreted as an indication that whites are at higher risk for Parkinson's disease. As shown in (Table 10-5), several hospital-based studies conducted in the United States and Africa found lower rates of Parkinson's disease in blacks. These observations are subject to biases, including those resulting from differences in use of health care, differences in perception of disease, and differences in survival. A door-to-door study conducted in Copiah County, Mississippi minimized the bias introduced by differences in use of health care. In this study, age-adjusted Parkinson's disease prevalence was not different in whites and blacks when the least stringent diagnostic criteria were used to define the disease.[28] The clarification of the true differences in disease risk associated with race require confirmation in prospective incidence studies in a racially diverse population.

TIME-SPECIFIC DISTRIBUTION

Whether the incidence of Parkinson's disease has changed since 1817 is unknown because of the paucity of longitudinal data. The only population-based data examine Parkinson's disease incidence in Olmsted County, Minnesota during the 50-year period from 1935 to 1988.[37] To minimize variability resulting from differences in diagnostic criteria over time, all cases were classified by a single neurologist, using extant diagnostic criteria. Estimated incidence increased from 9.2/100,000 annually for the interval from 1935 to 1944 to 16.3/100,000 for the interval from 1975 to 1984. In a meta-analysis using age- and gender-adjustment for comparison purposes, Zhang and Roman found no significant temporal fluctuations in the incidence and prevalence in Europe and the United States over the past 50 years.[38] Until other prospective studies are performed, it is not possible to determine whether there has been a true increase in disease frequency or simply a change in diagnostic pattern.

GEOGRAPHIC DISTRIBUTION

The reported rates of Parkinson's disease show marked geographic variation. For comparison, Zhang and Roman adjusted reported rates to the 1970 U.S. population.[38] Age-

TABLE 10-2 Estimated Crude Prevalence of Parkinson's Disease in Door-to-Door Surveys

Reference	Publication Year	Location	Ages (yr) Screened	Prevalence per 100,000
Li[27]	1985	China (six cities)	>50	44
Schoenberg[28]	1985	Mississippi	>39	347
Schoenberg[29]	1988	Igbo-ora, Nigeria	>39	59
Bharucha[30]	1988	Parsi community, Bombay, India	All ages	328
Acosta[31]	1988	Vejer de la Frontera Cadiz, Spain	All ages	270
Rocca[32]	1990	Terrasini, Santa Teresa di Riva Sicily, Italy	All ages	243
Wang[33]	1991	China (29 cities)	>50	15
Morgante[34]	1992	Sicily, Italy	>12	257
Wang[35]	1994	Kin-Hu, Kinmen	>50	170

TABLE 10-3 Age-Specific Prevalence of Parkinson's Disease

Reference	Location	PREVALENCE (PER 100,000) BY AGE GROUP IN YEARS					
		0–39	40–49	50–59	60–69	70–79	80–89
Marttila[13]	Turku, Finland	0.8	27.8	136.2	503.5	736.1	464.8 <79 yr
Rosati[14]	Sardinia, Italy	3.3	38.6	204.5	342.1	311.3	82.6
Harada[15]	Yonago, Japan	4.7	39.9	85.8	245.1	698.4	752.7
Sutcliffe[17]	Northampton, UK		3 <50 yr	4.0	277.0	702.0	1136 >79 yr
Li[27]*	China (6 cities)			92.0	145.0	615 >70 yr	
Mutch[19]	Aberdeen, Scotland	0.0	46.6	77.9	254.0	839.6	1925 >79 yr
Okada[22]	Izumo City, Japan	23.2	19.6	63.6	338.6	478.7	335.7
Mayeux[24]	New York, NY		23 <50 yr	45.7	234.8	525.6	1145 >80 yr
Morgante[34]*	Sicily, Italy		0.0	115.6	621.4	1978.3	3055
Svensen[26]	Alberta, Canada		46.6	77.9	254.0	839.6	1925 >79 yr
Wang[35]	Kin-Hu, Kinmen			0.0	780.0	1750	2500 >80 yr

*Door-to-door surveys.

adjusted incidence rates varied worldwide from 1.9/100,000 in China to 22.1/100,000 in Rochester, Minnesota. Age-adjusted prevalence ranged from 18/100,000 in China to 234/100,000 in Montevideo, Uruguay. When these differences reflect true variations in disease frequencies, rather than artifacts of study design or differences in medical care, they likely reflect differences in the distribution of etiologic risk factors for Parkinson's disease. For example, genetic or environmental risk factors could be more common in areas with higher disease frequency.

Any of the reported differences in Parkinson's disease frequency may simply be artifacts of differences in study design, including diagnostic criteria and case ascertainment. Socioeconomic factors likely have a greater impact on the estimated prevalence than on the incidence of Parkinson's disease. Lower prevalence rates may simply reflect poor socioeconomic conditions and, consequently, shortened survival. Because most reported rates are of prevalence, rather than incidence, this qualification is important.

MORTALITY

In the case of Parkinson's disease mortality rates (see Table 10-6) are more readily available than other measures of disease frequency (incidence and prevalence); nevertheless, even death rates do not accurately reflect the true distribution

TABLE 10-4 Prevalence of Parkinson's Disease Based on Gender

Reference	Location	PREVALENCE (PER 100,000)	
		Men	Women
Marttila[13]	Turku, Finland	98	140
Rosati[14]	Sardinia, Italy	74	58
Harada[15]	Yonago, Japan	63	97
Schoenberg[28]*	Mississippi	116	145
Sutcliffe[17]	Northampton, UK	102	114
Li[27]	China (6 cities)	32	12
Ashok[18]	Benghazi, Libya	33	30
Mutch[19]**	Aberdeen, Scotland	124	84
D'Alessandro[20]	San Marino, Italy	154	150
Bharucha[30]*	Bombay, India	375	296
Wang et al.[33]*	China (29 cities)	17	12
Okada[22]	Izumo City, Japan	47	114
Granieri[23]	Ferrara, Italy	160	219
Mayeux[24]	New York, U.S.	119	69
Svensen[26]	Alberta, Canada	269	225

*Door-to-door surveys.
**Age-adjusted prevalence.

TABLE 10-5 Crude Prevalence of Parkinson's Disease Based on Race and Gender

Location	PREVALENCE (PER 100,000)		
	Men	Women	Total
South Africa Johannesburg[36]			
Whites			159
Blacks			4
North America (U.S.) Baltimore[12]			
Whites	128	121	
Blacks	31	9	
Copiah County[28]			
Whites			159
Blacks			103

TABLE 10-6 Changes in Mortality in Parkinson's Disease Based on Age, Sex, and Time

Reference	Study Period	Location	MORTALITY RATE DIFFERENCES		
			Sex	Age**	Time (yr)***
Lilienfeld[39]	1962–1984	U.S.	M > F	Yes	NS
Williams[40]*	1959–1961	U.S.	M > F	Yes	NA
Svenson[41]	1979–1986	Canada	M > F	NA	Y
Riggs[42]	1955–1986	U.S.	M > F	Yes	Y (>75)
Kurtzke[43]	1980–1985	Denmark	M > F	Yes	Y (>75)
Treves[44,45]	1962–1985	U.S.	NA	Yes	Y (>74)
Vanacore[46]	1969–1987	Italy	NA	Yes	Y (>79)
Clarke[47]	1921–1989	England and Wales	M > F	Yes	Y (>75)
Chio[48]	1951–1987	Italy	M > F	Yes	Y (>75)
Imaizumi[49]	1950–1992	Japan	M > F	Yes	Y (>70)

NA, not assessed; NS, no significant change.
 * Included all forms of parkinsonism.
 ** Yes indicates increased mortality with advancing age.
*** Indicates increased mortality rate over time (applying only to age group indicated).

of disease. The reason is that Parkinson's disease is not a direct cause of death. Although in some cases it may be a contributing or underlying cause, Parkinson's disease is recorded on fewer than half of the death certificates of known cases.[49,50] This underreporting is compounded by variability in diagnostic accuracy and temporal and geographic differences in death statistics reporting. Nonetheless, mortality rate represents a unique population-based statistic, because the information is accrued over long time periods in virtually all communities.

In general, higher mortality rates have been reported for the United States and Northern Europe. Mortality rates for Parkinson's disease increase with increasing age in all reports, rising sharply after age 60 to rates of 100/100,000 or more in those age 80 or older at death. Mortality rates are slightly higher for men than for women. In the United States, overall mortality between 1962 and 1984 was estimated as 2/100,000 population for white men, 1/100,000 for nonwhite men and white women and less than 1/100,000 for nonwhite women.[38] Reported Parkinson's disease mortality increased from the early 1920s to the 1950s in all countries studied.[51,52] In subsequent years, rates increased in the older age groups but were decreased or stable at younger ages at death. Improved survival from antiparkinsonian therapy and decreased or delayed mortality from other disorders likely contribute to this reduction.[40] In a community-based 3.5 year follow-up of prevalent Parkinson's disease cases, death was predicted by dementia and later age at disease onset.[53]

RISK FACTORS

A variety of factors have been associated with altered risk of Parkinson's disease (Tables 10-7 and 10-8). Demographic factors such as age, gender, and race appear to influence the risk of developing Parkinson's disease. Increasing age is the factor most consistently associated with an increased risk of Parkinson's disease (see Tables 10-1 and 10-2). When considered as a clue to the cause of Parkinson's disease, this association may reflect age-related neuronal vulnerability. How-

TABLE 10-7 Factors Associated with Increased Risk for Parkinson's Disease

Aging, gender (men), and race (whites)
Family history of Parkinson's disease
Life experience
  Trauma
  Emotional stress
  Personality (shyness and depressiveness)
Environmental exposures
  Metals (manganese, iron)
  Drinking well water
  Farming
  Rural residence
  Wood pulp mills
  Steel alloy industries
  Herbicide and pesticide exposure (dieldrin)
  MPTP and MPTP-like compounds
Infectious agents

ever, other time-dependent factors, such as duration of exposure to a toxicant or the accumulation of a genetically determined biological defect, cannot easily be separated from age-related changes. Overall, men appear to be at slightly greater risk (about 1.5 times) of developing Parkinson's disease than women. Whether these reported differences reflect differences in ascertainment, inherent biological differences in susceptibility, or gender-associated behavioral differences resulting in greater toxicant exposures is unknown. Cauca-

TABLE 10-8 Factors Associated with Decreased Risk for Parkinson's Disease

Diet
  Vitamin E, supplemental multivitamins
  Cod liver oil
  Tocopherol
Life experience
  Cigarette smoking
  Drinking alcohol

TABLE 10-9 Putative Risk Factors for Parkinson's Disease Based on Ecological Studies

Reference	Location	Index/Method	Risk Factors
Barbeau[58]	Quebec, Canada	Prevalence based on drug sale	Vegetable farming, wood pulp, and paper manufacture
Rajput[59]	Saskatchewan, Canada	Case-control study	Rural residence, well water consumption
Aquilonius[60]	Sweden	Prevalence based on drug sale	Iron ore mining, steel manufacture
Tanner[61]	Midwestern U.S.	Case-control study	Rural residence, well water consumption
Kurtzke[43]	United States	Mortality rates	North-to-south disease distribution
Lilienfeld[62]	United States	Mortality rates	Higher rates in Rocky Mountain states
Svenson[42]	Canada	Mortality rates	Higher rates in Rocky Mountain states
Tanner[63]	International	Prevalence	Industrial exposure
Vanacore[46]	Italy	Mortality rates	Industrial & agricultural exposure
Rybecki[64]	Michigan	Mortality rates	Industrial exposure

sians appear to be at greater risk of Parkinson's disease than Asians or Africans, although these observations are controversial because of the inadequate design of most studies.

After the description of a cluster of toxicant-induced parkinsonism strikingly similar to Parkinson's disease,[54] interest in an environmental cause of Parkinson's disease burgeoned. The responsible compound, the pyridine 1-methyl-4-phenyl-1,2,3,6-tetrahydropyridine (MPTP), induces clinical, pathological, and biochemical changes in humans and primates remarkably like those of Parkinson's disease.[55–57] Although MPTP is unlikely to be environmentally present in sufficient quantities to cause most cases of Parkinson's disease, similar compounds more commonly present might theoretically be causative. Ecological or case-control studies seeking an association between environmental exposure and Parkinson's disease (Tables 10-9 and 10-10) have suggested an increased

risk associated with farming, rural residence, herbicide/pesticide exposure, and employment in industries manufacturing chemicals and wood pulp and paper, as well as iron mining and steel.[63–76] Chief among the many limitations of these studies are their inability to demonstrate causality and the nonspecific nature of the reported exposures. Two studies have implicated specific agents—dithiocarbamate herbicides in a Canadian case-control study[73,77] and the herbicide dieldrin in a comparison of postmortem brain tissue.[78] Replication of these observations in unselected prospectively followed populations will be important to the interpretation of their significance.

Other proposed risk factors include trauma, infection, premorbid personality, and emotional stress. Trauma (with or without loss of consciousness) is associated with Parkinson's disease in many case-control cross-sectional studies but not

TABLE 10-10 Putative Risk Factors for Parkinson's Disease Based on Case-Control Studies

Reference	Location	Number of Cases/Controls	ODDS RATIO			
			Rural Home	Farming	Well Water	Pesticides
Tanner[65]	China	100/200	0.57	0.17	NS	2.39
Ho[66]	Hong Kong	35/105	2.10	5.20	NA	3.60
Koller[67]	Kansas	150/150	1.90	NS	1.70	NS
Golbe[68]	New Jersey	106/106	2.00	NS	NS	7.00
Tanner[69]	Illinois	78/78	NS	3.00	NS	NS
Zayed[70]	Quebec, Canada	42/84	0.31	NS	NS	2.39
Hertzman[71]	British Columbia, Canada	57/122	NA	NA	NA	6.62
Campanella[72]	Italy	83/83	NA	NA	2.60	NA
Semchuk[73]	Calgary, Canada	130/260	NA	1.94	NA	3.06
Hubble[74]	Kansas	63/76	NS	NS	NS	3.15
Jimenez-Jimenez[75]	Madrid, Spain	128/256	NS	NS	1.77	NS
Rocca[76]	Sicily, Italy	62/124	NA	NS	NA	NA

NS, no significant differences in cases versus controls; NA, not assessed.

in the single prospectively conducted study, raising the question that this finding is an artifact, representing the tendency of patients to think more carefully about past injuries than healthy controls.[65,79–81]

Because infection (probably viral) resulted in an epidemic of parkinsonism after encephalitis early in this century, the belief that Parkinson's disease was the result of infection persisted for decades, despite the clear differences clinically and pathologically in the postencephalitic disease and Parkinson's disease.[82] Although an infectious agent has never been identified in Parkinson's disease,[83–87] and the insidious onset and slowly progressive course make traditional agents unlikely, the ubiquitous soil pathogen *Nocardia asteroides* has been reported to cause a parkinson-like disorder in animals and has been proposed as a cause of Parkinson's disease,[88] although evidence supporting this hypothesis was not found in a serological study in humans.[89] Emotional stress, which may cause increased dopamine turnover and resultant risk of oxidative nerve cell death,[90,91] has been associated with an increased disease risk in two studies of persons surviving extreme emotional and physical hardship.[92,93]

The inverse association between cigarette smoking and Parkinson's disease, a long-standing puzzle, has been reported in the majority of case-control studies.[70,71,80,81,94–101] A modest dose-response relationship has been recently confirmed in a large prospective study.[102] The significance of this inverse association remains elusive. Direct protective effects of nicotine may contribute[103] or nicotine may induce xenobiotic metabolizing enzymes, enabling a more speedy detoxification of a parkinsonism-causing toxicant.[104] Alternatively, this may be attributed to the so-called "parkinsonian personality," which is proposed to be a reflection of underlying dopaminergic deficiency contributing to avoidance of novelty-seeking behaviors such as smoking.[105]

Apart from increasing age, the strongest risk factor associated with Parkinson's disease is the presence of disease in a family member. The role of familial and genetic factors will be discussed in the next section.

Genetics of Parkinson's Disease

The potential role of heredity in the etiology of Parkinson's disease was initially implicated by clinical observations of the occurrence of secondary cases in families.[106] Large pedigrees have also been described in which multiple members in several generations of a single family have been affected with Parkinson's disease or parkinson-related syndrome[107,108] (see also Chap. 26). These reports suggest either an autosomal-dominant inheritance with a variable penetrance or multifactorial causation including genetic influences. However, twin studies have proven essentially negative with an overall low concordance rate and no clear difference in monozytic-versus-dizygotic twin pairs.[109] In the early 1980s, it was discovered that the mitochondrial toxin MPTP can cause clinical and experimental parkinsonism.[54–57] In addition, reports were issued describing mitochondrial abnormalities in brain and other body tissues in Parkinson's disease.[110] These findings opened the way for speculation that genetics of Parkinson's

disease may include maternal mitochondrial DNA inheritance patterns.[111]

More recently, the multifactorial etiologic hypothesis of interaction between environmental risk factors and genetic susceptibility in Parkinson's disease has gained interest (see also Chap. 12). This type of interactive causative mechanism has been implicated in a variety of complex disease processes, including diabetes, heart disease, and multiple sclerosis. Progress has been made in studying the relationship between Parkinson's disease and genetic polymorphisms related to xenobiotic enzymes and components involved in the sequence of events leading to degeneration of dopamine neurons.[112] This section will review the cumulative work examining genetic aspects of Parkinson's disease.

FAMILIAL PARKINSON'S DISEASE

FAMILIAL AGGREGATION OF PARKINSON'S DISEASE
The frequency of secondary Parkinson's disease cases among family members of probands varies across studies. As shown in Table 10-11, the estimated prevalence of secondary cases and positive family history range from 3–10 percent and 5–40 percent, respectively. In the beginning of this century, Gowers reported that about 15 percent of his patients with paralysis agitans had secondary cases in their families.[120] However, the first large-scale family study on Parkinson's disease was done by Mjones in 1949. He reviewed all possible Parkinson's disease cases from nine clinics in Sweden.[106] He identified 194 index cases, of whom 41 percent had affected family members. He concluded that Parkinson's disease was an autosomal-dominant disease with reduced penetrance.

A dominant inheritance model was also suggested by Maraganore et al.[117] Twenty families with two or more affected members were included. All family members over 44 years of age were examined. They observed a segregation ratio of 17 percent for siblings and 28 percent for parents and found a unilateral distribution of ancestral secondary cases, suggesting an autosomal-dominant inheritance of mutant gene(s) with reduced penetrance, although a polygenic inheritance pattern could not be excluded. Lazzarini et al. recently found that the cumulative risk for Parkinson's disease increased to about 50 percent in probands' siblings surviving to the 10th decade of life when a parent was also affected.[118] While in 80 pedigrees, an age-adjusted segregation ratio of about 45 percent was obtained for both siblings and parents. Again, these results were compatible with an autosomal-dominant mode of inheritance with reduced penetrance in at least a subset of Parkinson's disease.

Study results have also been used to argue for a multifactorial etiology or polygenic inheritance pattern. In the early 1970s, Kondo et al. surveyed patients at the Mayo Clinic in Minnesota and reported a positive family history in about 10 percent of the Parkinson's disease patients.[114] They used a multivariate statistical model to examine possible combined effects of risk factors and concluded that incomplete dominant transmission is untenable and that multifactorial etiology with a heritability of about 79 percent is more likely. They suggested that genetic predisposition and environmen-

TABLE 10-11 Family Studies in Parkinson's Disease

Reference	Cases	Controls	Cases	Controls	Diagnosis Confirmed by Exam	Comments
Mjones[106]	79/194		96/1062		Partially	Included cases of isolated tremor
Duvoisin[113]			4/146	3/145 spousal controls	Yes	
Kondo[114]	27/263		22/349		Partially	Included arteriosclerotic parkinsonism
Martin[115]	22/127	11/103	16/523	7/489 spousal controls	All PD cases	
Marttila[116]	27/429	19/443	4.4%	2.5% community controls	Partially	Included postencephalitic cases
Maraganore[117]			13/132		All family members	Selected on basis of positive family history
Semchuk[77]	14/128	13/255	8/128	3/255 community controls	Partially	
Lazzarini[118]	31/156		40/950		All PD cases	
Payami[119]	18/114	5/114	18/586	5/522 spouses & friends	Partially	

tal factors may interact and cause Parkinson's disease. This theory was supported by the study conducted by Martin and his colleagues, who found that the prevalence of secondary cases among proband siblings was only slightly higher than that among the spouse siblings.[115] In addition, they found that certain family members were at higher risk; this included relatives of probands with early-age disease onset, siblings of probands in families with additional secondary cases, and siblings of female probands and offspring of affected mothers. An overall 40 percent heritability rate was estimated by pooling Mjones data, together with their own. They suggest that a dominant inheritance pattern of a single causative gene does not offer a plausible explanation for their findings, arguing instead for a multifactorial or polygenic cause.

Young et al. reanalyzed the above-referenced data in terms of the distribution of ancestral second-degree relatives with Parkinson's disease.[121] They found that affected relatives were bilaterally distributed more often than would be expected for autosomal dominance and favored multifactorial inheritance, but they could not exclude autosomal dominance with reduced penetrance in certain families. In contrast, Maraganore et al.[117] and Lazzarini et al.[118] found a much higher ratio of unilateral versus bilateral ancestral cases (73:4 and 12:0, respectively), which favors autosomal-dominant inheritance.

Individuals with a positive family history are at a higher risk of developing Parkinson's disease. Usually, a twofold increase in risk over that of controls is suggested for first-degree relatives of random cases. Payami calculated an age-adjusted odds ratio of 3.5, suggesting that an overall threefold increase in risk for developing Parkinson's disease in the siblings of probands.[119] It is reported that the risk for Parkin-

son's disease in siblings of probands ranges from 12 to 24 percent, whereas the risk could be doubled when both a sibling and a parent is affected. Martin et al. observed that the risk of having Parkinson's disease for individuals whose parents were affected was 14 percent in the range from 55 to 64 years of age at onset and 29.7 percent in the range from 65 to 74 years age group.[115] When neither of the parents were affected, the risk of developing Parkinson's was about 2–3 percent overall. The risk for siblings was significantly increased when they had affected siblings with an early-onset age. As shown in Table 10-12, the risk ranged from about 8–35 percent when the proband's age of onset was greater than 55 years and from 20–62 percent if the proband's age of onset was less than 55 years.

There are large variations in the reported prevalence rate of familial cases in these studies. These discrepancies might be explained by different methods in case ascertainment.

TABLE 10-12 Cumulative Risk for Siblings and Parents of Probands Based on Onset Age of Parkinson's Disease in Probands

Reference	CUMULATIVE RISK FOR SIBLINGS AND PARENTS (%)	
	Onset Age ≤ 55 yr	Onset Age > 55 yr
Mjones[106]	36.6	34.8 for onset age 55–64 yr
		24.1 for onset age > 64 yr
Martin[115]	18.0	8.0
Maraganore[117]	62.0*	28.0*
Lazzarini[118]	No difference between two groups	

*Age-adjusted.

Most of the secondary cases were not diagnosed or verified by clinical examination but were based on either medical records or family description. Parkinson's disease can be easily confused with other neurodegenerative or movement disorders, including essential tremor. A high false-positive rate might be expected in historical family studies. The study by Maraganore et al. attempted to address this concern by examining all family members.[117] They found that only 2 of 42 (5 percent) reported affected members failed to fulfill diagnostic criteria when examined. Perhaps more importantly, these investigators found no examples of false-negative reports, that is, all reportedly unaffected family members were indeed without evidence of parkinsonism upon examination. Although "hands-on examination" is obviously the best approach to use in family Parkinson's disease studies, it is not always practical or possible. Furthermore, it does not address all the potential shortcomings of these endeavors. For example, some currently unaffected family members may subsequently develop clinical evidence of Parkinson's disease. In addition, there is an inherent case selection bias, as the families invited to participate usually have two or more known or suspected affected members. Applying resulting risk rates to family members of all Parkinson's patients should be done cautiously, if at all.

LARGE KINDREDS WITH PARKINSON'S DISEASE AND PARKINSONISM

The recent discovery of several large kindreds with Parkinson's disease or parkinson-related syndrome has sparked the interest in the genetics of Parkinson's disease (Table 10-13 and also Chap. 26). Spellman, in 1962[122] described a family in which nine members in four generations had atypical parkinsonism, with an average onset age of 30 years and rapid disease progression culminating in death in 2–12 years. Perry et al.[123,124] and Purdy et al.[125] reported three families in which patients had L-dopa-refractory parkinsonism, severe hypoventilation, and depression. Evident loss of dopamine neurons and gliosis in the substantia nigra were found. Either no or few atypical Lewy bodies were observed. All kindreds showed an autosomal-dominant inheritance pattern.

In 1988, Golbe et al. reported two large kindreds, with some members having immigrated to the New Jersey area from Contursi, a village in Salerno province, Italy.[107] In four generations, there were 27 affected individuals (15 male, 12 female) characterized by early age of disease onset (mean 47.5 years), rapid progression (with death at 56.1 years on the average), and rarity of tremor. Typical Lewy bodies were found on postmortem examination. Autosomal-dominant inheritance patterns were suggested, and penetrance was estimated at 96 percent. In a follow-up study of these kindreds, Golbe et al. found the number of affected persons increased to 41 in four generations in these two kindreds.[127] Patients had a good response to L-dopa. It was noted that the affected persons who spent most of their lives in Italy survived longer than their affected U.S. relatives and that a single causative gene was postulated. Subsequently, Golbe et al.[128] described a family with very slowly progressive Parkinson's disease with poor response to L-dopa and subjective visual difficulty. The clinical features were confirmed in four examined cases who had an early age of disease onset (average, 17 years). Autopsy showed typical loss of pigmented neurons and

TABLE 10-13 Large Kindred Studies of Parkinsonism with Autopsy Results

Reference	Generations Affected	Cases (M:F)	Clinical Features of Parkinsonism	Average Age of Onset	Mode of Inheritance	L-dopa Response	Autopsy Findings
Spellman[122]	4	9 (5:4)	Atypical	30	AD	NA	NL, GL in limbic region and brain stem
Perry[123,124]	3	8 (6:2)	Atypical with hypoventilation	50s	AD	No	No LB, NL, and GL in SN
Purdy[125]	2	4 (3:1)	Atypical with hypoventilation	40s	NA	No	Few LB, NL, and GL in SN
Inose[126]	3	4 (0:4)	Atypical with multisystems affected	37	AD	Good	Cortical LB and NL in multiple areas
Golbe[107,127]	4 and 3*	41 (23:18)	Atypical w/o tremor	46	AD	Good	Typical LB in SN and LC
Wszolek[108]	4	31 (13:18)	Atypical with multisystems affected	43	AD	No	No LB, NL, and GL in SN
Golbe[128]	5	7 (2:5)	Atypical	17	AD	Mild	Typical LB in SN and LC
Waters[129]	5	9 (4:5)	Atypical w/o tremor	30s	AD	Mild	Atypical LB in SN, LC, and cortex
Wszolek[130]	6	18 (6:12)	Typical	63	AD	Good	Typical LB in SN

*Two kindreds. AD, autosomal-dominant; NL, neuronal loss; GL, gliosis; LB, Lewy bodies; SN, substantia nigra; LC, locus ceruleus.

Lewy bodies. An autosomal-dominant inheritance was indicated. Recently, Waters and Miller[129] reported another kindred with autosomal-dominant Lewy body parkinsonism in four generations. The index case had typical clinical features of Parkinson's disease, except for an absence of rest tremor, and few atypical Lewy bodies were found.

Several large kindreds of parkinsonism were recently reported by Wszolek and colleagues.[108,130–132] Some of the kindreds ranged in size from 300 to 2000 family members. Clinically atypical parkinsonism was found with an autosomal-dominant inheritance pattern. However, they reported a single kindred with typical Parkinson's disease with 18 affected in four generations consisting of 188 family members total.[130] These cases were clinically characterized as manifesting the four cardinal signs of Parkinson's disease, no features of other nervous system involvement, late-onset age, and good response to L-dopa. PET scan showed a decreased striatal uptake of ^{18}F-dopa. Autopsy in one affected case showed typical Lewy bodies, loss of pigmented neurons, and gliosis in the substantia nigra pars compacta. The authors suggest that this kindred may represent a disease closely resembling, if not identical to, Parkinson's disease.

The above data indicate that an autosomal-dominant inheritance can explain the aggregation of familial parkinsonism in large kindreds. However, does this represent typical Parkinson's disease? Most of the reported kindreds have had clinically atypical parkinsonism or parkinson-plus syndrome, with most patients having no or mild response to L-dopa (see Table 10-13), although Lewy bodies and significant neuronal loss and gliosis may be found in the substantia nigra. Although an autosomal-dominant inheritance was indicated in almost all of the large kindreds, there were two families with a sex-determined transmission that may implicate a different inheritance pattern. These kindreds may help address some issues regarding the genetics of Parkinson's disease by exemplifying likely inheritance patterns or suggesting possible candidate genes, but it is unlikely that these large kindreds are affected by a condition clinically, pathologically, and etiologically identical to sporadic Parkinson's disease.

Linkage studies have been performed in three large kindred families described by Wszolek et al.[133,134] examining polymorphic markers associated with several candidate genes involving glutathione peroxidase, tyrosine hydroxylase, brain-derived neurotrophic factor (BDNF), catalase, amyloid precursor protein, copper-zinc superoxide dismutase, debrisoquine 4-hydrolase, manganese superoxide dismutase, dopamine transporter, basic fibroblast growth factor, and synaptic vesicle monoamine transporter. In addition, these investigators have examined markers spanning the entire chromosome 14, including the region bearing the genes for Machado-Joseph disease, early onset familial Alzheimer's disease, and dopa-responsive dystonia. No linkage has been demonstrated. In a recent study of families with multiple affected cases, another group[135] excluded the genes that encode the dopamine transporter, dopamine D2 receptor, monoamine oxidase A and B. However, genetic heterogeneity may significantly limit the efficiency of the linkage studies and complicate the analyses. The need for linkage analysis in multigenerational families or a large number of affected sib pairs is paramount.

TWIN STUDIES

Encouraged by the family studies, several investigations have been conducted to determine the concordance rate of Parkinson's disease in twin pairs. The study of twins provides a unique tool with which to study genetic factors in disease etiology. A higher concordance rate in monozygotic (MZ) twins, compared to that of dizygotic (DZ) twin pairs, offers strong evidence in support genetic causation.

MZ twin pairs discordant for Parkinson's disease were reported by Gudmundsson[3] and Pembrey.[136] Kissel and Andre[137] described female MZ twins who had a combination of parkinsonism and anosmia at the relatively early age of 36 years. In 1977, Duvoisin et al.[138] initiated a collaborative study of Parkinson's disease in twins. They initially identified 12 Parkinson's disease patients with MZ cotwins; none of the cotwins had evidence of parkinsonism on examination. There was a suggestion of premorbid personality differences between probands and cotwins dating back to late adolescence or early adult years. In a continuation of the study, they collected data on 43 MZ and 19 DZ twin pairs by 1983[139] and found that concordance for parkinsonism is no more frequent in twins than would be expected, given the general expected rate of disease occurrence (Table 10-14). On this basis, they concluded that the main factors in the etiology of Parkinson's disease must be nongenetic. However, in a follow-up review of the data, they have suggested that these results neither exclude nor prove a genetic role in Parkinson's disease. It is possible that cotwins seemingly unaffected at initial examination will have clinically evident disease later in life. In addition, low concordance rates in cotwins do not exclude the possibility of gene-environment variable interactions.

There is no biological marker for Parkinson's disease. Thus, premortal diagnostic accuracy is imperfect, and premorbid diagnosis is largely speculative. Functional brain imaging, such as PET scanning, may provide the means for early detection or confirmation of deficient function of the dopaminergic system in the nigrostriatal system. A recent study[143] found that 4 of 11 MZ and 2 of 7 DZ asymptomatic cotwins had abnormally low putamen ^{18}F-dopa uptake, whereas one from each MZ and DZ twin pair had a low normal value. The nonparkinsonian cotwins with abnormal PET findings had isolated posture tremor, possible bradykinesia, or both. Based on PET findings, disease concordance rates were estimated at 45 percent for MZ and 29 percent for DZ cotwins. These rates are much higher than those yielded by the earlier clinical twin studies (see Table 10-14) but offer no significant distinction between MZ and DZ states. Decreased striatal uptake of tracer radiolabeled F-fluorodopa (^{18}F-dopa) is only an indirect reflection of nigrostriatal function. Changes may occur in other basal ganglia neurodegenerative disorders or even in association with aging. Therefore, changes in ^{18}F-dopa uptake alone do not necessarily justify a diagnosis of Parkinson's disease, even in conjunction with isolated postural tremor or other subtle parkinsonian findings. Furthermore, it is likely that the reported Parkinson's twin study findings are confounded by case selection bias. Based on the extant twin data, the theory that a single gene is causative in Parkinson's disease is not supported. A cross-sectional twin study may help to clarify the role of genetics in Parkin-

TABLE 10-14 Concordance for Parkinson's Disease in Twin Pairs

Reference	MZ		DZ	
	Pairs	Concordance (%)	Pairs	Concordance (%)
Ward[139]				
A	43	1 (2.3)	19	0 (0.0)
B*	50	6 (12.0)	19	1 (5.3)
Marsden[140]	11	1 (9.1)	11	1 (9.1)
Marttila[141]	18	0 (0.0)	14	1 (7.1)
Vieregge[142]	9	3 (33.3)	12	3 (25.0)
Burn[143]	11	4 (45)**	7	2 (29.0)**
Others[3,136,144–147]	6	4	—	
Total	109	18 (16.5)	64	8 (12.5)

*Atypical cases included.
**Affected cotwins diagnosed on basis of PET scans (some with only isolated clinical features of parkinsonism).

son's disease. Such a study is under way, canvassing a cohort of approximately 20,000 U.S. military veteran twin pairs.

MITOCHONDRIAL INHERITANCE

Mitochondrial inheritance, a non-Mendelian transmission pattern, may be suggested by the lack of high concordance of Parkinson's disease in MZ twins. This hypothesis is further supported by studies demonstrating defective function of mitochondrial respiration resulting from exposure to the neurotoxin 1-methyl-4-phenyl-1,2,3,6-tetrahydropyridine (MPTP) in animal models of parkinsonism.[148] Mitochondrial defects have also been described in the nigrostriatal system of Parkinson's disease patients[149] (see also Chap 4). Specifically, the selective inhibition of mitochondrial complex I is suggested to be involved in the loss of nigral dopamine neurons.

When the disease is transmitted through a mitochondrial gene defect, it is expected that the disease phenotypes may follow a pattern of maternal transmission, because mitochondrial genes are maternally inherited. To compare the frequency of affected mother of probands with that of affected fathers, Zweig et al.[150] found that probands were about twice as likely to report an affected father as an affected mother, indicating that paternal transmission is more common. These data are consistent with other studies (Table 10-15). For example, Campanella et al.[151] found nine patients who reported affected fathers, as compared to only one case with the mother affected. These results do not suggest that Parkinson's disease is often transmitted through maternal inheritance and thus provide no direct evidence to support the hypothesis of mitochondrial inheritance.

SUSCEPTIBILITY GENES

Another approach in the study of genetic risk factors for developing Parkinson's disease is to attempt to identify phenotypic and genotypic markers with the hope that the precise genetic defect(s) will be subsequently elucidated. This strategy permits the hypothesis of a multifactorial etiology with either gene-gene or gene-environmental factor interactions.

Because of interest in the environmental etiologic hypothesis in Parkinson's disease, studies have been carried out, investigating the role of enzymes responsible for metabolizing xenobiotic substrates from exogenous compounds that may be directly or indirectly neurotoxic. It is hypothesized that a defective xenobiotic-metabolizing enzyme predisposes individuals to Parkinson's disease with subsequent environmental exposures, culminating in clinical expression. This hypothesis has led to investigations assessing the capacity of Parkinson's patients to metabolize endogenous and exogenous chemicals or toxins.

Barbeau et al.[152] first postulated that Parkinson's disease is the result of environmental factors acting on genetically susceptible individuals against a background of aging. Cytochrome P-450 enzymes catalyze many potential neurotoxic xenobiotics, and its association with Parkinson's disease has been studied. Barbeau and colleagues[152] studied cytochrome P-450 2D6 (CYP2D6), a subfamily of this enzymatic system that is responsible for the metabolism of debrisoquine and many drugs. In studying 40 parkinsonians and 40 controls, they found that more patients than controls had partially or totally defective debrisoquine metabolism. In particular, patients with earlier disease onset were most apt to be poor metabolizers. However, this finding was only partially confirmed in subsequent studies, with most reports claiming

TABLE 10-15 Distribution of Probands with Affected Father and Mother

Reference	No. of Probands	NUMBER OF PROBANDS WITH AFFECTED PROGENITOR	
		Father	Mother
Martin[115]	127	7	8
Duvoisin[113]	208	10	5
Campanella[151]	336	9	1
Zweig[150]	252	11	5
Lazzarini[118]	211	17	18
Total	1134	54	37

no relationship between poor debrisoquine metabolism and Parkinson's disease.[153-157]

More recently, three major variant CYP2D6 alleles have been defined and designated as CYP2D6 A, CYP2D6 B, and CYP2D6 D; the mutant alleles account for about 95 percent of the poor metabolizer phenotype.[158] An increased risk for Parkinson's disease has been associated with the CYP2D6 mutant allele,[159,160] but this could be a result of either a linkage dysequilibrium with a neighboring gene responsible for Parkinson's disease, a functional relationship, or other confounding differences between the comparison groups (cases and controls). This association between Parkinson's disease and the CYP2D6 locus has not been confirmed in other reports.[161] A new mutation with substitution of cytosine to thymine at position 2938 of exon 6 of the CYP2D6 gene, resulting in an exchange of amino acid arginine to cysteine at the protein position 296, has more recently been associated with Parkinson's disease in a Japanese study.[162] The overall relationship between the CYP2D6 alleles and Parkinson's disease remains unclear.

Both monoamine oxidase A (MAOA) and B (MAOB) play important roles in degrading biogenic amines, including dopamine, as well as in bioactivation of exogenous and endogenous neurotoxins such as MPTP and MPTP-like compounds. These enzymatic processes may generate toxic by-products, leading to neuronal death. It has been theorized that alterations in these oxidate enzyme systems, as determined by genetic mutations or polymorphisms, may lead to increased susceptibility to Parkinson's disease. Kurth et al.[163] identified polymorphic alleles in the MAOB gene in association with Parkinson's disease. However, in other studies, no association was found.[164] Hotamisligil et al.[165] compared the frequency of haplotypes at the MAOA and MAOB loci on the X chromosome in 91 male Parkinson's patients and 129 male controls. Although no association was observed between Parkinson's disease and MAOB alleles, two haplotypes at the MAOA locus were associated with altered risk for Parkinson's disease. The overall distribution of these MAOA alleles was different in Parkinson's disease and controls, suggesting that MAO genes may influence susceptibility of individuals to Parkinson's disease. Even when one assumes that CYP2D6, MAO, or both gene polymorphisms truly alter risk of development of Parkinson's disease, these genetic markers can only partially explain the cause of Parkinson's disease, as the allelic frequencies are relatively low among affected individuals, that is, less than 50 percent. Other candidate markers that appear to have no clear association with Parkinson's disease include the CAG trinucleotide repeat expansion and the genes encoding tyrosine hydroxylase, dopamine D2, D3 and D4 receptor genes.[166-168] Clearly, much work remains to be done regarding clarification of the putative role of genetics in Parkinson's disease.

Conclusions

Taken as a whole, the results of epidemiological studies of Parkinson's disease support two seemingly conflicting theories of causation. On the one hand, some work indicates a nongenetic environmental etiology. Other studies implicate a heritable cause. These disparate findings may not be mutually exclusive. Perhaps the disease results from one or more genetic defects made pathologically and clinically evident by nongenetic factors such as pesticide exposure. Alternatively, the condition now recognized as the single clinico-pathological entity Parkinson's disease may have several etiologies, both genetic and nongenetic. It is important to interpret extant data cautiously, as most are derived from case-control study populations or other select patient-family groups. Despite these reservations, this work may provide important clues to the etiology of Parkinson's disease. It should be used to provide direction to future epidemiological investigations exploring specific hypotheses in well-characterized study populations.

References

1. Parkinson J: *An Essay on the Shaking Palsy*. London: Sherwood, Neely and Jones, 1817.
2. Kurland LT: Epidemiology: Incidence, geographic distribution and genetic considerations, in Field W (ed): *Pathogenesis and Treatment of Parkinsonism*. Springfield, IL: Charles C Thomas, 1958, pp 5–43.
3. Gudmundsson KR: A clinical survey of parkinsonism in Iceland. *Acta Neurol Scand* 33:9–61, 1967.
4. Forno LS: The Lewy body in Parkinson's disease, in Parkinson's disease. *Adv Neurol* 45:35–43, 1986.
5. Koller WC, Hubble JP: Classification of parkinsonism, in Koller WC (ed): *Handbook of Parkinson's Disease*. New York: Marcel Dekker, 1992, pp 59–104.
6. Hughes AJ, Daniel SE, Kilford L, Lees AJ: The accuracy of the clinical diagnosis of Parkinson's disease: A clinico-pathological study of 100 cases. *J Neurol Neurosurg Psychiatry* 55:181–184, 1992.
7. Koller WC, Langston JW, Hubble JP, et al: Does a long preclinical period occur in Parkinson's disease? *Neurology* 45(5)(suppl 2):8–13, 1991.
8. Forno LS: Concentric hyalin intraneuronal inclusions of Lewy type in the brains of elderly persons (50 incidental cases): Relationship to parkinsonism. *J Am Geriatr Soc* 17:557–575, 1969.
9. Gibb WRG, Lees AJ: The relevance of the Lewy body of the pathogenesis of idiopathic Parkinson's disease. *J Neurol Neurosurg Psychiatry* 51:745–752, 1988.
10. Brewis M, Poskanzer DC, Rolland C et al: Neurological disease in an English city. *Acta Neurol Scand* 42(suppl 24):9–89, 1966.
11. Jenkins AC: Epidemiology of parkinsonism in Victoria. *Med J Aust* 2:497–502, 1966.
12. Kessler II: Epidemiologic studies of Parkinson's disease. III. A community-based survey. *Am J Epidemiol* 96:242–254, 1972.
13. Marttila RJ, Rinne UK: Epidemiology of Parkinson's disease in Finland. *Acta Neurol Scand* 43(suppl 33):9–61, 1976.
14. Rosati G, Granieri E, Pinna L, et al: The risk of Parkinson disease in Mediterranean people. *Neurology* 30:250–255, 1980.
15. Harada H, Nishikawa S, Takahashi K: Epidemiology of Parkinson's disease in a Japanese city. *Arch Neurol* 40:151–154, 1983.
16. Rajput AH, Offord KP, Beard CM, Kurland LT: Epidemiology of parkinsonism: Incidence, classification, and mortality. *Ann Neurol* 16:278–282, 1984.
17. Sutcliffe RLG, Prior R, Mawby B, McQuillan WJ: Parkinson's disease in the district of the Northampton Health Authority, United Kingdom. *Acta Neurol Scand* 72:363–379, 1985.
18. Ashok PP, Radhakrishan K, Sridharan R, et al: Parkinsonism in Benghazi, East Libya. *Clin Neurol Neurosurg* 88:109–113, 1986.

19. Mutch WJ, Dingwall-Fordyce I, Downie AW, et al: Parkinson's disease in a Scottish city. *Br Med J* 292:534–536, 1986.

20. D'Alessandro R, Gamberini G, Granieri E, et al: Prevalence of Parkinson's disease in the Republic of San Marino. *Neurology* 37:1679–1682, 1987.

21. Shi Y: Study on the prevalence of Parkinson's disease in Hongkou District, Shanghai. *Chin J Epidemiol* 4:205–209, 1987.

22. Okada K, Kobayashi S, Tsunematsu T: Prevalence of Parkinson's disease in Izumo City, Japan. *Gerontology* 36:340–344, 1990.

23. Granieri E, Carreras M, Casetta I, et al: Parkinson's disease in Ferrara, Italy, 1967 through 1987. *Arch Neurol* 48:854–857, 1991.

24. Mayeux R, Denaro J, Hemenegildo N, et al: A population-based investigation of Parkinson's disease with and without dementia: Relationships to age and gender. *Arch Neurol* 42:492–497, 1992.

25. Caradoc-Davies TH, Weatherall M, Dixon GS, et al: Is the prevalence of Parkinson's disease in New Zealand really changing? *Acta Neurol Scand* 86:40–44, 1992.

26. Svenson LW: Regional disparities in the annual prevalence rates of Parkinson's disease in Canada. *Neuroepidemiology* 10:205–210, 1991.

27. Li SC, Schoenberg BS, Wang CC, et al: A prevalence survey of Parkinson's disease and other movement disorders in the People's Republic of China. *Arch Neurol* 42:655–657, 1985.

28. Schoenberg BS, Anderson DW, Haerer AF: Prevalence of Parkinson's disease in the biracial population of Copiah County, Mississippi. *Neurology* 35:841–845, 1985.

29. Schoenberg BS, Osuntokun BO, Adeuja AOG, et al: Comparison of the prevalence of Parkinson's disease in black populations in the rural US and in rural Nigeria: Door-to-door community studies. *Neurology* 38:645–646, 1988.

30. Bharucha NE, Bharucha EP, Bharucha AE, et al: Prevalence of Parkinson's disease in the Parsi community of Bombay, India. *Arch Neurol* 45:1321–1323, 1988.

31. Acosta J: Epidemiology of Parkinson's disease: Record of patients in our rural medium: Verjel de la Frontera, 9th International Symposium on Parkinson's Disease, World Federation of Neurology, Jerusalem, 1988, p 57.

32. Rocca WA, Morgante L, Grigoletto F, et al: Prevalence of Parkinson's disease (Parkinson's disease) and other parkinsonisms: A door-to-door survey in two Sicilian communities. *Neurology* 40(suppl 1):422, 1990.

33. Wang Y and the Collaborative Group of Neuroepidemiology of the PLA: The incidence and prevalence of Parkinson's disease in the People's Republic of China. Chung-Hua Liu Hsing Ping Hsueh Tsa Chih. *Chin J Epidemiol* 12:363–365, 1991.

34. Morgante L, Rocca WA, Di Rosa AE, et al: Prevalence of Parkinson's disease and other parkinsonisms: A door-to-door survey in three Sicilian municipalities. *Neurology* 42:1901–1907, 1992.

35. Wang SJ, Fuh JL, Liu CY, et al: Parkinson's disease in Kin-Hu, Kinmen: A community survey by neurologists. *Neuroepidemiology* 13(1-2):69–74, 1994.

36. Reef HE: Prevalence of Parkinson's disease in a multiracial community, in Jage HWA, Bruyn GW, Heihstee APJ (eds): *Eleventh World Congress of Neurology*, Int Congr Ser 427. Amsterdam: Excepta Medica, 1977, p 125.

37. Tanner CM, Thelen JA, Offord KP, et al: Parkinson's disease incidence in Olmsted County, MN: 1935–1988. *Neurology* 42(suppl 3):194, 1992.

38. Zhang ZX, Roman GC: Worldwide occurrence of Parkinson's disease: An updated review. *Neuroepidemiology* 12:195–208, 1993.

39. Lilienfeld DE, Chan E, Ehland J, et al: Two decades of increasing mortality from Parkinson's disease among the US elderly. *Arch Neurol* 47:731–734, 1990.

40. Williams GR, Kurland LT, Goldberg ID: Morbidity and mortality with parkinsonism. *J Neurosurg* 24:138–143, 1966.

41. Svenson LW: Geographic distribution of deaths due to Parkinson's disease in Canada: 1979–1989. *Mov Disord* 5:322–324, 1990.

42. Riggs JE: Longitudinal Gompertzian analysis of Parkinson's disease mortality in the US, 1955–1986: The dramatic increase on overall mortality since 1980 is the natural consequent of deterministic mortality dynamics. *Mech Ageing Dev* 55:221–233, 1990.

43. Kurtzke JF, Goldberg ID: Parkinsonism death rates by race, sex and geography. *Neurology* 38:1558–1561, 1988.

44. Treves TA, Cuesta J: Time-space patterns in parkinsonism (PD) mortality in the US, 1971–78 (Abstr.). Presented at the 9th International Symposium on Parkinson's Disease, World Federation of Neurology, Jerusalem, 1988, pp 50–57.

45. Treves TA, de Pedro Cuesta J: Parkinsonism mortality in the US. 1: Time and space distribution. *Acta Neurol Scand* 84:389–397, 1991.

46. Vanacore N, Bonifati V, Bellatreccia A, et al: Mortality rates for Parkinson's disease and parkinsonism in Italy (1969–1987). *Neuroepidemiology* 11:65–73, 1992.

47. Clarke CE: Mortality from Parkinson's disease in England and Wales 1921–89. *J Neurol Neurosurg Psychiatry* 56(6):693–693, 1993.

48. Chio A, Magnani C, Tolardo G, Schiffer D: Parkinson's disease mortality in Italy, 1951 through 1987. Analysis of an increasing trend. *Arch Neurol* 50:149–153, 1993.

49. Imaizumi Y, Kaneko R: Rising mortality from Parkinson's disease in Japan, 1950–1992. *Acta Neurol Scand* 91(3):169–176, 1995.

50. Nobrega FT, Glattre E, Kurland LT, Okazaki H: Comments on the epidemiology of parkinsonism, including prevalence and incidence statistics for Rochester, Minnesota, 1935–1966, in Barbeau A, Brunette JR (eds): *Progress in Neurogenetics*. Amsterdam: Excerpta Medical Foundation, 1969, pp 474–485.

51. Bharucha NE, Chandra V, Schoenberg BS: Mortality data for the US for deaths due to and related to twenty neurologic diseases. *Neuroepidemiology* 3:149–168, 1984.

52. DeJong D: Parkinson's disease: Statistics. *J Neurosurg* 24:146–155, 1966.

53. Ebmeier KP, Calder SA, Crawford JR, et al: Parkinson's disease in Aberdeen: Survival after 3.5 years. *Acta Neurol Scand* 81:294–299, 1990.

54. Langston JW, Ballard PA, Tetrud JW, et al: Chronic parkinsonism in humans due to a product of meperidine-analog synthesis. *Science* 219:979–980, 1983.

55. Forno LS, Langston JW, DeLanney LE, et al: Locus coeruleus lesions and eosinophilic inclusions in MPTP-treated monkeys. *Ann Neurol* 20:449–455, 1986.

56. Ricaurte GA, DeLanney LE, Irwin I, Langston JW: Older dopaminergic neurons do not recover from the effects of MPTP. *Neuropharmacology* 26:97–99, 1987.

57. Davis GC, Williams AC, Markey SP, et al: Chronic parkinsonism secondary to intravenous injection of meperidine analogues. *Psychiatry Res* 1:249–259, 1979.

58. Barbeau A, Roy M: Uneven prevalence of Parkinson's disease in the province of Quebec. *Can J Neurol Sci* 12:169, 1985.

59. Rajput AH, Uitti RJ, Stern W, Laverty W: Early onset of Parkinson's disease in Saskatchewan–environmental considerations for etiology. *Can J Neurol Sci* 13:312–316, 1986.

60. Aquilonius SM, Hartvig P: A Swedish county with unexpectedly high utilization of anti-parkinsonian drugs. *Acta Neurol Scand* 74:379–382, 1986.

61. Tanner CM, Chen B, Wang W, et al: Environmental factors in the etiology of Parkinson's disease. *Can J Neurol Sci* 4:419–423, 1987.

62. Lilienfeld DE, Sekkor D, Simpson S, et al: Parkinsonism death rates by race, sex and geography: A 1980s update. *Neuroepidemiology* 9:243–247, 1990.

63. Tanner CM: The role of environmental toxins in the etiology of Parkinson's disease. *Trends Neurosci* 12:49–54, 1989.

64. Rybecki BA, Johnson CC, Uman J, Gorell JM: Parkinson's disease mortality and the industrial use of heavy metals in Michigan. *Mov Disord* 8:87–92, 1993.

65. Tanner CM, Chen B, Wang W, et al: Environmental factors and Parkinson's disease: A case-control study in China. *Neurology* 39:660–664, 1989.

66. Ho SC, Woo J, Lee CM: Epidemiologic study of Parkinson's disease in Hong Kong. *Neurology* 39:1314–1318, 1989.

67. Koller W, Vetere-Overfield B, Gray C, et al: Environmental risk factors in Parkinson's disease. *Neurology* 40:1218–1221, 1990.

68. Golbe LI, Farrell TM, Davis PH: Follow up study of early life protective and risk factors in Parkinson's disease. *Mov Disord* 5:66–70, 1990.

69. Tanner CM, Grabler P, Goetz CG: Occupation and the risk of Parkinson's disease: A case-control study in young onset patients. *Neurology* 40(suppl 1):422, 1990.

70. Zayed J, Ducic S, Campanella G, et al: Environmental factors in the etiology of Parkinson's disease. *Can J Neurol Sci* 17:286–291, 1990.

71. Hertzman C, Wiens M, Bowering D, et al: Parkinson's disease: A case-control study of occupational and environmental risk factors. *Am J Ind Med* 17:349–355, 1990.

72. Campanella G, Filla A, De Michele G, et al: Etiology of Parkinson's disease: Results of two case-control studies. *Mov Dis* 5(suppl 1):31, 1990.

73. Semchuk K, Love EJ, Lee RG: Parkinson's disease and exposure to agricultural work and pesticide chemicals. *Neurology* 42:1328–1335, 1992.

74. Hubble JP, Cao T, Hassanein RES, et al: Risk factors for Parkinson's disease. *Neurology* 43:1693–1697, 1993.

75. Jimenez-Jimenez FJ, Mateo D, Gimenez-Roldan S: Exposure to well-water and pesticides in Parkinson's disease: A case-control Study in the Madrid area. *Mov Disord* 7:149–152, 1992.

76. Rocca WA, Menenghini F, et al: Principal lifetime occupation in Parkinson's disease: A case-control study in an Italian population. *Neurology* 43:A239, 1993.

77. Semchuk KM, Love EJ, Lee RG: Parkinson's disease: A test of the multifactorial etiologic hypothesis. *Neurology* 43:1173–1180, 1993.

78. Fleming L, Mann JB, Bean J, et al: Parkinson's disease and brain levels of organochlorine pesticides. *Ann Neurol* 36(1):100–103, 1994.

79. Bharucha NE, Stokes L, Schoenberg BS, et al: A case-control study of twin pairs discordant for Parkinson's disease: A search for environmental risk factors. *Neurology* 36:284–288, 1986.

80. Dulaney E, Stern M, Hurtig H, et al: The epidemiology of Parkinson's disease: A case-control study of young-onset versus old onset patients. *Mov Disord* 5(suppl 1):12, 1990.

81. Rajput AH, Offord KP, Beard CM, Kurland LT: A case-control study of smoking habits, dementia, and other illnesses in idiopathic Parkinson's disease. *Neurology* 37:226–232, 1987.

82. Poskanzer DC, Schwab RS, Fraser DW: Further observations on the cohort phenomenon in Parkinson's syndrome, in Barbeau A, Brunette JR (eds): *Progress in Neurogenetics.* Amsterdam: Excerpta Medica Foundation, 1969, pp 497–505.

83. Mattock C, Marmot M, Stern G: Could Parkinson's disease follow intrauterine influenza? A speculative hypothesis. *J Neurol, Neurosurg Psychiatry* 51:753–756, 1988.

84. Ehmeier KP, Mutch WJ, Calder SA et al: Does idiopathic parkinsonism in Aberdeen follow intrauterine influenza? *J Neurol Neurosurg Psychiatry* 52:911–913, 1989.

85. Elizan TS, Casals J: The viral hypothesis in Parkinson's disease and Alzheimer's disease: A critique, in Kurstak E, Lipowski SJ, Morozov PV (eds): *Viruses, Immunity and Mental Disorders.* New York: Plenum Press, 1987, pp 47–59.

86. Marttila RJ, Halonen P, Rinne UK: Influenza virus antibodies in parkinsonism. *Arch Neurol* 34:99–100, 1977.

87. Fazzini E, Fleming J, Fahn S: Cerebrospinal fluid antibodies to coronaviruses in patients with Parkinson's disease. *Neurology* 40(suppl 1):169, 1990.

88. Kohbata S, Beaman BL: L-Dopa-responsive movement disorder caused by *Nocardia asteroides* localized in the brains of mice. *Infect Immun* 59:181–191, 1991.

89. Hubble JP, Cao T, Kjelstrom JA, et al: *Nocardia* species as an etiologic agent in Parkinson's disease: Serological testing in a case-control study. *J Clin Microbiol* 2768–2769, 1995.

90. Snyder AM, Stricker EM, Zigmond MJ: Stress-induced neurological impairments in an animal model of parkinsonism. *Ann Neurol* 18:554–551, 1985.

91. Spina MB, Cohen G: Dopamine turnover and glutathione oxidation: Implications for Parkinson's disease. *Proc Natl Acad Sci U S A* 86:1398–1400, 1989.

92. Treves TA, Rabey JM, Korczyn AD: Case-control study, with use of temporal approach, for evaluation of risk factors for Parkinson's disease. *Mov Disord* 5:11, 1990.

93. Gibberd FB, Simmons JP: Neurological disease in ex-Far-East prisoners of war. *Lancet* ii:135–138, 1980.

94. Kahn HA: The Dorn Study of smoking among US veterans, in National Cancer Institute: *Epidemiologic Approaches to the Study of Cancer and Other Diseases.* Washington, DC: US Government Printing Office, 1966, Monograph 19, pp 1–125.

95. Baumann RJ, Jameson HD, McKean HE, et al: Cigarette smoking and Parkinson's disease: I. A comparison of cases with matched neighbors. *Neurology* 30:839–843, 1980.

96. Burch PRJ: Cigarette smoking and Parkinson's disease. *Neurology* 31:500–503, 1981.

97. Godwin-Austin RB, Lee PN, Marmot MG, et al: Smoking and Parkinson's disease. *J Neurol Neurosurg Psychiatry* 45:577–581, 1982.

98. Haack DG, Baumann RJ, McKean HE, et al: Nicotine exposure and Parkinson's disease. *Am J Epidemiol* 114:119–200, 1981.

99. Kessler II, Diamond EL: Epidemiologic studies of Parkinson's disease. I. Smoking and Parkinson's disease: A survey and explanatory hypothesis. *Am J Epidemiol* 94:16–25, 1971.

100. Nefzinger MD, Quadfasel FA, Karl VC: A retrospective study of smoking and Parkinson's disease. *Am J Epidemiol* 88:149–158, 1968.

101. Tanner CM, Koller WC, Gilley DC, et al: Cigarette smoking, alcohol drinking and Parkinson's disease: Cross-cultural risk assessment. *Mov Disord* 5:11, 1990.

102. Grandinetti A, Morens DM, Reed D, MacEachern D: Prospective study of cigarette smoking and the risk of developing idiopathic Parkinson's disease. *Am J Epidemiol* 139:1129–1138, 1994.

103. Jansson B, Jankovic J: Low cancer rates among patients with Parkinson's disease. *Ann Neurol* 17:505–509, 1985.

104. Kirch DG, Alho AM, Wyatt RJ: Hypothesis: A nicotine-dopamine interaction linking smoking with Parkinson's disease and tardive dyskinesia. *Cell Mol Neurobiol* 8:285–291, 1988.

105. Menza M, Forman NE, Goldstein HE, Golbe LI: Parkinson's disease, personality and dopamine. *J Neuropsychiatry Clin Neurosci* 2:282–287, 1990.

106. Mjones H: Paralysis agitans: A clinical and genetic study. *Acta Psychiatr Neurol* 25(suppl 54):1–195, 1949.

107. Golbe LI, Di Iorio G, Bonavita V, et al: A large kindred with autosomal dominant Parkinson's disease. *Ann Neurol* 27(3):276–282, 1990.

108. Wszolek ZK, Pfeiffer RF, Bhatt MH, et al: Rapidly progressive autosomal dominant parkinsonism and dementia with pallidoponto-nigral degeneration. *Ann Neurol* 32(3):312–320, 1992.

109. Duvoisin RC: On heredity, twins, and Parkinson's disease. *Ann Neurol* 19(4):409–411, 1986.

110. Haas RH, Nasirian F, Nakano K, et al: Low platelet mitochondrial complex I and complex II/III activity in early untreated Parkinson's disease. *Ann Neurol* 37(6):714–722, 1995.

111. Schapira AH: Nuclear and mitochondrial genetics in Parkinson's disease. *J Med Genet* 32(6):411–414, 1995.

112. Williams A, Steventon G, Sturman S, Waring R: Xenobiotic enzyme profiles and Parkinson's disease. *Neurology* 41(5 suppl 2):29–32, discussion 32–33, 1991.

113. Duvoisin RC, Gearing FR, Schweitzer MD, Yahr MD: A family study of parkinsonism, in Barbeau A, Brunette JR (eds): *Proceedings of the 2nd International Congress of Neuro-Genetics and Neuro-Opthalmology, Montreal, 1967, International Congress Series.* Amsterdam: Excerpta Medica Foundation, 1969, pp 492–496.

114. Kondo K, Kurland LT, Schull WJ: Parkinson's disease: Genetic analysis and evidence of a multifactorial etiology. *Mayo Clin Proc* 48:465–475, 1973.

115. Martin WE, Young WI, Anderson VE: Parkinson's disease: A genetic study. *Brain* 96:495–506, 1973.

116. Marttila RJ, Rinne U: Epidemiology of Parkinson's disease in Finland. *Acta Neurol Scand* 53:81–102, 1976.

117. Maraganore DM, Harding AE, Marsden CD: A clinical and genetic study of familial Parkinson's disease. *Mov Disord* 6(3):205–211, 1991.

118. Lazzarini AM, Myers RH, Zimmerman TR Jr, et al: A clinical genetic study of Parkinson's disease: Evidence for dominant transmission. *Neurology* 44(3 Pt 1):499–506, 1994.

119. Payami H, Larsen K, Bernard S, Nutt J: Increased risk of Parkinson's disease in parents and siblings of patients. *Ann Neurol* 36(4):659–661, 1994.

120. Gowers WR: Paralysis agitans, in A manual of disease of the nervous system II. London: J & A Churchill, 1893, pp 636–639.

121. Young WI, Martin WE, Anderson VE: The distribution of ancestral secondary cases in Parkinson's disease. *Clin Genet* 11:189–192, 1977.

122. Spellman G: Report of familial cases of parkinsonism: Evidence of a dominant trait in a patient's family. *JAMA* 179:372–374, 1962.

123. Perry TL, Bratty P, Hansen S, et al: Hereditary mental depression and parkinsonism with taurine deficiency. *Arch Neurol* 32:108–113, 1975.

124. Perry TL, Wright J, Berry K, et al: Dominantly inherited apathy, central hypoventilation, and Parkinson's syndrome: Clinical, biochemical, and neuropathologic studies of 2 new cases. *Neurology* 49:1882–1887, 1990.

125. Purdy A, Hahn A, Barnett HJM, et al: Familial fatal parkinsonism with alveolar hypoventilation and mental depression. *Ann Neurol* 6:523–531, 1979.

126. Inose T, Miyakawa M, Miyakawa K, et al: Clinical and neuropathological study of a familial case of juvenile parkinsonism. *Jpn J Psychiatry Neurol* 42:265–276, 1988.

127. Golbe LI, Miller DC, Duvoisin RC: Autosomal dominant Lewy-body Parkinson's disease, in Parkinson's disease: anatomy, pathology and therapy. *Adv Neurol* 53:287–292, 1990.

128. Golbe LI, Lazzarini AM, Schwarz KO, et al: Autosomal dominant parkinsonism with benign course and typical Lewy-body pathology. *Neurology* 43:2222–2227, 1993.

129. Waters CH, Miller CA: Autosomal dominant transmission of Parkinson's disease in a four generation family. *Ann Neurol* 35:59–64, 1994.

130. Wszolek ZK, Pfeiffer B, Fulgham JR, et al: Western Nebraska family (family D) with autosomal dominant parkinsonism. *Neurology* 45(3 Pt 1):502–505, 1995.

131. Wszolek ZK, Cordes M, Calne DB, et al: Hereditary Parkinson disease: Report of 3 families with dominant autosomal inheritance. *Nervenarzt* 64(5):331–335, 1993.

132. Markopoulou K, Wszolek ZK, Pfeiffer RF: A Greek-American kindred with autosomal dominant, L-dopa-responsive parkinsonism and anticipation. *Ann Neurol* 38(3):373–378, 1995.

133. Gasser T, Wszolek ZK, Trofatter J, et al: Genetic linkage studies in autosomal dominant parkinsonism: Evaluation of seven candidate genes. *Ann Neurol* 36(3):387–396, 1994.

134. Supala A, Wszolek ZK, Trofatter J, et al: Genetic linkage studies in autosomal dominant parkinsonism: Evaluation of candidate genes. *Mov Disord* 9(suppl 1):32, 1994.

135. Taussig D, Plante-Bordeneuve V, Trassard O, et al: Genetic study of dopaminergic transmission in Parkinson's disease (PD). *Neurology* 45(suppl 4):316, 1995.

136. Pembrey ME: Discordant identical twins. II. Parkinsonism. *Practitioner* 209:240–243, 1972.

137. Kissel P, Andre JM: Parkinson's disease and anosmia in monozygotic twin sisters. *J Genet Hum* 24:113–117, 1976.

138. Duvoisin RC, Eldridge R, Williams A, et al: Twin study of Parkinson disease. *Neurology* 31:77–80, 1981.

139. Ward CD, Duvoisin RC, Ince SE, et al: Parkinson's disease in 65 pairs of twins and in a set of quadruplets. *Neurology* 33:815–824, 1983.

140. Marsden CD: Parkinson's disease in twins. *J Neurol Neurosurg Psychiatry* 50:105–106, 1987.

141. Marttila RJ, Kaprio J, Koskenvuo M, Rinne UK: Parkinson's disease in a nationwide twin cohort. *Neurology* 38:1217–1219, 1988.

142. Vieregge P, Schiffke A, Friedrich HJ, et al: Parkinson's disease in twins. *Neurology* 41(8):1453–1461, 1992.

143. Burn DJ, Mark MH, Playford ED, et al: Parkinson's disease in twins studied with 18F-dopa and positron emission tomography. *Neurology* 42(10):1894–1900, 1992.

144. Jankovic J, Reches A: Parkinson's disease in monozygotic twins. *Ann Neurol* 19(4):405–408, 1986.

145. Koller WC, O'Hara R, Nutt J, et al: Monozygotic twins with Parkinson's disease. *Ann Neurol* 19(4):402–405, 1986.

146. Pahwa R, Busenbark K, Gary C, Koller WC: Identical twins with similar onset of Parkinson's disease: A case report. *Neurology* 43(6):1159–1161, 1993.

147. Zimmerman TR, Bhatt MH, Calne DB, Duvoisin RC: Parkinson's disease in monozygotic twins: A follow-up. *Neurology* 41(suppl 1):255, 1991.

148. Nicklas WJ, Vyas I, Heikkila RE: Inhibition of NADH-linked oxidation in brain mitochondria by I-methyl-4-phenyl-1,2,3,6-tetrahydropyridine. *Life Sci* 36:2503–2508, 1985.

149. Mizuno Y, Ikebe S, Hattori N, et al: Role of mitochondria in the etiology and pathogenesis of Parkinson's disease. *Biochim Biophys Acta.* 1271(1):265–274, 1995.

150. Zweig RM, Singh A, Cardillo JE, Langston JW: The familial occurrence of Parkinson's disease—lack of evidence for maternal inheritance. *Arch Neurol* 49:1205–1207, 1992.

151. Campanella G, Idone M, De Michele G, Filla A: Paternal preponderance in familial Parkinson's disease. *Neurology* 34:1398–1400, 1984.

152. Barbeau A, Cloutier T, Roy M, et al: Ecogenetics of Parkinson's disease. 4-hydroxylation of debrisoquine. *Lancet* 2:1213–1216, 1985.

153. Poirier J, Roy M, Campanella G, et al: Debrisoquine metabolism in parkinsonian patients treated with antihistamine drugs. *Lancet* 2:386, 1987.

154. Benitez J, Ladero JM, Jiminez-Jiminez FJ, et al: Oxidative polymorphism of debrisoquine in Parkinson's disease. *J Neurol Neurosurg Psychiatry* 53:289–292, 1990.

155. Comella CL, Tanner CM, Goetz GC, et al: Debrisoquine metabolism in Parkinson's disease. *Neurology* 37:261–262, 1987.

156. Gudjonsson O, Sanz E, Alvan G, et al: Poor hydroxylator phenotypes of debrisoquine and S-mephenytoin are not over-represented in a group of patients with Parkinson's disease. *Br J Clin Pharmacol* 39:301–302, 1990.

157. Kallio J, Marttila RM, Rinne UK, et al: Debrisoquine oxidation in Parkinson's disease. *Acta Neurol Scand* 83:194–197, 1991.

158. Saxena R, Shaw GL, Relling MV, et al: Identification of a new variant CYP2D6 allele with a single base deletion in exon 3 and its association with the poor metabolizer phenotype. *Hum Molec Genet* 3(6):923–926, 1994.

159. Kurth MC, Kurth JH: Variant cytochrome P450 CYP2D6 allelic frequencies in Parkinson's disease. *Am J Med Genet* 48:166–168, 1993.

160. Armstrong M, Daly AK, Cholerton S, et al: Mutant debrisoquine hydroxylation genes in Parkinson's disease. *Lancet* 339(8800):1017–1018, 1992.

161. Plante-Bordeneuve V, Davis MB, Maraganore DM, et al: Debrisoquine hydroxylase gene polymorphism in familial Parkinson's disease. *J Neurol Neurosurg Psychiatry* 57(8):911–913, 1994.

162. Tsuneoka Y, Matsuo Y, Iwahashi K, et al: A novel cytochrome P-450IID6 mutant gene associated with Parkinson's disease. *J Biochem* 114(2):263–266, 1993.

163. Kurth JH, Kurth MC, Poduslo SE, Schwankhaus JD: Association of a monoamine oxidase B allele with Parkinson's disease. *Ann Neurol* 33(4):368–372, 1993.

164. Kurth JH, Hubble JP, Eggers EA, et al: Lack of association of CYP2D6 and MAO-B alleles with Parkinson's disease in a Kansas cohort. *Neurology* 45(suppl 4):A429, 1995.

165. Hotamisligil GS, Girmen AS, Fink JS, et al: Hereditary variations in monoamine oxidase as a risk factor for Parkinson's disease. *Mov Dis* 9(3):305–310, 1994.

166. Carero-Valenzuela R, Lindblad K, Payami H, et al: No evidence for association of familial Parkinson's disease with CAG repeat expansion. *Neurology* 45(9):1760–1763, 1995.

167. Plante-Bordeneuve V, Davis MB, Maraganore DM, et al: Tyrosine hydroxylase polymorphism in familial and sporadic Parkinson's disease. *Mov Disord* 9(3):337–339, 1994.

168. Nanko S, Ueki A, Hattori M, et al: No allelic association between Parkinson's disease and dopamine D2, D3, and D4 receptor gene polymorphisms. *Am J Med Genet* 54(4):361–364, 1994.

Chapter 11

NEUROCHEMISTRY AND NEUROPHARMACOLOGY OF PARKINSON'S DISEASE

G. FREDERICK WOOTEN

DOPAMINE
  General Metabolism
  Disposition of Dopamine Neurons in Brain
  Role of Dopamine in Parkinson's Disease
  Dopamine Receptors
NOREPINEPHRINE
SEROTONIN
GAMMA-AMINOBUTYRIC ACID
ACETYLCHOLINE
NEUROPEPTIDES
ENDOGENOUS FREE RADICAL SCAVENGERS AND
  GENERATORS
MITOCHONDRIAL FUNCTION
REGIONAL CEREBRAL GLUCOSE UTILIZATION
NEUROCHEMICAL ANALYSIS OF LEWY BODIES
SIGNIFICANCE OF NEUROCHEMICAL STUDIES OF
  PARKINSON'S DISEASE

The motor signs and symptoms of Parkinson's disease result primarily from dysfunction of the basal ganglia. The central mechanism for the physiological dysfunction of the basal ganglia in Parkinson's disease is a progressive decline in the concentration of dopamine. In the past 25 years, much progress has been made in identifying the anatomic connections and in characterizing the regional neurochemistry of the basal ganglia. The major intrinsic and extrinsic connections of the several cell groups that compose the basal ganglia and identified neurotransmitters for each pathway are summarized in Figure 11-1. Probably the first findings to support the relationship between Parkinson's disease and the basal ganglia were the clinical-pathological correlations of Wilson,[1] coupled with the observations made by neuropathologists of neuronal loss and depigmentation of the substantia nigra in the brains of parkinsonian patients.[2] The subsequent discovery of profound reductions in the concentration of the monoamine neurotransmitter dopamine in the caudate nucleus and putamen of parkinsonian patients[3] and the recognition that pigmented neurons of the substantia nigra project to the striatum and provide it with dopaminergic input strengthened the evidence that Parkinson's disease is primarily a disease of the basal ganglia.[4] Later observations that the neurotoxic opiate derivative 1-methyl-4-phenyl-1,2,3,6-tetrahydropyridine (MPTP) produced parkinsonism in humans and other primates, with resultant neuropathological changes restricted primarily to the substantia nigra and large decrements in the striatal concentration of dopamine, pro-

vided further substantiation for the pathophysiological basis of Parkinson's disease.[5]

The following structures are considered to comprise the basal ganglia: the putamen, caudate, globus pallidus (external and internal segments), subthalamic nucleus, and substantia nigra (pars reticulata and pars compacta). The major sources of afferents to basal ganglia structures arising from extrinsic neuronal groups include the neocortex to the caudate and putamen (collectively referred to as the striatum), the nonspecific nuclei of the thalamus to the striatum, the locus ceruleus to the substantia nigra, and the raphe nuclei to the substantia nigra and the striatum. The major efferent pathways from the basal ganglia structures to the extrinsic neuronal groups include the substantia nigra pars reticulata and the globus pallidus internal segment to the thalamus, as well as the substantia nigra pars reticulata to the deep layers of the superior colliculus, the brain stem reticular formation, and the spinal cord. The various nuclear groups of the basal ganglia are interconnected intimately. The striatum and substantia nigra have prominent reciprocal connections. The striatum also projects to both segments of the globus pallidus. The subthalamic nucleus receives afferents from the external segment of the globus pallidus and projects to both the substantia nigra pars reticulata and the internal segment of the globus pallidus. In addition, the striatum contains numerous interneurons that do not project outside the striatum. (For an extensive review of basal ganglia anatomy, see Ref. 6.) The neurotransmitters that have been identified for each projection pathway are depicted in Fig. 11-1, but the entirety of a particular projection may not be represented. For example, glutamate is used as a transmitter by neurons projecting from the neocortex to the stratum but other as yet unidentified neurotransmitters may also be present in this extensive projection. The neurotransmitters used by many of the basal ganglia projection pathways are known; this provides the potential for selective modification of activity in specific basal ganglia circuits by drugs.

Dopamine

GENERAL METABOLISM

Dopamine is synthesized in the brain from the amino acid L-tyrosine via the intermediate compound, L-3,4-dihydroxyphenylalanine (L-dopa). Tyrosine hydroxylase (TOH), the enzyme that catalyzes the conversion of L-tyrosine to L-dopa, is the rate-limiting step in dopamine synthesis. Because TOH is highly localized in catecholamine neurons, it is often used by investigators as a specific marker for dopamine neurons. L-Aromatic amino acid decarboxylase (L-AAAD), the enzyme that catalyzes the conversion of L-dopa to dopamine, has a relatively low substrate specificity and is thought to be present not only in dopamine neurons but also in other cells not specialized to synthesize catecholamines. Once synthesized, dopamine is concentrated in storage vesicles; the membranes of these cytoplasmic organelles contain a high-affinity, energy-dependent, carrier-mediated transport system that concentrates dopamine within the vesicle against a concentration gradient.

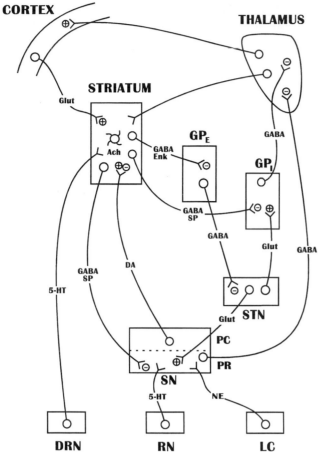

FIGURE 11-1 Simplified version of the major anatomic pathways within the basal ganglia, including identification of known neurotransmitters, when such information is available. Names and initials in upper case identify anatomically distinct nuclear groups within the basal ganglia; lower case abbreviations and contractions denote neurotransmitters. GPE, globus pallidus external segment; GPI, globus pallidus internal segment; STN, subthalamic nucleus; SN, substantia nigra (PC, pars compacta; PR, pars reticulata); DRN, dorsal raphé nucleus; RN, raphé nuclei; LC, locus ceruleus; Glut, glutamate; ACh, acetylcholine; Enk, enkephalin; GABA, gamma-aminobutyric acid; SP, substance P; 5-HT, serotonin; NE, norepinephrine.

Under physiological conditions, dopamine is released by a calcium-dependent mechanism from dopaminergic neurons. Dopamine released thus into the synaptic cleft is inactivated primarily by a high-affinity, stereospecific, carrier-mediated reuptake process. After reuptake, dopamine may be sequestered again in storage vesicles for rerelease. Released dopamine in the synaptic cleft may bind to specific cell surface dopamine receptors on the same neuron from which it is released (autoreceptor) or on another neuron (postsynaptic receptor). Some dopamine receptors are linked positively to a dopamine-sensitive adenylate cyclase enzyme activity. When dopamine occupies this receptor, the rate of synthesis of cyclic adenosine monophosphate (cyclic AMP) is increased. Other cell surface dopamine receptors appear to be linked negatively to adenylate cyclase. When these receptors are occupied by dopamine, there is a reduction in the rate

of cyclic AMP synthesis.[7] At least five different dopamine receptors have been cloned and sequenced, with each one fitting into one of the two large families, based on the nature of the linkage to adenylate cyclase (see Chap. 7).

Dopamine is inactivated enzymatically by the action of both monoamine oxidase (MAO), an enzyme associated with mitochondria and present in two forms, termed A and B, and catechol-*O*-methyltransferase (COMT), an enzyme localized primarily in glial cells in the brain. The resultant deamination and 3-*O*-methylation of dopamine produces homovanillic acid (HVA), the principal metabolite of dopamine (Fig. 11-2).

DISPOSITION OF DOPAMINE NEURONS IN BRAIN

There are several identified dopaminergic neuronal cell groups in the central nervous system.[8] The most prominent group is the mesotelencephalic group. This group is composed of the *nigrostriatal system*, with cell bodies in the substantia nigra pars compacta that project primarily to the striatum, and the *mesocortical system*, with cell bodies in the ventral tegmental area that project to the mesial frontal, anterior cingulate, and entorhinal cortices; olfactory bulb; anterior

FIGURE 11-2 Enzymatic synthesis and inactivation of dopamine.

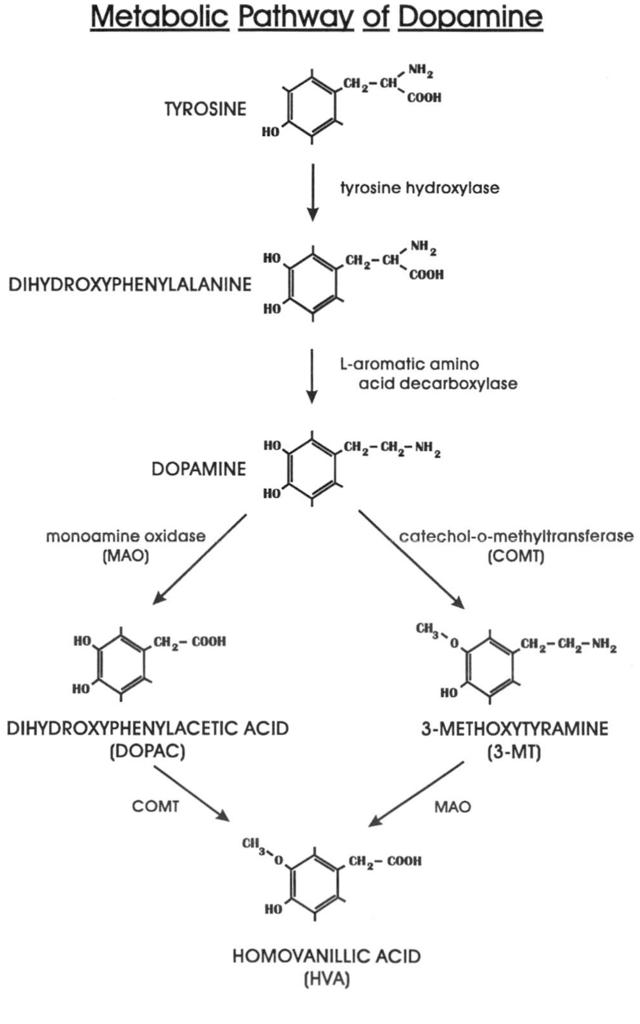

olfactory nucleus; olfactory tubercle; piriform cortex; nucleus accumbens; and amygdaloid complex. The *tuberohypophysial system* projects from the arcuate and periventricular hypothalamic nuclei to the intermediate lobe of the pituitary gland and the median eminence. The *incertohypothalamic system* projects from the zona incerta and posterior hypothalamus to the dorsal hypothalamic area and septum. Finally, the *periventricular system* contains cell bodies in the periventricular region of the medulla that project to the periventricular and periaqueductal gray, tegmentum, tectum, thalamus, and hypothalamus. The regional "fallout" of dopaminergic neurons in the subsantia nigra of patients with Parkinson's disease appears to be rather specific and selective.[9] Loss of pigmented neurons appears to be greatest in the lateral ventral tier, followed by the medial ventral tier and the dorsal tier. This contrasts dramatically with the pattern of pigmented neuron loss during normal aging in the substantia nigra. In normal aging the lateral ventral tier is relatively spared, compared to the cell loss in other regions of the substantia nigra.

ROLE OF DOPAMINE IN PARKINSON'S DISEASE

The first findings to suggest a role for dopamine in Parkinson's disease were the observations that reserpine treatment produced both the clinical and pathophysiological (i.e., depletion of striatal dopamine) pictures of parkinsonism.[10] Subsequently, Carlsson and his colleagues[10] showed that treatment with the dopamine precursor L-dopa reversed the behavioral effects of reserpine and partially restored brain dopamine levels in laboratory animals. These observations, coupled with early histofluorescence data showing very high concentrations of dopamine in the striatum, led Hornykiewicz to study the concentration of dopamine in postmortem brain material from patients who had died with Parkinson's disease.[3]

The discovery of marked reductions in the concentration of dopamine and HVA in the caudate, putamen, and substantia nigra of parkinsonian patients opened the door to a new era in the diagnosis and treatment of brain disease (Table 11-1).[3, 11-13] Furthermore, there was a strong positive correlation between the severity of the premorbid parkinsonian clinical syndrome and the degree of dopamine depletion in the striatum. The data, which are summarized in Table 11-1, showed a reduction in dopamine concentration in all basal ganglia structures. A more recent study of the postmortem striatal dopamine deficit in subregions of the parkinsonian basal ganglia found nearly complete depletion of dopamine in all segments of the putamen.[14] The greatest reduction was found in the caudal portion of the putamen, where dopamine levels were less than 1 percent of those in control postmortem brains.

Interestingly, the degree of reduction in dopamine concentration was much greater than the reduction in HVA concentration in brains of parkinsonian patients (see Table 11-1). Thus, the ratio of dopamine to HVA was much lower in these brains than in those of controls. Similar changes in the dopamine to HVA ratio have been noted following partial lesions of the nigrostriatal pathway in experimental animals and as a consequence of treatment with dopamine antagonist drugs. These changes in the dopamine to HVA ratio may reflect both an increase in the metabolic activity of the few remaining dopamine neurons and a reduced capacity for reuptake and storage of released dopamine.[15]

Another postmortem study focused on enzymatic markers of dopamine neurons and dopamine metabolism (Table 11-2). This study revealed marked reductions in the activities of TOH and L-AAAD in the caudate, putamen, and substantia nigra of patients with Parkinson's disease, but no changes were found in the levels of activity of MAO and COMT. These results reflect the high degree of localization of TOH and L-AAAD in dopamine neurons in the striatum, compared

TABLE 11-1 DA and HVA Concentrations in Discrete Brain Regions from Controls and Parkinson's Disease Patients

Brain Region	DA (μg/g wet wt)	HVA (μg/g wet wt)	DA/HVA
Putamen[a]			
Control	5.06 ± 0.39 (17)	4.92 ± 0.32 (16)	1.03
Parkinsonian patient	0.14 ± 0.13 (3)	0.54 ± 0.13 (3)	0.26
Caudate nucleus[a]			
Control	4.06 ± 0.47 (18)	2.92 ± 0.37 (19)	1.39
Parkinsonian patient	0.20 ± 0.19 (3)	1.19 ± 0.10 (3)	0.17
Substantia nigra[b,c]			
Control	0.46 (13)[b]	2.32 (7)[c]	0.20
Parkinsonian patient	0.07 (10)[b]	0.41 (9)[c]	0.17
Nucleus accumbens[d]			
Control	3.79 ± 0.82 (8)	4.38 ± 0.64 (8)	0.86
Parkinsonian patient	1.61 ± 0.28 (4)	3.13 ± 0.13 (3)	0.51

Results are expressed as mean ± SEM. Number in parentheses is number of cases.
[a] Ref. 11.
[b] Ref. 3.
[c] Ref. 12.
[d] Ref. 13.

TABLE 11-2 Activities of TOH, L-AAAD, COMT, and MAO in Discrete Brain Regions from Controls and Parkinson's Disease Patients

Brain Region	TOH (nmol CO_2/30 min/100 mg protein)	L-AAAD (nmol CO_2/2 h/ 100 mg protein)	COMT (nmol NMN/h/ 100 mg protein)	MAO (nmol PPA/30 min/100 mg protein)
Putamen				
Control	17.4 ± 2.4 (3)	432 ± 109 (18)	24.1 ± 2.5 (11)	1520 ± 127 (11)
Parkinsonian patient	3.1 ± 1.2 (3)[a]	32 ± 7 (13)[b]	19.8 ± 3.7 (9)	1648 ± 128 (10)
Caudate nucleus				
Control	18.7 ± 2.0 (3)	364 ± 95 (19)	25.4 ± 2.8 (10)	1726 ± 149 (10)
Parkinsonian patient	3.2 ± 0.5 (2)[a]	54 ± 14 (13)[b]	17.8 ± 3.8 (9)	1742 ± 197 (10)
Substantia nigra				
Control	17.4 (1)	549 ± 294 (15)	26.4 ± 4.7 (5)	1828 ± 200 (5)
Parkinsonian patient	6.1 ± 1.5 (3)	21 ± 6 (10)	21.7 ± 10.2 (9)	1477 ± 284 (4)

Results are expressed as mean ± SEM. Number in parentheses is number of patients.
[a] Differs from control $p < .02$.
[b] Differs from control $p < .01$.
SOURCE: Data derived from Ref. 11.

to the more general distribution of MAO and nonneuronal distribution of COMT activities.

Radiolabeled cocaine has been used as a ligand marker for the neuronal membrane transport site responsible for the reuptake of catecholamines into catecholaminergic neurons. The binding of cocaine to striatal membranes in patients who died with Parkinson's disease was greatly reduced, compared to that of controls.[16] Similar findings have been obtained with ligands more selective for the dopamine reuptake site, such as GBR-12935.[17] These results support previous evidence of a large reduction in all measurable neuronal markers for nigrostriatal dopaminergic neurons in the brains of patients with Parkinson's disease.

DOPAMINE RECEPTORS

The principal molecular site of action of dopamine in the brain is at dopamine receptors. Dopamine receptors are divided into two main families or categories, D1-like (positively linked to adenylate cyclase) and D2-like (negatively linked to adenylate cyclase).[7] Five different dopamine receptors have now been cloned and sequenced, but each of the five falls into one of the two main "families." Thus, D1-like receptors include D1 and D5, whereas D2, D3, and D4 are D2-like receptors. The D1 and D2 types are expressed predominantly in the basal ganglia, whereas D3, D4, and D5 have a low level of expression there (see Chap. 7).

D1 receptors in the basal ganglia appear to be expressed predominantly by striatonigral and striatopallidal (to medial pallidum) neurons that are GABAergic and also express substance P and dynorphin. In contrast, D2 receptors appear to be expressed primarily by substantia nigra dopaminergic neurons (autoreceptors), cholinergic interneurons in the striatum (i.e., some large aspiny neurons), and striatopallidal neurons projecting to the lateral segment of the globus pallidus that are GABAergic and coexpress enkephalin. Physiologically, the striatonigral and striato-medial pallidal pathways appear to be activated by the action of dopamine,

whereas the striato-lateral pallidal pathway appears to be tonically inhibited by the action of dopamine. Yet, the capacity of dopamine to reverse optimally the bradykinesia, rigidity, and tremor caused by dopamine depletion appears to require the action of dopamine at both receptor types. For a brief review of this subject, see Ref. 18.

Numerous studies of dopamine receptor number and density have been carried out in the brains of patients with Parkinson's disease and in experimental animal models of the disease. Yet, these studies have contributed little to our understanding of the mechanism of side effects of L-dopa and dopamine agonists such as psychosis and dyskinesia, nor have they yet resulted in improvement in the management of patients with Parkinson's disease.

Norepinephrine

The principal source of noradrenergic afferents to the forebrain is the locus ceruleus.[19] The locus ceruleus is one of the pigmented brain stem nuclei that is characteristically abnormal in the brains of parkinsonian patients. Specifically, these brains show depigmentation and loss of neurons, with Lewy bodies in the locus ceruleus. Several investigators described reductions of norepinephrine concentration and dopamine-beta-hydroxylase activity (a specific enzymatic marker of noradrenergic neurons) in forebrain regions.[20,21] Data are conflicting about whether norepinephrine levels are affected in the hypothalamus of patients with Parkinson's disease.[20,22] Studies of dopamine-beta-hydroxylase activity in the A1 and A2 noradrenergic areas of the brain stem of parkinsonian patients did not reveal any changes, suggesting that these nuclear groups, which also have rostral projections, are spared in Parkinson's disease.[23] Because levels of norepinephrine were rarely below 50 percent of those of controls in the brains of parkinsonian patients and, apparently, because certain noradrenergic cell groups of the lower brain stem were spared completely, it is unlikely that Parkinson's disease is associated with a generalized central catecholaminergic deficiency. The consequences of reduced norepinephrine levels in the adult brain are not clear, although evidence for both motor and cognitive functions of noradrenergic systems has been presented.[19]

Serotonin

The principal locations of cell bodies of serotonergic neurons are the raphe nuclei of the brain stem. There is no neuropathological evidence to suggest that these cell groups are specifically affected in Parkinson's disease. Nevertheless, serotonin levels were reduced throughout the forebrain in patients with Parkinson's disease, particularly in the striatum, substantia nigra, and hippocampus.[21,24] The mechanism and significance of the reduction in brain serotonin levels are not known; however, reduced serotonin levels may represent regulation of serotonergic neuronal activity in response to reduced activity of dopaminergic and/or noradrenergic neurons.

Gamma-Aminobutyric Acid

Gamma-aminobutyric acid (GABA) is a neurotransmitter found in several prominent basal ganglia projection pathways. There are probably GABA-releasing interneurons in the striatum, as well as GABAergic striatopallidal, striatonigral, nigrocollicular, and pallidothalamic projections.[6] No studies suggested that these neurons are affected primarily by the pathological process in Parkinson's disease. It is possible, however, that up- or down-regulation of GABA activity might occur as a consequence of dopamine depletion in the striatum.

Two specific markers for GABAergic neurons have been studied in postmortem brain material from patients with Parkinson's disease. These include direct measurement of brain GABA levels and assay of the activity of glutamic acid decarboxylase (GAD), the enzyme that catalyzes the conversion of glutamic acid to GABA. Perry et al. found that GABA levels were elevated significantly in the putamen of parkinsonian patients,[25] whereas Laaksonen et al. found reduced GABA levels in cerebral and cerebellar cortices but no change in GABA levels in any other brain region.[26] Lloyd and Hornykiewicz found reduced GAD activity (approximately 50 percent of that of controls) in the striatum, globus pallidus, and substantia nigra,[27] a finding confirmed by Laaksonen.[26] Subsequently, Perry et al. reported, however, that GAD activity in the putamen of parkinsonian patients does not differ from that in controls.[25]

Thus, there is controversy about whether GAD activity is altered in the brains of patients with Parkinson's disease. Nevertheless, the critical issue is whether GABA turnover is altered and, if so, in which neuronal groups. The development of pharmacological means to manipulate GABA neurotransmission is a potential avenue for new therapeutic strategies in the management of Parkinson's disease.

Acetylcholine

The principal site of action of cholinergic neurons in basal ganglia circuitry is thought to be the numerous cholinergic interneurons identified in the striatum.[6] Measurement of the activity of choline acetyltransferase (ChAT), the enzyme that catalyzes the one-step synthesis of acetylcholine, is the most frequently used marker for the cholinergic neurons. Lloyd et al. reported a significant reduction in ChAT activity in the putamen, caudate nucleus, globus pallidus, and substantia nigra in the brains of parkinsonian patients.[28] These changes in activity, again, may reflect regulation in response to reduced dopamine levels, rather than primary pathological involvement. Ruberg et al. found reduced ChAT activity in cerebral cortex and hippocampus in brains of patients with Parkinson's disease, which perhaps relates to the dementing process in these patients.[29]

Neuropeptides

Several of the neuropeptides that are putative neurotransmitters or neuromodulators are present in rather high concentrations in some nuclear groups of the basal ganglia. Their distribution has been mapped by immunocytochemical techniques, and radioimmunoassays (RIAs) have been used to quantify regional concentrations of various neuropeptides.

Using RIA techniques, Mauborgne et al. discovered reduced substance P levels in the substantia nigra, putamen, and globus pallidus external segment.[30] Immunocytochemical studies of patients with Parkinson's disease, however, did not confirm a change in substance P concentration in any basal ganglia area.[31]

Methionine-enkephalin concentration quantified by RIA was found to be diminished in the substantia nigra and ventral tegmental area.[32] Also, RIA studies showed reductions in both leucine- and methionine-enkephalin in the putamen and pallidum.[32] In contrast, immunocytochemical studies did not confirm any changes in enkephalin levels in the globus pallidus.[31] The discrepant findings using RIA and immunocytochemical techniques remain to be explained.

Some investigators suggested that cholecystokinin-8 (CCK-8) coexists with dopamine in dopaminergic neurons.[33] However, using RIA methods, Studler et al. found reduced CCK-8 levels in the substantia nigra but not in striatal or corticolimbic areas innervated by dopaminergic neurons.[34] These results from postmortem brains of parkinsonian patients cast doubt on the coexistence of dopamine and CCK-8 in nigral neurons.

Somatostatin levels in the basal ganglia of nondemented patients with Parkinson's disease did not differ from those of controls.[35] Somatostatin levels in the frontal cortex, hippocampus, and entorhinal cortex of demented parkinsonian patients were reduced, compared to levels in nondemented parkinsonian patients.[35]

As more information is accumulated about the cellular localization and physiological function of neuropeptides, the significance of these various changes in Parkinson's disease may be recognized. Currently, it appears that these changes represent secondary consequences of striatal dopamine depletion.

Endogenous Free Radical Scavengers and Generators

Studies aimed at elucidating the mechanism of MPTP-induced neuronal toxicity focused much attention on the possibility that the oxidative metabolism of MPTP generates cytotoxic free radical species. Cohen speculated that the generation of free radical species by MAO activity may contribute to dopaminergic neuronal death in Parkinson's disease.[36] In primates, the dopaminergic nigrostriatal neurons contain high concentrations of the pigment neuromelanin. Graham argued that Parkinson's disease may result from cytotoxicity of the products of catecholamine and melanin oxidation.[37] Furthermore, the concentration of iron is now known to be increased and that of ferritin reduced in the brains of patients with Parkinson's disease.[38] Iron catalyzes the production of hydroxyl radicals from hydrogen peroxide. Thus, the higher concentrations of free iron in the parkinsonian brain may predispose this disease state to a high rate of free radical production.[38] Whether the high concentration of iron in the parkinsonian brain is a primary or secondary event in the disease process is not known.

Free radicals are generated constantly in all living tissue. When their intracellular concentrations become too high, damage to cellular elements (e.g., lipid, protein, deoxyribonucleic acid [DNA]) may occur. Such damage is minimized by endogenous agents such as glutathione, ascorbate, beta-carotene, and tocopherol,[39] which are free radical "scavengers." Also, enzymatic defenses exist that "scavenge" free radicals; these enzymes include superoxide dismutase, catalase, and glutathione peroxidase (which requires reduced glutathione).[39] Perry et al. reported that reduced glutathione levels were lower in the substantia nigra than in any other human brain region and that reduced glutathione levels were absent virtually from the substantia nigra of patients dying with Parkinson's disease.[40] Because reduced glutathione is an important endogenous antioxidant, as well as a cofactor for the free radical-scavenging enzyme, glutathione peroxidase, it is interesting to speculate that the substantia nigra may be that region of the brain most susceptible to the toxic effects of free radicals. The activity of catalase has also been reported to be reduced in the brains of patients with Parkinson's disease.[41]

Increased products of lipid peroxidation have been found in the substantia nigra in Parkinson's, and this was associated with a decrease in polyunsaturated fatty acids, which are the substrates for lipid peroxidation.[42] Another investigator has reported a 10-fold increase in lipid hydroperoxides in the parkinsonian brain.[43]

Each of the above observations provides circumstantial evidence to support a role for excessive free radical production in the pathogenesis of Parkinson's disease.

Mitochondrial Function

In 1989, Parker et al. reported a selective reduction in the activity of complex I of the mitochondrial electron transport chain in platelets of patients with Parkinson's disease.[44] This finding was confirmed by several laboratories (e.g., the authors of Ref. 45). Subsequently, Schapira and his colleagues reported a selective reduction of NADH-CoQ1 reductase activity (an activity specific for complex I) in the substantia nigra of patients with Parkinson's disease.[46] Furthermore, such abnormality was not found in postmortem material from patients with multiple-system atrophy. It is thus a remarkable coincidence that MPP$^+$, the active toxic metabolite of MPTP, appears to exert its cytotoxic effects by inhibiting complex I of the mitochondrial electron transport chain. Several groups have failed to identify deletions of mitochondrial DNA in patients with Parkinson's disease.[47] Again, whether these changes in complex I activity are primary or secondary and whether they are genetically transmitted or acquired remains to be shown.

Regional Cerebral Glucose Utilization

Using fluorine-18-labeled fluorodeoxyglucose and positron emission tomographic (PET) imaging techniques, it is possible to estimate in vivo the regional rate of glucose utilization in brains of parkinsonian patients. Because glucose is a primary substrate for brain energy production and the major expenditure of energy in the brain is for pumping ions across membranes, estimates of regional cerebral glucose utilization represent an estimate of regional brain physiological activity.

In studies to date of patients with both unilateral and bilateral parkinsonism, strikingly little change in glucose has been measured in cortical areas or in the caudate-putamen region of the basal ganglia.[48–50] Martin et al. found increased glucose utilization in the inferomedial portion of the basal ganglia, probably corresponding to the globus pallidus, in patients with Parkinson's disease.[50] Similar changes also were reported using oxygen-15 imaging with PET techniques in parkinsonian patients.[51] Such an increase in glucose utilization in the globus pallidus was seen in experimental animals with lesions of the substantia nigra and may represent increased physiological activity in striatal efferents to the globus pallidus as a consequence of reduced dopamine neurotransmission in the striatum.[52]

Another advance in the field of in vivo neurochemistry using PET technology was the development of a method to image dopamine neurons, using radiolabeled L-dopa.[53] Garnett et al. reported that fluorine-18 accumulation, associated with [^{18}F]6-fluoro-L-dopa, was reduced in the striatum contralateral to the side of involvement in patients with unilateral parkinsonism, particularly in the putamen.[54] Others found that nonparkinsonian patients exposed to MPTP had decreased levels of ^{18}F accumulation in the striatum, compared to those of controls.[55] The accumulation of carbon-11-labeled nomifensine, a drug that binds rather selectively to dopamine reuptake sites on the neuronal membranes of dopaminergic neurons, was reduced in the striata of patients with Parkinson's disease to approximately the same extent as [^{18}F]6-fluoro-L-dopa accumulation.[56] These PET techniques have made possible the first reliable in vivo marker for the neurochemical deficit in Parkinson's disease. Unfortunately, the methods are extremely expensive and are available only as a research tool in a few centers around the world (see also Chap. 3).

Neurochemical Analysis of Lewy Bodies

The presence of Lewy bodies is a histological hallmark of Parkinson's disease. These intraneuronal cytoplasmic inclusions were found first in neurons of the substantia innominata and dorsal motor nucleus of the vagus.[57] Subsequently, Lewy bodies were found also in pigmented cells of the substantia nigra, as well as in the hypothalamus, locus ceruleus, raphe nuclei of the midbrain and rostral pons, sympathetic ganglia, and spinal cord.[58] Current opinion still favors evidence suggesting that the Lewy body is a highly specific marker of neuronal degeneration in Parkinson's disease.[58]

Despite the apparently unique appearance of Lewy bodies in degenerating neurons in the brains of parkinsonian patients, very little is known about their biochemical composition, and nothing is known of their genesis. Histological reactions suggest that Lewy bodies have a proteinaceous nature.[59,60] The dense core of Lewy bodies is composed of tightly packed aggregates of filaments, vesicular profiles, and other granular material; at the periphery, filamentous structures emerge radially and are mixed with granular and vesicular material. Immunocytochemical studies using polyclonal antibodies to neurofilament polypeptides have demonstrated specific staining of Lewy bodies.[61] These data suggest that abnormal organization of the neuronal cytoskeleton may be a pathological feature of Parkinson's disease. It is now well established that Lewy bodies contain the protein ubiquitin. Ubiquitin immunostaining is considered to be the method of choice for specific labeling of Lewy bodies, particularly those found in cortical areas of the brain. Further biochemical characterization of the composition of Lewy bodies may provide new insights into the mechanism(s) of neuronal degeneration in Parkinson's disease. It must be noted, however, that Lewy bodies may represent simply a cellular response to some other primary insult (see also Chap. 18).

Significance of Neurochemical Studies of Parkinson's Disease

Selective degeneration of the dopaminergic nigrostriatal pathway is the central pathological process in Parkinson's disease. The resulting reduction in striatal dopamine concentration is a condition sufficient for the emergence of the signs and symptoms of parkinsonism. The development of L-dopa therapy and newer direct-acting dopamine agonists in the treatment of Parkinson's disease grew out of the recognition of this relationship between dopamine deficiency and parkinsonian symptoms.

The changes in levels of other neurotransmitters, in neuronal markers, and in regional brain metabolism probably represent regulatory responses to the decrement in striatal dopamine neurotransmission. Future neurochemical studies holding the greatest promise of benefit to parkinsonian patients may be divided into two categories: (1) studies aimed at understanding the effects of dopamine depletion on other neurons and neurotransmitter systems that allow the symptoms of parkinsonism to emerge may form the basis for new therapeutic strategies to supplement dopamine replacement and (2) studies aimed at identifying the source of the selective vulnerability of dopamine neurons in patients with Parkinson's disease could result in therapeutic strategies to arrest the progression of, or actually prevent, Parkinson's disease.

References

1. Wilson SAK: Progressive lenticular degeneration: A familial nervous disease associated with cirrhosis of the liver. *Brain* 34:295–489, 1912.
2. Hassler R: Zur pathologie der paralysis agitans und des postenzephalitischen parkinsonismus. *J Psychol Neurol* 48:387–476, 1938.
3. Hornykiewicz O: Die Topische Lokalisation und das verhalten von noradrenalin und dopamin (3-Hydroxytyramin) in der substantia nigra des normalen und parkinsonkranken menschen. *Wien Klin Wochenschr* 75:309–312, 1963.
4. Hornykiewicz O: Dopamine (3-hydroxytyramine) and brain function. *Pharmacol Rev* 18:925–962, 1966.
5. Langston JW, Ballard P, Tetrud JW, Irwin I: Chronic parkinsonism in humans due to a product of meperidine analog synthesis. *Science* 291:979–980, 1983.
6. Carpenter MB: Anatomy of the corpus striatum and brainstem integrating systems, in Brooks VB (eds): *Handbook of Physiology.* Bethesda, MD: American Physiological Society, 1981, pp 947–995.
7. Stoof JC, Kebabian JW: Two dopamine receptors: Biochemistry, physiology and pharmacology. *Life Sci* 35:2281–2296, 1984.
8. Moore RY, Bloom FE: Central catecholamine neuron systems: Anatomy and physiology of the dopamine systems. *Annu Rev Neurosci* 1:129–169, 1978.
9. Fearnley JM, Lees AJ: Aging and Parkinson's disease: Substantia nigra regional selectivity. *Brain* 114:2283–2301, 1991.
10. Carlsson A, Lindquist M, Magnusson T: 3,4-Dihydroxyphenylalanine and 5-hydroxytryptophan as reserpine antagonists. *Nature* 180:1200–1201, 1957.
11. Lloyd KG, Davidson L, Hornykiewicz O: The neurochemistry of Parkinson's disease: Effect of L-dopa therapy. *J Pharmacol Exp Ther* 195:453–464, 1975.
12. Bernheimer H, Hornykiewicz O: Herabgesetzte konzentration der homovanillinsäure im gehirn von parkinsonkranken menschen als ausdruck der störung des zentralen opaminstoffwechsels. *Klin Wochenschr* 43:711–715, 1965.
13. Price KS, Farley IJ, Hornykiewicz O: Neurochemistry of Parkinson's disease: Relation between striatal and limbic dopamine. *Adv Biochem Psychopharmacol* 19:293–300, 1978.
14. Kish SJ, Shannak K, Hornykiewicz O: Uneven pattern of dopamine loss in the striatum of patients with idiopathic Parkinson's disease. *N Engl J Med* 318:876–880, 1988.
15. Zigmond MJ, Stricker EM: Parkinson's disease: Studies with an animal model. *Life Sci* 35:5–18, 1984.
16. Pimoule C, Schoemaker H, Javoy-Agid F, et al: Decrease in [3H] cocaine binding to the dopamine transporter in Parkinson's disease. *Eur J Pharmacol* 95:145–146, 1983.
17. Maloteaux J-M, Vanisberg M-A, Laterre C, et al: [3H]GBR 12935 binding to dopamine uptake sites: Subcellular localization and reduction in Parkinson's disease and progressive supranuclear palsy. *Eur J Pharmacol* 156:331–340, 1988.
18. Trugman JM, Leadbetter R, Zolis ME, et al: Treatment of severe axial dystonia with clozapine: Case report and hypothesis. *Mov Disord* 9:441–446, 1994.
19. Moore RY, Bloom FE: Central catecholamine neuron systems: Anatomy and physiology of the norepinephrine and epinephrine systems. *Annu Rev Neurosci* 2:113–168, 1979.

20. Farley IJ, Hornykiewicz O: Noradrenaline in subcortical brain regions of patients with Parkinson's disease and control subjects, in Birkmayer W, Hornykiewicz O (eds): *Advances in Parkinsonism.* Basel: Editiones Roche, 1976, pp 178–185.

21. Scatton B, Javoy-Agid F, Rouquier L, et al: Reduction of cortical dopamine, noradrenaline, serotonin, and their metabolites in Parkinson's disease. *Brain Res* 275:321–328, 1983.

22. Javoy-Agid F, Rubert M, Taquet H, et al: Biochemical neuropathology of Parkinson's disease, in Hassler RG, Christ JF (eds): *Advances in Neurology.* New York: Raven Press, 1984, vol 40, pp 189–198.

23. Kopp N, Denoroy L, Thomasi M, et al: Increase in noradrenaline-synthesizing enzyme activity in medulla oblongata in Parkinson's disease. *Acta Neuropathol* 56:17–21, 1982.

24. Bernheimer H, Birkmayer W, Hornykiewicz O: Verteilung des 5-hydroxytryptamins (serotonin) in gehirn des menschen und sein verhalten bei patienten mit Parkinson-syndrom. *Klin Wochenschr* 39:1056–1059, 1961.

25. Perry TL, Javoy-Agid F, Agid Y, Fibiger HC: Striatal gabaergic neuronal activity is not reduced in Parkinson's disease. *J Neurochem* 40:1120–1123, 1983.

26. Laaksonen H, Rinne UK, Sonninen V, Riekkinen P: Brain GABA neurons in Parkinson's disease. *Acta Neurol Scand* 57(suppl 67):282–283, 1978.

27. Lloyd KG, Hornykiewicz O: L-Glutamic acid decarboxylase in Parkinson's disease: Effect of L-dopa therapy. *Nature* 243:521–523, 1973.

28. Lloyd KG, Möhler H, Hertz P, Bartholini G: Distribution of choline acetyltransferase and glutamate decarboxylase within the substantia nigra and in other brain regions from control and parkinsonian patients. *J Neurochem* 25:789–795, 1975.

29. Ruberg M, Ploska A, Javoy-Agid F, Agid Y: Muscarinic binding and choline acetyltransferase activity in parkinsonian subjects with reference to dementia. *Brain Res* 232:129–139, 1982.

30. Mauborgne A, Javoy-Agid F, Legrand JC, et al: Decrease of substance P-like immunoreactivity in the substantia nigra and pallidum of parkinsonian brains. *Brain Res* 268:167–170, 1983.

31. Grafe MR, Forno LS, Eng LF: Immunocytochemical studies of substance P and metenkephalin in the basal ganglia and substantia nigra in Huntington's, Parkinson's and Alzheimer's diseases. *J Neuropathol Exp Neurol* 44:47–59, 1985.

32. Taquet H, Javoy-Agid F, Hamon H, et al: Parkinson's disease affects differently met5- and leu5-enkephalin in the human brain. *Brain Res* 280:379–382, 1983.

33. Hökfelt T, Skirboll L, Rehfeld JF, et al: A subpopulation of mesencephalic dopamine neurons projecting to limbic areas contains a cholecystokinin-like peptide: Evidence from immunohistochemistry combined with retrograde tracing. *Neuroscience* 5:2093–2124, 1980.

34. Studler JM, Javoy-Agid F, Cesselin F, et al: CCK-8-immunoreactivity distribution in human brain: Selective decrease in the substantia nigra from parkinsonian patients. *Brain Res* 243:176–179, 1982.

35. Epelbaum J, Ruberg M, Moyse E, et al: Somatostatin and dementia in Parkinson's disease. *Brain Res* 278:376–379, 1983.

36. Cohen G: The pathobiology of Parkinson's disease: Biochemical aspects of dopamine neuron senescence. *J Neural Trans* 19(suppl):89–103, 1983.

37. Graham DG: Catecholamine toxicity: A proposal for the molecular pathogenesis of manganese neurotoxicity and Parkinson's disease. *Neurotoxicology* 5:83–96, 1984.

38. Fahn S, Cohen G: The oxidant stress hypothesis in Parkinson's disease: Evidence supporting it. *Ann Neurol* 32:804–812, 1992.

39. Freeman BA, Crapo JD: Biology of disease: Free radicals and tissue injury. *Lab Invest* 47:412–426, 1982.

40. Perry TL, Godin DV, Hansen S: Parkinson's disease: A disorder due to nigral glutathione deficiency? *Neurosci Lett* 33:305–310, 1982.

41. Ambani LM, Van Woert MH, Murphy S: Brain peroxidase and catalase in Parkinson's disease. *Arch Neurol* 32:114–118, 1975.

42. Dexter DT, Carter CJ, Wells FR: Basal lipid peroxidation in substantia nigra is increased in Parkinson's disease. *J Neurochem* 52:381–389, 1989.

43. Jenner P: Oxidative stress as a cause of Parkinson's disease. *Acta Neurol Scand* 84:6–15, 1991.

44. Parker WD, Boyson SJ, Parks JK: Abnormalities of the electron transport chain in idiopathic Parkinson's disease. *Ann Neurol* 26:719–723, 1989.

45. Benecke R, Strumper P, Weiss H: Electron transfer complexes I and IV of platelets are abnormal in Parkinson's disease but normal in Parkinson-plus syndromes. *Brain* 116:1451–1463, 1993.

46. Schapira AH, Mann VM, Cooper JM: Anatomic and disease specificity of NADH CoQ1 reductase (complex I) deficiency in Parkinson's disease. *J Neurochem* 55:2142–2145, 1990.

47. Lestienne P, Nelson J, Riederer P, et al: Normal mitochondrial genome in brain from patients with Parkinson's disease and complex I defect. *J Neurochem* 55:1810–1812, 1990.

48. Kuhl DE, Metter EJ, Riege WR: Patterns of local cerebral glucose utilization determined in Parkinson's disease by the [18F] fluorodeoxyglucose method. *Ann Neurol* 15:419–424, 1984.

49. Rougemont D, Baron JC, Collard P, et al: Local cerebral glucose utilization in treated and untreated patients with Parkinson's disease. *J Neurol Neurosurg Psychiatry* 47:824–830, 1984.

50. Martin WRW, Beckman JH, Calne DB, et al: Cerebral glucose metabolism in Parkinson's disease. *Can J Neurol Sci* 11(suppl 1):169–173, 1984.

51. Leenders K, Wolfson L, Gibbs J, et al: Regional cerebral blood flow and oxygen metabolism in Parkinson's disease and their response to L-dopa. *J Cerebral Blood Flow Metab* 3(suppl 1):S488–S489, 1983.

52. Wooten GF, Collins RC: Metabolic effects of unilateral lesion of the substantia nigra. *J Neurosci* 1:285–291, 1981.

53. Garnett ES, Firnau G, Nahmias C: Dopamine visualized in the basal ganglia of living man. *Nature* 305:137–138, 1983.

54. Garnett ES, Nahmias C, Firnau G: Central dopaminergic pathways in hemiparkinsonism examined by positron emission tomography. *Can J Neurol Sci* 11(suppl 1):174–179, 1984.

55. Calne DB, Langston JW, Martin WRW, et al: Positron emission tomography after MPTP: Observations relating to the cause of Parkinson's disease. *Nature* 317:246–248, 1985.

56. Aquilonius S-M, Bergstrom K, Eckernas S-A, et al: In vivo evaluation of striatal dopamine reuptake sites using 11C-nomifersine and positron emission tomography. *Acta Neurol Scand* 76:283–287, 1987.

57. Lewy FH: Paralysis agitans. I. Pathologische anatomie, in Lewandowski M (ed): *Handbuck der Neurologie.* Berlin: Springer, 1912, pp 920–933.

58. Greenfield JG, Bosanquet FD: The brainstem lesion in parkinsonism. *J Neurol Neurosurg Psychiatry* 16:213–226, 1953.

59. Bethlem J, den Hartog Jager WA: The incidence and characteristics of Lewy bodies in idiopathic paralysis agitans (Parkinson's disease). *J Neurol Neurosurg Psychiatry* 23:74–80, 1960.

60. Issidorides MR, Mytilineou C, Whetsell WO, Yahr MD: Protein-rich cytoplasmic bodies of substantia nigra and locus ceruleus. *Arch Neurol* 35:633–637, 1978.

61. Goldman JE, Yen S-H, Chiu F-C, Peress NS: Lewy bodies of Parkinson's disease contain neurofilament antigens. *Science* 221:1082–1084, 1983.

Chapter 12 _____

ETIOLOGY OF PARKINSON'S DISEASE

YOSHIKUNI MIZUNO, SHIN-ICHIROU IKEBE, NOBUTAKA
HATTORI, HIDEKI MOCHIZUKI, YUKO NAKAGAWA-
HATTORI, and TOMOYOSHI KONDO

HISTORICAL ASPECTS
DEVELOPMENTS IN THE MODERN ERA
    MPTP-Induced Parkinsonism
    Structure and Function of Mitochondria
    Mitochondria in Parkinson's Disease
    Oxidative Stress in Parkinson's Disease
    Mitochondrial Respiratory Failure and Oxidative
      Stress: Which Comes First?
    Environmental Factors and Neurotoxins in
      Parkinson's Disease
    Genetic Predisposition
    Other Factors
SUMMARY AND CONCLUSION

Historical Aspects

The etiology of Parkinson's disease has long been discussed since the original description of the disease by James Parkinson in 1817;[1] as a potential cause of this disease, Parkinson mentioned the possibility of chronic injury to the cervical cord, which gave rise to nerves to the upper extremities, as the disease often had started in the upper extremities. However, he did not make any definite statement on the etiology and pathogenesis.

As parkinsonism was the frequent sequel of Economo's encephalitis, it had been postulated that a viral infection might have been a cause of nigral degeneration in Parkinson's disease. Von Economo's encephalitis started with the epidemics in Vienna in 1917[2] and resulted in worldwide pandemics until 1926 with high morbidity (up to 80 percent).[3] The incidence of parkinsonism among recovered patients was quite high (up to 80 percent or more) by the 10th year after the acute episode of encephalitis.[4] The pathological hallmark of postencephalitic parkinsonism is the presence of Alzheimer's neurofibrillary tangles in the remaining neurons of the substantia nigra,[5,6] in contrast to the presence of Lewy bodies in Parkinson's disease. It is unlikely that Economo's encephalitis plays any etiologic role in the pathogenesis of Parkinson's disease.[7] Parkinsonism may be seen as a sequel of various kinds of encephalitis other than Economo's encephalitis; parkinsonism has been reported after infections of Japanese B encephalitis,[8] Western equine encephalitis,[9,10] Coxsackie B type 2 encephalitis,[11] and central European tick-borne encephalitis.[12] However, parkinsonism after these en-

cephalitides is usually nonprogressive, and it is unlikely that these infections play any etiologic role in Parkinson's disease.

As herpes simplex viruses have affinity to monoamine neurons in the brain stem[13] and they can stay in the nervous system for a long period without causing inflammation or symptoms,[14] it was once postulated that a specific form of infection with herpes simplex viruses might cause Parkinson's disease. Increases in antibody titers against herpes simplex virus components have been reported in the literature, including complement-fixing antibody,[15] antibodies against herpes simplex capsid antigen, envelope antigen, and excreted antigen.[16] However, herpes simplex virus particles[17] or herpes simplex DNA[18] have never been found in the brains of patients who died of Parkinson's disease. Another virus that was considered in relation to the etiology of Parkinson's disease was influenza virus. As a pandemic of influenza occurred simultaneously with Economo's encephalitis from 1918 to 1919,[19] possible association of influenza virus infection and Parkinson's disease was also investigated;[17,18,20,21] however, researchers could not demonstrate any causal association between influenza infection and Parkinson's disease. Thus, it seems unlikely that infections with any known agents are playing a role in the etiology of Parkinson's disease.

Another possibility that was once considered was chronic metal intoxication. Chronic manganese intoxication produces parkinsonism,[22,23] and manganese and aluminum contents in the water consumed by Guamanian people who had developed parkinsonism-dementia complex were high.[24] However, the clinical picture and pathological changes in chronic manganese intoxication are different from those of Parkinson's disease. Clinically, psychiatric manifestations such as mental irritability, compulsive actions, and hallucinations are not uncommon in the early stage of manganese intoxication.[22] In the fully developed stage, parkinsonism dominates the clinical picture; however, tremor tends to be more postural,[22] and dystonia is more common.[23] Pathological changes are most prominent in the internal segment of globus pallidus and the subthalamic nucleus,[25] although other basal ganglia structures may also be involved. Furthermore, brain manganese levels are not elevated in Parkinson's disease[26] and, unless heavily exposed, people do not usually develop symptoms of metal intoxication. Thus, it seems unlikely that chronic metal intoxication plays a role in the etiology and pathogenesis of Parkinson's disease. Recently, increases in cerebral iron and aluminum have been reported in Parkinson's disease, which will be discussed later.

Another possibility once discussed was the MIF (melanocyte-stimulating hormone [MSH]-release inhibiting factor) deficiency theory.[27] MIF is a tripeptide synthesized in the hypothalamus and released into pituitary portal vessels inhibiting MSH release from the anterior pituitary gland.[28] This theory was postulated based on three observations. First, serum MSH levels were reported to be elevated in Parkinson's disease patients.[29] Second, MSH was found to aggravate parkinsonism.[30] Third, MIF showed marginal improvement in parkinsonism.[31,32] However, disturbance of MIF secretion or degeneration of MIF-producing neurons has never been proved in the brain of patients who died of Parkinson's disease, and this hypothesis appears to have been abandoned.

Developments in the Modern Era

MPTP-INDUCED PARKINSONISM

The modern era of research on the etiology and pathogenesis of Parkinson's disease was opened by the discovery of parkinsonism induced by MPTP (1-methyl-4-phenyl-1,2,3,6-tetrahydropyridine).

MPTP was found as a contaminant of illicit narcotics. In 1979, Davis et al.[33] reported a patient who developed severe parkinsonism after injecting a home-made illicit narcotic; the principal component, which had a narcotic action, is thought to have been MPPP (1-methyl-4-phenyl-4-propionoxypiperidine), a potent meperidine analogue (Fig. 12-1), which has a heroin-like action. MPTP was thought to have been produced as a by-product of the synthesis of MPPP. This patient was examined by neurologists at NIH and was treated with L-dopa and bromocriptine with marked improvement. However, 18 months later he was found dead, apparently from an overdose of narcotics. Postmortem examination revealed extensive degeneration and loss of pigmented neurons in the substantia nigra.[33] However, only one Lewy body-like inclusion is said to have been found in the substantia nigra, in contrast to Parkinson's disease, in which many Lewy bodies can be seen in the remaining nigral neurons.

In 1982, several young adults in northern California developed a parkinsonian syndrome after intravenous use of what was purported to be "synthetic heroin."[34,35] Analysis of the drug samples that those patients had taken identified MPTP as a probable toxin responsible for their parkinsonism.[34] The clinical picture of human MPTP-induced parkinsonism is very much like that of Parkinson's disease, although, resting tremor is less frequent; Ballard et al.[35] noted resting tremor in four of seven MPTP-induced parkinsonian patients. Interestingly, five of their seven patients experienced dyskinesias or on-off fluctuations within months of L-dopa treatment,[35]

indicating that severity of neuronal degeneration in the nigrostriatal dopaminergic terminals is a more important denominator of motor fluctuations than the duration of L-dopa treatment.

Animal models of MPTP-induced parkinsonism were successfully made not only in monkeys[36–38] but also in rodents;[39,40] Nigral neuronal cell death was only modest in mouse MPTP models, although striatum showed striking loss of dopamine;[40,41] rats are relatively insensitive to MPTP toxicity.[42] Thus it has been firmly established that MPTP can induce parkinsonism both in human beings and experimental animals; since then, MPTP-induced parkinsonism has been considered as the best animal model now available of Parkinson's disease. In contrast to Parkinson's disease, pathological change of MPTP-induced parkinsonism is more selective in the substantia nigra, with less involvement of locus ceruleus.[36,38]

Regarding intracerebral metabolism and transport, MPTP is taken up into astrocytes in the brain, and it is oxidized to MPP+ (1-methyl-4-phenylpyridinium ion) by monoamine oxidase B,[43] and MPP+ is actively taken up into nigrostriatal neurons[44,45] through dopamine transporters[46] with marked concentration within dopaminergic neurons;[47] this is the mechanism of selective toxicity of MPTP against dopaminergic neurons. MPTP-induced parkinsonism can be prevented by pretreatment of animals with monoamine oxidase B inhibitors[48] or dopamine uptake blockers.[41,49,50]

Regarding the mechanism of cytotoxicity of MPP+, inhibition of mitochondrial respiration and resultant energy crisis play the central role. MPP+ is actively taken up into mitochondria, depending on the gradient of electrical potential between the inside and the outside of the mitochondrial inner membrane.[51,52] As mitochondria respire, the inside of the mitochondria becomes negatively charged because of proton (H+) translocation from the inside of mitochondria to the intermembrane space, coupled with the electron transfer

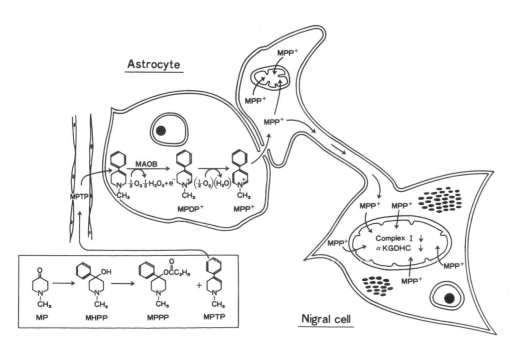

FIGURE 12-1 Schematic representation of biosynthetic pathway of MPTP synthesis and the mechanism of selective degeneration of the substantia nigra in MPTP-induced parkinsonism. MPP+ is actively taken up into dopaminergic neurons through the dopamine transporter and actively transported further into mitochondria. MPPP, 1-methyl-4-phenyl-4-propionoxypiperidine; MAOB, monamine oxidase type B; KGDHC, α-ketoglutarate dehydrogenase complex.

along the respiratory chain; thus positively charged MPP^+ is actively taken up into mitochondria with marked concentration within mitochondria as many other lipophilic cations are concentrated within mitochondria[53] in response to the electrical gradient.[54] Not all of the positively charged molecules can be concentrated within mitochondria; the size and structure of the molecule and relative solubility in the lipid bilayer appear to influence the active transport of charged molecules into mitochondria.

Within mitochondria, MPP^+ inhibits mitochondrial complex I and NADH-linked state 3 respiration.[51,52,55–58] MPP^+ can inhibit complex I, probably because of its structural similarity to NAD^+, as shown in Fig. 12-2. The inhibition of mitochondrial respiration results in loss of oxidative phosphorylation and rapid fall in the ATP level,[59] which may be fatal to respiring cells when loss of ATP reaches a certain critical level.

Table 12-1 shows our previous study on the inhibition of NADH-linked state 3 inhibition and the complex I activity by MPP^+. In this experiment, we measured NADH-linked state 3 respiration, using intact mitochondria in the presence of 50 micromolars of MPP^+, together with glutamate and malate; mitochondrial respiration was inhibited to approximately 10 percent of that of the control. The activity of complex I was then assayed, using the same mitochondria without freeze thawing. Although maximum activity of complex I could not be measured in this setting, the activity of complex I was inhibited to 50 percent of that of the corresponding control.[60] When inhibition of complex I by MPP^+ is measured using mitochondria with disrupted membranes with freeze thawing, millimolar order of MPP^+ is necessary to obtain 50 percent inhibition.[61] This would mean that while intact mitochondria were incubated with MPP^+ together with glutamate and malate as substrates to support mitochondrial respiration, the concentration of MPP^+ inside the mitochondria would have reached millimolar order while the outside was still in the micromolar order. Actually, Ramsay et al.[62] estimated that MPP^+ would be concentrated up to 800-fold within mitochondria, compared to the external medium.

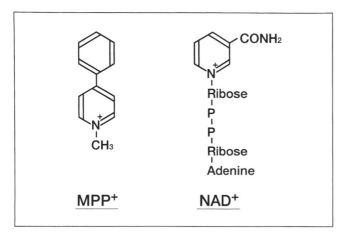

FIGURE 12-2 Structural similarity between MPP^+ and NAD^+. NAD^+ is a cofactor of dehydrogenases, including those within mitochondria.

TABLE 12-1 Effect of MPP^+ on Mitochondrial Respiration, Complex I Activity, and ATP Synthesis

	Control	MPP^+
State 3[a]	180 ± 25	21 ± 4*
State 4[a]	30 ± 5	11 ± 3*
Complex I[b]	57 ± 13	27 ± 6*
ATP formed[c]	637 ± 23	210 ± 31*

Glutamate and malate were used as substrates, MPP^+ = 50 micromolar, mean ± SEM, n = 9, *, $p < 0.001$.
[a] Nanoatom oxygen per minute per milligram of protein.
[b] Nanomole of NADH oxidized per minute per milligram of protein.
[c] Nanomoles of ATP formed from 750 nanomoles of ADP.
SOURCE: *From Mizuno et al.[60] Used with permission.*

Thus MPP^+ produces marked impairment of mitochondrial respiration and ATP synthesis; however, there is evidence to indicate that inhibition of complex I alone would not suffice to account for the marked inhibition of state 3 respiration. As shown in Table 12-1, while mitochondrial state 3 respiration was reduced to 10 percent of that of the control by 50 micromolars of MPP^+, the activity of complex I of those mitochondria was reduced only to 50 percent of the corresponding control.[60] We thought there must be another enzyme that would be inhibited by MPP^+ within mitochondria. Therefore, we studied the effect of MPP^+ on nicotinamide adenine dinucleotide-plus (NAD^+)-linked dehydrogenases in the tricarboxylic acid cycle. As shown in Table 12-2, the alpha-ketoglutarate dehydrogenase complex of the tricarboxylic acid cycle was also inhibited by MPP^+.[60,63] The IC_{50} of MPP^+ to inhibit the alpha-ketoglutarate dehydrogenase complex was 3.65 mM, which was in the same order of the IC_{50} of MPP^+ (3.2 mM) to inhibit complex I.[61] This dual inhibition of complex I and the alpha-ketoglutarate dehydrogenase complex by MPP^+ would account for the marked inhibition of mitochondrial state 3 respiration by MPP^+. The alpha-ketoglutarate dehydrogenase complex has been postulated to be the rate-limiting enzyme of the tricarboxylic acid (TCA) cycle,[64] and it provides nicotinamide adenine dinucleotide (NADH) for complex I and catalyzes the oxidation of alpha-ketoglutarate to succinate; the latter becomes a substrate for complex II. Thus inhibition of the alpha-ketoglutarate dehydrogenase complex would impair the electron transfer via complex II because of insufficient supply of succinate for complex II.

TABLE 12-2 Effect of MPP^+ on Dehydrogenases in the Tricarboxylic Acid (TCA) Cycle

	Control	MPP^+
Isocitrate dehydrogenase (DH)	285 ± 37	266 ± 35
Glutamate DH	556 ± 50	545 ± 52
α-ketoglutarate dehydrogenase complex (KGDHC)	34 ± 5	19 ± 3*
Malate DH	4760 ± 530	4870 ± 690

DHC, dehydrogenase complex. MPP^+ = 2 mM, mean ± SEM, n = 8, nanomole NADH oxidized per minute per milligram of protein. *, $p < 0.001$.
SOURCE: *From Mizuno et al.[60] Used with permission.*

Although respiratory failure is the major cause of nigral cell death in MPTP-induced parkinsonism, recently MPP[+] was reported to induce apoptosis;[65,66] the question is whether or not this apoptosis may be a consequence of respiratory failure.

STRUCTURE AND FUNCTION OF MITOCHONDRIA

Mitochondria are intracellular organelles of about 0.4–4 μm in length. They are essential for cellular respiration; more than 90 percent of oxygen in the body is consumed within mitochondria. Although the external membrane is permeable to many substances the inner mitochondrial membrane is relatively impermeable to anions. Therefore, a considerable proportion of the energy resulting from the proton concentration gradient is stored as membrane electric potential.[67] The internal membrane has many indentations, called cristae, toward the inside. The space inside of the inner membrane is called matrix, in which many important enzymes, including those of the TCA cycle, are located. The TCA cycle provides NADH as a substrate for complex I and succinate for complex II. Within the cristae, five electron transfer complexes are located, as schematically shown in Fig. 12-3; they are named as complex I, complex II, complex III, complex IV, and complex V. Each complex consists of hydrophilic and hydrophobic proteins called subunits; each complex has a finite number of subunits, as shown in Table 12-3, and some of them are encoded by mitochondrial DNA. Complex I is the largest subunit, consisting of more than 40 subunits,[68] and 7 of them are encoded by mitochondrial DNA;[69,70] Complex II does not have a mitochondrially encoded subunit. There are two electron transfer pathways, that is, from NADH via complex I to ubiquinone (coenzyme Q) and from succinate via complex II to ubiquinone (Fig. 12-4). Ubiquinone is reduced to ubiquinol in these reactions; the subsequent pathway is the same, that is, from ubiquinol via complex III to ferricytochrome C; ferricytochrome C is reduced to ferrocytochrome C and from ferrocytochrome C via complex IV to molecular oxygen; oxygen is reduced to water in the last reaction. Whereas electrons are transferred from either NADH or succinate to molecular oxygen, protons are translocated from the matrix side to the intermembrane space, and ATP is synthesized by the action of complex V, using the translocated protons. ATP synthesis is coupled with the reaction mediated by complex I, complex III, and complex IV but not by complex II; three molecules of ATP are synthesized when one equivalent of electrons is transferred from NADH to molecular oxygen.

The site of action of MPP[+] within the complex I molecule was reported to be the junction of NADH dehydrogenase and ubiquinone, that is, the Fe-S cluster of highest potential and ubiquinone[71] or ubiquinone binding site,[72] the same binding site as that of rotenone and piericidin, the classical specific inhibitors of complex I.[72,73]

Iron-sulfur clusters denote clusters of iron and sulfur atoms arranged either in the form of a cube or in the form of a square; in the former cluster, four iron atoms and four sulfur atoms take alternately the apex positions of a cube; this type of cluster is called a tetranuclear cluster [4Fe-4S]. In the latter cluster, they take the apex positions of a square; this type is called binuclear cluster [2Fe-2S], and usually cysteine residues in the subunits of the electron transfer complexes serve as ligands for these clusters.[74–76] Those subunits

TABLE 12-3 Number of Subunits of Electron Transfer Complexes

	Total	Nuclear Coded	Mitochondrially Coded
Complex I	41	34	7
Complex II	4	4	0
Complex III	10	9	1
Complex IV	12	9	3
Complex V	18	16	2

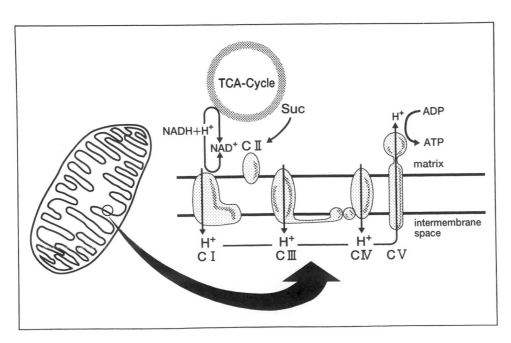

FIGURE 12-3 Schematic representation of mitochondria and the electron transfer complexes. Five electron transfer complexes are located within the inner membrane of mitochondria. Protons are translocated into the intermembrane space from the matrix; these protons are used by complex V to synthesize ATP from ADP.

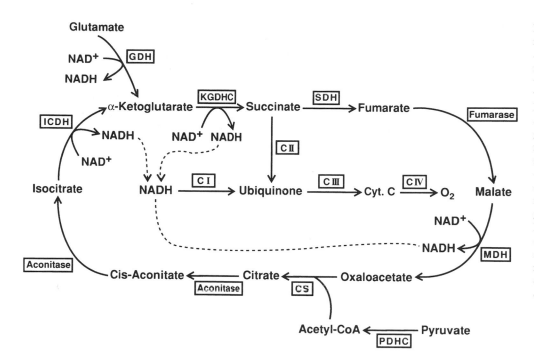

FIGURE 12-4 Schematic representation of the TCA cycle and the electron transfer chain in the center. Two electron transfer pathways are present with ubiquinone, that is, from NADH and from succinate. The alpha-ketoglutarate dehydrogenase complex provides not only NADH but also succinate. PDHC, pyruvate dehydrogenase complex; CS, citrate synthase; ICDH, isocitrate dehydrogenase; GDH, glutamate dehydrogenase; KGDHC, alpha-ketoglutarate dehydrogenase complex; SDH, succinate dehydrogenase; MDH, malate dehydrogenase; CI, complex I; CII, complex II; CIII, complex III; CIV, complex IV.

that have an iron-sulfur cluster are called iron-sulfur proteins, and usually they are hydrophilic. Complex I is thought to have four [4Fe-4S] clusters and two [2Fe-2S] clusters;[76] these iron sulfur clusters are considered to play a role in the electron transfer within complexes, as iron atoms can undergo redox cycling.[77]

Each mitochondrion has 2 to 10 copies of double-stranded circular DNA, consisting of 16,569 base pairs[78] (Table 12-4). Mitochondrial DNA encodes 13 subunits of the electron transfer complexes, 22 transfer RNAs, and 2 ribosomal RNAs. Mitochondrially encoded proteins are synthesized within mitochondria; mitochondria are equipped with all the necessary devices to synthesize proteins. Mitochondrial DNA is more vulnerable than nuclear DNA, particularly to oxidative stress, as will be discussed later in more detail.

One of the most important functions of mitochondria is synthesis of ATP, which has a high-energy phosphate bond in each molecule; ATP is essential for maintenance of cellular integrity and for many important biochemical reactions.

MITOCHONDRIA IN PARKINSON'S DISEASE

COMPLEX I

Since the discovery of MPP[+] toxicity on mitochondria, interest has been focused on mitochondrial functions in Parkinson's disease. Thus Schapira's group first reported a decrease in complex I activity in the substantia nigra of Parkinson's disease;[79,80] the complex I activity was reduced to approximately two-thirds of that of the control. We analyzed complex I subunits by Western blotting and reported a decrease in the lower molecular weight complex I subunits between 24 and 30 K, using striatal mitochondrial preparations.[81] Then we analyzed the nigral neurons by means of an immunohistochemical method, using specific antibodies against complex

I, II, III, and IV.[82] Immunostaining of the nigral neurons for complex II, III, and IV was well retained, despite marked degenerative changes. Immunostaining intensity of nigral neurons for complex I was not uniform from one neuron to another. In other words, nigral neurons were a mixture of well stained to poorly stained neurons with various degrees of reduction in the immunostaining intensity in between; the number of neurons that lost immunoreactivity to complex I was significantly increased in Parkinson's disease (Fig. 12-5). Such neurons with reduced immunostaining for complex I were also seen in the control patients in smaller numbers. This mosaicism in the immunostaining intensity for complex I fits well into the energy mosaicism theory proposed as a mechanism of neuronal cell death associated with aging.[83] Energy mosaicism theory postulates that neurons die one after another when the energy level within the individual neuron decreases to a certain critical level. Nigral change in Parkinson's disease may be regarded as localized accelerating aging. As neuronal death in neurodegenerative disease and in aging is a slow process not taking place simultaneously in all neurons, this concept of energy mosaicism fits well into what appears to be going on in Parkinson's disease.

TABLE 12-4 Demographic Data on Mitochondria and Mitochondrial DNA (mtDNA)

No. of mitochondria/cell	100–500
No. of mtDNA/mt	2–10 copies
No. of mtDNA/cell	1000/cell
No. of base pairs/mtDNA	16,569
No. of proteins encoded	13
No. of tRNA encoded	22
No. of rRNA encoded	2

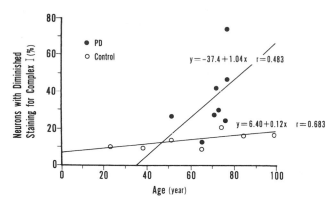

FIGURE 12-5 Proportions of nigral neurons that showed reduction in immunoreactivity to complex I and its relation to the age of the patients. Open circles represent the control patients; closed circles represent patients with Parkinson's disease (PD). A positive correlation was noted between the age and the proportion of neurons which showed decreased immunoreactivity in the control patients. Patients with Parkinson's disease showed significant increase in the proportions of neurons which showed reduced immunoreactivity. *(From Hattori et al.*[82] *Used with permission.)*

The reason why this localized "aging" process is accelerated in Parkinson's disease has to be studied further.

Regarding the specificity of complex I deficiency in Parkinson's disease, Schapira et al.[84] reported that this decrease in the complex I activity was specific for the substantia nigra of Parkinson's disease and not seen in other areas nor seen in the substantia nigra of other neurodegenerative disorders that affected the substantia nigra.[84]

Then complex I activity was measured in tissues other than those of the brain by several groups, however, controversies exist among those reports.[85] In platelets, decreased activity was reported by Parker et al.,[86] Kriege et al.,[87] and Yoshino et al.[88] In the skeletal muscle, decreased activity was reported by Bindoff et al.,[89,90] Nakagawa-Hattori et al.,[91] and Cardellach et al.[92] Furthermore, Blin et al.[93] reported abnormal mitochondrial respiration in the skeletal muscle from patients with Parkinson's disease, and Shoffner et al.[94] reported reduced oxidative phosphorylation in the skeletal muscle of patients with Parkinson's disease. Regarding complex IV, Bindoff et al.[89] and Cardellach et al.[92] reported decreased activity in the skeletal muscle. These observations would mean that patients with Parkinson's disease may have a subtle systemic abnormality that would cause reduction in the activity of complex I. The reason why patients with Parkinson's disease may have a systemic abnormality of complex I is not known; however, if it is true, two possibilities can be considered. First, patients with Parkinson's disease may be exposed to neurotoxins that would inhibit complex I. Second, patients with Parkinson's disease may have lower activities of enzymes that would metabolize substances toxic to complex I.

Contrary to the above results, Mann et al.[95] reported that complex I activity in tissues other than the substantia nigra, including platelets and the skeletal muscles, was not reduced

in Parkinson's disease, and Anderson et al.[96] and DiDonato et al.[97] also did not find abnormality in skeletal muscle mitochondria in Parkinson's disease. Furthermore, recently Przedborski et al.[98] postulated that loss of complex I might be a secondary phenomenon to L-dopa treatment, as chronic treatment of experimental animals with L-dopa resulted in reversible loss of complex I activity.[99] However, Cooper et al.[100] opposed this notion, because striatal complex I activity, in which complex I would be exposed to a high concentration of dopamine, was not reduced in Parkinson's disease. Thus controversy still exists in the complex I activity in systemic organs. However, it is not surprising to see marginal decreases in the complex I activity or mitochondrial respiration in systemic organs, because it has been postulated that Parkinson's disease may be caused by environmental neurotoxins in genetically susceptible persons.

MITOCHONDRIAL DNA

As 7 of 41 subunits of complex I are encoded by mitochondrial DNA,[69,70] mutations in mitochondrial DNA may cause a decrease in complex I activity. Thus we studied mitochondrial DNA for large deletions and point mutations.[101,102] By means of the polymerase chain reaction (PCR) method, Ikebe et al.[101] found mitochondria with a 5-kb deletion, using striatal DNA preparation. This deletion was located between the 13 base pair direct-repeat sequences, encompassing the ND 5 (NADH dehydrogenase subunit 5) gene and the ATPase 6/8 gene; between these two genes, genes for ND 3, ND4L, ND 4, and cytochrome c oxidase 3 (CCO3) are located (Fig. 12-6). This deletion is most commonly seen in the skeletal muscles of progressive external ophthalmoplegia.[103–105] The amount of deleted mitochondrial DNA was rather small in Parkinson's disease,[106,107] and it could not be detected by the Southern blotting.[108,109] Furthermore, it has been shown that the same 5-kb deletion increases with age; this deletion has been reported in the aged organs, including the brain,[110–112] cardiac muscle,[113,114] skeletal muscle,[115,116] and liver.[116,117] Even if it is an aging process, it may play a role in the progression of the nigral neuronal degeneration, as generally Parkinson's disease is a disease of elderly people. If patients with Parkinson's disease have certain genetic predisposition, then the addition of the aging process to the genetic predisposition may impair energy production.

Regarding point mutations of mitochondrial DNA, Ikebe et al.[102] sequenced total mitochondrial DNA on 5 patients with Parkinson's disease and compared those sequences with those of more than 30 control subjects. Each one of those five patients had at least a point mutation that would cause amino acid substitution in at least one of the subunits of complex I. However, the locations of the mutations were different from one patient to another; in other words, no single mutation common to Parkinson's disease was found. These point mutations may modify the hydrophobicity profiles or the secondary structures of complex I subunits. Whether or not these mutations constitute a genetic risk factor of Parkinson's disease should be studied further. Shoffner et al.[118] reported higher incidence of A to G mutation at nucleotide 4336 of tRNA[gln] gene in Parkinson's disease; however, we could not reproduce their results.

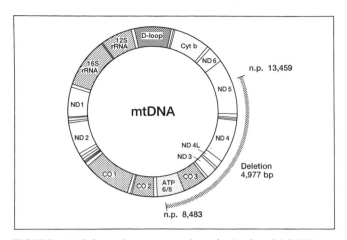

FIGURE 12-6 Schematic representation of mitochondrial DNA and the location of the common 5-kb deletion *(From Ikebe et al.[101] Used with permission.)*

ALPHA-KETOGLUTARATE DEHYDROGENASE COMPLEX

As the loss of complex I is only modest in Parkinson's disease both biochemically[79,80] and immunohistochemically,[82] we raised a question as to whether or not loss of complex I alone could account for nigral degeneration in Parkinson's disease. In mitochondrial encephalomyopathies, usually 50 percent or more loss of complex I is necessary to see muscle pathology;[119–122] more severe loss is usually necessary to see severe muscle degeneration.[120,121] As the alpha-ketoglutarate dehydrogenase complex of the TCA cycle was also inhibited by MPP^+ in addition to complex I,[63] we thought this enzyme complex might also be defective in Parkinson's disease. Initially we wanted to measure biochemical activity of this enzyme complex using autopsy materials; however, apparently the enzyme complex was not stable enough post or ante mortem, and we could not recover the enzyme activity. Therefore, we studied this enzyme complex by means of an immunohistochemical method. Details have been reported elsewhere.[123] Briefly there was a marked reduction in the immunoreactive alpha-ketoglutarate dehydrogenase complex in severely affected areas of the substantia nigra of Parkinson's disease. Usually, the lateral part of the substantia nigra is the most affected region, and this part showed the most extensive loss of immunoreactivity. The less affected medial part showed a relatively mild loss of immunoreactivity. The other NAD^+-linked dehydrogenases in the TCA cycle, that is, isocitrate dehydrogenase, glutamate dehydrogenase, and malate dehydrogenase, were not reduced in Parkinson's disease.[124]

The alpha-ketoglutarate dehydrogenase complex is probably the most important enzyme in the tricarboxylic acid cycle; it has been assumed that it is the rate-regulating enzyme of the TCA cycle,[64] and it has the lowest activity among the four dehydrogenases of the TCA cycle.[63] It provides not only NADH for complex I but also succinate for complex II, as shown in Fig. 12-4; electron transfer from succinate to ubiquinone via complex II is the alternate electron transfer pathway for the NADH to ubiquinone pathway. Therefore,

when complex I is reduced, the alternate pathway from succinate to ubiquinone becomes more important than usual; however, for the effective electron transfer via this pathway, supply of succinate is mandatory. Thus dual loss of complex I and the alpha-ketoglutarate dehydrogenase complex will deleteriously impair electron transfer and ATP synthesis. We believe loss of these two enzyme complexes plays a significant role in the nigral degeneration in Parkinson's disease. The NAD^+-linked dehydrogenases of the TCA cycle, including the alpha-ketoglutarate dehydrogenase complex, are believed to be located in close approximation to complex I[125]; therefore, noxious stimuli to the alpha-ketoglutarate dehydrogenase complex may have some influence on complex I, or vice versa.

CONSEQUENCE OF MITOCHONDRIAL RESPIRATORY FAILURE

Mitochondrial respiratory failure and resultant loss of ATP will cause protean changes in the respiring cells. Neurons are particularly vulnerable to lack of oxygen. This means that maintenance of ATP supply is essential for the integrity of neurons. Many enzymatic reactions require ATP; for instance, a group of enzymes with the general name "kinase" transfers the high-energy phosphate bond of ATP to other molecules of that enzyme reaction; examples are tyrosine kinase, protein kinase C, and phosphofructokinase, among others. Another group of enzyme with the general name "ATPase" uses the energy of the high-energy phosphate bond of ATP for the enzyme reaction; examples include Na-K ATPase, Ca-ATPase, and Mg-ATPase among others.

One of the most important enzymes that is essential for excitable cells such as neurons and muscles that uses ATP is Na-K ATPase. Normally, intracellular Na^+ concentration is lower than that in the extracellular space, and intracellular K^+ concentration is much higher than that in the extracellular space. Maintenance of this concentration gradient is achieved by the action of Na-K ATPase. When neurons or muscle cells undergo excitation, influx of Na^+ and outflow of K^+ occur; as the excitation goes away, Na^+ has to be expelled out against the concentration gradient between the inside and the outside of the cells by exchange with K^+. This is achieved using the energy of ATP by means of Na-K ATPase. When cellular level of ATP goes down, the activity of Na-K ATPase decreases, and Na^+ transport from the inside to outside diminishes. Then extra Na^+ has to be expelled out by exchange with Ca^{2+} in the extracellular space.[126,127] Thus intracellular Ca^{2+} will increase. Normally, intracellular Ca^{2+} is very low under the millimolar range, compared to the outside of the cell that is in micromolar range.[128] This Ca^{2+} gradient is maintained by calcium channel and ATPase coupled with the channel using the energy of ATP.[129] Increase in intracellular Ca^{2+} will induce protean adverse reactions.

Certain degradation enzymes are activated by increase in intracellular Ca^{2+} concentration. Ca^{2+}-activated neutral proteases (calpines) are a group of nonlysosomal enzymes activated by Ca^{2+}; cytoskeletal proteins may be attacked by these enzymes.[130] Ca^{2+}-activated phospholipases catalyze the hydrolysis of membrane phospholipids; activation of these enzymes may stimulate membrane breakdown or generate toxic metabolites.[131] Ca^{2+}-activated endonucleases mediate cleavage of nuclear DNA in oligonucleosome-length fragments; activation of an endogenous endonuclease is involved in programmed cell death and apoptosis in many systems.[132,133] Thus, increase in cellular Ca^{2+} level may induce apoptosis.[130] Interestingly, mitochondrial respiratory inhibitors can induce apoptotic cell death,[134,135] and we observed evidence to indicate an apoptotic process in the substantia nigra of patients who died of Parkinson's disease, using the nick end-labeling method.[136]

Calcium homeostasis is also important for normal mitochondrial functions. Mitochondria can sequester a large amount of Ca^{2+}.[137] Maintenance of Ca^{2+} homeostasis within mitochondria is dependent on the transmembrane electric potential induced by proton translocation; the inner mitochondrial membrane possesses a uniport carrier, which allows the electronic entry of Ca^{2+} in response to the negative transmembrane potential.[137] Cellular Ca^{2+} overload for any reason induces collapse of the mitochondria membrane potential, which will result in the failure of ATP synthesis.[131,138] Furthermore, the matrix-free Ca^{2+}-concentration regulates the activities of pyruvate dehydrogenase, alpha-ketoglutarate dehydrogenase, and isocitrate dehydrogenase and thus determines the rate of acetyl-CoA, NADH, and ATP synthesis.[139] In addition, when mitochondrial respiration goes down, mitochondria become unable to hold Ca^{2+} because of decrease in the membrane potential, and release Ca^{2+} into cytoplasm, thus, further increasing the cytosolic Ca^{2+} level.

Another adverse effect of mitochondrial respiratory failure is an increase in the formation of cytotoxically activated oxygen species within mitochondria, discussed in more detail in the following section.

OXIDATIVE STRESS IN PARKINSON'S DISEASE

DEFINITION OF OXIDATIVE STRESS AND FREE RADICALS

Oxidative stress denotes a state in which formation of free radicals is abnormally increased. Free radicals include any molecules and species that contain one or more unpaired electrons. Normally, each orbital of atoms and molecules can hold two electrons that have opposite spins; if an orbital contains only one electron, that electron is said to be unpaired.[140] The diatomic oxygen molecule has two unpaired electrons both spinning in the same direction; this is called triplet oxygen, and it is relatively stable as an oxidant because of its spin direction.[140] Singlet oxygen is an activated oxygen species; it does not have unpaired electrons, and thus it is not a radical. The pair of electrons in singlet oxygen has antiparallel spins; thus, spin restriction is removed, making singlet oxygen more reactive as oxidant than triplet oxygen.[141] When triplet oxygen undergoes one electron reduction, the superoxide anions are formed (Fig. 12-7). Superoxide anions are metabolized by superoxide dismutase to yield hydrogen peroxide (Fig. 12-7); in the presence of iron, hydroxyl radicals may be formed from hydrogen perioxide (Fig. 12-7). Activated oxygen species include superoxide anions, hydrogen peroxide, hydroxyl radical, and singlet oxygen, among which superoxide anions and hydroxyl radical are radicals by defi-

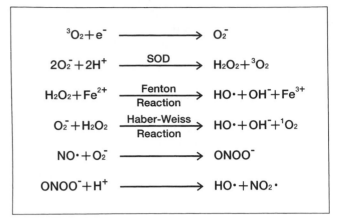

FIGURE 12-7 Activated oxygen species and the relationship among activated oxygen species. Nitric oxide and peroxynitrite are also shown. In the presence of ferric iron in the Haber-Weiss reaction, triplet oxygen is formed instead of singlet oxygen (iron-catalyzed Haber-Weiss reaction). $^3O_2$, triplet oxygen; O_2^-, superoxide anion, $HO\cdot$, hydroxyl radical; $^1O_2$, singlet oxygen; NO, nitric oxide; $ONOO^-$, peroxynitrite; SOD, superoxide dismutase.

nition. Among the activated oxygen species, the hydroxyl radical is most toxic, and hydrogen peroxide is relatively stable. These activated oxygen species are being formed in every respiring cell.

Generally, free radicals are highly reactive, oxidizing other substances by extracting an electron. They may nonselectively oxidize various substances, cause cross-linkage of sulfhydryl bonds of proteins, inactivate certain enzymes, may cause DNA breakdown, induce point mutations in DNA (which will be mentioned later), or cause lipid peroxidation. Particularly, unsaturated fatty acids are made liable to peroxidation by activated oxygen species; as unsaturated fatty acids are important components of various membrane systems, free radicals may have deleterious effects on cellular functions.

As respiring cells are exposed to free radicals, numbers of scavenging systems are present, protecting respiring cells. For instance, superoxide dismutase metabolizes superoxide anions to hydrogen peroxide and oxygen; catalase and glutathione peroxidase destroy hydrogen peroxide; and glutathione peroxidase breaks down other peroxides, and it may prevent lipid peroxidation.[142,143] Numbers of substances can scavenge hydroxyl radicals, for instance, vitamin E, metalothioneine, uric acid, ascorbate, glutathione, carotenoids, flavonoids, ubiquinone, salicylate, dimethyl sulfoxide, γ-oryzanol, phenolic compounds, urea compounds, and sugar compounds, including mannitol and others. Interestingly, 5-hydroxytryptophan, 5-hydroxyindole, and L-dopa were reported to have inhibited microsomal lipid peroxidation in the presence of vitamin E.[144] Fortunately, the life span of activated oxygen species is very short—less than 1 second, except for hydrogen peroxide.

Nitric oxide is a recently identified free radical;[145] it was found as a relaxation factor acting on vascular smooth muscles released from endothelial cells on stimulation by acetylcholine.[146] Nitric oxide is synthesized by nitric oxide synthase from L-arginine.[145] Nitric oxide synthase protein and mRNA have widespread distribution in the brain and the spinal cord and colocalize with NADPH diaphorase.[147,148] In addition to vasodilating action, nitric oxide has protean actions in neural transmission, particularly as a second messenger in glutamate neurotransmission.[149,150] Nitric oxide reacts with superoxide anion to produce peroxynitrite;[151] peroxynitrite is an unstable molecule at physiological pH and decomposes to nitrogen dioxide and hydroxyl radical[152] (Fig. 12-7). Half-life in the living organs is estimated to be 6–50 seconds.[153,154] Peroxynitrite is highly reactive, and it may play a role in neurodegeneration; for instance, mitochondrial electron transport is inhibited by peroxynitrite,[155,156] and nitric oxide inhibits complex I of the mitochondrial electron transfer chain.[149] Interestingly, nitric oxide positive neurons in the hippocampus are relatively spared in Alzheimer's disease;[157] therefore, the role of nitric oxide in neurodegeneration is not so simple. In Parkinson's disease, plasma levels of nitrates, an oxidation product that provides an indirect estimation of nitric oxide level, were reported to be normal.[158] Whether or not nitric oxide plays a role in Parkinson's disease has to be studied further.

FREE RADICAL SCAVENGING ENZYMES IN PARKINSON'S DISEASE

An interest in the possible involvement of free radicals in the etiology of Parkinson's disease dates back to 1975, when Ambani et al.[159] reported significant reduction in the activity of catalase and peroxidase in the substantia nigra and in the striatum. Reduction in peroxidase would result in reduced breakdown of peroxides that may injure neurons. Thus this was a very interesting observation; however, their results have never been confirmed by later studies. Later on, interest appears to have been focused on superoxide dismutase in Parkinson's disease. Dismutation means one of the substrate molecules is oxidized whereas another molecule of the same substrate is reduced; in the reaction catalyzed by superoxide dismutase while one superoxide molecule is oxidized to oxygen, another superoxide molecule is reduced to hydrogen peroxide. This is the most important enzyme for detoxification of superoxide anions.

Three isozymes are known for superoxide dismutase; one is cytosolic copper-zinc superoxide dismutase (Cu-Zn SOD); the second is mitochondrial manganese superoxide dismutase (Mn SOD), and the third one is extracellular superoxide dismutase (EC SOD). Cu-Zn SOD was found by McCord and Fridovich;[160] it is localized in the cytoplasm, and the gene locus is on chromosome 21;[161] cDNA was cloned in 1982.[162] Mn SOD was found by Weisinger and Fridovich;[163] it is localized in the matrix space of mitochondria, and the gene locus is on chromosome 6;[164] cDNA was cloned in 1988.[165] EC SOD is a secretory copper- and zinc-containing glycoprotein;[166] most of EC SOD exists in the intercellular spaces of tissues including plasma; one of the differences from Cu-Zn SOD is that while Cu-Zn SOD is a dimeric protein, EC SOD is a tetrameric enzyme;[167,168] the gene locus is also different from Cu-Zn SOD and is localized on the long arm of chromosome 4.[169]

In 1988, Marttila et al.[170] reported slight but significant increase in Cu-Zn SOD but not in Mn SOD in the substantia nigra of Parkinson's disease, whereas Saggu et al.[171] reported an increase in Mn SOD but not in Cu-Zn SOD. Although their results did not agree, increase in SOD activity was interpreted as a reaction to increased formation of superoxide anions. An increase in SOD activity will result in an increase in the formation of hydrogen peroxide; in the presence of iron, more cytotoxic hydroxyl radicals will be formed from hydrogen peroxide by Fenton reaction and iron-catalyzed Haber-Weiss reaction, as shown in Fig. 12-7.[172] Hydroxyl radicals enhance lipid peroxidation, and Dexter et al.[173] reported an increase in lipid peroxidation in the substantia nigra of patients with Parkinson's disease. Thus increase in SOD activity may induce an increase in hydroxyl radical formation and lipid peroxidation; thus SOD may be cytoprotective or cytotoxic, depending on the situation.

GLUTATHIONE IN PARKINSON'S DISEASE

Other evidence to suggest oxidative stress in the substantia nigra of Parkinson's disease is the reduction in reduced glutathione; 30–60 percent reduction in the reduced form of glutathione has been reported in the substantia nigra of Parkinson's disease.[174–177] Regarding oxidized form of glutathione, controversy exists, and one paper reported its marginal but significant elevation.[177] As most of tissue glutathione exists in the reduced form (GSH:GSSG > 50:1),[178] the significance of a small amount of increase in oxidized form probably awaits further research. Reduction in glutathione was also reported in MPTP-induced experimental parkinsonism.[179] Interestingly, glutathione was not reduced in the substantia nigra of multisystem degeneration and progressive supranuclear palsy.[180]

Glutathione is a tripeptide consisting of glutamate, cysteine, and glycine (γ-glutamylcysteinylglycine) (Fig. 12-8) synthesized by two enzymes, γ-glutamylcysteine synthase and glutathione synthase, with the former considered to be the rate-limiting step of glutathione synthesis.[180] Glutathione is a natural antioxidant, and it serves as a substrate for glutathione peroxidase. Glutathione is consumed when glutathione peroxidase catalyzes peroxidase reaction; reduced glutathione is oxidized to glutathione disulfide. In the central

FIGURE 12-8 Structure of glutathione and its synthetic pathways.

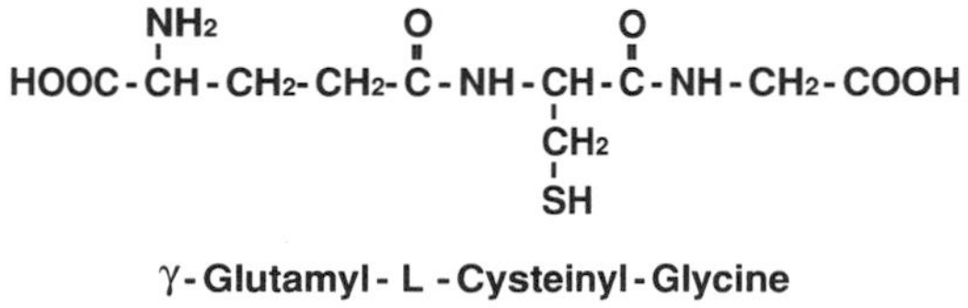

$$HOOC-\underset{\underset{NH_2}{|}}{CH}-CH_2-CH_2-\overset{\overset{O}{\|}}{C}-NH-\underset{\underset{CH_2}{|}}{\underset{\underset{SH}{|}}{CH}}-\overset{\overset{O}{\|}}{C}-NH-CH_2-COOH$$

γ- Glutamyl- L -Cysteinyl-Glycine

(Glutathione)

Glutamic acid + Cysteine + ATP $\xrightarrow{Mg^{2+}}$ γ-Glutamylcysteine + ADP + Pi

(γ-Glutamylcysteine synthatase)

γ-Glutamylcysteine + Glycine + ATP $\xrightarrow{Mg^{2+}}$ Glutathione + ADP + Pi

(Glutathione synthatase)

nervous system, glutathione is believed to be synthesized mainly in glia cells;[181,182] thus most of neuronal glutathione is probably transported from glia cells. A reduced level of glutathione is indirect evidence of oxidative stress.

Loss of glutathione is most likely a secondary change to oxidative stress, because glutathione-synthesizing enzymes were reported to be normal;[180] the activity of glutathione peroxidase was only slightly reduced (19 percent)[183] or normal,[180] and glutathione transferase was also normal.[180]

IRON IN PARKINSON'S DISEASE

Another line of evidence that suggests the presence of oxidative stress in Parkinson's disease has come from observations of iron. In Parkinson's disease, an increase in nigral iron has been confirmed by many studies.[175,184–190] Initially, iron was thought to be accumulated mainly in astrocytes and microglia; however, later observation, using x-ray microanalysis[188] and laser microprobe mass analysis,[190] revealed association of iron with melanin containing nigral neurons and with neuromelanin granules.

Iron exists in two forms, Fe^{3+} and Fe^{2+}, and most of the tissue iron is believed to be in the form of Fe^{3+}. However, a small amount of iron may exist in the form of Fe^{2+}.[191] In the presence of reducing substance, Fe^{3+} may be reduced to Fe^{2+}; Fe^{2+} is highly reactive, and it may induce free radical reactions; Fe^{2+} catalyzes Fenton reaction and Fe^{3+} mediates iron-catalyzed Haber-Weiss reaction (Fig. 12-7).[172] Both reactions produce hydroxyl radicals from hydrogen peroxide. Neuromelanin has high-affinity binding sites for iron[192] and in the presence of neuromelanin, Fe^{3+} is believed to be reduced to Fe^{2+}.[193] Thus iron accumulation would augment free radical formation. Toxicity of iron on cultured mesencephalic dopaminergic neurons is well established.[194–196]

The mechanism of iron accumulation in the substantia nigra in Parkinson's disease is not known. Iron in the plasma is bound to transferrin, the carrier protein for iron, and it is believed that the iron-transferrin complex bounds to transferrin receptors in the capillary endothels and that iron is incorporated into endothelial cells;[197,198] probably, plasma transferrin does not enter the brain. Iron transport within the brain is mediated by transferrin synthesized within the brain. Transferrin mRNA and transferrin protein are expressed in oligodendrocytes.[199] Iron not used immediately is stored as ferritin-bound iron in astrocytes and in microglia; ferritin is a storage protein for iron. There is a controversy as to the amount of ferritin in Parkinson's disease; both increases[186] and decreases[175,200] have been reported in the substantia nigra. Transferrin receptors were reported to be decreased in the putamen of Parkinson's disease and MPTP-induced mouse parkinsonism.[201]

Iron accumulation is also seen in MPTP-induced nigral degeneration;[202] therefore, it is not specific for Parkinson's disease. Elimination of iron out of the substantia nigra may be disturbed once neurons die; however, the exact mechanism of iron elimination is not known. Although the mechanism of iron accumulation in Parkinson's disease has to be studied further, once iron accumulates, it will play a role in the progression of the disease.

In addition to iron, aluminum was also reported to be increased in the substantia nigra of Parkinson's disease.[187,190]

Aluminum may also accelerate membrane lipid peroxidation in the presence of Fe^{2+}.[203]

DOPAMINE-DERIVED FREE RADICALS

In addition to the loss of glutathione and an increase in iron, dopamine itself has been implicated as a source of activated oxygen species. Hydrogen peroxide is formed by the oxidation of dopamine catalyzed by monoamine oxidase. As discussed above, hydroxyl radicals will be formed from hydrogen peroxide in the presence of iron. Dopamine in the storage vesicles is not attacked by monoamine oxidase; however, dopamine released and reuptaken in the terminals may be attacked by monoamine oxidase and may become a source of oxygen-free radicals. This was effectively shown experimentally in a metamphetamine-induced nigral toxicity model. Metamphetamine releases dopamine from the storage site,[204] which will result in increased uptake of dopamine to the terminals. Treatment of mice with metamphetamine resulted in an increase in the hydroxyl radical formation in the striatum.[205] Furthermore, dopamine may undergo autoxidation to quinoid forms; meanwhile, superoxide anions are formed.[206] Thus dopaminergic neurons are predisposed to free radical damage. Because of the potential neurotoxicity of dopamine, at one time it was postulated that L-dopa treatment might augment the degenerative process;[207] however, chronic treatment of mice with a large amount of L-dopa did not produce nigral degeneration[208] and our clinical experience do not support the idea that L-dopa is toxic.[209] Thus, some system must be present in the substantia nigra protecting them from dopamine toxicity.

OXIDATIVE DNA DAMAGE

One of the important aspects of oxidative damage is damage to DNA. Hydroxyl radicals would interact with guanine molecules of DNA to yield 8-hydroxydeoxyguanosine, which may be read as thymine at the time of DNA duplication; thus GC pair to AT pair mutation will be induced, as shown in Fig. 12-9.[210] The vulnerability of mitochondrial DNA to oxidative stress is based on its poor repair system[210–214] and high turnover rate.[215] The poor repair system of mitochondrial DNA comes from the absence of pyrimidine dimer repair mechanism,[210] the lack of a histone-like protein coating,[212] and a higher error rate of DNA polymerase-gamma,[213,214] which mediates duplication of mitochondrial DNA. In addition, mitochondrial DNA does not have introns. Mitochondrial DNA suffers 10 times more of the oxidative damage, as compared to nuclear DNA, because of lack of a repair system.[216] Therefore, many "normal" polymorphic base substitutions have been found in mitochondrial DNA.[217,218]

Furthermore, a marked increase in age-related 8-hydroxydeoxyguanosine in mitochondrial DNA has been reported in human diaphragm as well as in heart muscles[219,220] and in the brain;[221] the authors of the latter study reported a significant 10-fold increase in the amount of 8-hydroxydeoxyguanosine in mitochondrial DNA, as compared to that of nuclear DNA. Interestingly, Sanchez-Ramos et al.[222] reported increase in 8-hydroxydeoxyguanosine in the nigrostriatum of Parkinson's disease brain. These observation would suggest that

HO·+Guanosine ┈┈┈┈┈> 8-Hydroxyguanosine

G-C ┈┈┈┈> 8 OHG-C

8 OHG will be read as T

8 OHG-C ┈┈┈ duplication ┈┈> T-A+G-C

Net: Heteroplasmic transversion mutation from G-C to T-A

FIGURE 12-9 Formation of 8-hydroxydeoxyguanosine and the induction of the GC to AT transversion mutation.

acquired mutation of nuclear, as well as mitochondrial, DNA may occur under oxidative stress.

MITOCHONDRIAL RESPIRATORY FAILURE AND OXIDATIVE STRESS: WHICH COMES FIRST?

Mitochondrial respiratory failure and oxidative stress are two major contributors to nigral cell death in Parkinson's disease. The interesting question is: Which occurs first within the substantia nigra? It has been shown that glutathione deficiency leads to mitochondrial damage in brain.[223] Free radicals will impair the electron transfer components and ATPase[224] and as discussed above, oxidative stress may cause mitochondrial DNA mutations. Therefore, oxidative stress may occur first, and mitochondrial respiratory failure may follow oxidative stress. However, to prove that this is the case in Parkinson's disease, one has to answer this question: What may be the primary cause of oxidative stress? There is no good answer to this question. Glutathione synthesis is normal,[180] and iron is not increased in the early stage of Parkinson's disease.[175]

On the other hand, it has been shown that mitochondria produce free radicals such as superoxide anions,[225,226] hydrogen peroxide,[227,228] hydroxyl radicals, and semiubiquinone.[229,230] The origin of hydrogen peroxide is superoxide anions generated within mitochondria.[225,226] Furthermore, when mitochondrial electron transport slows down, a significant increase in the formation of oxygen-free radicals takes place;[231] this was also shown to be the case in MPP⁺-treated mitochondria, as revealed in the increase in superoxide formation and lipid peroxidation in the bovine heart submitochondrial particles.[232] Thus, oxidative stress may be the secondary phenomenon to the mitochondrial respiratory failure.

Jenner et al.[233] and Dexter et al.[234] tried to determine whether oxidative stress or mitochondrial respiratory failure occurred first in Parkinson's disease. They compared glutathione content and complex I activity in the substantia nigra of incidental Lewy body disease. Incidental Lewy body disease represents those patients who die from diseases other than Parkinson's disease without clinical evidence of parkinsonism or postmortem evidence to indicate dopaminergic cell degeneration, such as decrease in striatal dopamine or

homovanillic acid (HVA). They show Lewy bodies in the neurons of the substantia nigra, however. This condition has been considered to represent a preclinical state of Parkinson's disease.[235] In this condition, Jenner et al.[233] found a significant loss of glutathione in the substantia nigra; however, complex I activity, although it was reduced, did not reach statistical significance, and the loss of complex I activity was slightly less than that of glutathione.[233] Based on these findings, they concluded that oxidative stress would occur first in Parkinson's disease and that the respiratory failure was secondary to oxidative stress.

We view it another way. Suppose complex I is the only enzyme that is decreased in Parkinson's disease; then their conclusion may be right. However, not only complex I but also the alpha-ketoglutarate dehydrogenase complex is reduced in Parkinson's disease.[123] As discussed before, this is the most important enzyme in the TCA cycle, and dual loss of complex I and the alpha-ketoglutarate dehydrogenase complex would impair the mitochondrial electron transport seriously. Therefore, we believe that mitochondrial respiratory failure occurs first and that oxidative stress follows respiratory failure. We have to answer the question as to what may be the primary cause of mitochondrial respiratory failure. In this respect, epidemiological studies on environmental risk factors for Parkinson's disease and neurotoxicological studies on potential nigral neurotoxins will become very important.

ENVIRONMENTAL FACTORS AND NEUROTOXINS IN PARKINSON'S DISEASE

ENVIRONMENTAL FACTORS

As this subject has been discussed in detail in Chap. 10, only pertinent points will be discussed briefly here. Environmental factors that have been reported to increase the risk of developing Parkinson's disease include rural living and well water use,[236–240] exposure to pesticides and herbicides,[240–243] and industrial chemicals.[244] Although well water was implicated as a risk factor, analysis of 23 metals in the well water that Parkinson's disease patients had used showed no difference compared with analysis of other well water that control subjects had used.[245]

Although reports contrary to the above results do exist,[238,246] it is interesting to note that herbicides and pesticides, as well as some agricultural products, may contain substances that inhibit mitochondrial complex I activity. Rotenone, the classical inhibitor of complex I, was once used as an insecticide.

SMOKING AND PARKINSON'S DISEASE

Smoking has been inversely associated with Parkinson's disease in numerous surveys.[243,246–248] It has been assumed that the risk of parkinsonism in smokers is reduced to 20–70 percent of nonsmokers.[248] Pharmacological actions of nicotine have been studied extensively in the past. Nicotine increases the firing rate of dopaminergic nigrostriatal neurons[249,250] and causes an increase in striatal dopamine release;[251,252] thus, nicotine may have some symptomatic effect on parkinsonism, although the effect is not related to neuroprotection.

Regarding the neuroprotective role of cigarette smoking, Calne and Langston[253] postulated that carbon monoxide, which is produced in cigarette smoking, might have a scavenging action on free radicals that are produced in nigral neurons. Inhibition of monoamine oxidase B by cigarette smoking[254] is also an interesting possibility if a bioactivated nigral neurotoxin such as an MPTP-like compound is involved in the etiology Parkinson's disease.

However, in other studies, the incidence of previous exposure to smoking was not significantly different between Parkinson's disease patients and control subjects.[242,244,255] It is possible that because of a premorbid personality change people who eventually develop Parkinson's disease tend not to smoke habitually.

POTENTIAL ENDOGENOUS AND EXOGENOUS NEUROTOXINS

Discovery of MPTP has stimulated extensive studies on endogenous and exogenous neurotoxins that may accumulate in the substantia nigra and cause nigral cell death. Among these substances, tetrahydroisoquinolines (TIQs) and beta-carbolines have most extensively been studied. Tetrahydroisoquinolines are a group of compounds that are formed by condensation of aldehyde and phenylethylamine or its derivatives. Some of the representative compounds are shown in Fig. 12-10. Beta-carbolines are derived from indolamines and aldehydes. These substances are structurally similar to MPTP or MPP[+]. Monkeys chronically treated with TIQ showed a clinical syndrome similar to parkinsonism,[256] and dopamine content, biopterine level, and tyrosine hydroxylase activities in the striatum of those animals were reduced.[257] Some TIQs have been found endogenously,[258,259] and some of them are contained in certain foods.[260,261] Exogenously introduced TIQ, the prototype of TIQ compounds, can easily be transported into the brain.[262] Furthermore, TIQ was found toxic to mice[263] and to cultured mesencephalic dopaminergic neurons.[264,265] The mechanism of toxicity of TIQ on dopaminergic neurons has not yet been well elucidated; however, mitochondrial toxicity appears to be one of the possibilities, as TIQ inhibits complex I activity[266] and mitochondrial state 3 respiration.[267] In contrast to these findings, 1-methyl-derivative of TIQ prevented MPTP-induced parkinsonism in mice[268] and, interestingly enough, 1-methyl-TIQ was reduced in the striatum of Parkinson's disease.[269] Thus, structurally related less toxic compounds may prevent nigral lesion induced by more toxic substances.

In vivo metabolism of TIQ has also been studied rather extensively. Naoi et al.[270] found S-adenosylmethionine-mediated TIQ-N-methyltransferase in the human brain, and N-methylated TIQ was further oxidized to N-methylisoquinolinium ion by monoamine oxidase A and B or by autoxidation.[271] This N-methylisoquinolinium ion inhibited tyrosine hydroxylase, aromatic L-amino acid decarboxylase, and monoamine oxidase;[272] thus, N-methylated and oxidized compounds of TIQ appear to be more toxic to dopaminergic neurons, compared to the original compound.[272–274]

A dopamine-derived tetrahydroisoquinoline, that is, salsolinol was also found in human brains.[275,276] Salsolinol is also N-methylated in brain,[277] and both salsolinol and N-methylsalsolinol inhibit tyrosine hydroxylase.[278] Furthermore, oxidized N-methylsalsolinium ion binds to neuromela-

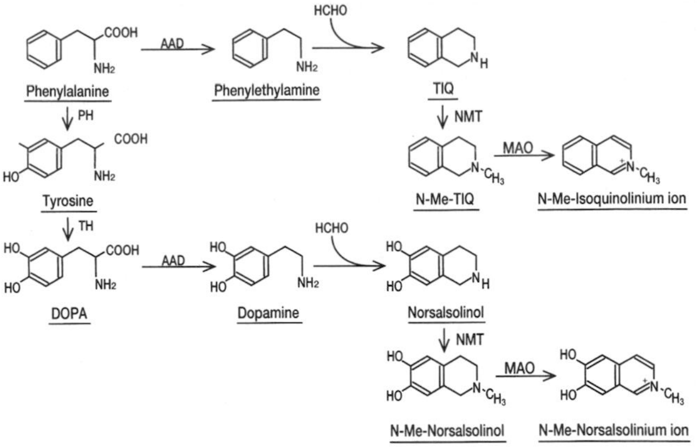

FIGURE 12-10 Structures of representative tetrahydroisoquinolines. Tetrahydroisoquinolines are formed by the condensation of phenylethylamine or its derivatives with an aldehyde. Tetrahydroisoquinolines may be N-methylated and may be further oxidized to ionic forms. PH, phenylalanine hydroxylase; TH, tyrosine hydroxylase; AAD, aromatic L-amino acid decarboxylase; NMT, N-methyltransferase; MAO, monoamine oxidase.

nin and may induce free radical reactions.[279] Beta-carbolines are another interesting class of endogenous compounds structurally similar to MPP[+].[280–282] Derivatives of beta-carbolines show differential toxicity on PC12 cells.[283] Some derivatives of beta-carbolines inhibit monoamine oxidase,[284] dopamine uptake,[285] and mitochondrial respiration.[286]

As no single toxin has yet been found to be definitely increased in Parkinson's disease, it seems possible that the detoxifying system for these compounds may be defective in patients with Parkinson's disease. Further studies on the enzymatic detoxifying system are needed to elucidate the etiology of Parkinson's disease.

GENETIC PREDISPOSITION

Although recently there has been a notion that Parkinson's disease may be an autosomal-dominant disease with low penetrance,[287,288] most of the sporadic patients who have Parkinson's disease do not appear to have a genetic disorder in the usual sense, as revealed by the low concordance rate in twin studies.[289] Nonetheless, genetic predisposition appears to be important for the acquisition of the disease. The risk of developing Parkinson's disease increases when a family member is affected with the disease.[242,243]

Genetic predispositions may be encoded in a subtle difference in the base sequences of some of the important proteins and enzymes as a form of DNA polymorphism. They may not produce a significant disturbance in the neuronal metabolism; however, when they are combined with environmental exposure to toxic substances, or when multiple mutations in different genes occur simultaneously in the same patients, Parkinson's disease may develop. Based on this concept, many candidate genes have been explored to find genetic predispositions for Parkinson's disease. Those genes include genes for enzymes that would detoxify exogenous toxic compounds; genes for proteins; and enzymes that are necessary to synthesize, transport, and metabolize dopamine and mitochondrial DNA.

The first enzyme studied was debrisoquine hydroxylase. Debrisoquine has a structure similar to that of tetrahydroisoquinoline and is metabolized by one of the hepatic cytochrome P-450 enzymes by the name of CYP2D6 (debrisoquine hydroxylase). The activity level of debrisoquine hydroxylase is genetically determined by the CYP2D6 gene as extensive metabolizers and poor metabolizers and inherited by mendelian inheritance,[290–293] and the incidence of poor metabolizers has been studied in Parkinsons disease. Barbeau et al.[294] reported a significant increase in the proportion of debrisoquine poor metabolizers compared to that of controls; however, this increase was later ascribed to antihistamine drugs that those Parkinson's disease patients were taking.[295] Since then, many studies have been reported; however, controversy exists regarding the results. Positive results were reported by Benitez et al.,[296] and negative results were reported by Marttila et al.[297] and by Liu et al.[298] in Chinese patients.

This question can be addressed by analyzing the gene for CYP2D6 by means of PCR.[299] Armstrong et al.[300] and Smith et al.[301] reported a significantly higher incidence of mutations of the gene for CYP2D6, which would result in debrisoquine-poor metabolizers among patients with Parkinson's disease, and the risk of developing Parkinson's disease was estimated as twice that in those without mutations. Kurth and Kurth[302] reported a similar result. However, the proportion of the Parkinson's disease patients who harbored the mutations resulting in a poor metabolizer was only 11.8 percent in one of the studies,[301] and mutation of this gene alone cannot explain the etiology of Parkinson's disease. Furthermore, the mutant gene frequency among Japanese patients with Parkinson's disease was not significantly different from that of the control population.[303] Recently, Tsuneoka et al.[304] found a new mutation in the CYP2D6 gene, which would result in a debrisoquine-poor metabolizer; 11.1 percent of Parkinson's disease patients and 2.2 percent of control subjects had this mutation, and the risk factor for the mutant homozygote was estimated to be 5.56.

Thus, although further studies are necessary to determine whether or not hepatic detoxifying systems play a role in the etiology of Parkinson's disease, it is interesting to note that MPTP inhibits debrisoquine hydroxylase,[305] and poor metabolizers of debrisoquine among rats showed a more pronounced and more sustained reduction of their motor activity after treatment with MPTP.[306] In addition, poor metabolizers of debrisoquine rats accumulated more TIQ in the brain.[307]

S-methylation is another detoxifying system for exogenous substances, and Waring et al.[308] reported reduced activity of erythrocyte S-methyltransferase in Parkinson's disease; however, we could not reproduce this result in Japanese Parkinson's disease patients.[309]

Possible association of Parkinson's disease with other genes has also been studied. Genes for enzymes regulating metabolism of monoamines, free radicals, and neurotoxins are targets of investigation. Kurth et al.[310] reported association of a monoamine oxidase B allele with Parkinson's disease; however, this finding was not confirmed by a subsequent study.[311] Hotamisligil et al.[312] reported association of Parkinson's disease with a MAO A allele. Association between

Parkinson's disease and genes for glutathione peroxidase, tyrosine hydroxylase, brain-derived neurotrophic factor, catalase, amyloid precursor protein, and copper-zinc superoxide dismutase have all been ruled out.[313]

Regarding mitochondrial DNA, Shoffner et al.[118] reported a higher incidence of A to G mutation in the tRNA^{gln} gene in Parkinson's disease; however, we could not reproduce this result in Japanese Parkinson's disease patients (unpublished data). As mentioned earlier, Ikebe et al.,[102] after using a sequence whole mitochondrial DNA in five patients with Parkinson's disease, found no disease-specific mutation in mitochondrial DNA of Parkinson's disease patients and no association of Parkinson's disease with certain mitochondrial genes.

Molecular genetic studies of familial Parkinson's disease are also important to find a molecule that is essential for the survival of nigral neurons. We recently found a new polymorphic mutation in the gene for the signal peptide of manganese superoxide dismutase in which valine at 9 position is replaced by alanine.[313a] Using this polymorphism and nearby DNA markers, we proved linkage of an autosomal recessive Lewy body-negative familial parkinsonism to the long arm of chromosome 6.[313b] Cloning of the causative gene for this type of familial parkinsonism would give a clue to investigate the pathogenesis of more common sporadic Parkinson's disease. Furthermore, we found that the incidence of the alanine allele was slightly but significantly higher among sporadic PD patients compared with a control group.[313a]

OTHER FACTORS

GLUTAMATE TOXICITY

Glutamate is a major excitatory neurotransmitter in the central nervous system, but it may play a role in excitotoxic neuronal damage. The most famous example is delayed neuronal death of the CA1 neurons of the hippocampus.[314] This can be completely prevented by pretreatment of experimental animals with one class of glutamate receptor antagonists, that is, N-methyl-D-aspartate (NMDA) receptor antagonists. Glutamate receptors are classified into three types, kainate, quisiqualate, and NMDA types.[315] These three classes are linked to membrane cation channels. The NMDA receptor is best defined, and it is believed that the NMDA receptor is particularly important in mediating excitotoxic cell injury.[316] When the NMDA receptor is stimulated by an agonist, influx of calcium follows the opening of the calcium channel, which is linked to the NMDA receptor. When the NMDA receptors are overstimulated, calcium homeostasis breaks down, and adverse reactions take place.[317] Glutamate receptors are believed to be present in nigral dopaminergic neurons, because the substantia nigra receives fibers from the cerebral cortex and the subthalamic nucleus.[318] In addition, intranigral injection of NMDA receptor antagonists has provided temporary relief from MPP$^+$-toxicity in experimental animals.[319] NMDA receptor antagonists show antiparkinsonian effects in animal models of parkinsonism;[320,321] however, these effects are attributable to antagonistic action on globus pallidus neurons. Also, the question of the role of glutamate receptors in the etiology of Parkinson's disease needs further studies.

NEUROTROPHIC FACTORS

In recent years, dopaminotrophic growth factors have been discovered, including brain-derived neurotrophic factor (BDNF) and glial cell line-derived neurotrophic factor (GDNF), and it has been postulated that deficiency of a dopaminotrophic factor may be a cause of Parkinson's disease; however, no such trophic factor deficiency that is specific for Parkinson's disease has yet been discovered. Nonetheless, dopaminotrophic factors are interesting and appear to be an important subject of investigation in relation to etiology and treatment of Parkinson's disease.

BDNF is present in minute amounts in the adult central nervous system[322] and promotes the survival of embryonic dopamine neurons in culture.[323,324] GDNF is a recently found neurotrophic factor that is expressed in the developing striatum[325,326] and promotes survival of cultured fetal mesencephalic dopamine neurons.[327] Pretreatment of mice or rats with intrastriatal injection of GDNF offered protection from nigral cell damage induced by MPP$^+$[328] and nigral damage by axotomy of the nigral afferent was protected by peripheral injection of GDNF.[329]

Other neurotrophic factors that have been reported to promote survival of dopaminergic neurons include neurotrophin-3 and neurotrophin-4/5,[330] basic fibroblast growth factor,[331] epidermal growth factor,[332] and a recently discovered soluble factor released from nigral type I astrocytes.[333] Interestingly, basic fibroblast growth factor was reported to be decreased in the substantia nigra of Parkinson's disease.[334]

Thus, dopaminotrophic factors may play a role in the pathogenesis of Parkinson's disease and may play a role in the treatment of Parkinson's disease, including transplantation.

Summary and Conclusion

There is ample evidence indicating that there is loss of complex I out of proportion to other electron transfer complexes in the substantia nigra of Parkinson's disease. Complex I appears to be one of the most vulnerable of the electron transfer complexes, and mitochondria appear to be the target of the initial attack in Parkinson's disease. Once mitochondrial respiration decreases, protean adverse reactions will be induced, including a decrease in ATP synthesis, disruption of mitochondrial as well as cytoplasmic calcium homeostasis, leakage of free radicals from the electron transfer chain with resultant decrease in glutathione, free radical damage to the electron transfer components as well as to other macromolecules, and DNA damage and mutations. Another important finding is the presence of oxidative stress in the substantia nigra, as revealed by a loss of reduced glutathione, an increase in lipid peroxidation, and an increase in magnesium superoxide dismutase activity. Mitochondria are considered to be the sites most intensively exposed to oxidative stress, as 90 percent of oxygen is used within mitochondria; leakage of superoxide anions and semiubiquinone radicals has been demonstrated; this is particularly true when mitochondrial electron transport decreases and leakage of free radicals increases. Thus mitochondrial respiratory failure and oxidative stress are closely related abnormalities, and once one of the two takes place, the other one will also be induced, starting a vicious cycle (Fig. 12-11).

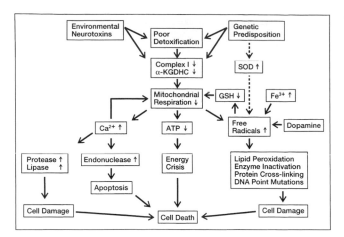

FIGURE 12-11 A schematic representation of the mechanism of nigral neuronal death in Parkinson's disease. SOD, superoxide dismutase.

One question is what the initial event is that induces this vicious cycle within mitochondria. Exogenous or endogenous toxins that may accumulate in the substantia nigra, if they exist, explain well the pathophysiological changes within nigral neurons so far reported in the literature. However, no such single neurotoxin has ever been identified in Parkinson's disease. Thus, interaction of genetic predisposition and environmental factors may play a role in the etiology of nigral cell death. With the long-term accumulation of noxious substances in genetically predisposed persons, together with the aging process, ultimately nigral neurons will die one after the other. In this respect, both epidemiological and molecular genetic studies are very important in finding the real cause of Parkinson's disease. So far no single gene mutation has ever been found to be etiologically related to Parkinson's disease; however, as Parkinson's disease is probably a heterogenous group of diseases, combinations of certain polymorphisms may eventually explain the development of the disease. Such a possibility should be pursued further to elucidate the etiology and pathogenesis of Parkinson's disease.

Acknowledgments

This study was supported in part by Grant-in-Aid for Priority Areas and Grant-in-Aid for Neuroscience Research from the Ministry of Education, Science, and Culture, Japan; Grant-in-Aid for Research on Intractable Disorders from the Ministry of Health and Welfare, Japan; and a Center of Excellence project grant from the National Parkinson Foundation, Miami, Florida.

References

1. Parkinson J: *An Essay on the Shaking Palsy.* London: Sherwood, Neely, and Jones, 1817.
2. Economo CV: Encephalitis lethargica. *Wien Klin Wochenschr* 30:581–585, 1917.
3. Duvoisin RC, Yahr MD: Encephalitis and parkinsonism. *Arch Neurol* 12:227–239, 1965.
4. Holt WL Jr: Epidemic encephalitis. A follow-up study of two hundred and sixty-six cases. *Arch Neurol Psychiatry* 38:1135–1144, 1937.

5. Hallervorden J: Anatomische Untersuchungen zur Pathogenese des postencephalitischen Parkinsonismus. *Deut Z Nervenheilk* 136:68–77, 1935.

6. Hirano A, Zimmerman HM: Alzheimer's neurofibrillary changes: A topographic study. *Arch Neurol* 7:227–242, 1962.

7. Duvoisin RC, Yahr MD: Encephalitis and parkinsonism. *Arch Neurol* 12:227–329, 1955.

8. Goto A: A long duration follow-up study of encephalitis japonica. *Folia Psychiatry Neurol Jpn* 17:326–334, 1963.

9. Mulder DW, Parrott M, Thaler M: Sequelae of Western equine encephalitis. *Neurology* 1:318–327, 1951.

10. Schultz DR, Barthal JS, Garrett C: Western equine encephalitis with rapid onset of parkinsonism. *Neurology* 27:1095–1096, 1977.

11. Walters JH: Post-encephalitic Parkinson syndrome after meningoencephalitis due to Coxsackie virus B, type 2. *N Engl J Med* 263:744–747, 1960.

12. Henner K, Hanzal F: Les encéphalites européennes à tiques. *Rev Neurol* 108:697–752, 1963.

13. Lycke E, Modigh K, Roos BE: The monoamine metabolism in viral encephalitides of the mouse. I. Virological and biochemical results. *Brain Res* 23:235–246, 1970.

14. Knotts FB, Cook ML, Stevens JG: Latent herpes simplex virus in the central nervous system of rabbits and mice. *J Exp Med* 138:740–744, 1973.

15. Marttila RJ, Arstila P, Nikoskelainen J, et al: Viral antibodies in the sera from patients with Parkinson's disease. *Eur Neurol* 15:25–33, 1977.

16. Marttila RJ, Kalimo KOK, Ziola BR, et al: Herpes simplex virus subunit antibodies in patients with Parkinson's disease. *Arch Neurol* 35:668–671. 1978.

17. Schwartz J, Elizan TS: Search for viral particles and virus-specific products in idiopathic Parkinson's disease brain material. *Ann Neurol* 6:261–263, 1979.

18. Wetmur JG, Schwartz J, Elizan TS: Nucleic acid homology studies of viral nucleic acids in idiopathic Parkinson's disease. *Arch Neurol* 36:462–464, 1979.

19. Rinne UK: Recent advances in research on parkinsonism. *Acta Neurol Scand* 57(suppl 67):77–113, 1978.

20. Marttila RJ, Halonen P, Rinne UK: Influenza virus antibodies in parkinsonism. *Arch Neurol* 34:99–100, 1977.

21. Elizan TS, Madden DL, Noble GR, et al: Viral antibodies in serum and CSF of parkinsonian patients and controls. *Arch Neurol* 36:529–534, 1979.

22. Mena I, Marin O, Fuenzalida S, Cotzias GC: Chronic manganese poisoning. Clinical picture and manganese turnover. *Neurology* 17:128–136, 1967.

23. Cotzias GC: Metabolic modification of some neurologic disorders. *JAMA* 210:1255–1262, 1969.

24. Yase Y: The pathogenesis of amyotrophic lateral sclerosis. *Lancet* 2:292–296, 1972.

25. Pentschew A, Ebner FF, Kovatch RM: Experimental manganese encephalopathy in monkeys. A preliminary report. *J Neuropathol Exp Neurol* 22:488–499, 1963.

26. Larsen NA, Pakkenberg H, Damsgaard E, et al: Distribution of arsenic, manganese, and selenium in the human brain in chronic renal insufficiency, Parkinson's disease, and amyotrophic lateral sclerosis. *J Neurol Sci* 51:437–446, 1981.

27. Barbeau A: Parkinson's disease: Etiological considerations. *Res Publ Assoc Res Nerv Ment Dis* 55:281–292, 1976.

28. Nair RMG, Kastin AJ, Schally AV: Isolation and structure of hypothalamic MSH release-inhibiting hormone. *Biochem Biophys Res Commun* 43:1376–1381, 1971.

29. Shuster S, Burton JL, Thody AJ, et al: Melanocyte-stimulating hormone in parkinsonism. *Lancet* 1:463–464, 1973.

30. Cotzias GC, Van Woert MH, Schiffer LM: Aromatic amino acids and modification of parkinsonism. *N Engl J Med* 27:374–379, 1967.

31. Katin AJ, Barbeau A: Preliminary clinical studies with L-prolyl-L-leucyl-glycine amide in Parkinson's disease. *Can Med Assoc J* 107:1079–1081, 1972.

32. Chase TN, Woods AC, Lipton MA, et al: Hypothalamic releasing factors and Parkinson's disease. *Arch Neurol* 31:55–56, 1974.

33. Davis GC, Williams AC, Markey SP, et al: Chronic parkinsonism secondary to intravenous injection of meperidine analogues. *Psychiatry Res* 1:249–254, 1979.

34. Langston JW, Ballard P, Tetrud JW, Irwin I: Chronic parkinsonism in humans due to a product of meperidine-analog synthesis. *Science* 219:979–980, 1983.

35. Ballard PA, Tetrud JW, Langston JW: Permanent human parkinsonism due to 1-methyl-phenyl-1,2,3,6-tetrahydropyridine (MPTP): Seven cases. *Neurology* 35:949–956, 1985.

36. Burns RS, Chiueh CC, Markey S, et al: A primate model of Parkinson's disease: Selective destruction of substantia nigra, pars compacta dopaminergic neurons by N-methyl-4-phenyl-1,2,3,6-tetrahydropyridine. *Proc Natl Acad Sci USA* 80:4546–4550, 1983.

37. Langston JW, Forno L, Rebert CS, Irwin I: Selective nigral toxicity after systemic administration of 1-methyl-4-phenyl-1,2,5,6-tetrahydropyridine (MPTP) in the squirrel monkey. *Brain Res* 292:390–394, 1984.

38. Forno LS, Langston JW, DeLanney LE, et al: Locus ceruleus lesions and eosinophilic inclusions in MPTP-treated monkeys. *Ann Neurol* 20:449–455, 1986.

39. Heikkila RE, Hess A, Duvoisin RC: Dopaminergic neurotoxicity of 1-methyl-4-phenyl-1,2,5,6-tetrahydropyridine in mice. *Science* 224:1451–1453, 1984.

40. Hallman H, Lange J, Olson I, et al: Neurochemical and histochemical characterization of neurotoxic effects of 1-methyl-4-phenyl-1,2,3,6-tetrahydropyridine on brain catecholamine neurons in the mouse. *J Neurochem* 44:117–127, 1985.

41. Ricaurte GA, Langston JW, Delanney LE, et al: Fate of nigrostriatal neurons in young mature mice given 1-methyl-4-phenyl-1,2,3,6-tetrahydropyridine: A neurochemical and morphological reassessment. *Brain Res* 376:117–124, 1986.

42. Matsuda L, Schmidt CJ, Hanson GR, Gibb JW: Effect of 1-methyl-4-phenyl-1,2,3,6-tetrahydropyridine (MPTP) on striatal tyrosine hydroxylase and tryptophan hydroxylase in rat. *Neuropharmacology* 25:249–255, 1986.

43. Chiba K, Trevor AJ, Castagnoli N Jr: Metabolism of the neurotoxic tertiary amine, MPTP, by brain monoamine oxidase. *Biochem Biophys Res Commun* 120:574–578, 1984.

44. Chiba K, Trevor A, Castagnoli N Jr: Active uptake of MPP+, metabolite of MPTP, by brain synaptosomes. *Biochem Biophys Res Commun* 128:1228–1232, 1985.

45. Javitch JA, D'Amato RJ, Strittmatter SM, Snyder SH: Parkinsonism-inducing neurotoxin, N-methyl-4-phenyl-1,2,3,6-tetrahydropyridine: Uptake of the metabolite N-methyl-4-phenylpyridine by dopamine neurons explains selective toxicity. *Proc Natl Acad Sci USA* 82:2173–2177, 1985.

46. Ricaurte GA, Langston JW, Delanney LE, et al: Dopamine uptake blockers protect against the dopamine depleting effect of 1-methyl-4-phenyl-1,2,3,6-tetrahydropyridine (MPTP) in the mouse striatum. *Neurosci Lett* 59:259–264, 1985.

47. Irwin I, Langston JW: Selective accumulation of MPP+ in the substantia nigra: A key to neurotoxicity? *Life Sci* 36:207–212, 1985.

48. Heikkila RE, Manzino L, Cabbat FS, Duvoisin RC: Protection against the dopaminergic neurotixicity of 1-methyl-4-phenyl-1,2,5,6-tetrahydropyridine by monoamine oxidase inhibitors. *Nature* 311:467–469, 1984.

49. Melamed E, Rosenthal J, Globus M, et al: Suppression of MPTP-induced dopaminergic neurotoxicity in mice by nomifensine and L-dopa. *Brain Res* 342:401–404, 1985.

50. Saitoh T: Suppression of 1-methyl-4-phenyl-1,2,3,6-tetrahydropyridine (MPTP)-induced dopaminergic neurotoxicity in

mouse brain by piroheptine and trihexyphenidyl. *J Neurol Sci* 83:161–166, 1988.

51. Frei B, Richter C: N-Methyl-4-phenylpyridine (MMP⁺) together with 6-hydroxydopamine or dopamine stimulates Ca²⁺ release from mitochondria. *FEBS Lett* 198:99–102, 1986.

52. Ramsay RR, Singer TP: Energy-dependent uptake of N-methyl-4-phenylpyridinium, the neurotoxic metabolite of 1-methyl-4-phenyl-1,2,3,6-tetrahydropyridine, by mitochondria. *J Biol Chem* 261:7585–7587, 1986.

53. Hoppel CL, Greenblatt D, Kwok HC, et al: Inhibition of mitochondrial respiration by analogs of 4-phenylpyridine and 1-methyl-4-phenylpyridinium cation (MPP⁺), the neurotoxic metabolite of MPTP. *Biochem Biophys Res Commun* 148:684–693, 1987.

54. Ramsay RR, Dadgar J, Trevor A, Singer TP: Energy-driven uptake of N-methyl-4-phenylpyridine by brain mitochondria mediates the neurotoxicity of MPTP. *Life Sci* 39:581–588, 1986.

55. Nicklas WJ, Vyas I, Heikkila RE: Inhibition of NADH-linked oxidation in brain mitochondria by 1-methyl-4-phenyl-pyridine, a metabolite of the neurotoxin, 1-methyl-4-phenyl-1,2,5,6-tetrahydropyridine. *Life Sci* 36:2503–2508, 1985.

56. Heikkila RE, Nicklas WL, Vyas I, Duvoisin RC: Dopaminergic toxicity of rotenone and the 1-methyl-4-phenylpyridinium ion after their stereotaxic administration to rats: Implication for the mechanism of 1-methyl-4-phenyl-1,2,5,6-tetrahydropyridine toxicity. *Neurosci Lett* 62:389–394, 1985.

57. Ramsay RR, Salach JI, Dadgar J, Singer TP: Inhibition of mitochondrial NADH dehydrogenase by pyridine derivatives and its possible relation to experimental and idiopathic parkinsonism. *Biochem Biophys Res Commun* 135:269–275, 1986.

58. Mizuno Y, Saitoh T, Sone N: Inhibition of mitochondrial NADH-ubiquinone oxidoreductase activity by 1-methyl-4-phenylpyridinium ion. *Biochem Biophys Res Commun* 143:294–299, 1987.

59. Mizuno Y, Suzuki K, Sone N, Saitoh T: Inhibition of ATP synthesis by 1-methyl-4-phenylpyridinium ion (MPP⁺) in isolated mitochondria from mouse brains. *Neurosci Lett* 81:204–208, 1987.

60. Mizuno Y, Sone N, Suzuki K, Saitoh T: Studies on the toxicity of 1-methyl-4-phenylpyridinium ion (MPP⁺) against mitochondria of mouse brain. *J Neurol Sci* 86:97–110, 1988.

61. Mizuno Y, Sone N, Saitoh T: Effects of 1-methyl-4-phenyl-1,2,3,6-tetrahydropyridine and 1-methyl-4-phenylpyridinium ion on activities of the enzymes in the electron transport system in mouse brain. *J Neurochem* 48:1787–1793, 1987.

62. Ramsay RR, McKeown KA, Johnson EA, et al: Inhibition of NADH oxidation by pyridine derivatives. *Biochem Biophys Res Commun* 146:53–60, 1987.

63. Mizuno Y, Saitoh T, Sone N: Inhibition of mitochondrial alpha-ketoglutarate dehydrogenase by 1-methyl-4-phenylpyridinium ion. *Biochem Biophys Res Commun* 143:971–976, 1987.

64. Lai JCK, Walsh JM, Dennis SC, Clark JB: Synaptic and nonsynaptic mitochondria from rat brain: Isolation and characterization. *J Neurochem* 28:625–631, 1977.

65. Dipasquale B, Marini M, Youl RJ: Apoptosis and DNA degradation by 1-methyl-4-phenylpyridinium in neurons. *Biochem Biophys Res Commun* 181:1442–1448, 1991.

66. Mochizuki H, Nakamura N, Nishi K, Mizuno Y: Apoptosis is induced by 1-methyl-4-phenylpyridinium ion (MPP⁺) in a ventral mesencephalic-striatal co-culture. *Neurosci Lett* 170:191–194, 1994.

67. Chen LB: Mitochondrial membrane potential in living cells. *Annu Rev Cell Biol* 4:155–181, 1988.

68. Walker JE, Arimendi JM, Dupuis A, et al: Sequences of 20 subunits of NADH:ubiquinone oxidoreductase from bovine heart mitochondria: Application of a novel strategy for sequencing proteins using the polymerase chain reaction. *J Mol Biol* 226:1051–1072, 1992.

69. Chomyn A, Mariottini P, Cleeter MWJ, et al: Six unidentified reading frames of human mitochondrial DNA encode components of the respiratory-chain NADH dehydrogenase. *Nature* 314:592–597, 1985.

70. Chomyn A, Cleeter MWJ, Ragan CI, et al: URF6, last unidentified reading frame of human mtDNA codes for an NADH dehydrogenase subunit. *Science* 234:614–618, 1986.

71. Krueger MJ, Singer TP, Casida JE, Ramsay RR: Evidence that the blockade of mitochondrial respiration by the neurotoxin 1-methyl-4-phenylpyridinium (MPP⁺) involves binding at the same site as the respiratory inhibitor, rotenone. *Biochem Biophys Res Commun* 169:123–128, 1990.

72. Singer TP, Ramsay RR: The reaction sites of rotenone and ubiquinone with mitochondrial NADH-dehydrogenase. *Biochim Biophys Acta* 1187:198–202, 1994.

73. Horgan DJ, Singer TP, Cassida J: Studies on the respiratory chain-linked NADH dehydrogenase XIII. Binding sites of rotenone, piericidin A, and amytal in the respiratory chain. *J Biol Chem* 243:834–843, 1968.

74. Ohnishi T, Blum H, Galante YM, Hatefi Y: Iron-sulfur clusters studied in NADH-ubiquinone oxidoreductase and in soluble NADH-dehydrogenase. *J Biol Chem* 256:9216–9220, 1981.

75. Ragan CI, Galante YM, Hatefi Y: Purification of three iron-sulfur proteins from the iron-protein fragment of mitochondrial NADH-ubiquinone oxidoreductase. *Biochemistry* 21:2518–2514, 1982.

76. Walker JE: The NADH:ubiquinone oxidoreductase of respiratory chains. *Q Rev Biophys* 25:253–324, 1992b.

77. Weiss H, Friedrich T: Redox linked proton translocation by NADH-ubiquinone reductase (complex I). *J Bioenerg Biomembr* 23:743–754, 1991.

78. Anderson S, Bankier AT, Barrell BG, et al: Sequence and organization of the human mitochondrial genome. *Nature* 90:457–465, 1981.

79. Schapira AHV, Cooper JM, Dexter D, et al: Mitochondrial complex I deficiency in Parkinson's disease. *Lancet* 1:1269, 1989.

80. Schapira AHV, Cooper JM, Dexter D, Clark JB, Jenner P, Marsden CD: Mitochondrial Complex I deficiency in Parkinson's disease. *J Neurochem* 54:823–827, 1990.

81. Mizuno Y, Ohta S, Tanaka M, et al: Deficiencies in complex I subunits of the respiratory chain in Parkinson's disease. *Biochem Biophys Res Commun* 163:1450–1455, 1989.

82. Hattori N, Tanaka M, Ozawa T, Mizuno Y: Immunohistochemical studies on complex I, II, III, and IV of mitochondria in Parkinson's disease. *Ann Neurol* 30:563–571, 1991.

83. Linnane AW, Marzuki S, Ozawa T, Tanaka M: Mitochondrial DNA mutations as an important contributor to ageing and degenerative diseases. *Lancet* 1:642–645, 1989.

84. Schapira AHV, Mann VM, Cooper JM, et al: Anatomic and disease specificity of NADH CoQ1 reductase (complex I) deficiency in Parkinson's disease. *J Neurochem* 55:2142–2145, 1990.

85. DiMauro S: Mitochondrial involvement in Parkinson's disease: The controversy continues. *Neurology* 43:2170–2178, 1993.

86. Parker WD Jr, Boyson SJ, Parks JK: Abnormalities of the electron transport chain in idiopathic Parkinson's disease. *Ann Neurol* 26:719–723, 1989.

87. Kriege D, Carroll MT, Cooper JM, et al: Platelet mitochondrial function in Parkinson's disease. *Ann Neurol* 32:782–788, 1992.

88. Yoshino H, Nakagawa-Hattori Y, Kondo T, Mizuno Y: Mitochondrial complex I and II activities of lymphocytes and platelets in Parkinson's disease. *J Neural Transm* 4:27–34, 1992.

89. Bindoff LA, Birch-Machin M, Cartlidge NEF, et al: Mitochondrial function in Parkinson's disease. *Lancet* 2:49, 1989.

90. Bindoff LA, Birch-Machin M, Cartlidge NEF, et al: Respiratory chain abnormalities in skeletal muscle from patients with Parkinson's disease. *J Neurol Sci* 104:203–208, 1991.

91. Nakagawa-Hattori Y, Hoshino H, Kondo T, et al: Is Parkinson's disease a mitochondrial disorder? *J Neurol Sci* 107:29–33, 1992.

92. Cardellach F, Martí MJ, Fernández-Solá J, et al: Mitochondrial respiratory chain activity in skeletal muscle from patients with Parkinson's disease. *Neurology* 43:2258–2262, 1993.

93. Blin O, Dsnuelle C, Rascol O, et al: Mitochondrial respiratory failure in skeletal muscle from patients with Parkinson's disease and multiple system atrophy. *J Neurol Sci* 125:95–101, 1994.

94. Shoffner JM, Watts RL, Juncos JL, et al: Mitochondrial oxidative phosphorylation defects in Parkinson's disease. *Ann Neurol* 30:332–339, 1991.

95. Mann VM, Cooper JM, Krige D, et al: Brain, skeletal muscle and platelet homogenate mitochondrial function in Parkinson's disease. *Brain* 115:333–342, 1992.

96. Anderson JJ, Ferrari R, Davis TL, et al: No evidence for altered muscle mitochondrial function in Parkinson's disease. *J Neurol Neurosurg Psychiatry* 56:477–480, 1993.

97. DiDonato S, Zeviani M, Giovannini P, et al: Respiratory chain and mitochondrial DNA in muscle and brain in Parkinson's disease patients. *Neurology* 43:2262–2268, 1993.

98. Przedborski S, Jackson-Lewis V, Fahn S: Antiparkinsonian therapies and brain mitochondrial complex I activity. *Mov Disord* 10:312–317, 1995.

99. Przedborski S, Jackson-Lewis V, Muthane U, et al: Chronic L-dopa administration alters cerebral mitochondrial respiratory chain activity. *Ann Neurol* 34:715–723, 1993.

100. Cooper JM, Daniel SE, Marsden CD, Schapira AHV: L-Dihydroxyphenylalanine and complex I deficiency in Parkinson's disease brain. *Mov Disord* 10:295–297, 1995.

101. Ikebe S, Tanaka M, Ohno K, et al: Increase of deleted mitochondrial DNA in the striatum in Parkinson's disease and senescence. *Biochem Biophys Res Commun* 170:1044–1048, 1990.

102. Ikebe S, Tanaka M, Ozawa T: Point mutations of mitochondrial genome in Parkinson's disease. *Mol Brain Res* 28:281–295, 1995.

103. Holt IJ, Harding AE, Mogan-Hughes JA: Deletions of muscle mitochondrial DNA in patients with mitochondrial myopathies. *Nature* 331:717–719, 1988.

104. Ohno K, Yamamoto T, Ozawa T: Direct sequencing of deleted mitochondrial DNA in myopathic patients. *Biochem Biophys Res Commun* 164:156–163, 1989.

105. Tanaka M, Sato W, Ohno K, Yamamoto T, Ozawa T: Direct sequencing of deleted mitochondrial DNA in myopathic patients. *Biochem Biophys Res Commun* 184:156–163, 1989.

106. Ozawa T, Tanaka M, Ikebe S, et al: Quantitative determination of deleted mitochondrial DNA relative to normal DNA in parkinsonian striatum by a kinetic PCR analysis. *Biochem Biophys Res Commun* 172:483–489, 1990.

107. Mann VM, Cooper JM, Schapira AHV: Quantitation of a mitochondrial DNA deletion in Parkinson's disease. *FEBS Lett* 299:218–222, 1992.

108. Schapira AHV, Holt IJ, Sweeney M, et al: Mitochondrial DNA analysis in Parkinson's disease. *Mov Disord* 5:294–297, 1990.

109. Lestienne P, Nelson J, Riederer P, et al: Normal mitochondrial genome in brain from patients with Parkinson's disease and complex I defect. *J Neurochem* 55:1810–1812, 1990.

110. Simonetti S, Chen X, DiMauro S, Schon EA: Accumulation of deletions in human mitochondrial DNA during normal aging: Analysis by quantitative PCR. *Biochim Biophys Acta* 1180:113–122, 1992.

111. Corral-Debrinski M, Horton T, Lott MT, et al: Mitochondrial DNA deletions in human brain: Regional variability and increase with advanced age. *Nature Genetics* 2:324–329, 1992.

112. Soon K, Hinton DR, Cortopassi G, Arnheim N: Mosaicism for a specific somatic mitochondrial DNA mutation in adult human brain. *Nature Genetics* 2:318–323, 1992.

113. Cortopassi GA, Arnheim N: Detection of a specific mitochondrial DNA deletion in tissues of older humans. *Nucleic Acids Res* 18:6927–6933, 1990.

114. Hattori K, Tanaka M, Sugiyama S, et al: Age-dependent increase in deleted mitochondrial DNA in the human heart: Possible contributory factor to presbycardia. *Am Heart J* 121:1735–1742, 1991.

115. Cooper JM, Mann VM, Schapira AHV: Analyses of mitochondrial respiratory chain function and mitochondrial DNA deletion in human skeletal muscle: Effect of ageing. *J Neurol Sci* 113:9–98, 1992.

116. Zhang C, Baumer A, Maxwell R, et al: Multiple mitochondrial DNA deletions in an elderly human individual. *FEBS Lett* 297:34–38, 1992.

117. Yen T-C, Su J-H, King K-L, Wei J-H: Ageing-associated 5 kb deletion in human liver mitochondrial DNA. *Biochem Biophys Res Commun* 178:124–131, 1991.

118. Shoffner JM, Brown MD, Torroni A, et al: Mitochondrial DNA variants observed in Alzheimer disease and Parkinson's disease patients. *Genomics* 17:171–184, 1993.

119. Yorifuji S, Ogasawara S, Takahashi M, Tarui S: Decreased activities in mitochondrial inner membrane electron transport system in muscle from patients with Kearns-Sayre syndrome. *J Neurol Sci* 71:65–75, 1985.

120. Kobayashi M, Morishita H, Sugiyama N, et al: Mitochondrial myopathy, encephalopathy, lactic acidosis and stroke-like episodes syndrome and NADH-CoQ reductase deficiency. *J Inherit Metab Dis* 9:301–304, 1986.

121. Nishizawa M, Tanaka K, Shinozawa K, et al: A mitochondrial encephalomyopathy with cardiomyopathy. A case revealing a defect of complex I in the respiratory chain. *J Neurol Sci* 78:189–201, 1987.

122. Moraes CT, DiMauro S, Zeviani M, et al: Mitochondrial DNA deletions in progressive external ophthalmoplegia and Kearns-Sayre syndrome. *N Engl J Med* 320:1293–1299, 1989.

123. Mizuno Y, Matuda S, Yoshino H, et al: An immunohistochemical study on α-ketoglutarate dehydrogenase complex in Parkinson's disease. *Ann Neurol* 35:204–210, 1989.

124. Mizuno Y, Suzuki K, Ohta S: Postmortem changes in mitochondrial respiratory enzymes in brain and a preliminary observation in Parkinson's disease. *J Neurol Sci* 96:49–57, 1990.

125. Porpaczy Z, Sumegi B, Alkonyi I: Interaction between NAD-dependent isocitrate dehydrogenase, α-ketoglutarate dehydrogenase complex, and NADH:ubiquinone oxidoreductase. *J Biol Chem* 262:9509–9514, 1987.

126. Stys PK, Waxman SG, Ransom BR: Na$^+$-Ca^{2+} exchanger mediates Ca^{2+} influx during anoxia in mammalian central nervous system white matter. *Ann Neurol* 30:375–380, 1990.

127. Reeves JP: Molecular aspects of sodium-calcium exchange. *Arch Biochem Biophys* 292:329–334, 1992.

128. Carafoli E: Intracellular Ca^{2+} homeostasis. *Annu Rev Biochem* 56:395–433, 1987.

129. Carafoli E: The Ca^{2+} pump of the plasma membrane. *J Biol Chem* 267:2116–2117, 1992.

130. Orrenius S, McConkey DJ, Nicotera F: Role of calcium in toxic and programmed cell death. *Adv Exp Med Biol* 283:419–425, 1991.

131. Nicotera P, Bellomo G, Orrenius S: The role of Ca^{2+} in cell killing. *Chem Res Toxicol* 3:484–494, 1990.

132. Wyllie AH: Glucocorticoid-induced thymocyte apoptosis is associated with endogenous endonuclease activation. *Nature* 280:555–556, 1980.

133. Arends MJ, Morris RG, Wyllie AH: Apoptosis: The role of the endonuclease. *Am J Pathol* 136:593–608, 1990.

134. Wolvetang EJ, Johnson KL, Krauer K, et al: Mitochondrial respiratory chain inhibitors induce apoptosis. *FEBS Lett* 339:40–44, 1994.

135. Hartley A, Stone JM, Heron C, et al: Complex I inhibitors induce dose-dependent apoptosis in PC12 cells: Relevance to Parkinson's disease. *J Neurochem* 63:1987–1990, 1994.

136. Mochizuki I I, Goto K, Mori H, Mizuno Y: Histochemical detection of apoptosis in Parkinson's disease. *J. Neurol Sci* 137:120–123, 1996.

137. Nicholls DJ: Intracellular Ca^{2+} homeostasis. *Br Med Bull* 42:353–358, 1986.

138. Gunther TE, Pfeiffer DR: Mechanisms by which mitochondria transport calcium. *Am J Physiol* 258:C755–C786, 1990.

139. McCormack JG, Halestrap AP, Denton RM: Role of calcium ions in regulation of mammalian intramitochondrial metabolism. *Physiol Rev* 70:391–425, 1990.

140. Halliwell B: Oxidants and the central nervous system: Some fundamental questions. *Acta Neurol Scand* 126:23–33, 1989.

141. Halliwell B, Gutteridge MC: Oxygen toxicity, oxygen radicals, transition metals and disease. *Biochem J* 219:1–14, 1984.

142. Younes M, Siegers CP: Lipid peroxidation as a consequence of glutathione depletion in rat and mouse liver. *Res Commun Chem Pathol Pharmacol* 27:119–128, 1980.

143. McCay PBM, Gibson DD, Hornbrook KR: Glutathione-dependent inhibition of lipid peroxidation by a soluble, heat-labile factor not glutathione peroxidase. *Fed Proc* 40:199–205, 1981.

144. Cadenas E, Simic MG, Sies H: Antioxidant activity of 5-hydroxytryptophan, 5-hydroxyindole, and dopa against microsomal lipid peroxidation and its dependence on vitamin E. *Free Radic Res Commun* 6:11–17, 1989.

145. Moncada S, Palmer RM, Higgs EZ: Biosynthesis of nitric oxide from L-arginine. *Biochem Pharmacol* 38:1709–1715, 1989.

146. Furchgott RF, Zawaldzki JV: The obligatory role of endothelial cells in the relaxation of arterial smooth muscle by acetylcholine. *Nature* 288:373–376, 1980.

147. Bredt DS, Glatt CE, Hwang PM, et al: Nitric oxide synthase protein and mRNA are discretely localized in neuronal populations of the mammalian CNS together with NADPH diaphorase. *Neuron* 7:615–624, 1991.

148. Hashikawa T, Leggio MG, Hattori R, Yui Y: Nitric oxide synthase immunoreactivity colocalized with NADPH-diaphorase histochemistry in monkey cerebral cortex. *Brain Res* 641:341–349, 1994.

149. Dawson TM, Dawson VL, Snyder SH: A novel neuronal messenger molecule in brain: The free radical, nitrix oxide. *Ann Neurol* 32:297–311, 1992.

150. Schuman EM, Madison DV: Nitric oxide and synaptic function. *Annu Rev Neurosci* 17:153–183, 1994.

151. Wang JF, Komorov P, Sies H, de Groot H: Contribution of nitric oxide synthase to luminol-dependent chemiluminescence generated by phorbol-ester-activated Kupffer cells. *Biochem J* 279:311–314, 1991.

152. Beckman JS, Beckman TW, Chen J, et al: Apparent hydroxyl radical production by peroxynitrite: Implications for endothelial injury from nitric oxide and superoxide. *Proc Natl Acad Sci U S A* 87:1620–1624, 1990.

153. Palmer RM, Ashton DS, Moncada S: Vascular endothelial cells synthesize nitric oxide from L-arginine. *Nature* 333:664–666, 1988.

154. Galthwaite J: Glutamate, nitric oxide and cell-cell signaling in the nervous system. *Trends Neurosci* 14:60–67, 1991.

155. Radi R, Rodriguez M, Castro L, Telleri R: Inhibition of mitochondrial electron transport by peroxynitrite. *Arch Biochem Biophys* 308:89–95, 1994.

156. Bolaños JP, Peuchen S, Heales SJR, et al: Nitric oxide-mediated inhibition of mitochondrial respiratory chain in cultured astrocytes. *J Neurochem* 63:910–916, 1994.

157. Hyman BT, Marzloff K, Wenninger JJ, et al: Relative sparing of nitric oxide synthase-containing neurons in the hippocampal formation in Alzheimer's disease. *Ann Neurol* 32:818–820, 1992.

158. Molina JA, Miménez-Miménez FJ, Navarro JS, et al: Plasma levels of nitrates in patients with Parkinson's disease. *J Neurol Sci* 127:87–89, 1994.

159. Ambani LM, Van Woert H, Murphy S: Brain peroxidase and catalase in Parkinson's disease. *Arch Neurol* 32:114–118, 1975.

160. McCord JM, Fridovich I: Superoxide dismutase. An enzymatic function for erythrocuprein (hemocuprein). *J Biol Chem* 244:6049–6055, 1969.

161. Tan YH, Tischfield J, Ruddle FH: The linkage of genes for the human interferon-induced antiviral protein and indophenol oxidase-B traits to chromosome G-21. *J Exp Med* 137:317–330, 1973.

162. Lieman-Hurwitz J, Dafni N, Lavie V, Groner Y: Human cytoplasmic superoxide dismutase cDNA clone: A probe for studying the molecular biology of Down syndrome. *Proc Natl Acad Sci USA* 79:2808–2811, 1982.

163. Weisinger RA, Fridovich I: Superoxide dismutase. Organelle specificity. *J Biol Chem* 248:3582–3592, 1973.

164. Creagen R, Rischfield J, Ricciuti F, Ruddle FH: Chromosome assignments of genes in man using mouse-human somatic cell hybrids: Mitochondrial superoxide dismutase (indophenol oxidase-B, tetrameric) to chromosome 6. *Humangenetik* 20:203–209, 1973.

165. Ho YS, Crapo JD: Isolation and characterization of complementary DNAs encoding human manganese-containing superoxide dismutase. *FEBS Lett* 229:256–260, 1988.

166. Marklund SL: Human copper-containing superoxide dismutase of high molecular weight. *Proc Natl Acad Sci USA* 79:7634–7638, 1982.

167. Marklund SL, Holme E, Hellner L: Superoxide dismutase in extracellular fluids. *Clin Chim Acta* 126:41–51, 1982.

168. Marklund SL: Extracellular superoxide dismutase and other superoxide dismutase isoenzymes in tissues from nine mammalian species. *Biochem J* 222:649–655, 1984.

169. Hendrickson DJ, Fisher JH, Jones C, Ho YS: Regional localization of human extracellular superoxide dismutase gene to 4pter-q21. *Genomics* 8:736–738, 1990.

170. Marttila RJ, Lorentz H, Rinne UK: Oxygen toxicity protecting enzymes in Parkinson's disease: Increase of superoxide dismutase-like activity in the substantia nigra and basal nucleus. *J Neurol Sci* 86:321–331, 1988.

171. Saggu H, Cooksey J, Dexter D, et al: A selective increase in particulate superoxide dismutase activity in parkinsonian substantia nigra. *J Neurochem* 53:692–697, 1989.

172. Burkitt ML, Bilbert BC: Model studies of the iron-catalyzed Haber-Weiss cycle and the ascorbate-driven Fenton reaction. *Free Radic Res Commun* 10:265–280, 1990.

173. Dexter DT, Carter CJ, Wells FR, et al: Basal lipid peroxidation in substantia nigra is increased in Parkinson's disease. *J Neurochem* 52:381–389, 1989.

174. Perry TL, Yong VW: Idiopathic Parkinson's disease, progressive supranuclear palsy and glutathione metabolism in the substantia nigra of patients. *Neurosci Lett* 67:269–274, 1986.

175. Riederer P, Sofic E, Rausch WD, et al: Transition metals, ferritin, glutathione, and ascorbic acid in parkinsonian brains. *J Neurochem* 52:515–520, 1989.

176. Sofic E, Lange KW, Jellinger K, Riederer P: Reduced and oxidized glutathione in the substantia nigra of patients with Parkinson's disease. *Neurosci Lett* 142:128–130, 1992.

177. Sian J, Dexter DT, Lees AJ, et al: Alterations in glutathione levels in Parkinson's disease and other neurodegenerative disorders affecting basal ganglia. *Ann Neurol* 36:348–355, 1994.

178. Adams JD, Kalaidman LK, Odunze IN, et al: Alzheimer's and Parkinson's disease brain levels of glutathione, glutathione disulfide, and vitamin E. *Mol Chem Neuropathol* 14:213–226, 1991.

179. Yong VW, Perry TL, Krisman AA: Depletion of glutathione in brain stem of mice caused by N-methyl-4-phenyl-1,2,3,6-

tetrahydropyridine is prevented by antioxidant pretreatment. *Neurosci Lett* 63:56–60, 1986.

180. Sian J, Dexter DT, Lees AJ, et al: Glutathione-related enzymes in brain in Parkinson's disease. *Ann Neurol* 36:356–361, 1994.

181. Slivka A, Mytilineou C, Cohen C: Histochemical evaluation of glutathione in human and monkey brain. *Brain Res* 409:275–284, 1987.

182. Raps SP, Lai JC, Hertz L, Cooper AJ: Glutathione is present in high concentrations in cultured astrocytes but not in cultured neurons. *Brain Res* 493:398–401, 1989.

183. Kish SJ, Morito C, Hornykiewicz O: Glutathione peroxidase activity in Parkinson's disease. *Neurosci Lett* 58:343–346, 1985.

184. Youdim MBH, Ben-Shachar D, Riederer P: Is Parkinson's disease a progressive siderosis of substantia nigra resulting in ion and melanin induced neurodegeneration? *Acta Neurol Scand* 126:47–54, 1989.

185. Dexter DT, Wells FR, Lees AJ, et al: Increased nigral iron content and alterations in other metal ions occurring in brain in Parkinson's disease. *J Neurochem* 52:1830–1836, 1989.

186. Jellinger K, Paulus W, Grundke-Iqbal P, et al: Brain iron and ferritin in Parkinson's and Alzheimer's disease. *J Neural Transm Park Dis Dement* 2:327–340, 1990.

187. Hirsch EC, Brandel JP, Galle P, et al: Iron and aluminum increase in the substantia nigra of patients with Parkinson's disease: An X-ray microanalysis. *J Neurochem* 56:446–451, 1991.

188. Jellinger K, Kienzl E, Rumpelmair G, et al: Iron-melanin complex in substantia nigra parkinsonian brains: An X-ray microanalysis. *J Neurochem* 59:1168–1171, 1992.

189. Sofic E, Paulus W, Jellinger K, et al: Selective increase of iron in substantia nigra zona compacta of parkinsonian brains. *J Neurochem* 56:978–982, 1991.

190. Good PF, Olanow CW, Perl DP: Neuromelanin-containing neurons of the substantia nigra accumulate iron and aluminum in Parkinson's disease: A LAMMA study. *Brain Res* 593:343–346, 1992.

191. Gutteridge JNC: Iron and oxygen radicals in brain. *Ann Neurol* 32:S16–S21, 1992.

192. Ben-Shachar D, Riederer P, Youdim MBH: Iron-melanin interaction and lipid peroxidation: Implications for Parkinson's disease. *J Neurochem* 57:1609–1614, 1991.

193. Youdim MBH, Ben-Shachar, Riederer P: Review: The possible role of iron in the etiopathology of Parkinson's disease. *Mov Disord* 8:1–12, 1993.

194. Tanaka M, Sotomatsu A, Kanai H, Hirai S: Combined histochemical and biochemical demonstration of nigral vulnerability to lipid peroxidation induced by DOPA and iron. *Neurosci Lett* 140:42–46, 1992.

195. Michel PP, Vyas S, Agid Y: Toxic effects of iron for cultured mesencephalic dopaminergic neurons derived from rat embryonic brains. *J Neurochem* 59:118–127, 1992.

196. Mochizuki H, Nishi K, Mizuno Y: Iron-melanin complex is toxic to dopaminergic neurons in a nigrostriatal co-culture. *Neurodegeneration* 2:1–7, 1993.

197. Pardridge WM, Eisenberg J, Yang J: Human blood-brain barrier transferrin receptor. *Metabolism* 36:892–895, 1987.

198. Roberts R, Sandra A, Siek GC, et al: Studies of the mechanism of iron transport across the blood-brain barrier. *Ann Neurol* 32:S43–S50, 1992.

199. Connor JR, Benkovic ST: Iron regulation in the brain: Histochemical, biochemical, and molecular considerations. *Ann Neurol* 32:S51–S61, 1992.

200. Dexter DT, Carayon A, Vidailhet M, et al: Decreased ferritin levels in brain in Parkinson's disease. *J Neurochem* 55:16–20, 1990.

201. Mash DC, Pablo J, Buck B, et al: Distribution and number of transferrin receptors in Parkinson's disease and in MPTP-treated mice. *Exp Neurol* 114:73–81, 1991.

202. Mochizuki H, Imai H, Endo K, et al: Iron accumulation in the substantia nigra of 1-methyl-4-phenyl-1,2,3,6-tetrahydropyridine (MPTP)-induced hemiparkinsonian monkeys. *Neurosci Lett* 168:251–253, 1994.

203. Gutteridge JM, Quinlan GJ, Clark I, Halliwell B: Aluminum salts accelerate peroxidation of membrane lipids stimulated by iron salts. *Biochim Biophys Acta* 835:441–447, 1985.

204. Schmidt CJ, Ritter JK, Sonsalla PK, et al: Role of dopamine in the neurotoxic effects of methamphetamine. *J Pharmacol Exp Ther* 233:539–544, 1985.

205. Kondo T, Ito T, Sugita Y: Bromocriptine scavenges methamphetamine-induced hydroxyl radicals and attenuates dopamine depletion in mouse striatum. *Ann NY Acad Sci* 738:222–229, 1994.

206. Graham DG, Tiffany SM, Bell WR, Gutknecht WF: Autoxidation versus covalent binding of quinones as the mechanism of toxicity of dopamine, 6-hydroxydopamine, and related compounds toward C1300 neuroblastoma cells in vitro. *Mol Pharmacol* 14:644–653, 1978.

207. Melamed E: Initiation of L-dopa in parkinsonian patients should be delayed until the advanced stages of the disease. *Arch Neurol* 43:402–405, 1986.

208. Hefti F, Melamed E, Bhawan J, Wurtman RJ: Long-term administration of L-DOPA does not damage dopaminergic neurons in the mouse. *Neurology* 31:1194–1195, 1981.

209. Diamond SG, Markham CH, Hoehn MM, McDowell FH: Multicenter study of Parkinson mortality with early versus later dopa treatment. *Ann Neurol* 22:8–12, 1987.

210. Cheng KC, Cahill DS, Kasai H, et al: 8-Hydroxyguanine, an abundant form of oxidative DNA damage, cause G→T and A→C substitutions. *J Biol Chem* 267:166–172, 1992.

211. Clayton DA, Doda JN, Friedberg EC: The absence of a pyrimidine dimer repair mechanism in mammalian mitochondria. *Proc Natl Acad Sci USA* 71:2777–2781, 1974.

212. Caron F, Jacq C, Rouviere-Yaniv: Characterization of a histone-like protein extracted from mitochondria. *Proc Natl Acad Sci USA* 76:4265–4269, 1979.

213. Kunkel TA, Loeb LA: Fidelity of mammalian DNA polymerase. *Science* 213:765–767, 1981.

214. Clayton DA: Replication of animal mitochondrial DNA. *Cell* 28:693–705, 1982.

215. Gross NJ, Getz GS, Rubinowitz M: Apparent turnover of mitochondrial deoxyribonucleic acid and mitochondrial phospholipids in the tissue of rat. *J Biol Chem* 244:1552–1562, 1969.

216. Richter C, Park J-W, Ames BN: Normal oxidative damage to mitochondrial and nuclear DNA is extensive. *Proc Natl Acad Sci USA* 85:6465–6467, 1988.

217. Brown WM: Polymorphism in mitochondrial DNA of humans as revealed by restriction endonuclease analysis. *Proc Natl Acad Sci USA* 77:3605–3609, 1980.

218. Horai S, Hayasaka K: Intraspecific nucleotide sequence differences in the major noncoding region of human mitochondrial DNA. *Am J Hum Genet* 46:828–842, 1990.

219. Hayakawa M, Torii K, Sugiyama S, et al: Age-associated accumulation of 8-hydroxydeoxyguanosine in mitochondrial DNA of human diaphragm. *Biochem Biophys Res Commun* 179:1023–1029, 1991.

220. Hayakawa M, Hattori K, Sugiyama S, Ozawa T: Age-associated oxygen damage and mutations in mitochondrial DNA in human hearts. *Biochem Biophys Res Commun* 189:979–985, 1992.

221. Mecocci P, NacGarvey U, Kaufman AE, et al: Oxidative damage to mitochondrial DNA shows marked age-dependent increases in human brain. *Ann Neurol* 34:609–616, 1993.

222. Sanchez-Ramos JR, Övervik E, Ames BN: A marker of oxyradical-mediated DNA damage (8-hydroxy-2'-deoxyguanosine) is increased in nigro-striatum of Parkinson's disease brain. *Neurodegeneration* 3:197–204, 1994.

223. Jain A, Martensson J, Stole E, et al: Glutathione deficiency leads to mitochondrial damage in brain. *Proc Natl Acad Sci USA* 88:1913–1917, 1991.

224. Zhang Y, Marcillat O, Giulvi C, et al: The oxidative inactivation of mitochondrial electron transport chain components and AT-Pase. *J Biol Chem* 165:16330–16336, 1990.

225. Loschen G, Azzi A, Richter C, Flohe L: Superoxide radicals as precursors of mitochondrial hydrogen peroxide. *FEBS Lett* 42:68–72, 1974.

226. Boveris A, Cadenas E: Mitochondrial production of superoxide anions and its relationship to the antimycin-insensitive respiration. *FEBS Lett* 54:311–315, 1975.

227. Loschen G, Flohe L, Chance B: Respiratory chain linked H_2O_2 production in pigeon heart mitochondria. *FEBS Lett* 18:262–264, 1971.

228. Boveris A, Chance B: The mitochondrial generation of hydrogen peroxide. *Biochem J* 134:707–716, 1973.

229. Wei YH, Scholes CP, King TW: Ubisemiquinone radicals from the cytochrome b-c1 complex of mitochondrial electron transport chain demonstration of QP-S radical formation. *Biochem Biophys Res Commun* 99:1411–1419, 1981.

230. Turrens JF, Alexandre A, Lehninger AL: Ubisemiquinone is the electron donor for superoxide formation by complex III of heart mitochondria. *Arch Biochem Biophys* 237:408–414, 1985.

231. Chance B, Sies H, Boveris A: Hydroperoxide metabolism in mammalian organs. *Physiol Rev* 59:527–605, 1979.

232. Hasegawa E, Takeshige K, Oishi T, et al: 1-Methyl-4-phenylpyridinium (MPP^+) induces NADH dependent superoxide formation, and enhances NADH-dependent lipid peroxidation in bovine heart submitochondrial particles. *Biochem Biophys Res Commun* 170:1049–1055, 1990.

233. Jenner P, Dexter DT, Sian J, et al: Oxidative stress as a cause of nigral cell death in Parkinson's disease and incidental Lewy body disease. *Ann Neurol* 32:S82–S87, 1992.

234. Dexter DT, Sian J, Rose S, et al: Indices of oxidative stress and mitochondrial function in individuals with incidental Lewy body disease. *Ann Neurol* 35:38–44, 1994.

235. Gibb WRG, Lees AJ: The relevance of the Lewy body to the pathogenesis of idiopathic Parkinson's disease. *J Neurol Neurosurg Psychiatry* 51:745–752, 1988.

236. Rajput AH, Uitti RJ, Stern W, Laverty W: Early onset Parkinson's disease in Saskatchewan—environmental considerations for etiology. *Can J Neurol Sci* 13:312–316, 1986.

237. Tanner CM, Langston JW: Do environmental toxins cause Parkinson's disease? A critical review. *Neurology* 40(suppl 3):17–31, 1990.

238. Koller W, Vetere-Overfield B, Gray C, et al: Environmental risk factors in Parkinson's disease. *Neurology* 40:1218–1221, 1991.

239. Wong GF, Gray CS, Hassanein RS, Koller WC: Environmental risk factors in siblings with Parkinson's disease. *Arch Neurol* 48:287–289, 1991.

240. Hubble JP, Cao T, Hassanein RES, et al: Risk factors for Parkinson's disease. *Neurology* 43:1693–1697, 1993.

241. Schoenberg BS: Environmental risk factors for Parkinson's disease: The epidemiologic evidence. *Can J Neurol Sci* 14:407–413, 1987.

242. Semchuck KM, Love EJ, Lee RG: Parkinson's disease: A test of the multifactorial etiologic hypothesis. *Neurology* 43:1173–1180, 1993.

243. Butterfield PG, Valanis BG, Spencer PS, et al: Environmental antecedents of young-onset Parkinson's disease. *Neurology* 43:1150–1158, 1993.

244. Tanner CM, Chen B, Wang W, et al: Environmental factors and Parkinson's disease: A case-control study in China. *Neurology* 39:660–664, 1989.

245. Rajput AH, Uitti RJ, Stern W, et al: Geography, drinking water chemistry, pesticides and herbicides and the etiology of Parkinson's disease. *Can J Neurol Sci* 14:414–418, 1987.

246. Stern M, Dulaney E, Gruber SB, et al: The epidemiology of Parkinson's disease: A case-control study of young-onset and old-onset patients. *Arch Neurol* 48:903–907, 1991.

247. Godwin-Austen RB, Lee PN, Marmot MG, Stern GM: Smoking and Parkinson's disease. *J Neurol Neurosurg Psychiatry* 45:577–581, 1982.

248. Baron JA: Cigarette smoking and Parkinson's disease. *Neurology* 36:1490–1496, 1986.

249. Lichtensteiger W, Felix D, Lienhart R, Hefti F: A quantitative correlation between single unit activity and fluorescence intensity of dopamine neurons in zona compacta of substantia nigra, as demonstrated under the influence of nicotine and physostigmine. *Brain Res* 117:85–103, 1976.

250. Anderson K, Fuxe K, Agnati LF: Effects of single injections of nictotine on the ascending dopamine pathways in the rat. *Acta Physiol Scand* 112:345–347, 1981.

251. Arqueros L, Naquira D, Zunino E: Nicotine-induced release of catecholamines from rat hippocampus and striatum. *Biochem Pharmacol* 27:2667–2674, 1978.

252. Giorguieff-Chesselet MF, Kemel ML, Wandscheer D, Glowinski J: Regulation of dopamine release by presynaptic nicotine receptors in rat striatal slices: Effect of nicotine in a low concentration. *Life Sci* 25:1257–1262, 1979.

253. Calne DB, Langston JW: Aetiology of Parkinson's disease. *Lancet* 2:1457–1459, 1983.

254. Oreland L, Fowler CJ, Schalling D: Low platelet monoamine oxidase activity in cigarette smokers. *Life Sci* 29:2511–2518, 1981.

255. Rajput AH, Offord KP, Beard CM, Kurland LT: A case-control study of smoking habits, dementia, and other illnesses in idiopathic Parkinson's disease. *Neurology* 37:226–232, 1987.

256. Yoshida M, Niwa T, Nagatsu T: Parkinsonism in monkeys produced by chronic administration of an endogenous substance of the brain, tetrahydroisoquinoline: The behavioral and biochemical changes. *Neurosci Lett* 119:109–113, 1990.

257. Nagatsu T, Yoshida M: An endogenous substance of the brain, tetrahydroisoquinoline, produces parkinsonism in primates with decreased dopamine, tyrosine hydroxylase and biopterine in the nigrostriatal regions. *Neurosci Lett* 87:178–182, 1988.

258. Kohno M, Ohta S, Hirobe M: Tetrahydroisoquinoline and 1-methyl-tetrahydroisoquinoline as novel endogenous amines in rat brain. *Biochem Biophys Res Commun* 140:448–454, 1986.

259. Niwa T, Takeda N, Kaneda N, et al: Presence of tetrahydroisoquinoline and 2-methyl-tetrahydroisoquinoline in parkinsonian and normal human brains. *Biochem Biophys Res Commun* 144:1084–1089, 1987.

260. Makino Y, Ohta S, Tachikawa O, Hirobe M: Presence of tetrahydroisoquinoline and 1-methyltetrahydro-isoquinoline in foods: Compounds related to Parkinson's disease. *Life Sci* 43:373–378, 1988.

261. Niwa T, Yoshizumi H, Tatematsu A, et al: Presence of tetrahydroisoquinoline, a parkinsonism-related compound, in foods. *J Chromatogr* 493:347–352, 1989.

262. Niwa T, Takeda N, Tatematsu A, et al: Migration of tetrahydroisoquinoline, a possible parkinsonian neurotoxin, into monkey brain from blood as proved by gas chromatography-mass spectrometry. *J Chromatogr* 452:85–91, 1988.

263. Ogawa M, Araki M, Nagatsu I, et al: The effect of 1,2,3,4-tetrahydroisoquinoline (TIQ) on mesencephalic dopaminergic neurons in C57BL/6J mice: Immunohistochemical studies—tyrosine hydroxylase. *Biog Amines* 6:427–436, 1989.

264. Niijima K, Araki M, Ogawa M, et al: N-methylisoquinolinium ion ($NMIQ^+$) destroys cultured mesencephalic dopamine neurons. *Biog Amines* 8:61–67, 1991.

265. Nishi K, Mochizuki H, Furukawa Y, et al: Neurotoxic effects of 1-methyl-4-phenylpyridinium (MPP+) and tetrahydroisoquinoline derivatives on dopaminergic neurons in ventral mesencephalic-striatal co-culture. *Neurodegeneration* 3:33–42, 1994.

266. Suzuki K, Mizuno Y, Yoshida M: Inhibition of mitochondrial NADH-ubiquinone oxidoreductase activity and ATP synthesis by tetrahydroisoquinoline. *Neurosci Lett* 86:105–108, 1988.

267. Suzuki K, Mizuno Y, Yoshida M: Inhibition of mitochondrial respiration by 1,2,3,4-tetrahydroisoquinoline-like endogenous alkaloids in mouse brain. *Neurochem Res* 15:705–710, 1990.

268. Tasaki Y, Makino Y, Ohta S, Hirobe M: 1-Methyl-1,2,3,4-tetrahydroisoquinoline, decreasing in 1-methyl-4-phenyl-1,2,3,6-tetrahydropyridine-treated mouse, prevents parkinsonism-like behavior abnormalities. *J Neurochem* 57:1940–1943, 1991.

269. Ohta S, Kohno M, Makino Y, et al: Tetrahydroisoquinoline and 1-methyl-tetrahydroisoquinoline are present in the human brain: Relation to Parkinson's disease. *Biomed Res* 8:453–456, 1987.

270. Naoi M, Matuura S, Takahashi T, Nagatsu T: A N-methyltransferase in human brain catalyzes N-methylation of 1,2,3,4-tetrahydroisoquinoline into N-methyl-1,2,3,4-tetrahydroisoquinoline, a precursor of a dopaminergic neurotoxin N-methylisoquinolinium ion. *Biochem Biophys Res Commun* 161:1213–1219, 1989.

271. Naoi M, Matsuura S, Parvez H, et al: Oxidation of N-methyl-1,2,3,4-tetrahydroisoquinoline into the N-methyl-isoquinolinium ion by monoamine oxidase. *J Neurochem* 52:653–655, 1989b.

272. Naoi M, Takahashi T, Parvez H, et al: N-methylisoquinolinium ion as an inhibitor of tyrosine hydroxylase, aromatic L-amino acid decarboxylase and monoamine oxidase. *Neurochem Int* 15:315–320, 1989.

273. Fukuda T: 2-Methyl-1,2,3,4-tetrahydroisoquinoline does dependently reduce the number of tyrosine hydroxylase-immunoreactive cells in the substantia nigra and locus ceruleus of C57BL/6J mice. *Brain Res* 639:325–328, 1994.

274. Suzuki K, Mizuno Y, Yamauchi Y, et al: Selective inhibition of complex I by N-methylisoquinolinium ion and N-methyl-1,2,3,4-tetrahydroisoquinoline in isolated mitochondria prepared from mouse brain. *J Neurol Sci* 109:219–223, 1992.

275. Sandler M, Carter SB, Hunter KR, Stern GM: Tetrahydroisoquinoline alkaloids: In vivo metabolites of L-dopa in man. *Nature* 241:439–443, 1973.

276. Sasaoka T, Kaneda N, Niwa T, et al: Analysis of salsolinol in human brain using high-performance liquid chromatography with electrochemical detection. *J Chromatogr* 428:152–155, 1988.

277. Maruyama W, Nakahara D, Ota M, et al: N-methylation of dopamine-derived 6,7-dihydroxy-1,2,3,4-tetrahydroisoquinoline, (R)-salsolinol, in rat brains: In vivo microdialysis study. *J Neurochem* 59:395–400, 1992.

278. Minami M, Takahashi T, Maruyama W, et al: Inhibition of tyrosine hydroxylase by R and S enantiomers of salsolinol, 1-methyl-6,7-dihydroxy-1,2,3,4-tetrahydroisoquinoline. *J Neurochem* 58:2097–2101, 1992.

279. Naoi M, Maruyama W, Dostert P: Binding of 1,2(N)-dimethyl-6,7-dihydroxy-isoquinolinium ion to melanin: Effects of ferrous and ferric ion on the binding. *Neurosci Lett* 171:9–12, 1994.

280. Collins MA, Neafsey E: β-Carboline analogues of N-methyl-4-phenyl-1,2,5,6-tetrahydropyridine (MPTP): Endogenous factors underlying idiopathic parkinsonism? *Neurosci Lett* 55:179–184, 1985.

281. Collins MA, Neafsey EJ, Matsubara K, et al: Indo—N-methylated β-carbolinium ions as potential brain-bioactivated neurotoxins. *Brain Res* 570:154–160, 1992.

282. Matsubara K, Collins MA, Akane A, et al: Potential bioactivated neurotoxins, N-methylated β-carbolinium ions, are present in human brain. *Brain Res* 610:90–96, 1993.

283. Cobuzzi RJ Jr, Neafsey EJ, Collins MA: Differential cytotoxicities of N-methyl-beta-carbolinium analogues of MPP+ in PC12 cells: Insights into potential neurotoxicants in Parkinson's disease. *J Neurochem* 62:1503–1510, 1994.

284. Kojima T, Naoi M, Wakabayashi K, et al: 3-Amino-1-methyl-5H-pyrido[4,3-β]indole(Trp-P-2) and other heterocyclic amines as inhibitors of mitochondrial monomania oxidases separated from human brain synaptosomes. *Neurochem Int* 16:51–57, 1990.

285. Drucker G, Raikoff K, Neafsey EJ, Collins MA: Dopamine uptake inhibitory capacities of beta-carboline and 3,4-dihydro-beta-carboline analogs of N-methyl-4-phenyl-1,2,3,6-tetrahydropyridine (MPTP) oxidation products. *Brain Res* 509:125–133, 1990.

286. Albores R, Heafsey EJ, Drucker G, et al: Mitochondrial respiratory inhibition by N-methylated beta-carboline derivatives structurally resembling N-methyl-4-phenylpyridine. *Proc Natl Acad Sci U S A* 87:9368–9372, 1990.

287. Lazzarini AM, Myers RH, Zimmerman TR Jr, et al: A clinical genetic study of Parkinson's disease: Evidence for dominant transmission. *Neurology* 44:499–506, 1994.

288. Payami H, Bernard S, Larsen K, et al: Genetic anticipation in Parkinson's disease. *Neurology* 45:135–138, 1995.

289. Ward CD, Duvoisin RC, Ince SE, et al: Parkinson's disease in 65 pairs of twins and in a set of quadruplets. *Neurology* 33:815–824, 1983.

290. Ishizaki T, Eichelbaum M, Horai Y, et al: Evidence for polymorphic oxidation of sparteine in Japanese subjects. *Br J Clin Pharmacol* 23:482–485, 1987.

291. Skoda R, Gonzalez FJ, Demierre A, Meyer UA: Two mutant alleles of the human cytochrome P-450db1 gene (*P 450C2D1*) associated with genetically deficient metabolism of debrisoquine and other drugs. *Proc Natl Acad Sci USA* 85:5240–5243, 1988.

292. Kagimoto M, Heim M, Kagimoto K, et al: Multiple mutations of the human cytochrome P450IID6 gene (CYP2D6) in poor metabolizers of debrisoquine: Study of the functional significance of individual mutations by expression of chimeric genes. *J Biol Chem* 265:17209–17217, 1990.

293. Eichelbaum M, Gross AS: The genetic polymorphism of debrisoquine/sparteine metabolism: Clinical aspects. *Pharmacol Ther* 46:377–394, 1990.

294. Barbeau A, Cloutier T, Roy M, et al: Ecogenetics of Parkinson's disease: 4 hydroxylation of debrisoquine. *Lancet* 2:1213–1215, 1985.

295. Poirier J, Roy M, Campanella G, et al: Debrisoquine metabolism in parkinsonian patients treated with antihistamine drugs. *Lancet* 2:386–387, 1987.

296. Benitez J, Ladero JM, Jimenez-Jimenez C, et al: Oxidative polymorphism of debrisoquine in Parkinson's disease. *J Neurol Neurosurg Psychiatry* 53:289–292, 1990.

297. Marttila KJ, Rinne UK, Sonninen V, Syvälahti E: Debrisoquine oxidation in Parkinson's disease. *Acta Neurol Scand* 83:194–197, 1991.

298. Liu TY, Chi CW, Yang JC, et al: Debrisoquine metabolism in Chinese patients with Alzheimer's and Parkinson's diseases. *Mol Chem Neuropathol* 17:31–37, 1992.

299. Heim M, Meyer UA: Genotyping of poor metabolizers of debrisoquine by allele-specific PCR amplification. *Lancet* 2:529–532, 1990.

300. Armstrong M, Daly AK, Cholerton S, et al: Mutant debrisoquine hydroxylation genes in Parkinson's disease. *Lancet* 339:1017–1018, 1992.

301. Smith CA, Gough AC, Leigh PN, et al: Debrisoquine hydroxylase gene polymorphism and susceptibility to Parkinson's disease. *Lancet* 339:1375–1377, 1992.

302. Kurth MC, Kurth JH: Variant cytochrome P450 CYP2D6 allelic frequencies in Parkinson's disease. *Am J Med Genet* 48:166–168, 1993.

303. Kondo I, Kanazawa I: Association of Xba 1 allele (Xba I 44kb) of the human cytochrome P-450dbI(CYP2D6) gene in Japanese patients with idiopathic Parkinson's disease, in Nagatsu T, Narabayashi H, Yoshida M (eds): *Advance in Neurology. Parkinson's Disease: from Clinical Aspects to Molecular Basis.* Wien: Springer-Verlag, 1991, vol 60, pp 111–117.

304. Tsuneoka Y, Matsuo Y, Iwahashi K, et al: A novel cytochrome P-450IID6 gene associated with Parkinson's disease. *J Biochem* 114:263–266, 1993.

305. Fonne-Pfister R, Bargetzi MJ, Meyer UA: MPTP, the neurotoxin inducing Parkinson's disease, is a potent competitive inhibitor of human and rat cytochrome P450 isozymes (P450bufI, P450db1) catalyzing debrisoquine 4-hydroxylation. *Biochem Biophys Res Commun* 148:1144–1150, 1987.

306. Jiménez-Jiménez FJ, Tabernero C, Mena MA, et al: Acute effects of 1-methyl-4-phenyl-1,2,3,6-tetrahydropyridine in a model of rat designated a poor metabolizer of debrisoquine. *J Neurochem* 57:81–87, 1991.

307. Ohta S, Tachikawa O, Makino Y, et al: Metabolism and brain accumulation of tetrahydroisoquinoline (TIQ), a possible parkinsonism inducing substance, in an animal model of a poor debrisoquine metabolizer. *Life Sci* 46:599–605, 1990.

308. Waring RH, Steventon GB, Sturman SG, et al: S-Methylation in motoneuron disease and Parkinson's disease. *Lancet* 2:356–357, 1989.

309. Nakagawa-Hattori Y, Hattori T, Kondo T, Mizuno Y: S-methylation in Parkinson's disease. *Neurology* 45:2279–2281, 1995.

310. Kurth JH, Kurth MC, Poduslo SE, Schwankhaus JD: Association of a monoamine oxidase B allele with Parkinson's disease. *Ann Neurol* 33:68–372, 1993.

311. Ho SL, Kapadí AL, Ramsden DB, Williams AC: An allelic association study of monoamine oxidase B in Parkinson's disease. *Ann Neurol* 37:403–405, 1995.

312. Hotamisligil GS, Girmen AS, Fink JS, et al: Hereditary variations in monoamine oxidase as a risk factor for Parkinson's disease. *Mov Disord* 9:305–310, 1994.

313. Gasser T, Wszolek ZK, Trofarter J, et al: Genetic linkage studies in autosomal dominant parkinsonism: Evaluation of seven candidate genes. *Ann Neurol* 36:387–396, 1994.

313a.Shimoda-Matsubayashi S, Matsumine H, Kobayashi T, et al. Structural dimorphism in the mitochondrial targeting sequence in the human MnSOD gene. A predictive evidence for conformational change to influence mitochondrial transport and a study of allelic association in Parkinson's disease. *Biochem Biophys Res Commun* 226:561–565, 1996.

313b.Matsumine H, Saito M, Shimoda-Matsubayashi S, et al. Localization of a gene for autosomal recessive form of juvenile parkinsonism (AR-JP) to chromosome 6q25.2-27. *Am J Hum Genet,* in press.

314. Simon RP, Swan JH, Griffiths T, Meldrum BS: Blockade of N-methyl-D-aspartate receptors may protect against ischemic damage in the brain. *Science* 226:850–852, 1984.

315. Watkins JC, Olverman HJ: Agonists and antagonists for excitatory amino acid receptors. *Trends Neurosci* 10:265–272, 1987.

316. Choi DW: Glutamate neurotoxicity and disease of the nervous system. *Neuron* 1:623–634, 1988.

317. Olney JW: Excitotoxic amino acids and neuropsychiatric disorders. *Ann Rev Pharmacol* 30:47–71, 1990.

318. Parent A: Extrinsic connections of the basal ganglia. *Trends Neurosci* 13:254–258, 1990.

319. Turski L, Bressier K, Rettig KJ, et al: Protection of substantia nigra from MPP+ neurotoxicity by N-methyl-D-aspartate antagonists. *Nature* 349:414–418, 1991.

320. Carlsson M, Carlsson A: Interactions between glutamatergic and monoaminergic systems within the basal ganglia—implications for schizophrenia and Parkinson's disease. *Trends Neurosci* 10:272–276, 1990.

321. Greenamyre JE, Eller RV, Zhang Z, et al: Antiparkinsonian effects of ramacemide hydrochloride, a glutamate antagonist, in rodent and primate models of Parkinson's disease. *Ann Neurol* 35:655–661, 1994.

322. Barde YA, Edgar D, Thoenen H: Purification of a new neurotrophic factor from mammalian brain. *EMBO J* 1:549–553, 1982.

323. Hyman C, Hofer M, Barde Y-A, et al: BDNF is a neurotrophic factor for dopaminergic neurons of the substantia nigra. *Nature* 350:230–232, 1991.

324. Altar CA, Boylyn CB, Fritsche M, et al: Efficacy of brain-derived neurotrophic factor and neurotrophin-3 on neurochemical and behavioral deficits associated with partial nigrostriatal lesions. *J Neurochem* 63:1021–1032, 1994.

325. Strömberg I, Björklund L, Johansson M, et al: Glial cell line-derived neurotrophic factor is expressed in the developing but not adult striatum and stimulates developing dopamine neurons *in vivo. Exp Neurol* 124:401–412, 1993.

326. Schaar DG, Sieber BA, Dreyfus CF, Black IB: Regional and cell-specific expression of GDNF in rat brain. *Exp Neurol* 124:368–371, 1993.

327. Lin L-F, Doherty DH, Lile JD, et al: GDNF: A glial cell line-derived neurotrophic factor for midbrain dopaminergic neurons. *Science* 260:1130–1132, 1993.

328. Tomac A, Lindqvist E, Lin LFH, et al: Protection and repair of the nigrostriatal dopaminergic system by GDNF in vivo. *Nature* 373:335–339, 1995.

329. Beck KD, Valverde J, Alexi T, et al: Mesencephalic dopaminergic neurons protected by GDNF from axotomy-induced degeneration in the adult brain. *Nature* 373:339–341, 1995.

330. Hyman C, Juhasz M, Jackson C, et al: Comparison of the effects of NT-3 and NT-4/5 on dopaminergic and GABAergic neurons of the ventral esencephalon. *J Neurosci* 14:335–347, 1994.

331. Park TH, Mytilineou C: Protection from 1-methyl-4-phenylpyridinium (MPP+) toxicity and stimulation of regrowth of MPP+ -damaged dopaminergic fibers by treatment of mesencephalic cultures with EGF and basic FGF. *Brain Res* 599:83–97, 1992.

332. Pezzoli G, Zecchinelli A, Ricardi S, et al: Intraventricular infusion of epidermal growth factor restores dopaminergic pathway in hemiparkinsonian rats. *Mov Disord* 6:281–287, 1991.

333. O'Malley EK, Sieber BA, Morrison RS, et al: Nigral type I astrocytes release a soluble factor that increases dopaminergic neuron survival through mechanisms distinct from basic fibroblast growth factor. *Brain Res* 647:83–90, 1994.

334. Tooyama I, Kawamata T, Walker D, et al: Loss of basic fibroblast growth factor in substantia nigra neurons in Parkinson's disease. *Neurology* 43:372–376, 1993.

Chapter 13

CLINICAL MANIFESTATIONS OF PARKINSON'S DISEASE

HENRY L. PAULSON and MATTHEW B. STERN

DEFINITIONS
DISEASE ONSET
CARDINAL MANIFESTATIONS
    Tremor
    Rigidity
    Akinesia
    Postural Instability
SECONDARY MANIFESTATIONS
    Cognitive Dysfunction
    Ocular Dysfunction
    Facial and Oropharyngeal Dysfunction
    Musculoskeletal Deformities
    Pain and Sensory Symptoms
    Autonomic Dysfunction
    Dermatologic Problems
ATYPICAL FEATURES AND DIFFERENTIAL
    DIAGNOSIS
    Young-Onset Patient
    Absent or Atypical Tremor
    Predominant Postural Instability
    Early Dementia
    Persistent Asymmetry
TREATMENT-RELATED MANIFESTATIONS
    Dyskinesias
    Motor Fluctuations
    Cognitive and Behavioral Disturbances
    Orthostatic Hypotension
CLINICAL RATING SCALES

James Parkinson's original 1817 description of the "shaking palsy" remains a remarkably accurate account of the disease now bearing his name.[1] Although the cardinal manifestations of Parkinson's disease (PD) are no different today, our understanding of the full array of parkinsonian signs and symptoms has grown immeasurably. Because of continuing advances in therapy, it is increasingly important that clinicians recognize PD in its earliest stages. Equally critical, PD must be distinguished from less common forms of parkinsonism, because prognosis and treatment may differ. In this chapter we discuss the primary and secondary clinical manifestations of PD, then address ways in which clinical signs can help distinguish it from other parkinsonian syndromes.

Definitions

Parkinsonism is a clinical syndrome characterized by specific motor deficits: tremor, akinesia (or bradykinesia), rigidity, and postural instability. At least two of these should be present to make the diagnosis. A wide variety of unrelated disease states can result in parkinsonism. The common thread linking these disorders is an underlying disruption of the dopaminergic nigrostriatal pathways that play a central role in controlling voluntary movements. This disruption can take one of many forms. It may be chemical, as is seen with drugs that deplete dopamine from intraneuronal storage sites (reserpine, tetrabenazine) or block striatal dopamine receptors (the phenothiazine and butyrophenone neuroleptics, as well as metaclopramide). Alternatively, it may stem from acute or chronic metabolic insults that cause destruction of neurons within the striatum or substantia nigra. Less commonly, the disruption may be structural, as with hydrocephalus and brain tumors. Finally, many inherited neurodegenerative disorders cause parkinsonism when the degenerative process involves the substantia nigra or striatum (as well as, depending on the particular disease, other brain regions). Causes of parkinsonism can be grouped into primary (or idiopathic), secondary (or symptomatic), the parkinsonism-plus syndromes, and hereditary neurodegenerative diseases (Table 13-1).

In contrast to parkinsonism, *Parkinson's disease* is a distinct clinical and pathological entity. It is the most common form of parkinsonism, accounting for approximately 75 percent of all cases seen in a movement disorders clinic. The *pathological* definition of PD includes massive loss of pigmented neurons in the substantia nigra and the presence of Lewy bodies.[2] Although a uniform *clinical* definition of PD has not been established, most movement disorder specialists consider the presence of two of three cardinal motor signs (tremor, rigidity, bradykinesia) and a consistent response to levodopa to indicate clinical PD.[3] The fourth clinical feature of parkinsonism, postural instability, is not included in this definition because of its frequent occurrence in other forms of parkinsonism (for example, multiple-system atrophy and progressive supranuclear palsy). Because of the broad phenotypic variability in PD, the lack of a precise and rigid clinical definition may be inevitable and, perhaps, even appropriate. A definition relying too heavily on any one clinical feature runs the risk of excluding legitimate cases. For example, one could argue that rest tremor should always be present, because this is the single most reliable sign of PD. However, a small percentage of patients *without* tremor will have a good response to L-dopa and display, at autopsy, the pathological hallmarks of PD. Also, response to L-dopa is not unique to PD, as other forms of parkinsonism may also improve with L-dopa.[4,5] Any clinical definition of PD must be flexible enough to accommodate such exceptions to the general rule.

PD is also defined, in part, by the absence of other causes of parkinsonism. Proposed exclusionary criteria for the diagnosis of PD include more than one affected relative, a remitting course, neuroleptic use within the past year, a history of encephalitis lethargica or repeated head trauma, oculogyric crisis, cerebellar signs, autonomic neuropathy, dementia from the onset of symptoms, pyramidal tract signs not explained by other focal neurological disease, and evidence of cerebrovascular disease. Some of these criteria (the use of neuroleptics, for example) make the diagnosis of PD untena-

TABLE 13-1 Classification of Parkinsonism

Primary (idiopathic)
  Parkinson's disease
Secondary (symptomatic)
  Drug-induced (phenothiazines, butyrophenones,
    metoclopramide, reserpine, alpha-methyldopa)
  Infectious (postencephalitic, syphilis)
  Metabolic (hepatocerebral degeneration, hypoxia, parathyroid
    dysfunction)
  Structural (brain tumor, hydrocephalus, trauma)
  Toxin (carbon monoxide, carbon disulphide, cyanide,
    manganese, MPTP)
  Vascular
Parkinsonism-plus syndromes
  Cortical-basal ganglionic degeneration
  Hemiparkinsonism-hemiatrophy
  Dementia syndromes
    Alzheimer's disease
    Diffuse Lewy body disease
  Multiple-system atrophy
    Parkinsonism-amyotrophy
    Shy-Drager syndrome
    Sporadic olivopontocerebellar degeneration
    Striatonigral degeneration
  Parkinsonism-dementia-ALS complex of Guam
    (Lytico-Bodig)
  Progressive supranuclear palsy
Hereditary degenerative diseases
  Autosomal-dominant cerebellar ataxias (includes Machado-
    Joseph disease)
  Hallervorden-Spatz disease
  Huntington's disease
  Mitochondriopathies
  Neuroacanthocytosis
  Wilson's disease

ble. Others, however, do not entirely rule out the possibility of PD. There may, for example, be a strong familial tendency in a subset of PD, and autonomic dysfunction is quite common among PD patients. In such cases, exclusionary criteria should weigh heavily, but not solely, in deciding whether a patient has PD. As a case in point, the patient who initially presents with disabling and overwhelming autonomic dysfunction is unlikely to have PD, but the tremulous and bradykinetic patient with minor autonomic complaints may well have it.

Its wide clinical variability has led some investigators to group PD into several subtypes,[6,7] including *juvenile* and *young-onset* forms, *tremor-dominant* versus *postural instability*-dominant forms, and *benign* versus *malignant* forms of PD. Whether these clinically defined subtypes correspond to differences at the biochemical or pathophysiological levels is unknown. Regardless, making such distinctions seems valid and useful. Studies indicate, for example, that young-onset patients are more likely to display exquisite sensitivity to L-dopa and develop drug-related dyskinesias sooner than do older patients.[8–10] Likewise, tremor-dominant PD tends to follow a more slowly progressive, benign course than postural instability-dominant disease.[7]

Disease Onset

PD is one of the most common causes of neurological disability, affecting 1 percent of the population over age 55. It is typically a disease of the middle to late years, beginning at a mean age of 50–60 years and progressing slowly over a 10- to 20-year period.[11–13] The age of onset assumes a broad bell-shaped distribution, with roughly 5 percent of cases beginning before age 40 (by definition, young-onset PD).

The underlying pathology of PD, the loss of nigral neurons, is believed to occur slowly in the decades preceding the onset of symptoms. Up to 80 percent of dopaminergic neurons are lost before the cardinal signs and symptoms of PD first appear. It is not surprising, then, that PD usually begins insidiously and is heralded by a prodrome of nonspecific symptoms.[14] Easy fatiguability, malaise, or personality changes may appear years before the first motor sign. Patients frequently first experience motor signs in subtle ways, such as a feeling of weakness, mild incoordination ("My golf game is off"), or difficulty writing. The "sudden weakness" that some patients describe may prove, after questioning, to be sudden awareness of weakness. Many will also complain of pain or tension confined to the muscles of one shoulder or arm, prompting a visit to an orthopedist before a neurologist. Asymmetric onset is typical in PD and has even been proposed as a defining criterion.[15]

Diagnosing PD in this earliest stage is difficult. The nonspecific nature of the symptoms and signs suggests a broad differential diagnosis, including myasthenia gravis, cerebrovascular disease, and multiple sclerosis. Mild parkinsonian features on examination—an intermittent tremor confined to one or several fingers, subtle cogwheel rigidity—may be the first clue that PD is the underlying problem. In many cases the diagnosis will only become apparent as motor signs develop in the ensuing years.

Cardinal Manifestations

TREMOR

The rest tremor of PD, the "involuntary tremulous motion" first noted by Parkinson, remains the best-known and most readily identifiable sign of disease (Table 13-2). In 75 percent of patients it is the first motor manifestation, usually beginning unilaterally in the distal limb, in most cases an arm. In some patients the tremor may be confined to a single finger for years before the appearance of other signs. The tremor often involves rhythmic, alternating opposition of the forefinger and thumb in the classic, stereotypic "pill-rolling" tremor. In others, it takes the form of a simple to-and-fro motion of the hand or arm. Occasionally, patients will complain that their tremor is felt internally, with only subtle external signs. In all cases, it oscillates with a characteristic frequency of 3–5 cycles/second. Over the course of several years, tremor usually spreads proximally in the affected arm before involving the ipsilateral leg and, finally, the contralat-

TABLE 13-2 Manifestations of Parkinson's Disease

Cardinal manifestations
  Rest tremor
  Rigidity
  Akinesia/bradykinesia
  Postural instability
Secondary manifestations
  Cognitive/neuropsychiatric
    Anxiety
    Bradyphrenia
    Dementia
    Depression
    Sleep disturbance
  Cranial nerve/facial
    Blurred vision (impaired upgaze, blepharospasm)
    Dysarthria
    Dysphagia
    Glabellar reflex (Myerson's sign)
    Masked facies
    Olfactory dysfunction
    Sialorrhea
  Musculoskeletal
    Compression neuropathies
    Dystonia
    Hand and foot deformities
    Kyphoscoliosis
    Peripheral edema
  Autonomic (including gastrointestinal and genitourinary
     symptoms)
    Constipation
    Lightheadedness (orthostatic hypotension)
    Increased sweating
    Sexual dysfunction (impotence, loss of libido)
    Urinary dysfunction (frequency, hesitancy or urgency)
  Sensory
    Cramps
    Pain
    Paresthesias
  Skin
    Seborrhea

eral limbs. Although tremor is bilateral in advanced disease, it often maintains some asymmetry throughout the course. In later stages, an accompanying tremor of the face, lips, or chin is not uncommon.

The tremor of PD is termed a rest tremor because it is present at rest and usually abates when the affected limb performs a motor task. Not uncommonly, at the same time that tremor decreases in an affected arm during voluntary movement, it increases asynchronously in the resting contralateral limb. When lower limbs are involved, tremor will be present in the legs when the patient is supine or sitting but disappears when the patient bears weight. Tremor often increases in the arms during walking; hence, the clinician should watch the arms as closely as the legs when examining a patient's gait. In the course of a day, tremor will occur intermittently and vary in intensity. It disappears in sleep and worsens with stress or anxiety. It is important to note that patients commonly also have a postural or kinetic component to their tremor, as well as an exaggerated physiological tremor. A moderate degree of action tremor is consistent

with PD, particularly in more advanced stages of disease.[16] However, a pronounced action tremor at disease onset should suggest other diagnoses.

The pathophysiological basis of the parkinsonian tremor is unknown.[17] It probably is centrally generated, as the frequency of tremor is the same in limbs as in the face and lips. Microelectrode recordings in patients and monkeys indicate that cells in the ventrolateral thalamus may serve as tremorigenic pacemakers. Delwaide and Gonce have proposed a dual mechanism to explain the tremor, whereby a thalamic pacer triggers the oscillation and is in turn influenced by peripheral kinesthetic input.[17] Currently, it is unclear how the selective loss of nigrostriatal dopaminergic input leads to hyperactivity in this putative long-loop reflex. That tremor can be affected by emotional state, motor activity, and general health suggests that the involved circuitry is linked to, and modulated by, a wide array of circuits within the nervous system.

RIGIDITY

The stiffness of PD is caused by an involuntary increase in muscle tone that can affect all muscle groups—axial and limb muscles, flexor as well as extensor muscles. On examination, rigidity is noted as increased resistance to passive movement of a limb segment. The amount of resistance remains fairly constant through the entire range of motion, both flexion and extension, and is not greatly influenced by the speed or force with which the movement is performed. This distinguishes it from spasticity, which displays a velocity-dependent increase in tone and variable resistance through the range of motion (clasp-knife phenomenon). Spasticity is further distinguished from PD by its associated pathological reflexes, weakness, and silent electromyogram at rest; in PD the EMG resembles ordinary tonic voluntary muscle activity.[18] Likewise, rigidity can be distinguished from the gegenhalten tone seen in a variety of encephalopathic conditions, because gegenhalten is intermittent and tends to increase in opposition to an applied force.

The rigidity of PD can be either smooth (lead pipe) or rachety (cogwheel). Cogwheeling is thought to reflect the superimposed rest tremor. Both rigidity and cogwheeling can be brought out (reinforced) by voluntary movement in the contralateral limb. As with tremor, rigidity frequently begins unilaterally, may vary during the course of the day, and is influenced by mood, stress, and medications.

Although the rigidity of PD likely limits the speed of voluntary movements, it is unclear to what degree it contributes to motor impairment. Some patients with prominent rigidity have relatively unimpeded motor function. Coincident akinesia probably plays a greater role than rigidity in determining a patient's degree of disability.

As with tremor, the pathophysiological basis of rigidity is not fully understood.[17] Afferent impulses must play a role, because sectioning of dorsal roots or application of local anesthetic in the epidural or subarachnoid space decreases rigidity.[17,19] Competing theories explaining rigidity—not necessarily mutually exclusive—have invoked either increased activity in long-loop reflex pathways or abnormalities in spinal interneuron function because of altered input from descending tracts. There may be changes intrinsic to the muscle as well. The rigidity of PD usually responds to dopaminergic therapy.

AKINESIA

In the strictest sense, akinesia means the absence of movement. Yet, it is also the term used to define the difficulty PD patients have in initiating and executing a motor plan. It is often the most disabling sign of PD, experienced by virtually all patients and manifested in a variety of ways (see Table 13-3). As a general rule, the nature and severity of akinesia worsen over the course of illness. Early on, hypokinesia (falling short of the mark when executing a movement) is nearly always present, later progressing to bradykinesia (slowed movements) and, finally, to akinesia. Early signs may be confined to distal muscles (micrographia, decreased dexterity, impaired sequential finger movements) but, eventually, all muscle groups can be affected. Particularly difficult for patients are sequential motor acts, such as alternating pronation-supination of the hand, and complex motor acts, such as buttoning a shirt. Quick repetitive movements, such as repeated opposition of the forefinger and thumb, typically will show a rapid decrease in both amplitude and frequency. In more advanced stages, patients have difficulty rising from a chair and display a generalized slowing of voluntary movements. Facial and vocal manifesations of akinesia (hypomimia, hypophonia, dysarthria, and sialorrhea) are often apparent to the clinician before the formal examination has even begun.

The pathophysiology of motor control in PD is a field unto itself. Researchers generally agree that patients with PD have little or no trouble "planning" a motor task. The problem lies in initiating and executing the sequential motor acts that comprise a particular motor program.[20,21] When a simple movement at one joint is attempted, the initial burst of agonist activity is inappropriately small; hence, the resulting movement is too slow and falls short of the intended target. The problem is further exacerbated in complex motor acts, as it is particularly difficult for PD patients to execute two motor programs simultaneously. Because these are the kinds of movements necessary for performing normal daily activities, it is understandable why akinesia is usually the most disabling sign of PD.

It is increasingly clear that dopamine plays a central role in modulating the striatal pathways that control motor initiation, execution, and adaptation.[22] Fortunately for patients, dopaminergic therapy is often quite effective in treating the varied manifestations of akinesia.

POSTURAL INSTABILITY

Postural instability with associated gait disorder is usually the last of the four cardinal signs to appear. Yet it often proves to be the most disabling, least treatable manifestation of the disease and represents the major contributing factor in progression from mild bilateral disease (Hoehn and Yahr stage 2) to wheelchair confinement (stage 5).[23] No single factor is alone responsible for postural instability and gait disturbance. Rather, it stems from a combination of deficits, including changes in postural adjustment, the loss of postural reflexes, rigidity, and akinesia.

Loss of postural reflexes often occurs early but is rarely disabling until years later. The patient adopts a stooped posture with flexion of the neck and trunk. The arms are held in an adducted position with elbows flexed. Once a patient starts to lose the ability to make rapid postural corrections, a tendency to fall forward or backward becomes evident. The examiner can elicit this finding with the "pull test," standing behind the patient and pulling backward on the shoulders: Patients with decreased righting reflexes will take more than two steps backward before catching themselves (retropulsion), whereas others with more advanced disease will fall unless caught.

The earliest sign of gait disturbance is often decreased arm swing, but over time patients also begin to walk with a short, shuffling, uncertain step. Gait initiation and turning become particularly difficult. Once walking has begun, the loss of postural reflexes and stooped posture combine to produce a *festinating gait:* In an effort to retain balance, the patient walks faster and faster in a shuffling manner, as the legs try to catch up with the body's forward momentum. In many cases, stopping is accomplished only by grabbing onto an object or running into a wall. Although the gait is unsteady, the base is usually minimally or not at all widened, and truncal ataxia is absent. Falls become increasingly common over time, in many cases resulting in hip fracture.

Freezing is a phenomenon distinct from other forms of akinesia. We discuss this poorly understood phenomenon here in relation to the gait disorder, because it is during ambulation that freezing proves most troublesome.[24] Patients freeze especially when starting to walk (start-hesitation), attempting to turn, or approaching a narrow or crowded space (doorways, corners, closets, a sidewalk with heavy traffic). Also called "motor blocks," freezing may occur just before

TABLE 13-3 Signs of Akinesia in Parkinson's Disease

General
    Delayed motor initiation
    Slowed voluntary movements (bradykinesia)
    Diminution in voluntary movements (hypokinesia)
    Rapid fatigue with repetitive movements
    Difficulty executing sequential actions
    Inability to perform simultaneous actions
    Decreased dexterity
    Freezing
Specific
    Masked facies (hypomimia)
    Decreased blink
    Hypometric saccades
    Hypophonia
    Dysarthria
    Sialorrhea
    Micrographia
    Dysdiadochokinesia
    Difficulty rising from a chair
    Shuffling gait, short steps
    Decreased arm swing

a patient reaches an intended target, for example, a chair or bed. Sitting "en bloc" represents a special form of freezing in which a patient literally falls into a chair. Freezing more often occurs in advanced disease and after years of levodopa therapy.[24]

The opposite of freezing can also occur in PD. *Kinesia paradoxica* is the term used to describe sudden short periods of relatively effortless mobility experienced by some patients. These episodes are unrelated to medication and should not be confused with the "on-off" phenomenon that occurs in advanced patients on dopaminergic therapy.

The mechanisms that control normal locomotion and postural stability are complex, involving neural structures from cerebral cortex to proprioceptive sensory afferents. The pathophysiological basis of gait and postural abnormalities in PD is not well understood but is almost certainly multifactorial. Its multifactorial origin may help explain why postural instability and gait disturbance are the least treatable signs of PD.

Secondary Manifestations

Many secondary manifestations[25] actually represent special cases of one of the four cardinal signs, yet are common and distinct enough to merit separate discussion (see Table 13-2).

COGNITIVE DYSFUNCTION

Although prodromal symptoms of PD can include changes in mood or personality, the mental status remains relatively intact in early PD. Tests of cognitive function demonstrate mild-to-moderate deficits, including visuospatial impairment, attentional set-shifting difficulties, and poor executive function, as demonstrated in the Wisconsin Card Sorting and verbal fluency tests (reviewed in Ref. 26; see also Refs. 27–29).[26–29] Patients demonstrate slowed thinking and slow responses to questions (bradyphrenia) but usually get the answers right.[30] Bradyphrenia may represent the cognitive analogue of bradykinesia but does not correlate with the degree of motor deficits and may, in part, reflect disruption of nondopaminergic pathways. Signs of dementia, if present at the onset of illness, should suggest diseases other than PD, including Alzheimer's disease, diffuse Lewy body disease, progressive supranuclear palsy (PSP), and Creutzfeldt-Jakob disease.

Although not an early finding in PD, dementia eventually occurs in 20–30 percent of PD patients, making it the third most common cause of dementia in the elderly.[31,32] Affected patients perform poorly on visuospatial and perceptual motor tests, but language function is typically spared (although grammatic complexity is reduced, aphasia is not present). Delayed recall memory is not impaired to the degree it is in Alzheimer's disease.[33] The dementia of PD has been called a "subcortical" dementia, although there is considerable overlap with cortical forms of dementia, such as Alzheimer's disease.[26,33] Subcortical features of PD dementia include bradyphrenia, psychomotor retardation and depression, the absence of aphasia, and relatively mild memory impairment. Many patients will nonetheless develop dementia that is indistinguishable from Alzheimer's disease. Risk factors for dementia include older age and masked facies at onset of PD, depression, levodopa-induced hallucinations, and akinetic-rigid predominant features.[34,35]

As PD progresses, patients often become passive and apathetic, relying on others to make decisions or do their talking. Many will become reclusive, fearful of going outside. Depression is common in PD, affecting up to one-half of patients.[36,37] It is generally mild to moderately severe and can take the form of chronic major depression or fluctuating dysthymia. Serotonin metabolites are reduced in depressed PD patients, suggesting an endogenous form of depression that may be intrinsic to the parkinsonian disease process. However, depression also can occur in reaction to chronic motor disability. Antidepressants prove helpful for both reactive and endogenous depression in PD.

OCULAR DYSFUNCTION

Oculomotor function is generally preserved in PD, in contrast to what is found in many parkinsonism-plus syndromes. Some patients will complain of blurred vision or difficulty reading, which may be a result of weakened convergence. Limited upgaze is common in PD patients but can also be seen in the asymptomatic elderly. Vertical gaze paresis *downward* is not seen in PD; if it is present, one should consider the diagnosis of PSP or multiple-system atrophy. Although slow saccades and jerky ocular pursuits are often seen in PD, ophthalmoparesis does not occur, and lid retraction is relatively uncommon.

The frequency of spontaneous eye blinking is reduced. A typical feature of PD is persistent eye blinking when the forehead is repeatedly tapped, called the glabellar reflex or Myerson's sign. This primitive reflex is intrinsic to the disease process and does not indicate dementia. Other primitive reflexes can also be seen in PD without associated dementia, most commonly, the snout reflex.[38]

FACIAL AND OROPHARYNGEAL DYSFUNCTION

Facial akinesia leads to a mask-like, staring expression (masked facies). The speech of PD is a hypokinetic dysarthria, typically monotonal, hypophonic, and muffled. The first syllable may be repeated (pallilalia), and words and phrases may rush together. Excessive saliva with drooling occurs in up to 80 percent of patients and is a consequence of decreased transfer of saliva to the pharynx.[39] Dysphagia, a consequence of pharyngeal akinesia, usually occurs later in disease and may prove life threatening. Early and prominent dysphagia should suggest other forms of parkinsonism (PSP, MSA).

Decreased olfactory function is an early sign in PD.[40,41] Reduced ability to smell is not something patients complain about unless specifically asked; even then, only 25 percent will have noticed a change. However, testing indicates that decreased smelling is a significant and widespread manifestation, occurring early in disease and bilaterally. It neither correlates with motor signs nor progresses over the course of illness. Olfactory dysfunction may help distinguish PD from other forms of parkinsonism, because patients with PSP and essential tremor do not show similar changes.

MUSCULOSKELETAL DEFORMITIES

Deformities of the hands and feet are common in PD. The parkinsonian hand displays ulnar deviation, flexion of the metacarpophalangeal and distal interphalangeal joints, and extension of the proximal interphalangeal joints (so-called striatal hand). Likewise, the great toe can be tonically extended, with the remaining toes curled clawlike. Dystonic cramps, particularly of the feet, may be troublesome. These can occur before medication or as a side effect of dopaminergic therapy.

Coincident with rigidity, changes occur in the curvature of the spine. Early on, mild scoliosis may be seen, concave contralateral to the affected side. As a result the patient may walk tilted away from the affected side. Later, kyphosis becomes prominent and contributes to the disabling postural changes of advanced disease.

Many patients complain of swelling in the extremities. This is probably a consequence of immobility, representing peripheral edema from venous stasis. Measures taken to improve mobility will often reduce the swelling. Rarely, the profoundly immobile patient will develop compression neuropathies.

PAIN AND SENSORY SYMPTOMS

Although peripheral nerve disease is not associated with PD, pain and sensory complaints are surprisingly common. In a random group of parkinsonians, approximately 50 percent complained of pain directly related to their parkinsonism.[42] Pain is often proportional to the degree of motor dysfunction and may take the form of muscle cramps, stiffness, dystonia, radiculopathy, or arthralgias.

Sensory complaints, also very common, are not associated with signs of peripheral neuropathy.[43,44] Numbness, burning, or tingling may occur at any stage of the disease, independent of medications and the degree of motor deficits and, in some cases, even precedes motor manifestations. Paresthesias were noted in 40 percent of patients in one series, more commonly occurring on the affected side in hemiparkinsonians.[43] The basis of sensory disturbance in PD is unknown but possibly reflects a role for the basal ganglia in sensory processing. One postulated mechanism is altered striatal input to sensory centers in the thalamus.

AUTONOMIC DYSFUNCTION

Although autonomic signs are more closely associated with multiple-system atrophy, nearly all PD patients experience some degree of autonomic dysfunction during the course of illness.[45] Careful measurements of autonomic function in PD (pulse variability, orthostatic blood pressure, response to Valsalva maneuver, and cold pressor stimuli) indicate that the underlying disease does cause mild autonomic insufficiency.[46]

By far the most frequent complaints referable to autonomic insufficiency are bowel and bladder symptoms. Constipation is an exceedingly common problem that can become quite serious, occasionally leading to intestinal pseudoobstruction or megacolon.[39] The basis of constipation is reduced colonic motility, possibly a direct consequence of PD as Lewy body neuropathology has been described within the myenteric plexus. Other factors exacerbate the problem, including poor diet, fluid depletion, reduced physical activity, and antiparkinsonian medications. Urinary difficulties include hesitancy, urgency, and increased frequency. Rarely, catheterization is required for an atonic bladder.

Sexual dysfunction is a frequent complaint and may involve both loss of libido and impotence. The cause of sexual problems is likely multifactorial, with possible contributing factors including a depressed mood, chronic motor disability, and partial or complete loss of autonomic innervation. Episodic sweating occurs in some patients. Frank orthostatic hypotension is uncommon in PD and is more likely a result of medications (particularly dopamine agonists) rather than the underlying disease.

DERMATOLOGIC PROBLEMS

Chronic seborrhea is a common finding. This leads to greasy skin, particularly on the face, that can be associated with erythema and scaly patches in skin creases.

Atypical Features and Differential Diagnosis

Recognizing classic cases of PD should not be difficult. The 60-year-old man who presents with a unilateral rest tremor and whose examination reveals masked facies, hypophonic dysarthria, generally slowed movements, and cogwheel rigidity almost certainly has Parkinson's disease. A good response to L-dopa will clinch the diagnosis. Yet many cases are not so straightforward. When the history is suggestive but the signs not obvious, every effort should be made to bring out cardinal features—for example, subtle cogwheel rigidity in a limb might only be present with reinforcement, and a hand tremor may appear only when a patient walks. Atypical features, either at onset or during the course of disease, should raise suspicion of other forms of parkinsonism (see Table 13-4).[47]

A complete history remains critical in establishing the correct diagnosis. The physician must enquire thoroughly about medications, possible environmental exposures, and family history of neurological disease, including essential tremor and dominantly inherited progressive ataxia, as well as parkinsonism. Careful attention should be paid to the precise sequence of symptoms experienced by the patient. For example, did tremor or rigidity begin unilaterally, as is typically the case in PD? In the patient on L-dopa, which symptoms improved in response to medication, by how much and for how long? Accurately reconstructing a patient's disease history may be difficult, given the insidious onset of PD, but well worth the effort if atypical features are uncovered.

YOUNG-ONSET PATIENT

Most movement disorder specialists define patients whose symptoms begin before age 40 as "young-onset PD."[48,49] "Juvenile-onset" is a separate term used by many authors to

TABLE 13-4 Atypical Features in Parkinsonism

Early or Predominant Feature	Disease
Young onset	Juvenile PD, HS, WD
Minimal or absent tremor	SND, PSP, SDS
	Vascular parkinsonism
	Hydrocephalic parkinsonism
Atypical tremor	CBGD, OPCD
Postural instability	PSP, MSA (all forms)
	Vascular parkinsonism
	Hydrocephalic parkisonism
Ataxia	MSA (particularly OPCD)
Pyramidal signs	MSA (particularly SND), CBGD
	Vascular or hydrocephalic parkinsonism
Neuropathy	MSA (particularly parkinsonism-amyotrophy)
Marked motor asymmetry	Hemiparkinsonism-hemiatrophy CBGD
Symmetric onset	SND
	Vascular or hydrocephalic parkinsonism
Myoclonus	CBGD, CJD
Dementia	LBD, AD, CJD, MID, PSP
Focal cortical signs	CBGD
Alien limb sign	CBGD
Oculomotor deficits	PSP, OPCA, CBGD
Dysautonomia	MSA (particularly SDS)

AD, Alzheimer's disease; CBGD, cortical-basal ganglionic degeneration; CJD, Creutzfeldt-Jakob disesae; HS, Hallervorden-Spatz disease; LBD, diffuse Lewy body disease; MID, multi-infarct dementia; MSA, multiple-system atrophy; OPCD, olivopontocerebellar degeneration; PSP, progressive supranuclear palsy; SDS, Shy-Drager syndrome; SND, striatonigral degeneration; WD, Wilson's disease.

refer to patients whose parkinsonism begins in childhood (before age 20). Disease in the former group resembles older-onset PD in most respects, and probably represents the tail end of the bell-shaped distribution for PD on the younger-age side. In contrast, juvenile-onset disease, although also resembling adult-onset PD in many ways,[50] may represent a distinct entity. Juvenile-onset patients are more likely to have a family history of PD and to display dystonic features as part of their parkinsonism. It is important not to confuse dystonia in juvenile-onset parkinsonism with dopa-responsive dystonia, another juvenile-onset disease.

Parkinsonism in the adolescent or young adult should never be assumed to be PD until other causes have been ruled out. Wilson's disease must be excluded by a slit-lamp examination and laboratory tests of copper, ceruloplasmin, and hepatocellular enzymes. A family history of neurological disease should raise concern about triplet repeat disorders, such as Huntington's and Machado-Joseph disease, both of which show anticipation in families and can present as juvenile parkinsonism. Signs of spasticity and retinal degeneration suggest Hallervorden-Spatz disease,[51] a diagnosis that is further supported by magnetic resonance imaging (MRI) evidence of symmetric signal abnormalities in the globus pallidus.

ABSENT OR ATYPICAL TREMOR

The absence of rest tremor, both by history and examination, makes the diagnosis of PD difficult. If the patient also fails to respond to L-dopa, the diagnosis is in serious doubt. A careful search, once again, for symptomatic causes of parkinsonism must be undertaken. The patient should be reexamined with a close look for downgaze paresis and facial dystonia (PSP), orthostatic hypotension (Shy-Drager syndrome), bulbar dysfunction with truncal ataxia (sporadic olivopontocerebellar degeneration and the autosomal-dominant hereditary ataxias), and pyramidal signs (cerebrovascular disease and hydrocephalus, among other disorders).

In the patient without tremor, risk factors for cerebrovascular disease should raise concern of *vascular parkinsonism*. In rare cases, the vascular parkinsonian will fulfill clinical criteria for PD, but most patients will have minimal tremor, poor response to L-dopa, and, occasionally, pyramidal signs and a stepwise progression. Brain MRI or computed tomography (CT) supports the diagnosis, demonstrating widespread small-vessel ischemic changes. The MRI is frequently helpful in other forms of parkinsonism as well: Symmetric abnormal signal in the basal ganglia suggests manganese or iron deposition, and atrophy within the brain stem, cerebellum, or striatum suggests several different parkinsonism-plus conditions (see Chap. 25).

Parkinsonism-plus syndromes frequently present with minimal or no tremor. Of these, *striatonigral degeneration* (SND)[52] most closely resembles PD and is often confused with it, especially when patients respond to L-dopa.[53] Like other disorders falling under the heading multiple-system atrophy, SND frequently presents with an early and pronounced gait disorder. Other features helpful in distinguishing it from PD include symmetrical onset, severe dysarthria or dysphonia, respiratory stridor, rapid progression, pyramidal signs, and a poor or transient response to L-dopa[54] (see Chap. 20).

Essential tremor is often mistaken for the rest tremor of PD. The patient with a pronounced kinetic or postural tremor, minimal or no signs of rigidity and bradykinesia, and a strong family history of tremor is much more likely to have essential tremor than PD. However, it is important to remember that many patients with PD have, as part of their disease, a superimposed kinetic tremor that may be indistinguishable from essential tremor. PD patients rarely display the tremulous voice that is characteristic of familial essential tremor, and this may serve as a clue. It is important to remember that cogwheeling is not pathognomonic for PD; essential tremor can also cause ratcheting during passive movement of the limb, although without rigidity. Because both PD and essential tremor are common disorders, a small number of PD patients will inherit the trait for familial tremor as well (see Chap. 28).

A coarse kinetic tremor originating proximally in the limb is probably not parkinsonian, because the rest tremor of PD typically originates distally. Degenerative diseases affecting the cerebellum and its outflow tracts can cause a coarse kinetic ("rubral") tremor associated with other cerebellar signs.

A markedly asymmetric tremor with myoclonic features suggests *cortical-basal ganglionic degeneration* (CBGD). Initially described by Rebeiz and colleagues,[55] this rare disorder is characterized by progressive asymmetric motor impairment and both cortical and basal ganglionic dysfunction.[56,57] Typical features include asymmetric parkinsonism with dystonia and myoclonus, apraxia, cortical sensory loss, the alien-limb phenomenon, ocular motility disturbance, and late-onset dementia. The tremor of CBGD often begins as an action tremor in an arm that, over time, becomes increasingly rigid and contracted. By late stages of disease, stimulus-induced myoclonus in the affected arm is usually apparent. Although stimulus-induced myoclonus is also seen in Creutzfeldt-Jakob disease and, occasionally, in SND, the combination of focal cortical and extrapyramidal signs usually distinguishes CBGD from these two diseases (see Chap. 45).

PREDOMINANT POSTURAL INSTABILITY

Although it is one of the cardinal features of PD, postural instability is rarely prominent early in disease. When initial signs include pronounced postural instability out of proportion to other manifestations, the clinican should look hard for other forms of parkinsonism. In particular, several parkinsonism-plus syndromes can present with postural instability and gait disorder, including progressive supranuclear palsy and the various forms of multiple-system atrophy.

Progressive supranuclear palsy (PSP)[58,59] may be the most common parkinsonism-plus syndrome, accounting for 7.5 percent of cases of parkinsonism in one series.[47] In early PSP, pronounced postural instability is a clue to the diagnosis, because the disease otherwise can resemble PD. Instead of the stooped, shuffling gait of PD, patients with PSP typically walk stiffly with extended trunk and knees. It is important to note that in early stages of disease, the most characteristic feature of PSP, vertical and (later) horizontal ophthalmoparesis, may be absent or manifested only by abnormal vertical optokinetic nystagmus. The vestibulo-ocular reflex remains intact, even in advanced disease, hence, the designation supranuclear. Other early clues distinguishing PSP from PD include a less prominent tremor, more prominent cognitive deficits, and a poor or transient response to L-dopa. Additional features include axial and nuchal rigidity with opisthotonic neck posturing and a fixed facial expression with dystonic features such as blepharospasm. Dementia is more common in PSP than in PD, and the cognitive disturbance of PSP tends to have more frontal lobe features.[60] These differences, however, are not reliable enough to be diagnostic (see Chap. 19).

The *multiple-system atrophies* (MSA) also frequently present with marked postural instability. MSA represents a spectrum of related clinical syndromes characterized by deficits in the extrapyramidal and pyramidal systems, cerebellum, and autonomic nervous system.[61] Particular forms of MSA are identified by the predominant involvement of one of these neural systems: the cerebellum in sporadic olivopontocerebellar degeneration (OPCD), the autonomic nervous system in Shy-Drager syndrome (SDS), the extrapyramidal and pyramidal systems in striatonigral degeneration (SND), and lower motor neurons in parkinsonism-amyotrophy. Still, there is considerable overlap between them, and parkinsonism is common to all. In addition to postural instability, the

parkinsonism of MSA typically shows features of an akinetic-rigid form of disease. Clues to the diagnosis of OPCD include progressive truncal and gait ataxia, ophthalmoparesis, and bulbar dysfunction. If a strong family history is present, the patient may have dominantly inherited cerebellar ataxia instead of sporadic OPCD. The dominant cerebellar ataxias include at least two known triplet-repeat diseases, spinocerebellar ataxia 1 and Machado-Joseph disease, as well as several other genetically distinct spinocerebellar ataxias.[62] In SDS,[63] the diagnosis is supported by evidence of autonomic dysfunction, including orthostatic hypotension, sexual dysfunction, urinary urgency or frequency, and anhydrosis. Frequent falls in the SDS patient may be the result of orthostatic hypotension rather than postural instability (see Chap. 20).

Marked postural instability with parkinsonism also occurs in *normal pressure hydrocephalus,* in which it is usually accompanied by urinary incontinence and dementia.[64] When attempting to walk, patients with normal pressure hydrocephalus may find it difficult to raise their leg from the floor (magnetic gait). The gait is slow, apraxic, and characterized by short, mincing, irregular steps ("march à petits pas"). Leg function usually improves markedly in the recumbent position. Hydrocephalic parkinsonism is not limited to normal pressure hydrocephalus, as noncommunicating hydrocephalus has also been reported with parkinsonian features.[4] Clinical features suggesting hydrocephalic parkinsonism include a history of head trauma, subarachnoid hemorrhage or meningitis, symmetrical onset involving the lower extremities, prominent gait disturbance, early cognitive or urinary symptoms, minimal or absent tremor, position-dependent bradykinesia (less when lying down), and brisk leg reflexes. A similar clinical picture may be seen in multi-infarct dementia. CT or MRI can distinguish between hydrocephalus and multi-infarct dementia, as the former typically shows prominent dilated ventricles and, on MRI, an aqueductal flow void.

Finally, it is important to remember that the differential diagnosis of early postural instability includes PD itself. Early postural instability in PD is of prognostic importance, because evidence suggests that postural instability-dominant disease tends to progress more rapidly and show a less effective response to medication than tremor-dominant PD.[7]

EARLY DEMENTIA

Dementia at the onset of illness argues strongly against PD, suggesting instead primary dementia with parkinsonian features. Forms of dementia associated with parkinsonism include Alzheimer's (AD), diffuse Lewy body (LBD), and Creutzfeldt-Jakob (CJD) diseases. Early cognitive changes are also common in *PSP,* which may be misdiagnosed as AD. Although parkinsonism is not a classic feature of AD, 25 percent of patients will have subtle bradykinesia and rigidity. LBD is a relatively recently identified pathological entity that may be an underdiagnosed cause of dementia with parkinsonism. Early psychiatric disturbance is said to be more common in LBD but, in fact, there is no sure way of distinguishing the dementia of Alzheimer's from that of diffuse Lewy body disease, except that the latter more often displays parkinsonian features. Creutzfeldt-Jakob disease typically progresses rapidly, over months instead of years, and usually can be identified by the presence of startle myoclonus and periodic complexes on the electroencephalogram; 5–10 percent of CJD patients will have a long duration variant in which disease may last greater than 2 years. There is considerable overlap in the clinical, and even pathological, features of the various dementia syndromes, meaning that the diagnosis in some patients cannot be made until autopsy.[65]

It is important to recognize that PD can exist concurrently with depression, masquerading as dementia, so-called pseudodementia. Compared to PD patients who are not depressed, those with depression show greater cognitive deficits and are more likely to show a rapid decline in global function.[34,66] Formal neuropsychological testing may distinguish bona fide dementia from PD associated with depression.

PERSISTENT ASYMMETRY

Although usually unilateral in onset, PD typically becomes bilateral within several years. A patient whose disease persists in a markedly asymmetric manner may have CBGD, discussed earlier, or *hemiparkinsonism-hemiatrophy* (HPHA). The latter is a rare condition characterized by unilateral body atrophy (face, arm, or leg), ipsilateral parkinsonism often accompanied by dystonia, and poor response to L-dopa.[67,68] Parkinsonism in this condition may represent a late manifestation of hypoxic-ischemic injury during brain development. Although imaging studies in CBGD and HPHA may demonstrate similar focal brain metabolic abnormalities, the two are distinguishable by the younger onset, slower progression, and focal body atrophy in HPHA, as well as the prominence of cortical signs in CBGD (see Chap. 24).

Just as persistent asymmetry is unusual, so is symmetrical onset of disease. It is more commonly seen in forms of parkinsonism other than PD, including vascular and hydrocephalic parkinsonism and several parkinsonism-plus syndromes.

Treatment-Related Manifestations

Our aim in this section is not to list all of the potential side effects of antiparkinsonian drugs, which most patients will experience, in one form or another, during the course of their illness. Instead, we will discuss specific treatment-related manifestations that can be mistaken for, or cloud the interpretation of, motor and cognitive deficits intrinsic to the disease. These include dyskinesias, motor fluctuations, cognitive and behavioral disturbances, and orthostatic hypotension.[69]

DYSKINESIAS

Most parkinsonian patients experience L-dopa-induced dyskinesias at some point in their illness.[69–71] Dyskinesias typically begin later in the course of disease and are greatest on the side most affected with parkinsonism. A variety of dyskinesias can be seen, including chorea, athetosis, ballismus, myoclonus, dystonia, and akathisia. Their relationship to medication dosage is often clear, falling under one of three temporal patterns: peak-dose, biphasic (onset and end-of-dose), and off-period dyskinesias. Peak-dose dyskine-

sias are usually choreic movements, whereas end-of-dose or off-period dyskinesias are typically dystonic. Frequently, patients do not notice or are not bothered by choreic movements, even when they are obvious and distressing to other family members. In contrast, off-period dystonia (for example, early-morning foot dystonia) can be quite painful and disabling. Akathisia is another common form of dyskinesia, occurring in 40 percent of patients.[72]

The severity of peak-dose dyskinesias is dose-dependent and correlates with higher plasma levels of L-dopa. Dyskinesias can be decreased by lowering the dosage of levodopa. Doing so, however, runs the risk of worsening parkinsonian symptoms. Many patients thus accept mild-to-moderate dyskinesias as the price to pay for increased mobility. Adding a dopamine agonist while decreasing the dose of L-dopa may allow better control of parkinsonism without inducing dyskinesias.

MOTOR FLUCTUATIONS

Motor fluctuations, such as kinesia paradoxica and freezing, are an intrinsic feature of PD that can occur prior to any dopaminergic therapy. Yet, fluctuations do not usually become a significant problem until after years of L-dopa therapy.[69,73–75] At first, most patients derive sustained and fairly steady benefit from L-dopa throughout the day. As PD advances, however, the duration of benefit shortens for each dose. L-dopa takes longer to "kick in" and "works" for a shorter length of time. Patients may start to experience extreme fluctuations from an "on" to an "off" state. These can occur suddenly and unpredictably, and the transition from "on" to "off" is often accompanied by a short period of severe dyskinesias. Measures to alleviate fluctuations include using more frequent dosings of L-dopa, switching to controlled-release L-dopa, or adding a dopamine agonist. Despite these measures, fluctuations may persist and, for many patients, may prove to be one of the most disabling aspects of disease.

In advanced disease, drug-resistant off periods also may occur. Most often a late-afternoon or early-evening phenomenon, these off periods fail to respond to increasing doses of L-dopa and dopamine agonists.

COGNITIVE AND BEHAVIORAL DISTURBANCES

L-dopa can cause a number of psychiatric side effects.[69] Although these typically do not occur until after several years of treatment, they may happen sooner in patients with dementia or prior psychiatric history. Early effects include disruption of the sleep cycle, vivid dreams, and nightmares. Over time these may progress to daytime visual hallucinations, a common and disabling side effect of L-dopa.[76] These are typically formed, stereotyped images of people or animals that are not threatening. However, a small percentage of patients will develop a paranoid psychosis. Hallucinations are dose-related; hence, efforts should be made to lower dopaminergic stimulation in affected patients. Adding the atypical neuroleptic clozapine may control hallucinations while permitting continued L-dopa therapy. Because of the rare side effect of agranulocytosis, weekly blood tests are required with this medication.

Panic attacks have also been described in late PD.[77] These tend to occur during "off" periods in patients experiencing fluctuations and dyskinesias and are relieved by additional dopaminergic therapy.

ORTHOSTATIC HYPOTENSION

Although more characteristic of MSA, autonomic dysfunction can cause postural hypotension in some untreated PD patients. More commonly in PD, however, postural hypotension occurs as a side effect of dopaminergic therapy, particularly dopamine agonists. In one study of the dopamine agonists pergolide and bromocriptine, one-third of patients had postural hypotension.[78] Measures to treat this drug-related effect are the same as for dysautonomia: increased salt and fluid intake, fitted elastic stockings, fludrocortisone or other drugs to correct orthostatic hypotension, and rising slowly to the standing position.

Clinical Rating Scales

In order to evaluate the efficacy of new pharmacotherapies for PD, it is crucial to have standardized methods to quantify disease severity, motor manifestations, and quality of life. Rating scales serve this purpose. Moreover, they prove useful in evaluating an individual patient's response to medication changes, as well as in assessing the contribution of treatment-related fluctuations and dyskinesias to a patient's disability. For these reasons a variety of PD rating scales have been developed. Here we will discuss three of the most commonly used scales. Other ways of assessing manifestations of PD are available, including videotape analysis (routinely used in movement disorders centers), patient diaries to assess on-off status, and simple timed maneuvers such as walking a defined distance. For a more detailed discussion, we refer the reader to Lang's thorough review.[79]

The *Hoehn and Yahr Staging Scale*[11] is a widely adopted and useful scale designed to give a rough estimate of disease severity. Its developers designated five stages of disease severity:

1. Unilateral disease only
2. Bilateral mild disease, with or without axial involvement
3. Mild-to-moderate bilateral disease, with first signs of deteriorating balance
4. Severe disease requiring considerable assistance
5. Confinement to wheelchair or bed unless aided

Stage 3 is distinguished from stage 2 by the appearance of postural instability. The stage 3 patient remains fully independent, whereas the stage 4 patient is unable to live alone without assistance. Interrater correlation with the Hoehn and Yahr Staging Scale is excellent. It was not designed for use in therapeutic trials and is clearly inadequate for such purposes when used in isolation. However, it has been incorporated into several recent rating scales as one arm in patient assessment, including the Unified Parkinson's Disease Rating Scale. Two additional stages, 1.5 and 2.5, have been added to the UPDRS (Table 13-5).

The *Schwab and England Capacity for Daily Living Scale* is the most widely used scale to assess patient disability in performing activities of daily living. It has a 10-point scoring system, with 100 percent representing completely normal function and 0 percent total helplessness. The UPDRS has incorporated the Schwab and England Capacity for Daily Living Scale as the sixth and final arm of patient assessment (Table 13-5). It provides an accurate assessment of disability and has the highest interrater concordance rate of the six stages in the UPDRS.[80]

In the 1980s in response to the need for standardized assessment of PD, Dr. Stanley Fahn led a group of clinical investigators in creating the *Unified Parkinson's Disease Rating Scale* (UPDRS, see Ref. 80). Now widely used, the UPDRS has undergone several revisions (see Table 13-5 for the current version). Its major strength is that it provides a detailed and accurate assessment of PD in a variety of respects. This also may be its greatest weakness, because completing the entire scale can prove somewhat cumbersome in a routine clinical practice. Several recent studies confirm the high interrater reliability of the UPDRS and suggest possible ways of further shortening the scale without compromising detail and accuracy.[81-83]

The UPDRS contains six sections. The first is a limited assessment of mood and cognition which, in some patients, will need to be supplemented with other tests for depression or cognitive disturbance. The second is an assessment of activities of daily living in both the "on" and "off" state, as determined by history. The third is a detailed motor examination based on the widely used Columbia scale. The fourth is a questionaire assessing complications of therapy, focussing principally on fluctuations and dyskinesias. The fifth and sixth sections are, respectively, a modified Hoehn and Yahr scale and the Schwab and England scale. Added stages to the Hoehn and Yahr scale take into account axial involvement (stage 1.5) and mild postural instability (stage 2.5). Taken together, the six stages provide a detailed and acccurate assessment of a patient's global function, level of disability, mood, and both disease-related and treatment-releated manifestations of PD.

TABLE 13-5 Unified Parkinson's Disease Rating Scale (UPDRS)

I. MENTATION, BEHAVIOR, AND MOOD

1. Intellectual Impairment:
   0 = None.
   1 = Mild. Consistent forgetfulness with partial recollection of events and no other difficulties.
   2 = Moderate memory loss, with disorientation and moderate difficulty handling complex problems. Mild but definite impairment of function at home with need of occasional prompting.
   3 = Severe memory loss with disorientation for time and often place. Severe impairment in handling problems.
   4 = Severe memory loss with orientation preserved to person only. Unable to make judgments or solve problems. Requires much help with personal care. Cannot be left alone at all.

2. Thought Disorder (Due to dementia or drug intoxication):
   0 = None.
   1 = Vivid dreaming.
   2 = "Benign" hallucinations with insight retained.
   3 = Occasional to frequent hallucinations or delusions; without insight; could interfere with daily activities.
   4 = Persistent hallucinations, delusions, or florid psychosis. Not able to care for self.

4. Depression:
   0 = Not present.
   1 = Periods of sadness or guilt greater than normal, never sustained for days or weeks.
   2 = Sustained depression (1 week or more).
   3 = Sustained depression with vegetative symptoms (insomnia, anorexia, weight loss, loss of interest).
   4 = Sustained depression with vegetative symptoms and suicidal thoughts or intent.

4. Motivation/Initiative:
   0 = Normal.
   1 = Less assertive than usual; more passive.
   2 = Loss of initiative or disinterest in elective (non-routine) activities.
   3 = Loss of initiative or disinterest in day to day (routine) activities.
   4 = Withdrawn, complete loss of motivation.

II. ACTIVITIES OF DAILY LIVING (DETERMINE FOR "ON/OFF")

5. Speech:
   0 = Normal.
   1 = Mildly affected; no difficulty being understood.
   2 = Moderately affected; sometimes asked to repeat statements.
   3 = Severe affected; frequently asked to repeat statements.
   4 = Unintelligible most of the time.

6. Salvation:
   0 = Normal.
   1 = Slight but definite excess of saliva in mouth; may have nighttime drooling.
   2 = Moderately excessive saliva; may have minimal drooling.
   3 = Marked excess of saliva with some drooling.
   4 = Marked drooling, requires constant tissue or handkerchief.

7. Swallowing:
   0 = Normal.
   1 = Rare choking,
   2 = Occasional choking.
   3 = Requires soft food.
   4 = Requires NG tube or gastrostomy feeding.

8. Handwriting:
   0 = Normal.
   1 = Slightly slow or small.
   2 = Moderately slow or small; all words are legible.
   3 = Severely affected; not all words are legible.
   4 = The majority of words are not legible.

9. Cutting Food and Handling Utensils:
   0 = Normal.
   1 = Somewhat slow and clumsy, but no help needed.
   2 = Can cut most foods, although clumsy and slow; some help needed.
   3 = Food must be cut by someone, but can still feed slowly.
   4 = Needs to be fed.

10. Dressing:
    0 = Normal.
    1 = Somewhat slow, but no help needed.
    2 = Occasional assistance with buttoning, getting arms in sleeves.
    3 = Considerable help required, but can do some things alone.
    4 = Helpless.

11. Hygiene:
    0 = Normal.
    1 = Somewhat slow, but no help needed.
    2 = Needs help to shower or bathe; or very slow in hygienic care.
    3 = Requires assistance for washing, brushing teeth, combing hair, going to bathroom.
    4 = Foley catheter or other mechanical aids.

12. Turning in Bed and Adjusting Bed Clothes:
    0 = Normal.
    1 = Somewhat slow and clumsy, but no help needed.
    2 = Can turn alone or adjust sheets, but with great difficulty.
    3 = Can initiate, but not turn or adjust sheets alone.
    4 = Helpless.

13. Falling (Unrelated to Freezing):
    0 = None.
    1 = Rare falling.
    2 = Occasionally falls, less than once per day.
    3 = Fall an average of once daily.
    4 = Falls more than once daily.

14. Freezing When Walking:
    0 = None.
    1 = Rare freezing when walking; may have start-hesitation.
    2 = Occasional freezing when walking.
    3 = Frequent freezing; occasionally falls from freezing.
    4 = Frequent falls from freezing.

TABLE 13-5 Unified Parkinson's Disease Rating Scale (UPDRS) *(Continued)*

15. Walking:
    0 = Normal.
    1 = Mild difficulty; may not swing arms or may tend to drag leg.
    2 = Moderate difficulty, but requires little or no assistance.
    3 = Severe disturbance of walking, requiring assistance.
    4 = Cannot walk at all, even with assistance.

16. Tremor:
    0 = Absent.
    1 = Slight and infrequently present.
    2 = Moderate; bothersome to patient.
    3 = Severe; interferes with many activities.
    4 = Marked; interferes with most activities.

17. Sensory Complaints Related to Parkinsonism:
    0 = None.
    1 = Occasionally has numbness, tingling, or mild aching.
    2 = Frequently has numbness, tingling, or aching; not distressing.
    3 = Frequent painful sensations.
    4 = Excruciating pain.

III. MOTOR EXAMINATION (DETERMINE FOR "ON/OFF")

18. Speech:
    0 = Normal.
    1 = Slight loss of expression, diction and/or volume.
    2 = Monotone, slurred but understandable; moderately impaired.
    3 = Marked impairment, difficult to understand.
    4 = Unintelligible.

19. Facial Expression:
    0 = Normal.
    1 = Minimal hypomimia, could be normal "poker face."
    2 = Slight but definitely abnormal diminution of facial expression.
    3 = Moderate hypomimia; lips parted some of the time.
    4 = Masked or fixed facies with severe or complete loss of facial expression; lips parted 1/4 inch or more.

20. Tremor at Rest:
    0 = Absent.
    1 = Slight and infrequently present.
    2 = Mild in amplitude and persistent. Or moderate in amplitude but only intermittently present.
    3 = Moderate in amplitude and present most of the time.
    4 = Marked in amplitude and present most of the time.

21. Action or Postural Tremor of Hands:
    0 = Absent.
    1 = Slight; present with action.
    2 = Moderate in amplitude, present with action.
    3 = Moderate in amplitude with posture holding as well as action.
    4 = Marked in amplitude; interferes with feeding.

22. Rigidity (Judged on passive movement of major joints with patient relaxed in sitting position. Cogwheeling to be ignored):

    0 = Absent.
    1 = Slight or detectable only when activated by mirror or other movements.
    2 = Mild to moderate.
    3 = Marked, but full range of motion easily achieved.
    4 = Severe, range of motion achieved with difficulty.

23. Finger Taps (Patient taps thumb with index finger in rapid succession with widest amplitude possible, each hand separately):
    0 = Normal ($\geq$ 15/5 seconds)
    1 = Mild slowing and/or reduction in amplitude (11–14/5 seconds)
    2 = Moderately impaired. Definite and early fatiguing. May have occasional arrests in movement (7–10/5 seconds)
    3 = Severely impaired. Frequent hesitation in initiating movements or arrests in ongoing movement (3–6/5 seconds)
    4 = Can barely perform the task (0–2/5 seconds)

24. Hand Movements (Patient opens and closes hands in rapid succession with widest amplitude possible, each hand separately):
    0 = Normal.
    1 = Mild slowing and/or reduction in amplitude.
    2 = Moderately impaired. Definite and early fatiguing. May have occasional arrests in movement.
    3 = Severely impaired. Frequent hesitation in initiating movements or arrests in ongoing movement.
    4 = Can barely perform the task.

25. Rapid Alternating Movements of Hands: (Pronation-supination movements of hands, vertically or horizontally, with as large an amplitude as possible, both hands simultaneously):
    0 = Normal.
    1 = Mild slowing and/or reduction in amplitude.
    2 = Moderately impaired. Definite and early fatiguing. May have occasional arrests in movement.
    3 = Severely impaired. Frequent hesitation in initiating movements or arrests in ongoing movement.
    4 = Can barely perform the task.

26. Leg Agility (Patient taps heel on ground in rapid succession, picking up entire leg; amplitude should be about 3 in.):
    0 = Normal.
    1 = Mild slowing and/or reduction in amplitude.
    2 = Moderately impaired. Definite and early fatiguing. May have occasional arrests in movement.
    3 = Severely impaired. Frequent hesitation in initiating movements or arrests in ongoing movement.
    4 = Can barely perform the task.

27. Rising from Chair (Patient attempts to rise from a straightbacked wood or metal chair, with arms folded across chest):
    0 = Normal.
    1 = Slow; or may need more than one attempt.
    2 = Pushes self up from arms of seat.
    3 = Tends to fall back and may have to try more than one time, but can get up without help.
    4 = Unable to rise without help.

TABLE 13-5 Unified Parkinson's Disease Rating Scale (UPDRS) *(Continued)*

28. Posture:
    0 = Normal erect.
    1 = Not quite erect, slightly stooped posture; could be normal for older person.
    2 = Moderately stooped posture, definitely abnormal; can be slightly leaning to one side.
    3 = Severely stooped position with kyphosis; can be moderately leaning to one side.
    4 = Marked flexion with extreme abnormality of posture.

29. Gait:
    0 = Normal.
    1 = Walks slowly, may shuffle with short steps, but not festination or propulsion.
    2 = Walks with difficulty, but requires little or no assistance; may have some festination, short steps, or propulsion.
    3 = Severe disturbance of gait, requiring assistance.
    4 = Cannot walk at all, even with assistance.

30. Postural Stability (Response to sudden posterior displacement produced by pull on shoulders while patient erect with eyes open and feet slightly apart. Patient is prepared):
    0 = Normal.
    1 = Retropulsion, but recovers unaided.
    2 = Absence of postural response, would fall if not caught by examiner.
    3 = Very unstable, tends to lose balance spontaneously.
    4 = Unable to stand without assistance.

31. Body Bradykinesia and Hypokinesia (Combining slowness, hesitancy, decreased armswing, small amplitude, and poverty of movement in general):
    0 = None.
    1 = Minimal slowness, giving movement a deliberate character; could be normal for some persons. Possibly reduced amplitude.
    2 = Mild degree of slowness and poverty of movement which is definitely abnormal. Alternatively, some reduced amplitude.
    3 = Moderate slowness, poverty or small amplitude of movement.
    4 = Marked slowness, poverty or small amplitude of movement.

IV. COMPLICATIONS OF THERAPY (In the past week)

A. DYSKINESIAS

32. Duration: What Proportion of the Walking Day Are Dyskinesias Present? (Historical information):
    0 = None.
    1 = 1–25% of day.
    2 = 26–50% of day.
    3 = 51–75% of day.
    4 = 76–100% of day.

33. Disability: How Disabling Are the Dyskinesias? (Historical information; may be modified by office examination):
    0 = Not disabling.
    1 = Mildly disabling.
    2 = Moderately disabling.
    3 = Severely disabling.
    4 = Completely disabled.

34. Painful Dyskinesias: How Painful Are the Dyskinesias?
    0 = No painful dyskinesias.
    1 = Slight.
    2 = Moderate.
    3 = Severe.
    4 = Marked.

35. Presence of Early Morning Dystonia (Historical information):
    0 = No
    1 = Yes

B. CLINICAL FLUCTUATIONS

36. Are Any "Off" Periods Predictable as to Timing After a Dose of Medication?
    0 = No
    1 = Yes

37. Are Any "Off" Periods Unpredictable as to Timing After a Dose of Medication?
    0 = No
    1 = Yes

38. Do any of the "Off" Periods Come on Suddenly (e.g., over a few seconds)?
    0 = No
    1 = Yes

39. What Proportion of the Walking Day Is the Patient "Off" on Average?
    0 = None.
    1 = 1–25% of day.
    2 = 26–50% of day.
    3 = 51–75% of day.
    4 = 76–100% of day.

C. OTHER COMPLICATIONS

40. Does the Patient Have Anorexia, Nausea, or Vomiting?
    0 = No
    1 = Yes

41. Does the Patient Have Any Sleep Disturbances (e.g., Insomnia or Hypersomnolence)?
    0 = No
    1 = Yes

42. Does the Patient Have Symptomatic Orthostasis?
    0 = No
    1 = Yes

Record the Patient's Blood Pressure, Pulse, and Weight on the Scoring Form

V. MODIFIED HOEHN AND YAHR STAGING

Stage 0   = No signs of disease.
Stage 1   = Unilateral disease.
Stage 1.5 = Unilateral plus axial involvement.
Stage 2   = Bilateral disease, without impairment of balance.
Stage 2.5 = Mild bilateral disease, with recovery on pull test.
Stage 3   = Mild to moderate bilateral disease; some postural instability; physically independent.

TABLE 13-5 Unified Parkinson's Disease Rating Scale (UPDRS) *(Continued)*

Stage 4 = Severe disability; still able to walk or stand unassisted.

Stage 5 = Wheelchair bound or bedridden unless aided.

VI. SCHWAB AND ENGLAND ACTIVITIES OF DAILY LIVING SCALE

100%—Completely independent. Able to do all chores without slowness, difficulty, or impairment. Essentially normal. Unaware of any dificulty.

90%—Completely independent. Able to do all chores with some degree of slowness, difficulty, and impairment. Might take twice as long. Beginning to be aware of difficulty.

80%—Completely independent in most chores. Takes twice as long. Conscious of difficulty and slowness.

70%—Not completely independent. More difficulty with some chores. Three to four times as long in some. Must spend a large part of the day with chores.

60%—Some dependency. Can do most chores, but exceedingly slowly and with much effort. Errors; some impossible.

50%—More dependent. Help with half, slower, etc. Difficulty with everything.

40%—Very dependent. Can assist with all chores, but few alone.

30%—With effort, now and then does a few chores alone or begins alone. Much help needed.

20%—Nothing alone. Can be a slight help with some chores. Severe invalid.

10%—Totally dependent, helpless, Complete invalid.

0%—Vegetative functions such as swallowing, bladder, and bowel functions are not functioning. Bedridden.

UNIFIED PARKINSON'S DISEASE RATING SCALE

Name: _____ Unit Number: _____

Dates:

	On	Off	On	Off	On	Off	On	Off
1. Mentation								
2. Thought disorder								
3. Depression								
4. Motivat./Initiat.								
SUBTOTAL #1–4								
5. Speech								
6. Salivation								
7. Swallowing								
8. Handwriting								
9. Cutting food								
10. Dressing								
11. Hygiene								
12. Turning in bed								
13. Falling								
14. Freezing								
15. Walking								
16. Tremor								
17. Sensory symptoms								
SUBTOTAL #5–17								
18. Speech								

UNIFIED PARKINSON'S DISEASE RATING SCALE *(Continued)*

Name: _____   Unit Number: _____

Dates:

	On	Off	On	Off	On	Off	On	Off
19. Facial express.								
20. Tremor-at-rest face, lips, chin								
R/L hands								
R/L feet								
21. Action tremor R/L								
R/L UE								
R/L LE								
23. Finger taps R/L								
24. Hand grips R/L								
25. Hand pron-sup R/L								
26. Leg agility R/L								
27. Arise from chair								
28. Posture								
29. Gait								
30. Postural stabil.								
31. Body bradykinesia								
TOTAL POINTS: #1–31								
32. Dyskinesia—durat.								
33. Dyskinesia—disab.								
34. Dyskinesia—pain								
35. Early morn. dyston.								
36. "Offs"—predict.								
37. "Offs"—unpredict.								
38. "Offs"—sudden								
39. "Offs"—duration								
40. Anorexia, N, V								
41. Sleep disturbance								
42. Sympt. orthostasis								
BP—sit/supine								
BP—standing								
Weight								
Pulse—sit/stand								

Scores at patient's:	Best	Worst	Best	Worst	Best	Worst	Best	Worst
Hoehn & Yahr Stage								
S&E ADL Score								

References

1. Parkinson J: *An Essay on the Shaking Palsy.* London: Sherwood, Neely, and Jones, 1817.
2. Gibb WR: The neuropathology of Parkinson disorders, in Jankovic J, Tolosa E (eds): *Parkinson's Disease and Movement Disorders.* Baltimore: Williams and Wilkins 1993, pp 205–233.
3. Stern MB, Koller WC: Parkinson's disease, in Stern MB, Koller WC (eds): *Parkinsonian Syndromes.* New York: Marcel Dekker, 1993.
4. Curran T, Lang AE: Parkinsonian syndromes associated with hydrocephalus: Case reports, a review of the literature, and pathophysiological hypotheses. *Mov Disord* 9:508–520, 1994.
5. Rajput AH, Rozdilsky B, Rajput A, Ang L: Levodopa efficacy and pathologic basis of Parkinson's disease. *Clin Neuropharmacol* 13:553–558, 1990.
6. Zetusky WJ, Jankovic J, Pirozzolo FJ: The heterogeneity of Parkinson's disease: Clinical and prognostic implications. *Neurology* 35:522–526, 1985.
7. Jankovic J, McDermott N, Carter J, et al: Variable expression of Parkinson's disease: A baseline analysis of the DATATOP cohort. *Neurology* 40:1529–1534, 1990.
8. Gibb WRG, Lees AJ: A comparison of clinical and pathologic features of young- and old-onset Parkinson's disease. *Neurology* 38:1402–1408, 1988.
9. Goetz CG, Tanner CM, Stebbins GT, Buchman AS: Risk factors for progression in Parkinson's disease. *Neurology* 38:1841–1844, 1988.
10. Kostic V, Przedborski S, Flaster E, Sternic N: Early development of levodopa induced dyskinesias and response fluctuations in young-onset Parkinson's disease. *Neurology* 41:202–205, 1991.
11. Hoehn MM: The natural history of Parkinson's disease in the pre-levodopa and post-levodopa eras. *Neurol Clin* 10:331–339, 1992.
12. Hoehn MM, Yahr MD: Parkinsonism: Onset progression and mortality. *Neurology* 17:427–442, 1967.
13. Rajput AH, Offord KP, Beard CM, Durland LT: Epidemiology of parkinsonism: Incidence, classification and mortality. *Ann Neurol* 16:278–282, 1984.
14. Koller WC: When does Parkinson's disease begin? *Neurology* 42:27–31, 1992.
15. Hughes AJ, Ben-Schlomo Y, Daniel SE, Lees AJ: What features improve the accuracy of clinical diagnosis in Parkinson's disease? *Neurology* 42:1142–1146, 1992.
16. Lance JW, Schwab RS, Peterson EA: Action tremor and the cogwheel phenomenon in Parkinson's disease. *Brain* 86:95–110, 1963.
17. Delwaide PJ, Gonce M: Pathophysiology of Parkinson's signs, in Jankovic J, Tolosa E, (eds): *Parkinson's Disease and Movement Disorders.* Baltimore: Williams & Wilkins, 1993.
18. Hoefer PF, Putnam TJ: Action potentials of muscles in rigidity and tremor. *Arch Neurol Psychiatry* 43:704–725, 1940.
19. Foerster O: Zur analyse und Pathophysiologie der striaten Bewegungstorungen. *Z Neurol Psychiatrie* 73:1–169, 1921.
20. Bloxham CA, Mindall TA, Frith CD: Initiation and execution of predictable and unpredictable movements in Parkinson's disease. *Brain* 107:371–384, 1984.
21. Marsden CD: Defects of movement in Parkinson's disease, in Delwaide PJ, Agnoli A (eds): *Clinical Neurophysiology in Parkinsonism.* Amsterdam: Elsevier Science Publishers, 1985.
22. Graybiel AM, Aosaki T, Flaherty AW, Kimura N: The basal ganglia and adaptive motor control. *Science* 265:1826–1831, 1994.
23. Klawans HL: Individual manifestations of Parkinson's disease after ten or more years of levodopa. *Mov Disord* 1:187–192, 1986.
24. Giladi N, McMahon D, Przedbovski S, et al: Motor blocks in Parkinson's disease. *Neurology* 42:333–339, 1992.
25. Stern M: The clinical characteristics of Parkinson's disease and parkinsonian syndromes: Diagnosis and assessment, in Stern MB, Hurtig HI (eds): *The Comprehensive Management of Parkinson's Disease.* New York: PMA Publishing Corporation, 1988.
26. Levin BE, Tomer R, Rey G: Cognitive impairments in Parkinson's disease. *Neurol Clin* 10:471–485, 1992.
27. Boller F, Passarfiume D, Keefe N, et al: Visuospatial impairment in Parkinson's disease. Role of perceptual and motor factors. *Arch Neurol* 41:485–490, 1984.
28. Cooper JA, Sagar HJ, Jordan N, et al: Cognitive impairment in early, untreated Parkinson's disease and its relationship to motor disability. *Brain* 114:2095–2122, 1991.
29. Stam CJ, Visser SL, Op de Coul AA, et al: Disturbed frontal regulation of attention in Parkinson's disease. *Brain* 116:1139–1158, 1993.
30. Pate DS, Margolin DI: Cognitive slowing in Parkinson's and Alzheimer's patient: Distinguishing bradyphrenia from dementia. *Neurology* 44:669–674, 1994.
31. Brown RG, Marsden DC: How common is dementia in Parkinson's disease? *Lancet* 2:1262–1265, 1984.
32. Mayeux R, Chen J, Mirabello E, et al: An estimate of the incidence of dementia in idiopathic Parkinson's disease. *Neurology* 40:1513–1517, 1990.
33. Stern Y, Richards M, Sano M, Mayeux R: Comparison of cognitive changes in patients with Alzheimer's and Parkinson's diseases. *Arch Neurol* 50:1040–1045, 1993.
34. Stern Y, Marder K, Tang MX, Mayeaux R: Antecedent clinical features associated with dementia in Parkinson's disease. *Neurology* 43:1690–1692, 1993.
35. Starkstein SE, Mayberg HS, Leiguarda R, et al: A prospective longitudinal study of depression, cognitive decline, and physical impairments with Parkinson's disease. *J Neurol Neurosurg Psychiatry* 55:377–382, 1992.
36. Gotham AM, Brown RG, Marsden CD: Depression in Parkinson's disease: A quantitative and qualitative analysis. *J Neurol Neurosurg Psychiatry* 49:381–389, 1986.
37. Taylor AE, Saint-Cyr JA, Lang AE, Kenney FT: Parkinson's disease and depression: A critical re-evaluation. *Brain* 109:279–292, 1986.
38. Vreeling FW, Verhey FR, Houx PJ, Jolles J: Primitive reflexes in Parkinson's disease. *J Neurol Neurosurg Psychiatry* 56:1323–1326, 1993.
39. Edwards LL, Quigley EMM, Pfeiffer RF: Gastrointestinal dysfunction in Parkinson's disease: Frequency and pathophysiology. *Neurology* 42:726–732, 1992.
40. Doty RL, Golbe LI, McKeown DA, et al: Olfactory testing differentiates between progressive supranuclear palsy and Parkinson's disease. *Neurology* 43:962–965, 1993.
41. Stern MB, Doty RL, Dotti M, et al: Olfactory function in Parkinson's disease. *Neurology* 44:266–268, 1994.
42. Goetz CG, Tanner CM, Levy M, et al: Pain in idiopathic Parkinson's disease. *Mov Disord* 1:45–50, 1986.
43. Koller WC: Sensory symptoms in Parkinson's disease. *Neurology* 34:957–959, 1984.
44. Snider SR, Fahn S, Isgreen WP, Cote LJ: Primary sensory symptoms in Parkinson's disease. *Neurology* 26:423–429, 1976.
45. Appenzeller O, Gross JE: Autonomic deficits in Parkinson's disease. *Arch Neurol* 24:50–57, 1971.
46. Goetz CG, Lutge W, Tanner C: Autonomic dysfunction in Parkinson's disease. *Neurology* 36:73–75, 1986.
47. Stacy M, Jankovic J: Differential diagnosis of Parkinson's disease and the parkinsonism plus syndromes. *Neurol Clinics* 10:341–359, 1992.
48. Giovanni P, Piccolo I, Genitrini S, et al: Early-onset Parkinson's disease. *Mov Disord* 6:36–42, 1991.

49. Quinn N, Critchley P, Marsden CD: Young onset Parkinson's disease. *Mov Disord* 2:73–91, 1987.
50. Muthane UD, Swamy HS, Satishchandra P, et al: Early onset Parkinson's disease: Are juvenile- and young-onset different? *Mov Disord* 9:539–544, 1994.
51. Hallervorden J, Spatz H: Eigenartige erkrangung im extrapyramidalen system mit besonderer beiteiligung des globus pallidus und der substantia nigra. *Z Neurol Psychiatry* 79:254–302, 1922.
52. Adams RD, van Bogaert L, Ecken HV: Striato-nigral degeneration. *J Neuropathol Exp Neurol* 23:589–608, 1964.
53. Fearnley JM, Lees AJ: Striatonigral degeneration. A clinicopathological study. *Brain* 113:1823–1842, 1990.
54. Gouider-Khouja N, Vidhailhet M, Bonnet A-M, et al: "Pure" striatonigral degeneration and Parkinson's disease: A comparative clinical study. *Mov Disord* 10:288–294, 1995.
55. Rebeiz JL, Kolodny EH, Richardson EP: Corticodentatonigral degeneration with neuronal achromasia. *Arch Neurol* 18:20–33, 1968.
56. Brunt ERP, Weerden TWv, Pruim J, Lakke JWPF: Unique myoclonic pattern in corticobasal degeneration. *Mov Disord* 10:132–142, 1995.
57. Riley DE, Lang AE, Lewis A, et al: Cortico-basal ganglionic degeneration. *Neurology* 40:1203–1212, 1990.
58. Gearing M, Olsen DA, Watts RL, Mirra SS: Progressive supranuclear palsy: Neuropathologic and clinical heterogeneity. *Neurology* 44:1015–1024, 1994.
59. Steele JC, Richardson JC, Olszewski J: Progressive supranuclear palsy: A heterogeneous degeneration involving the brainstem, basal ganglia and cerebellum with vertical gaze and pseudobulbar palsy, nuchal dystonia and dementia. *Arch Neurol* 10:333–359, 1964.
60. Pillon B, Dubois B, Ploska A, Agid Y: Severity and specificity of cognitive impairment in Alzheimer's, Huntington's, and Parkinson's diseases and progressive supranuclear palsy. *Neurology* 41:634–643, 1991.
61. Penney JB: Multiple systems atrophy and nonfamilial olivopontocerebellar atrophy are the same disease. *Ann Neurol* 37:553–554, 1995.
62. Rosenberg R: The genetic basis of ataxia, in "Advances in the Inherited Ataxias." *Clin Neurosci* 3:1–4, 1995.
63. Shy GM, Drager GA: A neurologic syndrome associated with orthostatic hypotension: A clinical-pathologic study. *Arch Neurol* 2:511–527, 1960.
64. Knutsen E, Lying-Tunell V: Gait apraxia in normal-pressure hydrocephalus: Patterns of movement and muscle activation. *Neurology* 35:155–160, 1985.
65. Wojcieszek J, Lang AE, Jankovic J, et al: Case 1, 1994: Rapidly progressive aphasia, apraxia, dementia, myoclonus, and parkinsonism. *Mov Disord* 9:358–366, 1994.
66. Troster AI, Paolo AM, Lyons KE, et al: The influence of depression on cognition in Parkinson's disease. *Neurology* 45:672–676, 1995.
67. Giladi N, Burke RE, Kostic V, et al: Hemiparkinsonism-hemiatrophy syndrome: Clinical and neuroradiologic features. *Neurology* 40:1731–1734, 1990.
68. Klawans HL: Hemiparkinsonism as a late complication of hemiatrophy: A new syndrome. *Neurology* 31:625–628, 1981.
69. Koller WC: Adverse effects of levodopa and other symptomatic therapies: Impact on quality of life of the Parkinson's disease patient, in Stern MB (ed): *Beyond the Decade of the Brain*. Kent, UK: Wells Medical Limited, 1994.
70. Nutt JC: Levodopa induced dyskinesias. *Neurology* 40:340–345, 1990.
71. Marconi R, Lefebure-Caparros D, Bonnet AM, et al: Levodopa induced dyskinesia in Parkinson's disease: Phenomenology and pathophysiology. *Mov Disord* 9:212, 1994.
72. Comella CL, Goetz CG: Akathisia in Parkinson's disease. *Mov Disord* 9:545–549, 1994.
73. Fahn S: On-off phenomenon with levodopa therapy in parkinsonism. *Neurology* 24:431–441, 1974.
74. Marsden CD, Parkes JP, Quinn N: Fluctuations of disability in Parkinson's disease, in Marsden CD, Fahn S (eds): *Movement Disorders*. London: Butterworth, 1982.
75. Nutt JG, Woodward WD, Hammerstad JP, et al: The "on-off" phenomenon in Parkinson's disease: Relationship to L-dopa absorption and transport. *N Engl J Med* 310:484–488, 1984.
76. Tanner CM, Vogel C, Goetz CG, et al: Hallucinations in Parkinson's disease. A population study. *Ann Neurol* 14:136, 1983.
77. Vasquez A, Jimenez-Jimenez FJ, Garcia-Ruiz P, Garcia-Urre D: "Panic attacks" in Parkinson's disease: A long-term complication of levodopa therapy. *Acta Neurol Scandinavia* 87:14–18, 1993.
78. LeWitt PA, Ward CD, Larsen TA, et al: Comparison of pergolide and bromocriptine therapy in parkinsonism. *Neurology* 33:1009–1014, 1983.
79. Lang AE: Clinical rating scales and videotape analysis, in Paulson GW, Koller WC (eds): *Therapy of Parkinson's Disease*. New York: Marcel Dekker, 1995.
80. Fahn S, Elton RL, and Members of the UPDRS Development Committee: Unified Parkinson's disease rating scale, in Fahn S, Marsden CD, Goldstein M, Calne DB (eds): *Recent Developments in Parkinson's Disease*. New York: Macmillan, 1987.
81. Hilton JJ, van der Zwan AD, Zwimmerman AH, Roos RAC: Rating impairment and disability in Parkinson's disease: Evaluation of the unified Parkinson's disease rating scale. *Mov Disord* 9:84–88, 1994.
82. Martinez-Martin P, Gil-Nagel A, Gracia LM, et al: Unified Parkinson's disease rating scale characteristics and structure. *Mov Disord* 9:76–83, 1994.
83. Richards M, Marder KM, Cote L, Mayeux RM: Interrater reliability of the unified Parkinson's disease rating scale motor examination. *Mov Disord* 9:89–91, 1994.

Chapter 14

PHARMACOLOGICAL TREATMENT OF PARKINSON'S DISEASE

WERNER POEWE and R. GRANATA

SYMPTOMATIC TREATMENT
    Pharmacology of Dopamine Receptors
    Dopaminergic Agents
    Nondopaminergic Agents
NEUROPROTECTIVE TREATMENT
    Mechanisms of Nigral Cell Loss in IPD
    Candidate Drugs for Neuroprotective Treatment of
        IPD
PRACTICAL TREATMENT DECISIONS IN IPD
    Treatment of De Novo Patients
    Treatment of Advanced IPD

The first empirical attempts of a pharmacological treatment of Parkinson's disease (PD) were made in the 1860s by Ordenstein and Charcot in Paris by using extracts from *Hyscyamus niger*, *Atropa belladonna*, and *Datura stramonium* containing the anticholinergic compounds hyoscine and scopolamine.[1,2] The development of synthetic anticholinergic drugs in the 1940s[3] led to their becoming the mainstay of antiparkinsonian drug treatment, but even though they improved tremor and rigidity, they had little effect on akinesia.[4]

The classical experiments on reserpinized animals by Carlsson in 1957, which showed that the akinesia of catecholamine-depleted animals could be reversed by D,L-dopa administration,[5] led to the hypothesis of a dopaminergic disorder as the pathophysiological basis of PD. Shortly afterward, the finding in postmortem studies of dopamine deficiency in the striatum of PD patients by Ehringer and Hornykiewicz in Vienna in 1960[6] and the observation of reduced dopamine excretion in the urine of PD patients made by Barbeau et al.[7] marked the beginning of a new "era" in the treatment of PD. In 1961, two groups in Vienna and Montreal independently reported positive results of open-label, small-scale clinical trials with L-dopa in parkinsonian patients.[8,9] Five years later, Cotzias and colleagues demonstrated striking efficacy of high-dose oral L-dopa,[10] the potentiation of its effects and the improvement of side effects with coadministration of peripheral dopa decarboxylase inhibitors (DCIs),[11] and the long-term side effects of L-dopa treatment.[12]

Until today L-dopa substitution has remained the gold standard of antiparkinsonian drug therapy, although important advances have been made, including the introduction of direct-acting dopamine agonists, MAO-B inhibitors, L-dopa slow-release formulations, and the experimental use of catechol-*O*-methyltransferase (COMT) inhibitors. In addition, new concepts of "neuroprotection" have led to the search for drugs that may halt or slow down the progression of nigral cell death in PD. So far, however, none of the agents tested have proven to be unequivocally neuroprotective. This chapter will first review the clinical pharmacology of currently available agents for the symptomatic treatment of PD, followed by a brief review of the present status of "neuroprotective" therapies. The final section will deal with the clinically most important practical treatment decisions in the course of PD.

Symptomatic Treatment

PHARMACOLOGY OF DOPAMINE RECEPTORS

Studies of molecular biology have revealed increasing details about human dopamine receptors, in particular, their amino-acid sequence, their secondary and tertiary configuration, their phyisiological and pharmacological action, and their localization within the CNS. Five human dopamine receptor subtypes have been cloned. They are divided into the D1-like (D1 and D5) and the D2-like (D2, D3, and D4) receptor families, based on their capability to stimulate or to inhibit adenylate cyclase, respectively. The presence or absence of stimulation of adenylate cyclase reflects their different interaction with the guanosine triphosphate (GTP)-dependent regulatory G_i/G_o and G_s-proteins.[13] Dopamine receptors are encoded by genes localized on different chromosomes (the D1 receptor gene is localized on chromosome 5, both D2 and D4 receptor genes on chromosome 11, the D3 on chromosome 3, and D5 on chromosome 4).[14-18] Dopamine receptors share some homologous amino acid sequences, probably reflecting common characteristics, whereas different sequences may reflect the different coupling of each subtype with one particular G protein (G_s or G_i/G_o), and their different drug specificity. Binding studies and, recently, in situ hybridization studies have shown the anatomic distribution of each dopamine receptor subtype, summarized in Table 14-1.

D1 and D2 receptors are mainly found in the striatum and substantia nigra, and they are thought to have a largely postsynaptic localization. D2 receptors can also function as autoreceptors, which have a feedback regulatory role at the presynaptic level, modulating dopamine synthesis and release and neuronal firing rate.[19] The dopaminergic denervation occurring in PD causes changes of these receptors at both the postsynaptic and the presynaptic levels. Experimental MPTP-induced destruction of the nigrostriatal pathway leads to a decrease of the presynaptic D2 receptor population in the substantia nigra at the initial stage of denervation (<90 percent dopaminergic cell loss), without interfering with the postsynaptic D1/D2 receptor population in the striatum. At higher degrees of denervation (>90 percent dopaminergic cell loss), upregulation of these postsynaptic receptors occurs[20] and can be reversed by treatment with L-dopa or other dopaminergic drugs.

The discovery of agonist and antagonist drugs selective for different receptor subtypes (Table 14-1) has enhanced understanding of their respective functions. Animal studies have shown that the D2-like receptors are involved in motor behavior, and the antiparkinsonian effect of dopaminergic

TABLE 14-1 Characteristics of Human Dopamine Receptors

	Chromosome Localization	G Protein Coupling Aden. cycl. stim.	Main Localization in the CNS	Neuronal Localization	Affinity for Dopamine	Specific Agonist	Specific Antagonist
D1	5 q31-q34	G_s Adenyl cyclase ↑	Neostriatum, nucleus accumbens, olfactory tubercle, substantia nigra pars reticulata, globus pallidus, entopeduncular and subthalamic, nuclei, lateral septum, dorsal thalamus	Postsynaptical	Micromolar	SKF 38393 SKF-82526	SCH 23390
D2	11 q22-q23	G_iG_o Adenyl cyclase ↓	Caudate-putamen, nucleus accumbens, olfactory tubercle, island of Calleja, claustrum, olfactory bulb, frontal cortex, pituitary gland	Pre- and postsynaptical	Micromolar	Bromocriptine	Haloperidol
D3	3 q13.3	?	Nucleus accumbens, islands of Calleja, olfactory tubercle, cingulate cortex, medial mammilaris nucleus (posterior part), septal nuclei	Pre- and postsynaptical	Nanomolar	Quinpirole Pergolide	UH232
D4	11 p	?	Medulla, frontal cortex	?	Submicromolar		Clozapine
D5	4 p16	G_s Adenyl cyclase ↑	Lateral mammillary nuclei, anterior pretectal nuclei, some hippocampal layers	?	Submicromolar		

drugs appears to be mainly a result of the D2-like receptor stimulation. Costimulation of D1 receptors, however, is also important for reversal of parkinsonian motor deficits.[21] D1 receptors are expressed on gamma-aminobutyric acid (GABA) neurons of the so-called direct striatal outflow pathway whereas the indirect striopallidal GABAergic pathway expresses the D2 receptor.

Dopamine has a differential effect on those two striatopallidal and striatonigral outflow systems, with inhibition of D1 receptor expressing neurons of the direct pathway and stimulation of D2 neurons of the indirect pathway (Fig. 14-1*A* and *B*). As a consequence, striatal dopamine deficiency of PD leads to underactivity in the direct pathway and hyperactivity in the indirect pathway.[22,23] Ideally, antiparkinsonian drugs should reverse both changes in a balanced way, which would appear to require mixed D1 and D2 agonism. So far, however, none of the available dopaminergic drugs seems to be capable of restoring normal striatal function on a long-term basis. More basic research has to be done in order to fully understand the function of dopamine receptors in PD, in particular the possible subtype differences within the same dopamine receptor class, their interaction, and their differential effect on the dopaminergic system itself or on other systems (cholinergic, serotoninergic, adrenergic).

FIGURE 14-1 A and B Schematic diagram of the "indirect" and the "direct" striatopallidal pathways with their neurotransmitters and neuropeptides. Striatal neurons forming the "indirect" pathway contain enkephalin (ENK) and the D2 dopamine (DA) receptor, those of the "direct" pathway contain substance P (SP) and the D1 dopamine receptor. Normally, there is balanced activity of the "indirect" and the "direct" pathways (*A*). DA denervation leads to overactivity of the "indirect" and underactivity of the "direct" pathway. As a result, there is overactivity of inhibitory efferents projecting from the internal globus pallidus segment (GPi) to the motor thalamus, reducing thalamocortical drive (*B*). GPe, global pallidus external segment; GLU, glutamate.

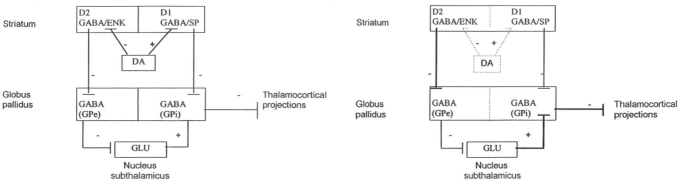

DOPAMINERGIC AGENTS

L-DOPA

Basic Pharmacology and Mechanisms of Action

L-dopa is absorbed in the gastrointestinal tract at the level of the small bowel, using the large neutral amino acid (LNAA) transport system. L-dopa is then rapidly distributed into other tissues, mainly muscle, with a half-life of 5–10 minutes.[24,25] It crosses the blood-brain barrier via the LNAA transport system, competing with the normal concentration of plasma amino acids. Peripherally, L-dopa is rapidly catabolized by aromatic amino acid decarboxylase (AADC) and COMT (Fig. 14-2) and eliminated from plasma with a half-life of approximately 60 minutes (Table 14-2).[24–26] The amount of L-dopa that eventually reaches the brain after ingestion of an oral dose is dependent on a number of variables that may interfere with absorption and transport of the drug.[25–28] The speed of gastric emptying is crucial for the time interval to reach plasma levels, as absorption sites for L-dopa are in the intestinal wall. Food may delay gastric transit time, and in the case of protein-rich meals, competition between L-dopa and dietary LNAA for transmucosal transport further contributes to erratic intestinal absorption (Fig. 14-3). L-dopa versus LNAA transport competition may also significantly reduce the amount of plasma L-dopa crossing the endothelial blood-brain barrier.[29,30] The stomach mucosa, as well as the bowel and the liver, are rich in AADC and COMT. Those enzymes convert L-dopa into dopamine and O-methyldopa, reducing the bioavailability of L-dopa.[31,32] For this reason commonly used L-dopa preparations contain inhibitors of the peripheral AADC (benserazide or carbidopa; see Table 14-3),[33,34] and inhibitors of COMT are currently undergoing clinical testing (see below).

Coadministration of peripherally acting AADC inhibitors doubles the bioavailability of L-dopa without significant effects on elimination half-life.[35] Consequently, therapeutically effective L-dopa doses are much lower when administered in combination with decarboxylase inhibitors (DCI) and the incidence of peripheral side effects like nausea, vomiting and hypotension is markedly reduced. The exact central mechanisms of L-dopa action are disputed. The classical hypothesis assumes that L-dopa is taken up by residual dopaminergic neurons, decarboxylated by AADC in these surviving cells, and finally synaptically released.[36] According to this hypothesis there should be a continuous loss of L-dopa efficacy with

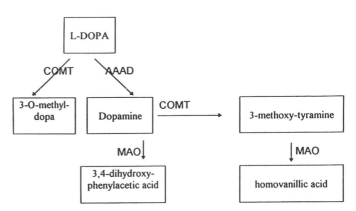

FIGURE 14-2 Schematic diagram of the two major avenues of enzymatic handling of L-dopa. AAAD, aromatic amino acid decarboxylase; COMT, catechol-O-methyltransferase; MAO, monoamine oxidase.

disease duration which is clearly not observed in some PD patients. This suggests alternative mechanisms of presynaptic handling of L-dopa, and the exact site of decarboxylation of exogenous L-dopa to dopamine remains unknown.[37] In the striatum, dopamine is mainly deaminated by a MAO-B and methylated by a central COMT, with production of 3-O-methyldopa (3-OMD).[38] There is clinical and animal experimental evidence to suggest that nigral cell loss results in secondary upregulation of postsynaptic D2 receptors (supersensitivity), accounting for the dramatic initial response to L-dopa substitution in untreated PD patients. It remains a matter of debate as to whether clinical problems of long-term treatment with L-dopa, such as response oscillations and dyskinesias, are related to treatment-induced downregulation of D2 receptors.[26] The role of D1 receptors in the pathogenesis of sensitivity changes is also obscure.

Regardless of these uncertainties concerning its exact mechanism of action, L-dopa is still the most effective and best tolerated of all antiparkinsonian drugs.

Current Indications

Despite numerous advances in the development of dopaminergic drugs, L-dopa substitution continues to be regarded as the gold standard of antiparkinsonian pharmacotherapy. L-dopa responsiveness is considered one of the diagnostic criteria differentiating idiopathic PD (IPD) from other parkinsonian syndromes (multiple-system atrophy, progressive su-

TABLE 14-2 L-dopa Pharmacokinetic Parameters: Summary of Human Studies

Study	Apparent Volume of Distribution	Plasma Clearance (liters/h)	T$_{1/2}$ Alpha (min)	T$_{1/2}$ Beta (h)
Hardie et al., 1986	83.1 liters	36.2	5.5	1.6
Sasahara et al., 1980	87.8 liters	96.6		0.6
Fabbrini et al., 1987	0.26 liters/h	0.13		1.4
Nutt et al., 1985	0.67 liters/h	0.3		1.4
Poewe et al. (unpublished data)	3 liters/h	1.4	5.4	1.5

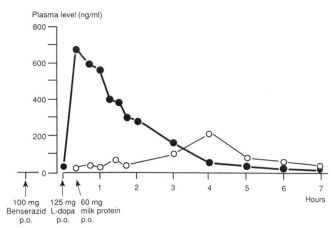

Plasma level (ng/ml)

100 mg Benserazid p.o. 125 mg L-dopa p.o. 60 mg milk protein p.o.

FIGURE 14-3 L-dopa plasma levels after a standard oral (p.o.) dose of 125 mg, given on an empty stomach (filled symbols) or with a 60-mg milk protein drink (open symbols). Note delayed plasma peak and reduced area under the curve when the drug was taken with protein.

TABLE 14-3 Commonly Used L-Dopa Preparations

Substance	Commercial Name	Dosage (mg)
L-dopa/carbidopa	Sinemet (tablets)	100/10
		100/25
		250/25
L-dopa/carbidopa slow-release	Sinemet CR (tablets)	100/25
		200/50
L-dopa/benserazide*	Madopar (capsule)	50/12.5
		100/25
		200/50
	Madopar (tablets)	100/25
		200/50
L-dopa/benserazide slow-release*	Madopar CR (capsule)	100/25
	Madopar HBS (capsule)	100/25
L-dopa/benserazide dispersible*	Madopar-dispersible (tablets)	100/25

*Not available in the United States.

pranuclear palsy, or secondary parkinsonism),[39] although some patients with multiple-system atrophy may initially respond to L-dopa.[40]

There is, however, controversy as to when in the course of Parkinson's disease L-dopa treatment should be started. It is currently accepted that the early use of L-dopa should be avoided in young onset IPD (before the age of 40), because these patients are at particular risk for early development of abnormal involuntary movements and response fluctuations (see below). On the other hand, L-dopa treatment is indicated in those patients in whom symptoms cause significant disability and/or interfere with performance at work and in whom alternative strategies fail to produce sufficient benefit.[41] Although it has been shown that low-dose L-dopa therapy is associated with fewer long-term complications, the L-dopa dose and the number of doses per day should be adjusted according to the individual needs.[42] The current available formulations of L-dopa in association with a peripheral AADC inhibitors are shown in Table 14-3.

Side Effects and Late L-Dopa Failure

Despite coadministration of AADC some patients initially experience nausea and vomiting when L-dopa treatment is started. Most patients, however, develop tolerance to these side effects within days. In severe cases they may be controlled outside the United States by coadministration of domperidone (10–20 mg) one hour before dosing. The same is true for postural hypotension induced by L-dopa.[43] In the United States, the use of extra carbidopa (25 mg, Lodosyn) or Tigan (trimethobenzamide) 100 mg–200 mg with each L-dopa dosage helps alleviate nausea and vomiting until tolerance develops (weeks or months). Long-term L-dopa administration is associated with the development of late complications, including a fluctuating motor response, drug-induced abnormal involuntary movements, and increasing psychiatric morbidity. Despite the short half-life of L-dopa of only about 60 minutes, patients early in the course of their

treatment experience a sustained motor response during the day with three or four oral doses. This "long-duration response" has been linked to presynaptic storage of dopamine derived from exogenous L-dopa in surviving striatal dopaminergic terminals. After several years of treatment plus disease progression, this "buffering" capacity decreases giving rise to "end-of-dose" deterioration and a predictable pattern of response oscillations related to the timing of oral L-dopa. A minority of patients progress to develop more malignant and unpredictable "on-off" swings with sudden changes of parkinsonian symptoms without apparent relation to their L-dopa-dosing schedule. This latter type of response oscillation has been linked to postsynaptic changes in receptor pharmacodynamics induced by long-term pulsatile stimulation.[44] This pathophysiological classification into presynaptic pharmacokinetic changes giving rise to predictable wearing-off effects and postsynaptic pharmacodynamic alterations producing sudden on-off swings may be too simplistic, because even the "long duration" response to L-dopa is likely to involve postsynaptic mechanisms.[45]

The emergence of response oscillations is usually associated with the appearance of L-dopa induced abnormal involuntary movements. According to their relation to L-dopa response cycles, they are commonly divided into three main types: (a) "peak dose" or "interdose" dyskinesias occur when there is a full L-dopa motor response and are characterized by phasic (choreic or ballistic) asymmetric limb movements but may also involve facial grimacing, as well as trunk and neck rotations. (b) "Diphasic" dyskinesias are clinically linked to transition periods (onset or wearing-off of benefit from an individual dose) and frequently contain phasic and dystonic elements causing bizarre twisting movements of the trunk and extremities. Again, limb involvement may be asymmetric. (c) "Off-period" dystonia occurs after the motor response has worn off and may initially be linked to the early morning hours ("early morning dystonia"). It characteristically consists of unilateral distal painful dystonic limb cramps, most often involving one foot.[46] The exact pathophysiology of dyskinesias is not fully understood, but they are probably related to striatal dopamine receptor changes after dopaminergic denervation and chronic exposure to L-dopa. These receptor alterations include changes of sensitivity, relative balance between different dopamine receptor subtypes, and different translational and neuromodulatory system responses.[47,48] The denervation-induced imbalance between the D1 and D2 receptor-controlled direct and indirect outflow pathways appears to be sustained by L-dopa, perhaps through its predominant action on the D1 receptor.[49]

Motor fluctuations and dyskinesias occur in about 50 percent of patients after 5 years of therapy and in 80 percent after 10 years.[50] Mood swings are commonly associated with "on-off periods" and are believed to be related to mesolimbic denervation with poorly understood postsynaptic receptor imbalance. Thus, depression, anxiety, or panic attacks may be associated with severe "off" states whereas euphoria, hypersexuality, hypomania, or mania may be noted during "on" periods. In addition, L-dopa is known to trigger a variety of psychiatric symptoms, particularly in elderly people or in patients with a history of psychiatric disease. Unusually vivid dreams may represent the first signs of L-dopa psychotoxicity, which may progress to visual hallucinations, delusions, and paranoid psychosis (see Chap. 17).

L-Dopa Slow-Release Preparations

Recently L-dopa slow-release preparations have been introduced in an attempt to produce prolonged clinical effects from each individual dose and thereby smooth out response oscillations. Several preparations have been tested for this purpose, and two are currently available: Sinemet CR and Madopar CR (Madopar HBS). Sinemet CR is either a combination of 200 mg L-dopa and 50 mg carbidopa or 100 mg L-dopa and 25 mg carbidopa, embedded in a slowly eroding matrix.[51,52] A rate-controlled erosion and dissolution takes place as the preparation passes along the duodenal-jejunal mucosa. Madopar CR contains 100 mg of L-dopa and 25 mg of benserazide which, upon gastric contact, are transformed into a gelatinous diffusion body that floats on the fluid contents of the stomach.[53] Both of these controlled-release preparations cause a delayed onset of peak L-dopa concentrations (Tmax); a prolonged decline of plasma levels, as compared to conventional preparations; and have been described as effective for "wearing-off" and other type of motor fluctuations.[54–57] Further pharmacokinetic features of L-dopa slow-release preparations include reduced-peak plasma levels and decreased bioavailability of about 25 percent, compared to that with conventional L-dopa formulations.[56] These pharmacokinetic characteristics have several clinical consequences: (1) the delay in Tmax causes delayed "on" effects, particularly after the first morning dose. (2) With multiple daily doses, L-dopa plasma levels during the day are generally more stable, compared to those of standard L-dopa, thereby reducing end-of-dose response swings. (3) In patients with mild wearing-off type motor fluctuations, interdose intervals can be stretched, resulting in a decreased dosing frequency, although this is usually not dramatic. (4) The decreased bio-availability of slow-release L-dopa requires greater total daily doses, compared to those used in standard preparations.

The combined use of slow-release plus standard L-dopa formulations may overcome delayed "on" effects and generally increase the predictability of onset of clinical effects for the patients. Not all patients with fluctuating IPD, however, are helped by controlled-release preparations.[58,59] The main reason for failure are a lack of predictability of onset of clinical effects and increased peak-dose or prolonged biphasic dyskinesias.[60]

L-dopa slow-release preparations have also been advocated as first-time treatment in de novo patients in the hope that this approach may prevent some aspects of late L-dopa failure. Appropriate studies to test this hypothesis are currently under way (see below).

COMT-Inhibitors

After continued administration of L-dopa with dopa decarboxylase inhibitors, the major catabolism of the drug is shifted to conversion to 3-OMD by the action of COMT (Fig. 14-2). 3-OMD, because of its long half-life of approximately 15 hours, accumulates during chronic L-dopa treatment and competes with L-dopa for intestinal absorption and active transport through the blood-brain barrier. By inhibiting COMT, it is possible to prolong the pharmacological half-life of L-dopa in plasma and brain. Two COMT inhibitors, entacapone and tolcapone, are currently in phase III clinical trials.

Entacapone acts as a peripheral COMT inhibitor[61] with a half-life of 1.5–3.5 hours[62] and inhibits erythrocyte COMT activity in a dose-dependent fashion.[63] Clinical pharmacokinetic studies have shown that coadministration of 200 mg of entacapone prolongs the elimination half-life and increases the mean area under the plasma concentration curve (AUC) of L-dopa because of significantly reduced metabolic loss of L-dopa into 3-OMD[64–68] (Table 14-4). Plasma 3-OMD levels from a given dose of L-dopa are reduced by 40–60 percent. ^{18}F-fluoro-dopa positron emission tomography (PET) studies have shown a significant increase in striatal signal after coadministration of entacapone.[69,70] Recent clinical short-term studies have shown that this compound is able to prolong the duration of action of L-dopa and increase "on" time in fluctuating PD patients.[66–68]

Tolcapone differs from entacapone in that it is a reversible inhibitor of both peripheral and central COMT. Therefore, it not only acts as a peripheral L-dopa enhancer by reducing 3-OMD production, but also it impairs the 3-O-methylation of dopamine in the brain.[70,71] Theoretically this might be a further advantage in fluctuating IPD. Another interesting aspect of cerebral COMT inhibition is the resultant increase in brain S-adenosyl-L-methionine, because decreased levels of S-adenosyl-L-methionine have been linked to depression.[72]

Initial data from small-scale acute single-dose studies in fluctuating IPD patients have shown that tolcapone is well tolerated and prolongs the L-dopa response by up to 65 percent, with a tendency to prolonged "on" latencies. Dyskinesias can be increased in severity or prolonged in duration.[70,71] In summary, COMT inhibitors promise to be a useful adjunct to L-dopa in the therapeutic management of fluctuating PD patients.

TABLE 14-4 COMT Inhibitors: Clinical Pharmacology in Acute Studies

Study	COMT Inhibitor	Dose (mg)	L-dopa (mg)	AUC L-dopa (%)	Tmax	Cmax	Duration of L-dopa Response (%)
Kaakola et al., 1994	Entacapone	200	"Optimal" dose	↓ 38	=	−	NS
Nutt et al., 1994	Entacapone	200	100–200	+45	↓	=	+20–80
Merello et al., 1994	Entacapone	200 or 800	200	"Increased"	=	=	+27–30
Keränen et al., 1993	Entacapone	400	100	+65	↓	=	NS
Myllylä et al., 1993	Entacapone	200	100	+46	↓	↓	NS
Roberts et al., 1993[68b]	Tolcapone	50–400	"Optimal" dose	+53	=	=	+67
Limousin et al., 1993	Tolcapone	200–400	100–150	+100	=	=	+65–77

=, unchanged; ↓, slightly decreased; NS, not stated.

DOPAMINE AGONISTS

Clinical Pharmacology

Dopamine agonists act directly on postsynaptic dopamine receptors, thereby bypassing the need for metabolic conversion, storage, and release in degenerating nigrostriatal nerve terminals, as required for the action of L-dopa. Furthermore, dopamine agonists decrease endogenous dopamine turnover, which is even enhanced by L-dopa and may be one source of potentially neurotoxic free radical formation through auto-oxidation of accumulating dopamine. Despite the considerable theoretical advantages of dopamine agonists over those of L-dopa, they have so far failed to parallel L-dopa's clinical efficacy or tolerability. When introduced into the clinic in the 1970s, dopamine agonists were primarily used as add-on treatment to patients with a failing L-dopa response. The current debate on their clinical role, however, is focused on early treatment, alone or combined with L-dopa, in de novo patients (see below).

Three dopamine agonists are in current clinical use: bromocriptine, lisuride, and pergolide. They are ergot derivatives that share many effects but differ in their respective affinity to dopamine receptor subtypes and duration of action. Their clinical pharmacology is summarized in the Table 14-5.

Bromocriptine mesylate is completely absorbed via the oral route and extensively metabolized in the liver. It has a plasma half-life of 7 hours, approximately four times that of L-dopa.[87] It acts as a D2 agonist with a D1 antagonist activity in nanomolar concentration and as a partial D1 agonist in micromolar concentrations.[88] Its clinical efficacy as add-on treatment to L-dopa was shown in the seventies[89] and later studies confirmed its efficacy as monotherapy in early IPD, with a lower incidence of long-term complications compared to L-dopa.[90] This long-term advantage, however, is compromised by less antiparkinsonian efficacy and poorer tolerability compared to L-dopa, so that only a minority of patients (about 30 percent) can be satisfactorily controlled by monotherapy for more than 3 years.[90] When added to L-dopa, bromocriptine can reduce "wearing off" and "on-off" phenomena in patients with fluctuating PD,[75,91] while concomitantly decreasing L-dopa dose requirements by about 10 percent[92], which may in turn reduce preexisting L-dopa induced dyskinesias. The optimal dose of bromocriptine has been a matter of controversy. Some authors have proposed daily doses as low as 7.5–12.5 mg added to L-dopa. The vast majority of clinical trials, however, have come up with considerably higher doses and the current consensus is that the bromocriptine dose required for effective monotherapy lies between 20 and 40 mg/day,[92] whereas slightly smaller doses may suffice when given as an adjunct to L-dopa.

Lisuride hydrogen maleate is a semisynthetic ergot alkaloid with predominantly D2 dopaminergic activity while it behaves as a partial D1 antagonist. It has a relatively short duration of action (2–4 hours) and improves parkinsonian symptoms and reduces motor fluctuations when added to L-dopa in advanced stages of the disease.[78] Similar to bromocriptine, add-on therapy with lisuride allows for reduced L-dopa doses and amelioration of peak-dose dyskinesias. Unlike the other available dopamine agonists, lisuride is easily water-soluble, which makes it a suitable candidate for parenteral administration. Continuous subcutaneous infusions of lisuride via portable minipumps have been introduced in the late 1980s by Obeso and colleagues for PD patients with refractory response oscillations, but this approach is associated with an unacceptable incidence of drug-induced psychosis in the long term.[93] Some authors have reported evi-

TABLE 14-5 Pharmacologic Features of Currently Available Dopamine Agonists

Substance	Dopamine Receptor Interaction	Interaction with Other Receptors		t/2 [h]	Dosage (mg)		References
		NA	5-HT		Monotherapy	In combination	
Bromocriptine	D2	+	+	3–6	25–45	15–25	1–5
Lisuride	D2 (±D1)	+	+	2–3	0.8–1.6	0.6–1.2	6–8
Pergolide	D2 > D1	+	+	15	1.5–5.0	0.75–5.0	9–14

1. Lieberman et al., 1990; 2. Rinne, 1987; 3. Olanow, 1988; 4. Nakanishi et al., 1992; 5. Montastruc et al., 1994; 6. Rinne, 1989; 7. Gopinathan et al., 1981; 8. Giovanni et al., 1988; 9. Rinne, 1987; 10. Lieberman et al., 1982; 11. Goetz et al., 1983; Lang et al., 1982; 13. Olanow et al., 1994; 14. Pezzoli et al., 1995.

dence for pharmacodynamic dopamine receptor changes with increases of dyskinetic thresholds after subcutaneous lisuride infusions in patients with late L-dopa failure, arguing for continuous dopaminergic stimulation as the optimal treatment modality in PD.[94]

Pergolide mesylate is a semisynthetic ergot derivative that differs from the drugs previously described by its relative potency (it is about 10 times more potent than bromocriptine on a milligram-to-milligram basis) and its longer half-life (it reaches plasma peak concentrations in 1–3 hours, and a single dose is completely cleared within 7 days, with a half-life of 15–42 hours).[95] It stimulates both D2 and, to a lesser extent, D1 receptors, and molecular biological studies have shown that pergolide also has a very high affinity for the D3 receptor.[19] Studies using catecholamine synthesis inhibitors have shown that the dopaminergic action of pergolide is much less dependent on intact dopamine stores than that of bromocriptine, and this difference may be related to the mixed D1-D2 agonistic properties of pergolide.[96] Pergolide has been in general clinical use since 1989, and numerous studies in patients with fluctuating PD have shown that it can reduce motor fluctuations by at least 30 percent and that concomitant L-dopa dose requirements go down by more than 25 percent.[97] Studies comparing pergolide and bromocriptine as add-on drugs in L-dopa-treated patients with response oscillations and dyskinesias have revealed slight advantages for pergolide, both in terms of efficacy and tolerability.[85,98,99] Controlled studies comparing pergolide and L-dopa as monotherapy in early PD are in progress. Pergolide has been reported to prevent the age-associated loss of rat dopamine neurons, prompting speculation about possible neuroprotective action of the drug in PD. This hypothesis is also currently being assessed in clinical trials.

Current Indications

As indicated above, dopamine agonists are well established as add-on therapy to L-dopa when the latter begins to lose effect as a result of the occurrence of motor oscillations and dyskinesias. Their use is also favored by some authors as early monotherapy in young-onset patients with IPD, because these patients are particulary likely to develop early and severe dyskinesias in response to sustained L-dopa. However, the exact role of early dopamine agonist treatment in de novo IPD patients is still a matter of controversy (see below).

Side Effects

Currently available dopamine agonists share a wide range of side effects with L-dopa, although there are differences in their relative frequency. Nausea and vomiting, postural hypotension, dizziness, bradycardia, and other signs of autonomic peripheral stimulation are slightly more common with dopamine agonists than with L-dopa. Dyskinesias and motor response oscillations are significantly less common with sustained dopamine agonist therapy, compared to that of L-dopa. In a small number of patients, the first dopamine agonist dose can induce severe hypotensive reactions, so that small starting doses (e.g., 1.25 or 2.5 mg of bromocriptine or 0.05 mg of pergolide as a single bedtime dose) and slow titration schemes are recommended. Outside of the United

States, coadministration of the peripheral dopamine receptor blocker domperidone can be used to counteract these peripherally induced dopaminergic side effects if necessary.

Dopamine agonists appear to have a slightly greater potential than L-dopa to induce confusional states and hallucinosis or paranoid psychosis.[100] Elderly patients over 70, and those with concomitant cerebrovascular disease and cognitive decline or antecedent history of psychiatric complications, are at particular risk.

EXPERIMENTAL DA AGONISTS

Several new dopamine agonist drugs have shown promising results in clinical trials and appear likely candidates for entering the antiparkinsonian drug market. In addition, apomorphine, the first dopamine agonist ever used in PD, has now been licensed as an antiparkinsonian drug in several European countries.

Apomorphine was first described as an antiparkinsonian agent, reversing all cardinal features of PD in the early 1950s by R. Schwab,[101] followed by observations on its antitremor effect by Struppler and von Uexküll.[102] Lack of knowledge about the underlying mechanism of action and the need for parenteral application initially prevented the further pursuit of apomorphine as an antiparkinsonian drug. This negative attitude was later reinforced by findings of Cotzias et al.[103] of reversible azotemia in patients on high-dose oral apomorphine.

Apomorphine is now known to be a potent mixed D1- and D2-type DA receptor agonist with powerful antiparkinsonian effects. It has a poor bioavailability when administered orally because of extensive first-pass metabolism. It is readily absorbed via sublingual, intranasal, or rectal routes. With s.c. or intravenous (i.v.) injections, it has a half-life of about 30 minutes,[104] corresponding to a 45- to 60-minute duration of clinical effect. Following a s.c. bolus injection, maximal plasma concentrations are reached in about 8 minutes, and clinical effects have a latency of 10–20 minutes. Latencies are longer for the various transmucosal routes (Table 14-6).

Current Indications

Apomorphine's present role in the treatment of PD was pioneered by the group of A. J. Lees and G. M. Stern in London, who showed that s.c. bolus injections or continuous s.c. infusions of apomorphine were highly effective and reliable in reversing "off" periods in fluctuating PD.[115,116] A number of further studies have since confirmed their original findings. Intermittent s.c. apomorphine injections will reverse "off" periods within 10–15 minutes in most, if not all, patients. Doses needed vary between 2 and 5 mg, with occasional patients requiring 7 mg or above for a sufficient effect.[117–119] Special pen injection systems are available in several European countries and enable many patients to perform injections themselves whenever needed, thereby ensuring independence.

On demand use of sublingual apomorphine tablets has the disadvantage of a 20- to 30-minute delay of action, while intranasal apomorphine produces local inflammation with prolonged use.[105,106,110,112]

TABLE 14-6 Transmucosal Apomorphine in Fluctuating Parkinson's Disease

Study	Route	Dose (mg)	Latency of Effect (min)	Duration of Effect (min)
Lees et al., 1989	Sublingual	30 (tbsp)	43	73
Durif et al., 1990	Sublingual	18 (tbsp)	30	120
Goncher et al., 1991	Sublingual	9–18 (tbsp)	20–40	15–90
Panegyres et al., 1991	Sublingual	10–30 (sol)	19	65
Hughes et al., 1991	Sublingual	57 (tbsp)	25	118
Montastruc et al., 1991	Sublingual	30 (tbsp)	10–40	90
Kapoor et al., 1990	Intranasal	6	9	44
Kleedorfer et al., 1991	Intranasal	4.3	5–15	30–60
Hughes et al., 1991	Rectal	200 (supp)	32	195
van Laar et al., 1992	Rectal	15–25 (enema)	5–15	35–60

Patients suffering from complex unpredictable and frequent on-off swings are likely to benefit from continuous s.c. apomorphine infusions given during the waking day or even around the clock via portable minimpumps. Two groups have now presented extended follow-up data of up to 5 years showing sustained benefit over time.[120,121] Painful off-period dystonia can almost always be controlled by intermittent s.c. apomorphine,[122] and some patients on chronic continuous s.c. infusions have shown a marked decrease in the severity of preexisting L-dopa-induced interdose dyskinesias.[121]

Side Effects

Apomorphine's most prevalent side effects include nausea, vomiting, and hypotension, which can all be controlled by coadministration of 20 mg domperidone t.i.d., starting 24 to 48 hours before the first dose of apomorphine. Red itching nodules at injection sites are almost universal but are usually well tolerated and transient. Problems of local tolerability with large areas of inflammation or s.c. abscesses or necrosis have been registered and are often related to noncompliance with hygiene rules for needle use.[120,121] Sedation and other neuropsychiatric side effects are usually mild but, occasionally, clozapine treatment is needed in patients with apomorphine-induced visual hallucinations who are dependent on s.c. infusions to ensure mobility.[122] Another rare complication is apomorphine-induced autoimmune hemolytic anemia, requiring monthly blood counts in patients on s.c. continuous infusions.[122]

Ropinirole is a selective nonergot D2 agonist with weak activity on alpha-2-adrenoceptors and 5-HT2 receptors. In animal models of parkinsonism it has been shown to reverse parkinsonian symptoms.[123,124] In clinical studies, ropinirole has antiparkinsonian effects at daily doses between 1.2 and 4 mg,[125] but the optimum dose range may be as high as 4–8 mg a day.[126] Adverse effects are similar to those seen with other dopamine agonists and can be controlled by the coadministration of domperidone, if necessary. Phase III clinical trials are currently underway.

Cabergoline is an ergoline derivative with D2 receptor affinity. It is characterized by a very long half-life (more than 24 hours)[127,128] and is thus longer acting than bromocriptine,[128,129] allowing for single daily dose scheduling.[130] Controlled clinical trials have confirmed its efficacy as an add-on to L-dopa in treating parkinsonian symptoms and in controlling motor fluctuations.[131,132] Side effects are similar to other dopamine agonists.[133]

Pramipexole is a benzothiazole derivative (nonergot) with a high affinity to the dopamine D2 receptor and moderate alpha-2-adrenoceptor stimulation. The antiparkinsonian effect of this drug has been proven in 6-hydroxydopamine (6-OHDA)-lesioned rats, as well as in MPTP-treated monkeys.[134] Pharmacokinetic studies indicate that pramipexole is rapidly absorbed with peak plasma levels 1–3 hours after administration and a half-life of approximately 9–12 hours (unpublished reports). Completed studies and ongoing phase III clinical trials show that pramipexole (top daily dose, 3–5 mg) is effective in controlling parkinsonian symptoms in both early and advanced PD with side effects similar to those of other dopamine agonists.

MAO-B INHIBITORS

MAO-B plays an important role in the biotransformation of dopamine in the human brain. Inhibitors of this enzyme block the oxidative deamination of dopamine and increase its half-life in the brain. The selective and irreversible MAO-B inhibitor *selegiline (deprenyl)* potentiates the efficacy of L-dopa and improves motor fluctuations in one-half to two-thirds of patients.[135–137] At the dose commonly given in PD (10 mg/day) selegiline effects a complete and irreversible inhibition of MAO-B, with only minimal effects on MAO-A, an enzyme which oxidatively deaminates serotonin and noradrenaline. Selegiline has a half-life of approximately 40 hours, with cumulative MAO inhibition at repeated doses; it has been shown that a 50 percent restoration of MAO-B activity in the rat brain occurs within approximately 10 days after discontinuation of the drug via de novo synthesis of the enzyme.[138] Selegiline is metabolized to metamphetamine and, to a lesser extent, to amphetamine,[139] which blocks dopamine reuptake and releases dopamine and may account for some of the dopaminergic effects. Although a clear antidepressant and amphetamine-like action has not been demonstrated in humans, the partial anti-MAO-A activity, as well as the effects exerted by its amphetamine metabolites, may explain some of the mood-brightening and mood-stimulating properties that can be observed in individual patients. Increased dyskinesias, nausea, hypotension, insomnia, and hallucinations constitute the most common side effects when selegiline is added to preexisting L-dopa treatment. In addition to its well established L-dopa potentiating efficacy, selegiline's role as a neuroprotective drug has more recently been subject to large-scale clinical trials and intensive scientific debate (see below).

Because it is not clear how much of the action of selegiline is really a result of its anti-MAO-B activity, as opposed to other potential mechanisms (including metabolites, MAO-A inhibition, or neurotrophic effects), the recent availability of novel, more selective MAO-B inhibitors may offer the opportunity to study more extensively the dopaminergic effect of the MAO-B inhibition. One of these, *lazabemide (Ro 19-6327)*, is a complete and reversible MAO-B inhibitor, with no effect on the MAO-A isoenzyme. Moreover, lazabemide is not metabolized into other pharmacologically active compounds. Experimentally, it has been shown that lazabemide potentiates the antiparkinsonian effect of L-dopa in MPTP marmosets.[140] The potential role of lazabemide in clinical practice has to be determined by ongoing clinical trials.

NONDOPAMINERGIC AGENTS

ANTICHOLINERGICS

The interaction of dopaminergic and acetycholine-containing neurons in the striatum has been extensively documented. For example, D2 dopamine receptor stimulation inhibits the release of acetylcholine in the striatum,[141,142] whereas D1 dopamine receptor stimulation has the opposite effect.[143] In animal experiments cholinergic muscarinic agonists have been shown to block dopamine reuptake into presynaptic dopaminergic terminals[144] and also to influence the regulation of striatal neuropeptide expression.[145]

The effect of striatal dopamine deficiency in human PD on these various aspects of dopaminergic-cholinergic interaction are not entirely clear, but it is commonly assumed that there is a relative cholinergic muscarinic overactivity.[146] From the first empirical use of the anticholinergic drug hyoscine in PD by Charcot in the nineteenth century, it took more than 60 years to develop the first synthetic anticholinergic drugs. At present a wide range of anticholinergic drugs with relative central nervous system (CNS) selectivity are available (Table 14-7). Their central role in antiparkinsonian drug therapy in the first half of this century quickly faded after the introduction of the much more effective L-dopa. Growing awareness about their detrimental effects on cognitive performance has further restricted their use, particularly in elderly patients. At present anticholinergics are mainly used in de novo patients when a delay in L-dopa treatment is indicated, especially when tremor is the predominant complaint. Their use is also recommended in neuroleptic-induced parkinsonism. Clinical studies suggest that anticholinergic drugs improve rigidity and tremor by 10–25 percent,[43] with little effect on akinesia. Because most of these drugs produce a clinical response of 2–4 hours in duration, they are commonly given three times a day, with the dosages dependent on side effects. The latter include dry mouth, constipation, dizziness, and nausea. Anticholinergics can cause blurred vision because of pupillary dilatation and should be avoided in patients with narrow-angle glaucoma. In patients with prostatic hypertophy, they can provoke acute urinary retention, although

TABLE 14-7 Commonly Available Anticholinergic Drugs

Substance	Recommended Daily Dose (mg)
Benztropine-mesylate	3–6
Biperiden-HCl/lactate	4–8
Trihexyphenidyl-HCl	4–8
Orphenadrine-HCl	150–300
Procyclidine-HCl	10–15

they may help in case of detrusor hyperreflexia. Patients showing choreiform dyskinesias as a result of long-term L-dopa treatment may experience an exacerbation of dyskinesias, whereas those with dystonic dyskinesias may benefit from anticholinergics. In elderly people or patients with dementia, anticholinergic drugs may worsen cognitive function and induce confusional states, with or without visual hallucinations.[147]

GLUTAMATE ANTAGONISTS

Current concepts of the pathophysiology of PD imply that the degeneration of nigrostriatal neurons results in increased activity of the internal pallidal segment that is further enhanced by a concomitant disinhibition of glutamatergic drive from the subthalamic nucleus. This overactivity of inhibitory GABAergic drive from the internal pallidal segment causes inhibition of the motor thalamus and its cortical output, which is believed to be responsible for the akinesia and rigidity that characterize IPD.[148] On the theoretical basis of an increased glutamatergic neurotransmission driving the internal pallidum to inhibit the motor thalamus and cause akinesia, some authors have recently reported beneficial effects of glutamate antagonists in animal models of parkinsonism. For example, N-methyl-D-aspartate (NMDA) receptor antagonists like MK-801, 3-[(±)-2-carboxypiperazin-4-yl-]propyl-1-phosphonate (CPP) and remacemide can potentiate the ability of L-dopa to reverse akinesia in monoamine-depleted rats[149,150]; non-NMDA antagonists, such as 2,3-dihydroxy-6-nitro-7-sulfamoyl-benzo(f)quinoxaline (NBQX), have also been reported to improve parkinsonian symptoms and to potentiate the effect of L-dopa in animal models of parkinsonism.[151] It has also been shown that specific stimulation of either NMDA or non-NMDA glutamate receptors by stereotactic injection in different subcortical targets induces parkinsonian features in rodents in a regionally specific manner.[152] The application of glutamate antagonists in PD, therefore, may require both receptor specificity plus regional selectivity. In addition to these experimental symptomatic antiparkinsonian effects, glutamate antagonists also have a neuroprotective potential via blockade of excitatory amino acid receptors (EAA) that can mediate excitotoxic neuronal cell death.[153]

At present, none of the NMDA glutamate antagonists showing an antiparkinsonian effect in animal experiments are clinically available. However, it is possible that the principal mode of action of the classical antiparkinsonian agent *amantadine* is via glutamate antagonism. Amantadine was first discovered as an antiparkinsonian drug in the 1970s by means of serendipity, and its mechanism of action has long been uncertain. Indirect dopaminergic and anticholinergic actions have been discussed, and only recently amantadine was shown to possess moderate NMDA receptor-blocking properties. Amantadine reaches peak plasma concentrations after 2–8 hours, with a clinical duration of action of up to 8 hours. A dose of 200 to 300 mg given in two to three individual doses (i.e., 100 mg BID-TID) offers moderate antiparkinsonian effects. About two-thirds of PD patients benefit from the administration of amantadine, in monotherapy or in combination with L-dopa. The beneficial effect of amantadine may, however, wear off after 6–12 weeks because of the occurrence of tolerance, but a proportion of patients continue to derive long-term benefit.[154] The drug is generally well tolerated, with livedo reticularis and ankle edema the most frequent side effects. Amantadine should be used with caution in patients with azotemia because of its largely renal elimination. The same applies to elderly patients with cognitive decline in whom amantadine administration may induce confusional states or hallucinosis.

Neuroprotective Treatment

MECHANISMS OF NIGRAL CELL LOSS IN IPD

PET studies have shown that the neurodegenerative process in PD is characterized by a long presymptomatic phase of dopaminergic cell loss, as shown in twin studies.[155] Rapid dopaminergic denervation occurs during the early stage of symptomatic PD, followed by a relatively moderate decline later on.[156] The exact pathogenetic mechanism underlying neuronal degeneration in PD remains unknown; however, a number of hypotheses have been made.

The "oxidative stress" hypothesis is largely based on observations made in the MPTP model of PD. MPTP crosses the blood-brain barrier and accumulates in glial cells in striatum and substantia nigra, where it is successively converted, by MAO-B, to MPDP+ and MPP+. MPP+ crosses the glial cell membrane and is taken up in dopaminergic striatal neurons by means of the dopamine uptake system. It is then retrogradely transported to the substantia nigra, where it blocks the mitochondrial respiratory chain by inhibiting complex I activity, resulting in adenotriphosphate (ATP) depletion and, finally, in cell death.[157] The action of MPTP on mitochondria may be biphasic: initally complex I inhibition causes a transient and reversible effect on mitochondrial respiratory function, then, if this action is sustained, an increase of free radicals ensues, leading to cell damage via oxidative stress. Why MPTP exerts its toxicity selectively on dopaminergic neurons is a matter of debate. A possible explanation is the presence of neuromelanin in dopaminergic neurons, because it can bind MPP+ and may store it, allowing influx of the toxin into the mitochondrial compartment.[158] It is unknown why nonmesencephalic dopaminergic neurons or those of lower phylogenetic species have a reduced sensitivity to MPTP. Recent studies using cloned sequences of cDNA for plasma and vesicular amine transporters have shown that dopaminergic neurons located in the ventral tegmental area express less mRNA encoding of such transporters than cells located in the substantia nigra. This could explain some selective vulnerability of monoamine neurons.[159] The discovery of complex I inhibition in experimental MPTP-induced parkinsonism stimulated the search for similar abnormalities in idiopathic PD. There is a strong body of evidence suggesting a disease-specific loss of complex I activity in the substantia nigra of PD patients that has not been observed in other neurodegenerative conditions associated with parkinsonism, such as multiple system atrophy or progressive supranuclear palsy.[160]

There have been a number of post-mortem studies implicating oxidative stress in the pathogenesis of PD. Increased formation of free radicals and lipid peroxidation of cell membranes have been demonstrated and are thought to result in inhibition of key enzymes, as well as structural damage of intracellular organs leading to cell death.

In early PD there is a selective depletion of the reduced form of glutathione, the natural free radical "scavenger."[161] Therefore, cytotoxic hydrogen peroxide and semiquinones representing the normal products of oxidation of dopamine are not sufficiently neutralized by the deficient reduced glutathione, resulting in the formation of a neurotoxic cascade. Increased free iron and decreased ferritin in the substantia nigra of PD patients, as well as cytoplasmic calcium accumulation, constitute other mechanisms of cytotoxicity that probably represent secondary phenomena related to impaired detoxification capacity and damaged cytoplasmic neuronal structures.

CANDIDATE DRUGS FOR NEUROPROTECTIVE TREATMENT OF IPD

Although the exact pathogenesis of nigral cell degeneration in IPD remains unknown, the presence of oxidative stress and mitochondrial abnormalities in parkinsonian substantia nigra provides interesting targets for neuroprotective treatment. Thus, clinical trials with antioxidant drugs have been initiated in order to halt or slow down disease progression. The finding that the MAO-B inhibitor selegiline (deprenyl) can prevent MPP+ formation and the onset of parkinsonism in MPTP-treated primates[162,163] suggested that this drug might also prevent neurotoxicity of hypothetical MPTP-like toxins in human IPD. This has inspired two important double-blind, placebo-controlled trials, the Tetrud-Langston and the DATATOP (Deprenyl and Tocopherol Antioxidative Therapy of Parkinsonism) studies, which reported on the effect of selegiline as monotherapy on the progression of disability in a large number of patients with early IPD. Both studies showed a significant delay of the onset of disabling symptoms that required symptomatic L-dopa therapy,[164,165] suggesting a neuroprotective role of selegiline. The methods of these studies were subsequently criticized, and it remains unknown whether the symptomatic effect of selegiline masked, rather than delayed, the parkinsonian disabilities. In order to differentiate protective versus symptomatic effects of deprenyl, data from the Tetrud-Langston and DATATOP studies were examined by means of performing wash-in and wash-out analyses.[166] In the Tetrud-Langston study no symptomatic effect of selegiline could be identified with the wash-in and wash-out examination, whereas in the DATATOP study a symptomatic effect was detected only with the wash-in analysis. The small number of patients included in the Tetrud-Langston study and the short follow-up period of the DATATOP study represent other "weak points" of these trials.[167] Recently, a prospective double-blind study (SINDEPAR) designed to control for the symptomatic effect of selegiline provided further evidence that this drug may actually retard the natural progression of the disease, as judged by clinical wash-out studies.[168] Although such studies can never offer direct evidence for increased numbers of nigral dopaminergic neurons, selegiline is presently widely used in IPD, a tendency that is supported by its excellent tolerability (see below).

Further compounds with antioxidant properties, such as alpha-tocopherol (vitamin E), ascorbic acid (vitamin C), and beta-carotene have also been proposed as possible neuroprotective agents for IPD. All of them provide protection against lipid peroxidation by acting as free radical scavengers, but only a-tocopherol has been used in controlled clinical trials because of its lipophilic properties and, consequently, its capacity to penetrate the CNS. However, in the DATATOP study, alpha-tocopherol failed to show neuroprotective properties.[169]

Other mechanisms of cytotoxicity, for example, free iron as well as cytoplasmic calcium accumulation observed in the substantia nigra of patients with IPD, constitute further targets for neuroprotective strategies. Glutamate antagonists, such as MK-801, also may have a potential neuroprotective effect, as discussed above.

Increased dopamine turnover itself produces oxidative stress, generating a pool of free radicals. Therefore, it has been postulated that L-dopa might accelerate nigral cell death by further increasing dopamine turnover and, conversely, that dopamine agonists might have a neuroprotective effect by decreasing dopamine turnover. Although a neuroprotective role of the dopamine agonist pergolide has been shown in one rat study,[170] there are no clinical data to support either the harmful effects of L-dopa or protective effects of dopamine agonists on the progression of IPD.

Recent studies of catecholaminergic cell transplants to the brain have pointed out the importance of trophic factors for the survival of transplanted cells and the sprouting of host cells. Some in vitro studies, as well as in vivo studies in animal models of parkinsonism, have shown that the administration of these compounds can reduce the degeneration of neuronal cells. From these observations it has been postulated that IPD could be caused by a deficiency of neurotrophic factors, and that their administration in the early stage of the disease could halt the progression of symptoms. Among the several trophic factors known only a few act specifically on mesencephalic dopaminergic cells and are, therefore, considered possible candidates for neuroprotective antiparkinsonian therapy (see Table 14-8). Because they do not readily cross the blood-brain barrier, it is at present a matter of investigation regarding how these compounds can best be delivered to the brain (e.g., by means of intraventricular infusion with micropump-controlled release systems or genetically engineered cells). Clinical trials are being planned with glial-derived neurotrophic factor (GDNF), which is currently regarded as potentially the most effective and dopamine-specific growth factor.

Practical Treatment Decisions in IPD

Beyond the presenting motor symptoms treatment of IPD has to take into account a number of additional issues, including age of the patient, employment status, associated nonmotor symptoms, and concomitant nonparkinsonian morbidity. Because treatment options include pharmacological as well as nonpharmacological interventions, treatment decisions in IPD are usually highly individualized and can reach a high degree of complexity.

The best way to guide clinicians through practical pharmacological treatment decisions is referral to controlled clinical trials, assessing the potential and risk of candidate drugs for the various clinical indications. Unfortunately, for IPD clinical trials have not yet provided sufficient data to rule out conflicting opinions between experts. Nevertheless, some generally accepted principles for rational pharmacotherapy of IPD at certain clinically relevant stages have emerged, and these will be summarized below.

TREATMENT OF DE NOVO PATIENTS

Although medical and psychosocial counseling, together with group support and physiotherapy, may for a limited time in a limited number of patients be sufficient as treatment of early IPD, there is generally no advantage in withholding effective pharmacotherapy from an IPD patient with subjectively or objectively disabling motor symptoms. The optimal time point at which to start effective symptomatic pharmacotherapy, however, not only depends on objective parameters in terms of severity of motor symptoms but also has to take into account an individual patient's psychological and socioeconomic status. Interference with performance at work usually is a powerful argument for starting rigorous antiparkinsonian drug therapy. Similar to the decision about when to treat the individual, choice of drugs for starting treatment in PD is based on additional individual factors beyond objective motor impairment. Depending on these variables, several monotherapy options exist.

NONDOPAMINERGIC DRUGS

Amantadine
The principal mechanism of action of amantadine has not yet been established with certainty. Although it is known to increase dopamine release and dopamine reuptake, it has also been shown to possess weak NMDA receptor antagonistic properties. There is a paucity of controlled clinical trials

TABLE 14-8 Neurotrophic Factors That Act on Mesencephalic Dopaminergic Cells

Glial-derived neurotrophic factor (GNDF)
Brain-derived neurotrophic factor (BDNF)
Platelet-derived growth factor (PDGF)
Epidermal growth factor (EGF)
Basic fibroblast growth factor (bFGF)
Acidic fibroblast growth factor (aFGF)
Insulin-like growth factors (IGF-I/IGF-II)
Neurotrophin 3

assessing amantadine monotherapy of PD, but it appears to affect all cardinal symptoms in at least two-thirds of patients. The clinical benefit from amantadine is often transient, with about one-third of patients showing slight-to-moderate loss of improvement within the first months of treatment, but some studies have reported sustained benefit for more than a year. Amantadine is, therefore, best used as short-term monotherapy in early PD with mild functional impairment. Doses of 100–300 mg/day, given in two or three divided doses, are usually well tolerated and may delay the need for levodopa for up to 1 year. Once symptom progression makes the introduction of L-dopa necessary, amantadine should be gradually discontinued to avoid unnecessary polypharmacy.

Anticholinergic Drugs

Age and cognitive status are important factors in deciding for or against anticholinergic monotherapy in early IPD. Generally, patients above 60 years of age or those exhibiting clinical signs of cognitive impairment should be excluded from anticholinergic therapy. Because anticholinergic drugs mainly influence tremor and rigidity without much effect on akinesia, tremor-dominant patients with mild-to-moderate functional impairment are the best candidates for this type of treatment. Clinically, there is little difference between the various available anticholinergic agents, but trihexyphenidyl and benztropine are the two most widely used candidates worldwide.

Generally, it is not recommended to use anticholinergic drugs in patients older than 60, even in the absence of specific signs of cognitive impairment. They may, however, be occasionally considered for use if resting tremor has proved resistant to other forms of treatment.

DOPAMINERGIC AGENTS

L-Dopa

L-Dopa continues to be the single most-effective and best-tolerated drug for the treatment of IPD. An excellent response to oral L-dopa with motor improvement exceeding 70 percent is one of the diagnostic criteria differentiating IPD from other parkinsonian disorders. However, long-term exposure to oral L-dopa will lead to motor complications and "late L-dopa failure" in some 50 percent of patients after 5 years or more of treatment (see above). This number further increases year by year so that, after 10 or more years of treatment most patients probably will develop fluctuations in motor response and L-dopa-induced dyskinesias. Although disease progression contributes to these aspects of "late L-dopa failure," many clinicians are concerned about the role of L-dopa in producing these motor complications. In addition, recent experimental studies have produced evidence that L-dopa exposure might contribute to oxidative stress mechanisms possibly underlying nigral neuronal damage in PD (see above). Although there is no clear clinical evidence after more than 25 years of large-scale use of L-dopa for the treatment of IPD that it would exert deleterious effects on the progression of PD, there is some controversy regarding the following aspects of L-dopa replacement therapy.

WHEN SHOULD L-DOPA BE STARTED? Concern about induction of motor fluctuations and dyskinesias has led many clinicians to delay L-dopa treatment for as long as possible and to initially use either nondopaminergic agents or dopamine agonists (see below). There is general consensus, however, that once a patient's disability has become significant and is interfering with activities of daily living and/or performance at work, L-dopa should be started. The decision about what constitutes significant disability has to be made on an individual basis, and the two major elements in the process are age of the patient and employment status. Patients under age 50 are particularly likely to develop disabling motor complications after a few years of L-dopa treatment, so L-dopa-sparing strategies are particularly important in this patient group. On the other hand, they are frequently the ones for whom the disease poses the greatest risk of unemployment, so that it is often impossible to come by without levodopa, leading to the use of early combined treatment with dopamine agonists (see below).

There are no prospective controlled trials that assess the effect of L-dopa dose on the development of late motor complications in IPD patients. Retrospective analyses of the prevalence of dyskinesias and motor fluctuations in patient groups receiving different doses of L-dopa have produced conflicting results, although there is a tendency for "high-dose treatment" with more than 500 mg of L-dopa per day to produce a greater incidence of side-effects.[42] Therefore, most clinicians will try to obtain sufficient symptomatic relief with the lowest dose of L-dopa possible. For many de novo patients this means treatment with daily doses between 300 and 500 mg of L-dopa plus carbidopa or benserazide. On the other hand, L-dopa responsiveness in a de novo patient with IPD is one of the diagnostic criteria for IPD versus other forms of neurodegenerative parkinsonism. In this diagnostic situation it may be necessary to administer 1000 mg or more of L-dopa for up to 3 months before a definite conclusion about L-dopa responsiveness can be reached.

L-DOPA STANDARD VERSUS SUSTAINED RELEASED PREPARATIONS Several experimental studies have shown differential effects of continuous versus intermittent dopaminergic stimulation on striatal dopamine receptor sensitivity and adaptive changes in the direct and indirect striatal outflow pathways.[171] In addition, there is clinical evidence of increased dyskinetic thresholds induced by intermittent dopaminergic treatment, which can be partially reversed by continuous dopaminergic drug delivery.[94] This has led some authors to believe that the mode of administration of L-dopa and other dopaminergic drugs plays a pathophysiological role in the development of motor complications and that continuous, as opposed to intermittent delivery, can not only smooth out motor oscillations but also prevent dyskinesias. Preliminary 2-year results from a small European study comparing standard versus sustained release L-dopa as initial treatment in de novo PD patients have produced some evidence along these lines. Larger-scaled prospective clinical trials are in progress, so that at present no sufficient data exist to demonstrate a clear advantage of initiating L-dopa treatment with slow-release preparations over use of standard formulations.

Dopamine Agonists

Three ergot dopamine agonists are currently available for the treatment of IPD worldwide. Although bromocriptine and pergolide are both marketed in the United States, Europe, and other countries, lisuride is not marketed in the United States. Bromocriptine and lisuride are D2 receptor agonists with pre- and postsynaptic effects, while pergolide stimulates both D1 and D2 receptors.

All currently available dopamine agonists are, however, less potent than L-dopa in reversing parkinsonian signs and symptoms and, at the same time, impose greater risks of side effects. Nevertheless, there is a growing tendency to use dopamine agonists in the treatment of early IPD, as opposed to their original indication as an add-on strategy when L-dopa treatment begins to fail. This is because the results of several open prospective studies show that bromocriptine monotherapy of IPD is associated with a much lower incidence of motor fluctuations and dyskinesias in the long term, as compared to that for treatment with L-dopa.[90] Similarly, uncontrolled prospective studies with lisuride and levodopa have shown that early combined treatment of IPD patients with L-dopa plus a dopamine agonist may also be associated with fewer long-term side effects after 5 and more years of follow-up, compared to L-dopa monotherapy.[74] Although this has not been reproduced in a small double-blind randomized prospective study comparing early combination therapy with L-dopa plus bromocriptine to L-dopa alone for four years,[172] many clinicians now advocate the treatment of early IPD with a combination of small doses of L-dopa plus a dopamine agonist.

For practical purposes the age of the patient may again be a useful clinical parameter on which to base the decision about using early dopamine agonist treatment. Early onset IPD patients below the age of 40 are at greatest risk of developing disabling motor oscillations and dyskinesias after 3–5 years of L-dopa therapy. It is therefore plausible to withhold L-dopa for as long as possible in this patient group, and some clinicians will define the age border for starting dopamine replacement with dopamine agonists as 60 years or younger.

Selegiline

The MAO-B inhibitor selegiline (formerly called deprenyl) has been shown to prevent MPTP neurotoxicity to nigral dopamine neurons in experimental animals. The concept of possible neuroprotective agents of this mild dopaminergic drug, originally introduced as an adjunct to potentiate L-dopa in the late 1970s, was subsequently reinforced by further accumulation of data suggesting a pathophysiological role of oxidative stress in the nerve cell degeneration of IPD (see "Mechanisms of Nigral Cell Loss in IPD"). If proven to be neuroprotective, selegiline should be given to all patients with IPD, once a diagnosis has been made. However, to date there is no compelling clinical evidence that selegiline does, indeed, exert such effects. Five prospective controlled studies have uniformly shown that selegiline monotherapy or combined selegiline plus L-dopa or selegiline plus bromocriptine can indeed slow the rate of symptom progression, as assessed by either a delay in the need for L-dopa treatment or a smaller degree of motor deterioration after a drug wash-out period in those patients on deprenyl.[164,165,168,169,173] However, there is

no consensus whether these effects reflect symptomatic or neuroprotective effects of the MAO-B inhibitor. Despite this uncertainty, the lack of side effects from selegiline treatment presently lead many clinicians to use it as the first-line drug in initiating pharmacotherapy in de novo patients with IPD. Further, nondopaminergic or dopaminergic agents are then introduced as progressing symptoms and disability make this necessary.

TREATMENT OF ADVANCED IPD

With advancing disease, pharmacotherapy of IPD becomes increasingly more complex and difficult as a result of motor complications of prolonged levodopa treatment, progressive gait and balance problems, increasing neuropsychiatric morbidity, and other nonmotor complications.

MANAGEMENT OF LATE L-DOPA FAILURE

With advancing IPD and prolonged exposure to L-dopa, more than 50 percent of patients will develop fluctuations in their motor response and drug-induced involuntary movements.[42,174,175] While motor response oscillations can often be controlled by a variety of drug strategies, certain types of drug-induced dyskinesias can be quite refractory to pharmacological approaches.

Management of L-Dopa Response Oscillations

Motor fluctuations in L-dopa treated PD belong to two pathophysiologically distinct categories: a progressive shortening of the duration of action of individual doses of L-dopa leads to end-of-dose failure or wearing-off effects, frequently first noted by patients as reemerging parkinsonism in the early morning after the drug-free interval of the night. This problem is closely linked to the pharmacokinetics of L-dopa. With progressive loss of nigral striatal neurons that can metabolize exogenous L-dopa and store it as dopamine, gastrointestinal absorption, blood-brain barrier transport and drug half-life become critical for the onset and duration of effect of each individual dose.[29,176] Wearing-off oscillations, therefore, respond to all measures that will maintain striatal dopaminergic tone (see Table 14-9). Which of the different options listed

TABLE 14-9 Pharmacologic Management Options in Fluctuating IPD

1. Improve L-dopa absorption and transport
   Dietary protein reduction (<1 g/kg per day)
   Enhance gastric motility (cisapride)
   Duodenal L-dopa infusions*
2. Stabilize L-dopa plasma levels
   Increase dosing frequency
   Introduce sustained-release formulations
   Add COMT inhibitors*
3. Enhance striatal dopamine concentration
   Add MAO-B inhibitors
   Add centrally active COMT inhibitors*
4. Add dopamine agonists
   Add bromocriptine or pergolide
   s.c. apomorphine* (continuous or intermittent)

*Experimental.

in Table 14-9 is used depends on the preexisting regimen and on individual patient factors. Shortening interdose intervals by introducing additional levodopa doses is a logical step to take with someone developing wearing-off effects on a t.i.d. or q.i.d. L-dopa regimen. Alternatively, such patients may be switched to L-dopa slow-release preparations or receive adjunct treatment with a MAO-B inhibitor at this point. Individuals younger than 60 years of age who first experience wearing-off effects at daily doses of 500 mg of L-dopa or more will be candidates for add-on treatment with dopamine agonists in order to avoid further increases in L-dopa intake.

A subgroup of patients on sustained L-dopa treatment will develop response oscillations not clearly linked to absorption transport and pharmacokinetics of L-dopa. Such complex fluctuations are often refractory to changes in L-dopa dosing schemes, dietary measures, L-dopa-sustained release preparations, or addition of MAO-B-inhibitors or dopamine agonists.[120,121,177] Pergolide, a D1-D2 mixed agonist with a long half-life, may smooth out response swings in some cases, whereas continuous dopaminergic drug delivery may be the only alternative in others. The available options are all experimental and presently include intraduodenal infusions of L-dopa or L-dopa methylester, as well as subcutaneous continuous infusions of apomorphine via portable minipumps (see above).

Management of Drug-Induced Dyskinesias

L-dopa-induced dyskinesias most often consist of choreic movements involving the trunk and extremities at times of peak effect.[178] Some 30 percent of patients additionally suffer from painful dystonic cramps, particularly involving the foot and leg at times of wearing-off of levodopa effects (off-period dystonia).[43] Still another variety of L-dopa-induced involuntary movements is linked to the phases of onset or waning of a motor response to an individual dose of L-dopa.[179,180] These biphasic dyskinesias also may contain prominent dystonic elements intermingled with jerky and ballastic limb movements (mobile dystonia, as opposed to the fixed painful cramps in off-period dystonia). These three main types of L-dopa induced dyskinesias require different pharmacological approaches (Table 14-10).

Off-period dystonia can be controlled in most patients by strategies preventing off periods. These include nighttime slow-release L-dopa preparations or bedtime doses of a dopamine agonist in those mainly suffering from nighttime or early morning off-period cramps, whereas intermittent subcutaneous apomorphine bolus injections, administered using an automatic pen-ject device, may be a useful strategy for those experiencing short intermittent off-period cramps during the day. Add-on treatment with a long-acting dopamine agonist, like pergolide, will also be helpful for off-period dystonia by reducing motor oscillations.

Disabling *interdose choreic dyskinesias* usually require L-dopa dose reductions with the introduction or increase of a dopamine agonist. Some patients become intolerant even to small L-dopa doses, so agonist monotherapy may be tried. Subcutaneous continuous apomorphine infusions with a discontinuation of all oral treatment have been reported to control dyskinesias in individual cases.[121] Sometimes, it may be necessary to combine L-dopa plus dopamine agonist treat-

TABLE 14-10 Pharmacological Management of L-Dopa-Induced Dyskinesias

1. Interdose dyskinesias
   Reduce L-dopa
   Add/increase dopamine agonists
   Switch to dopamine agonist monotherapy
   Use continuous drug delivery (duodenal L-dopa, s.c. apomorhine)
   Add atypical neuroleptics (sulpiride, clozapine)
2. Biphasic dyskinesias
   Avoid sustained-release L-dopa
   Increase individual L-dopa dose size
   Switch to dopamine agonist monotherapy
   Use s.c. apomorphine bolus injections
3. Early morning/off period dystonia
   Bedtime L-dopa-sustained release preparations
   Bedtime dopamine agonists
   Add baclofen, lithium
   Inject botulinum toxin type A into dystonic leg muscles
   Smooth out response oscillations (see Table 14-9)

ment with small doses of atypical neuroleptics (sulpiride or clozapine) to control disabling peak dose chorea. Recent reports about beneficial effects of medial pallidotomies in patients with refractory L-dopa-induced dyskinesias point to a possible nonpharmacological solution (see Chapter 16).[181]

Biphasic dyskinesias are equally difficult to control. Again, strategies coincide with those aiming at the prevention of on-off swings (see Table 14-9). Sustained release L-dopa preparations, however, are not helpful and may be counterproductive by inducing prolonged semi-"on" states with severe and sustained biphasic dyskinesias.

Management of Drug-Induced Psychosis

About 15–20 percent of patients with IPD develop signs of cognitive decline, leading on to dementia in the course of their illness.[182,183] Although this is very rare in patients with young-onset disease,[184] elderly individuals with PD have about twice the risk of becoming demented, compared to that of the general population. These patients are also at particular risk to develop acute toxic confusional states or paranoid hallucinosis in response to L-dopa or dopamine agonists. Confusion is frequently dose-related and occurs more frequently with agonists than with L-dopa treatment. Although drug-related, the occurrence of confusion and hallucinosis in a patient receiving ongoing interparkinsonian medication should initially prompt a search for intercurrent illnesses, particularly infections or metabolic disturbances. Dopaminergic-induced psychosis in response to L-dopa may be preceded by the patient's report about unusually vivid dreaming, followed by hallucinations at night. At first patients may see familiar human beings or animals without a sense of being threatened. In such situations, as in florid paranoid drug-induced psychosis, the first step is to reduce polypharmacy. In patients on combined regimens containing anticholinergics and/or amantadine, in addition to L-dopa or dopamine agonists, the former should be discontinued first. In combined treatment with L-dopa plus a dopamine agonist, the latter should be reduced or discontinued first

**TABLE 14-11 Pharmacological Management Options in
L-Dopa-Induced Psychosis**

1. Correction of triggering factors (infections, dehydration)
2. Reduction of antiparkinsonian drugs (aim: minimal effective
   monotherapy)
   Reduction/discontinuation of anticholinergics or amantadine
   In case of association L-dopa-dopamine agonists, dopamine
     agonists should be reduced first
   Reduction of L-dopa at the minimal effective dose
3. Administration of antipsychotics
   Clozapine   12.5–25 mg in the evening in case of mild
                 psychosis
               Up to 100–200 mg in 2–4 dosages/day in severe
                 psychosis
   Classic neuroleptics (i.e., Haldol) only in case of florid
     paranoid psychosis for a brief period
   Ondansetron

before reducing L-dopa to the minimum effective dose. Those
patients continuing to hallucinate despite antiparkinsonian
drug reductions have to be treated with antipsychotic agents
(Table 14-11). Clozapine is the drug of choice in this situation.[185,186] Recent reports have suggested that the serotonin
antagonist ondansetron[187] may also be effective as an antipsychotic agent without extrapyramidal side effects but, so far,
this drug is not widely available.

References

1. Ordestein L: Sur la paralysie agitante et la sclérose en plaque
   géneralisée. Doctoral thesis, Martinet, Paris, 1867.
2. Charcot J-M: Leçons sur les maladies du système nerveux. A
   Delahaye, Paris: 1872–1873.
3. Schwab RS, Leigh D: Parpanit in the treatment of Parkinson's
   disease. *JAMA* 139:629–634, 1939.
4. Corbin KB: Trihexyphenidyl (Artane): The evaluation of a new
   agent in the treatment of parkinsonism. *JAMA* 141:377–382,
   1949.
5. Carlsson A, Lindqvist M, Magnusson T: 3,4,dihydroxyphenylal-
   anine and 5-hydroxitriptophan as reserpine antagonists. *Nature*
   180:1200–1201, 1957.
6. Ehringer H, Hornykiewicz O: Verteilung von Noradrenalin und
   dopamin (3-Hydroxytyramin) im Gehirn des Menschen und
   ihr Verhalten bei Erkrangungen des extrapyramidalen Systems.
   Klin Wochenschr 38:1236–1239, 1960.
7. Barbeau A, Murphy CF, Sourkes TL: Excretion of dopamine in
   diseases of basal ganglia. *Science* 133:1706–1707, 1961.
8. Birkmayer W, Hornykiewicz O: Der l-3,4,Dioxyphenylalanin
   (=DOPA)- Effekt bei der Parkinson-Akinese. *Wien Klin Wochenschr* 73:787–788, 1961.
9. Barbeau A, Sourkes TL, Murphy CF: Les catécholamines dans
   la maladie de Parkinson, in J de Ajuriaguerra (ed): *Monoamines
   et Systéme Nerveaux Central*. Geneva: Georg, 1962, pp 247–262.
10. Cotzias GC, Van Woert MH, Schiffer L: Aromatic amino acids
    and modification of parkinsonism. *N Engl J Med* 276:374–379,
    1967.
11. Papavasiliou PS, Cotzias GC, Duby S, et al: Levodopa in parkin-
    sonism: Potentiation of central effects with a peripheral inhibi-
    tor. *N Engl J Med* 285:814, 1972.
12. Cotzias GC, Papavasiliou PS, Gellene R: Modification of parkin-
    sonism: Chronic treatment with L-DOPA. *N Engl J Med* 280:337–
    345, 1969.

13. Schwartz J-C, Giros B, Martres M-P, Sokoloff P: The dopamine
    receptor family: Molecular biology and pharmacology. *Sem
    Neurosci* 4:99–108,1992.
14. Grandy DK, Marchionni MA, Makan H, et al: Cloning of the
    cDNA and gene for a human D2 dopamine receptor. *Proc Natl
    Acad Sci USA* 84:9762–9766, 1989.
15. Sunahara RK, Niznik HB, Weiner DM, et al: Human dopamine
    D1 receptor encoded by an intronless gene on chromosome 5.
    Nature 347:80–83, 1990.
16. Van Tol HHM, Bunzow JR, Guan HC, et al: Cloning of the
    gene for a human dopamine D4 receptor with high affinity for
    the antipsychotic clozapine. *Nature* 350:610–614, 1991.
17. Tiberi M, Jarvie KR, Silvia C, et al: Cloning, molecular character-
    ization, and chromosomal assignment of a gene encoding a
    second D1 dopamine receptor subtype: Differential expression
    pattern in rat brain compared with the D1A receptor. *Proc Natl
    Acad Sci USA* 88:7491–7495, 1991.
18. Le Coniat M, Sokoloff P, Hillion J, et al: Chromosomal localiza-
    tion of the human D3 dopamine receptor gene. *Hum Genet*
    87:618–620, 1991.
19. Sokoloff P, Giros B, Martres M-P, et al: Molecular cloning and
    characterization of a novel dopamine receptor (D3) as a target
    for neuroleptics. *Nature* 347:146–151, 1990.
20. Gnanalingham KK, Smith LA, Hunter AJ, et al: Alteration in
    striatal and extrastriatal D1 and D2 dopamine receptors in the
    MPTP-treated common marmoset: An autoradiographic study.
    Synapse 14:184–194, 1993.
21. Haverstick D, Rubestein A, Bannon M: Striatal tachykinin gene
    expression regulated by interaction of D1 and D2 dopamine
    receptors. *J Pharmacol Exp Ther* 248:858–862, 1989.
22. Graybiel AM: Neurotransmitters and neuromodulators in the
    basal ganglia. *TINS* 13:244–254, 1990.
23. Gerfen CR, Engber TM, Mahan LC, et al: D1 and D2 dopamine
    receptor-regulated gene expression of striatonigral and striato-
    pallidal neurons. *Science* 250:1429–1432, 1990.
24. Hardie RJ, Malcom SL, Lees AJ, et al: The pharmacokinetics of
    intravenous and oral levodopa in patients with Parkinson's
    disease who exhibit on-off fluctuations. *Br J Pharmacol* 22:429–
    436, 1986.
25. Sasahara K, Habara T, Morioka T, Nakajima E: Bioavailability
    of marketed levodopa preparations in dogs and parkinsonian
    patients. *J Pharm Sci* 69:261–265, 1980.
26. Fabbrini G, Mouradian MM, Juncos JL, et al: Motor fluctuations
    in Parkinson's disease: Central pathophysiological mecha-
    nisms, part I. *Ann Neurol* 24:366–371, 1988.
27. Nutt JG, Fellman JH: Pharmacokinetics of levodopa. *Clin Neuro-
    pharmacol* 7:35–49, 1984.
28. Rivera-Calimin L, Duyovne CA, Morgan JP, et al: Absorbtion
    and metabolism of L-dopa by the human stomach. *Eur J Clin
    Invest* 1:313–320, 1971.
29. Nutt JG, Woodward WR, Hammerstad JP, et al: The "on-off"
    phenomenon in Parkinson's disease: Relation to levodopa ab-
    sorption and transport. *N Engl J Med* 310:483–488, 1984.
30. Leenders KL, Poewe W, Palmer AJ, et al: Inhibition of [18f]flu-
    orodopa uptake into human brain by amino acids demonstrated
    by positron emission tomography. *Ann Neurol* 20:258–262, 1986.
31. Nutt JG, Woodward WR, Anderson JL: The effect of carbidopa
    on the pharmacokinetics of intravenously administered levo-
    dopa: The mechanism of action in the treatment of Parkinson-
    ism. *Ann Neurol* 18:537–543, 1985.
32. Schultz E: Cathecol-O-methyltransferase and aromatic L-amino
    acid decarboxylase activities in human gastrointestinal tissues.
    Life Sci 49:721–725, 1991.
33. Barbeau A, Gillo-Joffroy L, Mars H: Treatment of Parkinson's
    disease with levodopa and Ro 4-4602. *Clin Pharmacol Ther*
    12:353–359, 1971.

34. Calne DB, Reid JL, Vakil SD, et al: Idiopathic parkinsonism treated with an extra-cerebral decarboxylase inhibitor in combination with levodopa. *Br Med J* 3:279–732, 1971.

35. Nutt JG, Woodward WR, Anderson JL: Effect of carbidopa on pharmacokinetics of intravenously administered levodopa: Implications for mechanism of action of carbidopa in the treatment of parkinsonism. *Ann Neurol* 13:537–544, 1985.

36. Hefti F, Melamed E, Wurtman RJ: The site of dopamine formation in rat striatum after L-dopa administration. *J Pharmacol Exp Ther* 217:189–197, 1980.

37. Poewe W: L-dopa in Parkinson's disease: Mechanisms of action anf pathophysiology of late failure, in Jankovic J, Tolosa E (eds): *Parkinson's Disease and Movement Disorders*. Baltimore: Williams & Wilkins, 1993, pp 103–113.

38. Kuruma I, Bartholini G, Tissot R, Pletscher A: The metabolism of 3-O methyldopa, a precursor of dopa in man. *Clin Pharmacol Ther* 12:678–682, 1971.

39. Hughes AJ, Daniel SE, Kilford L, Lees AJ: Accuracy of clinical diagnosis of idiopathic Parkinson's disease: a clinico-pathological study of 100 cases. *J Neurol Neurosurg Psychiatry* 55:181–184, 1992.

40. Wenning GK, Ben Shlomo Y, Magalhães, et al: Clinical features and natural history of multiple system atrophy. An analysis of 100 cases. *Brain* 117:835–845, 1994.

41. Marsden: Parkinson's disease. *J Neurol Neurosurg Psychiatry* 57:672–681, 1994.

42. Poewe WH, Lees AJ, Stern GM: Low-dose L-dopa therapy in Parkinson's disease: A 6-year follow-up study. *Neurology* 36:1528–1530, 1986.

43. Quinn NP: Anti-parkinsonian drugs today. *Drugs* 28:236–262, 1984.

44. Mouradian MM, Juncos JL, Fabbrini G, et al: Motor fluctuations in Parkinson's disease: Central pathophysiological mechanisms, part II. *Ann Neurol* 24:372–378, 1988.

45. Nutt JG, Woodward WR: Levodopa pharmacokinetics and pharmacodynamics in fluctuating parkinsonian patients. *Neurology* 36:739–744,1986.

46. Poewe W, Lees AJ, Stern GM: Dystonia in Parkinson's disease: Clinical and pharmacological features. *Ann Neurol* 23:73–78, 1988.

47. Savasta M, Dubois A, Feuerstein C, et al: Denervation supersensitivity of striatal D2 receptors is restricted to the ventro- and dorsolateral regions of the striatum. *Neurosci Lett* 74:180–186, 1987.

48. Chase TN, Engber TM, Mouradian MM: Striatal dopaminoceptive system changes and motor response complications in L-dopa-treated patients with advanced Parkinson's disease. *Adv Neurol* 60:181–185, 1993.

49. Jenner P: The rationale for the use of dopamine agonists in Parkinson's disease. *Neurology* 45(suppl 3):S6–S12, 1995.

50. Marsden CD: Late levodopa failure-pathophysiology and management, in Poewe W, Lees AJ (eds): 20 years of Madopar-new avenues. Basel, Switzerland: Editiones Roche, 1993, pp 65–76.

51. LeWitt PA, Nelson MV, Berchou RC, et al: Controlled-release carbodopa/levodopa (Sinemet 50/200 CR4): Clinical and pharmacokinetic studies. *Neurology* 39(suppl 2):45–53, 1989.

52. Yeh KC, August TF, Bush DF, et al: Pharmacokinetics and bioavailibility of Sinemet CR: A summary of human studies. *Neurology* 39:25–38, 1989.

53. Erni W, Held K: The hydrodynamically balanced system: A novel principle of controlled drug release. *Eur Neurol* 27(suppl 1):21–27, 1987.

54. Goetz CG, Tanner CM, Shannon KM, et al: Controlled-release carbidopa/levodopa (CR4-Sinemet) in Parkinson's disease patients with and without motor fluctuations. *Neurology* 38:1143–1146, 1988.

55. Cedarbaum JM, Breck L, Kutt H, McDowell FH: Controlled-release levodopa/carbidopa. II. Sinemet CR4 treatment of response fluctuations in Parkinson's disease. *Neurology* 37:1607–1612, 1987.

56. Koller W, Pahwa R: Treating motor fluctuations with controlled-release levodopa preparations. *Neurology* 44(suppl 6):S23–S28, 1994.

57. Rinne UK: Madopar HBS in the long-term treatment of parkinsonian patients with fluctuations in disability. *Eur Neurol* 27(suppl 1):120–125, 1987.

58. Poewe WH, Lees AJ, Stern GM: Treatment of motor fluctuations in Parkinson's disease with an oral sustained-release preparation of L-dopa: Clinical and pharmacological observations. *Clin Neuropharmacol* 9:430–439, 1986.

59. Kleedorfer B, Poewe W: Comparative efficacy of two oral sustained-release preparations of L-dopa in fluctuating Parkinson's disease. Preliminary findings in 20 patients. *J Neural Transm Park Dis Dement Sect* 4:173–178, 1992.

60. Le Witt PA: Clinical studies with and pharmacokinetic considerations of sustained-release levodopa. *Neurology* 42(suppl 1):28–31, 1992.

61. Kaakkola S, Wurtman RJ: Effects of COMT inhibitors on striatal dopamine metabolism: A microdialysis study. *Brain Res* 587:241–249, 1992.

62. Keränen T, Gordin A, Karlsson M, et al: Inhibition of solubile catechol-O-methyltransferase and single-dose pharmacokinetics after oral and intravenous administration of entacapone. *Eur J Clin Pharmacol* 46:151–157, 1994.

63. Nissinen E, Lindén IB, Schultz E, Pohto P: Biochemical and pharmacological properties of a peripherally acting catechol-O-methyltransferase inhibitor Entacapone. *Naunyn Schmiedebergs Arch Pharmacol* 346:262–266, 1992.

64. Myllyla VV, Sotaniemi KA, Illi A, et al: Effect of entacapone, a COMT inhibitor, on the pharmacokinetics of levodopa and on cardiovascular responses in patients with Parkinson's disease. *Eur J Clin Pharmacol* 45:419–423, 1993.

65. Keränen T, Gordin A, Harjola VP, et al: The effect of catechol-O-methyl transferase inhibition by entacapone on the pharmacokinetics and metabolism of levodopa in healthy volunteers. *Clin Neuropharmacol* 16:145–156, 1993.

66. Sawle GV, Burn DJ, Morrish PK, et al: The effect of entacapone (OR-611) on brain [18F]-6-L-fluorodopa metabolism: Implications for levodopa therapy of Parkinson's disease. *Neurology* 44:1292–1297, 1994.

67. Kaakkola S, Teräväinen H, Ahtila S, et al: Effect of entacapone, a COMT inhibitor, on clinical disability and levodopa metabolism in parkinsonian patients. *Neurology* 44:77–80, 1994.

68. Merello M, Lees AJ, Webster R, et al: Effect of entacapone, a peripherally acting catechol-O-methyltransferase inhibitor, on the motor response to acute treatment with levodopa in patients with Parkinson's disease. *J Neurol Neurosurg Psychiatry* 57:186–189, 1994.

68b. Roberts JW, Cora-Locatelli G, Bravi D, Amantea MA, Mouradian MM, Chase TN: Catechol-O-methyltransferase inhibitor Tolcapone prolongs levodopa/carbidopa action in parkinsonian patients. *Neurology* 43:2685–2688, 1993.

69. Nutt JG, Woodward WR, Beckner RM, et al: Effect of peripheral catechol-O-methyltransferase inhibition on the pharmacokinetics and pharmacodynamics of levodopa in parkinsonian patients. *Neurology* 44:913–919, 1994.

70. Limousin P, Pollak P, Gervason-Tournier CL, et al: Ro 40-7592, a COMT inhibitor, plus levodopa in Parkinson's disease. *Lancet* 341:1605, 1993.

71. Davis TL, Roznoski M, Burns RS: Effects of tolcapone in Parkinson's patients taking L-dihydroxyphenylalanine/carbidopa and selegiline. *Mov Disord* 10:349–351, 1995.

72. S-adenosyl-L-methionine as antidepressant: A meta-analysis of clinical studies: Bressa GM. *Acta Neurol Scand Suppl* 154:7–14, 1994.

73. Lieberman A, Gopinathan G, Neophydites A, et al: Dopamine agonists in Parkinson's disease, in Stern G (ed): *Parkinson's Disease.* London: Chapman Hall, 1990, pp 509–557.

74. Rinne UK: Early combination of bromocriptine and levodopa in the tratment of early Parkinson's disease: A 5-year follow up. *Neurology* 37:826–828, 1987.

75. Olanow CW: Single blind double observer-controlled study of carbidopa/levodopa vs bromocriptine in untreated Parkinson patients *Arch Neurol* 45:206, 1988.

76. Nakanishi T, Iwata M, Goto I, et al: Nation-wide collaborative study on the long-term effects of bromocriptine in the treatment of parkinsonian patients. *Eur Neurol* 32(suppl):9–22, 1992.

77. Montastruc JL, Rascol O, Senard JM, Rascol A: A randomised controlled study comparing bromocriptine to which levodopa was added later, with levodopa alone in previously untreated patients with Parkinson's disease: A five year follow up. *J Neurol Neurosurg Psychiatry* 57:1034–1038, 1994.

78. Rinne UK: Lisuride a dopamine agonist in the treatment of early Parkinson's disease. *Neurology* 39:336–339, 1989.

79. Gopinathan G, Teravainen H, Dambrosia JM, et al: Lisuride in parkinsonism. *Neurology* 31:371–376, 1981.

80. Giovannini P, Scigliano G, Piccolo I, et al: Lisuride in Parkinson's disease. *Clin Neuropharmacol* 11:201–211, 1988.

81. Rinne UK: Dopamine agonists as primary treatment in Parkinson's disease. *Adv Neurol* 456:519–524, 1987.

82. Lieberman A, Goldstein M, Gopinathan G: Further studies with pergolide in Parkinson's disease. *Neurology* 32:1181–1184, 1982.

83. Goetz CG, Tanner ZM, Glantz R: Pergolide in Parkinson's disease. *Arch Neurol* 40:785–787, 1983.

84. Lang AE, Quinn N, Brincat S: Pergolide in late stage Parkinson's disease. *Ann Neurol* 12:243–247, 1982.

85. Olanow CW, Fahn S, Muenter M, et al: A multicenter double-blind placebo-controlled trial of pergolide as an adjunct to Sinemet in Parkinson's disease. *Mov Disord* 9:40–47, 1994.

86. Pezzoli G, Martignoni E, Pacchetti C, et al: A crossover, controlled study comparing pergolide with bromocriptine as an adjunct to levodopa for the treatment of Parkinson's disease. *Neurology* 45(suppl 3):S22–27, 1995.

87. Olanow C: Dopamine agonists in early Parkinson's disease, in Stern MB, Hurtig HI (eds): *The Comprehensive Management of Parkinson's disease.* New York: PMA Publishing Co, 1988, pp 89–100.

88. Schachter M, Bedard P, Debona AG, et al: The role of D-1 and D-2 receptors. *Nature* 286:157–159, 1980.

89. Calne DB, Teychenne PF, Claveria LE, et al: Bromocriptine in parkinsonism. *Br Med J* 4:442–444, 1974.

90. Lees AJ, Stern GM: Sustained bromocriptine therapy in previously untreated patients with Parkinson's disease. *J Neurol Neurosurg Psychiatry* 44:1020–1023, 1981.

91. Lieberman A, Gopinathan G, Neophytides A: Management of levodopa failures: The use of dopamine agonists. *Clin Neuropharmacol* 9(suppl 2):S9–S21, 1986.

92. Lieberman AN, Neophytides A, Leibowitz M, et al: Comparative efficacy of pergolide and bromocriptine in patients with advanced Parkinson's disease. *Adv Neurol* 37:95–108, 1983.

93. Vaamonde J, Luquin MR, Obeso JA: Subcutaneous lisuride infusion in Parkinson's disease. Response to chronic administration in 34 patients. *Brain* 114:601–617, 1991.

94. Baronti F, Mouradian M, Davis LT: Continuous lisuride effects on central dopaminergic mechanisms in Parkinson's disease. *Ann Neurol* 32:776–781, 1992.

95. Rubin A, Leneberger L, Dhahir P: Physiologic disposition of pergolide. *Clin Pharmacol Ther* 30:258–265, 1981.

96. Duvoisin RC, Hekkila RE: Pergolide-induced circling in rats with 6-hydroxydopamine lesions of the nigro-striatal pathway. *Neurology* 31(suppl 2):133, 1981.

97. Langtry HD, Clissold SP: Pergolide: A review of its pharmacological properties and therapeutic potential in Parkinson's disease. *Drugs* 39:491–506, 1990.

98. Lieberman AN, Neophytides A, Leibowitz M, et al: Comparative efficacy of pergolide and bromocriptine in patients with advaced Parkinson's disease. *Adv Neurol* 37:95–108, 1983.

99. Goetz CG, Tanner CM, Glantz RH, Klawans HL: Chronic agonist therapy for Parkinson's disease: A five year study of bromocriptine and pergolide. *Neurology* 35:749–751, 1985.

100. Serby M, Angrist D, Lieberman A: Mental disturbancies during bromocriptine and lergotrile treatment of Parkinson's disease. *Am J Psychiatry* 135:1227–1229, 1978.

101. Schwab RS, Amador LV, Lettvin JY: Apomorphine in Parkinson's disease. *Trans Am Neurol Assoc* 76:251–253, 1951.

102. Struppler A, von Uexküll T: Untersuchungen über die Wirkungsweise des Apomorphin auf Parkinsonstremor. *Z Klin Med* 152:46–57, 1953.

103. Cotzias GC, Papavasiliou PS, Tolosa ES, et al: Treatment of Parkinson's disease with apomorphine: Possible role of growth hormone. *N Engl J Med* 294:567 572, 1976.

104. Gancher ST, Woodward WR, Boucher B, Nutt JG: Peripheral pharmacokinetics of apomorphine in humans. *Ann Neurol* 26:232–238, 1989.

105. Lees AJ, Montastruc JL, Turjanski N, et al: Sublingual apomorphine and Parkinson's disease. *J Neurol Neurosurg Psychiatry* 52:1440, 1989.

106. Durif F, Deffond D, Tournilhac M: Efficacy of sublingual apomorphine in Parkinson's disease. *J Neurol Neurosurg Psychiatry* 53:1150, 1990.

107. Gancher ST, Nutt JG, Woodward WR: Absorption of apomorphine by various routes in parkinsonism. *Mov Disord* 6:212–216, 1991.

108. Panegyres PK, Graham SJ, Williams BK, et al: Sublingual apomorphine solution in Parkinson's disease. *Med J Aust* 155:648, 1991.

109. Hughes AJ, Webster R, Bovingdon M, et al: Sublingual apomorphine in the treatment of Parkinson's disease complicated by motor fluctuations. *Clin Neuropharmacol* 14:556–561, 1991.

110. Montastruc JL, Rascol O, Senard JM, et al: Sublingual apomorphine in Parkinson's disease: A clinical and pharmacokinetic study. *Clin Neuropharmacol* 14:432–437, 1991.

111. Kapoor R, Turjanski N, Frankel J, et al: Intranasal apomorphine: A new treatment in Parkinson's disease. *J Neurol Neurosurg Psychiatry* 53:1015, 1990.

112. Kleedorfer B, Turjanski N, Ryan R, et al: Intranasal apomorphine in Parkinson's disease. *Neurology* 41:761–762, 1991.

113. Hughes AJ, Bishop S, Lees AJ, et al: Rectal apomorphine in Parkinson's disease. *Lancet* 337:118, 1991.

114. van Laar T, Jansen EN, Essink AW, et al: Rectal apomorphine: A new treatment modality in Parkinson's disease. *J Neurol Neurosurg Psychiatry* 55:737–738, 1992.

115. Stibe CM, Lees AJ, Kempster PA, Stern GM: Subcutaneous apomorphine in Parkinsonian on-off oscillations. *Lancet* 1:403–406, 1988.

116. Frankel JP, Lees AJ, Kempster PA Stern GM: Subcutaneous apomorphine in the treatment of Parkinson's disease. *J Neurol Neurosurg Psychiatry* 53:96–101, 1990.

117. Poewe W, Kleedorfer B, Gerstenbrand F, Oertel WH: Die Behandlung von Parkinsonpatienten mit L-dopa-Wirkungsfluktuation mittels subkutanen Apomorphingaben. *Akt Neurol* 16:73–77, 1989.

118. Poewe W, Kleedorfer B, Wagner M, et al: Side effects of subcutaneous apomorphine in Parkinson's disease. *Lancet* 1:1084–1085, 1989.

119. Pollak P, Champay AS, Gaio JM, et al: Subcutaneous administration of apomorphine in motor fluctuations in Parkinson's disease. *Rev Neurol (Paris)* 146:116–122, 1990.

120. Hughes AJ, Bishop S, Kleedorfer B, et al: Subcutaneous apomorphine in Parkinson's disease: Response to chronic administration for up to five years. *Mov Disord* 8:165–170, 1993.

121. Poewe W, Kleedorfer B, Wagner M, et al: Continuous subcutaneous apomorphine infusions for fluctuating Parkinson's disease: Long term follow-up in 18 patients. *Adv Neurol* 60:656–659, 1993.

122. Poewe W, Kleedorfer B, Gerstenbrand F, Oertel W: Subcutaneous apomorphine in Parkinson's disease. *Lancet* 1:943, 1988.

123. Eden RJ, Costell B Domeney AM, et al: Preclinical pharmacology of ropinirole (SK&F 101468-A), a novel dopamine D2 agonist. *Pharmacol Biochem Behav* 38:147–154, 1991.

124. Costall B, Domeney AM, Eden RJ, et al: The antiparkinsonian potential of SK&F 101468—a revealed in rodent and primate tests. *Br J Pharmacol* 96(suppl):90P, 1989.

125. Kapoor R, Pirtosek Z, Frankel JP, et al: Treatment of Parkinson's disease with novel dopamine D2 agonist SK&F 101468. *Lancet* 1:1445–1446, 1989.

126. Kleedorfer B, Stern GM, Lees JA: Ropinirole (SK&F 101468) in the treatment of Parkinson's disease. *J Neurol Neurosurg Psychiatry* 54:938, 1991.

127. Obeso JA, Lera G, Vaamonde J, et al: Cabergoline for the treatment of motor complications in PD. *Neurology* 41(Suppl 1):172, 1991.

128. Ferrari C, Barbieri C, Caldara R: Long-lasting prolactin lowering effect of cabergoline, a new dopamine agonist, in hyperprolactinemic pationets. *J Clin Endocrinol Metab* 63:941–945, 1986.

129. Webster J, Piscitelli G, Polli A, et al: A comparison of cabergoline and bromocriptine in the treatment of hyperprolactinemic amenorrhea. Cabergoline Comparative Study Group. *N Engl J Med* 331:904–909, 1994.

130. Lera G, Vaamonde J, Rodriguez M, Obeso JA: Cabergoline in Parkinson's disease. *Neurology* 43:2587–2590, 1993.

131. Lieberman A, Imke S, Muenter M, et al: Multicenter study of cabergoline, a long-acting dopamine receptor agonist, in Parkinson's disease patients with fluctuating responses to levodopa/carbidopa. *Neurology* 43:1981–1984, 1993.

132. Hutton JT, Morris JL, Melaine A: Controlled study of the antiparkinsonian activity and tolerability of cabergoline. *Neurology* 43:613–616, 1993.

133. Ahlskog JE, Muenter MD, Maraganore DM, et al: Fluctuating Parkinson's disease. Treatment with the long-acting dopamine agonist cabergoline. *Arch Neurol* 51:1236–1241, 1994.

134. Mierau J, Schingnitz G: Biochemical and pharamacological studies on pramipexole, a potent selective D2 receptor agonist. *Eur J Pharmacol* 215:161–170, 1992.

135. Birkmayer W, Riederer P, Youdim MBH, Linauer W: The potentiation of the anti-akinetic effect after levodopa treatment by an inhibitor of MAO-B, deprenyl. *J Neural Transm* 36:303–326, 1975.

136. Rinne UK, Siirtola T, Sonninen V: L-deprenyl treatment of on-off phenomena in Parkinson's disease. *J Neural Transm* 43:253–262, 1978.

137. Golbe LI, Lieberman AN, Muenter MD: Deprenyl in the treatment of symptom fluctuations in advanced Parkinson's disease. *Clin Neuropharmacol* 11:45–55.

138. Turkish S, Tu PH Grenshaw AJ: Monoamine oxidase-B inhibition: A comparison of in vivo and ex vivo measures of reversible effects *J Neural Transm* 74:141–148, 1988.

139. Reynolds GP, Elsworth JD, Blau K: Deprenyl is metabolized to methamphetamine and amphetamine in man. *Br J Clin Pharmacol* 6:542–544, 1978.

140. Nomoto M, Fukada T: A selective MAO-B inhibitor Ro 19-6327 potentiates the effects of levodopa on parkinsonism induced by MPTP in the common marmoset. *Neuropharmacology* 32:473–477, 1993.

141. Stoof JC, Kebabian JW: Indepentent in vitro regulation by the dopamine-stimulated efflux of cyclic AMP and K+-stimulated release of acetylcholine from rat neostriatum. *Brain Res* 250:263–270, 1982.

142. Friedman E, Wang H-Y, Butkerait P: Decreased striatal release of acetylcholine following withdrawal from long-term treatment with haloperidol: Modulation by cholinergic, dopamine D1, D2 mechanisms. *Neuropharmacology* 29:537–544, 1990.

143. Damsma G, Tham CS, Robertson GS, Fibiger HC: Dopamine D1 receptor stimulation increases striatal acetylcholine release in the rat. *Eur J Pharmacol* 186:335–338.

144. Coyle JT, Snyder SH: Antiparkinsonian drugs: Inhibition of dopamine uptake in the corpus striatum as a possible mechanism of action. *Science* 166:899–901, 1969.

145. Pollack AE, Wooten GF: D2 dopaminergic regulation of striatal preproenkephalin mRNA levels is mediated at least in part through cholinergic interneurons. *Mol Brain Res* 13:35–41, 1992.

146. Duvoisin RC: Cholinergic-anticholinergic antagonism in parkinsonism. *Arch Neurol* 17:124–136, 1967.

147. Dubois B, Danze F, Pillon B, et al: Cholinergic-dependent cognitive deficits in Parkinson's disease. *Ann Neurol* 22:26–30, 1987.

148. Albin RL, Young AB, Penney JP: The functional anatomy of basal ganglia disorders. *Trend Neurosci* 12:366–375, 1989.

149. Klockgether T, Turski L: NMDA antagonists potentiate antiparkinsonian actions of L-dopa in monoamine-depleted rats. *Ann Neurol* 28:539–546, 1990.

150. Greenamyre JT, Eller RV, Zhang Z, et al: Antiparkinsonian effects of ramacemide hydrochloride, a glutamate antagonist, in rodent and primate models of Parkinson's disease. *Ann Neurol* 35:655–661, 1994.

151. Klockgether T, Turski L, Honoré T, et al: The AMPA receptor antagonist NBQX has antiparkinsonian effects in monoamine-depleted rats and MPTP-treated monkeys. *Ann Neurol* 30:717–723, 1991.

152. Klockgether T, Turski L: Toward an understanding of the role of glutamate in experimental parkinsonism: Agonist-sensitive sites in the basal ganglia. *Ann Neurol* 34:585–593, 1993.

153. Albin RL, Greenamyre JT: Alternative excitotoxic hypotheses. *Neurology* 42:733–738, 1992.

154. Parkes JD: Clinical pharmacology of amantadine and derivatives, in Przuntek H, Riederer P (eds): *Early Diagnosis and Preventive Therapy in Parkinson's Disease.* Wien: Springer-Verlag, 1989, pp 335–341.

155. Burn DJ, Mark MN, Playford ED, et al: Parkinson's disease in twins studied with 18F-dopa and positron emission tomography. *Neurology* 42:1894–1900, 1992.

156. Fearnley JM, Lees AJ: Ageing and Parkinson's disease: Substantia nigra regional selectivity. *Brain* 144:2283–2301, 1991.

157. Cleeter MW, Cooper JM, Schapira AH: Irreversible inhibition of mitochondrial complex I by 1-methyl-4-phenylpyridinium: Evidence for free radical involvement. *J Neurochem* 58:786–789, 1992.

158. D'Amato RJ, Lipman ZP, Snyder SH: Selectivity of the parkinsonian neurotoxin MPTP: Toxic metabolite MPP+ binds to neuromelanin. *Science* 231:897–899, 1986.

159. Shimada S, Kitayama S, Walther D, Uhl G: Dopamine transporter mRNA: Dense expression in ventral midbrain neurons. *Mol Brain Res* 13:359–362, 1992.

160. Schapira AH, Mann VM, Cooper JM, et al: Mitochondrial function in Parkinson's disease. *Ann Neurol* 32(suppl):S116–124, 1992.

161. Sian J, Dexter DT, Lees AJ, et al: Alterations in glutathione levels in Parkinson's disease and other neurodegenerative disorders affecting basal ganglia. *Ann Neurol* 36:348–355, 1994.

162. Cohen G, Pasik P, Cohen B, et al: Pargyline and deprenyl prevent the neurotoxicity of 1-methyl-4-phenyl-1,2,3,6-tetrahydropyridine (MPTP) in monkeys. *Eur J Pharmacol* 106:209–210, 1984.

163. Langston JW, Irwin I, Langston EB, Forno LS: Pargyline prevents MPTP-induced parkinsonism in primates. *Science* 225:1480–1482, 1984.

164. The Parkinson's Study Group: Effect of deprenyl on the progression of disability in early Parkinson's disease. *N Engl J Med* 321:1364–1371, 1989.

165. Tetrud JW, Langston JW: The effect of deprenyl (Selegiline) on the natural history of Parkinson's disease. *Science* 245:519–522, 1989.

166. Shoulson I and the Parkinson Study Group: Deprenyl and early Parkinson's disease: Symptomatic versus protective efficacy. *Neurology* 40(suppl 1):153, 1990.

167. Olanow CW: Protective therapy for Parkinson's disease, in Olanow CW, Lieberman AN (eds): *The scientific basis for the treatment of Parkinson's disease.* NJ: The Parthenon Publishing Group, 1992.

168. Olanow CW, Calne D: Does selegiline monotherapy in Parkinson's disease act by symptomatic or protective mechanisms? *Neurology* 42(suppl 4):13–26, 1992.

169. Parkinson Study Group: Effect of tocopherol and deprenyl on the progression of disability in early Parkinson's disease. *N Engl J Med* 328:176–183, 1993.

170. Felten DL, Felten SY, Fuller RW, et al: Chronic dietary pergolide preserves nigrostriatal neuronal integrity in aged Fischer-344 rats. *Neurobiol Aging* 13:339–351, 1992.

171. Chen JF, Aloyo VJ, Weiss B: Continuous treatment with the D2 dopamine receptor agonist quinpirole decreases D2 dopamine receptors, dopamine receptor messenger RNA and proenkephalin messenger RNA, and increases MU opioid receptors in mouse striatum. *Neuroscience* 54:669–680, 1993.

172. Weiner WJ, Factor SA, Sanchez-Ramos RJ, et al: Early combination therapy (bromocriptine and levodopa) does not prevent motor fluctuations in Parkinson's disease. *Neurology* 43:21–27, 1993.

173. Myllyla VV, Sotaniemi KA, Vuorinen JA: Selegiline as initial treatment in de novo parkinsonian patients. *Neurology* 42:339–343, 1992.

174. Marsden CD, Parkes JD: Success and problems of long term levodopa therapy in Parkinson's disease. *Lancet* 1:345–349, 1977.

175. Hardie RJ: Problems and unanswered questions concerning levodopa treatment in Parkinson's disease. *Acta Neurol Scand* 126(suppl):77–82, 1989.

176. Mouradian MM, Juncos JL, Fabbrini G, Chase TN: Motor fluctuations in Parkinson's disease: Pathogenetic and therapeutic studies. *Ann Neurol* 22:475–479, 1987.

177. Sage JI, Trooskin S, Sonsalla PK, et al: Long-term duodenal infusion of levodopa for motor fluctuations in parkinsonism. *Ann Neurol* 24:87–89, 1988.

178. Nutt GJ: Levodopa-induced dyskinesia: Review, observations and speculations. *Neurology* 40:340–345, 1990.

179. Muenter MD, Sharpless NS, Tyce GM, Darley FL: Patterns of dystonia ("I-D-I" and "D-I-D") in response to L-dopa therapy for Parkinson's disease. *Mayo Clin Proc* 52:163–174, 1977.

180. Marsden CD, Parkes JD, Quinn N: Fluctuations of disability in Parkinson's disease: Clinical aspects, in Marsden CD, Fahn S (eds): *Movement Disorders.* London: Butterworth, 1981, pp 96–122.

181. Laitinen LV, Begenheim AT, Hariz MI: Ventroposterolateral pallidotomy can abolish all parkinsonian symptoms. *Stereotact Funct Neurosurg* 58:14–21, 1992.

182. Brown RG, Marsden CD: How common is dementia in Parkinson disease. *Lancet* 2:1262–1265, 1984.

183. Mayeux R, Chen J, Mirabello E, et al: An extimate of the incidence of dementia in idiopathic Parkinson's disease. *Neurology* 40:1513–1517, 1990.

184. Quinn N, Critchley P, Marsden CD: Young onset Parkinson's disease. *Mov Disord* 2:73–91, 1987.

185. Wolters EC, Hurwitz TA, Mak E, et al: Clozapine in the treatment of parkinsonian patients with dopaminomimetic psychosis. *Neurology* 40:832–834, 1990.

186. Friedman JH, Lannon MC: Clozapine in the treatment of psychosis in Parkinson's disease. *Neurology* 39:1219–1221, 1989.

187. Zoldan J, Friedberg G, Golbergstern H, Melamed E: Ondansetron for hallucinosis in advanced Parkinson's disease. *Lancet* 341:562–563, 1993.

Chapter 15

TRANSPLANTATION STRATEGIES FOR PARKINSON'S DISEASE

C. WARREN OLANOW, THOMAS B. FREEMAN,
and JEFFREY H. KORDOWER

FETAL NIGRAL TRANSPLANTATION—PRECLINICAL
   ISSUES
      Tissue Acquisition
      Donor Age
      Method of Tissue Storage
      Type of Transplant
      Site of Implant
      Volume of Tissue
      Tissue Distribution
FETAL NIGRAL TRANSPLANTATION—CLINICAL
   ISSUES
      Patient Selection
      Infectious Disease Issues
      Immunosuppression
      Clinical Evaluations
      Drug Management
FETAL NIGRAL TRANSPLANTATION—CLINICAL
   RESULTS
FETAL NIGRAL TRANSPLANTATION—
   NEUROANATOMIC CONSIDERATIONS
FETAL NIGRAL TRANSPLANTATION—FUTURE
   DIRECTIONS

Parkinson's disease (PD) is an age-related neurodegenerative disorder characterized by loss of melanin-containing neurons in the substantia nigra pars compacta (SNc) and a reduction in striatal dopamine.[1] Treatment in the United States primarily consists of L-dopa coupled with the peripheral decarboxylase inhibitor carbidopa (Sinemet). Initially, this treatment provides substantial antiparkinsonian benefit, but long-term treatment is frequently complicated by debilitating side effects, such as motor fluctuations, dyskinesia, and neuropsychiatric problems.[2] Furthermore, disease progression is frequently associated with the development of postural instability, freezing episodes, and autonomic disturbances that do not respond to L-dopa replacement. Other therapies, such as sustained-release formulations of L-dopa, dopamine agonists, selegiline, catechol-O-methyltransferase (COMT) inhibitors, dietary manipulation, and atypical neuroleptics may provide some benefit in the later stages of the disease, but the majority of advanced PD patients experience disability that can not be satisfactorily controlled with available therapies. Accordingly, there has been a search for alternative treatments that can restore function to this population of patients.

Neural transplantation is a rational consideration for treating PD patients because (1) PD is associated with a relatively specific dopamine neuronal degeneration. (2) Dopaminergic neurons provide tonic, rather than phasic innervation to postsynaptic receptors. (3) Dopamine replacement provides dramatic clinical benefit. (4) There are well-defined target areas for neural transplantation. Based on this hypothesis, fetal nigral dopaminergic grafts have been extensively tested in animal models of PD. It has now been demonstrated that fetal mesencephalic neurons can survive, manufacture and secrete dopamine, form synaptic connections, and reduce motor and sensory abnormalities in 6-hydroxy dopamine (6-OHDA)-lesioned rats[3-7] and 1-methyl-4-phenyl-1,2,3,6-tetrahydropyridine (MPTP)-treated primates.[8-13] Grafts can be transplanted as either solid pieces or cell suspensions. Fetal dopaminergic allografts have also been shown to form normal-appearing graft-host interconnections and to reinnervate the striatum in an organotypic pattern.[14,15] These grafts also exhibit normal electrical firing patterns and spontaneous dopamine synthesis and release.[16,17] Functional benefits can be long-lasting and have been observed to persist in rodents for more than 2 years.[18] Human fetal nigral grafts transplantated into immunocompromised rats also survive and form synaptic connections with host cells.[19-22] They more completely reinnervate the host striatum, but neuritic outgrowth and functional recovery occur over a more protracted period of time. Similarly, fetal nigral allografts transplanted into MPTP-treated primates have been demonstrated to survive, reinnervate the host striatum, and improve motor disability.[8-13] Benefits after fetal nigral transplantation are dependent on the continued presence of donor mesencephalic cells and are lost after their removal or destruction.[23] Behavioral effects are dependent on the type of tissue transplanted and the site of implantation. Benefits are not seen with intrastriatal grafts of nondopaminergic tissue or when dopaminergic grafts are implanted into nonstriatal regions.[24]

These studies illustrate that grafting of fetal nigral cells can provide functional benefits in rodent and primate models of dopamine deficiency and suggest that this strategy may be beneficial in patients with PD. Alternate sources of dopamine-producing cells have also been studied. Sympathetic ganglia, carotid body glomus cells, PC-12 cells, and neuroblastoma cells do not produce behavioral effects that are as prominent or as long-lasting as those observed with embryonic nigral grafts.[25-29] There has been considerable interest in the chromaffin cells of the adrenal medulla. These cells normally produce epinephrine and norepinephrine but only small amounts of dopamine. However, dopamine levels are increased when medullary cells are separated from the overlying adrenal cortex and removed from the influence of glucocorticoids. Grafts of adrenal medulla placed into the denervated striatum or lateral ventricle of 6-OHDA-lesioned rats or MPTP-treated primates provide some behavioral improvement[30-33]; however, these effects are neither as great in magnitude nor in duration as those observed with fetal nigral implants. Initial trials of stereotactic implantation of cell suspensions of autologous adrenal medullary cells into the putamen of PD patients did not provide significant clinical benefit.[34,35] Subsequently, Madrazo and coworkers reported "dramatic amelioration" of symptoms in two PD patients after transplantation of solid grafts of autologous adrenal medullary tissue into the head of the caudate nucleus, using an open microsurgical procedure.[36] This report was widely covered in the media and generated considerable public interest. However, other investigators, using a similar technique, failed to replicate these dramatic effects.[37-40] Most studies did note a reduction in percent "off" time and a modest improvement in motor function during "off" periods, but benefits tended to be modest and transient.[38] Furthermore, the procedure was associated with significant morbidity and mortality, reflecting the need for a craniotomy and laporotomy in a patient with advanced PD.[41] It is now generally felt that the benefits obtained do not justify the risks, and the procedure has largely been abandoned. The lack of a dramatic benefit after adrenal medullary transplantation may reflect the fact that chromaffin cells survive poorly after transplantation.[42] Furthermore, because adrenal chromaffin cells do not send out neurites or form well-defined synaptic contacts with host neurons, it remains difficult for them to secrete dopamine throughout the large volume of the human striatum (see below). Attempts to enhance chromaffin cell viability by infusion of trophic factors[31] or cografting of trophic factor-secreting cells[43] still do not provide benefits comparable to those observed after fetal transplantation.

Of all dopaminergic cells tested to date, fetal nigral cells provide the best behavioral results in animal models of PD. Fetal nigral transplantation also obviates the need for laparotomy and is accordingly associated with less surgical morbidity and mortality than procedures such as adrenal medullary transplantation. Thus, of the dopaminergic cells currently available, fetal dopamine-producing cells currently offer PD patients the best possibility of obtaining a good clinical response with the least morbidity. Based on these considerations, trials of fetal nigral grafting in PD patients have now begun.

Fetal Nigral Transplantation— Preclinical Issues

In considering a fetal nigral transplantation program, it is important to appreciate that many variables related to the transplantation procedure can influence the likelihood that implanted cells will survive, innervate the target region, and provide optimal clinical benefits. Those variables that the authors consider to be most important are: (1) the manner in which tissue is acquired; (2) the age of the donor tissue; (3) the method of storage; (4) the type of transplant; (5) the site of implant; (6) the distribution of tissue; (7) the risk of transferring a contagious agent; and (8) the need for immunosuppressants. Decisions as to how to manage these transplant variables are likely to impact on clinical results.

TISSUE ACQUISITION

Fetal tissue can be obtained from women undergoing spontaneous or elective abortion. It has been argued that fetal cells for transplantation can be derived from spontaneous abortions,[44] based on studies demonstrating that these grafts provide functional benefits in rodent models of parkinsonism.[45]

However, most research centers have chosen to use fetal tissue derived from elective abortions.[46] This is because spontaneously aborted fetal tissue is more likely to: (1) contain genetic or CNS defects; (2) be infected; (3) be disrupted, making it difficult to identify landmarks, stage tissue, and dissect dopaminergic cells; and (4) provide a nonviable graft.

In addition, it is more difficult to obtain donors from spontaneous abortions in such a way as to permit the use of multiple grafts or to schedule the timing of surgery reliably. To ensure that women will not become pregnant solely to provide tissue for transplantation, we use the following guidelines: (1) consent for the use of donor fetuses is requested only after surgical consent for the abortion has been signed; (2) there is no monetary or other inducement provided to either the mother or the physician; (3) we do not advertise for donors; (4) patients are not denied medical care for refusal to donate tissue for transplantation; (5) confidentiality of donor and recipient are maintained; (6) donation of embryonic tissue is made without restriction as to the recipient; and (7) no assurance is provided that donated tissue will be used for clinical or animal research.

It is highly unlikely that the decision to have an abortion will be influenced by the prospects of participating in fetal research. During the 30-year history of fetal tissue research in the United States, there is no evidence that this reseach has influenced the demographics of abortion. At the present time, voluntary abortion is permitted under U.S. laws. More than 1 million abortions are performed annually, and it is estimated that tissue from less than 0.01 percent of these is used for research purposes.[47] In addition, there is no alteration in the timing or indication for the abortion; the abortion is performed in a routine manner; and the fetus is pronounced dead by a physician not related to the transplantation process. The research study involves only the use of otherwise-discarded fetal tissue. Recipients are informed that they are receiving transplanted fetal tissue derived from an elective abortion. All involved hospital staff are also fully informed as to the nature of the procedure.

DONOR AGE

The optimal donor age for graft survival is considered to be from the time dopaminergic cells are first detected in the subventricular zone until they differentiate and extend neuritic processes. Once neuritic processes are formed, cells are thought to be less likely to survive transplantation, possibly because they may be axotomized during preparation. To determine the optimal "window" for fetal nigral transplantation, the authors performed a study of the ontogeny of human embryonic dopamine-producing cells.[48] Tyrosine hydroxylase immunoreactive (TH-IR) dopaminergic neurons were first detected in the subventricular floor at approximately $5^{1}/_{2}$–$6^{1}/_{2}$ weeks postconception (PC). Neuritic processes were first identified at approximately 8 weeks PC and extended to reach the striatum at 9 weeks PC. By approximately 11 weeks PC, all TH-IR cells had migrated from the subventricular zone toward their adult location in the ventral portion of the mesencephalon. These observations suggest that the ideal donor age for transplantation of human embryonic mesencephalic dopamine cells is between 5¹/₂ and 9 weeks PC (Fig. 15-1). Human-to-rodent nigral xenografts confirm these assumptions, demonstrating that optimal survival is between 5¹/₂ and 8 weeks PC for suspension grafts and between 6¹/₂ and 9 weeks PC for solid grafts.[49]

FIGURE 15-1 Low-power (*A* and *B*) and medium-power (*C*) photomicrographs of TH-immunostained sections through the striatum of 6-OHDA-lesioned immunosuppressed rats receiving fetal human nigral xenografts from the optimal donor window. Grafted TH-ir neurons survived in an organotypic manner and extensively innervated the surrounding host striatum. Tissue was stored for 4 days in "hibernation" medium before transplantation. Scale bar in *A* represents the following magnifications: *A* and *B*, 250 μm; *C*, 100 μm.

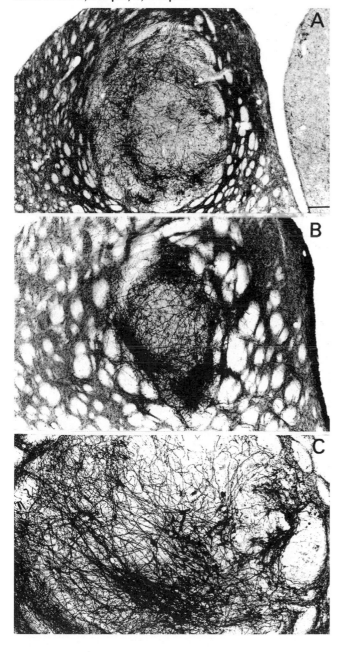

METHOD OF TISSUE STORAGE

It is necessary to store embryonic tissue in order to permit time for transportation to the medical center, screening for infectious agents, acquisition of multiple donors, and elective scheduling of surgery. Redmond and coworkers used cryopreservation to store fetal tissue before grafting.[50] However, cryopreservation of cells for 1 year is associated with a significant reduction in cell viability and neuritic outgrowth after transplantation in vivo,[51] even though there is no fall in dopamine levels in vitro.[52] Tissue has been stored in human amniotic fluid with reports of good clinical benefit.[53] We use a chemically defined "hibernation medium" containing gentamycin in which tissue is stored at 8°C. Using this cold-storage medium, the authors have demonstrated robust cell survival after transplantation in animal models after storage for up to 4 days (Fig. 15-1) without degradation in either the viability or number of transplanted neurons.[54] Using cells stored in this manner, the authors have demonstrated consistent clinical benefits in PD patients[55] and robust survival at postmortem.[75]

TYPE OF TRANSPLANT

Fetal mesencephalic cells can be transplanted as either a cell suspension or solid graft. Most studies performed to date have used a cell suspension graft. This provides more homogeneous tissue distribution but necessitates pooling of tissue. Accordingly, infection or rejection in any one donor could adversely affect all graft deposits. Additionally, cells are more likely to be injured during graft preparation. Solid grafts have an extended donor window, are easier to prepare, and preserve cytoarchitectural relationships. We have demonstrated comparable suvival after transplantation of solid or suspension grafts of human ventral mesencephalon into immunosuppressed rats[54] and, for reasons described above, use solid grafts in our clinical studies.

SITE OF IMPLANT

Although the striatum is separated anatomically into a distinct putamen and caudate nucleus, functional relationships are not based on these anatomic boundaries (Fig. 15-2). Embryologically, development of the posterior two-thirds or the postcommissural portion of the putamen differs from that of the anterior putamen, which is more closely linked spatially and temporally to the caudate nucleus.[56] The postcommissural putamen also differs from the anterior putamen-caudate nucleus complex in its anatomic connections. The postcommissural putamen has reciprocal connections with the precentral motor fields,[57,58] and microstimulation studies in this area evoke discrete movements of contralateral body parts.[59] In contrast, the caudate nucleus and anterior putamen are less related to primary motor circuitry and have extensive neuronal interconnections with the prefrontal cortex and frontal eyefields.[60] Functional recovery after dopamine neuronal grafting is also site-specific in both rodent and primate models of parkinsonism. Grafts placed into the dorsal striatum of 6-OHDA-lesioned rats ameliorate drug-induced rota-

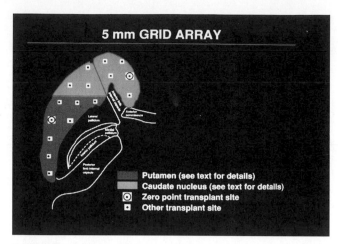

FIGURE 15-2 Schematic representation of putamen and caudate nucleus. Although the putamen and caudate nucleus are anatomically distinct, we divide the striatum into the postcommissural putamen (shown in darker gray) and the anterior putamen and caudate nucleus (shown in lighter gray), because they are more related functionally and embryologically. The postcommissural putamen is more affected in PD and is the target of our transplant procedure. We implant tissue at 5-mm intervals in three dimensions (as illustrated in this diagram) in order to ensure dopaminergic innervation to the entire extent of the target region.

tional asymmetries whereas those placed in the ventrolateral striatum ameliorate sensorimotor attentional deficits.[61,62] Similarly, the pattern of behavioral improvement in MPTP-primates is different after grafting into the caudate and putamen.[63]

It is important to determine which target site is associated with maximal clinical benefit because of the risks involved with multiple needle passes through the brain and difficulties in obtaining multiple fetal donors. There are several reasons to consider the postcommissural putamen as the primary site for neural grafting in PD. Both autopsy and positron emission tomography (PET) scan studies demonstrate greater dopamine depletion within the posterior putamen than in the anterior putamen-caudate nucleus complex in PD patients.[64–67] In addition, degeneration of the substantia nigra pars compacta in PD preferentially occurs in regions that project to the posterior putamen.[68] Experiments in MPTP-lesioned primates demonstrate that dopamine grafts placed exclusively into the putamen induce significant improvement of motor function.[12,63]

There is also evidence suggesting that the anterior putamen-caudate nucleus may be an important target for transplantation in PD. Hemiparkinsonism can be induced by MPTP injection into the caudate nucleus,[69] and fetal nigral grafts placed into the caudate nucleus of MPTP-treated monkeys can induce significant functional recovery, with benefits different from those associated with neural grafting into the posterior putamen.[10,13] Indeed, the best clinical results may ultimately be associated with grafting into both caudate and putamen. Further testing is also required to evaluate the possibility of benefits from grafting into other potential target areas, such as the substantia nigra pars compacta and the nucleus accumbens.

VOLUME OF TISSUE

The volume of tissue that is required to provide optimal results after fetal nigral grafting is not known at this time. A scientifically based determination of this issue is complicated by the fact that dopamine neurons comprise only about 5–10 percent of the cells in a mesencephalic graft and only 5–10 percent of transplanted cells survive in 6-OHDA lesioned rats.[70] Behavioral improvement can be observed in rodents after transplantation of a fragment of a single human embryonic ventral mesencephalon.[19] The smallest number of transplanted dopaminergic neurons demonstrated to provide behavioral improvement is 120 in the rodent[70] and 2000 in the marmoset (S. Dunnett). The human striatum is substantially larger than the rat or primate striatum, and it is therefore likely that transplantation of a significantly greater number of nigral neurons will be required to achieve meaningful clinical benefit. There are approximately 500,000 dopamine neurons in the human substantia nigra, of which an estimated 60,000 project to the putamen.[71] Approximately 20,000–40,000 dopamine neurons from a single human fetus have been shown to be able to survive transplantation into immunosuppressed rodents.[19,72] It may thus be necessary to transplant mesencephalic tissue from three or more donors into each putamen in order to completely restore the normal number of dopaminergic neurons, and both clinical and PET studies show enhanced improvement after implantation of multiple versus single donors.[73,74] In our autopsy patient, more than 200,000 tyrosine hydroxylase (TH)-positive cells survived after transplantation of six embryonic donors.[75] This suggests that approximately 5 percent of human nigral neurons survive transplantation and corresponds to estimates based on animal studies. Complete replacement of dopamine cells may also not be required to reverse disability in PD, as clinical features do not emerge until there has been a 60–80 percent reduction in nigral neurons and striatal dopamine. It is possible that the number of dopaminergic neurons that survive transplantation may overestimate the number capable of re-innervating the striatum. Nigral grafts include neurons from the ventral tegmental area (VTA) that can be recognized because they colocalize cholecystokinin (CCK). These cells do not normally project to the striatum or provide innervation after transplantation.[76] It may also be that excess dopamine neurons are necessary to compensate for neuronal degeneration that occurs as a result of immune rejection or an ongoing neurodegenerative process. Ultimately, a dose-response study will be required to determine the optimal number of donors for fetal nigral grafting in PD.

TISSUE DISTRIBUTION

The human striatum is approximately 500 times larger in volume than the striatum of the rodent. This presents a significant technical challenge for neural transplantation. Even when the correct number of donor cells is transplanted, improper distribution may result in a suboptimal clinical response. Based on our preclinical experiments, we estimate that implanted human fetal nigral neurons uniformly innervate a region of the striatum with a radius of approximately 2.5 mm, although more extensive fiber outgrowth may occur in a single direction. Dopamine diffusion from genetically engineered cells or after intracerebral microperfusion also appears to be limited.[77,78] To achieve confluent dopamine innervation of the target region, it may thus be necessary to distribute deposits of embryonic nigral cells at no more than 5-mm intervals throughout its 3-dimensional configuration. This can be accomplished in the postcommisural putamen or in the anterior putamen-caudate complex by placing four deposits in each of six to eight needle tracts (Fig. 15-2). Using such a protocol, we have observed confluent dopaminergic reinervation after transplantation on autopsy studies.[55,75]

Fetal Nigral Transplantation— Clinical Issues

PATIENT SELECTION

It is not yet known which PD patients are the best candidates for a neural transplantation procedure. At the present time, it is easiest to justify performing an experimental procedure on patients with advanced PD who can not be satisfactorily controlled with available medical therapy. However, these patients have greater perioperative risk. In addition, they are more likely to have clinical features that do not respond to L-dopa and, accordingly, they may not be capable of responding to grafted dopaminergic neurons. These problems may be less significant in patients with early PD. These patients may also not require drug therapy, thereby avoiding issues relating to the potential toxic effects of L-dopa metabolites on graft viability.[79]

INFECTIOUS DISEASE ISSUES

RECIPIENT

The authors routinely screen all patients who are candidates for a transplantation procedure for the following laboratory studies: complete blood count (CBC), Chem 18, HIV I (Ab, Ag), HIV II (Ab), Hepatitis B (HBsAg, HBcAb), Hepatitis C (HCV Ab), cytomegalovirus (CMV IgG), toxoplasma (TOXO IgG), syphilis VDRL or RPR, and Herpes simplex (HSV IgG). Patients are excluded when they test positive for HIV. In the past we have restricted participation to patients who are CMV- and TOXO-positive in order to minimize the risk of infection with one of these contagious agents in a naive recipient. PCR studies in our laboratories suggest that this may not be necessary in the case of CMV, as infection with this organism has not been detected in any of the donors we have tested to date. All patients receive antibiotic coverage while awaiting final reports of donor bacterial cultures. When the cultures are negative, antibiotics are discontinued; when positive, patients receive a full course of the appropriate antibiotic.

DONOR

In our protocol,[55] each donor is screened using maternal blood for CBC, HIV I (Ab, Ag), HIV II (Ab), HTLV-I (Ab), Hepatitis A (HAV IgM), Hepatitis B (HBsAg, HBcAb), Hepa-

titis C (HCV Ab), CMV (IgM), toxoplasma (IgM), syphilis (VDRL or RPR), and Herpes simplex (HSV IgM). In addition, fetal tissue is cultured for aerobic and anaerobic bacteria, as well as yeast. Donors are excluded when there is evidence of infection with HIV-I, HIV-II, HTLV-I, syphilis, hepatitis B transmissibility, or hepatitis C. In addition, donors are not used from mothers who have been the recipient of multiple blood transfusions, have a temperature of greater than 100.5°F, a white blood cell (WBC) count greater than 15,000, a history of prostitution, or evidence of active genital Herpes simplex.

As there is little information at the present time regarding the risk of transmitting an infectious organism during the fetal transplantation procedure, the authors meticulously evaluate donors for the possibility of contagious agents. As infection can stimulate rejection, this approach may not only reduce the risk of transmitting infection but also improve patient outcome.

IMMUNOSUPPRESSION

The central nervous system is an immunologically privileged site, and it may be that immunosuppression is not essential for successful nigral grafting. Fetal allografts have been observed to survive for extended periods of time without immunosuppression in rodents and nonhuman primates.[9,80] Furthermore, clinical improvement is reported to have been observed in patients who received fetal grafts without immunosuppression.[81,82] However, graft rejection in transplanted patients who do not receive immunosuppression might preclude development of a graft-related clinical benefit. Surgical trauma or the graft itself could disrupt the blood-brain barrier and permit the immune system access to graft antigens within the brain.[83] This is particularly relevant to protocols using multiple immunologically unrelated donors. Immunosuppression has been shown to improve survival of xenografts in rodent models of parkinsonism,[70,84] and allograft rejection has been described in immunologically disparate rodents.[85] Furthermore, immunosupresion was not used by the group reporting the highest proportion of clinical failures.[86] For these reasons, most transplant groups have used immunosupresion with cyclosporine (CsA) in studies performed to date. In our own studies, we treat patients with CsA (6 mg/kg) for approximately 1 month. Thereafter, the dose of CsA is reduced to 2 mg/kg, and the drug is discontinued after 6 months, at which time the blood-brain barrier is expected to be closed. Using this treatment protocol, the authors have noted robust survival of implanted neurons without evidence of immune rejection 18 months after transplantation and 12 months after discontinuation of CsA.[75] This suggests that prolonged treatment with CsA may not be necessary. It remains to be determined whether CsA can be withheld entirely from the transplant protocol.

When CsA is to be used, it is reasonable to consider the possibility that it may affect PD signs and symptoms and confound interpretation of transplant benefits. Sanberg et al. have shown that CsA induces increased spontaneous and dopamine agonist-induced motor activity in rodents.[87] There is also evidence of inflammation in the substantia nigra pars compacta of PD patients,[88] raising the possibility that an inflammatory reaction may contribute to the pathogenesis of cell degeneration in PD and be attenuated by CsA administration. These factors must be considered in interpreting study results and determining the benefit of a transplant procedure in comparison to unoperated PD controls. Further studies to define the role of CsA in PD are warrented.

CLINICAL EVALUATIONS

MOTOR ASSESSMENT

The Core Assessment Protocol for Intracerebral Transplantation (CAPIT) is a standardized evaluation of parkinsonian features that has been developed to facilitate comparison of results among different transplant centers.[89] Clinical evaluations include measures of disability, motor function, and timed motor tasks during "on" and "off" stages. The CAPIT also includes self-administered calendar determination of percent "on" time while awake and percent "on" time with dyskinesia. Many centers also perform a L-dopa response test, neurophysiological determination of motor function, neuropsychological measures of cognitive function, and standardized videotape evaluations.

COGNITIVE FUNCTION

Changes in cognitive function can frequently be detected even in nondemented PD patients. Specific impairments are most frequently seen in strategic cognitive abilities, such as effortful recall of information,[90] dual-process tasks,[91] memory for temporal order,[92] and switching of cognitive sets.[93] These deficits are thought to be a result of impairment of the caudate outflow to the frontal lobes.[93] Two studies have presented data on changes in cognitive functioning after adrenal medullary implantation in PD. One found marked improvements in strategic cognitive functioning in seven patients 3 months after surgery,[94] but in another study using the same surgical technique no significant change in cognitive functioning was detected in seven patients after 1 year.[95] No data have yet been presented on the effect of fetal nigral transplant surgery on cognitive function but, clearly, such studies are important both from the standpoint of detecting putative site-specific benefits of transplantation and assessing possible adverse effects of the transplant procedure.

PET

Striatal fluorodopa (FD) uptake on PET is useful as a measure of striatal dopaminergic terminals.[96] FD is decarboxylated to fluorodopamine in the brain and retained in the striatum, probably within nigrostriatal dopaminergic nerve terminals. A steady-state striatal FD uptake rate constant can be calculated by the graphic method of Patlak and Blasberg[97] and has been shown to correlate with dopamine cell counts and levels.[98] There are several reports of increased striatal FD uptake on PET after fetal nigral grafting in PD or MPTP-parkinsonism.[55,77,99–101] As illustrated in Fig. 15-3, the authors have observed consistent increases in striatal FD uptake in each of our transplanted patients,[55] and Remy et al have noted that change in striatal FD uptake correlates with clinical improvement.[74] After unilateral transplantation, striatal FD uptake has been observed to increase on the transplanted side but decrease on the contralateral (unoperated) side, pos-

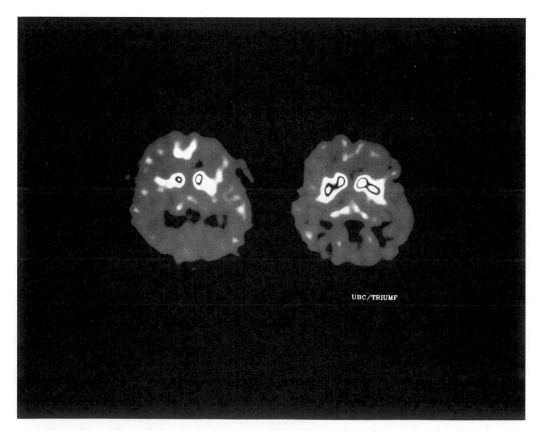

UBC/TRIUMF

FIGURE 15-3 PET scan showing decreased striatal fluorodopa (FD) uptake preoperatively, particularly in the region of the postcommissural putamen (*left*). Note the dramatic increase in striatal FD uptake bilaterally in the target region of transplantation (*right*). This magnitude of improvement has been seen in each of our transplanted patients.

sibly because of disease progression.[102] A progressive increase in striatal FD uptake has been observed in a few patients who have undergone sequential postoperative PET studies.[74,77,102] It is likely that increased striatal FD uptake on PET after transplantation reflects graft survival with neuritic outgrowth based on pathological confirmation in two cases[74,103] and the positive correlation between PET changes and clinical response.[74] It is unlikely that increased FD uptake is a result of surgical trauma and/or a trophic effect, as PET changes were not seen after adrenal transplantation, despite a greater degree of trauma,[104] and host-derived sprouting has not been reported to occur in the putamen, where PET changes have been most prominent. There has been interest recently in the use of PET and single-photon emission tomography (SPECT) to measure ligands for the dopamine transporter as a marker of dopaminergic terminals. These techniques offer considerable promise for evaluating transplantation in an objective fashion, as well as for better understanding the nature of the pathophysiological defect in PD.

DRUG MANAGEMENT

There are several concerns about the use of L-dopa after a transplantation procedure for PD. Breakdown of the blood-brain barrier after transplantation can theoretically permit carbidopa administered with L-dopa to inhibit central decarboxylase activity. However, L-dopa has not been shown to be more effective than L-dopa/carbidopa, and carbidopa was not identified in the ventricular cerebrospinal fluid (CSF) of L-dopa/carbidopa-treated PD patients 6 months after adrenal transplantation.[105] L-dopa has been shown to be capable of inducing degeneration of both cultured and transplanted fetal nigral cells,[80,106] possibly because of its capacity to promote free radical formation. However, clinical benefits and increased FD uptake on PET have been demonstrated to persist for more than 3 years after transplantation in L-dopa-treated patients,[107] and our postmortem study revealed large numbers of healthy-appearing nigral neurons, despite con-

tinued L-dopa therapy.[75] Finally, there are clinical trial issues with regard to the management of L-dopa. Lowering the L-dopa dose can, paradoxically, lead to symptomatic improvement in some PD patients and confound interpretation of transplant benefits. Accordingly, caution must be exercised in using a decrease in L-dopa dosage as an index of clinical improvement after transplantation. On the other hand, elimination of the need for L-dopa in a patient with advanced PD would be clear evidence of a transplant effect. Although total drug withdrawal is a desirable goal, only a single patient has been completely withdrawn from L-dopa after a transplant procedure.[107]

Fetal Nigral Transplantation—Clinical Results

Several studies have demonstrated the feasability of performing fetal nigral transplantation in PD, and it is estimated that more than 150 transplant procedures have been performed to date.[73] Published results on fetal grafting in PD, using a variety of transplant variables, have been reported from Sweden,[99,107–109] Colorado,[53,82] Yale,[110] France,[111] Mexico,[112,113] Czechoslovakia,[114] Spain,[115] Poland,[116] United Kingdom,[81,86] China,[117] Cuba,[118] and our own program at the University of South Florida and the Mount Sinai School of Medicine.[55,75,119] Results have been inconsistent and difficult to compare because of variations in patient selection, transplant variables, rating systems, level of scrutiny, and clinical expertise. Selected examples derived from peer-reviewed reports are described more fully below and summarized in Table 15-1 (adapted from Ref. 119). Numerous unreported transplant procedures have also been performed.

Lindvall and coworkers were the first to report clinical benefit from fetal nigral grafting in PD.[108] Fetal nigral tissue from four fetuses aged 7–9 weeks PC was implanted unilaterally into the caudate and anterior putamen of two PD patients. A small, but significant, improvement in motor perfor-

TABLE 15-1 Published Outcomes of Fetal Transplantation[119]

Reference	No. of Patients	CSA	Type of Transplant	Donor Age (PC, wks)	No. of Donors	Bilateral Grafts	Site	BENEFIT None	Mild	Moderate	Marked	% decrease L-dopa	F-D PET
Lindvall et al., 1989	2	Yes	Susp.	7–9	4	No	Anterior P+C	0	2	0	0	0	
Lindvall et al., 1990, 1992	2	Yes	Susp.	6–7	4	No	P	0	0	2	0	0	+
Freed et al., 1992	2	4 of 7	Solid	5–6	1	No	C+P	1	0	1	0	39	
	5		Solid	5–6	1	Yes	P	0	2	3	0		
Spencer et al., 1992	4	Yes	Solid	5–9	1	No	C	1	3	0	0	24	−
Widner et al., 1992	2	Yes	Susp.	6–8	6–8	Yes	C+P	0	0	0	2		+
Freeman et al., 1994	4	Yes	Solid	6.5–9	6–8	Yes	Posterior	0	0	2	2	0	+ +

−, no benefit; + increased uptake; + +, markedly increased uptake.

mance during "off" periods was detected during the first 6 months. However, there was no change in the duration of response to a dose of L-dopa, and striatal FD uptake on PET was not significantly increased. This group subsequently performed a unilateral transplant procedure, which differed from the original in that mesencephalic tissue was derived from fetuses aged 6–7 weeks PC, a smaller-gauge transplant needle was used, and tissue was implanted exclusively into the putamen.[99,109] These patients experienced a greater degree of clinical improvement, beginning 6–12 weeks after surgery. Clinical benefits were observed bilaterally but were more pronounced on the side contralateral to the transplant. Improvement was noted in motor performance during "off" episodes, percent "off" time, and the number of daily "off" periods. Benefits progressively increased during the first year of follow-up. A progressive increase in striatal FD uptake was observed within the grafted putamen consistent with graft survival. In contrast, striatal FD uptake declined on the unoperated side, suggesting disease progression.[102] Benefits have persisted over several years, and at least one patient has been able to be taken off of L-dopa.[107] Similar results have been reported by Peschanski et al., using a related protocol.[111]

Seven patients have undergone a transplantation procedure at the University of Colorado. Ventral mesencephalon derived from a single 6- to 7-week PC embryo was implanted as a solid graft or "noodle" into the caudate and putamen on the side opposite maximal parkinsonian deficit in two patients and into the putamen bilaterally in the others.[53,82] Immunosuppression was not used in some cases. Modest but statistically significant improvement was observed in activities of daily living in both "on" and "off" states. Improvement was also noted in scores of facial expression, postural control, gait and bradykinesia. One patient did not improve, and two were improved "in some respects." The mean L-dopa dose was reduced by 39 percent. This group is presently carrying out an NIH-sponsored prospective double-blind, surgical placebo-controlled study with a protocol that includes bilateral transplantation.

At Yale University, four patients diagnosed as having severe PD underwent transplantation into the right caudate nucleus of cryopreserved fragments of embryonic mesencephalic tissue.[112] Tissue was derived from a single 5- to 9-week PC fetal cadaver. Three patients were reported to be mildly improved at 18 months, but they were not significantly different from a group of preselected, medically treated control patients. A postmortem study in one patient demonstrated striatonigral degeneration, rather than PD, and the presence of only a few surviving neurons.[121] The lack of consistent benefit in this study may have related to the use of cryopreserved tissue and the inability of patients with basal ganglia dysfunction associated with widespread neurodegeneration to respond to a dopaminergic transplant.

Benefits of fetal mesencephalic grafting have also been reported in two patients with MPTP-parkinsonism.[101] In these patients, fetal tissue derived from three to four embryos per side aged 6–8 weeks PC were bilaterally implanted into both the putamen and caudate nucleus. The patients experienced progressive improvement in motor function, beginning 3–4 months after transplantation, with some motor functions returning to a near normal level. Striatal fluorodopa uptake on PET scan was unchanged at 6 months but was noted to be increased bilaterally at 1 and 2 years postoperatively. The extent of benefit observed in these patients may be related to the relatively large quantity of fetal tissue that was implanted, the use of bilateral transplants, and target sites in both the putamen and caudate nucleus. In addition, patients with MPTP parkinsonism may be better candidates for a neural transplant procedure than PD patients, because of differences in the nature of the underlying degenerative process and their effects on grafted cells, as well as the young age of these patients.

We have studied six patients with relatively advanced PD using solid grafts derived from four donors per side, aged 6.5 to 9 weeks PC.[55,75,119] Tissue was implanted bilaterally into the postcommissural putamen. Six to eight needle tracts with four deposits per tract were used to ensure that nigral deposits were seperated by no more than 5 mm throughout the 3-dimensional configuration of the posterior putamen. Immunosuppression with CsA was used for 6 months. Each of the patients who underwent transplantation according to this protocol experienced clinically meaningful benefit 6 months after the transplantation procedure.[55] Significant benefit was observed for UPDRS scores during "off" time, percent "on" time, percent "on" time without dyskinesia, and Schwab/ England score when "off." Benefits were also seen in measures of "on" and "off" period dystonia, walking, falling, and freezing. Clinical improvement was maintained during 18 months of follow-up in all but one patient. Striatal FD uptake on PET at 6 months was increased bilaterally in each patient and was significantly increased for the group as a whole. PET scan benefits persisted at 12 months, and in some individuals striatal FD uptake continued to improve, returning to near normal levels. Interestingly, one patient in our study experienced clinical worsening in conjunction with a flu-like episode. This was associated with a fall in striatal FD uptake and raises the interesting possibility that deterioration may have been related to an immune assault directed at one or more transplant deposits induced by this flu-like event. It is noteworthy that all other patients experienced sustained improvement in "on" time, as well as in percent "on" time without dyskinesia, despite the fact that efforts were made to maintain L-dopa doses at preoperative levels. We postulate that this may be because of a transplant-related increase in dopamine terminals with a renewed capacity to store dopamine and to regulate dopamine neurotransmission more physiologically. The magnitude and consistency of the benefits observed in our cases may relate to (1) the use of larger quantities of more diffusely distributed nigral tissue within our target region than has been used by other centers to date; (2) the targeting of the postcommissural putamen; and (3) the exclusive use of solid grafts derived from donors aged $6^{1}/_{2}$ to 9 weeks PC. Based on these preliminary data, we are now conducting an NIH-sponsored trial to evaluate the safety and efficacy of fetal nigral grafting in a placebo-controlled study, as well as to compare the effects of transplatating one versus four donors per side. This study is a prospective, double-blind, surgical placebo-controlled clinical trial in which patients are randomized to receive a fetal nigral transplant procedure or a sham operation that consists of a partial burr hole to simulate the transplant procedure but does not involve penetration of the brain with needle tracts. The sham procedure will control for the placebo effect. In addition, the comparison of one versus four donors per side will control for the effects of the trauma associated with the surgical procedure, as the only difference in the two protocols is the concentration of tissue in each deposit. Although there is controversy regarding the use of surgical placebo controls to evaluate surgical procedures, it is clear that surgery can induce a prominent placebo response that confounds interpretation of any procedure-derived benefit.[120] Furthermore, there are examples of surgical procedures that have been used in routine practice, only to be found lacking when held to the light of a controlled trial.[121]

Fetal Nigral Transplantation— Neuroanatomic Considerations

In rodent and nonhuman primate models of PD, grafts of fetal nigral neurons have been shown to consistently survive, produce dopamine, form synaptic connections, and ameliorate motor dysfunction resulting from lesions of the nigrostriatal pathway. However, results of fetal grafting in PD patients have, to date, been variable. Some studies report significant clinical benefit after nigral grafting[55,107] whereas others describe little if any improvement.[86,110] This variability may relate to differences in the survival of implanted dopaminergic neurons, a factor that is critical in achieving functional recovery in animal models of PD. FD-PET has been used as a measure of putative graft viability, and recent studies demonstrated a good correlation between clinical benefit and increased striatal FD uptake on PET.[74] However, FD-PET cannot distinguish between grafted neurons and sprouting of host dopaminergic terminals. To this end, direct anatomic confirmation that implanted cells survive and reinnervate the striatum is required. Early pathological studies did not show survival of meaningful numbers of implanted neurons,[81,122] and some of the cells contained extraordinarily large amounts of neuromelanin, suggestive of pathological dopamine auto-oxidation. We recently had the opportunity to examine the brain of a 59-year-old man who expired from unrelated causes 18 months after a transplant procedure.[75] Following the grafting procedure, he enjoyed substantial clinical benefit with virtual elimination of both "off" time and dyskinesia. At autopsy, large viable transplants were observed bilaterally in grafted regions (Fig. 15-4). More than 200,000 TH-staining transplanted neurons were detected in the grafted putamen.[123] Abundant neuritic processes extended from graft deposits into the neighboring striatum and were seamlessly integrated into the host. Innervation of the striatum was continuous between graft deposits and organized in a classic patch-matrix fashion. This was in stark contrast to ungrafted regions, which demonstrated virtually no TH-immunoreactive staining. Electron microscopy demonstrated normal-appearing synaptic connections between implanted cells and host neurons. Cytochrome oxidase stain-

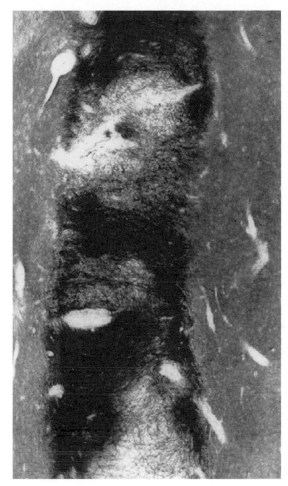

FIGURE 15-4 Low-power photomicrograph showing a TH immunostained graft deposit, demonstrating robust cellular survival with extensive and seamless innervation to the surrounding striatum.

ing, an index of metabolic activity, was markedly increased in transplanted regions. Similarly, there was extensive TH-mRNA expression and staining for dopamine transporter protein in grafted regions of the putamen, in contrast to nongrafted regions of the striatum and the host substantia nigra. No evidence for graft-mediated host sprouting or immune rejection was detected.

This case represents the first demonstration that grafted fetal nigral neurons can survive, reinnervate the striatum, and lead to clinically meaningful benefits in the absence of host-derived sprouting. We have recently examined the brain from a second patient who died from unrelated causes approximately 18 months after a transplant procedure. Once again, there was evidence of robust graft survival and striatal reinnervation. As such, these cases provide strong support for the notion that the clinical benefits observed in transplanted PD patients are dependent on the survival of implanted dopaminergic neurons. The correlation between cell survival and striatal FD uptake in this patient also provide support for the notion that this technique provides a good index of graft viability. The robust survival of grafted nigral neurons in our patient is in contrast to previous observations made after transplantation in PD patients. Redmond and coworkers reported negligible survival, using transplanted cells derived from a fetus aged 10 weeks PC that had been cryopreserved before the grafting procedure.[122] Hitchcock et al. also noted poor survival of grafted nigral neurons that had been derived from second trimester (>12 week PC) fetuses.[81] The few TH-immunoreactive-grafted neurons that were identified were atrophic, had minimal neuritic extension, and had massive accumulation of neuromelanin. The donor age and the method of storage used in these cases may have mitigated against optimal cell survival. It is noteworthy that poor cell survival in these cases was associated with little, if any, clinical benefit.

The authors' patients both displayed progressive and bilateral increases in putaminal FD uptake on PET scan at 6 and 12 months after transplantation. Others have observed a similar increase in FD uptake and have interpreted this finding to be a representation of graft viability.[102] However, sprouting of host dopaminergic fibers because of local trauma or implanted trophic factors can theoretically account for these PET scan findings, as well as for the clinical benefits in transplanted patients.[124] Host-derived sprouting has been observed in PD patients, as well as in rodent and primate models of PD after adrenal medullary transplant procedures.[42,125,126] In our patients, sprouting of host fibers was carefully sought but was not detected. Clearly in these cases, increased putaminal FD uptake was associated with graft survival. Interestingly, we also noted increased FD uptake in the right caudate nucleus of one patient that was not the target of any transplant deposits.[55,75] At post mortem in this case, we observed that grafts placed within the medial right putamen extended processes across the internal capsule to innervate the caudate nucleus and likely account for the increased FD uptake in this region. These findings, coupled with the failure of adrenal transplant to induce PET changes despite more extensive trauma[104] and the failure to detect sprouting in the putamen in preclinical studies, support the concept that the increased FD uptake observed after fetal nigral grafting procedures represents graft survival.

The need for immunosuppression after fetal transplantation remains controversial. Although long-term survival of fetal allografts is routinely observed experimentally, the same is not known to occur in humans. The authors used a low-dose regimen of CsA to increase the likelihood that grafted cells would survive during the period when the blood-brain barrier was most likely to be disrupted. A number of factors suggest that immune rejection did not occur in the authors' patient, even though CsA had been discontinued for 12 months before death. Grafted cells displayed the normal morphological features of healthy dopaminergic neurons; macrophages were rarely observed within graft deposits; and the patient experienced sustained clinical benefit and progressive improvement on PET. These findings suggest that long-term immunosuppression is not required after fetal grafting and that studies to determine whether immunosuppression can be totally eliminated are warranted.

Fetal Nigral Transplantation—Future Directions

Our finding of robust survival of TH-ir neurons with striatal reinnervation in two PD patients who had undergone a fetal nigral transplant procedure provides essential confirmation of the hypothesis that fetal nigral grafts can survive and mediate clinical recovery, as predicted by animal studies. As exciting as these observations are, enthusiasm is tempered by the fact that despite excellent graft survival and impressive striatal innervation, no patient has yet been cured of parkinsonism. We observed the survival of supranormal numbers of dopamine-containing neurons within the putamen of both of our transplant cases that came to autopsy, but patients only displayed partial recovery. The most parsimonious explanation is that, despite supranormal numbers of grafted nigral neurons, there was a subnormal pattern of innervation. In our first case, the graft provided dopaminergic innervation to only 53 percent and 28 percent of the right and left putamen, respectively.[123] It is possible that this innervation pattern might have continued to increase over time, as progressive increases in fluorodopa uptake were seen on PET scan in both of these cases. Furthermore, grafted patients from other centers have continued to show clinical improvement over prolonged periods of time.[107] However, more immediate clinical benefits are required. In this regard, it is noteworthy that even though we observed an impressive number of surviving dopaminergic neurons after transplant, it still represents a small fraction (5–10 percent) of the original population of grafted TH-ir cells. Enhanced survival or larger numbers of donors might provide better clinical results. It is thus possible that there is a window of opportunity to improve upon the transplantation procedure and improve on clinical results by manipulation of transplant variables.

Additionally, improving neurite outgrowth from the graft might enhance the magnitude of functional benefit and the speed with which recovery occurs. One method for improving neurite outgrowth from grafted dopamine neurons is to expose them in vitro or in vivo to trophic factors. Many different neurotrophic factors support the viability and/or phenotypic expression of dopaminergic neurons,[127] including brain-derived neurotrophic factor (BDNF), basic fibroblast growth factor (β-FGF), and glial-derived neurotrophic factor (GDNF) (see also Chapter 8). BDNF has been demonstrated to enhance neurite outgrowth from BDNF-producing cells in vitro.[128] We have genetically modified oligodendroglia to secrete BDNF and have shown that when these cells are cocultured with fetal nigral neurons, neurite outgrowth and neuron viability can be enhanced (Fig. 15-5). After grafting fetal nigral tissue to the dopamine-depleted striatum, rats treated with chronic intraventricular infusions or daily intrastriatal injections of BDNF display a significant reduction in ipsiversive rotations after amphetamine administration.[129] Similarly, functional recovery in dopamine-lesioned rodents is enhanced when fetal nigral neurons are cografted with BDNF-secreting oligodendroglia (JH Kordower, unpublished data). BDNF has been demonstrated to enhance neurite outgrowth from fetal nigral neurons and to potentiate

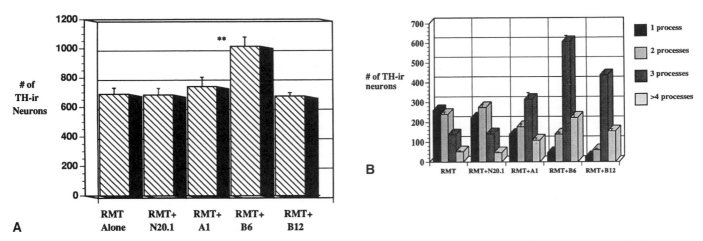

FIGURE 15-5 *A.* Cell cultures containing rostral mesencephalon (RMT) cultures alone, with a non-BDNF-secreting parental oligodendroglial cell line (N20.1), or with one of three oligodendroglial cell lines that have been genetically modified to secrete BDNF (A1, B6, and B12). Note that TH-ir RMT neurons cultured alone or with the N20.1 parental cell line preferentially display only one to two neurites, with fewer cells displaying three to four neurites. In contrast, the number of TH-ir neurons displaying three to four neurites is increased when RMT cells are cocultured with any of the three BDNF-secreting oligodendroglial cell lines. *B.* Viability of TH-ir rostral mesencephalic neurons was enhanced when cells were cocultured with the BDNF-secreting B6 cells. The number of TH-ir RMT neurons was unchanged when cocultured with the A1 or B12 BDNF-secreting cell lines relative to coculture with the parental (N20.1) non-BDNF-producing cells or RMT cells alone. Additional studies reveal that the B6 cell line produced the highest titers of BDNF, which may be responsible for this selective effect.

the functional effects of fetal grafts in rodent models of PD.[130] However, BDNF has not been shown to have a significant effect on cell survival, suggesting that BDNF may act as a tropic, rather than a trophic, factor for implanted fetal nigral neurons.

Other trophic factors can also influence the effects of fetal nigral grafting. GDNF has also been shown to promote the survival and phenotypic differentiation of fetal rat midbrain dopaminergic neurons in culture.[131] After intraocular transplantation, GDNF treatment increases the number of TH-immunoreactive cells and increases neuritic outgrowth from these cells.[132] More recently, it has been demonstrated that GDNF enhances the viability and neurite outgrowth of grafted nigral neurons and potentiates functional recovery in unilateral 6-OHDA lesioned rats.[133] Ultimately, the use of these trophic factors, either alone or in combination, may optimize graft viability, neurite outgrowth and, hopefully, functional recovery.

The entrance of molecular biology into the field of neural transplantation has greatly extended our ability to manipulate and generate cell lines that may be candidates for transplantation in PD. Ex vivo and in vivo gene therapy approaches have now become commonplace methods of inducing the expression of a particular gene product. In a relatively straightforward manner, genes encoding specific proteins can be transfected into dividing cells using retroviral vectors and then transplanted into the brain, where these proteins will hopefully continue to be expressed. In some circumstances, cells manipulated in this manner have been shown to induce anatomic and/or functional changes after grafting in a manner comparable to that seen after direct infusion of the specific protein. Gage and coworkers,[134,135] as well as others,[136] have used genetically modified fibroblasts

as donor cells for transplantation. There are many advantages to using fibroblasts as parental cells for genetic modifications. First, they readily divide in culture, thus providing a large population of cells for transplantation. Additionally, these donor cells can easily be obtained from the host, making the graft autologous and minimizing the potential of graft rejection. Genetically modified fibroblasts have been used in two different model systems. Fibroblasts have been infected with the gene encoding nerve growth factor (NGF) and then grafted into rats with unilateral fimbria-fornix transections.[137] These grafts rescue cholinergic septal-diagonal band neurons that would normally degenerate after axotomy. Fibroblasts secreting NGF can also reduce the area of necrosis after intrastriatal lesions of quinolinic acid and selectively protect cholinergic interneurons from degenerating.[136] Fibroblasts have also been infected with the gene to produce TH and grafted into rats with unilateral nigrostriatal lesions.[135] These TH-producing fibroblasts survive grafting and produce high levels of L-dopa, although virtually no dopamine. Even so, these grafts are capable of reversing apomorphine-induced rotation.

Other groups have used different cell types for gene transfection. For instance, Jiao and colleagues[138] have transfected muscle cells with TH and have reversed apomorphine-induced rotation in unilateral nigrostriatal-lesioned rats. In addition to grafting cells for direct functional enhancement of host systems, a number of groups have used genetically engineered cells to provide trophic support for *other grafted cells.* Astrocytes[139] and fibroblasts[140] have been transfected with the gene-producing NGF. These cells have then been cografted with NGF-sensitive adrenal chromaffin cells, augmenting their survival and potentiating their functional effects.[139] We have begun to use retroviral vectors aimed at genetically modifying fetal neurons in such a way that they become immortal at a permissive temperature, yet remain amitotic and differentiate at a second higher temperature.[141] Specifically, ventral mesencephalon are dissected from embryonic day 13 rats, and dopaminergic cells are infected with the simian virus (SV 40) large T antigen. This renders these cells immortal at 33°C but permanently amitotic at 38°–39°C. Once differentiated, these cells do not revert to a mitotic state, even if they are returned to the lower permissive temperature. Once they are transfected, clonal lines of dopamine-producing cells can be established. The end result is a limitless supply of neuronal-like progenitors, all of which express TH and synthesize dopamine, the deficient neurotransmitter in PD. The levels of dopamine produced by these cells can be further augmented by infecting these cells with the TH cDNA found in PC-12 cells, a cell line that synthesizes high levels of dopamine. After grafting into unilateral nigrostriatal-lesioned rats, these cells survive, express TH, and reverse apomorphine-induced rotation. Furthermore, these cells survive transplantation into hemiparkinsonian monkeys. Grafts placed into the dopamine-deficient striatum have yet to display evidence of tumor formation. These data indicate that neurons can be rendered immortal by transfecting these cells with the SV 40 large T antigen and that clonal dopaminergic cell lines can be generated that will survive transplantation and reverse lesion-induced motor deficits. Although our recent data indicate that grafting of genetically modified neurons is encouraging, a number of fundamental issues still need to be resolved before this approach can be considered for clinical use. Although grafts of SV40-infected dopaminergic cells survive grafting, express TH immunoreactivity, and mediate functional recovery for up to 1 month, long-term studies are required to validate the usefulness of this donor tissue for transplantation studies. Furthermore, it is essential that long-term studies ensure that these cells do not revert to a mitotic state. Finally, it is also possible to change the phenotype of in vivo neurons and glia in specific brain regions through the use of adeno, adeno-associated, and lentiviruses. In preliminary studies, long-term improvement has been attained in parkinsonian rats after intrastriatal injection of an HSV vector designed to induce TH expression in endogenous cells.[142]

In summary, transplantation for PD has a bright future. Today, we can get large numbers of fetal neurons to survive grafting, reinnervate the striatum, and mediate clinically relevant benefit in patients with PD. This can be accomplished with only 5–10 percent of transplanted cells surviving and incomplete reinnervation. In the future, modern molecular biological techniques and trophic factor adjunctive therapy will likely fill the large gap available for improvement in this technology. Hopefully, these modifications will bring us to our goal; a long-term effective treatment for patients with PD.

References

1. Olanow CW: Parkinson's disease: Clinical crossroads. *J Am Med Assoc* 275:716–722, 1996.
2. Fahn S: Adverse effects of L-dopa. In Olanow CW, Lieberman AN, (eds): *The Scientific Basis for the Treatment of Parkinson's Disease.* Lancs, UK: Parthenon Publishing Group, 1992, pp 89–112.
3. Bjorklund A, Stenevi U: Reconstruction of the nigrostriatal dopamine pathway by intracerebral nigral transplants. *Brain Res* 177:555–560, 1979.
4. Dunnett SB, Bjorklund A, Stenevi U, Iversen SD: Behavioral recovery following transplantation of substantia nigra in rats subjected to 6-OHDA lesions of the nigrostriatal pathway. *Brain Res* 215:147–161, 1981.
5. Perlow MJ, Freed WJ, Hoffer BJ, et al: Brain grafts reduce motor abnormalities produced by destruction of nigro-striatal dopamine system. *Science* 204:643–647, 1979.
6. Bjorklund A, Stenevi U, Dunnett SB, et al: Functional reactivation of the deafferented neostriatum by nigral transplants. *Nature* 289:497–499, 1981.
7. Brundin P, Bjorklund A: Survival, growth and function of dopaminergic neurons grafted to the brain. *Prog Brain Res* 71:293–308, 1987.
8. Sladek JR Jr, Collier TC, Haber SN, et al: Survival and growth of fetal catecholamine neurons transplanted into the primate brain. *Brain Res Bull* 17:809–818, 1986.
9. Sladek JR Jr, Redmond DE, Collier TC, et al: Fetal dopamine neural grafts: Extended reversal of methylphenyltetrahydropyridine-induced parkinsonism in primates: Transplantation into the mammalian CNS. *Prog Brain Res* 78:497–506, 1988.
10. Redmond DE, Roth RH, Elsworth JD, et al: Fetal neuronal grafts in monkeys given methyl-phenyl-tetrahydro-pyridine. *Lancet* May:1125–1127, 1986.
11. Bakay RAE, Barrow DL, Fiandaca MS, et al: Biochemical and behavioral correction of MPTP-like syndrome by fetal cell transplantation. *Ann NY Scad Sci* 495:623–640, 1987.
12. Fine A, Hunt SB, Oertel WH, et al: Transplantation of embryonic dopaminergic neurons to the corpus straitaum of marmosets rendered parkinsonian by 1-methyl-4-phenyl-1,2,3,6 tetrahydropyridine. Transplantation into the mammalian CNS. *Prog Brain Res* 78:479–490, 1988.
13. Bankiewicz KS, Plunkett RJ, Jacobawitz DM, et al: The effect of fetal mesencephalon implants on primate MPTP-induced parkinsonism. *J Neurosurg* 72:231–244, 1990.
14. Mahalick TJ, Finger TE, Stromberg I, et al: Substantia nigra transplants into denenervated striatum of the rat: Ultrastructure of graft-host interconnections. *J Comp Neurol* 240:60–70, 1985.
15. Bjorklund A, Stenevi U, Schmidt RH, et al: Intracerebral grafting of neuronal cell suspensions. II: Survival and growth of nigral cell suspensions implanted in different brain sites. *Acta Physiol Scand* 522:9–18, 1983.
16. Wuerthele SM, Freed WJ, Olson L, et al: Effects of dopamine agonists and antagonists on the electrical activity of substantia nigra neurons transplanted into the lateral ventricle of the rat. *Exp Brain Res* 44:1–10, 1981.
17. Schmidt RH, Ingvar M, Lindvall O, et al: Functional activity of substantia nigra grafts reinnervating the striatum: Neurotransmitter metabolism and (14C)-2-deoxy-D-glucose autoradiography. *J Neurochem* 38:737–748, 1982.
18. Freed WJ, Perlow MJ, Karoum F, et al: Restoration of dopamine brain function by grafting fetal substantia nigra to the caudate nucleus: Long term behavioral, biochemical, and histological studies. *Ann Neurol* 8:510–523, 1980.
19. Brundin P, Strecker RE, Widner H, et al: Human fetal dopamine neurons grafted in a rat model of Parkinson's disease: Immunological aspects, spontaneous and drug-induced behavior, and dopamine release. *Exp Brain Res* 70:192–208, 1988.
20. Stromberg I, Almqvist P, Bygdeman M, et al: Human fetal mesencephalic tissue grafted to dopamine-denervated striatum of athymic rats: Light and electron microscopic histochemical and in vivo chronoamperometric studies. *J Neurosci* 614–624, 1989.

21. van Horne CG, Mahalik T, Hoffer B, et al: Behavioral and electrophysiological correlates of human mesencephalic dopamine xenograft function in the rat striatum. *Brain Res Bull* 25:325–334, 1990.

22. Clarke DJ, Brundin P, Strecker RE, et al: Human fetal dopamine neurons grafted in a rat model of Parkinson's disease: Ultrastructural evidence for synapse formation using tyrosine hydroxylase immunocytochemistry. *Exp Brain Res* 73:115–126, 1988.

23. Brundin P, Widner H, Nilsson OG, et al: Intracerebral xenografts of dopamine neurons: The role of immunosuppression and the blood-brain barrier. *Exp Brain Res* 75:195–207, 1989.

24. Dunnett SB, Hernandez TD, Summerfield A, et al: Graft-derived recovery from 6-OHDA lesions: Specificity of ventral mesencephalic graft tissues. *Exp Brain Res* 71:411–424, 1988.

25. Itakura T, Kamei I, Nakai K, et al: Autotransplantation of the superior cervical ganglion into the brain: A possible therapy for Parkinson's disease. *J Neurosurg* 68:955–959, 1988.

26. Pasik P, Martinez JF, Yahr MD, et al: Grafting of human sympathetic ganglia into the brain of MPTP-treated monkeys. *Soc Neurosci Abstr* 1988:5–6.

27. Hefti F, Hartikka J, Schlumpf M: Implantation of PC12 cells into the corpus striatum of rats with lesions of the dopaminergic nigrostriatal neurons. *Brain Res* 348:283–288, 1985.

28. Freed WJ, Patel-Vaidya U, Geller HM: Properties of PC12 pheochromocytoma cells transplanted to the adult rat brain. *Exp Brain Res* 63:557–566, 1986.

29. Jaeger CB: Morphological and immunocytochemical characteristics of PC12 cell grafts in rat brain. *Ann NY Acad Sci* 495:334–349, 1987.

30. Freed WJ, Morihisa JM, Spoor E, et al: Transplanted adrenal chromaffin cells in rat brain reduce lesion-induced rotational behavior. *Nature* 292:351–352, 1981.

31. Stromberg I, Herrera-Marschitz M, Ungerstedt U, et al: Chronic implants of chromaffin tissue into the dopamine-denervated striatum: Effects of NGF on graft survival, fiber growth and rotational behavior. *Exp Brain Res* 60:335–349, 1985.

32. Freed WJ, Cannon-Spoor HE, Krauthamer E: Intrastriatal adrenal medulla grafts in rats: Long-term survival and behavioral effects. *J Neurosurg* 65:664–670, 1986.

33. Bankiewicz KS, Plunkett RJ, Jacobowitz DM, et al: Fetal nondopaminergic neural implants in parkinsonian primates. *J Neurosurg* 74:97–104, 1991.

34. Backlund EO, Granberg PO, Hamberger B, et al: Transplantation of adrenal medullary tissue to striatum in parkinsonism: First clinical trials. *J Neurosurg* 62:169–173, 1985.

35. Lindvall O, Backlund EO, Farde L, et al: Transplantation in Parkinson's disease: Two cases of adrenal medullary grafts to the putamen. *Ann Neurol* 22:457–468, 1987.

36. Madrazo I, Drucker-Colin R, Diaz V, et al: Open microsurgical autograft of adrenal medulla to right caudate nucleus in two patients with intractable Parkinson's disease. *N Engl J Med* 316:831–834, 1987.

37. Goetz CG, Olanow CW, Koller WC, et al: Multicenter study of autologous adrenal medullary transplantation to the corpus striatum in patients with advanced Parkinson's disease. *N Engl J Med* 320:337–341, 1989.

38. Olanow CW, Koller W, Goetz CG, et al: Autologous transplantation of adrenal medulla in Parkinson's disease. *Arch Neurol* 47:1286–1289, 1990.

39. Allen GS, Burns RS, Tulipan NB, Parker RA: Adrenal medullary transplantation to the caudate nucleus in Parkinson's disease: Initial clinical results in 18 patients. *Arch Neurol* 46:487–491, 1989.

40. Jankovic J, Grossman R, Goodman C, et al: Clinical, biochemical, and neuropathologic findings following transplantation of adrenal medulla to the caudate nucleus for treatment of Parkinson's disease. *Neurology* 39:1227–1234, 1989.

41. Goetz CG, Stebbins GT, Klawans HL, et al: United Parkinson foundation neurotransplantation registry on adrenal medullary transplants: Presurgical, and 1-and 2-year follow-up. *Neurology* 41:1719–1722, 1991.

42. Kordower JH, Cochran E, Penn R, et al: Putative chromaffin cell survival and enhanced host derived TH-fiber innervation following a functional adrenal medulla autograft for Parkinson's disease. *Ann Neurol* 29:405–412, 1991.

43. Kordower JH, Fiandaca MS, Notter MFD, et al: NGF-like trophic support from peripheral nerve for grafted rhesus adrenal chromaffin cells. *J Neurosurg* 73:418, 1990.

44. Branch DW, Ducat L, Fantel A, et al: Suitability of fetal tissue from spontaneous abortions and from ectopic pregnancies for transplantation. *JAMA* 273:64–65, 1995.

45. Kondoh T, Blount JP, Conrad JA, et al: Functional effects of transplanted human fetal ventral mesencephalic brain tissue from spontaneous abortions into a rodent model of Parkinson's disease. *Transplant Proc* 26:335, 1994.

46. Freeman TB, Olanow CW: Fetal homotransplants. *Arch Neurol* 40:1529–1534, 1990.

47. Centers for Disease Control: 1985 Abortion surveillance, Atlanta, 1981. US DHHS Public Health Service, 1985.

48. Freeman TB, Spence MS, Boss BD, et al: Development of dopaminergic neurons in the human substantia nigra. *Exp Neurol* 113:344–353, 1991.

49. Freeman TB, Sanberg PR, Nauert GM, et al: The influence of donor age on the survival of solid and suspension intraparenchymal human embryonic nigral grafts. *Cell Transplant* 4:141–154, 1995.

50. Redmond DE Jr, Naftolin F, Collier TJ, et al: Cryopreservation, culture, and transplantation of human fetal mesencephalic tissue in monkeys. *Science* 242:820–822, 1988.

51. Collier TJ, Gallagher MJ, Sladek CD: Cryopreservation and storage of embryonic rat mesencephalic dopamine neurons for one year: Comparison to fresh tissue in culture and neural grafts. *Brain Res* 623:249–256, 1993.

52. Kontur PJ, Leranth C, Redmond DE Jr, et al: Tyrosine hydroxylase immunoreactivity and monoamine metabolite levels in cryopreserved human fetal ventral mesencephalon. *Exp Neurol* 121:172–180, 1993.

53. Freed CR, Breeze RE, Rosenberg Nl, et al: Survival of implanted fetal dopamine cells and neurologic improvement 12 to 46 months after transplantation for Parkinson's disease. *N Engl J Med* 327:1549–1555, 1992.

54. Freeman TB, Kordower JH: Human cadaver embryonic substantia nigra grafts: Effects of ontogeny, pre-operative graft preparation and tissue storage. In Lindvall O, Bjorklund A, Widner H (eds): *Intracerebral Transplantation in Movement Disorders.* New York: Elsevier Science Publishers, 1991, pp 163–184.

55. Freeman TB, Olanow CW, Hauser RA, et al: Bilateral fetal nigral transplantation as a treatment for Parkinson's disease. *Ann Neurol* 38:379–388, 1995.

56. Bayer, SA: Neurogenesis in the rat neostriatum. *Int J Dev Neurosci* 2:163–175, 1984.

57. Kunzle H: Bilateral projections from precentral motor cortex to the putamen and other parts of the basal ganglia: An autoradiographic study in Maca fascucularis. *Brain Behav Evol* 88:195–209, 1975.

58. Alexander GE, Crutcher MD, DeLong MR: Basal ganglia-thalamocortical circuits: Parallel substrates for motor, oculomotor, 'prefrontal' and 'limbic' functions. *Prog Brain Res* 85:119–146, 1990.

59. Alexander GE, DeLong MR: Microstimulation of the primate neostriatum. II. Somatotopic organization of striatal microexci-

table zones and their relation to neuronal response properties. *J Neurophysiol* 53:1417–1430, 1985.

60. Kunzle H: An autoradiographic analysis of the efferent connections from premotor and adjacent prefrontal regions (areas 6 and 9) in Macaca fascicularis. *Brain Behav Evol* 15:185–234, 1978.

61. Dunnett SB, Bjorklund A, Stenevi U, Iversen SD: Behavioral recovery following transplantation of substantia nigra in rats subjected to 6-OHDA lesions of the nigrostriatal pathway. *Brain Res* 215:147–161, 1981.

62. Dunnett SB, Bjorklund A, Schmidt RH, et al: Intracerebral grafting of neuronal cell suspensions IV. Behavioral recovery in rats with unilateral 6-OHDA lesions following implantation of nigral cell suspensions in different forebrain sites. *Acta Physiol Scand* 522:29–37, 1983.

63. Dunnett SB, Annett LE: Nigral transplants in primate models of parkinsonism. In Lindvall O, Bjorklund A, Widner H (eds): *Intracerebral Transplantation in Movement Disorders.* New York: Elsevier Science Publishers, 1991, pp 27–50.

64. Bernheimer H, Birkmayer W, Hornykiewicz O, et al: Brain dopamine and the syndromes of Parkinson and Huntington: Clinical, morphological and neurochemical correlations. *J Neurol Sci* 20:415–455, 1973.

65. Kish SJ Shannak K, Hornykiewicz O: Uneven pattern of dopamine loss in the striatum of patients with idiopathic Parkinson's disease: Pathophysiologic and clinical implications. *N Engl J Med* 318:876–880, 1988.

66. Nyberg P, Nordberg A, Webster P: Dopaminergic deficiency is more pronounced in putamen than in nucleus caudatus in Parkinson's disease. *Neurochem Pathol* 1:193–202, 1983.

67. Leenders KL, Salmon EP, Tyrrell P, et al: The nigrostriatal dopaminergic system assessed in vivo by positron emission tomography in healthy volunteer subjects and patients with Parkinson's disease. *Arch Neurol* 47:1290–1297, 1990.

68. Szabo J: Organization of the ascending striatal afferents in monkeys. *J Comp Neurol* 189:307–321, 1980.

69. Imai H, Nakamura T, Endo K, et al: Hemiparkinsonism in monkeys after unilateral caudate nucleus infusion of 1-methyl-4-phenyl-1,2,3,6-tetrahydropyridine (MPTP): Behavior and histology. *Brain Res* 474:327–332, 1988.

70. Brundin P, Isacson O, Bjorklund A: Monitoring of cell viability in suspensions of embryonic CNS tissue and its use as a criterion for intracerebral graft survival. *Brain Res* 331:251–259, 1985.

71. Pakkenberg B, Moller A, Gunderson HJG, et al: The absolute number of nerve cells in substantia nigra normal subjects and in patients with Parkinson's disease estimated with an unbiased stereological method. *J Neurol Neurosurg Psychiatry* 54:30–33, 1991.

72. Frodl EM, Duan WM, Sauer H, et al: Human embryonic dopamine neurons xenografted to rat: Effect of cryopreservation and varying regional source of donor cells on transplant survival and morphology. *Brain Res* 647:286–298, 1994.

73. Lindvall O: Neural transplantation in Parkinson's disease, in Dunnet SB, Bjorklund A (eds): *Functional Neural Transplantation.* New York: Raven Press, 1994, pp 103–137.

74. Remy P, Samson Y, Hantraye P, et al: Clinical correlates of [^{18}F] fluorodopa uptake in five grafted Parkinsonian patients. *Ann Neurol* 38:580–588, 1995.

75. Kordower JH, Freeman TB, Snow BJ, et al: Neuropathological evidence of graft survival and striatal reinnervation after the transplantation of fetal mesencephalic tissue in a patient with Parkinson's disease. *N Engl J Med* 332:1118–1124, 1995.

76. Schultzberg M, Dunnett SB, Bjorklund A, et al: Dopamine and cholecystokinin immunoreactive neurones in mesencephalic grafts reinnervating the neostriatum: Evidence for selective growth regulation. *Neuroscience* 12:17–32, 1984.

77. Horellou P, Brundin P, Kalen P, et al: In vivo release of DOPA and dopamine from genetically engineered cells grafted to the denervated rat striatum. *Neuron* 5:393–402, 1990.

78. Sendeldeck SL, Urquhart J: Spatial distribution of dopamine, methotrexate, and antipyrine during continuous intracerebral microperfusion. *Brain Res* 328:251–258, 1985.

79. Yurek DM, Steece-Collier K, Collier TJ, Sladek JR Jr: Chronic L-dopa impairs the recovery of dopamine agonist-induced rotational behavior following neural grafting. *Exp Brain Res* 86:97–107, 1991.

80. Fiandaca MS, Kordower JH, Hansen JT, et al: Adrenal medullary autografts into the basal ganglia of Cebus monkeys: Injury-induced regeneration. *Exp Neurol* 102:76–91, 1988.

81. Hitchcock ER, Clough C, Hughes R, Kenny B: Embryos and Parkinson's disease. *Lancet* 1:12–74, 1988.

82. Freed CR, Breeze RE, Rosenberg NL, et al: Transplantation of human fetal dopamine cells for Parkinson's disease: Results at one year. *Arch Neurol* 47:505–512, 1990.

83. Wekerle H, Linington C, Lassmann H, Meyerman R: Cellular reactivity within the CNS. *Trends Neurosci* 6:271, 1986.

84. Inoue H, Kohsaka S, Yoshida K, et al: Cyclosporin A enhances the survivability of mouse cerebral cortex grafted into the third ventricle of rat brain. *Neurosci Lett* 54:85, 1985.

85. Nicholas MK, Antel JP, Stefansson K, Arnason BGW: Rejection of fetal neocortical neural transplants by H-2 incompatible mice. *J Immunol* 139:2275–2283, 1987.

86. Henderson BTH, Clough CG, Hughes Rc, et al: Implantation of human ventral mesencephalon to the right caudate nucleus in advanced Parkinson's disease. *Arch Neurol* 48:822–827, 1991.

87. Borlongan CV, Freeman TB, Sorcia TA, et al: Cyclosporine A increases spontaneous and dopamine agonist-induced locomotor behavior in normal rats. *Cell Transplant* 4:65–73, 1995.

88. McGeer PL, Itagaki S, Boyes BE, McGeer EG: Reactive microglia are positive for HLA-DR in the substantia nigra of Parkinson and Alzheimer's disease brains. *Neurology* 38:1285–1291, 1988.

89. Langston JW, Widner H, Brooks D, et al: Core assessment program for intracerebral transplantations (CAPIT). *Mov Disord* 7:2–13, 1992.

90. Pirrozzolo FJ, Hansch EC, Mortimer JA, et al: Dementia in Parkinson's disease: A neuropsychological analysis. *Brain Cogn* 1:71–83, 1982.

91. Brown RG, Marsden CD: Dual tasks performance and processing resources in normal subjects and patients with Parkinson's disease. *Brain* 114:1215–1231, 1991.

92. Sagar HJ, Sullivan EV, Gabrieli JDE, et al: Temporal ordering and short-term memory deficits in Parkinson's disease. *Brain* 111:525–539, 1988.

93. Taylor AE, Saint-Cyr JA, Lang AE: Frontal lobe dysfunction in Parkinson's disease. *Brain* 109:845–883, 1986.

94. Ostrosky-Solis F, Quintanar L, Madrazo I, et al: Neuropsychological effects of brain autograft of adrenal medullary tissue for the treatment of Parkinson's disease. *Neurology* 38:1442–1450, 1988.

95. Goetz CG, Tanner CM, Penn RD, et al: Adrenal medullary transplant to the striatum of patients with advanced Parkinson's disease: 1-year motor and psychomotor data. *Neurology* 40:273–276, 1990.

96. Martin WRW, Palmer MR, Patlak CS, Calne DB: Nigrostriatal function in man studied with positron emission tomography. *Ann Neurol* 26:535–542, 1989.

97. Patlak CS, Blasberg RG: Graphical evaluation of blood-to-brain transfer constants from multiple-time uptake data: Generalizations. *J Cereb Blood Flow Metab* 5:584–590, 1985.

98. Snow BJ, Tooyama I, McGeer EG, et al: Human positron emission tomographic {18F}-fluorodopa studies correlate with dopamine cell counts and levels. *Ann Neurol* 34:324–330, 1993.

99. Lindvall O, Brundin P, Widner H, et al: Grafts of fetal dopamine neurons survive and improve motor fucntion in Parkinson's disease. *Science* 247:574–577, 1990.

100. Sawle GV, Bloomfield PM, Bjorklund A, et al: Transplantation of fetal dopamine neurons in Parkinson's disease: PET [18F]-6-L-fluorodopa studies in two patients with putaminal implants. *Ann Neurol* 31:166–173, 1992.

101. Widner H, Tetrud JW, Rehncrona S, et al: Bilateral fetal mesencephalic grafting in two patients with MPTP-induced parkinsonism. *N Engl J Med* 327:1556–1563, 1992.

102. Sawle GV, Myers R: The role of positron emission tomography in the assessment of human neurotransplantation. *Trends Neurosci* 16(5):172–176, 1993.

103. Kordower JH, Rosenstein JM, Collier TJ, et al: Functional fetal nigral grafts in a second patient with Parkinson's disease: A post mortem analysis. *Soc Neurosci Abst.* In Press.

104. Guttman M, Burns RS, Martin WRW, et al: PET studies of parkinsonian patients treated with autologous adrenal transplants. *Can J Neurol Sci* 16:305–309, 1989.

105. Olanow CW, Gauger LL, Cedarbaum J: Temporal relationships between plasma and CSF pharmacokinetics of L-dopa and clinical effect in Parkinson's disease. *Ann Neurol* 29:556–559, 1991.

106. Mytilineou C, Han S-K, Cohen G: Toxic and protective effects of L-dopa on mesencephalic cell cultures. *J Neurochem* 61:1470–1478, 1993.

107. Lindvall O, Sawle G, Widner H, et al: Evidence for long-term survival and function of dopaminergic grafts in progressive Parkinson's disease. *Ann Neurol* 35:172–180, 1994.

108. Lindvall O, Rehncrona S, Brundin P, et al: Human fetal dopamine neurons grafted into the striatum in two patients with Parkinson's disease: A detailed account of methodology and 6 month follow-up. *Arch Neurol* 46:615–631, 1989.

109. Lindvall O, Widner H, Rehncrona S, et al: Transplantation of fetal dopamine neurons in Parkinson's disease: One-year clinical and neurophysiological observations in two patients with putaminal implants. *Ann Neurol* 31:155–165, 1992.

110. Spencer DD, Robbins RJ, Naftolin F, et al: Unilateral transplantation of human fetal mesencephalic tissue into the caudate nucleus of patients with Parkinson's disease. *N Engl J Med* 327:1541–1548, 1992.

111. Peschanski M, Defer G, N'Guyen JP, et al: Bilateral motor improvement and alteration of L-dopa effect in 2 patients with Parkinson's disease following intrastriatal transplantation of foetal ventral mesencephalon. *Brain* 117:487–499, 1994.

112. Madrazo I, Franco-Bourland R, Ostrosky-Solis F, et al: Neural transplantation (auto-adrenal, fetal nigral and fetal adrenal) in Parkinson's disease: The Mexican experience. *Prog Brain Res* 82:593–602, 1990.

113. Madrazo I, Franco-Bourland R, Ostrosky-Solis F, et al: Fetal homotransplants (ventral mesencephalon and adrenal tissue) to the striatum of parkinsonian subjects. *Arch Neurol* 47:1281–1285, 1990.

114. Subrt O, Tichy M, Vladyka V, Hurt K: Grafting of fetal dopamine neurons in Parkinson's disease: The Czech experience with severe akinetic patients. *Acta Neurochir Suppl (Wien)* 52:51–53, 1991.

115. Lopez-Lozano JJ, Bravo G, et al: Can an analogy be drawn between the clinical evolution of Parkinson's disease patient who undergo autoimplantation of adrenal medulla and those of fetal ventral mesencephalon transplant recipients? in Bjorklund A, Widner H (eds): *Transplantation in Movement Disorders.* New York: Elsevier Science Publishers, 1993, pp 87–98.

116. Dymecki J, Zabek M, Mazurowski W, et al: 30-month results of foetal dopamine cell transplantation into the brains of parkinsonian patients. *J Neural Transplant Plast* 3:325–326, 1992.

117. Huang S, Pei G, Kang FA, et al: Transplant operation of human fetal substantia nigra tissue to caudate nucleus in Parkinson's disease: First clinical trials. *Chin J Neurosurg* 5:210–213, 1989.

118. Molina H, Quinones R, Alvarez L, et al: Transplantation of human fetal mesencephalic tissue in caudate nucleus as treatment for Parkinson's disease: The Cuban experience, in Lindvall O, Bjorklund A, Widner H (eds): *Intracerebral Transplantation in Movement Disorders: Experimental Basis and Clinical Experiences.* Amsterdam: Elsevier, 1991, pp 99–110.

119. Olanow CW, Freeman TB, Kordower JH: Fetal nigral transplantation as a therapy for Parkinson's disease. *Trends Neurosci* 19:102–109, 1996.

120. Beecher HK: Surgery as placebo. *J Am Med Assoc* 176:1102–1107, 1961.

121. The EC/IC Bypass Study Group: Failure of extracranial/intracranial arterial bypass to reduce the risk of ischemic stroke. *N Engl J Med* 313:1191–1200, 1985.

122. Redmond DE Jr, Leranth C, Spencer DD, et al: Fetal neural graft survival. *Lancet* 336:820–822, 1990.

123. Kordower JH, Rosenstein JM, Collier TM, et al: Functional fetal nigral grafts in a patient with Parkinson's disease: Chemoanatomic, quantitative, ultrastructural, and metabolic studies. *J Comp Neurol* 370:203–230, 1996.

124. Miletich RS, Bankiewicz KS, Plunkett G, et al: 6-[18F] fluoro-L-dopa PET imaging of catecholaminergic fiber sprouting. *J Cereb Blood Flow Metab* 9:725, 1989.

125. Bohn MC, Cupit L, Marciano F, et al: Adrenal medulla grafts enhance recovery of striatal dopaminergic fibers. *Science* 237:913–915, 1987.

126. Bohn MC, Cupit L, Marciano F, et al: Adrenal medulla autografts into the basal ganglia of cebus monkeys: Injury-induced regeneration. *Exp Neurol* 102:76–91, 1988.

127. Lindsay RM, Wiegand SJ, Altar CA, Distephano PS: Neurotrophic factors: From molecule to man. *Trends Neurosci* 17:182–190, 1994.

128. Hyman C, Hofer M, Barde Y-A, et al: BDNF is a neurotrophic factor for dopaminergic neurons of the substantia nigra. *Nature* 350:230–232, 1991.

129. Sauer H, Fischer W, Nikkah G, et al: Brain derived neurotrophic factors enhance function rather than survival of intrastriatal dopamine cell-rich grafts. *Brain Res* 626:37–44, 1993.

130. Yurek DM, Altar CA, Ventimiglia R, et al: Optimal effects of exogenous BDNF on grafts of fetal dopaminergic neurons coincides with the ontogenic period when dopamine content and BDNF expression increase within the striatum. *Soc Neurosci Abstr* 21:1562, 1995.

131. Lin L-F, Doherty DH, Lile JD, et al: A glial cellline-derived neurotrophic factor for midbrain dopaminergic neurons. *Science* 260:1130–1132, 1993.

132. Johansson M, Friedemann M, Hoffer B, Stromberg I: Effects of glial cell line-derived neurotrophic factor on developing and mature ventral mesencephalic grafts in oculo. *Exp Neurol* 134:25–34, 1995.

133. Granholm A-C, Mott JL, Hoffer BJ, et al: Neurotrophic treatment of intraocular and intracranial fetal brain tissue transplants. *American Society Neural Transplatation Abstracts* 3:13, 1996.

134. Rosenberg MB, Friedmann T, Robertson RC, et al: Grafting genetically modified cells to the damaged brain: Restorative effects of NGF expression. *Science* 242:157, 1988.

135. Wolff JA, Fisher LJ, Xu L, et al: Grafting fibroblasts genetically modified to produce L-dopa in a rat model of Parkinson's disease. *Proc Natl Acad Sci USA* 86:9011, 1989.

136. Frim DM, Short MP, Rosenberg UC, et al: Local protective effects of nerve growth factor secreting fibroblasts against excitotoxic lesions in the rat striatum. *J Neurosurg* 78:267, 1993.

137. Stromberg I, Wetmore CJ, Ebendal T, et al: Rescue of basal forebrain cholinergic neurons after implantation of genetically modified cells producing recombinant NGF. *J Neurosci Res* 25:405, 1990.

138. Jiao S-S, Williams P, Wolff J: Intracerebral transplantation of genetically engineered muscle cells reduces experimental parkinsonism in rats. *Soc Neurosci Abstr* 18:782, 1992.

139. Cunningham LA, Hansen JT, Short MP, Bohn MC: The use of genetically altered astrocytes to provide nerve growth factor (NGF) to adrenal chromaffin cells grafted into the striatum. *Brain Res* 561:192, 1991.

140. Chalmers GR, Niijima K, Patterson PH, et al: Chromaffin cells cografted with NGF-producing fibroblasts exhibit neuronal features. *Soc Neurosci Abstr* 18:782, 1992.

141. Anton R, Kordower JH, Manaster JS, et al: Neural-targeted gene therapy for rodent and primate hemiparkinsonism. *Exp Neurol* 127:199–206, 1994.

142. During MJ, Naegele JR, O'Malley KL, Geller AI: Long-term behavioral recovery in parkinsonian rats by a HSV vector expressing tyrosine hydroxylase. *Science* 11(269):856–857, 1995.

Chapter 16

STEREOTAXIC SURGERY AND DEEP BRAIN STIMULATION FOR PARKINSON'S DISEASE AND MOVEMENT DISORDERS

JERROLD L. VITEK

PATHOPHYSIOLOGICAL BASIS OF HYPO- AND
    HYPERKINETIC MOVEMENT DISORDERS
        Organization of Basal Ganglia and Thalamocortical
            Circuits
        Pathophysiology Underlying Hypo- and Hyperkinetic
            Movement Disorders
SURGICAL ABLATIVE APPROACHES TO THE
    TREATMENT OF HYPO- AND HYPERKINETIC
    MOVEMENT DISORDERS
        Parkinson's Disease
        Dystonia
        Essential and Intention Tremor
        Hemiballismus
RADIOGRAPHIC AND MICROELECTRODE MAPPING
    TECHNIQUES FOR TARGET LOCALIZATION
        Radiographic Techniques
        Microelectrode Mapping Technique for Physiological
            Localization of the Target Site
        Semimicroelectrode Technique
ELECTRICAL STIMULATION IN THE TREATMENT OF
    HYPO- AND HYPERKINETIC MOVEMENT
    DISORDERS
        Applications
        Potential Mechanism(s) Underlying the Beneficial
            Effect of DBS
        Alternative Sites

Stereotaxic surgical procedures for the treatment of Parkinson's disease (PD) and other movement disorders have increased significantly over the last several years. Part of this resurgence stems from an improved understanding of the pathophysiological basis underlying these movement disorders. This improved understanding of the underlying pathophysiology has occurred, in large part, as a result of the development and study of physiological models of hypokinetic and hyperkinetic movement disorders (see also Chap. 6). These discoveries have now led to the selection of surgical

targets based on scientific principle, rather than serendipitous discovery or "seek and destroy" tactics. Functional neurosurgical procedures, using the knowledge gained from physiological and pathophysiological studies, are now incorporating electrophysiological recording techniques to refine old and develop new and innovative approaches to the treatment of movement disorders.

In this chapter the role of stereotaxic surgery and deep brain stimulation for the treatment of movement disorders will be examined, focusing on the treatment of PD, tremor, dystonia, and hemiballismus. The various subcortical sites that are now being targeted, the basis for their selection, and the application of electrophysiological recording techniques that have been used to physiologically define and improve target localization will be discussed.

The history of the development of stereotaxic surgery for the treatment of movement disorders is replete with different approaches to different targets in an attempt to ameliorate a variety of movement disorders. Reports of remarkable successes are mixed with complete failures after the same stereotaxic intervention.[1,2] The earliest approaches were generally not based on sound scientific principles but were empirically driven or based on simplistic rationales that led to what often appears as a desperate search for an effective target. The first known attempts to treat PD surgically were based on the presumed relationship between the motor symptoms and the foci of infection in patients with encephalitis lethargica. These consisted of removing the various organs suspected of harboring the infection evolving to sympathetic ramisectomies and cervical ganglionectomies. In 1930 Pollack and Davis,[3] in a failed attempt to relieve parkinsonian tremor, sectioned the dorsal roots of one patient. Although the rigidity was lessened, the tremor remained. Subsequent attempts included anterolateral cordotomies,[4,5] dentatectomy,[6] and extirpation of the precentral cortex.[7] These were generally unsuccessful and were associated with considerable morbidity. Meyers[2] subsequently reported improvements in some patients in which various parts of the basal ganglia, including the caudate, putamen, and globus pallidus or its outflow tracts, the ansa lenticularis or fascicularis lenticularis, were removed or sectioned, respectively. However, there remained significant morbidity and mortality associated with these procedures. In 1952 Cooper observed alleviation of Parkinsonian motor signs after accidental ligation of the anterior choroidal artery, which led to a number of unpredictable outcomes after subsequent ligations in other PD patients.[8] A variety of approaches were subsequently used to interrupt the pallidofugal pathways, including heating, freezing, and injections of procaine oil into the pallidum. Results, however, were inconsistent. Was it a problem of appropriate target selection, or an inability to consistently reach the chosen target that led to such a wide variation in the results for different patients with similar movement disorders? With the development of stereotaxis by Spiegel and Wycis,[9] there was an opportunity to improve target localization. Yet results, although somewhat improved, were still quite variable. This led to the report by Svennilson et al., who described the effect of pallidotomy on 81 patients operated on by Lars Leksell.[10] Leksell, varying the lesion site within the globus pallidus pars interna (GPi), observed a clear difference in outcome that was correlated with lesion location. In the last 20 patients with lesions placed in the posteroventral portion of GPi, 19 were substantially improved. With the advent of L-dopa, however, surgical treatment of PD became less frequent. Subsequent approaches were focused on thalamotomy for parkinsonian tremor, because most surgeons, at that time, felt that this was a better target for tremor alleviation.[11] Although Svennilson et al. had reported that more than 80 percent of patients experienced complete tremor alleviation after pallidotomy, the target site was moved to the thalamus.

Thalamotomy, although effective for tremor, rigidity, and L-dopa-induced dyskinesia, was ineffective for akinesia and, oftentimes, it worsened gait or speech disorders. It remained the target of choice, however, until recently, when pallidotomy was favorably reexplored by Lauri Laitinen.[12] Laitinen's report of significant improvement in parkinsonian motor signs, as well as amelioration of drug-induced dyskinesias after posteroventral pallidotomy, together with separate reports of successful improvement of parkinsonian motor signs after ablation or inactivation of the subthalamic nucleus (STN) and GPi in animal models of PD, has led to a resurgence of stereotaxic pallidotomy for PD. Several centers have now corroborated earlier reports[10,12] of amelioration of parkinsonian motor signs after stereotaxic pallidotomy.[13–17] Results, however, are not uniformly successful across centers, with some reporting minimal improvement[18,19] whereas others, like to Svennilson et al. and Laitinen, report significant improvement across the vast majority of patients.[13–17] The reasons for these differences are, as in the past, likely dependent on a variety of clinical variables, including lesion location and size, the patient's age and cognitive state, and other, as yet unidentified variables, including the presence of cerebral atrophy, response to medication, associated medical problems, and varied brain pathology. These variables, of which lesion location, age, and etiology of the movement disorder will likely play a central role, may also account, in part, for the variable success rates of stereotaxic intervention in other movement disorders.

Like earlier surgical approaches for PD, the surgical treatment of dystonia and tremor has also met with mixed success. Dystonia, both generalized and multisegmental, has been alleviated by both thalamotomy and pallidotomy, with similar success rates reported for both.[20–22] Yet, the overall results have been quite variable for both procedures, with approximately 25 percent of patients reported as showing marked improvement, 50 percent mild-to-moderate improvement, and 25 percent little or no benefit[21–23] Thalamotomy has a longer track record and has been used more frequently than pallidotomy, whereas pallidotomy, although reportedly effective in relieving various types of dystonia, has not been used with as much frequency, and the experience is more limited. Given the substantial phenotypic variability of dystonia, the underlying pathophysiological basis for dystonia may incorporate a variety of cortical and subcortical structures and vary for different types of dystonia. Thus, depending on the underlying pathophysiology for the particular type of dystonia being treated, one approach may prove more effective than another.

Parkinsonian, essential, and intention tremor have also proven amenable to surgical ablative therapy, although to

differing degrees. Parkinsonian tremor has met with the most consistent improvement, successfully abolished or significantly reduced in over 80–90 percent of cases after Vim thalamotomy.[22,24] Success after pallidotomy has been reported in over 80 percent of patients,[10,12] and this author has observed similar success rates.[13,14] Although initial reports are promising, the long-term outcome of pallidotomy for Parkinsonian tremor has not been as clearly defined as that for thalamotomy.

Essential and intention tremors have also been successfully treated with thalamotomy, although neither as effectively as Parkinsonian tremor, with many of these patients subsequently experiencing a recurrence of their tremor in the weeks or months to follow. Those tremors most difficult to treat and most likely to recur after thalamotomy are those involving proximal limb regions. The reasons for this may lie, in part, in the somatotopic organization of the motor thalamus, as recently described in the monkey, in which proximal limb regions occupy a larger region of the motor thalamus than more distal portions of the limb.[25] Thus, successful amelioration of proximal limb tremors will likely require ablation of a larger portion of the motor thalamus. In support of this argument, Hirai et al.[26] described a correlation between lesion volume and clinical outcome, which differed for the three tremor types. In this study Hirai et al. reported that larger lesions were more likely to reduce or abolish tremor that involved more proximal muscles, i.e., intention and severe essential tremor. They pointed out that effective lesions for intention tremor were more than three times the volume of those that were effective in abolishing tremor that included more distal muscles, i.e., PD and less severe essential tremors.

The importance of lesion location and size is being increasingly underscored in light of past[10,26] and present[27] studies reporting a dependence of clinical outcome on lesion location within the targeted structure. The reasons for this dependence in determining clinical outcome are strongly supported by the results of physiological studies. Specific regions within the pallidum, STN, and thalamus have been identified in which sensorimotor responses are found, underscoring their role in motor control.[28] Furthermore, these responses are somatotopically organized, and inactivation of these, but not adjacent, sites leads to improvement in the motor signs of PD.[29] Thus, although development of the stereotaxic frame offered improved methods of localization and was critical to the development of surgical therapies in the treatment of movement disorders, little was known about the functional organization of these subcortical targets, and the importance of lesioning specific regions within these targets was, therefore, not fully appreciated. Even if it had been, the problems inherent in locating the precise area to be lesioned could be formidable, with errors of a few millimeters leading to partial or no benefit.[30] Most surgeons generally relied on identification of the anterior and posterior commissures, using ventriculography and, more recently, computed tomography (CT) or magnetic resonance imaging (MRI) locate and identify the target to be ablated. Electrophysiological mapping of neural activity to determine the target physiologically was performed at only a few centers,[31–35] with most relying on conventional techniques of the time. With improved understanding of the importance of lesion placement, it has become increasingly clear that electrophysiological mapping techniques, when combined with conventional radiographic methods, provide an important tool for improving target delineation and localization.

With the resurgence of surgical approaches for the treatment of movement disorders, new applications are also being developed. Electrical stimulation, used predominantly for parkinsonian tremor, is now increasingly being used for the treatment of PD and will soon be extended to evaluate its potential role in the treatment of other movement disorders as well.

Pathophysiological Basis of Hypo- and Hyperkinetic Movement Disorders

ORGANIZATION OF BASAL GANGLIA AND THALAMOCORTICAL CIRCUITS

Based on our understanding of the anatomy and physiology of the basal ganglia and related structures, a scheme for

the functional organization of the basal ganglia has been developed (Fig. 16-1)[36] (see also Chaps. 5 and 6). This scheme views the basal ganglia as a family of larger segregated circuits involving specific portions of the thalamus and cerebral cortex. These circuits take origin from different cortical areas, project to separate portions of the basal ganglia, which in turn project to separate portions of the thalamus, then return to the same areas of the frontal cortex from which they took origin. One of these circuits, the "motor" circuit, has been considered most important in the pathogenesis of hypo- and hyperkinetic movement disorders, including PD, dystonia, hemiballismus, and Huntington's chorea (HC)[37] (see also Chapter 6). Parkinsonian tremor, although more recently implicated in this circuit, may have a more diverse etiology,[38,39] whereas essential and intention tremor are most likely a result of alterations in cerebellothalamic pathways.[40–42]

The motor circuit takes origin from precentral motor and postcentral somatosensory cortical areas and projects to motor areas of the basal ganglia and thalamus en route to its return to motor and premotor cortical areas (Fig. 16-2). This circuit is somatotopically organized throughout the different

FIGURE 16-1 Basal ganglia-thalamocortical circuits. ACA, anterior cingulate area; APA, arcuate premotor area; CAUD, caudate, (b) body, (h) head; DLC, dorsolateral prefrontal cortex; EC, entorhinal cortex; FEF, frontal eye fields; GPi, internal segment of the globus pallidus; HC, hippocampal cortex; ITG, inferior temporal gyrus; LOF, lateral orbitofrontal cortex; MC, motor cortex; MDpl, medialis dorsalis pars paralamellaris; MDmc, medialis dorsalis pars magnocellularis; MDpc, medialis dorsalis pars parvocellularis; PPC, posterior parietal cortex; PUT, putamen; SC, somatosensory cortex; SMA, supplementary motor area; SNr, substantia nigra pars reticulata; STG, superior temporal gyrus; VAmc, ventralis anterior pars magnocellularis; VApc, ventralis anterior pars parvocellularis; VLm, ventralis lateralis pars medialis; VLo, ventralis lateralis pars oralis; VP, ventral pallidum; VS, ventral striatum; cl-, caudolateral; cdm-, caudal dorsomedial; dl-, dorsolateral; l-, lateral; ldm-, lateral dorsomedial; m-, medial; mdm-, medial dorsomedial; pm, posteromedial; rd-, rostrodorsal; rl-, rostrolateral; rm-, rostomedial; vm-, ventromedial; vl-, ventrolateral.

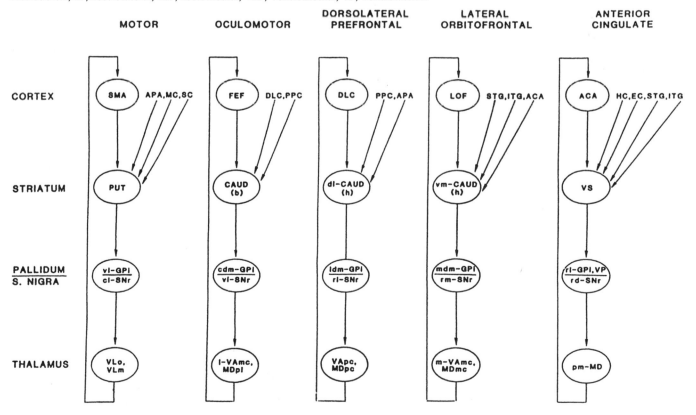

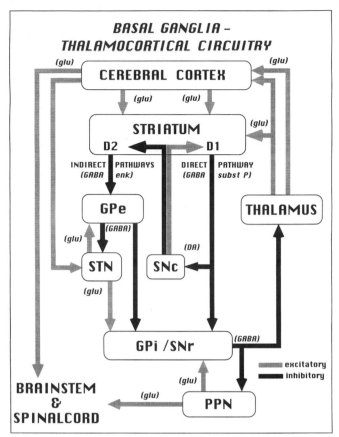

FIGURE 16-2 Schematic illustration of the basal ganglia-thalamocortical "motor" circuit and its neurotransmitters. "Indirect" and "direct" pathways from the striatum to basal ganglia output nuclei are represented by the arrows. GPe, globus pallidus pars externa; GPi, globus pallidus pars interna; STN, subthalamic nucleus; SNr, substantia nigra pars reticulata; SNc, substantia nigra pars compacta; PPN, pedunculopontine nucleus; glu, glutamate; GABA, gammaaminobutyric acid; enk, enkephalin; subst P, substance P. Dopamine (DA) receptor subtypes 1 and 2 are represented as D1 and D2, respectively.

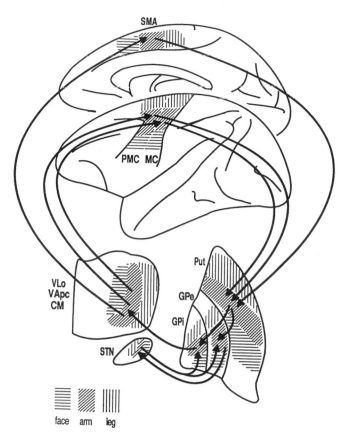

FIGURE 16-3 Somatotopic organization of the "motor" circuit. Arrows illustrate the projections from each cortical motor area to the striatum and within the basal ganglia-thalamocortical "motor" circuit. Different body parts are represented by different shading. See Fig. 16-2 for abbreviations, except for the following additions: MC, motor cortex; SMA, supplementary motor area; PMC, premotor cortex; VLo, ventralis lateralis pars oralis; VApc, ventralis anterior pars parvocellularis; CM, centromedian; Put, putamen.

cortical and subcortical motor areas (Fig. 16-3). Cortical input to the subcortical portions of the motor circuit occur via their projections to the putamen. Putaminal output arrives at the two major output routes from the basal ganglia, the GPi and the substantia nigra pars reticulata (SNr) via two pathways, termed the "direct" and the "indirect" pathways (see Fig. 16-2). The "direct" pathway takes origin from medium spiny neurons with presumed dopaminergic excitatory responses and monosynaptic projections to GPi and SNr. The "indirect" pathway takes origin from medium spiny neurons with presumed dopaminergic inhibitory responses that project, via GPe and STN, to the GPi and SNr. In addition, there are return projections from the STN to globus pallidus pars externa, (GPe) as well as direct projections from GPe to GPi, SNr, and the reticularis nucleus of the thalamus.[43]

The primary projection site from GPi is to the "motor" thalamus, ventralis lateralis pars oralis (VLo), and ventralis anterior (VA).[44–48] These areas project predominantly to the supplementary motor area and premotor areas, respectively,

but also have projections to the primary motor and arcuate premotor areas.[49–51] The SNr projects predominantly to ventralis anterior magnocellularis (VAmc) which projects to the prefrontal[52] cortex. GPi and SNr also have smaller projections to the midbrain tegmentum and the superior colliculus.[53,54] All intrinsic and output projections from the basal ganglia (putamen, GPe, GPi, SNr), with the exception of the STN, which is glutaminergic and excitatory, are gamma-aminobutyric acid (GABA)ergic and inhibitory. Projections from the cortex to putamen, and from the thalamus to the cortex, are excitatory.

More recently it has been discovered, through the use of retrograde transynaptic tracers, that within the motor circuit there may be a series of segregated circuits, each taking origin in different motor and premotor cortical areas (motor cortex, supplementary and arcuate premotor cortex), involving different portions of the basal ganglia and thalamus.[55,56] The proposal that these subcircuits may differentially affect movement receives some support from the differential role these cortical areas are proposed to play in motor control,[57–60] as well as from observations that neurons in different portions of GPi, electrophysiologically identified to project to different thalamic and cortical motor areas, have characteristic patterns of activity related to different components of the behavioral task.[56] Thus, it appears likely that these subcircuits may indeed be differentially involved in motor control and when altered in a particular fashion, may lead to the development of specific motor signs, i.e., rigidity, tremor, akinesia, dystonia, and dyskinesias.

PATHOPHYSIOLOGY UNDERLYING HYPO- AND HYPERKINETIC MOVEMENT DISORDERS

PARKINSON'S DISEASE

Based on our understanding of the pathophysiological changes that occur in the basal ganglia thalamocortical circuit in the parkinsonian monkey, a model for PD has been developed (Fig. 16-4). Loss of dopamine in the substantia nigra pars compacta (SNc) is proposed to lead to differential changes in neuronal activity of striatal cells in the direct and indirect pathway. In the direct pathway, loss of dopamine leads to a decrease of inhibitory activity from the putamen to GPi, whereas in the indirect pathway, activity in GPe is

reduced as a result of loss of excitation from the putamen. The decrease in inhibitory output from GPe to STN leads to excessive excitation from the STN to the GPi. Thus, there is an increase in inhibitory activity from the GPi to the thalamus and brain stem, which occurs via both the direct and indirect pathways.

Inhibition of thalamocortical and midbrain projections in the motor circuit has been proposed as the primary cause of the development of parkinsonian motor signs and the hypokinetic features associated with PD.[37] Similarly, the model predicts that a loss or lowering of inhibitory input from GPi to the thalamus may result in the hyperkinetic movements associated with drug-induced dyskinesias.[11,61,62] Changes in mean firing rates of neurons in GPe, GPi, STN, and VLo in the 1-methyl-4-phenyl-1,2,3,6-tetrahydropyridine (MPTP) monkey model of PD, and in GPe and GPi in patients with idiopathic PD, are consistent with those predicted by the model, that is, a decrease in mean discharge rates in GPe and VLo and an increase in mean discharge rates in STN and GPi.[30,37,63–66] Furthermore, positron emission tomography (PET) studies in PD patients have shown increased activity in cortical motor areas after pallidotomy, consistent with disinhibition of thalamocortical pathways.[67]

Contrary to the observed changes in mean firing rates in GPe, GPi, STN, and VLo in the monkey model and humans with idiopathic PD, the observed effect of lesions on parkinsonian motor signs both support and refute the model. Lesions within STN and GPi have been reported to ameliorate the major motor signs of PD, including akinesia, rigidity, and tremor. Lesions within the motor thalamus, however, do not exacerbate or induce parkinsonian motor signs, as predicted by the model but, instead, are reported to improve or abolish parkinsonian tremor, rigidity, and drug-induced dyskinesias,[61,68,69] suggesting that a decrease in activity of thalamic neurons cannot by itself account for the development of parkinsonian motor signs. Alternatively, these motor signs may occur, in part, because of an altered pattern of neuronal activity. This altered pattern of thalamocortical activity may, in turn, disrupt the normal operation of cortico-cortical circuits involved in motor control. Our observations of increased bursting and rhythmic oscillatory patterns of activity within the thalamus in parkinsonian monkeys, together with the clear improvement in most parkinsonian motor signs after thalamotomy, lend support to this hypothesis.[66,70,71] The actual role and relative contribution of altered patterns of activity versus changes in mean rates, or the potential relationship between levels of neuronal activity and the development of altered patterns of neuronal activity, in the genesis of parkinsonian motor signs and the altered motor behavior in PD, however, remains to be characterized.

Although altered patterns and rates of neuronal activity within the pallidothalamocortical motor circuit likely provide a significant contribution to the development of the motor signs associated with PD, the contribution of other pathways should not be disregarded, either in terms of their role in the underlying pathophysiology or in our approach to treatment. Perhaps the best example of the role of alternative pathways in the development of parkinsonian motor signs is the potential role of the cerebellothalamocortical pathway in the development of parkinsonian tremor. In previous ani-

FIGURE 16-4 Schematic representation of the motor circuit in hypokinetic disorders. The width of the lines relative to those in Fig. 16-2 represents the relative change in neuronal activity from the normal state. Wider lines represent an increase while thinner lines represent a decrease in neuronal activity. See Fig. 16-2 for abbreviations.

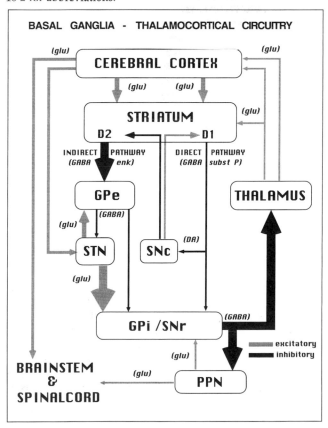

mal models of parkinsonian tremor, in which a portion of the midbrain tegmentum was ablated, it was necessary to include cerebellothalamic projections in order for tremor to develop.[72] Furthermore, whereas lesions in the sensorimotor portion of GPi are effective in improving or ameliorating parkinsonian tremor, lesions within the pallidal receiving area of the thalamus (Vop and Voa) have not generally been reported to be as effective as those within the cerebellar receiving area (Vim).[73–75] Although Hassler et al. reported that lesions within Vop were effective for parkinsonian tremor, he considered Vop to be a cerebellar receiving area not associated with pallidothalamic input.[11,76] The importance of interrupting the cerebellothalamic pathway in alleviating tremor was emphasized in his report of postmortem material obtained after thalamotomy. In patients with complete tremor arrest, he reported "coagulations either in the Vop or in the dentato-thalamic fibers, which end in the Vop." The discrepancy between the observations of Hassler et al. and others concerning the most effective site in the thalamus for alleviation of parkinsonian tremor may be no more than a difference in nomenclature or may be the result of a difference in interpretation of the cytoarchitectonic boundaries of thalamic subnuclei. Both groups, however, argue that the most effective lesions for relief of parkinsonian tremor lie in the cerebellar receiving area of the motor thalamus.

Additional support for a role of the cerebellothalamic pathway in the pathogenesis of parkinsonian tremor are the observations of rhythmic activity of neurons in Vim strongly correlated with tremor, as well as reports that the optimal location for lesions to alleviate such tremor appears to be within or includes significant portions of this region within Vim.[26,75,77–79] Other potentially important pathways in PD involve the role of brain stem regions, that is, the pedunculopontine nucleus (PPN) and midbrain extrapyramidal area (MEA), which receive projections from GPi and SNr and project to the thalamus, as well as the locus ceruleus (LC), which has widespread projections to the thalamus, cerebellum, and brain stem and may suffer significant cellular loss in PD.

Another potentially significant pathway in the development of parkinsonian motor signs is the projection from GPe to the nucleus reticularis (Rt) of the thalamus.[43,80] Other than through its effect on the STN, the role of GPe in the development of the motor signs associated with PD has been largely disregarded. Given the significant decrease in mean firing rates in GPe in PD, and the diffuse projections of reticularis neurons within and across thalamic subnuclei, the projection from GPe to Rt may serve an important role in the underlying pathophysiology of PD. Other potentially important pathways in the pathogenesis of parkinsonian signs are those from the GPi and SNr to the MEA and the PPN. The MEA sends projections back to the GPi and SNr, as well as to the brain stem and spinal cord, whereas the PPN has extensive projections to the thalamus.[81–84] Cholinergic projections from the PPN have a differential effect on thalamic relay and reticular neurons, depolarizing relay neurons and hyperpolarizing reticular neurons.[85–88] Thus, cholinergic brain stem projections from the PPN are generally excitatory to thalamic relay neurons and inhibitory to reticular neurons. Therefore, in addition to the direct effect of GPi and PPN projections on thalamic relay cells, there are likely indirect effects on these cells from GPe and PPN projections to the Rt. The extensive projections from Rt and PPN throughout the motor thalamus may explain the observed changes in neuronal activity reported in both pallidal and cerebellar receiving areas in animal models of PD.[66,81–84] Such a diffuse change in both the rate and pattern of neuronal activity in the motor thalamus is hard to account for without considering the potential role of GPe and/or brain stem thalamic projections in mediating them (Fig. 16-5).

DYSTONIA

Dystonia is a movement disorder characterized by sustained muscle contractions, leading to twisting, repetitive movements and abnormal postures. Clinicopathological studies in patients with dystonia indicate that the most common site in which a lesion can be identified is in the basal ganglia, that is, caudate, putamen, or pallidum. Thalamic lesions, although less common, have also been observed in patients with dystonia[89,90] (see also Chapter 33).

In mapping the receptive fields of thalamic neurons in patients with dystonia undergoing microelectrode-guided thalamotomy, we have observed an increased area of representation of the affected body part, compared to that in those patients without dystonia, that is, patients with essential or intention tremor (JL Vitek, unpublished observations). In addition, in a recent study in hemidystonic patients,[91,92] the incidence of somatosensory responses in Vop and Vim was significantly greater than that in a control group comprised of chronic pain or tremor (non-PD) patients. In this study, the percentage of sensory cells in the motor thalamus (22 percent) was significantly greater than that observed in control patients (9.5 percent). Notably, the number of sensory cells responding to movement of more than one joint was significantly higher in dystonic (23 percent) than in control patients (9 percent), an observation similar to that made in the MPTP monkey model of parkinsonism.[93] In addition, microstimulation in and around Vim produced simultaneous contraction of multiple muscles in the forearm of dystonic patients, with the activity of many neurons in Vop and Vim showing peaks of activity at the frequency of the dystonic movements, which were significantly correlated with electromyogram (EMG) activity in the affected limb segment.[91,92] A small lesion, presumably involving Vop and part of Vim, produced an immediate and dramatic decrease in the involuntary movements of these dystonic patients. These observations provide compelling evidence that Vop and Vim, receiving areas of the motor thalamus, are both involved in the pathogenesis of some types of dystonia.

Further evidence for a role of the pallidothalamic "motor" circuit in the pathogenesis of dystonia may be gleaned from observations in parkinsonian monkeys, in which dystonia has been reported to develop after high continuous doses of dopamine.[94] Furthermore, in patients with PD, in whom the pallidothalamic pathway is clearly altered, dystonia may occur as a presenting symptom or, develop as a consequence of medical therapy, that is, L-dopa-induced dystonia. The observation that some dystonic patients respond to low doses of L-dopa (Segawa variant), together with reports that lesions within the pallidum or thalamus alleviate dystonia,[20,21,95] also

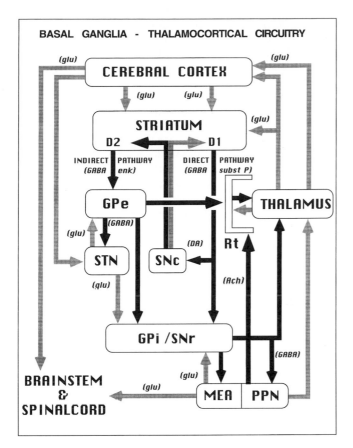
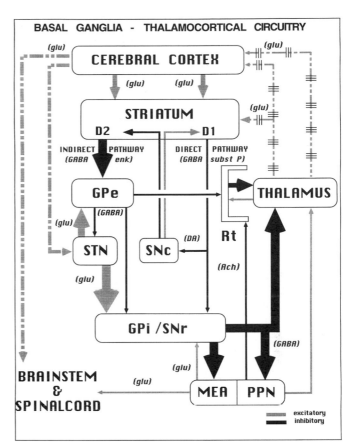

FIGURE 16-5 *A* and *B*. Schematic representation of the motor circuit in the normal (*A*) and hypokinetic (*B*) models, including those projections from the PPN to the Rt and thalamus. See Fig. 16-2 for abbreviations, except for the following additions: MEA, midbrain extrapyramidal area; Ach, acetylcholine. As in Figs. 16-2 and 16-4, wider lines represent a relative increase while thinner lines represent a relative decrease in neuronal activity.

suggests that alterations in neuronal activity within these structures may be the underlying basis for the development of the abnormal movements that occur in dystonia.

Pathophysiologically, dystonia may be a presenting symptom in parkinsonian patients who are not taking antiparkinsonian medications or alternatively may appear as a consequence of L-dopa treatment (peak dose dystonia), dystonia can be viewed as either a hypo- or hyperkinetic movement disorder. Whether this reflects etiologically different "types" of dystonia or merely represents a variation along the same general pathophysiological scheme is unclear. Although both types of dystonia likely reflect an alteration in the neural activity in the pallidothalamocortical and, probably, the cerebellothalamocortical circuit, the exact relationship between changes (rate and pattern) in neural activity in these regions and the development of dystonia remains unclear. In addition, pallidal projections to the brain stem are also likely to contribute to the pathogenesis of some "types" of dystonia. As with the pallido- and cerebellothalamic pathways, the particular changes in neural activity in these areas and their relationship to the development of dystonia is unclear.

ESSENTIAL AND ACTION TREMOR

Cerebellothalamic pathways, although likely contributing to the development of parkinsonian tremor, may also play a significant role in the development of essential and intention tremors. In both disorders tremor-related activity has been identified in Vim, and lesions within this area can significantly reduce or abolish both benign essential and cerebellar outflow tremors.

The physiological basis for the development of these tremors has been a much-debated issue. Neurons in the "cerebellar" thalamus in patients with either essential or cerebellar tremor have rhythmic bursting activity at tremor frequency.[96] Whether this occurs as a result of inherent neuronal rhythmicity expressed secondarily to conditions particular to these disorders and results in tremor, or occurs secondarily to or coincident with the development of these tremors, remains unclear. Thus, although the central mechanisms underlying the development of these tremors is not well defined, they clearly appear to involve thalamic neurons given the resolution of such tremors after thalamotomy.

The contribution of peripheral afferent mechanisms to the development of these tremors is also unclear. Some investigators have argued that the contribution of peripheral afferent mechanisms could be assessed by determining the degree of phase resetting of bursting neuronal activity in the thalamus after unexpected perturbations to the tremulous limb, and they termed this the resetting index.[97] An index of 0 suggested that there was no resetting whereas an index of 1 implied complete resetting. The resetting index for essential tremor was high, suggesting a significant peripheral contribution. It can be argued, however, that the index simply describes the degree to which tremor-related activity may be altered by peripheral input and not necessarily whether it underlies tremor genesis. Support implicating peripheral afferent mechanisms in the genesis of cerebellar tremor was provided by Vilis and Hore, who cooled the deep cerebellar nuclei and examined the change in response of motor cortical neurons, as well as the charge in timing and duration of agonist and antagonist EMG responses to torque pulses applied to the upper limb.[42,98,99] They concluded that cerebellar tremor occurred secondary to disordered reflex loops involving the motor cortex, because the delay in the response of motor cortex cells related to agonist-antagonist EMG activity was correlated with the delay observed in these EMG responses to controlled perturbation.[42,98,99] These data, although suggestive of a peripheral contribution to the pathogenesis of cerebellar tremor, however, do not address the role of inherent oscillatory mechanisms in the development of cerebellar tremor. Given the reports of rhythmically bursting neuronal activity in the motor thalamus in patients with cerebellar tremor who undergo thalamotomy, there is likely a significant central component underlying the genesis of this tremor.[68,100] One explanation for the development of cerebellar tremor lies in the inherent tendency for hyperpolarized thalamic neurons to burst after a depolarizing pulse.[88,101,102] Interruption of excitatory cerebellar projections to thalamic neurons could put these neurons into a hyperpolarized "burst-promoting" state. With initiation of movement, depolarizing corticothalamic projections may produce synchronous bursting activity of a population of thalamic neurons. When a critical population of thalamic neurons bursts synchronously, it may lead to the development of rhythmic bursting activity which, when transmitted to a critical number of alpha-motoneurons via the motor cortex induces an action tremor. Thus, although both peripheral and central tremorgenic mechanisms likely contribute to the development of cerebellar tremor, the relative contribution remains unclear.

HEMIBALLISMUS

Hemiballism consists of involuntary, often violent, movements of the contralateral limbs. These movements are most closely associated with inactivation or destruction of the STN or its efferent pathway.[103] A fiber-sparing neurotoxin has been observed in humans after vascular lesions restricted to the STN, as well as in monkeys after selective lesioning of the STN with ibotenic acid.[104,105] Although initially thought to occur secondary to release of inhibition from the STN to GPi, hemiballismus is now thought to occur predominantly as a result of disinhibition of the thalamus, occurring as a result of decreased excitatory drive from the STN to the GPi, leading to decreased inhibitory drive from GPi to the thalamus.

This model receives support from both experimental studies in the monkey and studies of patients with intractable hemiballismus[103–108] who undergo microelectrode-guided pallidotomy.[108] In both the human and the monkey, there is a significant reduction in the tonic discharge rate in GPi

after an STN lesion and the development of hemiballismus. Consistent with this observation, monkeys with hemiballismus after inactivation of STN show decreased metabolic activity in both GPi and the ventral lateral thalamus.[109]

SUMMARY

Our understanding of the pathophysiological basis of hypo- and hyperkinetic movement disorders has increased significantly over the last decade. Current models of these disorders have focused on alterations in tonic and phasic neuronal activity in the pallidothalamocortical "motor" circuit. Generally, it has been argued that excessive output from the STN and GPi leads to inhibition of thalamocortical pathways and the behavioral disturbances observed in these hypokinetic disorders. On the other hand, hyperkinetic movement disorders have been argued to arise from a release of thalamocortical activity, occurring as a result of decreased output from the STN and GPi. Support for this model comes from recordings throughout the motor circuit in monkey models of these hypo- and hyperkinetic disorders, as well as from patients with idiopathic PD and hemiballismus.

Given the observation in humans that thalamic lesions do not induce parkinsonism or that pallidal lesions do not induce chronic dyskinesia, the predictions of the model do not entirely hold up. However, given observations of altered neuronal activity in the thalamus in both the monkey model of PD and in patients with PD or dystonia, it is likely that the motor symptoms observed in these patients arise as a result of alterations in both the rate and pattern of activity in thalamic, as well as pallidal, brain stem and cortical neurons. Furthermore, the altered responsiveness of neurons throughout the motor circuit to peripheral input suggests that processing of sensory information is also significantly altered in these disorders. Thus, alterations in spontaneous patterns, tonic rates, and response to peripheral input may lead to an alteration of thalamocortical and cortical-cortical signal transmission and contribute to or underlie the development of the observed changes in motor behavior associated with these movement disorders.

Surgical Ablative Approaches to the Treatment of Hypo- and Hyperkinetic Movement Disorders

PARKINSON'S DISEASE

TARGET SELECTION

Based on the hypokinetic model, lesions in either the sensorimotor portion of the GPi or the STN should be effective in reducing or alleviating the motor signs associated with PD. Lesions that lie outside or involve only a portion of this circuit are likely to result in no or only a partial benefit.[27] Fig. 16-6 is an example of a patient in whom a radiologically guided lesion was made in the anteromedial "nonmotor" portion of GPi. This patient experienced transient improvement in motor symptoms for approximately 1 week, after which her symptoms returned. A subsequent lesion, made with microelectrode guidance, was placed posteriorly and

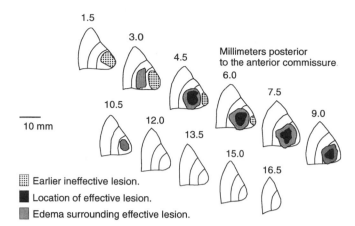

1.5

3.0

4.5

Millimeters posterior
to the anterior commissure

6.0

7.5

9.0

10.5

10 mm

12.0

13.5

15.0

16.5

▦ Earlier ineffective lesion.

■ Location of effective lesion.

▨ Edema surrounding effective lesion.

FIGURE 16-6 Serial MRI reconstruction illustrating the lesion location in a patient who underwent conventional radiologically guided pallidotomy, subsequently followed several months later by a microelectrode-guided pallidotomy.

laterally to the first, in the sensorimotor portion of the GPi. The latter lesion has led to significant long-lasting improvement (more than 2 years at the time of this writing) in all motor symptoms, including tremor, rigidity, bradykinesia, and lower extremity dystonia. Thus, although lesions that encroach on the motor circuit may lead to some benefit in terms of parkinsonian motor signs, this benefit may be transient and partial. Optimal benefit is most likely to occur with lesions that most completely interrupt the motor circuit.[10,27] The optimal location and size of the lesion within the GPi, although not yet fully defined, should involve as much of the sensorimotor portion of GPi as possible without infringing on nearby critical structures, including the GPe, nucleus basalis, internal capsule, and the optic tract. Clinical trials to assess clinical outcome and to identify and ascertain the relative strength of clinical variables in predicting those outcomes are currently under way and will be critically important in defining the role of pallidotomy in the treatment of patients with PD.

The STN is another potential target in the treatment of parkinsonian motor signs. Although STN lesions in monkeys have been highly successful in ameliorating parkinsonian motor signs,[110–112] there is significant concern over the application of this technique in humans because of the association of such lesions with the development of hemiballismus.[103–107] Although transient in most cases, intractable hemiballismus may occur after subcortical lesions involving the STN.[113] In addition, although the intensity of hemiballism has been reported to decrease over time, in animal experiments it has been reported to persist to some degree for the duration of the experiments (8 months) and may become intensified after administration of dopaminergic drugs.[110,112,114] Monkeys in which these observations were made, however, had not been on chronic L-dopa therapy, and the effect of subthalamotomy on dopa-induced dyskinesia in patients with long-term dopaminergic drug use is unclear. These observations, the location of the STN near the internal capsule, together with its rich blood supply, have, for the present time, made this a less desirable target for an ablative lesion in the treatment of

parkinsonian motor signs. Alternative treatment approaches directed at this target include the use of glutaminergic antagonists to reduce excessive excitatory activity from the STN or the use of implantable stimulation devices. The use of deep-brain stimulation will be discussed in more detail in a subsequent section.

Contrary to the palliative effect of ablation of the sensorimotor portion of GPi and STN, based on the current model of hypokinetic disorders, ablation of the motor thalamus should induce or worsen the motor signs of PD. There are numerous reports, however, with histological verification of lesion location, improvement in parkinsonian tremor, rigidity, and drug-induced dyskinesia after lesions in Vim, Vop, and Voa.[11,115] The thalamus has been targeted predominantly for its benefit on tremor. Lesions within Vim are highly effective in alleviating parkinsonian tremor in more than 85 percent of patients,[24,73] and if extended anteriorly to include Vop, and possibly portions of Voa, they also improve rigidity and dopa-induced dyskinesia.[61] Thalamic lesions generally have not been reported to improve bradykinesia or akinesia and have been reported to exacerbate speech and gait disorders in some patients.[116,117]

The observation that tremor, rigidity, and drug-induced dyskinesias improve after thalamotomy is consistent with the theory that altered patterns of thalamic neuronal activity may play a significant role in the development of parkinsonian motor signs[13] and provides new insight into the mechanism underlying the beneficial effect of thalamotomy in parkinsonian patients with these motor signs. Indeed, previous observations of the differential effect of lesions within pallidal (Voa, Vop) versus cerebellar (Vim) receiving areas of the motor thalamus on rigidity and tremor, respectively,[61,62,118,119] suggest that these circuits may play a differential role in mediating the development of parkinsonian motor signs. In this regard, it is compelling to consider the potential role of other thalamocortical circuits in the development of akinesia. Previous observations of transient akinesia induced in monkeys after lesions within the VA of the motor thalamus[120] suggest that more anteriorly located pallidothalamocortical circuits may be implicated in the pathogenesis of akinesia in humans with idiopathic PD. Such regions are not currently regarded as targets of stereotaxic surgeons and have not been intentionally lesioned in the past. Only a few studies have quantitatively examined patients' movement times after thalamotomy and those that have often reported some improvement.[11,117,121] It is possible that patients in whom akinesia was reported to improve after thalamotomy had lesions placed slightly more anteriorly than those who did not. Because most previous reports in humans have not correlated the location of thalamic lesions with the improvement or lack of improvement in akinesia, the potential role of this pallidothalamocortical circuit in mediating akinesia remains untested.

PATIENT SELECTION

Patients with medically intractable idiopathic PD with at least two of the four cardinal motor symptoms, that is, tremor, rigidity, bradykinesia/akinesia, or difficulty with gait and postural instability (freezing, festination), are considered candidates for pallidotomy. Motor fluctuations, on-off phenomenon, dystonia (off or on) and drug-induced dyskinesia are also responsive to pallidotomy and may be the predominant feature in some patients' PD, for which they are undergoing surgery. Patients should have demonstrated a clear and long-lasting benefit from antiparkinsonian medication, in particular L-dopa preparations and dopamine agonists. Patients with multiple-system atrophy, striatonigral degeneration, progressive supranuclear palsy, or olivopontocerebellar atrophy are not candidates for pallidotomy. Medical management of patients with idiopathic PD should be optimized before surgery; depression should be treated; and the cognitive state of patients should be thoroughly assessed. Patients with significant cognitive decline appear less likely to have long-lasting improvement after pallidotomy and may be unable to cooperate with motor and visual field testing during the procedure.[14,30,122]

Thalamotomy, although extremely effective in relieving parkinsonian tremor, rigidity, and drug-induced dyskinesia, has not generally been reported to be effective in alleviating akinesia and may even worsen gait or speech in some patients. Thus, in patients with significant akinesia/bradykinesia, or in whom there are significant problems with gait, postural stability, or speech, pallidotomy is recommended. However, in tremor-predominant patients, there is still considerable controversy over which procedure, pallidotomy or thalamotomy, is better. Several points need to be considered when making this decision. First is the relative efficacy of each procedure in effectively alleviating tremor. Thalamotomy has been reported as effective in approximately 80–90 percent of patients.[22,24] Pallidotomy is reported as effective in alleviating tremor in more than 80 percent of patients.[10,12,14] Thalamotomy patients have been studied in more detail and for longer periods of time, as compared to those who underwent pallidotomy, which has recently been investigated more closely for its long-term effect on tremor and other parkinsonian motor signs. In this regard, thalamotomy has a longer track record, and these numbers are less likely to change when compared to those of patients who had pallidotomy. It is likely, however, that both procedures may be equally effective for tremor alleviation when the appropriate portion of the thalamus or pallidum is lesioned. One must also consider, however, that all patients with PD generally progress; therefore, one must weigh the potential for that patient developing functionally disabling akinesia/bradykinesia, freezing, and motor fluctuations against the likelihood and relative degree of improvement in tremor after thalamotomy versus pallidotomy. More experience and longer follow-up with tremor-predominant patients after pallidotomy will be forthcoming and should help make these decisions easier in the future.

DYSTONIA

TARGET SELECTION
Both thalamotomy and pallidotomy have been successful in the treatment of various types of dystonia. The degree of benefit after these procedures, however, as with earlier surgical approaches to PD, is often inconsistent and unpredictable. Overall success rates (greater than 50 percent reduction in dystonic movements) generally vary from 25–50 percent.[21,23,95,123] However, there is a considerable amount of variability in the methods used for assessing the degree of improvement, the types of dystonia patient studied, and the length of follow-up. Many patients experience a reoccurrence of symptoms requiring a second surgery to expand the lesion. Cooper, in his series of 226 patients with genetic or acquired dystonia muscularum deformans, reported an average of two operations per patient, with the majority of patients having two, but the number per patient actually ranging from one to seven. Thus, lesion location and size were probably quite variable across these patients and studies and likely contributed significantly to the variable success rates reported across various centers.

Thalamic lesions for dystonia have generally been directed at the ventrolateral "motor" thalamus with some targeting regions more anterior in the pallidal receiving area (Vop, Voa),[69] whereas, others focus their lesions more posteriorly at the cerebellar receiving area (Vim).[23] Still others attempt to place their lesions to involve portions of both Vop and Vim.[92] Other thalamic sites have included CM, zona incerta (zi), anterior portions of ventralis caudalis (Vc), and the pulvinar.[23] In trying to decide on the best place to place lesions in the thalamus for dystonia, one must reexamine the hypo/hyperkinetic model. In PD it appears likely that altered neuronal activities in *both* Vop and Voa and in Vim, as described above, are related to the development of parkinsonian motor signs. Based on our observation that baseline firing rates of neurons are decreased and somatosensory responses are broadened in both Vop and Vim,[92] which is similar to that made in the MPTP model of parkinson's disease, and the observation that many parkinsonian patients develop "off" dystonia, at least some types of dystonia can be viewed pathophysiologically as a hypokinetic movement disorder. Using this premise as a model for the treatment of dystonia, along with the previous observation that the most effective thalamic lesions involved a large portion of the motor thalamus,[23] one would predict that dystonia, like PD, may result from altered neuronal activities throughout the motor thalamus[13,92] (JL Vitek, unpublished observations).

If one accepts the hypothesis that altered neuronal activity in both Vop and Vim contributes to the development of dystonia, then one would predict that thalamic lesions that remove this altered activity would be effective in improving dystonia. Thus, in order to alleviate dystonia, thalamic lesions may need to include both Vop and Vim. Previous studies in humans with small lesions placed, presumably, in specific subnuclei (i.e., in Vim, Vop, or Voa) have not been reported to consistently (in more than 50 percent of cases) or significantly (in more than 50 percent improvement) alleviate dystonia.[21,23] Larger lesions in the Vop and Vim nuclei, however, have been reported to produce more consistent and significantly better improvement.[124]

In placing lesions in the thalamus one must take into consideration the functional organization of these areas. Individual body regions in the monkey thalamus are represented in a series of lamellae, organized in a partial onionskin-like arrangement. In this arrangement the leg is represented in the outermost lamella, and the trunk, arm, and orofacial regions are represented in successively deeper lamella, with proximal limb portions forming the outer lamellae and occupying a relatively greater area than distal limb regions.[25] Given this organization, and the involvement of multiple subnuclei, it is easy to see why small lesions that do not include the affected body segments and are restricted to a single subnucleus are unlikely to provide significant improvement in multisegmental or generalized dystonia. Thus, if thalamic lesions are to be effective in alleviating multisegmental or generalized dystonias they should encompass the full extent of both Vop and Vim and, possibly, Voa.

Pallidotomy, although used less frequently than thalamotomy, has also been successful in alleviating dystonia in some patients. In one study examining the relative benefit of pallidotomy versus thalamotomy for patients with focal or generalized dystonia, there was no significant difference in clinical outcome between the two procedures.[20] Given the somatotopic organization of the pallidum,[65] a similar argument concerning lesion location and size may be made for pallidotomy. That is, lesions must include the somatotopic region of the affected body part, if they are to be effective. Part of the explanation for the variable results previously reported may lie in the inherent problem of target localization. To date, however, there have been no systematic studies correlating lesion location and/or size to long-term clinical outcome, assessed through objective clinical means, in determining the effectiveness of thalamotomy or pallidotomy for dystonia.

PATIENT SELECTION
Patients with generalized or focal dystonias, either primary or secondary, have been considered candidates for stereotaxic thalamotomy or pallidotomy. Currently, there are no clear guidelines describing the best candidates or whether different types of patients may respond better to one procedure versus another. Although all groups of patients have been reported as responding to ablative lesions in the thalamus or pallidum, the reported benefits from surgery are quite different, both in terms of the types of patients that respond and the consistency of their response to intervention. The types of patients, characteristics of the lesion in terms of size and location, as well as the method of clinical assessment and time of follow-up, differ significantly from study to study making comparison between studies difficult. The fact that many patients with generalized dystonia have shown such remarkable improvement after thalamotomy or pallidotomy whereas others do not, however, suggests that among these patients there are clinical variables, that is, differences in lesion characteristics (location, size,) etiology of the dystonia, or some as yet unidentified factors which, if better characterized (in terms of predicting clinical outcome), could be used to improve patient selection criterion. Generally, however, those patients with secondary hemi, or focal limb dystonias, are reported to benefit the most, whereas those with primary generalized and axial dystonias benefit the least. Treatment of spasmodic torticollis, a focal dystonia involving predominantly neck and paraspinal cervical muscles, has a reported success rate of approximately 60 percent across several studies[20,23,95]; however, the relatively high incidence, varying from 20–56 percent, of dysphonia after thalamotomy is a major factor when one is deciding whether or not to recommend thalamotomy for these patients. Although Cooper reported

remarkable successes in some patients with torticollis, fully one-third did not show any improvement after thalamotomy. The reasons for the variable response and associated complications in some patients after thalamotomy is unclear, but they may be secondary to the lesion involving different portions of the thalamus, involvement of different muscle groups, or a slightly different underlying or associated pathology. Patients with axial (trunk and neck) involvement are less likely to benefit to the same degree as those with limb dystonia after a unilateral lesion and are more likely to require bilateral procedures to show a similar degree of benefit. Patients undergoing bilateral thalamotomy, however, are at considerable greater risk of developing problems with speech, and the potential benefit must be weighed against the risks before proceeding with a second procedure on the other side. Thus, although some investigators report significant benefit among all groups of patients after stereotaxic thalamotomy,[23] most have reported significantly less benefit among primary generalized dystonia, whereas the patient group reported most likely to improve is those with hemidystonia after unilateral brain damage.[95]

ESSENTIAL AND INTENTION TREMOR

TARGET SELECTION
The cerebellar receiving area of the motor thalamus, Vim, has been the site most frequently targeted for the surgical treatment of essential and cerebellar outflow tremors.[24,26,75] Neurons in this area have been shown to respond to passive manipulations of the tremulous limb, to have tremor-synchronous neuronal activity,[31,60,75,77,125–127] and to respond with short latency to electrical stimulation of the peripheral nerve in the affected limb.[125] Although a detailed somatotopic map of this region has not been developed for humans, a well-defined somatotopic map has been developed for the monkey.[25] Details of this somatotopic organization are particularly important when targeting tremors involving the proximal limb, because proximal limb regions appear to occupy a larger area within Vim, enveloping distal limb regions anteriorly, laterally, and dorsally.[25] It is well accepted in the neurosurgical literature that proximal tremors, that is, intention and severe essential tremor, are much more difficult to treat than distal tremors. Many patients require several procedures, and some never experience significant long-lasting benefit. Details of the somatotopic organization of the cerebellar receiving area in the monkey, analogous to Vim in the human, offer an explanation for this observation. Because the shoulder and elbow area extend over a considerable distance in the medial-lateral and anterior-posterior direction, small lesions involving only a portion of the proximal limb area are less likely to be effective in abolishing cerebellar intention tremors, as they do not involve a large enough area of the proximal arm representation. Thus, the lesion must be placed so that it includes as much of the region in the thalamus that represents the affected body part as possible.

PATIENT SELECTION
Patients with medically intractable essential or cerebellar intention tremors are considered candidates for surgical inter-

vention. Patients with essential tremor should have been on maximal doses of inderal and mysoline alone and in combination before recommending surgical intervention. Patients with predominant head and voice tremor without significant limb tremor are not considered good candidates for surgery, because head and voice tremor have not been consistently demonstrated to improve significantly after surgery. Part of the explanation for this may again lie in the somatotopic organization of Vim. Head and orofacial structures lie in the most medial portion of Vim, adjacent to midline thalamic subnuclei. Lesions most likely to benefit head and voice tremor would need to be placed medially and would likely be associated with a greater incidence of dysphonia, making these tremors much more difficult to treat.

Those patients with essential tremor who are most likely to benefit from thalamotomy are those with predominantly distal limb tremor. Patients with tremor involving more proximal limbs may also receive significant benefit but require a larger lesion. Improvement is contralateral to the side of the lesion, with little or no improvement in the ipsilateral side. Those patients with bilateral tremor should have the side operated on which, in the patient and surgeon's view, will give them the most functional benefit. A second thalamotomy can be performed but entails a higher risk of complication in the form of dysarthria, aphasia, or cognitive changes. Restricting lesions to the motor thalamus, minimizing the size, and avoiding encroachment on midline structures may help to reduce this risk. In no case should bilateral procedures be performed at the same time. Generally, a minimum of 3–6 months should elapse before a second procedure is performed.

Patients with cerebellar outflow tremors, often patients with multiple sclerosis or post-traumatic brain injury, are less likely to benefit from medical therapy. However, surgical intervention is often the only hope these patients have. Success among this group of patients has been highly variable, with many undergoing several procedures, only to have their tremor return. Larger lesions are required for these tremors and should involve as much of the affected limb region within Vim as possible. Patients with bilateral tremor should be assessed for asymmetry and have the most severe side operated on. Some patients may prefer to have the dominant side operated on, even if it is less severely affected. Bilateral thalamotomy can be done but, as above, entails a greater risk of complication, particularly in this patient group, who will require a larger lesion and may have associated problems with dysarthria, gait, or other impaired motor or cognitive function. Generally, such procedures should be avoided unless deemed necessary by both the physician and patient and unless the risks are well understood by the patient and their family.

HEMIBALLISMUS

TARGET SELECTION
Both thalamotomy and pallidotomy have been reported to be effective in the surgical treatment of intractable hemiballismus.[71,103,108] Although there are few cases with histological confirmation of lesion location, the effective lesions in GPi are reported to lie in the posterior pallidum.[71] Those in the thalamus are placed in the ventrolateral thalamus and would appear to include portions of what is now termed Vop and Vim. These lesions, however, likely involved surrounding subnuclei and, in some histologically verified cases, involved portions of the zona incerta and reticular nucleus of the thalamus.[23,128]

PATIENT SELECTION
Patients in whom medical therapy has been unsuccessful and/or whose health is at risk secondary to continuous excessive hemiballistic movements should be considered candidates for pallidotomy or thalamotomy.

Radiographic and Microelectrode Mapping Techniques for Target Localization

RADIOGRAPHIC TECHNIQUES

Initial target coordinates are obtained by conventional radiographic techniques using CT, MRI, and/or ventriculography. The location of the anterior and posterior commissures relative to fiducial markers on the stereotaxic frame are used to calculate the X, Y, and Z coordinates of the target. For pallidotomy the coordinates are 21 mm lateral, 3 mm anterior, and 3–6 mm ventral to the midcommissural line. Based on physiological data gathered during microelectrode-guided pallidotomies, these coordinates target the sensorimotor portion of GPi.[30] For thalamotomy a good starting point is approximately 3–5 mm anterior to the posterior commissure at lateral 15, depth just at the ac-pc line. These coordinates should allow the first pass with the recording electrode to penetrate portions of the sensory thalamus which, combined with determination of the receptive fields of neurons in the adjacent motor thalamus, provides a highly reliable landmark for subsequent penetrations. Because of individual variation in the length of the ac-pc line, size of the third ventricle, and radiographic distortion inherent in these techniques, these coordinates should serve only as a starting point, with the final target dependent on the result of physiological mapping with the microelectrode. The lesion should be placed based on the type of movement disorder being treated, the somatotopic organization of the structure to be lesioned, the portion of the body involved, and the relative location of nearby critical structures to be avoided. The region to be lesioned will generally encompass a considerably larger portion of the thalamus or pallidum than can be involved with a single lesion, based on one set of target coordinates. This information cannot be obtained by conventional radiographic means alone and requires the use of electophysiological mapping techniques.

MICROELECTRODE MAPPING TECHNIQUE FOR PHYSIOLOGICAL LOCALIZATION OF THE TARGET SITE

Microelectrode recording techniques used in conjunction with radiographic methods facilitate identification and localization of the target structure to be ablated. This approach enhances the ability of the surgeon to locate and place the lesion within the identified target and sculpt the lesion to involve as much or as little of the target as deemed necessary to provide the optimal outcome, while avoiding adjacent structures, that is, internal capsule, midline, and sensory thalamus for thalamotomy, as well as the internal capsule, optic tract, GPe, and nucleus basalis for pallidotomy.

TECHNICAL COMMENTS AND ELECTROPHYSIOLOGICAL EQUIPMENT

A variety of electrodes can be used for electrophysiologic recording; however, platinum-iridium glass-coated microelectrodes with a tip diameter of 2–4 μm and an impedance of 0.5–2.0 Mohms (at 1000 Hz), provide excellent recording characteristics that do not deteriorate after microstimulation. The electrode is protected in a stainless steel "carrier" tube attached to a microdrive assembly, which is adapted to fit onto the stereotaxic frame and manually zeroed so that the tip of the electrode is even with the end of the carrier tube when the microdrive is at zero. The microelectrode in its carrier tube is lowered into a protective guide tube and comes to rest at the level of the tip of the guide tube, which is approximately 45 mm from the radiographically determined target. The recording electrode is connected to standard electrophysiological equipment for amplification, filtering, and discrimination of electrophysiological signals.

PALLIDOTOMY

Microelectrode penetrations are made in the parasagittal plane, proceeding from the anterodorsal to posteroventral direction at an angle of approximately 30 degrees from vertical. As the microelectrode is advanced, patterns of neural activity are noted throughout the track. The major structures that are identified using this plane of approach are the white matter, striatum (caudate and putamen), the GPe and GPi, the optic tract, and the internal capsule. The nucleus basalis may be encountered with anteriorly placed penetrations. Each cellular region has a characteristic pattern of neural

activity similar to that described in the monkey[129] (Fig. 16-7). Low spontaneous discharge rates that increase transiently as the electrode is advanced typify neural activity from the striatum, whereas units that consist of high-frequency discharges separated by pauses (HFD-P) and units that are active in bursts separated by periods of single-spike discharges at low frequency (LFD-B) typify those found within GPe. High-frequency tonic activity characterizes the majority of neural activity within GPi, although a variety of other patterns may be present, including bursts with little pause between them, emitting a "chugging" sound, or lower-frequency bursting in the range of 4–6 Hz. Within the laminae of the pallidum (i.e., between the GPe and GPi, as well as laminae within GPi), neurons with slower rates of tonic neural activity ("border" cells) may be encountered. These cells help identify border regions of the pallidal segments.

Once through the pallidum, the optic tract or the internal capsule can be identified by microstimulation. In the optic tract, microstimulation typically results in brief flashes of light (phosphenes). In the internal capsule microstimulation induces movement of the limbs or orofacial structures. The relative proximity of these structures (i.e., optic tract and internal capsule) can be ascertained by the stimulation threshold at which these phosphenes are noted or muscle contraction occurs. The optic tract can also be identified by flashing a light in the patient's eyes and listening for high-frequency modulation of the background audio signal coincident with the light stimulus.

The target region within GPi is determined by identifying neurons with responses to passive manipulations and active movement of the extremities and orofacial structures of the patient. The presence of bursting activity and its relationship to tremor, if present, is noted, along with each type of neural activity. The presence and somatotopic location of neuronal responses in the GPi to passive or active movement, as well as the relative location of the optic tract and internal capsule (noting the thresholds), are used to generate a topographic map of this subcortical region. This topographic map is, in turn, used to determine the location within GPi and guide lesion placement.

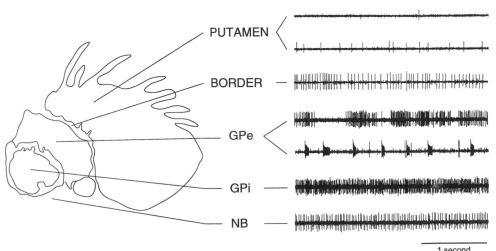

FIGURE 16-7 Different patterns of neural activity encountered in the basal ganglia during a single penetration with the microelectrode. St, striatal; HFD-P, high-frequency discharge pause; LFD-B, low-frequency discharge burst; B, border. Abbreviations for the neural structures in which they are encountered are the same as those for figures 16-2 and 16-3 with the addition of nucleus basalis (NB).

PUTAMEN

BORDER

GPe

GPi

NB

1 second

Neurons within the sensorimotor portion of the pallidum are characterized by increased activity to deep-muscle palpation, passive joint movement, or active movement of specific body parts. These responses are predominantly contralateral and specific to a single joint, although neurons with responses to multiple joints or limbs or even the ipsilateral limb may be encountered.[30] More importantly, there is somatotopic organization within the sensorimotor region of GPi with the leg found medial, posterior, and dorsal to the arm area and the face ventral.[25]

Sensorimotor responses are found predominantly in the posterolateral portions of GPi, whereas neurons in regions more anterior and medial do not respond to active or passive manipulations of the limbs or orofacial structures and are likely related to nonmotor "associative" functions. Lesions in this region alone will likely result in no or partial improvement in the motor symptoms of PD (see Fig. 16-6). Lesions placed in this portion of GPi are likely to produce similar results for dystonia or hemiballismus.

THALAMOTOMY

A similar, although somewhat different, strategy is used for thalamotomy. The thalamus contains 50–60 different subnuclei. The targeted subnuclei lie adjacent to regions that, when lesioned, may lead to significant cognitive, language, or sensory impairment. It is important, therefore, to map precisely the boundaries of the region(s) to be included within the lesion to obtain the maximal benefit while minimizing potential complications as a result of lesion encroachment on adjacent subnuclei.

The microelectrode and electrophysiological equipment used for thalamotomy are the same as those used for pallidotomy. The parasagittal approach is also the same, except for cases in which one wants to include Vop or portions of Voa, in which case one may choose an angle of 45 degrees from vertical. A sharper angle allows one microelectrode penetration to cross a greater portion of adjacent thalamic subnuclei and provides a better approximation of the borders between thalamic subnuclei.

As the microelectrode is passed into the thalamus, a characteristic rhythmic activity is found. Just before this, one may encounter neurons with broad receptive fields responding to passive or active movement, confrontational hand gestures, or changes in attention. These types of responses are typical of neurons in the reticular nucleus of the thalamus. This nucleus is only a few hundred micrometers thick and is followed by a thin laminae of similar diameter before the rhythmic discharge of thalamic neurons in the motor thalamus is encountered. At this point single units are discriminated throughout the track. Neuronal responses to passive and active movement of individual body parts are sought, and microstimulation is carried out at a maximum of 40–50 μA, with trains of symmetric biphasic pulse pairs at a frequency of 300–400 Hz. The patient is instructed to report any change in sensation that occurs with microstimulation, describing its location, quality, and intensity. At each stimulation site, when changes in sensation occur with stimulation, sensory thresholds are determined by decreasing the current intensity progressively, until the stimulus no longer elicits a sensory response. For each microelectrode penetration response to microstimulation, sensory thresholds, spontaneous activity patterns, and the response of each isolated cell to sensorimotor examination are plotted on plastic overlays, then fitted to computer-generated maps of the human thalamus taken from the Schaltenbrand and Bailey Atlas and scaled to the patients ac-pc coordinates.

Lateral, anterior, and ventral boundaries of the motor (Voa, Vop, and Vim) and sensory (Vc) thalamus are determined based on microstimulation effects, the presence or absence of neuronal activity, and neuronal response properties to sensorimotor examination. Penetrations through more lateral portions of the thalamus are characterized by neuronal responses that occur at deeper locations over shorter distances because of its lateral convexity. In addition, because the lateral border of the thalamus is adjacent to the internal capsule, where microstimulation results in short latency-evoked movements, this region is easily identified. The anterior border of the sensory thalamus, Vc, is identified by the presence of neurons with small, well-defined fields receptive to tactile sensation in a body region in which low threshold (5–10 μA), stimulation-induced paresthesias occur. The relative distance of the recording electrode from the anterior border of Vc can be approximated by the sensory threshold at which microstimulation induces paresthesias. Sites sufficiently anterior to Vc are characterized by a lack of microstimulation-induced paresthesias, even at current intensities of 40–50 μA. Because of the somatotopic organization of these regions, penetrations near the lateral border of the sensory thalamus are characterized by microstimulation-induced paresthesias of somatosensory responses predominately restricted to the leg. Penetrations made progressively more medially will have responses largely restricted to the arm and face, respectively. As one moves rostrally from Vc to Vim, Vop, and Voa, there is a gradation of cell responses to sensorimotor examination: cells in Vc respond to tactile stimuli whereas those in Vim, Vop, and Voa do not; cells in Vim respond readily to passive manipulations of the limbs and orofacial structures, whereas cells in Vop and Voa tend to respond more selectively to voluntary movement and less to passive manipulations, which is similar to the case described in the monkey for homologous subnuclei.[25,130]

SEMIMICROELECTRODE TECHNIQUE

An alternative recording technique for physiological localization of target sites involves the use of a bipolar concentric semimicroelectrode with a tip diameter of approximately 0.6 mm and an interpole distance of 0.3–0.6 mm. Although the basic technique is the same as that used for the microelectrode, the type of information provided differs significantly. The semimicroelectrode gives a broader, more integrated sampling of multicellular activity, whereas the microelectrode allows characterization of the response properties of single units. Basically, the semimicroelectrode is better suited to locate and differentiate individual subnuclei, whereas the microelectrode is more precise, allowing for the determination of spontaneous activity patterns and sensorimotor response properties of single units.

Electrical Stimulation in the Treatment of Hypo- and Hyperkinetic Movement Disorders

APPLICATIONS

PARKINSONIAN AND OTHER TREMORS

Chronic deep-brain stimulation has been used for treatment of parkinsonian, essential, and cerebellar outflow tremors. The greatest experience with thalamic stimulation for tremor is that of Benabid and Pollack, who reported that approximately 88 percent of patients with parkinsonian tremor and 68 percent with essential tremor demonstrate complete or marked tremor alleviation with thalamic stimulation.[131] In contrast to those patients with parkinsonian or essential tremor, only about 10–20 percent of patients with an intention tremor show a similar degree of benefit. The generally poor effect of electrical stimulation for intention tremors may occur as a result of the somatotopic organization of the thalamus, in which proximal limb regions occupy a relatively larger territory.[25] As with ablative lesions, which must be significantly larger for action/proximal tremor,[26] electrical stimulation must, in turn, affect a relatively larger portion of Vim for alleviation of tremor involving proximal versus distal limb segments. It is important that the somatotopic organization of these regions be taken into account when implanting deep-brain stimulation devices in order to optimize their efficacy.

Electrical stimulation offers several advantages over traditional ablative therapies. A variety of pulse widths, stimulation frequencies, current intensities, and lead combinations (using a multipolar lead) can be used to optimize the beneficial effect. Similarly, if untoward side effects occur, stimulation parameters can be adjusted to minimize them. Generally stimulation frequencies greater than 130 Hz and pulse widths of 60–90 μs have been reported as being most beneficial.[132] However, these parameters can be modified to obtain the desired effect.

PARKINSON'S DISEASE

In addition to parkinsonian tremor, deep-brain stimulators have more recently been implanted in the GPi and STN to treat other motor signs of PD.[133–135] GPi stimulation in patients with PD has been reported to improve all of the cardinal motor symptoms, including tremor, rigidity, bradykinesia, and gait, as well as drug-induced dyskinesias and motor fluctuations.[133] Similarly, stimulation in the STN has also been reported as highly successful in alleviating the major motor signs of PD.[134] Although stimulation in the STN improves motor fluctuations and freezing, it may actually induce dyskinesias at higher current intensities.[134] At present, experience with the use of electrical stimulation for the treatment of PD, although promising, is limited. Larger numbers of patients in well-controlled studies will be required to assess the benefits and improve our understanding of this technique in order to optimize its use in the treatment of PD.

POTENTIAL MECHANISM(S) UNDERLYING THE BENEFICIAL EFFECT OF DBS

The physiological basis underlying the beneficial effect of deep-brain stimulation (DBS) in Vim, GPi, or STN on parkinsonian motor signs is unclear, however, a number of possibilities have been proposed. Because both DBS and lesions in Vim alleviate tremor, it has been argued that stimulation may act by inactivating the region in which the stimulation is applied. This can occur through a mechanism termed depolarization block, in which neurons are depolarized and put into an absolute or relative refractory period blocking subsequent neuronal action potentials, essentially putting cells into a dormant electrical state. There is some evidence that a single pulse from a microelectrode can inhibit neurons surrounding the electrical stimulus[136]; however, the effect of continuous high-frequency stimulation on neuronal activity is unclear. Alternatively, it has been argued that DBS may activate neurons, but in such a way as to block tremorgenic activity by inhibiting or "jamming" rhythmic neuronal activity. This could occur by desynchronizing[137] or blocking transmission of neuronal activity by interfering with neuronal loops responsible for thalamic-bursting activity.[138] Alternatively, this could also occur through an as yet unknown mechanism on cerebellar and brain stem circuits via anti- or orthodromic activation of cells or fibers of passage.[130–140] This argument receives some support from PET studies in which regional cerebral blood flow in the cerebellar nuclei, as well as in the precentral and accessory motor cortex, was decreased during DBS in the thalamus.[141]

The effects of GPi stimulation on parkinsonian motor signs may be mediated by mechanisms similar to those proposed for thalamic stimulation. Assuming the improvement in parkinsonian motor signs reported coincident with GPi stimulation most likely occurs as a result of decreased GPi output, such decreases can occur either through inhibition or blocking of neuronal activity, directly via depolarization block, or via activation of other circuits inhibitory to GPi neurons, that is, antidromic activation of GPe. STN stimulation, similar to that of GPi stimulation, has a host of possible mechanisms that underlie its beneficial effects on parkinsonian motor signs. These include (1) inactivation of STN directly by electrical stimulation, (2) activation of STN in a fashion that alters neuronal activity in GPi, either decreasing it, blocking its transmission, or normalizing its pattern, (3) antidromic activation of GPe, leading to inhibition of STN, GPi, and /or reticularis neurons in the thalamus, which then leads to normalization of thalamic neuronal activity.[66,142]

Thus, the mechanism(s) underlying the effect of electrical stimulation in these subcortical structures are likely multifactorial and are most certainly dependent on stimulation parameters and location of the stimulating electrode.[143] The effect of electrical stimulation on neuronal activity is complex, likely activating some cells while inhibiting others,[136] and antidromically and orthodromically activating some fibers, while blocking still others. Together with the effects on fibers of passage and local-circuit neurons, electrical stimulation provides a host of possibilities for the mechanisms that underlie its beneficial effect(s). Given its reversibility and reported low incidence of side effects, it is a technique with important therapeutic applications. It is critically important to understand the mechanisms that underlie the beneficial effects of DBS in order to develop this potentially powerful technique to its full potential for the treatment of PD and to fully explore its potential for the treatment of other movement disorders, that is, dystonia, intention tremor, etc.

ALTERNATIVE SITES

Other sites where electrical stimulation may prove equally or more effective for the treatment of parkinsonian motor symptoms have yet to be explored. Acute stimulation within GPe in parkinsonian patients undergoing pallidotomy has been reported to be effective in improving bradykinesia.[143] This effect was critically dependent on the stimulation parameters used, with higher frequencies (>100 Hz) more effective than lower frequencies in alleviating bradykinesia.[143] Given this dependence, it is likely that cells and fibers are differentially activated or inhibited in varying combinations dependent on the stimulation parameters, geometric configuration, and location of the stimulation device being used. If stimulation can be used to activate projection neurons, stimulation within the GPe could potentially be more effective than that observed for STN or GPi. Given the projection of GPe to the reticularis nucleus of the thalamus, as well as to both GPi and STN, which project, in turn, to SNr, PPN, and MEA, normalization of activity within GPe would theoretically have a far greater effect on amelioration of parkinsonian motor signs, because it can potentially affect all of the major output areas, as opposed to only a few, such as with ablation or stimulation of STN or GPi.

A potential concern with ablative techniques is the possibility of sprouting, which may occur at target sites of degenerating axons after ablation of their projection neurons.[144] Such sprouting can lead to the functional reorganization of these structures and contribute to the recurrence of some motor symptoms. Although there are some reports of sprouting with DBS,[145] the relative amount and contribution to the functional reorganization that may occur after ablative lesions could likely be minimized, using DBS. In this regard, stimulation within the pallidum and/or thalamus for movement disorders such as dystonia[146] and intention tremor, which have a history of recurrence after ablative techniques, offers new promise for a consistently effective treatment of these disorders with potentially greater efficacy and reduced morbidity.

References

1. Cooper IS: A review of surgical approaches to the treatment of parkinsonism, in Cooper IS (ed): *Parkinsonism: Its Medical and Surgical Therapy.* Springfield, Illinois: Charles C Thomas, 1960, pp 14–128.
2. Meyers R: Surgical interruption of the pallidofugal fibres: Its effect on the syndrome paralysis agitans and technical considerations in its application. *N Y State J Med* 42:317–325, 1942.
3. Pollack LT, Davis L: Muscle tone in parkinsonian states. *Arch Neurol Psychiatry* 23:303–319, 1930.
4. Putnam TJ: Treatment of unilateral paralysis agitans by section of the lateral pyramidal tract. *Arch Neurol Psychiatry* 44:950–976, 1940.
5. Foerster O, Gagel O: Die Vorderseitenstrangdurchschneidung beim Menschen. *Ztschr Neurol Psychiat* 138:1, 1932.
6. Delmas-Marsalet P, Van Bogaert L: Sur un cas de myoclonies rhythmique continues par une intervention chirurgicale sur le tronc cerebral. *Rev Neurol* 64:728–740, 1935.
7. Bucy JC: Cortical extirpation in the treatment of involuntary movement. *Arch Neurol Psychiatry* 21, 1942.
8. Cooper IS: Ligation of the anterior choroidal artery for involuntary movements of parkinsonism. *Arch Neurol* 75:36–48, 1952.
9. Spiegel EA, Wycis HT, Marks M, Lee AJ: Stereotaxic apparatus for operations on the human brain. *Science* 106:349–350, 1946.
10. Svennilson E, Torvik A, Lowe R, Leksell L: Treatment of Parkinsonism by stereotactic thermolesions in the pallidal region: A clinical evaluation of 81 cases. *Acta Psychiatr Neurol Scand* 35:358–377, 1960.
11. Hassler R, Mundinger F, Riechert T: *Stereotaxis in Parkinsonian Syndromes.* Berlin: Springer-Verlag, 1979.
12. Laitinen LV, Bergenheim AT, Hariz MI: Leksell's posteroventral pallidotomy in the treatment of Parkinson's disease. *J Neurosurg* 76:53, 1992.
13. Vitek JL, Bakay RAE, DeLong MR: GPi pallidotomy for medically intractable Parkinson's disease. *Adv Neurol* In Press.
14. Baron MS, Vitek JL, Bakay RAE, et al: Treatment of advanced parkinson's disease with microelectrode-guided pallidotomy: 1 year pilot-study results. (pallidotomy for advanced PD). *Ann Neurol* 40:355–366, 1996.
15. Dogali M, Fazzini E, Kolodny E, et al: Stereotactic ventral pallidotomy for Parkinson's disease. *Neurology* 45:753–761, 1995.
16. Lozano AM, Lang AE, Galvez-Jimenez N, et al: Effect of GPi pallidotomy on motor function in Parkinson's disease. *Lancet* 346:1383–1387, 1995.
17. Vitek JL, Baron M, Kaneoke Y, et al: Microelectrode-guided pallidotomy is an effective treatment for medically intractable Parkinson's disease. *Neurology* 44(4):P703, 1994.
18. Sutton JP, Couldwell W, Lew MF, et al: Ventroposterior medial pallidotomy in patients with advanced Parkinson's disease. *Neurosurgery* 36:1112–1117, 1995.
19. Roberts JW, Nicholson DE, Heilbrun MP: Ventroposterolateral pallidotomy improves motor signs of Parkinson's disease. *Neurology* 45(4):A377, 1995.
20. Burzaco J: Stereotactic pallidotomy in extrapyramidal disorders. *Appl Neurophysiol* 48:283–287, 1985.
21. Tasker RR, Doorly T, Yamashiro K: Thalamotomy in generalized dystonia. *Adv Neurol* 50:615–631, 1988.
22. Andrew J, Capildeo R: Surgical treatment of tremor, in Findley LJ (ed): *Movement Disorders: Tremor.* New York: Oxford University Press, 1984.
23. Cooper IS: 20-Year followup study of the neurosurgical treatment of dystonia musculorum deformans. *Adv Neurol* 14:423–452, 1976.
24. Kelly PJ, Ahlskog JE, Goerss SJ, et al: Computer-assisted stereotactic ventralis lateralis thalamotomy with microelectrode recording in patients with Parkinson's disease. *Mayo Clin Proc* 62:655–664, 1987.
25. Vitek JL, Ashe J, DeLong MR, Alexander GE: Physiologic properties and somatotopic organization of the primate motor thalamus. *J Neurophysiol* 71:1498–1513, 1994.
26. Hirai T, Miyazaki M, Nakajima H, et al: The correlation between tremor characteristics and the predicted volume of effective lesions in stereotaxic nucleus ventralis intermedius thalamotomy. *Brain* 106:1001–1018, 1983.
27. Vitek JL, Hashimoto T, Baron MS, et al: Lesion location related to outcome in microelectrode-guided pallidotomy. *Ann Neurol* 36(2):279, 1994.

28. DeLong MR, Crutcher MD, Georgopoulos AP: Primate globus pallidus and subthalamic nucleus: Functional organization. *J Neurophysiol* 53:530–543, 1985.

29. Wichmann T, Baron MS, DeLong MR: Local inactivation of the sensorimotor territories of the internal segment of the globus pallidus and the subthalamic nucleus alleviates parkinsonian motor signs in MPTP treated monkeys, in Percheron JS, McKenzie JS, Feger J (eds): *The Basal Ganglia IV: New Ideas and Data on Structure and Function.* New York: Plenum Press, 1994, pp 357–364.

30. Vitek JL, Bakay RAE, Hashimoto T, et al: Microelectrode-guided pallidotomy: Technical approach and application for treatment of medically intractable Parkinson's disease. Unpublished.

31. Albe-Fessard D, Rocha-Miranda C, Oswaldo-Cruz E: Activites evoquees dans le noyau caude du chat en response a des types divers d'afferences. II. Etude microphysiologique. *Electroencephalogr Clin Neurophysiol* 12:649–661, 1960.

32. Jasper HH, Bertrand G: Thalamic units involved in somatic sensation and voluntary and involuntary movements in man, in Purpura DP, Yahr MD (eds): *The Thalamus.* New York: Columbia University Press, 1966, pp 365–390.

33. Narabayashi H, Okuma T: Procaine oil blocking of the globus pallidus for the treatment of rigidity and tremor of parkinsonism. *Proc Japan Acad* 29:134–137, 1953.

34. Bertrand G, Jasper H: Microelectrode recording of unit activity in the human thalamus. *Confin Neurol* 26:205–208, 1965.

35. Ohye C, Kubota K, Hooper HE, et al: Ventrolateral and subventrolateral thalamic stimulation. *Arch Neurol* 11:427–434, 1964.

36. Alexander GE, Crutcher MD, DeLong MR: Basal ganglia-thalamocortical circuits: Parallel substrates for motor, oculomotor, 'prefrontal' and 'limbic' functions. *Prog Brain Res* 85:119–146, 1990.

37. DeLong MR: Primate models of movement disorders of basal ganglia origin. *Trends Neurosci* 13:281–285, 1990.

38. Vitek JL, Wichmann T, DeLong MR: Current concepts of basal ganglia neurophysiology with respect to tremorgenesis, in Findley LJ, Koller W (eds): *Handbook of Tremor Disorders.* New York: Marcel Dekker, 1994, pp 37–50.

39. Lamarre Y, Joffroy AJ: Experimental tremor in monkey: Activity of thalamic and precentral cortical neurons in the absence of peripheral feedback. *Adv Neurol* 24:109–122, 1979.

40. Lamarre Y: Tremorogenic mechanisms in primates. *Adv Neurol* 10:23–34, 1975.

41. Llinas RR: Rebound excitation as the physiological basis for tremor: A biophysical study of the oscillatory properties of mammalian central neurones in vitro, in Findley LJ, Capildeo R (eds): *Movement Disorders: Tremor.* New York: Oxford University Press, 1984, pp 165–182.

42. Vilis T, Hore J: Central neural mechanisms contributing to cerebellar tremor produced by limb perturbations. *J Neurophysiol* 43:279–291, 1980.

43. Hazrati L-N, Parent A: Projection from the external pallidum to the reticular thalamic nucleus in the squirrel monkey. *Brain* 550:142–146, 1991.

44. Ilinsky I, Kultas-Ilinsky K: Sagittal cytoarchitectonic maps of the macaca mulatta thalamus with a revised nomenclature of the motor-related nuclei validated by observations on their connectivity. *J Comp Neurol* 262:331–364, 1987.

45. Asanuma C, Thach T, Jones EG: Distribution of cerebellar terminations in the ventral lateral thalamic region of the monkey. *Brain Res Rev* 5:237–265, 1983.

46. Asanuma C, Thach WT, Jones EG: Anatomical evidence for segregated focal grouping of efferent cells and their terminal ramifications in the cerebellothalamic pathway of the monkey. *Brain Res Rev* 5:267–297, 1983.

47. Asanuma C, Thach WT, Jones EG: Cytoarchitectonic delineation of the ventral lateral thalamic region in the monkey. *Brain Res Rev* 5:219–235, 1983.

48. DeVito JL, Andersen ME: An autoradiographic study of the efferent connections of the globus pallidus in macaca mullata. *Brain Res* 46:107–117, 1982.

49. Schell GR, Strick PL: The origin of thalamic inputs to the arcuate premotor and supplementary motor areas. *J Neurosci* 4:539–560, 1984.

50. Jones EG, Coulter JD, Burton H, Porter R: Cells of origin and terminal distribution of corticostriatal fibers arising in the sensory-motor cortex of monkeys. *J Comp Neurol* 173:53–80, 1977.

51. Darian-Smith C, Darian-Smith I, Cheema SS: Thalamic projections to sensorimotor cortex in the macaque monkey: Use of multiple retrograde fluorescent tracers. *J Comp Neurol* 299:17–46, 1990.

52. Ilinsky IA, Jouandet ML, Goldman-Rakic PS: Organization of the nigrothalamocortical system in the rhesus monkey. *J Comp Neurol* 236:315–330, 1985.

53. Harnois C, Filion M: Pallidofugal projections to the thalalmus and midbrain: A quantitative antidromic activation study in monkeys and cats. *Exp Brain Res* 47:277–285, 1982.

54. Parent A, DeBellefeuille L: Organization of efferent projections from the internal segment of globus pallidus in primate as revealed by fluorescence retrograde labeling method. *Brain Res* 245:201–213, 1982.

55. Hoover JE, Strick PL: Multiple output channels in the basal ganglia. *Science* 259:819–821, 1993.

56. Jinnai K, Nambu A, Yoshida S, Tanibuchi I: The two separate neuron circuits through the basal ganglia concerning the preparatory or execution processes of motor control, in Mano N, Hamada I, DeLong MR (eds): *Role of the Cerebellum and Basal Ganglia in Voluntary Movement.* New York: Elsevier Science Publishers, 1993, pp 153–161.

57. Tanji J: Comparison of neuronal activities in the monkey supplementary and precentral motor areas. *Behav Brain Res* 18:137–142, 1985.

58. Tanji J, Kurata K: Contrasting neuronal activity in supplementary and precentral motor cortex of monkeys. I. Responses to instructions determining motor responses to forthcoming modalities. *J Neurophysiol* 53:129–141, 1985.

59. Tanji J, Okano K, Sato KC: Relation of neurons in the nonprimary motor cortex to bilateral hand movement. *Nature* 327:618–620, 1987.

60. Wise SP, Godschalk M: Functional fractionation of frontal fields. *Trends Neurosci* 10:449–450, 1987.

61. Narabayashi H, Yokochi F, Nakajima Y: L-dopa–induced dyskinesia and thalamotomy. *J Neurol Neurosurg Psychiatry* 47:831–839, 1984.

62. Ohye C: Depth microelectrode studies, in Walker AE (ed): *Stereotaxy of the Human Brain.* New York: 1982, pp 372–389.

63. Miller WC, DeLong MR: Altered tonic activity of neurons in the globus pallidus and subthalamic nucleus in the primate MPTP model of parkinsonism, in Carpenter MB, Jayaraman A (eds): *The Basal Ganglia II.* New York: Plenum Press, 1987, pp 415–427.

64. Filion M, Tremblay L: Abnormal spontaneous activity of globus pallidus neurons in monkeys with MPTP-induced parkinsonism. *Brain Res* 547:142–151, 1991.

65. Vitek JL, Kaneoke Y, Turner R, et al: Neuronal activity in the internal (GPi) and external (GPe) segments of the globus pallidus (GP) of parkinsonian patients is similar to that in the MPTP-treated primate model of parkinsonism. *Soc Neurosci* 19:1584, 1993.

66. Vitek JL, Ashe J, Kaneoke Y: Spontaneous neuronal activity in the motor thalamus: Alteration in pattern and rate in parkinsonism. *Soc Neurosci* 20:561, 1994.

67. Ceballos-Bauman AO, Obeso JA, Vitek JL, et al: Restoration of thalamocortical activity after posteroventrolateral pallidotomy in Parkinson's disease. *Lancet* 344:814, 1994.

68. Narabayashi H: Tremor mechanisms, in Schaltenbrand G, Walker AE (eds): *Stereotaxy of the Human Brain*. Stuttgart: Thieme, 1982, pp 510–514.

69. Hassler R, Dieckmann G: Stereotactic treatment of different kinds of spasmodic torticollis. *Confin Neurol* 32:135–143, 1970.

70. Tasker RR, Yamashiro K, Lenz F, Dostrovsky JO: Thalamotomy in Parkinson's disease: Microelectrode techniques, in Lundsford D (ed): *Modern Stereotactic Surgery*. Norwell, MA: Academic Press, 1988, pp 297–313.

71. Kaneoke Y, Vitek. The motor thalamus in the parkinsonian primate: Enhanced burst and oscillatory activities. *Soc Neurosci* 21(part 2):1428, 1995.

72. Nakaoka T: Experimental tremor produced by ventromedial tegmental lesion in monkeys. *Appl Neurophysiol* 46:92–106, 1983.

73. Narabayashi H: Surgical approach to tremor, in Marsden CD (ed): *Neurology 2: Movement Disorders*. London: Butterworth, 1982.

74. Ohye C, Nakamura R, Fukamachi A, Narabayashi H: Recording and stimulation of the ventralis intermedius nucleus of the human thalamus. *Conf Neurol* 37:258, 1975.

75. Ohye C, Narabayashi H: Physiological study of presumed ventralis intermedius neurons in the human thalamus. *J Neurosurg* 50:290–297, 1979.

76. Hassler R, Mundinger F, Riechert T: Correlations between clinical and autopsy findings in stereotactic operations of parkinsonism. *Confin Neurol* 26:282–290, 1965.

77. Lenz FA, Schnider S, Tasker RR, et al: The role of feedback in the tremor frequency activity of tremor cells in patients with parkinsonian tremor. *Acta Neurochir* (Wien) In Press.

78. Narabayashi H: Tremor: Its generation mechanism and treatment. *Handbook Clin Neurol* 5:597–607, 1986.

79. Lenz FA, Kwan HC, Martin RL, et al: Single unit analysis of the human ventral thalamic nuclear group: Tremor-related activity in functionally identified cells. *Brain* 117:531–543, 1994.

80. Asanuma C: Organization of the external pallidal projection upon the thalamic reticular nucleus in squirrel monkeys. *Soc Neurosci* 20:332, 1994.

81. Hallanger AE, Levey AI, Lee HJ, et al: The origins of cholinergic and other subcortical afferents to the thalamus in the rat. *J Comp Neurol* 262:105–124, 1987.

82. Levey AI, Hallanger AE, Wainer BH: Cholinergic nucleus basalis neurons may influence the cortex via the thalamus. *Neurosci Lett* b-74:7–13, 1987.

83. Pare D, Smith Y, Parent A, Steriade M: Projections of brainstem core cholinergic and non-cholinergic neurons of cat to intralaminar and reticular thalamic nuclei. *Neuroscience* 25:69–86, 1988.

84. Steriade M, Pare D, Parent A, Smith Y: Projections of cholinergic and non-cholinergic neurons of the brainstem core to relay and associational thalamic nuclei in the cat and macaque monkey. *Neuroscience* 25:47–67, 1988.

85. McCormick DA, Prince DA: Acetylcholine induces burst firing in thalamic reticular neurones by activating a potassium conductance. *Nature* a-319:402–405, 1986.

86. McCormick DA, Prince DA: Actions of acetylcholine in the guinea-pig and cat medial and lateral geniculate nuclei, in vitro. *J Physiol* 392:147–165, 1987.

87. McCormick DA, Pape H: Acetylcholine inhibits identified interneurons in the cat lateral geniculate nucleus. *Nature* 334:246–248, 1988.

88. McCormick DA: Cholinergic and noradrenergic modulation of thalamocortical processing. *Trends Neurosci* 12(6):215–221, 1989.

89. Lee MS, Marsden CD: Movement disorders following lesions of the thalamus or subthalamic region. *Mov Disord* 9:493–507, 1994.

90. Marsden CD, Obeso JA, Zarranz JJ, Lang AE: The anatomical basis of symptomatic hemidystonia. *Brain* 108:463–483, 1985.

91. Lenz FA, Jaeger CJ, Seike MS, et al: Cross-correlation analysis of thalamic single neuron and EMG activities in patients with dystonia. Unpublished.

92. Lenz FA, Seike MS, Jaeger CJ, et al: Single neuron analysis of thalamic activity in patients with dystonia. In Press.

93. Vitek JL, Ashe J, DeLong MR, Alexander GE: Altered somatosensory response properties of neurons in the 'motor' thalamus of MPTP treated parkinsonian monkeys. *Soc Neurosci* 16:425, 1989.

94. Mitchell IJ, Luquin R, Boyce S, et al: Neural mechanisms of dystonia: Evidence from a 2-deoxyglucose uptake study in a primate model of dopamine agonist-induced dystonia. *Mov Disord* 5:49–54, 1990.

95. Andrew J, Fowler CJ, Harrison MJG: Stereotaxic thalamotomy in 55 cases of dystonia. *Brain* 106:981–1000, 1983.

96. Narabayashi H, Ohye C: Importance of microstereoencephalotomy for tremor alleviation. *Appl Neurophysiol* 43:222–227, 1980.

97. Lee RG, Stein RB: Resetting of tremor by mechanical perturbations: A comparison of essential tremor and parkinsonian tremor. *Ann Neurol* 10:523–531, 1981.

98. Vilis T, Hore J: Effects of changes in mechanical state of limb on cerebellar intention tremor. *J Neurophysiol* 40:1214–1224, 1977.

99. Hore J, Flament D: Changes in motor cortex neural discharge associated with the development of cerebellar limb ataxia. *J Neurophysiol* 60:1285–1302, 1988.

100. Narabayashi H: A consideration of intention tremor, in Ito M, et al (eds): *Integrative Control Function of the Brain*. Tokyo: Kodansha, 1979, vol 2, pp 185–187.

101. Steriade M, Jones EG, Llinas RR: *Thalamic Oscillations and Signaling*. New York: Wiley-Interscience, 1990.

102. Llinas RR: The intrinsic electrophysiological properties of mammalian neurons: Insights into central nervous system function. *Science* 242:1654–1664, 1988.

103. Carpenter MB, Whittier JR, Mettler FA: Analysis of choreoid hyperkinesia in the rhesus monkey: Surgical and pharmacological analysis of hyperkinesia resulting from lesions in the subthalamic nucleus of Luys. *J Comp Neurol* 92:293–332, 1950.

104. Hamada I, DeLong MR: Excitotoxic acid lesions of the primate subthalamic nucleus result in reduced pallidal neuronal activity during active holding. *J Neurophysiol* 68:1859–1866, 1992.

105. Hamada I, DeLong MR: Excitotoxic acid lesions of the primate subthalamic nucleus result in transient dyskinesias of the contralateral limbs. *J Neurophysiol* 68:1850–1858, 1992.

106. Whittier JR, Mettler FA: Studies of the subthalamus of the rhesus monkey. II. Hyperkinesia and other physiologic effects of subthalamic lesions with special references to the subthalamic nucleus of Luys. *J Comp Neurol* 90:319–372, 1949.

107. Martin JP: Hemichorea (hemiballismus) without lesions in the corpus luysii. *Brain* 80:1–10, 1957.

108. Vitek JL, Kaneoke Y, Hashimoto T, et al: *Neuronal Activity in the Pallidum of a Patient with Hemiballismus* (abstract). American Neurological Association, 1995.

109. Crossman AR, Mitchell IJ, Sambrook MA: Regional brain uptake of 2-deoxyglucose in N-methyl-4-phenyl-1,2,3,6-tetrahydropyridine (MPTP)-induced parkinsonism in the macaque monkey. *Neuropharmacology* 24:587–591, 1985.

110. Bergman H, Wichmann T, DeLong MR: Reversal of experimental parkinsonism by lesions of the subthalamic nucleus. *Science* 249:1436–1438, 1990.

111. Guridi J, Luquin MR, Herrero MT, Obeso JA: The subthalamic nucleus: A possible target for stereotaxic surgery in Parkinson's disease. *Mov Disord* 8:421–429, 1993.

112. Aziz TZ, Peggs D, Sambrook MA, Crossman AR: Lesion of the subthalamic nucleus for the alleviation of 1-methyl-4-phenyl-1,2,3,6-tetrahydropyridine (MPTP)-induced parkinsonism in the primate. *Mov Disord* 6:288–292, 1991.

113. Lang AE: Persistent hemiballismus with lesions outside the subthalamic nucleus. *Can J Neurol Sci* 12:125–128, 1985.

114. Guridi J, Luquin MR, Guillen J, et al: Antiparkinsonian effect of subthalamotomy in MPTP-exposed monkeys. *Mov Disord* 8:415, 1993.

115. Smith MC: Location of stereotactic lesions confirmed at necropsy. *Br Med J* 1962, pp 900–906.

116. Selby G: Stereotactic surgery for the relief of Parkinson's disease. I. A critical review. *J Neurol Sci* 5:315–342, 1967.

117. Speelman JD: *Parkinson's Disease and Stereotaxic Surgery.* Amsterdam: Elsevier Science Publishers, 1991.

118. Hassler R, Reichert T, Mundinger F, et al: Physiological observations in stereotaxic operations in extrapyramidal motor disturbances. *Brain* 83:337–350, 1960.

119. Tasker RR, Lenz F, Yamashiro K, et al: Microelectrode techniques in localization of stereotactic targets. *Neurosci Res* 9:105–112, 1987.

120. Canavan AG, Nixon PD, Passingham RE: Motor learning in monkeys (Macaca fascicularis) with lesions in motor thalamus. *Exp Brain Res* 77:113–126, 1989.

121. Webster DD: Dynamic evaluation of thalamotomy in Parkinson's disease: Analysis of 75 consecutive cases, in Gillingham FJ, Donaldson IML (eds): *Third Symposium on Parkinson's disease.* Edinburgh: E&S Livingstone, 1969, pp 266–271.

122. Vitek JL, Baron MS, Bakay RAE, et al: Microelectrode-guided pallidotomy for Parkinson's disease: Clinical response and determinants of clinical outcome. Unpublished.

123. Gross C, Frerebeau PH, Perez-Dominguez E, et al: Long term results of stereotaxic surgery for infantile dystonia and dyskinesia. *Neurochirurgia* 19:171–178, 1976.

124. Yamashiro K, Tasker RR: Stereotactic thalamotomy for dystonic patients. *Stereotact Funct Neurosurg* 60:81–85, 1993.

125. Ohye C, Shibazaki T, Hirai T, et al: Further physiologic observations on the ventralis intermedius neurons in the human thalamus. *J Neurophysiol* 61(3):488–500, 1989.

126. Lenz FA, Vitek JL, DeLong MR: Role of the thalamus in parkinsonian tremor: Evidence from studies in patients and primate models. *Stereotact Funct Neurosurg* 60:94–103, 1993.

127. Lenz FA, Tasker RR, Kwan HC, et al: Cross-correlation analysis of thalamic neurons and EMG activity in parkinsonian tremor. *Appl Neurophysiol* 48:305–308, 1985.

128. Gioino GG, Dierssen G, Cooper IS: The effect of subcortical lesions on production and alleviation of hemiballic or hemichoreic movements. *J Neurol Sci* 3:10–36, 1966.

129. DeLong MR: Activity of pallidal neurons during movement. *J Neurophysiol* 34:414–427, 1971.

130. Hirai T, Jones EG: A new parcellation of the human thalamus on the basis of histochemical staining. *Brain Res Rev* 14:1–34, 1989.

131. Benabid AL, Pollak P, Seigneuret E, et al: Chronic VIM thalamic stimulation in Parkinson's disease, essential tremor and extrapyramidal dyskinesias. *Acta Neurochir* 58:39–44, 1993.

132. Benabid AL, Pollak P, Gervason C, et al: Long-term suppression of tremor by chronic stimulation of the ventral intermediate thalamic nucleus. *Lancet* 337:403–406, 1991.

133. Siegel J, Lippitz B: Bilateral chronic electrostimulation of ventroposterolateral pallidum: A new therapeutic approach for alleviating all parkinsonian symptoms. *Neurosurgery* 35:1126–1130, 1994.

134. Limousin P, Pollak P, Benazzouz A, et al: Bilateral subthalamic nucleus stimulation for severe Parkinson's disease. *Mov Disord* 10:672–674, 1995.

135. Galvez-Jimenez N, Lang AE, Lozano AM, et al: Deep brain stimulation in Parkinson's disease: New methods of tailoring functional surgery to patient needs and response. *Neurology* 48:A402, 1996.

136. Schlag J, Villablanca J: A quantitative study of temporal and spatial response patterns in a thalamic cell population electrically stimulated. *Brain Res* 8:255–270, 1968.

137. Blond S, Caparros-Lefebvre D, Parker F, et al: Control of tremor and involuntary movement disorders by chronic stereotactic stimulation of the ventral intermediate thalamic nucleus. *J Neurosurg* 77:62–68, 1991.

138. Deiber M, Pollak P, Passingham R, et al: Thalamic stimulation and suppression of parkinsonian tremor: Evidence of as cerebellar deactivation using positron emission tomography. *Brain* 116:267–279, 1993.

139. Ohye C, Shibaaki T, Hirai T, et al: Possible descending pathways mediating spontaneous tremor in monkeys. *Adv Neurol* 40:181–188, 1984.

140. Caparros-Lefebvre D, Blond S, Vermersch P, et al: Chronic thalamic stimulation improves tremor and L-dopa induced dyskinesias in Parkinson's disease. *J Neurol Neurosurg Psychiatry* 56:268–273, 1993.

141. Caparros-Lefebvre D, Ruchoux MM, Blond S, et al: Long-term thalamic stimulation in Parkinson's disease: Postmortem anatomoclinical study. *Neurology* 44:1856–1860, 1994.

142. Kaneoke Y, Vitek. The motor thalamus in the parkinsonian primate: Enhanced burst and oscillatory activities. *Neuroscience* 21(part 2):1428 (#560.5), 1995.

143. Vitek JL, Hashimoto T, Kaneoke Y, et al: Improvement of parkinsonian motor signs during electrical stimulation of the pallidum. *Mov Disord* 9(suppl 1):102 (#P421), 1994.

144. Kultas-Ilinsky K, DeBoom T, Ilinsky IA: Synaptic reorganization in the feline ventral anterior thalamic nucleus induced by lesions in the basal ganglia. *Exp Neurol* 116:312–329, 1992.

145. Keller A, Arissian K, Asanuma H: Synaptic proliferation in the motor cortex of adult cats after long-term thalamic stimulation. *J Neurophysiol* 68:295–308, 1992.

146. Sellal F, Hirsch E, Barth P, et al: A case of symptomatic hemidystonia improved by ventrosposterolateral thalamic electrostimulation. *Mov Disord* 4:515–518, 1993.

Chapter 17

NEUROBEHAVIORAL ABNORMALITIES IN PARKINSON'S DISEASE

ELDAD MELAMED

DEPRESSION
IS THERE A SPECIFIC PARKINSONIAN PERSONALITY
   TRAIT?
ANXIETY DISORDERS
SLEEP DISORDERS
PSYCHOSIS

Although Parkinson's disease is best known and mostly considered a disorder affecting movement, it is by no means limited to the motor domain. In addition to the nonmotor autonomic and cognitive impairments, such as dementia (see Chap. 2), there are also important neurobehavorial abnormalities that affect and are in turn affected by the illness (see Table 17-1). These mainly include depression, personality changes, anxiety and panic attacks, a variety of sleep alterations (including vivid dreams), and psychosis. The problems may be related to the basic pathology of Parkinson's disease, to the effect of antiparkinsonian drugs, or to both. Sometimes, the neurobehavorial impairments become dominating and influence motor function, functional disability, cognition, and the response to L-dopa and other medications.

Depression

Depression is by far the most common psychiatric or neurobehavioral problem in Parkinson's disease.[1-6] Its prevalence varies among the different series but generally is estimated to be within the range of 25–40 percent.[1-6] It is not unlikely that part of the depression may be reactive to the presence of a chronic progressive illness and particularly to the incapacitating movement abnormalities.[6-8] However, it is now commonly accepted that most of the depression in Parkinson's disease is endogenous and represents an important and common aspect within the spectrum of disease symptomatology. This is based on several observations: (1) Quite often, depression (in 15–25 percent) develops before the first emergence of the motor signs and symptoms,[1-6] and it may precede the motor manifestations by a year to even several years. (2) Depression is relatively more prevalent in patients with Parkinson's disease than in subjects with chronic disorders involving similar disability.[6] (3) It is not necessarily correlated directly with the severity of the disease.[8] In general, parkinsonian depression is mild-to-moderate and, sometimes, it may be revealed only by direct questioning or the use of various neuropsychological tests and scales. Only in a small percentage of patients is depression severe, and it is only rarely associated with suicidal attempts.[6-9] When present, depression may be permanent and chronic in some patients and relapsing-remitting in others. There seems to be no direct association with sex, age, duration of disease, and the various antiparkinsonian drugs. However, the presence and severity of depression may have an impact on several aspects of the disease. It may adversely affect the basic parkinsonian symptomatology and even the response to drugs. In a patient starting on L-dopa, a good objective motor improvement without parallel satisfaction should draw the attention of the treating neurologist to the possiblity of overt or masked depression. Likewise, in a patient with a more advanced illness who is optimally managed, a sudden motor deterioration without an obvious cause, such as infection, physical trauma, stroke, noncompliance, or inappropriate medication, may be a result of the development of depression. Depression may affect sleep and contribute to insomnia. It may have a negative effect on cognition, particularly on the memory of the patients.[11-14] It may amplify the basic fatigue and lack of energy that are quite common in Parkinson's disease and reduce the patient's general drive and desire to engage in physical activities. Depression commonly leads to loss of appetite and reduced caloric intake. Hence, depression-associated anorexia is an important cause of loss of weight, leading even to emaciation, particularly in the more advanced stages of the disease.

The pathogenic mechanisms responsible for the common occurrence of depression in Parkinson's disease are unknown. One possibility is that this particular type of depression may be a result of the loss of dopaminergic innervation in specific parts of the basal ganglia or, more likely, in the limbic system. There is evidence of major degeneration of the nigromesolimbic dopaminergic neurons emanating from the A10 region within the midbrain. Reserpine, a drug that depletes dopamine in its vesicular storage sites, causes both parkinsonism and depression as its most common adverse reactions. In patients with response fluctuations associated with chronic L-dopa administration, "off" periods are commonly associated with severe depression that rapidly disappears when a dose of L-dopa successfully turns them "on".[15,16] However, there is crucial evidence against dopamine depletion as a cause of parkinsonian depression. Administration of L-dopa increases dopamine concentrations and restores dopaminergic transmission in the striatum (caudate and putamen nuclei) and also in the limbic system (e.g., nucleus accumbens and hippocampus). However, although treatment with L-dopa (and also other antiparkinsonian drugs) is beneficial for the motor phenomena, it does not improve the depression significantly. Another possibility is that serotonergic mechanisms are involved.[17] There is evidence that serotonergic projections originating from the brain stem raphe nuclei are variably involved in the degeneration process of Parkinson's disease. Generally, in depression and also in depressed parkinsonians, there is a reduction of the major metabolite of serotonin, 5-hydroxyindoleacetic acid (5-HIAA), in the cerebral spinal fluid (CSF), indicating reduced central serotonergic neurotransmission.[6] It is mandatory that depression should be looked for and diagnosed in patients

TABLE 17-1 Neurobehavioral Abnormalities in Parkinson's Disease

Depression
Personality changes
Anxiety and panic attacks
Sleep alterations
Psychosis

with Parkinson's disease. When present, it should be brought to the attention of patients and families and properly treated. Sometimes, reassurance with or without supplementary psychotherapy is sufficient. More often than not, patients with parkinsonian depression need to be placed on antidepressant medications. Tricyclic and serotonin uptake inhibitory (e.g., fluoxetine) antidepressants are usually effective.[6,17–19] These drugs rarely cause drug-induced parkinsonism, aggravation of existing Parkinson's disease, or blockade of antiparkinsonian efficacy of L-dopa.[19] Electroconvulsive therapy (ECT) is not contraindicated and may be used successfully in selected severely depressed patients or in those not responding well to pharmacotherapy.[20,21]

Is There a Specific Parkinsonian Personality Trait?

There have been many attempts to define a characteristic premorbid personality type in Parkinson's disease.[22–24] Results of these studies are inconclusive, but it seems that subjects who are passive, anxious, moody, insecure, and morally rigid and prudish show more tendency to develop the disease. For instance, refraining from or stopping smoking, common in Parkinson's disease, may simply be related to a premorbid personality trait and not necessarily to an antiparkinsonian protective effect of cigarette smoke.

Anxiety Disorders

Anxiety is extremely common in Parkinson's disease and may adversely affect the basic parkinsonian symptomatology.[6,25] A sudden unexplained deterioration in a patient who is well-balanced on optimal antiparkinsonian medications should alert the treating neurologist to the possibility of first emergence or exacerbation of anxiety. Anxiety particularly increases the parkinsonian tremor. Severity of the tremor may often serve as an index for anxiety, rather than for the basic Parkinson's disease. Many patients claim that their tremor is aggravated, even when they just think that others are looking at their hands. An increase in anxiety can also dramatically enhance the frequency and severity of freezing gait. It also can amplify L-dopa-induced dyskinesias. Anxiety adversely affects sleep, appetite, and general function. Recurrent or persistent side effects of various antiparkinsonian drugs, for example, nausea, may be of psychogenic origin because of anxiety. Patients with anxiety may develop various phobic disorders, including fear of gait, fear of falling, fear of being alone, and fear of open places or crowds,[6] leading to reluctance to leave home and, sometimes, even to

severe social withdrawal. Anxiety and depression are commonly interrelated.

Most devastating within the scope of anxiety disorders are panic attacks.[26,27] These are manifested by the sudden extreme enhancement of anxiety and unexplained fear associated with sympathetic overactivity, including palpitations, sweating, heat waves, and dry mouth. They may be rare or frequent, occurring several times during the day. In patients with response fluctuations, panic attacks commonly coincide with "off" phases, particularly those linked to "wearing off" or "on-off" phenomena, and they subside when an "on" is achieved by a successful dose of L-dopa. Panic attacks can be totally dissociated from the motor fluctuations, even occurring abruptly without any obvious cause at the peak of a good motor response to L-dopa. In a fluctuating patient, a panic attack can often prematurely terminate an "on" period. Anxiety can cause certain patients to take an excessive amount of L-dopa and thus aggravate dyskinesias and induce hallucinosis. In others, it may lead to inadvertent cessation of medications, resulting in a parkinsonian crisis. Because of the above, anxiety should be vigorously treated by reassurance, psychotherapy, and drugs (including benzodiazepines such as alprazolam). The latter rarely exacerbate parkinsonian symptoms or reduce the efficacy of L-dopa.

Sleep Disorders

Sleep problems are very common in Parkinson's disease[28–31] (see also Chap. 51). Many patients suffer from "paradoxical sleep," that is, they do not sleep well or remain awake at nights and are hypersomnolent during the day. The presence of anxiety, depression, or psychosis (particularly if associated with agitation) may aggravate insomnia.[32] Nocturnal akinesia and rigidity, and the resultant discomfort in bed linked to inadequate L-dopa coverage at night, may be an important factor contributing to sleep difficulties. Polysomnographics show that in untreated patients with Parkinson's disease there are reductions in slow-wave sleep, frequent nocturnal awakenings, and decreased rapid eye movement (REM) sleep duration with normal REM percentage. The effect of L-dopa and other antiparkinsonian treatments on sleep parameters is inconclusive.[28,29,31] Fragmentation of sleep, that is, repeated arousals, may be more common in treated patients.

Tremors and dyskinesias usually disappear during sleep. Nocturnal foot dystonia and leg cramps may occur when the patient is asleep, and the associated pain and discomfort can cause premature awakening. Paradoxically, there may be an increase in nocturnal myoclonic phenomena and periodic sleep movements. Patients sometimes toss and turn excessively in bed, particularly during REM sleep, and have violent thrashing movements. They may unknowingly beat or kick their bed partners, subsequently leading them to seek other sleeping quarters.

Many patients, particularly those being treated with L-dopa, develop the phenomenon of vivid dreaming. They are sometimes colorful, friendly, and pleasant but, more often, the dreams are frightening, menacing, and associated with past unpleasant and threatening experiences. Patients frequently report dreaming about long-deceased family members (particularly parents) or friends, and they may exhibit nocturnal vocalizations and sleep talking. Excessive body movements are also associated with such vivid dreams, and they can become extremely frightening, taking the form of night terrors (pavor nocturnus). Patients may shout, cry, and show signs of intense fear during these episodes, sometimes resulting in their awakening. It is commonly believed that the presence of vivid dreams, particularly the night terror type, herald the development of parkinsonian psychosis.

Treatment is complicated and should be tailored according to the problems and requirements of the individual patient. Sleep problems associated with nocturnal akinesia respond favorably to the addition of a slow-release L-dopa preparation (e.g., Sinemet CR), taken immediately before sleep. It may be necessary sometimes to administer a regular, immediate-release L-dopa preparation at this time to enable entry into bed and falling asleep. Nocturnal insomnia, excessive periodic sleep movements, and vivid dreams may improve after the administration of benzodiazepines or alprazolam. Caution should be advocated, however, because these drugs may sometimes cause or increase awakening, confusion, and instability and lead to the loss of balance and falling, particularly in males who need to urinate frequently during the night. Selegiline (L-deprenyl) may cause sleep difficulties in some patients and, if necessary, should be discontinued or taken only in the morning. Reduction of L-dopa dosage and intake of the last dose in the early evening can prevent or reduce vivid dreams and night terrors, but it may be intolerable because of a resultant increase in nocturnal akinesia and rigidity. Excessive daytime somnolence should be treated mainly by increasing physical and mental activity and only rarely with mild psychostimulants, such as methylphenidate.

In a small percentage of patients, particularly those in the advanced stage of the illness who already have motor response fluctuations, individual L-dopa doses (particularly the first morning dose) may cause narcolepsy-like irresistible somnolence. Episodes of L-dopa-induced sleep may last for 30–60 minutes and represent an additional disabling side effect of chronic L-dopa therapy. It is of interest to note that in certain patients, an "on" response to a single dose of L-dopa is heralded by grotesque involuntary yawning. This phenomenon is more commonly seen after apomorphine injections, used as a rescue from "off" situations. The mechanisms responsible for L-dopa-induced somnolence and yawning are unknown and may involve serotonergic or cholinergic abnormalities within the reticular activating system.

Psychosis

Parkinsonian psychosis is one of the most disabling complications of long-term L-dopa treatment in patients with advanced illness.[6,33–36] It is rather a spectrum of disorders consisting of illusions and hallucinosis, predominantly of the visual type; paranoid delusions; agitation; aggression; confusion; and even delirium. It develops in approximately 8–15 percent of Parkinson's disease patients and is more frequent in elderly parkinsonians, who show signs of impaired cognition and have a longer duration of illness and L-dopa treatment.[37] It is associated mainly with chronic L-dopa administration, but it may first be caused or aggravated by all other antiparkinsonian drugs, including selegiline (L-deprenyl), anticholinergics, and dopamine agonists. It may be triggered sometimes by a very small drug dose, but its development and severity are more commonly a dose-dependent event. A combination of several antiparkinsonian drugs makes patients more susceptible to this adverse reaction. The presence of vivid dreams and night terrors may herald a transition into psychosis. It may suddenly appear in an otherwise optimally managed patient after infection, physical or mental trauma, and surgery, particularly after administration of general anesthesia. It usually, but not always, emerges first after an attempt to increase the dose of L-dopa or to initiate or add other antiparkinsonian drugs. It rarely occurs after abrupt discontinuation of L-dopa associated with, for instance, the patient's noncompliance or with a planned L-dopa "holiday." Very seldom there are de novo patients with Parkinson's disease who, for unknown reasons, are extremely sensitive and develop psychosis in response to the initiation of even small L-dopa doses. In some, this early and usually unexpected adverse reaction is transitory and does not recur when L-dopa is reinitiated after a brief interval. In others, this early intolerance to small L-dopa doses may indicate the presence of dementia.

The development of psychosis in the later stages of the disease is a grave milestone indicating further deterioration and bad prognosis. It represents the most common cause for transferring a Parkinson's disease patient from home to a nursing home.[38] Family members who, despite great difficulties, may continue to cope with the many incapacitating aspects of this chronic disease, including decline in L-dopa efficacy, response fluctuations, dyskinesias, and postural instability, break down and become helpless and discouraged when psychosis emerges and deteriorates. Much more importantly, parkinsonian psychosis is the predominant limiting factor in providing the patient with the optimal antiparkinsonian drug therapy. Its presence prevents the increases in L-dopa dosage or the addition of other drugs that are very much required to improve motor function, particularly in advanced stages of illness. Such attempts are almost invariably associated with intolerable worsening of the psychotic phenomena. On the other hand, when L-dopa is discontinued or reduced, psychosis may improve or even subside, but the parkinsonian motor signs and symptoms, and especially bradykinesia and rigidity, soon deteriorate, and the patient may develop a catastrophic and life-threatening parkinsonian crisis.

The *clinical features* are varied and complex, yet quite stereotypical. The central symptom is hallucinosis, which is mainly of the visual type (see Table 17-2). Occasionally, there are hallucinations of "presence," that is, a physical sensation that someone or something is standing at the side or behind the patient. Auditory hallucinations are rare. When they are predominating, other types of psychosis should be considered. Visual hallucinations are usually those of human images, single or many, males or females, adults or children, whole or partial, colorless, dressed or naked, normal-appearing or distorted (sometimes, faceless or demoniacal),

TABLE 17-2 Manifestations of Psychosis in Parkinson's Disease

Vivid dreams/illusions
Benign visual hallucinosis
Visual, auditory, or tactile hallucinations that are threatening or
  disturbing
Paranoid delusions
Agitated delirium

usually, but not always, unfamiliar to the patient, located in various parts of the house. They may be threatening, indifferent, or even invited and welcome. Hallucinations may take the form of inhuman images, such as dogs, cats, rodents, lizards, snakes, worms, and various insects (e.g., ants, scorpions, cockroaches). Patients may even stop eating and lose weight, imagining that insects or worms are in their food, making it repulsive and inedible. Visual hallucinations may consist less often of plant-like images (trees, flowers), colorful tapestry and, sometimes, monstrous mythological apparitions. The hallucinations may occur only at night (e.g., when waking up, during the lingering of a dream into a state of wakefulness when turning on the lights, etc.), or during the whole day. They may occur only rarely or become established as a common regular daily phenomenon. The frequency and intensity of hallucinosis may increase or decrease in a given subject. Sometimes, the hallucinations are of a "benign" nature, occurring only sporadically and as nonthreatening in nature. When they are this type, patients have partial or complete insight. The visual hallucinations may seem very real, and the patient finds it difficult initially to believe that they are imaginary. However, patients can be convinced that they are experiencing hallucinations and should not be intimidated by them. Most people learn "how to live" with the hallucinations, mainly by developing a type of tolerance in order to disregard them. Some deny their existence, even though they continue to appear, because they are ashamed to admit their presence. When the visual hallucinations are of the "benign" type, nothing much should be done. However, their presence should curtail any increases in antiparkinsonian medications, because they carry the potential of becoming malignant rapidly.

Psychosis becomes malignant and truly incapacitating when the hallucinations are frequent and frightening and when paranoid delusions emerge. These paranoid delusions may include or be associated with persecutory thoughts, suspiciousness, negativism, agitation, aggression, hypersexuality, or abnormal sexual behavior and confusion (with disorientation as to time and place). Patients feel threatened by malignant hallucinations and paranoid delusions. They accuse family members and other individuals of cheating, stealing, adultery, or other aggressive motives. They sometimes do not recognize their spouses as such and invent imaginary or so-called "real" husbands or wives. They become fearful and restless, have no insight, and cannot be convinced otherwise. Patients wake up in the middle of the night and, in confusion, partially dress themselves and try to go out. Nightmares may become a frequent phenomenon. It is at this stage that the situation at home may become intolerable, and the family finds it extremely difficult to cope

with. When therapeutic attempts fail, the patient may then have to be placed in a nursing home.

The mechanisms responsible for the development of psychosis in Parkinson's diseases are not yet completely elucidated. One of the major theories proposes that the psychosis is mainly because of an impairment in central dopaminergic neurotransmission.[39] In Parkinson's disease, there is a progressive degeneration not only of the nigrostriatal dopaminergic neurons but also of the nigromesolimbic and nigrocortical projections.[40] Such denervation may render the postsynaptic dopaminergic receptors supersensitive in the limbic system and cortex. Treatment with exogenous L-dopa increases dopamine formation not only in the striatum but also in the limbic and cortical regions. This theory is supported by the fact that the psychosis may be attenuated by reduction or withdrawal of L-dopa or the addition of typical (phenothiazines or butyrophenones) or atypical (clozapine) dopamine receptor-blocking neuroleptics.

Another emerging hypothesis is that the psychosis may be because of abnormalities in central serotonergic (5-hydroxytryptamine (5-HT)) neurotransmission.[41,42] The 5-HT raphe nuclei in the brain stem can be involved in the degenerative process of Parkinson's disease.[42] Exogenous L-dopa enters the brain and can be taken up by 5-HT nerve terminals, where it can be inadvertently metabolized to dopamine by the enzyme dopa decarboxylase (aromatic amino acid decarboxylase).[43,44] This enzyme normally catalyzes the conversion of L-dopa to dopamine in dopaminergic nerve terminals and L-5-hydroxytryptophan to 5-HT in serotonergic nerve endings.[43] Acute and chronic treatment with L-dopa decreases 5-HT levels and increases 5-HIAA concentrations in various brain regions, indicating increased 5-HT turnover.[42] Therefore, it is possible that the psychosis is a result of nonphysiological serotonin release or displacement from its nerve terminals in the cortex and limbic systems caused by the dopamine generated from the exogenous L-dopa. Such serotonin molecules may reach and activate 5-HT receptors, which are supersensitive because of previous raphe degeneration. There is evidence for both 5-HT and dopaminergic innervation within the mammalian visual cortex. It is theoretically possible that the visual hallucinosis characteristic of parkinsonian psychosis is a result of 5-HT receptor overstimulation by forced 5-HT release within the occipital cortex induced by L-dopa administration. It should be noted also that dopamine agonists and dopamine-blocking neuroleptics (including clozapine) are not entirely selective and may interact with 5-HT receptors in brain.

Treatment of parkinsonian psychosis, particularly when it is fully developed and incapacitating, is both difficult and frustrating.[45] The first step should be correction of possible triggering factors (see Table 17-3), then the reduction and possible discontinuation of non-L-dopa antiparkinsonian medications, including anticholinergics, amantadine, selegiline, and dopamine agonists should be attempted. At this stage, they may not be particularly useful for the motor signs and may aggravate the psychosis. When this is not helpful, the total L-dopa daily dose and the number of doses should be reduced to a tolerable minimum. This may lead to the deterioration of parkinsonism. When such worsening is disabling, L-dopa should again be slowly increased. Some de-

TABLE 17-3 Treatment Approach for Psychosis in Parkinson's Disease

1. Correction of triggering factors (infections, dehydration, change of medications)
2. Reduction of antiparkinsonian drugs (aim: minimal effective monotherapy)
   —reduction/discontinuation of anticholinergics or amantadine
   —reduction of selegiline
   —in case of combined L-dopa/dopamine agonists the latter should be reduced first
   —reduction of L-dopa at the minimal effective dose
3. Administration of antipsychotics
   —clozapine: 12.5–25 mg in the evening in case of mild psychosis, up to 100–200 mg in 2–4 dosages/day in severe psychosis
   —resperidone, 0.5–2.0 mg in the evening (1 or 2 daytime doses of 0.5–1 mg may be required in more serious cases; watch for worsening of PD above 1–2 mg/day)
   —classic neuroleptics (i.e., haliperidol) only in case of florid paranoid psychosis for a brief period
   —ondansetron or other 5-HT receptor antagonists

*Adapted from Poewe and Granata, Table 14-11, in Chapter 14 of this book.

gree of psychosis may persist in order to keep the patient partially mobile. As mentioned above, the addition of classical dopamine receptor-blocking neuroleptics of the phenothiazine (e.g., chlorpromazine) or butyrophenone (e.g., haloperidol) subtypes may attenuate the psychosis, but they also aggravate parkinsonian signs and inhibit the efficacy of L-dopa. When there is no choice, thioridazine, a less potent member of this family of drugs, can be given at dosages of 10–25 mg one to three times daily, in the hope that it will improve the psychosis without causing deterioration of the parkinsonian signs.

Clozapine is an atypical neuroleptic agent in that it is a D4 dopamine receptor antagonist and has little effect on the D2 receptor, which is crucial in motor control. It exerts its inhibitory activity principally within the limbic system, where the D4 receptors are abundant. Because the striatum is lacking D4 receptors, administration of clozapine in schizophrenics may lead to an antipsychotic effect without causing drug-induced parkinsonism. The dose required for treatment of psychosis in schizophrenia is in the range of hundreds of milligrams daily. Several studies have now shown that small doses of clozapine, e.g., 10–50 mg daily, in one to three divided doses, can satisfactorily attenuate parkinsonian psychosis without exacerbating motor disability or blocking L-dopa efficacy.[45–49] However, 1–2 percent of patients may develop drug-induced neutropenia, which necessitates weekly white blood counts during treatment. Other side effects are hypersomnolence, orthostatic hypotension, sialorrhea, and paradoxical worsening of confusion in moderately to severely demented patients.

Because serotonergic overactivity may be partly responsible for the parkinsonian psychosis, Zoldan et al. recently tried treating such patients with ondansetron, a selective 5-HT3 receptor antagonist.[49] This drug is used as a novel antiemetic treatment in cancer patients receiving chemotherapy. In an open protocol (a controlled study is ongoing), ondansetron, at an average daily dose of 18 mg, was effective against the visual hallucinosis and paranoid delusions without causing any worsening in the parkinsonian motor signs or suppressing efficacy of L-dopa. The drug was well-tolerated with only minimal side effects. When the results are borne out in the controlled trial, it may become possible to treat parkinsonian psychosis with new pharmacological strategies, such as the use of 5-HT receptor antagonists. Such treatment may permit increases of daily L-dopa dosage without risking psychotic relapses, thus improving the patient's quality of life and enabling him or her to remain at home with his or her families.

References

1. Cummings JL: Depression and Parkinson's disease: A review. *Am J Psychiatry* 149:443–454, 1992.
2. Doonreief G, Mirabello E, Bell K, et al: An estimate of the incidence of depression in idiopathic Parkinson's disease. *Arch Neurol* 49:305–307, 1992.
3. Starkstein SE, Preziosi TJ, Berthier ML, et al: Depression and cognitive impairment in Parkinson's disease. *Brain* 112:1141–1153, 1983.
4. Gotham AM, Brown RG, Marsden CD: Depression in Parkinson's disease: A quantitative and qualitative analysis. *J Neurol Neurosurg Psychiatry* 49:381–389, 1986.
5. Mayeux R, Williams JBW, Stern Y, Cote L: Depression and Parkinson's disease. *Adv Neurol* 40:241–250, 1984.
6. Mayeux R: Mental state. In Koller WC (ed): *Handbook of Parkinson's disease*. New York: Marcel Dekker, 1987, pp 127–143.
7. Mindham RHS, Marsden CD, Parkes JD: Psychiatric symptoms during L-dopa therapy for Parkinson's disease and their relationship to physical disability. *Psychiatr Med* 6:23–33, 1976.
8. Huber SJ, Paulson GW, Shuttleworth EC: Relationship of motor symptoms, intellectual impairment and depression in Parkinson's disease. *J Neurol Neurosurg Psychiatry* 51:855–858, 1988.
9. Santamaria J, Tolosa E, Valles A: Parkinson's disease with depression: A possible subgroup of idiopathic parkinsonism. *Neurology* 36:1130–1133, 1986.
10. Taylor AE, Saint-Cyr JA, Lang AE, Kenny FT: Parkinson's disease and depression: A critical re-evaluation. *Brain* 109:279–292, 1986.
11. Mayeux R, Stern Y, Rosen J, Leventhal J: Depression, intellectual impairment and Parkinson's disease. *Neurology* 31:645–650, 1981.
12. Starkstein SE, Bolduc PL, Mayberg HS, et al: Cognitive impairments and depression in Parkinson's disease: A follow-up study. *J Neurol Neurosurg Psychiatry* 53:594–602, 1990.
13. Wertman E, Speedie L, Shemesh Z, et al: Cognitive disturbances in parkinsonian patients with depression. *Neuropsychiatry Neuropsychol Behav Neurol* 6:31–37, 1993.
14. Troster AI, Paolo AM, Lyons KE, et al: The influence of depression on cognition in Parkinson's disease: A pattern of impairment distinguishable from Alzheimer's disease. *Neurology* 45:672–676, 1995.
15. Menza MA, Sage J, Marshall E, et al: Mood changes and "on-off" phenomena in Parkinson's disease. *Mov Disord* 5:148–151, 1990.
16. Nissenbaum H, Quinn NP, Brown RG, et al: Mood swings associated with the "on-off" phenomenon in Parkinson's disease. *Psychol Med* 17:899–904, 1987.
17. Mayeux R: The serotonin hypothesis for depression in Parkinson's disease. *Adv Neurol* 53:163–166, 1990.
18. Anderson J, Aabro E, Gulman N, et al: Anti-depressant treatment of Parkinson's disease. *Acta Neurol Scand* 62:210–219, 1980.

19. Montastruc JL, Fabre N, Blin O, et al: Does fluoxetine aggravate Parkinson's disease? A pilot prospective study. *Mov Disord* 10:355–357, 1995.
20. Lebensohn Z, Jenkins RB: Improvement of parkinsonism in depressed patient with ECT. *Am J Psychiatry* 132:283–285, 1975.
21. Asnis G: Parkinson's disease, depression and ECT: A review and case study. *Am J Psychiatry* 134:191–195, 1977.
22. Sands JJ: The type of personality susceptible to Parkinson's disease. *J Mt Sinai Hosp* 9:752–801, 1942.
23. Poewe W, Gerstenbrand F, Ransmyr G, Plorer S: Premorbid personality in Parkinson patients. *J Neurol Trans* 19:215–224, 1983.
24. Todes CJ, Lees AJ: The premorbid personality of patients with Parkinson's disease. *J Neurol Neurosurg Psychiatry* 48:97–100, 1983.
25. Henderson R, Kurlan R, Kersun JM, Como P: Preliminary examination of the co-morbidity of anxiety and depression in Parkinson's disease. *J Neuropsychiatry Clin Neurosci* 4:257–264, 1992.
26. Vazquez A, Jimenez-Jimenez FJ, Garcia-Ruiz P, Garcia-Urra D: "Panic attacks" in Parkinson's disease: A long-term complication of L-dopa therapy. *Acta Neurol Scand* 87:14–18, 1993.
27. Maricle RA, Nutt JG, Carter JH: Mood and anxiety fluctuation in Parkinson's disease associated with L-dopa infusion. Preliminary findings. *Mov Disord* 10:329–332, 1995.
28. Nausieda PA: Sleep disorders. In Koller WC (ed): *Handbook of Parkinson's disease.* New York: Marcel Dekker, 1987, pp 371–380.
29. Kales A, Ansel RD, Markham CH: Sleep in patients with Parkinson's disease and in normal subjects prior to and following L-dopa administration. *Clin Pharmacol Ther* 12:397–406, 1971.
30. Mourert J: Differences in sleep in patients with Parkinson's disease. *Electroencephalogr Clin Neurophysiol* 38:653–657, 1975.
31. Wyatt RJ, Chase TN, Scott J, Snyder F: Effect of L-dopa on the sleep of man. *Nature* 228:999–1001, 1976.
32. Comella CL, Tanner CM, Ristanowic RK: Polysomnographic sleep measures in Parkinson's disease patients with treatment-induced hallucinations. *Ann Neurol* 34:710–714, 1993.
33. Celesia GC, Barr AN: Psychosis and other psychiatric manifestations of L-dopa therapy. *Arch Neurol* 23:193–200, 1970.
34. Tanner CM, Vogel C, Goetz CG, Klawans HL: Hallucinations in Parkinson's disease: A population study. *Ann Neurol* 14:136–139, 1983.
35. Klawans HL: Psychiatric side effects during treatment of Parkinson's disease. *J Neurol Trans* 27(suppl):117–122, 1988.
36. Nausieda PA, Glantz R, Weber S, et al: Psychiatric complications of L-dopa therapy of Parkinson's disease. *Adv Neurol* 40:271–277, 1984
37. Fahn S: Adverse effects of L-dopa. In Olanow CW, Lieberman AN (eds): The scientific basis of the treatment of Parkinson's diseases. New York: Parthenon Publishing Group, 1992, pp 89–112.
38. Goetz CG, Stebbins GT: Risk factors for nursing home placement in advanced Parkinson's disease. *Neurology* 43:2227–2229, 1993.
39. Goetz CG, Tanner CM, Klawans HL: Pharmacology of hallucinations induced by long-term drug therapy. *Am J Psychiatry* 139:494–497, 1982.
40. Agid Y, Javoy-Agid F, Ruberge M: Biochemistry of neurotransmitters in Parkinson's disease. In Marsden CD, Fahn S (eds): *Movement Disorders.* London: Butterworth, 1987, pp 166–230.
41. Nausieda PA, Tanner CW, Klawans HL: Serotonergically active agents in L-dopa-induced psychiatric toxicity reactions. *Adv Neurol* 37:23–32, 1983.
42. Melamed E, Zoldan J, Friedberg G, Weizmann A: Involvement of serotonin in clinical features of Parkinson's disease and complications of L-dopa therapy. *Adv Neurol* 69:545–550, 1996.
43. Melamed E, Hefti F, Wurtman RJ: L-3,4-dihydroxyphenylalanine and L-5-hydroxytryptophan decarboxylase activities in rat striatum: Effect of selective destruction of dopaminergic and serotonergic inputs. *J Neurochem* 34:1753–1756, 1980.
44. Melamed E, Hefti F, Wurtman RJ: Non-aminergic striatal neurons convert exogenous L-dopa to dopamine in parkinsonism. *Ann Neurol* 8:558–563, 1980.
45. Friedman JH: The management of L-dopa psychosis. *Clin Neuropharmacol* 14:283–295, 1991.
46. Kahn N, Freeman A, Juncos JL, et al: Clozapine is beneficial for psychosis in Parkinson's disease. *Neurology* 41:1699–1700, 1991.
47. Pfeiffer RF, Kang J, Grabler B, et al: Clozapine for psychosis in Parkinson's disease. *Mov Disord* 5:239–242, 1990.
48. Factor SA, Brown D, Molho ES, Podskalny GD: Clozapine: A 2-year open trial in Parkinson's disease patients with psychosis. *Neurology* 44:544–546, 1994.
49. Zoldan J, Friedberg G, Livneh M, Melamed E: Psychosis in advanced Parkinson's disease: Treatment with ondansetron, a 5-HT3 receptor antagonist. *Neurology* 45:1305–1308, 1995.

Chapter 18

PARKINSON'S DISEASE: NEUROPATHOLOGY

JULIAN FEARNLEY and ANDREW J. LEES

NEURONAL INCLUSIONS OF PARKINSON'S DISEASE
    Lewy Body
    Lewy Body-Like Material
    Acidophilic Granules
    Pale Body
    Spheroid Bodies
ANATOMY OF THE SUBSTANTIA NIGRA
CELLULAR ASPECTS OF PARKINSON'S DISEASE
    Substantia Nigra
    Corpus Striatum
MOLECULAR BIOLOGY
    Substantia Nigra
    Striatal Output Studies
PRESYMPTOMATIC PARKINSON'S DISEASE
PROGRESSION OF PARKINSON'S DISEASE
ETIOLOGY OF PARKINSON'S DISEASE
    Aging and Parkinson's Disease
    The Role of Neuromelanin
    Iron and Oxidative Stress
    MPTP and Mitochondrial Function
FAMILIAL PARKINSONISM
    Dopa-Responsive Dystonia/Parkinsonism
    Familial Parkinsonism with Apathy and Central
      Hypoventilation
    Familial LB Parkinsonism
    LB Negative Familial Parkinsonism
LEWY BODY DEMENTIA
BENIGN PARKINSON'S DISEASE
JUVENILE PARKINSON'S DISEASE
ARTERIOSCLEROTIC PARKINSONISM

A clinically definite diagnosis of Parkinson's disease (PD) can never be made, and even pathological examination is fallible. In those patients diagnosed by neurologists as having PD, about 15 percent have a different pathological diagnosis.[1] During life there is no specific diagnostic test, and there are a number of other causes of parkinsonism that can be confused with PD, the most challenging of which is multiple-system atrophy (MSA). Clinical features suggesting a diagnosis other than PD include a negative or poorly sustained response to L-dopa, stroke-like episodes, early falls, early bulbar involvement, supranuclear down-gaze palsy, and early autonomic failure. However, significant autonomic dysfunction,[2] supranuclear gaze palsies,[3,4] and a poor response to L-dopa[5] may occur in patients with Lewy body (LB) pathology, and patients with MSA may have a sustained response to L-dopa.[6,7] Neuroimaging can be helpful when it shows cerebellar and/or brain stem atrophy suggestive of MSA with olivopontocerebellar atrophy or, more specifically, altered MR T2 signals in the striatum, or a reduced N-acetyl-aspartate/creatine ratio with magnetic resonance (MR) spectroscopy.[8] In any event, the pathological hallmarks of PD and their relevance to current etiologic theories will be covered in this chapter.

Neuronal Inclusions of Parkinson's Disease

LEWY BODY

The Lewy body (LB) is a hyaline intraneuronal inclusion, and its presence is essential for pathological confirmation of PD.[9] Unfortunately, the LB is not specific to PD, as it is found in a number of disparate conditions, including Hallervorden-Spatz disease, ataxia telangiectasia, and subacute sclerosing panencephalitis. In the elderly it is also a frequent incidental finding thought to represent presymptomatic disease (Table 18-1). LBs also coexist with other central nervous system (CNS) pathologies, such as Alzheimer's-type change and glial cytoplasmic inclusions. It was first described by the German pathologist Lewy and then given its eponymous title by Tretiakoff.[10,11] It measures 5–25 μm and classically has three layers of varying eosinophilia: a core which is infrequently present, a body and a halo[12] (Fig. 18-1). Generally, the more central the layer, the greater its eosinophilia, but in the very occasional LB with more than three layers, there may be alternating degrees of eosinophilia and the core can have a paler center.[13] LBs may be divided into a brain stem type, as described above, and a cortical type.[14] The cortical type tends to be more homogeneous and less eosinophilic and argyrophilic. In the dorsal vagal motor nucleus, hypothalamus, and sympathetic ganglia, LBs can be multiple and overlapping, merging to form an elongated serpiginous inclusion. The LB is widely distributed and can be found in sites ranging from the cerebral cortex to the myenteric plexus of the intestine (Table 18-2).

The histochemical staining properties of the LB are given in Table 18-3. Basically, it contains protein, free fatty acids, sphingomyelin, and polysaccharides. Markers for secretory vesicles, synaptophysin, and chromogranin A suggest that the lipid component is derived from secretory vesicle membrane.[15] Electron probe microanalysis has shown the LB to contain calcium, phosphate, and sulphur.[16]

Immunocytochemistry of the LB is outlined in Table 18-4. The LB stains for all three subunits of neurofilament with no evidence of missing portions.[17] However, there is evidence that the neurofilament in the LB is altered. In the normal neuron, neurofilament in the cell body is nonphosphorylated, but as it moves outward into the axon it becomes progressively phosphorylated and, as a result, more compact and resistant to proteolytic degradation.[18,19] The outer part of the LB body immunostains for phosphorylated high and medium molecular weight neurofilament,[17,20] and it has been suggested that Ca^{2+}/calmodulin-dependent protein kinase II immunoreactivity found in the outer LB halo is important in this process.[21] It is unclear what happens to neurofilament more centrally within the LB. Immunologically, there is an absence of staining for the tail region of high and medium molecular weight neurofilament,[17] which could either be because of alteration of the neurofilament itself or compacting of the neurofilament and masking of epitopes. Electron mi-

TABLE 18-1 Lewy Bodies and Other Diseases

Multiple system atrophy (10% of patients[150])
Progressive supranuclear palsy syndrome (4%[151,152])
Parkinsonian-dementia complex of Guam (10%[153])
Hallervorden-Spatz disease (15%[154])
Ataxia telangiectasia (rare[155-157])
Neuroaxonal dystrophy[158]
Subacute sclerosing panencephalitis (two patients[159])
Machado-Joseph disease (two patients[160])
Familial Alzheimer's disease (occasional[161,162])
Beçhet's disease (one patient[163])

TABLE 18-2 Distribution of Lewy Bodies in Idiopathic PD[117,164-171]

Cerebral cortex	
Mesial temporal	
Insular	
Anterior cingulate	
Neocortex	
Diencephalon	
Substantia innominata	Hypothalamus
Thalamus	Subthalamus
N. mammiloinfundibularis	Olfactory bulb
Midbrain	
Substantia nigra	Ventral tegmental area
Oculomotor nucleus	Edinger-Westphal nucleus
Periaqueductal gray	Pedunculopontine nucleus
N. darkschewitsch	Dorsal tegmental nucleus
Pons	
Locus ceruleus	N. pontis centralis
N. subceruleus	Central superior raphe nucleus
Pontine nucleus	Central pontine gray
Medulla	
Dorsal motor vagal nucleus	Perihypoglossal nucleus
Inferior olive	
Spinal cord	
Intermediolateral column	
Vertebral sympathetic ganglia	
Gastrointestinal tract	
Esophagus	Colon and rectum

croscopy has shown that the halo and body are composed of similar filaments and that the core is made up of dense granular material[22] (Fig. 18-2). In the halo the filaments are less densely packed and radially arranged and measure 7.5–20 nm in diameter whereas in the body the filaments are more densely packed, sometimes forming rings and measuring 7–8 nm in diameter (neurofilament measures 7–8 nm). In another ultrastructural study it was speculated that the LB resulted from neurofilament degradation.[13] LBs also stain intensely with monoclonal antiubiquitin antibody (Fig. 18-2), and this method is particularly sensitive in demonstrating cortical LBs.[23] Ubiquitin is a 76-amino acid protein that conjugates with abnormal proteins and normal but short-lived proteins, targeting them for nonlysosomal adenosine triphosphatase-(ATP) dependent proteolysis.[24]

LBs in the substantia nigra are invariably accompanied by neuronal loss, and in other brain regions the presence of LBs is believed usually to indicate associated neuronal damage. However, no significant neuronal loss was found in the lateral tuberal nucleus of the hypothalamus of seven cases with PD, despite the presence of LBs.[25] Although in only three of these cases were LBs in the cell bodies, and most appeared to be intraneuritic, possibly originating from the tuberomamillary body. Conversely, death of pigmented neurons in PD can occur in the absence of LB formation (J Fearnley and A Lees, personal observation, using serial sections), and it

seems unlikely that these instances represent cell death resulting from other causes, such as aging. It is not known whether LBs may be present without detectable cell loss in the earliest phase of PD.

LEWY BODY-LIKE MATERIAL

Gibb et al. have made the distinction between the pale body and LB-like matter, which is found in the cerebral cortex, limbic system, dorsal motor vagal nucleus, and sympathetic ganglia.[26] It has a glassy appearance and immunostains for

FIGURE 18-1 Substantia nigra of a patient with PD. H&E, ×450. *A.* Classic trilaminar Lewy body, demonstrating an outer halo, body, and inner core. *B.* Bilaminar Lewy body in neuron to the right and a pale body showing marked eosinophilic granularity in the neuron to the left. See Color Plates 4 and 5.

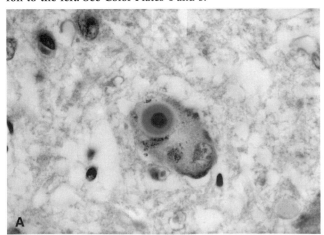

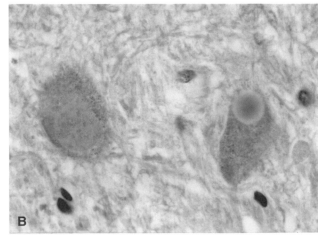

TABLE 18-3 Lewy Body Histochemical Staining[164,175]

		LEWY BODY	
Stain	Element Stained	Core	Body
Hematoxylin & eosin	Connective tissue	Dark pink	Pale pink
Nissl's method (cresyl violet)	Nucleoprotein	Pale blue	
Luxol fast blue	Phospholipid	Blue	Pale blue
Periodic acid-Schiff	Carbohydrate		
Bielschowsky's method	Neurofilament	Black	Brown
Masson's trichrome		Red	Green
Phosphotungstic hematotoxylin	Protein		Pink
Congo red	Amyloid		
Sudan black B	Phospholipid		
Nile blue sulfate	Phospholipid		Positive
OsO$_4$-alpha-naphthylamine	Phospholipid		
NaOH-OsO$_4$-alpha-naphthylamine	Spingomyelin		Positive

neurofilament and ubiquitin. It probably represents an immature form of the LB peculiar to these areas.

ACIDOPHILIC GRANULES

Acidophilic granules are eosinophilic bodies which, under electron microscopy, commonly arise within mitochondria and are composed of histone-like protein rich in arginine.[27,28] These inclusions appear to fall in number in the substantia nigra of PD, and it has been proposed that this may be integrally related to the formation of LBs.[29]

PALE BODY

Tretiakoff was the first to describe areas of granular degeneration within neurons of PD, which have since been variously termed glassy degeneration, pale bodies, and hyaline or colloid inclusion bodies[11,26,30] (Fig. 18-1). It is a round granular area within the cell body of varying eosinophilia, which displaces neuromelanin in nigral neurons. Adjacent to the pale body there is often a single large LB or multiple small LBs (J Fearnley and A Lees, personal observations). They appear to be confined to the substantia nigra and locus ceruleus.[26] They seem to be relatively specific for PD in that they have not been reported in normal aging, MSA, progressive supranuclear palsy syndrome (PSP), corticobasal degeneration, Pick's disease, Alzheimer's disease, or amyotrophic lateral sclerosis.[26,30] Electron microscopy has shown the pale body to be made up of a sparse collection of thin short branching filaments, vacuoles, and granular material.[26,30] Immunohistochemically, most stain with ubiquitin (69 percent) and a minority stain with neurofilament (15 percent)[31] (Fig. 18-2). The pale body when adjacent to an LB is usually in close continuity with the LB halo, which also stains weakly

FIGURE 18-2 Locus ceruleus of a patient with PD. Pigmented neuron (demonstrated by serial sections). Stained with H&E and then decolorized and stained for ubiquitin, ×575. *A.* H&E. Two trilaminar Lewy bodies with cores, demonstrating central pallor, and an adjacent pale body. *B.* Ubiquitin. Lewy bodies: circumferential staining of the halo-body junction and focal staining of the body-core junction. Pale body: diffuse reticular-granular staining, which is contiguous with one of the Lewy bodies. See Color Plates 6 and 7.

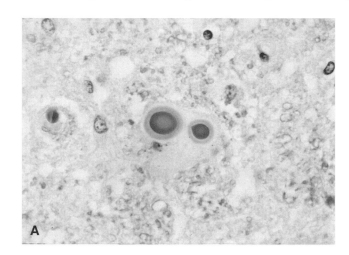
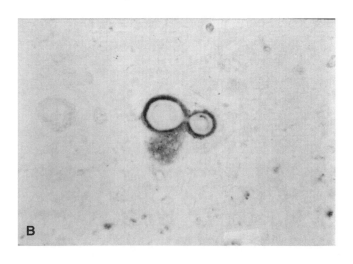

TABLE 18-4 Immunocytochemistry of the Lewy Body

Phosphorylated neurofilament[20]
Tubulin[172]
Microtubular associated protein[172]
Ubiquitin[173]
TH[174,175]
Vasoactive intestinal protein[170]
Substance P[175]
Neuropeptide Y[175]
Adrenaline[175]
Serotonin[175]

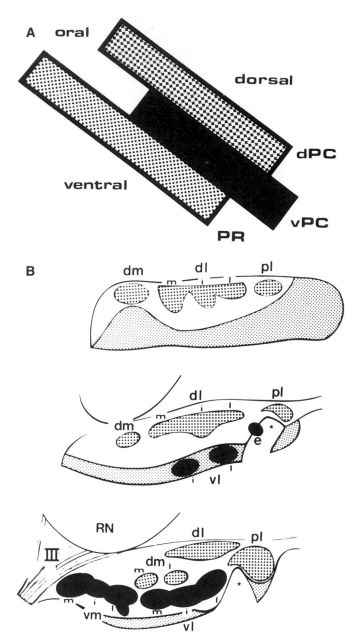

FIGURE 18-3 Diagrammatic illustration of substantia nigra regional anatomy.[34] *A*. Saggital section of the substantia nigra. PR, pars reticularis; vPC, pars compacta ventral tier; dPC, pars compacta dorsal tier. *B*. Transverse sections taken from oral (top) to caudal (bottom). ventral tier: vm, medial part; vl, lateral part; dorsal tier: dm, medial part; dl, lateral part; pl, pars lateralis.

with neurofilament, but it is unresolved, whether the two inclusions are related or whether the pale body might represent an LB precursor.

SPHEROID BODIES

Spheroid bodies are swellings within neuronal processes, which can be seen in a variety of neurodegenerative conditions and normal aging. In PD, they have been classified into two types: dendritic and axonal.[32] The dendritic type is seen in the pars compacta of the substantia nigra and tends to be fusiform in shape measuring 10–25 μm. It is difficult to visualize with conventional stains, but it does immunostain for ubiquitin, TH, and microtubule associated protein 1 (MAP1), but not MAP2 or neurofilament.[32] The axonal type is less specific for PD. It is found in the distal nigrostriatal tract and is smaller and unlike the dendritic type stains with neurofilament.[32]

Anatomy of the Substantia Nigra

The complex microarchitecture of the substantia nigra has been extensively studied by Hassler,[33] who divided the substantia nigra into a large number of discrete nuclear groups. The basic anatomy can be divided into a pars reticularis and pars compacta with the latter further subdivided into ventral and dorsal tiers. These divisions form staggered columns along the orocaudal axis (Fig. 18-3). The bulk of the dorsal tier and the pars reticularis are rostrally situated, whereas the ventral tier is located in the caudal part of the substantia nigra. Hassler divided the substantia nigra into rostral and caudal halves, ignoring the continuity of the dorsal tier and essentially doubling the number of groups.[34] Within each tier there are medial and lateral divisions, which have distinct groupings of neurons. In the nonhuman primate the substantia nigra can be divided by tracing techniques into alternating clusters of caudate and putamen-projecting neurons[35] and it is probable that the complex anatomic groupings in the human substantia nigra have some as yet unknown functional significance.

Cellular Aspects of Parkinson's Disease

SUBSTANTIA NIGRA

Golgi studies of the substantia nigra and locus ceruleus have shown significant changes in the dendrites and somatic ap-

pendages of pigmented neurons in PD. Patt and colleagues[36,37] demonstrated loss of dendritic length, diminished arborization, and a reduced number of dendritic spines. They also found varicosities within the dendrites that were thought to be intraneuritic LBs but could also have been dendritic spheroids. In an ultrastructural study, the size of the excitatory cholinergic terminals synapsing with the dendrites of nigral neurons is increased by nearly 40 percent, and the number of noncholinergic terminals, presumably inhibitory gamma-aminobutyric acid (GABAergic), was reduced by about 50 percent.[38]

Duffy and Tennyson[22] commented that surviving nigral neurons in PD showed depigmentation on electron microscopy; however, this was not verified in a later study.[39]

The pars reticulata neurons of the substantia nigra of PD often have increased amounts of lipofuscin (J Fearnley and A Lees, personal observation) and have been shown to be hypertrophic with a greater cross-sectional area, which has been interpreted as possible increased GABAergic output to the ventromedial nucleus of the thalamus.[40]

CORPUS STRIATUM

Secondary changes have been found in the corpus striatum with the loss of medium spiny neuron dendrites, which receive the dopaminergic output from the substantia nigra.[41] Whether there is actual neuronal cell loss in the corpus striatum is still unclear, although variably reduced cell counts have been described in two semiquantitative studies.[42,43] In support of striatal involvement are the electron microscopic findings of dystrophic neurites in two parkinsonian patients in whom material from the caudate nucleus was obtained during adrenomedullary transplantation.[44] However, there was no pathological confirmation of the diagnosis of PD, and the presence of hypertrophic astrocytes in the caudate raised the possibility of MSA. Furthermore, an earlier electron microscopic study showed no changes in the striatum.[45]

Molecular Biology

SUBSTANTIA NIGRA

Javoy-Agid et al.[46] found variable expression of tyrosine hydroxylase (TH) mRNA among pigmented neurons in the substantia nigra of both control and PD brains. However, there was a significant reduction of TH mRNA in PD[46] with proportional reduction of TH.[47] This is compatible with the previous finding of TH-negative immunoreactivity in some pigmented neurons.[48] Of note, there were no neurons overexpressing TH mRNA, which would seem to be at variance with the increased turnover of dopamine in PD.[49] This may reflect increased breakdown of mRNA, rather than reduced expression or increased tyrosine hydroxylation by conversion of inactive to active forms of TH.[46] Dopa decarboxylase mRNA is also reduced,[50] so it is likely that these changes are not primary events. Furthermore, there is a 57 percent reduction of dopamine transporter mRNA in the substantia nigra of PD.[51] These changes probably represent widespread cellular dysfunction, rather than specific abnormalities. It is possible that PD is a disease of the cytoskeleton and its organization, and it is interesting that neurofilament mRNA expression is diminished in the substantia nigra.[52]

STRIATAL OUTPUT STUDIES

There are two striatal output pathways: direct and indirect. In the direct pathway, striatal neurons project directly to the medial (or internal) globus pallidus. In the indirect pathway striatal neurons project to the medial pallidum via the lateral (or external) pallidum and subthalamic nucleus. In experimental models of PD, there is underactivity of the lateral pallidum and overactivity of the medial pallidum. The in situ work of Nisbet and colleagues has lent considerable support to this notion.[53,54] The lateral pallidum exerts its effect on the subthalamic nucleus by an inhibitory GABAergic projection. Glutamic acid decarboxylase (GAD) is necessary in the synthesis of GABA. GAD mRNA has been shown to be reduced by 50 percent in postmortem material of PD cases.[54] Furthermore, enkephalin immunoreactive fibers project from the striatum to the lateral pallidum (inhibitory), and there is an increase in striatal preproenkephalin mRNA, which encodes enkephalin.[53] Substance P immunoreactive fibers project from the striatum to the medial pallidum, and from animal studies one would expect downregulation of this direct pathway, but in human material there was no significant reduction of preprotachykinin mRNA.[53] However, it was suggested that this may be because of L-dopa therapy, and this finding may be important in the genesis of L-dopa-induced dyskinesia.[53] A novel finding has been the demonstration of increased expression of nitric oxide synthase mRNA in the cholinergic neurons of the medial medullary lamina of the globus pallidus.[55] It has been suggested that these neurons might project back to the striatum and possibly increase striatal dopamine release, thereby acting as a compensatory mechanism.

Presymptomatic Parkinson's Disease

LBs found at post mortem in patients who die without clinical signs of parkinsonism are termed incidental. The prevalence of incidental LBs increases with age (see Fig. 18-4). Whether a proportion of these cases had undetected clinical signs is uncertain, as early parkinsonism is often difficult to diagnose, particularly in the elderly. Clinical signs do not occur until there is an 80 percent depletion of striatal dopamine and a 50 percent loss of pigmented neurons in the caudal substantia nigra.[34,56] There must therefore be a presymptomatic phase, during which there is active neuronal loss without any clinical features of PD.[57] This is supported by evidence that there

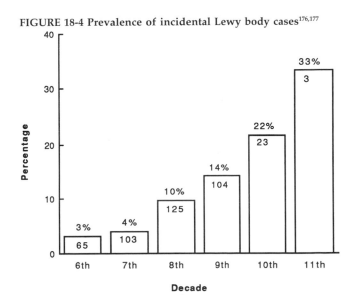

FIGURE 18-4 Prevalence of incidental Lewy body cases[176,177]

is significant cell loss in the substantia nigra of incidental LB cases in a pattern similar to that of PD, with predilection for the lateral ventral tier,[34] raising the possibility that incidental LBs represent this presymptomatic phase in individuals dying of other causes before PD could manifest clinically. There is some evidence that some patients with drug-induced parkinsonism may be a result of the unmasking of incidental LB disease.[58]

Progression of Parkinson's Disease

The rate of clinical progression in PD is not always uniform. In the majority of patients it is slow, but in a very few patients with so-called benign PD it is extremely slow.[59] Furthermore, prodromal symptoms extending back 10 years are occasionally noted by observant patients.[60] These nonspecific symptoms may be subtle indicators of the presymptomatic phase between the onset of neuronal death and the appearance of definite parkinsonism. It is likely that parkinsonism features occur as a result of both potentially reversible neuronal malfunction and irreversible neuronal death, and there may be an early period when there is minimal neuronal loss but significant malfunction. There is a striking difference in the amount of cell loss between PD and postencephalitic parkinsonism patients, in whom only a very few cells are left, yet the degree of disability is not necessarily greater. This would argue in favor of a greater degree of cellular dysfunction in PD.

There is very little pathological data on the rate of neuronal death in PD. In our own study we found an exponential loss of neurons with a relatively rapid loss of neurons early in the disease, followed by much smaller losses later on.[34] We also found a differential neuronal loss within different regions of the substantia nigra. Losses were greatest in the lateral ventral tier, followed by those in the medial tier; the least loss was in the dorsal tier. The duration of the presymptomatic phase was calculated as being on average 4.6 years, but this relates to neuronal death and would not include any period of prior neuronal dysfunction.

Etiology of Parkinson's Disease

Current thinking suggests that PD results from a combination of genetic susceptibility and an exogenous toxin. A genetic marker for PD has yet to be found, but investigation of familial cases may provide an important clue.

AGING AND PARKINSON'S DISEASE

PD is an illness of later life, with an average age of onset of 60 years and an increasing prevalence with age.[61,62] There is significant neuronal attrition in the substantia nigra as a direct result of aging, estimated to be in the order of 33–48 percent between the ages of 20 and 90 years.[34,63–65] To explore the possibility that aging is an important component in the pathogenesis of PD, two theories have been proposed.[66] First, PD may be a form of accelerated aging, and, second, an initial insult causes a depletion of neuronal reserve and parkinson-

ism, then appears once further attrition secondary to aging ensues (biphasic theory). Evidence against the accelerated aging theory has been found by looking at the regional selective loss within the substantia nigra for both aging and PD.[34] Aging has a predilection for the dorsal tier of the substantia nigra, which is the most heavily pigmented region, whereas losses in PD start and are greatest in the lateral part of the ventral tier. Regarding the biphasic theory, the rate of cell loss in the first 10 years of PD is 10 times greater than that of normal aging,[34] and the number of pigmented neurons being phagocytosed is about six times greater.[66]

THE ROLE OF NEUROMELANIN

PD has a predilection for pigmented nuclei—the substantia nigra, locus ceruleus, and dorsal motor vagal nucleus—and for this reason it has been claimed that neuromelanin may be important in the pathogenesis of the disease. Melanin is generated by the auto-oxidation of catecholamines, and neuromelanin is formed by the incorporation of melanin into lipofuscin derived from lysosomes.[67] It has been postulated that neuromelanin may be pivotal in the destruction of cells, either by mechanical disruption related to a mass effect, free radical formation during the process of neuromelanin production, or binding by neuromelanin of putative neurotoxins. However, the point has been made that in PD nonpigmented neurons, such as those in the nucleus basalis of Meynert, also undergo degeneration.[67] On the basis of the available evidence, it seems more likely that neuromelanin plays a more important role in the loss of neurons because of aging in the substantia nigra.[34]

In a study of PD substantia nigra using neuronal counts and a cytophotometric assessment of neuronal pigmentation, there was an 80 percent fallout of neurons, and a 15 percent reduction in the mean neuronal pigmentation.[68] These findings were interpreted as evidence that there was preferential fallout of the more heavily pigmented neurons. However, the method of selecting cells for measurement of neuromelanin was not specified. Furthermore, in the band of the most heavily melanized neurons, there seemed to be no difference in the number in the PD and control group. Similar results were obtained in another study, which sampled all pigmented neurons on a single section of the substantia nigra and ventral tegmental area.[69] There was a 59 percent loss of pigmented neurons and a 6 percent reduction in the mean optical density of neuromelanin within the remaining neurons. Looking at subgroups of pigmentation there was a predicted loss of about 40 percent for the most lightly melanized neurons and 65 percent for the most heavily melanized neurons. However, subregional analysis, using the divisions of Olszewski and Baxter,[70] was contradictory. Pars α which sustained the heaviest losses, had virtually no lightly or heavily melanized neurons. In pars β the proportions of lightly and heavily melanized neurons were unchanged. Only in pars lateralis and pars γ was there an increase in the proportion of lightly melanized neurons, and these regions were outside the areas of maximum predilection for nigral damage in PD; therefore, these findings are of less significance.

Within the caudal substantia nigra, the lateral part of the ventral tier is the least melanized but sustains the greatest cell loss in PD,[33,34,71,72] whereas the dorsal tier is the most melanized and suffers the greatest losses with aging. Furthermore, although the degree of pigmentation is greater in the locus ceruleus than in the substantia nigra, as judged by the ratio of pigmented neurons to TH positive neurons, the actual percentage cell loss in PD is less.[48]

IRON AND OXIDATIVE STRESS

Iron has been implicated in the pathogenesis of PD by enhancing free radical formation and, thereby causing lipid peroxidation and, ultimately, cell death.[73] MPTP infused into the striatum of the monkey results in increased iron staining of the pars compacta.[74] In a postmortem study of PD, MSA, and PSP, iron was increased in the substantia nigra in all three conditions, in the putamen in PSP (values for globus pallidus were not given), and in both the putamen and caudate in MSA.[75] This would suggest that the increase in iron was purely a secondary phenomenon resulting from neuronal death, rather than a primary cause. However, the amount of immunoreactive ferritin in PD was significantly reduced in the substantia nigra, and it was suggested that this reflected a reduced iron binding capacity and subsequent iron overload. Ferritin was also reduced in areas believed to be unaffected in PD, such as the corpus striatum, globus pallidus, and cerebellum. The controls for the PD group had a considerably increased ferritin content compared to that for the MSA and PSP control groups. In early PD, ferritin has been found to be normal,[76] suggesting that ferritin is not important in the initial stages of the disease.

Histochemically, excess iron in the substantia nigra in PD is confined to astrocytes, macrophages, and microglia in the pars compacta and in nonpigmented neurons in both the pars compacta and reticulata.[77] Iron staining is directly related to the presence of free pigment, and similar findings can be found in MSA and PSP (J Fearnley and A Lees, personal observation; see Fig. 18-5).

Hirsch et al.[78] used x-ray microanalysis to assess iron in the midbrain of PD. Measurements in the substantia nigra were confined to neuromelanin aggregates, areas without neuromelanin (no further delineation), and LBs identified by an indirect method using coordinates. There was a 35 percent decrease of iron in neuromelanin, and 340 percent increase in nonmelanized areas, and a 200 percent increase in LBs. Two possible explanations were put forward for the apparent reduction of neuromelanin iron observed. First, the pigmented neurons that were measured had survived as a consequence of their low iron content, whereas those with high content had already died. Alternatively, the reduction in iron may have been part of the pathological process. Conflicting data, however, have been reported, using energy-dispersive x-ray microanalysis[79] and laser microprobe mass analysis,[80] in which a 45 percent increase in neuromelanin iron was observed. Furthermore, these studies were able to measure iron in specific areas by direct visualization, and there was no significant increase in the cytoplasm of pigmented neurons, in LBs, or in the neuropil.

No significant change in iron or ferritin has been found in incidental LB cases.[81] In PD it is the lateral part of the ventral tier in the substantia nigra, which is most vulnerable

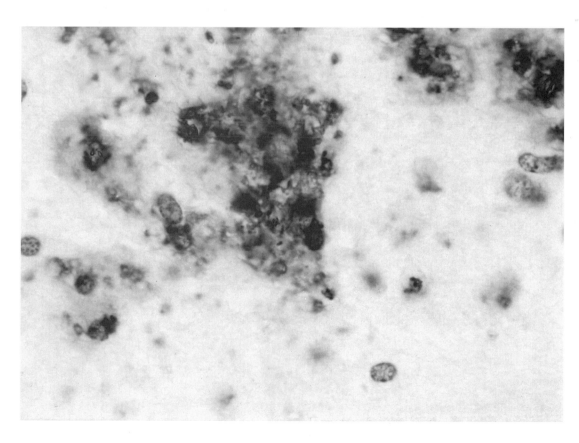

FIGURE 18-5 Incidental Lewy body case. Perl's stain, demonstrating iron in the vicinity of free pigment and macrophages. ×1250. See Color Plate 8.

and sustains the greatest neuronal loss.[34] In the incidental cases, roughly 50 percent of the neurons remain in this area, as opposed to 10 percent in PD.[34] Therefore, one would have expected a metabolic defect to be more easily detected in incidental LB cases. Furthermore, the lateral ventral tier is the least melanized region of the substantia nigra, the dorsal tier the most heavily melanized area.[33,72] If the trapping of iron by neuromelanin is pivotal in the pathogenesis of PD, then the lateral ventral tier should be spared relative to the dorsal tier, which is opposite to the pattern of cell loss seen in PD. In contrast, significantly decreased levels of reduced glutathione levels have been found in incidental LB cases indicative of oxidative stress.[81]

MPTP AND MITOCHONDRIAL FUNCTION

N-methyl-4-pheayl-1, 2, 3, 6-tetrahydropyridine (MPTP), a by-product in the manufacture of a synthetic narcotic meperidine, caused a small outbreak of parkinsonism in California drug addicts during the early 1980s. Relatively selective damage to the substantia nigra without LB formation occurs,[82,83] although in the nonhuman primate experimental model, diffuse inclusion bodies have been found in elderly cases in a similar distribution to the LB in human PD.[84] MPTP is a protoxin that is converted by the mitochondrial enzyme monoamine oxidase B, probably in astrocytes, to N-methyl-4-phenylpyridine (MPP$^+$) and is then taken up by nigral neurons through the dopamine reuptake system.[85] Neuromelanin binds MPP$^+$ and may act as a reservoir that slowly releases the toxin,[86] although there is no evidence for progression after initial exposure in the experimental model,[84] and partial recovery of function may occur. MPP$^+$ is felt to exert its effect by inhibiting the activity of complex I in oxidative phosphorylation.[87] In PD, a 37 percent reduction of complex I activity has been demonstrated in homogenates of the substantia nigra, which does not occur in MSA.[88–90] This is for all cell types within the nigra and not just pigmented neurons and, therefore, this finding may represent a generalized cellular abnormality. If this were a primary abnormality affecting pigmented neurons, then one would expect a significant if not greater reduction in incidental LB cases in which there is relative preservation of neuronal numbers in the most vulnerable areas. In a study by Dexter and colleagues,[81] six incidental LB cases had a 29 percent reduction in rotenone-sensitive NADH CoQ$_1$ activity (complex I), but this did not reach statistical significance. There was a longer postmortem delay, averaging 7 hours in the incidental LB group, compared to that of the control group. However, there was no correlation in the control group between postmortem delay and complex I activity, although in rats there is a roughly a 30 percent reduction over a 13-hour period.[91] Parkinsonism is extremely rare in primary mitochondrial disease,[92,93] and it remains to be determined whether a disturbance of mitochondrial function is an important factor in PD.

Familial Parkinsonism

DOPA-RESPONSIVE DYSTONIA/PARKINSONISM

This condition usually presents in childhood, with lower limb dystonia starting in the legs. In about three-quarters of reported cases there is marked diurnal variation, with the patient better in the morning and after rest and worse after exercise. It is exquisitely responsive to small doses of L-dopa, and this striking therapeutic response is not complicated by dyskinesia or on-off fluctuations, even after decades of treatment. The condition may be misdiagnosed as cerebral palsy, particularly when there are associated brisk reflexes and Babinski signs. The most important alternative diagnosis is juvenile parkinsonism, which has a less favorable prognosis. Elderly relatives may develop late-onset parkinsonism indistinguishable from PD, sometimes with a dramatic response to L-dopa and no motor fluctuations.[94] Striatal fluorodopa uptake is near normal.[95]

The condition is autosomal-dominant (chromosome 14q) with incomplete penetrance, especially in males (male to female ratio 1:2). The responsible gene has been found and encodes guanosine triphosphate (GTP) cyclohydrolase I, which is the rate-limiting step in the synthesis of tetrahydrobiopterin, an important cofactor for TH.[96]

There has been a single case report of a juvenile patient dying at the age of 19 in a road accident.[94] In the substantia nigra, the neurons of the ventral tier appeared hypopigmented, but there were no cell loss and no LBs. Dopamine was diminished in the striatum (putamen 8 percent of normal, caudate 18 percent), and reductions were greatest dorsally.

FAMILIAL PARKINSONISM WITH APATHY AND CENTRAL HYPOVENTILATION

A distinctive form of familial parkinsonism has been described in four families affecting 26 members, including an incidental patient diagnosed at autopsy,[97–101] in whom inheritance appears to be autosomal-dominant. It usually begins in middle age (mean age of onset, 50 years; range, 44–56) with a malignant course (mean age at death, 53 years; range, 49–61; mean duration, 5 years; range, 2–10) and is characterized by early profound apathy, weight loss, and central hypoventilation. It is not clear whether the apathy is a result of respiratory failure and/or depression. Dyspnea, ataxic breathing with apnea, gasping, sleep apnea, daytime hypersomnolence, respiratory arrest, and sudden death may all occur. Respiratory involvement was reported in 75 percent of cases, and an additional 10 percent died suddenly. Patients may also become confused, cognitively blunted, and they may experience visual hallucinations. Nocturnal and intermittent daytime-assisted ventilation in a single case[100] was highly effective, leading to resolution of the depression and weight gain. In one case there was a partial response of depression with very high doses of amitriptyline (250 mg/day), with only partial weight gain and persistent lethargy.[98] Another patient committed suicide very early in the illness, before developing the syndrome.[97]

Parkinsonism occurs in 88 percent, but may be delayed in its appearance and mild. In particular the family of Perry et al.[97] had subtle signs and predominant tremor. In all cases with parkinsonism, tremor occurred in 70 percent, bradykinesia in 55 percent, and rigidity in 50 percent. L-dopa was tried in nine cases, and five had a dramatic response to low doses (all confined to the family described by Roy et al.[100]), but only one of the cases of Lechevalier et al.[101] had a transient response. Severe bulbar problems occurred in 60 percent. In the family of Perry et al.[97] there were accompanying visuospatial problems with difficulty judging distances.

The pathology in nine cases,[97–101] including one presymptomatic,[98] has shown severe neuronal loss in the substantia nigra and possibly less so in the locus ceruleus. LBs have been present in 4/9, but only in very small numbers, and in one case this was limited to a single LB in the median raphe. Probable pale bodies with saccular cytoplasmic clearings were reported in a single case.[97] The basal ganglia were affected by neuronal loss and gliosis, but this was usually mild. The striatum was involved in four cases (two caudate and putamen[101]; two caudate[99]). The globus pallidus was affected in two cases.[99] A pathological correlate of the respiratory failure is lacking, although gliosis has been reported in other brain stem structures.[99]

Bhatia and colleagues[102] have reported a family of three generations with a similar disorder but no documented respiratory failure. Three members had parkinsonism and severe depression; three had isolated parkinsonism; and two had depression. The mean age of onset of parkinsonism was 42 years old (range, 35–51), and duration was 5 years (range, 3–10). Response to L-dopa was poor. In the proband, adequate pathology was available and showed severe neuronal depletion of the substantia nigra and locus ceruleus with few LBs in the remaining neurons. There was also gliosis with no appreciable neuronal loss in the head of the caudate and the globus pallidus. Unlike PD, there were no demonstrable cortical LBs.

FAMILIAL LB PARKINSONISM

This group comprises four families with inherited parkinsonism and pathology identical to PD.[103–107] In all of the families, autosomal-dominant inheritance seemed likely, and in Golbe's second family there was anticipation,[106] raising the possibility of a trinucleotide repeat. The clinical features are listed in Table 18-5.

Compared to PD, all four families had a younger age of onset, and progression was rapid, except for Golbe's second

family.[106] The parkinsonian features were similar to PD, although there was a lower incidence of tremor in Golbe's first family.[104] In half the families there was cognitive involvement compatible with Lewy body dementia (LBD). An unusual feature in Golbe's second family[106] was the presence of unexplained visual disturbance, which could have been the result of an oculomotor defect or cortical problem, and it caused difficulty with reading and depth perception.

Pathological examination was performed in an unspecified number of Muenter's patients[103] and one patient each from the other three families.[104,106,107] In the latter three families, there were neuronal loss and LBs in the substantia nigra, locus ceruleus, nucleus basalis of Meynert and, usually, in the dorsal motor vagal nucleus (2/3), which is typical of PD. In Waters & Miller's[107] study of family with associated dementia, there were cortical LBs and CA2-3 dystrophic neurites, compatible with LBD. In Muenter's family it is implied that the pathology was identical to that of LBD/PD.[103]

LB NEGATIVE FAMILIAL PARKINSONISM

INCLUSION NEGATIVE

There have been two kindreds recently reported with familial parkinsonism without intraneuronal inclusions[108,109] and a third family with additional severe pallidal involvement.[110] The clinical features of the first two kindreds are outlined in Table 18-5.

In the family of Dwork et al[108] inheritance appeared to be autosomal-dominant. Pathology was present in a single patient, and relevant abnormalities were confined to the substantia nigra with severe neuronal loss, where the remaining neurons were poorly pigmented. There was no neuronal attrition in the other areas affected in PD.

The family of Takahashi and others[109] was the result of a consanguineous marriage and inheritance appeared autosomal-recessive. There were similarities to dopa-responsive dystonia, with juvenile onset, early gait disorder with dystonic features, and profound sleep benefit. However, unlike dopa-responsive dystonia, there was a relatively poor response to L-dopa. Pathological examination in a single patient

TABLE 18-5 LB and LB Negative Familial Parkinsonism

Family	Inheritance	n	Autopsy	Onset	Duration	Motor Features	L-dopa Response	Dystonia	Dementia
Lewy body									
Muenter[103]	AD	12	?	10–30	4–11	art			Severe
Golbe[104,105]	AD+	44	1++	22–68	2–18	ar(t)	Good		±Mild late
Golbe[106]	AD	8	1	6–35*	31*	art	Poor-moderate	Foot**	Absent
Waters[107]	AD	9	1	36–45	6–7	art	Moderate	Toe	Late
Inclusion negative									
Dwork[108]	AD	14	1	2–39	11–16	art	Unsustained	Foot	Absent
Takahashi[109]	AR	4	1	8–10	19–57	art	Moderate	Foot	Absent
Ballooned neurons									
Mizutani[111]	AD	6	2	24–59	6–11	art	Poor	Absent	Severe
Neurofibrillary tangle									
Mata[112]	AR	3	1	23	?8	ar	Absent	Absent	Severe

a, akinetic; r, rigid; t, tremor; (t), 20% had tremor; +, anticipation; ++, additional patient with incomplete autopsy not included; *information available on only one patient; **members with juvenile onset.

showed neuronal depletion in the substantia nigra and locus ceruleus, and in the remaining neurons it was felt that there was a reduction in the amount of intraneuronal pigmentation.

BALLOONED NEURONS

Mizutani and colleagues[111] have reported a kindred with an autosomal-dominant pattern of inheritance. The syndrome was characterized in most members by early onset, aggressive course, parkinsonism with early postural instability, severe dementia with variable myoclonus and seizures, and poor response to L-dopa (see Table 18-5). Pathologically, there was atrophy of frontotemporal cortex (especially the anterior temporal) and depigmentation of the substantia nigra and locus ceruleus. Ballooned achromatic neurons, accompanied by granulovacuolar degeneration with neuronal loss and gliosis, were distributed widely in the affected cortex, nucleus basalis of Meynert, parahippocampus, amygdala, posterior hypothalamus, substantia nigra, locus ceruleus, and dorsal motor vagal nucleus. There were only occasional LBs and no Pick cells. The authors cited pathological similarities to corticobasal degeneration but felt it probably represented a unique disorder.

NEUROFIBRILLARY TANGLE POSITIVE

Mata et al[112] have described three siblings with a dementia-parkinsonism syndrome with supranuclear gaze palsy (see Table 18-5). Notably, one of the patients experienced oculogyric crises. In the single autopsied patient, there was cell loss in the substantia nigra and locus ceruleus, with gliosis in the periaqueductal gray and superior colliculi. Neurofibrillary tangles were found in the neurons of these areas, in the hippocampus and, to a lesser extent, the globus pallidus, which had minimal cell loss. There were no LBs and no neuritic plaques. The pathology was felt to be similar in some respects to both parkinson-dementia of Guam and PSP. The point has been made that these conditions and postencephalitic parkinsonism overlap pathologically and may be indistinguishable.[113]

Lewy Body Dementia

Lewy body dementia (LBD) was first described in 1961 by Okazaki and colleagues,[114] but it was not until the mid-1980s that it was recognized in the English literature as a common cause of dementia.[115] There are good arguments that it forms a continuum with PD.[116] It may present with parkinsonism identical to PD or with a temporoparietal dementia indistinguishable from Alzheimer's disease.[117] However, frequently in the early stages of LBD there are characteristic fluctuations in cognitive functioning from day to day[115] and prominent psychiatric features, such as anxiety, depression, hallucinations, and paranoid delusions.[115,117]

Pathologically, cortical LBs are best demonstrated by anti-ubiquitin immunostaining[23] and are most frequently found in the limbic system (entorhinal, inferior temporal, parahippocampus, insular, and anterior cingulate cortex) and, to a lesser extent, in the neocortex,[118] mainly in the small- and medium-sized pyramidal neurons of the deeper fifth and sixth layers. Beta amyloid plaques are frequently found in LBD, and in one study they correlated with the number of cortical LBs.[118] Unlike Alzheimer's disease, they are not usually accompanied by neuritic degeneration.[119] Neurofibrillary tangles are absent in the majority of patients but can occur, and in these cases they may well indicate coexistent Alzheimer's disease. It has been claimed that the presence of dystrophic neurites in the CA2-3 sector of the hippocampus are specific for LBD.[120] Other areas have been implicated in the dementia of PD, particularly the cholinergic nucleus basalis of Meynert[121] and the noradrenergic locus ceruleus.[120]

In late-onset familial and sporadic Alzheimer's disease, the apolipoprotein ∈4 gene has been associated with increased risk of developing the disease and an earlier age of onset.[122,123] Apolipoprotein ∈4 may be important in the development of β amyloid plaques and neuritic degeneration.[124] However, there is no evidence that apolipoprotein E is a susceptibility gene for PD with or without dementia.[125,126] To some extent apolipoprotein ∈4 may affect the pathological features of cortical LB disease. In a small study of cases, the majority of which had β amyloid plaques, there were greater numbers of β amyloid plaques with apolipoprotein ∈2 and ∈4 and greater CA2-3 neuritic degeneration in ∈4.[127]

Benign Parkinson's Disease

This disorder was defined by Scott and Brody[59] and as a very slowly progressive unilateral parkinsonian disorder. Twenty-one patients with a mean age of onset of 14–56. Even after 10 years, these patients were relatively free of axial involvement. As yet, this group of patients has not been pathologically defined, although some may represent postencephalitic cases.

Juvenile Parkinson's Disease

Early-onset PD can be divided into juvenile parkinsonism, with onset <21 years old and young-onset PD beginning between 21 and 40 years of age.[128] Young-onset PD is clinically similar to late-onset PD but with earlier motor fluctuations and dyskinesia and a low incidence of dementia. Dystonic features are frequent in juvenile parkinsonism and can be difficult to distinguish from dopa-responsive dystonia; however, the requirement for larger doses of L-dopa, the early appearance of motor fluctuations and dyskinesia, and the reduced fluorodopa uptake on PET scanning help make the clinical distinction.[129,130] Juvenile parkinsonism can be divided into an LB type, which is probably a subgroup of PD, and a non-LB type (see LB negative familial parkinsonism). A positive family history is relatively common in both juvenile parkinsonism and young-onset PD.[131] As a result, the distinction between juvenile and familial PD can be arbitrary.

There are few pathological reports of juvenile PD, reflecting the rarity of this condition. In one recent report there were LBs in the substantia nigra without any demonstrable neuronal loss and apparently reduced intraneuronal pigmentation. It was speculated that the clinical effects were secondary to an abnormality of the nigrostriatal terminals.[129] However, in the same case Gibb et al. were able to show devastation of the lateral part of the ventral tier of the nigra, which could only be recognized by a dense glial scar.[132] The remainder of the substantia nigra appeared untouched, apart from some neurons with LBs and pale bodies (shown in a later ultrastructural study to have plentiful cored vesicles[133]), and there was no extraneuronal pigment to suggest continuing neuronal death. Again, there was poor melanization of nigral neurons, raising the possibility of a metabolic defect. These are remarkable findings in respect to the extreme regional selectivity of juvenile PD, even if there was some minor undetected cell loss outside the lateral ventral tier. In another case there was severe neuronal loss within the substantia nigra and locus ceruleus with LBs in the few remaining neurons.[134]

Arteriosclerotic Parkinsonism

In 1929, Critchley[135] gave prominence to an arteriosclerotic form of parkinsonism, based on a clinical study without the benefit of any pathological correlation. Subsequently, the diagnosis was often proposed solely on the coexistence of associated cardiovascular disease or cerebrovascular disease in an elderly parkinsonian patient. However, this notion fell into disrepute,[136,137] and in recent years the term has been used in a much more restricted way to describe patients with multi-infarct cerebrovascular disease or diffuse white matter subcortical ischemia on neuroimaging and so-called lower-body parkinsonism.[138] Cases of parkinsonism may also follow infarcts of the substantia nigra but are very rare.[137,139] It is not clear whether lacunar infarction of the basal ganglia can cause true parkinsonism,[140] and this is confounded by the frequent presence of both lacunar disease and LB pathology in the elderly patient. In the literature, there have been three patients without pathology who developed either akinesia or akinesia and rigidity after basal ganglia infarction, with some improvement in two patients that was suggestive of a vascular cause.[141] A further patient with polyarteritis nodosa developed a transient asymmetrical akinetic-rigid syndrome and a left striatal infarct on CT scanning, which then resolved with immunosuppressive therapy.[142]

Attempts have been made to propose operational criteria for the clinical diagnosis of arteriosclerotic parkinsonism. Parkes and others[143] defined it as those patients with a past history of completed stroke who had rigidity greatest in the legs, compared to the arms (lower-body parkinsonism), paratonia, infrequent tremor, no response to L-dopa, normal CSF homovanillic acid levels, and electroencephalogram (EEG) slow-wave activity. Friedman et al[144] have suggested the following criteria: sudden onset of parkinsonian signs, subsequent improvement, and exclusion of other causes of parkinsonism on clinical and pathological assessment. Unfortunately, in both studies no clinicopathological correlations were made. The concept of lower-body parkinsonism encompasses those patients presenting primarily with gait difficulties, such as start hesitation, shuffling, and postural instability, and those who have variable lower-limb rigidity and akinesia unresponsive to L-dopa and associated hypertension and subcortical white matter lesions on magnetic resonance imaging (MRI).[145]

In a recent study of 100 parkinsonian patients in a movement disorder clinic, 20 patients had basal ganglia lacunes on computed tomography (CT) scanning, and of these seven had had clinical stroke.[146] There was no difference between the lacunar and nonlacunar groups, apart from a lower incidence of tremor in the former. In particular, there was no lower-body parkinsonism, no correlation between the asymmetry of the parkinsonian signs and side of the lacune, no stepwise deterioration to suggest a vascular basis, and no differential L-dopa response.

Pathological case reports are scarce and do not lend sufficient evidence to support the concept of arteriosclerotic parkinsonism. Parkinsonism attributed to vascular disease has been reported occasionally. One patient[147] died at the age of 74, having had a 20-year history of slowly progressive asymmetric parkinsonism with rigidity, bradykinesia, tremor, and a good response to L-dopa. There was also a long history of uncontrolled hypertension, and there were diffuse white matter ischemic lesions apparent on CT scanning. Histological examination of the brain revealed microscopic lacunar infarcts throughout the basal ganglia and substantia nigra. There was no cell loss in the substantia nigra or extracellular pigment, but there was an average of one LB per section of the substantia nigra and two to three per section of the locus ceruleus. LBs are usually associated with cell loss, and occasionally significant cell loss can be overlooked. In another case,[148] there was no substantia nigra pathology, and in particular, no LBs, but there were lacunes in the putamen of one side, cortical scarring, and amyloid angiopathy. However, the patient was felt not to have PD clinically in that the main problem was a shuffling gait, with only slight akinesia and rigidity and periodic rest tremor in the presence of essential tremor. Nisbet et al.[149] have been able to review nine cases from the UK Parkinson's Disease Society Brain Bank, who were diagnosed in life as having PD and/or cerebrovascular disease and then found at autopsy to have cerebral small vessel disease in the absence of any alternative pathology. Hypertension was present in seven and a past history of stroke in six. In at least four cases the clinical features bore sufficient semblance to parkinsonism to justify the notion of an arteriosclerotic form. Unlike typical PD, the illness usually started with a shuffling gait, frequently accompanied by falls. Resting tremor occurred in one case, which may have been an essential or dystonic tremor; bradykinesia was relatively infrequent; and response to L-dopa was often absent or poor. Compared to PD, deficits were often greater in the lower than upper limbs, but only three cases had lower body parkinsonism. Notably in a proportion of cases, pyramidal signs were absent or minimal. Pathological examination revealed extensive damage to the striatum with microinfarction (9/9) and lacunar infarction (6/9). A single case had an infarct in the rostral substantia nigra. Binswanger-type white matter changes were present in 8/9, and in all cases the lateral ventricles were dilated to some degree. (See also Chap. 25.)

References

1. Hughes AJ, Daniel SE, Blankson S, et al: A clinicopathological study of 100 cases of Parkinson's disease. *Arch Neurol* 50:140–148, 1993.

2. Quinn NP: Multiple system atrophy—The nature of the beast. *J Neurol Neurosurg Psychiatry* 52 (special suppl):78–89, 1989.

3. Fearnley JM, Revezs T, Frackowiak RSJ, et al: Diffuse Lewy body disease presenting with a progressive supranuclear gaze palsy. *J Neurol Neurosurg Psychiatry* 54:159–161, 1991.

4. de Bruin VM, Lees AJ, Daniel SE: Diffuse Lewy body disease presenting with supranuclear gaze palsy, parkinsonism, and dementia: A case report. *Mov Disord* 7:355–358, 1992.

5. Mark MH, Sage JI, Dickson DW, et al: L-dopa-nonresponsive Lewy body parkinsonism: Clinicopathological study of two cases. *Neurology* 42:1323–1327, 1992.

6. Fearnley JM, Lees AJ: Striatonigral degeneration: A clinicopathological study. *Brain* 113:1823–1842, 1990.

7. Wenning GK, Ben Shlomo Y, Magalhães M, et al: Clinical features and natural history of multiple system atrophy: An analysis of 100 cases. *Brain* 117:835–845, 1994.

8. Davie CA, Wenning GK, Barker GJ, et al: Differentiation of multiple system atrophy from idiopathic Parkinson's disease using proton magnetic resonance spectroscopy. *Ann Neurol* 37:204–210, 1995.

9. Gibb WRG, Lees AJ: The significance of the Lewy body in the diagnosis of idiopathic Parkinson's disease. *Neuropathol Appl Neurobiol* 15:27–44, 1989.

10. Lewy FH: Zur pathologischen Anatomie der Paralysis agitans. *Dsch Z Nervenheilkd* 50:50–55, 1914.

11. Tretiakoff C: Contribution a l'étude de l'anatomie pathologique du locus niger de Soemmering avec quelques déductions relatives à la pathogénie des troubles du tonus musculaire et de la maladie de Parkinson. Thesis, University of Paris, 1919.

12. Gibb WRG: Idiopathic Parkinson's disease and the Lewy body disorders. *Neuropathol Appl Neurobiol* 12:223–234, 1986.

13. Roy S, Wolman L: Ultrastructural observations in parkinsonism. *J Pathol* 99:39–44, 1969.

14. Kosaka K: Lewy bodies in the cerebral cortex: Report of three cases. *Acta Neurol (Berl)* 42:127–134, 1978.

15. Nishimura M, Tomimoto H, Suenaga T, et al: Synaptophysin and chromogranin A immunoreactivities of Lewy bodies in Parkinson's disease brains. *Brain Res* 634:339–344, 1994.

16. Kimula Y, Utsuyama M, Yoshimura M, et al: Element analysis of Lewy and adrenal bodies in Parkinson's disease by electron probe microanalysis. *Acta Neuropathol (Berl)* 59:233–236, 1983.

17. Hill WD, Lee VM, Hurtig HI, et al: Epitopes located in spatially separate domains of each neurofilament subunit are present in Parkinson's disease Lewy bodies. *J Comp Neurol* 309:150–160, 1991.

18. Sternberger LA, Sternberger NH: Monoclonal antibodies distinguish phosphorylated and non-phosphorylated forms of neurofilaments in situ. *Proc Natl Acad Sci USA* 80:6126–6130, 1983.

19. Kuzuhara S, Mori H, Izumiyama N, et al: Lewy bodies are ubiquinated: A light and electron microscopic immunocytochemical study. *Acta Neuropathol (Berl)* 75:345–353, 1988.

20. Forno LS, Sternberger LA, Sternberger NH, et al: Reaction of Lewy bodies with antibodies to phosphorylated and non-phosphorylated neurofilaments. *Neurosci Lett* 64:253–258, 1986.

21. Iwatsubo T, Nakano I, Fukunaga K, et al: Ca2 + /calmodulin-dependent protein kinase II immunoreactivity in Lewy bodies. *Acta Neuropathol (Berl)* 82:159–163, 1991.

22. Duffy PE, Tennyson VM: Phase and electron microscopic observations of Lewy bodies and melanin granules in the substantia nigra and locus ceruleus in Parkinson's disease. *J Neuropathol Exp Neurol* 24:398–414, 1965.

23. Lennox G, Lowe J, Morrell K, et al: Anti-ubiquitin immunocytochemistry is more sensitive than conventional techniques in the detection of diffuse Lewy body disease. *J Neurol Neurosurg Psychiatry* 52:67–71, 1989.

24. Anonymous: Ubiquitin, protein degradation and dynamic neuropathology. *Lancet* ii:319–320, 1988.

25. Kremer HPH, Bots GTAM: Lewy bodies in the lateral hypothalamus: Do they imply neuronal loss? *Mov Disord* 8:315–320, 1993.

26. Gibb WR, Scott T, Lees AJ: Neuronal inclusions of Parkinson's disease. *Mov Disord* 6:2–11, 1991.

27. Panayotacopoulou MT, Issidorides MR: Arginine-rich proteins in spherical inclusions of human locus ceruleus neurons demonstrated by benzil modifications. *J Histochem Cytochem* 32:1192–1196, 1984.

28. Sekiya S, Tanaka M, Hayashi S, et al: Light- and electronmicroscopic studies of intracytoplasmic acidiphilic granules in the human locus ceruleus and substantia nigra. *Acta Neuropathol (Berl)* 56:78–80, 1982.

29. Issidorides MR, Mytilineou C, Whetsell WO, et al: Protein-rich cytoplasmic bodies of substantia nigra and locus ceruleus: A comparative study in parkinsonian and normal brain. *Arch Neurol* 35:633–637, 1978.

30. Pappolla MA, Shank DL, Alzofon J, et al: Colloid (hyaline) inclusion bodies in the central nervous system: Their presence in the substantia nigra is diagnostic of Parkinson's disease. *Hum Pathol* 19:27–31, 1988.

31. Dale GE, Probst A, Luthert P, et al: Relationships between Lewy bodies and pale bodies in Parkinson's disease. *Acta Neuropathol (Berl)* 83:525–529, 1992.

32. Yamada T, Akiyama H, McGeer PL: Two types of spheroid bodies in the nigral neurons in Parkinson's disease. *Can J Neurol Sci* 18:287–294, 1991.

33. Hassler R: Zur Normalanatomie der Substantia Nigra. *J Psychol Neurol* 48:1–55, 1937.

34. Fearnley JM, Lees AJ: Aging and Parkinson's disease: Substantia nigra regional selectivity. *Brain* 114:2283–2301, 1991.

35. Parent A, Mackey A, De Bellefeuille L: The subcortical afferents to caudate nucleus and putamen in primate: A flourescence retrograde double-labeling study. *Neuroscience* 10:1137–1150, 1983.

36. Patt S, Gertz HJ, Gerhard L, et al: Pathological changes in dendrites of substantia nigra neurons in Parkinson's disease: A Golgi study. *Histol Histopathol* 6:373–380, 1991.

37. Patt S, Gerhard L: A Golgi study of human locus ceruleus in normal brains and in Parkinson's disease. *Neuropathol Appl Neurobiol* 19:519–523, 1993.

38. Anglade P, Tsuji S, Javoy-Agid F, et al: Plasticity of nerve afferents to nigrostriatal neurons in Parkinson's disease. *Ann Neurol* 37:265–272, 1995.

39. Forno LS, Alvord EC: Depigmentation in the nerve cells of the substantia nigra and locus ceruleus in parkinsonism. *Adv Neurol* 5:195–202, 1974.

40. Neal JW, Pearson RC, Cole G, et al: Neuronal hypertrophy in the pars reticulate of the substantia nigra in Parkinson's disease. *Neuropathol Appl Neurobiol* 17:203–206, 1991.

41. Freund TF, Powell JF, Smith AD: Tyrosine hydroxylase-immunoreactive boutons in synaptic contacts with identified striatonigral neurons, with particular reference to dendritic spines. *Neuroscience* 13:1189–1215, 1984.

42. Bugiani O, Perdelli F, Salvarani S, et al: Loss of striatal neurons in Parkinson's disease: A cytometric study. *Eur Neurol* 19:339–344, 1980.

43. Bockelmann R, Wolf G, Ransmayr G, et al: NADPH-diaphorase/nitric oxide synthase containing neurons in normal and

Parkinson's disease putamen. *J Neural Transm Park Dis Dement Sect* 7:115–121, 1994.

44. Lach B, Grimes D, Benoit B, et al: Caudate nucleus pathology in Parkinson's disease: Ultrastructural and biochemical findings in biopsy material. *Acta Neuropathol (Berl)* 83:352–360, 1992.

45. Forno LS, Norville RL: Ultrastructure of neostriatum in Huntington's and Parkinson's disease. *Adv Neurol* 23:123–135, 1979.

46. Javoy-Agid F, Hirsch EC, Dumas S, et al: Decreased tyrosine hydroxylase messenger RNA in the surviving dopamine neurons of the substantia nigra in Parkinson's disease: An in situ hybridization study. *Neuroscience* 38:245–253, 1990.

47. Kastner A, Hirsch EC, Agid Y, et al: Tyrosine hydroxylase protein and messenger RNA in the dopaminergic nigral neurons of patients with Parkinson's disease. *Brain Res* 606:341–345, 1993.

48. Hirsch E, Graybiel AM, Agid YA: Melanized dopaminergic neurons are differentially susceptible to degeneration in Parkinson's diseae. *Nature* 334:345–348, 1988.

49. Agid Y, Javoy-Agid F, Ruberg M: Biochemistry of neurotransmitters in Parkinson's disease, in Marsden CD, Fahn S (eds): *Movement Disorders*. London: Butterworth, 1987, pp 166–230.

50. Ichinose H, Ohye T, Fujita K, et al: Quantification of mRNA of tyrosine hydroxylase and aromatic L-amino acid decarboxylase in the substantia nigra in Parkinson's disease and schizophrenia. *J Neural Transm Park Dis Dement Sect* 8:149–158, 1994.

51. Uhl GR, Walther D, Mash D, et al: Dopamine transporter messenger mRNA in Parkinson's disease and control substantia nigra neurons. *Ann Neurol* 35:494–498, 1994.

52. Hill WD, Arai M, Cohen JA, et al: Neurofilament mRNA is reduced in Parkinson's disease substantia nigra pars compacta neurons. *J Comp Neurol* 329:328–336, 1993.

53. Nisbet AP, Foster OJF, Kingsbury A, et al: Preproenkephalin and preprotachykinin messenger RNA expression in normal human basal ganglia and in Parkinson's disease. *Neuroscience* 66:361–376, 1995.

54. Nisbet AP, Eve DJ, Kingsbury AE, et al: Glutamic acid decarboxylase-67 mRNA (GAD67 mRNA) expression in normal human basal ganglia and in Parkinson's disease. *Neuroscience* 75:389–406, 1996.

55. Nisbet AP, Foster OJF, Kingsbury A, et al: Nitric oxide synthase mRNA expression in human subthalamic nucleus, striatum and globus pallidus: Implications for basal ganglia function. *Brain Res Mol Brain Res* 22:329–332, 1994.

56. Bernheimer H, Birkmayer W, Hornykiewicz O, et al: Brain dopamine and the syndromes of Parkinson and Huntington: Clinical, morphological and neurochemical correlations. *J Neurol Sci* 20:415–455, 1973.

57. Forno LS: Concentric hyalin intraneuronal inclusions of Lewy type in the brains of elderly persons (50 incidental cases): Relationship to parkinsonism. *J Am Geriatr Soc* 17:557–575, 1969.

58. Rajput AH, Rozdilsky B, Hornykiewicz O, et al: Reversible drug-induced parkinsonism: Clinicopathological study of two cases. *Arch Neurol* 39:644–646, 1982.

59. Scott RM, Brody JA: Benign early onset of Parkinson's disease: A syndrome distinct from classic post-encephalitic parkinsonism. *Neurology* 21:366–368, 1971.

60. Lees AJ: When did Ray Kennedy's Parkinson's disease begin? *Mov Disord* 7:110–116, 1992.

61. Hoehn MD, Yahr MM: Parkinsonism: Onset, progression and mortality. *Neurology* 17:427–442, 1967.

62. Mutch WJ, Dingwall-Fordyce I, Downie AW, et al: Parkinson's disease in a Scottish city. *BMJ* 292:534–536, 1986.

63. Hirai S: Histochemical study on the regressive degeneration of the senile brain with special reference to the aging of the substantia nigra. *Adv Neurol Sci* 12:845–849, 1968.

64. McGeer PL, McGeer EG, Suzuki JS: Aging and extrapyramidal function. *Arch Neurol* 34:33–35, 1977.

65. Mann DMA, Yates PO, Marcyniuk B: Monoaminergic neurotransmitter systems in presenile Alzheimer's disease and in senile dementia of Alzheimer type. *Clin Neuropathol* 3:199–205, 1984.

66. McGeer PL, Itagaki S, Akiyama H, et al: The rate of cell death in parkinsonism indicates active neuropathological process. *Ann Neurol* 24:574–576, 1988.

67. Marsden CD: Neuromelanin and Parkinson's disease. *J Neural Transm* 19:121–141, 1983.

68. Mann DMA, Yates PO: Possible role of neuromelanin in the pathogensis of Parkinson's disease. *Mech Aging Dev* 21:193–203, 1983.

69. Kastner A, Hirsch EC, Lejeune O, et al: Is the vulnerability of neurons in the substantia nigra of patients with Parkinson's disease related to their neuromelanin content? *J Neurochem* 59:1080–1089, 1992.

70. Olszewski J, Baxter D: *Cytoarchitecture of the Human Brainstem*. New York: S. Karger, 1954.

71. Hassler R: Zur Pathologie der Paralysis agitans und des postenzephalitischen Parkinsonismus. *J Psychol Neurol* 48:387–476, 1938.

72. Gibb WRG, Lees AJ: Anatomy, pigmentation, ventral and dorsal subpopulations of the substantia nigra and differential cell death in Parkinson's disease. *J Neurol Neurosurg Psychiatry* 54:388–396, 1991.

73. Dexter DT, Carter CJ, Wells FR, et al: Basal lipid peroxidation in the substantia nigra is increased in Parkinson's disease. *J Neurochem* 52:381–389, 1989.

74. Mochizuki H, Imai H, Endo K, et al: Iron accumulation in the substantia nigra of 1-methyl-4-phenyl-1,2,3,6-tetrahydropyridine (MPTP)-induced hemiparkinsonian monkeys. *Neurosci Lett* 168:251–253, 1994.

75. Dexter DT, Carayon A, Javoy-Agid F, et al: Alterations in the levels of iron, ferritin and other trace metals in Parkinson's disease and other neurodegenerative diseases affecting the basal ganglia. *Brain* 114:1953–1975, 1991.

76. Riederer P, Sofic E, Rausch W-D, et al: Transition metals, ferritin, glutathione, and ascorbic acid in parkinsonian brains. *J Neurochem* 52:515–520, 1989.

77. Jellinger K, Paulus W, Grundke-Iqbal I, et al: Brain iron and ferritin in Parkinson's and Alzheimer's diseases. *J Neural Transm Park Dis Dement Sect* 2:327–340, 1990.

78. Hirsch EC, Brandel J-P, Galle P, et al: Iron and aluminum increase in the substantia nigra of patients with Parkinson's disease: An x-ray microanalysis. *J Neurochem* 56:446–451, 1991.

79. Jellinger K, Kienzl E, Rumpelmair G, et al: Iron-melanin complex in substantia nigra of parkinsonian brains: An X-ray microanalysis. *J Neurochem* 59:1168–1171, 1992.

80. Good PF, Olanow CW, Perl DP: Neuromelanin-containing neurons of the substantia nigra accumulate iron and aluminum in Parkinson's disease: A LAMMA study. *Brain Res* 593:343–346, 1992.

81. Dexter DT, Sian J, Rose S, et al: Indices of oxidative stress and mitochondrial function in individuals with incidental Lewy body disease. *Ann Neurol* 35:38–44, 1994.

82. Davis GC, Williams AC, Markey SP, et al: Chronic parkinsonism secondary to intravenous injection of meperidine analogues. *Psychiatry Res* 1:249–254, 1979.

83. Ballard PA, Tetrud JW, Langston JW: Permanent human parkinsonism due to MPTP. *Neurology* 35:949–956, 1985.

84. Forno LS, DeLanney LE, Irwin I, et al: Similarities and differences between MPTP-induced parkinsonism and Parkinson's disease: Neuropathological considerations. *Adv Neurol* 60:600–608, 1993.

85. Javitch JA, D'Amato RJ, Strittmatter SM, et al: Parkinsonism inducing neurotoxin, N-methyl-4-phenyl-1,2,3,6-tetrahydropyridine: Uptake of the metabolite N-methyl-4-phenylpyridine by dopamine neurons explains selective toxicity. *Proc Natl Acad Sci USA* 82:2173–2177, 1985.

86. D'Amato RJ, Lipman ZP, Snyder SH: Selectivity of the parkinsonian neurotoxin MPTP: Toxic metabolite MPP$^+$ binds to neuromelanin. *Science* 231:987–989, 1986.

87. Nicklas WJ, Vyas I, Heikkila RE: Inhibition of NADH-linked oxidation in brain mitochondria by 1-methyl-4-phenylpyridine, a metabolite of the neurotoxin, 1-methyl-4-phenyl-1,2,3,6-tetrahydropyridine. *Life Sci* 36:2503–2508, 1985.

88. Schapira AHV, Cooper JM, Dexter D, et al: Mitochondrial complex I deficiency in Parkinson's disease. *J Neurochem* 54:823–827, 1990.

89. Schapira AHV, Mann VM, Cooper JM, et al: Anatomic and disease specificity of NADH CoQ$_1$ reductase (complex I) deficiency in Parkinson's disease. *J Neurochem* 55:2142–2145, 1990.

90. Mann VM, Cooper JM, Krige D, et al: Brain, skeletal muscle and platelet homogenate mitochondrial function in Parkinson's disease. *Brain* 115:333–342, 1992.

91. Mizuno Y, Suzuki K, Ohta S: Postmortem changes in mitochondrial respiratory enzymes in brain and a preliminary observation in Parkinson's disease. *J Neurol Sci* 96:49–57, 1990.

92. Troung DD, Harding AE, Scaravelli F, et al: Movement disorders in mitochondrial myopathies. *Mov Disord* 5:109–117, 1990.

93. Djaldetti R, Ziv I, Achiron A, et al: Parkinson's disease in a patient with mitochondrial myopathy: Is there a causative relationship? *Mov Disord* 7:382–383, 1992.

94. Rajput AH, Gibb WRG, Zhong XH, et al: Dopa-responsive dystonia: Pathological and biochemical observations in a case. *Ann Neurol* 35:396–402, 1994.

95. Turjanski N, Bhatia K, Burn DJ, et al: Comparison of striatal ^{18}F-dopa uptake in adult onset dystonia-parkinsonism, Parkinson's disease, and dopa-responsive dystonia. *Neurology* 43:1563–1568, 1993.

96. Ichinose H, Ohye T, Takahashi E, et al: Hereditary progressive dystonia with marked diurnal fluctuation caused by mutations in GTP cyclohydrolase I gene. *Nature Genet* 8:236–242, 1994.

97. Perry TL, Bratty JA, Hansen S, et al: Hereditary mental depression and parkinsonism with taurine deficiency. *Arch Neurol* 32:108–113, 1975.

98. Perry TL, Wright JM, Berry K, et al: Dominantly inherited apathy, central hypoventilation, and Parkinson's syndrome: Clinical, biochemical and neuropathological studies of 2 new cases. *Neurology* 40:1882–1887, 1990.

99. Purdy A, Hahn A, Barnett JM, et al: Familial fatal parkinsonism with alveolar hypoventilation and mental depression. *Ann Neurol* 6:523–531, 1979.

100. Roy EP, Riggs JE, Martin JD, et al: Familial parkinsonism, apathy, weight loss, and central hypoventilation: Successful long-term management. *Neurology* 38:637–639, 1988.

101. Lechevalier B, Schupp C, Fallet-Bianco C, et al: Syndrome parkinsonien familial avec athymhormie et hypoventilation. *Rev Neurol (Paris)* 148:39–46, 1992.

102. Bhatia KP, Daniel SE, Marsden CD: Familial parkinsonism with depression: A clinicopathological study. *Ann Neurol* 34:842–847, 1993.

103. Muenter MD, Howard FM, Okazaki H, et al: A familial parkinson-dementia syndrome. *Neurology* 36(Suppl 1):115, 1986.

104. Golbe LI, Di Iorio G, Bonavita V, et al: A large kindred with autosomal dominant Parkinson's disease. *Ann Neurol* 27:276–282, 1990.

105. Golbe LI, Dilorio G, Bonavita V, et al: A large kindred with Parkinson's disease (PD): Onset age, segregation ratios and anticipation. *Mov Disord* 7(Suppl 1):24, 1992.

106. Golbe LI, Lazzarini AM, Schwarz KO, et al: Autosomal dominant parkinsonism with benign course and typical Lewy-body pathology. *Neurology* 43:2222–2227, 1993.

107. Waters CH, Miller CA: Autosomal dominant Lewy body parkinsonism in a four-generation family. *Ann Neurol* 35:59–64, 1994.

108. Dwork AJ, Balmaceda C, Fazzini EA, et al: Dominantly inherited early-onset parkinsonism: Neuropathology of a new form. *Neurology* 43:69–74, 1993.

109. Takahashi H, Ohama E, Suzuki S, et al: Familial juvenile parkinsonism: Clinical and pathologic study in a family. *Neurology* 44:437–441, 1994.

110. Wszolek ZK, Pfeiffer RF, Bhatt MH, et al: Rapidly progressive autosomal dominant parkinsonism and dementia with pallido-ponto-nigral degeneration. *Ann Neurol* 32:312–320, 1992.

111. Mizutani T, Inose T, Nakajima S, et al: Familial parkinsonism and dementia with "ballooned neurons." *Adv Neurol* 60:613–617, 1993.

112. Mata M, Dorovini-Zis K, Wilson M, et al: New form of familial Parkinson-dementia syndrome: Clinical and pathological findings. *Neurology* 33:1439–1443, 1983.

113. Geddes JF, Hughes AJ, Lees AJ, et al: Pathological overlap in cases of parkinsonism with neurofibrillary tangles: A study of recent cases of post-encephalitic parkinsonism and comparison with progressive supranuclear palsy and Guamanian parkinsonism-dementia complex. *Brain* 116:281–302, 1993.

114. Okazaki H, Lipkin LE, Aronson SM: Diffuse intracytoplasmic ganglionic inclusions (Lewy type) associated with progressive dementia and quadriparesis in flexion. *J Neuropathol Exp Neurol* 20:237–244, 1961.

115. Byrne EJ, Lennox G, Lowe J, et al: Diffuse Lewy body disease: Clinical features in 15 cases. *J Neurol Neurosurg Psychiatry* 52:709–717, 1989.

116. Lennox G: Lewy body dementia. *Bailliere's Clin Neurol* 1(3):653–676, 1992.

117. Gibb WRG, Esiri MM, Lees AJ: Clinical and pathological features of diffuse cortical Lewy body disease (Lewy body dementia). *Brain* 110:1131–1153, 1987.

118. Lennox G, Loew J, Landon M, et al: Diffuse Lewy body disease: Correlative neuropathology using anti-ubiquitin immunocytochemistry. *J Neurol Neurosurg Psychiatry* 52:1236–1247, 1989.

119. Lippa CF, Smith TW, Swearer J: Alzheimer's disease and Lewy body disease: A comparative clinicopathological study. *Ann Neurol* 35:81–88, 1994.

120. Dickson D, Ruan D, Crystal H, et al: Hippocampal degeneration differentiates diffuse Lewy body disease (DLBD) from Alzheimer's disease: Light and electron microscopic immunocytochemistry of CA2-3 neurites specific to DLBD. *Neurology* 41:1402–1409, 1991.

121. Whitehouse PJ, Hedreen JC, White CJ, et al: Basal forebrain neurons in the dementia of Parkinson's disease. *Ann Neurol* 13:243–248, 1983.

122. Corder EH, Saunders AM, Strittmater WJ, et al: Gene dose of apolipoprotein E type 4 allele and risk of Alzheimer's disease in late onset families. *Science* 261:921–923, 1993.

123. Saunders AM, Strittmatter WJ, Schmechal D, et al: Association of apolipoprotein E allele ϵ4 with late-onset familial and sporadic Alzheimer's disease. *Neurology* 43:1467–1472, 1993.

124. Schmechel DE, Saunders AM, Strittmatter WJ, et al: Increased amyloid β-peptide deposition as a consequence of apolipoprotein E genotype in late-onset Alzheimer's disease. *Proc Natl Acad Sci USA* 90:9649–9653, 1993.

125. Marder K, Maestre G, Cote L, et al: The apolipoprotein ε4 allele in Parkinson's disease with and without dementia. *Neurology* 44:1330–1331, 1994.

126. Koller WC, Glatt SL, Hubble JP, et al: Apolipoprotein E genotypes in Parkinson's disease with and without dementia. *Ann Neurol* 37:242 245, 1995.

127. Lippa CF, Smith TW, Saunders AM, et al: Apolipoprotein E genotype and Lewy body disease. *Neurology* 45:97–103, 1995.

128. Quinn N, Critchley P, Marsden CD: Young onset Parkinson's disease. *Mov Disord* 2:73–91, 1987.

129. Yokochi M, Narabayashi H, Iizuka R, et al: Juvenile parkinsonism—Some clinical, pharmacological, and neuropathological aspects. *Adv Neurol* 40:407–413, 1984.

130. Snow BJ, Nygaard TG, Takahashi H, et al: Positron emission tomographic studies of dopa-responsive dystonia and early onset idiopathic parkinsonism. *Ann Neurol* 34:733–738, 1993.

131. Muthane UB, Swamy HS, Satishchandra P, et al: Early onset Parkinson's disease: Are juvenile- and young-onset different? *Mov Disord* 9:539–544, 1994.

132. Gibb WR, Narabayashi H, Yocochi M, et al: New pathologic observations in juvenile onset parkinsonism with dystonia. *Neurology* 41:820–822, 1991.

133. Hayashida K, Oyanagi S, Mizutani Y, et al: An early cytoplasmic change before Lewy body maturation: An ultrastructural study of the substantia nigra from an autopsy case of juvenile parkinsonism. *Acta Neuropathol (Berl)* 85:445–448, 1993.

134. Olsson JE, Brunk U, Lindvall B, et al: Dopa-responsive dystonia with depigmentation of the substantia nigra and formation of Lewy bodies. *J Neurol Sci* 112:90–95, 1992.

135. Critchley M: Arteriosclerotic parkinsonism. *Brain* 52:23–83, 1929.

136. Eadie MJ, Sutherland JM: Arteriosclerosis in parkinsonism. *J Neurol Neurosurg Psychiatry* 27:237–240, 1964.

137. Schwab RS, England AC: Parkinson syndromes due to various specific causes, in Vinkin PJ, Bruyn GW (eds): *Handbook in Clinical Neurology*. Amsterdam: North Holland, 1968, pp 227–247.

138. Thompson PD, Marsden CD: Gait disorder of subcortical arteriosclerotic encephalopathy: Binswanger's disease. *Mov Disord* 2:1–8, 1987.

139. Hunter R, Smith J, Thomson T, et al: Hemiparkinson with infarction of the ipsilateral substantia nigra. *Neuropathol Appl Neurobiol* 4:297–301, 1978.

140. Denny-Brown D: The basal ganglia and their relation to disorders of movement. Oxford: Oxford University Press, 1962.

141. Tolosa ES, Santamaria J: Parkinsonism and basal ganglia infarcts. *Neurology* 34:1516–1518, 1984.

142. Mayo J, Arias M, Leno C, et al: Vascular parkinsonism and periarteritis. *Neurology* 36:874–875, 1986.

143. Parkes JD, Marsden CD, Rees JE, et al: Parkinson's disease, cerebral arteriosclerosis, and senile dementia. *Q J Med* 43:49–61, 1974.

144. Friedman A, Kang UJ, Tatemichi TK, et al: A case of parkinsonism following striatal lacunar infarction. *J Neurol Neurosurg Psychiatry* 49:1087–1088, 1986.

145. Fitzgerald PM, Jankovic J: Lower body parkinsonism: Evidence for vascular etiology. *Mov Disord* 4:249–260, 1989.

146. Inzelberg R, Bornstein NM, Reider I, et al: Basal ganglia lacunes and parkinsonism. *Neuroepidemiology* 13:108–112, 1994.

147. Murrow RW, Schweiger GD, Kepes JJ, et al: Parkinsonism due to basal ganglia lacunar state: Clinicopathological study. *Neurology* 40:897–900, 1990.

148. Quinn N, Parkes D, Janota I, et al: Preservation of the substantia nigra and locus ceruleus in a patient receiving L-dopa (2 kg) plus decarboxylase inhibitor over a four-year period. *Mov Disord* 1:65–68, 1986.

149. Nisbet AP, Daniel SE, Lees AJ: Arteriosclerotic parkinsonism. *Brain*. In press, 1996.

150. Gibb WRG: The Lewy body in autonomic failure, in Bannister R (eds): *Autonomic Failure:* Oxford: Oxford University Press, 1988, pp 484–497.

151. Jellinger K, Riederer P, Tomonaga M: Progressive supranuclear palsy: clinico-pathological and biochemical studies. *J Neural Transm* 16 (Suppl):111–128, 1980.

152. Gomori AJ, Sima AAF: An atypical case of progressive supranuclear palsy. *Can J Neurol Sci* 11:48–52, 1984.

153. Iwata K, Hirano A: Current problems in the pathology of amyotrophic lateral sclerosis, in Zimmerman HM (eds): *Progress in Neuropathology*. London: Grune & Stratton, 1979, pp 227–298.

154. Gibb WRG: Neuropathology of movement disorders. *J Neurol Neurosurg Psychiatry* 52 (special suppl):55–67, 1989.

155. DeLeon GA, Grover WD, Huff DS: Neuropathological changes in ataxia-telangiectasia. *Neurology* 26:947–951, 1976.

156. Agamanolis DP, Greenstein JI: Ataxia telangiectasia: Report of a case with Lewy bodies and vascular abnormalities within cerebral tissue. *J Neuropathol Exp Neurol* 38:475–489, 1979.

157. Monaco S, Nardelli E, Moretto G, et al: Cytoskeletal pathology in ataxia telangiectasia. *Clin Neuropathol* 7:44–46, 1988.

158. Hayashi S, Akasaki Y, Morimura Y, et al: An autopsy case of late infantile and juvenile neuroaxonal dystrophy with diffuse Lewy bodies and neurofibrillary tangles. *Clin Neuropathol* 11:1–5, 1992.

159. Gibb WRG, Scaravilli F, Michaud J: Lewy bodies and subacute sclerosing panencephalitis. *J Neurol Neurosurg Psychiatry* 53:710–711, 1990.

160. Sachdev HS, Forno LS, Kane CA: Joseph disease. A multisystem degenerative disorder of the nervous system. *Neurology* 32:192–195, 1982.

161. Gibb WRG, Mountjoy CQ, Mann DMA, et al: A pathological study of the association between Lewy body disease and Alzheimer's disease. *J Neurol Neurosurg Psychiatry* 52:701–708, 1989.

162. Lantos PL, Luthert PJ, Hanger D, et al: Familial Alzheimer's disease with the amyloid precursor protein position 717 mutation and sporadic Alzheimer's disease have the same cytoskeletal pathology. *Neurosci Lett* 137:221–224, 1992.

163. Iihara K, Abe J, Murakami T: Neuronal hyaline inclusions observed in an autopsy case of Behcet's disease. *Acta Pathol Jpn* 42:432–438, 1992.

164. Greenfield JG, Bosanquet FD: The brainstem lesions in parkinsonism. *J Neurol Neurosurg Psychiatry* 16:213–226, 1953.

165. Hartog Jager den WA, Bethlem J: The distribution of Lewy bodies in the central and autonomic nervous systems in idiopathic paralysis agitans. *J Neurol Neurosurg Psychiatry* 23:283–290, 1960.

166. Forno LS, Norville RL: Ultrastructure of Lewy bodies in the stellate ganglion. *Acta Neuropathol (Berl)* 34:183–197, 1976.

167. Langston JW, Forno LS: The hypothalamus in Parkinson's disease. *Ann Neurol* 3:129–133, 1978.

168. Qualman SJ, Haupt HM, Yang P, et al: Esophageal Lewy bodies associated with ganglion cells in achalasia. Similarity to Parkinson's disease. *Gastroenterology* 87:848–856, 1984.

169. Zweig RM, Jankel WR, Hedreen JC, et al: The pedunculopontine nucleus in Parkinson's disease. *Ann Neurol* 26:41–46, 1989.

170. Wakabayashi K, Takahashi H, Ohama E, et al: Parkinson's disease: An immunohistochemical study of Lewy body-containing neurons in the enteric nervous system. *Acta Neuropathol (Berl)* 79:581–583, 1990.

171. Daniel SE, Hawkes CH: Preliminary diagnosis of Parkinson's disease by olfactory bulb pathology. *Lancet* 340:186, 1992.

172. Galloway PG, Grundke I, Iqbal K, et al: Lewy bodies contain epitopes both shared and distinct from Alzheimer neurofibrillary tangles. *J Neuropathol Exp Neurol* 47:654–663, 1988.

173. Kuzuhara S, Mori H, Izumiyama N, et al: Lewy bodies are ubiquinated: A light and electron microscopic immunocyto-chemical study. *Acta Neuropathol (Berl)* 75:345–353, 1988.
174. Nakashima S, Ikuta F: Tyrosine hydroxylase protein in Lewy bodies of parkinsonian and senile brains. *J Neurol Sci* 66:91–96, 1984.
175. Halliday GM, Li YW, Blumbergs PC, et al: Neuropathology of immunohistochemically identified brainstem neurons in Parkinson's disease. *Ann Neurol* 27:373–385, 1990.
176. Gibb WRG, Lees AJ: The relevance of the Lewy body to the pathogenesis of idiopathic Parkinson's disease. *J Neurol Neurosurg Psychiatry* 51:745–752, 1988.
177. Tomonaga M: Neuropathology of the locus ceruleus: A semi-quantitative study. *J Neurol* 230:231–240, 1983.
178. Harkog Jager den WA: Sphingomyelin, in Lewy inclusion bodies in Parkinson's disease. *Arch Neurol* 21:615–619, 1969.

Chapter 19.

PROGRESSIVE SUPRANUCLEAR PALSY

LAWRENCE I. GOLBE

OVERVIEW
HISTORY
    Description
    Previous Descriptions and Nomenclature
DIAGNOSTIC CRITERIA
    Pathological Diagnostic Criteria
    Clinical Diagnostic Criteria
    Differential Diagnosis
NEUROPATHOLOGY, NEUROCHEMISTRY, AND THEIR
   CLINICAL CORRELATES
    Lesion Description
    Anatomic Distribution of Degeneration
EPIDEMIOLOGY AND ETIOLOGY
    Descriptive Epidemiology
    Analytic Epidemiology
    Is There a Hereditary Component?
TREATMENT
    Pharmacotherapy
    Nonpharmacological Therapy
PATIENT RESOURCES

Overview

The first clinicopathological descriptions of progressive supranuclear palsy (PSP) to draw widespread attention were published in 1963 and 1964.[1-3] Since then, PSP has evolved from a condition interesting or accessible to few researchers except for neuropathologists to one that intrigues every neurology resident and can be recognized by every practicing neurologist. However, PSP has yet to emerge from the realm of "degenerative" disorders with mysterious etiology, unclear pathogenesis, and elusive treatment.

Part of the fascination of PSP is its clinical phenomenology. The full-blown, typical case is at once unusually complex in its combination of motor and behavioral features and so distinctive that the diagnosis is unmistakable at a glance. PSP is also biologically intriguing, because it is both a disorder of basal ganglia dopaminergic function, like Parkinson's disease (PD), and a neurofibrillary tangle (NFT) disorder, like Alzheimer's disease (AD). Indeed, much of our knowledge of PSP has been gleaned from studies that used PSP as a foil against which to study the far more prevalent PD or AD.

This chapter, when possible, will emphasize differential diagnosis and clinicopathological correlation. Rather than catalogue present scientific knowledge of PSP, it will empha-

size that which is most germane to current attempts to untangle the etiology and pathogenesis of the condition.

PRESENTING FEATURES

Gait disturbance, often with unheralded falls, is the presenting feature in more than 60 percent of cases.[4-5] In contrast, PD presents with gait disturbance in only 11 percent.[6] The falls may prompt a workup for vestibulopathy, myelopathy, basilar artery ischemia, cardiac syncope, or epilepsy. In most cases, the gait disturbance is accompanied by enough bradykinesia and/or rigidity to prompt a misdiagnosis of PD.

Perhaps the next most common presenting feature is a nonspecific change in personality. Mental and physical slowness, irritability, social withdrawal, or fatigability[7] are usually interpreted by the patient as normal aging. The rare patients for whom medical attention is sought at this point typically receive a diagnosis of primary depression or AD.

In the minority of patients who present with gaze palsy, dysarthria, or dysphagia, the initial workup may embark on a search for myasthenia gravis, progressive bulbar palsy, or local causes of esophageal dysmotility. Cataract extraction may be performed in a futile effort to correct the nonrefractible visual deficit of early, unrecognized supranuclear gaze fixation instability.

FULL-BLOWN PICTURE

In its full-blown clinical picture, PSP will not be confused with other illnesses. There can be little diagnostic doubt in a patient with a progressive syndrome of astasia, erect posture with retrocollis, contracted facial muscles, predominantly proximal rigidity and bradykinesia, predominantly vertical supranuclear gaze abnormality, spastic dysarthria, dangerous dysphagia, and behavioral abnormalities referable disproportionately to frontal lobe dysfunction. The illness progresses to an immobile state over less than a decade in most patients.[4,5]

PSP VERSUS PD

The most important points by which PSP can be differentiated from PD in the clinic, sometimes at a glance, are the contracted rather than flaccid facies, undirected rather than staring gaze, erect rather than flexed posture, dysarthria that is spastic and ataxic rather than hypophonic, and absence of rest tremor. Careful history and examination typically reveal a history of poor response to dopaminergic treatment (a common reason for the patient's referral), pseudobulbar affect, prominent square-wave jerks, slow or hypometric saccades in the upward or downward directions, unexpectedly mild rigidity in the wrists and elbows, and unexpectedly mild bradykinesia of the fingers (Table 19-1).

ATYPICAL FEATURES

Cases departing from this typical picture are common. Some patients with PSP have prominent dementia suggestive of AD.[8] Others have asymmetric apraxia or dystonia suggestive of cortical basal ganglionic degeneration,[9,10] and others resemble PD or striatonigral degeneration until late in the illness, when clear vertical supranuclear gaze abnormalities finally

TABLE 19-1 Median Actuarially Adjusted Interval from Initial Symptom to Onset of Disease Milestones in PSP

Initial Symptom	Years
Initial gait difficulty	0.3
Cane or helper needed to walk	3.1
Dysarthria	3.4
Visual symptoms	3.9
Dysphagia	4.4
Confined to bed or wheelchair	8.2
Death	9.7

SOURCE: Data obtained by retrospective interview of patient and family (from Golbe et al.[4]).

appear. Even findings such as moderate asymmetry and mild rest tremor, claimed by earlier authors to virtually exclude PSP, occurred in 2 of 12 pathologically confirmed cases in a recent series.[11] Another autopsy series[12] found asymmetric onset in 3 of 16 cases.

History

DESCRIPTION

The seminal 1964 description of Steele et al.[3] arose in the clinical experience of J. Clifford Richardson at Toronto's Sunnybrook Military Hospital during the 1950s and later at Toronto General Hospital. Jerzy Olszewski of Toronto's Banting Institute contributed the pathological observations. Richardson encouraged his resident, John C. Steele, to assist in gathering and reporting the data on the seven autopsied patients.[13]

After the initial public presentation of the cases of 1963 by Steele et al.,[1] authorities such as Merritt, Schwab, Denny-Brown, and others admitted that they had never seen similar cases (R.C. Duvoisin, personal communication). Within a few years, however, patients with PSP were being recognized at many centers, and by 1972, Steele[14] was able to review 73 reported cases from many parts of the world.

PREVIOUS DESCRIPTIONS AND NOMENCLATURE

In retrospect, 13 cases, 6 of which included autopsy confirmation, were published between 1904 and 1964.[15] Steele et al. cite many of these[3] and acknowledge that many earlier patients with PSP, even those with autopsy, may have been misinterpreted as clinical variants of postencephalitic parkinsonism (PEP). The remoteness of the 1960s from the encephalitis lethargica epidemics of earlier decades may have allowed recognition of PSP as a new disease. The eponym "Steele-Richardson-Olszewski syndrome" was first applied to PSP in 1965 by a fellow Canadian, Barbeau,[16] who chose the order of authors in the last of the three publications[1–3] describing virtually the same patients. This eponym has since become the standard term for PSP in much of Europe. Its failure to reach more widespread use may be the result not only of its multiplicity of syllables, but also of a desire not to minimize the contributions of those who described the illness earlier.[15]

Diagnostic Criteria

PATHOLOGICAL DIAGNOSTIC CRITERIA

An international workshop of eight neuropathologists, convened by Litvan in 1993,[17] reached consensus on neuropathological criteria for the diagnosis of PSP. The deliberations were based in part on the results of 104 autopsies of patients with detailed clinical histories suggestive of PSP or of competing considerations, such as multiple-system atrophy (MSA), PD, diffuse Lewy body disease, cortical basal ganglionic degeneration (CBDG), Pick's disease, Creutzfeldt-Jakob disease, AD, dentatorubropallidoluysian atrophy, Parkinson-dementia complex of Guam and PEP. They formulated criteria that would delineate a reasonably unitary clinicopathological group.

The autopsy criteria[17] for "typical PSP" and "atypical PSP" appear in Table 19-2. One may argue that the latter would be more appropriately called "possible," rather than "atypical." The major departure of these pathological criteria from those used informally in the literature is the recognition that discriminating PSP from the other diagnostic possibilities requires not only a qualitative presence of neurofibrillary tangles (NFTs) and neuropil threads in certain parts of the basal ganglia and brain stem but also a semiquantitative assessment of their density in those areas.

CLINICAL DIAGNOSTIC CRITERIA

Several sets of clinical diagnostic criteria have been published, none validated by formal correlation with autopsy results, even in retrospect. Diagnostic criteria to be used in an epidemiological study must balance sensitivity and specificity, but a treatment trial demands very high specificity, even at the cost of loss of some patients with true but atypical PSP. A set that was formulated for use in settings that permit detailed examination of patients appears in Table 19-3. This would be suitable for drug trials or for small epidemiological studies in which an experienced neurologist visits each patient. It would not be suitable when only medical records, possibly from inexperienced examiners, are available.

DIFFERENTIAL DIAGNOSIS

COMPETING CONSIDERATIONS
Every published or proposed set of diagnostic criteria specifies or assumes that patients with positive evidence for competing diagnostic entities be disqualified from a diagnosis of PSP. This leaves much to the examiner's judgment. For a neuropathologist with access to the full range of modern, but routine, histopathological techniques, the principal entities competing with PSP are only cortical basal ganglionic degeneration (CBGD), PEP, and PDC. Only the first of these is a realistic possibility, given a history compatible with PSP. The clinician must contend with a longer list that includes some cases of PD, CBGD,[18] MSA (principally striatonigral degeneration but also olivopontocerebellar atrophy),[19] progressive subcortical gliosis,[20] Creutzfeldt-Jakob disease,[21] AD with

TABLE 19-2 Pathological Criteria for the Diagnosis of PSP

A. Typical PSP

at ×250 magnification:

1) At least two neurons with NFTs or neuropil threads must occur in the same field in at least three of the following four areas:
   Pallidum
   Subthalamic nucleus
   Substantia nigra
   Pons

and

2) At least one such neuron in at least three of the following four areas:
   Striatum
   Oculomotor complex
   Medulla
   Dentate

B. Atypical PSP

At least one such neuron in at least five of the following six areas:
   Pallidum
   Subthalamic nucleus
   Substantia nigra
   Pons
   Medulla
   Dentate

C. To exclude other conditions, the stains must include at least the following:

   Hematoxylin-eosin *plus* a silver stain
   or
   Hematoxylin-eosin *plus* tau *plus* ubiquitin

SOURCE: *From Hauw et al.[17] Used with permission.*

parkinsonism, diffuse Lewy-body disease,[22] Pick's disease, and the primary pallidal atrophies, including dentatorubro-pallidoluysian atrophy.[23] Some clinical points by which PSP can be differentiated from some of the most common of these entities appears in Table 19-4.

Perhaps the most difficult differentiation of PSP is from MSA. One recent study[17] found that certain clinical features could distinguish MSA from PD with acceptable certainty, but that they could not distinguish MSA from PSP in the absence of specific signs such as downgaze palsy or extensor axial dystonia.

Nondegenerative diseases that can mimic PSP are a multi-infarct state, the most common such condition; Whipple's disease, which can cause vertical supranuclear gaze abnormality and parkinsonism; mitochondrial myopathies, which can cause eye muscle weakness and a variety of movement abnormalities;[24] Wilson's disease, which generally occurs at a younger age than PSP; and adult-onset Niemann-Pick disease type C, which can cause gaze palsies, rigidity, loss of manual dexterity, and dementia in young adults.

CLINICAL EVALUATION
A thorough clinical examination and history will generally reveal PEP, PDC, myasthenia gravis (as a cause of gaze palsy, dysarthria, and dysphagia), mitochondrial myopathy (as a cause of gaze palsy), and bulbar amyotrophic lateral sclerosis. Magnetic resonance imaging (MRI) or x-ray computed to-

mography (CT) will reveal, although not necessarily incriminate, mimics such as hydrocephalus,[25] midbrain tumors, and a multi-infarct state. Lacunar states can reproduce virtually the full range of clinical features of PSP, as they can the features of AD and PD.[26–28] This may be suspected in the patient with stepwise progression, marked pyramidal signs, focal weakness and, as mentioned, ischemic changes on MRI or CT.

RADIOLOGICAL EVALUATION
Positron emission tomography (PET), using ^{18}F-fluorodopa, distinguished 90 percent of patients with clinically diagnosed PSP, in which both caudate and putamen showed decreased tracer uptake, from a group with PD, in which the abnormality was largely confined to putamen.[29] However, the sensitivity and specificity of PET in distinguishing patients with clinically equivocal or early PSP from other conditions has not been assessed. For this reason, fluorodopa PET is not yet considered a standard diagnostic tool in PSP. The cost of that technology is a separate problem that would limit the use of PET in PSP to research settings for the foreseeable future.

MRI and CT imaging are nonspecific in most cases of PSP (Table 19-5). In the moderate-to-advanced stages, they may reveal thinning of the anteroposterior diameter of the midbrain tectum and tegmentum with atrophy of the colliculi and disproportionate enlargement of the sylvian fissures and posterior third ventricle.[30–35] MRI may show high signal in

TABLE 19-3 Proposed Diagnostic Criteria for PSP

All of these:
  Onset at age 40 or later
  Progressive course
  Bradykinesia
  Supranuclear gaze palsy, per criteria below
Plus any three of these:
  Dysarthria or dysphagia
  Neck rigidity (to flexion/extension) greater than limb rigidity
  Neck in a posture of extension
  Minimal or absent tremor
  Frequent falls or gait disturbance early in course
Without any of these:
  Early or prominent cerebellar signs
  Unexplained polyneuropathy
  Prominent noniatrogenic dysautonomia other than isolated
    postural hypotension

Criteria for Supranuclear Gaze Palsy:
EITHER:
Both of these:
  Voluntary downgaze less than 15 degrees (tested by instructing
    patient to "look down" without presenting a specific
    target; accept the best result after several attempts)
  Preserved horizontal oculocephalic reflexes (except in very
    advanced stages)
OR all three of these:
  Slowed downward saccades (defined as slow enough for the
    examiner to perceive the movement itself)
  Impaired opticokinetic nystagmus with the stimulus moving
    downward
  Poor voluntary suppression of vertical vestibulo-ocular reflex

With relatively high specificity for use in studies in which subjects can be examined by a neurologist experienced in evaluating eye movements.

the periaqueductal gray compatible with gliotic change, a nonspecific finding in the parkinsonian syndromes. As is the case with PET imaging, the value of MRI and CT in the early, diagnostically doubtful case is not established, except to rule out nondegenerative pathology or to rule out cerebellar atrophy that would direct suspicion toward olivopontocerebellar atrophy as the diagnosis.

A similar challenge faces the use of single-photon emission computed tomography (SPECT), using markers of cerebral blood flow and/or metabolism. Such studies show bifrontal hypometabolism in established PSP[36-38] and have yet to be evaluated in equivocal cases. However, SPECT imaging of D2 receptor sites, using ^{123}I-iodobenzamide (IBZM) is promising as a means of differentiating PSP, where there is often detectable striatal D2 loss, from PD, where there is not.[39,40]

Neuropathology, Neurochemistry, and Their Clinical Correlates

PSP is one of the NFT diseases. This group's best-known member is AD, but it also includes Pick's disease, PEP, PDC, CBGD, Down's syndrome, and dementia pugilistica. The distribution and morphology of the NFT's and the distribution of accompanying neuronal loss and gliosis help the patholo-

TABLE 19-4 Clinical Points Differentiating PSP from Some Other Parkinsonian Disorders

	PSP	PD	MSA (SD)	CBGD
Symmetry of deficit	+ + +	+	+ + +	−
Axial rigidity	+ + +	+ +	+ +	+ +
Limb dystonia	+	+	+	+ + +
Postural instability	+ + +	+ +	+ +	+
Vertical supranuclear gaze restriction	+ + +	+	+ +	+ +
Frontal behavior	+ + +	+	+	+ +
Dysautonomia	−	+	+ +	−
L-dopa response early in course	+	+ + +	+	−
L-dopa response late in course	−	+ +	+	−
Asymmetric cortical atrophy on MRI	−	−	−	+ +

SD, Shy-Drager; −, absent or rare; +, occasional, mild, or late; + +, usual, moderate; + + +, usual, severe, or early.

gist differentiate these diseases. However, wide variability in PSP and the other conditions produces overlap in the pathological pictures. This overlap suggests commonalities of pathogenesis among these conditions and may even raise questions regarding their separation as unitary diseases, if we define "disease" at the histopathological and histochemical level. Definitive nosology awaits analysis at the molecular and etiologic levels.

Dopaminergic damage in the nigrostriatal pathway and cholinergic damage in many areas are the most consistent, severe neurotransmitter-related changes in PSP.[41-44] Gamma-aminobutyric acid (GABAergic) function of the basal ganglia (in striatum and globus pallidus pars interna (GPi) and globus pallidus pars externa (GPe)) is moderately but widely impaired.[45] Unlike the case in PD, the peptidergic systems and the mesolimbic and mesocortical dopaminergic systems are intact.[46] Serotonergic receptor sites are somewhat reduced in the cortex, but unlike in PD, are normal in basal ganglia.[46] The loss of adrenoceptors is widespread,[47] reflecting the wide projections of the often severely damaged locus ceruleus.

LESION DESCRIPTION

NEUROFIBRILLARY TANGLES
Although neuronal loss and gliosis are the most prominent microanatomic features of PSP and their characteristic anatomic distribution can produce suspicion of PSP, the diagnosis cannot be made in the absence of NFTs. Although most of the NFTs of most brains with PSP have a rounded ("globose") shape, a few are "flame-shaped." This situation is reversed in AD and seems to relate more closely to the structure of the neuron containing the NFT than to the disease producing the damage.[48]

Ultrastructure
The filaments composing the NFTs of PSP are unpaired straight filaments 15–18 nm in diameter, comprised of at

TABLE 19-5 MRI Features of PSP and Some Other Conditions

	PSP	PD	MSA (OPCA)	MSA (SD)	CBGD	AD
Cortical atrophy	+ +	+	+ / −	+	+ + / −	+ +
Putaminal atrophy	−	−	−	+ +	−	−
Pontine atrophy	+	−	+ + +	−	+ / −	−
Midbrain atrophy	+ +	−	+	−	+ / −	−
Cerebellar atrophy	−	−	+ + / −	−	−	−
High putaminal iron	−	−	+ / −	+ / −	−	−

OPCA, olivopontocerebellar atrophy; −, absent or rare; +, occasional, mild or late; + +, usual, moderate; + + +, usual, severe, or early.

least six protofilaments 2–5 nm in diameter.[49–53] Filaments of AD, by contrast, are mostly paired helical filaments 22 nm in diameter with a minor component of straight filaments similar to that of PSP.[54] A few cortical areas in PSP, or even subcortical nuclei, may display paired helical filaments of the Alzheimer type.[55,56] Paired straight filaments and unpaired twisted filaments, which may be a sign of a more advanced stage of filament formation, also occur occasionally in PSP.[56]

The immunostaining and ultrastructural properties of the filaments of PSP tangles are nearly identical to those of CBGD.[56,57] However, the white matter tangles of CBGD occur in oligodendroglia, rather than in astrocytes, as in most[58] but not all[59] cases of PSP.

Tau Protein
Cortical FTs of PSP appear to be antigenically identical to those of AD, most notably with regard to the presence of abnormally phosphorylated tau protein.[60–63] Tau is a low-molecular-weight component of microtubule-associated protein. The latter is involved in axonal transport of vesicles. PSP tau exhibits bands on Western blot of 64 and 69 kD, whereas AD and Down's syndrome tau has those two bands, plus one of 55 kD.[64,65] In CBGD, tau is chemically similar to that of PSP but is located in the axon, rather than in the cell body as in PSP (DW Dickson, personal communication).

Staining with anti-tau antibody greatly aids the identification of NFTs in PSP and has largely replaced silver stains and hematoxylin and eosin for this purpose, at least in the research setting. Anti-tau staining has revealed the existence of neuropil threads, also known as curly fibers, in the same neurons that include NFTs and in oligodendroglia of white matter tracts connecting affected areas of subcortical gray matter.[66–68] Most neuropil threads of AD, on the other hand, occur in neurons, sparing glia. Staining for ubiquitin, a peptide involved in proteolysis and occurring in NFTs of AD and Lewy bodies of PD, is weak or variable in the NFTs of PSP.[69]

OTHER CHANGES
Grumose degeneration, in which eosinophilic material surrounds degenerating neurons, accompanied by spherical argentophilic components, occurs in a significant minority of cases with PSP, particularly in the cerebellar dentate nucleus.[2,70,71] It appears to be comprised of abnormally regenerated synaptic terminal material of Purkinje cells. Grumose degeneration of the dentate occurs also in dentatorubropallidoluysian atrophy, a condition with more obvious ataxia than occurs in PSP.

The swollen, achromatic neurons characteristic of CBGD and Pick's disease occur in a few cases of otherwise typical PSP, generally in tegmental and inferior temporal areas.[72]

Although amyloid or senile plaques do not occur in PSP, another hallmark of AD, granulovacuolar degeneration, does occur to a mild extent. The overlap of PSP with AD is further illustrated by a recent series of 13 autopsies with the full pathological picture of PSP.[73] Of the 13, 4 also exhibited pathological changes of "definite AD," and 2 had "probable AD." A primary clinical diagnosis of AD with memory loss as the first neurological symptom was present in two of these six and in three of the seven without AD pathology.

ANATOMIC DISTRIBUTION OF DEGENERATION

The major areas of primary involvement in PSP, together with an oversimplified but convenient scheme of their clinical correlates, are the cerebral cortex, producing cognitive and behavioral changes; the nigrostriatopallidal area, producing rigidity, bradykinesia, and postural instability; the cholinergic pontomesencephalic nuclei area, producing gaze palsies, sleep disturbances, and axial motor abnormalities; and the hindbrain area, producing dysarthria and dysphagia. The daunting complexity of this syndrome, the interactions of its parts, and its tremendous interpatient variability may be the principal reason for the continuing resistance of PSP to pathophysiological understanding and pharmacological intervention.

CEREBRAL CORTEX

Pathoanatomy
The marked central and cortical atrophy of cerebrum seen on gross postmortem examination in AD is only mild in PSP. Early studies of PSP found little microscopic pathology in cerebral cortex, but the advent of tau immunostaining has permitted identification of the motor strip (Area 4) and a partly ocular motor association area (Area 39) as the most important sites of pathology.[74–76] Many other cortical areas are affected but much less severely. The least affected area appears to be the primary visual cortex (Area 17), as is the case in AD.[77] The affection of the motor area of cortex may be secondary to the severe degeneration of subcortical areas, such as the subthalamic nucleus, which project to cortex.[78]

PSP affects the large pyramidal and small neurons of layers V and VI, whereas AD affects the medium-sized neurons of layers III and V.[74,79,80] Cortical involvement in PSP, therefore, differs importantly from that in AD at the gyral, laminar, cytological, ultrastructural, and biochemical levels.

Frontal Lobes

Behavioral changes were the initial symptom of PSP in 22 percent of patients in one series[4] that used family interview data and in 2 of 24 (8 percent) in a series with autopsy confirmation and good clinical records (I. Litvan, personal communication). Disabling mental changes eventually occur in 80 percent or more of cases.[5,81]

ANATOMIC AND EUROCHEMICAL CHANGES The prefrontal areas, which are the most obviously affected by behavioral testing and by measures of cerebral blood flow,[36–38,82–85] display relatively little neurofibrillary pathology or neuronal loss in PSP.[74,77] This suggests that in PSP, secondary cortical dysfunction is caused by subcortical pathology, as in the cholinergic nucleus basalis of Meynert and the cholinergic pedunculopontine nucleus (PPN), both important and relatively constant sites of involvement.[86–88] The situation is not quite that simple, however, because in PSP, unlike in PD, clinical dementia does not correlate with the degree of reduction in choline acetyltransferase activity.[42,89] Damage to the striatopallidal complex may also contribute to dementia via reduction of its output to the frontal lobes.[14,78,90]

CLINICAL CORRELATES The clinical frontal lobe dysfunction of PSP can be striking. Intellectual slowing and impairment of "executive" functions, related to slowed central sensory processing, are consistent, albeit nonspecific findings.[91–92] Tests of reaction time that control for motor slowing show that the cognitive component of such tasks is greatly prolonged in PSP, approximately 50 percent longer than in PD.[93] It is a common clinical observation that the patient with PSP can supply correct answers to complex questions after a delay of several minutes.

Examples of the executive dysfunction are difficulty shifting between mental tasks and in tests of sorting and of verbal fluency.[94–97] Other examining room tasks that can reveal a frontal defect are the ability to perform an action (e.g., tapping once) when the examiner performs a slightly different one (e.g., tapping twice), as well as the ability, when confronted by the examiner's widely separated hands, to direct horizontal gaze toward the hand that does not wave, the "antisaccade task."

Spontaneous frontal motor behaviors can also be dramatic in some patients with PSP.[95,98] When combined with symmetric, nontremorous parkinsonism, they may be relatively specific for PSP. Most obvious are palilalia,[96] imitative behavior (such as mimicking the examiner's hand movements), and motor perseveration (as when unable to cease clapping after being asked to imitate the examiner's three handclaps—the "applause sign"), motor grasping (often for the arm or clothing of the examiner), and visual grasping (often mimicking gaze palsy).

Hippocampus

The hippocampus, a primary site of pathology in AD, is involved in only one-half of patients with PSP.[99] This probably explains the relative preservation of memory, except

for tasks requiring frontally mediated memory searching.[8,100] The qualitative anatomic pattern of involvement of the hippocampus in PSP, however, is similar to that in AD and PD.[76] The qualitative clinical pattern of memory impairment is similar to that of PD and Huntington's disease and different from that in AD, where forgetting is more rapid than in PSP.[101]

NIGROSTRIATAL SYSTEM

Distribution of Pathology

Damage to the pigmented neurons of the zona compacta of the substantia nigra, the most consistent abnormality in PSP, occurs in a different distribution than is the case in PD.[102] In PSP, the damage is relatively uniform, except for relative sparing of a small, extreme lateral portion, whereas in PD, both the dorsal and extreme lateral portions are relatively spared. The dorsal portion projects principally to the caudate, the ventral to the putamen. This probably explains the relative sparing of presynaptic caudate dopamine reuptake in PD and its involvement in PSP, as measured by 18F-fluoro-dopa PET.[29,103]

In the striatum, there is also severe loss of acetylcholinergic activity,[43] although the majority of affected striatal cells appear to be astrocytes, rather than neurons ("tufted" astrocytes).[63] They include tau-positive, argyrophilic NFTs, and neuropil threads similar to those in affected neurons. Such astrocytic pathology may be unique to PSP.

Most of the few affected striatal neurons are probably cholinergic interneurons.[44,104,105] It is unclear whether the poor response of the parkinsonian components of PSP to dopamine replacement therapy and the relative resistance of PSP to the hyperkinetic side effects of such therapy are the result of pathology in the striatum or further downstream in the striatal system. It is also unclear whether the loss of the cholinergic striatal interneurons explains the failure of anticholinergic treatment (relative to its success in PD) and the hints of improvement from cholinergic treatment.[106]

As one would predict given the paucity of striatal neuronal damage, there is no loss of postsynaptic dopamine D1 receptors, as measured by binding studies and by D1 receptor mRNA levels.[46] Similarly, density of D2 receptors is probably normal or only slightly decreased.[46,107,108]

Clinical Course

Postural instability, often with falls ("paroxysmal dysequilibrium"), is the initial symptom in approximately two-thirds of patients with PSP.[4,5] It starts a mean of 1.8 years after disease onset[80] and often has a more irregular, ataxic quality than the gait of PD. Occasionally, the initial or only gait abnormality is severe gait "freezing" or "apraxia"[109–112] with no rigidity.

The postural instability is usually the most disabling feature of later PSP. The median intervals from initial symptom, corrected by the Kaplan-Meier lifetable method, are 3.1 years until assistance is required and 8.2 years until wheelchair confinement.[4]

Contrary to widespread impression, rest tremor does occur in PSP, in about 5 to 10 percent of patients, usually early in the course.[113,114] Action or postural tremor occurs in about 25 percent. The limb rigidity and distal bradykinesia are mild relative to axial rigidity and bradykinesia. The rigidity tends to increase from wrist to elbow to shoulder.

OTHER BASAL GANGLIA

Subthalamic Nucleus

Damage to the subthalamic nucleus ranks beside that of the substantia nigra as a constant in PSP and is far more specific to PSP. Subthalamic neuronal depletion is so severe that the posteroinferior portion of the third ventricle may be disproportionately dilated on CT or MRI.[30] This can give the third ventricle the shape of a bowling pin on axial imaging, contrasting with the cigar shape characteristic of AD.

GPi

The basal ganglia damage furthest "downstream" and, therefore, perhaps the most relevant therapeutically is in the GPi. This structure acts as the common outflow pathway from the basal ganglia to the thalamus. This lesion is not quite as constant as that of the substantia nigra or subthalamic nucleus, but it probably explains the failure of stereotactic GPi lesions, which are therapeutic in PD, to ameliorate PSP (E Fazzini, personal communication). Similarly, the outflow function of the GPi probably explains the therapeutic failure of fetal mesencephalic implantation into the striatum in PSP.

Pedunculopontine Nucleus

Despite the status of the GABAergic GPi (and the partly GABAergic substantia nigra reticulata) as the final outflow from the basal ganglia, and despite low GABAergic activity in many parts of the basal ganglia, efforts to treat PSP with the GABAergic drug valproic acid have failed.[115] Part of the explanation as to why this is so may be that the GPi projects not only to the thalamus, which is nearly intact in PSP, but also to the cholinergic PPN, which is severely affected.[87,88,116] There is evidence that lesions of the PPN alone can cause severe postural instability.[117] Nevertheless, GABA agonists more selective for basal ganglia function should be tested in PSP.

Others

The GPe, ventral tegmental area, red nucleus, intralaminar nuclei of the thalamus, and locus ceruleus are also involved in PSP, although not as constantly or severely as the foregoing areas. The reported slight therapeutic benefit (mostly to gait) of a noradrenergic drug, idazoxan,[118] suggests that the locus ceruleus pathology may play a pivotal role.

Experimental lesions of the interstitial nucleus of Cajal in monkeys produce extensor rigidity at the neck and postural instability,[119] and this nucleus is characteristically affected in PSP.[120] However, the severe damage in the striatopallidal pathway could also help explain the unusual extensor tone of PSP.[121]

MESENCEPHALIC AND PONTINE OCULAR MOTOR AREAS

Pathoanatomy

The predominantly vertical supranuclear gaze palsy presumably originates in the rostral midbrain, where there is variable involvement of the interstitial nucleus of Cajal, the nucleus of Darkshewitsch, the rostral interstitial nucleus of the medial longitudinal fasciculus, and the mesencephalic reticular formation.[78,87,120,122] Their relative contributions to the clinical deficit have not been sorted out. There have been cases of damage to some of these nuclei in patients without clinical supranuclear gaze abnormality.[123–126] Conversely, there is one report of PSP-like gaze palsy in idiopathic calcification of basal ganglia in which the dorsal midbrain was spared.[127]

Some of the vertical paresis may result from subselective involvement of these nuclei themselves, followed by nuclear ocular paresis at the end stage of PSP in some cases. The horizontal gaze palsy that appears eventually in most cases is attributable to degeneration of nuclei of the pontine base.[128] The ocular motor cranial nerve nuclei are perhaps the sole example of cholinergic nuclei to escape important involvement in PSP.

Clinical Phenomenology

VOLUNTARY GAZE   Symptomatic eye movement difficulty does not begin until a median of 3.9 years after disease onset, nearly half of the clinical course.[4] Before that time, however, most patients with otherwise diagnosable PSP will exhibit slowing of vertical saccades, saccadic pursuit, breakdown of opticokinetic nystagmus in the vertical plane, disordered Bell's phenomenon, poor convergence, and subtle square-wave jerks (SWJs).[129–131] (Table 19-6) The last finding has perhaps the greatest sensitivity for PSP, occurring in all or nearly all patients with PSP.[131,132] SWJs occur in very few patients with PD but are sufficiently common in MSA and other conditions that they cannot be used to differentiate them from PSP.[132]

The frontal dysfunction[133] is expressed via such ocular motor phenomena as visual prehension and poor performance on the antisaccade task. Here, the patient quickly directs the gaze to the examiner's hand that does *not* move. An altitudinal visual attentional deficit,[134] arising from damaged tectal centers, may contribute to overloading the fork, poor aim of the urinary stream, and poor attention to dress out of

TABLE 19-6 Sensitivity and Specificity of Some Ocular Motor Abnormalities in Early PSP

Symptom	Sensitivity	Specificity
Supranuclear downgaze paresis alone	+	+ +
Supranuclear upgaze paresis alone	+	−
Slow downward saccades alone	+ +	+ +
Square-wave jerks	+ + +	+ +
Poor voluntary suppression of horizontal VOR (vertical normal)	+ + +	−
Poor voluntary suppression of vertical VOR (horizontal normal)	+	+ + +
"Apraxia" of lid opening	−	+ + +
Blepharospasm	+	−

Sensitivity is the percentage of patients with PSP who exhibit the sign; specificity is the percentage of patients without PSP who do not exhibit the sign. −, minimally or not useful; +, slightly useful; + +, moderately useful; + + +, highly useful.

proportion to dementia. In addition, patients with PSP seem less aware of their postural instability than do patients with other causes of the same degree of instability.

Later in the course, the patient loses range of vertical gaze, with downgaze usually, but far from always, worse than upgaze. Voluntary gaze without a specific target (i.e., "look down") is usually worse than command gaze to target, which is worse than pursuit, and reflex gaze is by far the least affected.

REFLEX GAZE   From the earliest stages, most patients also suffer loss of the ability to voluntarily suppress the horizontal vestibulo-ocular reflex (VOR).[135] This may be tested by seating the patient in a swivel chair or wheelchair and asking him to extend the arms at the level of the eyes, clasp his hands, and fixate on one thumbnail as the examiner slowly rotates the chair and patient en bloc. Patients with PSP (and many other basal ganglia disorders) are unable to suppress the opticokinetic nystagmus produced by relative movement of the environment. Disproportionate difficulty in suppressing vertical VOR (if the axial rigidity allows it to be tested) may be a valuable clue to the presence of very early PSP.

EYELID MOVEMENT   Eyelid movement abnormalities, particularly apraxia of eyelid opening and blepharospasm occur in about one-third of patients and can cause functional blindness.[136–139] Apraxia of lid closing and the very slow blink rate of PSP (often less than 5 blinks/minute) can allow conjunctival drying with annoying reactive inflammation and lacrimation.

Brain Stem Centers Controlling Sleep and Arousal

SLEEP DISTURBANCE   Sleep disturbance is a prominent abnormality in PSP. It is presumably related principally to damage to the (serotonergic) raphe nuclei, the (cholinergic) PPN and others, the (noradrenergic) locus ceruleus, and the periaqueductal gray. The most important clinical component is a severe reduction in rapid eye movement (REM) sleep.[140] There is a loss of sleep spindles and K complexes. During what REM sleep remains, there are abnormal slow waves and absence of normal sawtooth waves.[141]

THE AUDITORY STARTLE AND AUDITORY BLINK REFLEXES The auditory startle and auditory blink reflexes are absent or severely impaired in PSP,[142] despite normal auditory evoked potentials[143] and electrical blink reflex.[142] Startle is mediated via the lower pontine reticular formation, in particular the nucleus reticularis pontis caudalis, which degenerates in PSP.

BRAIN STEM CENTERS CONTROLLING SPEECH AND SWALLOWING

Dysarthria

Steele et al.[3] were referring to the lower brain stem functions as much as to the eye movements in applying the term "supranuclear palsy." Indeed, degeneration of the cranial nerve nuclei in PSP is generally mild.[144] Likewise, the dysarthria of PSP features no lower motor neuron components. Rather,

it is a variable combination of, in descending order of importance, spasticity, hypophonia, and ataxia.[145] The combination is unique among the competing diagnostic considerations, at least from a statistical standpoint (Table 19-7). The slow rate of speech with a strained and strangled quality and some hyperkinetic, ataxic components is highly specific for PSP.

Dysarthria can be an early symptom that often brings the patient to a physician.[5] Within 2 years after disease onset, 41 percent of patients (or their families) have detected dysarthria. By the 5th year, the figure is 68 percent.[4]

Dysphagia

Relative to the morbidity it causes, the dysphagia of PSP has received only little and belated research attention. Aspiration pneumonia is a major risk in advanced PSP, but only 18 percent of patients report symptomatic dysphagia within 2 years after PSP onset, and 46 percent do so by 5 years.[4]

In one study[146] that performed videofluoroscopy in 22 patients with mild-to-moderate PSP with symptomatic dysphagia, at least 80 percent of patients exhibited abnormalities attributable to parkinsonian rigidity of the oral and pharyngeal muscles. Esophageal problems occurred in fewer than one-half of patients, and nasal reflux occurred in none. Only one patient (4.5 percent) aspirated contrast material, but 27 percent coughed or choked.

It is common for patients with PSP, but not with PD, to exaggerate the effects of dysphagia by overloading the fork, probably through a combination of poor downgaze, frontal disinhibition, and inferior-field visual inattention.[147] The neck hyperextension that occurs eventually in some patients with PSP may decrease the ability of the epiglottis to protect the airway. However, relative to patients with PD, those with PSP appear more aware of their dysphagia and have less rigidity and tremor of the tongue, major causes of dysphagia in PD.[146]

SPINAL AND AUTONOMIC CENTERS

PSP includes less dysautonomia than PD,[148] a point useful in its clinical differentiation from MSA. Nevertheless, there can be disabling bladder dysfunction,[149] which is probably the result of the mild gray matter tract degeneration in the spinal cord.[78] In one series,[80] urinary incontinence occurred in 42 percent of patients, beginning a mean of 3.5 years into the disease course.

TABLE 19-7 Components of Dysarthria in PSP and Some Related Conditions

	Hypokinesia	Ataxia	Spasticity
PSP	+ +	+	+ + +
PD	+ + +	−	−
MSA (striatonigral degeneration)	+ + +	+ +	+
MSA (olivoponto-cerebellar atrophy)	+	+ + +	+ +

−, absent; +, mild; + +, moderate; + + +, marked.
SOURCE: *Data are from Kluin et al.*[145]

Epidemiology and Etiology

The multiplicity of pathoanatomic lesions in PSP makes prevention or arrest of the disease process unlikely to be found at that level. A more fruitful avenue is probably to identify a necessary etiologic agent, be it genetic or environmental, or to identify a basic molecular mechanism. The pathological similarities between PSP and PEP point to a postviral etiology, and the similarities to PDC suggest an environmental toxin.[150] Either agent could interact with a genetic factor.

DESCRIPTIVE EPIDEMIOLOGY

ONSET AGE

In most series, PSP begins, on average, in the late 50s to mid-60s, as is the case for PD. The earliest-onset autopsy-proven case began at age 43,[15] and about one-third of cases begin before age 60.[4] The standard deviation of the onset age is typically 6–7 years,[4] far less than the 10 to 12 years typical for PD. Age-specific onset data, far more useful for understanding the cause of a late-life condition, are not available for PSP.

SURVIVAL

Death occurred at an actuarially corrected median of 9.7 years after onset in one survey[4] and 5.9 years in another.[5] It is usually related to pneumonia and other inevitable complications of immobility, but frank aspiration, head trauma as a result of a fall, and complications of hip fracture are important preventable causes of death in PSP. There is no relationship of survival in PSP to onset age, presence of dysphagia at diagnosis, or degree of dementia.[5]

PREVALENCE

A study of the prevalence of PSP in two counties with a population of 800,000 in central New Jersey in 1986 surveyed medical records of neurologists, hospitals, and chronic-care facilities. Six men and five women in the two counties were confirmed by the authors' examination as having PSP, according to the diagnostic criteria in Table 19-3. The age-adjusted prevalence ratio was 1.4 per 100,000. PSP may, therefore, be considered approximately 1 percent as common as PD.

The prevalence figure for PSP must be considered a minimal prevalence, as the median delay from symptom onset to a diagnosis of PSP was 3 years in one study and 5 years in another, amounting to approximately one-half the duration of the disease.[151] An unknown number of additional cases are never correctly diagnosed.

INCIDENCE

For a chronic disease, incidence, the number of new cases in a defined population per year, gives a more valid measure than prevalence of the intensity of the etiologic agent in the population or environment. The incidence of PSP has been measured directly in two populations: Perth, Australia (population 1 million) over 2 years and Rochester, Minnesota (population 50,000) over 13 years, giving crude incidences of 3.1–4.0 per million per year.[152,153] The incidence of PSP, then, lies very close to that of some better-recognized neurological conditions (Table 19-8).[154]

SEX RATIO

Published cases of PSP reveal a sex ratio (M to F) of approximately 2:1.[15] The finding of six men and five women in the survey in New Jersey, the closest so far to a community-based rather than referral-based survey, is not statistically different from this ratio. The absence of so asymmetric a ratio in other highly referred neurodegenerative disorders is a point against gender-related referral bias as the explanation and points to an occupational toxin as a factor in the cause of PSP.

ANALYTIC EPIDEMIOLOGY

The sole case-control study of risk factors in PSP to date administered an 85-item questionnaire to 50 patients and 100 matched controls in New Jersey.[155] It revealed that patients were 3.1 times more likely than controls to have completed high school and 2.9 times as likely to have completed college. Patients were also 2.4 times more likely to have lived as an adult over age 40 in a locality of population less than 10,000. These both reached statistical significance but were interpreted by the authors as probable effects of ascertainment bias or referral bias. Items that gave statistically nonsignificant results concerned living overseas, occupations implicated in other neurological illnesses, potential exposure to occupational toxins, smoking, alcohol, caffeine, contact sports, head trauma, type A personality, early menopause, estrogen supplementation, multiparity, various medical conditions, surgical history, psychiatric history, animal exposure, maternal age, birth order, and family neurological history.

Anecdotal reports from one investigator in Canada suggest greater-than-expected exposure to hydrocarbons in a small series of patients with PSP.[156,157] This may help explain the asymmetric sex ratio but has not yet been specifically examined in a controlled study.

TABLE 19-8 Approximate Incidence Rates of PSP and Some Other Neurological Disorders[151,154]

	Incidence Rate
PD	20
ALS	10–20
Guillain-Barre syndrome	10
All muscular dystrophies	7
Polymyositis	5
Tourette syndrome	5
Huntington's disease	5
PSP	3–4
Myasthenia gravis	3–4
Syringomyelia	3
Charcot-Marie-Tooth	2
Wilson's disease	2

New cases per million population per year. ALS, amyotrophic lateral sclerosis.

A TRANSMISSIBLE AGENT?

The profound pathological resemblance (and superficial clinical resemblance) of PSP to PDC aroused suspicion that a slow virus may be their cause, as it is in Kuru, another neurodegenerative disease of the western Pacific. However, after a mean of 9.1 years' observation (range, 3–24) of 29 chimpanzees given intracerebral inoculation of brain tissue from 10 patients with PSP, results are negative.[158] An attempt to detect prion protein in PSP and other parkinsonian disorders, despite the pathological similarities between PSP and Creutzfeldt-Jakob disease, was also negative.[159]

In PD and AD, but not in PSP,[160] there is a deficit in the sense of smell, the function of which involves dopaminergic transmission. This is evidence against the hypothesis that in all three conditions an etiologic agent gains entry to the central nervous system via the olfactory epithelium.

IS THERE A HEREDITARY COMPONENT?

EPIDEMIOLOGICAL SURVEYS AND MULTICASE FAMILIES

In reviewing the records of 104 patients with PSP, Jankovic et al.[161] found no allegations of secondary cases of PSP among their 409 relatives, and the frequency of PD, tremor, and dementia among the relatives was only that expected in the population. A retrospectively controlled survey from the same clinic[162] found a family history of tremor in relatives of patients with (nonfamilial) PSP (2.6 percent) to be similar to that among relatives of controls (2.2 percent). However, in a formal case-control study,[123] the question inquiring into the presence of PD among parents, siblings, grandparents, aunts, uncles, and first cousins elicited a positive answer 5.0 times as frequently in those with PSP as in controls. For "Alzheimer's or dementia," the ratio was 3.6. These were statistically nonsignificant because of the small numbers involved but suggest that the question remains unresolved.

Recent reports of families with more than one member with PSP give additional reason to reconsider the issue of a genetic factor in the cause of PSP. Six such reports with autopsy confirmation in at least one member have appeared, all most compatible with autosomal-dominant transmission[163–168] (Table 19-9). Paternal transmission was evident in most of these families, a strong point against a mitochondrial gene as the culprit. It is intriguing that some of these families include additional members with reports of typical PD or essential tremor.

POSSIBLE MOLECULAR MECHANISMS

There has been little molecular genetic study of PSP. One candidate locus, the Apo E locus, which exhibits a disproportionate prevalence of the ε4 allele in AD, exhibits only the normal distribution of alleles in PSP.[169–171] Other candidate genes could be subjected to similar allelic association studies in PSP, but there are as yet too few multiplex families or affected sibling pairs to perform linkage analysis.

A more promising lead arises from the finding[172] that skeletal muscle mitochondrial respiratory function, assessed at the biochemical level, is reduced by about 30 percent in PSP. Although that study found normal muscle histopathology, one other patient with PSP (LI Golbe, unpublished data) did show ragged red fibers compatible with mitochondrial myopathy. Mitochondrial function of brain tissue in PSP has not been examined.

Although there is abundant evidence for oxidative damage (altered brain iron, high reduced glutathione to oxidized glutathione (GSH to GSSG) ratio) as the mechanism of cell death in PD, these changes are absent in PSP.[173]

Treatment

PHARMACOTHERAPY

As is the case for most other degenerative disorders, neurotransmitter replacement or receptor stimulation in PSP has met little or none of the success it has in PD (Table 19-10).

DOPAMINERGICS

The extent and nature of the benefit of L-dopa in PSP has not been adequately studied in double-blind fashion, but any benefit is nearly always mild and/or brief. In two retrospec-

TABLE 19-9 Families with Adult-Onset Autopsy-Confirmed PSP

First Author (Year)	No. Clearly Affected	Generations Affected	Relationship	Others Possibly Affected
Ohara[164] (1992)	2	1	Brother-sister	None
Brown[163] (1993)	2	1	Female first cousins	Mother of one had parkinsonism and dementia.
Tetrud[166] (1996)	2	1	Brother-sister	Parkinsonism in their mother and maternal grandfather. Isolated tremor in four other close relatives.
Gazeley[167] (1994)	2	1	Sisters	None
Golbe[165] (1995)	2	2	Father-son	Parkinsonism in father's sister and father's nephew
García de Yebenes[168] (1995)	7	4	Autosomal-dominant pattern	Six others with possible PSP

TABLE 19-10 Benefit and Adverse Effects of Some Drugs in PSP

	N	BENEFIT (%)				ADVERSE EFFECT (%)		
		No effect	Minimal	Moderate	Marked	Minimal	Moderate	Marked
Amantadine	13	39	38	0	0	15	8	0
Amitriptyline	28	18	18	14	0	32	14	4
Bromocriptine	23	35	22	0	0	26	17	0
Desipramine	20	20	20	0	0	20	35	5
Fluoxetine	31	42	13	3	0	26	16	0
Imipramine	14	7	14	7	7	29	29	7
L-dopa/carbidopa	82	40	30	7	0	17	6	0
Methysergide	17	59	12	6	0	23	18	0

SOURCE: *From Nieforth and Golbe.*[115] *Used with permission.*

tive, uncontrolled studies, 51 percent[174] and 38 percent[115] of patients responded, most of them minimally. (The placebo response rate in PD drug trials is generally about 30 percent.) Only the rigidity and bradykinesia, including those components of dysarthria and dysphagia attributable to them, may respond more than would be expected from placebo. Therefore, there is no reason to prescribe dopaminergic treatment for patients whose activities are not impaired by those specific abnormalities.

Although hyperkinetic side effects and response fluctuations of L-dopa are very rare in PSP, agitation (0 of 82 patients in one survey[115]), confusion and/or hallucinations are less rare (5 of 82, 6 percent[115]). Still, it is the author's practice to prescribe for PSP approximately twice the L-dopa/carbidopa dosages used for PD with the equivalent degree of parkinsonism. Dopamine receptor agonists provide similar benefit with additional risks.[115,175,176]

CHOLINERGICS AND ANTICHOLINERGICS

It is perhaps symptomatic of our state of knowledge of PSP therapy that opposite direction in cholinergic intervention have been advocated. Anticholinergics have been used by analogy with PD but are far less efficacious than L-dopa.[115,174,177] An exception may be amantadine, which has dopaminergic and antiglutamatergic properties as well, and was found to be a close second to L-dopa in risk to benefit ratio.[115]

Trials of cholinergics have been inspired by the severe and widespread degeneration of acetylcholinergic systems in PSP. The cholinesterase inhibitor physostigmine reportedly improved PET evidence of prefrontal dysfunction, long-term verbal memory, and visuospatial attention, all very slightly,[92,106] but a subsequent trial by one of these groups gave negative results, with worsening of gait.[178] There are no data on the use of tacrine, a commercially available cholinergic drug, in PSP, but scopolamine is of no benefit.[178] The benefits of RS-86, another cholinergic agent, were limited to some aspects of sleep.[179]

ANTIDEPRESSANTS AND ANTISEROTONERGICS

In a double-blind trial,[180] amitriptyline improved gait and rigidity in three of four patients, and desipramine improved apraxia of eyelid opening in both of two patients. In a retrospective series,[115] amitriptyline gave a risk to benefit ratio that was slightly less favorable than those of L-dopa and amantadine. Amitriptyline is generally started at 25 mg at bedtime, increasing by that amount each week, given in two divided doses. If 50 mg twice daily proves ineffective, higher dosages are unlikely to do otherwise. Imipramine confers a slightly less favorable risk to benefit ratio than amitriptyline,[115] and desipramine confers a quite unfavorable ratio.

Fluoxetine, a nontricyclic antidepressant that blocks serotonin reuptake, appears valueless against the motor deficits of PSP,[115] but a similar drug, trazodone, helped one atypical patient to a moderate degree.[181] The antiserotonergic drug methysergide was found moderately efficacious in a controlled trial published in 1981,[147] but subsequent informal experience has not confirmed this benefit.[115,182]

NORADRENERGICS

In a controlled trial, idazoxan, an experimental blocker of presynaptic alpha-2 receptors, modestly improved ambulation and manual dexterity in five of nine patients.[118] However, other deficits did not improve, and sympathomimetic side effects proved sufficiently severe and frequent enough to render clinical use of the drug impractical. An analogue that may be better tolerated, efaroxan, is under clinical evaluation in Europe.

Yohimbine, a well-tolerated drug with a similar noradrenergic mechanism, has long been approved for use in male impotence. In 20 of the author's patients, it occasionally provided a modest energizing effect without other discernible objective motor or mental benefit.

BOTULINUM TOXIN

Blepharospasm in PSP responds well to botulinum A injections.[183] Preliminary personal observations suggest that even apraxia of lid opening may respond to botulinum A. Torticollis or retrocollis in PSP may also respond, but the occasional occurrence of mild dysphagia after botulinum injection for idiopathic spasmodic torticollis dictates caution in the case of PSP, in which slight exacerbation of dysphagia could allow aspiration. Botulinum toxin may also be useful in focal dystonia of PSP.[184]

NONPHARMACOLOGICAL THERAPY

GAZE AND LID PARESES

Blepharospasm or lid levator inhibition may be overcome if a family member presents a finger-counting task. Some patients can overcome the voluntary downgaze palsy that impairs eating by using their remaining pursuit downgaze ability to follow the fork from eye level to the plate. When downgaze palsy or inattention to the lower half of space is present, low-lying objects, such as children's toys, throw rugs, and coffee tables, should be removed from the patient's path. Although prisms are not usually useful in correcting the patient's inability to attend to the lower half of space, they may help diplopia related to dysconjugate gaze.

The chronic conjunctivitis and reactive lacrimation caused by the low blink rate may be treated by instillation of methylcellulose or polyvinyl alcohol drops when the patient is awake and a petrolatum-based ointment or mineral oil at bedtime.

PHYSICAL, SPEECH, AND SWALLOWING THERAPY

Physical therapy seems to be of little or no benefit against the postural instability of PSP, but instruction for the family in the physical care of the poorly ambulant patient may be useful, and regular exercise provides clear psychological benefit.[185] Similarly, speech therapy has proved of little benefit in most patients, but the speech pathologist may be able to arrange adjunctive means of communication, such as electronic typing devices or simple pointing boards.

The family of the dysphagic patient may be instructed in the preparation of foods of proper consistency, using a blender or cornstarch-based thickeners as necessary. A barium swallow radiograph, using boluses of varying consistency, will guide this advice. The speech pathologist can teach the patient safer swallowing techniques and can monitor the patient for the need for a feeding gastronomy. The high morbidity and mortality related to aspiration in advanced PSP has led the author to recommend endoscopic placement of a feeding gastrostomy after the first episode of aspiration pneumonitis, when the patient requires more time to finish a meal than the household can practically provide, when there is significant weight loss because of reduced intake, or when a minor degree of aspiration occurs with every mouthful (K Kluin, personal communication).

SURGICAL STRIATAL IMPLANTS

A trial of autograft of adrenal medullary tissue to striatum in three patients with PSP produced only modest and transient improvement in postural stability in one and no change in the others, with important postoperative morbidity.[186] Current data, therefore, does not recommend this procedure. Fetal nigral cell striatal allografts have not been attempted in PSP, but the advanced state of degeneration of centers downstream from the striatum, contrasting with the situation in PD, suggests that such procedure is unlikely to be of benefit.

ELECTROCONVULSIVE THERAPY (ECT)

Two personal cases and one from the literature[187] have markedly worsened with ECT with regard to both motor and cognitive functioning. All three patients improved nearly to baseline over subsequent weeks. This contrasts with the benefit of ECT in PD.[188]

Patient Resources

The Society for Progressive Supranuclear Palsy (SPSP) is headquartered in Baltimore and serves North America. The Progressive Supranuclear Palsy Association (PSPA) is based in the UK and serves all of Europe (Table 19-11). They are patient service and advocacy organizations offering support meetings and lay-language literature. Just as important is these organizations' implicit message to patients that their having an "orphan disease" does not mean that they are ignored by the medical world.

The SPSP and PSPA serve as a professional resource for clinicians and as referral sources of study subjects for researchers. They can help organize multicenter trials and prospective data banks and can help support a brain bank. Perhaps only a multidisciplinary, multi-institutional research effort under the aegis of such organizations can solve so unusual and complex a puzzle as PSP.

TABLE 19-11 Lay Organizations Dedicated to PSP

The Society for Progressive Supranuclear Palsy, Inc.
Johns Hopkins Hospital
5065 Outpatient Center
601 N. Caroline Street
Baltimore, MD 21287

The Progressive Supranuclear Palsy Association
21 Church Street
Mears Ashby
Northampton 6 OD United Kingdom

References

1. Richardson JC, Steele J, Olszewski J: Supranuclear ophthalmoplegia, pseudobulbar palsy, nuchal dystonia and dementia: A clinical report on eight cases of "heterogeneous system degeneration." *Trans Am Neurol Assoc* 88:25–29, 1963.
2. Olszewski J, Steele J, Richardson JC: Pathological report on six cases of heterogeneous system degeneration. *J Neuropathol Exp Neurol* 23:187–188, 1963.
3. Steele JC, Richardson JC, Olszewski J: Progressive supranuclear palsy: A heterogeneous degeneration involving the brain stem, basal ganglia and cerebellum, with vertical gaze and pseudobulbar palsy, nuchal dystonia and dementia. *Arch Neurol* 10:333–359, 1964.
4. Golbe LI, Davis PH, Schoenberg BS, Duvoisin RC: Prevalence and natural history of progressive supranuclear palsy. *Neurology* 38:1031–1034, 1988.
5. Maher ER, Lees AJ: The clinical features and natural history of the Steele-Richardson-Olszewski syndrome (progressive supranuclear palsy). *Neurology* 36:1005–1008, 1986.
6. Hoehn MM, Yahr MD: Parkinsonism: Onset, progression, and mortality. *Neurology* 17:427–442, 1967.
7. Duvoisin RC: Clinical diagnosis, in Litvan I, Agid Y (eds): *Progressive Supranuclear Palsy: Clinical and Research Approaches.* New York: Oxford University Press, 1992, pp 15–33.

8. Milberg W, Albert M: Cognitive differences between patients with progressive supranuclear palsy and Alzheimer's disease. *J Clin Exp Neuropsychol* 11:605–611, 1989.

9. Rivest J, Quinn N, Marsden CD: Dystonia in Parkinson's disease, multiple system atrophy, and progressive supranuclear palsy. *Neurology* 40:1571–1578, 1990.

10. Gibb WRG, Luthert PJ, Marsden CD: Corticobasal degeneration. *Brain* 112:1171–1192, 1989.

11. Collins SJ, Ahlskog JE, Parisi JE, Maraganore DM: Progressive supranuclear palsy: Neuropathologically based diagnostic clinical criteria. *J Neurol Neurosurg Psychiatry* 58:167–173, 1995.

12. Colosimo C, Albanese A, Hughes AJ, et al: Some specific clinical features differentiate multiple system atrophy (striatonigral variety) from Parkinson's disease. *Arch Neurol* 52:294–298, 1995.

13. Steele JC: Introduction, in Litvan I, Agid Y (eds): *Progressive Supranuclear Palsy: Clinical and Research Approaches.* New York: Oxford University Press, 1992, chap 2, pp 3–14.

14. Steele JC: Progressive supranuclear palsy. *Brain* 95:693–704, 1972.

15. Brusa A, Peloso PF: *An Introduction to Progressive Supranuclear Palsy.* Rome: John Libby, 1993.

16. Barbeau A: Degenerescence plurisystematisee du nevraxe: Syndrome de Steele-Richardson-Olszewski. *Union Med Can* 94:715–718, 1965.

17. Hauw J-J, Daniel SE, Dickson D, et al: Preliminary NINDS neuropathologic criteria for Steele-Richardson-Olszewski syndrome (progressive supranuclear palsy). *Neurology* 44:2015–2019, 1994.

18. Duvoisin RC, Golbe LI, Lepore FE: Progressive supranuclear palsy. *Can J Neurol Sci* 14:547–554, 1987.

19. Robbins TW, James M, Owen AM, et al: Cognitive deficits in progressive supranuclear palsy, Parkinson's disease, and multiple system atrophy in tests sensitive to frontal lobe dysfunction. *J Neurol Neurosurg Psychiatry* 57:79–88, 1994.

20. Will RG, Lees AJ, Gibb W, Barnard RO: A case of progressive subcortical gliosis presenting clinically as Steele Richardson Olszewski syndrome. *J Neurol Neurosurg Psychiatry* 51:1224–1227, 1988.

21. Bertoni J, Label LS, Sackellares C, Hicks SP: Supranuclear gaze palsy in familial Creutzfeldt-Jakob disease. *Arch Neurol* 40:618–622, 1983.

22. Fearnley JM, Revesz T, Brooks DJ, et al: Diffuse Lewy body disease presenting with a supranuclear gaze palsy. *J Neurol Neurosurg Psychiatry* 54:159–161, 1991.

23. Pahwa R, Koller WC, Stern MB: Primary pallidal atrophy, in Stern MB, Koller WC (eds): *Parkinsonian Syndromes.* New York: Marcel Dekker, 1993, chap 26, pp 433–440.

24. Truong DD, Harding AE, Scaravilli F, et al: Movement disorders in mitochondrial myopathies: A study of nine cases with two autopsy studies. *Mov Disord* 5:109–117, 1990.

25. Curran T, Lang AE: Parkinsonian syndromes associated with hydrocephalus: Case reports, a review of the literature, and pathophysiological hypotheses. *Mov Disord* 9:508–509, 1994.

26. Tanner CM, Goetz CG, Klawans HL: Multi-infarct PSP. *Neurology* 37:1819, 1987.

27. Winikates J, Jankovic J: Vascular progressive supranuclear palsy. *J Neural Transm Suppl* 42:189–201, 1994.

28. Dubinsky RM, Jankovic J: Progressive supranuclear palsy and a multi-infarct state. *Neurology* 37:570–576, 1987.

29. Burn DJ, Sawle GV, Brooks DJ: Differential diagnosis of Parkinson's disease, multiple system atrophy, and Steele-Richardson-Olszewski syndrome: Discriminant analysis of striatal ^{18}F-dopa PET data. *J Neurol Neurosurg Psychiatry* 57:278–284, 1994.

30. Schonfeld SM, Golbe LI, Safer J, et al: Computed tomographic findings in progressive supranuclear palsy: Correlation with clinical grade. *Mov Disorder* 2:263–278, 1987.

31. Drayer BP, Olanow W, Burger P, et al: Parkinson plus syndrome: Diagnosis using high field MR imaging of brain iron. *Radiology* 159:493–498, 1986.

32. Savoiardo M, Strada L, Girotti F, et al: MR imaging in progressive supranuclear palsy and Shy-Drager syndrome. *J Comput Assist Tomogr* 13:555–560, 1989.

33. Saitoh H, Yoshii F, Shinohara Y: Computed tomographic findings in progressive supranuclear palsy. *Neuroradiology* 29:168–171, 1987.

34. Yuki, Sato S, Yuasa T, et al: Computed tomographic findings of progressive supranuclear palsy compared with Parkinson's disease. *Jpn J Med Sci Biol* 29:506–511, 1990.

35. Stern MB, Braffman BH, Skolnick BE, et al: Magnetic resonance imaging in Parkinson's disease and parkinsonian syndromes. *Neurology* 39:1524–1526, 1989.

36. Timmons JH, Bonikowski FW, Harshorne MF: Iodoamphetamine-123 brain imaging demonstrating cortical deactivation in a patient with progressive supranuclear palsy. *Clin Nucl Med* 14:841–842, 1989.

37. Habert MO, Spampinato U, Mas JL, et al: A comparative technetium 99m hexamethylpropylene amine oxime SPECT study in different types of dementia. *Eur J Nucl Med* 18:3–11, 1991.

38. Neary D, Snowdon JS, Shields RA, et al: Single photon emission tomography using ^{99}mTc-HM-PAO in the investigation of dementia. *J Neurol Neurosurg Psychiatry* 50:1101–1109, 1987.

39. von Royen E, Verhoeff F, Speelman JD, et al: Multiple system atrophy and progressive supranuclear palsy: Diminished striatal D2 dopamine receptor activity demonstrated by ^{123}I-IBZM single photon emission computed tomography. *Arch Neurol* 50:513–516, 1993.

40. Schwarz J, Tatsch K, Arnold G, et al: ^{123}Iodobenzamide-SPECT predicts dopaminergic responsiveness in patients with de novo parkinsonism. *Neurology* 42:556–561, 1992.

41. Jellinger K, Riederer P, Tomonaga M: Progressive supranuclear palsy: Clinicopathological and biochemical studies. *J Neural Transm* (Suppl)16:111–128, 1980.

42. Kish SJ, Chang LJ, Mirchandani L, et al: Progressive supranuclear palsy: Relationship between extrapyramidal disturbances, dementia and brain neurotransmitter markers. *Ann Neurol* 18:530–536, 1985.

43. Ruberg M, Javoy-Agid F, Hirsch E, et al: Dopaminergic and cholinergic lesions in progressive supranuclear palsy. *Ann Neurol* 18:523–529, 1985.

44. Young AB: Progressive supranuclear palsy: Postmortem chemical analysis. *Neurology* 18:521–522, 1985.

45. Levy R, Ruberg M, Herrero MT, et al: Alterations of GABAergic neurons in the basal ganglia of patients with progressive supranuclear palsy: An in situ hybridization study of GAD_{67} messenger RNA. *Neurology* 45:127–134, 1995.

46. Landwehrmeyer B, Palacios JM: Neurotransmitter receptors in PSP. *J Neural Transm Suppl* 42:229–246, 1994.

47. Pascual J, Berciano J, Gonzalez AM, et al: Autoradiographic demonstration of loss of alpha-2-adrenoceptors in progressive supranuclear palsy: Preliminary report. *J Neurol Sci* 114:165–169, 1993.

48. Ishino H, Otsuki S: Frequency of Alzheimer's neurofibrillary tangles in the cerebral cortex in progressive supranuclear palsy. *J Neurol Sci* 28:309–316, 1976.

49. Powell HC, London GW, Lampert PW: Neurofibrillary tangles in progressive supranuclear palsy. *J Neuropath Exp Neurol* 33:98–106, 1974.

50. Roy S, Datta CK, Hirano A, et al: Electron microscopic study of neurofibrillary tangles in Steele-Richardson-Olszewski syndrome. *Acta Neuropathol (Berl)* 45:175–179, 1979.

51. Tellez-Nagel I, Wisniewski HM: Ultrastructure of neurofibrillary tangles in Steele-Richardson-Olszewski syndrome. *Arch Neurol* 29:324–327, 1973.

52. Tomonaga M: Ultrastructure of neurofibrillary tangles in progressive supranuclear palsy. *Acta Neuropathol (Berl)* 37:1771–1781, 1977.

53. Montpetit V, Clapin DR, Guberman A: Substructure of 20 nm filaments of progressive supranuclear palsy. *Acta Neuropathol* 63:311–318, 1985.

54. Dickson DW, Kress Y, Crowe A, Yen S-H: Monoclonal antibodies to Alzheimer neurofibrillary tangles (ANT): 2. Demonstration of a common antigenic determinant between ANT and neurofibrillary degeneration in progressive supranuclear palsy. *Am J Pathol* 120:292–303, 1985.

55. Ghatak R, Nochlin D, Hadfield MG: Neurofibrillary pathology in progressive supranuclear palsy. *Acta Neuropathol (Berl)* 52:73–76, 1980.

56. Ikeda K, Akiyama H, Haga C, et al: Argyrophilic thread-like structure in corticobasal degeneration and supranuclear palsy. *Neurosci Lett* 174:157–159, 1994.

57. Mori H, Nishimura M, Namba Y, Oda M: Corticobasal degeneration: A disease with widespread appearance of abnormal tau and neurofibrillary tangles, and its relation to progressive supranuclear palsy. *Acta Neuropathol (Berl)* 88:113–121, 1994.

58. Wakabayashi K, Oyanagi K, Makifuchi T, et al: Corticobasal degeneration: Etiopathological significance of the cytoskeletal alterations. *Acta Neuropathol (Berl)* 87:545–553, 1994.

59. Inagaki T, Ishino H, Seno H, et al: An autopsy case of PSP with astrocytic inclusions. *Jpn J Psychiatry Neurol* 48:85–89, 1994.

60. Pollock J, Mirra SS, Binder LI, et al: Filamentous aggregates in Pick's disease, progressive supranuclear palsy, and Alzheimer's disease share antigenic determinants with microtubule-associated protein, tau. *Lancet* 2:1211, 1986.

61. Love S, Saitoh T, Quijada S, et al: Alz-50, ubiquitin and tau immunoreactivity of neurofibrillary tangles, Pick bodies and Lewy bodies. *J Neuropathol Exp Neurol* 47:393–405, 1988.

62. Tabaton M, Whitehouse PJ, Perry G, et al: Alz 50 recognizes abnormal filaments in Alzheimer's disease and progressive supranuclear palsy. *Ann Neurol* 24:407–413, 1988.

63. Yamada T, Calne DB, Akiyama H, et al: Further observations on tau-positive glia in the brains with progressive supranuclear palsy. *Acta Neuropathol* 85:308–315, 1993.

64. Flament S, Delacourte A, Verny M, et al: Abnormal tau proteins in progressive supranuclear palsy. *Acta Neuropathol (Berl)* 81:591–596, 1991.

65. Vermersch P, Robitaille Y, Bernier L, et al: Biochemical mapping of neurofibrillary degeneration in a case of progressive supranuclear palsy: Evidence for general cortical involvement. *Acta Neuropathol* 87:572–577, 1994.

66. Probst A, Langui D, Lautenschlager C, et al: Progressive supranuclear palsy: Extensive neuropil threads in addition to neurofibrillary tangles. *Acta Neuropathol (Berl)* 77:61–68, 1988.

67. Nelson SJ, Yen S-H, Davies P, Dickson DW: Basal ganglia neuropil threads in progressive supranuclear palsy. *J Neuropathol Exp Neurol* 48:324, 1989.

68. Iwatsubo T, Hasegawa M, Ihara Y: Neuronal and glial tau-positive inclusions in diverse neurologic diseases share common phosphorylation characteristics. *Acta Neuropathol (Berl)* 88:129–136, 1994.

69. Lennox G, Lowe J, Morrell K, et al: Ubiquitin is a component of neurofibrillary tangles in a variety of neurodegenerative diseases. *Neurosci Lett* 94:211–217, 1988.

70. Arain: "Grumose degeneration" of the dentate nucleus: A light and electron microscopic study in PSP and dentatorubropallidoluysian atrophy. *J Neurol Sci* 90:131–145, 1987.

71. Cruz-Sanchez FF, Rossi ML, Cardozo A, et al: Immunohistological study of grumose degeneration of the dentate nucleus in progressive supranuclear palsy. *J Neurol Sci* 110:228–231, 1992.

72. Giaccone G, Tagliavini F, Street JS, et al: Progressive supranuclear palsy with hypertrophy of the olives: An immunohistochemical study of argyrophilic neurons. *Acta Neuropathol (Berl)* 77:14–20, 1988.

73. Gearing M, Olson DA, Watts RL, Mirra SS: Progressive supranuclear palsy: Neuropathologic and clinical heterogeneity. *Neurology* 44:1015–1024, 1994.

74. Hauw J-J, Verny M, Delaere P, et al: Constant neurofibrillary changes in the neocortex in progressive supranuclear palsy: Basic differences with Alzheimer's disease and aging. *Neurosci Lett* 119:182–186, 1990.

75. Hof PR, Delacourte A, Bouras C: Distribution of cortical neurofibrillary tangles in progressive supranuclear palsy: A quantitative analysis of six cases. *Acta Neuropathol (Berl)* 84:45–51, 1992.

76. Braak H, Jellinger K, Braak E, Bohl J: Allocortical neurofibrillary changes in progressive supranuclear palsy. *Acta Neuropathol* 84:478–483, 1992.

77. Verny M, Duyckaerts C, Delaére P, et al: Cortical tangles in progressive supranuclear palsy. *J Neural Transm Suppl* 42:179–188, 1994.

78. Jellinger KA, Bancher C: Neuropathology, in Litvan I, Agid Y (eds): *Progressive Supranuclear Palsy: Clinical and Research Approaches*. New York, Oxford University Press, 1992, chap 4, pp 44–88.

79. Cruz-Sanchez FF, Rossi ML, Cardozo A, et al: Clinical and pathological study of two patients with progressive supranuclear palsy and Alzheimer's changes: Antigenic determinants that distinguish cortical and subcortical neurofibrillary tangles. *Neurosci Lett* 136:43–46, 1992.

80. Fenelon G, Guillard A, Romatet S, et al: Les signes parkinsoniens du syndrome de Steele-Richardson-Olszewski. *Rev Neurol* 149:30–36, 1993.

81. Jankovic J, Van der Linden C: Progressive supranuclear palsy, in Chokroverty S (ed): *Movement Disorders*. New York: PMA, 1990, pp 267–286.

82. D'Antona R, Baron JC, Sanson Y, et al: Subcortical dementia: Frontal cortex hypometabolism detected by positron tomography in patients with progressive supranuclear palsy. *Brain* 108:785–799, 1985.

83. Foster L, Gilman S, Berent S, et al: Cerebral hypometabolism in progressive supranuclear palsy studied with positron emission tomography. *Ann Neurol* 24:399–406, 1988.

84. Leenders KL, Frackowiak RSJ, Lees AJ: Steele-Richardson-Olszewski syndrome: Brain energy metabolism, blood flow and fluorodopa uptake measured by positron emission tomography. *Brain* 111:615–630, 1988.

85. Goffinet AM, De Volder AG, Guillain C, et al: Positron tomography demonstrates frontal lobe hypometabolism in progressive supranuclear palsy. *Ann Neurol* 25:131–139, 1989.

86. Tagliavini F, Pilleri G, Bouras C, Constantinidis J: The basal nucleus of Meynert in patients with progressive supranuclear palsy. *Neurosci Lett* 44:37–42, 1984.

87. Zweig RM, Whitehouse PJ, Casanova MF, et al: Loss of pedunculopontine neurons in progressive supranuclear palsy. *Ann Neurol* 22:18–25, 1987.

88. Jellinger K: The pedunculopontine nucleus in Parkinson's disease, progressive supranuclear palsy and Alzheimer's disease. *J Neurol Neurosurg Psychiatry* 52:540–543, 1988.

89. Perry RH, Tomlinson BE, Candy JM, et al: Cortical cholinergic deficit in mentally impaired parkinsonian patients. *Lancet* 2:789–790, 1983.

90. Agid Y, Graybiel AM, Ruberg M, et al: The efficacy of L-dopa treatment declines in the course of Parkinson disease: Do nondopaminergic lesions play a role? *Adv Neurol* 53:83–100, 1990.

91. Johnson R, Litvan I, Grafman J: Progressive supranuclear palsy: Altered sensory processing leads to degraded cognition. *Neurology* 41:1257–1262, 1991.

92. Kertzman C, Robinson DL, Litvan I: Effects of physostigmine on spatial attention in patients with progressive supranuclear palsy. *Arch Neurol* 47:1346–1350, 1990.

93. Dubois B, Pillon B, Legault F, et al: Slowing of cognitive processing in progressive supranuclear palsy. *Arch Neurol* 45:1194–1199, 1988.

94. Pillon B, Gouider-Khoujan, Deweer B, et al: Neuropsychological pattern of striatonigral degeneration: Comparison with Parkinson's disease and progressive supranuclear palsy. *J Neurol Neurosurg Psychiatry* 58:174–179, 1995.

95. Grafman J, Litvan I, Gomez C, Chase T: Frontal lobe function in progressive supranuclear palsy. *Arch Neurol* 47:553–558, 1990.

96. Podoll K, Schwarz M, Noth J: Language functions in progressive supranuclear palsy. *Brain* 114:1457–1472, 1991.

97. Rosser A, Hodges JR: Initial letter and semantic category fluency in Alzheimer's disease, Huntington's disease, and progressive supranuclear palsy. *J Neurol Neurosurg Psychiatry* 57:1389–1394, 1994.

98. Cambier J, Masson M, Viader F, et al: Le syndrome frontal de paralysie supranucleaire progressive. *Rev Neurol (Paris)* 141:528–536, 1985.

99. Agid Y, Javoy-Agid F, Ruberg M, et al: Progressive supranuclear palsy: Anatomo-clinical and biochemical considerations. *Adv Neurol* 45:191–206, 1987.

100. Pillon B, Dubois B: Cognitive and behavioral impairments, in Litvan I, Agid Y (eds): *Progressive Supranuclear Palsy: Clinical and Research Approaches*. New York: Oxford University Press, 1992, chap 12, pp 223–239.

101. Pillon B, Deweer B, Michon A, et al: Are explicit memory disorders of progressive supranuclear palsy related to damage to striatofrontal circuits? Comparison with Alzheimer's, Parkinson's and Huntington's diseases. *Neurology* 44:1264–1270, 1994.

102. Fearnley JM, Lees AJ: Ageing and Parkinson's disease: Substantia nigra regional selectivity. *Brain* 114:2283–2301, 1991.

103. Brooks DJ, Ibanez V, Sawle GV, et al: Differing patterns of striatal ^{18}F-dopa uptake in Parkinson's disease, multiple system atrophy, and progressive supranuclear palsy. *Ann Neurol* 28:547–555, 1990.

104. Villares J, Strada O, Faucheux B, et al: Loss of striatal high affinity GF binding sites in progressive supranuclear palsy but not in Parkinson's disease. *Neurosci Lett* 182:59–62, 1994.

105. Oyanaki K, Takahashi H, Wakabayashi K, Ikuta F: Large neurons in the neostriatum in Alzheimer's disease and progressive supranuclear palsy: A topographic, histologic and ultrastructural investigation. *Brain Res* 544:221–226, 1991.

106. Litvan I, Gomez C, Atack JR, et al: Physostigmine treatment of progressive supranuclear palsy. *Ann Neurol* 26:404–407, 1989.

107. Baron JC, Mazière B, Loc'h C, et al: Loss of striatal [^{76}Br] bromospiperone binding sites demonstrated by positron emission tomography in progressive supranuclear palsy. *J Cereb Blood Flow Metab* 6:131–136, 1986.

108. Brooks DJ, Ibanez V, Sawle GV, et al: Striatal D$_2$ receptor status in patients with Parkinson's disease, striatonigral degeneration, and progressive supranuclear palsy. *J Cereb Blood Flow Metab* 6:131–136, 1986.

109. Matsuo H, Takashima H, Kishikawa M, et al: Pure akinesia: An atypical manifestation of progressive supranuclear palsy. *J Neurol Neurosurg Psychiatry* 54:397, 1991.

110. Imai H, Nakamura T, Kondo T, Narabayashi H: Dopa-unresponsive pure akinesia or freezing: A condition with a wide spectrum of PSP? *Adv Neurol* 60:622–625, 1993.

111. Mizusawa H, Mochizuki A, Ohkoshin, et al: Progressive supranuclear palsy presenting with pure akinesia. *Adv Neurol* 60:618–621, 1993.

112. Riley DE, Fogt N, Leigh RJ: The syndrome of "pure akinesia" and its relationship to progressive supranuclear palsy. *Neurology* 44:1025–1029, 1994.

113. Masucci EF, Kurtzke JF: Tremor in progressive supranuclear palsy. *Acta Neurol Scand* 80:296–300, 1989.

114. Jankovic J, Van der Linden C: Progressive supranuclear palsy (Steele-Richardson-Olszewski syndrome), in Chokroverty S (ed): *Movement Disorders*. New York: PMA Publishing, 1990, chap 12, pp 267–286.

115. Nieforth KA, Golbe LI: Retrospective study of drug response in 87 patients with progressive supranuclear palsy. *Clin Neuropharmacol* 16:338–346, 1993.

116. Moriizumi T, Hattori T: Separate neuronal populations of the rat globus pallidus projecting to the subthalamic nucleus, auditory cortex and pedunculopontine tegmental area. *Neuroscience* 46:701–710, 1992.

117. Masdeu JC, Alampur U, Cavaliere R, Tavoulareas G: Astasia and gait failure with damage of the pontomesencephalic locomotor region. *Ann Neurol* 35:619–621, 1994.

118. Ghika J, Tennis M, Hoffman E, et al: Idazoxan treatment in progressive supranuclear palsy. *Neurology* 41:986–991, 1991.

119. Carpenter MB, Harbison JW, Peter P: Accessory oculomotor nuclei in the monkey: Projections and effects of discrete lesions. *J Comp Neurol* 140:131–147, 1970.

120. Fukushima-Kudo J, Fukushima K, Tahiro K: Rigidity and dorsi flexion of the neck in progressive supranuclear palsy and the interstitial nucleus of Cajal. *J Neurol Neurosurg Psychiatry* 50:1197–1203, 1987.

121. Lees AJ: The Steele-Richardson-Olszewski syndrome (progressive supranuclear palsy). *Mov Disord* 2:272–287, 1987.

122. Juncos JL, Hirsch EC, Malessa S, et al: Mesencephalic cholinergic nuclei in progressive supranuclear palsy. *Neurology* 41:25–30, 1991.

123. Davis PH, Bergeron C, McLachlan DR: Atypical presentation of progressive supranuclear palsy. *Ann Neurol* 17:337–343, 1985.

124. Dubas F, Gray F, Escourolle R: Maladie de Steele-Richardson-Olszewski sans ophthalmoplégie; 6 cas anatomo-cliniques. *Rev Neurol* 139:407–416, 1992.

125. Nuwer MR: Progressive supranuclear palsy despite normal eye movements. *Arch Neurol* 38:784, 1981.

126. Kida E, Barcikowska M, Niemszewska M: Immunohistochemical study of a case with progressive supranuclear palsy without ophthalmoplegia. *Acta Neuropathol* 83:328–332, 1992.

127. Saver JL, Liu GT, Charness ME: Idiopathic striopallidodentate calcification with prominent supranuclear abnormality of eye movement. *J Neuro-Ophthalmol* 14:29–33, 1994.

128. Malessa S, Gaymard B, Rivaud S, et al: Role of pontine nuclei damage in smooth pursuit impairment of progressive supranuclear palsy: A clinical-pathologic study. *Neurology* 44:716–721, 1994.

129. Pfaffenbach DD, Layton DD, Kearns TP: Ocular manifestations in progressive supranuclear palsy. *Am J Ophthalmol* 74:1179–1184, 1972.

130. Chu FC, Reingold DB, Cogan DG, Williams AC: The eye movement disorders of progressive supranuclear palsy. *Ophthalmology* 86:422–428, 1979.

131. Troost BT, Daroff RB: The ocular motor defects in progressive supranuclear palsy. *Ann Neurol* 2:397–403, 1977.

132. Rascol O, Sabatini U, Simonetta-Moreau M, et al: Square wave jerks in parkinsonian syndromes. *J Neurol Neurosurg Psychiatry* 54:599–602, 1991.

133. Pierrot-Deseilligny C, Rivaud S, Pillon B, et al: Lateral visually-guided saccades in progressive supranuclear palsy. *Brain* 112:471–487, 1989.

134. Rafal RD, Posner MI, Friedman JH, et al: Orienting of visual attention in progressive supranuclear palsy. *Brain* 111:267–280, 1988.

135. Rascol OJ, Clanet M, Senard JM, et al: Vestibulo-ocular reflex in Parkinson's disease and multiple system atrophy. *Adv Neurol* 60:395–397, 1993.

136. Lepore FE, Duvoisin RC: "Apraxia" of eyelid opening: An involuntary levator inhibition. *Neurology* 35:423–427, 1985.

137. Dehaene I: Apraxia of eyelid opening in progressive supranuclear palsy. *Neurology* 15:115–116, 1984.

138. Jankovic J: Apraxia of eyelid opening in progressive supranuclear palsy: Reply. *Neurology* 15:116, 1984b.

139. Golbe LI, Davis PH, Lepore FE: Eyelid movement abnormalities in progressive supranuclear palsy. *Mov Dis* 4:297–302, 1989.

140. Aldrich MS, Foster L, White RF, et al: Sleep abnormalities in progressive supranuclear palsy. *Ann Neurol* 25:577–581, 1989.

141. Leygonie F, Thomas J, Degos JD, et al: Troubles du sommeil dans la maladie de Steele-Richardson: Etude polygraphique de 3 cas. *Rev Neurol* 132:125–136, 1976.

142. Vidailhet M, Rothwell JC, Thompson PD, et al: The auditory startle response in the Steele-Richardson-Olszewski syndrome and Parkinson's disease. *Brain* 115:1181–1192, 1992.

143. Tolosa ES, Zeese JA: Brainstem auditory evoked responses in progressive supranuclear palsy. *Ann Neurol* 6:369, 1979.

144. De Bruin VMS, Lees AJ: Subcortical neurofibrillary degeneration presenting as Steele-Richardson-Olszewski and other related syndromes: A review of 90 pathologically verified cases. *Mov Disord* 9:381–389, 1994.

145. Kluin KJ, Foster L, Berent S, Gilman S: Perceptual analysis of speech disorders in progressive supranuclear palsy. *Neurology* 43:563–566, 1993.

146. Sonies BC: Swallowing and speech disturbances, in Litvan I, Agid Y (eds): *Progressive Supranuclear Palsy: Clinical and Research Approaches.* New York: Oxford University Press, 1992, chap 13, pp 240–254.

147. Rafal RD, Grimm RJ: Progressive supranuclear palsy: Functional analysis of the response to methysergide and antiparkinsonian agents. *Neurology* 31:1507–1518, 1981.

148. Gert van Dijk J, Haan J, Koenderink M, Roos RAC: Autonomic nervous function of progressive supranuclear palsy. *Arch Neurol* 48:1083–1084, 1991.

149. Sakakibara R, Hattori T, Tojo M, et al: Micturitional disturbance in progressive supranuclear palsy. *J Autonomic Nerv Sys* 45:101–106, 1993.

150. Geddes JF, Hughes AJ, Lees AJ, Daniel SE: Pathological overlap in cases in parkinsonism associated with neurofibrillary tangles: A study of recent cases of postencephalitic parkinsonism and comparison with progressive supranuclear palsy and Guamanian parkinsonism-dementia complex. *Brain* 116:281–302, 1993.

151. Golbe LI: The epidemiology of progressive supranuclear palsy. *Neurol* 69:25–32, 1996.

152. Mastaglia FL, Grainger K, Kee F, et al: Progressive supranuclear palsy (the Steele-Richardson-Olszewski syndrome): Clinical and electrophysiological observations in eleven cases. *Proc Austral Assoc Neurol* 10:35–44, 1973.

153. Rajput AH, Offord KP, Beard CM, Kurland LT: Epidemiology of parkinsonism: Incidence, classification, and mortality. *Ann Neurol* 16:278–282, 1984.

154. Kurtzke JF, Kurland LT: Neuroepidemiology: A summation, in Kurland LT, Kurtzke JF, Goldberg ID (eds): *Epidemiology of Neurologic and Sense Organ Disorders.* Cambridge, MA: Harvard University Press, 1973, chap 14, pp 305–332.

155. Davis PH, Golbe LI, Duvoisin RC, Schoenberg BS: Risk factors for progressive supranuclear palsy. *Neurology* 38:1546–1552, 1988.

156. McCrank E: PSP risk factors. *Neurology* 40:1637, 1990.

157. McCrank E, Rabheru K: Four cases of progressive supranuclear palsy in patients exposed to organic solvents. *Can J Psychiatry* 34:934–935, 1989.

158. Brown P, Gibbs CJ, Rodgers-Johnson P, et al: Human spongiform encephalopathy: The National Institutes of Health series of 300 cases of experimentally transmitted disease. *Ann Neurol* 35:513–529, 1994.

159. Jendroska K, Hoffmann O, Schelosky L, et al: Absence of disease related prion protein in neurodegenerative disorders presenting with Parkinson's syndrome. *J Neurol Neurosurg Psychiatry* 57:1249–1251, 1994.

160. Doty RL, Golbe LI, McKeown DA, et al: Olfactory testing differentiates between progressive supranuclear palsy and Parkinson's disease. *Neurology* 43:962–965, 1993.

161. Jankovic J, Friedman DI, Pirozzolo FJ, McCrary JA: Progressive supranuclear palsy: Motor, neurobehavioral, and neuro-ophthalmic findings. *Adv Neurol* 53:293–304, 1990.

162. Jankovic J, Beach J, Schwartz K, Contant C: Tremor and longevity in relatives of patients with Parkinson's disease, essential tremor, and control subjects. *Neurology* 45:645–468, 1995.

163. Brown J, Lantos P, Stratton M, et al: Familial progressive supranuclear palsy. *J Neurol Neurosurg Psychiatry* 56:473–476, 1993.

164. Ohara S, Kondo K, Morita H, et al: Progressive supranuclear palsy-like syndrome in two siblings of a consanguineous marriage. *Neurology* 42:1009–1014, 1992.

165. Golbe LI, Dickson DW: Familial autopsy-proven progressive supranuclear palsy. *Neurology* 45(suppl 4):A255, 1995.

166. Tetrud JW, Golbe LI, Farmer PM, Forno LS: Autopsy-proven progressive supranuclear palsy in two siblings. *Neurology* 46:931–934, 1996.

167. Gazely S, Maguire J: Familial progressive supranuclear palsy. *Brain Pathol* 4:534, 1994.

168. García de Yébenes J, Sarasa JL, Daniel SE, Lees AJ: Familial progressive supranuclear palsy: Description of a pedigree and review of the literature. *Brain* 118:1094–1103, 1995.

169. Anouti A, Golbe L, Schmidt K, et al: Apo E genotypes in progressive supranuclear palsy. *Neurology* 45(suppl 4):A255, 1995.

170. Tabaton M, Masturzo P, Angelini G, et al: Apolipoprotein E4 allele frequency is not increased in progressive supranuclear palsy. *Neurology* 45(suppl 4):A470, 1995.

171. Schneider JA, Gearing M, Robbins RS, et al: Apolipoprotein E genotype in diverse neurodegenerative disorders. *Ann Neurol* 38:131–135, 1995.

172. Di Monte CA, Harati Y, Jankovic J, et al: Muscle mitochondrial ATP production in progressive supranuclear palsy. *J Neurochem* 62:1631–1634, 1994.

173. Sian J, Dexter DT, Lees AJ, et al: Alterations in glutathione levels in Parkinson's disease and other neurodegenerative disorders affecting basal ganglia. *Ann Neurol* 36:348–355, 1994.

174. Jankovic J: Progressive supranuclear palsy: Clinical and pharmacologic update. *Neurol Clin* 2:473–486, 1984.

175. Neophytides A, Lieberman A, Goldstein M, et al: The use of lisuride, a potent dopamine and serotonin agonist, in the treatment of progressive supranuclear palsy. *J Neurol Neurosurg Psychiatry* 45:261–263, 1982.

176. Jankovic J: Controlled trial of pergolide mesylate in Parkinson's disease and progressive supranuclear palsy. *Neurology* 33:505–507, 1983.

177. Jackson JA, Jankovic J, Ford J: Progressive supranuclear palsy: Clinical features and response to treatment in 16 patients. *Ann Neurol* 13:273–278, 1983.

178. Litvan I, Blesa R, Clark K, et al: Pharmacological evaluation of the cholinergic system in progressive supranuclear palsy. *Ann Neurol* 36:55–61, 1994.

179. Foster L, Aldrich MS, Bluemlein L, et al: Failure of cholinergic agonist RS-86 to improve cognition and movement in PSP despite effects on sleep. *Neurology* 39:257–261, 1989.

180. Newman GC: Treatment of progressive supranuclear palsy with tricyclic antidepressants. *Neurology* 35:1189–1193, 1985.

181. Kato E, Takahashi S, Abe T, et al: A case of progressive supranuclear palsy showing improvement of rigidity, nuchal dystonia and autonomic failure with trazodone. *Rinsho Shinkeigaku* 34:1013–1017, 1994.

182. Gaudet RJ, Kessler II: Transparently blinded trials of methysergide. *N Engl J Med* 316:279–280, 1987.

183. Lepore FE: Progressive supranuclear palsy, in Tusa RJ, Newman SA (eds): *Neuro-Ophthalmological Disorders: Diagnostic Workup and Management.* New York: Marcel Dekker, 1995, pp 537–542.

184. Polo KB, Jabbari B: Botulinum toxin-A improves the rigidity of progressive supranuclear palsy. *Ann Neurol* 35:237–239, 1994.

185. Sosner J, Wall GC, Sznajder J: Progressive supranuclear palsy: Clinical presentation and rehabilitation of two patients. *Arch Phys Med Rehab* 74:537–539, 1993.

186. Koller WC, Morantz R, Vetere-Overfield B, Waxman M: Autologous adrenal medullary transplant in progressive supranuclear palsy. *Neurology* 39:1066–1068, 1989.

187. Hauser RA, Trehan R: Initial experience with electroconvulsive therapy for progressive supranuclear palsy. *Mov Disord* 9:466–468, 1994.

188. Rasmussen K, Abrams R: Treatment of Parkinson's disease with electroconvulsive therapy. *Psychiatr Clin North Am* 14:925–933, 1991.

Chapter 20

MULTIPLE-SYSTEM ATROPHY

LISA M. SHULMAN and WILLIAM J. WEINER

HISTORICAL BACKGROUND AND NOSOLOGY
CLINICAL DIAGNOSIS
    Extrapyramidal Features
    Autonomic Failure
    Cerebellar Dysfunction
    Pyramidal Signs
    Cognitive Function and Behavior
DIAGNOSTIC INVESTIGATIONS
NEUROPATHOLOGY
DIFFERENTIAL DIAGNOSIS

The topic multiple-system atrophy (MSA) alerts the reader that a description of a subset of neurodegenerative disorders characterized by predominant involvement of the extrapyramidal, cerebellar, and autonomic pathways (Fig. 20-1) follows. The uninitiated may be understandably misled by the broad inference of the term MSA. We later describe the historical derivation of this appellation, although perhaps we should not dismiss the impulse to reexamine the congruity of this diagnostic subset with the range of patients seen in the clinical setting. The sharp distinction of MSA from the other neurodegenerative processes, as depicted in discrete chapters of this textbook, belies the challenge facing the clinician when diagnosing the individual patient. Despite the prodigious advances in medicine, MSA and the neurodegenerative disorders as a group remain clinical diagnoses, and the heterogeneity of our patients defies simple classification.

Historical Background and Nosology

The conceptualization of the diagnosis MSA emerged from a series of publications that each describe fragments of a larger picture. Dejerine and Thomas[1] first coined the term olivopontocerebellar atrophy (OPCA) in 1900 to describe two sporadic cases of progressive cerebellar degeneration with parkinsonism. Sixty years later, Shy and Drager[2] published the first clinical pathological study of a patient with idiopathic orthostatic hypotension. They recognized the association of orthostatic hypotension with a primary degenerative disorder of the nervous system involving the intermediolateral cell column of the spinal cord, medulla, pons, midbrain, cerebellum, and basal ganglia. The full clinical syndrome comprised "orthostatic hypotension, urinary and rectal incontinence, loss of sweating, iris atrophy, external ocular palsies, rigidity, tremor, loss of associated movement, impotence, the findings of an atonic bladder and loss of the rectal sphincter tone, fasciculations, wasting of distal muscles, and evidence of a neuropathic lesion."[2]

Also in 1960, van der Eecken et al.[3] described a unique pathological subgroup among a large number of patients with paralysis agitans. Striatopallidonigral degeneration was identified with "virtual disappearance of the small cells of the caudate nucleus and putamen" in a few patients with extrapyramidal rigidity but minimal tremor. The full clinical pathological study was published the following year.[4] In addition to parkinsonism, the diagnostic signs of brisk reflexes, extensor plantar responses, ataxia, dysarthria, syncope, incontinence, and impotence were described among the three patients reported. Neurodegeneration was also identified in the cerebellum, olivary nuclei, and pons.

The conceptual threads of the three disorders, OPCA, Shy-Drager syndrome (SDS), and striatonigral degeneration (SND), were tied together in a seminal paper by Graham and Oppenheimer[5] in 1969:

> What is needed is a general term to cover this collection of overlapping progressive presenile multisystem degenerations. As the causes of this group of conditions are still unknown, such a general term would merely be a temporary practical convenience. . . . What we wish to avoid is the multiplication of names for 'disease entities' which in fact are merely the expressions of neuronal atrophy in a variety of overlapping combinations. We therefore propose to use the term multiple system atrophy to cover the whole group.

Graham and Oppenheimer also identified two subgroups of patients with idiopathic orthostatic hypotension, those with Lewy body pathology and those without. This latter group comprised the patients with MSA. Bannister and Oppenheimer[6] again highlighted this distinction in their clinical pathological review of 16 patients in 1972. Although parkinsonian features and lesions of the pigmented nuclei were common to both groups, MSA was distinguished by an earlier mean age of onset than idiopathic paralysis agitans (49 years, as compared to 65) and a worsened prognosis.

Although the existence of MSA as a unique pathological disorder remains unproven, we believe that the term retains clinical usefulness. The usage of the terms SND, OPCA, or SDS confers additional information about the predominant clinical presentation. Nevertheless, the close relationship between these three subgroups is implicit. Although either parkinsonism, autonomic failure, or cerebellar dysfunction may mark the beginning of the disease, the emergence of the other two syndromes can be predicted when the patient survives long enough.

Familial associations of SND or SDS are rarely observed; however, OPCA is distinguished in this regard. Although nonfamilial idiopathic cerebellar degeneration is more common, much of the medical literature regarding OPCA has focused on the hereditary, autosomal-dominant cerebellar ataxias. In fact, familial cerebellar ataxia was initially described by Menzel[7] in 1891, before the introduction of the term OPCA by Dejerine and Thomas. Greenfield[8] initially subdivided OPCA into the familial Menzel-type and the sporadic Dejerine and Thomas type. It is unclear whether or not both types are properly classified as MSA. In a recent editorial, Penny pointed out that there is a growing body of evidence from positron emission tomography (PET) studies and pathology to indicate that sporadic OPCA of the Dejerine

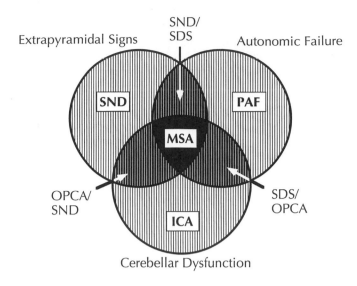

ICA: idiopathic cerebellar ataxia	PAF: pure autonomic failure
MSA: multiple system atrophy	SDS: Shy-Drager syndrome
OPCA: olivopontocerebellar atrophy	SND: striatonigral degeneration

FIGURE 20-1 Cardinal features of multiple-system atrophy. Diagnostic representation of the overlapping combination of signs and symptoms in MSA.

and Thomas type is MSA and is distinct from the dominantly inherited cerebellar degenerations.[9] In a further comparison of the clinical features of sporadic and familial OPCA by Harding,[10] retinal degeneration was confined to the familial cases. Also, both optic atrophy and ophthalmoplegia occurred with far greater frequency in the familial cases. Patients with familial history developed their initial symptoms at a younger age.

We use the term MSA to refer to a gradually progressive, idiopathic neurodegenerative process of adult onset characterized by varying proportions of cerebellar dysfunction, autonomic failure, and parkinsonism that is poorly responsive to L-dopa therapy. The clinical syndrome is dominated but not confined to these features. Familial presentations will heretofore be excluded from the discussion. It is understood that these lines are currently drawn more to conform with precedent and practicality than to reflect genuine and fundamental attributes of pathophysiology.

Clinical Diagnosis

The initial evaluation of a patient with MSA is simply a "snapshot" of the evolving neurodegenerative process. Although the initial presentation may suggest the diagnosis, often the full picture will remain obscured for some time. In fact, the akinetic-rigid patient who is poorly responsive to L-dopa therapy has a broad differential diagnosis. The impression will be later refined by the emerging signs: a vertical supranuclear ophthalmoparesis suggests progressive supranuclear palsy, whereas prominent orthostatic hypotension suggests MSA. Ironically, an initial evaluation of a patient

with an advanced neurodegenerative disorder may also be difficult to sort out, particularly when historical data regarding the order and time frame of the symptoms is lacking. For example, cerebellar signs may be difficult to appreciate in the wheelchair-bound patient with profound rigidity and bradykinesia. Therefore, diagnostic accuracy requires either long-term follow-up of the individual patient or the good fortune to be confronted by the patient when all the diagnostic pieces of the puzzle are in place. Even then, confidence in our diagnostic impression is tempered by the inability to confirm our clinical intuition.

Quinn,[11] expanding on his earlier work detailing the clinical features and natural history of 100 patients diagnosed with MSA,[12] compiled the clinical data of 231 cases of pathologically proven MSA from the medical literature. There was a slight male predominance among these patients (1.4:1), and the median age of onset was 53 years. Greater than 90 percent of the patients were between 40 and 69 years of age. In Berciano's review of 65 cases of pathologically verified sporadic OPCA patients, the gender ratio was 1:1, and the average age of onset was 50.[13] Median survival after diagnosis was between 5 and 6 years, and it has been suggested that earlier and more severe involvement of the autonomic nervous system shortens survival.[14] Although MSA patients can manifest any combination of extrapyramidal, autonomic, and cerebellar features, extrapyramidal signs are the most common. Quinn reported that parkinsonism was present in 89 percent of MSA case reports at some point in the course of their illness. Autonomic failure occurred in 78 percent and cerebellar signs in 55 percent. Pyramidal involvement is also very common, occurring in 61 percent. Twenty-eight percent of MSA patients developed the full clinical spectrum (i.e., parkinsonism, autonomic failure, cerebellar signs, pyramidal signs) before death.

As parkinsonism appears in the large majority of MSA patients, the vague terminology of "atypical parkinsonism" or "Parkinson plus" is often applied. The subgroups of SND, SDS, and OPCA correlate with the number of patients who are initially identified with L-dopa nonresponsive parkinsonism, dysautonomic parkinsonism, and cerebellar parkinsonism, respectively.

Quinn[15] proposed a set of clinical diagnostic criteria for MSA. *Definite* MSA is restricted to patients with postmortem pathological confirmation. A *possible* diagnosis may be conferred in patients with either parkinsonism with poor L-dopa responsiveness or cerebellar parkinsonism. Lastly, a *probable* diagnosis of MSA applies to patients presenting with the many possible permutations of the designated clinical syndromes (i.e., extrapyramidal, pyramidal, cerebellar, and autonomic). Exclusionary criteria include age less than 30 years, a family history, or the presence of another identifiable cause.

It is difficult to assess the incidence of MSA because of the inaccuracy of clinical diagnosis. Pathological surveys of the incidence of MSA among parkinsonians have also resulted in widely varying results. MSA has been identified in as many as 22 percent of brains from parkinsonian patients in two recent reports.[16,17] Although incidence and prevalence data remain inadequate, the increasing sophistication of the practice of medicine continues to expand the usage of this diagnosis in clinical practice.

EXTRAPYRAMIDAL FEATURES

Progressive akinesia, rigidity, and postural instability are common features of MSA. Tremor may occur, although it is less frequent than in idiopathic Parkinson's disease (PD). Bilateral onset of symptoms favors MSA over PD, although unilateral presentations do occur.[18] Diminished facial expressivity, micrographia, and a narrowly based shuffling gait with flexion posture appear. The primary distinguishing factors between PD and MSA presenting with isolated extrapyramidal signs are early postural instability, rapid progression, and a poor or atypical response to dopaminergic therapy.[19]

An adequate trial of L-dopa assumes a central role in identifying patients with MSA, although one can be misled. One-third of early MSA patients reported by Rajput et al.[20] experienced a moderate-to-marked improvement with L-dopa therapy, and Quinn[11] similarly observed a moderate-to-good response in one third. Hughes et al.[21] reported that 65 percent of pathologically confirmed MSA patients had an initial response to L-dopa, and 35 percent remained partially responsive until death. The benefits are generally less impressive than that observed in PD and tend to decline over 1–2 years of treatment. L-dopa-induced dyskinesias occur in MSA. They may appear unusually early and with an atypical predilection for the face and neck. Dyskinesias may be observed without concomitant symptomatic improvement. It is uncommon to obtain symptomatic relief from other antiparkinsonian agents in the absence of a response to L-dopa. Although the benefits are less gratifying than in PD, this should not discourage the clinician from attempting an adequate trial of high-dose L-dopa (1500 mg/day) in MSA patients with parkinsonism. We also try to treat these patients with dopamine agonists (e.g., bromocriptine or pergolide).

AUTONOMIC FAILURE

Autonomic failure was present in 78 percent of MSA patients during the course of their illness.[11] Autonomic symptoms such as postural hypotension, urinary involvement, and impotence in men are frequently the first indications of the disorder. From the perspective of a neurological clinic, where the neurological history and examination are more intensive than the autonomic evaluation, the prevalence, severity, and time frame of the dysautonomia is often underestimated. Although orthostasis and genitourinary difficulties are most likely to be brought to the attention of the physician, problems of thermoregulation and gastrointestinal and respiratory function are not uncommon.

Autonomic dysfunction may also occur in idiopathic PD and, therefore, this array of symptoms and signs in a patient with an akinetic-rigid syndrome does not immediately imply a diagnosis of MSA. Magalhaes et al.,[22] in a retrospective review of autonomic dysfunction in pathologically confirmed cases of MSA and PD, identified certain distinctions regarding prevalence and severity that may prove useful in differentiating MSA and PD when autonomic signs and symptoms are present. All patients with MSA had some autonomic involvement, whereas 24 percent of PD had none. Autonomic dysfunction in MSA involved more autonomic functions and was more severe than that seen in PD, particularly with regard to inspiratory stridor. Although this investigation concluded that autonomic disturbance alone does not distinguish among MSA and PD in individual patients, the presence of severe autonomic dysfunction, autonomic dysfunction that precedes parkinsonism, or inspiratory stridor are all suggestive of MSA.

On initial evaluation of the patient with autonomic signs, the distinction between the primary autonomic failure of MSA and secondary autonomic dysfunction should be considered. Common medical disorders, including diabetes mellitus, autoimmune disease, neoplasia, and renal failure, may give rise to autonomic dysfunction. A variety of medications, including antihypertensives, cardiovascular agents, diuretics, tricyclic antidepressants, and antiparkinsonian drugs, may contribute to postural hypotension.

Orthostatic hypotension (OH) is the most commonly recognized symptom of autonomic dysfunction and develops in nearly all patients with autonomic failure. OH is generally defined as a fall of more than 20 mm Hg systolic blood pressure when the patient stands from a seated position. Not infrequently, significant orthostasis is documented in asymptomatic patients, as gradually progressive and chronic autonomic failure promotes compensatory adjustments of cerebral autoregulation. The symptoms related to postural hypotension are variable, ranging from vague descriptions of lethargy or weakness to full syncope. Other complaints include dizziness, visual disturbances, and craniocervical discomfort, although patients rarely relate their symptoms to changes of position without direct questioning.

Postural hypotension is exacerbated after prolonged recumbency, mealtime, and physical exertion. Other contributory factors are heat, alcohol, coughing, and defecation.[23,24] Management of OH involves a number of prophylactic measures. As nocturnal diuresis in the elderly contributes to inadequate blood volume and OH upon arising, recommendations are designed to improve intravascular volume and diminish peripheral edema. Liberalizing salt and water intake, the application of elastic stockings before arising, elevation of the legs periodically during the day, and elevation of the head at night may be helpful (Table 20-1). Physical exertion should be delayed until the afternoon and should not closely follow mealtime. Pharmacotherapy of OH may include the use of fludrocortisone, midodrine, recombinant human erythropoietin, phenylpropanolamine, indomethacin, dihydroxyphenylserine, caffeine, and ergots.[25]

Genitourinary dysfunction in MSA is very common. Beck et al.[26] studied neurourological features of 62 patients clinically diagnosed with MSA. All patients had abnormal urethral or anal sphincter electromyograms, a finding the authors considered diagnostic in the appropriate clinical setting. Impotence was the presenting symptom in 37 percent of men and occurred in 96 percent with progression of the illness. Frequent spontaneous penile erections may antedate erectile failure. The absence of penile erection upon awakening in the morning favors a neurogenic rather than a functional etiology for impotence. Therapeutic alternatives include penile implants, intracavernosal papaverine injections, and the administration of yohimbine. Urinary symptoms resulted from a combination of detrusor hyperreflexia, urethral

TABLE 20-1 Management and Symptomatic Treatment of MSA

Extrapyramidal Features
  Administration of carbidopa/L-dopa (up to 1500 mg
    L-dopa/day)
  Administration of bromocriptine (up to 60 mg/day)
  Administration of pergolide (up to 6 mg/day)
  Physical therapy, occupational therapy, speech therapy
Autonomic Failure
  Orthostatic hypotension
    Liberalizing salt and water intake
    Application of elastic stockings
    Elevation of the head of the bed at night
    Elevation of the legs periodically during the day
    Delay physical exertion until the afternoon
    Exercise caution upon arising in the morning and
      immediately after meals or physical exertion
    Fludrocortisone administration (0.1–1.0 mg/day)
    Trials of midodrine, recombinant human erythropoietin,
      phenylpropanolamine, ephedrine, indomethacin,
      dihydroxyphenylserine, caffeine, and ergots
  Male impotence
    Administration of yohimbine
    Intracavernosal papaverine injection
    Placement of a penile implant
  Urinary difficulties
    Treatment of concurrent prostatism in men or pelvic floor
      muscle laxity in women
    Treatment of concurrent urinary tract infection
    Urinary acidification
    Administration of anticholinergic agents
    Intermittent or continuous urinary catheterization
  Constipation
    Encourage dietary fiber and liquid intake
    Encourage physical activity
    Administration of bulk agents, laxatives, and suppositories
  Dysphagia
    Barium swallow study with video fluoroscopy
    Introduce a soft mechanical diet
    Percutaneous gastrostomy placement
  Respiratory stridor
    Laryngoscopy and/or sleep study
    Tracheostomy placement

sphincter weakness and, finally, failure of detrusor contraction. The urinary symptoms simulated outflow obstruction in men, and 43 percent underwent prostatic or bladder neck surgery. Fifty-seven percent of the women had stress incontinence, and one-half had undergone surgical bladder repair. The results of operative procedures in both sexes was poor. Nonsurgical treatment with intermittent catheterization, anticholinergic medication, and desmopressin spray improved continence in over one-half of the patients. Anticholinergic medication may result in urinary retention, and intermittent catheterization may result in recurrent infection.

Sakakibara et al. also studied micturitional disturbance in 86 patients with clinically diagnosed MSA.[27] The authors subdivided their MSA patients into those with SDS, SND, and OPCA to further classify urinary dysfunction. Micturitional symptoms were found in more than 90 percent of patients, regardless of MSA subdivision. Urinary symptoms

appeared earlier and were more severe in SDS than in SND or OPCA. Urinary symptoms progressed with disease progression.

Constipation is the most common gastrointestinal symptom. Straining during evacuation or micturition elevates intrathoracic pressure and may result in symptomatic hypotension. Daily use of dietary fiber, adequate liquid intake, and laxatives is helpful. Fecal incontinence occasionally occurs, although it is less common than urinary incontinence. Dysphagia is not uncommon in more advanced stages of the disorder. Respiratory stridor also often occurs with progression because of laryngeal muscle paresis. The advisability of either gastrostomy or tracheostomy should be approached on an individual basis with a realistic appraisal of the patient's general quality of life.

CEREBELLAR DYSFUNCTION

Whereas the majority of MSA patients present with bradykinetic parkinsonian signs, in others a cerebellar syndrome heralds the development of multisystem involvement. The initial manifestation is frequently gait ataxia with eventual involvement of the upper limbs.[13] Dysarthria is nearly universal, although its nature may vary. Speech may be scanning, bulbar, pseudobulbar, monotone, slow, or hypophonic. Kinetic tremor with dysmetria may occur. Other cerebellar features include hypotonia and exaggerated rebound with loss of checking response. Myoclonus is less common. Ocular motor signs frequently emerge, although they are more common in the familial form of OPCA than in the sporadic form. Supranuclear ophthalmoplegia occurs primarily in familial OPCA[13] or, of course, progressive supranuclear palsy (PSP), whereas nystagmus, jerky pursuit, ocular dysmetria, fixation instability, and slowing of saccades are common in MSA patients.[28] Mild limitations of gaze are also common. However, Quinn believes that a prominent downgaze palsy is an exclusion criterion for a clinical diagnosis of MSA.[11]

Therapeutics for cerebellar signs remains a disappointing and frustrating area for the clinician. When tremor or myoclonus are prominent, trials of clonazepam or valproate may prove worthwhile. Patients with isolated cerebellar dysfunction are frequently diagnosed with cerebellar degeneration. The later emergence of autonomic, extrapyramidal, and pyramidal signs is often overlooked for some time, delaying both appropriate diagnosis as well as therapeutic opportunities for parkinsonian or autonomic symptoms. A clinicopathological study of 35 patients with MSA revealed that 88 percent had evidence of OPCA, with the cerebellar vermis usually more involved than the cerebellar hemispheres. Surprisingly, the presence of cerebellar pathology was unrelated to the presence of cerebellar signs in life.[29]

PYRAMIDAL SIGNS

Exaggerated deep tendon reflexes, extensor plantar responses, pseudobulbar palsy, and spasticity are present in the majority of MSA patients, oftentimes early in the disorder. The presence of prominent extrapyramidal rigidity and bradykinesia often masks both pyramidal spasticity and cerebellar incoordination.

COGNITIVE FUNCTION AND BEHAVIOR

Although progressive dementia is not a feature of MSA, cognitive deficits and alterations of personality and mood are common. When the cognitive performance of 16 patients with probable MSA of the striatonigral type (mean Hoehn and Yahr stage 3.7) was studied and compared to that of normal controls, the MSA group showed significant deficits on tests of frontal lobe function.[30] Specifically, attentional set shifting and speed of thinking were impaired, although there was no consistent evidence of intellectual deterioration, as measured by the Wechsler Adult Intelligence Scale. Cognitive deficits were not correlated with either the duration or severity of disease. The pattern of deficits was distinctive, markedly in contrast to Alzheimer's dementia, less in contrast to PD. Personality alterations include apathy, passivity, emotional lability, and depression. This confluence of impaired executive functions, apathy, and impulsivity is characteristic of frontal-subcortical circuit dysfunction.[31] Treatment of associated psychotic disturbances is often complicated and unsuccessful. A single patient with OPCA and neuroleptic-resistant depression was treated successfully with clozapine without compromise of neurological function.[32]

Diagnostic Investigations

Neuroradiographic evaluation is routinely performed in the investigation of a patient with progressive neurological deficits. Cranial computed tomography (CT) may reveal infratentorial atrophy. When CT images of 33 MSA patients and 40 age-matched controls were blindly analyzed by neuroradiologists, atrophy of the cerebellar hemispheres, vermis, pons, midbrain, and cerebral hemispheres, as well as enlargement of the basilar cisterns and fourth ventricle, were differentially discriminated between the two groups.[33] However, in no case did CT imaging confirm cerebellar or brain stem involvement that was not clinically evident. Wenning et al. concluded that CT is of limited diagnostic use in MSA.

Magnetic resonance imaging (MRI) of the brain reveals abnormally hypointense signal in the putamen with T_2-weighted images of many patients with atypical parkinsonism,[34] in addition to the previously described findings of atrophy. The sensitivity and specificity of the finding of abnormal putaminal signal has not yet been sufficiently clarified to use it for reliable diagnosis. Testa et al.[35] reported that 9 of 9 patients with SND all had MRI putaminal abnormalities, and 13 of 13 patients with OPCA all had posterior fossa abnormalities consistent with OPCA. Infratentorial atrophy may be seen more readily with MRI than with CT and may assist in differentiating idiopathic PD from MSA/OPCA before the full clinical picture is apparent (Figs. 20-2 to 20-5).

PET studies have been performed with ^{18}F-6-fluorodopa (FD), ^{11}C-raclopride (RAC), and ^{11}C-diprenorphine in order to examine both the pre- and postsynaptic segments of the dopaminergic pathway. Reduced putaminal uptake of FD has been reported in MSA, as well as reduced striatal binding of diprenorphine and RAC.[36-38] Abnormalities of striatal glucose metabolism have also been demonstrated with ^{18}F-flu-

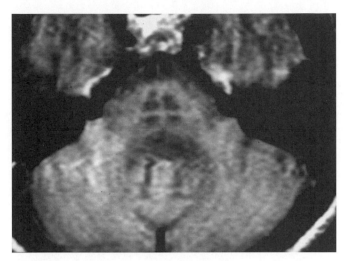

FIGURE 20-2 MRI proton density image demonstrating increased signal in the brain stem involving the midline raphe and transverse pontine fibers and sparing the tegmentum, pyramidal tracts, and superior cerebellar peduncles. *(Courtesy of Dr. Brian Bowen.)*

orodeoxyglucose PET studies.[39-41] These results suggest that selective metabolic reduction in the putamen and cerebellum may be a marker for MSA. In addition, PET studies have contributed to the evidence that sporadic OPCA is MSA, whereas dominantly inherited OPCA is a separate entity. ^{123}I-iodobenzamide single-photon emission computed tomography (SPECT) scanning may be useful in assessing the integrity of striatal dopamine receptors in early parkinsonians.[42] Proton magnetic resonance spectroscopy has been reported to differentiate MSA from PD.[43] In patients with the SND form of MSA the N-acetylaspartate (NAA) to creatine ratio and the choline to creatine ratio were significantly reduced in the putamen and globus pallidus, compared to the preserved ratio in patients with PD. OPCA patients showed a significant but less marked reduction in these ratios. The

FIGURE 20-3 OPCA. Increased signal on MRI in the middle cerebellar peduncles. *(Courtesy of Dr. Brian Bowen.)*

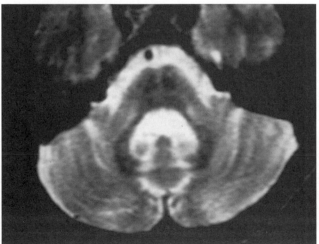

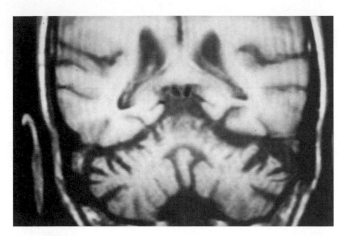
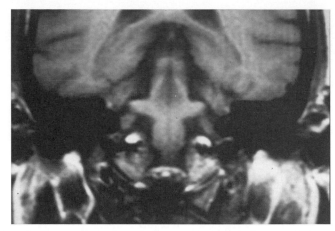

FIGURE 20-4 and 20-5 OPCA. MRI T₁-weighted coronal images showing the brain stem and cerebellar atrophy. Cerebellar atrophy is often worse for the hemispheres than the vermis. Atrophy of the middle cerebellar peduncles results in a "cross" or "t" appearance on the coronal image. *(Courtesy of Dr. Brian Bowen.)*

reduced ratio probably reflects neuronal loss occurring predominantly in the putamen. It is suggested that proton magnetic resonance spectroscopy may prove to be a useful noninvasive technique to diagnose MSA. However, whether or not this technique can differentiate MSA from PSP or other akinetic-rigid syndromes is unknown. Experience is currently insufficient to state whether any of these studies will reliably distinguish MSA from the spectrum of neurological disorders.

Electrophysiological studies are not useful for the diagnosis or management of MSA with the exception of the urethral or rectal sphincter electromyogram (EMG). Although this study is not widely used, Eardley et al.[44] reported that EMG parameters of denervation and reinnervation (large, prolonged, polyphasic motor unit action potentials) are recorded at the urethral and rectal sphincters as a result of anterior horn cell loss from Onuf's nucleus in the sacral region of the spinal cord. This test may be helpful in the differentiation of MSA and PD, although the correlation of these findings with the presence of urinary or fecal incontinence is uncertain. Electroencephalographic studies are normal in MSA, and evoked responses yield widely varying results.

Although autonomic failure is commonly diagnosed in the setting of the appropriate history and the demonstration of a significant drop in blood pressure upon arising, there are a number of sophisticated investigations of autonomic function available.[24] Postural hypotension is best evaluated with the use of a tilt table. Plasma norepinephrine responses to postural change may provide a quantitative biochemical assessment of the sympathetic nervous system. In individual patients, barium swallowing studies for dysphagia, urodynamic studies for urinary difficulties and laryngoscopy, or sleep studies for respiratory stridor may be useful for both diagnosis and management.

In summary, although diagnostic investigations are routinely pursued, their major contribution is in the exclusion of diagnoses that are more amenable to therapy than MSA. The accumulated data may add to the clinical impression; however, no diagnostic study can reliably distinguish the autonomic failure, electrophysiology, or neuroradiology of MSA from the other possible etiologies in this setting.

Neuropathology

Postmortem brains of MSA patients demonstrate cell loss and gliosis in an assortment of the following regions: striatum, substantia nigra, locus ceruleus, pontine nuclei, middle cerebellar peduncles, cerebellar Purkinje cells, inferior olives, and intermediolateral cell columns (Fig. 20-6 to 20-8).[11] However, the clinicopathological correlation of MSA is not high, particularly in the early stages of the disorder. A distinctive glial cytoplasmic inclusion (GCI) was initially described by Papp et al.[45] in 11 patients with SND, OPCA, or SDS; it was not present in 284 brains of adults with other neurological disorders including PD, AD, PSP, and vascular parkinsonism (Fig. 20-9). GCIs surround the nuclei of oligodendroglia with a crescent or flame-shaped morphology. They are found in large numbers in many regions of the central nervous system, with a particular predilection for the white matter tracts. Papp and Lantos[46] reported later that these inclusion bodies can be demonstrated in the cytoplasm and nucleus of both neuronal and oligodendroglial cells and in the neuronal processes by means of silver staining, immunochemistry and electron microscopy. These inclusions were stained only by antiubiquitin antibody.[46,47] Tubular structures forming the inclusion bodies are similar to the linear structures described in motor neuron disease. This work demonstrates that the accumulation of abnormal tubular structures in both oligodendrocytes and neurons is the pathological marker for MSA. Recent work[48] involving the semiquantitative mapping of GCIs in MSA revealed that a system-bound extensive degeneration of interfascicular, perineuronal, and perivascular oligodendrocytes exists. GCIs occur in the primary motor and higher motor areas of the cerebral cortex (pyramidal, extrapyramidal, corticocerebellar systems), in the supraspinal autonomic system, and in their targets. In contrast, the visual and auditory pathways, somatosensory system, olfactory structures, association and limbic cortical areas, and subcortical limbic structures contain no or few GCIs. Papp and Lantos[48] conclude that there is a striking preponderance of oligodendroglial degeneration, compared to that of neuronal alteration in the same area, and that degeneration of neurons

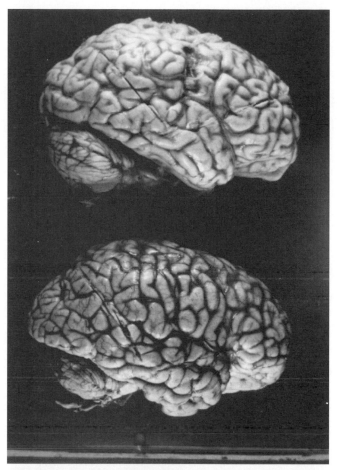

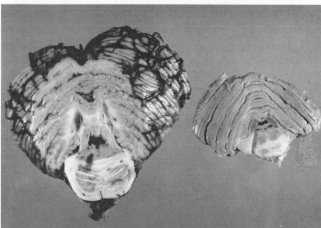

FIGURE 20-6 *Top:* OPCA *below* with the control brain *above.* *(Courtesy of Dr. Michael Norenberg.) Bottom:* OPCA on *right,* control on *left. (Courtesy of Dr. Michael Norenberg.)*

is not a prerequisite for the development of GCIs. This raises the possibility that oligodendroglial degeneration may cause or contribute to the manifestation of clinical symptomatology in structures with GCI accumulation without convincing neuronal alterations.

As with other CNS cellular inclusions (neurofibrillary tangles, Lewy bodies) the relationship of GCIs to the mechanism of the disorder has yet to be elucidated. GCIs may represent glial reaction to neuronal injury or evidence of a primary

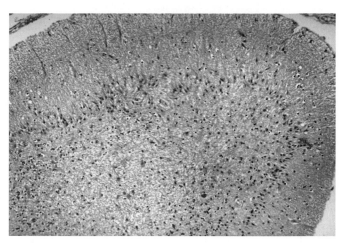

FIGURE 20-7 OPCA with loss of Purkinje and granule cells associated with Bergmann gliosis. *(Courtesy of Dr. Michael Norenberg.)*

oligodendroglia cell disease.[45,49] Nevertheless, Quinn[11] believes that the presence of GCIs is essential to the pathological diagnosis of MSA and has furthermore proposed the concept of "minimal change MSA,"[50] neuronal loss restricted to the pigmented brain stem nuclei associated with GCIs.

Differential Diagnosis

The most instrumental tool currently available to the clinician to make the diagnosis of MSA is the passage of time. Indeed, we all have congratulated ourselves for diagnosing MSA in patients with previous misdiagnoses of idiopathic PD or cerebellar ataxia, when we simply have been the beneficiary of information unavailable to our predecessors. There is considerable similarity between the neurological signs that appear in the various neurodegenerative disorders (Table 20-2). The particular vulnerability of the substantia nigra and striatum to neuronal injury is borne out by the presence of moderate-to-severe parkinsonism in the full range of disorders. Autonomic failure, cognitive dysfunction, oculomotor

FIGURE 20-8 OPCA. Biotin stain showing loss of Purkinje cells. A torpedo is indicated by the arrow. *(Courtesy of Dr. Michael Norenberg.)*

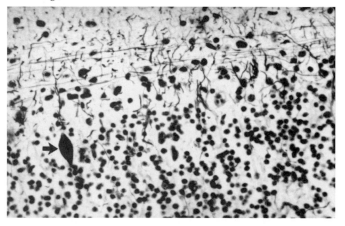

TABLE 20-2 Neurological Signs of the Neurodegenerative Disorders

	MSA			PSP	PD	DLBD	CBD	AD
	SND	SDS	OPCA					
Parkinsonism	+ + + +	+ + +	+ +	+ + + +	+ + + +	+ + + +	+ + + +	+ +
Cerebellar signs	+ +	+	+ + + +	+	0	0	+	+
Autonomic failure	+ +	+ + + +	+ +	+	+ +	+ +	+	+
Pyramidal signs	+ +	+	+ +	+ +	0	+	+ +	+
Cognitive dysfunction	+ +	+	+ +	+ + +	+ +	+ + + +	+ +	+ + + +
Oculomotor impairment	+	+	+ + +	+ + + +	+ +	+ +	+ +	+
Dysarthria	+ + +	+	+ + +	+ + +	+ +	+ +	+ + +	+ +
Dysphagia	+ +	+	+ +	+ + +	+ +	+ +	+	+ +
Peripheral neuropathy	+	+	+ +	+	0	0	+ +	+
Involuntary movements	+	+	+ +	+	+ + +	+ + +	+ +	+

0, none; +, uncommon or unusual; + +, common or moderate; + + +, frequent or marked; + + + +, present in nearly all cases or severe. DLBD, diffuse Lewy body disease; CBD, corticobasal degeneration; AD, Alzheimer's disease.

impairment, dysarthria, dysphagia, and involuntary movements are also pervasive. The clinical impression is formed by the relative proportions of a similar array of neurological signs, tempered by knowledge of the natural history of the individual disorders. Nonetheless, the astute clinician can be sensitized to clues or idiosyncrasies that suggest the presence of one disorder over another.

MSA is most commonly confused with PD, although PSP often bears the greatest similarity. Corticobasal degeneration (CBD) also deserves consideration in the differential diagnosis of atypical parkinsonism, especially in the early years before the fully developed clinical picture emerges. In a prospective clinical pathological study of diagnostic accuracy in parkinsonism, the initial diagnosis of idiopathic PD was correct in 65 percent of cases, and improved to 76 percent with follow-up.[17] The diagnostic accuracy for MSA with at least 5 years of follow-up was 69 percent. SND and SND/SDS were misdiagnosed as idiopathic PD in 31 percent, whereas OPCA was accurately identified in this study.

The major clinical features that raise suspicion about a diagnosis of idiopathic PD are a poor response to L-dopa;

the presence of pyramidal, cerebellar, or autonomic signs; early postural instability; and rapid clinical deterioration. Questions are also raised by the absence of rest tremor, the presence of a symmetrical onset of signs, a severe dysarthria, disproportionate antecollis, and respiratory stridor. PSP is most frequently distinguished from MSA by the appearance of a prominent supranuclear vertical ophthalmoparesis with associated visual impairment (see also Chap. 19). Hyperextension of the head or unusually erect posture, lid retraction associated with a surprised facial expression, disproportionate nuchal and axial rigidity, and apraxia of eyelid opening also suggest the presence of PSP. CBD is most frequently distinguished from MSA by the presence of early signs of cortical dysfunction (especially apraxia and cortical sensory loss), prominent myoclonus, and asymmetric perirolandic frontoparietal cortical atrophy on CT or MRI scans (see also Chap. 45). Vascular parkinsonism may be confused with MSA; however, a good history, the association of hypertension or other stroke risk factors, and modern neuroimaging help the clinician distinguish between them (see also Chap. 25).

Our current knowledge of MSA and other neurodegenerative disorders that have similar presentations is fragmentary, and the conundrum of where to draw the lines that define and compartmentalize "unique" disorders remains an ongoing challenge. Clinical description, diagnostic investigations, and neuropathology are insufficient. Advances in cellular biochemistry and molecular biology will ultimately identify the fundamental distinguishing attributes of these disorders.

Acknowledgment

Supported in part by the National Parkinson Foundation.

References

1. Dejerine J, Thomas A: L'atrophie olivo-ponto-cerebelleuse. *Nouv Iconogr Salpet* 13:330–370, 1900.
2. Shy GM, Drager GA: A neurological syndrome associated with orthostatic hypotension. *Arch Neurol* 2:511–527, 1960.

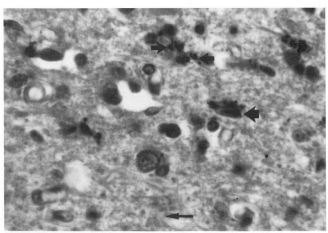

FIGURE 20-9 The arrows indicate pigmented inclusions in glial cells within the striatum in a patient with nigrostriatal degeneration. H&E stain. *(Courtesy of Dr. Michael Norenberg.)*

3. van der Eecken H, Adams RD, van Bogaert L: Striopallidal-nigral degeneration: A hitherto undescribed lesion in paralysis agitans. *J Neuropathol Exp Neurol* 19:159–161, 1960.

4. Adams RD, vonBogaert L, van der Eecken H: Degeneres cences nigro-striees et cerebello-nigro-striees. *Psychiatr Neurol* 142:219–259, 1961.

5. Graham JG, Oppenheimer DR: Orthostatic hypotension and nicotine sensitivity in a case of multiple system atrophy. *J Neurol Neurosurg Psychiatry* 32:28–34, 1969.

6. Bannister R, Oppenheimer DR: Degenerative diseases of the nervous system associated with autonomic failure. *Brain* 95:457–474, 1972.

7. Menzel P: Beitrag zur kenntniss der hereditaren ataxie und klein-hirnatrophie. *Arch Psychiatrie Nervenkrankheiten* 22:160–190, 1891.

8. Greenfield JG: The spino-cerebellar degenerations. Springfield, IL: Charles C Thomas, 1954.

9. Penney JB: Multiple systems atrophy and nonfamilial olivopontocerebellar atrophy are the same disease. *Ann Neurol* 37:553–554, 1995.

10. Harding AE: 'Idiopathic' late onset cerebellar ataxia, in Harding AE (ed): The *Hereditary Ataxias and Related Disorders*. New York: Churchill Livingstone, 1984, pp 166–173.

11. Quinn NP: Multiple system atrophy, in Marsden CD, Fahn S (eds): *Movement Disorders 3*. Oxford: Butterworth-Heinemann, 1994, pp 262–281.

12. Wenning GK, Ben Shlomo Y, Magalhaes M, et al: Clinical features and natural history of multiple system atrophy: An analysis of 100 cases. *Brain* 117:835–845, 1994.

13. Berciano J: Olivopontocerebellar atrophy, in Jankovic J, Tolosa E (eds): *Parkinson's Disease and Movement Disorders*. Baltimore: Williams & Wilkins, 1993, pp 163–189.

14. Saito Y, Matsuoka Y, Takahashi A, Ohno Y: Survival of patients with multiple system atrophy. *Intern Med* 33:321–325, 1994.

15. Quinn N: Multiple system atrophy—the nature of the beast. *J Neurol Neurosurg Psychiatry* (suppl.)1989, pp 78–89.

16. Fearnley JM, Lees AJ: Striatonigral degeneration: A clinicopathological study. *Brain* 113:1823–1842, 1990.

17. Rajput AH, Rodzilsky B, Rajput A: Accuracy of clinical diagnosis in parkinsonism—a prospective study. *Can J Neurol Sci* 18:275–278, 1991.

18. Adams RD, Salam-Adams M: Striatonigral degeneration, in Vinken PJ, Bruyn GW, Klawans HL (eds): *Extrapyramidal Disorders*. Amsterdam: Elsevier Science Publishers, 1986, pp 205–212.

19. Gouider-Khouja N, Vidailhef M, Bonnef AM, et al: "Pure" striatonigral degeneration and Parkinson's disease: A comparative clinical study. *Mov Disord* 10:288–294, 1995.

20. Rajput AH, Rodzilsky B, Rajput A, Ang L: L-dopa efficacy and pathological basis of Parkinson syndromes. *Clin Neuropharmacol* 13:553–558, 1990.

21. Hughes AJ, Colosimo C, Kleedorfen B, et al: The dopaminergic response in multiple system atrophy. *J Neurol Neurosurg Psychiatry* 55:1009–1013, 1992.

22. Magalhaes M, Wenning GK, Daniel SE, Quinn NP: Autonomic dysfunction in pathologically confirmed multiple system atrophy and idiopathic Parkinson's disease—a retrospective comparison. *Acta Neurol Scand* 91:98–102, 1995.

23. Mathias CJ: Orthostatic hypotension: Causes, mechanisms and influencing factors. *Neurology* 45:S6–S11, 1995.

24. Robertson D, Davis TL: Recent advances in the treatment of orthostatic hypotension. *Neurology* 45:S26–S32, 1995.

25. Mathias CJ, Williams AC: The Shy-Drager syndrome and multiple system atrophy, in Calne DB (ed): *Neurodegenerative Diseases*. Philadelphia: WB Saunders, 1994, pp 743–767.

26. Beck RO, Betts CD, Fowler CJ: Genitourinary dysfunction in multiple system atrophy: Clinical features and treatment in 62 cases. *J Urol* 151:1336–1341, 1994.

27. Sakakibara R, Hattori T, Tojo M, et al: Micturitional disturbance in multiple system atrophy. *Jpn J Psychiatry Neurol* 47:591–598, 1993.

28. Duvoisin RC: The olivopontocerebellar atrophies, in Marsden CD, Fahn S (eds): *Movement Disorders 2*. London: Butterworth, 1987, pp 249–271.

29. Wenning GK, Ben-Shlomo Y, Magalhaes M, et al: Clinicopathological study of 35 cases of multiple system atrophy. *J Neurol Neurosurg Psychiatry* 58:160–166, 1995.

30. Robbins TW, James M, Lange KW, et al: Cognitive performance in multiple system atrophy. *Brain* 115:271–291, 1992.

31. Cummings JL: Frontal-subcortical circuits and human behavior. *Arch Neurol* 50:873–880, 1993.

32. Parsa MA, Simon M, Dubrow C, et al: Psychiatric manifestations of olivopontocerebellar atrophy and treatment with clozapine. *Int J Psychiatry Med* 23:149–156, 1993.

33. Wenning GK, Jager K, Kendall B, et al: Is cranial computerized tomography useful in the diagnosis of multiple system atrophy? *Mov Disord* 9:333–336, 1994.

34. Drayer BP, Olanow W, Burger P, et al: Parkinson plus syndrome: Diagnosis using high field MR imaging of brain iron. *Radiology* 159:493–498, 1986.

35. Testa D, Savoiardo M, Fetoni V, et al: Multiple system atrophy. Clinical and MR observations on 42 cases. *Ital J Neurol Sci* 14:211–216, 1993.

36. Brooks DJ, Ibanez V, Sawle GV, et al: Differing patterns of striatal 18F-dopa uptake in Parkinson's disease, multiple system atrophy, and progressive supranuclear palsy. *Ann Neurol* 28:547–555, 1990.

37. Sawle GV, Playford ED, Brooks DJ, et al: Asymmetrical presynaptic and post-synaptic changes to the striatal dopamine projection in dopa naive parkinsonism: Diagnostic implications of the D2 receptor status. *Brain* 116:853–867, 1993.

38. Rinne JO, Burn DJ, Mathias CJ, et al: Positron emission tomography studies on the dopaminergic system and striatal opioid binding in the olivopontocerebellar atrophy variant of multiple system atrophy. *Ann Neurol* 37:568–573, 1995.

39. Eidelberg D, Takikawa S, Moeller JR, et al: Striatal hypometabolism distinguishes striatonigral degeneration from Parkinson's disease. *Ann Neurol* 33:518–527, 1993.

40. Perani D, Bressi S, Testa D, et al: Clinical/metabolic correlations in multiple system atrophy: A fluorodeoxyglucose F 18 positron emission tomographic study. *Arch Neurol* 52:179–185, 1995.

41. Gilman S, Koeppe RA, Junck L, et al: Patterns of cerebral glucose metabolism detected with positron emission tomography differ in multiple system atrophy and olivopontocerebellar atrophy. *Ann Neurol* 36:166–175, 1994.

42. Schwarz J, Taksen K, Arnold G, et al: 123I-iodobenzamide SPECT predicts dopaminergic responsiveness in patients with de novo parkinsonism. *Neurology* 42:556–561, 1992.

43. Davie CA, Wenning GK, Barker GJ, et al: Differentiation of multiple system atrophy from idiopathic Parkinson's disease using proton magnetic resonance spectroscopy. *Ann Neurol* 37:204–210, 1995.

44. Eardley I, Quinn NP, Fowler CJ, et al: The value of urethral sphincter electromyography in the differential diagnosis of parkinsonism. *Br J Urol* 64:360–362, 1989.

45. Papp MI, Kahn JE, Lantos PL: Glial cytoplasmic inclusions in the CNS of patients with multiple system atrophy (striatonigral degeneration, olivopontocerebellar atrophy and Shy-Drager syndrome). *J Neurol Sci* 94:79–100, 1989.

46. Papp MI, Lantos PL: Accumulation of tubular structures in oligodendroglial and neuronal cells as the basic alteration in multiple system atrophy. *J Neurol Sci* 107:172–182, 1992.

47. Kato S, Nakamura H, Hirano A, Ito H, et al: Agryophilic ubiquitinated cytoplasmic inclusions of leu-7-positive glial cells in olivo-

pontocerebellar atrophy (multiple system atrophy). *Acta Neuro-pathol (Berl)* 82:488–493, 1991.

48. Papp MI, Lantos PL: The distribution of oligodendroglial inclusions in multiple system atrophy and its relevance to clinical symptomatology. *Brain* 117:235–243, 1994.

49. Costa C, Duyckaerts C: Oligodendroglial and neuronal inclusions in multiple system atrophy. *Curr Opin Neurol* 6:865–871, 1993.

50. Wenning GK, Quinn NP, Magalhaes M, et al: "Minimal change" multiple system atrophy. *Mov Disord* 9:161–166, 1994.

Chapter 21

INFECTIOUS AND POSTINFECTIOUS PARKINSONISM

PUIU NISIPEANU, DIANA PALEACU, and AMOS D. KORCZYN

CLINICAL FEATURES OF ENCEPHALITIS
  LETHARGICA
POSTENCEPHALITIC PARKINSONISM
    Clinical Features
    Pathophysiology
    Pathology
    Treatment
PARKINSONISM RESULTING FROM OTHER
  INFECTIOUS CAUSES
    Acquired Immune Deficiency Syndrome (AIDS)
    Nonviral Infections
    Syphilis
    Fungal and Parasitic Infections
    Creutzfeldt-Jakob Disease (CJD)
SUMMARY

Parkinsonian features can develop during or after various infectious diseases (Table 21-1). A major cause of parkinsonism in earlier decades of this century, fortunately only of historical interest at the present time, is *encephalitis lethargica* (EL). This disease, also called von Economo's disease, appeared as an epidemic during World War I, and many new cases were reported for more than 10 years. In Austria and France, EL was first described in 1917 by von Economo[1] and by Cruchet et al.[2] By 1918 the disease had spread throughout Europe to England and Germany, and later it spread to North America and the Chinese province of Younnanfou.[3] By 1919 it had overrun Europe and disseminated to Central America, India and, later, Japan, Africa and Australia.[4,5] However, the number of new cases was negligible after 1935, and the disease essentially disappeared from public health reports and mortality data in 1940, when the term EL was replaced by the more inclusive "infectious encephalitides" on the International List of the Causes of Death.[6]

Postencephalitic parkinsonism (PEP), first delineated by Souques,[7] was a frequently seen variant of parkinsonism in the 1920s, and probably the best estimates were provided by Dimsdale's review of the patients seen in London clinics between 1900 and 1942. Her data indicate that EL accounted for two-thirds of the cases of parkinsonism seen in the period from 1920–1930 and for one-half of the cases seen during the following decade.

In a later retrospective study, conducted in 1959 and 1960, a history suggesting EL was obtained from 13 percent of 107 consecutive patients with parkinsonism and other encephalitides from a further 16 percent.[5] A progressive decline of PEP was seen over time; whereas in 1955 20 percent of the parkinsonian population was diagnosed as suffering from PEP, 10 years later, PEP contributed only 6.6 percent of patients, and no new patients were diagnosed as having the disease after 1967. In 1968, Duvoisin[9] noted that PEP represented less than 1 percent of patients. Nevertheless, considering the prior high frequency of PEP, it was suggested that many cases of "idiopathic" Parkinson's disease (PD) were actually caused by the pandemic EL during the 1920s, in which these subjects were affected subclinically. It was further suggested that as the cohort of patients who had undergone subclinical infection died, the frequency of PD would decrease dramatically, so that PD would cease to exist as a major entity.[10] This theory, known as the cohort theory, was supported by the observation that the mean age at onset of parkinsonism rose progressively during the calendar years from 1920 to 1955.[11] However, an alternative interpretation may be more valid, namely, that the increasing age of onset of PD could be a result of the increasing number of elderly people, and several decades later, the cohort theory is obsolete. There is no trend toward a decrease in PD prevalence, although PEP has almost totally disappeared.

Clinical Features of Encephalitis Lethargica

The initial clinical features of EL were of a nonspecific viral infection. Von Economo's description of EL was as follows: "The patients all showed a slight influenza like a prodromal condition with pharyngeal symptoms, a slight rise of temperature which was soon followed by a variety of nervous system symptoms of which generally one or another pointed to the midbrain as the source."[12]

Most patients exhibited a persistent pathological somnolence, or sleep lasting for days to weeks (a feature giving the disease its name), from which they could be aroused briefly by vigorous stimulation. Another prominent feature was ophthalmoplegia, usually in combination with somnolence (the "somnolent ophthalmoplegic" form). Wilson, one of the leading neurologists of the period, remarked that every type of internal or external ophthalmoplegia could be found.[13] This common somnolent ophthalmoplegic form suggested inflammatory involvement of the upper midbrain to von Economo. Signs of cortical dysfunction, such as aphasia, convulsions, psychosis, and sensory impairment, including disorders of hearing and vision, were notably rare. A small percentage of patients were overactive, rather than somnolent, and an even smaller fraction exhibited movement disorders like chorea or myoclonus on a cataplectic background. Bradykinesia and mutism were predominant in a remainder group smaller yet. As in other viral encephalitides, fever was a constant feature, whereas elevated CSF protein level with lymphocytic pleocytosis was seen in about one-half of the patients.

The clinical, laboratory, and pathological features of EL were highly suggestive of a viral infection. Von Economo even reported successful transmission to nonhuman primates. However, no virus was ever convincingly identified.

TABLE 21-1 Infectious Agents Associated with Parkinsonism

Measles
Japanese B encephalitis
Western equine encephalitis
Tick-borne encephalitis
Poliomyelitis
Cytomegalovirus
HIV
Influenza A

Attempts to establish a link between EL/PEP and a number of viruses, notably influenza strains A and B and herpes viruses, were unsuccessful.[14–16] The hypothesis[17,18] that influenza virus was the responsible agent is more attractive than that of a one-time unidentified virus, as it may explain—at least for those who believe that PD is caused by viral exposure—the occurrence of PD before the EL pandemic.[11] The role of retroviruses was discussed recently by Elizan and Casals,[19] who found in EL and PEP brain specimens white matter astrogliosis, similar to the astrogliosis seen in human ummunodeficiency virus-1 HIV-1 encephalopathy. The addition of polymerase chain reaction techniques that may be applied to detect viral genomes in paraffin-embedded tissues could provide new impetus to continue the search for a viral etiology of EL.

The onset of EL was acute or subacute; the disease lasted for several weeks; and the mortality in some areas was as high as 30–40 percent. Many of those who survived the acute phase of the illness were left with a wide variety of symptoms, including mental impairment; difficulty in reestablishing a normal sleep-wake cycle; myoclonus; dystonia; tics and other bizarre movements, postures, or gait; bulimia and obesity; sociopathic behavior in adults; and personality changes in children with compulsive behavior.[20] However, three very peculiar delayed features became evident: (1) Oculogyric crises (OGC); (2) Central respiratory irregularities, including increased respiratory rate, apneic episodes, myoclonic jerks of the diaphragm, and cluster breathing resulting in hypoxia; and (3) parkinsonism.

OGC apparently were not seen during the epidemic of EL,[13,21–23] and they were first reported by Oecknighaus[24] in 1921, consisting of forceful deviation of the eyes, almost always upward or upward and laterally, seldom in a horizontal or downward direction, and rarely, convergence. Most attacks were of a sustained tonic nature (usually continuing for minutes or hours and disappearing during sleep), but instances of repeated clonic spasms of ocular deviation also occurred. Almost always OGC appeared in patients who had already developed parkinsonism, although rarely they preceded it by a short period. Their prevalence was probably close to 20 percent of PEP patients.[25] Once present, OGC tended to persist, possibly later decreasing in intensity.

In some patients with OGC, deviation of the head; blepharospasm; contractions of muscles of the tongue and jaws; cranial dystonia similar to that in Meige's syndrome; or dystonia of the limbs also occurred. Remarkably, patients frequently complained of fear, anxiety, depression, or suicidal ideation that preceded or accompanied OGC.

The only other encephalitic patient with OGC unrelated to

EL who developed parkinsonism after acute Western Equine Encephalitis was followed by Mulder et al.[26] They only mentioned two short episodes of upward deviation of the eyes in a 6-month period. More recently, few patients were reported with OGC during acute encephalitis considered to represent sporadic EL.[27]

The pathophysiology of OGC and of thought changes was recently discussed by Leigh et al.[28] Because OGCs were well controlled by anticholinergic medication, they may be caused by a transient disequilibrium between increased cholinergic and low dopaminergic activity. In contrast to postencephalitic OGC, the acute drug-induced OGC usually is not associated with parkinsonism.

Postencephalitic Parkinsonism

CLINICAL FEATURES

Dating the onset of PEP was obviously difficult because of the insidious development of symptomatology. A few of the survivors of acute EL probably went on to develop parkinsonism immediately. Reviewing the available data, Duvoisin and Yahr[6] found that in about one-half of the patients who developed parkinsonism, this feature was present 5 years after EL, in 80 percent or more at 10 years, and that by 1950 most of the long-term survivors had already developed parkinsonism. As some patients never developed a clear-cut episode of EL but exhibited features typical of PEP, it was accepted that PEP may occur without overt infection and that its occurrence is not related to the severity of EL. The symptom-free period may have variable lengths, presumably depending on the extent of cell destruction, compensatory hyperactivity of those neurons which survive, and supersensitivity of postsynaptic dopamine receptors to dopamine.

It seems, however, that some EL epidemics were "bad for parkinsonism," according to Wilson.[13] von Economo stated that he knew of only two patients in whom parkinsonism had occurred that suffered from EL in 1916 and 1917, but that many of those who were acutely ill in 1920 and 1921 developed PEP.[12]

The extrapyramidal features, which appeared after a variable latent "parkinsonism-free" period, included rigidity, mask face, bradykinesia, impaired gait, and dysarthria, but clinicians were impressed by differences between PEP and "cryptogenic" parkinsonism. Wilson noted not only that PEP patients were usually much younger but also that they had many features unseen in idiopathic parkinsonism, such as myoclonus, chorea, tics or spasms, OGC, respiratory disturbances, pupillary dysfunction, ocular palsies, and behavioral disorders.[13] Interestingly, the study of PEP patients contributed to the delineation of bradyphrenia, as Naville[29] termed the slowing of cognitive processing in these patients.

When present, the resting "coarse" or typical pill rolling tremor was less prominent than rigidity ("paralysis agitans without agitation"); sometimes, a disabling rigidity of neck extension was encountered. Many patients manifested catatonic akinesia, whereas others were embarrassed by akathisia. Another notable feature was that some PEP patients demonstrated a striking fluctuation of their rigidity and motor impairment.

Once it had appeared, the evolution of PEP was difficult to predict. Wilson expressed the view that "the course of residua and sequelae is difficult to foretell" and that "among the sequelae parkinsonism seems least likely to alter," whereas Duncan[30] mentioned the worsening of parkinsonian symptomatology. This view was confirmed by Duvoisin and Yahr who, in a retrospective study in the early 1960s, observed that on the whole the encephalitic sequelae had been rather mild and remarkably stable but also that in the previous 10 years, there had been definite slow and insidious progression in less than one-half of the patients.[6] Two more recent studies[31,32] have shown late progression of PEP patients, most of whom were in their 70s. Motor deterioration exceeded changes naturally seen in normal elderly populations.

Vierrege et al.[32] studied retrospectively 10 autopsied PEP cases and found that four of them had motor worsening before death but no intellectual decline. It is of interest to emphasize that generally dementia was rare among PEP patients, in contrast to its high incidence in PD.

PATHOPHYSIOLOGY

In a clinicopathological study of eight cases of PEP with long survival, Geddes et al.[33] found that seven had slowly progressive disease. This progression manifested, as was noted also by Calne and Lees,[31] by increased bradykinesia, rigidity, and postural instability. In a brief reference, however, Agid[14] considered motor decline in PEP patients to be related to aging and not to progression of the disease. The issue of whether PEP patients manifest delayed exacerbation of the parkinsonism may be important, because it may provide clues to the hypothesis of interaction between acute environmental damage and age-related neuronal attrition.[35] When this late progression exists, is it phenomenologically different from the initial development of parkinsonism after years of "PEP-free" period? How consistent is this difference with the hypothesis that a one-time exposure to a very aggressive agent will be followed by a short presymptomatic period, as happened in MPTP-induced acute parkinsonism? Or is the long presymptomatic phase the expression of a continuous or intermittent but mildly potent inducer of dopaminergic neuronal death, by different mechanisms, possibly autoimmune, because there is some experimental evidence suggesting that autoimmunity may be relevant to the pathogenesis of parkinsonism[36]? Unfortunately, most EL survivors have now died, so that more answers as to the progression of PEP are unlikely to be forthcoming. The demonstration of immunoglobulin G oligoclonal bands in the cerebrospinal fluid (CSF) of PEP patients[37] may provide additional evidence of an intrathecal immune response. The nature of the antigen provoking the response, or even whether the response is directly triggered by a virus, is not known, and the persistence of oligoclonal bands does not necessarily signify a response to an active infection.

There are contradictory data concerning the role of genetic factors in the development of PEP, as in the report of Elizan et al.,[38] which found that an increased frequency of human leukocyte antigen-B_4 (HLA-B_4) antigen in PEP patients, compared with that of matched controls, and which was not replicated.[39]

PATHOLOGY

Brain weight and macroscopic cortical atrophy were similar in long-standing PEP and an age-matched control group.[40] The earlier reports concentrated on basal ganglia and brain stem pathology, with less emphasis on other brain structures.[41,42] The characteristic macroscopic change is depigmentation of the substantia nigra and, to a lesser degree, of the locus ceruleus.

The microscopic examination was typical for severe and diffuse neuronal loss and gliosis in the substantia nigra, and inflammatory perivascular lymphocytic cuffing, such as was seen in EL, was present also in PEP brains examined shortly after disease onset. Gibbs and Lees[40] have found that the loss of pigmented nigral cells is significantly higher than that in PD, exceeding 90 percent. The locus ceruleus was less affected than in PD. No Lewy bodies were found.

An important pathological feature of PEP is the presence of neurofibrillary tangles (NFT).[43,44] Notably, NFTs are not found in PD. NFTs are widely distributed and are usually present not only in the substantia nigra and locus ceruleus, but also in the nuclei of the reticular formation, hippocampus, nucleus basalis of Meynert, and variably in other structures, including neocortex and spinal cord. A detailed analysis of NFTs allowed Geddes et al.[33] to suggest that PEP was an active degenerative process, rather than the expression of delayed cell decompensation and aging after an initial acute illness. They found that the few surviving neurons in which NFTs were already present showed granular cytoplasmic staining. The NFTs of the substantia nigra in PEP reacted positively with anti-τ antibodies and with antisera raised against a purified human brain microtubule fraction.[45] The accumulation of abnormal tau protein starts in neuronal soma, and the gradual formation of mature NFTs is followed after neuronal death by extracellular NFT "ghosts".

The presence of granular cytoplasmic staining for tau protein was believed to represent then an early stage in NFT formation, which would be unexpected after many years during which the disease process was apparently inactive. Furthermore, relatively few extracellular "ghosts" were seen, again in contrast to the expected total extracellular occurrence after a very long disease duration.

NFTs are found in a diversity of genetic and acquired conditions, such as Alzheimer's disease, progressive supranuclear palsy, Guam parkinsonism-dementia complex (GPDC), subacute sclerosing panencephalitis, and myotonic dystrophy, and thus it may constitute a final common pathway for different types of cellular injury. Moreover, the NFT distribution, morphology, and antigenic profile are essentially the same in PEP and GPDC, suggesting a common pathogenesis, if not etiology, in these disorders. Although GPDC is a disease that affects mainly the Chamorro population and its etiology is still elusive, an environmental risk factor is highly suspected.[46] As happened in some PEP patients, GPDC was reported to be present or to progress decades after withdrawal from the exposure to the presumed environmental risk factor.

It must be emphasized that Geddes et al.,[33] in contrast to Viarregi et al.,[32] failed to find inflammatory changes involving nigral dopaminergic cells, accepted as markers of an active pathological process.[47]

There was no correlation between clinical symptomatology and the abovementioned pathological findings (neuronal loss, gliosis, or NFT severity and distribution).[33]

TREATMENT

Amphetamines were widely used to treat patients with PEP. Initially recommended for their alerting effect, amphetamines were found not only to produce subjective improvement but but also to reduce slightly motor disability.[48]

Before the introduction of L-dopa, the belladonna alkaloids proved to be most effective.[49] The anticholinergic drugs continued to be used extensively for decades, because their long-term tolerance was better than that of L-dopa (see below). Tics, OGC and, sometimes, behavioral disturbances were influenced in addition to objective improvement of extrapyramidal symptomatology. Surprisingly, in the long-term use of anticholinergics dystonia was probably the most prominent adverse effect.[50]

The introduction of L-dopa as therapy for idiopathic parkinsonism was extended to PEP, and it was proven to be of some benefit. The first double-blind controlled trial of L-dopa in PEP was conducted by Calne et al.[51] They administered for more than 6 weeks maximally tolerated doses of L-dopa to a group of 20 institutionalized PEP "active" patients. The maximum tolerated dose was 2.5 g daily (without decarboxylase inhibitors), much lower than the doses used in the same period for idiopathic parkinsonism. Ten patients improved, five did not, and five were withdrawn because of side effects. The main improvement occurred in walking, but OGC crises and drooling were also alleviated. Side effects included disturbing dyskinesias and pathological restlessness.

An open extension of the trial was reported by Hunter et al.[52] Of 50 patients, 16 continued to benefit; 16 showed no change; and 18 were unable to tolerate L-dopa. The conclusion of this study was that the majority of PEP patients do not benefit or tolerate L-dopa for extended periods of time. The observation of limited tolerance of L-dopa was confirmed by Krasner and Cornelius[53] and by Sacks et al.,[54] who were also concerned about the high incidence of side effects, especially respiratory crises, respiratory or phonatory tics, and exacerbation of OGC.

Duvoisin et al. generally supported the results of Calne et al. regarding the overall effect on parkinsonism symptomatology, OGC crises, and drooling. In their latest study of long-term PEP,[55] Duvoisin et al. entered 30 patients. Twenty-six patients who remained on therapy for at least 4 months (mean, 16.8 months) were evaluated. It was concluded that PEP patients may respond as well to L-dopa as PD patients, but both the improvement and the adverse effects tend to appear at lower dosage. The somewhat surprising greater responsiveness of PEP patients—with a more severe depletion of dopaminergic neurons—to L-dopa was speculated to

be because of additional changes of the dopamine receptors that were rendered supersensitive to dopamine. However, Calne and Lees[31] recently noted that no patient was able to tolerate sustained treatment with L-dopa.

Parkinsonism Resulting from Other Infectious Causes

Although EL ceased to occur, at least in an epidemic form, in the 1930s, parkinsonian syndromes were infrequently described in association with acute encephalitic illness, sometimes supposed to represent sporadic cases of EL. More often they appeared during or following an episode of poorly documented febrile illness or after an encephalitis not resembling EL.

Duvoisin and Yahr[6] concluded that "the rare association of a progressive parkinsonian syndrome such as is understood by the term PD with any known type of viral encephalitis (except for EL) had not been shown to be more than coincidental." A similar approach was expressed by Schwab and England.[56] Extrapyramidal features, such as hypomimia, rigidity, tremor, impaired posture, and gait, that are somewhat similar to PD may occur during the acute phase of various encephalitides, notably Japanese B encephalitis and Western Equine Encephalitis. Parkinsonian symptomatology in such cases is most often transient, mild, and nonprogressive, and the free period after the infection, characteristic for EL and PEP, is not seen.

Single-patient reports or small series of patients have been added by Bojinov,[57] Herishanu and Noah,[58] Rail et al.,[59] Howard and Lees,[60] Blunt et al.,[61] Wu-Chung Shen et al.,[62] among others. Both Rail et al.[59] and Howard and Lees[60] were concerned with a strict definition of EL diagnostic criteria. They opted for an episode of acute or subacute encephalitis, presence of extrapyramidal signs, ocular palsies, oculogyric crises, and behavioral disturbances. Undoubtedly, in the absence of a specific diagnostic test for EL, and because of the variability of EL manifestations, many of the reported cases remain controversial.

An extended list of viral infections, other than Japanese B and Western equine encephalitis, reported to be associated with parkinsonism generally compliant to the conclusions expressed by Duvoisin and Yahr, includes coxsackie B type 2, measles, Murray Valley encephalitis, poliomyelitis, influenza inoculation with vaccinia virus and, possibly, herpes simplex.[61-66]

A particularly interesting patient was recently reported on by Lin et al.[69] This young patient developed a pure extrapyramidal syndrome that followed after 1 week of headache and intermittent fever, attributed to a probable viral (herpes simplex type 1) infection of the brain. The MRI evaluation showed hyperintense (T_2-weighted) signals bilaterally within substantia nigra that almost disappeared 2 months later. Clinical improvement occurred and, after 8 months, when she was asymptomatic, positron emission tomography scanning with fluorodopa and raclopride revealed a pattern similar to that seen in idiopathic parkinsonism. This may represent isolated involvement of substantia nigra by means of an external agent inducing a reduction of fluorodopa uptake more marked in the putamen than in the caudate and opening again the discussion of an infectious etiology for idiopathic parkinsonism.

ACQUIRED IMMUNE DEFICIENCY SYNDROME (AIDS)

Extrapyramidal features may occur in HIV-1 encephalopathy. Bradykinesia, cogwheel rigidity, hypomimia, postural impairment, and gait instability were found in patients with established AIDS-dementia complex.[70] However, the occurrence of distinctive parkinsonism seems to be extremely rare.[71,72]

De Mattos et al.[73] found three other cases of parkinsonism among 1086 AIDS patients, of whom 36 percent had neurological dysfunction. In contrast to patients having the chorea who are said to be virtually pathognomic of cerebral toxoplasmosis,[70] their AIDS patients were apparently free of opportunistic brain infections. Some AIDS-dementia complex patients develop acute extrapyramidal symptomatology when treated with low doses of neuroleptics. This susceptibility may be a result of subclinical neuronal loss in the pars compacta of the substantia nigra, according to Reyes et al., and of neuronal loss in the globus pallidum.[75]

NONVIRAL INFECTIONS

Nonviral infections were also found to induce acute parkinsonism. Several children developed extrapyramidal features associated with proven or probable *Mycoplasma pneumoniae*.[76–78] The symptomatology included bradykinesia, rigidity, dystonia, and choreic movements and was reversible. In one patient, brain MRIs showed bilateral lesions in the basal ganglia with hemiparkinsonism that later disappeared in parallel with resolution of midbrain MRI enhancement.

SYPHILIS

Because meningovascular syphilis involves the midbrain, it is conceivable that parkinsonian features may be induced or precipitated. However, most cases that were reported when neurosyphilis was a more common disease[79] probably reflected the coincidence of two independent diseases.

A more stringent link can be made to a 43-year-old patient with active neurosyphilis, described by Neill,[80] who developed typical parkinsonism insidiously. Penicillin treatment was followed by definite improvement. Another recent report mentioned a 66-year-old male with general paresis who developed bradykinesia and rigidity much later and in whom autopsy findings were similar to those found in PEP.[81]

FUNGAL AND PARASITIC INFECTIONS

Cryptococcal infection in the mesencephalon and specifically in the substantia nigra was sometimes demonstrated on autopsy.[82] Bilateral, small, hyperintense signals in basal ganglia were shown on MRI (on long T_2-weighted images) in a patient with AIDS and cryptococcal meningitis.[83] However, the development of subacute parkinsonism in patients with crypto-coccal meningoencephalitis or cryptococcal granulomata is probably exceedingly rare.

The permanent parkinsonian syndrome that appeared in a young patient with cryptococcal meningitis after intraventricular administration of amphotericin B was considered to be a result of amphotericin B rather than the infection.[84]

Another reported patient developed parkinsonian features before the onset of meningoencephalitic symptoms, but they worsened dramatically thereafter and improved after anticryptococcal therapy. No basal ganglia lesions were seen on cranial computed tomography (CT).[85] The role of cryptococcal infection remained unclear, as the period of observation was too short before the patient's death, and no autopsy was performed.

A more impressive correlation between parkinsonism and fungal infection was shown in a patient reported by Adler et al.[86] The patient, a young IV drug user, developed subacute, aymmetric, severe parkinsonism, including pharyngeal akinesia. MRI revealed bilateral striatal abscesses which, at biopsy, showed the presence of hyphae, consistent with either aspergillus or mucor. After systemic amphotericin B therapy, the parkinsonism improved, together with shrinkage of the striatal lesions.

Interestingly, in an experimental model, mice injected with *Nocardia asteroides* developed a L-dopa-responsive extrapyramidal disorder, associated with hyaline inclusion bodies that resembled Lewy bodies, suggesting that *Nocardia* may localize and grow within the brain.[87]

Neurocysticercosis as a cause of acute-onset parkinsonism was reported in a single case. During an abrupt aggravation of known neurocysticercosis treated with praziquantel, this patient developed asymmetric parkinsonism that was attributed to cysticercus cysts located by magnetic resonance imaging within the midbrain. The extrapyramidal symptoms were entirely reversible.[88]

CREUTZFELDT-JAKOB DISEASE (CJD)

Although CJD is not strictly an infectious disease, it is potentially transmissible.[89] The symptomatology is diverse and, even in one subtype, the genetic form related to the codon 200 mutation in the prion protein gene, there is phenotypic variability.[90–92] The main features are mental deterioration, cerebellar ataxia, and involuntary movements. The characteristic pathology, spongiform changes, predominates within the cortex and basal ganglia. Rigidity very rarely occurs at onset but later is quite common. Brown et al.[89] have found that 56 percent of patients with sporadic CJD developed extrapyramidal symptomatology during the course of the disease, as compared with 9 percent on their first examination.

Summary

Several etiologies can result in parkinsonism. These include degenerative (as in idiopathic PD) or toxic (as in manganese or MPTP poisoning). Infectious causes are extremely rare, with the obvious exception of PEP. Although the cause of EL is unknown, clinical data are highly suggestive of a viral agent. The identity of the virus is still unknown and may never be known with certainty. It is remarkable that the EL epidemic, reaching dimensions that justify referring to it as a pandemic, has all but completely disappeared. The rare cases that have appeared lately, in which an agent was identified, may or may not be related to the EL agent. Although the EL agent has disappeared, it could well reappear. It is possible, but not proven, that this agent changes its genetic code frequently, as does that of the influenza virus. When this is the case, we may expect reappearance when a mutation of the virus occurs.

References

1. Von Economo C: Encephalitis lethargica. *Wien Klin Wochnschr* 30:581, 1917.
2. Cruchet JR, Montier J, Calmettes R: Quarante cas d'encephalomyelite subaigue. *Bull Soc Med Hop (Paris)* 41:814, 1917.
3. Neal JB: Lethargic encephalitis. *Arch Neurol Psychiatry* 2:271, 1919.
4. Watson AJ: Encephalitis lethargica. *Lancet* 19:1396, 1981.
5. Eadie MJ, Sutherland JM, Doherty RL: Encephalitis in the etiology of parkinsonism in Australia. *Arch Neurol* 12:240, 1965.
6. Duvoisin RC, Yahr MD: Encephalities and parkinsonism. *Arch Neurol* 12:227, 1965.
7. Souques AA: Rapport sur les syndromes parkinsoniens. *Rev Neurol* 28:534, 1921.
8. Dimsdale H: Changes in Parkinson syndrome in the 20th century. *Q J Med* 15:155, 1946.
9. Duvoisin RC: Genetics of Parkinson's disease. *Adv Neurol* 45:447–480, 1986.
10. Poskanzer DC, Schwab RS: Studies in the epidemiology of Parkinson's disease predicting its disappearance as a major clinical entity by 1980. *Trans Am Neurol Assoc* 86:234, 1961.
11. Martilla RJ: Epidemiology, in Koller WC (ed): *Handbook of Parkinson's disease.* New York: Marcel Dekker, 1987, pp 35–50.
12. Von Economo C: *Encephalitis Lethargica: Its Sequelae and Treatment.* New York: Oxford University Press, 1931.
13. Wilson SAK: Epidemic encephalitis, in AN Bruce (ed): *Neurology* London: Arnold, 1940, vol I, pp 99–144.
14. Martilla RJ, Halonen P, Rinne UK: Influenza virus antibodies in parkinsonism: Comparison of postencephalitic and idiopathic Parkinson patients and matched controls. *Arch Neurol* 34:99, 1977.
15. Esiri MK, Swash M: Absence of herpes simplex virus antigen in brain in encephalitis lethargica. *J Neurol Neurosurg Psychiatry* 47:1049, 1984.
16. Elizan TS, Madden DL, Noble GR, et al: Viral antibodies in serum and CSF of parkinsonian patients and controls. *Arch Neurol* 36:529, 1979.
17. Ravenholt RT, Foege WH: 1918 influenza, encephalitis lethargica, parkinsonism. *Lancet* 2:860, 1982.
18. Mattock C, Marmoty M, Stern G: Could Parkinson's disease follow intrauterine influenza? A speculative hypothesis. *J Neurol Neurosurg Psychiatry* 51:753, 1988.
19. Elizan TS, Casals J: Astrogliosis in von Economi's and postencephalitic Parkinson's disease supports probable viral etiology. *J Neurol Sci* 105:131, 1991.
20. Krusz JC, Koller WC, Ziegler DK: Historical review: Abnormal movements associated with epidemic encephalitis lethargica. *Mov Disord* 2:137, 1987.
21. Medical Research Council: *The Sheffield Outbreak of Epidemic Encephalitis in 1924.* London: His Majesty's Stationery Office, 1926.
22. Grinker RR, Bucy PC: *Epidemic Encephalitis in Neurology*, 4th ed. Oxford, England: Blackwell Scientific Publications, 1949, pp 651–663.
23. Walshe FMR: *Diseases of the Nervous System*, 8th ed. Baltimore: Williams & Wilkins, 1955, p 162.
24. Oecknighaus W: Encephalitis epidemica und Wilsonsches Krankleithild. *Dtsch Z Nervenkr* 72:294, 1921.
25. McCowan PK, Cook LC: Oculogyric crises in chronic epidemic encephalitis. *Brain* 51:285, 1928.
26. Mulder DW, Parrott M, Thaler M: Sequelae of western equine encephalitis. *Neurology* 318, 1950.
27. Clough CG, Plaitakis A, Yahr MD: Oculogyric crises and parkinsonism. *Arch Neurol* 40:36, 1983.
28. Leigh RJ, Foley JM, Remler BF, Civil RH: Oculogyric crisis: A syndrome of thought disorder and ocular deviation. *Ann Neurol* 22:13, 1987.
29. Naville F: Etudes sur les complications et les sequelles menteles de l'encephalité pidemique: La bralyphrenie. *Encephale* 17:423, 1922.
30. Duncan AG: The sequelae of encephalitis lethargica. *Brain* 47:76, 1924.
31. Calne DB, Lees AJ: Late progression of postencephalitic Parkinson's syndrome. *Can J Neurol Sci* 15:135–138, 1988.
32. Vierrege P, Reinhardt V, Höft B: Is progression in postencephalitic Parkinson's disease late and age-related? *J Neurol* 238:299–303, 1991.
33. Geddes JF, Hughes A, Lees AJ, Damtl SE: Pathological overlap in cases of parkinsonism associated with neurofibrillary tangles—a study of recent cases of postencephalitic parkinsonism and comparison with supranuclear palsy and Guamanian Parkinson dementia complex. *Brain* 116:281, 1993.
34. Agid Y: Parkinson's disease: Paths physiology. *Lancet* 337:1321–1324, 1991.
35. Calne DB: Is idiopathic parkinsonism the consequence of an event or a process? *Neurology* 44:5–10, 1994.
36. Appel SH, Le WD, Taijti J, et al: Nigral damage and dopaminergic hypofunction in mesencephalon-immunized guinea pigs. *Ann Neurol* 32:494, 1992.
37. Williams A, Houff S, Lees A, Cahil DB: Oligoclonal banding in the cerebrospinal fluid of patients with postencephalitic parkinsonism. *J Neurol Neurosurg Psychiatry* 42:790, 1979.
38. Elizan TS, Terasky PL, Yahr MD: HLA-B14 antigen and postencephalitic Parkinson's disease, their association in an American Jewish ethnic group. *Arch Neurol* 37:542, 1980.
39. Lees AJ, Stern GM, Compston DAS: Histocompatibility agents and postencephalitic parkinsonism. *J Neurol Neurosurg Psychiatry* 45:1060, 1982.
40. Gibb SRG, Lees AJ: The progression of idiopathic Parkinson's disease is not explained by age-related changes: Clinical and pathological comparisons with postencephalitic parkinsonian syndrome. *Acta Neuropathol* 73:195–201, 1987.
41. Greenfield JG, Bosanquet FD: The brain stem lesions in parkinsonism. *J Neurol Neuropsych Neurosurg* 16:213–226, 1963.
42. Forno LS: Pathology of parkinsonism: A preliminary report of 24 cases. *J Neurosurg* 1:266–271, 1966.
43. Hallervorden J: Zur pathogenese des postencepalitis Parkinsonisms. *Klin Wchnschr* 12:692, 1933.
44. Hallervorden J: Anatomische Untersuchungen zur pathogenese des postencephalitischen parkinsonisms. *Dtsch Zeitschrift Nervenheilkunde* 136:68, 1935.
45. Yen SH, Houroupian DS, Terry RD: Immunocytochemical comparison of neurofibrillary tangles in Alzheimer type dementia, progressive supranuclear palsy and postencephalitic parkinsonism. *Ann Neurol* 13:172, 1982.
46. Hudson AY, Rice GPA: Similarities of Guamanian ALS/PD to postencephalitic parkinsonism/ALS: Possible viral cause. *Can J Neurol Sci* 17:427, 1990.
47. McGeer PL, Itagaki S, Akiyama H, McGeer EG: Rate of cell death in parkinsonism indicates active neuropathological process. *Ann Neurol* 24:574, 1988.

48. Parkes JD, Tarsy D, Marsden CD, et al: Amphetamines in the treatment of Parkinson's disease. *J Neurol Neurosurg Psychiatry* 38:232, 1975.

49. Mark MH, Duvoisin RC: The history of the medical therapy of Parkinson's disease, in Koller WC, Paulson G (eds): *Therapy of Parkinson's Disease*, 2d ed. New York: Marcel Dekker, 1995, pp. 1–20.

50. Solomon P, Mitchell RS, Prinzmetal M: The use of benzedrine sulfate in postencephalitic Parkinson's disease. *J Am Med Assoc* 108:1765, 1937.

51. Calne DB, Stern GM, Laurence DR, et al: L-Dopa in postencephalitic parkinsonism. *Lancet* 12:744, 1969.

52. Hunter KR, Stern GM, Sharkey J: L-dopa in postencephalitic parkinsonisms. *Lancet* 2:1366, 1970.

53. Krasner N, Cornelius JM: L-dopa for postencephalitic parkinsonism. *Br Med J*, 4:496, 1970.

54. Sacks OW, Kohl M, Schwartz W, Messeloff C: Side effects of L-dopa in postencephalitic parkinsonism. *Lancet* 1:1006, 1970.

55. Duvoisin RC, Antunes JL, Yahr MD: Response of patients with postencephalitic parkinsonism to L-dopa. *J Neurol Neurosurg Psychiatry* 35:487, 1977.

56. Schwab RS, England AC: Parkinsonian syndrome due to various specific causes, in Vinken PY, Bruya GW (eds): *Handbook of Clinical Neurology*, vol. 6, Amsterdam: North Holland, 1968, pp 227–245.

57. Bojinov S: Encephalitis with acute parkinsonism syndrome and bilateral inflammatory necrosis of substantia nigra. *J Neurol Sci* 12:383, 1971.

58. Herishanu Y, Noah Z: On acute encephalitic parkinsonism syndrome. *Eur Neurol* 10:117, 1973.

59. Rail D, Scholtz C, Swash M: Postencephalitic parkinsonism: Current experience. *J Neurol Neurosurg Psychiatry* 44:670, 1981.

60. Howard RS, Lees AJ: Encephalitis lethargica: A report of four recent cases. *Brain* 110:19, 1987.

61. Blunt SB, Lane RJM, Perkin GD: Encephalitis lethargica: Clinical features and management. *Mov Disord* 9:(Suppl 1): 73, 1994.

62. Shen WC, Ho YJ, Lee SK, Lee KR: MRI of transient postencephalitic parkinsonism. *J Comput Assist Tomogr* 18:155, 1994.

63. Poser CM, Huntley CJ, Poland JD: Paraencephalitic parkinsonism: Report of an acute case due to coxsackie virus type B and re-examination of the aetiologic concepts of post-encephalitic parkinsonism. *Acta Neurol Scand* 45:199, 1969.

64. Isgreen WP, Chutorian AM, Fahn S: Sequential parkinsonism and chorea following mild influenza. *Trans Am Neurol Assoc* 101:56, 1976.

65. Walters JH: Postencephalitic parkinsonism syndrome after meningoencephalitis due to coxsackie virus group B, type 2. *N Engl J Med* 263:746, 1960.

66. Solbrig M, Nashuf L: Acute parkinsonism in suspected herpes simplex encephalitis. *Mov Disord* 8:233, 1993.

67. Alves RSC, Barbosa ER, Scaff M: Postvaccinal parkinsonism. *Mov Disord* 7:178, 1992.

68. Thieffry S: Enterovirus (Poliomyelite, Coxsackie, ECHO) et maladies du systeme nerveux: Revision critique et experience personnelle. *Rev Neurol* 105:753, 1963.

69. Lin SK, Lu CS, Vingerhoets F, et al: Isolated involvement of substantia nigra in acute transient parkinsonism: MRI and PET observations. *Parkinsonism Related Disord* 1:367–372, 1995.

70. Berger JR, Levy RM: The neurologic complications of human immunodeficiency virus infection. *Med Clin North Am* 77:1, 1993.

71. Nath A, Jankovic J, Pettigrew LC: Movement disorders and AIDS. *Neurology* 37:37–41, 1987.

72. Trujillo R, Garcia-Ramos G, Nowark IS, et al: Neurologic manifestations of AIDS: A comparative study of two populations from Mexico and the United States. *J Acquir Immune Defic Syndr Hum Retrovirol* 8:23, 1995.

73. De Mattos JP, Rosso AL, Correa RB, Novis S: Involuntary movements and AIDS. Report of seven cases and review of the literature. *Arq Neuropsiquiatr* 51:491, 1993.

74. Reyes MG, Faraldi A, Senseng CS, Flowers C, et al: Nigral degeneration in acquired immune deficiency syndrome (AIDS). *Acta Neuropathol* 82:39, 1991.

75. Factor SA, Podskalny GD, Barron KD: Persistent neuroleptic-induced rigidity and dystonia in AIDS dementia complex: A clinicopathological case report. *J Neurol Sci* 127:114, 1994.

76. Al Mateen M, Gibbs M, Dietrich R, et al: Encephalitis lethargica-like illness in a girl with mycoplasma infection. *Neurology* 38:1155, 1988.

77. Saitoh S, Wada T, Narita M, et al: Mycoplasma pneumoniae infection may cause striatal lesions leading to acute neurologic dysfunction. *Neurology* 43:2150, 1993.

78. Kim JS, Choi IS, Lee MC: Reversible parkinsonism and dystonia following probable Mycoplasma pneumoniae infection. *Mov Disord* 10:510, 1995.

79. Denny-Brown D: Syphilitic parkinsonism, in *Diseases of the Basal Ganglia and Subthalamic Nucleus*. New York: Oxford University Press, 1945, pp 299.

80. Neill KJ: An unusual case of syphilitic parkinsonism. *Br Med J* 2:320, 1953.

81. Matsuyama Y, Fukunaga H, Takayama S: Parkinson's disease of postencephalitic type following general paresis—An autopsied case. *Folia Psychiatr Neurol Jpn* 37:85, 1983.

82. Weenink HR, Bruyn GW: Cryptococcosis of the nervous system, in Vinken PJ, Bruyn GW, Klawans HL (eds): *Handbook of Clinical Neurology*, Amsterdam: Elsevier North Holland, 1978, vol 35, pp 459–502.

83. Balakrishnau J, Becker PS, Jumar AY, et al: Acquired immune deficiency syndrome: Correlation of radiologic and pathologic findings in the brain. *Radiographics* 10:201–216, 1990.

84. Fisher JF, Dewald J: Parkinsonism associated with intraventricular amphotericin B. *J Antimicrob Chemother* 12:97–99, 1983.

85. Wszolek Z, Monsour H, Smith P, Pfeiffer R: Cryptococcal meningoencephalitis with Parkinsonian features. *Mov Disord* 3:271–273, 1988.

86. Adler CH, Stern MB, Brooks ML: Parkinsonism secondary to bilateral striatal fungal abscesses. *Mov Disord* 4:333–337, 1989.

87. Kohbata S, Beaman BL: L-Dopa-responsive movement disorder caused by Nocardia asteroides localized in the brains of mice. *Infect Immun* 59:1871, 1991.

88. Verma A, Berger JR, Bower BC, Sanchez-Ramos J: Reversible parkinsonism syndrome complicating cysticercus midbrain encephalitis. *Mov Disord* 10:215, 1995.

89. Brown P, Gibbs CY Jr, Rodgers-Johnson P, et al: Human spongiform encephalopathy: The NIH series of 300 cases of experimentally transmitted disease. *Ann Neurol* 35:513, 1994.

90. Korczyn AD: Creutzfeldt-Jakob disease among Libyan Jews. *Eur J Epidemiol* 7:490, 1991.

91. Chapman J, Korczyn AD: Genetic and environmental factors determining the development of Creutzfeld-Jakob disease in Libyan Jews. *Neuroepidemiology* 10:228, 1991.

92. Chapman J, Brown P, Rabey JM, et al: Transmission of spongiform encephalopathy from a familial Creutzfeldt-Jakob disease patient of Jewish Libyan origin carrying the PRNP codon 200 mutation. *Neurology* 42:1249, 1992.

Chapter 22

TOXIN-INDUCED PARKINSONIAN SYNDROMES

RAJESH PAHWA

MPTP-INDUCED PARKINSONISM
   History
   Clinical Features
   Pathology
   Mechanism of Toxicity
   Treatment
MANGANESE
   Clinical Features
   Pathology
   Mechanism of Toxicity
   Treatment
CARBON MONOXIDE
   Clinical Features
   Pathology
   Mechanism of Toxicity
   Treatment
CARBON DISULFIDE
   Clinical Features
   Pathology
   Mechanism of Toxicity
   Treatment
CYANIDE
   Clinical Features
   Pathology
   Mechanism of Toxicity
   Treatment
METHANOL
   Clinical Features
   Pathology
   Mechanism of Toxicity
   Treatment
SUMMARY

A parkinsonian syndrome characterized by rigidity and bradykinesia can be induced by a variety of toxins, including manganese, carbon monoxide, carbon disulfide, and cyanide. In 1837, manganese was the first toxin reported to cause parkinsonism.[1] The discovery of the neurotoxin MPTP (1-methyl-4-phenyl-1,2,3,6-tetrahydropyridine) as a cause of parkinsonism has benefited almost every aspect of Parkinson's disease (PD) research.[2] MPTP-induced parkinsonism in laboratory animals is currently regarded as the best animal model for PD.[2] In this chapter, we will discuss the various toxins that can induce parkinsonism (Table 22-1).

MPTP-Induced Parkinsonism

HISTORY

In 1947, Ziering and coworkers[3] synthesized the compound 1-methyl-4-phenyl-4-propionoxypiperidine (MPPP). This compound underwent testing as a possible antiparkinsonian drug.[4] Primates who received this compound became rigid and unable to move, and two humans died during or shortly after the study, and this agent was abandoned as a possible therapeutic agent.[4]

In 1979, Davis et al[5] reported a 23-year-old college student who became parkinsonian after injecting a compound that he had synthesized. It is believed that the offending agent was a mixture of MPPP and MPTP.[6] The parkinsonian symptoms responded to L-dopa and bromocriptine, and at autopsy there was neuronal loss in the substantia nigra and eosinophilic inclusion bodies similar to Lewy bodies.[5]

In 1982 an illicit chemist in northern California synthesized and distributed MPPP as a heroin substitute.[7] Because of shortcuts in the synthesis, he produced a mixture of MPPP and MPTP that resulted in a number of young addicts being admitted with acute parkinsonism. Samples of the substance used by the addicts were analyzed; MPPP and MPTP were identified in the samples, and in one batch MPTP was the only compound identified.[8] Subsequent animal studies confirmed that MPTP was the neurotoxin that caused selective damage to the substantia nigra and produced clinical characteristics similar to those of PD.[9]

CLINICAL FEATURES

Although the majority of the 400 intravenous (IV) drug users estimated to be exposed to MPTP[10] have remained asymptomatic, there are reports of patients who developed mild-to-severe parkinsonism.[11–13] In the seven patients reported to have developed moderate-to-severe parkinsonism, the acute reactions associated with IV use of MPTP included a burning sensation at the site of the injection, followed by a "high" sensation and visual changes with hallucinations.[11] The majority of these patients experienced generalized jerking movements, and one patient reported twisting postures of arms, legs, and neck. Within a few days, patients developed drooling, oily face, slow generalized movements, low-volume speech, and tremor.

All seven patients developed rapidly progressive parkinsonian symptoms within 2 weeks. The patients had the cardinal signs of PD, namely, bradykinesia, rigidity, resting tremor, and postural instability. Other features of PD, including flexed posture, shuffling gait, micrographia, loss of associated movements, masked facies, freezing, and akinesia paradoxica, were also present. None of the patients had dementia[14] or associated cortical spinal tract, cerebellar, or sensory findings.[11] All patients had a dramatic response to L-dopa. The long-term complications of L-dopa therapy, namely, dyskinesias, motor fluctuations, and psychiatric disturbances, occurred within weeks to months,[15] in comparison to PD, in which it usually takes years. The side effects related to L-dopa therapy did worsen over time.[2]

Tetrud and Langston[2] reported mild parkinsonism in 22 individuals who were exposed to MPTP. These individuals demonstrated parkinsonian features similar to those of patients with early PD. In addition, they examined 150 individuals who were exposed to MPTP but were asymptomatic. Worsening of parkinsonian symptoms occurs in patients with moderate-to-severe MPTP-induced parkinsonism.[2]

TABLE 22-1 Various Toxins That Can Induce Parkinsonism

MPTP
Manganese
Carbon monoxide
Carbon disulfide
Cyanide
Methanol

Asymptomatic or mildly affected individuals have developed symptoms over time that are similar to those of patients with early PD.[2] Two surveys carried out in a group of MPTP-exposed individuals have supported the findings of symptom progression.[10,16] One of the surveys was a retrospective chart review of individuals who complained of typical PD symptoms,[16] and the second was a survey of 83 individuals exposed to MPTP who developed parkinsonian symptoms about 1 year after exposure.[10] Although these surveys suggest symptom progression, they cannot be considered definite, as they relied on patient reports.

PATHOLOGY

In the human postmortem study of MPTP-induced parkinsonism,[5] there was a selective loss of neurons in the substantia nigra. Unlike in PD, the lesions in MPTP-induced parkinsonism were restricted to the substantia nigra. A Lewy body-like inclusion was reported in the autopsied case.

In nonhuman primates, MPTP also causes selective pathological changes. There is extensive damage to the tyrosine hydrolase-positive dopamine cells of the substantia nigra.[17–19] The cells in the centrolateral area of the zona compacta are more extensively damaged than the cells in the medial portion of the substantia nigra,[20] which is similar to the findings in PD.

MECHANISM OF TOXICITY

MPTP is a protoxin and is converted to MPP^+, which is the toxin responsible for cell damage in the substantia nigra.[21,22] MPTP is metabolized by extraneuronal monoamine oxidase B (MAO-B) located in the glial cells[23] to 1-methyl-4-phenyl-2,3-dihydropyridinium ($MPDP^+$), which is converted to MPP^+ or MPTP.[24] Pretreatment of animals with a MAO-B inhibitor blocks the toxicity of MPTP.[25,26]

MPP^+ enters the neurons through the dopamine uptake systems.[27] It is not exactly known why the toxicity is limited to the dopaminergic neurons in the substantia nigra; however, Langston and Irwin[28] proposed the following hypothesis:

TABLE 22-2 Clinical Features That Are Common to MPTP-Induced Parkinsonism and PD

Resting tremor
Bradykinesia
Rigidity
Dramatic response of motor disabilities to L-dopa
Development of motor fluctuations and dyskinesias
Progression of symptoms over time

TABLE 22-3 Clinical Features in MPTP-induced Parkinsonism That Differentiate It from PD

Young-age of onset (less than 40 years of age)
History of intravenous drug abuse
Rapidly progressive symptoms and complications of L-dopa therapy

When the presence of a dopamine uptake system is a prerequisite for MPTP toxicity, there are three primary dopaminergic projection systems in the brain: hypothalamic dopaminergic system, ventral tegmental system, and the nigrostriatal system. The hypothalamic dopaminergic system is less avid[29] and, hence, would be more resistant to the toxicity of MPTP. The glia surrounding the substantia nigra but not the ventral tegmental area are rich in MAO-B[28]; hence, only the substantia nigra has all of the requirements for the generation of toxic MPP^+.

Previously it was believed that once MPP^+ enters the neuron, it might kill cells through a process of free radical generation. The reason for this speculation was that MPP^+ has structural similarities to paraquat, which is an herbicide. Paraquat generates highly reactive oxygen species by a process called redox cycling.[30] However, with the use of isolated hepatocyte preparations, investigators have shown that MPP^+ alone neither undergoes redox cycling nor produces free radicals.[31,32]

Once it is within the cell, MPP^+ is accumulated by the mitochondria.[33] This process is dependent on the mitochondrial membrane gradient and appears to be driven by the mitochondrial membrane potential. In the mitochondria, MPP^+ appears to act by interfering with the mitochondrial energy metabolism and inhibiting nicotinamide adenine dinucleotide (NAD^+)-linked oxidation in complex I,[34–36] thereby interrupting the process of cellular energy production. Despite lack of definitive evidence, most investigators believe that this energy depletion is the ultimate cause of cell death.[33]

TREATMENT

Patients with MPTP-induced parkinsonism have a dramatic and unequivocal response to L-dopa and dopamine agonists.[8,11,15] Unfortunately, they develop the long-term complications of L-dopa therapy, such as end-of-dose "wearing-off," peak-dose dyskinesias, on-off phenomenon, and psychiatric complications, including hallucinations and agitation.[15] However, these L-dopa complications occur much more rapidly than is seen with PD (Tables 22-2 and 22-3).

In 1992, Widner et al[37] reported the outcome after grafting human fetal tissue bilaterally to the caudate and putamen in two immunosuppressed patients with MPTP-induced parkinsonism. The patients were assessed 18 months preoperatively and 22–24 months after the surgery. Both patients had substantial, sustained improvement in motor function. Striatal uptake of fluorodopa, as measured by positron emission tomography (PET) scans, showed a marked increase in uptake on both sides, paralleling the patients' clinical improvement. However, this surgical technique is still investigational.

Manganese

Manganese is the twelfth most common element in the earth's crust and the fourth most widely used metal in the world.[38] It is used for the manufacture of steel and dry batteries. Potassium permanganate, which is used industrially for bleaching resins and fabrics, in printing fabrics, for dyeing wood, for tanning leather, and for water purification, can also be a source of manganese intoxication.[39] Maneb, a fungicide, also contains manganese.

CLINICAL FEATURES

In 1837, Couper[40] was the first researcher to describe the effects of chronic manganese intoxication. He described five patients who worked in a manganese ore-crushing plant and developed clinical features similar to PD. The clinical syndrome has since been reported in miners, smelters, and workers involved in the manufacture of dry batteries.[41–44] The clinical syndrome of manganese intoxication has an insidious onset after 1–2 years of exposure. The miners have a different onset, compared to that of patients with industrial exposure. The major difference is the psychiatric prodome ("manganese madness" or "locura manganesa") reported in the miners.[45,46] In manganese miners, the syndrome usually begins with mild and transient psychiatric disturbances, such as irritability, emotional instability, illusions, and hallucinations.[45,46] This usually lasts for 1–3 months. The motor symptoms are similar in miners and industrially exposed patients. A majority of the symptoms are similar to PD and include seborrhea, increased sweating, soft speech, clumsiness with impaired dexterity, and gait problems.[47] Generalized weakness, headaches, and impotence occur occasionally. Bradykinesia and rigidity are the predominant signs. The patients often have a peculiar gait, "cock walk," in which patients swagger on their toes. Limb and truncal dystonia is often present, resulting in painful cramps.[48,49] Other neurological signs include dementia and cerebellar dysfunction. There may be progression of signs and symptoms, even after withdrawal from the exposure.[47] Lack of tremor as a predominant feature, early dystonia, postural impairment early in the course of the illness, and failure to have a sustained response to dopaminomimetic agents help to differentiate it from PD.[38]

PATHOLOGY

Pathological changes with manganese intoxication result in neuronal loss and gliosis in the globus pallidus.[50,51] The changes are more extensive in the medial segment of the globus pallidus, as compared to the lateral segment. Changes in the other basal ganglia are less prominent. Bernheimer et al.[52] reported a case of depigmentation and cell damage in the substantia nigra with Lewy bodies; however, the case is atypical, and the patient may have had PD.[38]

In primates exposed to manganese, postmortem studies have shown widespread lesions in the caudate and putamen,[53] as well as no significant atrophy in the pallidum or striatum.[54] There is a report of degeneration and depigmentation of the substantia nigra in primates after 18 months of exposure to manganese.[55]

MECHANISM OF TOXICITY

Normally, manganese functions in carbohydrate metabolism and gluconeogenesis. However, overexposure to manganese will result in neurotoxicity, possibly a result of increased auto-oxidation of dopamine by a higher-valence manganese (Mn^{3+}) ion causing increased generation of free radicals.[56,57] However, manganese in its Mn^{2+} form or in complexes such as superoxide dismutase is normally a scavenger of free radicals.[58,59] Barbeau[49] proposed that brain regions with high concentrations of oxidative enzymes, such as the nuclei of basal ganglia, promote the oxidation of Mn^{2+} to Mn^{3+}, which causes increased auto-oxidation of dopamine to toxic quinones and hydroxyl radicals. However, manganese toxicity also results in degeneration of nondopaminergic neurons in the pallidum, caudate, and putamen. It is postulated that the rich dopaminergic innervation of the striatum results in high extracellular concentrations of dopamine, which in the presence of Mn^{3+} are sufficient to injure the adjacent neurons.[46,60]

TREATMENT

Administration of the chelating agent ethylenediaminetetraacetic acid (EDTA) has not resulted in significant clinical improvement.[61] Open-label studies with L-dopa have reported some response to L-dopa.[48,62] Mena et al.[48] reported dramatic improvement of rigidity, hypokinesia, postural reflexes, and balance in five patients and dystonia in two patients. One of the patients had L-dopa aggravation of weakness, postural impairment, tremor, hypokinesia, and hypotonia but improved with 5 hydroxytryptophan. There is another report of improvement of cognition and bradykinesia but not of dystonia in one patient.[62] Cook et al.[61] and Greenhouse[63] reported patients that had a range of no to some benefit with L-dopa. However, in a placebo-controlled study of L-dopa there was no change in motor scores, finger tapping, gait, or dystonia in six patients.[64] There is one report of para-aminosalicylic acid improving the condition of two patients with chronic manganese poisoning.[65]

Carbon Monoxide

Carbon monoxide is a colorless, odorless, nonirritating gas that can cause central nervous system damage. Approximately 2–26 percent of afflicted individuals die from acute intoxication with carbon monoxide,[66–70] and 2–40 percent of the survivors develop sequelae.[66,70–73] The recovery in patients with sequelae is 53–75 percent, the morbidity is 17–21 percent, and mortality is 8–25 percent.[66,72]

CLINICAL FEATURES

The sequelae of carbon monoxide intoxication are divided as progressive and delayed relapsing.[74] In the progressive type, acute encephalopathy from carbon monoxide intoxication progresses directly into the vegetative state, whereas in the delayed relapsing type, neurological deficits develop after a period of recovery from the acute poisoning. Lee and Marsden[74] described eight patients with progressive-type sequelae. The patients opened their eyes spontaneously 2–15 days after recovery from coma but remained in a mute vegetative state. The patients were nonresponsive, rigid, spastic, bedbound, and exhibiting little or no spontaneous movement. In patients with delayed relapsing type of carbon monoxide intoxication, after the initial coma they recovered completely after a period of days to weeks.[72,75] The delayed symptoms may be parkinsonian or akinetic-mute. The parkinsonian patients have slow shuffling gait, loss of armswing, retropulsion, bradykinesia, rigidity, masked face and, occasionally, resting tremor.[76] There may be fixed dystonia of the hands and feet.[74] Emotional change, confusion, memory disturbances, anxiety, and depression may occur.[66,72,74,77] In the akinetic-mute patients, initial mental changes progress to apathy and mutism along with motor deterioration. Incontinence, rigidity, and primitive responses to painful stimuli may be present.[74] The delayed deterioration may progress, may stop at any time during the progression, or may improve subsequently.[74,78]

Rare patients with tremor,[74,79] chorea,[80,81] myoclonus,[74,82] and Gilles de la Tourette syndrome[83] have also been described as sequelae of carbon monoxide intoxication. Patients with carbon monoxide intoxication may have a normal computed tomography (CT) scan, white matter low-density lesions, bilateral globus pallidus lesions, or both white matter and globus pallidus lesions.[74,84–86] Follow-up CT scans may show new lesions or progression of white matter and globus pallidus lesions.[74,87–89]

PATHOLOGY

The most prominent pathological changes with carbon monoxide poisoning are white matter changes and necrosis of the globus pallidus.[90–92] When death occurs a few hours after acute intoxication, the pathological changes are similar to those seen with asphyxia. The brain appears swollen with congestion of the capillaries and veins along with petechial hemorrhages.[93] Three types of white matter damage have been reported: small multifocal necrotic lesions with fragmentation of axis cylinders, extensive diffuse necrotic lesions with severe axis cylinder damage, and diffuse demyelination with sparing of axis cylinders.[92,94] These changes may be because of the differences in the severity of poisoning.[95]

Unilateral or bilateral necrosis of the globus pallidus is the most striking finding.[93,96] The hemorrhage or necrosis of the globus pallidus is limited to the anterior and superior parts of the inner pallidium.[90,92,93] Rarely, the pallidum may be spared in cases of carbon monoxide encephalopathy when the predominant finding is white matter lesions.[93,97]

MECHANISM OF TOXICITY

Carbon monoxide is an asphyxiant that has a much greater affinity for hemoglobin oxygen-binding sites, compared to that of oxygen. It enters the blood, where it binds with the ferrous ion complex of protoporphyrin IX in hemoglobin and, hence, blocks the binding of oxygen.[39] This results in anoxia that leads to tissue damage. The globus pallidus is vulnerable to anoxic injury, which could be a result of intrin-

sic metabolic susceptibility,[98] such as high oxygen consumption[99] and high iron content.[100] Carbon monoxide also blocks adenotriphosphatase (ATP) production by binding to the cytochrome oxidase of the mitochondrial chain,[39] which potentiates the injury because of anoxia.

TREATMENT

There have been some reports that L-dopa and anticholinergics have been helpful in a few patients.[101,102] Lee and Marsden[74] used anticholinergic drugs and carbidopa/L-dopa (375–750 mg/day) in 23 patients. Because of spontaneous improvement of the symptoms, they found it difficult to evaluate the benefits of these medications. None of their patients had a dramatic response, nor was there any deterioration after the medications were discontinued.

Carbon Disulfide

Carbon disulfide is a colorless and highly volatile liquid used in different industries. It is used in the production of cellophane and viscose rayon; as a solvent for resins, fats, and rubber; and in the manufacture of carbon tetrachloride. It is also used as a fumigant in combination with carbon tetrachloride to treat corn, wheat, rye, and other grains.

CLINICAL FEATURES

Nervousness, irritability, confusion, disorientation, insomnia, memory problems, and hallucinations are mental changes that can be seen with carbon disulfide intoxication.[103] Neurological findings associated with carbon disulfide exposure include peripheral sensorimotor neuropathy, cranial nerve and brain stem abnormalities, pyramidal and extrapyramidal dysfunction and, rarely, dystonia and choreoathetosis.[103–105] Resting tremor, gait abnormalities, decreased associated movements, and rigidity are the common parkinsonian features.[106,107] MRI may be normal or show a pattern consistent with central demyelination.[104]

PATHOLOGY

There have been very few reports of pathological findings after chronic carbon disulfide intoxication. The pathological changes in the brain show diffuse neuronal damage with focal lesions in the globus pallidus and striatum.[108] In a rhesus monkey, after chronic exposure to carbon disulfide, bilateral necrosis of the globus pallidus and zona reticulata of the substantia nigra have been reported.[109]

MECHANISM OF TOXICITY

Carbon disulfide may induce neurotoxicity by formation of dithiocarbamate metabolites.[110] Dithiocarbamate complexes are capable of chelating metal ions, such as copper and zinc, which are of physiological importance.[111] It is also possible that carbon disulfide inhibits cytochrome oxidase and brain tissue respiration,[112] which induces lesions of the striatopallidum.

TREATMENT

There are no reports of dramatic improvement in parkinsonian features with L-dopa.

Cyanide

CLINICAL FEATURES

Cyanide poisoning may result from accidental or suicidal exposure through ingestion, injection, or asphyxiation with hydrocyanic fumes. Acute intoxication results in dizziness, headaches, coma, convulsions, and death, usually within seconds to minutes.[46] The mortality rate with acute cyanide poisoning is 95 percent.[113] Although survival after acute intoxication is rare, in those who recover consciousness parkinsonian features develop over a period of days.[113–115] Gait abnormalities, masked facies, infrequent blinking, rigidity, and weak hypophonic voice are the common parkinsonian features.[113–115] Mild postural and resting tremor has been reported.[113,114] Dystonia and dementia are other features that may occur.[113,115,116]

Immediately after acute intoxication, neuroimaging studies are unremarkable; however, after 3–6 months, bilateral symmetric lesions in the globus pallidus and posterior putamen are reported.[114–116] 6-Fluorodopa PET scan has revealed diffusely decreased activity in the posterior regions of the basal ganglia, similar to that in patients with PD.[114]

PATHOLOGY

Pathological changes after acute cyanide intoxication have demonstrated selective destruction of the basal ganglia, especially the globus pallidus.[117,118] Pathological findings in a patient with cyanide-induced parkinsonism demonstrated destruction of the putamen and globus pallidus.[113] There was also atrophy of the cerebellum, subthalamic nucleus, and complete nerve cell loss along with marked fibrous gliosis in the zona reticularis of the substantia nigra.[113] In experimental animals, multifocal lesions in the basal ganglia, cerebral cortex, cerebellum, and white matter are reported after a single large dose[119–121] or many small doses of cyanide.[121]

MECHANISM OF TOXICITY

As with the other neurotoxins discussed in this chapter, cyanide radicals inactivate cytochrome oxidase and other oxidative enzymes, which leads to cell death from tissue anoxia.[122]

TREATMENT

Amantadine, anticholinergics, and carbidopa/L-dopa have been used in patients with cyanide-induced parkinsonism.[113–115] None of the patients had a dramatic response to these medications.

Methanol

CLINICAL FEATURES

Methanol poisoning occurs after its ingestion as a substitute for ethanol or when it is used as an adulterant with ethanol. Acute intoxication with methanol results in severe acidosis, confusion, and coma.[122] Blindness from retinal degeneration and subsequent optic atrophy is the most common deficit in patients who survive the acute intoxication.[122,123] There are multiple reports of parkinsonism developing a few days after acute intoxication with methanol.[122–125] Soft voice, tremulousness, rigidity, bradykinesia, and slow shuffling gait are the common parkinsonian features reported. CT scans demonstrate bilateral putaminal abnormalities.[122,123]

PATHOLOGY

Bilateral necrosis of the putamen optic atrophy and widespread lesions in the cerebral cortex, anterior horn, and other gray matter nuclei are lesions often induced by methanol intoxication.[93,122,124] Although the duration of survival after methanol ingestion determines the severity of the lesions, bilateral putaminal necrosis has been reported after survival of at least 24 hours.[125]

MECHANISM OF TOXICITY

The exact pathogenesis of methanol intoxication is controversial. Methanol is metabolized to formaldehyde and formic acid by liver alcohol dehydrogenase.[126] Formic acid is believed to be largely responsible for the severe systemic acidosis.[127,128] Because formaldehyde and formic acid achieve high concentrations within the putamen,[129] it is believed to have selective toxicity to the putamen. Toxicity of methanol is delayed in monkeys who receive 4-methylpyrazole, an inhibitor of liver alcohol dehydrogenase, as formic acid is not produced.[128]

TREATMENT

There is a report of L-dopa showing dramatic improvement in rigidity, tremor, and hypokinesia in a patient with methanol-induced parkinsonism[123]; however, other reports have not confirmed this finding.[122]

Summary

Parkinsonism (especially rigidity and bradykinesia) after exposure to toxins is rare but can be present. MPTP-induced parkinsonism has clinical characteristics similar to those of PD (Tables 22-2 and 22-3). Unlike parkinsonism induced by MPTP, the other toxins usually cause rigidity and bradykinesia and usually do not respond to L-dopa (Table 22-4). These cases have lesions primarily in the pallidostriatum. Better understanding of toxin-induced parkinsonism may help elucidate the cause(s) of PD.

TABLE 22-4 Clinical Features Associated with PD and Various Toxin-Induced Parkinsonian Syndromes

Clinical Features	PD	MPTP	MN	CO	CS	CN	Methanol
Tremor	+ +	+ +	±	±	+	±	+
Bradykinesia	+ +	+ +	+ +	+ +	+ +	+ +	+ +
Rigidity	+ +	+ +	+ +	+ +	+ +	+ +	+ +
Gait abnormality	+ +	+ +	+ +	+ +	+ +	+ +	+ +
Dystonia	±	±	+ +	+	±	±	±
Mental changes	+	±	+ +	+	−	+	−
L-dopa response	+ +	+ +	±	±	−	±	+
Motor fluctuations	+ +	+ +	−	−	−	−	−

PD, Parkinson's disease; MPTP, 1-methyl-4-phenyl-1,2,3,6-tetrahydropyridine induced parkinsonism; MN, manganese-induced parkinsonism; CO, carbon monoxide-induced parkinsonism; CS, carbon disulfide-induced parkinsonism; CN, cyanide-induced parkinsonism; methanol, Methanol-induced parkinsonism; −, not present; ±, may be present; +, rarely present; + +, commonly present.

References

1. Crouper J: Sur les effets du peroxide de managanese. *J Chim Med Pharm Toxicol* 3:223–225, 1837.
2. Tetrud JW, Langston JW: MPTP and Parkinson's disease: One decade later, in Stern MB, Koller WC (eds): *Parkinsonian Syndromes*. New York: Marcel Dekker, 1993, pp 173–193.
3. Ziering A, Berger L, Heineman SD, Lee J: Piperidine derivatives. Part III. 4-arylpiperidines. *J Org Chem* 12:911–914, 1947.
4. Langston JW, Langston EB, Irwin I: MPTP-induced parkinsonism in human and non-human primates—Clinical and experimental aspects. *Acta Neurol Scand* 70:49–54, 1984.
5. Davis GC, Williams AC, Markey SP, et al: Chronic parkinsonism secondary to intravenous injection of meperidine analogues. *Psychiatry Res* 1:249–254, 1979.
6. Markey SP: MPTP: A new tool to understand Parkinson's disease. *Discuss Neurosci* 3:11–51, 1986.
7. Langston JW: MPTP: The promise of a new neurotoxin, in Marsden CD, Fahn S (eds): *Movement Disorders 2*. London: Butterworth, 1987, pp 73–90.
8. Langston JW, Ballard P, Tetrud J, Irwin I: Chronic parkinsonism in humans due to a product of meperidine—Analog synthesis. *Science* 219:979–980, 1983.
9. Langston JW, Forno LS, Rebert CS, Irwin I: Selective nigral toxicity after systemic administration of 1-methyl-4-phenyl-1,2,5,6-tetrahydropyridine (MPTP) in the squirrel monkey. *Brain Res* 292:390–394, 1984.
10. Ruttenber AJ, Garbe PL, Kalter HD, et al: Meperidine analog exposure in California narcotics abusers: Initial epidemiologic findings, in Markey SP, Castagnoli N Jr, Trevor AJ, Kopin IJ (eds): *MPTP: A Neurotoxin Producing a Parkinsonian Syndrome*. New York: Academic Press, 1986, pp 339–353.
11. Ballard PA, Tetrud JW, Langston JW: Permanent parkinsonism in humans due to 1-methyl-4-phenyl-1,2,3,6-tetrahydropyridine (MPTP): Seven cases. *Neurology* 35:949–956, 1985.
12. Tetrud JW, Langston JW, Redmond DE Jr, et al: MPTP-induced tremor in human and non-human primates. *Neurology* 36:308, 1986.
13. Tetrud JW, Langston JW, Garbe PL, Ruttenber JA: Early parkinsonism in persons exposed to 1-methyl-4-phenyl-1,2,3,6-tetrahydropyridine (MPTP). *Neurology* 39:1483–1487, 1989.
14. Stern Y, Langston JW: Intellectual changes in patients with MPTP-induced parkinsonism. *Neurology* 35:1506–1509, 1985.
15. Langston JW, Ballard PA: Parkinsonism induced by 1-methyl-4-phenyl-1,2,3,6-tetrahydropyridine (MPTP): Implications for treatment and the pathogenesis of Parkinson's disease. *Can J Neurol Sci* 11:160–165, 1984.
16. Langston JW: MPTP-induced parkinsonism: How good a model is it?, in Fahn S, Marsden CD, Teychenne P, Jenner P (eds): *Recent advances in Parkinson's Disease*. New York: Raven Press, 1986, pp 119–126.
17. Burns RS, Chiueh CC, Markey SP, et al: A primate model of parkinsonism: Selective destruction of dopaminergic neurones in the pars compacta of the substantia nigra by N-methyl-4-phenyl-1,2,3,6-tetrahydropyridine. *Proc Natl Acad Sci U S A* 80:4546–4550, 1983.
18. Langston JW, Forno LS, Rebert SC, Irwin I: Selective nigral toxicity after systemic administration of 1-methyl-4-phenyl-1,2,3,6-tetrahydropyridine (MPTP) in the squirrel monkey. *Brain Res* 292:390–394, 1984.
19. Waters CM, Hunt SP, Bond AB, Jenner P, et al: Neuropathological, immunohistochemical and receptor changes seen in marmosets treated with MPTP, in Markey SP, Castagnoli N Jr, Trevor AJ, Kopin IJ (eds): *MPTP: A Neurotoxin Producing Parkinsonian Syndrome*. New York: Academic Press, 1986, pp 637–642.
20. Gibb WRG, Lees AJ, Jenner P, Marsden CD: Effects of MPTP in the mid-brain of the marmoset, in Markey SP, Castagnoli N Jr, Trevor AJ, Kopin I (eds): *MPTP: A Neurotoxin Producing a Parkinsonian Syndrome*. New York: Academic Press, 1986, pp 607–614.
21. Langston JW, Irwin I, Langston EB, Forno LS: 1-methyl-4-phenyl-pyridinium ion (MPP+): Identification of a metabolite of MPTP, a toxin selective to the substantia nigra. *Neurosci Lett* 48:87–92, 1984.
22. Sanchez-Ramos JR, Barrett JN, Goldstein M, Weiner WJ, et al: 1-methyl-4-phenylpyridinium (MPP+) but not 1-methyl-4-phenyl-1,2,3,6-tetrahydropyridine (MPTP) selectively destroys dopaminergic neurons in cultures of dissociated rat mesencephalic neurons. *Neurosci Lett* 72:215–220, 1986.
23. Uhl GR, Javitch JA, Snyder SH: Normal MPTP binding in parkinsonian substantia nigra: Evidence for extraneuronal toxin conversion in human brain. *Lancet* 1:956–957, 1985.
24. Chiba K, Trevor AJ, Castagnoli N Jr: Metabolism of the neurotoxic tertiary amine, MPTP, by brain monoamine oxidase. *Biochem Biophys Res Commun* 120:574–578, 1984.
25. Langston JW, Irwin I, Langston EB, Forno LS: Pargyline prevents MPTP-induced parkinsonism in primates. *Science* 225:1480–1482, 1984.
26. Cohen G, Pasik P, Cohen B, Leist A, et al: Pargyline and deprenyl prevent the neurotoxicity of 1-methyl-4-phenyl-1,2,3,6-tetrahydropyridine (MPTP) in monkeys. *Eur J Pharmacol* 106:209–210, 1985.

27. Javitch DA, D'Amato RJ, Strittmatter SM, Snyder SH: Parkinsonism-inducing neurotoxin, N-methy-4-phenyl-1,2,3,6-tetrahydropyridine: Uptake of the metabolite N-methyl-4-phenylpyridine by dopamine neurones explains selective toxicity. *Proc Natl Acad Sci U S A* 82:2173–2177, 1985.

28. Langston JW, Irwin I: MPTP: Current concepts and controversies. *Clin Neuropharmacol* 9:485–507, 1986.

29. Demarest KT, Moore KE: Lack of high affinity transport system for dopamine in the median eminence and posterior pituitary. *Brain Res* 171:545–551, 1979.

30. Bus JS, Aust SD, Gibson JE: Paraquat: Model for oxidant-initiated toxicity. *Environ Health Perspect* 55:37–46, 1984.

31. Di Monte D, Jewell SA, Ekstrom G, Sandy MS, et al: 1-methyl-4-phenyl-1,2,3,6-tetrahydropyridine (MPTP) and 1-methyl-4-phenylpyridine (MPP$^+$) cause rapid ATP depletion in isolation hepatocytes. *Biochem Biophys Res Commun* 137:310–315, 1986.

32. Smith MT, Ekstrom G, Sandy MS, Di Monte D: Studies on the mechanism of 1-methyl-4-phenyl-1,2,3,6-tetrahydropyridine cytotoxicity in isolated hepatocytes. *Life Sci* 40:747–748, 1987.

33. Di Monte DA: Mitochondrial DNA and Parkinson's disease. *Neurology* 4(suppl 2):38–42, 1991.

34. Nicklas WJ, Vyas I, Heikkila RE: Inhibition of NADH-linked oxidation in brain mitochondria by 1-methyl-4-phenyl-1,2,3,6-tetrahydropyridine. *Life Sci* 36:2503–2508, 1985.

35. Poirier J, Barbeau A: 1-methyl-4-phenyl-pyridinium-induced inhibition of nicotinamide adenosine dinucleotide cytochrome c reductase. *Neurosci Lett* 62:7–11, 1985.

36. Mizuno Y, Suzuki K, Sone N, Saitoh T: Inhibition of ATP synthesis by 1-methyl-4-phenylpyridinium ion (MPP$^+$) in isolated mitochondria from mouse brains. *Neurosci Lett* 81:204–208, 1987.

37. Widner H, Tetrud J, Rehncrona S, Snow B, et al: Bilateral fetal mesencephalic grafting in two patients with parkinsonism induced by 1-methyl-4-phenyl-1,2,3,6-tetrahydropyridine (MPTP). *N Engl J Med* 327:1556–1563, 1992.

38. Calne DB, Chu NS, Huang CC, Lu CS, et al: Manganism and idiopathic parkinsonism: Similarities and differences. *Neurology* 44:1583–1586, 1994.

39. Spencer PS, Butterfield PG: Environmental agents and Parkinson's disease, in Ellenberg JH, Koller WC, Langston JW (eds): *Etiology of Parkinson's Disease.* New York: Marcel Dekker, 1995, pp 319–365.

40. Couper J: On the effects of black oxide of manganese when inhaled into the lungs. *Br Ann Med Pharm* 1:41–42, 1987.

41. Canavan MM, Cobb S, Drinker CK: Chronic manganese poisoning. *Arch Neurol Psychiatry* 32:501–512, 1934.

42. Flinn RH, Neal PA, Fulton WB: Industrial manganese poisoning. *J Ind Hyg Toxicol* 23:374–387, 1941.

43. Rodier J: Manganese poisoning in Moroccan miners. *Br J Ind Med* 12:21–35, 1955.

44. Emara AM, El-Shawabi SH, Madkour OI, El-Samra GH: Chronic manganese poisoning in the dry battery industry. *Br J Ind Med* 28:78–82, 1971.

45. Mena I, Marin O, Fuenzalida S, Cotzias GC: Chronic manganese poisoning: Clinical picture and manganese turnover. *Neurology* 17:128–136, 1967.

46. Sanchez-Ramos JR: Toxin-induced parkinsonism, in Stern MB, Koller WC (eds): *Parkinsonian Syndromes.* New York: Marcel Dekker, 1993, pp 155–172.

47. Huang CC, Chu NS, Song C, Wang JD: Chronic manganese intoxication. *Arch Neurol* 46:1104–1112, 1989.

48. Mena I, Court J, Fuenzalida S, Papavasilious PS, et al: Modification of chronic manganese poisoning-treatment with L-dopa or 5-OH tryptophane. *N Engl J Med* 282:5–10, 1970.

49. Barbeau A: Manganese and extrapyramidal disorders. *Neurotoxicology* 5:13–36, 1984.

50. Canavan M, Cobb S, Drinker CK: Chronic manganese poisoning: Report of a case with autopsy. *Arch Neurol Psychiatry* 32:500–505, 1934.

51. Yamada M, Ohno S, Okayasu I, Okeda R, et al: Chronic manganese poisoning: A neuropathological study with determination of manganese distribution. *Acta Neuropathol* 71, 1976.

52. Bernheimer H, Birkmayer W, Hornykiewicz O, Jellinger K, et al: Brain dopamine and the syndromes of Parkinson and Huntington: Clinical, morphological and neurochemical correlations. *J Neurol Sci* 20:415–425, 1973.

53. Mella H: The experimental production of basal ganglia symptomatology in macaque rhesus. *Arch Neurol Psychiatry* 11:405–417, 1923.

54. Van Bogaert L, Dallemagne MJ: Approaches expérimentales des troubles nerveux du manganisme. *Monatsschr Psychiatr Neurol* II:60–89, 1943.

55. Gupta SK, Murthy RC, Chandra SV: Neuromelanin in manganese-exposed primates. *Toxicol Lett* 6:17–20, 1980.

56. Donaldson J, Labaella FS, Gesser D: Enhanced autoxidation of dopamine as a possible basis of manganese neurotoxicity. *Neurotoxicity* 2:53–64, 1981.

57. Donaldson J: The pathophysiology of trace metal: Neurotransmitter interaction in the CNS. *Trends Pharmacol Sci* 1:75–77, 1981.

58. Kono Y, Takahashi M, Asada K: Oxidation of manganous pyrophosphate by superoxide radicals and illuminated spinach chloroplasts. *Arch Biochem Biophys* 174:454–461, 1976.

59. Archibald FS, Fridovich I: Manganese, superoxide dismutase and oxygen tolerance in some lactic acid bacteria. *J Bacteriol* 146:928–936, 1981.

60. Graham DG: Catecholamine toxicity: A proposal for the molecular pathogenesis of manganese neurotoxicity and Parkinson's disease. *Neurotoxicology* 5:83–96, 1984.

61. Cook DG, Fahn S, Brait KA: Chronic manganese intoxication. *Arch Neurol* 30:59–64, 1974.

62. Rosenstock HA, Simons DG, Meyer JS: Chronic manganism: Neurologic and laboratory studies during treatment with L-dopa. *J Am Med Assoc* 217:1354–1358, 1971.

63. Greenhouse AH: Manganese intoxication in the United States. *Trans Am Neurol Assoc* 96:248–249, 1971.

64. Lu CS, Huang CC, Chu NS, Calne DB: L-dopa failure in chronic manganism. *Neurology* 44:1600–1602, 1994.

65. Ky S, Deng H, Xie P, Hu W: A report of two cases of chronic serious manganese poisoning treated with sodium paraaminosalicylic acid. *Br J Ind Med* 49:66–69, 1992.

66. Shillito JH, Drinker CK, Shaughnessy TJ: The problem of nervous and mental sequelae in carbon monoxide poisoning. *J Am Med Assoc* 106:669–674, 1936.

67. Meigs JW, Hughes JPW: Acute carbon monoxide poisoning. *Arch Ind Hyg Occup Med* 6:344–356, 1952.

68. Richarson JC, Chambers RA, Heywood PM: Encephalopathies of anoxia and hypoglycemia. *Arch Neurol* 1:178–182, 1959.

69. Bour H, Tutin M, Pasquier P: The central nervous system and carbon monoxide poisoning. I. Clinical data with reference to 20 fatal cases. *Prog Brain Res* 24:1–30, 1967.

70. Smith J, Brandon S: Morbidity from acute carbon monoxide poisoning at three year follow up. *Br Med J* 1:318–320, 1970.

71. Norkool DM, Kirkpatrick JN: Treatment of acute carbon monoxide poisoning with hyperbaric oxygen: A review of 115 cases. *Ann Emerg Med* 14:1168–1171, 1985.

72. Choi IS: Delayed neurological sequelae in carbon monoxide intoxication. *Arch Neurol* 40:433–435, 1983.

73. Mathieu D, Nolf M, Durocher A, et al: Acute carbon monoxide poisoning: Risk of late sequelae and treatment by hyperbaric oxygen. *Clin Toxicol* 23:315–324, 1985.

74. Lee MS, Marsden CD: Neurological sequelae following carbon monoxide poisoning: Clinical course and outcome according to the clinical types and brain computed tomography scan findings. *Mov Disord* 9:550–558, 1994.

75. Siesjö BK: Carbon monoxide poisoning: Mechanism of damage, late sequelae and therapy. *Clin Toxicol* 23:247–248, 1985.

76. Min SK: A brain syndrome associated with delayed neuropsychiatric sequelae following acute carbon monoxide intoxication. *Acta Psychiatr Scand* 73:80–86, 1986.

77. Lacey DJ: Neurological sequelae of acute carbon monoxide intoxication. *Am J Dis Child* 135:145–147, 1981.

78. Ginsberg MD: Delayed neurological deterioration following hypoxia. *Adv Neurol* 26:21–43, 1979.

79. Raskin N, Mullaney OC: The mental and neurological sequelae of carbon monoxide asphyxia in a case observed for fifteen years. *J Nerv Ment Dis* 92:640–659, 1940.

80. Schwarz A, Hennerici M, Wegener OH: Delayed choreoathetosis following carbon monoxide poisoning. *Neurology* 35:98–99, 1985.

81. Davous P, Rondot P, Marion MH, Guerguen B: Severe chorea after carbon monoxide poisoning. *J Neurol Neurosurg Psychiatry* 49:206–208, 1986.

82. Kim JS, Lee SA, Kim JS: Myoclonus, delayed sequelae of carbon monoxide poisoning: Piracetam trial. *Yonsei Med J* 28:231–233, 1987.

83. Pulst SM, Walshe TM, Rovero JA: Carbon monoxide poisoning with features of Gilles de la Tourette's syndrome. *Arch Neurol* 40:443–444, 1983.

84. Sawada Y, Takahashi M, Ohashi N, et al: Computed tomography as an indication of long-term outcome after acute carbon monoxide poisoning. *Lancet* 1:783–784, 1980.

85. Miura T, Mitomo M, Kawai R, Harada: CT of the brain in acute carbon monoxide intoxication: Characteristic features and prognosis. *AJNR* 6:739–742, 1985.

86. Hayashi R, Hayashi K, Inoue K, Yanagiasawa N: A serial computerized tomographic study of the interval form of CO poisoning. *Eur Neurol* 33:27–29, 1993.

87. Destee A, Courteville V, Devos PH, Besson P, et al: Computed tomography and acute carbon monoxide poisoning. *J Neurol Neurosurg Psychiatry* 48:281–282, 1985.

88. Jaeckle RS, Nasrallah HA: Major depression and carbon monoxide-induced parkinsonism: Diagnosis, computerized axial tomography, and response to L-dopa. *J Nerv Ment Dis* 173:503–508, 1985.

89. Vieregge P, Klostermann W, Blümm RG, Borgis KJ: Carbon monoxide poisoning: Clinical, neurophysiological, and brain imaging observations in acute disease and follow-up. *J Neurol* 236:478–481, 1989.

90. Garland I I, Pearce J: Neurological complication of carbon monoxide poisoning. *Q J Med* 36:445–475, 1967.

91. Gordon EB: Carbon monoxide encephalopathy. *Br Med J* 1:1232, 1965.

92. Lapresle J, Fardeau M: The central nervous system and carbon monoxide poisoning. II Anatomical study of brain lesion following intoxication with carbon monoxide, in Bour H, Ledingham IM (eds): *Progress in Brain Research*. Amsterdam: Elsevier, 1967, pp 31–74.

93. Jellinger K: Exogenous lesions of the pallidum, in Vincken PJ, Bruyn GW (eds): *Handbook of Clinical Neurology*. New York: Elsevier, 1986, pp 465–491.

94. Kobayashi K, Isaki K, Fukutani Y, et al: CT findings of the interval form of carbon monoxide poisoning compared with neuropathological findings. *Eur Neurol* 23:34–43, 1984.

95. Jefferson JW: Subtle neuropsychiatric sequelae of carbon monoxide intoxication: Two case reports. *Am J Psychiatry* 133:961–964, 1976.

96. Shiraki H: The neuropathology of carbon monoxide poisoning in humans with special reference to the change of globus pallidus. *Adv Neurol Sci* 13:25–32, 1969.

97. Ginsberg MD, Hedley-White ET, Richardson EP Jr: Hypoxic-ischemic leukoencephalopathy in man. *Arch Neurol* 33:5–14, 1976.

98. Vogt C, Vogt O: Erkrandungen der Grosshirnrunde im Lichte der Topistik, Pathoklise und Pathoarchitektonik. *J Psychol Neurol* 28:1–171, 1922.

99. Friede RL: Chemoarchitecture and neuropathology. *Proceedings of the 4th International Congress on Neuropathology*. Stuttgart: G Thieme, 1962, pp 70–75.

100. Dexter DT, Wells FR, Lees AJ, Agid Y, et al: Increased nigral iron content in post-mortem parkinsonian brain. *Lancet* 2:1219–1220, 1967.

101. Ringel RW, Klawans HL: Carbon monoxide induced parkinsonism. *J Neurol Sci* 16:245–251, 1972.

102. Klawans HL, Stein RW, Tanner CM, Goetz CG: A pure parkinsonian syndrome following acute carbon monoxide poisoning. *Arch Neurol* 39:302–304, 1982.

103. Lewey FH: Neurological, medical and biochemical signs and symptoms indicating chronic industrial carbon disulfide absorption. *Ann Intern Med* 15:869–883, 1941.

104. Peters HA, Levine RL, Matthews CG, Chapman LJ: Extrapyramidal and other neurological manifestations associated with carbon disulfide fumigant exposure. *Arch Neurol* 45:537–540, 1988.

105. Pentschew A: Intoxications, in Menckler J (ed): *Pathology of Nervous System*. New York: McGraw-Hill, 1971, pp 1618–1650.

106. Peters HA, Levine RL, Mattews CG, et al: Carbon disulfide-induced neuropsychiatric changes in grain storage workers. *Am J Ind Med* 3:373–391, 1982.

107. Peters HA, Levine RL, Mattews CG, et al: Synergistic neurotoxicity of carbon tetrachloride/carbon disulfide (80/20 fumigants) and other pesticides in grain storage workers. *Acta Pharmacol Toxicol* 59(suppl 7):535–546, 1986.

108. Alpers BJ, Lewy FH: Changes in the nervous system following carbon disulfide poisoning in animals and in man. *Arch Neurol Psychiatry* 44:725–726, 1940.

109. Richter R: Degeneration of the basal ganglia in monkeys from chronic carbon disulfide poisoning. *J Neuropathol Exp Neurol* 4:324–353, 1945.

110. Bus JS: The relationship of carbon disulfide metabolism to development of toxicity. *Neurotoxicology* 4:73–80, 1985.

111. Barbeau A, Pourcher E: New data on the genetics of Parkinson's disease. *Can J Neurol Sci* 9:53–60, 1982.

112. Seppalainen AKM, Haltia M: Carbon disulfide, in Spencer RS, Schaumburg HM (eds): *Experimental Clinical Neurotoxicology*. Baltimore, Williams & Wilkins, 1980, pp 356–373.

113. Uitti RJ, Rajput AH, Ashenhurst EM, Rozkilsky B: Cyanide-induced parkinsonism: A clinicopathologic report. *Neurology* 35:921–925, 1985.

114. Rosenberg NL, Myers JA, Wayne WR: Cyanide-induced parkinsonism: Clinical, MRI, and 6-fluorodopa PET studies. *Neurology* 39:142–144, 1989.

115. Feldman JL, Feldman MD: Sequelae of attempted suicide by cyanide ingestion: A case report. *Int J Psychiatry Med* 20:173–179, 1990.

116. Grandas F, Artieda J, Obesco JA: Clinical and CT scan findings in a case of cyanide intoxication. *Mov Disord* 4:188–193, 1989.

117. Edelman F: Ein Beitrag zur Vergiftung mit gasformiger Blausäure insbesondere zu den dabei auftretenden Geheinveränderungen. *Dtsch Z Nervenheilkd* 72:259–287, 1921.

118. Schmorl G: Demonstrationen 3. Gehirn bei Blausäurevergiftung. *Muench Med Wochenschur* 67:913, 1920.

119. Meyer A: Experimentelle Vergiftungsstudien. III. Über Gehirnveränderungen bei experimenteller Blausäurevergiftung. *Z Gesamte Neurol Psychiatr* 143:333–348, 1933.

120. Hurst EW: Experimental demyelination of the central nervous system. I. The encephalopathy produced by potassium cyanide. *Aust J Exp Biol Med Sci* 18:210–223, 1940.

121. Haymaker W, Ginzler AM, Ferguson RL: Residual neuropathological effects of cyanide poisoning: A study of the central nervous system of 23 dogs exposed to cyanide compounds. *Milit Surg* 111:231–246, 1952.

122. Mclean DR, Jacobs H, Mielke BW: Methanol poisoning: A clinical and pathological study. *Ann Neurol* 8:161–167, 1980.

123. Guggenheim MA, Couch JR, Weinberg W: Motor dysfunction as a permanent complication of methanol ingestion. *Arch Neurol* 24:550–554, 1971.

124. Potts AM, Praglin J, Farkas J, Orbison J, et al: Studies on the visual toxicity of methanol. *Am J Ophthalmol* 40:76–83, 1955.

125. Erlanson P, Frisz H, Hagstram K: Severe methanol intoxication. *Acta Med Scand* 117:393–408, 1965.

126. Ritchie JM: The aliphatic alcohols, in Goodman LS, Gelman A (eds): *The Pharmacological Basis of Therapeutics.* London: Macmillan, 1970, pp 135–150.

127. Clay KL, Murphy RC, Watkins WD: Experimental methanol toxicity in the primates: analysis of metabolic acidosis. *Toxicol Appl Pharmacol* 34:49–61, 1975.

128. McMartin KE, Makar AB, Martin A, et al: Methanol poisoning. I. The role of formic acid in the development of metabolic acidosis of the monkey and the reversal by 4-methylpyrazole. *Biochem Med* 13:319–333, 1975.

129. Symon L, Pasztor E, Dorsch NWC: Physiological responses of local areas of the cerebral circulation in experimental primates determined by the method of hydrogen clearance. *Stroke* 4:632–634, 1973.

Chapter 23

DRUG-INDUCED PARKINSONISM

JEAN P. HUBBLE

NEUROLEPTIC-INDUCED PARKINSONISM
    Background
    Specific Neuroleptic Agents
    Clinical Features
    Pathogenesis
    Treatment of Neuroleptic-Induced Parkinsonism
DOPAMINE STORAGE AND TRANSPORT INHIBITORS
CALCIUM-CHANNEL BLOCKERS
OTHER MEDICATIONS
SUMMARY

Neuroleptic-Induced Parkinsonism

BACKGROUND

Many drugs can produce parkinsonism. The antipsychotic drugs or neuroleptics are well-recognized in this regard. In the early 1950s, after its introduction for the treatment of psychiatric illness, reports were issued linking the neuroleptic chlorpromazine with various neurological side effects, including parkinsonism.[1,2] In these early series, the incidence of drug-induced parkinsonism (DIP) varied from 4–40 percent.[3–5] Whereas investigators agreed on the clinical manifestations of the syndrome, they varied in their opinions regarding causative mechanism and identification of at-risk individuals. A clear dose-response was lacking, that is, there was no correlation between occurrence of parkinsonian signs and amount of chlorpromazine administered.[5] It was initially hypothesized that DIP may be related to chlorpromazine-induced liver damage. In their study of DIP, Hall et al. found no relationship between liver function tests and the occurrence of this syndrome.[5] Similarly, these investigators were unable to corroborate the claim, made by others, that patients with the most pronounced antipsychotic drug benefit were most apt to develop DIP.

In subsequent years, additional neuroleptic compounds were developed and marketed. As the number of individuals exposed to this class of drugs grew, several distinct adverse reactions involving abnormalities in movement and tone were described. In 1961, Ayd reported extrapyramidal reactions, including DIP, dyskinesia, and akathisia in 39 percent of 3775 neuroleptic-treated patients.[6] In searching for clues to the cause of DIP, Ayd found that the syndrome developed

over a shorter time period in individuals treated with the piperazine and fluorinated phenothiazine compounds.

SPECIFIC NEUROLEPTIC AGENTS

It is now recognized that parkinsonism can result from the use of numerous drugs among the various types of neuroleptics (Table 23-1). Certain neuroleptics, such as thioridazine and molindone, have fewer reported extrapyramidal side effects; thus, the risk of DIP may be less with their use. However, well-controlled comparison studies substantiating this notion are lacking. In one series, thioridazine was the third most common offending drug, after haloperidol and amitriptyline/perphenazine among 125 patients followed for drug-induced movement disorders at a referral specialty clinic.

The atypical neuroleptic, clozapine, has a low incidence of extrapyramidal side effects, including parkinsonism.[7] This is attributed to the relative specificity of clozapine's dopamine receptor blockade. The introduction of clozapine offered particular promise for the treatment of psychosis in patients with Parkinson's disease (PD).[8,9] Confusion, agitation, and hallucinations can occur in PD as a result of dopaminergic drug therapy, the primary disease process, or unrelated psychiatric disorders. Conventional antipsychotics are poorly tolerated in the PD patient because of the propensity of these drugs to exacerbate parkinsonian symptoms. In addition to its reported efficacy in the control of psychosis, clozapine may reduce tremor and motor fluctuations in PD.[10,11] However, clozapine at higher doses (75–250 mg/day) in PD patients has been associated with sedation, delirium, and worsening of motor signs and symptoms.[12] The association of this drug with hematologic abnormalities, including fatal agranulocytosis, has necessitated weekly blood counts in all treated individuals.[13] The concern over the potential for neutropenia, coupled with the cost and inconvenience of frequent blood tests, has limited the use of this agent. As a result of the development of clozapine, it is hoped that similar agents with less potential toxicity will be forthcoming.

Although neuroleptics are used primarily as antipsychotic agents, it is important to recognize their other nonpsychiatric uses. These drugs are sometimes prescribed for depression, anxiety, and insomnia. Typically used to control nausea and vomiting, prochlorperazine and related agents belong to the neuroleptic class of drugs and can produce DIP.[14] Metoclopramide, an atypical neuroleptic belonging to the benzamide class, is used to ameliorate gastric stasis and is used as an antiemetic; various extrapyramidal reactions, including parkinsonism, have been associated with its use.[15–17] In one series, 5 of 2557 metoclopramide-treated patients developed parkinsonism; all affected individuals were over 40 years of age.[18]

CLINICAL FEATURES

Clinical descriptions of neuroleptic-induced parkinsonism date back to the original reports in the 1960s. In 1961, Ayd reported on DIP's responsiveness to anticholinergic medications, noted its usual abatement with the discontinuation of the offending drug and distinguished it clinically from PD.[6] Ayd also reported it to be more common in women and in the

---

*In part, text and tables modified and reproduced with publisher's permission from Hubble: Drug-induced parkinsonism, in Koller WC, Stern M (eds): *Parkinsonian Syndromes*. New York: Marcel Dekker, 1993, pp 111–122.

TABLE 23-1 Neuroleptics and Related Agents

Trade Name	Generic Name
Phenothiazines	
Compazine	Prochlorperazine
Etrafon (Triavil)	Perphenazine and amitriptyline
Levoprome	Methotrimeprazine
Mellaril	Thioridazine
Phenergan	Promethazine
Prolixin	Fluphenazine
Norzine	Thiethylperazine
Serentil	Mesoridazine
Sparine	Promaxine
Stelazine	Trifluoperazine
Thorazine	Chlorpromazine
Torecan	Thiethylperazine
Trilafon	Perphenazine
Butyrophenones	
Haldol	Haloperidol
Fentanyl	Droperidol
Thioxanthenes	
Navane	Thiothixene
Taractran	Chlorprothixene
Benzamides	
Reglan	Metoclopramide
Dihydroindolone	
Moban	Molindone
Dibenzoxazepine	
Loxitane	Loxapine
Dibenzodiazepine	
Clozaril	Clozapine

TABLE 23-2 Clinical Features That May Distinguish Drug-Induced Parkinsonism from Idiopathic PD

	Drug-Induced Parkinsonism	PD
Symptom onset	Bilateral and symmetric	Unilateral or asymmetric
Course	Acute or subacute	Insidious, chronic
Tremor type	Bilateral symmetric postural or rest tremor	Unilateral or asymmetric rest tremor
Anticholinergic drug response	May be pronounced	Usually mild to moderate
Withdrawal of suspected offending drug	Remittance within weeks to months	Symptoms and signs slowly progress

elderly. It was initially suggested that neuroleptic-induced parkinsonism resembled postencephalitic parkinsonism, rather than PD.[19] However, subsequent work suggests that the clinical manifestation of this syndrome is quite similar to that of PD.[20] Akinesia, rigidity, postural abnormalities, and tremor may occur. Bradykinesia is the earliest, most common and, frequently, the only manifestation of DIP, accounting for the expressionless face, loss of associated movements, slow initiation of motor activity, and disturbed speech. Rigidity of the extremities, neck, or trunk, usually without a "cogwheel" phenomenon, may occur after the onset of bradykinesia. Although the characteristic parkinsonian "pill-rolling" tremor at rest may be present, postural tremor resembling essential tremor may also be seen.[21,22]

Although DIP may be clinically indistinguishable from PD, some differentiating characteristics may occur[23] (Table 23-2). The signs and symptoms of PD usually begin insidiously on one side of the body; with time, the opposite side is also affected but to a lesser degree. The manifestations of neuroleptic-induced parkinsonism are frequently bilateral and symmetric and often develop acutely or subacutely. In one series, the signs of parkinsonism emerged within a few days of neuroleptic treatment with a gradual increase in incidence so that 50–70 percent of cases appeared by 1 month and 90 percent of cases within 3 months.[20] It is often stated that tolerance develops to neuroleptic-induced parkinsonism. However, prospective studies to verify this phenomenon are lacking. The only clinical basis for this assumption is the observation that withdrawal of anticholinergic drugs,

coadministered for several months with neuroleptics, is followed by the appearance of relatively few cases of DIP.

After discontinuation of neuroleptics, the majority of patients are free of parkinsonian signs within a few weeks. However, the effects may last longer, in some cases for up to several years.[23] Metoclopramide-induced parkinsonism has been reported to take several months to resolve completely.[24,25] The potentially long duration of neuroleptic-induced parkinsonism is important to appreciate so that one can avoid diagnostic error. DIP will usually improve slowly over time with reduction or discontinuation of the drug, whereas the signs and symptoms of PD will progressively worsen.

Neuroleptic-induced movement disorders, including DIP, frequently go unrecognized.[25] This lack of recognition on the part of treating physicians is suggested by Miller and Jankovic in their review of metoclopramide-induced movement disorders; they found that the offending drug was continued for an average of 6 months after the onset of extrapyramidal symptoms.[17] Hansen et al. found that psychiatry resident physicians diagnosed DIP in 11 percent of neuroleptic-treated patients, whereas researchers determined the prevalence to be 26 percent in this study population.[26] The work of Albanese et al. further emphasizes that the proper diagnosis of DIP depends on a high index of suspicion.[27] These authors detail three cases in which individuals developed parkinsonism while unwittingly ingesting neuroleptics being surreptitiously administered to them by their consorts.

PATHOGENESIS

The primary neurochemical determinant of PD is striatal dopamine depletion.[28] Because neuroleptic drugs function as dopamine receptor blockers, it is not surprising that clinical features of parkinsonism can result from their use. It is not plausible that DIP is simply the result of dopamine receptor blockade. If this were true, then the incidence and severity of DIP should correlate with drug dosage and length of exposure. Attempts to link total drug dosage with the occurrence of parkinsonism have failed to show a clear relationship[5]; furthermore, plasma neuroleptic drug levels do not correlate with the severity of DIP.[29] Parkinsonism appearing within several days of treatment with relatively small drug doses is a common clinical experience; yet, other patients are successfully maintained on relatively high doses for several years without developing parkinsonism. It had been suggested that DIP was simply idiopathic PD occurring by chance in neuroleptic-treated individuals, as in the general population. The reported prevalence of neuroleptic-induced parkinsonism varies, but clinically significant parkinsonism reportedly occurs in 10–15 percent of treated individuals.[30,31] These rates of DIP are probably underestimates[32]; thus, coincidental idiopathic PD could not account for all cases of DIP, because the occurrence rate of parkinsonism in neuroleptic-treated individuals is much greater than estimates of PD in the general populace.

The mechanisms determining individual susceptibility to DIP remain unclear. Some studies suggest that women are at an increased risk for the development of neuroleptic-induced movement disorders, including tardive dyskinesia[33,34] and DIP.[6,30] Estrogen-related dopamine receptor blockade has been offered as the explanation for this female preponderance.[35] Others have not substantiated a gender influence[36,37]; these discrepancies could be explained by disparities in case ascertainment and by differences in medication prescription and usage based on sex. In one report, low urinary levels of free dopamine were associated with the subsequent development of phenothiazine-induced parkinsonism suggesting an inherent metabolic defect may be causative.[38] Human leukocyte antigen B44 (HLA B44) is reported to be common in DIP, suggesting a genetic influence.[39] In one series, 5 of 16 patients with metoclopramide-induced movement disorders had family members with reported parkinsonism, tremor, or chorea.[17] However, the precise role of genetics in DIP remains uncertain.

The possibility that increased susceptibility to DIP might be related to subclinical PD has also been considered.[40,41] In some instances, it appears that PD becomes clinically overt during neuroleptic therapy and then subsides when the drug is discontinued, only to reappear years later; at least nine such cases have been documented in the medical literature.[42–44] In addition, Rajput et al. described two patients with drug-induced parkinsonism that completely remitted upon drug withdrawal; postmortem examination ultimately revealed pathological changes consistent with PD.[45] Brooks reported reduced putamen ^{18}F-dopa uptake on positron emission tomography (PET) in two of seven individuals with DIP[46]; four of the five patients with normal PET scans recovered fully with cessation of drug therapy. The two patients with abnormal scans had persistent evidence of parkinsonism requiring levodopa therapy, suggesting underlying PD.

The relationship of DIP to other neuroleptic-induced extrapyramidal syndromes is intriguing. Like DIP, tardive dyskinesia is reported to occur more frequently in the elderly.[47–49] Saltz et al.[50] followed 215 patients over 55 years of age after the initiation of neuroleptic therapy. Evidence of parkinsonism was found in 103 patients by week 43; tardive dyskinesia developed in 40 percent of the parkinsonian patients, compared to 12 percent of nonparkinsonian subjects. The coexistence of DIP and tardive dyskinesia has been reported by others.[51–53] The occurrence of both hypokinetic and hyperkinetic drug-induced side effects in a common patient population is difficult to explain. In reviewing the effects of neuroleptics, Seeman et al. postulated action at the presynaptic site as causative in both DIP and tardive dyskinesia.[54] This may reflect the differential effects of neuroleptics on dopamine receptor subtypes; the geriatric patient population may be especially vulnerable to such effects because of diminished drug metabolism, dopaminergic neuronal loss, or alterations in dopamine receptors.[35,55,56]

TREATMENT OF NEUROLEPTIC-INDUCED PARKINSONISM

Withdrawal of the offending drug when possible is the obvious treatment of choice. This, however, is done at the risk of exacerbating the underlying condition for which the drug was initially prescribed. This is a particular difficulty in the instance of psychosis associated with schizophrenia. It is prudent to weigh the benefits that the patient derives from the drug against the severity and disability of DIP. Mild nondisabling DIP occurring in individuals who have achieved good control of psychotic symptoms on a stable dose of neuroleptic may require only observation and no intervention. Alternatively, the patient can be switched to a neuroleptic with less potential side effects, such as thioridazine or clozapine. As described above, the atypical antipsychotic clozapine is an effective antipsychotic, having virtually no parkinsonian side effects but requiring weekly blood tests and close follow-up. In lieu of the antiemetics metoclopramide and chlorpromazine, the peripherally acting dopamine antagonist, domperidone, is sometimes used.[57] Domperidone is not commercially available within the United States. Despite its reportedly low central nervous system penetration, drug-induced movement disorders have occasionally been associated with the use of domperidone.[58] Antiemetics that do not act via dopamine blockade, such as ondansetron and benzquinamide hydrochloride, can be used in some instances.

Standard antiparkinsonian drugs can be used to treat DIP. Anticholinergic compounds are frequently used in this regard. Anticholinergic drugs reportedly decrease the signs and symptoms of neuroleptic-induced parkinsonism to a greater degree than in PD. This drug response is touted to be of use as a means of distinguishing between DIP and PD.[59] Dopaminergic drugs, including levodopa, can ameliorate DIP but may provoke the very symptoms for which the neuroleptic drug was prescribed, such as nausea and hallucinations.[60] In a single case report, pyridoxine was reported to ameliorate DIP and tardive dyskinesia in an individual with neuroleptic-treated schizophrenia.[61]

Dopamine Storage and Transport Inhibitors

Reserpine, an antihypertensive, depletes brain dopamine and other biogenic amines by interfering with presynaptic vesicular storage mechanisms. It can produce both clinical and experimental parkinsonism.[62] With numerous other antihypertensives now available, reserpine is rarely used to control blood pressure but is sometimes prescribed to treat tardive dyskinesia.[63,64] Because individuals with tardive dyskinesia may be at increased risk for DIP, close monitoring of these patients is warranted if treatment with reserpine is used. Tetrabenazine, a synthetic analogue of reserpine, also depletes amines and may also block postsynaptic dopamine receptors.[65] Not currently marketed in the United States, tetrabenazine, like reserpine, may be useful in the treatment of hyperkinetic disorders.[66,67] Jankovic and Orman reported parkinsonism as the most common side effect of tetrabenazine exposure, affecting 53 of 217 patients receiving the drug for hyperkinesia.[67]

Two cases of PD exacerbated by alpha-methyldopa have been observed, as well as several cases of parkinsonism reported to be induced by the drug.[68,69] Theorized as acting as a "false" neurotransmitter, alpha-methyldopa has been used as an antihypertensive drug and has even been used in the treatment of PD.[70] Therefore, the significance of the few reported cases of alpha-methyldopa-induced parkinsonism is unclear.

Calcium-Channel Blockers

Available in Europe and Latin America, the piperazine derivatives, flunarizine and cinnarizine, act as calcium-entry blockers and have been prescribed for various disorders, including vertigo, migraine, and tinnitus.[71,72] Extrapyramidal reactions, including DIP and exacerbation of PD, have been associated with their use.[73,74] A primate model of cinnarizine-induced parkinsonism has also been described.[75] Parkinsonism is thought to be a result of the antidopaminergic effects of these compounds, which may be pre- or postsynaptic.[76,77] Garcia-Ruiz et al. reported persistence of parkinsonian signs, particularly in the aged, many months after the cessation of the offending drug.[78] Negrotti et al. suggested that DIP resulting from calcium-channel blockers may have a genetic component, because they found a relatively higher occurrence of other movement disorders among relatives of affected individuals.[79] Calcium-channel blockers, widely available in the United States, are rarely associated with parkinsonism,[80] although the antidopaminergic effect of one such agent, nimodipine, has been demonstrated experimentally.[81]

Other Medications

Drugs of various types have occasionally been associated with parkinsonism (Table 23-3). The cardiac antiarrhythmic agent, amiodarone, may cause sundry neurological side effects, including tremor. Amiodarone-induced tremor is typically of the postural type, resembling essential tremor; however, parkinsonian signs and symptoms have also been described.[82–84]

In single case reports, parkinsonism has been ascribed to cholinergic drugs, including bethanechol and the cholinesterase inhibitor pyridostigmine.[85,86] This side effect is theorized to be a result of drug-induced cholinergic overactivity, that is, an imbalance of striatal acetylcholine-dopamine activity. In one instance of bethanechol-induced parkinsonism, post-

TABLE 23-3 Miscellaneous Drugs Associated with Parkinsonism

Reserpine
  Tetrabenazine
Alpha-methyldopa
Calcium-channel blockers (cinnarizine, flunarizine)
Amiodarone
Bethamechol
Pyridostigmine
Lithium
Diazepam
Fluoxetine
Phenelzine
Procaine
Meperidine
Amphotericin B
Cephaloridine
5-Fluorouracil
Vincristine-Adriamycin

mortem analysis demonstrated pathological changes consistent with PD, suggesting that the drug made clinically manifest the underlying nigrostriatal pathology.[85] However, it is more difficult to explain parkinsonism secondary to pyridostigmine, because this drug appears to penetrate the blood-brain barrier poorly, and central nervous system effects would not be anticipated.

Lithium commonly produces a postural tremor, but whether it can induce parkinsonism is not firmly established. Cogwheel rigidity has been found on examination in a small percentage of patients taking lithium.[87] Two patients were reported to develop parkinsonian symptoms after lithium therapy but both had prior exposure to neuroleptics.[88] Lutz described transient parkinsonism in an individual with elevated lithium blood levels who had been taking a liquid protein diet.[89]

DIP was reported in four patients on high dose (≥ 100 mg/day) diazepam in the treatment of schizophrenia.[90] Fluoxetine, alone and in conjunction with neuroleptics or carbamazepine, has been associated with parkinsonism.[91–93] Isolated instances of parkinsonism have been ascribed to sundry other agents, including phenelzine,[94] procaine,[95] meperidine,[96] amphotericin B,[97] cephaloridine,[98] 5-fluorouracil,[99] and vincristine combined with Adriamycin.[100]

Summary

In summary, parkinsonism secondary to drug ingestion is common particularly in the elderly. Dopamine receptor blockers, used primarily as antipsychotics and antiemetics, are the most frequent offending agents. Other pharmacological classes of medications have also been impugned, although the mechanism of DIP in such instances is less certain. The susceptibility of the individual to developing DIP has not been established, but it may represent latent PD or a heritable trait, in some instances. Further scrutiny of the occurrence and characteristics of DIP would yield a better understanding of this phenomenon and may also provide greater insight into the cause and pathogenesis of PD.

References

1. Anton-Stephens D: Preliminary observations on the psychiatric uses of chlorpromazine (Largactil). *J Mental Sci* 100:543–545, 1954.

2. Lehmann HE, Hanrahan GE: Chlorpromazine: New inhibiting agent for psychomotor excitement and manic states. *Arch Neurol Psychiatry* 71:227, 1954.

3. Kinross-Wright V: Chlorpromazine—A major advance in psychiatric treatment. *Postgrad Med* 16:297, 1954.

4. Goldman D: Treatment of psychotic states with chlorpromazine. *J Am Med Assoc* 157:1274–1277, 1955.

5. Hall RA, Jackson RB, Swain JM: Neurotoxic reactions resulting from chlorpromazine administration. *J Am Med Assoc* 161:214–218, 1956.

6. Ayd FJ Jr: A survey of drug-induced extrapyramidal reactions. *J Am Med Assoc* 175:1054–1060, 1961.

7. Baldessarini RJ, Frankenburg FR: Clozapine: A novel antipsychotic agent. *N Engl J Med* 324:746–754, 1991.

8. Scholz E, Dichgans J: Treatment of drug-induced exogenous psychosis in parkinsonism with clozapine and fluperlapine. *Eur Arch Psychiatry Neurol Sci* 235:60–64, 1985.

9. Friedman JH, Lannon MC: Clozapine in the treatment of psychosis in Parkinson's disease. *Neurology* 39:1219–1221, 1989.

10. Bennett JP, Landow ER, Schuh LA: Suppression of dyskinesias in advanced Parkinson's disease. II. Increasing daily clozapine doses suppress dyskinesias and improve parkinsonism symptoms. *Neurology* 43:1551–1555, 1993.

11. Friedman JH, Lannon MC: Clozapine treatment of tremor in Parkinson's disease. *Mov Disord* 5(suppl 1):50, 1990.

12. Wolters EC, Hurwitz TA, Mak E, et al: Clozapine in the treatment of parkinsonian patients with dopaminometic psychosis. *Neurology* 40:832–834, 1990.

13. Kane J, Honigfeld G, Singer J, et al: Clozapine for the treatment-resistant schizophrenic. *Arch Gen Psychiatry* 45:789–796, 1988.

14. Bateman DN, Rawlins MC, Simpson JM: Extrapyramidal reactions to prochlorperazine and haloperidol in the United Kingdom. *Q J Med* 59:549–556, 1986.

15. Grimes D, Hassan MN, Preston DN: Adverse neurologic effects of metoclopramide. *Can Med Assoc J* 126:23–25, 1982.

16. Sethi KD, Patel B, Meador KJ: Metoclopramide-induced parkinsonism. *South Med J* 82:1581–1582, 1989.

17. Miller LG, Jankovic J: Metoclopramide-induced movement disorders. *Arch Intern Med* 149:2486–2492, 1989.

18. Bateman DN, Darling WM, Boys R, Rawlins MD: Extrapyramidal reactions to metoclopramide and prochlorperazine. *Q J Med* 71:307–311, 1989.

19. Steck H: Le syndrome extra-pyramidal et diencephalique au cours des traitements au forgactil au Serpasil. *Ann Med Psychol* 1/2:737–743, 1954.

20. Marsden CD, Tarsy D, Baldessarini RJ: Spontaneous and drug-induced movement disorders, in Benson DF, Blumer D (eds): *Psychiatric Aspects of Neurologic Disease.* New York: Grune & Stratton, 1975.

21. Indo T, Ando K: Metoclopramide induced parkinsonism: Clinical characteristics of ten cases. *Arch Neurol* 39:494–496, 1982.

22. Hershey LA, Gift T, Rivera-Calminlin L: Not Parkinson disease. *Lancet* 2:49, 1982.

23. Klawans HL, Bergen D, Bruyn GW: Prolonged drug-induced parkinsonism. *Cont Neurol* 35:368–377, 1973.

24. Yamamoto M, Ujike H, Ogawa N: Metoclopramide-induced parkinsonism. *Clin Neuropharmacol* 10:287–289, 1987.

25. Weiden PJ, Mann JJ, Hass G, et al: Clinical nonrecognition of neuroleptic-induced movement disorders: A cautionary study. *Am J Psychiatry* 144:1148–1153, 1987.

26. Hansen TE, Brown WL, Weigel RM, Casey DE: Underrecognition of tardive dyskinesia and drug-induced parkinsonism by psychiatric residents. *Gen Hosp Psychiatry* 14:340–344, 1992.

27. Albanese A, Colosimo C, Bentivoglio AR, Bergonzi P: Unsuspected, surreptitious drug-induced parkinsonism. *Neurology* 42:459, 1992.

28. Ehringer H, Hornykiewicz O: Verteilung von noradrenalin und dopamin (3-hydroxytyramin) im Gehirn des Menschen und ihr Verhalten bei Erkrankungen des extrapyramidalen Systems. *Klin Wochenschr* 38:1236–1260, 1960.

29. Crowley TJ, Hoehn MM, Rutledge CD, et al: Dopamine excretion and vulnerability to drug-induced parkinsonism. *Arch Gen Psychiatry* 35:97–104, 1978.

30. Korczyn AD, Goldberg GJ: Extrapyramidal effects of neuroleptics. *J Neurol Neurosurg Psychiatry* 39:866–869, 1976.

31. Moleman P, Janzen G, von Bargen BA, et al: Relationship between age and incidence of parkinsonism in psychiatric patients treated with haloperidol. *Am J Psychiatry* 143:232–234, 1986.

32. McClelland HA: Discussion on assessment of drug-induced extrapyramidal reactions. *Br J Clin Pharmacol* 3:401–403, 1976.

33. Kane JM, Smith JM: Tardive dyskinesia: Prevalence and risk factors, 1959–1979. *Arch Gen Psychiatry* 39:473–481, 1982.

34. Jus A, Pineau R, Lachance R, et al: Epidemiology of tardive dyskinesia. Part I. *Dis Nerv Syst* 37:210–214, 1976.

35. Glazer WM, Naftolin F, Moore DL, et al: The relationship of circulating estradiol to tardive dyskinesia in men and postmenopausal women. *Psychoneuroendocrinology* 8:429–434, 1983.

36. Moleman P, Schmitz PJM, Ladee GA: Extrapyramidal side effects and oral haloperidol: An analysis of explanatory patient and treatment characteristics. *J Clin Psychiatry* 43:492–496, 1982.

37. Kennedy PF, Hershon HI, McGuire RJ: Extrapyramidal disorders after prolonged phenothiazine therapy. *Br J Psychiatry* 118:509–518, 1971.

38. Crowley TJ, Rutledge CO, Hoehn MM, et al: Low urinary dopamine and prediction of phenothiazine induced parkinsonism: A preliminary report. *Am J Psychiatry* 133:703–706, 1976.

39. Metzer WS, Newton JEO, Steele RW, et al: HLA antigens in drug-induced parkinsonism. *Mov Disord* 4:121–128, 1989.

40. Gelay J, Deniker P: Drug-induced extrapyramidal syndromes, in Vinken PJ, Bruyn GW (eds): *Handbook of Clinical Neurology: Diseases of the Basal Ganglia.* Amsterdam: North-Holland, 1968, vol 6.

41. Duvoisin RC: Problems in the treatment of parkinsonism. *Adv Exp Med Biol* 90:131–155, 1977.

42. Goetz CG: Drug-induced parkinsonism and idiopathic Parkinson's disease. *Arch Neurol* 40:325–326, 1983.

43. Stephen PJ, Williamson J: Drug-induced parkinsonism in the elderly. *Lancet* 2:1082–1083, 1984.

44. Hardie RJ, Lees AJ: Neuroleptic-induced Parkinson's syndrome: Clinical features and results of treatment with levodopa. *J Neurol Neurosurg Psychiatry* 8:850–854, 1988.

45. Rajput AH, Rozdilsky B, Hornykiewicz O, Shannak K, et al: Reversible drug-induced parkinsonism: Clinicopathologic study of two cases. *Arch Neurol* 39:644–646, 1982.

46. Brooks DJ: Detection of preclinical Parkinson's disease with PET. *Neurology* 41(5, Suppl 2):24–27, 1991.

47. Jeste DV, Wyatt RJ: *Understanding and Treating Tardive Dyskinesia.* New York: Guilford Press, 1982.

48. Crane GE, Smeets RA: Tardive dyskinesia and drug therapy in geriatric patients. *Arch Gen Psychiatry* 30:314–343, 1974.

49. Woerner MG, Kane JM, Lieberman JA, et al: The prevalence of tardive dyskinesia. *J Clin Psychopharmacol* 11:34–42, 1991.

50. Saltz BL, Woerner MG, Kane JM, et al: Prospective study of tardive dyskinesia incidence in the elderly. *J Am Med Assoc* 266:2402–2406, 1991.

51. De Fraites EG, Davis KL, Berger PA: Coexisting tardive dyskinesia and parkinsonism: A case report. *Biol Psychiatry* 12:267–272, 1977.

52. Fann WE, Lake CR: On the co-existence of parkinsonism and tardive dyskinesia. *Dis Nerv Syst* 35:325–326, 1974.

53. Rao JM, Cowie VA, Mathew B: Tardive dyskinesia in neuroleptic medicated mentally handicapped subjects. *Acta Psychiatr Scand* 76:507–513, 1987.

54. Seeman P, Staiman A, Lee T, et al: The membrane action of tranquilizers in relation to neuroleptic-induced parkinsonism and tardive dyskinesia, in Forrest IS, Carr CJ, Usdin E (eds): *The Phenothiazines and Structurally Related Drugs.* New York: Raven Press, 1974.

55. Finch CE: Catecholamine metabolism in the brains of aging male mice. *Brain Res* 52:261–276, 1973.

56. Goetz CG, Weiner WJ, Nausieda PA, Klawans HL: Tardive dyskinesia: Pharmacology and clinical implications. *Clin Neuropharmacol* 5:3–22, 1983.

57. Parkes JD: Domperidone and Parkinson's disease. *Clin Neuropharmacol* 9:517–532, 1986.

58. Debontridder O: Dystonic reactions after domperidone. *Lancet* 2:1259, 1980.

59. Hornykiewicz O: Parkinsonism induced by dopaminergic antagonists. *Adv Neurol* 9:155–164, 1975.

60. Hausner RS: Amantadine-associated recurrence of psychosis. *Am J Psychiatry* 137:240–242, 1980.

61. Sandyk R, Pardeshi R: Pyridoxine improves drug-induced parkinsonism and psychosis in a schizophrenic patient. *Int J Neurosci* 52:225–232, 1990.

62. Carlsson A, Lindquist M, Magnusson T: 3,4-Dihydroxyphenylalanine and 6-hydroxytryptophan as reserpine antagonists. *Nature* 180:1200–1201, 1957.

63. Fahn S: Treatment of tardive dyskinesia: Use of dopamine-depleting agents. *Clin Neuropharmacol* 6:151–157, 1983.

64. Klawans HL, Tanner CM: The reversibility of permanent tardive dyskinesia. *Neurology* 33(Suppl 2):163, 1983.

65. Reches A, Burke RE, Kahn C, Fahn S: Tetrabenazine, an amine depleting agent, also blocks dopamine receptors in rat brain. *J Pharmacol Exp Ther* 225:515–521, 1983.

66. Jankovic J: Tetrabenazine in the treatment of hyperkinetic movement disorders. *Adv Neurol* 37:227–289, 1983.

67. Jankovic J, Orman J: Tetrabenazine therapy of dystonia, chorea, tics, and other dyskinesias. *Neurology* 38:391–394, 1988.

68. Rosenblum AM, Montgomery EB: Exacerbation of parkinsonism by methyldopa. *J Am Med Assoc* 244:2727–2728, 1980.

69. Gillman MA, Sandyk R: Parkinsonism inducing by methyldopa. *S Afr Med J* 65:194, 1984.

70. Fermaglich J, Chase TN: Methyldopa or methyldopahydrazine as levodopa synergists. *Lancet* 1:1261–1262, 1973.

71. Godfrain T, Towse G, Van Nueten JM: Cinnarizine: A selective calcium entry blocker. *Drugs Today* 18:27–42, 1982.

72. Holmes B, Brogden RN, Heel RC, et al: Flunarizine: A review of its pharmacodynamic and pharmacokinetic properties and therapeutic use. *Drugs* 27:6–44, 1984.

73. Micheli F, Pardal MF, Gatto M, et al: Flunarizine- and cinnarizine-induced extrapyramidal reactions. *Neurology* 37:881–884, 1987.

74. Micheli FE, Pardal MMF, Giannaula R, et al: Movement disorders and depression due to flunarizine and cinnarizine. *Mov Disord* 4:139–146, 1989.

75. Marti Masso JF, Obeso JA, Carrera N, Martinez-Lage JM: Aggravation of Parkinson's disease by cinnarize. *J Neurol Neurosurg Psychiatry* 50:804–805, 1987.

76. Fadda F, Gessa GL, Mosca E, Stefanini E: Different effects of the calcium antagonists nimodipine and flunarizine on dopamine metabolism in the rat brain. *J Neural Transm* 75:195–200, 1989.

77. De Vries DJ, Beart PM: Competitive inhibition of [^{3}H]spiperone binding to D-2 dopamine receptors in striatal homogenates by organic calcium-channel antagonists and polyvalent cations. *Eur J Pharmacol* 106:133–139, 1985.

78. Garcia-Ruiz PJ, de Yebenes JG, Jimenez-Jimenez FJ, Vazquez A, et al: Parkinsonism associated with calcium channel blockers: A prospective follow-up study. *Clin Neuropharmacol* 15:19–26, 1992.

79. Negrotti A, Calzetti S, Sasso E: Calcium-entry blockers-induced parkinsonism: Possible role of inherited susceptibility. *Neurotoxicology* 13:261–264, 1992.

80. Dick RS, Barold SS: Diltiazem-induced parkinsonism. *Am J Med* 87:95–96, 1989.

81. Pileblad E, Carlsson A: In vivo effects of the Ca^{++} antagonist nimodipine on dopamine metabolism in mouse brain. *J Neural Transm* 66:171–187, 1986.

82. LeMaire JF, Autret A, Biziere K, et al: Amiodarone neuropathy: Further arguments for human drug-induced neurolipidosis. *Eur Neurol* 21:65–68, 1982.

83. Palakurthy PR, Iyer V, Meckler RJ: Unusual neurotoxicity associated with amiodarone therapy. *Arch Intern Med* 147:881–884, 1987.

84. Werner EG, Olanow CW: Parkinsonism and amiodarone therapy. *Ann Neurol* 25:630–632, 1989.

85. Fox JH, Bennett DA, Goetz CG, et al: Induction of parkinsonism by intraventricular bethanechol in a patient with Alzheimer's disease. *Neurology* 39:1265, 1989.

86. Iwasaki Y, Wakata N, Kinoshita M: Parkinsonism induced by pyridostigmine. *Acta Neurol Scand* 78:236, 1988.

87. Kane J, Rifkin A, Quitkin F, Klein D: Extrapyramidal side effects with lithium treatment. *Am J Psychiatry* 135:851–853, 1978.

88. Tyrer P, Alexander MS, Regan A, Lee I: An extrapyramidal syndrome after lithium therapy. *Br J Psychiatry* 136:191–194, 1980.

89. Lutz EG: Acute lithium-induced parkinsonism precipitated by liquid protein diet. *J Med Soc NJ* 75:165–166, 1978.

90. Suranyi-Cadotte BE, Nestoros JN, Nair NPV, et al: Parkinsonism induced by high doses of diazepam. *Biol Psychiatry* 20:451–460, 1985.

91. Bouchard RH, Pourcher E, Vincent P: Fluoxetine and extrapyramidal side effects (letter). *Am J Psychiatry* 146:1352–1353, 1989.

92. Tate JL: Extrapyramidal symptoms in a patient taking haloperidol and fluoxetine (letter). *Am J Psychiatry* 146:399–340, 1989.

93. Gernaat HBPE, Van de Woude J, Touw DJ: Fluoxetine and parkinsonism in patients taking carbamazepine (letter). *Am J Psychiatry* 148:1604–1605, 1991.

94. Teusink JP, Alexopoulos GS, Shamoian CA: Parkinsonian side effects induced by a monoamine oxidase inhibitor. *Am J Psychiatry* 141:118–119, 1984.

95. Gjerris F: Transitory procaine-induced parkinsonism. *J Neurol Neurosurg Psychiatry* 34:20–22, 1971.

96. Lieberman AN, Goldstein M: Reversible parkinsonism related to meperidine. *N Engl J Med* 8:509, 1985.

97. Fisher JF, Dewald J: Parkinsonism associated with intraventricular amphotericin B. *J Antimicrob Ther* 12:97–99, 1983.

98. Mintz U, Liberman UA, Vries A: Parkinsonism syndrome due to cephaloridine. *J Am Med Assoc* 216:1200, 1971.

99. Bergevin PR, Patwardhan VC, Weissman J, et al: Neurotoxicity of 5-fluorouracil. *Lancet* i:410, 1975.

100. Boranic M, Raci F: A parkinson-like syndrome as side effect of chemo-therapy with vincristine and Adriamycin in a child with acute leukaemia. *Biomedicine* 31:124–125, 1979.

Chapter 24

OTHER DEGENERATIVE SYNDROMES THAT CAUSE PARKINSONISM

WOLFGANG H. OERTEL and J. C. MÖLLER

DISINHIBITION-DEMENTIA-PARKINSONISM-
  AMYOTROPHY COMPLEX (DDPAC)
HALLERVORDEN-SPATZ DISEASE (HSD)
HEMIPARKINSON-HEMIATROPHY SYNDROME (HPHA)
DIFFUSE LEWY BODY DISEASE (DLBD)
X-LINKED DYSTONIA-PARKINSONISM SYNDROME
  (LUBAG)
NEUROACANTHOCYTOSIS
PALLIDAL, PALLIDONIGRAL, AND
  PALLIDOLUYSIONIGRAL DEGENERATIONS
FAMILIAL L-DOPA-RESPONSIVE PARKINSONIAN-
  PYRAMIDAL SYNDROME
RETT SYNDROME

Disinhibition-Dementia-Parkinsonism-Amyotrophy Complex (DDPAC)

CLINICAL DEFINITION

Several descriptions of sporadic or familial syndromes with the common occurrence of dementia, parkinsonism, and amyotrophy have been published. Probably the best known example is the dementia-parkinsonism amyotrophic lateral sclerosis (ALS) complex of Guam.[1,2] There is an ongoing discussion about the classification of this kind of neurodegenerative disorder, thereby reflecting the problem of defining a new clinical and pathological entity, in contrast to an overlap of common neurodegenerative diseases. Other familial parkinsonism-dementia syndromes are, for example, the rapidly progressive autosomal-dominant parkinsonism and dementia with pallidopontonigral degeneration,[3] the dominantly inherited dementia and parkinsonism with non-Alzheimer amyloid plaques[4] or the syndrome described by Mata et al.[5] Because of their inhereditability, they will be discussed elsewhere (see Chap. 26). This chapter provides details on an additional parkinsonism-dementia syndrome, the DDPAC.[6] Its clinical definition resembles the above mentioned syndromes. However, this disorder is defined by its presentation with disinhibition, the subsequent development of varying degrees of frontal lobe dementia, parkinsonism, and amyotrophy, and its familial aggregation.

EPIDEMIOLOGY

Until now only one family with 33 members was studied; therefore, no data regarding the incidence or the prevalence are available.

NEUROGENETICS

Linkage analyses were performed, and lod scores consistent with linkage were obtained for microsatellite polymorphisms associated with the HOX2B (Lod_{max}3.03 with $\Theta_{Lodmax} = 0$) and GP3A (Lod_{max}3.28 with $\Theta_{Lodmax} = 0$) loci on chromosome 17q21-23.[6] Furthermore, the pedigree of the examined family shows that 10 of 21 affected parents had symptoms by the age of 50. This is compatible with a highly penetrant, autosomal-dominant trait.

PATHOGENESIS

Nothing is known about the underlying etiopathogenesis.

NEUROPATHOLOGY

Six brains and two spinal cords from affected individuals were analyzed postmortem.[6] Macroscopically, moderate-to-severe frontal and temporal lobe atrophy was seen. Microscopically, the number of the pigmented, as well as the non-pigmented, cell populations of the substantia nigra were markedly reduced. Nerve cell loss and astrocytosis in the amygdala were severe. The superficial neocortical laminae showed modest neuronal attrition and patchy astrocytosis. Furthermore, there was a spongy rarefaction of the neuropil confined to the inner border of the plexiform layer and the second cortical layer with reduction in the number of small pyramidal cells. Virtually no large multipolar nerve cells remained in the second layer of the entorhinal cortex. Pyramidal cell loss was substantial in the broad third layer. No Lewy bodies, neurofibrillary tangles, or senile plaques were found. Anterior horn cell loss and astrocytosis were present in both spinal cords examined.

CLINICAL MANIFESTATIONS

The clinical manifestations consist of the occurrence of psychiatric symptoms at a mean age at 45 years, before onset of subsequently developing neurological manifestations and neuropsychological alterations. The full clinical picture developed over 5–10 years and average duration was 13 years.[6]

CENTRAL NERVOUS SYSTEM (CNS) MANIFESTATIONS

Normally, a personality change heralded the onset of the neurological symptoms.[6] Neuropsychological alterations were composed of memory loss, anomia, poor general knowledge, and poor constructions. Inappropriate behavior was seen during testing and, ultimately, the neurobehavioral pattern was consistent with frontal lobe dementia. Interestingly, all patients had at least two of the symptoms of the Klüver-Bucy syndrome: prominent oral tendencies, emotional blunting, a tendency to react to environmental stimuli as soon as they are noticed, hypersexuality, and altered dietary habits. These clinical signs have prompted the term disinhibition. Six of seven examined patients showed frontal lobe release signs. Rigidity and bradykinesia were observed in all affected and examined family members; only one had no postural instability. Muscle wasting, weakness, ankle clonus, and fasciculations developed in the late stages in one patient; two others showed hyperreflexia, but in only one of these patients were Babinski signs observed.

NEUROLOGICAL CARDINAL SYMPTOMS

The designation of the disorder reflects the cardinal symptoms: frontal lobe dementia, parkinsonism, and amyotrophy.

PSYCHIATRIC SYMPTOMS

Twelve of thirteen affected persons were analyzed regarding their psychiatric symptoms. The personality change heralded the onset of the neurological manifestation. Prodromal symptoms consisted of the following: alcohol abuse in five, hypersexuality in four, and hyperreligiosity in three persons. There was a progression from "childish" disinhibited behavior to a withdrawn state with emotional blunting in all. A typical feature appears to be a craving to eat sweets. Aggressive behavior was noticed in two patients; depression and a stereotyped obsessive routine were found in three persons.

DIAGNOSIS/DIFFERENTIAL DIAGNOSIS

It was proposed[6] that at least two of the following four criteria were required for considering a person affected: (1) personality change, including aggression; change in sexual habits; alcohol abuse; hyperreligiosity; disinhibited "childish" egocentric behavior; apathetic and stereotyped behavior; emotional blunting; and impairment of judgment, including shoplifting, irritability, callousness, or excessive eating; (2) profound memory loss; (3) parkinsonism progressing to akinetic mutism; and (4) clinical evidence of motor neuron disease. With neurogenetic methods it would be possible to prove the suspected diagnosis; this may be valid also for presymptomatic diagnosis of children of affected families.

All other sporadic and familial parkinsonism-dementia syndromes must be considered as possible differential diagnoses. The dementia-parkinsonism-ALS complex of Guam or related disorders might present with a similar combination of clinical features. Pick's disease exhibits a high degree of similarity to the beginning of DDPAC, particularly regarding the neuropsychological and psychiatric findings. Also, Alzheimer's disease (AD) should be considered in the differential diagnosis.

BIOCHEMICAL CRITERIA

No biochemical criteria exist.

NEUROIMAGING

Computed tomography (CT) and magnetic resonance imaging (MRI) in five cases showed moderate-to-severe atrophy and ventricular dilatation with prominent cortical sulci. Bilateral hypoactivity in the frontal lobes was found in three cases, using regional cerebral blood flow measurements or fluorodeoxyglucose positron emission tomography (PET).

THERAPY

A specific therapy is not known. The patients showed no significant response to L-dopa. Data about other drug therapies are not available at present. Depending on the individual case, L-dopa or other antiparkinsonian agents should be tried. Psychiatric treatment may be necessary.

Hallervorden-Spatz Disease (HSD)

CLINICAL DEFINITION

Hallervorden and Spatz reported in 1922 for the first time a sibship affected by a new disease entity characterized by impairment of gait resulting from rigidity of legs and feet deformity and mental deterioration with juvenile onset.[7] The neuropathological picture consisted of a rusty-brown discoloration of globus pallidus and pars reticulata of substantia nigra and the occurrence of so-called spheroids. There is still an ongoing discussion about the nosological classification of this disease. According to Seitelberger,[8] HSD can be classified among the neuroaxonal dystrophies. Although spheroid formation is reminiscent of alterations in infantile neuroaxonal dystrophy, there is no proven clinical or genetic relationship between these two groups of patients.[9] Furthermore, it was proposed to distinguish between HSD and Hallervorden-Spatz syndrome (HSS), considering the multitude of conditions presenting with iron accumulation in basal ganglia and regarding the high degree of variation in the clinical picture of cases reported as HSD.[10] Depending on age of onset, Gross et al. classified HSD into three categories: late-infantile, juvenile, and adult type.[11]

EPIDEMIOLOGY

The disease is very rare. No sufficient epidemiological data are available.

NEUROGENETICS

The mode of inheritance appears to be autosomal-recessive. This is consistent with the observations made in familial cases and with the occurrence of some apparently sporadic cases.[9] Nothing is known about a gene locus associated with any form of HSD.

PATHOGENESIS

The pathogenesis of HSD remains unclear. Two cases of HSD were reported with decreased activity of cysteine dioxygenase in globus pallidus, suggesting a role of lipid peroxidation in the etiology of HSD.[12] Apart from this, other investigators have proposed a possible deficiency of fatty acid membrane components and an abnormality of cyclic guanosine monophosphate (cGMP) metabolism in the pathogenesis of HSD. At present, iron accumulation in pallidal structures is the most robust neuropathological finding. A disturbance of iron metabolism possibly facilitates lipid peroxidation or modulates neurotransmitter activities.[9]

NEUROPATHOLOGY

Macroscopically, the most striking neuropathological feature is the rust-brown pigmentation of globus pallidus and pars reticulata of substantia nigra. On the microscopic level, iron granules were found in neurons, microglial cells, and astrocytes. Also, some iron was localized extracellularly. Furthermore, "mulberry" concretions were observed in tissue and regarded as so-called pseudocalcium. A further prominent finding of the disease is a widely distributed distal axonal swelling in affected structures of brain. These swellings may be surrounded by glial cells and may contain pigment granules, particularly when located in globus pallidus or pars reticulata of substantia nigra. Apart from these regions, they are especially observed in the subthalamic nucleus of Luys. These structures have become known as spheroid bodies.[7,9] These spheroids resemble those found in neuroaxonal dystrophy,[8] but in the latter the spheroids in the pallidum store fatty material and not pigments. These neuropathological alterations are accompanied by some loss of neurons and of myelinated fibers, as well as by gliosis.

CLINICAL MANIFESTATIONS

Apart from CNS manifestations, foot deformities were frequently observed and skin pigmentation was noted in some cases.[10] Moreover, tapetoretinal degeneration was found in 10 of 42 patients.[13] As mentioned below, abnormal cytosomes in circulating lymphocytes and sea-blue histiocytes in the bone marrow have been reported.

CNS MANIFESTATIONS

Dooling et al.[14] examined 42 patients who fulfilled both clinical and neuropathological criteria for HSD. Onset of disease occurred in 24 patients before age of 10 years, and 39 patients were ill before age 22. The mean duration of disease was 11 years. Gait difficulty and postural impairment were noted as initial symptoms in 37 patients. This may be a result of spasticity secondary to involvement of corticospinal tracts, whereas symptoms of extrapyramidal dysfunction may be delayed by one to several years. However, the usual course included progression of rigidity and presence of postural abnormalities. Other basal ganglia signs were observed, including dystonia in 23 patients, choreoathethosis in 19 patients, and tremor without any distinctive character in 15 patients. Additionally, mental impairment was common, and in 9 of 42 patients, seizures occurred. Generally, there was a wide spectrum of variation in the clinical manifestations of HSD. It is noteworthy that one case of late onset HSD was reported, presenting as familial parkinsonism. The patient died at the age of 68.[15]

NEUROLOGICAL CARDINAL SYMPTOMS

The neurological cardinal symptoms consist of an extrapyramidal movement disorder, mainly presenting with rigidity and dystonia, intellectual impairment, and pyramidal tract signs, with onset mostly after early childhood.

PSYCHIATRIC SYMPTOMS

Apart from mental deterioration, psychiatric symptoms do not accompany this disorder.

DIAGNOSIS/DIFFERENTIAL DIAGNOSIS

To establish a diagnosis of HSD, so-called obligatory features and at least two of the corroborative symptoms should be present.[9] The obligatory features are (1) onset during the first 2 decades of life, (2) a progressive course and (3) evidence of extrapyramidal dysfunction. The corroborative symptoms include (1) pyramidal tract signs, (2) progressive mental deterioration, (3) hypodensities in basal ganglia on MRI, (4) occurrence of seizures, (5) opthalmological symptoms in the form of retinitis pigmentosa or optic atrophy, (6) positive family history and (7) abnormal cytosomes in circulating lymphocytes and sea-blue histiocytes in bone marrow. Differential diagnostic considerations include Wilson's disease, Huntington's disease, neuroacanthocytosis, and neurometabolic disorders, particularly neuronal ceroid-lipofuscinosis. Finally, definite diagnosis depends on postmortem analysis. The combination of neurological signs and appropriate MRI findings allows the probable diagnosis of HSD in living patients.[16]

BIOCHEMICAL CRITERIA

Laboratory investigations do not reveal any distinctive abnormalities. Hematologic studies have shown vacuolated circulating lymphocytes containing abnormal cytosomes and the occurrence of sea-blue histiocytes in bone marrow in some patients.[17]

NEUROIMAGING

CT in patients with HSD has been reported to show atrophy and low-density lesions in basal ganglia.[18] In contrast, one case was described with high-density lesions in basal ganglia on CT.[19] MRI, using a high field-strength unit (1.5 Tesla) showed decreased signal intensity in globus pallidus and pars reticulata of substantia nigra in T_2-weighted images, which is compatible with heavy metal (iron) deposits, and a small area of hyperintensity in the internal segment of pallidum, constituting the so-called "eye of the tiger" sign.[20,21] In addition, there have been reports of delayed iron clearance over the basal ganglia after an injection of ^{59}Fe.[22]

THERAPY

There is no specific therapy for HSD. However, symptomatic management, such as that using L-dopa and dopamine agonists, may be beneficial to patients.[9] With the occurrence of epileptic seizures, antiepileptic therapy is necessary.

Hemiparkinson-Hemiatrophy Syndrome (HPHA)

CLINICAL DEFINITION

The HPHA syndrome is defined by the occurrence of a body hemiatrophy with features of a highly asymmetric, L-dopa-responsive parkinsonism more prominent on the side of the hemiatrophy.[23,24] Other characteristics are an early age of onset, ipsilateral premedication dystonia, and a slowly progressive course. An association with contralateral brain atrophy was also shown.[25]

EPIDEMIOLOGY

There are no epidemiological data available.

NEUROGENETICS

Investigations regarding a possible role of genetic factors have not been performed.

PATHOGENESIS

Up to the present time, no brains were subjected to a postmortem examination. It has been reported that lesions of the postcentral gyrus before age 3 are associated with a relative smallness of the contralateral parts of the body.[26] Therefore, it was suggested that the occurrence of parkinsonism in these patients is related to an accompanying subcortical lesion.[23] In support of this point of view, Giladi et al. presented neuroradiological evidence of a contralateral brain hemiatrophy in 64 percent of their patients.[25] In patients with HPHA, a history of birth injury was frequently observed,[24] but history of brain insult was lacking. Therefore, diagnosis of a "primary" brain hemiatrophy[27] as a result of perinatal brain damage was suggested. Interestingly, there is an association between perinatal asphyxia, brain hemiatrophy, and delayed onset hemidystonia.[28] Correspondingly, HPHA could represent an example of a movement disorder with a delayed onset as a consequence of neonatal brain injury.[25] Finally, investigations using PET led to the hypothesis that nigral and extranigral dysfunction causes HPHA.[29,30]

NEUROPATHOLOGY

No postmortem analysis has been performed.

CLINICAL MANIFESTATIONS

In addition to the CNS manifestations, patients suffer from a body hemiatrophy with small and narrow extremities on one side. There is a wide variation in the degree of hemiatrophy: in some patients the face, arm, and a leg were affected, whereas in other patients only the hand seemed to be affected. The most likely part of the hand to demonstrate hemiatrophy was the thumb. It has to be kept in mind that there is "normal" asymmetry of the two halves of the human body. The term "normal" asymmetry can be applied only to differences in opposite limb length that are not visually apparent in the absence of measurements.[31] Interestingly, one patient[25] showed no body hemiatrophy, but an enlarged lateral ventricle was the sign of brain hemiatrophy.

CNS MANIFESTATIONS

With respect to the CNS manifestations, Buchman et al.[24] reported that the mean age of onset of parkinsonism was 43.7 years. The course of the disease is slowly progressive, i.e., the mean duration of disease until initiation of L-dopa therapy was 14.2 years. In contrast, in patients suffering from idiopathic PD, L-dopa treatment was started after 4.1 years.[24] Furthermore, no progression to Hoehn and Yahr stage IV of V (H&Y) was observed. Interestingly, 8 of 15 patients remained asymmetric after the development of bilateral disease. Giladi et al. found a more variable clinical course; for instance, one patient progressed from H and Y stage I to IV when "off" within 2.5 years.[25] Ipsilateral dystonic movements, sometimes presenting as the first symptom, often occur early in the course of the disease before exposure to L-dopa. Ten of 15 patients showed tremor as their initial symptom. Apart from the parkinsonian features, pyramidal tract dysfunction ipsilateral to the side of HPHA was present in 8 of 15 patients.[24]

NEUROLOGICAL CARDINAL SYMPTOMS

The neurological cardinal symptoms include early age of onset of unilateral parkinsonism, as well as ipsilateral dystonia occurring prior to L-dopa therapy.

PSYCHIATRIC SYMPTOMS

Psychiatric symptoms are not a major feature of this syndrome.

DIAGNOSIS/DIFFERENTIAL DIAGNOSIS

In the differential diagnosis a benign, early-onset parkinsonism has to be considered. Common features are the early age of onset and the unilateral symptoms with mild progression. The main differences are the evidence of ipsilateral hemiatrophy and the prominence of early dystonia by HPHA patients. Therefore, the diagnosis depends on a thorough physical examination. Neuroradiological methods might be helpful: 64 percent of the patients examined by Giladi et al. showed a brain asymmetry on CT or MRI. Furthermore, ^{18}F-fluorodeoxyglucose and PET may be helpful in differentiating HPHA from typical asymmetric Parkinson's disease (PD). Moreover, early on the differential diagnosis may include cortical-basal ganglionic degeneration, because HPHA may mimic its early stage.[32]

BIOCHEMICAL CRITERIA

Because of involvement of the nigrostriatal dopaminergic system, the level of homovanillic acid in the cerebrospinal fluid can be reduced.[25]

NEUROIMAGING

CT and MRI showed contralateral brain asymmetry in 64 percent of the investigated patients.[25] However, Buchman et al. found in 11 of 12 patients no evidence of cerebral hemiatrophy (cortical or ventricular asymmetry).[24] Studies using ^{18}F-fluorodeoxyglucose and PET showed a focal hypometabolism in the basal ganglia and the medial frontal cortex of the contralateral side, whereas ^{18}F-fluorodopa and PET revealed a reduction in the striatal ^{18}F-fluorodopa uptake. Hence the former examination might be useful to distinguish HPHA from typical unilateral idiopathic PD.[29,30] Recently, a case of HPHA was reported with an area of altered MRI signal intensity in the mesencephalon.[33]

THERAPY

Of the investigated patients, seven of nine showed a good response to L-dopa therapy, either alone or in combination with anticholinergics or amantadine, whereas the latter were mainly ineffective when given alone. Of eight patients, seven responded well to the combination of amantadine and anticholinergics.[24] Other investigators found a good response to L-dopa treatment in 7 of 11 patients.[25]

Diffuse Lewy Body Disease (DLBD)

CLINICAL DEFINITION

There is still an ongoing discussion of whether DLBD is a variant form of PD or a disease entity. If the latter is correct, then DLBD is a chronic progressive neuropsychiatric disorder distinguished by parkinsonian symptoms, mostly of presenile or senile onset, with or without dementia. However, progressive dementia might be the first and predominant symptom. With respect to the neuropathological findings two distinct forms of DLBD are defined: (1) the pure form presenting with Lewy bodies in cortical and subcortical structures and (2) the common form characterized by Lewy bodies accompanied by senile plaques and neurofibrillary tangles.[34-36] In contrast, some authors, for example, Quinn, emphasize the overlap between the pathologies of PD and AD without the need to invent new terms or new diseases, and they regard DLBD as a variant of PD.[37]

EPIDEMIOLOGY

More than 90 autopsy cases were reported until 1989 and were reviewed by Kosaka.[36] The disorder occurred in Japan, in Europe, and in American countries. Fifteen cases were observed during a single year in one health district in the UK, indicating that this disease is not an extremely rare condition.[38]

NEUROGENETICS

No familial predisposition for DLBD has so far been reported. Because of the close relationship with PD, the same considerations regarding possible neurogenetic implications might hold true for both conditions.

PATHOGENESIS

It has been proposed that DLBD might represent the extended form of PD, suggesting that the brain stem type of DLBD is identical to idiopathic PD.[36] Despite the uncertainty concerning the classification of DLBD as a disease entity, the common pathological hallmark of PD and DLBD, the so-called Lewy body, suggests a closely related pathogenesis of these two conditions.

NEUROPATHOLOGY

Lewy bodies are characteristic of both PD and DLBD.[34,39] Lewy bodies are rounded eosinophilic inclusion bodies (containing ubiquitin as a main component) that are found within brain stem nuclei in PD. In PD they are mainly seen in the surviving neurons of the substantia nigra (SN). In contrast, in DLBD they are widely spread throughout the cerebral cortex and are seen in SN and other subcortical regions. The cortical Lewy bodies are usually found in small neurons of the deeper layers of temporal, frontal, and insular cortex, but all lobes are more or less affected. Interestingly, cortical Lewy bodies can also be detected in PD,[40] yet to a lesser degree. Therefore, it was suggested that the presence of more than five cortical Lewy bodies in each visual field at a magnification of $100\times$ is necessary for the diagnosis of DLBD.[36] Cortical atrophy is not prominent in DLBD. Additionally, in the common form of DLBD senile plaques and neurofibrillary tangles of the AD type, partly restricted to the hippocampus and parahippocampal gyrus, are present widely.

CLINICAL MANIFESTATIONS

Manifestations apart from CNS neurological and psychiatric signs and symptoms are not known.

CNS MANIFESTATIONS

The CNS manifestations of DLBD resemble those of PD. Kosaka et al.[36] pointed out that there might be dependence of the presenting symptom on the form of DLBD: in the common form of DLBD, 57 percent of patients presented initially with memory disturbance, whereas in the pure form of DLBD 78 percent of patients showed parkinsonism as their initial symptom. It is also noteworthy that about one-fifth of cases of common form had no parkinsonism.[41] Moreover, in Japan an early mean age of onset of 33 years was observed in pure form.[36] However, juvenile cases of pure form are only rarely reported in European or American countries. With respect to cognitive impairment, memory disturbance is usually the most apparent symptom. Detailed neuropsychological assessment revealed other cortical deficits, including dysphasia, dyscalculia, and visuospatial, constructional, and ideomotor dyspraxia.[38] Additionally, marked cognitive fluctuation at some point during illness was found. Also, impairment of both vertical and horizontal gaze has been reported as a prominent feature of DLBD in rare cases.[42] All of these statements stem from retrospective analyses of clinical data.

NEUROLOGICAL CARDINAL SYMPTOMS

Generally, DLBD may present within the range of parkinsonism with subsequent dementia or dementia with subsequent parkinsonian features.

PSYCHIATRIC SYMPTOMS

A psychotic state was found to be the presenting symptom in approximately 20 percent of patients.[36] Byrne et al. observed in 53 percent of patients the occurrence of psychiatric changes, mainly depression, auditory and visual hallucinations, and paranoid ideation.[38]

DIAGNOSIS/DIFFERENTIAL DIAGNOSIS

The most important differential diagnosis is between PD and DLBD. DLBD shows an earlier mean age of onset than PD, but the two diseases are similar with respect to both the male to female ratio and the mean disease duration. Psychiatric alterations or cognitive impairment were more frequently reported in DLBD (100 percent) than in PD (65 percent). Rest tremor was specifically mentioned in 29 percent of DLBD versus 56 percent of PD; meanwhile, bradykinesia was less common in PD (56 percent versus 86 percent in DLBD). Considering DLBD patients presenting first with parkinsonism, there were only small differences between DLBD and PD with respect to the frequency of cognitive or psychiatric changes, bradykinesia, rest tremor, and age of onset.[43] These slight differences do not allow a reliable distinctive diagnosis. If dementia develops first, then it is likely DLBD. In this case, other causes of dementia, especially AD in combination with PD, have to be strongly considered. However, currently there is no reliable way to distinguish DLBD from AD with PD, except perhaps by brain biopsy,[44] and the correct diagnosis has to be confirmed by postmortem analysis.

BIOCHEMICAL CRITERIA

There are no known biochemical criteria.

NEUROIMAGING

There are, to our knowledge, no typical neuroradiological findings in DLBD.

THERAPY

The parkinsonian features are reported to benefit from L-dopa in a substantial proportion of patients.[38,41]

X-Linked Dystonia-Parkinsonism Syndrome (Lubag)

CLINICAL DEFINITION

Lubag is an x-linked recessive form of movement disorder, prevalent among Filipino men born on Panay island (see also Chap. 33). This entity was first reported by Lee et al.[45] Onset occurs at 30–45 years of age with focal dystonia, subsequently generalizing within approximately 6 years. Parkinsonism may be the only manifestation of this disorder in late-onset cases, or it develops frequently after the onset of dystonia.[46]

EPIDEMIOLOGY

Lubag occurs endemically in the Philippines. In the province of Capiz on Panay island, the frequency of dystonia is approximately 1/4000 males.[47] Presumably, the disease originated from a common ancestor on this island, suggesting a single gene mutation. The neuropathological similarity between a patient with lubag and a non-Filipino patient with dystonia suggests that this mutation may not be restricted to the Filipino population.[48]

NEUROGENETICS

An X-linked recessive mode of inheritance was proposed. Linkage was established between the phenotype lubag and DNA markers that span the pericentromeric region Xp11.22–Xq21.3, defining an interval of about 20 centimorgans as the most likely site of the disease locus, called XDPD (X-linked dystonia-parkinsonism).[49] This finding was confirmed by other authors.[50] Recently, haplotype association analysis has suggested that the gene responsible for lubag is located within the Xq13 region.[51] However, it should be pointed out that it is also possible for women to be affected.[52] This led to the hypothesis that lubag may be a codominant disorder.

PATHOGENESIS

The gene responsible for lubag is still not identified. The pathogenesis of this disease is at present unknown.

NEUROPATHOLOGY

A subtle astrocytosis in a mosaic pattern was found in the caudate and putamen. The lateral part of the putamen was the most severely gliotic. Gliotic areas also exhibited neuronal loss, whereby no part of the striatum appeared to be spared. However, the gliosis and the neuronal loss were less extensive in the caudate nucleus. These observations were made in a single case,[48] but they are in agreement with the neuropathological findings in two other patients with dystonia, suggesting that this might be the neuropathology of lubag.

CLINICAL MANIFESTATIONS

There are no other clinical manifestations beyond the CNS signs and symptoms.

CNS MANIFESTATIONS

Forty-two patients were assessed and clinically investigated.[46] The mean age of onset of dystonia was 35+/−6 years. Initial symptoms in 12 percent involved the head, in

29 percent the axial musculature, in 23 percent the upper extremities, and in 36 percent the lower extremities. Other initial symptoms included tremor of unknown etiology or paresthesias. Focal dystonia progressed to either multifocal or generalized involvement in all cases. The mean duration of illness until generalization occurred was approximately 5 years. The most commonly observed symptoms were an abnormal gait (mostly from leg dystonia), oromandibular dystonia, blepharospasm, and neck and truncal dystonia. As a complication, aspiration pneumonia caused by associated dysphagia occurred in some cases. A case of a Filipino man who presented in severe respiratory distress as a result of adductor laryngeal breathing "dystonia" was reported.[53] Thirty-six percent of patients displayed one or more concurrent parkinsonian features, whereby the age of onset of patients with parkinsonian symptoms was signicantly higher, compared to that of those with pure dystonia. Additionally, it was postulated that an early report of sex-linked dystonia parkinsonism in a Filipino kindred described the same syndrome with parkinsonism as the predominant symptom.[54] Frequent reports of tremor as an initial symptom have occurred; therefore, it is conceivable that parkinsonian features may precede the onset of dystonia. In conclusion, lubag has to be considered as one nosological entity that may present with parkinsonian symptoms but always in association with adult-onset progressive dystonia.

NEUROLOGICAL CARDINAL SYMPTOMS

The neurological cardinal symptoms are focal, multifocal, or generalized dystonia, as well as parkinsonism.

PSYCHIATRIC SYMPTOMS

Primary psychiatric symptoms have not been reported.

DIAGNOSIS/DIFFERENTIAL DIAGNOSIS

This syndrome can be diagnosed by its typical clinical features. In the differential diagnosis, any of the dystonias associated with parkinsonism should be considered; for example, Wilson's disease, HSD, neuroacanthocytosis, and dopa-responsive dystonia. Significant differences between the latter and lubag are the age of onset, the sex predominance, and the distinct response to L-dopa therapy. In the future, diagnosis of lubag will likely be made by the detection of elements of the consensus haplotype, using a neurogenetic approach.[51]

BIOCHEMICAL CRITERIA

With the exception of an elevated manganese value obtained in the serum of affected Filipino men, laboratory studies showed no abnormalities.[45]

NEUROIMAGING

CT may reveal mild cerebral atrophy. Using ^{18}F-fluorodeoxyglucose and PET, a selective reduction of striatal glucose metabolism was determined, whereas the ^{18}F-fluorodopa uptake was found to be in the normal range.[55]

THERAPY

Some patients were treated with trihexyphenidyl, L-dopa, lorazepam, diazepam, or diphenhydramine, either alone or in combination; however, the course of the disease was not reported to be affected by any medication regimen.[46]

Neuroacanthocytosis

CLINICAL DEFINITION

Acanthocytes are erythrocytes with changed morphology bearing spicules of variable length and breadth.[56] They occur in association with three different neurological syndromes. First, they are observed in abetalipoproteinemia, the so-called Bassen-Kornzweig syndrome[57] and in familial hypobetalipoproteinemia.[58] Second, they are detectable in choreoacanthocytosis, also known as neuroacanthocytosis.[59–62] Third, the McLeod syndrome features a further entity with the occurrence of acanthocytes and neurological symptoms.[63,64] Moreover, there are some other conditions in which a sporadic association with acanthocytes has been described, that is, HSD and mitochondrial encephalomyopathies.[65] Here, the focus will be on neuroacanthocytosis. This is a disorder characterized by chorea, oromandibular dyskinesias, dementia, seizures, and peripheral neuropathy (see also Chap. 38). Additionally, parkinsonism may occur either with chorea or as a subsequent feature when the hyperkinetic movement disorder subsides.[66,67] In contrast to the Bassen-Kornzweig syndrome and to the familial hypobetalipoproteinemia, decreased serum lipid levels are not found in neuroacanthocytosis. Because of this and its distinct neurological manifestations, it represents an independent entity manifested primarily as a movement disorder.

EPIDEMIOLOGY

Sufficient epidemiological data are not available.

NEUROGENETICS

The pattern of inheritance remains unclear. There is evidence of autosomal-recessive inheritance, because parenteral consanguinity could be traced in some familial cases, but the occurrence of cases of acanthocytosis associated with neurological deficits in two consecutive generations suggests a possibly dominant transmission.[65]

PATHOGENESIS

The etiology of this syndrome is not known. It is believed that the underlying mechanism consists of a membrane abnormality that gives the acanthocyte its striking appearance. In the absence of any major differences in lipid constitution, changes in membrane fluidity or conformational defects of the membrane proteins are conceivable.[65] The suggested occurrence of the clinical syndrome of neuroacanthocytosis without acanthocytes may indicate that the basic defect can be variably expressed in different tissues and may cause neurological abnormalities alone.[68]

NEUROPATHOLOGY

Macroscopically the brains showed enlargement of the ventricles, particularly of the frontal horns. Caudate nucleus and putamen were the most severely affected brain areas showing atrophy, neuronal loss, and gliosis. Depletion of small- and medium-sized striatal neurons was most apparent. Involvement of globus pallidus was also present, and in some cases thalamus and the anterior horns of spinal cord showed neuronal loss and mild gliosis.[69] The SN of three patients with neuroacanthocytosis was investigated in more detail[70]: In neuroacanthocytosis with parkinsonism a reduced neuronal density (particularly in the ventrolateral region) of SN was determined, whereas in one patient with neuroacanthocytosis but without parkinsonian features the number of neurons was at the lower limit of the control range.

CLINICAL MANIFESTATIONS

The salient clinical features are mainly characterized by the neurological symptoms.

CNS MANIFESTATIONS

The mean age of onset was 32 years, but it ranged from 8 to 62 years. The most striking symptoms were involuntary movements affecting the orofacial region and the limbs presenting as orofacial dyskinesias and limb chorea.[71] The former can cause tongue and lip biting and interferes very often with speech and swallowing. Accordingly, involuntary vocalizations were frequently observed. In some cases, the predominant manifestation was dystonia, rather than chorea, and tics were noticed. Additionally, hypo- or areflexia was repeatedly found. In many cases muscle wasting occurred, and an axonal neuropathy was demonstrated.[72] Moreover, one-third of patients suffered from seizures and in more than one-half of the cases cognitive impairment, psychiatric features and personality change were seen.[65,73] Spitz et al. reported two cases of neuroacanthocytosis presenting as tics, but these were subsequently and progressively replaced or masked by progressive parkinsonism.[67] Furthermore, Yamamoto et al.[66] and Hardie et al.[73] described the occurrence of akinetic-rigid features simultaneously with the appearance of hyperkinetic disorders in 2 of 2 and 5 of 19 cases, respectively. However, in 2 of 19 patients, no movement disorder could be established, indicating that this might not be a necessary condition.[73]

NEUROLOGICAL CARDINAL SYMPTOMS

A movement disorder presenting mainly with orofacial dyskinesias and as limb chorea is most frequently observed.

PSYCHIATRIC SYMPTOMS

Of 19 examined patients, 11 showed psychiatric symptoms.[73] The most consistent symptom was a personality change with impulsive and distractable behavior, apathy, and loss of insight. Additionally, depression, anxiety, paranoid delusions, and obsessive-compulsive features were seen.

DIAGNOSIS/DIFFERENTIAL DIAGNOSIS

The correct diagnosis depends on the combination of significant acanthocytosis with normal plasma lipoproteins and neurological abnormalities. In this context, the clinical picture of neuroacanthocytosis with a movement disorder, personality change, and cognitive impairment may resemble that of Huntington's disease. Therefore, in any suspected case of Huntington's disease acanthocytosis should be excluded. Significant acanthocytosis is defined by >3 percent acanthocytes in dried blood smears. In this context acanthocytes have to be thoroughly distinguished from echinocytes. Scanning electron microscopy may be helpful in measuring the extent of the erythrocyte morphological abnormalities when in doubt.[73]

BIOCHEMICAL CRITERIA

Apart from acanthocytosis, only modestly elevated creatine kinase levels have been reported.[71] Other laboratory parameters, especially plasma lipoproteins, show no abnormalities.

NEUROIMAGING

CT revealed cortical or occasional caudate atrophy as significant features.[72,73] MRI showed nonspecific focal and symmetric signal abnormalities in the caudate and lentiform nuclei in three of four cases.[73] PET revealed the following alterations: mean posterior putamen ^{18}F-fluorodopa uptake was reduced to 42 percent of normal; depressed frontal and striatal blood flow was seen; and a loss of caudate and putamen D2-receptors were observed.[74]

THERAPY

Because there is no specific treatment known, therapy remains symptomatic. However, parkinsonian symptoms did not respond to high dosages of L-dopa,[67] and the response of the involuntary movements to drug treatment was generally poor.[65]

Pallidal, Pallidonigral, and Pallidoluysionigral Degenerations

CLINICAL DEFINITION

The pallidal, pallidonigral, and pallidoluysionigral degenerations include a number of familial or sporadically occurring movement disorders clinically defined by a slowly progressive course and a wide variety of extrapyramidal symptoms. Morphologically, a degeneration of the pallidum alone or in association with the substantia nigra and/or the nucleus subthalamicus (of Luys) is found. The first four sporadic cases were described by Hunt.[75] Today, this category of disorders with predominant affection of the pallidoluysionigral system is classified into four distinct groups[76]: (a) pure pallidal atrophy, (b) pure pallidoluysian atrophy, (c) extended forms of pallidal degeneration, that is, the pallidonigral and the pallidoluysionigral atrophy and (d) variable forms of these mentioned subtypes with other cerebrospinal degenerations. For instance, the separately described familial parkinsonian-pyramidal syndrome (see below) can be considered as a member of this group.[77] Furthermore, the relation of the familial pallidonigral system degeneration with cystic damage reported by McCormick et al.[78] to the disease entity discussed here in is not known. Finally, in a small number of cases there is evidence of a possibly different movement disorder, characterized by the isolated degeneration of the external pallidum or status marmoratus of the basal ganglia in association with the occurrence of intraneuronal polyglucosan (Bielschowsky) bodies.[79]

EPIDEMIOLOGY

No epidemiological data are available because of the small number of investigated cases.

NEUROGENETICS

In most of the reported families to date the condition appears to be of autosomal-recessive inheritance.[77]

PATHOGENESIS

The pathogenesis of this disorder(s) is not known. Recently, it was proposed that the deposition of iron in a case of pallidoluysionigral atrophy was related to the causative mechanisms of the observed lesions.[80]

NEUROPATHOLOGY

A progressive loss of nerve cells and fibers accompanied by proportional gliosis, particularly in the globus pallidus and the subthalamic nucleus, has been found.[77] The changes may vary in their extent. In rare instances they might be associated with further degenerative lesions in other extrapyramidal, motor neuron, or spinocerebellar systems. A pure pallidal atrophy with gliosis and locally differing neuronal loss was demonstrated by Lange et al.[81] The neurons of some brain areas not primarily affected showed an increased lipofuscin content.

Recently, in another case of pure pallidal atrophy of adult onset,[82] morphometric analysis revealed a shrinkage of the globus pallidus externus to 59 percent and the globus pallidus internus to 37 percent of normal, but the neuron density seemed not to be affected. Accordingly, bilateral symmetrical loss of neurons and myelin with gliosis mainly in the outer pallidum was combined with pallor of the ansa lenticularis and atrophy of subthalamic nucleus in a case of pure pallidoluysian atrophy.[83] These changes are consistent with the findings observed in the various extended forms of this group of neurodegenerative disorders. Additionally, in a case of pallidoluysionigral atrophy[84] a massive occurrence of corpora amylacea throughout the CNS was reported. Recently, three autopsied cases of pallidonigroluysian atrophy were presented in which brown granular deposits showing a positive reaction for iron were found in the degenerated nuclei and the striatum.[80]

CLINICAL MANIFESTATIONS

Except for the CNS and psychiatric symptoms (see below), no other clinical manifestations are known.

CNS MANIFESTATIONS

The disorders demonstrate an insidious onset and a slowly progressive course. Onset of illness in familial cases was between ages 5 and 40 and in sporadic cases between ages 30 and 64. Depending on the variable pattern of morphological alterations, there may be distinct predominant symptoms. In pure pallidal degeneration the clinical picture is characterized by the development of a progressive choreoathetotic hyperkinesia with axial dystonia, followed by the appearance of progressive rigidity. Finally, the involuntary movements are overcome by permanent rigidity, and the patients become bedridden.[77] In contrast, Aizawa et al. reported one case of pure pallidal degeneration with an extreme slowness of movement without rigidity as the main symptom.[82] In pallidoluysian atrophy, additional symptoms are torticollis, head tremor, and distal movements with or without a ballistic component.[77] Recently, another case of pure pallidoluysian atrophy was reported, presenting with 20 years of progressive generalized dystonia, dysarthria, gait disorder, vertical gaze palsy, and bradykinesia.[85] However, in pallidoluysionigral degeneration the most apparent symptoms are progressive akinesia and rigidity with little or no tremor.[77] Additionally, upward gaze palsy or Parinaud's syndrome has also been observed. In conclusion, a wide spectrum of different clinical manifestations exists, depending on the spatial and temporal pattern of affection of the distinct brain areas. Consequently, because of their rarity, the clinical correlates of the distinct forms of pallidal, pallidoluysian, and pallidoluysionigral degeneration are still not well described.

NEUROLOGICAL CARDINAL SYMPTOMS

Familial occurrence of the combination of progressive rigidity and choreoathethosis or torsion dystonia with an early onset may suggest pallidal degeneration.

PSYCHIATRIC SYMPTOMS

These disorders might be accompanied by mental deterioration, but intellectual impairment may be absent, even in advanced disease stages.[77] A history of psychosis was also reported in several cases.[80,84]

DIAGNOSIS/DIFFERENTIAL DIAGNOSIS

The diagnosis of these rare conditions can only be proven by means of postmortem examination. Possible differential diagnoses include juvenile parkinsonism, idiopathic torsion dystonia, HSD, dentatorubropallidoluysian atrophy, progressive supranuclear palsy, striatonigral degeneration, corticobasal degeneration, and others.

BIOCHEMICAL CRITERIA

Routine laboratory data are unremarkable.[77]

NEUROIMAGING

CT in younger patients was normal[77]; minimal atrophy of the brain stem and dilatation of the sylvian fissure were seen in a single case.[82] MRI of the brain in a patient with pallidoluysian atrophy showed no abnormalities.[85]

THERAPY

Treatment with L-dopa has produced only equivocal improvement of the movement disorder.[82,86] However, one patient with dystonic symptoms was reported to benefit from baclofen.[85]

Familial L-Dopa-Responsive Parkinsonian-Pyramidal Syndrome

CLINICAL DEFINITION

The familial L-dopa-responsive parkinsonian-pyramidal syndrome is thought to be an autosomal-recessive disease with onset in the second or early third decade, with a clinical picture consisting of parkinsonism (akinesia, rigidity, and rest tremor) and pyramidal tract signs.[87–90] Recently, a syndrome, probably new, was reported that is closely related but not identical to the parkinsonian-pyramidal syndrome. It is called Kufor-Rakeb syndrome and is characterized additionally by supranuclear upgaze paresis and dementia.[91]

EPIDEMIOLOGY

Until now only 10 familial and 2 nonfamilial cases have been described.

NEUROGENETICS

It has been suggested that this condition is recessively inherited.[90]

PATHOGENESIS

The pathogenesis of this syndrome is unknown.

NEUROPATHOLOGY

Until now only one autopsy in a nonfamilial patient 50 years after onset has been performed.[87] A pallor of the pallidal segments, slight shrinkage and cellular change of the SN, a thinning of the ansa lenticularis, and early demyelination of the pyramids and crossed pyramidal tracts were observed. The latter extended from the lower parts of the medulla oblongata into the spinal cord.

CLINICAL MANIFESTATIONS

The parkinsonian-pyramidal syndrome is characterized by its CNS symptoms and signs.

CNS MANIFESTATIONS

In general, disease onset was in the second or the early third decade. However, the two siblings reported on by Horowitz and Greenberg[88] developed their first symptoms in the first decade of life. The classical parkinsonian features were observed in all cases. Pyramidal tract signs, consisting of hyperreflexia, spastic muscle tone, and bilateral extensor plantar responses, were found. In the patients described by Nisipeanu et al. the occurrence of pyramidal tract signs preceded the appearance of extrapyramidal symptoms.[90] Only a slow progression of the disorder was noted, for example, the two patients investigated by Horowitz et al.[88] were still ambulatory after 10–13 years of disease. No diurnal variation was noted. Some patients examined by Davison showed additional symptoms; among which were horizontal nystagmus, intention tremor, and poor memory and impaired intelligence.[87]

CARDINAL NEUROLOGICAL SYMPTOMS

The cardinal neurological symptoms are featured by the co-occurrence of young-onset parkinsonism and pyramidal tract signs.

PSYCHIATRIC SYMPTOMS

Psychiatric symptoms have not been seen in this syndrome. However, one patient reported by Davison had impaired intelligence. Furthermore, three of the five patients with Kufor-Rakeb syndrome[91] were demented.

DIAGNOSIS

The diagnostic possibilities are limited. Evidence of isolated extrapyramidal and pyramidal signs and normal laboratory and neuroradiologic investigations in a young adult are suggestive of the parkinsonian-pyramidal syndrome. Possible differential diagnoses are juvenile parkinsonism and L-dopa-responsive dystonia.

BIOCHEMICAL CRITERIA

No biochemical criteria for diagnosis are known.

NEUROIMAGING

Three of the four patients examined by Nisipeanu et al. were subjected to cranial CT and MRI. No abnormalities were found. Interestingly, patients suffering from the so-called Kufor-Rakeb syndrome showed, in contrast, generalized atrophy on MRI with pronounced atrophy of the lentiform nuclei and the pyramids.[89] PET with fluorodeoxyglucose was performed in one patient with parkinsonian-pyramidal syndrome, and the result was normal.[88]

THERAPY

Extrapyramidal symptoms improved with L-dopa therapy. Typically, the pyramidal symptoms were not influenced by this treatment. However, Tranchant et al. reported a worsening of pyramidal tract signs because of the medication regimen.[89] Response to L-dopa was somewhat variable; most patients responded rapidly to low doses, with improvement persisting for a long period. After many years of treatment, "wearing off" phenomena occurred. The daily dose of L-dopa used in the patients reported by Nisipeanu et al.[90] amounted to 500–1000 mg plus 50–100 mg of carbidopa.

Rett Syndrome

CLINICAL DEFINITION

Rett syndrome is a progressive neurodegenerative disorder, which is reported only in females and characterized by a wide spectrum of motor and behavioral abnormalities. It was first described by Rett in 1966[92,93] and subsequently was investigated by other authors.[94–97] The most typical symptoms are stereotyped movements and gait disturbance. Furthermore, parkinsonism and hyperkinetic disorders are frequently associated with Rett syndrome.

EPIDEMIOLOGY

The prevalence of Rett syndrome is estimated to be about 0.44/10,000.[98]

NEUROGENETICS

It has been proposed that Rett syndrome is the result of an X-linked-dominant mutation with mortality for hemizygous males, whereby each case represents a new mutation.[99] In one patient with Rett syndrome a de novo X; 3, translocation with the chromosomal breakpoint at Xp21.3 was detected, possibly causing this disorder.[100] However, there is also evidence that Rett syndrome is not a consequence of an X mutation.[101]

PATHOGENESIS

The cause of this syndrome is still poorly defined. Recent investigations suggest that an increased tendency to chromosome breakage may be part of a genetically determined disorder in Rett syndrome patients.[102]

NEUROPATHOLOGY

Autopsy studies showed diffuse cerebral atrophy with a decrease in brain weight of 13.8–33.8 percent, compared to that of age-matched controls, with increased amounts of lipofuscin and, occasionally, mild astrocytosis seen microscopically. Moreover, mild but inconsistent spongy changes of white matter were found. Most apparent was a low level of pigmentation of the substantia nigra, whereas the number of nigral neurons was normal.[103] Recently, selective dendritic alterations in the cortex of patients with Rett syndrome were reported.[104]

CLINICAL MANIFESTATIONS

Rett syndrome leads not only to neurological abnormalities but also to dysfunction of other organ systems.[105] Gastroenterological complaints include constipation and weight loss. Swallowing difficulties are also common. Furthermore, an unusual breathing pattern with central apnea intermixed with hyperventilation is frequently observed. Scoliosis occurs often. Girls with Rett syndrome have significantly longer corrected QT intervals and T-wave abnormalities on electrocardiograms that might explain the sudden death that is seen in Rett syndrome.[106]

CNS MANIFESTATIONS

A four-stage model for the description of Rett syndrome was proposed.[95] Stage 1 is defined by developmental stagnation, hypotonia, and deceleration of head growth (onset age, 6 months to 1.5 years). Stage 2 is characterized by loss of functional hand use, stereotypic hand-wringing, loss of expressive language, rapid developmental regression, and occasional seizures (onset age, 1–3 or 4 years). Stage 3 is termed a pseudostationary period because of some restitution of communication, but increasing ataxia, hyperreflexia, and rigidity, as well as breathing dysfunction and bruxism, are observed. After several years stage 4 develops with the so-called late motor deterioration and growth retardation. With respect to extrapyramidal dysfunction, bruxism (97 percent), oculogyric crises (63 percent), and parkinsonism and dystonia (59 percent) are common features. Myoclonus and choreoatheosis were only seen infrequently. In younger patients the hyperkinetic disorders were more evident, whereas in older patients the bradykinetic syndrome tended to predominate.[97] Drooling (75 percent), rigidity (44 percent), and bradykinesia (41 percent) were the most often observed parkinsonian findings.

NEUROLOGICAL CARDINAL SYMPTOMS

The neurological cardinal symptoms and signs are featured by developmental stagnation followed by dementia, autism, loss of purposeful hand movements, and jerky truncal ataxia in a stage-dependent manner.[94] It has been suggested that the jerky truncal ataxia represents a combination of cerebellar ataxia and myoclonus.[97]

PSYCHIATRIC SYMPTOMS

Sleep disturbances, mainly in the early stages, are frequently present in Rett syndrome. They are characterized by an overall increase in daytime sleep and a delayed onset of sleep at night. Despite their mental retardation and their loss of expressive language, these patients tend to appear happy and enjoy close physical contact.

DIAGNOSIS/DIFFERENTIAL DIAGNOSIS

The Rett syndrome diagnostic criteria work group[96] proposed that the diagnosis be based on the following clinical manifestations: Necessary criteria are normal prenatal and perinatal periods, normal psychomotor development through the first 6 months of life, normal head circumference at birth with subsequent deceleration of head growth, loss of purposeful hand skills, severely impaired expressive and receptive language, apparent severe mental retardation and gait and truncal apraxia. Supportive criteria include breathing dysfunction, seizures, spasticity, scoliosis, and growth retardation. Infantile autism is one of the most important differential diagnoses. At the current time there are no specific cytogenetic, biochemical, or molecular markers for this disorder.

BIOCHEMICAL CRITERIA

It was proposed that hyperammonemia could be an essential sign of this condition,[92,93] but further investigations did not reproduce the findings of hyperammonemia in most patients.[94] Significant reductions in the metabolites of norepinephrine, dopamine, and serotonin, as well as an elevation of biopterin in the cerebrospinal fluid, constituted the first detected biochemical alterations.[107] Additionally, there is evidence of elevation of lactate, pyruvate, alpha-ketoglutarate, and malate,[108] as well as of glutamate,[109] in the cerebrospinal fluid.

NEUROIMAGING

MRI indicated a global hypoplasia of brain and progressive cerebellar atrophy increasing with age.[110] An increased density of D2 receptors in striata of patients suffering from Rett syndrome using single-photon emission spectroscopy (SPECT) imaging was found.[111] ^{18}F-fluorodeoxyglucose PET showed several areas of hypometabolism, with markedly lower metabolism in the occipital lobes.[112]

THERAPY

There is no specific treatment established. Recent studies revealed that naltrexone appears to provide clinical benefit in the treatment of breathing dysfunction and cognitive impairment.[113] Furthermore, in one case of Rett syndrome L-carnitine was successfully used.[114] Symptomatic therapeutic approaches also include physio- and music therapy.[104]

References

1. Hirano A, Kurland LT, Krooth RS, Lessell S: Parkinsonism-dementia complex: An endemic disease on the island of Guam. I. Clinical features. *Brain* 84:642–661, 1961.
2. Hirano A, Malamud N, Kurland LT: Parkinsonism-dementia complex: An endemic disease on the island of Guam. II. Pathologic features. *Brain* 84:662–679, 1961.
3. Wszolek ZK, Pfeiffer RF, Bhatt MH, et al: Rapidly progressive autosomal dominant parkinsonism and dementia with pallido-ponto-nigral degeneration. *Ann Neurol* 32:314–320, 1992.
4. Rosenberg RN, Green JB, White CL III, et al: Dominantly inherited dementia and parkinsonism, with Non-Alzheimer amyloid plaques: A new neurogenetic disorder. *Ann Neurol* 25:152–158, 1989.
5. Mata M, Dorovini-Zis K, Wilson M, Young AB: New form of familial parkinson-dementia syndrome: clinical and pathologic findings. *Neurology* 33:1439–1443, 1983.
6. Lynch T, Sano M, Marder KS, Bell MD, et al: Clinical characteristics of a family with chromosome 17-linked disinhibition-dementia-parkinsonism-amyotrophy complex. *Neurology* 44:1878–1884, 1994.
7. Hallervorden J, Spatz H: Eigenartige Erkrankung im extrapyramidalen System mit besonderer Beteiligung des Globus pallidus und der Substantia nigra. *Z Gesamte Neurol Psychiatr* 79:254–302, 1922.
8. Seitelberger F: Zur Morphologie und Histochemie der degenerativen Axonveränderungen vom Zentralnervensystem, in *Proceedings of the 3rd International Congress of Neuropathology 1957*, pp 127–147.
9. Swaiman KF: Hallervorden-Spatz syndrome and brain iron metabolism. *Arch Neurol* 48:1285–1293, 1991.
10. Wigboldus JM, Bruyn GW: Hallervorden-Spatz disease, in Vinken PJ, Bruyn GW (eds): *Diseases of the Basal Ganglia: Handbook of Clinical Neurology*, 1968, vol 6, pp 604–631.
11. Gross H, Kaltenbäck E, Uiberrak B: Über eine spätinfantile Form der Hallervorden-Spatzschen Krankheit: Klin.-anatomische Befunde. *Dtsch Z Nervenheilkd* 176:77–103, 1957.
12. Perry TL, Norman MG, Young VW, et al: Hallervorden-Spatz disease: Cysteine accumulation and cysteine dioxygenase deficiency in the globus pallidus. *Ann Neurol* 18:482–489, 1985.
13. Newell FW, Johnson RO II, Huttenlocher PR: Pigmentary degeneration of the retina in the Hallervorden-Spatz syndrome. *Am J Ophthalmol* 88:467–471, 1979.
14. Dooling EC, Schoene WC, Richardson EP: Hallervorden-Spatz syndrome. *Arch Neurol* 30:70–83, 1974.
15. Jankovic J, Kirkpatrick JB, Blomquist KA, et al: Late-onset Hallervorden-Spatz disease presenting as familial parkinsonism. *Neurology* 35:227–234, 1985.
16. Angelini L, Nardocci N, Rumi V, et al: Hallervorden-Spatz disease: Clinical and MRI study of 11 cases diagnosed in life. *J Neurol* 239:417–425, 1992.
17. Swaiman KF, Smith SA, Trock GL, Siddiqui AR: Sea-blue histiocytes, lymphocytic cytosomes and ^{59}Fe-studies in Hallervorden-Spatz syndrome. *Neurology* 33:301–305, 1983.
18. Dooling EC, Richardson EP, Davis KR: Computed tomography in Hallervorden-Spatz disease. *Neurology* 30:1128–1130, 1980.
19. Tennison MB, Bouldin TW, Whaley RA: Mineralization of the basal ganglia detected by CT in Hallervorden-Spatz syndrome. *Neurology* 38:154–155, 1988.
20. Rutledge JN, Hilal SK, Silver AJ, Defendini R, et al: Study of movement disorders and brain iron by magnetic resonance. *Am J Roentgenol* 149:365–379, 1987.
21. Sethi KD, Adams RJ, Loring DW, El Gammal T: Hallervorden-Spatz syndrome: Clinical and magnetic resonance imaging correlations. *Ann Neurol* 24:692–694, 1988.
22. Szanto J, Gallyas F: A study of iron metabolism in neuropsychiatric patients. *Arch Neurol* 14:438–442, 1966.
23. Klawans HL: Hemiparkinsonism as a late complication of hemiatrophy: A new syndrome. *Neurology* 31:625–628, 1981.
24. Buchman AS, Christopher GG, Goetz MD, Klawans HL: Hemiparkinsonism with hemiatrophy. *Neurology* 38:527–530, 1988.
25. Giladi N, Burke RE, Kostic V, et al: Hemiparkinson-hemiatrophy syndrome: Clinical and neuroradiologic features. *Neurology* 40:1731–1734, 1990.
26. Penfield W, Robertson JSM: Growth asymmetry due to lesions of the post central cortex. *Arch Neurol Psychiatry* 50:405–430, 1943.
27. Alpers BJ, Dear RB: Hemiatrophy of the brain. *J Nerv Ment Dis* 89:653–669, 1939.
28. Burke RE, Fahn S, Gold AP: Delayed onset dystonia in patients with "static" encephalopathy. *J Neurol Neurosurg Psychiatry* 48:650–657, 1985.
29. Przedborski S, Goldman S, Levivier M, et al: Brain glucose metabolism and dopamine D_2 receptor analysis in a patient with hemiparkinsonism-hemiatrophy syndrome. *Mov Disord* 8:391–395, 1993.
30. Przedborski S, Giladi N, Takikawa S, et al: Metabolic topography of the hemiparkinsonism-hemiatrophy syndrome. *Neurology* 44:1622–1628, 1994.

31. Halperin G: Normal asymmetry and unilateral hypertrophy. *Arch Intern Med* 48:676–684, 1931.

32. Giladi N, Fahn S: Hemiparkinson-hemiatrophy syndrome may mimic early-stage cortical-basal ganglionic degeneration. *Mov Disord* 7(4):384–385, 1992.

33. Costa B, Zanette G, Bertolasi L, Fiaschi A: Hemiparkinson-hemiatrophy syndrome: Neuroradiological and neurophysiological findings. *Eur Neurol* 34:107–109, 1994.

34. Okazaki H, Lipkin LE, Aronson SM: Diffuse intracytoplasmic ganglionic inclusions (Lewy type) associated with progressive dementia and quadriparesis in flexion. *J Neuropathol Exp Neurol* 20:237–244, 1961.

35. Kosaka K, Yoshimura M, Ikeda K, Budka H: Diffuse type of Lewy body disease: Progressive dementia with abundant cortical Lewy bodies and senile changes of varying degree—A new disease? *Clin Neuropathol* 3:185–192, 1984.

36. Kosaka K: Diffuse Lewy body disease in Japan. *J Neurol* 237:197–204, 1990.

37. Quinn NP: Dementia and Parkinson's disease, in Wolters EC, Scheltens P (eds): *Mental Dysfunction and Parkinson's Disease, Proceedings of the European Congress on Mental Dysfunction in PD.* Amsterdam: Elsevier, 1993, pp 113–121.

38. Byrne EJ, Lennox G, Lowe J, Godwin-Austin RB: Diffuse Lewy body disease: Clinical features in 15 cases. *J Neurol Neurosurg Psychiatry* 52:709–717, 1989.

39. Gibb WRG, Esiri MM, Lees AJ: Clinical and pathological features of diffuse Lewy body disease (Lewy body dementia). *Brain* 110:1131–1153, 1985.

40. Hughes AJ, Daniel SE, Kilford L, Lees AJ: The accuracy of clinical diagnosis of idiopathic Parkinson's disease: A clinicopathological study of 100 cases. *J Neurol Neurosurg Psychiatry* 55:181–184, 1992.

41. Kosaka K: Dementia and neuropathology in Lewy body disease. *Adv Neurol* 60:456–463, 1993.

42. De Bruin VMS, Lees AJ, Daniel SE: Diffuse Lewy body disease presenting with supranuclear gaze palsy, parkinsonism and dementia: A case report. *Mov Disord* 7:355–358, 1992.

43. Louis ED, Goldman JE, Powers JM, Fahn S: Parkinsonian features of eight pathologically diagnosed cases of diffuse Lewy body disease. *Mov Disord* 10: 188–194, 1995.

44. Crystal HA, Dickson DW, Lizardi JE, et al: Antemortem diagnosis of diffuse Lewy body disease. *Neurology* 40:1523–1528, 1990.

45. Lee LV, Pascasio FM, Fuentes FD, Viterbo GH: Torsion dystonia in Panay, Philippines. *Adv Neurol* 14:137–151, 1976.

46. Lee LV, Kupke KG, Caballargonzaga F, et al: The phenotype of the x-linked dystonia-parkinsonism syndrome—An assessment of 42 cases in the Philippines. *Medicine* 70:179–187, 1991.

47. Kupke K, Lee LV, Viterbo GH, et al: X-linked recessive torsion dystonia in the Philippines. *Am J Med Genet* 36:237–242, 1990.

48. Waters CH, Faust PL, Powers J, et al: Neuropathology of lubag (X-linked dystonia parkinsonism). *Mov Disord* 8:387–390, 1993.

49. Wilhelmsen KC, Weeks DE, Nygaard TG, et al: Genetic mapping of "lubag" (X-linked dystonia-parkinsonism) in a Filipino kindred to the pericentromeric region of the X chromosome. *Ann Neurol* 29:124–131, 1991.

50. Kupke KG, Graeber MB, Muller U: Dystonia-parkinsonism syndrome (XDP) locus: Flanking markers in Xq12-q21.1. *Am J Hum Genet* 50:808–815, 1992.

51. Wilhelmsen KC, Neystat M, Weeks DE, et al: Progress in positional cloning of the gene responsible for lubag: Implications for presymptomatic diagnosis. *Mov Disord* 9(S1):151, 1994.

52. Waters CH, Takahashi H, Wilhelmsen KC, et al: Phenotypic expression of X-linked dystonia-parkinsonism (lubag) in two women. *Neurology* 43:1555–1558, 1993.

53. Lew MF, Shindo M, Moskowitz CB, et al: Adductor laryngeal breathing dystonia in a patient with lubag (X-linked dystonia-parkinsonism syndrome). *Mov Disord* 9:318–320, 1994.

54. Johnston AW, McKusick VA: Sex-linked recessive inheritance in spastic paraplegia and parkinsonism in *Proceedings of the Second International Congress of Human Genetics,* Rome, 1961, vol 3, pp 1652–1654.

55. Eidelberg D, Takikawa S, Wilhelmsen K, et al: Positron emission tomographic findings in Filipino X-linked dystonia-parkinsonism. *Ann Neurol* 34:185–191, 1993.

56. Brecher G, Bessis M: Present status of spiculated red cells and their relationship to the discocyte-echinocyte transformation: A critical review. *Blood* 40:333–344, 1972.

57. Kornzweig AL, Bassen FA: Retinitis pigmentosa, acanthocytosis and heredodegenerative neuromuscular disease. *Arch Ophthalmol NY* 58:183–187, 1957.

58. Young SG, Bertics SJ, Curtiss LK, et al: Genetic analysis of a kindred with familial hypobetalipoproteinemia: Evidence for two separate gene defects. *J Clin Invest* 79:1842–1851, 1987.

59. Aminoff MJ: Acanthocytosis and neurological disease. *Brain* 95:749–760, 1972.

60. Bird TD, Cedarbaum S, Valpey RW, et al: Familial degeneration of the basal ganglia with acanthocytosis: A clinical, neuropathological and neurochemical study. *Ann Neurol* 3:253–258, 1978.

61. Levine IM, Estes JW, Looney JM: Hereditary neurological disease with acanthocytosis. *Arch Neurol* 19:403–409, 1968.

62. Critchley EMR, Clark DB, Wikler A: Acanthocytosis and neurological disorder without hypobetalipoproteinemia. *Ann Neurol* 18:134–140, 1968.

63. Allen FH, Krabbe SMR, Corcoran PA: A new phenotype (McLeod) in the Kell blood group system. *Vox Sang* 6:555–560, 1961.

64. Swash M, Schwartz MS, Carter ND, et al: Benign X-linked myopathy with acanthocytes (McLeod syndrome): Its relationship to X-linked muscular dystrophy. *Brain* 106:717–733, 1983.

65. Hardie RJ: Acanthocytosis and neurological impairment—A review. *Q J Med* 71:291–306, 1989.

66. Yamamoto T, Hirose G, Shimazaki K, et al: Movement disorders of familial neuroacanthocytosis syndrome. *Arch Neurol* 39:298–301, 1982.

67. Spitz MC, Jankovic J, Killian JM: Familial tic disorder, parkinsonism, motor neuron disease and acanthocytosis: A new syndrome. *Neurology* 35:366–370, 1985.

68. O'Brien CF, Schwarz H, Kurlan R: Neuroacanthocytosis without acanthocytes. *Mov Disord* 5 (suppl. 1):353, 1990.

69. Rinne JO, Daniel SE, Scaravilli F, et al: The neuropathological features of neuroacanthocytosis. *Mov Disord* 9:297–304, 1994.

70. Rinne JO, Daniel SE, Scaravilli F, et al: Nigral degeneration in neuroacanthocytosis. *Neurology* 44:1629–1632, 1994.

71. Sakai T, Mawatari S, Iwashita H, et al: Choreoacanthocytosis: Clues to clinical diagnosis. *Arch Neurol* 38:335–338, 1981.

72. Serra S, Xerra A, Scribano E, et al: Computerized tomography in amyotrophic choreo-acanthocytosis. *Neuroradiology* 29:480–482, 1987.

73. Hardie RJ, Pullon HW, Harding AE, et al: Neuroacanthocytosis: A clinical, haematological and pathological study of 19 cases. *Brain* 114:13–49, 1991.

74. Brooks DJ, Ibanez V, Playford ED, et al: Presynaptic and postsynaptic striatal dopaminergic function in neuroacanthocytosis: A positron emission tomographic study. *Ann Neurol* 30:166–171, 1991.

75. Hunt JR: Progressive atrophy of the globus pallidus (primary atrophy of the pallidal system): A system disease of the paralysis agitans type, characterized by atrophy of the motor cells of the corpus striatum. A contribution to the functions of the corpus striatum. *Brain* 40:58–148, 1917.

76. Jellinger K: Progressive pallidumatrophie. *J Neurol Sci* 6:19–44, 1968.

77. Jellinger K: Pallidal, pallidonigral and pallidoluysionigral degenerations including association with thalamic and dentate degenerations, in Vinken PJ, Brun GW, Klawans HL (eds): *Handbook of Clinical Neurology*, vol. 49 (rev. ser. 5), 1986, pp 445–463.

78. McCormick WF, Lemmi H: Familial degeneration of the pallidonigral system. *Neurology* 15:141–153, 1965.

79. Yagishita S, Itoh Y, Nakano T, et al: Pleomorphic intraneuronal polyglucosan bodies mainly restricted to the pallidum. *Acta Neuropathol* 62:159–163, 1983.

80. Kawai J, Sasahara M, Hazama F, et al: Pallidonigroluysian degeneration with iron deposition: A study of three autopsy cases. *Acta Neuropathol* 86:609–616, 1993.

81. Lange E, Poppe W, Scholtze P: Familial progressive pallidum atrophy. *Eur Neurol* 3:265–267, 1970.

82. Aizawa H, Kwak S, Shimizu T, et al: A case of adult onset pure pallidal degeneration. I. Clinical manifestations and neuropathological observations. *J Neurol Sci* 102:76–82, 1991.

83. Van Bogaert L: Aspects cliniques et pathologiques des atrophies pallidales et pallido-luysiennes progressives. *J Belge Neurol Psychiatr* 47:268–286, 1947.

84. Kosaka K, Matsushita M, Oyanagi S, et al: Pallido-nigro-luysial atrophy with massive appearance of corpora amylacea in the CNS. *Acta Neuropathol* 53:169–172, 1981.

85. Wooten GF, Lopes MB, Harris WO, et al: Pallidoluysian atropy: Dystonia and basal ganglia dysfunction. *Neurology* 43:1764–1768, 1993.

86. Yamamoto T, Kawamura J, Hashimoto S, et al: Pallido-nigro-luysian atrophy, progressive supranuclear palsy and adult onset Hallervorden-Spatz disease: A case of akinesia as a predominant feature of parkinsonism. *J Neurol Sci* 101:98–106, 1990.

87. Davison C: Pallido-pyramidal disease. *J Neuropathol Exp Neurol* 13:50–59, 1954.

88. Horowitz G, Greenberg J: Pallido-pyramidal syndrome treated with L-dopa. *J Neurol Neurosurg Psychiatry* 38:238–240, 1975.

89. Tranchant C, Boulay C, Warter JM: The pallido-pyramidal syndrome: An unrecognized entity. *Rev Neurol (Paris)* 147(4):308–310, 1991.

90. Nisipeanu P, Kuritzky A, Korczyn AD: Familial L-dopa-responsive parkinsonian-pyramidal syndrome. *Mov Disord* 9:673–675, 1994.

91. Najim Al-Din AS, Wriekat A, Mubaidin A, et al: Pallido-pyramidal degeneration, supranuclear upgaze paresis and dementia: Kufor-Rakeb syndrome. *Acta Neurol Scand* 89:347–352, 1994.

92. Rett A: Über ein eigenartiges hirnatrophisches Syndrom bei Hyperammonaemie im Kindesalter. *Wien Med Wochenschr* 116:723–728, 1966.

93. Rett A: Cerebral atrophy with hyperammonaemia, in Vinken PJ, Bruyn GW (eds): *Handbook of Clinical Neurology*, 1977, vol 29, pp 305–329.

94. Hagberg B, Aicardi J, Dias K, et al: A progressive syndrome of autism, dementia, ataxia and loss of purposeful hand use in girls: Rett's syndrome: Report of 35 cases. *Ann Neurol* 14:471–479, 1983.

95. Hagberg B, Witt-Engerstrom I: Rett syndrome: A suggested staging system for describing impairment profile with increasing age towards adolescence. *Am J Med Genet* 24:47–59, 1986.

96. The Rett Syndrome Diagnostic Criteria Work Group: Diagnostic criteria for Rett syndrome. *Ann Neurol* 23:425–428, 1988.

97. FitzGerald PM, Jankovic J, Percy AK: Rett syndrome and associated movement disorders. *Mov Disord* 5:195–202, 1990.

98. Kozinetz CA, Skender ML, MacNaughton N, et al: Epidemiology of Rett syndrome: A population-based registry. *Pediatrics* 91:445–450, 1993.

99. Comings DE: The genetics of Rett syndrome: The consequences of a disorder where every case is a new mutation. *Am J Med Genet* 24:383–388, 1986.

100. Ellison KA, Roth EJ, McCabe ER, et al: Isolation of a yeast artificial chromosome contig spanning the X chromosomal translocation breakpoint in a patient with Rett syndrome. *Am J Med Genet* 47:1124–1134, 1993.

101. Migeon BR, Dunn MA, Thomas G, et al: Studies of X inactivation and isodisomy in twins provide further evidence that the X chromosome is not involved in Rett syndrome. *Am J Hum Genet* 56:647–653, 1995.

102. Telvi L, Leboyer M, Chiron C, et al: Is Rett syndrome a chromosome breakage syndrome? *Am J Med Genet* 15:602–605, 1994.

103. Jellinger K, Seitelberger F: Neuropathology of Rett syndrome. *Am J Med Genet* 24:259–288, 1986.

104. Armstrong D, Dunn JK, Antalffy B, et al: Selective dendritic alterations in the cortex of Rett syndrome. *J Neuropathol Exp Neurol* 54:195–201, 1995.

105. Braddock SR, Braddock BA, Graham JM: Rett syndrome: An update and review for the primary pediatrician. *Clin Pediatr* 32:613–626, 1993.

106. Sekul EA, Moak JP, Schultz RJ, et al: Electrocardiographic findings in Rett syndrome: An explanation for sudden death? *J Pediatr* 125:80–82, 1994.

107. Zoghbi HY, Milstien S, Butler IJ, et al: Cerebrospinal fluid biogenic amines and biopterin in Rett syndrome. *Ann Neurol* 25:56–60, 1989.

108. Matsuishi T, Urabe F, Percy AK, et al: Abnormal carbohydrate metabolism in cerebrospinal fluid in Rett syndrome. *J Child Neurol* 9:26–30, 1994.

109. Hamberger A, Gillberg C, Palm A, et al: Elevated CSF glutamate in Rett syndrome. *Neuropediatrics* 23:212–213, 1992.

110. Murakami JW, Courchesne E, Haas RH, et al: Cerebellar and cerebral abnormalities in Rett syndrome: A quantitative MR analysis. *Am J Roentgenol* 159:177–183, 1992.

111. Chiron C, Bulteau C, Loch C, et al: Dopaminergic D2 receptor SPECT imaging in Rett syndrome: Increase of specific binding in striatum. *J Nucl Med* 34:1717–1721, 1993.

112. Naidu S, Wong DF, Kitt C, et al: Positron emission tomography in the Rett syndrome: Clinical, biochemical and pathological correlates. *Brain Dev* 14:S75–79, 1992.

113. Levin JR, Valentine CL, Bierwaltes P: Clinical efficacy of naltrexone in Rett syndrome. *Mov Disord* 5(S1):68, 1990.

114. Plioplys AV, Kasnicka I: L-carnitine as treatment for Rett syndrome. *South Med J* 86:1411–1412, 1993.

OTHER CENTRAL NERVOUS SYSTEM CONDITIONS THAT MAY CAUSE OR MIMIC PARKINSONISM

JACOB I. SAGE

VASCULAR PARKINSONISM
TRAUMA AS A CAUSE OF PARKINSONISM
PARKINSONISM AND HYDROCEPHALUS
STRUCTURAL LESIONS PRODUCING PARKINSONISM
CALCIFICATION OF THE BASAL GANGLIA,
    DISORDERS OF CALCIUM METABOLISM, AND
    PARKINSONISM
NEUROLEPTIC MALIGNANT SYNDROME
    (PARKINSONISM HYPERPYREXIA SYNDROME)

This chapter will cover parkinsonian syndromes caused by vascular disease, hydrocephalus, trauma, structural lesions, disorders of calcium metabolism, and the neuroleptic-malignant syndrome. For the most part, these entities present with atypical findings in that the complete clinical syndrome associated with most cases of Lewy body Parkinson's disease (PD) (rest tremor, rigidity, bradykinesia, and postural instability) is not present. Generally, but not always, rest tremor and L-dopa responsiveness are not features of these forms of parkinsonism. More importantly, however, it is the historical setting, associated clinical and laboratory findings, and disease course that lead to a diagnosis of one of these conditions rather than PD.

Vascular Parkinsonism

Vascular parkinsonism is a condition whose nosology is still under debate. Our concept of its contribution in terms of numbers to the parkinsonian disorders, even its distinctness as a separate entity, has changed over the past 100 years and continues to change. Therefore, it is useful to review briefly the history of this syndrome.[1]

Near the end of the nineteenth century, an arteriosclerotic disorder was delineated that resembled the disease described by James Parkinson, most prominently as a disorder of gait in the elderly. To this short-stepped gait, which came to be known as *march a petit pas,* were added the additional characteristics of dementia, pyramidal signs and symptoms, including mild hemiparesis, urinary and emotional incontinence, and dysarthria. This clinical syndrome was correlated

with multiple basal ganglia cavitations (*etat crible*) and infarcts (*etat lacunaris*). By the 1920s parkinsonism was defined by the anatomic site of the lesion in the basal ganglia for which a number of causes could be found, one of which was vascular.

Despite the lack of a clear pathological substrate defining PD in the late 1920s, there was a feeling that PD was a separate entity from other possible causes of parkinsonism. In 1929, this underlying sense that PD was different from vascular parkinsonism led to Critchley's monograph on arteriosclerotic parkinsonism.[2] Despite nearly 70 years of technological advances and debate, this paper remains the single most useful contribution delineating vascular parkinsonism from PD. To the features of vascular parkinsonism described in the previous paragraph, he adds gegenhalten, pseudobulbar palsy, a shuffling gait with persistent freezing but *without* festination, diminished arm swing, tremor, or associated seborrhea. Signs are usually symmetrical in vascular parkinsonism. Cerebellar system involvement is seen in some cases. There is a history of hypertension and stepwise progression with distinct plateaus in the clinical course. In contrast, patients with PD tend to be younger at disease onset, have cogwheel rigidity, asymmetrical findings, festination but only transient freezing, diminished arm swing, and a rest tremor. Today, we must add that a good response to L-dopa strongly favors a diagnosis of PD[3] (see also Chap. 13).

Because of Critchley's paper, attempts to redefine the limits of vascular parkinsonism have led to the concept of "lower body parkinsonism."[4,5] Such refinement occurred partly because substantia nigra degeneration with Lewy bodies was now accepted as the pathological substrate of PD,[6] and L-dopa responsiveness was taken as convincing evidence in favor of that diagnosis during life. This knowledge eliminated some of the confusion facing neurologists and pathologists before the 1960s and 1970s in that it largely separated PD from other forms of parkinsonism. A lower-body gait disorder, different but not entirely distinct from senile gait[7,8] without apparent cause, came to be associated with vascular brain pathology and not with Lewy body disease.

The evolving definition of vascular parkinsonism also came about because the advent of computerized axial tomography during the 1970s revealed changes suggesting deep white matter vasculopathy in a group of patients presenting predominantly with disorders of gait.[9] White matter periventricular low-density changes correlated with gait apraxia and poor balance. These patients exhibited a wide-based ataxic gait, which was presumably similar to the cerebellar gait alluded to in Critchley's description. This gait was dissimilar from the narrow-based gait seen in patients with PD. The periventricular location of these radiographic abnormalities presumably accounted for lower-body parkinsonism by disrupting pathways to the legs in preference to those to the upper body. Subsequent studies in the magnetic resonance imaging (MRI) era support but by no means prove these speculations.[10]

The idea that lower-body parkinsonism is primarily from arteriosclerotic cerebral vascular disease has been extended to include clinical syndromes suggesting progressive supranuclear palsy (PSP).[5,9] In one study, 19 of 58 patients with a clinical diagnosis of PSP had radiographic evidence of multiple small infarcts in the brain stem and deep white matter.[9] These patients were more likely to be hypertensive than those with PD. As with many diagnoses relying on imaging studies in elderly patients, it remains to be seen whether the white matter changes and small infarcts are truly indicative of the underlying pathology or are simply a finding seen with increasing frequency in the aged.[10] White matter changes in older patients may turn out to be unrelated to the cause of their parkinsonism.

In a number of patients, however, it is impossible not to relate widespread abnormalities in the deep cerebral white matter to neurological deterioration. This subcortical arteriosclerotic encephalopathy (Binswanger's disease) is usually characterized by a gradually worsening dementia in the setting of vascular risk factors.[11] Atypical gait, often having elements of both parkinsonism and ataxia, may be the initial symptom. Criteria to aid in the diagnosis of Binswanger's disease recently have been proposed.[12] They include dementia, abnormalities on imaging studies suggestive of rarefaction bilaterally in the deep white matter, and any two of the following findings: vascular risk factor, focal cerebral vascular disease, or subcortical cerebral dysfunction (parkinsonism). Some patients may present with a PSP like syndrome. Although most patients are L-dopa-unresponsive, cases have been reported that did improve with L-dopa. Furthermore, at least one pathologically documented case did not have dementia during life.[13] Binswanger's disease remains difficult to diagnose with certainty before death.

Hurtig has outlined a set of criteria for the diagnosis of vascular parkinsonism which it seems prudent to follow.[1] They include the acute or subacute (preferably stepwise) evolution of an akinetic-rigid syndrome in the setting of documented vascular risk factors (hypertension, previous strokes, lipid abnormalities, sytemic arteriosclerotic vascular disease). Imaging studies should show at least two infarcts in the basal ganglia. To this may be added widespread and severe white matter disease on MRI consistent with Binswanger's pathology. There should be improvement in clinical signs without the use of L-dopa therapy or after it has been withdrawn, if given acutely. Adherence to these criteria may miss some cases of bona fide vascular parkinsonism but will minimize confusion among the various forms of parkinsonism not attributable to Lewy body disease. Treatment is directed at control of underlying risk factors, as with other forms of cerebral vascular disease.

Trauma as a Cause of Parkinsonism

The exact relationship between trauma and parkinsonism has been a subject of debate[14] since James Parkinson first speculated that it might be responsible for the syndrome he described in 1817. By the late nineteenth century, traumatic parkinsonism, resulting from everything from emotional stress to moral lapses, became a fashionable diagnosis with no solid clinical or pathological basis.[15] In particular, peripheral limb trauma was thought to be causative if parkinsonism subsequently developed in the same extremity. In retrospect, many cases were clearly misdiagnosed, and in others evidence for the relation between the trauma and parkinsonism

was weak.[16] By the early decades of the twentieth century, only concussion remained as a significant cause of post-traumatic parkinsonism. Experience during the great war made many neurologists skeptical even of this relation, because parkinsonism was not a noticeable sequela of hundreds and thousands of concussions from combat wounds.

In the years after the war, however, as neurologists sought to delineate postencephalitic from other types of parkinsonism, cases of post-traumatic parkinsonism with more specific clinical and pathological characteristics began to accumulate.[17] With these cases in mind, neurologists developed specific criteria for the diagnosis of post-traumatic parkinsonism that are still relevant today. They include the onset of a bradykinetic-rigid syndrome (often unilateral, with variable degree of tremor), which slowly becomes generalized. Postural instability, gait disorders, headache, psychiatric and cognitive dysfunction, and pyramidal signs are often present. More recently, post-traumatic parkinsonism resembling PSP[18] and the hemiparkinsonism-hemiatrophy syndrome[19] also have been described. The latter disorder includes such features as slow progression, dystonia, and pyramidal dysfunction (see also Chap. 24).

Diagnostic criteria to justify a diagnosis of post-traumatic parkinsonism include a short duration of time from the trauma to the onset of clinical symptoms and a sufficiently violent blow to cause a concussion. Pathological evidence for necrosis or hemorrhage in the basal ganglia or midbrain should be found at autopsy. At present, in the absence of postmortem examinations, imaging studies showing structural damage in the basal ganglia or midbrain after concussion may be taken as evidence in favor of a diagnosis of traumatic parkinsonism.[20] Midbrain injury occurs either by direct damage from basilar skull fractures, hemorrhage, and infarction or indirectly by the effects of herniation from supratentorial or infratentorial mass lesions. Shearing injury with axonal damage may occur in the midbrain as it rotates from the impact of a blow to the head.[21] A diagnosis of post-traumatic parkinsonism should not be made in the absence of evidence for structural damage to basal ganglia or midbrain.

Dementia pugilistica represents a somewhat different form of post-traumatic parkinsonism.[22] It usually results from a long career of blows to the head and is insidious in onset. Ataxia, dysarthria, personality changes, psychosis, and rest tremor frequently accompany the cognitive decline and other features of parkinsonism.[23,24] Imaging studies show generalized brain atrophy and, frequently, a cavum septum pellucidum.[25,26] Pathological studies correlate well with the clinical syndrome, showing loss of cells in the substantia nigra, hippocampal gyrus, and amygdala. Neurofibrillary tangles are seen. Cerebellar infarctions and loss of Purkinje cells have been noted.[27] L-dopa may be of benefit and should be tried in most patients who have traumatic parkinsonism.

Although head trauma does not cause PD, there is some controversy about the effect of head trauma on the onset and progression of Lewy body PD. A number of retrospective studies support the notion that head trauma is a risk factor for the subsequent development of PD;[28,29] others do not.[30] A single prospective study of 821 patients did not a show a relationship between previous head trauma and PD, suggesting that other studies supporting the opposite position may suffer from recall bias.[31] What is clear from a prospective study of patients with already diagnosed PD is that trauma may worsen existing symptoms.[32] This worsening, however, is generally reversible by 3 months after the injury. Therefore, it is possible that head trauma may precipitate symptoms of PD in patients with nigral loss just below the threshold for symptoms to appear. In this sense, PD may appear after head injury, with the assumption being that it would have occurred anyway, just a little later.

Parkinsonism and Hydrocephalus

Although hydrocephalus from any cause may include parkinsonian symptoms and signs, normal pressure hydrocephalus (NPH) has received the most attention since it was described in 1965.[33] The clinical picture of the complete syndrome includes the gradual onset of dementia, gait ataxia, and urinary incontinence, although all three components of this picture are not always present. The description of the gait disorder has variously been described as magnetic, apraxic, or ataxic. More often, it appears to include elements of all three gait types with a tendency to lurch and fall. All of the typical features of parkinsonism have been described in one or another patient, including rest tremor, hypophonia, hypomimia, bradykinesia, and rigidity.[34] Occasionally, altered levels of consciousness, oculomotor dysfunction or headache may be present. Corticospinal signs, nystagmus, and even seizures have been reported.

The pathophysiology of NPH is still obscure. The initial event may be a deficiency of cerebrospinal fluid absorption at the arachnoid villi, making this entity one of the types of extraventricular obstructive hydrocephalus, a term preferred by some authors.[34] This obstruction to cerebrospinal fluid (CSF) flow results in transient high-pressure hydrocephalus with subsequent ventricular enlargement. As the ventricles enlarge, the intraventricular pressure may return to normal, but the force generated at the ventricular surface may increase (Pascal's law), leading to further increases in ventricular size.[35] This enlargement of the ventricles compromises corticospinal pathways, especially those to the legs, leading to the characteristic gait abnormalities. Parkinsonism from basal ganglia compromise and dementia and incontinence from frontal lobe dysfunction may also be explained in part from this mechanism.

Although some patients with parkinsonian features have responded to L-dopa,[36] surgical shunting remains the main mode of therapy.[37] A major unresolved issue is that of predicting which patients will respond favorably to shunting. Imaging studies reveal enlargement of the ventricular system without significant cortical atrophy. In the appropriate clinical setting described above, this radiographic picture is sufficient to suggest the diagnosis of NPH. All other radiological signs and clinical tests must be considered as possibly helpful but not clearly diagnostic. These include a CSF flow void in the acqueduct of Sylvius.[38] The absence of this finding may be suggestive of hydrocephalus not associated with NPH. Isotope cisternography with reversal of CSF flow into the lateral ventricles and delayed clearance from the subarachnoid space have not proven a reliable indicator of success after shunting procedures. Removal of 50 cc of CSF from lumbar puncture, with subsequent clinical improvement over the next few hours or days or with increases in cerebral blood flow, may be more helpful.[39] Removal of lumbar CSF temporarily abolishes bladder hyperactivity in some patients with NPH and may predict a good outcome from shunting.[40] Continuous external lumbar drainage of CSF has reportedly produced amelioration of symptoms and may give some indication as to the effect of a more permanent shunting procedure.[41] In one study, a ratio of cerebral blood flow from anterior to posterior of greater than 1.05 correctly predicted surgical outcome.[42]

Making the correct diagnosis and predicting outcome is of paramount importance, because the results of shunting procedures are not stunning and the complications are frequent. Early reports of universal success, usually from neurosurgical centers, were clearly unreliable, but led to surgery for many patients with various forms of dementia. In fact it may be precisely this lack of an exact diagnosis that is responsible for the low percentage of patients who improved after shunting. In a recent retrospective but reliable multicenter study, marked improvement was seen in only 21 percent of patients.[43] The complication rate was nearly 30 percent. Thus, it seems prudent to resort to shunting only in patients with a relatively complete clinical picture compatible with NPH and one or more imaging and other studies consistent with that diagnosis. Some patients can be treated with repeated lumbar puncture without resorting to the use of intracranial shunting procedures.

As reviewed by Shannon, features of more or less typical parkinsonism are seen with intraventricular obstructive hydrocephalus as well.[34] Most prominent are parkinsonian gait disorders with small shuffling steps. Rigidity and bradykinesia are not infrequent, and rest tremor is present in as many as one-half of the reported cases. It must be kept in mind, however, that all cases also have signs to suggest dysfunction of brain areas other than the basal ganglia, most frequently, pyramidal and cerebellar systems. Etiology of the hydrocephalus includes aqueductal stenosis, posterior fossa tumors, Paget's disease, head trauma, and encephalitis.

Parkinsonism resulting from extraventricular hydrocephalus related to specific causes other than NPH has been reported. The clinical syndromes are similar to those described above for intraventricular hydrocephalus, again with the emphasis that signs suggesting involvement of systems other than the basal ganglia are almost always present.[34] Head trauma, subarachnoid hemorhage, and subdural hematoma have all been implicated in small numbers of patients. A few patients responded to L-dopa, suggesting that two disease processes (PD and hydrocephalus) were involved.[36] Although this may be possible, it need not be the case, because L-dopa could benefit parkinsonian symptoms related to midbrain dysfunction caused by entities other than PD.

Structural Lesions Producing Parkinsonism

Structural lesions associated with cases of parkinsonism in which at least two of the four cardinal signs and symptoms were present have been catalogued by Waters in a recent review.[44] Tumors comprise most of the documented cases. Somewhat surprisingly, tumors of the striatum presenting with parkinsonian features are rare. Tumors in other brain areas (frontal, parietal, temporal, thalamus, midbrain, and third ventricle) presumably are responsible for parkinsonian features resulting from compression of the basal ganglia or by means of compression, or direct involvement, of the midbrain. As expected, gliomas and menigiomas are the most frequently noted tumors. The few additional cases are of metastatic tumor, lymphoma, and fibrosarcoma.

Subdural hematoma may also cause parkinsonism, presumably by compression of the basal ganglia or midbrain depending on location and type of herniation. These symptoms have generally been reversible with evacuation. It should be remembered that in most cases, additional clues were present that led to the correct diagnosis, most prominently, headache, decreased level of consciousness, and confusion.

Striatal abscess, midbrain tuberculoma, vascular malformations, and posterior fossa cysts have all been reported to include features of parkinsonism in the clinical picture.

Calcification of the Basal Ganglia, Disorders of Calcium Metabolism, and Parkinsonism

Since the advent of computerized axial tomography, it has been possible to ascertain the prevalence of basal ganglia calcification (sometimes called Fahr's disease) in large, if selected, groups of patients undergoing imaging studies for various reasons. In these studies, basal ganglia calcification is noted in fewer than 0.7 percent of patients, in whom less than 7 percent had a clinical disorder related to the basal ganglia.[45–47] Even fewer of these patients had parkinsonism. From these studies and from reports of families with familial basal ganglia calcification, it is clear that calcification of the basal ganglia (from whatever cause) is not sufficient in and of itself to cause symptoms of parkinsonism.[48]

Although case reports of basal ganglia calcification have been described in numerous diseases, it is most frequently associated with hypoparathyroidism. Basal ganglia calcification is reported in over 70 percent of patients with indiopathic hypoparathyroidism[49] and in nearly all patients with pseudo-hypoparathyroidism.[50] Most descriptions of parkinsonism with hypoparathyroidism have been anecdotal, although one study notes that nearly one-quarter of patients with hypoparathyroidism may have some features of parkinsonism along with a picture of more diffuse neurological involvement.[49] Secondary hypoparathyroidism is much less likely to be associated with calcification, presumably because of the shorter duration of disease before treatment begins in this disorder. Symptoms of parkinsonism generally improve after treatment of hypocalcemia, but this favorable outcome is not universal.[51] L-dopa is of little benefit.[52] Other neurological abnormalities seen in all three major types of hypoparathyroidism include tetany, chorea, psychiatric symptoms,

and seizures, all of which may in fact be more common than parkinsonism in these disorders.

Neuroleptic Malignant Syndrome (Parkinsonism Hyperpyrexia Syndrome)

Neuroleptic malignant syndrome (NMS) is a rare condition that occurs in the setting of either withdrawal of dopaminergic drugs in patients with PD or in patients receiving central dopamine-blocking agents. It can be considered, therefore, a state of acute dopamine deficiency. It has been argued that the obligate clinical characteristics of NMS are hyperpyrexia and a parkinsonian picture consisting, most prominently, of severe rigidity; hence, the term parkinsonism-hyperpyrexia syndrome.[53] Other clinical features include autonomic dysfunction (diaphoresis, incontinence, tachycardia, blood pressure changes), tremor, akinesia, and an altered level of consciousness.[54] Leukocytosis may occur. The clinical course usually begins with rigidity and autonomic changes, followed by fever within several hours of onset. Medical complications of NMS include aspiration pneumonia, myocardial infarction, rhabdomyolysis, and subsequent renal failure. Hemodialysis may be required. The duration of NMS typically is between 1 and 2 weeks. Much has been made of concomitant elevations in creatine kinase (CK), although this finding may be present in only about one-half the cases.[55]

Although the incidence of NMS in patients taking neuroleptics is probably less than 1 in 1000,[56] a number of factors that increase risk emerge from epidemiological and case studies. Men are more commonly affected than women.[57] Dehydration, exposure to heat, and organic brain disease seem to put patients at increased risk for NMS.[58] Multiple neuroleptics, depot forms of neuroleptics, and the additional use of lithium confer particular risk.[55,59] Lithium may even adversely affect outcome.[60] All types of dopamine-blocking agents have been associated with NMS, including compazine and metoclopramide.[61]

There are a number of other medical and psychiatric conditions that may mimic NMS and must be excluded. Lethal catatonia usually begins with agitation and fever, followed shortly by catatonia.[62] Muscle rigidity may be difficult to distinquish from catatonia. A prior history of catatonia in the absence of neuroleptic treatment favors this diagnosis rather than NMS. When there is doubt, it is probably prudent to treat for NMS (see below).[53] Both systemic and CNS infections must be considered early in the differential diagnosis; evaluations by lumbar puncture and cultures are mandatory. Drug withdrawal syndromes may cause fever, altered consciousness, and autonomic instability that might be confused with NMS. Rigidity can occur in alcohol and benzodiazepine withdrawal states, but they are not likely to cause full-blown parkinsonism. An accurate history should clarify the situation. Heat stroke (fever and altered consciousness) also is generally obvious from the setting. Neuroleptic drugs, however, by altering sweating, may contribute to the risk of hot humid conditions and may confuse the diagnosis. The same is true of malignant hyperthermia (fever and rigidity), in which a genetic risk factor predisposes some patients to this condition, which occurs shortly after exposure to inhalation anesthetics.[63] Despite reports that tricyclic antidepressants, phenytoin, and cocaine may cause NMS, it is unlikely that these agents by themselves are responsible for more than drug-induced fever associated with other nonspecific neurological signs and symptoms.[53]

Treatment of NMS depends on recognition and immediate stoppage of neuroleptic drugs. Patients should be hydrated, fever reduced, and medical support instituted. Hemodialysis should be started in those in acute renal failure. Therapy with bromocriptine (2.5–10 mg t.i.d.) is aimed at reducing parkinsonism.[64] It may be used alone or in combination with dantrolene (up to 3 mg/kg/day), which acts directly at the sarcoplasmic reticulum to reduce muscle rigidity.[65] Fever also responds to dantrolene, presumably by decreasing that component of fever caused by peripheral heat production. There is some evidence suggesting that combination therapy (bromocriptine and dantrolene) shortens the course of illness,[66] although either therapy alone has been shown to be effective. Other antiparkinsonian therapy, particularly L-dopa, would be expected to work although the number of patients treated with this approach has been far fewer than with either bromocriptine or dantrolene. Electroconvulsive therapy (ECT) may be effective in some cases[67] but should not be used as primary treatment for NMS. Once an episode of NMS is over, only patients absolutely requiring neuroleptics should be restarted on these drugs. Waiting 2 weeks before rechallenge is a prudent absolute minimum, and close monitoring is necessary to look for recurrence of symptoms.[68]

References

1. Hurtig HI: Vascular parkinsonism, in Stern MB, Koller WC (eds): *Parkinsonian Syndromes*. New York: Marcel Dekker, 1993, pp 81–93.
2. Critchley M: Arteriosclerotic parkinsonism. *Brain* 52:23–83, 1929.
3. Parkes JD, Marsden CD, Rees JE, et al: Parkinson's disease: Cerebral arteriosclerosis and senile dementia. *Q J Med* 43:49–61, 1974.
4. Thompson PD, Marsden CD: Gait disorder of subcortical arteriosclerotic encephalopathy: Binswanger's disease. *Mov Disord* 2:1–8, 1987.
5. Fitzgerald PM, Jankovic J: Lower body parkinsonism: Evidence for a vascular etiology. *Mov Disord* 4:249–260, 1989.
6. Greenfield JG, Bosanquet FD: Brainstem lesions in parkinsonism. *J Neurol Neurosurg Psychiatry* 16:213–226, 1953.
7. Critchley M: On senile disorders of gait including the so-called senile paraplegia. *Geriatrics* 3:364–370, 1948.
8. Sudarsky L: Gait disorders in the elderly. *N Engl J Med* 322:1441, 1990.
9. Dubinsky RM, Jankovic J: Progressive supranuclear palsy and a multi-infarct state. *Neurology* 37:570–576, 1987.
10. Fazekas F, Niederkorn K, Schmidt R, et al: White matter signal abnormalities in normal individuals: Correlation with carotid ultrasound, cerebral blood flow measurements, and cerebrovascular disease risk factors. *Stroke* 19:1285–1288, 1988.
11. Pellissier JF, Poncet M: Binswanger's encephalopathy, in Toole JF (ed): *Vascular Diseases*, vol. 2. *Handbook of Clinical Neurology:* Amsterdam: Elsevier Science Publishers, 1989, vol 54, pp 221–233.
12. Bennett DA, Wilson RS, Gilley DW, Fox JH: Clinical diagnosis of Binswanger's disease. *J Neurol Neurosurg Psychiatry* 53:961–965, 1990.
13. Mark MH, Sage JI, Walters AS, et al: Binswanger's disease presenting as L-dopa-responsive parkinsonism: Clinicopathologic study of three cases. *Mov Disord* 10:450–454, 1995.
14. Factor SA: Posttraumatic parkinsonism, in Stern MB, Koller WC (eds): *Parkinsonian Syndromes*. New York: Marcel Dekker, 1993, pp 95–110.
15. Factor SA, Sanchez-Ramos J, Weiner WJ: Trauma as an etiology of parkinsonism: A historical review of the concept. *Mov Disord* 3:30–36, 1988.
16. Grimberg L: Paralysis agitans and trauma. *J Nerv Ment Dis* 79:14–42, 1934.
17. Crouzan O, Justin-Besancon L: Le Parkinsonisms traumatique. *Presse Med* 37:1325–1327, 1929.
18. Koller WC, Wong GF, Lang A: Posttraumatic movement disorders: A review. *Mov Disord* 4:20–36, 1989.
19. Giladi N, Burke RE, Kostic V, et al: Hemiparkinsonism-hemiatrophy syndrome: Clinical and neuroradiologic features. *Neurology* 40:1731–1734, 1990.
20. Nayernouri T: Posttraumatic parkinsonism. *Surg Neurol* 24:263–264, 1985.
21. Peerless SJ, Rewcastle NB: Shear injuries of the brain. *Can Med Assoc J* 96:577–582, 1967.
22. Martland HS: Punch drunk. *J Am Med Assoc* 91:1103–1107, 1928.
23. Critchley M: Medical aspects of boxing, particularly from a neurological standpoint. *Br Med J* 1:357–362, 1957.
24. Johnson J: Organic psychosyndromes due to boxing. *Br J Psychiatry* 115:45–53, 1969.
25. Casson IR: Neurologic syndromes in boxers. *Neuroview* 1:1–3, 1985.
26. Jordan BD: Neurologic aspects of boxing. *Arch Neurol* 44:453–459, 1987.
27. Lampert PW, Hardman JM: Morphological changes in brains of boxers. *JAMA* 251:2676–2679, 1984.
28. Factor SA, Weiner WJ: Prior history of head trauma in Parkinson's disease. *Mov Disord* 6:225–229, 1991.
29. Stern M, Dulaney E, Gruber SB, et al: The epidemiology of Parkinson's disease: A case-control study of young onset and old onset patients. *Arch Neurol* 48:903–907, 1991.
30. Ward CD, Duvoisin RC, Ince RE, et al: Parkinson's disease in 65 pairs of twins and in a set of quadruplets. *Neurology* 33:815–824, 1983.
31. Williams DB, Anneyers JF, Kohmen E, et al: Brain injury and neurologic sequelae: A cohort study of dementia, parkinsonism and amyotrophic lateral sclerosis. *Neurology* 41:1554–1557, 1991.
32. Goetz CG, Stebbins GT: Effects of head trauma from motor vehicle accidents on Parkinson's disease. *Ann Neurol* 29:191–193, 1991.
33. Hakim S, Adams RD: The special clinical problem of symptomatic hydrocephalus with normal cerebrospinal fluid pressure: Observations on cerebrospinal fluid hydrodynamics. *J Neurol Sci* 2:307–327, 1965.
34. Shannon KM: Hydrocephalus and parkinsonism, in Stern MB, Koller WC (eds): *Parkinsonian Syndromes*. New York: Marcel Dekker, 1993, pp 123–136.
35. Prockop LD: Hydrocephalus, in Rowland LP (ed): *Merritt's Textbook of Neurology*. Baltimore: Williams & Wilkins, 1995, pp 294–302.
36. Jacobs L, Conti D, Kinkel WR, Manning EG: "Normal pressure" hydrocephalus: Relationship of clinical and radiographic findings to improvement following shunt surgery. *JAMA* 235(5):510–512, 1976.

37. Sage JI, Duvoisin RC: The Parkinson plus syndromes: Current opinion in neurology and neurosurgery 2:314–318, 1989.
38. Jack CR Jr, Mokri B, Laws ER Jr, et al: MR findings in normal-pressure hydrocephalus: Significance and comparison with other forms of dementia. *J Comput Assist Tomogr* 11:923–931, 1987.
39. Mamo HL, Meric PC, Ponsin JC, et al: Cerebral blood flow in normal pressure hydrocephalus. *Stroke* 18:1074–1080, 1987.
40. Ahlberg J, Norlen L, Blomstrand C, Wikkelso C: Outcome of shunt operation on urinary incontinence in normal pressure hydrocephalus predicted by lumbar puncture. *J Neurol Neurosurg Psychiatry* 51:105–108, 1988.
41. Haan J, Thomeer RTWM: Predictive value of temporary external lumbar drainage in normal pressure hydrocephalus. *Neurosurgery* 22:388–391, 1988.
42. Graff-Radford NR, Rezai K, Godersky JC, et al: Regional cerebral blood flow in normal pressure hydrocephalus. *J Neurol Neurosurg Psychiatry* 50:1589–1596, 1987.
43. Vanneste J, Augustijn P, Dirven C, et al: Shunting normal-pressure hydrocephalus: Do the benefits outweigh the risks? A multicenter study and literature review. *Neurology* 42:54–59, 1992.
44. Waters CH: Structural lesions and parkinsonism, in Stern MB, Koller WC (eds): *Parkinsonian Syndromes*. New York: Marcel Dekker, 1993, pp 137–144.
45. Comella CL: Bilateral striopallidodentate calcinosis, in Stern MB, Koller WC (eds): *Parkinsonian Syndromes*. New York: Marcel Dekker, 1993, pp 483–501.
46. Murphy MJ: Clinical correlations of CT scan-detected calcifications of the basal ganglia. *Ann Neurol* 6:507–511, 1979.
47. Brannan TS, Burger AA, Chaudhary MY: Bilateral basal ganglia calcification visualized on CT scan. *J Neurol Neurosurg Psychiatry* 40:403–406, 1980.
48. Okada J, Takeuchi K, Ohkado M, Hoshina K: Familial basal ganglia calcifications visualized by computed tomography. *Acta Neurol Scand* 64:273–279, 1981.
49. Sachs C, Sjoberg HE, Ericson K: Basal ganglia calcification on CT: Relation to hypoparathyroidism. *Neurology* 32:779–782, 1982.
50. Illum F, Dupont E: Prevalence of CT-detected calcification in the basal ganglia in idiopathic hypoparathyroidism and pseudohypoparathyroidism. *Neuroradiology* 27:32–37, 1985.
51. Muenter MD, Whisnant JP: Basal ganglia calcification, hypoparathyroidism, and extrapyramidal motor manifestations. *Neurology* 18:1075–1082, 1968.
52. Klawans HL, Lupton M, Simon L: Calcification of the basal ganglia as a cause of L-dopa-resistant parkinsonism. *Neurology* 26:221–225, 1976.
53. Granner MA, Wooten GF: Neuroleptic maligant syndrome or parkinsonism hyperpyrexia syndrome. *Semin Neurol* 11:228–234, 1991.
54. Buckley PF, Hutchinson M: Neuroleptic malignant syndrome. *J Neurol Neurosurg Psychiatry* 59:271–273, 1995.
55. Kurlan R, Hamill R, Shoulson I: Neuroleptic malignant syndrome. *Clin Neuropharmacol* 7:109–120, 1984.
56. Keck PE, Pope HG, McElroy SL: Declining frequency of neuroleptic malignant syndrome in a hospital population. *Am J Psychiatry* 148:880–882, 1991.
57. Caroff SN: The neuroleptic malignant syndrome. *J Clin Psychiatry* 41:79–83, 1980.
58. Guze BH, Baxter LR: Current concepts: Neuroleptic malignant syndrome. *N Engl J Med* 313:163–166, 1985.
59. Kirkpatrick B, Edelsohn GA: Risk factors for the neuroleptic malignant syndrome. *Psychiatr Med* 2:371–381, 1985.
60. Cohen WJ, Cohen NH: Lithium carbonate, haloperidol, and irreversible brain damage. *J Am Med Assoc* 230:1283–1287, 1974.
61. Friedman LS, Weinrauch LA, D'Elia JA: Metoclopramide-induced neuroleptic malignant syndrome. *Arch Intern Med* 147:1495–1497, 1987.
62. Mann SC, Caroff SN, Bleier HR, et al: Lethal catatonia. *Am J Psychiatry* 143:1374–1381, 1986.
63. Heiman-Patterson TD: Neuroleptic malignant syndrome and malignant hyperthermia. *Med Clin North Am* 71:477–492, 1993.
64. Sakkas P, Davis JM, Jancak PG, Wang Z: Drug treatment of the neuroleptic malignant syndrome. *Psychopharmacol Bull* 27:381–384, 1991.
65. Nisijima K, Ishiguro I: Does dantrolene influence central dopamine and serotonin metabolism in the neuroleptic malignant syndrome? A retrospective study. *Biol Psychiatry* 33:45–48, 1993.
66. Rosenberg MR, Green M: Neuroleptic malignant syndrome: Review of response to therapy. *Arch Intern Med* 149:1927–1931, 1989.
67. Davis JM, Janicak PG, Sakkas P, et al: Electroconvulsive therapy in the treatment of neuroleptic malignant syndrome. *Convulsive Therapy* 7:111–120, 1991.
68. Wells AJ, Sommi RW, Crismon ML: Neuroleptic rechallenge after neuroleptic malignant syndrome: Case report and literature review. *Drug Intelligence Clin Pharm* 22:475–480, 1988.

Chapter 26 _____

HEREDOFAMILIAL PARKINSONIAN SYNDROMES

ZBIGNIEW K. WSZOLEK and RONALD F. PFEIFFER

HISTORICAL BACKGROUND: PRE–L-DOPA ERA
KINDRED EVALUATIONS: L-DOPA ERA
    Kindreds with "Typical" IP Phenotype (Type I)
    Kindreds with PPS Phenotype (Type II)
    Kindreds with Neurodegenerative Phenotype and
        Some Parkinsonian Features (Type III)
SUMMARY

The possible role of genetic factors in the etiology of idiopathic parkinsonism (IP) and parkinsonism-plus syndromes (PPS) has received considerable attention.[1-3] Patients with IP display various combinations of bradykinesia, rigidity, rest tremor, and postural instability. Treatment with L-dopa alleviates their symptoms. To qualify as IP, there also should be no cerebellar or lower motor neuron deficits, no paresis of conjugate gaze beyond impaired upgaze, no autonomic failure, and no pyramidal dysfunction.[4] IP is a slowly progressive disorder with typical age of onset between the ages of 50 and 70, although younger-onset and even juvenile forms have also been identified.[5,6] Depigmentation of the substantia nigra and locus ceruleus is present on gross pathological examination. These abnormalities are substantiated under the microscope with the findings of pigmented neuronal loss, gliosis, and the presence of Lewy bodies in surviving neurons.[7] As defined, the etiology of IP is unknown (Chaps. 10 and 12). Environmental factors may be important, but genetic influences play an unquestionable role in recently described well-studied kindreds.

In specialized movement disorder clinics, up to 25 percent of patients presenting with parkinsonian features do not fit the IP definition because of identifiable causes, such as trauma, infections, tumors, strokes, medications, illicit drug use, or toxin exposure, or their parkinsonism is part of a well-defined PPS, such as progressive supranuclear palsy (Chap. 19), multiple-system atrophy (Chap. 20), Wilson's disease (Chap. 46), cortical basal ganglionic degeneration (Chap. 45), cerebellar disorders (Chaps. 43 and 44), and others.[8]

Patients affected with PPS are usually younger than those affected with IP. PPS patients' disease follows a more aggressive course, and death often occurs at a younger age. Treatment with L-dopa brings only minimal or no improvement in clinical symptoms. Affected patients may present with cardinal features of parkinsonism but, frequently, rest tremor is absent and rigidity is expressed more prominently in axial, rather than appendicular, muscles. Pyramidal signs, eye movement abnormalities, sensory disturbances, sphincter incontinence, autonomic dysfunction, respiratory difficulties, dementia, personality changes, depression, lower motor neuron involvement, and other signs frequently occur in PPS, either alone or in combination. Pathological findings of PPS also differ from those of IP. Neuronal loss and gliosis involve not only substantia nigra and locus ceruleus but also many other subcortical and brain stem nuclei, as well as cerebral and cerebellar cortices. The locus ceruleus, however, may be spared. Lewy bodies may not be present in surviving substantia nigra neurons or, alternatively, they may be widespread throughout the brain. Frequently, neurofibrillary tangles, senile plaques, amyloid deposits, and ballooned neurons are seen.[8]

There is also a group of PPS clearly hereditary in nature. These familial PPS are often difficult to classify fully at the present time, but with the explosion of genetic analysis, this will eventually be accomplished, and chromosomal abnormalities will be described. Review of the literature also indicates that extrapyramidal features, including cardinal parkinsonian signs, are frequently described in kindreds predominantly presenting with dementia, personality changes, amyotrophy, and dystonia. In fact, some believe that IP, Alzheimer's disease, and amyotrophic lateral sclerosis (ALS) have a common etiology.[9,10]

Historical Background: Pre–L-Dopa Era

Hereditary factors were not mentioned by James Parkinson in his monograph published in 1817.[11] However, in his 1888 classic textbook, Gowers stated that a hereditary basis may be "traced" in up to 15 percent of IP.[12] Bell and Clark, in a review of the literature in 1926, described 10 kindreds with "shaking palsy" believed to exist on a hereditary basis and provided 20 references of earlier accounts of familial paralysis agitans.[13] Allen, in 1937, detailed 25 kindreds with inherited parkinsonism and speculated that in approximately two-thirds of these kindreds, the inheritance was autosomal-dominant and the result of a "single autosomal gene."[14] Van Bogaert described in 1954 a kindred containing individuals with ALS, parkinsonism, or a combination of the two.[15] The extensive monograph of Mjönes in 1949 detailed eight pedigrees with inherited parkinsonism, some with atypical features.[16] In 1955, Biemond and Sinnege reported a multigeneration pedigree of young-onset atypical parkinsonism with six affected individuals and pathological findings that included nigral depigmentation, astrocytic gliosis, and "phagocytosing microglia."[17] A second, smaller kindred was reported by Biemond and Beck, also in 1955.[18] Šercl and Kovařík in 1963 reported several ALS kindreds, with extrapyramidal features noted in one of them.[19] Two additional pedigrees were initially described in the pre-L-dopa era but have been subsequently re-examined and are discussed below.[20,21]

Kindred Evaluations: L-Dopa Era

Review of the kindreds with parkinsonian features published since the introduction of L-dopa permits classification into three major categories, depending on clinical, pathological, and partly genealogical and genetic characteristics:

KINDREDS WITH "TYPICAL" IP PHENOTYPE (TYPE I)

Affected family members usually present with cardinal parkinsonian signs, such as bradykinesia, rigidity, postural instability, and rest tremor; L-dopa responsiveness is the rule. Autopsy material, when available, demonstrates the presence of neuronal loss, gliosis, and Lewy bodies in substantia nigra.

KINDREDS WITH PPS PHENOTYPE (TYPE II)

Affected family members usually display more than two, if not all, cardinal parkinsonian signs but with additional features such as amyotrophy, dementia, dystonia, ataxia, eye movement abnormalities, and others. L-dopa responsiveness is usually absent. Autopsy findings, when available, demonstrate rather generalized abnormalities with involvement not only of substantia nigra, locus ceruleus, and other brain stem nuclei but also cerebral cortex, thalamus, corpus striatum, hippocampus, and others. Lewy bodies (typical and atypical) may be absent, or they can be seen in widespread distribution. Neurofibrillary tangles, senile plaques, amyloid deposits, and ballooned neurons are also frequently present.

KINDREDS WITH NEURODEGENERATIVE PHENOTYPE AND SOME PARKINSONIAN FEATURES (TYPE III)

Affected members present with dementia, personality changes, amyotrophy, pyramidal signs, and dystonia occurring in combination or alone. However, review of these published kindreds indicates that extrapyramidal features, including one or more parkinsonian cardinal signs, are also frequently present. L-dopa responsiveness may not be discussed at all.

Autopsy findings, when available, may indicate substantia nigra involvement as part of the pathological picture. Lewy bodies, typical or atypical, may also been seen.

All three types of kindreds are summarized in Tables 26-1–26-3, which are constructed by the year of publication. Only papers with published pedigrees were considered for our review.

KINDREDS WITH "TYPICAL" IP PHENOTYPE (TYPE I)

A total of 16 kindreds have been described in 13 publications (Table 26-1) in which the clinical presentation consisted of more or less typical features of IP.[2,3,20,22–31] However, in 9 of the 16 kindreds no autopsy description is provided, and in an additional three, it was not possible to correlate the clinical and autopsy findings because of the manuscript format. Of the remaining four kindreds, all show the pathological features of neuronal loss, gliosis, and Lewy body formation in the substantia nigra, but in two of the kindreds, additional pathological features (widespread neurofibrillary tangles in one, widespread Lewy body formation in one) were present. Of the two remaining kindreds with typical autopsy-proven pathology, the extensive Contoursi kindred described by Golbe et al.[23] is characterized clinically by typical IP features,

but without rest tremor and with a relatively young age of onset and unusually rapid course. Thus, data about only one kindred have been published to date in which both pathological and clinical features are fully compatible with sporadic IP.[31] Longitudinal clinical observations and follow-up investigations are planned on this family. It may well be that with accumulation of additional information, even this kindred will be reclassified. In none of these kindreds has the abnormal gene been identified at the time of this writing, although some candidate genes (GPX1, TH, BDNF, CAT, APP, SOD1, CYP2D6) have been excluded in two of the kindreds.[32]

KINDREDS WITH PPS PHENOTYPE (TYPE II)

Forty-six kindreds have been described that fit this category and are listed in Table 26-2.[3,21,28,33–71] Families in this category develop clinical features of parkinsonism but also a variety of other neurological abnormalities. Therefore, they can be sub-classified according to these nonparkinsonian features, although this type of subclassification is somewhat artificial, because overlapping features frequently exist, and kindreds may display multiple nonparkinsonian findings. Widespread pathological abnormalities—with or without Lewy body formation—are also characteristic of this group of kindreds.

PPS—AMYOTROPHY

Five kindreds have been reported with predominant parkinsonism, in which amyotrophy was also noted.[3,28,34,44,47,68,69] The parkinsonism was characterized by bradykinesia and rigidity in all kindreds, but typical parkinsonian rest tremor was also described in three of the five families. Only one kindred, however, displayed consistent L-dopa responsiveness. A variety of other nonparkinsonian features were described in these kindreds (Table 26-2). Adequate autopsy information is available in only three of the kindreds; depigmentation, gliosis, and neuronal loss in the substantia nigra were present in each kindred, but Lewy body formation was observed in only one. Axonal spheroids in anterior horn cells were described in two of the kindreds. An autosomal-dominant inheritance pattern was present in three of the five kindreds; in the other two, an autosomal-recessive mode was suspected.

PPS—DEMENTIA

In all, 11 kindreds with predominant parkinsonism have also displayed progressive dementia as a part of the clinical picture.[21,33,35,36,39,44,49,51,53,60,61,65,68,69,71] The parkinsonism was characterized by bradykinesia in all 11 kindreds and rigidity in 10 of 11, and rest tremor was present in five kindreds. L-dopa responsiveness was noted in three kindreds, only one of which displayed rest tremor. Once again, a variety of other nonparkinsonian features was present in these kindreds, including amyotrophy in two (Table 26-2). Neuronal loss and gliosis were described in the substantia nigra in all 10 kindreds in which autopsy results were reported. Lewy bodies were present in six kindreds; they were limited to brain stem nuclei in three kindreds, and were widespread in both brain stem and cerebrum in three kindreds. Neurofibrillary tangles, senile plaques, ballooned neurons, amyloid plaques, and spongiform changes, occurring alone or in combination,

TABLE 26-1 Kindreds with "Typical" IP Phenotype (Type I)*

First Author/ Year of Publication	No. of Affected Generations	Mode of Inheritance	Atypical Features	Autopsy Findings
Branger[20]/1956, Otto[22+]/ 1983	5	AD	None	None
Golbe et al.[23]/1990	4	AD	Relatively young onset, no rest tremor, rapid course	LBs in SN, LC, NL, and GL of SN, LC, and NB
Mauri et al.[24]/1990	4	AD	None	None
Maraganore et al.[25]/1991				
Kindred a	4	AD	None	None
Kindred b	3	AD	None	None
Sawle et al.[26]/1992 Irish kindred	1	Unknown	Relatively young onset, postural tremor	None
Petelin[27]/1993	3	AD	None	None
Wszolek et al.[3,28**]/1993/ 1995				
Family B	3	AD	Dementia, dementia alone	NL, GL, and LBs in SN, widespread neurofibrillary tangles, and senile plaques
Family C	3	AD	None	None
Waters and Miller[29]/1994	5	AD	Young onset, rapid course	NL and LBs in SN, HC, and neocortex
Lazzarini et al.[2]/1994				Unable to correlate clinical and autopsy findings because of the manuscript format
Family I	3	AD	None	
Family II	3	AD	None	
Family III	2	Probably AD	None	
Bonifati et al.[30]/1994	3	Probably AD	None	None
Wszolek et al.[3,31**]/1995 Family D	4	AD	None	NL, GL and LBs in SN
Denson and Wszolek[3]/1995 Family F	2	Probably AD	Dementia	None

*, affected family members present with cardinal parkinsonian features. +, initial report by Branger with follow-up investigations performed by Otto.
**, description of the same family. AD, autosomal dominant inheritance; LB, Lewy body; SN, substantia nigra; LC, locus ceruleus; NL, neuronal loss; GL, gliosis; NB, nucleus basalis of Meynert; HC, hippocampus.

were seen in seven of the kindreds. Eight families displayed an autosomal-dominant inheritance pattern; in two an autosomal-recessive pattern was suspected, and in one the pattern of inheritance was unclear.

PPS—PSYCHIATRIC DISTURBANCES

In all, 14 kindreds with predominant parkinsonism in which psychiatric dysfunction also developed have been described.[35–38,40–43,50–52,55–57,59–61,63,65,68,69] Depression was present in eight of the kindreds, manic-depressive illness in two, psychosis in two, and personality changes in four. In one kindred both depression and personality changes were described. Bradykinesia was present in all 14 kindreds, rigidity in 13, and rest tremor in 8. L-dopa responsiveness was noted in 5 of the 14 kindreds; each of these displayed rest tremor. In four of the five L-dopa-responsive kindreds the associated psychiatric disturbance was depression. As with the previous subgroups, a variety of other nonparkinsonian features was identified in these kindreds. Autopsy information was available in 10 of the 14 kindreds. Depigmentation, neuronal loss, and gliosis were present in the substantia nigra of all 10. Lewy bodies were present in six kindreds, confined to brain stem structures in four and widespread in two. Ballooned neurons were described in two kindreds and spongiform changes in one, but neurofibrillary tangles and senile plaques were not described in any of these kindreds. Thirteen of the kindreds displayed an autosomal-dominant inheritance pattern; in one an autosomal-recessive pattern was suspected.

PPS—DYSTONIA

In six kindreds with predominant parkinsonism, dystonia was also described as part of the clinical picture.[48,53,54,60–62,70] Bradykinesia and rigidity were present in all kindreds but rest tremor in only two. Rest tremor did not predict L-dopa responsiveness. As with other subgroups, a variety of other nonparkinsonian features was also described (Table 26-2). Autopsy descriptions were noted in only two kindreds; nei-

TABLE 26-2 Kindreds with PPS Phenotype (Type II)*

First Author/Year of Publication	No. of Affected Generations	No. of Affected Individuals (Male:Female)	Mode of Inheritance	Mean Age Of Onset (Years)	Cardinal Parkinsonian Features	Additional Features	Autopsy Findings
Spellman[21]/1962, Muenter et al.[33+]/1986	4	12(8:4)	AD	20-30	B, R, RT, PI	Ataxia, seizures, dementia, dysarthria, rapid weight loss	NL, GL and LBs in limbic areas and pigmented nuclei of brain stem
Ziegler et al.[34]/1972	4	31(18:13)	AD	42	B, R, RT	Ataxia, fasciculations, muscle wasting, postural tremor, pyramidal signs, sensory changes, dysarthria, nystagmus, variable response to L-dopa	Normal SN in one affected patient who did not display parkinsonian signs
Perry, et al.[35,36*]/1975 and 1990	3	8(6:2)	AD	45-50	B, RT	Depression, dementia, hypoventilation, weight loss, sleep disorders, no response to L-dopa	Depigmentation, NL, GL, and rare LBs in SN
Purdy et al.[37]/1979	3	5(3:2)	AD	40s	B, R	Depression, apathy, lethargy, hypoventilation, weight loss, postural tremor, dysphagia, no response to L-dopa	Depigmentation, NL GL, and scarce LBs in SN; NL and GL of BG; GL of medulla
Tune et al.[38]/1982	3	5(3:2)	AD	60s	B, R, RT, PI, LD-R	Manic-depressive illness	None
Mata et al.[39]/1983	1	3(2:1)	Unknown	20s	B, R, PI	Dementia, ophthalmoparesis, pyramidal signs, kyphoscoliosis, dysphagia, postural tremor but no RT, no response to L-dopa therapy	Depigmentation, NL, GL, NFTs in SN and LC; LBs and NFTs in HC and brain stem nuclei
Roy et al.[40]/1983 Barbeau et al.[41]/1984 Barbeau and Roy[42]/1984 Barbeau[43*]/1986							
Pedigree 002	3	6(5:1)	AD	Unknown	Akinetic parkinsonism only in 1 patient	Essential tremor	None
Pedigree 007	4	7(4:3)	AD	Unknown	"Mixed" parkinsonism only in 1 patient	Essential tremor, thyroidopathy	None
Pedigree 023	2	5(0:5)	Unkown (pseudo-dominant?)	Unknown	B, R	Severe parkinsonism	None
Pedigree 026	1	2(0:2)	AR	Unknown	B, R	Rapid progression, no RT	None
Pedigree 029	1	2(2:0)	AR	Unknown	B, R	Essential tremor	None
Pedigree 301	4	6(5:1)	AD	Unknown	B, R	Essential tremor, depressive illness	None
Pedigree 309	1	2(2:0)	AR	Unknown	B, R	No RT	None
Pedigree 315	3	3(1:2)	AD	Unknown	"Mixed" parkinsonism only in 1 patient	Essential tremor	None

Reference/Year		No. (M:F)	Inheritance	Onset age	Signs	Clinical features	Neuropathology
Pedigree DCD-2	4	9(4:5)	AR	Unknown	B, R	Essential tremor, Gaucher's disease	None
Schmitt et al.[44]/1984	2	10(6:4)	Unclear (AR?)	50	B, R, RT	Dementia, amyotrophy, pyramidal signs, dysphagia, dysarthria, unknown if responsive to L-dopa	NL, GL in SN, no LBs; diffuse cortical NL; NFTs in LC, SN, substantia innominata; NL and axonal spheroids in anterior horn cells
Laxova et al.[45] 1985, Gregg et al.[46,100] 1991 Pedigree	3	14(13:1)	X-linked recessive	10s	B, R, RT, PI	Mental retardation, frontal lobe release, signs, seizures, choreoathetosis strabismus, no response to L-dopa	None
Spitz et al.[47] 1985	1	2(2:0)	Unclear (AR?)	24.5	B, R, PI	Tourettism, amyotrophy, dysarthria, dysphagia, vertical gaze paresis, acanthocytosis, atypical tremor, no response to L-dopa	None
Nygaard and Duvoisin[48] 1986	5	12(5:7)	AD	9	B, R, PI, LD-R	Lower limb and axial dystonia, spinal scoliosis, frontal lobe release signs, dysarthria, "jerky" ocular pursuit, nystagmus, postural tremor	None
Giménez-Roldán et al.[49]/1986	2	4(1:3)	Probably AD	68	B, R, PI, LD-R	Dementia, dementia alone, no RT	NL, GL, and few LBs in SN; NL and GL in HC, parahippocampal gyrus, and neocortex; abundant NFTs in amygdala, HC, and parahippocampal gyrus
Roy et al.[50]/1988	2	6(3:3)	Probably AD	50	B, R, RT, PI, LD-R	Depression, lethargy, weight loss, hypoventilation	NL, GL in SN, no LBs
Inose, et al.[51]/1988	3	4(0:4)	AD	37	B, R, RT, PI, LD-R	Dementia, psychosis, myoclonus, generalized seizures, eye movement abnormalities, pyramidal signs, urinary incontinence, rapid course, young onset	Depigmentation and NL in SN; NL, GL, typical and atypical LBs in cerebral cortex, HC, amygdala, striatum, claustrum, NB, hypothalamus, LC, dorsal vagal nucleus; ballooned neurons in widespread distribution
Degl'Innocenti et al.[52]/1989	2	8(4:4)	Probably AD	57	B, R, RT, LD-R	Anxiety, depression, postural tremor, syncope	None
Rosenberg et al.[53]/1989	5	14(4:10)	AD	40s	B, R, RT, PI	Dementia, dystonia, progressive speech impairment, pyramidal signs, no response to L-dopa	Depigmentation of SN; extracellular hyaline eosinophillic, congophillic amyloid plaques in cerebral cortex, basal ganglia, thalmus, SN; atrophy and GL of SN; no LBs

TABLE 26-2—(continued)

First Author/ Year of Publication	No. of Affected Generations	No. of Affected Individuals (Male : Female)	Mode of Inheritance	Mean Age Of Onset (Years)	Cardinal Parkinsonian Features	Additional Features	Autopsy Findings
Ishikawa et al.[54]/1990	3	7(3:4)	AR	23	B, R, PI, LD-R	Dystonia, nystagmus, brisk deep tendon reflexes, postural tremor	None
Sage, et al.[55]/ 1990 Duvoisin[56]/ 1991 Nova Scotia Family	2	15(3:12)	Probably AD	69	B, R, PI	Depression, myoclonus, oligosymptomatic individuals included, no RT, no response to L-dopa	Depigmentation, NL, GL and LBs in SN; LBs in hypothalamus; GL and LBs in NB
Takei et al.[57]/ 1990	2	6(3:3)	Unclear (AR?)	39	B, R, PI	Manic-depressive illness, psychosis, L-dopa response not discussed	None
Tanaka et al.[58]/ 1991 Family 1 Family 2 Family 3 Family 4 Family 5 Family 6 Family 7	1 1 1 1 1 1 1	2(2:0) 1(0:1) 1(0:1) 3(1:2) 1(0:1) 2(0:2) 1(0:1)	Unknown (AR?) for all families	In 30s for all families	Unable to determine because of the paper presentation	Unable to determine because of the paper presentation	None
Lechevalier et al.[59]/1992	2	5(2:3)	Probably AD	51.5	B, R, RT, PI, LD-R	Central respiratory disorder, personality changes, insomnia, anxiety, apathia, depression, anorexia	NL in SN, LC, dorsal motor nucleus of vagus nerve, nucleus of the tractus solitarius, striatum, pallidum, and frontal cortex; no LBs
Wszolek et al.[60]/ 1992; Wszolek and Pfeiffer[61]**/ 1993 PPND Family	4	34(14:20)	AD	43	B, R, PI	Personality changes, dementia, dysarthria, pyramidal signs, eye movement abnormalities, eyelid opening and closing apraxia, weight loss, dysphagia, dystonia, mutism, urinary incontinence, sensory impairment, no rest tremor, rapid course, no response to L-dopa	Depigmentation, NL, and GL in SN; NL and GL in subcortical cerebral white matter, HC, entorhinal cortex, amygdala, caudate nucleus, globus pallidus, putamen, mesencephalic/pontine tegmentum, and subthalamic nucleus; no LBs
Dobyns et al.[62]/ 1993	3	14(10:4)	AD	23	B, R, PI	Dystonia, rapid progression, oculogyric crisis, no rest tremor, minimal response to L-dopa	None
Bhatia et al.[63]/ 1993	3	8(4:4)	AD	30s–40s	B, R, RT, PI	Severe depression, depression alone, rapid course, short response to L-dopa	Depigmentation, NL and GL in SN and LC; LBs in SN
Golbe et al.[64]/ 1993	5	7(2:5)	AD	29	B, R, RT, PI	Subjective visual difficulties, myoclonus, encephalopathy, poor response to L-dopa	Depigmentation, NL, GL, and LBs in SN, LC, and NB

Reference/year	No. of families	Inheritance	Affected family members	Parkinsonian features	Clinical description	Neuropathology
Mizutani et al.[65]/1993	3	AD	6(2:4)	B, R, RT, PI	Personality changes, sexual delinquency, delusions, dementia, myoclonus, marked orthostatic hypotension with reactive tachycardia, syncope, dysphagia, postural tremor, pyramidal signs, generalized convulsions, urinary incontinence	Depigmentation, NL, GL, and ballooned neurons in SN and LC; NL, GL, and ballooned neurons also in cerebral cortex, amygdala, parahippocampal gyrus, hypothalamus, dorsal vagal nucleus, NB; few LBs in LC, dorsal vagal nucleus, and Edinger-Westphal nucleus
Wszolek et al.[3,28]/1993 and 1995 Family A	3	AD	7(4:3)	B, R, RT, PI, LD-R	Amyotrophy	Depigmentation, NL, GL, and LBs in SN, widespread SPs and NFTs, enlarged axonal spheroids in anterior horn cells of spinal cord
Yamamura et al.[66]/1993 Family MS	1	Unknown	3(0:3)	"Parkinsonism", LD-R	Marked diurnal fluctuation of symptoms	Marked depigmentation and NL in SN, no LBs; NL in LC and ventral tegmental area
Nisipeanu et al.[67]/1994 Family I	1	Unknown	2(1:1)	B, R, RT, PI, LD-R	Spasticity	None
Family II	1	Unknown	2(2:0)	B, R, RT, PI, LD-R	Spasticity	None
Lynch et al.[68]/1994; Wilhelmsen et al.[69]/1994 Family Mo/DDPAC	3	AD	13(4:9)	B, R, PI	Personality changes, dementia, amyotrophy, pyramidal signs, slow saccades, no response to L-dopa	Depigmentation, NL and GL in SN, no LBs, spongiform changes in frontotemporal corticis
Sasaki et al.[70]/1994	2	Probably AD	4(2:2)	B, R, RT, PI, LD-R	Foot dystonia, marked diurnal fluctuations in some affected patients	None
Najim Al-Din et al.[71]/1994	1	Uncertain (AR?)	5(4:1)	B, R, PI, LD-R	Dementia, supranuclear upgaze paresis, anarthria, pyramidal signs, no rest tremor	None

*, affected family members present with at least two cardinal parkinsonian features (except pedigree 007, see Ref. 38; only RT seen). +, both reports are on the same family, as discussed in Ref. 60; **, description of the same family. AD, autosomal dominant inheritance; RT, rest tremor; GL, gliosis; BG, basal ganglia; AR, autosomal-recessive inheritance; NFT, neurofibrillary tangles; B, bradykinesia; PI, postural instability; LB, Lewy body; HC, hippocampus; LD-R, L-dopa responsiveness; R, rigidity; NL, neuronal loss; SN, substantia nigra; SP, senile plaques; NB, nucleus basalis of Meynart.

TABLE 26-3 Kindreds with Neurodegenerative Phenotype and Some Parkinsonian Features*

First Author/ Year of Publication	No. of Affected Generations	Mode of Inheritance	Predominant Clinical Features	Comment: Parkinsonian Features with Autopsy Findings
Moya et al.[73]/1969 Family URC	2	Unknown	Amyotrophy, anal incontinence	Possibly postural instability; depigmentation, NL and GL in SN; lesions in anterior horn cells, medulla oblongata, corpus Luysii, pallidum and fasciculus gracilis
Arnould et al.[74]/1972	2	Probably AD	Amyotrophy	No clinical signs of PD, but on autopsy NL and GL in SN were noted
Finlayson et al.[75]/1973	2	Probably AD	Amyotrophy, dementia, personality changes	No clinical signs of parkinsonism, but in one autopsied patient, eosinophilic cytoplasmic inclusion believed to be an atypical LB was found in SN and LC
Alter and Schaumann[76]/1976 M Family	2	Probably AD	Amyotrophy, dementia, sensory deficits, sphincter incontinence	Rigidity and rest tremor were observed in 3 patients; depigmentation of SN in one autopsy; no LBs
Lee et al.[77]/1976				
Family 10	2	X-linked recessive	Dystonia	Rest tremor, relatives with parkinsonism in both families
Family 11	2	X-linked recessive	Dystonia	
Additional references pertinent to x-linked dystonia-parkinsonism, lubag disease[78-87+]	1–4	X-linked recessive (Xq12– Xq13.1)	Dystonia and parkinsonism (bradykinesia, rigidity, rest tremor, postural instability and, in some affected patients, positive response to L-dopa)	Normal SN; NL and GL in caudate and lateral putamen; no LBs
Allen and Knopp[88**]/1976	3	AD	Childhood onset of dystonia with later development of parkinsonism	Rigidity, bradykinesia, rest tremor, postural instability, marked improvement with L-dopa
Segawa et al.[90#]/1976			Progressive dystonia with marked diurnal fluctuation	Parkinsonian features such as rigidity, rest tremor, mask-like face, frozen gait, propulsion, marked improvement with L-dopa therapy
Family T	1	Unknown (AD?)		
Family AS	3	AD		
Family S	1	Unknown (AD?)		
Additional references pertinent to dopa-responsive dystonia, Segawa disease[89,92-101]		AD with sex-related, reduced penetrance mapped to 14q22.1–q22.2		
Kim et al.[102]/1981	1	Unknown	Dementia, personality changes, sphincter incontinence	Rigidity, mask-like facial expressions, shuffling gait in 3 of 5 affected patients, depigmentation of SN seen in 1 of 3 autopsies
Khoubesserian et al.[103]/1985	1	Unknown	Dementia	Rigidity, postural instability, rest tremor; no autopsy but biopsy showed swelling of astrocytes and subcortical gliosis
Jankovic et al.[104]/1985	1	Unknown	Dementia, rigidity, bradykinesia, mild tremor, dystonia, blepharospasm, eyelid opening apraxia, anarthria, sphincter incontinence	Family has been regarded as a late-onset Hallervorden-Spatz disease with parkinsonism. On autopsy generalized brain atrophy, iron deposits in globus pallidus, caudate and SN. No LBs

TABLE 26-3—(continued)

First Author/ Year of Publication	No. of Affected Generations	Mode of Inheritance	Predominant Clinical Features	Comment: Parkinsonian Features with Autopsy Findings
Constantinidis[105]/1987	3	AD	Dementia, personality changes, depression, amyotrophy, pyramidal signs, mutism	Rigidity seen in at least one affected individual; depigmentation, NL, GL, and LBs in SN; NL, GL in frontotemporal gyri and pallidum; ALS lesions in medulla oblongata and the spinal cord; ballooned cells present; no SPs or NFTs
Bird et al.[106,107]/1988 and 1989				
Family R	4	AD	Dementia	Rigidity; pyramidal and frontal lobe release signs; stimulus-induced myoclonus; diffuse cortical SPs and NFTs
Family L	3	AD	Dementia	Sparse NFTs in SN; striatal NL and GL
Family W	2	Probably AD	Dementia	Rigidity; NL and GL in SN
Family T	2	Probably AD	Dementia	Increased muscle tone and hand tremor; LBs in SN and LC
Family BK	3	AD	Dementia, personality changes	Rigidity, rest tremor, and mutism; a few NFTs in SN
Nygaard et al.[108]/1990 Family S	4	AD	Dystonia	Definite parkinsonism in 5 affected patients
Lanska et al.[109]/1994			Personality changes, dementia, mutism, Klüver-Bucy syndrome seen in both families	Extrapyramidal signs present in both families; autopsy performed on 7 patients from both families: depigmentation, NL and GL of SN, no LBs
Family A	4	AD		
Family B	3	AD		
Campion et al.[110]/1995	5	AD Genetic marker on chromosome 14q124.3	Dementia, depression, myoclonus, generalized tonic-clonic seizures	Rigidity, stooped posture, bradykinesia but no rest tremor in almost all patients, but most of them treated with neuroleptics; on autopsy, severe cortical atrophy; frequent SPs and NFTs in neocortex and HC; no LBs

*, affected family members present predominantly with dementia, personality changes, amyotrophic lateral sclerosis, and dystonia. However, detailed analysis of this published pedigree indicates the presence of extrapyramidal features, frequently including one or more parkinsonian cardinal signs. +, only papers with published pedigrees are cited. **, additional proband description in Ref. 89. #, earlier description in Ref. 91. NL, neuronal loss; HC, hippocampus; GL, gliosis; SN, substantia nigra; AD, autosomal-dominant inheritance pattern; LB, Lewy body; LC, locus ceruleus; ALS, amyotrophic lateral sclerosis; SP, senile plaques; NFT, neurofibrillary tangles.

ther demonstrated Lewy bodies. An autosomal-dominant pattern was present in five kindreds, an autosomal-recessive pattern in one.

PPS—EYE MOVEMENT ABNORMALITIES

In all, 12 kindreds displayed a variety of eye movement or visual difficulties, including vertical-gaze paresis, strabismus, nystagmus, "jerky" ocular pursuit, apraxia of eyelid opening and closing, oculogyric crisis, slow saccades, and "visual difficulties" of an unspecified nature.[34,39,45-48,51,54,60-62,64,68,69,71] The most frequently described abnormalities were vertical-gaze paresis and nystagmus. All kindreds displayed bradykinesia and rigidity. Only 4 of the 12 demonstrated rest tremor; 1 of these was L-dopa responsive. The other three L-dopa-responsive kindreds did not possess rest tremor as a charac-

teristic. Pathological material was published in only 6 of the 12 kindreds. Lewy bodies were described in three, confined to the brain stem in one and widespread in the other two. A recessive inheritance pattern was identified in four kindreds (three autosomal; one x-linked), an autosomal-dominant pattern was noted in seven; and in one the pattern of inheritance was unclear.

PPS—POSTURAL TREMOR

Postural tremor in a clinical setting characterized predominantly by parkinsonism was described in 13 kindreds.[34,37,39-43,48,52,54,65] Bradykinesia and rigidity were present in all kindreds whereas rest tremor was seen in three kindreds and did not necessarily correlate with L-dopa responsiveness. Autopsy material was available in only 3 of the 13 kindreds;

Lewy bodies were confined to the brain stem in 2 and more widespread in 1. Nine of the kindreds displayed an autosomal-dominant inheritance pattern, three were presumed to be autosomal-recessive, and in one the pattern could not be determined.

PPS—MYOCLONUS/SEIZURES

Six kindreds contained either myoclonus or seizures as part of their clinical spectrum but within a predominantly parkinsonian framework.[21,33,45,46,51,55,56,64,65] Bradykinesia and rigidity were characteristic of all six kindreds. Rest tremor was present in five of the six families, but only one of the six kindreds displayed L-dopa responsiveness. Autopsy examinations were performed in five kindreds. Lewy bodies were present in all kindreds and extended beyond brain stem structures in four of the five. Ballooned neurons were described in two kindreds. Five kindreds displayed an autosomal-dominant pattern; one showed an x-linked recessive pattern.

PPS—RESPIRATORY ABNORMALITIES

Four kindreds displayed a combination of depression, hypoventilation, and parkinsonism.[35–37,50,59] All displayed bradykinesia, and three of the four were characterized by rest tremor. L-dopa responsiveness was present in two kindreds; both displayed rest tremor. Lewy bodies were present in the brain stem in two kindreds; they were not seen in the other two. An autosomal-dominant inheritance pattern was present in all four kindreds.

PPS—MISCELLANEOUS ABNORMALITIES

A variety of other neurological features have been described in these kindreds. These include ataxia, pyramidal signs, choreoathetosis, tourettism, sleep disorders, dysarthria, dysphagia, anorexia, mutism, urinary incontinence, scoliosis, sensory abnormalities, and "encephalopathy." However, they have not been described in a sufficient number of kindreds to allow further characterization.

GENETIC STUDIES OF PPS

Genetic studies have been performed on some of the 46 kindreds in this heterogeneous group of disorders. The specific genetic abnormality has been identified in two kindreds: the disinhibition-dementia-parkinsonism-amyotrophy complex (family Mo/DDPAC) described by Lynch et al.[68] and Wilhelmsen et al.[69] and pallidopontonigral degeneration (PPND family) described by Wszolek et al.[60] and Wszolek and Pfeiffer.[61] The abnormal gene is located on chromosome 17q21-22 in both families, but most likely there are two different mutations (Wilhelmsen and Arwert, personal communication). Genetic studies in another kindred (family A) have examined seven candidate genes,[32,72] without positive findings and studies in yet another kindred have excluded DYT1 as a candidate gene in this family.[62]

KINDREDS WITH NEURODEGENERATIVE PHENOTYPE AND SOME PARKINSONIAN FEATURES (TYPE III)

A number of other kindreds have been published in the neurological literature that are characterized primarily by such neurodegenerative features as dementia, personality changes, ALS, or dystonia, but which also may include some parkinsonian signs as a part of the clinical syndrome. These kindreds are summarized in Table 26-3.[73–110] Some of these kindreds, such as X-linked dystonia-parkinsonism, lubag disease,[77–87] and dopa-responsive dystonia (Segawa's disease),[89–101] have been extensively characterized clinically and their genetic basis identified.

Summary

A daunting array of published kindreds confronts the clinician examining familial parkinsonian syndromes. Classification of the published kindreds is a most difficult task, and the one presented in this chapter is far from ideal. No clear-cut pathological patterns that might allow a meaningful anatomic classification are evident; a clinical classification format is compromised by considerable overlap of neurological features between kindreds. Moreover, phenotypes may also vary within kindreds themselves. Ultimately, order may come to the classification of familial parkinsonian syndromes as specific genetic abnormalities are identified.

It is clear, however, that the vast majority of currently described familial parkinsonian syndromes deviate significantly in their clinical and pathological characteristics from the typical features of sporadic IP. What implications these differences have for the question of an environmental-versus-genetic basis for sporadic IP is not clear, but further study of additional kindreds—and reexamination of previously described kindreds—is clearly warranted.

The frequent coexistence of parkinsonism, dementia, and motor neuron disease in the kindreds described in this chapter reinforces the suggestion by Calne and Eisen[9] that some common mechanism—genetic or otherwise—links the neuronal degeneration seen in each of these processes. As our knowledge of the specific genetic basis of these various familial syndromes expands, the solution to this riddle may also become clear.

References

1. Duvoisin RC: Research on the genetics of Parkinson's disease: Will it lead to the cause and a cure, in Stern MB (ed): *Beyond the Decade of the Brain*. Chapel Place, UK: Wells Medical Limited, 1994, pp 95–108.
2. Lazzarini AM, Myers RH, Zimmerman Jr TR, et al: A clinical genetic study of Parkinson's disease: Evidence for dominant transmission. *Neurology* 44:499–506, 1994.
3. Denson MA, Wszolek ZK: Familial parkinsonism: Our experience and review. *Parkinsonism Related Disord* 1:1–8, 1995.
4. Calne DB: Is idiopathic parkinsonism the consequence of an event or a process? *Neurology* 44:5–10, 1994.
5. Stern MB, Koller WC: Parkinson's disease, in Stern MB, Koller WC (eds): *Parkinsonian Syndromes*. New York: Marcel Dekker, 1993, pp 9–11.
6. Muthane UB, Swamy HS, Satishchandra P, et al: Early onset Parkinson's disease: Are juvenile and young-onset different? *Mov Disord* 9:539–544, 1994.

7. Fearnley J, Lees A: Pathology of Parkinson's disease, in Calne DB (ed): *Neurodegenerative Diseases*. Philadelphia: W.B. Saunders, 1994, pp 545–554.

8. Jankovic J: Parkinsonism-plus syndromes. *Mov Disord* 4(suppl 1):S95–S119, 1989.

9. Calne DB, Eisen A: The relationship between Alzheimer's disease, Parkinson's disease and motor neuron disease. *Can J Neurol Sci* 16:547–550, 1989.

10. Uitti RJ, Calne DB: Pathogenesis of idiopathic parkinsonism. *Eur Neurol* 33(suppl 1):6–23, 1993.

11. Parkinson J: *An Essay on the Shaking Palsy*. London: Whittingham and Rowland for Sherwood, Neely and Jones, 1817.

12. Gowers WR: *Diseases of the Nervous System*. Philadelphia: P. Blakiston, Son & Co, 1988, pp 996.

13. Bell J, Clark AJ: A pedigree of paralysis agitans. *Ann Eugenics* 1:455–462, 1926.

14. Allen W: Inheritance of the shaking palsy. *Arch Intern Med* 60:424–436, 1937.

15. Van Bogaert L, Radermecker MA: Scléroses latérales amyotrophiques typiques et paralysies agitantes héréditaires, dans une même famille, avec une forme de passage possible entre les deux affections. *Mschr Psychiatr Neurol* 127:185–203, 1954.

16. Mjönes H: Paralysis agitans: A clinical and genetic study. *Acta Psychiatr Neurol Scand* (suppl 54):1–195, 1949.

17. Biemond A, Sinnege JLM: Tabes of Friedreich with degeneration of the substantia nigra, a special type of hereditary parkinsonism. *Confin Neurol* 15:129–142, 1955.

18. Biemond A, Beck W: Neural muscle atrophy with degeneration of the substantia nigra. *Confin Neurol* 15:142–153, 1955.

19. Šercl M, Kovařík J: On the familial incidence of amyotrophic lateral sclerosis. *Acta Neurol Scand* 39:169–176, 1963.

20. Branger F: Une forme familiale de paralysie agitante dans une souche des grisons. *J Genet Hum* 5:261–270, 1956.

21. Spellman GG: Report of familial cases of parkinsonism. *J Am Med Assoc* 372–374, Feb. 3, 1962.

22. Otto FG: Ein beitrag zu familiär gehäuft auftretenden fällen von parkinsonismus. *Nervenarzt* 54:423–425, 1983.

23. Golbe LI, DiIorio G, Bonavita V, et al: A large kindred with autosomal dominant Parkinson's disease. *Ann Neurol* 27:276–282, 1990.

24. Mauri JA, Asensio M, Jiménez A, et al: Enfermedad de parkinson familiar. *Neurologia* 5:45–47, 1990.

25. Maraganore DM, Harding AE, Marsden CD: A clinical and genetic study of familial Parkinson's disease. *Mov Disord* 6:205–211, 1991.

26. Sawle GV, Wroe SJ, Lees AJ, et al: The identification of presymptomatic parkinsonism: Clinical and [^{18}F] dopa positron emission tomography studies in an Irish kindred. *Ann Neurol* 32:609–617, 1992.

27. Petelin LS: Clinical aspects and treatment of parkinsonism. *Neurology* 43;2(suppl 1):9, 1993.

28. Wszolek ZK, Cordes M, Calne DB, et al: Hereditärer morbus parkinson: Bericht über drei familien mit autosomal-dominantem Ebgang. *Nervenarzt* 64:331–335, 1993.

29. Waters CH, Miller CA: Autosomal dominant Lewy body parkinsonism in a four-generation family. *Ann Neurol* 35:59–64, 1994.

30. Bonifati V, Vanacore N, Meco, G: Anticipation of onset age of familial Parkinson's disease. *Neurology* 44:1978–1979, 1994.

31. Wszolek ZK, Pfeiffer B, Fulgham JR, et al: Western Nebraska family (family D) with autosomal dominant parkinsonism. *Neurology* 45:502–505, 1995.

32. Gasser T, Wszolek ZK, Trofatter J, et al: Genetic linkage studies in autosomal dominant parkinsonism: Evaluation of seven candidate genes. *Ann Neurol* 36:387–396, 1994.

33. Muenter MD, Howard FM Jr, Okazaki H, et al: A familial parkinson-dementia syndrome. *Neurology* 36(suppl 1):115, 1986.

34. Ziegler DK, Schimke RN, Kepes JJ, et al: Late onset ataxia, rigidity and peripheral neuropathy. *Arch Neurol* 27:52–66, 1972.

35. Perry TL, Bratty PJA, Hansen S, et al: Hereditary mental depression and parkinsonism with taurine deficiency. *Arch Neurol* 32:108–113, 1975.

36. Perry TL, Wright JM, Berry K, et al: Dominantly inherited apathy, central hypoventilation, and Parkinson's syndrome: Clinical, biochemical, and neuropathologic studies of 2 new cases. *Neurology* 40:1882–1887, 1990.

37. Purdy A, Hahn A, Barnett HJM, et al: Familial fatal parkinsonism with alveolar hypoventilation and mental depression. *Ann Neurol* 6:523–531, 1979.

38. Tune LE, Folstein M, Rabins P, et al: Familial manic-depressive illness and familial Parkinson's disease: A case report. *Johns Hopkins Med J* 151:65–70, 1982.

39. Mata M, Dorovin-Zis K, Wilson M, Young AB: New form of familial parkinson-dementia syndrome: Clinical and pathologic findings. *Neurology* 33:1439–1443, 1983.

40. Roy M, Boyer L, Barbeau A: A prospective study of 50 cases of familial Parkinson's disease. *Can J Neurol Sci* 10:37–42, 1983.

41. Barbeau A, Roy M, Boyer L: Genetic studies in Parkinson's disease. *Adv Neurol* 40:333–339, 1984.

42. Barbeau A, Roy M: Familial subsets in idiopathic Parkinson's disease. *Can J Neurol Sci* 11:144–150, 1984.

43. Barbeau A: Parkinson's disease: Clinical features and etiopathology, in Vinken PJ, Bruyn GW, Klawans HL (eds): *Handbook of Clinical Neurology*. New York: Elsevier Science Publishers, 1986, pp 87–152.

44. Schmitt HP, Emser W, Heimes C: Familial occurrence of amyotrophic lateral sclerosis, parkinsonism and dementia. *Ann Neurol* 16:642–648, 1984.

45. Laxova R, Brown ES, Hogan K, et al: An x-linked recessive basal ganglia disorder with mental retardation. *Am J Med Genet* 21:681–689, 1985.

46. Gregg RG, Metzenberg AB, Hogan K, et al: Waisman syndrome, a human x-linked recessive basal ganglia disorder with mental retardation: Localization to Xq27.3-qter. *Genomics* 9:701–706, 1991.

47. Spitz MC, Jankovic J, Killian JM: Familial tic disorder, parkinsonism, motor neuron disease, and acanthocytosis: A new syndrome. *Neurology* 35:366–370, 1985.

48. Nygaard TG, Duvoisin RC: Hereditary dystonia–parkinsonism syndrome of juvenile onset. *Neurology* 36:1424–1428, 1986.

49. Giménez-Roldán S, Mateo D, Escalona-Zapata J: Familial Alzheimer's disease presenting as L-dopa-responsive parkinsonism. *Adv Neurol* 45:431–436, 1986.

50. Roy EP III, Riggs JE, Martin JD, et al: Familial parkinsonism, apathy, weight loss, and central hypoventilation: Successful long-term management. *Neurology* 38:637–639, 1988.

51. Inose T, Miyakawa M, Miyakawa K, et al: Clinical and neuropathological study of a familial case of juvenile parkinsonism. *Jpn J Psychiatr Neurol* 42:265–276, 1988.

52. Degl'Innocenti F, Maurello MT, Marini P: A parkinsonian kindred. *Ital J Neurol Sci* 10:307–310, 1989.

53. Rosenberg RN, Green JB, White CL III, et al: Dominantly inherited dementia and parkinsonism with non-alzheimer amyloid plaques: A new neurogenetic disorder. *Ann Neurol* 25:152–158, 1989.

54. Ishikawa A, Tanaka K, Koyama A, Miyatake T: A patient presenting mainly dystonia in a family with juvenile parkinsonism, edited by T Nagatsu. New York: Plenum Press, 1990, vol 2, pp 227–233.

55. Sage JI, Miller DC, Golbe LI, et al: Clinically atypical expression of pathologically typical Lewy-body parkinsonism. *Clin Neuropharmacol* 13:36–47, 1990.

56. Duvoisin RC: The genetics of Parkinson's disease: A review, in Rinne UK, Nagatsu T, Horowski R (eds): *International Workshop Berlin Parkinson's disease.* The Netherlands: Medicom Europe, 1991, pp 38–57.

57. Takei A, Chiba S, Sato Y, Miyagishi T: Familial Parkinson's disease and familial manic-depressive illness, in Nagatsu T (ed): *Basic Clinical and Therapeutic Aspects of Alzheimer's and Parkinson's Diseases.* New York: Plenum Press, 1990, vol 2, pp 201–204.

58. Tanaka H, Ishikawa A, Ginns EI, et al: Linkage analysis of juvenile parkinsonism to tyrosine hydroxylase gene locus on chromosome 11. *Neurology* 41:719–722, 1991.

59. Lechevalier B, Schupp C, Fallet-Bianco C, et al: Syndrome parkinsonien familial avec athymhormie et hypoventilation. *Rev Neurol (Paris)* 148:39–46, 1992.

60. Wszolek ZK, Pfeiffer RF, Bhatt MH, et al: Rapidly progressive autosomal dominant parkinsonism and dementia with pallido-ponto-nigral degeneration. *Ann Neurol* 32:312–320, 1992.

61. Wszolek ZK, Pfeiffer RF: Rapidly progressive autosomal dominant parkinsonism and dementia with pallidopontonigral degeneration, in Stern MB, Koller WC (eds): *Parkinsonian Syndromes.* New York: Marcel Dekker, 1993, pp 297–312.

62. Dobyns WB, Ozelius LJ, Kramer PL, et al: Rapid-onset dystonia-parkinsonism. *Neurology* 43:2596–2602, 1993.

63. Bhatia KP, Daniel SE, Marsden CD: Familial parkinsonism with depression: A clinicopathological study. *Ann Neurol* 34:842–847, 1993.

64. Golbe LI, Lazzarini AM, Schwarz KO, et al: Autosomal dominant parkinsonism with benign course and typical Lewy-body pathology. *Neurology* 43:2222–2227, 1993.

65. Mizutani T, Inose T, Nakajima S, Gambetti P: Familial parkinsonism and dementia with "ballooned neurons." *Adv Neurol* 60:613–617, 1993.

66. Yamamura Y, Arihiro K, Kohriyama T, Nakamura S: Early-onset parkinsonism with diurnal fluctuation: Clinical and pathological studies. *Rinsho Shinkeigaku* 33:491–496, 1993.

67. Nisipeanu P, Kuritzky A, Korczyn AD: Familial L-dopa-responsive parkinsonian-pyramidal syndrome: *Mov Disord* 9:673–675, 1994.

68. Lynch T, Sano M, Marder KS, et al: Clinical characteristics of a family with chromosome 17-linked disinhibition-dementia-parkinsonism-amyotrophy complex. *Neurology* 44:1878–1884, 1994.

69. Wilhelmsen KC, Lynch T, Pavlou E, et al: Localization of disinhibition-dementia-parkinsonism amyotrophy complex to 17q21-22. *Am J Hum Genet* 55:1159–1165, 1994.

70. Sasaki R, Kuzuhara S, Taniguchi A, et al: A family of parkinsonism in which the clinical feature of constituents varied with the age of onset. *Clin Neurol* 34:736–738, 1994.

71. Najim Al-Din AS, Wriekat A, Mubaidin A, et al: Pallido-pyramidal degeneration, supranuclear upgaze paresis and dementia: Kufor-Rakeb syndrome. *Acta Neurol Scand* 89:347–352, 1994.

72. Supala A, Wszolek ZK, Trofatter J, et al: Genetic linkage studies in autosomal dominant parkinsonism: Evaluation of candidate genes. *Mov Disord* 9:32, 1994.

73. Moya G, Miranda-Nieves G, Perez Sotelo M: Un cas familial d'amyotrophie spinale progressive montrant une atteinte histologique, cliniquement muette, du pallidum, du locus niger, du noyau de Luys et du faisceau de Goll. *Acta Neurol Belg* 69:1002–1012, 1969.

74. Arnould G, Tridon P, Weber M, et al: Forme familiale d'amyotrophie spinale subaiguë. *Soc Fran Neurologie* 126:70–76, 1972.

75. Finlayson MH, Guberman A, Martin JB: Cerebral lesions in familial amyotrophic lateral sclerosis and dementia. *Acta Neuropathol (Berl)* 26:237–246, 1973.

76. Alter M, Schaumann B: Hereditary amyotrophic lateral sclerosis: A report of two families. *Eur Neurol* 14:250–265, 1976.

77. Lee LV, Pascasio FM, Fuentes FD, Viterbo GH: Torsion dystonia in Panay, Philippines. *Adv Neurol* 14:137–151, 1976.

78. Kupke KG, Lee LV, Viterbo GH, et al: X-linked recessive torsion dystonia in the Philippines. *Am J Med Genet* 36:237–242, 1990.

79. Kupke KG, Lee LV, Müller U: Assignment of the x-linked torsion dystonia gene to Xq21 by linkage analysis. *Neurology* 40:1438–1442, 1990.

80. Wilhelmsen KC, Weeks DE, Nygaard TG, et al: Genetic mapping of "lubag" (x-linked dystonia-parkinsonism) in a Filipino kindred to the pericentromeric region of the X chromosome. *Ann Neurol* 29:124–131, 1991.

81. Lee LV, Kupke KG, Caballar-Gonzaga F, et al: The phenotype of the x-linked dystonia-parkinsonism syndrome: An assessment of 42 cases in the Philippines. *Medicine* 70:179–187, 1991.

82. Graeber MB, Müller U: The x-linked dystonia-parkinsonism syndrome (XDP): Clinical and molecular genetic analysis. *Brain Pathol* 2:287–295, 1992.

83. Kupke KG, Graeber MB, Müller U: Dystonia-parkinsonism syndrome (XDP) locus: Flanking markers in Xq12-21.1. *Am J Hum Genet* 50:808–815, 1992.

84. Graeber MB, Kupke KG, Müller U: Delineation of the dystonia-parkinsonism syndrome locus in Xq13. *Proc Natl Acad Sci U S A* 89:8245–8248, 1992.

85. Waters CH, Faust PL, Powers J, et al: Neuropathology of lubag (x-linked dystonia parkinsonism). *Mov Disord* 8:387–390, 1993.

86. Waters CH, Takahashi H, Wilhelmsen KC, et al: Phenotypic expression of x-linked dystonia-parkinsonism (lubag) in two women. *Neurology* 43:1555–1558, 1993.

87. Müller U, Haberhausen G, Wagner T, et al: DXS106 and DXS559 flank the x-linked dystonia-parkinsonism syndrome locus (DYT3). *Genomics* 23:114–117, 1994.

88. Allen N, Knopp W: Hereditary parkinsonism-dystonia with sustained control by L-dopa and anticholinergic medication. *Adv Neurol* 14:201–213, 1976.

89. Nygaard TG, Marsden CD, Duvoisin RC: Dopa-responsive dystonia. *Adv Neurol* 50:377–384, 1988.

90. Segawa M, Hosaka A, Miyagawa F, et al:. Hereditary progressive dystonia with marked diurnal fluctuation. *Adv Neurol* 14:215–233, 1976.

91. Segawa M, Ohmi K, Itoh S, et al: Childhood basal ganglia disease with remarkable response to L-dopa, "hereditary basal ganglia disease with marked diurnal fluctuation." *Shinryo* 24:667–672, 1971.

92. Segawa M, Nomura Y, Kase M: Hereditary progressive dystonia with marked diurnal fluctuation: Clinicopathophysiological identification in reference to juvenile Parkinson's disease. *Adv Neurol* 45:227–234, 1987.

93. Segawa M, Nomura Y, Kase M: Diurnally fluctuating hereditary progressive dystonia, in Vinken PJ, Bruyn GW, Klawans HL (eds): *Handbook of Clinical Neurology.* New York: Elsevier Science Publishers, 1986, vol 5, pp 529–539.

94. Segawa M, Nomura Y, Tanaka S, et al: Hereditary progressive dystonia with marked diurnal fluctuation—consideration on its pathophysiology based on the characteristics of clinical and polysomnographical findings. *Adv Neurol* 50:367–376, 1988.

95. Ujike H, Nakashima M, Kuroda S, Otsuki S: Two siblings of juvenile Parkinson's disease dystonic type (Yokochi type 3) and hereditary progressive dystonia with marked diurnal fluctuation (Segawa). *Clin Neurol* 29:890–894, 1989.

96. Nygaard TG, Takahaski H, Heiman GA, et al: Long-term treatment response and fluorodopa positron emission tomographic scanning of parkinsonism in a family with dopa-responsive dystonia. *Ann Neurol* 32:603–608, 1992.

97. Nygaard T: Dopa-responsive dystonia—delineation of the clinical syndrome and clues to pathogenesis, in Narabayashi H, Nagatsu T, Yanagisawa N, Mizuno Y (eds): *Adv Neurol* 60:577–585, 1993.

98. Segawa M, Nomura Y: Hereditary progressive dystonia with marked diurnal fluctuation—pathophysiological importance of the age of onset. *Adv Neurol* 60:568–576, 1993.

99. Nygaard TG, Wilhelmsen KC, Risch NJ, et al: Linkage mapping of dopa-responsive dystonia (DRD) to chromosome 14q. *Nature Genet* 5:386–391, 1993.

100. Ichinose H, Ohye T, Takahaski EI, et al: Hereditary progressive dystonia with marked diurnal fluctuation caused by mutations in the GTP cyclohydrolase I gene. *Nature Genet* 8:236–242, 1994.

101. Tanaka H, Endo K, Tsuji S, et al: The gene for hereditary progressive dystonia with marked diurnal fluctuation maps to chromosome 14q. *Ann Neurol* 37:405–408, 1995.

102. Kim RC, Collins GH, Parisi JE, et al: Familial dementia of adult onset with pathological findings of a 'non-specific' nature. *Brain* 104:61–78, 1981.

103. Khoubesserian P, Davous P, Bianco C, et al: Démence familiale de type neumann. *Rev Neurol (Paris)* 141:706–712, 1985.

104. Jankovic J, Kirkpatrick JB, Blomquist KA, et al: Late-onset Hallervorden-Spatz disease presenting as familial parkinsonism. *Neurology* 35:227–234, 1985.

105. Constantinidis J: Syndrome familial: Association de maladie de pick et sclérale amyotrophique. *Encephale* 13:285–293, 1987.

106. Bird TD, Lampe TH, Nemens EJ, et al: Familial Alzheimer's disease in American descendants of the Volga Germans: Probably genetic founder effect. *Ann Neurol* 23:25–31, 1988.

107. Bird TD, Sumi SM, Nemens EJ, et al: Phenotypic heterogeneity in familial Alzheimer's disease: A study of 24 kindreds. *Ann Neurol* 25:12–25, 1989.

108. Nygaard TG, Trugman JM, deYebenes JG, Fahn S: Dopa-responsive dystonia: The spectrum of clinical manifestations in a large North American family. *Neurology* 40:66–69, 1990.

109. Lanska DJ, Currier RD, Cohen M, et al: Familial progressive subcortical gliosis. *Neurology* 44:1633–1643, 1994.

110. Campion D, Brice A, Hannequin D, et al: A large pedigree with early-onset Alzheimer's disease. *Neurology* 45:80–85, 1995.

Chapter 27

ESSENTIAL TREMOR

WILLIAM C. KOLLER and KAREN L. BUSENBARK

HISTORY
EPIDEMIOLOGY OF ESSENTIAL TREMOR
GENETICS
CLINICAL MANIFESTATIONS
    Classification
    Body Region Affected by ET
    Disease Onset and Progression
    Factors Influencing ET
    Disability
    Diagnostic Pitfalls
    Clinical Variants
ASSOCIATED CONDITIONS
PATHOPHYSIOLOGY
ASSESSMENT OF TREMOR
TREATMENT
    Alcohol
    Beta-Adrenergic Blockers
    Primidone
    Phenobarbital
    Benzodiazepines
    Carbonic Anhydrase Inhibitors
    Other Drugs
    Botulinum Toxin Injection
    Thalamotomy
    Thalamic Stimulation
    Behavioral Therapy
    Drugs of Choice
SUMMARY

Essential tremor (ET) is most likely the most common movement disorder. We will review the history, epidemiology, genetics, clinical features, pathophysiology, and therapy of ET and expand on previous reviews of ET.[1-5]

History

Historically, tremor as an affliction of the elderly has long been noted; however, tremor as an isolated symptom commencing before old age and occurring within families has been clearly described only within the past 2 centuries. Critchley[6] provided a detailed chronological review of the history of ET. He cites one of the earlier references to tremor: "The keepers of the house shall tremble" (*Ecclesiastes*, XII.3). Galen in the second century described tremor as "an involuntary alternating up-and-down motion" differentiating it from other movements in his treatise, *On Tremor, Palpitation, Spasm, and Rigor.*[7] In 1817 James Parkinson,[8] in his landmark monograph *An Essay on the Shaking Palsy,* distinguished se-

nile tremor as a separate entity from the tremor of paralysis agitans. In the late nineteenth century, Charcot[9] commented on the salient clinical features of familial and senile tremor. In addition, the variability of clinical expression in ET was recognized by Charcot[10]; he described head tremor in two elderly female patients well: "The head participates in the shaking, on its own account; the movements which are both vertical and horizontal succeed each other with regularity, and in these the patient seems, by her gesture, to say yes or no."

Credit for first noting the familial form of tremor is usually given to Most who, in 1836, reported briefly on several cases of tremor in a single family.[6,11,12] However, in 1887, Dana[12] wrote the first thorough account of familial tremor; he described three families with tremor, detailing 45 patients with tremor within a single pedigree. In addition to the excellent family history, Dana provided a thorough clinical description of ET. He noted the body parts affected, variability in severity and age of onset, remission during sleep, and lack of increased mortality. Regarding familial and senile tremor as two distinct entities, Dana wrote that senile tremor "generally affects first and entirely the head and neck." In addition, he considered ET to be associated with neuroses, psychoses, epilepsy, unique talents, and high intellect. He reported that ET "illustrates the fact that a neuropathic taint in a family may develop as a disease, or as some brilliant mental endowment."

The notion of the ET patient as having unique characteristics was shared by others. Critchley[6] reviewed the work of the Russian neurologist, Minor, who in the early 1920s proposed the concept of *status macrobioticus multiparus*—the trial of familial tremor, longevity, and fecundity. This association of tremor with long life and prolificacy has not been corroborated by others when examining families with ET.[13,14] Other traits have also been ascribed to ET patients over the years. Inebriety, nervousness, emotivity, and anxiety have been reported in association with ET.[15] Raymond[16] considered "neuropathic shock" to be the precipitant of ET. From the contrary viewpoint, Katzenstein[17] considered families affected with tremor to be unusually accomplished and highly intelligent. Critchley[6] observed that ET has been noted among individuals of great intelligence giving, as an example, Joseph Babinski. These divergent views of the ET patient have not been addressed in recent times. Detailed epidemiological and genetic studies performed within the past 25 years offer no substantiation of these notions.[14,18]

Epidemiology of Essential Tremor

The epidemiology of ET is only partly understood. ET has been described as "common," "not uncommon," and "rare."[6,19,20] Reports of ET have been issued from around the world, indicating a global occurrence.[21-26] Depending on the study methods,[21,23,26] prevalence estimates vary widely (0.0005 to 5.55 percent). As part of a door-to-door neuroepidemiological survey, Salemi et al.[27] investigated the frequency and distribution of ET in a Sicilian municipality. They administered a screening instrument for tremor to 7653 persons residing in Terrasini (Palermo province). Neurologists evaluated those subjects who had screened positively. They found 31 subjects affected by ET (17 men, 14 women); 11 patients (35.5 percent) reported a familial aggregation. The prevalence of ET was for the total population, and 1074.9 per 100,000 for those 40 years old or older. The prevalence increased with advancing age for both sexes and was slightly but consistently higher in men.[27] Epidemiological surveys are complicated by less-than-ideal case ascertainment. As ET is usually monosymptomatic and often minimally disabling, it is likely to be underrepresented in surveys of neurological disorders.[14] Only a small percentage of individuals with ET comes to medical attention; in the series of Rautakorpi et al.[23] only 10 percent of identified ET patients had sought treatment. Even if the patient seeks medical advice, the disorder may not be properly recognized. Mild forms of ET may be dismissed as incidental, particularly in the elderly; Critchley[6] noted that tremor is not simply a characteristic of aging when he cited Charcot's report of tremor in only 1–2 percent of the aged inmates of the Salpêtrière. The symptom of ET may also be ascribed incorrectly to other medical conditions, with severe tremor commonly misdiagnosed as Parkinson's disease (PD).[28] For these reasons, medical registries cannot be relied on in studying the epidemiology of ET. Instead, a population-based approach is suggested,[29] in which an entire community is surveyed for features of ET.

Several epidemiological surveys for ET have been undertaken (Table 27-1). Larsson and Sjögren[14] conducted a comprehensive epidemiological survey in an isolated region of northern Sweden (population, 7451) in which a high frequency of ET had been previously noted. The prevalence of the condition was 1.4 percent for the general population and rose to 3.7 percent in the over-40-year-old age group. Similarly, Hornabrook and Nagurney[24] examined a region in New Guinea in which a propensity for tremor had been

described. When five language groups in this area are considered, prevalence rates were reported of 0.35 percent in the general population and 1.64 percent in the over-40-year-old age group. However, in other nearby communities with distinct linguistic and ethnic features, ET was remarkably uncommon. The New Guinea study was distinctive in that over-40-year-old subjects comprised only 21 percent of the study population; in addition, a significantly greater prevalence of ET among females was found. The investigators speculated that tremor might be more frequently detected in females because of the heavy manual labor performed by the women of this society. Because of their restricted geographic, ethnic, and cultural features, the findings of the Swedish and New Guinea studies cannot easily be generalized to other more diversified populations.

Rautakorpi et al.,[23] in a two-phase population-based study, examined the occurrence of ET in over-40-year-old patients in two rural communities in Finland. In the first phase, community members with tremor were identified by questionnaire. Clinical examinations were performed in phase two. Based on their findings, a minimal prevalence rate of 5.55 percent for ET in the over-40-year-old age group was reported. The authors suggested that the actual prevalence of ET among over-40-year-old patients may be close to 10 percent, as their data did not consider cases lost as a result of nonparticipation or incorrect reporting. A male preponderance was seen, and ET occurred more frequently with advancing age; the peak prevalence (12.6 percent) was in the 70–79-year-old age group. In the United States, Haerer et al.[22] reported on the prevalence of ET derived from a survey of major neurological disorders in a biracial Mississippi county. A screening questionnaire was administered to Copiah County residents. Based on questionnaire responses, individuals suspected of having ET were examined. The minimal prevalence rate of ET in this population was 0.41 percent with the condition more common in whites than in blacks,

TABLE 27-1 Epidemiological Studies of Essential Tremor

Methodology	Reference (yr)	PREVALENCE (%)	
		Total Population	Over-40-Year-Old Population
Population survey	Larsson and Sjögren[14] (1960)	1.7	3.73
Population survey	Hornabrook and Nagurney[24] (1976)	0.35	1.64
			2.12 females
			1.03 males
Population survey	Rautakorpi[18] (1978)		5.55
			4.73 females
			6.62 males
Population survey	Haerer et al.[22] (1982)		0.45 white females
			0.41 white males
			0.41 black females
			0.33 black males
Medical record review	Rajput et al.[31] (1982)	0.31	
Medical record review	Aiyesiloju et al.[26] (1984)	0.0005	
Population survey	Bharucha et al.[30] (1988)	1.59	2.76
			2.81 females
			2.71 males

for either sex; it was more common in women than men, for either race. The occurrence of ET was approximately tenfold greater in the 70–79-year-old age group, as compared to the 40–69-year-old group (1.18 versus .12 percent). The lower prevalence rates obtained in this study may, at least in part, be attributed to more stringent diagnostic criteria. Only tremor that significantly interfered with activities of daily living was considered; in addition, a ten-or-more-year history of tremor or a positive family history was required. A similar population-based study was conducted in the Parsi community of Bombay, India.[30] The prevalence of ET in this group was 1.52 percent. Age-adjusted prevalence rates were similar for men and women. A second epidemiological study of ET in the United States was reported by Rajput et al.[21,31] Their findings were based on the retrospective review of medical records from a 45-year period in Rochester, Minnesota. The estimated prevalence rate was 0.31 percent. The incidence of ET rose sharply after age 49 years. No difference in the incidence rates between males and females was found. Survival of patients diagnosed as having ET was comparable to that of the sex- and age-matched control population. Interestingly, when the data was considered in 15-year intervals a progressive increase in the incidence rate of ET was noted, that is, the diagnosis of ET was being made more frequently with the passage of time. The authors attributed this rise to the greater availability of health care and increased physician awareness of ET in recent years.

A similar retrospective review of hospital records was conducted by Aiyesiloju et al. in Nigeria.[26] A strikingly low prevalence rate of 0.0005 percent for ET was found. Other inheritable neurodegenerative disorders were also noted to be quite rare in this population. Genetic, environmental, and cultural features unique to this populace may explain these findings. In addition, ET as a sole medical condition would be expected to result rarely in hospital admission, making case ascertainment quite limited in this survey. In a report from a Chinese clinic, 146 of 258 tremor patients were thought to have ET.[32] There were 96 males and 50 females, ranging from 14 to 89 years of age. The hands were affected in all cases. A familial tendency was obvious in 32 percent. Epidemiological studies reveal that ET is more common than PD. The marked difference in prevalence ratios for PD and ET is attributed to: (1) higher incidence of ET in the general population; (2) a greater possibility that most, if not all, ET patients would reside in the community, whereas a sizable proportion of elderly PD patients may be inionalized, and (3) shortened survival in PD but a normal life expectancy in ET.[33]

Age appears to be a risk factor for ET. Data from the Mayo clinic shows a dramatic increase in the prevalence of ET with aging.[21] Anecdotal experience in the clinic also indicates that postural tremors are common in the aging population. Therefore, ET can be viewed as a disorder that is closely linked to the aging nervous system. A better understanding of ET will undoubtedly increase our knowledge of nervous system changes that occur with aging.

In summary, despite the variability in data, epidemiological studies illustrate ET to be a frequently encountered disorder, especially among the elderly. Applying the prevalence rate of ET derived from the Finnish study to U.S. Census Bureau population statistics (1988), one can estimate that more than 5 million individuals over 40 years of age in the United States are affected. Essential tremor would, therefore, appear to be the most common movement disorder.[1,11,21]

Genetics

The tendency of ET to run in families has been recognized for many years. In the American medical literature Dana[12] reported on three families with tremor in 1887. In the intervening years authors reviewing ET have reaffirmed its heritable nature.[6,11,14,16] Family history positivity varies by report from 17 to 70%.[18,21,24,26,34] Pedigree charts have been published, providing details on families with ET. Although Critchley cautioned that "more than one type of inheritance may be concerned," the genealogical reports published to date support the assumption that familial ET is inherited in an autosomal-dominant manner.[6,12,35–37]

A comprehensive genetic population study was conducted in a region of northern Sweden by Larsson and Sjögren.[14] In this study, 210 cases of ET were traced to 9 ancestral families in this geographically and ethnically restricted area. The pattern of occurrence of ET in this study was consistent with autosomal-dominant transmittance. Despite reports by others to the contrary,[6,18] Larsson and Sjögren[14] reported no instance of familial ET skipping generations. In 10 families both parents were affected with ET; estimating that approximately one-third of the affected offspring could be expected to be homozygotes, the investigators could identify no clinical features distinguishing homozygotes from heterozygotes. The disease manifested itself by age 70 in virtually all patients, that is, complete penetrance by 70 years of age. Rautakorpi[18] reported a similar age of onset of familial ET, with virtually all patients becoming symptomatic by age 65 and more than 50 percent of patients having tremor by age 40. This relatively early age of onset may distinguish familial ET from sporadic cases in which the peak age of onset is later.[18] Critchley[6] remarked on the occurrence of "anticipation," that is, younger age of onset of tremor in each succeeding generation within a given family; this phenomenon was not observed by Larsson and Sjögren.[14] In keeping with the observations of others, our experience with familial ET indicates that remarkable variability in age of onset and clinical expression may occur within a given family.[14,36] The cause of sporadic ET is unclear. Many of these cases may, indeed, have a familial basis, as family history can be unreliable or unattainable.

It should be noted that for most studies the presence or absence of a family history of ET was ascertained simply by inquiring from the patient. Therefore, there is the strong possibility of underreporting. For instance, a mild postural tremor could be present in a family member, or an individual who has a tremor may deny its existence to others. Acknowledgment of a familial disease may even be socially unacceptable.[26] It is possible that all cases of ET have a genetic basis and that the existence of sporadic cases is an artifact related to the method of data collection. Indeed, a recent study suggests that most reported negative family histories are positive when investigated.[38]

Another problem related to the issue of heredity and ET is how to define the presence of familial occurrence. If ET does occur sporadically and ET is a very common condition, then how does one define familiar occurrence? Criteria need to be developed that clearly separate familial from sporadic cases. Also, investigation of possible clinical and pharmacological differences between hereditary and sporadic ET (if it exists) needs to be performed. There is a report of an association of ET and CAG repeats in the androgen receptor gene[39]; however, this needs to be confirmed. A tremor indistinguishable from ET may be observed in patients with autosomal-dominant idiopathic torsion dystonia (ITD), in which the disease locus has been mapped to 9q32-34 in some kindreds, tightly linked to the argininosuccinate synthetase (ASS) locus. Conway et al.[40] performed linkage analysis in 15 families with ET containing 60 definitely affected individuals, using dinucleotide repeat polymorphisms at the ASS locus and the Abelson locus (ABL). Cumulative lod scores were −19.5 for ASS and −10.8 for ABL at a recombination fraction of 0.01, and tight linkage to ASS was excluded individually in 11 of the families. These data indicate that the ET gene is not allelic to that causing ITD.

Additional genetic linkage analysis studies of ET have been initiated recently, and results from these investigations will clarify the issue of heredity and ET.

Clinical Manifestations

ET has as its sole clinical manifestation tremor. The diagnosis is made either incidentally or when the patient presents because of the mechanical or social disability resulting from the tremor. Other neurological signs or symptoms are typically absent.[6,11,36,41] Mild abnormalities of tone or gait are occasionally reported.[11,14] Singer et al.[42] found that 50 percent of ET patients exhibited tandem gait abnormalities, as compared to 28 percent of age-matched controls. Tremor, indistinguishable in appearance from ET, can be seen in association with other neurological disorders (see Associated Conditions).[6,11,43]

In general, tremor is rarely confused with other involuntary movements.[44] Its rhythmic, oscillating nature allows relatively easy recognition.[28,45] Physiologically, tremor has been defined as an "involuntary oscillation of a body part produced by alternating or synchronous contractions of reciprocally innervated antagonistic muscles."[45] Essential tremor is typically of the postural type, that is, the tremor is best seen with maintenance of a fixed posture.[11,28] It may be accentuated with goal-directed movement of the limbs (kinetic tremor) and, in some instances, may be present at rest.[6,11,46] The tremor may occur only during the maintenance of a specific position. Changing the angle of the position may significantly alter the severity of the tremor. Sanes and Hallet[47] examined the influence of limb positioning in ET and other pathological tremors and found that different postures of the arm affected the magnitude of the tremor. This phenomenon was more evident in instances of postural tremor other than in ET.

CLASSIFICATION

Critchley[6] noted that ET may occur in a wide range of frequencies (4–12 cycles/s) with an inverse relationship between amplitude size and tremor rate. It has been suggested that ET is simply exaggerated physiological tremor, following the same frequency pattern.[34] More recent electrophysiological data do not support this assumption.[48,49] With the recognition that ET is a heterogeneous condition, various classification schemes have been proposed. Findley and Gretsy[48] separated two types of ET on the basis of frequency analysis: those with frequencies between 7 and 11 Hz, having features of enhanced physiological tremor, and those with frequencies below 6.5 Hz. Categorizing ET on the basis of frequency alone, however, is not optimal, as it may vary within a single family or even in a given individual.[46] Marsden and colleagues[43] proposed a classification into four types, based on the presence or absence of a family history, response to alcohol, and response to beta-adrenergic-blocking drugs. Responsiveness to primidone was not addressed. Only types 2 and 3 of this classification should be considered ET. Currently, there are no data to support this classification, but this proposal does form the basis for future investigation. Deuschl and coworkers[50] have proposed another classification, based on pharmacological and electrophysiological properties. They tested 25 patients and found one group had normal long latency and synchronous tremor burst in antagonists or activity of antigravity muscles alone. The second group was characterized by abnormal long latency reflexes and reciprocal EMG activity in antagonists. It was further suggested that patients of the first group respond to propranolol, whereas those of the second group do not. However, pharmacological responsiveness was tested in only some subjects, and no objective measure of drug response was performed. Koller et al.[51] attempted to classify ET, using tremor frequency; tremor duration; family history of tremor; responsiveness to alcohol, propranolol, and primidone, muscle contraction pattern; and by using long-latency reflexes. They collected information from 61 patterns and found few correlations. It was concluded that ET could not be divided into subtypes using these characteristics. More investigation is needed to clarify the proper classification of ET.

BODY REGION AFFECTED BY ET

ET appears most frequently in the hands.[5,52,53] An adduction-abduction movement of the fingers and a flexion-extension movement of the hand is typical; less often, a pronation-supination movement (similar to the tremor of PD) is seen.[6,28] Frequently, the tremor is unilateral at the onset, but with time, both sides become involved.[6,14,54] With hand tremor, handwriting may become tremulous, and rounded letters take on a sharp angularity. Critchley[6] provided a handwriting example of both clinical and historical note when he reproduced the normal and tremor-affected signatures of Oliver Cromwell. The handwriting in ET does not become micrographic, distinguishing it from the script in PD.

The next most frequently affected body area is cranial musculature.[5,52] Although the tongue, head, or voice may be

COLOR PLATES

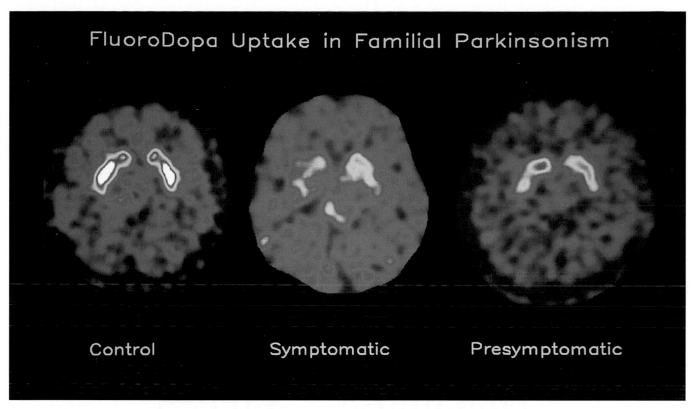

1 PET images of striatal ^{18}F-dopa uptake in a normal subject, a parkinsonian patient, and his presymptomatic relative. It can be seen that the relative has abnormal dopaminergic function. See also Figure 3-2. (Courtesy of Dr. GV Sawle.)

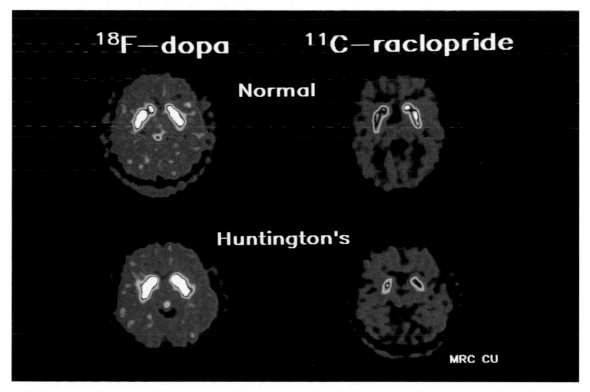

2 PET images of ^{18}F-dopa and ^{11}C-raclopride uptake in Huntington's disease. It can be seen that the presynaptic dopaminergic system is intact, but a profound loss of dopamine D2 receptors has occurred in HD. See also Figure 3-3. (Courtesy of Dr. N Turjanski.)

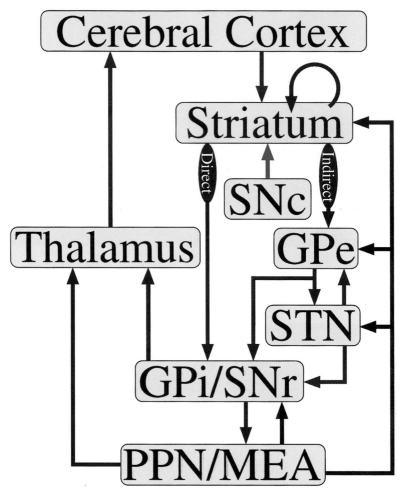

3 Schematic of basal ganglia circuitry model. Connectivity of basal ganglia and various related nuclei is color coded according to predominant neurotransmitter systems as follows: blue (GABA), red (glutamate), green (dopamine), purple (acetycholine), and black (unknown). Direct and indirect pathways originating from striatum are named according to the immediacy of their regulation of the basal ganglia output nuclei, GPi/SNr. The purple arrow originating from and looping back to striatum represents cholinergic interneurons.GPe, globus pallidus external segment; GPi/SNr, globus pallidus internal segment/substantia nigra pars reticulata; PPN/MEA, pedunculopontine nucleus/midbrain extrapyramidal area; SNc, substantia nigra pars compacta; STN, subthalamic nucleus. See also Figure 7-1.

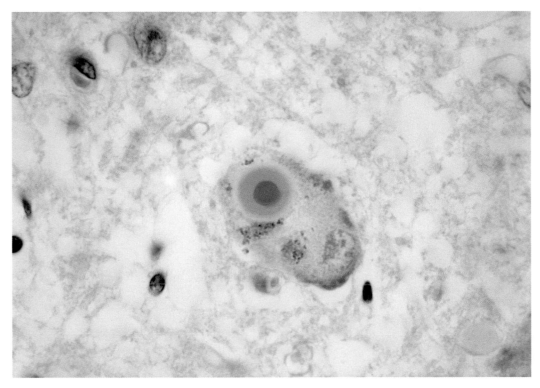

4 Substantia nigra of a patient with Parkinson's disease. H&E, × 450. Classic trilaminar Lewy body, demonstrating an outer halo, body, and inner core. See also Figure 18-1A.

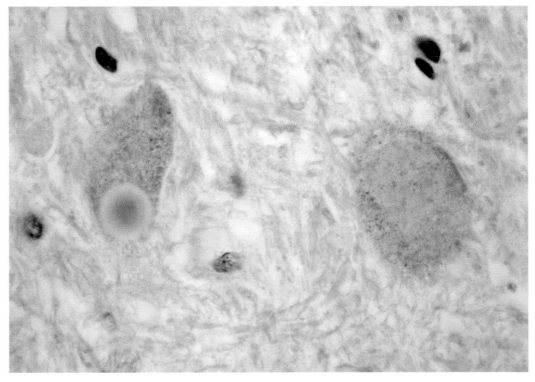

5 Substantia nigra of a patient with Parkinson's disease. H&E, × 450. Bilaminar Lewy body in neuron to the left and a pale body showing marked eosinophilic granularity in the neuron to the left. See also Figure 18-1B.

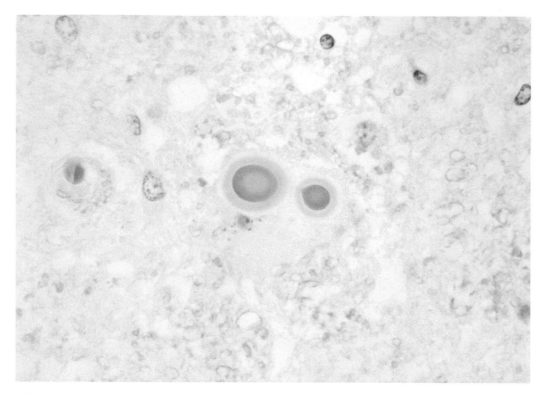

6 Locus ceruleus of a patient with Parkinson's disease. Pigmented neuron (demonstrated by serial sections). Stained with H&E, × 575. Two trilaminar Lewy bodies with cores, demonstrating central pallor, and an adjacent pale body. See also Figure 18-2A.

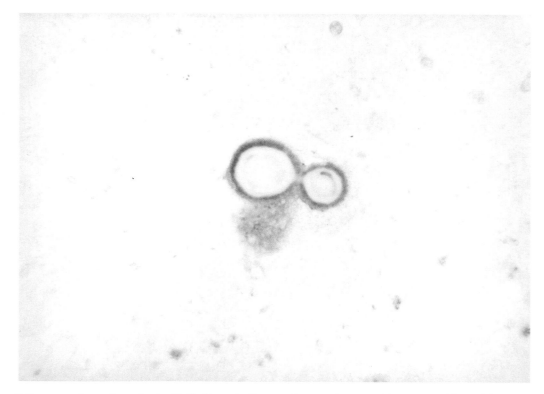

7 Locus ceruleus of a patient with Parkinson's disease. Pigmented neuron (demonstrated by serial sections), stained for ubiquitin, × 575. Lewy bodies: circumferential staining of the halo-body junction and focal staining of the body-core junction. Pale body: diffuse reticular-granular staining, which is contiguous with one of the Lewy bodies. See also Figure 18-2B.

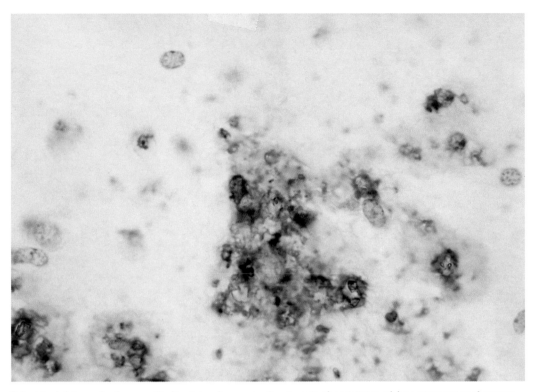

8 Incidental Lewy body case. Perl's stain, demonstrating iron in the vicinity of free pigment and macro-phages. × 1250. See also Figure 18-5.

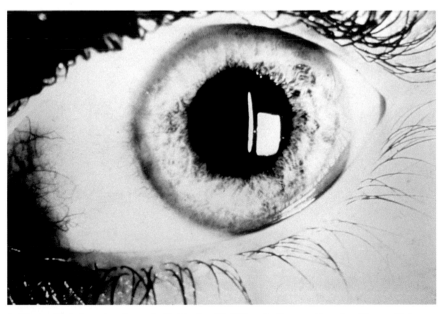

9 Kayser-Fleischer ring in an individual with Wilson's disease. See also Figure 46-1. (Courtesy of Rown Zetterman.)

affected in isolation (see Clinical Variants), it is most common for tremor in these regions to occur in association with hand tremor.[14,54,55] In advanced cases, tremor of the palate, voice, and tongue may result in dysarthric speech, but this infrequently occurs before 65 years of age.[14] The legs and trunk become affected infrequently and usually in the later stages of the illness.[28]

DISEASE ONSET AND PROGRESSION

ET may commence at any age, but its incidence rises with advancing years (see Epidemiology of ET). The onset of ET may be earlier in the familial form, as compared to the sporadic form.[14,18] It is rarely reported in infancy and childhood.[56] Categorizing ET by age of onset has not proved useful, as it does not assist in predicting clinical outcome or therapeutic response.[6,11,16] In the nineteenth century, Dana[12] distinguished between senile tremor and hereditary tremor, but this differentiation was soon recognized as arbitrary, and both entities are now considered to be manifestations of the same disease.[16,57]

ET is generally considered to be a slowly progressive disorder, but variability in its clinical course has been noted. The progression of this disease can be defined as an increase in tremor amplitude or extension of tremor to previously unaffected body parts. It is the former that impairs the patient's voluntary movements and results in disability. Critchley[6,37] characterized the illness as occurring in stages: In the initial 1–2 years a slow deterioration occurs, then little or no change in the tremor may be noted for several years, and then in later life the tremor may suddenly worsen. Larsson and Sjögren[14] in their study of familial ET suggest that the disease typically appears before age 50 with a fine rapid hand tremor of little consequence, by age 65 years the tremor is moderate, and at 70 years it is quite pronounced (increased in amplitude and diminished in frequency). Despite its progressive nature, it has long been recognized that the diagnosis of ET is not associated with increased mortality.[12]

FACTORS INFLUENCING ET

Tremor can be affected by a host of factors. Overall, it tends to progress with age, so that with advancing years, tremor frequency declines and amplitude increases.[34,36] Handedness may play a role in the expression and severity of ET; Biary and Koller[58] found a higher incidence of left-handedness among ET patients than controls; in addition, a direct relationship was found between hand dominance and tremor severity. It is not unusual for patients to associate the onset of tremor with a specific incident or circumstance, however, establishing causal relationship is difficult. Tremor, resembling ET, has been reported following head trauma;[59] it is unlikely that this phenomenon represents a form of ET, given the abruptness of onset, temporal link to the trauma, and refractoriness to therapy.

A number of elements can affect tremor in the short term. In 1887, Dana[12] remarked that "everything that produces excitement or nervousness" may increase ET. In the intervening years a number of specific factors that may exacerbate ET have been suggested: fatigue, extremes of temperature,

emotional upset, sexual arousal, central nervous system stimulants, and diurnal fluctuations in catecholamine levels.[6,11,60] Alcohol may produce a remarkable ameliorative effect on ET. In many patients tremor is lessened by ingesting even a small amount of alcoholic beverage. Intravenous alcohol infusion, but not local intra-arterial injection, decreases ET[61] and suggests that the effect of alcohol is centrally mediated. Indeed, alcohol is able to reverse the increase in cerebral or regional blood flow seen in ET (L Findley, personal communication). Although the therapeutic effect of alcohol is most typical of ET, it has been reported to occur rarely in other forms of tremor.[62] Caffeine is commonly considered to be a precipitant of tremor; however, in a formal study evaluating 50 ET patients, caffeine produced no discernible effect.[63] As is the case with most involuntary movements, ET typically remits during sleep; there are, however, rare reports of its persistence during slumber.[6,41]

In summary, the appearance of tremor in a given patient may vary, not only with the passage of years but even over the course of a single day.

DISABILITY

The patient with ET may be handicapped by the physical limitations that the tremor may create (e.g., writing, drinking liquids, etc.) or by the social embarrassment that it may cause. The physical disability is directly related to tremor amplitude; with aging or disease progression, amplitude increases, and the ability to execute fine, discrete movements may be impaired. Compromise of occupational skills may occur; approximately 15 percent of ET patients referred to a university clinic[18] were pensioned as a result of tremor. Cooper noted that in 1962, in rare cases, tremor is so severe as to warrant surgical intervention.[64] One cannot estimate to what extent ET alters quality of life, given the variability in social limitations that patients may impose on themselves because of embarrassment resulting from tremor. Although ET is sometimes preceded by the prefix "benign," the condition is clearly very disabling in some individuals. Busenbark and coworkers[65] analyzed the results of the Sickness Impact Profile, a standardized assessment tool that measures illness-related dysfunction, in 753 ET patients, 145 parkinsonians, and 87 controls. ET patients had greater dysfunction than the controls but less than the parkinsonians. Communication, work, emotional behavior, home management, and reactions and pastimes were particularly impaired in ET. The investigators concluded that significant disability can occur in ET and, compared to PD, ET tends to be less severe but causes relatively greater psychosocial dysfunction. Social phobia-like symptoms occur in ET,[66] and several recent surveys[5,52] have documented the high prevalence of disability in ET.

DIAGNOSTIC PITFALLS

ET can be misdiagnosed, being most commonly mislabeled as incipient PD.[28] The correct diagnosis of ET can also be clouded by the consideration of other neurological illnesses that may have tremor as a clinical manifestation. This would include multiple sclerosis, Wilson's disease, Huntington's chorea, and cerebellar degenerative diseases. In addition, tremor can be precipitated by drugs and toxins (e.g., lithium and volproic acid) and by systemic illness (e.g., thyrotoxicosis).[28] In an effort to minimize diagnostic errors, we have adopted the use of diagnostic criteria for ET. Such guidelines not only assist in individual case assessment but also are crucial to ensure validity in the clinical investigation of ET. The Tremor Research Investigation Group (TRIG), a committee of scientists studying ET, recently proposed a working definition of ET for research studies.[67]

DEFINITE ESSENTIAL TREMOR

1. Presence of postural tremor in the arms that worsens with action, in the absence of any condition or drug known to cause enhanced physiological tremor (listed below), in the absence of cerebellar symptoms and signs, and in the absence of PD dystonia, hyperthyroidism, chronic alcoholism, peripheral neuropathy, and an anxiety state. Medications known to be tremorgenic, such as (1) beta agonists, for example, terbutaline, (2) lithium, (3) neuroleptics, (4) valproate, (5) tricyclic antidepressants, (6) antihistamines, (7) anticholinergics, (8) corticosteroids, and (9) dopamine agonists.

OR

2. Postural tremor of arms without action tremor of arms, plus head (neck) tremor, in the absence of any condition or drug known to cause enhanced physiological tremor and in the absence of cerebellar symptoms and signs and in the absence of PD and dystonia.

PROBABLE ESSENTIAL TREMOR

1. Presence of both postural tremor and action tremor of arms, without an increase during action, in the absence of any condition or drug known to cause enhanced physiological tremor, in the absence of cerebellar symptoms and signs, and in the absence of PD and dystonia.

OR

2. Presence of action tremor alone, in the absence of any condition or drug known to cause enhanced physiological tremor, in the absence of cerebellar symptoms and signs, and in the absence of PD and dystonia.

OR

3. Postural tremor of arms that gets better with action, in the absence of any condition or drug known to cause enhanced physiological tremor, in the absence of cerebellar symptoms and signs, and in the absence of PD and dystonia.

OR

4. Postural tremor of arms and vocal tremor, in the absence of any condition or drug known to cause enhanced physiological tremor, in the absence of cerebellar symptoms and signs, and in the absence of PD and dystonia.

OR

5. Vocal and head or neck tremor without other known causes present, in the absence of any condition or drug known to cause enhanced physiological tremor, in the absence of cerebellar symptoms and signs, and in the absence of PD and dystonia.

POSSIBLE ESSENTIAL TREMOR

1. Postural tremor of arms and action tremor of arms, in the absence of any condition or drug known to cause enhanced physiological tremor and in the absence of cerebellar symptoms and signs but in the presence of PD or dystonia affecting those limbs.

OR

2. Postural tremor that goes away with action or remains unchanged with action, in the absence of any condition or drug known to cause enhanced physiological tremor and in the absence of cerebellar symptoms and signs but in the presence of PD or dystonia affecting those limbs.

OR

3. Leg or head or neck or lingual tremor alone, in the absence of any condition or drug known to cause enhanced physiological tremor and in the absence of cerebellar symptoms and signs but in the presence of PD or dystonia affecting those limbs.

CLINICAL VARIANTS

A variety of atypical tremor disorders exists that appears to be related to ET.[68] An association of these conditions with ET is suggested by a high occurrence of a family history of ET, frequent presence of a mild postural tremor, and tremor reduction with alcohol ingestion. In most patients with ET, varying degrees of postural and kinetic tremor are observed; however, in kinetic predominant tremor a marked dissociation occurs, with the postural component minimal or absent.[69] Cerebellar signs are absent. Disability may be severe in these patients. A resting tremor is not a defined component of ET, although it has been observed in severely affected or elderly patients.[11] Koller and Rubino[70] reported a group of patients with a combined resting and postural tremor with minimal kinetic tremor. A postural tremor often occurs in PD,[48] but the patients reported by Koller and Rubino[70] had no other parkinsonian features, despite a long duration of tremor. Tremor reduction did not occur with antiparkinsonian drugs in these patients. Several case reports of familial paroxysmal tremor with clinical features similar to ET exist.[71,72]

A task-specific or selective action tremor affecting the hands is primary writing tremor, in which pronation of the forearm elicits a pronation/supination tremor that is not seen during other movements of the arm.[73-75] Other activities involving pronation may also result in tremor; however, the major disability is impaired handwriting, which may be the patient's sole complaint. Tremor is present for the duration of writing, often making the task impossible. Postural and kinetic tremors, when present, are usually mild. EMG findings show an alteration of antagonist muscles, and there is no significant increase of reflex excitability or evidence of cortical hyperexcitability.[75] Primary writing tremor needs to be distinguished from a segmental dystonia of the hands, or writer's cramp.[76] Dystonic spasms are observed in writer's cramp, rather than in tremor. However, tremor may occur secondary to trying to control the dystonia, and some families have been reported as having different members who exhibit writer's cramp, ET, and primary writing tremor.[77] Elble and coworkers[78] studied five patients who had severe

5 to 7-Hz tremor when attempting to write or draw. They noted abnormal coactivation of the antagonistic muscles, which produced subtle dystonic posturing of the affected limb that was overshadowed by the tremor. The authors suggested that the nonspecificity of dystonia and postural tremor should be considered when discussing the pathophysiology of primary writing tremor.

ET can affect solely or predominantly one body part. Therefore, isolated tremors of the tongue, chin, and voice may occur. Tongue tremor is commonly found when the patient is tested for it in the postural position, although the patient is often unaware of any difficulty with the tongue. However, a tongue tremor can be a patient's chief complaint. Tongue shaking may interfere both with speaking and eating. An isolated chin tremor (geniospasm) not involving the lips may also occur. Isolated trembling of the chin may also occur in families, transmitted as an autosomal-dominant gene.[79,80] This hereditary condition is stimulus-sensitive, may begin at birth, and may improve with age. Quavering of the lower lip can occur in PD but is almost always associated with other parkinsonian signs. Speech involvement in ET is not uncommon and, occasionally, may be the predominant or sole symptom.[81,82] Riveat and Marsden[83] suggested that some of these tremors may be associated with dystonia. They studied five patients who had an isolated tremor of the trunk or neck and found that their clinical characteristics were similar to those of other patients who presented with tremors and eventually developed torticollis or arm dystonia. They concluded that isolated tremors of the trunk and head, especially when of slow frequency, for example, 2–3 Hz, may be the initial manifestation of a focal dystonia.

Truncal tremor is occasionally observed in ET patients with a long history of severe hand and head tremors. Truncal tremor occurring as a presenting symptom is rare. Heilman[84] first reported three patients with the sole symptom of orthostatic tremor of the trunk and the proximal legs. Wee and coworkers[85] described a family that had both typical ET of the hands and orthostatic trunk tremor. Koller and coworkers[68] and Pape and Gershanik[86] reported patients similar to those of Heilman. Tremor was present after standing for several seconds, increased with time, and could lead to falling. There was no tremor during sitting, walking, or leaning against a firm support. Gabellini et al.[87] described eight cases of orthostatic tremor; six were thought to be idiopathic; 1 was said to be a result of hydrocephalus; and 1 was a result of chronic relapsing polyradiculoneuropathy. They suggested a relationship between orthostatic tremor and ET. Pape and Gershanik[86] reported electromyogram (EMG) findings in orthostatic tremor that were similar to those of ET in the upper and lower limbs. However, standing or sustaining certain positions with the arms and legs would bring about dramatic changes in the pattern of rhythmic discharges, with a high-frequency activity of 15–16 Hz.[86,88] They thought that the clinical manifestations could be a result of instability caused by stiffness of the legs, depending on the high-frequency tremor, which is not clearly visible. Thompson and coworkers[89] described electrophysiological findings in one patient with orthostatic tremor. In this patient the tremor affected primarily the legs and was alternating between antagonist muscle groups and had a high frequency of 16 Hz. The tremor

was present only during certain postures. A tremor of the same frequency was also recorded in the arms during particular movements. It was suggested that orthostatic tremor is generated by spontaneous oscillations responsible for organizing the motor programs for standing.

An orthostatic tremor patient was described by Walker et al.[90] in which electromyography revealed tremor burst of 15 Hz in the lower extremities while standing and with isometric activation of the muscles, but the bursts disappeared with isotonic activation of muscles. Uncini and coworkers[91] reported two patients with orthostatic tremor with 10 to 12- and 16-Hz EMG bursts in antagonistic muscles. EMG activity was synchronous in corresponding muscles of both legs. They suggested that orthostatic tremor may be an exaggeration of physiological tremor resulting from synchronization of motor units by spontaneous oscillations in central structures. Lewitt[92] hypothesized that orthostatic tremor shares a similar mechanism with the entity of "paradoxical clonus" or shorting reaction (see also Chap. 29).

Associated Conditions

ET has been described in association with various disorders and conditions. The chance of simultaneous occurrence of such a common disorder with other diseases must be considered when one is reviewing the long list of "associated conditions." In an epidemiological study in Finland by Rautakorpi,[18] there was a significantly higher incidence of cardiovascular disorders, including arterial hypertension, coronary heart disease, and cerebrovascular disease in ET patients than in controls. He proposed that this association may depend on the occurrence of a selection bias in the control group or a genetic linkage between ET and certain risk factors of cardiovascular disease. Other studies have not substantiated this link between cardiovascular disorders and ET. In a 45-year retrospective study based on original medical records, Rajput et al.[21] reported that diagnosis of hypertension was made at some time or another in 30 percent of the cases. There was no significant difference between patients and controls for risk of hypertension subsequent to the diagnosis of ET. In their study of ET in Papua, New Guinea, Hornabrook and Nagurney[24] found that blood pressures and electrocardiographs of their ET population were comparable with those of a control series.

The incidence of nonspecific neurological abnormalities in ET patients has been studied with various conclusions. Larrson and Sjögren[14] described stiff gait, slight rigidity, or other nonspecific neurological abnormalities in 17 of the 81 cases. Hornabrook and Nagurney[24] also noted a certain stiffness in some patients, stating that it is "perhaps better described as a tenseness of the general musculature. This was qualitatively distinct from the akinetic rigidity so familiar in paralysis agitans . . . Patients appeared to hold themselves stiffly, perhaps in order to give themselves less opportunity for the involuntary tremors to become manifest." A study of 200 ET patients observed mild reduction of upper limb synkinetic movements during gait in four patients (2 percent) and hypomimic facies in two patients (1 percent).[93] The authors speculated that extrapyramidal impairment may be common in the normal aging population as a result of progressive loss of nigrostriatal neurons and brain dopamine.[94,95] Therefore, they concluded, it was not surprising to find similar signs in elderly ET patients. In a study of 247 ET patients in London and Chicago, mild extrapyramidal signs occurred in only 4.5 percent of ET patients and did not differ significantly from the findings in age-matched controls.[96]

The relationship of ET and PD has been controversial since James Parkinson (1817) first commented on the distinction between paralysis agitans and senile (essential) tremor in 1817.[8] Gowers[97] in 1888 did not make this distinction, but rather, he stated that "it is doubtful whether this senile tremor is essentially different from paralysis agitans. Some cases are met with a character intermediate between the two affections." He also described "simple" tremor and stated that "in spite of the occasional collateral relation to paralysis agitans, it seems to have little tendency to develop into the latter disease, and certainly is less closely connected with it than is senile tremor."[97] In 1949, Critchley[6] stressed that, because both disorders are relatively common, chance may account for the presence of ET or PD in family members and cases of concurrent ET-PD. In a clinical series, Duvoisin et al.[19] noted that the incidence of ET among the 85 index Parkinson's patients' siblings and spouses was the same.

In their study in New Guinea, Hornabrook and Nagurney[24] reported that there "is slight evidence from this series that the two conditions are in some way linked." In another epidemiological study, Marttila and Rinne[98] found no association, reporting that 5.8 percent of PD patients and 8.1 percent of control subjects had relatives with probable ET. More recent epidemiological studies have also concluded that ET and PD are genetically independent diseases.[21,99]

Barbeau and Pourcher[100] reported a strong family history of ET in early-onset PD. In a clinical series of 50 cases of familial PD, Roy et al.[101] proposed two main patterns of genetic transmission within parkinsonian patients, with one a parkinsonism related to hereditary ET. They reported a high prevalence of ET in families of PD patients who had tremor as their initial symptom. Geraghty et al.,[102] in a clinical series of 130 ET patients, concluded that the risk of PD is 24 times greater than in an age-matched, randomly selected population. In a recent report from the same clinic the clinical correlates of 350 ET patients were reported.[103] Twenty percent of patients were thought to have parkinsonism. However, this conclusion has been challenged because of methodological flaws of the study, which include the problem of dual reporting and unclear definition of postural tremors and ET.[104] Lang et al.[105] also found a higher incidence of familial tremor in PD patients than in controls but not the striking association reported by Geraghty et al.[102] Cleeves et al.[96] found no association or genetic link between ET and PD in their clinical series of 237 ET patients, 100 PD patients, and 100 normal controls. Frequency of family history of ET was higher among PD patients than controls but was not statistically significant. The authors propose that although there is no overall relationship, there may be an association between ET and a distinct subgroup of PD patients, as suggested earlier by Barbeau and Pourcher.[100] In a clinical series examining the occurrence of PD and ET in parents and siblings of early-onset parkinsonian patients, the incidence of PD or ET did

not differ significantly from the relevant expected incidence in any group.[106] In a study of several kindreds of ET Bain and colleagues[5] found no association with PD, and in an investigation of over 800 ET patients, only 7 percent were thought to have concomitant PD.[52]

The controversy over the relationship of PD and ET continues and is compounded by the frequent inability to distinguish the two disorders.[28] Parkinsonian signs, such as cogwheeling and tremor at rest, may be seen in ET,[107] and postural tremor is not uncommon in PD.[48] However, recent observations have further suggested that ET is unrelated to PD.[108,109] Rajput et al.[110] reported the postmortem results of six patients with ET. There was no neuronal loss in the substantia nigra, and Lewy bodies were not observed. Positron emission tomography (PET) scanning indicates that striatal fluorodopa uptake is normal in ET.[111] Olfaction function, measured by the University of Pennsylvania Smell Identification Test, was found to be normal in ET, whereas dysfunction in olfaction is a common and early sign in PD.[112]

The presence of a postural tremor in patients with focal or generalized dystonia is not uncommon. Whether this can truly be labeled "ET" is debatable. Yanagisawa et al.[113] described six generations of a Japanese family with 149 members, 5 of whom had dystonia musculorum deformans, another 12 of whom had a forme fruste of this disease, and all 17 of whom had a postural tremor. In their study of patients with torsion dystonia, Johnson et al.[114] found a large number of family members with tremor. In reviewing the records of 100 patients with the diagnosis of ET, familial, or senile tremor, Baxter and Lal[115] found dystonic symptoms in 12 cases. Other researchers have reported a 1–3 percent incidence of dystonia in their ET populations.[14,93] In 1949, Critchley[6] summarized the European literature on ET and reported individual cases of torticollis and ET. A strong association between spasmodic torticollis and ET was reported by Couch.[116] Of 30 patients with idiopathic spasmodic torticollis, 26 demonstrated tremor, "usually rhythmic" and resembling ET. A family history of tremor was present in 16 of the patients who had tremor with dystonia. Couch[116] proposed that ET is a forme fruste of dystonia but acknowledge the association of postural tremor with a wide variety of basal ganglia disorders. Duane[117] noted that although idiopathic spasmodic torticollis and essential head tremor may coexist, patients who have essential head tremor commonly tilt their head to one side in an effort to suppress the tremor. In the database of the Dystonia Clinic at the University of Kansas Medical Center for patients with dystonia and tremor, Dubinsky et al.[118] found that of 296 patients with idiopathic dystonia, 24 had dystonic tremor; 20 with cervical dystonia had an isolated head-nodding tremor; 2 with writer's cramp had ipsilateral hand tremor; and 2 with generalized dystonia had arm tremor. Eight patients, all with cervical dystonia, had essential tremor that preceded the onset of their dystonia.

Using surface EMG, Yanagisawa and Goto[119] showed that an irregular 1- to 6.5-Hz grouping of motor unit discharges is often associated with the involuntary dystonic contractions, but a more rhythmic 5- to 11-Hz grouping is seen during voluntary contraction. The rhythmic motor unit grouping is indistinguishable from that of ET, but the irregular 1- to 6.5-Hz tremor bears very little resemblance to ET, making a proposed relationship questionable.

The presence of tremor in writer's cramp has been recognized, but the specific relationship is unclear.[75,76] Ravits et al.[75] describes four patients with tremor upon writing that they consider to have a form of focal dystonia with tremor, noting similar physiological findings in a patient with myoclonic writer's cramp and in tremor patients. Klawans et al.[73] described six patients who had a tremor upon writing, five of whom responded to anticholinergic therapy and none of whom responded to propranolol. Sheehy and Marsden[74] proposed that patients who present clinically with primary writing tremor may have a variant of essential tremor that is responsive to alcohol and propranolol, or a tremulous form of dystonia, as described by Ravits et al.[75] and Klawans et al.[73] Rosenbaum and Jankovic[120] studied focal task specific tremor and dystonia and noted that the two disorders shared many clinical, genetic, physiological, and pharmacological features with the more common generalized movement disorders and suggested interrelationships between the focal and the generalized forms of tremor and dystonia. In one report 47 percent of ET patients were said to have some form of dystonia.[103] This observation is contrary to most clinicians' experience, and the findings may represent a referral bias to a specialty clinic.

Tremor may occur in familial and acquired peripheral neuropathies.[121-124] Roussy and Levy[121] provided the classic description of a hereditary neuropathy patient who had tremor as a clinical manifestation. In more recent years, it has been suggested that the Roussy-Levy syndrome does not represent a distinct entity but that tremor may be seen in hereditary motor-sensory neuropathies of both the hypertrophic and nonhypertrophic types.[125-127] This association of tremor with familial neuropathies has led to consideration as to whether this represents the expression of linked genetic material ("Charcot-Marie-Tooth gene" linked to the "ET gene" in a given family), the expression of a single genetic aberration (independent of Charcot-Marie-Tooth disease and ET), or that tremor may simply occur in hereditary neuropathies owing to pathophysiological circumstances within the peripheral nervous system.[127] The heterogeneous nature of such tremors is illustrated by the diversity of genetic, clinical, physiological, and pharmacological features in the reported cases.[127,128] Similarly, tremors of sundry natures have been associated with acquired peripheral neuropathies, including neuropathies of the chronic relapsing type and those attributed to dysgammaglobulinemia, diabetes, uremia, and amyloidosis.[122-124,129] It has been suggested that such tremor represents physiological tremor, enhanced by weakness or impaired stretch reflexes.[122,130] In summary, although neuropathic tremor remains an obscure entity in terms of its pathogenesis and nosological significance, it should be considered distinct from ET.

Baughman[131] and Pittman et al.[132] described several patients with concurrent Klinefelter's syndrome and ET. Baughman et al.[131] studied 13 males in a private neurology practice and 11 institutionalized male retardates, all with known sex chromosome abnormalities. ET was present in 5 from each group, 10 of 24 total. They concluded that "ET is a common and significant component of the male supernumerary X syndromes and probably supernumerary Y syndromes."

In short, postural and kinetic tremors are a common accompaniment of many illnesses, both systemic and neurological. Characteristics of these tremors are so nonspecific as to preclude firm conclusions regarding a pathophysiological relationship. Consequently, reported associations with other medical conditions must be interpreted with caution (see also Chap. 29).

Pathophysiology

Unfortunately, our knowledge regarding the anatomic localization of possible neural abnormalities in ET is minimal, and, likewise, there is almost no understanding of possible pathophysiological mechanisms. Is the pathogenesis of ET related to dysfunction of the peripheral or central nervous system? The anatomic basis of tremor could be a result of oscillation in the stretch reflex or in a centrally located network of neurons. It is clear that tremor can be modified by various maneuvers that perturb both the stretch reflex and cortical mechanisms, such as transcranial magnetic stimulation.[133-136] However, when ET is produced by a central oscillator, the tremor must be expressed through the neuromuscular machinery of the stretch reflex and limb mechanisms. Several observations suggest that ET does not result solely from peripheral mechanisms. There is no correlation between tremor frequency and nerve conduction velocities,[122] and the frequency of ET has no relationship to the reflex loop time.[54] Furthermore, there is a lack of tremor entrainment produced by peripheral rhythmic inputs.[43] A central site for the abnormality in ET is supported by the beneficial effect of thalamotomy[138] and by drugs that appear to act centrally.[28,61] ET has been reported to be alleviated unilaterally in two patients with strokes that involved the pyramidal tracts[138,139] and in one patient with homolateral cerebellar infarction.[140] Several brain areas are candidates for the exaggerated oscillations responsible for ET. Areas with inherent rhythmicity in the frequency range of ET included the inferior olivary and thalamic nuclei.[141-143] Hypermetabolism of the inferior olive can be observed on PET during tremor activation.[144] Colebatch and coworkers[145] also studied cerebral blood flow, using carbon-15-labeled carbon dioxide with PET technology in four ET patients and four controls. They found that the cerebellum was selectively activated in ET and suggested that the increased blood flow in the cerebellum represented neural activity involved in tremor generation. These investigators concluded that ET is the result of oscillation within the cerebello-olivary pathways that is relayed by way of the thalamus and motor cortex to the spinal cord. Increased activity of the cerebellum in ET, both at rest and when the tremor is advanced, has been observed in other PET studies.[146] A tremor disorder that resembles ET can be caused by vascular or traumatic insults to the brain stem, particularly around the area of the red nucleus.[147] Because of the lack of human data, animal models of ET would be important. Tremors can be induced by drugs such as harmaline and oxotremorine and by anatomic lesions.[148,149] However, the relevance of these conditions to ET is uncertain.

It would appear that ET may be a result of an abnormal oscillation of a central nervous system "pacemaker," the location of which is currently unknown. There have been only approximately 20 reported postmortem examinations of patients with ET.[3,137,150–154] These investigations have reported nonspecific changes, and it would appear that the gross anatomic change may not occur in ET. Studies of possible neurochemical changes in ET brains have not to date been performed. Drug trials with gamma-aminobutyric acid (GABA, progabide) and serotoninergic (trazodone) agonists, using these drugs as pharmacological probes, have not indicated a role for these neurotransmitters in ET.[155,156]

It can be concluded that ET is probably produced by a central oscillator that can be enhanced or suppressed by reflex pathways. Analysis of postmortem material from ET brains is needed if we are to further understand the pathophysiology of ET (see also Chap. 30).

Assessment of Tremor

A variety of means have been used in the assessment of ET.[5,157,158] One major difficulty with attempts to quantify ET is that the severity of tremor can fluctuate significantly over short periods of time. The changing intensity of tremor relates probably both to an inherent rhythm of ET and the influence of external factors.

Clinical rating scales have been used to assess tremor. One such scale that is currently in use is shown below:

TREMOR
0—No tremor perceived.
1—Slight (barely noticeable).
2—Moderate, noticeable, probably not disabling, less than 2 cm excursions of affected part.
3—Marked, probably partially disabling (2- to 4-cm excursions).
4—Severe, disabling (more than 4-cm excursion).

Tremor can be rated for the resting, postural, and kinetic positions and for the affected body part.

Self-assessment scales have also been developed to quantify the functional disability associated with ET.

SPEAKING PHONATION
0—Normal.
1—Mild speech difficulty and/or voice tremulousness when "nervous" only.
2—Mild speech difficulty and/or voice tremor, most of the time.
3—Moderate speech difficulty and/or voice tremor constant.
4—Severe speech difficulty and/or voice tremor. Most words or phrases difficult to understand.

FEEDING (OTHER THAN LIQUIDS)
0—Normal.
1—Mildly abnormal. Can bring all solids to mouth, spilling only rarely.
2—Moderately abnormal. Frequently spills peas and similar foods. May bring head at least halfway to meet food.
3—Markedly abnormal. Unable to cut or uses both hands to feed.
4—Severely abnormal. Needs help to feed.

BRINGING LIQUIDS TO MOUTH (DRINKING)
0—Normal.
1—Mildly abnormal. Can still use a spoon but spills if completely full.
2—Moderately abnormal. Unable to use a spoon. Still uses cup or glass but spills more frequently if more than half full.
3—Markedly abnormal. Can drink from cup or glass but needs both hands.
4—Severely abnormal. Must use a straw.

HYGIENE
0—Normal.
1—Mildly abnormal. Able to do everything but is more careful than average person.
2—Moderately abnormal. Able to do everything but with errors; for example, uses an electric shaver because of tremor.
3—Markedly abnormal. Unable to do most fine tasks, such as putting on lipstick or shaving (even with electric shaver), unless using both hands.
4—Severely abnormal. Unable to do any fine movement tasks.

DRESSING
0—Normal.
1—Mildly abnormal. Able to do everything but is clumsier than average person.
2—Moderately abnormal. Able to do everything but with difficulty.
3—Markedly abnormal. Needs some assistance with buttoning or tying shoelaces.
4—Severely abnormal. Requires assistance with most dressing activities.

WRITING
0—Normal.
1—Mildly abnormal. Legible. Continues to write letters.
2—Moderately abnormal. Legible but no longer writes letters.
3—Markedly abnormal. Illegible.
4—Severely abnormal. Unable to sign checks or other documents requiring signature.

WORKING
0—Tremor does not interfere with primary occupation.
1—Able to perform primary occupation but requires more effort than the average person.
2—Able to do everything but with errors. Poorer than usual performance because of tremor.
3—Unable to do primary occupation. Many have changed to a different job because of tremor. Tremor limits housework, such as ironing.
4—Unable to do outside job; housework very limited.

FINE MOVEMENTS

0—Normal.
1—Minimal impairment. Difficulty threading needles.
2—Moderate impairment. Difficulty buttoning shirt buttons.
3—Marked impairment. Difficulty placing a key in a lock.
4—Severe impairment. Requires both hands to put on glasses.

EMBARRASSMENT

0—None.
1—Minimal change in social activities, still socializes.
2—Moderate change in social activities, avoids encounters with strangers.
3—Marked change in social activities, avoids encounters with friends.
4—Severe change in social activities, avoiding public encounters.

Functional disability can also be assessed by scales when a rater scores the patient's ability to perform motor tasks.

HANDWRITING

Have the subject write the standard sentence "Today is a nice day" with dominant hand.

WITH STRATEGY (COMPENSATORY MANEUVERS)
Describe strategy:
0—Normal.
1—Mildly abnormal. Slightly untidy, tremulous.
2—Moderately abnormal. Legible but with considerable tremor.
3—Markedly abnormal. Illegible.
4—Severely abnormal. Unable to keep pencil or pen on paper without holding down with the other hand.

WITHOUT STRATEGY
0—Normal.
1—Mildly abnormal. Slightly untidy, tremulous.
2—Moderately abnormal. Legible but with considerable tremor.
3—Markedly abnormal. Illegible.
4—Severely abnormal. Unable to keep pencil or pen on paper without holding down with the other hand.

DRAWINGS

Ask the subject to draw the requested figures. Test each hand without leaning the hand or arm on the table. Use a ball point pen only.

SPIRAL
0—Normal.
1—Slightly tremulous.
2—Moderately tremulous.
3—Accomplishes the task with great difficulty. Figure still recognizable.
4—Unable to complete drawing. Figure not recognizable.

DRAW STRAIGHT LINE BETWEEN LINES (PATIENT WORKSHEET ATTACHED)
0—Normal.
1—Slightly tremulous.
2—Moderately tremulous.
3—Accomplishes the task with great difficulty. Figure still recognizable.
4—Unable to complete drawing. Figure not recognizable.

DRAW SINE WAVE BETWEEN LINES
0—Normal.
1—Slightly tremulous.
2—Moderately tremulous.
3—Accomplishes the task with great difficulty. Many errors.
4—Unable to complete drawing. Figure not recognizable.

POURING

USE FIRM PLASTIC CUPS (8 CM TALL, WITHOUT HANDLES) FILLED WITH WATER 1 CM FROM THE TOP. ASK PATIENT TO POUR WATER FROM ONE CUP TO ANOTHER.
0—Normal.
1—More careful than a person without tremor, but no water is spilled.
2—Spills a small amount of water (up to 10 percent of the total amount).
3—Spills a considerable amount of water (>10–50 percent).
4—Unable to pour without spilling most of the water.

The rhythmic, oscillatory kinetics of tremor make it suitable for quantification by objective means. Both acute and chronic recordings have been performed.[3,159] A variety of recording systems have been used. An accelerometer (velocity transducer), which is sensitive to movement (displacement), is attached to the hand or another body part. The signal is then amplified, and a summating technique such as spectral analysis is applied to an epoch of tremor, for example, 60 s. An amplitude measurement is then generated at a peak frequency.

Attempts have been made to develop an ambulatory tremor-recording device the size of a wrist watch which can be worn for a prolonged period of time, for example, days or weeks.[159] To date, none of these devices has been perfected. One difficulty is separating normal rhythmic movements from tremor. However, with new developments in technology, it is likely that such an ambulatory recording device will become commercially available in the near future.

Treatment

Magee[160] in 1965 stated that there was no effective therapy for ET. Recent advances have now resulted in successful treatment for ET. A variety of pharmacological approaches to ET is available, and new strategies are being studied. However, tremor of different body parts and various tremor variants may have different pharmacological responsiveness and some patients still cannot be effectively treated.[5,51]

ALCOHOL

Alcohol will temporarily cause a dramatic tremor reduction in the majority of patients.[61,161] Clinical observations suggest that with time, larger amounts of alcohol may be needed to cause tremor reduction. It is generally recommended that the judicious use of small amounts of alcoholic beverages before meals or other events to reduce tremor is reasonable.[4] Alcohol's mechanism of action is unknown; however, PET studies have shown that alcohol decreases the increase in regional cerebellar blood flow in ET (T Findley, personal communication). A better understanding of its action could lead to the development of other pharmacological agents for ET. Taräväinen and coworkers[162] investigated the alcohol derivative, methylpentynol, a 6-carbon alcohol, in ET and found its effect was not different from placebo. Critchley[6] warned that alcohol, when used in ET, "appeared only too often to have served as an excuse for habits of intemperance." The risk of addiction was considered a contraindication to the use of alcohol. However, the rate of chronic alcoholism in ET has only recently been defined. Schroeder and Nasrallah,[163] in a retrospective chart survey, found a 60 percent alcoholic rate in ET and concluded that ET is an important cause of alcoholism. However, Koller,[164] in a prospective study, found that the prevalence of pathological drinking in ET did not differ from other tremor disorders or chronic neurological disease without tremor. Likewise, similar surveys in Finland and Sweden found that ET patients neither used more alcohol nor had a higher prevalence of alcoholism than the general population.[164] Moreover, a recent study found that chronic alcoholism may itself result in a persistent postural tremor, lasting up to 1 year after complete abstinence.[165] It can be concluded that the occasional use of alcohol in ET is not contraindicated and that the risk of alcoholism is low.

BETA-ADRENERGIC BLOCKERS

Marshall,[166] in 1968, suggested that beta-adrenergic blockers may be useful in the treatment of ET. Winkler and Young[167] and Sevitt[168] both reported that propranolol decreased ET. Several subsequent studies reported a lack of effect of propranolol.[169,170] However, this may have been a result of inadequate doses, small sample size, or lack of objective measurements. Most investigations have confirmed the efficacy of propranolol in reducing postural hand tremor, using both subjective and objective (accelerometer recordings) evaluation.[167,171–173] Tremor amplitude is decreased, but tremor frequency is unchanged. Propranolol became the drug of choice for ET; however, the clinical response to propranolol is variable and often incomplete.[11,28] It is generally estimated that 50–70 percent of patients will have symptomatic relief. Dramatic improvement occurs in a much smaller percentage, and some patients will have no response. Average tremor reduction of 50–60 percent is suggested by some studies, but the number of patients investigated has been small. There are no well-defined factors that predict therapeutic responsiveness. Dupuis et al.[140] and Murray[172] found that the effect of chronic propranolol treatment was better in younger patients and in those with a shorter duration of disease. However,

Teräväinen et al.[174] and Larsen et al.[175] found propranolol treatment more effective in older patients and in those with lower frequency of tremor. Calzetti and coworkers[176] found a better response to a single oral dose of propranolol in patients with a larger tremor amplitude and a lower frequency. With chronic administration, they found no correlation with disease duration, patient's age, or degree of cardiac beta-blockage.[176] The number of patients in the above studies has been small, which may account for the variable findings. In a dose-response study of propranolol, 240–320 mg/day was found to be the optimal dose range.[177] Doses above 320 mg/day conferred no additional benefit. A sustained-release preparation of propranolol (propranolol long-acting) designed for once daily dosage has been reported to provide similar, or in some cases, greater tremor reduction than divided doses.[178,179] Many patients preferred propranolol long-acting for ease of administration.

Propanolol therapy is usually well-tolerated. Relative contraindications for propranolol use are (1) heart failure, especially if poorly controlled; (2) second- or third-degree atrioventricular block; (3) asthma or other bronchospastic disease; and (4) insulin-dependent diabetes, in which propranolol may block the adrenergic manifestations of hypoglycemia. Most side effects of propranolol are related to beta-blockage. The pulse rate will be lowered in most patients. A pulse of 60 beats/min is usually well-tolerated. Other less common adverse reactions include fatigue, weight gain, nausea, diarrhea, rash, impotency, and mental status alterations (for example, depression). It has been suggested that tolerance may develop to propranolol's effect[180]; however, several studies have found that the majority of patients do not lose any effect of propranolol after 1 year of therapy, although the dose had to be increased in some patients to maintain the same degree of efficacy.[181,182]

The mechanism of action of propranolol in ET is unknown. Young[183] proposed a central site of action, because they noted no effect of intravenous or intra-arterial propranolol and a delay in the effect of chronic oral therapy. However, several controlled studies have shown that propranolol causes an immediate and sustained reduction in tremor.[184,185] Jefferson colleagues[186] have proposed a peripheral site of action. Beta-blockers that enter the central nervous system with difficulty can reduce ET. Specific beta$_2$ antagonists (ICI 118551 and LI 32-468), which act predominantly peripherally, are effective in decreasing tremor, further supporting a peripheral beta$_2$ mechanism of action.[186,187]

Other orally active beta-adrenergic blocking drugs are available, such as metoprolol, nadolol, atenolol, timolol, and pindolol. The beta-blockers are classified according to the presence or absence of beta$_1$-adrenergic selectivity, intrinsic sympathomimetic activity (partial agonists), and membrane-stabilizing properties. Differences in potency, metabolism, half-life, protein binding, and excretion are recognized. Despite the therapeutic similarity of beta-blocking drugs, differences in their pharmacodynamic properties may be clinically important. The effectiveness of metoprolol in ET has been demonstrated in multiple case reports and a controlled study.[182,188–193] Metoprolol differs from propranolol in preferentially antagonizing beta$_1$-adrenergic receptors. The selectivity for beta$_1$ receptors is, however, only relative. With higher dosages beta$_2$-adrenergic receptors are also blocked. Some degree of beta$_2$-blockage appears in patients at daily doses above 100 mg. Metoprolol is beneficial in ET at divided doses of 100–200 mg/day. Patients who failed to respond to propranolol also did not respond to metoprolol.[193] It has been suggested that metoprolol is the preferred drug for use in patients with bronchospastic disease.[193] Because of its relative lack of beta$_2$-blocking properties, metoprolol should theoretically be better tolerated than propranolol, a nonspecific blocker. Several asthmatic patients with ET have been reported who could tolerate metoprolol but not propranolol. Metoprolol is, however, capable of causing respiratory distress and should be used with caution in bronchospastic disease. Nadolol, when administered once daily, at doses of 120 and 240 mg/day was found in a controlled study to significantly decrease ET in patients who also responded to propranolol.[194] Nadolol has a 24-hour half-life and can be taken once daily, avoiding inconveniences and compliance problems of multiple daily drug administration. Atenolol was reported to have no effect on tremor and to cause slight tremor reduction.[176,186,195] Timolol was found to decrease tremor,[195] and pindolol was found to be ineffective.[174] Pindolol because of its partial agonist activity may actually produce tremors.[196] Kuroda and coworkers[198] reported that arotinolol (30 mg/day), a peripherally acting beta-adrenergic blocker, significantly reduced ET in 15 patients.

The usefulness of other beta-adrenergic blockers is not much different from propranolol. Selective beta-blockers, like metoprolol, can be used at low doses in bronchospastic disease. When a side effect such as impotence occurs with propranolol, changing to a different beta-blocker may result in disappearance of the adverse affect without loss of beneficial action.

PRIMIDONE

O'Brien and coworkers in 1981[198] noted that primidone given to a patient with epilepsy and ET reduced tremor, and they gave the drug to 20 other patients, starting with 125 mg and increasing to 750 mg/day. Six patients, including four at the 125-mg dose, could not tolerate the drug because of vertigo, unsteadiness, and nausea. Twelve patients had a good clinical response. Addition of propranolol resulted in further improvement. It was concluded that primidone was more effective than propranolol, but ET patients did not tolerate primidone as well as seizure patients did. However, epileptic patients are often taking other drugs that cause hepatic enzyme induction, which may explain these perceived differences in toxicity. Chakrabarti and Pearce[199] gave primidone to five patients, starting at 125 mg for several days with a gradual increase of 750–1000 mg/day. Improvement was evident within a few days with increased functional capabilities. Findley et al.[200] studied 11 patients using objective recording techniques, starting primidone at 62.5 mg and increasing the dose to 750 mg/day. Side effects occurred in six patients, and only seven patients achieved the maximum dose. Tremor was decreased by an average of 66 percent (mean dose, 590 mg/day) and by more than 90 percent in two patients. Koller and Royse,[201] in a placebo-controlled study using objective recording techniques, found that primi-

done (50–1000 mg/day) significantly reduced the amplitude of essential hand tremor in both untreated and propranolol-treated patients. Low doses (i.e., 250 mg/day) were as effective as high doses. Primidone decreased tremor more than propranolol. There was no correlation between therapeutic response and serum levels. Acute reactions to the initial dose and side effects of higher dose caused drug intolerance. A single oral dose of 250 mg/day of primidone decreased tremor by 60 percent 1–7 hours after ingestion with stable serum primidone levels but no detectable phenobarbital. Tremor control was lost when primidone was replaced by phenobarbital. Gorman and coworkers[202] compared primidone, propranolol, and placebo in 14 patients. Both propranolol and primidone significantly reduced tremor, but there was no significant difference in improvement between the drugs. It has been suggested that tolerance to primidone may develop[203,204]; however, two studies that investigated the long-term effects of primidone have found that its antitremor effect was maintained for a 1-year period.[181,205]

The mechanism of action of primidone's antitremor effect is unknown. Primidone is converted to two active metabolites: phenyethylmalonamide (PEMA) with a half-life of approximately 30 hours and phenobarbital with a half-life of approximately 10 days. The administration of high doses of PEMA had no effect on tremor.[206] Findley and Calzetti[207] suggested that the beneficial effect was mediated by both primidone and phenobarbital. However, primidone decreased tremor when there was no detectable serum phenobarbital, and phenobarbital may have only minimal antitremor action.[201] Primidone itself or an unrecognized metabolite appears to be the responsible agent. It is important to note that with primidone monotherapy the ratio of primidone to phenobarbital in the serum is 1:2.

PHENOBARBITAL

Phenobarbital has been used in ET for many years, and generally its effect has been thought to be minimal. However, several studies have demonstrated a beneficial effect of phenobarbital. Procaccianti and coworkers[208] found that phenobarbital caused a significant reduction in tremor, as compared to that in placebo. The effect in 12 patients was comparable to that of propranolol. In a double-blind controlled study, Baruzzi and coworkers[209] found that both phenobarbital and propranolol were more effective than placebo with objective measures and patient self-assessment. However, clinical evaluation showed no difference between phenobarbital and placebo. Findley and Cleeves[210] gave phenobarbital (120 mg/day) to 12 patients and also found that the drug was better than placebo. They suggested that phenobarbital may be an alternate drug for the treatment of ET. It is possible, however, that the tremolytic effect of phenobarbital might be directly related to the degree of central sedation. Koller and Royse,[201] using objective measures, found no effect of phenobarbital (90 mg/day) in essential hand tremor in 12 patients. In a double-blind comparison of primidone and phenobarbital, Sasso and colleagues[211] found primidone superior to both placebo and phenobarbital in reducing tremor in 13 patients. Phenobarbital, at a dosage yielding levels greater than those seen with primidone, was not better than placebo. The effectiveness and role of phenobarbital in ET is controversial; however, the drug may be used in patients who do not respond well to propranolol or primidone. Cabrera-Valdivia et al.[212] reported that phenobarbital was a successful treatment in two patients with orthostatic truncal tremor.

BENZODIAZEPINES

Benzodiazepines and other sedative-hypnotic drugs have, for a long time, been used in the treatment of ET, perhaps in the mistaken belief that tremor was due to anxiety. Interestingly, there has been no investigation of the most commonly used drug, diazepam (Valium), in the treatment of ET. It is generally thought that these medications possess only limited efficacy, which is probably related to a reduction in tension and anxiety that can cause tremor enhancement. Several compounds have been investigated. The effect of clonazepam in ET was studied by Thompson and coworkers,[213] who found that the drug had no effect. Sedation was a frequent side effect. Clonazepam (1 to 3 mg/day) is, however, very effective in treating kinetic predominant tremor[69] and orthostatic truncal tremor.[84,86] Huber and Paulson[214] studied alprazolam, a triazole analogue of the benzodiazepines, in ET in a double-blind, placebo-controlled study of 24 patients. Significant improvement occurred, but transient mild fatigue or sedation occurred in one-half of patients. The contribution of the sedative or anxiolytic effect of alprazolam to tremor reduction is unknown but may be substantial. Further controlled studies of alprazolam are needed to establish its role in the therapy of ET.

CARBONIC ANHYDRASE INHIBITORS

Muenter and coworkers in 1991[215] reported that the carbonic anhydrase inhibitor, methazolamide, was highly effective in ET. They administered methazolamide to 28 ET patients in an open trial. Marked improvement was reported in 12 patients, moderate improvement in 4, mild improvement in 4, and no effect in 8 patients. It was noted that head and voice tremor were particularly improved. The mean maximum daily dose was 203 mg. Adverse reactions, including sedation, nausea, epigastric distress, anorexia, and numbness and paresthesias, were common. The authors suggest that perhaps the doses used were too high and that doses were increased too rapidly. Only 10 patients continued on the drug. Busenbark and coworkers[216] found that acetazolamide, another carbonic anhydrase, significantly decreased tremor on clinical rating scales, and a higher mean dose appeared to have more of an effect. However, no major change was reported by the patients on their assessment of functional disability, and ratings of motor function showed only modest improvement. Therefore, these investigations did not find the dramatic improvement reported with methazolamide. Head and voice tremor did not appear to be particularly sensitive to acetazolamide. A double-blind placebo-controlled study by Busenbark et al.[217] studied the effect of methazolamide in 25 patients with ET. Tremor assessment included patient self-reporting of functional disability, clinical rating of motor tasks and tremor

severity, and accelerometric measurements. There was no significant difference between methazolamide and placebo in any of the assessments. Side effects, paresthesias, sedation, headaches, and gastrointestinal symptoms were common. Only two patients elected to remain on the drug after the study. They concluded that methazolamide has only limited efficacy in the treatment of ET.[217]

OTHER DRUGS

ET patients are sometimes given antiparkinsonian drugs that are usually discontinued because they are ineffective. Therefore, clinical experience indicates that these drugs have no benefit, although there has been no formal study of L-dopa or anticholinergic treatment in ET. It has been suggested that L-dopa therapy may worsen ET.[154,218] Amantadine (Symmetrel), which possesses both dopaminergic and anticholinergic properties, was reported by Critchley[219] to improve tremor in 26 patients. However, this conclusion was based solely on clinical observations. Manyam,[220] using clinical scoring, found that amantadine (100 mg twice per day) caused improvement in five patients, had no effect in one, and worsened tremor in two others. Obeso and coworkers[221] observed one patient who had a dramatic response to amantadine therapy. Koller[222] evaluated six patients, using objective techniques, and found that amantadine exacerbated tremor in three patients and had no effect in the other three. It would appear that amantadine is not generally useful in ET, but an occasional patient may respond to the drug.

Caccia and Mangoni,[223] in an open trial study, suggested that clonidine might cause improvement of ET. Clonidine's ability to stimulate central alpha-adrenergic receptors was the proposed mechanism of action. Koller and coworkers[224] studied the effect of clonidine treatment (average dose, 0.4 mg/day) in 10 patients in a double-blind placebo-controlled investigation. Tremor amplitude was quantified by an accelerometer. Tremor was not significantly changed by clonidine therapy. Side effects (dry mouth, decreased urination, tiredness, and lightheadedness) were common and often dose-limiting. It was concluded that clonidine is not effective treatment for ET. Mai and Olsen[225] reported that the alpha-adrenergic-blocking drug, thymoxamine, given intravenously, significantly suppressed ET in nine patients. However, when Koller[226] studied in a controlled manner the alpha-adrenergic blocker, phenoxybenzamine, no effect on ET could be demonstrated. There is no evidence that alpha-adrenergic mechanisms are involved in the pathogenesis of ET, and alpha-adrenergic drugs, agonists or antagonists, appear to have no role in the treatment of ET. Morris and coworkers[227] found the serotoninergic precursor tryptophan, given with pyridoxine, was ineffective in ET patients. However, McLeod and White[228] observed "significant improvement" of ET in two patients with trazodone (150 mg/day), a serotonin agonist. Improvement was observed only after 3 weeks of treatment. No objective measures were made in these open-label observations. Discontinuation of trazodone in one patient was said to be associated with an increase in tremor. The authors suggested that serotoninergic neurotransmission may be important in ET, because trazodone stimulates serotonin receptors and blocks reuptake mechanisms. Koller[156] performed a double-blind placebo controlled investigation of trazodone in 24 patients and found that the drug was ineffective. Likewise Cleeves and Findley[229] found trazodone ineffective in ET. The selective serotonin receptor type 2 antagonist, ritanserin, was found to reduce parkinsonian tremor but to have no effect in ET.[230] Caccia et al.[231] found that the venous infusion of propranolol and clonidine, but not of urapidil or trazodone, reduced ET in 25 patients whose tremor was recorded by accelerometry. Pharmacological studies suggest no role for serotoninergic neurotransmission, even though the inferior olivary nucleus, which may be an important structure in the genesis of ET, receives serotoninergic input.

Several of the drugs effective in ET affect central gamma-aminobutyric (GABA) neurotransmission, suggesting a possible involvement of this neurotransmitter. However, Koller and coworkers[155] gave progabide, a GABA agonist (30 mg/kg/day) to 10 patients in a double-blind crossover study and found no effect of the drug on tremor.

Mephenesin, a centrally acting muscle relaxant, was touted to have a limited effect in reducing ET[219]; however, the drug never gained widespread use. Topakias and coworkers[232] studied the acute effects of two calcium channel blockers, nifedipine and verapamil, in ET. Nifedipine (10 mg) increased tremor intensity, and verapamil (80 mg) had no effect. However, in 14 patients with ET in a crossover study with nicardipine (1 mg/kg/day) and propranolol (160 mg/day), both drugs improved ET, with a nonsignificantly higher efficacy of propranolol. These results suggest that nicardipine might be efficacious for ET.[233] Curran and Lang[234] studied the effects of flunarizine in 10 patients with moderate-to-severe essential tremor. Tremor was evaluated after 6 weeks of treatment, using patient and physician assessment, as well as blinded video analysis. Only one patient had mild subjective transient improvement, and three experienced worsening of tremor. No patient elected to remain on treatment. They concluded that flumarizine is ineffective for moderate-to-severe ET and may actually worsen the symptoms in some patients. Biary and coworkers[235] investigated the effect of flunarizine (10 mg/day) in 17 ET patients in a double-blind placebo controlled trial. Of patients who completed the study, 13 of 15 showed improvement in both subjective and objective measures. The authors concluded that flunarizine is effective treatment for ET. This drug is, however, not available in North America at this time. Pakkenberg and Pakkenberg[236] found, in an open trial, that the atypical neuroleptic, clozapine, decreased ET in 9 of 12 patients. Tremor reduction may be related to sedation, which was a major side effect. McCarthy also reports efficacy of clozapine in ET.[237] McDowell[238] reported two patients who had suppression of their tremor with glutethimide (Doriden) at doses of 1000–4000 mg/day. One patient had taken the drug for 14 years without side effects.

Xanthines derivatives, such as theophylline, can induce tremor or appear to worsen ET in some patients. However, Mally and Stone[239] administered theophylline to 20 ET patients in a double-blind crossover study. Tremor was said to improve after 4 weeks of treatment. It was suggested that enhancement of GABA sensitivity may be responsible for the therapeutic effect.

BOTULINUM TOXIN INJECTION

Recently, a novel therapeutic approach to the treatment of ET has been reported, using botulinum toxin-A intramuscular injections.[240] Botulinum toxin causes some degree of muscle paresis by acting at peripheral nerve endings to block the release of acetylcholine. This agent has been shown to be effective in a variety of focal dystonias and has been suggested as the treatment of choice in these disorders.[241] Jankovic and Schwartz[240] found that injection of this chemical successfully reduced tremor in 67 percent of patients in an open-label trial of botulinum toxin in various tremor disorders. The duration of maximum response was 10.5 weeks. Hand weakness was the most common adverse reaction. In another open-label study, Trosch and Pullman[242] found botulinum toxin subjectively but not objectively improved ET in 14 patients. These initial encouraging results need to be scientifically assessed with a double-blind, placebo-controlled study. Many questions need to answered, such as: What is the optimal dose? What muscles should be injected? What is the time frame for reinjection? Hopefully, future studies will determine whether botulinum toxin injection is effective in ET and delineate the parameters for its use. Our anecdotal experience suggests that this form of therapy is only of minimal value.

THALAMOTOMY

Stereotaxic thalamotomy is an effective procedure in the treatment of parkinsonian, cerebellar, and essential tremors.[136,243–248] The technical aspects of the procedure have improved greatly in the last decade. Advances in the neurophysiological confirmation of the site of the lesion now allow for accurate placement. The site of the lesion selected is the ventral anterior or the ventral intermediate (Vim) nucleus of the thalamus. Stereotaxic thalamotomy can be performed with the use of mild sedation and local anesthesia.[249] The neurological status of the patients can, therefore, be monitored. Stereotaxic coordinates are generated by use of the CT head-scanning and computerized programs. A microelectrode with a recording tip is lowered into the brain, and the neuronal response further defines the anatomic site for the lesion. Heating of the electrode tip creates a small lesion. The reported results of thalamotomy in ET have been favorable.[249–251] Bertrand[243] stated that "the results are most satisfactory and one may expect a marked relief of tremor in 90% of cases, with a total relief in a high percentage of these." Ohye and coworkers[245] reported 15 patients successfully treated with small lesions in the Vim nucleus. No late relapse was noted. Andrew[246] treated 10 patients with thalamotomy. In three cases the tremor was improved, and in five patients there was almost total suppression of tremor. Functional abilities were said to be markedly improved in these patients. One patient had no change after the operation, and another patient suffered hemiplegia as a complication of the procedure. Stereotaxic thalamotomy currently has a mortality rate of less than 0.3 percent, mostly related to postoperative complications.[248] Temporary intellectual deficits and transitory hemiparesis may occur. A lasting weakness is unusual. Other uncommon adverse reactions include seizures, involuntary movements, and cerebellar signs. A transient deterioration of speech may be seen occasionally after unilateral thalamotomy that will return to normal after several weeks. Bilateral thalamotomy is associated with much more serious complications. In particular, a severe persistent dysarthria occurs. Permanent mental changes may also occur. Therefore, bilateral operations can be recommended only with reservation.

There is only minimal information regarding the long-term effects of thalamotomy for the treatment of ET. Mohadjer and coworkers[32] at the University of Freiburg in Germany reported follow-up from a group of 104 ET patients who were operated on from 1964 to 1984. Sixty-five patients were reexamined who had an average follow-up period of 8.6 years. Eighty percent were found to have evidence of a successful operation, with 69 percent having complete or substantial reduction of tremor and 11.9 percent having moderate improvement. Also, 11.9 percent of patients showed deterioration on the operated side, compared to 34 percent who showed deterioration on the unoperated side.

Thalamotomy appears to be a neglected therapeutic option. It should be reserved for those with (1) severe unilateral or asymmetrical tremor, (2) marked functional disability, and (3) a tremor that is unresponsive to maximally tolerated doses of propranolol, primidone, phenobarbital, and clonazepam.

THALAMIC STIMULATION

Benabid and colleagues[252] recently reported their results, using electrical stimulation of the thalamus as treatment for tremor disorders. They used high-frequency stimulation of the Vim nucleus of the thalamus in six ET patients with disabling tremor. Chronic stimulating electrodes were connected to a pulse generator implanted in the Vim. Tremor was assessed by accelerometry. The stimulator was on during the day and turned off at night in five of the six patients. Moderate-to-major improvement occurred in all patients. Adverse reactions were mild and could be eliminated by reduction or cessation of stimulation. This technique presumably causes an electrophysiological block similar to that of thalamic destructive surgery. Additional studies[253,254] have confirmed that deep brain stimulation of the Vim nucleus of the thalamus is an effective and safe means of treating severe, intractable ET.

BEHAVIORAL THERAPY

A variety of behavioral techniques, including psychotherapy, biofeedback, and hypnosis, have been used in the treatment of movement disorders. Any benefit from these procedures has been minimal and short-lived. There is one report of the beneficial effect of psychotherapy in ET.[255] The reported improvement of symptoms was thought to be a result of "mental stabilization" and relaxation of muscle tension.

DRUGS OF CHOICE

Propranolol and other beta-adrenergic blockers and primidone are currently the only two drugs that have been clearly shown to be effective in suppressing ET. It is unclear which should be the drug of first choice. As many as 20 percent of

patients will suffer side effects for several days after the first dose of primidone. When the patient is warned of these potential adverse reactions and encouraged to continue to take the drug, only a minority will discontinue primidone. Side effects with chronic therapy are uncommon with primidone but are much more of a concern with propranolol. Many elderly patients cannot take beta-adrenergic blockers. It appears that marked tremor reduction is more often achieved with primidone than with propranolol. Some patients may require both propranolol and primidone therapy. *We recommend the following treatment schedule:*

1. Start with primidone, 50 mg at nighttime. (Warn patient of possible side effects but recommend continuation of drug even when side effects occur).
2. Increase primidone to 125 mg at nighttime when necessary.
3. Increase primidone to 250 mg at nighttime when necessary.
4. Add or switch to propranolol-LA, 80 mg, in the morning.
5. Increase propranolol-LA to 160 mg in the morning, when necessary.
6. Increase propranolol-LA to 240 mg when necessary.
7. Increase propranolol-LA to 320 mg in the morning when necessary.

When the patient has no response to either primidone or propranolol, alprazolam should be tried. When this drug also fails, a trial of phenobarbital can be initiated. Hopefully, future research will find new therapeutic agents for those patients not responding to currently used drugs.

Summary

ET is the most common movement disorder, occurring most frequently in individuals over 40 years of age. A positive family history for tremor is obtained in approximately one-half of the cases. The affliction usually begins as a postural tremor in the hands but may later involve the head and other body parts. Typically, tremor amplitude increases, and frequency decreases with age. Disability results from impairment of fine motor skills or social withdrawal. The occurrence of tremor resembling ET in other neurological disorders may lead to misdiagnosis and clouding of nosological classification. The pathophysiological basis of ET is uncertain but is thought to be central in origin. Abnormal oscillation of a central nervous system pacemaker (presumably within the cerebellar-brain stem circuitry) has been hypothesized. Beta-adrenergic-blocking agents and primidone are medications with proven efficacy for the treatment of ET.

References

1. Findley LJ, Koller WC: Essential tremor: A review. *Neurology* 37:1194–1197, 1987.
2. Hubble JP, Busenbark KL, Koller WC: Essential tremor. *Clin Neuropharmacol* 12:453–482, 1989.

3. Elble R, Koller WC: *Tremor.* Baltimore: Johns Hopkins University Press, 1990.

4. Koller WC, Hubble J, Busenbark K: Essential tremor, in Calne DB (ed): *Neurodegenerative Disease.* Philadelphia: WB Saunders, 1994, pp 717–742.

5. Bain PG, Findley LJ, Thompson PD, et al: A study of hereditary essential tremor. *Brain* 117:805–824, 1994.

6. Critchley M: Observations on essential (heredofamilial) tremor. *Brain* 72:113–139, 1949.

7. Sider D, McVaugh M: Galen on tremor, palpitation, spasm, and rigor. *Trans Stud Coll Physicians Phila* 1:183–210, 1979.

8. Parkinson J: *An Essay on the Shaking Palsy.* London: Whittingham & Rowland, 1817.

9. Charcot JM: *Policlinique du Mardi: Lecons de Mardi.* Paris: 24 Juiller, 1888, pp 448–451.

10. Charcot JM: Clinical lectures on disease of the nervous system, vol III, lecture XV, translated by Thomas Savill. *The New Sydenham Society (Lond)* 128:183–197, 1889.

11. Larsen TA, Calne DB: Essential tremor. *Clin Neuropharmacol* 6:185–206, 1983.

12. Dana CL: Hereditary tremor, a hitherto undescribed form of motor neurosis. *Am J Med Sci* 94:386–393, 1887.

13. Pintus G: Sul tippo "macrobioticus multiparus" del tremor essenziale. *Riv Patol Nerv Ment* 51:114–124, 1938.

14. Larsson T, Sjögren T: Essential tremor. A clinical and genetic population study. *Acta Psychiatry Neurol Scand* 36(suppl 144):1–176, 1960.

15. Flatau J: Le tremblement essentiel héréditaire (abstr.). *Rev Neurol* 17:417, 1909.

16. Raymond F: Le tremblement essentiel héréditaire (abstr.). *Rev Neurol* 17:416–417, 1909.

17. Katzenstein E: Uber familiaren tremor. *Arch Suisses Neurol Psychiatry* 61:380–381, 1948.

18. Rautakorpi I: Essential Tremor: An Epidemiological, Clinical, and Genetic Study. Dissertation, Turku, Finland, 1978.

19. Duvoisin RC, Gearing FR, Schweitzer MD, Yahr MD: A family study of parkinsonism, in Barbeau A, Brunette JR (eds): *Progress in Neurogenetics.* Amsterdam: Excerpta Medica Foundation, 1969, pp 492–496.

20. McDowell FH, Lee JE, Sweet RD: Extrapyramidal disease, in Baker AB, Baker LH (eds): *Clinical Neurology.* Philadelphia: Harper & Row, 1938, pp 53–54.

21. Rajput AH, Offord KP, Beard CM, Kurland LT: Essential tremor in Rochester, Minnesota: A 45-year study. *J Neurol Neurosurg Psychiatry* 47:466–470, 1984.

22. Haerer AF, Anderson DW, Schoenberg BS: Prevalence of essential tremor: Results from the Copiah County study. *Arch Neurol* 39:750–751, 1982.

23. Rautakorpi I, Takala J, Marttila RJ, et al: Essential tremor in a Finnish population. *Acta Neurol Scand* 66:58–67, 1982.

24. Hornabrook RW, Nagurney JT: Essential tremor in Papua New Guinea. *Brain* 99:659–672, 1976.

25. Moretti G, Calzetti S, Quartucci G, et al: [Epidemiological study on tremor in the aged]. *Minerva Med* 74:1701–1705, 1983.

26. Aiyesiloju AB, Osuntodum BO, Bademosi O, Adeuja AO: Hereditary neurodegenerative disorders in Nigerian Africans. *Neurology* 34:361–362, 1984.

27. Salemi G, Savettieri G, Rocca WA, et al: Prevalence of essential tremor: A door-to-door survey in Terrasini, Sicily: Sicilian Neuro-Epidemiologic Study Group. *Neurology* 44:61–64, 1994.

28. Koller WC: Diagnosis and treatment of tremor. *Neurol Clin* 2:499–514, 1984.

29. Rautakorpi I, Marttila RJ, Rinne UK: Epidemiology of essential tremor, in Findley LJ, Capildeo R (eds): *Movement Disorders: Tremor.* London: Macmillan, 1984, pp 211–218.

30. Bharucha NE, Bharucha EP, Bharuch AE, et al: Prevalence of essential tremor in the Parsi community of Bombay, India. *Arch Neurol* 45:907–908, 1988.

31. Rajput AH, Offord KP, Kurland LT: Epidemiologic survey of essential tremor in Rochester, MN. *Neurology* 32:A128, 1982.

32. Mohadjer M, Goerke H, Milios E, et al: Long-term results of stereotaxy in the treatment of essential tremor. *Stereotact Funct Neurosurg* 54155:125–129, 1990.

33. Moghal S, Rajput AH, D'Arcy C, Rajput R: Prevalence of movement disorders in elderly community residents. *Neuroepidemiology* 13:175—178, 1994.

34. Marshall J: Observations on essential tremor. *J Neurol Neurosurg Psychiatry* 25:122–125, 1962.

35. Jager BV, King T: Hereditary tremor. *Arch Intern Med* 95:788–793, 1955.

36. Herskovits E, Figueroa E, Mangone C: Hereditary essential tremor in Buenos Aires (Argentina). *Arq Neuropsiquiatr* 46:238–247, 1988.

37. Buckley P: Familial tremor. *Proc R Soc Med* 31:297, 1938.

38. Busenbark K, Barnes P, Lyons K, et al: Accuracy of reported family history of essential tremor. *Neurology.* In Press.

39. Kaneko K, Igarashi S, Miyatake T, Tsuiji S: 'Essential tremor' and CAG repeats in the androgen receptor gene. *Neurology* 43:1618–1619, 1993.

40. Conway D, Bain PG, Warner TT, et al: Linkage analysis with chromosome 9 markers in hereditary essential tremor. *Mov Disord* 8:374–376, 1993.

41. Davis CH, Kunkle EC: Benign essential (heredofamilial) tremor. *Arch Intern Med* 87:808–816, 1951.

42. Singer C, Sanchez-Ramos J, Weiner WJ: Gait abnormality in essential tremor. *Mov Disord* 9:193–196, 1994.

43. Marsden CD, Obeso J, Rothwell JC: Benign essential tremor is no a single entity, in Yahr MD (ed): *Current Concepts in Parkinson's disease.* Amsterdam: Excerpta Medica, 1983, pp 31–46.

44. Hallett M: Differential diagnosis of tremor, in Vinken PJ, Bruyn GW, Klawans HL (eds): *Handbook of Clinical Neurology.* Amsterdam: Elsevier Publishers, 1989, pp 583–595.

45. Jankovic J, Fahn S: Physiologic and pathologic tremors: Diagnosis, mechanism and management. *Ann Intern Med* 93:460–465, 1980.

46. Elble RJ: Physiologic and essential tremor. *Neurology* 36:225–231, 1986.

47. Sanes JN, Hallet M: Limb positioning and magnitude of essential tremor and other pathological tremors. *Mov Disord* 5:304–309, 1990.

48. Findley LF, Gresty MA: Tremor. *Br J Hosp Med* 26:16–32, 1981.

49. Wade P, Gresty MA, Findley LJ: A normative study of postural tremor of the hand. *Arch Neurol* 39:358–362, 1982.

50. Deuschl G, Lücking CH, Schenk E: Essential tremor: Electrophysiological and pharmacological evidence for a subdivision. *J Neurol Neurosurg Psychiatry* 50:1435–1441, 1987.

51. Koller WC, Busenbark KL, Dubinsky R, Hubble J: Classification of essential tremor. *Clin Neuropharmacol* 15:81–88, 1992.

52. Koller WC, Busenbark K, Miner K: The relationship of essential tremor to other movement disorders: Report on 678 patients. Essential Tremor Study Group. *Ann Neurol* 35:717–723, 1994.

53. Borges V, Ferraz HB, de Andrade LA: Essential tremor: Clinical characterization in a sample of 176 patients. *Arq Neuropsiquiatr* 52:161–165, 1994.

54. Longe AC: Essential tremor in Nigerians: A prospective study of 35 cases. *East Afr Med J* 62:672–676, 1985.

55. Massey EW, Paulson GW: Essential vocal tremor: Clinical characteristics and response to therapy. *South Med J* 78:316–317, 1985.

56. Vanesse M, Bedard P, Andermann F: Shuddering attacks in children: An early clinical manifestation of essential tremor. *Neurology (Minneap)* 26:1027–1030, 1976.

57. Sutherland JM, Edwards VE, Eadie MJ: Essential (hereditary or senile) tremor. *Med J Aust* 2:44–47, 1975.

58. Biary N, Koller W: Handedness and essential tremor. *Arch Neurol* 42:1082–1083, 1985.

59. Biary N, Cleeves L, Findley L, Koller W: Post-traumatic tremor. *Neurology* 39:103–106, 1989.

60. Wake A, Takahashi Y, Onishi T, et al: Treatment of essential tremor through behaviour therapy—use of Jacobson's progressive relaxation method. *Jpn J Psychiatry Neurol* 76:509–517, 1974.

61. Growdon JH, Shahani BT, Young RR: The effect of alcohol on essential tremor. *Neurology* 28:259–262, 1975.

62. Rajput AH, Jamieson H, Hirsh S, Quraishi A: Relative efficacy of alcohol and propranolol in action tremor. *Can J Neurol Sci* 2:31–35, 1975.

63. Koller W, Cone S, Herbster G: Caffeine and tremor. *Neurology* 37:169–172, 1987.

64. Cooper IS: Heredofamilial tremor abolition by chemothalamectomy. *Arch Neurol* 7:129–131, 1962.

65. Busenbark KL, Nash J, Nash S, et al: Is essential tremor benign? *Neurology* 41:1982–1983, 1991.

66. George MS, Lydiard RB: Social phobia secondary to physical disability: A review of benign essential tremor (BET) and stuttering. *Psychosomatics* 35:520–523, 1994.

67. Findley LJ, Koller WC, De Witt P, et al: Classification and definition of tremor. Cited by Findley LJ, in Lord Walton of Detchant (ed): *Indications for and Clinical Implications of Botulinum Toxin Therapy.* London: Royal Society of Medicine, 1993, pp 22–23.

68. Koller WC, Glatt S, Biary N, Rubino FA: Essential tremor variants: Effect of treatment. *Clin Neuropharmacol* 10:342–350, 1987.

69. Biary N, Koller WC: Kinetic predominant tremor: Effect of clonazepam. *Neurology* 37:471–474, 1987.

70. Koller WC, Rubino FA: Combined resting-postural tremor. *Arch Neurol* 42:683–684, 1985.

71. Bain PG, Findley LJ: Familial paroxysmal tremor: An essential tremor variant (letter). *J Neurol Neurosurg Psychiatry* 57:1019, 1994.

72. Garcia-Albea E, Jimenez-Jimenez FJ, Ayuso-Peralta L, et al: "Familial paroxysmal tremor": An essential tremor variant? (letter). *J Neurol Neurosurg Psychiatry* 56:1329, 1993.

73. Klawans HL, Glantz R, Tanner CM, Goetz CG: Primary writing tremor: Selective action tremor. *Neurology* 32:203–206, 1982.

74. Rothwell JC, Traub MM, Marsden CD: Primary writing tremor. *J Neurol Neurosurg Psychiatry* 42:1106–114, 1979.

75. Ravits J, Hallet M, Baker M, Wilkins D: Primary writing tremor and myoclonic writer's cramp. *Neurology* 35:1387–1391, 1985.

76. Sheehy MP, Marsden CD: Writers' cramp—a focal dystonia. *Brain* 105:461–480, 1982.

77. Cohen LG, Hallett M, Sudarsky L: A single family with writer's cramp, essential tremor, and primary writing tremor. *Mov Disord* 2:109–116, 1987.

78. Elble RJ, Moody C, Higgins C: Primary writing tremor: A form of focal dystonia. *Mov Disord* 5:118–126, 1990.

79. Grossman BJ: Trembling of the chin—an inheritable dominant character. *Pediatrics* 19:453–455, 1957.

80. Lawrence BM, Matthews W, Diggle JA: Hereditary quivering of the chin. *Arch Dis Child* 43:249–254, 1968.

81. Brown JR, Simonson J: Organic voice tremor. *Neurology* 17:520–527, 1967.

82. Hachinski VC, Thomsen IV, Buch NH: The nature of primary vocal tremor. *Can J Neurol Sci* 2:195–197, 1975.

83. Riveat J, Marsden CD: Trunk and head tremor as isolated manifestations of dystonia. *Mov Disord* 5:60–65, 1990.

84. Heilman KM: Orthostatic tremor. *Arch Neurol* 4:880–881, 1984.

85. Wee AS, Subramony SH, Currier RD: Orthostatic tremor: A variant of essential tremor. *Neurology* 36:1241–1245, 1986.

86. Pape SM, Gershanik OS: Orthostatic tremor: An essential tremor variant. *Mov Disord* 3:97–108, 1988.

87. Gabellini AS, Martinelli P, Gulli MR, et al: Orthostatic tremor: Essential and symptomatic cases. *Acta Neurol Scand* 81:111–112, 1990.

88. McManis PG, Sharbrough FW: Orthostatic tremor: Clinical and electrophysiologic characteristics. *Muscle Nerve* 16:1254–1260, 1993.

89. Thompson RD, Rothwell JC, Day BL, et al: The physiology of orthostatic truncal tremor. *Arch Neurol* 43:584–587, 1986.

90. Walker FO, McCormick CM, Hunt VP: Isometric features of orthostatic tremor: An electromyographic analysis. *Muscle Nerve* 13:918–922, 1990.

91. Uncini A, Onofrj M, Basciani M, et al: Orthostatic tremor: Report of 2 cases and an electrophysiological study. *Acta Neurol Scand* 79:119–122, 1989.

92. Lewitt P: Orthostatic tremor: The phenomenon of "paradoxical clonus". *Arch Neurol* 47:501, 1990.

93. Martinelli P, Gabellini AS, Gulli MR, Lugaresi E: Different clinical features of essential tremor: A 200 patient study. *Acta Neurol Scand* 75:106–111, 1987.

94. Newman RP, Lewitt PA, Jaffe M, et al: Motor function in the normal aging population: Treatment with l-dopa. *Neurology* 35:571–573, 1985.

95. McGeer PL, McGeer EG, Siyuki JS: Aging and extrapyramidal function. *Arch Neurol* 34:33–35, 1977.

96. Cleeves L, Findley L, Koller WC: Lack of association between essential tremor and Parkinson's disease. *Ann Neurol* 24:23–26, 1988.

97. Gowers WR: *A Manual of Diseases of the Nervous System.* Philadelphia: P Blakiston, Son & Co., 1888, pp 995–1013.

98. Marttilla RJ, Rinne UK: Arteriosclerosis, heredity and some pervious infections in the etiology of Parkinson's disease: A case control study. *Clin Neurol Neurosurg* 79:45–56, 1976.

99. Marttilla RJ, Rautakorpi I, Rinne UK: The relation of essential tremor to Parkinson's disease. *J Neurol Neurosurg Psychiatry* 47:734–735, 1984.

100. Barbeau A, Pourcher E: New data on the genetics of Parkinson's disease. *Can J Neurol Sci* 9:53–60, 1982.

101. Roy M, Boyer L, Barbeau A: A prospective study of 50 cases of familial Parkinson's disease. *Can J Neurol Sci* 10:34–42, 1983.

102. Geraghty JJ, Jankovic J, Zetusky WJ: Association between essential tremor and Parkinson's disease. *Ann Neurol* 17:329–333, 1985.

103. Lou JS, Jankovic J: Essential tremor: Clinical correlates in 350 patients. *Neurology* 41:234–238, 1991.

104. Lang AE, Marsden CD, Findley LJ, et al: Clinical correlates of essential tremor. *Neurology*. In Press.

105. Lang AE, Kierans C, Blair RDG: Family history of tremor in Parkinson's disease compared with those of controls and patients with idiopathic dystonia. *Adv Neurol* 45:313–316, 1986.

106. Marttilla RJ, Rinne UK: Parkinson's disease and essential tremor in families of patients with early-onset Parkinson's disease. *J Neurol Neurosurg Psychiatry* 51:429–431, 1988.

107. Salisachs P, Findley LJ: Problems in the differential diagnosis of essential tremor, in Findley LJ, Capildeo R (eds): *Movement Disorders: Tremor.* London: Macmillan, 1984, pp 219–224.

108. Rajput AH, Rozdilsky B, Ang L, Rajput A: Significance of parkinsonian manifestations in essential tremor. *Can J Neurol Sci* 20:114–117, 1993.

109. Pahwa R, Koller WC: Is there a relationship between Parkinson's disease and essential tremor? *Clin Neuropharmacol* 16:30–35, 1993.

110. Rajput AH, Rozdilsky B, Ang L, Rajput A: Clinicopathological observations in essential tremor: Report of 6 cases. *Neurology* 41:1422–1424, 1991.

111. Brooks DJ: Detection of preclinical Parkinson's disease with PET. *Neurology* 41(suppl 2):24–28, 1991.

112. Busenbark K, Huber SJ, Greer G, et al: Olfactory function in essential tremor. *Neurology* 42:1631–1632, 1992.

113. Yanagisawa N, Goto A, Narabagashi H: Familial dystonia musculorum deformans and tremor. *J Neurol Sci* 16:125–136, 1971.

114. Johnson W, Schwartz G, Barbeau A: Studies on dystonia musculorum deformans. *Arch Neurol* 7:301–313, 1962.

115. Baxter DW, Lal S: Essential tremor and dystonia syndromes. *Adv Neurol* 24:373–377, 1979.

116. Couch JR: Dystonia and tremor in spasmodic torticollis. *Adv Neurol* 14:245–258, 1976.

117. Duane DD: Spasmodic torticollis. *Adv Neurol* 49:135–150, 1988.

118. Dubinsky RM, Gray CS, Koller WC: Essential tremor and dystonia. *Neurology* 43:2382–2384, 1993.

119. Yanagisawa N, Goto A: Dystonia musculoram deformans: Analysis with electromyography. *J Neurol Sci* 13:39–65, 1971.

120. Rosenbaum F, Jankovic J: Focal task-specific tremor and dystonia: Categorization of occupational movement disorders. *Neurology* 38:522–527, 1988.

121. Roussy G, Levy G: Sept cas d'une maladie familiale particuliere: Troubles de la march, pieds bots et areflexie tendineuse generalisee avec acessoirement maladresse des mains. *Rev Neurol (Paris)* 2:427–450, 1926.

122. Said G, Bathien N, Cesar P: Peripheral neuropathies and tremor. *Neurology* 32:480–485, 1982.

123. Thomas PK, Lascelles RG, Hallpike JF, Hewer RL: Recurrent and chronic relapsing Guillain-Barre polyneuritis. *Brain* 92:589–606, 1969.

124. Dalakas MC, TerävVäinen H, Engel WK: Tremor as a feature of chronic relapsing and dysgammaglobulinemic polyneuropathies: Incidence and management. *Arch Neurol* 41:711–714, 1984.

125. Delwaide PJ, Schoenen J: Non-hypertrophic familial neuropathy associated with intention tremor: A variety of Charcot-Marie-Tooth disease? *J Neurol Sci* 27:59–69, 1976.

126. Barbieri F, Filla A, Ragno M, et al: Evidence that Charcot-Marie-Tooth disease with tremor coincides with the Roussy-Levy syndrome. *Can J Neurol Sci* 11:534–540, 1984.

127. Salisachs P: Charcot-Marie-Tooth disease associated with "essential tremor": Report of 7 cases and a review of the literature. *J Neurol Sci* 28:17–40, 1976.

128. Shahani BT, Young RR, Adams RD: Neuropathic tremor. *Electroencephalogr Clin Neurophysiol* 34:800, 1973.

129. Mendell JR, Sahenk Z, Whitaker JN, et al: Polyneuropathy and IgM monoclonal gammopathy: Studies on the pathogenic role of anti-myelin-associated glycoprotein antibody. *Ann Neurol* 17:243–254, 1985.

130. Adams RD, Shahani BT, Young RR: Tremor in association with polyneuropathy. *Trans Am Neurol Assoc* 97:44–48, 1972.

131. Baughman FA: Klinefelter's syndrome and essential tremor. *Lancet* 2:545, 1969.

132. Pittman CS, Finley WH, Finley SC: Klinefelter's syndrome and essential tremor. *Lancet* 2:749, 1969.

133. Lee RG, Stein RB: Resetting of tremor by mechanical pertubations: A comparison of essential tremor and parkinsonian tremor. *Ann Neurol* 10:523–531, 1981.

134. Elble RJ, Higgens C, Moody CJ: Stretch reflex oscillations and essential tremor. *J Neurol Neurosurg Psychiatry* 50:691–698, 1987.

135. Britton TC, Thompson PD, Day BL, et al: "Resetting" of postural tremors at the wrist with mechanical stretches in Parkinson's disease, essential tremor and normal subjects mimicking tremor. *Ann Neurol* 31:507–514, 1992.

136. Pascual-Leone A, Valls-Sole J, Toro C, et al: Resetting of essential tremor and postural tremor in Parkinson's disease with transcranial magnetic stimulation. *Muscle Nerve* 17:800–807, 1994.

137. Koller WC: Treatment of essential tremor, in Marsden CD, Conrad B, Benecke N (eds): *Motor Disorders*. London: Academic Press, 1987, pp 55–62.

138. Mylle G, Van Bogaert L: Etudes anatomo-clinques de syndromes hypercinetiques complexes. I. Sur le tremblement familial. *Mschr Psychiatr Neurol* 103:28–43, 1940.

139. Laitinan F: Stereotaxic treatment of hereditary tremor. *Acta Neurol Scand* 41:74–79, 1965.

140. Dupuis MJM, Delwaide PJ, Boucqucy D, Gonsette RE: Homolateral disappearance of essential tremor after cerebellar stroke. *Mov Disord* 4:180–187, 1989.

141. Jahnsen H, Clinas R: Ionic basis for the electroresponsiveness and oscillatory properties of guinea pig thalamic neurons in vitro. *J Physiol* 349:227–247, 1986.

142. Deschenas M, Paradis M, Roy JP, Steriade N: Electrophysiology of neurons of lateral thalamic nucleus in cat: Resting properties and burst discharges. *J Neurophysiol* 51:1196–1219, 1984.

143. Armstrong DM, Harvey RJ: Responses in the inferior olive to stimulation of the cerebellum and cerebral cortex in the cat. *J Physiol* 187:553–574, 1966.

144. Dubinsky R, Hallet M: Glucose hypermetabolism of the inferior olive in patients with essential tremor. *Ann Neurol* 22:118, 1987.

145. Colebatch JG, Findley LJ, Frackowiak RSJ, et al: Preliminary report: Activation of the cerebellum in essential tremor. *Lancet* 336:1028–1030, 1990.

146. Jenkins IH, Bain PG, Colebatch JG, et al: A positron emission tomography study of essential tremor: Evidence for overactivity of cerebellar connections. *Ann Neurol* 34:82–90, 1993.

147. Samie MR, Selhorst JB, Koller WC: Post-traumatic midbrain tremors. *Neurology* 40:62–66, 1990.

148. Llinas R, Varon Y: Oscillatory properties of guinea pig inferior olivary neurones and their pharmacological modulation: An in vitro study. *J Physiol* 376:163–182, 1986.

149. Gunther H, Brunner R, Klussmann FN: Spectral analysis of tremorine and cold tremor electromyograms in animal species of different size. *Pflugers Arch* 399:180–185, 1983.

150. Frankl-Hochwart: *La Degenerescence Hepato-Lenticulaire (Maladies de Wilson, Pseudo-sclerose)*. Paris: Masson et Cie, 1903.

151. Hassler R: Zur pathologischen anatomie des senilen und des parkinsonistischen tremor. *J Psychol Neurol* 49:193–230, 1939.

152. Mylle G, Van Bogaert L: Du tremblement essential non familial. *Mschr Psychiatr Neurol* 115:80–90, 1948.

153. Herskovits E, Blackwood W: Essential (familial, hereditary) tremor: A case report. *J Neurol Neurosurg Psychiatry* 32:509–511, 1969.

154. Lapresle J, Rondot P, Said G: Tremblement idiopathique de repos, d'attitude et d'action. *Rev Neurol (Paris)* 130:343–348, 1974.

155. Koller WC, Gupta S: Pharmacologic probe with progabide of GABA mechanism in essential tremor. *Arch Neurol* 44:905–907, 1987.

156. Koller WC: Trazodone in essential tremor: Probe of serotoninergic mechanisms. *Clin Neuropharmacol* 12:134–137, 1987.

157. Fahn S, Tolosa E, Marin C: Clinical rating scale for tremor, in Jankovic J, Tolosa E (eds): *Parkinson's Disease and Movement Disorders*. Baltimore: Urban & Schwarzenberg, 1988.

158. Bain PG, Findley LJ, Atchison P, et al: Assessing tremor severity (see comments). *J Neurol Neurosurg Psychiatry* 56:868–873, 1993.

159. Bacher M, Scholz E, Diener AC: 24-hour continuous tremor quantification based on EMG recordings. *Electroencephalogr Clin Neurophysiol* 72:176–183, 1989.

160. Magee KR: Essential tremor: Diagnosis and treatment. *Clin Med* 72:33–41, 1965.

161. Koller WC, Biary N: Effect of alcohol on tremor: Comparison to propranolol. *Neurology* 34:221–222, 1984.

162. Teräväinen H, Huttunen J, Lewitt P: Ineffective treatment of essential tremor with an alcohol, methylpentynol. *J Neurol Neurosurg Psychiatry* 49:198–199, 1986.

163. Schroeder D, Nasrallah HA: High alcoholism rate in essential tremor patients. *Am J Psychiatry* 139:1471–1473, 1982.

164. Koller WC: Alcoholism in essential tremor. *Neurology* 33:1074–1076, 1983.

165. Koller WC, O'Hara R, Dorus W, Bauer J: Tremor in chronic alcoholism. *Neurology* 35:1660–1662, 1985.

166. Marshall J: Tremor, in Vinken PJ, Bruyn GW, eds. *Handbook of Clinical Neurology.* Amsterdam: North-Holland Publishing Co, 1968, vol 6, pp 809–825.

167. Winkler GF, Young RR: Efficacy of chronic propranolol therapy in action tremors of the familial, senile or essential varieties. *N Engl J Med* 290:984–988, 1974.

168. Sevitt I: The effect of adrenergic beta-receptor blocking drugs on tremor. *Practitioner* 207:677–678, 1971.

169. Foster JB, Longley BP, Stewart-Wynne EG: Propranolol in essential tremor. *Lancet* 1:1455, 1973.

170. Sweet RD, Blumberg J, Lee JE, McDowell FH: Propranolol treatment of essential tremor. *Neurology* 24:64–67, 1974.

171. Tolosa ES, Loewenson RB: Essential tremor: Treatment with propranolol. *Neurology* 25:1041–1044, 1975.

172. Murray TJ: Treatment of essential tremor with propranolol. *Can Med Assoc J* 107:984–986, 1972.

173. Barbeau A: Traitment du tremblement essentiel famial par le propranolol. *Union Med Can* 102:899–902, 1962.

174. Taräväinen H, Fogelholm R, Larsen A: Effect of propranolol on essential tremor. *Neurology* 26:27–30, 1976.

175. Larsen TA, Taräväinen H, Calne DB: Atenolol vs propranolol in essential tremor: A controlled, quantitative study. *Acta Neurol Scand* 66:547–554, 1982.

176. Calzetti S, Findley LJ, Gresty MA, et al: Effect of a single dose of propranolol on essential tremor: A double-blind controlled study. *Ann Neurol* 13:165–171, 1983.

177. Koller WC: Dose-response relationship of propranolol in essential tremor. *Arch Neurol* 35:42–43, 1986.

178. Koller WC: Long-acting propranolol in essential tremor. *Neurology* 36:106–108, 1985.

179. Cleeves L, Findley LJ, Koller W: Lack of association between essential tremor and Parkinson's disease. *Ann Neurol* 24:23–26, 1988.

180. Findley LJ, Cleeves L: Beta-adrenoreceptor antagonists in essential tremor. *Lancet* 29:856–857, 1984.

181. Koller WC, Vetere-Overfield B: Acute and chronic affects of propranolol and primidone in essential tremor. *Neurology* 39:1587–1588, 1989.

182. Calzetti S, Sasso E, Baratti M, Faua R: Clinical and computer-based assessment of long-term therapeutic efficacy of propranolol in essential tremor. *Acta Neurol Scand* 81:392–396, 1990.

183. Young RR: Essential-familial tremor and other action tremors. *Semin Neurol* 2:386–391, 1982.

184. Calzettii S, Findley LJ, Perucca E, Richens A: The response of essential tremor to propranolol: Evaluation of clinical variables governing the efficacy on prolonged administration. *J Neurol Neurosurg Psychiatry* 46:393–398, 1983.

185. Koller WC, Royse V: Time course of a single oral dose of propranolol in essential tremor. *Neurology* 35:1494–1499, 1985.

186. Jefferson D, Jenner P, Marsden CD: Beta-adrenoreceptor antagonists in essential tremor. *J Neurol Neurosurg Psychiatry* 42:904–909, 1979.

187. Huttunen J, Taräväinen H, Larsen A: Beta-adrenoreceptor antagonist in essential tremor. *Lancet* ii:857, 1984.

188. Britt CR, Peters BH: Metoprolol for essential tremor. *N Engl J Med* 301:31, 1979.

189. Ljung O: Treatment of essential tremor with metoprolol. *N Engl J Med* 301:1005, 1979.

190. Newman RP, Jacobs L: Metoprolol in essential tremor. *Arch Neurol* 37:596–597, 1980.

191. Riley T, Pleet AB: Metoprolol tartrate for essential tremor. *N Engl J Med* 301:663, 1979.

192. Turnbull DM, Shaw DA: Metoprolol in essential tremor. *Lancet* i:95, 1980.

193. Koller WC, Biary N: Metoprolol compared to propranolol in the treatment of essential tremor. *Arch Neurol* 41:171–172, 1984.

194. Koller WC: Nadolol in the treatment of essential tremor. *Neurology* 33:1074–1075, 1983.

195. Dietrichson P, Espen E: Effects of timolol and atenolol on benign essential tremor: Placebo-controlled studies based on quantitative tremor recordings. *J Neurol Neurosurg Psychiatry* 44:677–683, 1981.

196. Koller WC, Larsen L, Potempa K: Pindolol-induced tremor. *Clin Neuropharmacol* 10:449–460, 1987.

197. Kuroda Y, Kakigi R, Shilasaki H: Treatment of essential tremor with arotinolol. *Neurology* 38:650–651, 1988.

198. O'Brien MD, Upton AR, Toseland PA: Benign familial tremor treated with primidone. *Br Med J* 282:178–180, 1981.

199. Chakrabarti A, Pearce JMS: Essential tremor: Response to primidone. *J Neurol Neurosurg Psychiatry* 44:650, 1981.

200. Findley LJ, Cleeves L, Calzetti S: Primidone in essential tremor of the hands and head: A double-blind controlled clinical study. *J Neurol Neurosurg Psychiatry* 481:911–915, 1985.

201. Koller WC, Royse V: Efficacy of primidone in essential tremor. *Neurology* 36:121–124, 1986.

202. Gorman WP, Cooper R, Pocock P, Campbell MJ: A comparison of primidone, propranolol, and placebo in essential tremor using quantitative analysis. *J Neurol Neurosurg Psychiatry* 491:64–68, 1986.

203. Crystal HR: Duration of effectiveness of primidone in essential tremor. *Neurology* 36:1543, 1986.

204. Shale H, Fahn S: Response to essential tremor to treatment with primidone (abstr.). *Neurology* 37:123, 1987.

205. Sasso E, Perucca E, Fava N, Calzetti S: Primidone in the long-term treatment of essential tremor: A prospective study with computerized quantitative analysis. *Clin Neuropharmacol* 13:67–76, 1990.

206. Calzetti S, Findley L, Risani F, Richens A: Phenyethylmalonamide in essential tremor. *J Neurol Neurosurg Psychiatry* 44:932–934, 1981.

207. Findley LJ, Calzetti S: Double-blind controlled study of primidone in essential tremor: Preliminary results. *Br Med J* 285:608, 1982.

208. Procaccianti G, Baruzzi Λ, Martinclli P, ct al: Bcnign familial tremor treated with primidone. *Br Med J* 283:558, 1981.

209. Baruzzi A, Procaceranti G, Martinelle P: Phenobarbital and propranolol in essential tremor: A double-blind controlled clinical trial. *Neurology* 33:296–300, 1983.

210. Findley LJ, Cleeves L: Phenobarbital in essential tremor. *Neurology* 35:1784–1787, 1985.

211. Sasso E, Perucca E, Calzetti S: Double-blind comparison of primidone and phenobarbital in essential tremor. *Neurology* 38:808–810, 1988.

212. Cabrera-Valdivia F, Jimenez-Jimenez J, Albea EG, et al: Orthostatic tremor: Successful treatment with phenobarbital. *Clin Neuropharmacol* 14:438–441, 1991.

213. Thompson C, Lang A, Parkes JD, Marsden CD: A double-blind trial of clonazepam in benign essential tremor. *Clin Neuropharmacol* 7:83–88, 1984.

214. Huber SJ, Paulson GW: Efficacy of alprazolam for essential tremor. *Neurology* 38:241–243, 1988.

215. Muenter MD, Daube JR, Caviness JN, Miller PN: Treatment of essential tremor with methazolamide. *Mayo Clin Proc* 66:991–997, 1991.

216. Busenbark K, Hubble J, Pahwa P, Koller WC: The effect of acetazolamide on essential tremor. *Neurology* 42:1631–1632, 1992.

217. Busenbark K, Pahwa R, Hubble J, et al: Double-blind controlled study of methazolamide in the treatment of essential tremor. *Neurology* 43:1045–1047, 1993.

218. Barbeau A: L-Dopa therapy in Parkinson's disease: A critical review of nine years' experience. *Can Med Assoc J* 101:791–800, 1969.

219. Critchley E: Clinical manifestation of essential tremor. *J Neurol Neurosurg Psychiatry* 35:365–372, 1972.

220. Manyam BV: Amantadine in essential tremor. *Ann Neurol* 9:198–199, 1981.

221. Obeso JA, Luguin MR, Artieda J, Martinez-Lage JM: Amantadine may be useful in essential tremor. *Ann Neurol* 19:99–100, 1986.

222. Koller WC: Amantadine in essential tremor. *Ann Neurol* 15:508–509, 1984.

223. Caccia MR, Mangoni A: Clonidine in essential tremor: Preliminary observations from an open trial. *J Neurol* 232:55–57, 1985.

224. Koller WC, Herbster G, Cone S: Clonidine in the treatment of essential tremor. *Mov Disord* 1:235–237, 1986.

225. Mai J, Olsen RB: Depression of essential tremor by alpha-adrenergic blockade. *J Neurol Neurosurg Psychiatry* 44:1171, 1981.

226. Koller WC: Ineffectiveness of phenoxybenzamine in essential tremor. *J Neurol Neurosurg Psychiatry* 49:222, 1986.

227. Morris CE, Prange AJ, Hall CD, Weiss EA: Inefficacy of tryptophan/pyridoxine in essential tremor. *Lancet* 2:165–166, 1971.

228. McLeod NA, White LE: Trazodone in essential tremor. *J Am Med Assoc* 256.2675–2676, 1986.

229. Cleeves L, Findley LJ: Trazodone is ineffective in essential tremor. *J Neurol Neurosurg Psychiatry* 53:268–269, 1990.

230. Meert TF, De Beukelaar F, Geldera YG: Ritanserin, a thymosthenic drug in parkinsonism tremor and drug-induced EPS: A review of existing data. *Tremor 88*. Caesarea, Israel: 1988, p 38.

231. Caccia ML, Oslo M, Galimberti V, et al: Propranolol, clonidine, urapidil, and trazodone in essential tremor. *Acta Neurol Scand* 79:379–383, 1989.

232. Topakias S, Onur R, Dalkara S: Calcium channel blockers and essential tremor. *Eur Neurol* 27:114–119, 1987.

233. Jimenez-Jimenez FJ, Garcia Ruiz PJ, Cabrera-Valdivia F: Nicardipine versus propranolol in essential tremor. *Acta Neurol Napoli* 16:184–188, 1994.

234. Curran T, Lang AE: Flunarizine in essential tremor. *Clin Neuropharmacol* 16:460–463, 1993.

235. Biary N, Saleh M, Deeb A, Langenberg P: The effect of flunarizine on essential tremor. *Neurology* 41:311–312, 1991.

236. Pakkenberg H, Pakkenberg B: Clozapine in the treatment of tremor. *Acta Neurol Scand* 73:295–297, 1986.

237. McCarthy RH: Clozapine reduces essential tremor independent of its antipsychotic effect: A case report (letter). *J Clin Psychopharmacol* 14:212–213, 1994.

238. McDowell FH: The use of glutethimide for treatment of essential tremor. *Mov Disord* 4:75–80, 1989.

239. Mally J, Stone TW: The effect of theophylline on essential tremor: The possible role of GABA. *Pharmacol Biochem Behav* 39:345–349, 1991.

240. Jankovic J, Schwartz K: Botulinium toxin treatment of tremors. *Neurology* 41:1185–1188, 1991.

241. American Academy of Neurology Therapeutics and Technology Subcommittee: Assessment: The clinical usefulness of botulinum toxin-A in treating neurologic disorders. Special article. *Neurology* 40:1332–1336, 1990.

242. Trosch RM, Pullman SL: Botulinum toxin A injections for the treatment of hand tremors. *Mov Disord* 9:601–609, 1994.

243. Bertrand C: Stereotactic and peripheral surgery for the control of movement disorders, in Barbeau A (ed): *Disorders of Movement*. Lancaster PA: MTP Press, 1981, pp 191–208.

244. Blocher HM, Bertrand C, Martinez N, et al: Hypotonia accompanying the neurosurgical relief of essential tremor. *J Nerv Ment Dis* 147:49–55, 1968.

245. Ohye E, Hirai T, Miyazaki M, Shibazaki N: VIM thalamotomy for the treatment of various kinds of tremor. *Appl Neurophysiol* 451:275–280, 1981.

246. Andrew J: Surgical treatment of tremor, in Findley LJ, Capildeo R (eds): *Movement Disorders: Tremor*. London: MacMillan, 1984, pp 339–350.

247. Kelly PJ, Ahlekog JE, Goeres SJ, et al: Computer-assisted stereotactic ventralis lateralis thalamotomy with microelectrode recording in patients with Parkinson's disease. *Mayo Clin Proc* 62:655–664, 1987.

248. Selby G: Stereotaxic surgery, in WC Koller (ed): *Handbook of Parkinson's disease*. New York: Marcel-Dekker, 1987, pp 421–436.

249. Goldman MS, Kelly PJ: Stereotactic thalamotomy for medically intractable essential tremor. *Stereotact Funct Neurosurg* 58:22–25, 1992.

250. Niclot P, Pollin B, N'Guyen J, et al: Treatment of tremor by stereotactic surgery. *Rev Neurol (Paris)* 149:755–763, 1993.

251. Goldman MS, Ahlskog JE, Kelly PJ: The symptomatic and functional outcome of stereotactic thalamotomy for medically intractable essential tremor. *J Neurosurg* 76:924–928, 1992.

252. Benabid AL, Pollak P, Gervason L, et al: Long-term suppression of tremor by chronic stimulation of the ventral intermediate thalamic nucleus. *Lancet* 337:403–406, 1991.

253. Blond S, Caparros-Lefebvre D, Parker F, et al: Control of tremor and involuntary movement disorders by chronic stereotactic stimulation of the ventral intermediate thalamic nucleus. *J Neurosurg* 77:62–68, 1992.

254. Benabid AL, Pollak P, Seigneuret E, et al: Chronic VIM thalamic stimulation in Parkinson's disease, essential tremor and extrapyramidal dyskinesias. *Acta Neurochir Suppl (Wien)* 53:39–44, 1993.

255. Wake A, Takahashi Y, Onishi T, et al: Treatment of essential tremor by behavior therapy—use of Jacobsen's progressive relaxation method. *Psychiatr Neurol Jpn* 76:509–517, 1974.

Chapter 28

UNCOMMON FORMS OF TREMOR

BALA V. MANYAM

PHYSIOLOGICAL TREMOR
CEREBELLAR TREMOR
CORTICAL TREMOR
DYSTONIC TREMOR
FOOD- AND DRUG-INDUCED TREMOR
    Food and Beverages
    Stimulants
    Tranquilizers
    Dopamine Receptor-Blocking Drugs
    Antidepressants
    Antiepileptic Drugs
    Cardiac Drugs
    Immunosuppressants
MIDBRAIN TREMOR
TREMOR AS A RESULT OF NEUROTOXINS
    Heavy Metals
    Insecticides and Herbicides
    Solvents
ORTHOSTATIC TREMOR
SYMPTOMATIC PALATAL TREMOR
PERIPHERAL NEUROPATHY-ASSOCIATED TREMOR
PSYCHOGENIC TREMORS
REST TREMOR
STROKE-ASSOCIATED TREMOR
POSTTRAUMATIC TREMOR
VOCAL TREMOR
PRIMARY WRITING TREMOR

Tremor remains the most common of all movement disorders. The most accepted and simple definition is as follows: "Tremor is an involuntary, approximately rhythmic, and roughly sinusoidal movement."[1] Thus, in any part of the body where agonistic and antagonistic muscles function, tremor could occur. Tremor is most commonly seen in the upper extremities but tremor of the lower extremities, head, trunk, lips, chin, tongue, and vocal cords could also occur. Functionally, *rest tremor* is present when the affected part of the body is in repose and is fully supported against gravity, requiring no active muscle contraction.[2] Tremor seen in Parkinson's disease and other forms of Parkinsonism are typically rest tremors. This tremor typically disappears with onset of movement but, once partial stability is attained in the new position, the tremor returns. When tremor occurs with maintained posture such as holding arms perpendicular to the body, it is called *postural tremor*. Postural tremor is possibly the most common form of tremor and can be seen in physiological tremor, essential tremor, cerebellar postural tremor, and others. This tremor is often the most functionally disabling. When tremor occurs with movement from one point to another, it is referred to as *kinetic* or *intentional tremor*. Kinetic tremor that appears near termination of movement is known as *terminal tremor*. Kinetic tremor present during specific tasks but absent with other activities involving the same limb is referred to as *task specific tremor*. Examples include primary writing tremor, vocal tremor, and orthostatic tremor. Tremor may arise from several anatomic locations within the central nervous system or peripheral nervous system, including the cerebral cortex, white matter, basal ganglia, thalamus, midbrain, cerebellum, and peripheral nerves. In physiological tremor no known lesion is present. Alterations in neurotransmitters such as dopamine deficiency (as seen in Parkinson's disease), excess epinephrine as seen in anxiety, decreased level of substrate such as glucose (hypoglycemia), reduced level of electrolyte (hyponatremia), and excess level of a hormone such as thyroxin (thyrotoxicosis) can induce tremor leading to biochemical nonspecificity.

Frequency of tremor has often been given much importance and is used in classification. When the frequency is low (4–5 Hz), the diagnosis of Parkinson's disease is entertained and if the frequency is higher (8–12 Hz), Parkinson's disease is "ruled out." Amplitude of tremor is easily quantifiable and is classified as mild, moderate, and severe on various rating scales. The amplitude of the tremor in patients with the same disease may vary and can be exaggerated by physical and emotional stress. Treatment for tremor disorders is aimed at reducing tremor amplitude, which is what produces functional disability.

Although autosomal-dominant inheritance is the hallmark of essential tremor, there are considerable numbers of sporadic cases. Biary and Koller[3] defined essential tremor as a monosymptomatic, clinically uniform disorder involving mainly the hand and the head. Elble[4] suggested that essential tremor cannot be classified solely on the basis of phase relationships of electromyogram (EMG) bursts between agonist and antagonist muscles and may not represent a single clinical entity. Subsequently, the word "essential tremor variant" has been used.[3] In this chapter, tremor other than that strictly defined as essential tremor will be discussed. It is possible, however, there will be some degree of overlap of what may be considered "essential tremor variant" and "tremor other than essential tremor."

Physiological Tremor

Physiological tremor, the invisible mechanical vibration of body parts, is present in all normal people. However, it is barely visible to the naked eye and is symptomatic only during activities that require extreme precision. Physiological tremor has two distinct oscillations. The *8- to 12-Hz level*[5] is very resistant to frequency change. Internal loads,[6,7] elastic loads,[8] limb cooling,[5] and torque loads[9] produce less than a 1- to 2-Hz frequency change. This frequency invariability and the intense synchronous motor unit modulation suggests that the neuronal oscillator is responsible for the 8- to 12-Hz tremor.[5] It occurs during the maintenance of study limb postures and has a low amplitude. The functional significance of this tremor is not known. The *mechanical-reflex compo-*

nent is the larger of the two distinct oscillations of physiological tremor and is a result of the internal viscous and elastic properties of the limb or some other body part. The two oscillations are superimposed upon a background of irregular fluctuations in muscle force and limb displacement. The frequency of this mechanical reflex oscillation is determined largely by inertia and stiffness of the body part. Consequently, normal elbow tremors have a frequency of 3–5 Hz, wrist tremors 8–12 Hz, and metacarpophalangeal joint tremors 17–30 Hz. Mechanical reflex tremor is a passive oscillation that occurs in response to broad-frequency, irregular forces that are produced by asynchronous subtetanic motor unit firing. It has been considered that the component of the lower frequency originated from the central nervous system as a long loop, and that of the higher frequency originated from the muscle-spindle loop system as a short loop.[10] Although both oscillations should be considered together, from a practical standpoint the 8- to 12-Hz seem to have more practical implications. It has been considered that physiological tremor may be a protective measure against unusual limb posture.[11] Because the physiological tremor has 8- to 12-Hz and alpha rhythm in electroencephalogram (EEG) has a similar frequency (7 to 13), a common central origin was considered. No evidence for such a hypothesis has been found.[12] Tremor recording with an accelerometer in 1079 healthy subjects showed frequency peaks between 5.85 and 8.80 Hz. with spectral analysis. Chronic cigarette smoking and coffee drinking did not modify the tremor. Relaxation sessions decreased tremor significantly.[13]

Exaggeration of physiological tremor can occur under various conditions, including emotional stress, fatigue, exercise, hypoglycemia, thyrotoxicosis, pheochromocytoma, hypothermia, alcohol withdrawal, and by means of drugs such as valproic acid, lithium, neuroleptics, and tricyclic antidepressants. Ethanol can also cause a decrease in the amplitude of physiological tremor.[14] It has been considered that the stretch-reflex response to oscillation increases during fatigue and in anxiety and response to the several medications named above and to hormones that produce a modulation of motor unit activity. This is what results in an increase in amplitude, being referred to as "enhanced physiological tremor."[15,16] Physiological tremor was not altered by caffeine in controlled studies.[17] Studies with tremorolytic action of beta-adrenoceptor blockers in physiological and isoprenaline-induced tremor suggested that the tremor activity is exerted via the same beta$_2$-adrenoceptors located in a deep peripheral compartment that is thought to be in the muscle spindles.[18] Intravenous propranolol produces a 34–60 percent decrease in the amplitude of physiological tremor. There was a delay of about 10 minutes, suggesting that this was the result of formation of a highly specific, centrally acting metabolite of propranolol.[19]

Physiological tremor can interfere with fine coordinative movements, such as those required for performing microsurgery, watch repair, or diamond cutting. Although knowledge of factors that aggravate physiological tremor should be addressed, such as lack of sleep, fatigue, anxiety, etc., use of a single 40-mg dose of propranolol has been found to be effective.[20] Surgeons who perform microsurgery are known to take such a drug before the start of a procedure.

Cerebellar Tremor

The main anomaly of cerebellar movement is its discontinuity. When discontinuity in movement becomes rhythmic, the definition of tremor can be applied. Kinetic tremor could occur as the target is reached (as, for example, in the finger-to-nose test). This is referred to as *terminal tremor*. In the early part of the cerebellar disease (or if the cerebellar damage is minimal), mild degree of terminal tremor may be the only sign. As the disease advances, the tremor may be present during the entire course of finger-to-nose test. In the early phases, tremor can be present in the extremities, but as the disease advances, it can involve axial structures. Occasionally, tremor may start as head tremor, even though this is less common. The frequency and amplitude of cerebellar tremor are usually irregular. The frequency of cerebellar kinetic tremor is commonly described as being 3–5 Hz, but studies have shown that the frequency of cerebellar tremor is inversely proportional to limb inertia, resulting in frequency being dependent on the part of the body affected. In the upper extremities, kinetic tremor has a frequency of 3–8 Hz, whereas in the lower extremities it is usually around 3 Hz. The truncal tremor, which is a rhythmic partial sway, usually has a frequency of 2–4 Hz.[1] At times, cerebellar tremor is so irregular it may appear proximal. In cerebellar kinetic tremor the oscillations are of variable amplitude and are perpendicular to the direction of movement. Postural tremor of the head may be the first manifestation of cerebellar disease. Postural tremor of the limb can also occur. Cerebellar tremor is classically elicited by finger-to-nose and heel-to-shin tests. However, the tremor can also be recognized in a patient's handwriting. Each wave form in the halices drawn by a patient with tremor represents upward and downward deflection of a tremor.

Attempts to correlate tremor to cerebellar lesions often results in incomplete data. What is known is that in humans, lesions in the posterior funiculus aggravate cerebellar tremor, whereas stimulation of Ia fibers by application of vibrations to the tendon diminishes the tremor.[21] In experimental monkeys, damage to dentate, globase, and emboliform nuclei in the cerebellum or to the superior cerebellar peduncles produces tremor.[22] It is also known that in humans, damage to the superior cerebellar peduncles or to the dentate nucleus is defined as the most common site of focal pathology that leads to severe intention tremor.

The underlying complexity of the transcortical and transcerebellar loops is probably the principal reason why effective pharmacotherapy is not available for cerebellar tremors or, for that matter, cerebellar dysfunction.[1] Nevertheless, several drugs have been tested.[1,23,24] Reports emerge in the literature, from time to time, either single case reports or open trial in a small number of patients, indicating success with pharmacotherapy. However, sustained benefit or double-blind studies are few and often do not confirm the initial results. Stereotactic thalamotomy or stimulation in the contralateral ventralis intermedius nucleus is often effective in reducing the amplitude of the tremor but may result in deterioration of other aspects of motor function.[25–27]

Mechanical therapy, such as strapping lead weights to the wrist, has been used and was found to reduce kinetic tremor.[28] Use of weighted instruments during eating and other activities may be helpful,[1] but the mechanical load must be tailored to the need of each patient. Devices for reducing tremor are often cumbersome and may not necessarily improve a patient's functional ability. Overall treatment for cerebellar tremor remains unsatisfactory.

Cortical Tremor

The term "cortical tremor" was coined by Ikeda et al.[29] who described two patients with action and postural 9-Hz tremor with electrophysiological evidence of cortical myoclonus, were refractory to beta-blocker therapy but responded to a combination of valproic acid and clonazepam. The authors concluded that this tremor disorder represented a variant of action-induced myoclonus in the setting of cortical myoclonus. Subsequently, Toro et al.[30] described 10 additional cases. The common features of these 12 cases were shared by both males and females, with an age range of 16–75 years. The presenting symptom was often tremor or action myoclonus. In five the etiology was five idiopathic, in 3 baltac myoclonus, and in 1 each of Lafora body disease, postanoxic myoclonus, progressive myoclonic epilepsy of unknown etiology, and opsoclonus myoclonus syndrome. The features common to all patients were abnormal rhythmic bursts on the EMG during voluntary isometric contraction with synchronous activation of agonist and antagonist muscles, alternating periods of near silence, a peak burst frequency of 9–18 Hz with low levels of isometric activation, and an associated cortical potential on electroencephalogram (EEG) back averaging. In the 10 cases described by Toro et al., the rhythmic disturbance produced by isometric muscle activation was a source of disabling deception of skill in motor task, such as holding a pen for writing or holding a cup.

Dystonic Tremor

Oppenheim[31] described presence of tremor associated with dystonic movements. In a review of 42 patients with idiopathic torsion dystonia, tremor was found in 14 percent,[32] but occurrence of tremor before manifestation of dystonia is not uncommon.[33,34] In a series of 271 patients with cervical dystonia, 71 percent had associated tremor.[35] In another series of 308 patients, 10 percent of the patients with varieties of dystonia had tremor.[36] In an accidental toxic exposure to 2,3,7,8-tetrachlorodibenzo-*p*-dioxin, focal hand dystonia and intention tremor were present in 22 of the 45 patients.[37] Dystonic tremor is also described as postural, localized, and irregular in amplitude, with periodicity absent during muscle relaxation, exacerbated by smooth muscle contraction, and associated frequently with myoclonus. It is considered a distinct entity from essential tremor, as it is irregular, has a broad range of frequencies, and remains localized.[38] Thus, there is considerable confusion on this very nomenclature. Treatment of dystonia with botulinum often results in significant improvement of tremor as seen in cases of cervical dystonia.

Food and Drug-Induced Tremor

It has been said that "all drugs are poisons in large doses; all poisons are drugs in small doses." Tremor secondary to diet, drugs, and toxins can take many forms, including enhanced physiological tremor, precipitated essential tremor, rest tremor secondary to parkinsonism, tremor of cerebellar syndrome, or can be associated with peripheral neuropathy.

FOOD AND BEVERAGES

Coffee, tea, cocoa, and caffeinated soda are sources of caffeine, a stimulant. It is believed that caffeine can induce new onset of tremor or may exacerbate previously existing tremor.[39,40] In a survey of 4558 healthy individuals, 16 percent report that tremor was sometimes associated with coffee intake.[41] Although a double-blind study has not been done, measurement of tremor using an accelerometer after oral dose of 325 mg of caffeine did not increase physiological essential tremor or parkinsonian tremor at 1, 2, or 3 hours after ingestion.[17] However, individual sensitivity to caffeine may vary. Higher doses may precipitate tremor, but experimental evidence is lacking on the maximum tolerated level of caffeine in humans. There appears to be significant variation in drinking caffeinated beverages and in the symptoms attributed to caffeine. Some individuals drink up to 15 cups of coffee per day and still not have any symptoms attributable to caffeine, whereas others may complain after a single cup. The psychological overlay could also be a factor not only in tremor but in other symptoms attributed to caffeine, such as insomnia. Decaffeinated beverages may not be totally free of caffeine and whether other noncaffeine compounds exist that are tremorogenic has not been proven.

Alcohol, known to suppress essential tremor and a few other forms of tremor,[42] can itself induce tremor through different mechanisms. The most common tremulousness of hepatic encephalopathy, referred to as metabolic tremor, may simply be a less pronounced manifestation.[43] Tremor could also be associated with alcohol withdrawal. This is a postural tremor of the arms which, when severe, may spread to other parts of the body—face, tongue, larynx, muscles, and head.[44,45] The tremor from withdrawal may persist for more than 1 year in the absence of alcohol intake, even though amplitude may diminish.[45] Chronic alcoholism results in cerebellar degeneration, in which case a 3-Hz leg tremor and upper extremity tremor have been demonstrated.[46,47] A variety of movement disorders associated with cirrhosis of the liver occurs in chronic alcoholics and is complicated by posterosystemic shunts, resulting in *acquired hepatocerebral degeneration*. The symptoms include various forms of tremor.[48]

The Chamorro population of the western Pacific islands of Guam and Rota consume palm (*Cycas circinalis*) flour as a staple diet and are known to develop dementia-amyotrophic lateral sclerosis-parkinsonism, which includes rest tremor. The active compound beta-*N*-methylamino-L-alanine is considered the underlying cause,[49] but the exact cause is not fully established.

Intake of tobacco is accomplished by chewing, smoking, or sniffing. Nicotine affects both the peripheral and central nervous systems. Nicotine causes tremor in animals[50,51] and is also reported to produce tremor in normal individuals.[52,53] However, a controlled study failed to elicit any significant influence of nicotine on either physiological or pathological tremor.[54]

STIMULANTS

The enhancement of physiological tremor is often considered to be related to sympathomimetic effects of stimulants via stimulation of peripheral adrenergic receptors. Severe tremor has been reported with intravenous amphetamine abuse.[55] Stimulants may also be associated with increased postural tremor in the upper extremities.[47]

Drugs used in the treatment of asthma can often produce tremor as a common side effect. These include isoproterenol, terbutaline, aminophylline, and others.[56] Isotributyline produced occasional tremor in 31 percent of patients.[57] Theophylline has a narrow therapeutic margin, and when the serum level exceeds 15 mg/L, onset of tremor is not uncommon.[58]

TRANQUILIZERS

Tranquilizers, including the benzodiazapine group, are often used in treatment of tremor, because the calming effect on the central nervous system is considered to have therapeutic benefit on tremors. However, occurrence of tremor during diazepam withdrawal in patients who consumed 60–120 mg/day for 3–14 year is reported.[59]

DOPAMINE RECEPTOR-BLOCKING DRUGS

Neurological sequelae resulting from dopamine receptor-blocking medications (neuroleptics) is well recognized. Tremor as a complication of dopamine receptor-blocking therapy could manifest in the form of resting tremor in drug-induced parkinsonism, rabbit syndrome when there is tremor involving mainly the lips, and tremor associated with tardive dyskinesia or tardive tremor.

Tremor as result of drug-induced parkinsonism could occur because of either blockage of dopamine receptors[60] or depletion of dopamine stores in the nerve terminal.[61] Tremor is mainly manifested as resting tremor, but it is not uncommon to see partial tremor as well. Although tremor may be more predominant in the upper extremities, it is not uncommon to see head or even lower-extremity tremor. In a detailed study, the incidence of parkinsonian tremor were found to be greater than 13 percent with thioridazine, whereas the incidence with chlorpromazine was less than half of that.[62] However, in this study about 5 percent of the patients treated with placebo also exhibited tremor. Tremor is often the major concern in patients with drug-induced parkinsonism.[63] Metaclopramide, a drug used in the treatment of gastroparesis, symptomatic gastroesophageal reflux is known to produce parkinsonism with rest tremor.[64] On discontinuing treatment, the parkinsonism is fully reversible. Catecholamine-depletswing agents such as reserpine or tetrabenzine (which is less potent than reserpine) may also be capable of producing

tremor as part of drug-induced parkinsonism. Treatment of drug-induced parkinsonism is discussed in detail in Chapter 24 by Hubble.

In *Rabbit syndrome*, rest tremor affecting the periorbicularis oris muscle of the lips is seen. Similar to the movements seen in rabbit's mouth originally described by Villeneuve,[65] there is often a popping-like sound produced as the lips rapidly separate. The frequency is 4–6 Hz. There may be tremor of chin and extremities. Anticholinergics are considered to be effective in this disorder.

Tardive tremor is predominantly partial and kinetic tremor that interferes with writing, eating, and other activities of daily living. Little or no parkinsonian features were described in patients who were exposed to neuroleptic therapy. The tremor persisted even after 6 years of cessation of neuroleptic therapy. The tremor persisted at rest. Tardive tremor is a rare disorder in patients exposed to neuroleptics, as only 5 patients of 243 patients with drug-induced movement disorders were seen.[66] The mechanism of tardive tremor is not known and may not respond to conventional antitremor therapy. Tetrabenazine and other dopamine-depleting agents seem to be effective.

ANTIDEPRESSANTS

Lithium is widely accepted as a prophylactic therapy in recurrent affective disorders and is known to produce enhancement of physiological tremor. The incidence is considered to range from 33 percent to 65 percent,[67] and the occurrence rate increases with increasing serum lithium levels and manifests almost 100 percent in lithium toxicity. Centrally acting beta-blockers, such as propranolol, are effective when tremor occurs, even when lithium is maintained at therapeutic range.

Tricyclic antidepressants are known to produce high-frequency, low-amplitude postural tremor and are considered to represent enhanced physiological tremor.[68] Although specific treatment may not be required, reduction in the dose may be all that is required, as the tremors seem to correlate with the plasma levels of the drug.[69] However, in an occasional case, use of a beta blocker such as propranolol may be necessary.[70]

Monoamine oxide inhibitors are known to cause tremor. The incidence of tremor was 15 percent in a prospective study of phenelzine for depression.[71]

ANTIEPILEPTIC DRUGS

Valproic acid is the most common tremorogenic drug among antiepileptic drugs. In chronic valproic acid therapy, tremor incidence is considered to occur in about one-fourth of the patients.[72] Tremor is generally postural, and the frequency may range from 6 to 15 Hz.[72] Tremor may occur, even when the dose of valproic acid is within the therapeutic range. Onset of tremor could occur within the few weeks after treatment but generally begins anywhere between 3 and 14 months after the therapy is started.[73,74] Although no correlation between the severity of tremor and the serum levels of valproic acid is found, patients may note reduction in the amplitude of tremor when the drug is withheld or after a change in the bioavailability of the drug.[47] Most valproic acid-associated tremor may not require treatment unless the serum level of the drug is at a toxic level. When tremor is persistent, despite serum level of the drug being at a therapeutic level, use of beta-blocking agents such as propranolol may be needed.[47]

Occasional tremor has been reported with phenytoin[75] and carbamazepine.[76]

CARDIAC DRUGS

Amiodarone, a cardiac antiarrhythmic, in a study involving 70 consecutive patients showed tremor, along with ataxia, in 52 (74 percent) patients on a daily maintenance dose of 600 mg/a day.[77]

Calcium-channel blockers are reported to possess mild D2 receptor-blocking effects.[78,79] As a result, both parkinsonism and rabbit syndrome have been reported to be caused by cinnarizine and flunarizine associated with tremor.[47] Cinnarizine and flunarizine are known to cause tremor.[78] Nifedipine, another calcium-channel blocking agent, is reported to enhance physiological tremor.[79]

Beta-blockers were introduced for the treatment of hypertension, cardiac arrhythmias, and myocardial infarction. Subsequently, centrally acting beta-blockers were found to be effective in the treatment of essential tremor and other forms of tremor. Pindolol, a beta-blocker, possesses partial agonist activity. Beta-blockers with partial agonist activity in high doses may stimulate beta-2 musculoskeletal receptors. Development of pindolol-induced tremor during a double-blind, randomized, clinical trial is reported.[80]

Procainamide, another antiarrhythmic drug, is also known to produce tremor, but this is rare.[81]

IMMUNOSUPPRESSANTS

Cyclosporine-A, an important immunosuppressive agent that is used in organ transplantation and a variety of other immunological diseases, is known to produce tremor of low amplitude and high frequency.[82]

Midbrain Tremor

The term "rubral" tremor has been used since 1904, when Holmes described a tremor of the fingers with rotation at wrist and elbow, as he believed that the rubral spinal tract was involved in production of this tremor based on observation of a patient with involvement of the rubrospinal tract in the pons.[83] Subsequent observation showed that the superior cerebellar tract or another cerebellar outflow system may be involved.[84] Studies in experimental animals have demonstrated that this tremor is caused by combined lesion of the red nucleus and neighboring structures.[85,86] However, the red nucleus itself has not been shown to be the source of abnormal oscillation; concomitant damage to the cerebellothalamic fibers and nigrostriatal dopaminergic fibers may be necessary.[1] Most clinical pathological correlations of the midbrain tremor have described lesions in the upper brain stem. For this reason the term, *midbrain tremor* has been proposed[87] and accepted by most authors, even though for want of a better

description, the tremor is named on the anatomic site of the lesion.[1,88] It is now believed that the midbrain tremor most likely is a result of interruptions of a combination of pathways in the midbrain tegmentum, namely, rubro-olivocerebellorubral loop, rubrospinal fibers, dopaminergic nigrostriatal fibers, and the serotonergic brain stem telencephalic fibers.[88]

Midbrain tremor is described as a combination of rest and postural and kinetic tremor. The amplitude while resting may be small, but on attempting posture it becomes uncontrollable, and on attempting movement (kinetic) the amplitude may be at the peak degree. Occasionally, the tremor at rest can be quite large and irregular and may increase during certain sustained posture. During active movement there may be further terminal acceleration.[88] The frequency of midbrain tremor may vary from 2 to 5 Hz[1]. The proximal muscles may be affected more than the distal muscle, unlike in most other forms of tremor. In addition, there are almost always other signs of midbrain damage, such as hemiparesis and cranial nerve palsy. Positron emission tomography (PET) evaluation of D2-receptors with [75Br]bromolisuride showed no asymmetry of D2 binding, despite the important asymmetry of 18F-fluorodopa uptake, indicating involvement of the nigra dopaminergic system that appeared to be independent of postsynaptic dopamine receptors in production of midbrain tremor.[89] Table 28:1 lists various causes that produce midbrain tremor.

Treatment of midbrain tremor is generally considered difficult, and spontaneous improvement may occur. Of the various drug treatments tested, response to L-dopa, as reported by Findley and Gresty[89] and, more recently, by Ramy et al.[90] found that L-dopa with dopa decarboxylase inhibitor showed fair-to-significant improvement. Others found L-dopa disappointing.[91] Clonazepam,[92] a combination of valproic acid and propranolol,[87] anticholinergics,[63,93] and bromocriptine,[63] is reported to be effective. Unfortunately, these are all single case reports or open trials done on a small number of patients, and no controlled studies have been done because of the rarity of the disorder. Because of the nature of the underlying pathology, patients with midbrain tremor frequently have a shortened life expectancy.[1] Patients with a long-standing tremor and stable medical illness may be considered for stereotactic thalamotomy or thalamic stimulation in ventralis intermedius, as significant reduction of tremor has been reported as a result of this procedure.[25,94,95]

Tremor as a Result of Neurotoxins

The association of toxins causing tremor has long been known. Jean Fernel, in 1557, linked mercury poisoning to tremor.[96] There are more than 850 neurotoxic chemicals found in the workplace, of which 65 are the most common ones.[97] A conservative estimate of the number of workers exposed full time to one or more of these neurotoxins is considered to be 7.7 million.[98] Toxins such as harmaline and oxotremorine produce tremor and can be used in developing tremor animal models.[99] Naturally occurring tremorogenic mycotoxins are synthesized by aspergillus, penicillium, and claviceps species. Onset of tremor in cattle and other animals is known.

TABLE 28-1 Causes of Midbrain Tremor

Etiology	Location	Reference No.
Vascular	Occlusion of postcommunicating artery	88
	Embolic infarction of right thalamus and left cerebellum (vertebral/basilar artery distribution)	202
	Midbrain region ischemic infarct	156
	SCP, thalamus (hemorrhage)	89
	SCP (hemorrhage)	89
	SCP, thalamus (hemorrhage AVM)	89
	Subthalamus (hemorrhage)	203
Trauma	Midbrain	204
	SCP (gunshot injury)	88
	SCP and subthalamic region (hemorrhage)	89
	Midbrain	205
	Midbrain	204
	Multiple (punch-drunk syndrome)	89
	SCP/midbrain	93
	Closed-head injury, nonlocalized (tremor precipitated by neuroleptic)	63
Infection	Midbrain (tuberculoma)	206
	Midbrain (*Toxoplasma* abscess)	84
Multiple sclerosis	Midbrain (demyelination)	207
Neoplastic	Midbrain	207
Radiation	Irradiation of pineal region vascular hamartoma	218

SCP, superior cerebellar peduncle.

No convincing neurotoxic effects in humans are documented from the above tremorogens.[100]

HEAVY METALS

Neurotoxic effects from ingestion of metals such as mercury, lead, copper, arsenic, and aluminum are well known. However, few of these are known to cause tremor. Mercury was found useful in the treatment of syphilis in the sixteenth century, leading to increased demands for the mineral and, therefore, to heightened mining activities. Miners were said to remain at work rarely for more than a few years because they developed the "trembles" and vertigo. This was considered possibly a result of the toxicity of mercury.[101] Epidemics of inorganic mercury poisoning have occurred, usually manifested by the appearance of tremor. Chronic inorganic exposure to mercury may lead to fine rapid tremor that affects extremities, head, tongue, eyelids, and voice. The incidence of tremor in felt hat makers was found to be 20 percent when exposed for more than 20 years. However, in industrial accidents, the incidence has been 50–90 percent.[101] Organic mercury poisoning was rare before 1953, at which time industrial pollution in Minamata Bay, Japan, caused an epidemic of mercury poisoning. Ataxic tremor was one of the components. At autopsy, cerebellar atrophy, along with cerebral edema, was seen.[102] A similar syndrome in a single family from Alamagordo, New Mexico, who consumed meat from hogs that were accidentally fed with grain treated with methyl mercury fungicide, has been reported.[103] Onset of intention tremor along with cerebellar signs has been reported in an agricultural worker after the worker consumed cereal seeds treated with mercury derivative.[104] Accidental acute mercury vapor poisoning with high mercury levels in blood and urine in three patients, resulting in tremor, severe

pulmonary edema, and coma leading to death, has been reported.[105] Treatment of mercury intoxication is through the use of chelating agent-British anti-Lewisite (BAL). Use of N-acetyl-DL-penicillamine has been used.[106] Whether BAL alone is effective or and penicillamine alone or in combination is necessary is not established. Avoidance of further exposure is equally important.

Chronic exposure to manganese, usually among manganese miners or in an industry where manganese is processed, leads to rest tremor as part of parkinsonism that occurs. Experimental animals treated with manganese developed tremor, rigidity, and incoordination. Depletion of dopamine from the basal ganglia is considered to be the underlying cause. In Chilean manganese miners the incidence of extrapyramidal disease is considered to be 65 percent. In addition a small number of patients may manifest cerebellar findings. The absorption of manganese is through the lung and gastrointestinal tract.[101] Chelation is considered not to help in manganese intoxication.[107] Levodopa showed a varied response.

Lead neurotoxicity manifests mainly as encephalopathy with irritability, insomnia, memory loss, restlessness, confusion, and hallucinations. Leaded gasoline sniffing leading onto lead toxicity in Navajo adolescents resulted in 31 percent having tremor and ataxia. Also, their blood lead levels were elevated.[108] Another single case of postural tremor is reported in a 15-year-old boy who inhaled gasoline for its euphoric effects.[109] The treatment of choice in lead poisoning is chelation with calcium ethylenediaminetetraacetic acid (EDTA).

INSECTICIDES AND HERBICIDES

Chlordecone (kepone), an organochlorine pesticide, is used as an ant and roach pesticide. Exposure to this pesticide in industrial workers resulted in occurrence of tremor. In the severely affected workers, tremor was present, even at rest, whereas in those patients moderately affected, tremor was described as irregular and nonpurposive with a frequency of 12 Hz.[110] In addition, workers exhibited ataxia, weight loss, opsoclonus, pleuratic and joint pains, and abnormalities on liver function tests.[111] The tremors were reproducible in mice[112] and rats.[113] Studies showed that norepinephrine may be involved in the expression of tremor induced by chlordecone.[114] Treatment consists of use of cholestyramine, an anion exchange resin that would facilitate fecal excretion.[115]

Dichlorodiphenyltrichloroethane (DDT), a residual insecticide, was used worldwide to control mosquitoes, especially in endemic areas where malaria is prevalent, and banned in most places because of its carcinogenicity. DDT is known to produce tremor in experimental animals.[116,117] Inhaling the toxic fumigant-phosphine, 31 crew members aboard a grain freighter resulted in intention tremor, ataxia, diplopia, and other neurological manifestations.[118] Methylbromide is widely used as a fumigant and is known to produce tremor, ataxia, and myoclonus.[119] Herbicide dioxin (referred to as agent orange) exposure resulted in postural and intention tremor in 35 of 47 railroad workers during a chemical spillage after damage to a tank car filled with this chemical.[37] Carbon disulfide, along with carbon tetrachloride, is used as a fumigant. Exposure in 21 grain workers resulted in about one-half of them developing parkinsonian features, along with resting tremor, and the other half developed cerebellar syndrome associated with intention tremor.[120]

SOLVENTS

Exposure to solvents that contained toluene and methyl ethyl ketone during spray painting in a closed garage resulted in development of intention tremor and other cerebellar signs.[121] Toluene abuse in the form of lacquer sniffing in a 24-year-old man for 5 years resulted in development of tremor with cerebellar signs, with evidence of severe atrophy of cerebellar hemispheres, vermis and brain stem, as well as mild atrophy of cerebral hemispheres on computed tomography (CT) scan.[122] Irreversible cholinesterase inhibitor *soman*, used as a nerve gas, is known to produce tremor.[123]

Orthostatic Tremor

Orthostatic tremor, also referred to as "shaky leg syndrome," a disorder wherein patients find it almost impossible to remain standing for more than 10 seconds, was first described by Heilman.[124] Walking, sitting, and lying were unaffected. Standing involved a wide base, but gait was normal. Presence of fine tremor was felt better than it could be seen, in both the legs on standing or when the muscles are in isometric contraction. There are no other abnormal neurological signs or symptoms. Patients find it increasingly difficult to stand still, are unsteady, and are forced to take a step to regain balance. Falls and injuries are uncommon, as patients start moving as soon as the sense of imbalance occurs. The diagnosis is confirmed by surface electromyographic recordings that show rhythmic activation of lower limb muscles at a frequency of 14–18 Hz. Within any individual patient the frequency remains unchanged in all of the muscles examined.

This frequency is higher than for physiological tremor, which may show a frequency of 8–12 Hz[5,7] or essential tremor, which has a frequency of 5–8 Hz.[125] The age of onset may vary from the 3rd through 7th decades of life, with the majority of the patients developing the symptoms in the 6th or 7th decades of life. Men and women seem to be affected equally, and family history of tremor is present only in a small number of patients.[126] The condition is rare, as of 1992, 28 cases have been reported.[126] The etiology of this condition is unknown, and the question has been raised as to whether orthostatic tremor is a variant of essential tremor.[127,128] However, there is a considerable difference between the two forms of tremor (Table 28-2), and the general consensus is that the two are separate entities. Successful response to clonazoline, phenobarbital, primidone, and valproic acid has been reported, whereas response to propranolol and ethanol remain unsatisfactory.[129]

Symptomatic Palatal Tremor

What was formerly called palatal myoclonus (synonyms: rhythmic palatal myoclonus, oculopalatal myoclonus, palatal nystagmus, brain stem myorhythmia, and palatal myorhythmia) has been renamed palatal tremor. This reclassification more accurately describes the condition.[130] Palatal tremor is divided into two distinct clinical entities, *symptomatic palatal tremor* (SPT), in which patients are often unaware of the palatal movements but may complain of coincidental oscillopsia and have symptoms and signs of brain stem or cerebellar dysfunction associated with hypertrophic degeneration of inferior olive, and *essential palatal tremor*, in which patients often complain of a rhythmic ear clicks but do not have any symptoms.[131] Table 28-3 gives the criteria for symptomatic and essential forms of palatal tremor. In this section only the symptomatic form will be discussed. SPT often is a result of an underlying neurological abnormality, such as a previous brain stem stroke, multiple sclerosis, trauma, or degenerative disease. Thus, it is not surprising that the most consistent clinical finding in these patients is a unilateral or bilateral

TABLE 28-2 Differences between Othostatic Tremor and Essential Tremor

	Orthostatic Tremor	Essential Tremor
Age of onset	Late	Early (adult)
Family history of tremor	Rare	Common
Occurrence	Standing	Postural
Legs affected	Always	Rarely
Tremor frequency	14–16 Hz	6–8 Hz
Paraspinal muscle effected	Always	Rarely
Response to:		
Alcohol	0	+ + +
Propranolol	0	+ + +
Clonazepam	+ +	+
Phenobarbital	+ +	+ +
Primidone	+ +	+ +

0, absent; +, fair response; + +, good response; + + +, excellent response.
SOURCE: Data taken from Refs. 125, 128, and 208.

TABLE 28-3 Criteria for Symptomatic and Essential Forms of Palatal Tremor

Criteria	Symptomatic Palatal Tremor	Essential Palatal Tremor
Cause	Cerebrovascular disease, degenerative disease, encephalitis, multiple sclerosis, trauma	Unknown
Anamnestic or clinical evidence of brain stem or cerebellar disease	Present	Absent
Presenting symptoms	Oscillopsia and others related to brain stem or cerebellar disease	Ear clicks
Involvement of muscle groups other than soft palate	Frequently	Rarely
Involvement of eyes	Frequently	Never
Involvement of extremities	Rarely	Never
Involvement of soft palatal muscles	Levator veli palatini	Tensor veli palatini
Activation of brain stem motor nuclei	Ambiguous nucleus or facial nucleus	Trigeminal nucleus
Cessation of symptoms during sleep	No	Yes
Remote effects of palatal tremor on tonic EMG activity	Unilateral or bilateral	None
Brain stem reflexes	Often abnormal, indicating focal brain stem disease	Normal or nonspecific abnormalities
MRI	Inferior olive abnormality	Normal

SOURCE: *From Deuschl et al.[131] Used with permission.*

cerebellar syndrome. On magnetic resonance imaging (MRI) scan (provided it is done with a high-field scanner with specific proton density and a T_2-weighted series), unilateral or bilateral hyperintense signals in the upper medulla consistent with the gliosis representing olivary pseudohypertrophy,[131] which is considered hallmark for SPT, is seen. When unilateral olivary abnormality is seen, palatal tremor and cerebellar signs are present contralateral to the side of olivary hypertrophy. Sleep does not abolish SPT. SPT results from activation of levator veli palatini muscle, which is innervated by the 7th or 9th cranial nerves. Frequency of palatal tremor is 2 Hz, which is the range of normal firing frequency of inferior olive cells.[132] The tremor rhythm in SPT is highly resistant to both external and internal inferences[133,134] (see also Chap. 41)

Peripheral Neuropathy-Associated Tremor

A wide variety of tremors have been described in patients with peripheral neuropathy. These include rest tremors, postural tremors, and intention tremors.[135–137] The tremor seen in peripheral neuropathy has been described as irregular, rhythmic, proximal, or distal, with a frequency ranging from 3 to 10 Hz.[1] Peripheral neuropathies cause slowing of the nerve conduction. No relationship between the degree of conduction velocity and sensory loss has been found.[136,138] Slowing of nerve conduction would increase the delay in

stretch reflex, and this may lead to enhancement of tremor.[139] It was suggested that tremor associated with peripheral neuropathy may be an enhancement of physiological tremor secondary to weakness.[138] This hypothesis has been disputed.[140] It was hypothesized that generation of tremor in peripheral neuropathy may be the result of an abnormality in the central nervous system. However, most patients with peripheral neuropathy show normal CT/MRI scan and routine cerebrospinal fluid (CSF) examination. In dogs (Scottish terriers) with whole-body tremor and ataxia, widespread axonal changes, vacuolation, and gliosis in the white matter of central nervous system were seen at autopsy.[141] Such changes in humans with varieties of peripheral neuropathy have not been reported.

Table 28-4 lists tremor occurring in various peripheral neuropathies. Presence of tremor in Charcot-Marie-Tooth disease was named Roussy-Lévy syndrome. Currently, it is classified as hereditary motor sensory neuropathy (HMSN) type I. Marie observed presence of tremor in HMSN.[142] A detailed evaluation in HMSN type I revealed that tremor was present in 40 percent of patients. The time from appearance of tremor until onset of disease was 16 years, and the tremor involved mostly hand, followed by arms, legs, and head. Tremor was mostly postural, with rest components but no parkinsonian features. Some patients reported improvement of tremor with alcohol, and some indicated improvement with propranolol. The authors considered that the pattern of tremor seen in HMSN type I resembles essential tremor. Perhaps, HMSN type I and essential tremor are related by linkage of a common gene.[143]

TABLE 28-4 Tremor in Peripheral Neuropathy

1. Hereditary motor and sensory neuropathy type I (HMSN type I).
2. Chronic inflammatory demyelinating polyneuropathy (CIDP).
3. Immunoglobulin M (IgM) chronic paraproteinemic demyelinating polyneuropathy (IgM CPDP).
4. Guillain-Barré syndrome (recovery stage).
5. Diabetic neuropathy.
6. Uremic neuropathy.
7. Neuropathy associated with porphyria.
8. Amiodarone can cause both tremor and peripheral neuropathy.
9. Neuropathy associated with alcoholism.

SOURCE: *From Smith.*[139] *Used with permission.*

In chronic demyelinating polyneuropathy with IgM paraproteinemia, the incidence of tremor is considered to be 47 percent.[139] Tremor is often mild, postural, and seen in the hands. When the amplitude is prominent, tremor may be more disabling than weakness. A range of incidence (3–84 percent) of tremor in chronic sensorimotor neuropathy (CIDP) has been reported. Tremor may appear during relapse and disappear during remission. Tremor subsides with treatment of CIDP with corticosteroid therapy, either alone or in combination with cytotoxic drug, or plasma exchange.[139] In other conditions of peripheral neuropathy associated with tremor, symptomatic treatment with beta blockers and other drugs used in essential tremor can be tried.

Psychogenic Tremors

Occurrence of tremor as a manifestation of hysteria has been known for over a century.[144] Koller et al.[145] reported a more detailed study and established diagnostic criteria (Table 28-5). Not all of the criteria may be present in every patient. As with all of the psychogenic disorders, the incidence is higher in females than males, could occur at any age, but is seldom reported in children. The onset is often abrupt with fluctuating severity and is nonprogressive. Tremor is generally bilateral with a mixture of frequencies and patterns. Activities of daily living are not impaired; patients will appear well groomed, but when asked to demonstrate, significant changes in handwriting and other tasks can be seen. Symptoms present usually when attention is given to the patient, either during clinical examination or by family members, and disappears when attention is drawn to some other task or when the patient is alone. Tremor can be kinetic, postural, or resting but lack the physiological pattern; for example, postural tremor may be of higher amplitude than the kinetic tremor. The direction of tremor may change from supination-pronation orientation to one of flexion-extension.[145] On the other hand, the amplitude may be strikingly consistent in all positions—a pattern rarely encountered in tremor of organic origin. Often, there is a history of symptoms for a year or longer before the patient seeks medical attention, and location of the tremor and the pattern may vary from one visit to another. Additional nonphysiological neurological findings may or may not be present, such as split tuning-fork test, clearly detectable physiological weakness, or other

TABLE 28-5 Clinical Features of Psychogenic Tremor

1. Abrupt onset
2. Static course
3. Spontaneous remissions
4. Unclassifiable tremors (complex tremors)
5. Clinical inconsistencies (selective disabilities)
6. Changing tremor characteristics
7. Unresponsiveness to antitremor drugs
8. Tremor increases with attention
9. Tremor lessens with distractibility
10. Responsiveness to placebo
11. Absence of other neurological signs
12. Remission with psychotherapy
13. Multiple somatizations
14. Multiple undiagnosed conditions
15. Spontaneous remissions or cures of symptoms
16. Presence of unphysiological weakness or sensory complaints
17. No evidence of disease by laboratory or radiographic procedures
18. Presence of unwitnessed paroxysmal disorders
19. Employment in allied health professions
20. Litigation or compensation pending
21. Presence of secondary gain
22. Presence of psychiatric disease
23. Documented functional disturbances in the past

SOURCE: *From Koller et al. Used with permission.*

sensory changes. Tremorogram recording may reveal marked fluctuation in amplitude and frequency during the same run, a feature not seen in organic tremors. EMG recordings are of limited diagnostic utility as, for example, when tremor is voluntarily produced, an alternating pattern of antagonist muscle interaction can be produced. Pharmacological therapy in organic tremor may reduce amplitude, but seldom by 100 percent, and the psychogenic tremor may be totally suppressed (by placebo effect), especially when associated with the suggestion of a "cure." Some patients with psychogenic tremor may refuse to take medication or, after short trial, may stop medication with a complaint of side effects or ineffectiveness. Pharmacotherapy in organic tremor reduces amplitude but does not alter tremor frequency.[40,146] Diagnosis of psychogenic tremor is made by exclusion, and not all features described above may be present in a given patient. More than one visit may be necessary, or a detailed history may be lacking. Some patients respond to psychotherapy suggestion or placebo treatment. In a small number of patients, psychogenic tremor may be superimposed on other conditions with a preexisting disorder in which tremor is part of the disease, such as Parkinson's disease, and a clear distinction between the psychogenic segment and underlying disease segment may not always be easy to make. It is equally important to realize that all tremors can be exaggerated by anxiety.

Rest Tremor

Although rest tremor is a descriptive term, it is included in this section because, in addition to parkinsonism, rest tremor can occur in several other conditions (Table 28-6). Rest tremor

TABLE 28-6 Conditions That Can Cause Rest Tremor

	No. of Patients Studied	% with Rest Tremor	Reference No.
Idiopathic Parkinson's disease	81	83	209
Infarct in striatum			163
Infarct in the thalamus			160
Progressive supranuclear palsy	Lit. review + au's 5 patients	12–16	210
Postencephalopathic Parkinsonism			219
Multiple-system atrophy	100	29	211
Olivopontocerebellar atrophy			
Diffuse Lewy body disease	8	29	212
Chronic demyelinating polyneuropathy with benign IgM			139
Paraproteinemia			
Chronic inflammatory demyelinating neuropathy			135
Psychogenic			213
Brain stem infarction with palatal tremor	5	80	214
Midbrain hemorrhage	1		215
Orofacial dystonia	1		216
Large subdural hematoma	1		*
Large frontotemporal meningioma	1		217

*Author's unpublished observation. Blanks indicate that the number of patients not stated.

is present when the affected part of the body is in repose and is fully supported against gravity, requiring no active muscle contraction.[2] The most common anatomic site for rest tremor is in the distal parts of the upper limbs. It can also be seen in lower extremities and, less commonly, in lips, tongue, and jaw.[147] The characteristic upper limb rest tremor includes pronation-supination of the forearm, flexion-extension of the wrist, or "pill-rolling" movement of the thumb, producing a gliding movement across the first two or three fingers.[148] Frequency of rest tremor is 4–5.3 Hz, varying only by 0.2–0.3 Hz from person to person.[149] Rest tremor is produced by the alternate contraction of antagonistic muscles.[150] Experimental studies in lesioned monkeys suggest that for parkinsonism, rest tremor involves ascending nigrostriatal dopaminergic pathway, rubrotegmentospinal fibers, and rubro-olivodentatorubral loop that normally modifies the input into the ventrolateral nucleus of the thalamus.[151] Studies have shown that rest tremors are a social handicap but do not correlate with the disability or performance items when the tremor is mild-to-moderate; rather, when the tremor is severe, it can interfere with these items.

Parkinson rest tremor may be difficult to control. Controlled-release propranolol hydrochloride (160 mg) reduced the amplitude of rest tremor by 70 percent,[152] anticholinergics and carbidopa/levodopa by 50 percent, and amantadine by 25 percent.[153] Subcutaneous apomorphine is found to be effective in reducing amplitude by more than 50 percent.[154] Thalamotomy produces a sustained reduction in contralateral rest tremor in at least 85 percent of patients. The optimal site for lesioning is the vastus anterior medialis (Vam) of the thalamus. This may be treatment of choice when the tremor is severe and pharmacotherapy is not effective or not tolerated. It is also a treatment to be considered when tremor is unilaterally present in the hand.[1]

Stroke-Associated Tremor

Midbrain tremor, with its classical appearance secondary to stroke, is included in Table 28-1. Isolated tremor as a result of stroke is rare. In a review of 62 cases of movement disorders associated with focal lesion in the thalamus and subthalamus, no case of isolated tremor was found.[155] In lesions confined to thalamus, six cases of tremor with a postural and kinetic component have been described.[156–160] Moroo et al.[161] described three patients with postural and kinetic tremor with a frequency of 3–4 Hz whose MRIs showed an ischemic lesion in the midthalamus. Ferbert and Gerwig[162] described four patients with tremor, among whom three had associated dystonia and one hemiparesis. Dethy et al.[163] reported a patient with pure motor stroke associated with hemibody tremor involving right upper and lower extremities. Tremor frequency was 5–6 Hz. MRI scan showed ischemic lesion in the left centrum semiovale and the left caudate nucleus. PET scan showed glucose hypermetabolism in the ipsilateral sensory motor cortex. Thalamic ataxia syndrome, in which there are significant cerebellar signs may be associated with intention tremor.

Tremor occurring immediately after a stroke seems to have a better prognosis than tremor with delayed onset.[162] Because tremor is not usually an isolated phenomenon and there are associated neurological deficits, treatment needs to address all segments of a patient's disability. When there is an associated cerebellar component with the tremor, pharmacotherapy is often disappointing. In the absence of a cerebellar component, attempts at treatment may be made by using drugs that are used to treat essential tremor. No controlled studies have been done, so the only approach is to use one drug at a time, reaching the maximum dose and trying another when the previous one is not effective.

Posttraumatic Tremor

In recent times the definition of trauma has been broadened to include conditions other than those resulting from extrinsic physical injury. Thus, terms such as emotional trauma, metabolic trauma, psychic trauma, and intrinsic trauma (i.e., rupture of an aneurysm, ischemic infarct, etc.) are being used. In this section trauma will refer to physical trauma, such as injury to a structure that was previously intact. An artificial separation of central versus peripheral injury will also be made, even as we remain fully aware of the intimate relationship between the central and peripheral nervous systems. When tremor is noted with a past history of injury there is always an interval of days to years before onset of the tremor. Additionally, there are often associated neurological findings, such as rigidity, hemiparesis, reflex sympathetic dystrophy etc., so tremor generally does not occur in isolation. Tremor does not have a specific anatomic location in the nervous system, because it can occur from lesions of the cerebral cortex, basal ganglia, thalamus, midbrain, cerebellum, and peripheral nerves. Widespread possibilities exist. CT or MRI scan may not show lesions that are tiny and at a cellular or subcellular level. In light of these factors and limitations one can still find evidence in the literature of tremor being precipitated or caused by various injuries. For an excellent review the reader is referred to Curren and Lang.[164]

Most cases of tremor resulting from severe head injury are believed to result from damage to the midbrain but, in addition to the typical midbrain tremor discussed above, other forms of tremor are well recognized. The association of head trauma with parkinsonism was made in 1929.[165] A year earlier, parkinsonian symptoms, including rest tremor associated with "punch drunk" syndrome caused by multiple head injuries in boxers, were studied.[166] Subsequently, more clear cases of parkinsonism with known head injury were studied.[167–169] Tremor developing after minor head injury with no loss of consciousness or other neurological deficits was investigated.[92] Tremor was asymmetric with postural and kinetic components. Tremor occurred after sudden twisting of the neck that resulted in an intimal tear of the carotid artery, leading to an embolic infarct.[170] An 18-year-old girl, in a diving accident at a swimming pool, developed ipsilateral tremor in the right upper and lower extremities. The tremor had a kinetic component. The MRI scan showed a lesion in the left ventral lateral thalamus (Elble RJ, Neurology Grand Rounds case, SIU School of Medicine).

Tremor resulting from peripheral nerve injury is rare. There are often other associated neurological abnormalities, such as dystonia or reflex sympathetic dystrophy. In one study of 43 patients with movement disorders associated with reflex sympathetic dystrophy described by Schwartzman and Kerrigan,[171] only 38 demonstrated a history of injury. Deuschl et al.[172] found that 12 of their 21 patients showed a distal tremor with a mean frequency of 7.2 Hz, and those researchers considered it as enhanced physiological tremor. On treatment of reflex sympathetic dystrophy, the tremor completely disappeared. Only 4 of the 23 patients who had tremor did not have reflex sympathetic dystrophy, and 1 of 5 patients with reflex sympathetic dystro-

phy had tremor in a series reported by Jankovic and Van der Linden.[173] Entrapment of the ulnar nerve in Guyon's canal resulted in development of a tremor in the 4th and 5th fingers with disappearance of tremor after surgery in a secretary/typist subjected to repeated hand movement.[174] This has illustrated the possibility that peripheral trauma could induce tremor, but the exact mechanism remains unknown.

As far as treatment for tremor from central or peripheral trauma is concerned, treating the cause is the key. When the cause can be identified, treatment is often beneficial. Such is the case for compression neuropathy or reflex sympathetic dystrophy. However, where a cause can not be found or where other associated conditions are present, such as lesion of the midbrain, conventional (pharmacological) therapies have been less than satisfactory. Stereotactic thalamotomy has been tried with success.[94,170] In one long-term follow-up study of patients who developed tremor secondary to trauma, 88 percent showed spontaneous improvement over a period of time with no intervention, and the authors suggested that the surgery be restricted to select cases of disabling tremorously.[95]

Vocal Tremor

Vocal tremor (synonyms: tremulous voice, wavy voice, or tremulous, quivering speech) is defined as involuntary, rhythmic, oscillatory movements that affect the vocal musculature in patients with tremulous diseases. The muscles of the sound production mechanism may also be affected, and rhythm alterations in pitch and loudness may be generated.[175] The "prime generator" of voice tremor is central nervous system disturbance; the phonatory reflection is typically multifactorial, involving a combination of the extrinsic and intrinsic laryngeal muscles, pharyngeal muscles (including that of the supraglottic structure), and auxiliary respiratory muscles, including the intercostal abdominal muscles and the diaphragm.[175] The frequency of vocal tremor may range from 4 to 8 Hz, with amplitudes of oscillation ranging widely.[176–180] Acoustic analysis has been the primary noninvasive method for quantification of vocal tremor, with most acoustic data obtained by visual inspection of oscillographic displays of the waveform data or graphic record displays of amplitude contours of sustained oral phonation. As a result, the bulk of acoustic data on vocal tremor includes visual quantifiable amplitude oscillations without frequency modulation components.[175,176,179,181,182] Vocal tremor occurs in Parkinson's disease[183] at an incidence rate of 30.5 percent.[184] The tremor frequency is reported to range from 5–7 Hz.[185] Despite the recognition of vocal tremor in Parkinson's disease, hypophonia is often the major problem. Voice tremor is characterized by rhythmic alterations of pitch and loudness of vowels and in some cases with voice arrests, especially during vowel prolongation.[176,179,186]

Mild voice tremor may be masked during contextual speech[186] and is referred to as essential voice tremor. Eleven percent of patients with essential tremor are known to suffer from voice tremor.[187] In a double-blind study, clonazepam, propranolol, and diazepam treatments were effective for voice and hand tremor, based on clinical and electrophysiological examinations (Fig. 28-1), although hand tremor was more responsive to these drugs.[188] Koller et al. did not find propranolol beneficial in seven patients, compared to placebo.[189] Koda and Ludlow[188] found that the thyroarythenoid muscle was affected in voice tremor and suggested that botulinum toxin injections may be beneficial in treating this disorder.

In cerebellar diseases, dysarthria and vocal tremor occur simultaneously.[176,190] Voice tremor frequency in cerebellar diseases is reported to be 3 Hz, which is similar to that reported for cerebellar and kinetic postural tremor.[191]

In the differential diagnoses of vocal tremor, idiopathic spasmodic dysphonia of two types should be considered. In *abductor spasmodic dysphonia* caused by intermittent abduction of the vocal folds, patients exhibit a breathy effortful voice quality with abrupt termination of voicing, resulting in aphonic, whispered segments of speech. In *adductor spasmodic dysphonia* caused by irregular hyperabduction of the vocal folds, patients exhibit a choked, strained-strangled voice quality, with abrupt initiation and termination of voicing, resulting in short breaks in phonation. Some patients can have a combination of the two. Because many patients with spasmodic dysphonia present with a tremulous voice, differential diagnosis between essential voice tremor and spasmodic dysphonia may be difficult. Both respond to botulinum treatment (see also Chaps. 31 and 32).

Primary Writing Tremor

Primary writing tremor (PWT) was first described by Rothwell et al. in a 20-year-old man who presented with tremor while writing.[192] Active pronation of his hand produced several beats of pronation/supination tremor. A burst of tremor could also be elicited by tendon taps to the volar surface of the wrist, to the finger extensors, to pectoralis major, and by means of forcible supination of the wrist delivered by torte motor. The subject's writing difficulty and tremor were temporarily abolished by partial motor point anesthesia of pronator teres. The frequency of this tremor was 4–6 Hz, and EMG revealed tremor in the muscle toward the forearm and arm. PWT is the most common form of task-specific tremor in the upper extremities. Task-specific tremors involve skilled, highly learned motor acts. Examples include hair-cutting, shaving, putting on make-up, combing hair, use of tools, sewing, use of scissors, golf club swinging, playing a musical instrument, and other activities. The tremor is often not reduced by goal-directed movement or certain posture. Generally, no other associated neurological signs and symptoms are present. The frequency of tremor is 5–7 Hz.[193] EMG has shown both an alternating and roughly synchronous pattern in the antagonistic muscles, but the alternating pattern appears to be more common.[193]

Several authors have argued that PWT is a variant of essential tremor.[194–196] However, although essential tremor is generally inherited in an autosomal-dominant fashion, PWT is most often sporadic. Unlike PWT, clinical and neurophysiological characteristics of essential tremor are too varied. Essential tremor often responds to ethanol, propranolol, and others but not to anticholinergics, whereas these drugs are not as effective in PWT.

PWT is considered a form of focal dystonia.[193,196,197] The clinical characteristics of PWT and focal dystonia of hand (writer's cramp and other occupational cramp) are similar in several respects, as both conditions are more or less task

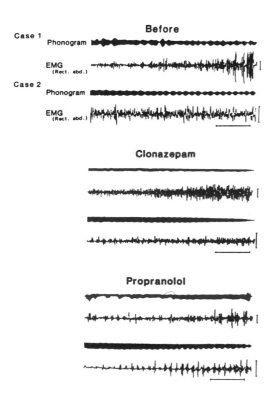

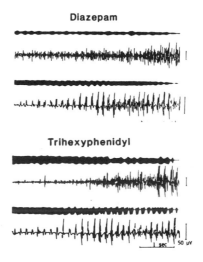

FIGURE 28-1 Phonogram and EMG from rectus abdominis muscle before and after drug administration in two patients. Improvement after treatment is noted with clonazepam, propranolol, and diazepam. Worsening with trihexyphenidyl. (From *Koda and Ludlow.*[188] *Used with permission.*)

specific and are not inherited. Patients with PWT often do not exhibit dystonia. On the other hand, tremor is known to occur in focal dystonia.[198] PET studies of regional cerebral blood flow on voluntary wrist oscillations of control subjects produced ipsilateral cerebellar activation. Patients with PWT displayed bilateral cerebellar activation only, whereas those with essential tremor displayed bilateral cerebellar activation and activation in red nucleus and thalamus.[199]

Pharmacological treatment for primary writing tremor is disappointing. Recently, botulinum toxin injections have been used.[200] Stereotactic selective thalamotomy centered mainly on the Vim has also been successfully used in treatment of this condition.[201]

References

1. Elble RJ, Koller WC: *Tremor.* Baltimore: The Johns Hopkins University Press, 1990.
2. Fahn S: Cerebellar tremor: Clinical aspects, in Findley LJ, Capildeo R (eds): *Movement Disorders: Tremor.* London: Macmillan Press, 1984, pp 355–363.
3. Bairy N, Koller WC: Kinetic predominant essential tremor: Successful treatment with clonazepam. *Neurology* 37:471–474, 1988.
4. Elble RJ: Physiologic and essential tremor. *Neurology* 36:225–231, 1986.
5. Elble RJ, Randall JE: Motor-unit activity responsible for 8- to 12-Hz component of human physiological finger tremor. *J Neurophysiol* 39:370, 1976.
6. Fox JR, Randall JE: Relationship between forearm tremor and the biceps electromyogram. *J Appl Physiol* 29:103, 1970.
7. Elble RJ, Randall JE: Mechanistic components of normal hand tremor. *Electroencephalogr Clin Neurophysiol* 44:72–82, 1978.
8. Matthews PBC, Muir RB: Comparison of electromyogram spectra with force spectra during human elbow tremor. *J Physiol (Lond)* 302:427, 1980.
9. Sutton GG, Sykes K: The variation of hand tremor with force in healthy subjects. *J Physiol (Lond)* 191:699, 1967.
10. Sakamoto K, Nishida K, Zhou L, et al: Characteristics of physiological tremor in five fingers and evaluations of fatigue of fingers in typing. *Ann Physiol Anthropol* 11:61–68, 1992.
11. Elke-Okoro ST: Explanation of physiological muscle tremor. *Electromyogr Clin Neurophysiol* 34:341–343, 1994.
12. Pizzuti GP, Byford GH, Cifaldi S, et al: Finger tremor and the central nervous system. *J Biomed Eng* 14:356–359, 1992.
13. Comby B, Chevalier G, Bouchoucha M: A new method for the measurement of tremor at rest. *Arch Int Physiol Biochim Biophys* 100:73–78, 1992.
14. Lakie M, Frymann K, Villagra F, Jakeman P: The effect of alcohol on physiological tremor. *Exp Physiol* 79:273–276, 1994.
15. Hagbarth K-E, Young RR: Participation of the stretch reflex in human physiological tremor. *Brain* 102:509, 1979.
16. Young RR, Hagbarth K-E: Physiological tremor enhanced by maneuvers affecting the segmental stretch reflex. *J Neurol Neurosurg Psychiatry* 43:248, 1980.
17. Koller W, Cone S, Herbster G: Caffeine and tremor. *Neurology* 37:169, 1987.
18. Abila B, Wilson JF, Marshall RW, Richens A: The tremorolytic action of beta-adrenoceptor blockers in essential, physiological and isoprenaline-induced tremor is mediated by beta-adrenoceptors located in a deep peripheral compartment. *Br J Clin Pharmacol* 20:369–376, 1985.
19. Zilm DH: The effect of propranolol on normal physiologic tremor. *Electroencephalogr Clin Neurophysiol.* 41:310–313, 1976.
20. Hallett M: Classification and treatment of tremor. *J Am Med Assoc.* 266:1115–1117, 1984.
21. Rondot P, Bathein N: Motor control in cerebellar tremor, in Findley LJ, Capideo R (eds): *Movement Disorders: Tremor.* London: Macmillan Press, 1984, pp 366–376.
22. Thach WT, Goodkin HP, Keating JG: The cerebellum and the adaptive coordination of movement. *Annu Rev Neurosci* 15:403–442, 1992.
23. Manyam BV: Recent advances in the treatment of ataxia. *J. Clin Neuropharmacol* 9:508–516, 1986.
24. Manyam BV: Ataxia, in Klawans HL, Goetz C, Tanner C (eds): *Textbook of Clinical Neuropharmacology.* New York: Raven Press, 1992, chap 23, pp 297–306.
25. Goldman MS, Kelly PJ: Symptomatic and functional outcome of stereotactic ventralis lateralis thalamotomy for intention tremor. *J Neurosurg* 77:223, 1992.
26. Wester K, Hauglie-Hanssen E: Stereotaxic thalamotomy—experiences from the levodopa era. *J Neurol Neurosurg Psychiatry* 53:427, 1990.
27. Nguyen JP, Degos JD: Thalamic stimulation and proximal tremor. *Arch Neurol* 50:498–500, 1993.
28. Hewer RL, Cooper R, Morgan MH: An investigation into the value of treating intention tremor by weighting the affected limb. *Brain* 95:570, 1972.
29. Ikeda A, Kakigi A, Funai N, et al: Cortical tremor: A variant of cortical reflex myoclonus. *Neurology.* 40:1561–1565, 1990.
30. Toro C, Pascual-Leone A, Deuschl G, et al: Cortical tremor: A common manifestation of cortical myoclonus. *Neurology* 43:2346–2353, 1993.
31. Oppenheim H: Uber eine eigenartige Kramfkrankheit des kindlichen und jungedichen Alters (Dybasia lordotica progressiva, dystonia musculorum deformans): *Neurologie Centralblatt* 30:1090, 1911.
32. Marsden CE, Harrison MJG: Idiopathic torsion dystonia (dystonia musculorum deformans): A review of forty-two patients. *Brain* 97:793, 1974.
33. Rivest J, Marsden CD: Trunk and head tremor as isolated manifestations of dystonia. *Mov Disord* 5:60, 1990.
34. Hughes AJ, Lees AJ, Marsden CE: Paroxysmal dystonia head tremor. *Mov Disord* 6:85, 1991.
35. Jankovic J, Leder S, Warner D, Schwartz K: Cervical dystonia: clinical findings and associated movement disorders. *Neurology* 41:1088, 1991.
36. Dubinsky RM: Tremor and dystonia, in Findley LJ, Koller WC (eds): *Handbook of Tremor Disorders.* New York: Marcel Dekker, 1995, chap 28, pp 405–410.
37. Klawans HL: Dystonia and tremor following exposure to 2,3,7,8-tetrachlorodibenzo-p-dioxin. *Mov Disord* 2:255, 1987.
38. Jedynak CP, Bonnet AM, Agid Y: Tremor and idiopathic dystonia. *Mov Disord* 6:230, 1991.
39. Jankovic J, Fahn S: Physiologic and pathologic tremors. *Ann Intern Med* 73:460, 1980.
40. Larsen TA, Calne DB: Essential tremor. *Clin Neuropharmacol* 6:185, 1983.
41. Shirlow MJ, Matheers CS: A study of caffeine consumption and symptoms: Indigestion, palpitations, tremor, headache, and insomnia. *Int J Epidemiol* 14:239, 1985.
42. Rajput AH, Jamison H, Hirsh S, Quraishi A: Relative efficacy of alcohol and propranolol in action tremor. *Can J Neurol Sci* 2:31–35, 1975.
43. Leavitt S, Tyler HR: Studies in asterixis. *Arch Neurol* 10:360, 1964.
44. Rondot P, Jedynak CP, Ferrey G: Pathological tremors: Nosological correlates. *Prog Clin Neurophysiol* 5:95, 1978.
45. Koller W, O'Hara R, Durus W, Bauer J: Tremor in chronic alcoholism. *Neurology* 35:1660, 1985.

46. Silverskoid BP: Romberg's test in the cerebellar syndrome occurring in chronic alcoholism. *Acta Neurol Scand* 45:292, 1969.

47. Lang AE: Miscellaneous drug-induced movement disorders, in Lang AE, Weiner WJ (eds): *Drug-Induced Movement Disorders.* Mt. Kisco, NY: Futura Publishing Co, 1992, chap 12, pp 339–381.

48. Victor M, Adams RD, Cole lM: The acquired (non-Wilsonian) type of chronic hepatocerebral degeneration. *Medicine (Baltimore)* 44:345, 1965.

49. Spencer PS, Nunn PB, Hu J, et al: Guam amyotrophic lateral sclerosis-parkinsonism-dementia linked to a plant exicitant. *Science* 237:517, 1987.

50. Bovet D, Longo VG: The action of nicotine-induced tremors of substances effective in parkinsonism. *J Pharmacol Exp Ther* 102:22, 1951.

51. Cahen RL, Thomas JM, Tvede KM: Nicotinolytic drugs. II: Action of adrenergic blocking agents on nicotine-induced tremors. *J Pharmacol Exp Ther* 107:424, 1953.

52. Stiffmaln SM, Fritz ER, Maltese J, et al: Effects of cigarette smoking and oral nicotine on hand tremor. *Clin Pharmacol Ther* 33:800, 1983.

53. Lippold OC, Williams EJ, Wilson CG: Finger tremor and cigarette smoking. *Br J Clin Pharmacol* 10:83, 1980.

54. Zdonczyk D, Royse V, Koller WC: Nicotine and tremor. *Clin Neuropharmacol* 11:282, 1988.

55. Kramer JC, Fischman VS, Littlefield DC: Amphetamine abuse: Patterns and effects of high doses taken intravenously. *J Am Med Assoc* 201:305, 1967.

56. LeWitt PA: Tremor induced or enhanced by pharmacological means, in Findley LJ, Koller WC (eds): *Handbook of Tremor Disorders.* New York: Marcel Dekker, 1995, chap 34, pp 473–481.

57. Formgren H: The therapeutic value of oral long-term treatment with terbutaline (Bricanyl) in asthma: A follow-up study of its efficacy and side effects. *Scand J Respir Dis* 56:321, 1975.

58. Heath A, Knudsen K: Role of extracorporeal drug removal in acute theophylline poisoning: A review. *Med Toxicol Adver Drug Exp* 2:294, 1987.

59. Mellor CS, Jain VK: Diazepam withdrawal syndrome: Its prolonged and changing nature. *Can Med Assoc J* 127:1093, 1982.

60. Hornykiewicz O: Parkinsonism induced by dopaminergic antagonists. *Adv Neurol* 9:155, 1975.

61. Freyhan FA: Psychomotility and parkinsonism in treatment with neuroleptic drugs. *Arch Neurol Psychiatry* 78:465, 1957.

62. National Instutute of Mental Health Psychopharmacology Service Center Collaborative Study Group: Phenothiazine treatment in acute schizophrenia. *Arch Gen Psychiatry* 10:246, 1964.

63. Friedman JH: "Rubral" tremor induced by a neuroleptic drug. *Mov Disord* 7:281, 1992.

64. Indo T, Ando K: Metoclopramide-induced parkinsonism: Clinical characteristics of ten cases. *Arch Neurol* 39:494, 1982.

65. Villeneuve A: The rabbit syndrome: A peculiar extrapyramidal reaction. *Can Psychiatr Assoc J Suppl* 2:SS69, 1972.

66. Stacy M, Jankovic J: Tardive tremor. *Move Disord* 7:53, 1992.

67. Vestergaard P: Clinically important side effects of long-term lithium treatment: A review. *Acta Psychiatr Scand* 67(suppl):11, 1983.

68. Young RR: Physiological and enhanced physiological tremor, in Findley LJ, 1984, Capildeo R (eds): *Movement Disorders: Tremor.* New York: Oxford University Press, pp 127–135.

69. Nelson JC, Jatlow PI, Quinlan DM: Subjective complaints during desipramine treatment. *Arch Gen Psychiatry* 41:55, 1984.

70. Kronfol Z, Greden JF, Zis AP: Imipramine-induced tremor: Effects of a beta-adrenergic blocking agent. *J Clin Psychopharmacol.* 44:225, 1983.

71. Evans DL, Davidson J, Raft D: Early and late side effects of phenelzine. *J Clin Psychopharmacol* 2:208, 1982.

72. Karas BJ, Wilder BJ, Hammond EJ, Bauman AW: Valproate tremors. *Neurology* 32:428, 1982.

73. Price DJI: The advantages of sodium valkproate in the neurosurgical practice, in Legg NJ (ed): *Clinical and Pharmacological Aspects of Sodium Valproate (Epilim) in the Treatment of Epilepsy.* Turnbridge Wells, England: MCS Consultants, 1976, pp 44–50.

74. Hyman NM, Dennis PD, Sinclair KGA: Tremor due to sodium valpropate. *Neurology* 19:1177, 1979.

75. Prensky AL, DeVivo DC, Palkes H: Severe bradykinesia as a manifestation of toxicity to anti-epileptic medications. *J Pediatr* 78:700, 1974.

76. Hajnsek F, Sartorius N: A case of intoxication with Tegretol. *Epilepsia* 5:371, 1964.

77. Greene HL, Graham EL, Werner JA, et al: Toxic and therapeutic effects of amiodarone in the treatment of cardiac arrhythmias. *J Am Coll Cardiol.* 2:1114, 1983.

78. Capella D, Laporte JR, Castel JM: Parkinsonism, tremor, and depression induced by cinnarizine and flunarizine. *Br Med J* 297:722–723, 1988.

79. Amery WK, Heykants J: Essential tremor and flunarizine. *Cephalalgia* 8:227, 1988

80. Koller W, Orebaugh C, Lawson L, Potempa K: Pindolol-induced tremor. *Clin Neuropharmacol* 5:449–452, 1987.

81. Rubinstein A, Cabili S: Tremor induced by procainamide. *Am J Cardiol* 57:340–341, 1986.

82. Palmer BF, Toto RD: Severe neurologic toxicity induced by cyclosporine A in three renal transplant patients. *Am J Kidney Dis* 18:116, 1991.

83. Holmes G: On certain tremors in organic cerebral lesions. *Brain* 27:327, 1904.

84. Koppel BS, Daras M: "Rubral" tremor due to midbrain toxoplasma abscess. *Mov Disord* 5:154, 1990.

85. Carpenter MB: A study of the red nucleus in the rhesus monkey. *J Comp Neurol* 105:195, 1956.

86. Ohye C, Shibazaki T, Hirai T, et al: Special role of the parvocellular red nucleus in lesion-induced spontaneous tremor in monkeys. *Behav Brain Res* 28:241, 1988.

87. Samie MR, Selhorst JB, Koller WC: Post-traumatic midbrain tremors. *Neurology* 40:62, 1990.

88. Hopfensperger KJ, Busenbark K, Koller WC: Midbrain tremor, in Findley LJ, Koller WC (eds): *Handbook of Tremor Disorders,* New York: Marcel Dekker, 1995, chap 32, pp 455–459.

89. Findley LF, Gresty MA: Suppression of "rubral" tremor with levodopa. *Br Med J* 28:1043, 1980.

90. Remy P, de Recondo A, Defer G, et al: Peduncular 'rubral' tremor and dopaminergic denervation: A PET study. *Neurology* 45:472, 1995.

91. Yuill GM: Suppression of "rubral" tremor with levodopa: Personal observation. *Br Med J* 281:1428, 1980.

92. Biary N, Cleeves L, Findley L, Koller W: Post-traumatic tremor. *Neurology* 39:103, 1989.

93. Krack P, Deuschl G, Kaps M, et al: Delayed onset of "rubral tremor" 23 years after brainstem trauma (Letter to the Editor). *Mov Disord* 9:240, 1994.

94. Andrew J, Fowler CJ, Harrison MJ: Tremor after head injury and its treatment by sterotaxic surgery. *J Neurol Neurosurg Psychiatry* 45:815, 1982.

95. Krauss JK, Mohadjer M, Nobbe F, Mundinger F: The treatment of posttraumatic tremor by stereotactic surgery: Symptomatic and functional outcome in a series of 35 patients. *J Neurosurg* 80:810, 1994.

96. Chang LW: Mercury, in Spencer PS, Schaumburg HH (eds): *Experimental and Clinical Neurotoxicology.* Baltimore: Williams & Wilkins, 1980, pp 508–526.

97. National Institute for Occupational Safety and Health: Leading work-related diseases and injuries—United States. *J Am Med Assoc* 255:1552–1559, 1986.

98. National Institute for Occupational Safety and Health: *National Occupational Hazard Survey, 1972–74*. National Institute for Occupational Safety and Health, Cincinnati, DHEW (NOISH) publication No. 78–114, 1977.

99. Iwata S, Nomoto M, Fukuda T: Effects of beta-adrenergic blockers on drug-induced tremors. *Pharmacol Biochem Behav* 44:611, 1993.

100. Ludolph AC, Spencer PS: Mycotoxins and tremorogens, in Chang LW, Dyer RS (eds): *Handbook of Neurotoxicology*. New York: Marcel Dekker, 1995, pp 601–603.

101. Greenhouse AH: Heavy metals and the nervous system. *Clin Neuropharmacol*. 5:45, 1982.

102. Kurland L, Faro S, Siedler H: Minamata disease: The outbreak of a neurologic disorder in Minamata, Japan and its relationship to the ingestion of seafood contaminated by mercuric compounds. *World Neurol* 1:370, 1960.

103. Nelson N, Byerly TC, Kolbye AC, et al: Hazards of mercury: Special report to the secretary's pesticide advisory committee, Department of Health, Education and Welfare. *Environ Res* 4:1, 1971.

104. Lefevre JP, Gil R: Encephalopathy due to organomercuric compounds (translated title). *Semaine Hopitaux* 53:165, 1977.

105. Jaeger A, Tempe JD, Haegy JM, Leroy M, Porte A, Mantz JM: Accidental acute mercury vapor poisoning. *Vet Hum Toxicol* 21 (suppl) 62, 1979.

106. Kark RA, Poskanzer D, Bullock J, Boylen G: Mercury poisoning and its treatment with N-acetyl-D,L-penicillamine. *N Engl J Med*. 185:10, 1971.

107. Mena I, Marin O, Fuenzalida S, Cotzias G: Chronic manganese poisoning: Clinical picture and manganese turnover. *Neurology* 17:128, 1967.

108. Coulehan JL, Hirsch W, Brillman J, et al: Gasoline sniffing and lead toxicity in Navajo adolescents. *Pediatrics* 71(1):113, 1983.

109. Goldings AS, Stewart RM: Organic lead encephalopathy: Behavioral change and movement disorder following gasoline inhalation. *J Clin Psychol* 43:70–72, 1982.

110. Gerhart JM, Hong JS, Uphouse LL, Tilson HA: Chlordecone-induced tremor: Quantification and pharmacological analysis. *Toxicol Appl Pharmacol* 66:234, 1982.

111. Taylor JR, Selhorst JB, Houff SA, Martinez AJ: Chlordecone intoxication of man. I: Clinical observations. *Neurology* 28:626, 1978.

112. Huang TP, Ho IK, Mehendale HM: Assessment of neurotoxicity induced by oral administration of chlordecone (Kepone) in the mouse. *Neurotoxicology* 2:113, 1981.

113. Reiter LW, Kidd K, Ledbetter G, et al: Comparative behavioral toxicology of mirex and kepone in the rat. *Toxicol Appl Pharmacol* 41:143, 1977.

114. Chen PH, Tilson HA, Marbury GD, et al: Effect of chlordecone (Kepone) on the rat brain concentration of 3-methoxy-4-hydroxyphenlglycol: Evidence for a possible involvement of the norepinephrine system in chlordecone-induced tremor. *Toxicol Appl Pharmacol* 77:158, 1985.

115. Cohn WJ, Boylan JJ, Blanke RV, et al: Treatment of chlordecone (Kepone) toxicity with cholestyramine. *N Engl J Med* 198:243, 1978.

116. Hietanen E, Vainio H: Effect of administration route on DDT on acute toxicity and on drug biotransformation in various rodents. *Arch Environ Contam Toxicol* 4:201, 1976.

117. Kashyap SK, Nigam SK, Karnik AB, et al: Carcinogenicity of DDT (dichlorodiphenyl trichloroethane) in pure inbred Swiss mice. *Int J Cancer* 19:725, 1977.

118. Wilson R, Lovejoy FH, Jaeger RJ, Landrigan PL: Acute phosphine poisoning aboard a grain freighter: Epidemiologic, clinical, and pathological findings. *J Am Med Assoc* 244:148, 1980.

119. Zatuchni J, Hong K: Methyl bromide poisoning seen initially as psychosis. *Arch Neurol* 38:529, 1981.

120. Peters HA, Levine RL, Matthews CG, Chapman LJ: Extrapyramidal and other neurologic manifestations associated with carbon disulfide fumigant exposure. *Arch Neurol* 45:537, 1988.

121. Welch L, Kirschner H, Heath A, et al: Chronic neuropsychological and neurological impairment following acute exposure to a solvent mixture of toluene and methyl ethyl ketone (MEK). *J Toxicol Clin Toxicol* 29:435, 1991.

122. Poungvarin N: Multifocal brain damage due to lacquer sniffing: The first case report of Thailand. *J Med Assoc Thailand* 74:296, 1991.

123. Buccafusco JJ, Heithold DL, Chon SH: Long-term behavioral and learning abnormalities produced by the irreversible cholinesterase inhibitor soman: Effect of a standard pretreatment regimen and clonidine. *Toxicol Lett* 52(3):319, 1990.

124. Heilman KM: Orthostatic tremor. *Arch Neurol* 41:880, 1984.

125. Thompson PD, Rothwell JC, Day BL, et al: The physiology of orthostatic tremor. *Arch Neurol* 43:584, 1986.

126. Thompson PD: Primary orthostatic tremor, in Findley LJ, Koller WC (eds): *Handbook of Tremor Disorders*. New York: Marcel Dekker, 1995, chap 26, pp 387–399.

127. Papa SM, Gershanik OS: Orthostatic tremor: An essential tremor variant? *Mov Disord* 3:97, 1988.

128. FitzGerald PM, Jankovic J: Orthostatic tremor: An association with essential tremor. *Mov Disord* 6:60, 1991.

129. Cabrera-Valdiva F, Jimenez-Jimenez FJ, Albea EG, et al: Orthostatic tremor: Successful treatment with phenobarbital. *Clin Neuropharmacol*. 14:438, 1991.

130. Hallett M, Shibasaki H, Obeso J: Criteria for the visual identification of myoclonus. *Mov Disord* 9:1994

131. Deuschl G, Toro C, Valls-Sole J, et al: Symptomatic and essential palatal tremor. *Brain* 117:775–788, 1994.

132. Thack WT: Discharge of cerebellar neurons related to two maintained postures and two prompt movements. I. Nuclear cell output. *J Neurophysiol* 33:527, 1970.

133. Schenck E: *Die Hirnnervenmyorhythmie, ihre Pathogenese and ihre Stellung im myoklonischen Syndrom*. Berlin: Springer Verlag, 1965.

134. Laprsle J: Palatal myoclonus. *Adv Neurol* 43:265, 1986.

135. Matthews WB, Howell DA, Hughes RC: Relapsing corticosteroid-dependent polyneuritis. *J Neurol Neurosurg Psychiatry* 33:330, 1970.

136. Smith IS, Furness P, Thomas PK: Tremor in peripheral neuropathy, in Findley LF, Capildeo R (eds): *Movement Disorders: Tremor*. London: Macmillan Press, 1984, chap 30, pp 399–406.

137. Thomas PK: Clinical features and differential diagnosis, in Dyck PJ, Thomas PK, Lambert EH, Bunge R (eds): *Peripheral Neuropathy*, 2d ed. Philadelphia: WB Saunders, 1984, chap 51.

138. Said G, Bathien N, Cesaro P: Peripheral neuropathies and tremor. *Neurology* 32:480, 1982.

139. Smith IS: Tremor in peripheral neuropathy, in Findley LJ, Koller WC (eds): *Handbook of Tremor Disorders*. New York: Marcel Dekker, 1995, chap 31 pp 443–454.

140. Elble RJ: Peripheral neuropathies and tremor. *Neurology* 33:1389, 1983.

141. Van Ham L, Vandevelde M, Desmidt M, et al: A tremor syndrome with a central axonopathy in Scottish terriers. *J Vet Intern Med* 8:290, 1994.

142. Marie MP: Forme speciale de nevrite interstitielle hypergrophique progressive de l'enfance. *Rev Neurol* (Paris) 14:557, 1906.

143. Cardoso, FEC, Jankovic J: Hereditary motor-sensory neuropathy and movement disorders. *Muscle Nerve* 16:904, 1993.

144. Gowers WR: Disease of the nervous system. Philadelphia, Blakiston, Son & Co, 1888.

145. Koller W, Lang A, Vetere-Overfield B, et al: Psychogenic tremors. *Neurology* 39:1094, 1989.

146. Koller WC: Diagnosis and treatment of tremors. *Neurol Clin* 2:499, 1984.

147. Hunker CJ, Abbs JH: Uniform frequency of parkinsonian resting tremor in the lips, jaw, tongue and index finger. *Mov Disord* 5:71, 1990.

148. Rajput AH: Clinical features of tremor in extrapyramidal syndromes, in Findley LJ, Koller WC (eds): *Handbook of Tremor Disorders*. New York: Marcel Dekker, 1995, chap 19, pp 275–291.

149. Findley LJ, Gresty MA, Halmagi GM: Tremor, the cogwheel phenomenon and clonus in Parkinson's disease. *J Neurol Neurosurg Psychiatry*. 44:534, 1981.

150. Shahani BT, Young RR: Physiological and pharmacological aids in the differential diagnosis of tremor. *J Neurol Neurosurg Psychiatry* 39:772, 1976.

151. Pechadre JC, Larochelle L, Poirier LJ: Parkinsonian akinesia, rigidity and tremor in the monkey. *J Neurol Sci* 28:147–157, 1976.

152. Koller WC, Herbster G: Adjuvant therapy of parkinsonian tremor. *Arch Neurol* 44:921, 1987.

153. Koller WC: Pharmacologic treatment of parkinsonian tremor. *Arch Neurol* 43:126, 1986.

154. Hughes AJ, Lees AJ, Stern GM: Apomorphine in the diagnosis and treatment of parkinsonian tremor. *Clin Neuropharmacol* 13:312, 1990.

155. Lee MS, Marsden CD: Movement disorders following lesions of the thalamus or subthalamic region. *Mov Disord* 9:493, 1994.

156. Berkovic SF, Bladin PF: Rubral tremor: Clinical Features and treatment of three cases. *Clin Exp Neurol* 20:119, 1984.

157. Marsden CD, Obeso JA, Zarranz JJ, Lang AE: The anatomical basis of symptomatic dystonia. *Brain* 108:463, 1985.

158. Pettigrew LC, Jankovic J: Hemidystonia: A report of 22 patients and a review of the literature. *J Neurol Neurosurg Psychiatry* 48:650, 1985.

159. Schlitt M, Brown JW, Zeiger HE, Galbraith JG: Appendicular tremor as a late complication of intracerebral hemorrhage. *Surg Neurol* 25:181, 1986.

160. Kim JS: Delayed onset of hand tremor caused by cerebral infarction. *Stroke* 23:292, 1992.

161. Moroo I, Hirayama K, Kohima S: Involuntary movements caused by thalamic lesion. Rinsho Shinkeigaku—Clin Neuroi. 34:805, 1994.

162. Ferbert, Gerwig M: Tremor due to stroke. *Mov Disord* 8:179, 1993.

163. Dethy S, Luxen A, Bidaut LM, Goldman S: Hemibody tremor related to stroke. *Stroke* 24:2094, 1993.

164. Curran TG, Lang AE: Trauma and tremor: in Findley LJ, Koller WC (eds): *Handbook of Tremor Disorders*. New York: Marcel Dekker, 1995.

165. Crouzon O, Justin-Besancon L: Le parkinsonisme traumatique. *Presse Med* 37:1325, 1929.

166. Martland HS: Punch drunk. *J Am Med Assoc* 91:1103, 1928.

167. Lindenberg R: Die schadigungmechanismen der substantia nigra bei hirntraumen und das problem des posttraumatischen parkinsonismus. *Dtsch Z Nervenheilkd* 185:637, 1964.

168. Nayernouri T: Postraumatic parkinsonism. *Surg Neurol* 24:263, 1985.

169. Bruetsch WL, DeArmond M: The parkinsonian syndrome due to trauma. A clinico-anatomical study of a case. *J Nerv Ment Dis* 81:531, 1935.

170. Andrew J, Fowler CJ, Harrison MJG, Kendall BE: Post-traumatic tremor due to vascular injury and its treatment by stereotactic thalamotomy. *J Neurol Neurosurg Psychiatry* 45:560, 1982.

171. Schwartzman RJ, Kerrigan J: The movement disorder of reflex sympathetic dystrophy. *Neurology* 40:57, 1990.

172. Deuschl G, Blumberg H, Lucking CH: Tremor in reflex sympathetic dystrophy. *Arch Neurol* 48:1247, 1991.

173. Jankovic J, Van der Linden C: Dystonia and tremor induced by peripheral trauma: Predisposing factors. *J Neurol Neurosurg Psychiatry* 5:1512, 1988.

174. Streib EW: Distal ulnar neuropathy as a cause of finger tremor: A case report. *Neurology* 40:153, 1990.

175. Brin MF, Bilitzer A: Vocal tremor, in Findley LJ, Koller WC (eds): *Handbook of Tremor Disorders*, New York: Marcel Dekker, 1995, chap 37, pp 495–520.

176. Brown JR, Simonson J: Organic voice tremor: A tremor of phonation. *Neurology* 13:520, 1963.

177. Lebrun Y, Devreux F, Rousseau JJ, Darimont P: Tremulous speech. *Folia Phoniatr (Basel)* 34:134, 1982.

178. Ludlow C. Bassich C, Connor N, Coulter D: Phonatory characteristics of vocal fold tremor. *J Phonet* 14:509, 1986.

179. Hachinski VC, Thomsen IV, Buch NH: The nature of primary vocal tremor. *Can J Neurol Sci* 2:195, 1975.

180. Ramig LA, Shipp T: Comparative measures of vocal tremor and vocal vibrato. *J Voice* 2:162, 1987.

181. Hartman DE, Overholt SL, Vishwanat B: A case of vocal cord nodules masking essential (voice) tremor. *Arch Otolaryngol* 108:52, 1982.

182. Massey EW, Paulson G: Essential vocal tremor: Response to therapy. *Neurology* 32:A113, 1982.

183. Seguier N, Spira A, Dordain M, et al: Relationship between speech disorders and other clinical manifestations of Parkinson's disease (translated title). *Folia Phoniatr (Basel)* 16:108, 1974.

184. Logemann J, Fisher H, Boshes B, Blonsky E: Frequency and cooccurrence of vocal tract dysfunctions in the speech of a large sample of Parkinson patients. *J Speech Hear Disord* 43:47, 1978.

185. Ramig LA, Scherer RC, Titze IR, Ringel SP: Acoustic analysis of voices of patients with neurologic disease: Rationale and preliminary data. *Ann Otol Rhinol Laryngol* 97:164, 1988.

186. Aronson AE: Organic (essential) voice tremor, in: Aronson AE (ed): *Clinical Voice Disorders*. New York: Thieme-Stratton, 1980, pp 108–111.

187. Findley LJ, Gresty MA: Head, facial, and voice tremor. *Adv in Neurol* 239–253, 1988.

188. Koda J, Ludlow CL: An evaluation of laryngeal muscle activation in patients with voice tremor. *Otolaryngol Head Neck Surg* 107:684, 1992.

189. Koller W, Graner D, Mlcoch A: Essential voice tremor: Treatment with propranolol. *Neurology* 35:106, 1985.

190. Ackerman H, Ziegler W: Cerebellar voice tremor: An acoustic analysis. *J Neurol Neurosurg Psychiatry* 54:74, 1991.

191. Silfverskiold BP: A 3 c/sec leg tremor in a "cerebellar" syndrome. *Acta Neurol Scand* 55:385, 1977.

192. Rothwell JC, Traub MM, Marsden CD: Primary writing tremor. *J Neurol Neurosurg Psychiatry* 42:1106, 1979.

193. Elble RJ, Moody C, Higgins C: Primary writing tremor. *Mov Disord* 5:118, 1990.

194. Kachi T, Rothwell JC, Cowan JMA, Marsden CD: Writing tremor: Its relationship to benign essential tremor. *J Neurol Neurosurg Psychiatry* 48:545, 1985.

195. Koller WC, Martyn B: Writing tremor: Its relationship to essential tremor. *J Neurol Neurosurg Psychiatry* 49:220, 1986.

196. Rosenbaum F, Jankovic J: Focal task-specific tremor and dystonia: Categorization of occupational movement disorders. *Neurology* 38:522, 1988.

197. Lang AE: Writing tremor and writing dystonia. *Mov Disord* 5:354, 1990.

198. Sheehy MP, Marsden CD: Writer's cramp—a focal dystonia. *Brain* 105:461, 1982.

199. Wills AJ, Jenkins IH, Thompson PD, et al: A positron emission tomography study of cerebral activation associated with essential and writing tremor. *Arch Neurol* 52:299, 1995.

200. Bain P: Task specific tremor. *ITF Newsletter* 5:3, 1993.

201. Ohye C, Miyazaki M, Hirai T, et al: Primary writing tremor treated by stereotactic selective thalamotomy. *J Neurol Neurosurg Psychiatry* 45:988, 1982.

202. Yamamoto M, Wakayama Y, Kawasaki H, et al: Symptomatological rubral tremor caused by vertebral-basilar artery embolism. *Rinsho Shinkeigaku* 3l:1110, 1991.

203. Mossuto-Agatiello L, Puccetti G, Castellano AE: "Rubral" tremor after thalamic haemorrhage. *J Neurol* 241:27, 1993.

204. Kremer M, Ritchie Russell W, Smyth GE: A midbrain syndrome following head injury. *J Neurol Neurosurg Psychiatry* 10:49, 1947.

205. De Recondo A, Rondot P, Loc'h C, et al: Positron-emission tomographic study of the dopaminergic system in a case of secondary unilateral tremor after mesencephalic hematoma (translated title). *Rev Neurol (Paris)* 149(1):46, 1993.

206. Benedikt M: Translated, in Wolf JK: *The Classical Brain Stem Syndromes.* Springfield, IL: Charles C Thomas, 1991, pp 103–109.

207. Deuschl G: Tremor-syndrome, in Hopf HC, Poeck K, Schliak H (eds): *Neurologie in Clinik und Praxis,* 2d ed. Stuttgart, Germany: Thieme, 1992, vol II, pp 53–61.

208. McManus PG, Sharbrough FW: Orthostatic tremor: clinical and electrophysiologic characteristics. Muscle Nerve 16:1254, 1993.

209. Zimmerman R, Deuschl G, Hornig A, et al: Tremors in Parkinson's disease: Symptom analysis and rating. *Clin Neuropharmacol* 17:303, 1994.

210. Masucci EF, Kurtzke JF: Tremor in progressive supranuclear palsy. *Acta Neurol Scand* 80:296, 1989.

211. Wenning GK, Ben Shlomo Y, Magalhaes M, et al: Clinical features and natural history of multiple system atrophy: An analysis of 100 cases. *Brain.* 117:835, 1994.

212. Louis ED, Goldman JE, Powers JM, Fahn S: Parkinsonian features of eight pathologically diagnosed cases of diffuse Lewy body diseases (Review). *Mov Disord* 10:188, 1995.

213. Moon SL, Koller WC: Psychogenic tremor, in Findley LJ, Koller WC (eds): *Handbook of Tremor Disorders.* New York: Marcel Dekker, 1995, chap 36, pp 491–494.

214. Masucci E, Kurtzke J: Palatal myoclonus associated with extremity tremor. *J Neurol* 236:474, 1989.

215. Defer GL, Remy P, Malapert D, et al: Rest tremor and extrapyramidal symptoms after midbrain haemorrhage: Clinical and 18F-dopa PET evaluation. *J Neurol Neurosurg Psychiatry* 57:987, 1994.

216. Bhatia K, Daniel SE, Marsden CD: Orofacial dystonia and rest tremor in a patient with normal brain pathology. *Mov Disord* 8:361, 1993.

217. Barbosa ER, Teixira MJ, Chaves CJ, Scaff M: Parkinson disease associated to a brain tumor: A case report *Arq Neuropsiquiatr* 49:338, 1991.

218. Pomeranz S, Shalit M, Sherman Y: "Rubral" tremor following radiation of a pineal region vascular hamartoma. *Acta Neurochir (Wien)* 103:79, 1990.

219. Rail D, Schlotz C, Swash M: Post-encephalitic parkinsonism: Current experience. *J Neurol Neurosurg Psychiatry* 44:670–676, 1981.

THE PATHOPHYSIOLOGY OF TREMOR

RODGER J. ELBLE

PHYSIOLOGICAL TREMOR
GENERAL PROPERTIES OF PATHOLOGICAL TREMORS
ESSENTIAL TREMOR
PARKINSONIAN TREMOR
CEREBELLAR TREMOR
RUBRAL (MIDBRAIN) TREMOR
PALATAL MYOCLONUS
STROKE-INDUCED TREMOR
TREMOR RESULTING FROM PERIPHERAL NERVE
  PATHOLOGY
TASK-SPECIFIC, FOCAL, AND DYSTONIC TREMORS
CORTICAL TREMOR
DRUG-INDUCED TREMOR
SUMMARY

Tremor is an approximately rhythmic, roughly sinusoidal involuntary movement. Despite nearly a century of modern clinical and laboratory investigations, no tremor is understood completely. The more common forms of tremor are reviewed in this chapter, and two basic questions are addressed for each form: What is the source of oscillation? Why does the oscillation occur?

Physiological Tremor

Physiological tremor is barely visible to the unaided eye and is symptomatic only during activities that require extreme precision. Physiological tremor consists of two distinct oscillations: a mechanical-reflex component and an 8- to 12-Hz component, which are superimposed on a background of irregular fluctuations in muscle force and limb displacement.[1,2] These background irregularities have a frequency of 0–15 Hz and are produced by motor units that fire near their threshold.[3-7] The low-pass filtering property of skeletal muscle attenuates the amplitude of these irregularities at frequencies above 3–5 Hz.[8]

The mechanical-reflex component of physiological tremor is much larger than the 8- to 12-Hz component and is exhibited by everyone. The mechanical-reflex component is a passive mechanical oscillation that is produced by the underdamped inertial, viscous, and elastic properties of the limbs and other body parts. Participation of the stretch reflex is evident only when physiological tremor is enhanced by fatigue, anxiety, or drugs.[9,10] The mechanical attributes of most body parts are such that damped oscillations occur in response to pulsatile perturbations. The frequency of these mechanical-reflex oscillations, ω, is determined largely by the inertia I and stiffness K of the body part, according to the formula $\omega = \sqrt{K/I}$. Consequently, normal elbow tremor has a frequency, 3–5 Hz, that is lower than the 8- to 12-Hz frequency of wrist tremor, because the forearm has much greater inertia than the hand. Similarly, the finger has even less inertia, so the frequency of metacarpophalangeal joint tremor is 17–30 Hz. Voluntary cocontraction of the muscles about a joint produces a slight increase in tremor frequency as a result of increased joint stiffness. Conversely, gradual relaxation of the joint causes the frequency of mechanical-reflex tremor to fall.

The mechanical properties of the body are not sufficient to cause tremor. One or more sources of mechanical energy are required to force or perturb a limb into oscillation at a frequency determined by limb inertia and stiffness. Voluntary muscle contraction contains irregularities in subtetanic motor unit firing that perturb the limb continuously and randomly. The ejection of blood at cardiac systole provides additional perturbations to the limbs. Such cardioballistics account for nearly all of physiological tremor at rest but only a fraction of physiological postural and kinetic tremor.[2,11,12]

Somatosensory receptors (e.g., muscle spindles) respond to the mechanical oscillations of physiological tremor, but the response is too weak to entrain motoneurons at the frequency of tremor, unless additional mechanical forcings are applied to the limb to increase the amplitude of mechanical oscillation.[13] Consequently, the power spectrum of rectified-filtered electromyogram (EMG) is essentially flat during normal steady muscle contraction (Fig. 29-1). The stretch-reflex response to oscillation increases during fatigue and anxiety and in response to some medications, producing a modulation of motor unit activity and so-called enhanced physiological tremor (Fig. 29-1).[9,10,14] This involvement of the stretch-reflex can increase tremor or suppress it, depending on the dynamics of the reflex loop and limb mechanics.[15] Thus, mechanical-reflex oscillation is minimized when the natural frequency of the mechanical system is far removed from the natural frequencies of associated stretch-reflex pathways.

In contrast to the mechanical-reflex oscillation, the 8- to 12-Hz component of physiological tremor is always associated with modulation of motor unit activity, even when the 8- to 12-Hz tremor is much smaller than the mechanical-reflex oscillation (Fig. 29-1). Participating motor units are entrained at 8-12 Hz, regardless of their mean frequency of discharge.[1] The 8- to 12-Hz and mechanical-reflex oscillations are easily distinguished by their response to inertial and elastic loads. The frequency of 8- to 12-Hz tremor exhibits little or no change when inertial or elastic loads are attached to the limb. By contrast, the frequency of mechanical-reflex oscillation is proportional to $\sqrt{K/I}$, where K is added stiffness and I is added inertia.[14,16] Furthermore, the frequency of 8- to 12-Hz tremor is independent of stretch-reflex loop time and muscle twitch properties.[17,18] For these reasons, the 8- to 12-Hz tremor probably originates from an unidentified oscillating neuronal network within the central nervous system. The spinal cord,[19] inferior olive,[20,21] thalamus,[22] and cerebral cortex[23,24] are only a few of the possible sources of 8- to 12-Hz tremor.

Mechanical

No Added Mass

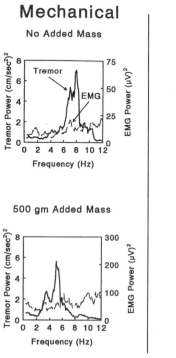

500 gm Added Mass

Enhanced

No Added Mass

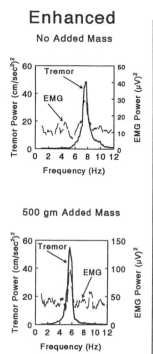

500 gm Added Mass

8- to 12-Hz

No Added Mass

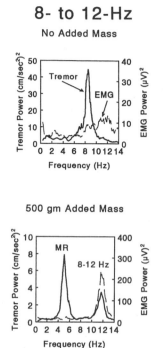

500 gm Added Mass

FIGURE 29-1 Fourier power spectra of normal mechanical-reflex tremor (Mechanical), enhanced physiological tremor because of thyrotoxicosis (Enhanced), and physiological tremor with a prominent 8- to 12-Hz component (8- to 12- Hz). Postural hand tremor was recorded with a miniature accelerometer, and rectified-filtered EMG of the extensor carpi radialis brevis was recorded with Ag-AgCl skin electrodes. Note how a 500-gm load on the hand reduces normal and enhanced mechanical-reflex (MR) tremor. By contrast, the 8- to 12-Hz tremor increases in amplitude, but its frequency does not change.

General Properties of Pathological Tremors

The segmental stretch-reflex and limb mechanics comprise the final common pathway for all forms of tremor (Fig. 29-2). Therefore, the stretch-reflex and limb mechanics can influence the frequency or amplitude of a tremor, depending on its origin. The frequency of normal mechanical-reflex tremor is largely a function of limb inertia and stiffness and is easily changed by added inertia or stiffness, because there is little involvement of segmental and long-loop reflexes. However, tremors with greater involvement of segmental and long-loop (e.g., transcortical) sensorimotor pathways have frequencies that are less dependent on limb mechanics and more dependent upon reflex loop dynamics (e.g., loop time).[25,26] Consequently, the frequencies of enhanced physiological tremor and cerebellar tremor are altered less by mechanical loads than the frequency of normal mechanical-reflex tremor.[14,27] Tremors orginating from central oscillators have frequencies that are independent of limb mechanics and reflex arc length. Parkinsonian tremor and essential tremor are common examples of central oscillation.[28,29]

Motor pathways are sufficiently integrated so that no source of tremor can be isolated completely from the effects of sensory feedback. Consequently, peripheral stretch reflex manipulations can reset the phase and entrain the frequency of tremors, even when they emerge from central sources of oscillation.[30] For example, essential tremor and parkinsonian tremor originate from central sources of oscillation. Nevertheless, the phase (timing) of these tremors can be altered predictably by pulsatile electrical and mechanical stretch-reflex perturbations, and the frequency of these tremors can

be entrained by sinusoidal forcings.[31–34] Similarly, a central oscillator can resonate with the mechanical-reflex system, when tremors' natural frequencies are similar.[33] For example, parkinsonian and essential hand tremors have frequencies

FIGURE 29-2 This simplified schematic diagram illustrates some of the pathways that have been implicated in the various tremors discussed in this chapter. Body mechanics are represented by a muscle with stiffness (spring), viscosity (dash pot) and mass. SMA, supplementary motor area; M1, motor cortex; PN, pontine nuclei; SNc, substantia nigra pars compacta; GPe and GPi, globus pallidus externa and interna; RN, red nucleus; RetN, reticular nuclei; VN, lateral vestibular nucleus; IO, inferior olive; Cereblm, cerebellum; Vop and Vim, ventralis oralis posterior and ventralis intermedius of the motor thalamus.

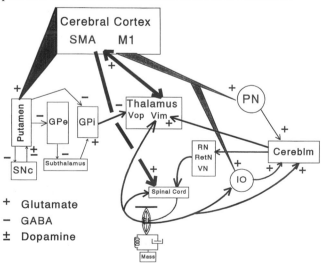

that are similar to the mechanical-reflex frequency of the wrist, so there is less mechanical limitation of the tremor than would occur if these tremors had much higher frequencies. The 14- to 18-Hz frequency of orthostatic tremor is much higher than the natural mechanical-reflex frequency of the lower limbs, so this tremor is not visible to the examiner until the tremor frequency undergoes subharmonic reduction to 7–9 Hz.[35–39] Similar dynamic interactions undoubtedly occur between the central oscillators of pathological tremors and the central neural pathways to which the oscillators are connected. Resonance between a tremor oscillator and other parts of the central nervous system is probably as important as the strength of the oscillator in determining the amplitude of pathological tremors.

Magnetic stimulation of the contralateral motor cortex can reset the phase of essential tremor, parkinsonian tremor and normal rapid alternating wrist movements.[40,41] These observations prove that the motor cortex can influence essential tremor and parkinsonian tremor but do not reveal the anatomic origin of tremor. Positron emission tomography (PET) has revealed increased cerebellar blood flow in patients with many forms of tremor, including parkinsonian tremor, writing tremor, orthostatic tremor, and essential tremor.[42] The cerebellum receives all forms of sensory feedback and projects directly or indirectly to nearly all parts of the motor system. Loops between the cerebellum and brain-stem nuclei (e.g., the dentato-rubro-olivo-cerebellar pathway) have a tendency to reverberate[43] and could therefore produce tremorogenic oscillation or simply promote oscillation originating elsewhere. Consequently, cerebellar hyperactivity could be a consequence of tremor, rather than its cause.

Nucleus ventralis intermedius of the ventrolateral thalamus receives inputs from the contralateral cerebellar nuclei and, possibly, from ascending somatosensory pathways.[43–46] Stereotactic lesions and high-frequency stimulation in ventralis intermedius are beneficial in the treatment of essential, parkinsonian, cerebellar, rubral, and task-specific tremors.[47–54] Although ventralis intermedius may not be the source of oscillation in any of these tremor disorders, the oscillatory properties and anatomic connections of ventralis intermedius could facilitate the transmission of oscillation from other sources throughout the motor system. Although the precise mechanism is unclear, ventralis intermedius is clearly a nonspecific Achilles heel for many forms of pathological tremor.

Many etiologies of tremor produce additional disturbances of motor control, such as bradykinesia, weakness, ataxia, and altered muscle tone. However, tremor alone can influence motor control by limiting the timing and frequency of voluntary movement. Strong entrainment of motor units by tremor restrict the timing of voluntary motor unit activity. For example, the volitional bursts of agonist and antagonist muscle activity emerge from the ongoing tremor rhythm during ballistic and rapidly alternating movements in patients with essential tremor and Parkinson's disease.[55–58] Consequently, the tremor oscillator could affect the coordination of movement by altering the timing and amplitude of muscle activity,[59] thereby creating an illusion of cerebellar ataxia.

Oscillations in the frequency range of tremor are involved in sensorimotor integration,[60] motor timing,[61] muscle coordination,[24,61] and sympathetic control.[62] The neural networks responsible for these oscillations are distributed throughout the central nervous system. Many of these physiological oscillators are potential sources of tremor. Thus, the pathology of tremor need not produce a *de novo* oscillation; rather, it could simply increase oscillation within a physiological oscillator or could promote entrainment of otherwise normal motor pathways. In general, tremor could originate from neurons with inherent rhythmical properties (pacemaker neurons) or could emerge from the interaction of neurons within and among neuronal networks. These two mechanisms of neuronal oscillation are not mutually exclusive. Neuronal networks in the sensorimotor cortex,[63] the thalamus,[64] the inferior olive (interacting with the cerebellum),[20,65–67] brain stem raphe and reticular nuclei,[62] globus pallidus,[68] and the spinal cord[19] are just a few of the many documented sources of physiological neuronal oscillation which, if pathologically altered, could produce an abnormal tremor.

Most neuronal oscillators have network properties that promote neuronal entrainment through recurrent inhibition, recurrent excitation, or dendrodendritic synapses. In addition, the principal neurons in these oscillators often exhibit membrane properties that produce oscillation by means of a mechanism known as inhibition-rebound excitation.[21] This mechanism involves a calcium-dependent, potassium-mediated membrane hyperpolarization that activates a low-threshold calcium spike, which leads to another action potential or burst of action potentials. This process perpetuates itself in a rhythmic fashion. The frequency of oscillation is determined by the duration of hyperpolarization. The inferior olive,[66,67] thalamus,[64] globus pallidus,[68] and spinal cord[69] exhibit these properties. Pathological tremor could result from increased entrainment of motor pathways by these oscillators, increased strength of oscillation within these oscillators, or both. Gamma-aminobutyric acid (GABA), acetylcholine, norepinephrine, glutamate (*N*-methyl-D-aspartate (NMDA) receptors), serotonin, and probably other neurotransmitters modulate these sources of oscillation, and alterations in these and other neurotransmitters can produce increased oscillation within a neuronal network or increased entrainment throughout the motor system. Treatment of tremor could suppress the oscillator or block the entrainment. Continuing investigations into the sites and mechanisms of physiological neuronal oscillation are crucial to the understanding of specific pathological tremors, which are now discussed.

Essential Tremor

Essential tremor is the most common form of pathological tremor. Essential tremor begins at any age but is most common in older people, having a prevalence of at least 0.4–1.1 percent in people over the age of 40.[70,71] Thirty to fifty percent of all cases are dominantly inherited, and most patients with essential tremor have no other abnormal neurological signs. Essential tremor most commonly affects the hands but also occurs in the head, voice, face, trunk, and lower extremities.[72,73] Essential tremor is a postural tremor with a variable kinetic component. Tremor in repose is uncommon and is observed only in the most advanced patients, who are typically older. The complex pill-rolling hand movements of parkinsonian tremor are not seen in essential tremor.

Tremor resembling essential tremor is seen in many other neurological disorders, including Parkinson's disease and dystonia, and pathophysiological relationships between essential tremor and these disorders are frequently debated. These debates will not be resolved until specific diagnositic tests for essential tremor are found. Essential tremor in the upper extremities does not have unique diagnostic features, and tremors resembling essential tremor are seen in many neurological disorders, particularly those that produce parkinsonism and dystonia. There is considerable clinical heterogeneity among and within families with hereditary essential tremor, and genetic markers have not been identified. Essential tremor may not be a single entity. Mild essential tremor is frequently dismissed as physiological tremor, particularly in the elderly, and mild parkinsonism and dystonia are easily overlooked. Therefore, anything short of a careful door-to-door population study is likely to be flawed by significant selection bias and diagnostic error. Currently, there is no compelling support for an etiologic relationship between essential tremor and other neurological disorders.[74–79]

The *sine qua non* of essential tremor is a rhythmic 4- to 12-Hz entrainment of motor unit discharge that forces the affected body part into oscillation. The neurophysiological properties of essential tremor are consistent with a central source of oscillation that is influenced by somatosensory reflex pathways. Mechanical loads have little effect on the frequency of essential tremor (Fig. 29-3), thereby distinguishing this tremor from enhanced physiological tremor.[28,29] Cooling the upper extremity reduces tremor amplitude but does not change tremor frequency.[80] Patients with essential tremor exhibit normal mechanical-reflex properties,[13] and mechanical-reflex oscillation and essential tremor can exhibit mutual frequency entrainment and resonance when their frequencies are similar (Fig. 29-3, no added mass). When a mechanical load separates the mechanical-reflex and essential tremors, resonance and entrainment are abolished, resulting in reduced tremor amplitude and a more clear demonstration of the frequency of essential tremor (best measured in the rectified-filtered EMG spectrum, Fig. 29-3).

Tremor amplitude bears a logarithmic relationship with the intensity and frequency of motor unit entrainment, according to the equation

$$\log (amplitude) = -2.3 \log(frequency) + 2.3 \log(intensity) + 10.^{[83]}$$

The frequency-amplitude relationship (slope is approximately -2) of essential tremor is predicted by the second-order, low-pass filtering properties of skeletal muscle.[81] This relationship also predicts that tremor amplitude can be significantly reduced by increasing tremor frequency. Thus far, no drug or surgical intervention has altered the frequency of essential tremor.[82]

Mild high-frequency essential tremor is qualitatively similar to the 8- to 12-Hz physiological tremor,[28] so these tremors could emerge from the same central oscillator. However, oscillators in the frequency range of essential tremor are found throughout the nervous system, and the similarities between essential tremor and physiological tremor might be fortuitous. Nevertheless, patients within the same family

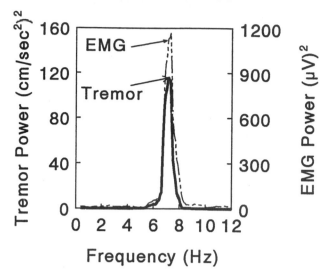

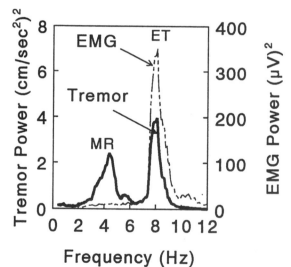

FIGURE 29-3 Fourier power spectral of postural hand tremor recorded from a 57-year-old woman with mild familial tremor. Hand tremor was recorded with a miniature accelerometer, and an extensor digitorum brevis EMG was recorded with skin electrodes. Note the single large spectral peak in tremor and EMG (no added mass). Mass loading reduced the frequency of the mechanical-reflex (MR) oscillation to 4 Hz, leaving the essential tremor (ET) at 8 Hz. This precluded any resonance between the two oscillations. Consequently, the overall amplitude of tremor was reduced (500 g, added mass).

commonly exhibit tremors with different frequencies, ranging from 4 to 12 Hz, and tremor frequency is strongly correlated with the patient's age (in years), according to the equation $frequency = -0.077age + 11.4.^{[83]}$ The frequency of essential tremor has little or no correlation with duration of illness.[83]

The origin of essential tremor is unknown. Routine postmortem examinations have revealed no abnormalities.[84] The inferior olive,[20,21] thalamus,[22] and cerebral cortex[23,24] comprise an abbreviated list of plausible candidates. The inferior olive is incriminated by the most experimental data, but the evidence is far from conclusive. The olivary hypothesis is based upon the similarities between essential tremor and the tremor induced by harmaline in laboratory primates. Harmaline enhances the inhibition-rebound properties of olivary neurons, resulting in increased rhythmicity and neuronal entrainment throughout the olive.[67] This harmaline-induced olivary oscillation produces in monkeys an action tremor with the frequency, EMG and drug-response characteristics of essential tremor.[20,30,65] The olivary hypothesis is also supported by PET studies that revealed increased olivary glucose use and cerebellar blood flow in patients with essential tremor.[85–87]

According to the olivary hypothesis, patients with essential tremor have enhanced synchronization and 4- to 12-Hz neuronal rhythmicity in their olives. This could result from altered olivary network properties (e.g., increased dendrodendritic connections), altered neuromodulation of the olivary network (e.g., serotonin),[88] abnormal enhancement of the membrane conductances that underlie the neuronal oscillations, or a combination of these mechanisms. Olivary oscillation can be amplified through the cerebellum, resulting in an entrainment of the thalamus, motor cortex, and brain stem nuclei (e.g., red nucleus and reticular nuclei).[66] Widespread entrainment of the motor system by olivary oscillation could explain why lesions in so many areas of the motor system suppress essential tremor.[30]

Thalamotomy probably suppresses tremor by reducing entrainment throughout the motor system by the tremor oscillator. An alternative possibility is that essential tremor originates in ventralis intermedius, motor cortex, or thalamocortical loop. The latter possibility seems unlikely, given the nonspecific beneficial effect of ventralis intermedius thalamotomy and thalamic stimulation on essential, parkinsonian, cerebellar, rubral, and task specific tremors.[47–54]

Ethanol, primidone, beta-adrenergic blockers, and thalamotomy in ventralis intermedius suppress essential tremor by mechanisms that are poorly understood.[89] Based on the harmaline model, ethanol and primidone could have direct actions on the neuronal oscillator or could uncouple the oscillation from segmental spinal pathways. Beta-blockers act peripherally, possibly by reducing the sensitivity of sensory receptors (e.g., muscle spindles) and by increasing the low-pass filtering properties of skeletal muscle. A central mode of action is also possible. None of these treatments is specific for essential tremor.

Parkinsonian Tremor

Rest tremor in the upper or lower extremities is the best-known and most specific feature of Parkinson's disease. In the upper extremities, rhythmic 3- to 5-Hz "pill-rolling" finger movements are superimposed upon rhythmic extension-flexion of the wrist and pronation-supination of the forearm. Voluntary muscle contraction typically suppresses parkinsonian rest tremor, but this is usually followed almost immediately by a mild-to-moderate action tremor. In many patients, the rest tremor simply persists during posture and movement,

with no change in frequency or EMG characteristics.[90] In other patients, the action tremor has a slightly higher frequency than the rest tremor. Postural tremor is occasionally the only tremor exhibited by a patient with Parkinson's disease. There is no compelling reason to hypothesize different sources of oscillation for Parkinson postural tremor and rest tremor, and both forms of tremor have neurophysiological properties that are consistent with a central source of oscillation.[29,91–93]

The principal pathology of Parkinson's disease is loss of dopaminergic cells in the substantia nigra pars compacta, and this abnormality is responsible for most, if not all, of the motor abnormalities, including tremor.[94] However, the source of oscillation in parkinsonian tremor is still uncertain. 1-Methyl-4-phenyl-1,2,3,6- tetrahydropyridine (MPTP)-treated monkeys have subthalamic and internal pallidal neurons that burst in correlation with tremor,[95–97] consistent with a role in tremorogenesis. The striatum is capable of similar phasic activity.[98,99] For decades, neurons in the ventral lateral thalamus have been known to exhibit phasic discharge in correlation with tremor[47,52–54,100] and are hypothesized to be the source of parkinsonian tremor.[101,102] Finally, the motor cortex and pyramidal tracts are necessary for the clinical expression of tremor,[103] and electrical stimulation of the motor cortex is capable of generating tremor.[104]

Is the ventral lateral thalamus the oscillator of Parkinson tremor? Ventralis intermedius (Vim) is the most effective stereotactic surgical site for treating parkinsonian tremor,[47,52–54,100] but this thalamic nucleus receives inputs from cerebellum and possibly from ascending spinal tracts, but not from the basal ganglia.[105,106] Furthermore, Vim thalamotomy is not an effective treatment for other aspects of parkinsonism but is an effective treatment of many other forms of tremor.[47,52–54,100] High-frequency electrical stimulation of Vim suppresses parkinsonian tremor,[50] and the suppression of tremor is associated with reduced blood flow in the cerebellum.[106–107] This observation suggests that transcerebellar pathways and Vim are entrained by the parkinsonian tremor oscillator. Vim thalamotomy probably interrupts this entrainment, thereby reducing tremor. However, Vim is an unlikely source of parkinsonian tremor.

Destruction of the posteroventrolateral internal pallidum or the subthalamus suppresses parkinsonian tremor and most other motor signs of Parkinson's disease.[108,109] Tremor-related phasic neuronal activity is known to occur in the internal pallidum and subthalamus of parkinsonian monkeys,[95–97] and either nucleus could be the origin of parkinsonian tremor. However, neither the internal pallidum nor the subthalamus projects to Vim, which is the most effective stereotactic target for the treatment of tremor. Instead, the motor portion of the internal pallidum projects to ventralis oralis posterior (Vop), which is adjacent to Vim.[46,105,110] Stereotactic destruction of Vop does not suppress tremor as well as Vim thalamotomy, but Vop thalamotomy is more effective in the treatment of rigidity and bradykinesia.[47] Nevertheless, Vop contains many neurons that fire in correlation with tremor,[111] and a striatopallidal-Vop pathway clearly plays some role in tremorogenesis.

Oscillation in motor cortex and its corticothalamic loop is also involved in the production of tremor, but it is unclear whether the motor cortex is the origin of tremor or merely an avenue for the spread of oscillation generated elsewhere.

Extirpation of motor cortex and section of the pyramidal tracts suppress parkinsonian tremor,[103] and electrical stimulation of the motor cortex of patients with and without Parkinson's disease can produce 5-Hz hand tremor.[104] Parkinsonian rest tremor suppresses the EEG mu rhythm in a manner similar to voluntary muscle contraction,[112] and the same motor and premotor cortical areas activated by voluntary repetitive hand movement are activated by parkinsonian rest tremor.[113] Posteroventral pallidotomy restores frontal cortical activity in parkinsonian patients as measured with H2[15O] positron emission tomography,[113] and the underactive parkinsonian state of frontal cortex might be conducive to oscillation. The increased, phasic internal pallidal activity in Parkinson's disease could modify ventrolateral thalamic function in such a way that the motor cortex and its corticothalamic loop become the principal source of tremorogenic oscillation.

A motor cortical or corticothalamic origin for parkinsonian tremor could explain why tremor-related thalamic neurons are found in both Vop and Vim. Both thalamic nuclei have reciprocal connections with motor cortex and with supplementary motor cortex.[114] These connections and those with the thalamic reticular nucleus[114,115] could mediate neuronal entrainment and the spread of oscillation originating in the cortex, basal ganglia, or thalamus. An oscillating corticothalamic loop can also explain the variable-phase relationships that tremor-related neurons in Vop and Vim have with tremor and could produce the variable firing relationships that tremor-related neurons in Vop and Vim have with active and passive movement.[111]

In sum, many anatomic structures are involved in parkinsonian tremor and are situated within multiple complex loops. These loops make the pathophysiology of parkinsonian tremor difficult to define. The hypotheses reviewed are not mutually exclusive.

Cerebellar Tremor

Gordon Holmes[116] used the terms "static tremor" and "intention tremor" to describe the tremors that he observed in patients with cerebellar lesions. This discussion is devoted to kinetic (intention) tremor, which is most common.

The rhythm and amplitude of cerebellar tremor are usually irregular, and proximal limb muscles are often more involved than distal ones. The frequency of cerebellar tremor is commonly cited as 3–5 Hz,[117–119] but animal and human studies have shown that tremor frequency is influenced by reflex arc length and by the inertia and stiffness of the body part, according to the equation $frequency \approx \sqrt{stiffness/inertia}$.[27,120] These observations are consistent with the mechanistic involvement of somatosensory feedback loops. However, instability in these loops is probably not the sole source of tremor, because upper extremity deafferentation in decerebellate monkeys does not eliminate the 2- to 4-Hz intention tremor that occurs with cerebellar ablation.[121] The preservation of tremor after somatosensory deafferentation is probably the result of participation of visual feedback in tremorogenesis,[122] but additional contribution from a central source of oscillation cannot be excluded.

A dramatic 3- to 5-Hz kinetic tremor in the ipsilateral extremities occurs in laboratory primates with lesions in the deep cerebellar nuclei (dentate, globose, and emboliform) or in the outflow tracts of these nuclei (superior cerebellar peduncle). The critical nuclear lesion is still debated, but damage to globose and emboliform (interpositus in monkeys) seems most likely.[123] Tremulous modulation of neuronal activity occurs in the motor cortex, somatosensory cortex, interpositus nucleus, and somatosensory afferents of monkeys but does not occur in the dentate nucleus, which receives no somatosensory feedback.[27,124] These observations are consistent with the hypothesis that cerebellar tremor is produced by abnormal oscillation in transcortical and transcerebellar sensorimotor feedback loops. Changes in stiffness and inertia influence the frequency of cerebellar tremor less than the frequency of physiological tremor (mechanical-reflex component), because transcortical and transcerebellar sensorimotor loops are heavily involved in cerebellar tremor but not in physiological tremor.

Normal rapid limb movements toward a target are stopped with a burst of antagonist muscle contraction. Target overshoot and limb oscillation occur when this antagonist activity is delayed or inappropriately sized. Patients with cerebellar damage exhibit delayed antagonist muscle activation and terminal oscillation.[124,125] Cerebellar damage impairs the feedforward control of movement, such that available sensory information and prior experience are not used effectively in the formulation of antagonist muscle activity before the target is reached. Instead, limb movement is guided more by sensory feedback control.[124] Vestibular, visual, and somatosensory feedback are the three principal sensory modalities in the control of posture and movement, but feedback control with these modalities is too slow and imprecise to prevent ataxia and tremor. Feed-forward control (e.g., anticipatory braking) of movement is necessary, and the cerebellum plays a critical role in this regard.

Many medications have been tried with little or no benefit in the treatment of cerebellar tremor.[126] This is not surprising, given the pathophysiological complexity of the oscillating transcortical and transcerebellar pathways. The added inertia of wrist weights attenuates cerebellar tremor and is useful in some patients.[127] Prostheses with mechanical damping may also prove useful.[128] Thalamotomy in the contralateral ventralis intermedius can be effective.[129] However, the surgical treatment of cerebellar tremor must be approached with great care and caution, because small lesions in the ventrolateral thalamus can produce increased ataxia and an intention tremor that is identical to cerebellar tremor (Fig. 29-4).

Rubral (Midbrain) Tremor

Rubral (midbrain) tremor is an unusual combination of 2- to 5-Hz rest, postural, and kinetic tremor of an upper extremity. This unusual tremor is caused by lesions in the vicinity of the red nucleus, hence, the name rubral tremor. Many clinicians prefer the term midbrain tremor, because isolated lesions in the red nucleus are not tremorogenic. A combination of damage to the neighboring cerebellothalamic, cerebello-olivary, and nigrostriatal fiber tracts is required and explains the peculiar rest, postural, and kinetic features.[130–134]

Hand Tremor (acceleration)

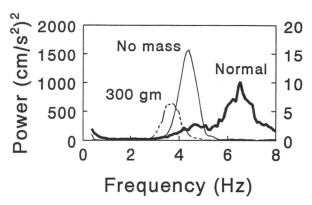

Ext. Carpi Radialis Brevis EMG

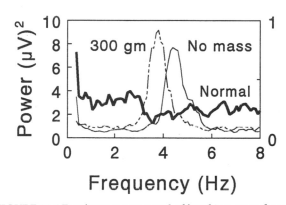

FIGURE 29-4 Fourier power spectral of hand tremor and rectified-filtered forearm EMG that were recorded from an 8-year-old girl who suffered a small infarct in the contralateral ventrolateral thalamus. With horizontal posture, she exhibited tremor with a normal amplitude (normal, right vertical axis) and no entrainment of motor units in the extensor carpi radialis brevis (statistically flat spectrum). However, her tremor increased substantially when she pointed at a fixed target without moving her hand, and prominent tremor-related bursts of EMG occurred in the forearm muscles, producing an EMG spectral peak at the frequency of tremor. The increased tremor occurred at a lower frequency (no mass), and the frequency of this abormal tremor decreased further with mass loading (300 g). However, the change in frequency with mass loading was not as great as that seen in normal people (see Fig. 29-1). Similar abnormal tremor was evident when writing, drawing, and performing finger-to-nose testing.

Rubral tremor most commonly begins weeks to months after brain stem trauma or stroke. Consequently, the pathophysiology of this tremor probably involves compensatory changes in nervous system function. Medications are nearly always ineffective. Stereotactic thalamotomy and high-frequency stimulation in ventralis intermedius suppress rubral tremor, but the mechanism is unknown.[129,135,136]

Palatal Myoclonus

Palatal myoclonus consists of vertical oscillations of the soft palate at 1–3 Hz. Higher frequencies are rarely encountered.

There are two forms of palatal myoclonus, symptomatic and essential, which differ clinically and pathophysiologically. Symptomatic palatal myoclonus is produced by damage, usually ischemic, in the dentato-olivary pathway, which causes secondary hypertrophic olivary degeneration.[137,138] This anatomical abnormality is often visible with magnetic resonance imaging.[139,140] The palatal movements of symptomatic palatal myoclonus are usually asymptomatic but can cause an ear click by moving the eustachian tube. Symptomatic palatal myoclonus is nearly always associated with other brain stem and cerebellar signs, depending on the nature and extent of underlying pathology.[137] Synchronous movements of the tongue, floor of the mouth, larynx, face, diaphragm, intercostal muscles, eyes, extremities, and trunk may also occur.[137,138] By contrast, essential palatal myoclonus causes an annoying ear click but no other neurological signs or symptoms, and the pathophysiology of essential palatal tremor is a complete mystery.[137] The ear click of essential palatal myoclonus is produced by movements of the eustachian tube that are caused by contraction of the tensor veli palatini,[141] which can be suppressed with botulinum toxin injection. The levator veli palatini muscle is rhythmically active in symptomatic palatal myoclonus.[141]

Clinicopathological studies have repeatedly found dentato-olivary pathway damage in patients with symptomatic palatal myoclonus.[137,138] This leads to secondary hypertrophic olivary degeneration. Because the olives are a normal source of oscillation,[66,67] hypertrophied olives might oscillate at 1–3 Hz, producing abnormal movements at the same frequency. However, the data supporting this hypothesis are largely inferential and inconclusive. One PET study revealed increased fluorodeoxyglucose uptake in the region of the hypertrophied olives,[142] but electrophysiological studies of olivary hypertrophy have not been done in laboratory animals or in humans. Other brain stem and cerebellar sources of 1- to 3-Hz oscillation, induced by olivary degeneration and dentato-olivary damage, are possible.

The similarities between palatal myoclonus and tremor have been noted for many decades,[138] and many specialists now prefer the synonymous term "palatal tremor".[137] Symptomatic palatal myoclonus is associated with at least three forms of extremity tremor. An asymptomatic tremor is produced by periodic inhibition of limb muscles at 1–3 Hz, time-locked to the palatal movements.[140] These brief periods of inhibition cause irregularities in muscle force that perturb the limb, producing an enhanced mechanical-reflex tremor. The other two forms of tremor are associated with palatal myoclonus, but it is not clear that these tremors emerge from the same source of oscillation. Masucci and Kurtzke[143] described five patients with symptomatic palatal myoclonus and a 2- to 4-Hz rest tremor of the limbs that persisted during posture and movement. All of their patients had signs of extensive brain stem damage, and only one of the five patients had tremor that appeared to be synchronous with the palatal movements. Rigorous cross-correlation or cross-spectral analyses were not performed. Masucci and coworkers[144] also described a 1- to 3-Hz mixed rest and action tremor, called myorhythmia, that can involve various combinations of one or more extremities, the trunk, head, face, pharynx, jaw, tongue, and eyes. These body parts can oscillate synchronously or asynchronously. The distribution of pathology is very similar to that seen in patients with palatal myoclonus, but some patients do not have palatal myoclonus and olivary hypertrophy.[144]

Stroke-Induced Tremor

Tremor frequently follows strokes in the midbrain, superior cerebellar peduncle, and cerebellum, but tremor is a surprisingly rare complication of strokes elsewhere in the nervous system. Stroke-induced tremor in the absence of other neurological signs is very rare. Tremor usually begins weeks to months after the ictus, so secondary neuronal changes are probably involved.[145–147] In this regard, the example of palatal myoclonus and olivary hypertrophy has been discussed.

A review of 240 published cases of focal lesions in the basal ganglia revealed only three cases of tremor,[148] one of which resembled parkinsonian rest tremor.[146] Strokes in the posteroventrolateral thalamus have produced a disabling contralateral 2.5- to 4.5-Hz action tremor[145,147] and a parkinsonian rest tremor.[146] Lee and Marsden[149] recently reviewed published reports of movement disorders associated with isolated thalamic lesions (33 cases) and with thalamic lesions that extended into the subthalamus (16 cases). Seven patients with isolated thalamic lesions had various combinations of rest, postural, and kinetic tremor, and all of these patients had coexistent dystonia.

Tremor Resulting from Peripheral Nerve Pathology

Patients with acquired and hereditary peripheral neuropathies frequently exhibit symptomatic 3- to 10-Hz action tremors. These tremors are usually less rhythmic than essential tremor, although some patients with hereditary neuropathy have tremor that is indistinguishable from 6- to 8-Hz essential tremor.[150] The action tremor in many patients behaves like an abnormal mechanical-reflex oscillation, resembling enhanced physiological tremor or cerebellar tremor.[151]

The frequency and amplitude of most neuropathic tremors bear no relationship to the degree of sensory loss or velocity of nerve conduction,[151–153] and the underlying illnesses in most patients do not cause damage to the central nervous system. However, compensatory changes in central nervous system function could cause abnormal oscillation to emerge from otherwise normal sensorimotor pathways, resulting in symptomatic tremor. Such central reorganization in response to altered peripheral sensorimotor function is hypothesized to cause the rare heterogeneous tremors that occur weeks to months after peripheral nerve trauma.[154]

Task-Specific, Focal, and Dystonic Tremors

Patients with *primary writing tremor* exhibit severe tremor during the act of writing but experience little or no tremor during other activities. The frequency of primary writing tremor is not altered by mechanical loads, suggesting a central source of oscillation.[155] It is unclear whether primary writing tremor is a symptom of focal dystonia, a variant of essential tremor, or a separate disease entity.[155–158] Dystonic muscle contractions are commonly tremulous, and writer's cramp is no exception.[159–161] Furthermore, the dystonia in patients with isolated writing tremor can be very subtle and difficult or impossible to distinguish from compensatory posturing aimed at stabilizing the hand.[155] Nevertheless, some patients with isolated writing tremor exhibit normal reciprocal inhibition of the median nerve H-reflex, whereas patients with typical writer's cramp exhibit reduced reciprocal inhibition.[162] Thus, some cases of isolated writing tremor are probably not focal dystonia. Essential tremor can be relatively task specific and frequently is most symptomatic during the act of writing. The relationship between primary writing tremor and essential tremor will not be resolved until a specific marker for essential tremor is found.

Orthostatic tremor is an unusual postural tremor that develops in the lower extremities and torso within seconds or more of assuming quiet erect stance.[35–39] Electromyography of the lower extremities and torso reveals rhythmic bursts of motor unit activity at 14–18 Hz. This activity often begins almost immediately upon standing and is usually symptomatic to the patient but barely visible to the examiner. Within seconds to minutes of continued standing, the frequency of body tremor changes into a 7- to 9-Hz subharmonic oscillation that is far more symptomatic and visible. In fact, the tremor can reach violent proportions before relief is obtained by walking, sitting, or lying. The 14- to 18-Hz frequency of orthostatic tremor is far too high to originate in a lower extremity reflex loop, so a central source of oscillation is hypothesized by most investigators. The precise location of this oscillator is unknown. Like many other tremors, orthostatic tremor is associated with increased cerebellar blood flow, as measured with $H_2^{15}O$ PET.[42]

Essential tremor and orthostatic tremor differ in several respects. Essential tremor affects the lower extremities in 30–45 percent of patients,[162] whereas orthostatic tremor invariably affects the lower extremities and torso.[163] The frequency of essential tremor is 4–12 Hz, which is much lower than the unusually high frequency of orthostatic tremor (14–18 Hz). Motor unit entrainment at 14–18 Hz can be elicited from the upper extremities of a minority of patients with orthostatic tremor and is present only when bearing body weight with the upper extremities or when standing.[163] By contrast, upper extremity tremor occurs in most patients with essential tremor and does not depend on body posture.[30,162] Finally, clonazepam is a very effective treatment for orthostatic tremor but is only occasionally beneficial to patients with essential tremor.

Isolated tremors of the voice, chin, tongue, and smile have been described, but these conditions are sufficiently rare that their proper nosology is unclear.[164,165] Like other focal and task-specific tremors, these tremors probably represent unusual presentations of focal dystonia, essential tremor, and other disorders. Remember that dystonic muscle contractions are commonly tremulous, and dystonia can present as a focal, task specific, or essential tremor.[159–161,166] The dystonia may be so subtle or obscured by tremor that it is not easily recognized. Similarly, mild postural tremor in the upper extremities can be mistaken for physiological tremor, particularly in older people.

Cortical Tremor

An irregular 7- to 14-Hz action tremor, resembling essential tremor, occurs in patients with cortical reflex myoclonus and is called cortical tremor. Major motor seizures, myoclonus, and a family history of these disorders and tremor are characteristic of cortical tremor.[23,167,168] Cortical tremor is suppressed by clonazepam and primidone. The enhanced C-reflex and giant sensory evoked potentials in most of these patients are consistent with the presence of enhanced cortical irritability and transcortical reflexes. Like essential tremor and parkinsonian tremor, cortical tremor can be reset by transcranial magnetic stimulation but is relatively refractory to peripheral electrical and mechanical stimuli. Thus, the 7- to 14-Hz oscillation of cortical tremor probably emerges from abnormal cortical oscillation, although participation by enhanced transcortical reflexes and subcortical nuclei cannot be excluded.

Drug-Induced Tremor

Many drugs[169] produce parkinsonian rest tremor (neuroleptics), postural tremor (beta-adrenergic agonists, valproic acid, thyroxin, tricyclic antidepressants, and methylxanthines), kinetic tremor (lithium), and combinations thereof (lithium, amiodarone, and valproic acid). Little is known about the mechanisms of these tremors. Amiodarone- and lithium-induced tremors are particularly noteworthy, because they are occasionally irreversible.[170-174] Persistent lithium-induced tremor and ataxia are caused by neuronal loss and gliosis of the cerebellar cortex and dentate nuclei.[175] It has long been suspected but never proven that people with subclinical essential tremor and subclinical Parkinson's disease are more susceptible to tremorogenic drugs.

Summary

The motor system contains a vast array of central and peripheral feedback loops, oscillating neuronal networks, and underdamped body mechanics. The complex integration of these sources of oscillation has made the elucidation of all tremors exceedingly difficult. Some tremors may emerge from the interaction of two or more anatomic structures, such that the identification of a single anatomic source of tremor is not possible. Nevertheless, considerable progress has been made, and many patients with disabling tremors are now the beneficiaries of a large and rapidly growing research effort.

Acknowledgment

Supported by NS20973 from the NINDS.

References

1. Elble RJ, Randall JE: Motor-unit activity responsible for 8- to 12-Hz component of human physiological finger tremor. *J Neurophysiol* 39:370–383, 1976.
2. Elble RJ, Randall JE: Mechanistic components of normal hand tremor. *Electroencephalogr Clin Neurophysiol* 44:72–82, 1978.
3. Allum JHJ, Dietz V, Freund H-J: Neuronal mechanisms underlying physiological tremor. *J Neurophysiol* 41:557–571, 1978.
4. Christakos CN, Lal S: Lumped and population stochastic models of skeletal muscle: Implications and predictions. *Biol Cybern* 36:73–85, 1980.
5. Dietz V, Bischofberger E, Wita C, Freund H-J: Correlation between the discharges of two simultaneously recorded motor units and physiological tremor. *Electroencephalogr Clin Neurophysiol* 40:97–105, 1976.
6. Freund H-J: Motor unit and muscle activity in voluntary motor control. *Physiol Rev* 63:387–436, 1983.
7. Marshall J, Walsh EG: Physiological tremor. *J Neurol Neurosurg Psychiatry* 19:260–267, 1956.
8. Partridge LD: Signal-handling characteristics of load-moving skeletal muscle. *Am J Physiol* 210:1178–1191, 1966.
9. Hagbarth K-E, Young RR: Participation of the stretch reflex in human physiological tremor. *Brain* 102:509–526, 1979.
10. Young RR, Hagbarth K-E: Physiological tremor enhanced by maneuvers affecting the segmental stretch reflex. *J Neurol Neurosurg Psychiatry* 43:248–256, 1980.
11. Brumlik J, Yap C-B: Normal tremor: A comparative study. Springfield, IL: Charles C Thomas, 1970, pp 3–15.
12. Marsden CD, Meadows JC, Lange GW, Watson RS: The role of the ballistocardiac impulse in the genesis of physiological tremor. *Brain* 92:647–662, 1969.
13. Elble RJ, Higgins C, Moody C. Stretch reflex oscillations and essential tremor. *J Neurol Neurosurg Psychiatry* 50:691–698, 1987.
14. Stiles RN: Mechanical and neural feedback factors in postural hand tremor of normal subjects. *J Neurophysiol* 44:40–59, 1980.
15. Rack PMH: Limitations of somatosensory feedback in control of posture and movement, in Brooks VB (ed): *Handbook of Physiology: The Nervous System: Motor Control*. Baltimore: Williams & Wilkins, 1981, pp 229–256.
16. Stiles RN, Randall JE: Mechanical factors in human tremor frequency. *J Appl Physiol* 23:324–330, 1967.
17. Brown TIH, Rack PMH, Ross HF: Different types of tremor in the human thumb. *J Physiol (Lond)* 332:113–123, 1982.
18. Elble RJ, Koller WC: The physiology of normal tremor, in Elble RJ, Koller WC (eds) *Tremor*. Baltimore: Johns Hopkins University Press, 1990, pp 37–53.
19. Koshland GF, Smith JL: Mutable and immutable features of pawshake responses after hindlimb deafferentation in the cat. *J Neurophysiol* 62:162–173, 1989.
20. Lamarre Y: Cerebro-cerebellar mechanisms involved in experimental tremor, in Massion J, Sasaki K (eds): *Cerebro-Cerebellar Interactions*. Amsterdam: Elsevier/North Holland Biomedical Press, 1979, pp 249–259.
21. Llinás R: Rebound excitation as the physiological basis for tremor: A biophysical study of the oscillating properties of mammalian central neurons, in Findley LJ, Capildeo R (eds): *Movement Disorders: Tremor*. London: Macmillan, 1984, pp 339–351.
22. Semba K, Szechtman H, Komisaruk BR: Synchrony among rhythmical facial tremor, neocortical 'alpha' waves, and thalamic non-sensory neuronal bursts in intact awake rats. *Brain Res* 195:281–298, 1980.

23. Toro C, Pascual-Leone A, Deuschl G, et al: Cortical tremor: A common manifestation of cortical myoclonus. *Neurology* 43:2346–2353, 1993.

24. Toro C, Cox C, Friehs G et al: 8-12 Hz rhythmic oscillations in human motor cortex during two-dimensional arm movements: Evidence for representation of kinematic parameters. *Electroencephalogr Clin Neurophysiol* 93:390–403, 1994.

25. Stein RB, Lee RG: Tremor and clonus, in Brooks V (ed): *Handbook of Physiology: The Nervous System: Motor Control*. Baltimore: Williams & Wilkins, 1981, pp 325–343.

26. Stein RB, Oguztöreli MN: Tremor and other oscillations in neuromuscular systems. *Biol Cybern* 22:147–157, 1976.

27. Elble RJ, Schieber MH, Thach WT: Activity of muscle spindles, motor cortex and cerebellar nuclei during action tremor. *Brain Res* 323:330–334, 1984.

28. Elble RJ: Physiologic and essential tremor. *Neurology* 1986:36:225–231, 1986.

29. Hömberg V, Hefter H, Reiners K, Freund H-J: Differential effects of changes in mechanical limb properties on physiological and pathological tremor. *J Neurol Neurosurg Psychiatry* 50:568–579, 1987.

30. Elble RJ, Koller WC: The diagnosis and pathophysiology of essential tremor, in Tremor 1990:54–89.

31. Britton TC, Thompson PD, Day BL, et al: "Resetting" of postural tremors at the wrist with mechanical stretches in Parkinson's disease, essential tremor, and normal subjects mimicking tremor. *Ann Neurol* 31:507–514, 1992.

32. Britton TC, Thompson PD, Day BL, et al: Modulation of postural tremors at the wrist by supramaximal electrical median nerve shocks in essential tremor, Parkinson's disease and normal subjects mimicking tremor. *J Neurol Neurosurg Psychiatry* 56:1085–1089, 1993.

33. Elble RJ, Higgins C, Hughes L: Phase resetting and frequency entrainment of essential tremor. *Exp Neurol* 116:355–361, 1992.

34. Rack PMH, Ross HF: The role of reflexes in the resting tremor of Parkinson's disease. *Brain* 109:115–141, 1986.

35. Britton TC, Thompson PD, van der Kamp W, et al: Primary orthostatic tremor: Further observations in six cases. *J Neurol* 239:209–217, 1992.

36. Heilman KM: Orthostatic tremor. *Arch Neurol* 41:880–881, 1984.

37. Thompson PD, Rothwell JC, Day BL, et al: The physiology of orthostatic tremor. *Arch Neurol* 43:584–587, 1986.

38. Kelly JJ, Sharbrough FW: EMG in orthostatic tremor. *Neurology* 37:1434, 1987.

39. van der Zwan A, Verwey JC, Van Gijn J: Relief of orthostatic tremor by primidone. *Neurology* 38:1332, 1988.

40. Britton TC, Thompson PD, Day BL, et al: Modulation of postural wrist tremors by magnetic stimulation of the motor cortex in patients with Parkinson's disease or essential tremor and in normal subjects mimicking tremor. *Ann Neurol* 33:473–479, 1993.

41. Pascual-Leone A, Valls-Solé J, Toro C, et al: Resetting of essential tremor and postural tremor in Parkinson's disease with transcranial magnetic stimulation. *Muscle Nerve* 17:800–807, 1994.

42. Wills AJ, Jenkins IH, Thompson PD, et al: Abnormal bilateral cerebellar activation in orthostatic tremor. *Neurology* 44(suppl 2):A369, 1994.

43. Houk JC, Keifer J, Barfo AG: Distributed motor commands in the limb premotor network. *Trends Neurosci* 16:27–33, 1993.

44. Apkarian AV, Hodge CJ: Primate spinothalamic pathways: III. thalamic terminations of the dorsolateral and ventral spinothalamic pathways. *J Comp Neurol* 288:493–511, 1989.

45. Asanuma C, Thach WT, Jones EG: Distribution of cerebellar terminations and their relation to other afferent terminations in the ventral lateral thalamic region of the monkey. *Brain Res Rev* 5:237–265, 1983.

46. Hirai T, Jones EG: A new parcellation of the human thalamus on the basis of histochemical staining. *Brain Res Rev* 14:1–34, 1989.

47. Bakay RAE, Vitek JL, DeLong MR: Thalamotomy for tremor. *Neurosurg Oper Atlas* 2:299–312, 1992.

48. Benabid AL, Pollak P, Gervason C, et al: Long-term suppression of tremor by chronic stimulation of the ventral intermediate thalamic nucleus. *Lancet* 337:403–406, 1991.

49. Blond S, Caparros-Lefebvre D, Parker F, et al: Control of tremor and involuntary movement disorders by chronic stereotactic stimulation of the ventral intermediate thalamic nucleus. *J Neurosurg* 77:62–68, 1992.

50. Caparros-Lefebvre D, Blond S, Vermersch P, et al: Chronic thalamic stimulation improves tremor and L-dopa induced dyskinesias in Parkinson's disease. *J Neurol Neurosurg Psychiatry* 56:268–273, 1993.

51. Goldman MS, Ahlskog JE, Kelly PJ: The symptomatic and functional outcome of stereotactic thalamotomy for medically intractable essential tremor. *J Neurosurg* 76:924–928, 1992.

52. Lenz FA, Tasker RR, Kwan HC, et al: Single unit analysis of the human ventral thalamic nuclear group: Correlation of thalamic 'tremor cells' with the 3-6 Hz component of parkinsonian tremor. *J Neurosci* 8:754–764, 1988.

53. Narabayashi H: Stereotactic Vim thalamotomy for treatment of tremor. *Eur Neurol* 29(suppl 1):29–32, 1989.

54. Narabayashi H: Striatal symptoms, in Gildenberg Phl (ed): *Stereotactic and Functional Neurosurgery*. Basel, Switzerland: Karger, 1989b, vol 52, pp 200–204.

55. Goodman D, Kelso JAS: Exploring the functional significance of physiological tremor: A biospectroscopic approach. *Exp Brain Res* 49:419–431, 1983.

56. Elble RJ, Higgins C, Hughes L: Essential tremor entrains rapid voluntary movements. *Exp Neurol* 126:138–143, 1994.

57. Logigian E, Hefter H, Reiners K, Freund H-J: Does tremor pace repetitive voluntary motor behavior in Parkinson's disease? Ann Neurol 30:172–179, 1991.

58. Wierzbicka MM, Staude G, Wolf W. Dengler R: Relationship between tremor and the onset of rapid voluntary contraction in Parkinson's disease. *J Neurol Neurosurg Psychiatry* 56:782–787, 1993.

59. Britton TC, Thompson PD, Day BL, et al: Rapid wrist movements in patients with essential tremor. *Brain* 117:39–47, 1994.

60. Nicolelis MAL, Baccala LA, Lin RCS, Chapin JK: Sensorimotor encoding by synchronous neural ensemble activity at multiple levels of the somatosensory system. *Science* 268:1353–1358, 1995.

61. Welsh JP, Lang EJ, Sugihara I, Llinás R: Dynamic organization of motor control within the olivocerebellar system. *Nature* 374:453–457, 1995.

62. Barman SM, Orer HS, Gebber GL: A 10-Hz rhythm reflects the organization of a brainstem network that specifically governs sympathetic nerve discharge. *Brain Res* 671:345–350, 1995.

63. Silva LR, Amitai Y, Connors BW: Intrinsic oscillations of neocortex generated by layer 5 pyramidal neurons. *Science* 251:432–435, 1991.

64. Steriade M, LLinás RR: The functional states of the thalamus and the associated neuronal interplay. *Physiol Rev* 68:649–742, 1988.

65. Lamarre Y: Tremorgenic mechanisms in primates. *Adv Neurol* 10:23–34, 1975.

66. Llinás R, Mühlethaler M: Electrophysiology of guinea-pig cerebellar nuclear cells in the in vitro brain stem-cerebellar preparation. *J Physiol (Lond)* 404:241–258, 1988.

67. Llinás R, Yarom Y: Oscillatory properties of guinea-pig inferior olivary neurones and their pharmacological modulations: an in vitro study. *J Physiol (Lond)* 376:163–182, 1986.

68. Nambu A, Llinás R: Electrophysiology of globus pallidus neurons in vitro. *J Neurophysiol* 72:1127–1139, 1994.

69. Murase K, Randic M: Electrophysiological properties of rat spinal dorsal horn neurons in vitro: calcium-dependent action potentials. *J Physiol (Lond)* 334:141–153, 1983.

70. Haerer AF, Anderson DW, Schoenberg BS: Prevalence of essential tremor: results from the Copiah county study. *Arch Neurol* 39:750–751, 1982.

71. Salemi G, Savettieri G, Rocca WA, et al: Prevalence of essential tremor: A door-to-door survey in Terrasini, Sicily. *Neurology* 44:61–64, 1994.

72. Findley LJ, Gresty MA: Head, facial, and voice tremor, in Jankovic J, Tolosa E (eds): *Facial Dyskinesias*. New York: Raven Press, 1988, pp 239–253.

73. Gerstenbrand F, Klingler D, Pfeiffer B: Der essentialle tremor, phanomenologie and epidemiologie. *Nervenarzt* 43:46–53, 1983.

74. Bain PG, Findley LJ, Thompson PD, et al: A study of hereditary essential tremor. *Brain* 117:805–824, 1994.

75. Conway D, Bain PG, Warner TT, et al: Linkage analysis with chromosome 9 markers in hereditary essential tremor. *Mov Disord* 8:374–376, 1993.

76. Dubinsky RM, Gray CS, Koller WC: Essential tremor and dystonia. *Neurology* 43:2383–2384, 1993.

77. Dürr A, Stevanin G, Jedynak CP, et al: Familial essential tremor and idiopathic torsion dystonia are different genetic entities. *Neurology* 43:2212–2214, 1993.

78. Koller WC, Busenbark K, Miner K: The Essential Tremor Study Group. The relationship of essential tremor to other movement disorders: Report on 678 patients. *Ann Neurol* 35:717–723, 1994.

79. Pahwa R, Koller WC: Is there a relationship between Parkinson's disease and essential tremor? *Clin Neuropharmacol* 16:30–35, 1993.

80. Lakie M, Walsh EG, Arblaster LA, et al: Limb temperature and human tremors. *J Neurol Neurosurg Psychiatry* 57:35–42, 1994.

81. Milner-Brown HS, Stein RB, Yemm R: The contractile properties of human motor units during voluntary isometric contractions. *J Physiol (Lond)* 228:285–306, 1973.

82. Lakie M, Arblaster LA, Roberts RC, Varma TRK: Effect of stereotactic thalamic lesion on essential tremor. *Lancet* 340:206–207, 1992.

83. Elble RJ, Higgins C, Hughes L: Longitudinal study of essential tremor. *Neurology* 42:441–443, 1992.

84. Rajput AH, Rozdilsky B, Ang L, Rajput A: Clinicopathologic observations in essential tremor: Report of six cases. *Neurology* 41:1422–1424, 1991.

85. Colebatch JG, Findley LJ, Frackowiak RSJ, Marsden CD, Brooks DJ: Preliminary report: activation of the cerebellum in essential tremor. *Lancet* 336:1028–1030, 1990.

86. Hallett M, Dubinsky RM: Glucose metabolism in the brain of patients with essential tremor. *J Neurol Sci* 114:45–48, 1993.

87. Jenkins IH, Bain PG, Colebatch JG, et al: A positron emission tomography study of essential tremor: Evidence for overactivity of cerebellar connections. *Ann Neurol* 34:82–90, 1993.

88. Wiklund L: Serotonergic innervation of the inferior olive and tremor generated in the olivocerebellar climbing fiber system, in Trouillas P, Fuxe K (eds): *Serotonin, the Cerebellum, and Ataxia*. New York: Raven Press, 1993, pp 113–119.

89. Elble RJ, Koller WC: Treatment of essential tremor, in: *Tremor* 1990, pp 90–105.

90. Henderson JM, Yiannikas C, Morris JGL, et al: Postural tremor of Parkinson's disease. *Clin Neuropharmacol* 17:277–285, 1994.

91. Lance JW, Schwab RS, Peterson EA: Action tremor and the cogwheel phenomenon in Parkinson's disease. *Brain* 86:95–110, 1963.

92. Hunker CJ, Abbs JH: Uniform frequency of parkinsonian resting tremor in the lips, jaw, tongue, and index finger. *Mov Disord* 5:71–77, 1990.

93. Elble RJ, Koller WC: Parkinson tremor, in: *Tremor* 1990, pp 118–133.

94. Tetrud JW, Langston JW: Tremor in MPTP-induced parkinsonism. *Neurology* 42:407–410, 1992.

95. Bergman H, Wichmann T, Karmon B, DeLong MR: The primate subthalamic nucleus. II. Neuronal activity in the MPTP model of parkinsonism. *J Neurophysiol* 72:507–520, 1994.

96. DeLong MR, Wichmann T: Basal ganglia—thalamocortical circuits in parkinsonian signs. *Clin Neurosci* 1:18–26, 1993.

97. Wichmann T, Bergman H, DeLong MR: The primate subthalamic nucleus. III. Chages in motor behavior and neuronal activity in the internal pallidum induced by subthalamic inactivation in the MPTP model of parkinsonism. *J Neurophysiol* 72:521–530, 1994.

98. Raeva SN: Unit activity of some deep nuclear structures of the human brain during voluntary movements, in Somjen G (ed): *Neurophysiology Studied in Man*. Amsterdam: Excerpta Medica, 1972, pp 64–78.

99. Raeva SN: Role of neurons of the neostriatum and nonspecific thalamus in the organization of goal-directed activity. *Hum Physiol* 3:972–984, 1977.

100. Fox MW, Ahlskog JE, Kelly PJ: Stereotactic ventrolateralis thalamotomy for medically refractory tremor in post-L-dopa era Parkinson's disease patients. *J Neurosurg* 75:723–730, 1991.

101. Buzsáki G: The thalamic clock: Emergent network properties. *Neuroscience* 41:351–364, 1991.

102. Paré D, Curro'Dossi R, Steriade M: Neuronal basis of the parkinsonian resting tremor: A hypothesis and its implications for treatment. *Neuroscience* 35:217–226, 1990.

103. Putnam TJ: The operative treatment of diseases characterized by involuntary movements (tremor, athetosis). *Assoc Res Nerv Ment Dis* 21:666–696, 1940.

104. Alberts WW: A simple view of parkinsonian tremor: electrical stimulation of cortex adjacent to the rolandic fissure in awake man. *Brain Res* 44:357–369, 1972.

105. Inase M, Tanji J: Thalamic distribution of projection neurons to the primary motor cortex relative to afferent terminal fields from the globus pallidus in the macaque monkey. *J Comp Neurol* 353:415–426, 1995.

106. Deiber MP, Pollak P, Passingham R, et al: Thalamic stimulation and suppression of parkinsonian tremor. Evidence of a cerebellar deactivation using positron emission tomography. *Brain* 116:267–279, 1993.

107. Friston K, Frackowiak R, Mauguière F, Benabid AL: Thalamic stimulation and suppression of parkinsonian tremor. Evidence of a cerebellar deactivation using positron emission tomography. *Brain* 116:267–279, 1993.

108. Dogali M, Fazzini E, Kolodny E, et al: Stereotactic ventral pallidotomy for Parkinson's disease. *Neurology* 45:753–761, 1995.

109. Guridi J, Luquin MR, Herrero MT, Obeso JA: The subthalamic nucleus: A possible target for stereotaxic surgery in Parkinson's disease. *Mov Disord* 8:421–429, 1993.

110. Bakay RAE, DeLong MR, Vitek JL: Posteroventral pallidotomy for Parkinson's disease. *J Neurosurg* 77:487–488, 1992.

111. Lenz FA, Kwan HC, Martin Rl, et al: Single unit analysis of the human ventral thalamic nuclear group: Tremor-related activity in functionally identified cells. *Brain* 117:531–543, 1994.

112. Mäkelä JP, Hari R, Karhu J: Suppression of magnetic μ rhythm during parkinsonian tremor. *Brain Res* 617:189–193, 1993.

113. Duffau H, Tzourio N, Caparros-Lafebvre D, et al: Tremor and voluntary repetitive movement in Parkinson's disease: Comparison before and after L-dopa with positron emission tomography. *Evp Brain Res* 349: 558–582, 1994.

114. Stepniewska I, Preuss TM, Kaas JH: Thalamic connections of the primary motor cortex (M1) of owl monkeys. *J Comp Neurol* 349:558–582, 1994.

115. Parent A, Hazrati L-N: Functional anatomy of the basal ganglia. I. The cortico-basal ganglia-thalamo-cortical loop. *Brain Res Rev* 20:91–127, 1995.

116. Holmes G: The symptoms of acute cerebellar injuries due to gunshot injuries. *Brain* 40:461–535, 1917.

117. Diener HC, Dichgans J, Bacher M, Gompf B: Quantification of postural sway in normals and patients with cerebellar diseases. *Electroencephalogr Clin Neurophysiol* 57:134–142, 1984.

118. Rondot P, Bathien M: Motor control in cerebellar tremor, in Findley LJ, Capildeo R (eds): *Movement Disorders: Tremor.* London: Macmillan, 1984, chap 27.

119. Silfverskiold BP: A 3c/sec leg tremor in a 'cerebellar' syndrome. *Acta Neurol Scand* 55:385–393, 1977.

120. Vilis T, Hore J: Effects of changes in mechanical state of limb on cerebellar intention tremor. *J Neurophysiol* 40:1214–1224, 1977.

121. Gilman S, Carr D, Hollenberg J: Kinematic effects of deafferentation and cerebellar ablation. *Brain* 99:311–330, 1976.

122. Sanes JN, LeWitt PA, Mauritz K-H: Visual and mechanical control of postural and kinetic tremor in cerebellar system disorders. *J Neurol Neurosurg Psychiatry* 51:934–943, 1988.

123. Thach WT, Goodkin HP, Keating JG: The cerebellum and the adaptive coordination of movement. *Ann Rev Neurosci* 15:403–442, 1992.

124. Hore J, Vilis T: A cerebellar-dependent efference copy mechanism for generating appropriate muscle responses to limb perturbations, in Bloedel JR, Dichgans J, Precht W (eds): *Cerebellar Functions.* Berlin: Springer-Verlag, 1984, pp 24–35.

125. Diener H-C, Dichgans J: Pathophysiology of cerebellar ataxia. *Mov Disord* 7:95–109, 1992.

126. Elble RJ, Koller WC: Cerebellar tremor, In *Tremor.* Baltimore: Johns Hopkins University Press, 1990, pp 106–117.

127. Hewer RL, Cooper R, Morgan MH: An investigation into the value of treating intention tremor by weighting the affected limb. *Brain* 95:570–590, 1972.

128. Aisen ML, Arnold A, Baiges I, et al: The effect of mechanical damping loads on disabling action tremor. *Neurology* 43:1346–1350, 1993.

129. Goldman MS, Kelly PJ: Symptomatic and functional outcome of stereotactic ventralis lateralis thalamotomy for intention tremor. *J Neurosurg* 77:223–229, 1992.

130. Carpenter MB: Brain stem and infratentorial neuraxis in experimental dyskinesia. *Arch Neurol* 5:58–78, 1961.

131. Carey JH: Certain anatomical and functional interrelations between the tegmentum of the midbrain and the basal ganglia. *J Comp Neurol* 108:57–89, 1957.

132. Denny-Brown D: Clinical symptomatology of diseases of the basal ganglia, in Vinker PJ, Bruyn GW (eds): *Handbook of Clinical Neurology: Diseases of the Basal Ganglia.* Amsterdam: North Holland, 1968, pp 162–164.

133. Holmes G: On certain tremors in organic cerebral lesions. *Brain* 27:327–375, 1904.

134. Ohye C, Shibazaki T, Hirai, T et al: A special role of the parvocellular red nucleus in lesion-induced spontaneous tremor in monkeys. *Behav Brain Res* 28:241–243, 1988.

135. Andrew J, Fowler CJ, Harrison MJG: Tremor after head injury and its treatment by stereotaxic surgery. *J Neurol Neurosurg Psychiatry* 45:815–819, 1982.

136. Broggi G, Brock S, Franzini A, Geminiani G: A case of posttraumatic tremor treated by chronic stimulation of the thalamus. *Mov Disord* 8:206–208, 1993.

137. Deuschl G, Mischke G, Schenck E, et al: Symptomatic and essential rhythmic palatal myoclonus. *Brain* 113:1645–1672, 1990.

138. Guillain G: The syndrome of synchronous and rhythmic palato-pharyngo-laryngo-oculo-diaphragmatic myoclonus. *Proc R Soc Med* 31:1031–1038, 1938.

139. Birbamer G, Gerstenbrand F, Kofler M, et al: Post-traumatic segmental myoclonus associated with bilateral olivary hypertrophy. *Acta Neurol Scand* 87:505–509, 1993.

140. Elble RJ: Inhibition of forearm EMG by palatal myoclonus. *Mov Disord* 6:324–329, 1991.

141. Deuschl G, Toro C, Hallett M: Symptomatic and essential palatal tremor. 2. Differences of palatal movements. *Mov Disord* 9:676–678, 1994.

142. Dubinsky RM, Hallett M, Di Chiro G, et al: Increased glucose metabolism in the medulla of patients with palatal myoclonus. *Neurology* 41:557–562, 1991.

143. Masucci E, Kurtzke J: Palatal myoclonus associated with extremity tremor. *J Neurol* 236:474–477, 1989.

144. Masucci EF, Kurtzke JF, Saini N: Myorhythmia: A widespread movement disorder. *Brain* 107:53–79, 1984.

145. Ferbert A, Gerwig M: Tremor due to stroke. *Mov Disord* 8:179–182, 1993.

146. Kim JS: Delayed onset hand tremor caused by cerebral infarction. *Stroke* 23:292–294, 1992.

147. Mano Y, Nakamuro T, Takayanagi T, Mayer RF: Ceruletide therapy in action tremor following thalamic hemorrhage. *J Neurol* 240:144–148, 1993.

148. Bhatia KP, Marsden CD: The behavioural and motor consequences of focal lesions of the basal ganglia in man. *Brain* 117:859–876, 1994.

149. Lee MS, Marsden CD: Movement disorders following lesions of the thalamus or subthalamic region. *Mov Disord* 9:493–507, 1994.

150. Shahani BT: Tremor associated with peripheral neuropathy, in: Findley LJ, Capildeo R (eds). *Movement Disorders: Tremor.* London: Macmillan, 1984, pp 389–398.

151. Smith IS, Kahn SN, Lacey BW, et al: Chronic demyelinating neuropathy associated with benign IgM paraproteinemia. *Brain* 106:169–195, 1983.

152. Said G, Bathien N, Cesaro P: Peripheral neuropathies and tremor. *Neurology* 32:480–485, 1982.

153. Dalakas MC, Teräväinen H, Engel WK: Tremor as a feature of chronic relapsing and dysgammaglobulinemic polyneuropathies. *Arch Neurol* 41:711–714, 1984.

154. Cardoso F, Jankovic J: Peripherally induced tremor and parkinsonism. *Arch Neurol* 52:263–270, 1995.

155. Elble RJ, Moody C, Higgins C: Primary writing tremor: A form of focal dystonia? Mov Disord 5:118–126, 1990.

156. Ravits J, Hallett M, Baker M, Wilkins D: Primary writing tremor and myoclonic writer's cramp. *Neurology* 35:1387–1391, 1985.

157. Rosenbaum R, Jankovic J: Focal task-specific tremor and dystonia: Categorization of occupational movement disorders. *Neurology* 38:522–527, 1988.

158. Rothwell JC, Traub MM, Marsden CD: Primary writing tremor. *J Neurol Neurosurg Psychiatry* 42:1106–1114, 1979.

159. Deuschl G, Heinen F, Kleedorfer B, et al: Clinical and polymyographic investigation of spasmodic torticollis. *J Neurol* 239:9–15, 1992.

160. Sheehy PM, Marsden CD: Writer's cramp—a focal dystonia. *Brain* 105:461–480, 1982.

161. Yanagisawa N, Goto A: Dystonia musculorum deformans: Analysis with electromyography. *J Neurol Sci* 13:39–65, 1971.

162. Bain PG, Findley LJ, Britton TC, et al: Primary writing tremor. *Brain* 118: 1461–1472, 1995.

163. McManis PG, Sharbrough FW. Orthostatic tremor: Clinical and electrophysiological characteristics. *Muscle Nerve* 16:1254–1260, 1993.

164. Elble RJ, Koller WC: Unusual forms of tremor, in: *Tremor* 1990, pp 143–157.

165. Danek A: Geniospasm: hereditary chin trembling. *Mov Disord* 8:335–338, 1993.

166. Rivest J, Marsden CD: Trunk and head tremor as manifestations of dystonia. *Mov Disord* 5:60–65, 1990.

167. Ikeda A, Kakigi R, Funai N, et al: Cortical tremor: A variant of cortical reflex myoclonus. *Neurology* 40:1561–1565, 1990.

168. Oguni E, Hayashi A, Ishii A, et al: A case of cortical tremor as a variant of cortical reflex myoclonus. *Eur Neurol* 35:63–64, 1995.

169. Elble RJ, Koller WC: Drug-induced tremor, In: *Tremor.* Baltimore: Johns Hopkins University Press, 1990, pp 134–142.

170. Charness ME, Morady F, Scheinman MM: Frequent neurologic toxicity associated with amiodarone therapy. *Neurology* 34:669–671, 1984.

171. Donaldson IM, Cuningham J: Persisting neurologic sequelae of lithium carbonate therapy. *Arch Neurol* 40:747–751, 1983.

172. Palakurthy PR, Iyer V, Meckler RJ: Unusual neurotoxicity associated with amiodarone therapy. *Arch Intern Med* 147:881–884, 1987.

173. Prien RF: Lithium in the treatment of affective disorders. *Clin Neuropharmacol* 3:113–131, 1978.

174. Werner EG, Olanow CW: Parkinsonism and amiodarone therapy. *Ann Neurol* 25:630–632, 1989.

175. Schneider JA, Mirra SS: Neurophysiologic correlates of persistent neurologic deficit in lithium intoxication. *Ann Neurol* 36:928–931, 1994.

Chapter 30

CHILDHOOD DYSTONIA

SUSAN B. BRESSMAN and STANLEY FAHN

CLINICAL FEATURES
EPIDEMIOLOGY
PATHOLOGY
BIOCHEMISTRY
GENETICS
    Inheritance Pattern of Early-Onset ITD
    Genetic Linkage Studies
    Linkage Disequilibrium of DYT1 with 9q Markers in
        Ashkenazi Jews
    Summary of Genetics and Counseling
        Recommendations
EVALUATION
DOPA-RESPONSIVE DYSTONIA (DRD)

Dystonia is a syndrome of sustained muscle contractions that produce twisting and repetitive movements and abnormal postures.[1,2] The extent and severity of muscle involvement are remarkably variable, ranging from intermittent contractions limited to a single body region (focal dystonia) to generalized dystonia involving the limbs and axial muscles (Table 30-1).

Dystonia may be a result of many different causes. Two broad etiologic categories have been proposed: idiopathic (or primary) and symptomatic (or secondary) (Table 30-2). The symptomatic dystonias encompass a host of disorders that are either inherited (e.g., Wilson's disease, Huntington's disease, the gangliosidoses) or are a result of exogenous factors (e.g., perinatal injury, neuroleptic medications, infection). In symptomatic dystonia, examination abnormalities other than dystonia (e.g., dementia, ataxia, optic atrophy, parkinsonism) are frequently present; often, there are pathological changes involving the basal ganglia, and laboratory findings usually help in diagnosis. In contrast, dystonia is the only examination abnormality in idiopathic dystonia; no consistent pathological changes are found (see below), and diagnostic studies are unrevealing.

Although reports describing dystonia date back to as early as 1652, when Tulpius described spasmodic torticollis,[2a] the word dystonia is a twentieth-century creation. Oppenheim[3] first used the word in 1911 in naming a childhood-onset syndrome he termed *dystonia musculorum deformans*. The syndrome consisted of twisted postures; muscle spasms; bizarre walking, with bending and twisting of the torso; rapid, sometimes-rhythmic jerking movements; and progression of symptoms eventually leading to sustained fixed postural deformities.[4] Many of the early descriptions of children with dystonia also described other affected family members,[5–8] and the condition was suspected to be inherited. Only recent studies, however, have elucidated the genetic basis of childhood and adolescent-onset idiopathic dystonia (also fre-

quently termed idiopathic torsion dystonia, or ITD). This chapter reviews the clinical features and genetics of ITD in children and adolescence, and the relationship of this early-onset form of ITD to adult- or late-onset ITD. Treatment of ITD is covered in Chap. 32.

Clinical Features

As mentioned above, the clinical range of ITD is remarkably variable. Studies over the years describe the clustering of certain clinical features with more or less distinct subtypes emerging. However, the category of ITD has been obfuscated by the inclusion of rare "variant" dystonic disorders that do not strictly meet the definition of ITD; namely, these disorders typically manifest clinical features other than dystonia, such as parkinsonism, hyperreflexia, and myoclonus (see Table 30-2) and are more appropriately classified as symptomatic dystonia. The variant disorders include dopa-responsive dystonia (also known as dystonia with diurnal variation and Segawa's disease),[9,10] myoclonic dystonia,[11] rapid-onset dystonia-parkinsonism,[12] X-linked dystonia-parkinsonism found in the Filipino population,[13–15] and dystonia with whispering dysphonia/Wilson's disease.[16] With the exception of Filipino dystonia-parkinsonism, which is X-linked, these variants are inherited in an autosomal-dominant fashion.

Based on their unique clinical features, the variant dystonias are each suspected to be the result of a different genetic defect. To date, linkage studies confirm this: the gene for dopa responsive dystonia (DRD) is localized to chromosome 14q,[17] and mutations in the GTP cyclohydrolase 1 gene[18] are thought to be responsible; Filipino dystonia-parkinsonism maps to Xq21; genes for the other variant subtypes, although not mapped, have been excluded from the known ITD locus, DYT1 (see below). Of the variant dystonias, DRD is the most common cause of dystonia in children, constituting about 5 percent of cases, and presenting signs of DRD are often difficult to distinguish from those of ITD. Because of this, and because the condition responds dramatically to L-dopa therapy, it will be discussed separately at the end of this chapter.

Clinical studies of ITD have long noted a relationship among the age at onset of symptoms, the body region first affected, and the progression of disease. There is a bimodal distribution in the age at onset, with modes at ages 9 (early-onset) and 45 (late-onset) years and a nadir at 27 years.[19] Early-onset dystonia usually first involves a leg or arm and, less commonly, starts in the neck or vocal cords.[20,21] The majority of early-onset patients progress to involve more than one limb, and about one-half eventually generalize to involve the legs and arms. Patients with leg onset have a somewhat earlier age at onset (8–9 years), compared to those with initial involvement of arm muscles (12–14 years); also, those with leg onset are more likely to evolve into generalized dystonia, compared to those patients with dystonia starting in an arm. Similarly, the rate of progression to generalized dystonia is faster in those with onset in a leg (mean, 4.7 years), compared to arm-onset cases (mean, 11.4 years).[21] In contrast to early-onset, late-onset ITD usually starts in the neck or cranial muscles and, less commonly, first involves an arm; onset in a leg is very rare. Late-onset ITD also usually

TABLE 30-1 Classification of Dystonia According to Distribution of Body Regions Affected

I. *Focal:* A single area is involved. These areas include upper face (or blepharospasm), oromandibular, vocal cords (or spasmodic dysphonia), an arm (or writer's cramp), and neck (or spasmodic torticollis).

II. *Segmental:* Two or more contiguous areas are affected. Common examples include cranial (e.g., face + jaw + tongue + vocal cords), cranial + cervical, cervical + brachial, bibrachial, and axial (neck + trunk).

III. *Multifocal:* Two or more noncontiguous body regions are involved. Examples include involvement of one or both arms + one leg, and cranial muscle involvement, such as blepharospasm + leg dystonia. Hemidystonia is a type of multifocal dystonia.

IV. *Generalized:* Both legs ± trunk are involved and at least one other region or one leg + trunk and at least one other region.

TABLE 30-2 Etiologic Classification of Dystonia

I. *Primary (Idiopathic) Dystonia*
  A. Childhood and adolescent onset
    1. Ashkenazi: Autosomal-dominant (penetrance = 0.3), most a result of single-founder mutation event in the DYT1 gene
    2. Non-Jewish: Autosomal-dominant (penetrance = 0.4), many a result of different mutation events in DYT1
  B. Adult onset
    ?autosomal-dominant, extent of DYT1 involvement unknown; not DYT1 in some non-Jewish families and not a result of common early-onset mutation in Ashkenazim

II. *Secondary (Symptomatic) Dystonia*
  A. Associated with hereditary neurologic syndromes
    Dopa-responsive dystonia (DRD)
    Myoclonic dystonia
    Rapid-onset dystonia-parkinsonism
    X-linked Filipino/lubag (XPD)
    Wilson's disease
    Gangliosidoses
    Metachromatic leukodystrophy
    Lesch-Nyhan syndrome
    Homocystinuria
    Hartnup disease
    Glutaric acidemia
    Leigh's disease
    Familial basal ganglia calcifications
    Hallervorden-Spatz disease
    Dystonic lipidosis (sea-blue histiocytosis)
    Ceroid lipofuscinosis
    Ataxia-telangiectasia
    Neuroacanthocytosis
    Intraneuronal inclusion disease
    Huntington's disease
    Machado-Joseph's disease/SCA3
    Mitochondrial encephalomyopathies/Leber's disease
  B. A result of known environmental cause
    Perinatal cerebral injury
    Encephalitis, infectious and postinfectious
    Head trauma
    Pontine myelinolysis
    Primary antiphospholipid syndrome
    Stroke
    Tumor
    Multiple sclerosis
    Cervical cord injury or lesion
    Peripheral injury
    Drugs
    Toxins
  C. Dystonia as part of parkinsonism
  D. Psychogenic dystonia

remains localized as focal or segmental dystonia, and spreading to involve the legs is rare.

The relationship between age at onset and clinical progression is illustrated in a large series of 2431 patients with ITD seen at the Dystonia Clinical Research Center in New York City; 20 percent of all patients had onset before 21 years of age, and 8.7 percent had generalized dystonia. However, generalized dystonia occurred in 47.5 percent of patients with childhood-onset ITD, in 13.5 percent with adolescent onset, and in only 1.9 percent with adult-onset (Table 30-3).

The relationship between age of onset and signs of dystonia is somewhat different for the symptomatic dystonias (Table 30-4). First of all, there are only about one-third as many patients with symptomatic dystonia, compared to those with ITD. A higher percentage of patients with symptomatic dystonia has early onset (53 percent) or generalized dystonia (25.2 percent); also, unlike ITD, symptomatic dystonia beginning in adults is more likely to generalize (13.5 percent). Another major distinction between idiopathic and symptomatic dystonias is that a much higher proportion of patients with symptomatic dystonia develop hemidystonia (8 percent versus 0.5 percent).

ITD in a limb commonly begins with a specific-action dystonia; that is, the abnormal movements appear while a patient is performing a special action and are not present at rest. For example, when idiopathic dystonia begins in a leg, it is seen only while walking. It is often absent with running or walking backward. As the dystonic condition progresses, less specific actions of the affected leg may activate the dystonia, e.g., tapping the floor. Also, actions in other parts of the body can induce dystonic movements of the involved leg, so-called "overflow." With still further worsening, the affected limb can develop dystonic movements while it is at rest. Eventually, the leg can have sustained posturing. Similarly, arm dystonia typically starts while the individual is performing a specific task, such as writing or playing a musical instrument. Over time, the dystonia may be apparent when another part of the body is engaged in voluntary activity or with less specific activities of the limb; finally, it may be present at rest. Thus, dystonia at rest is usually a more severe form than pure action dystonia.

Progression proceeds not only in terms of the severity of dystonic contractions in the limb first affected but also in terms of the spread of dystonia to involve other parts of the body. Usually, it first spreads to adjacent segments of the body and then more distally. Sometimes, the dystonia may affect the other ipsilateral limb, producing a hemidystonia. However, more than 90 percent of the time, hemidystonia indicates that the dystonia is symptomatic, rather than idiopathic.[22,23]

TABLE 30-3 Distribution of ITD as a Function of Age at Onset

Age at Onset (yr)	N	Generalized	Segmental and Multifocal	Focal	Hemidystonia
<13	318	151 (47.5%)	103	60	4
13–20	171	23 (13.5%)	59	86	3
>20	1942	37 (1.9%)	609	1291	5
Total	2431	211 (8.7%)	771	1437	12

Percentages represent the percent of generalized dystonia for the total of that age group.

Dystonic movements tend to increase with fatigue, stress, and emotional states, and they tend to be suppressed with relaxation, hypnosis, and sleep.[24] One of the characteristic features of dystonic movements is that they can be diminished by tactile or proprioceptive "sensory tricks" (geste antagoniste). Thus, touching the involved or adjacent body part can often reduce the muscle contractions. The most common type of dystonia to benefit from sensory tricks is cervical dystonia; typically, the patient places her hand on the chin, on the side of the face, or in back of the head to reduce nuchal contractions. Patients with generalized dystonia may also respond to analogous sensory tricks. Not uncommonly, the severe flexed trunk on walking can be overcome by the patient placing one hand on the back of the head.

Usually, dystonia is present continually throughout the day, whenever the affected body part is in use or, in more severe cases, at rest; it disappears with deep sleep. In contrast to dopa-responsive dystonia, marked diurnal patterns are not common in ITD, although mild variations may occur. Remissions are rare in early-onset ITD, and we have never encountered a patient with generalized ITD and a complete remission of dystonic signs. Complete remissions may occur in patients with cervical dystonia,[25,26] and, rarely, a patient with generalized dystonia may have a partial remission.[27]

Pain is uncommon in ITD, with the exception of cervical dystonia; 75 percent of patients with cervical dystonia (spasmodic torticollis) have pain.[28] Dystonia in most parts of the body rarely is accompanied by pain; when it is, it is not clear whether the pain is from painful contractions of muscles or some other factor. The high incidence of pain in cervical dystonia appears to be the result of muscle contractions, because this pain is usually relieved by injections of botulinum toxin.[29] It is believed that the posterior cervical muscles are rich in pain fibers and that continual contractions of these muscles result in pain. Tension headaches are similarly the result of chronic nuchal muscle contractions. Patients with generalized dystonia who have involvement of the nuchal muscles may have pain in this area. Another potential reason for pain in the cervical area is that dystonia there increases the likelihood of patients developing cervical osteoarthritis, which also produces pain.

Because the legs and trunk are so often affected in early-onset dystonia, most children and teens with ITD have an abnormal gait. The leg commonly swings abnormally when it is carried forward. There may be abduction at hip and, often, the foot will swing medially, almost striking the other leg. The knee tends to be abnormally elevated and the foot in an equinovarus posture, but other postures, such as knee extension and foot eversion, are not uncommon. When the trunk is affected, there is commonly a bent-over posture, so-called "dromedary gait," with the neck extended while there is flexion at the hips. This contrasts to the opisthotonic gait that fairly commonly occurs in patients with tardive dystonia. Some patients with generalized dystonia cannot walk or can walk only for a few steps before the dystonia overwhelms them. In the early stages of the disease, the trunk may not be dystonic when the patient is sitting or lying down. However, with time, there is a tendency for the trunk to become involved in these positions as well. It is helpful to quantify the severity of dystonia. The Fahn-Marsden scale for assessing generalized dystonia has been validated[30] and can be used to follow the course of the disease or the response to treatment. Videotaping patients is another important method of assessing patients.

Patients with primary torsion dystonia sometimes have rhythmic movements manifested as a tremor.[31,32] There are basically two types of tremor seen in dystonic patients: an accompanying tremor that resembles essential tremor and a tremor that is a rhythmic expression of rapid dystonic movements.[33] The latter can usually be distinguished from the former by showing that the tremor appears only when the affected body part is placed in a position of opposition

TABLE 30-4 Distribution of Symptomatic Torsion Dystonia as a Function of Age at Onset

Age at Onset (yr)	N	Generalized	Segmental and Multifocal	Focal	Hemidystonia
<13	239	126 (52.7%)	56	27	30
13–20	87	26 (29.9%)	30	22	9
>20	599	81 (13.5%)	243	243	32
Total	925	233 (25.2%)	329	292	71

Percentages represent the percent of generalized dystonia for the total of that age group.

to the major direction of pulling by the abnormal dystonic contractions. Dystonic tremor appears to be less regular than essential tremor.[34] Sometimes, it is very difficult to distinguish between the two types. Myorhythmia is a term that Herz[35] used to describe slow repetitive movements in patients with idiopathic torsion dystonia (which today would usually be called dystonic tremor). Myorhythmia refers to a slow oscillation (2-3 Hz) around a joint. It is present with the affected body part at rest and persists during action. Unfortunately, the term myorhythmia has also been used to refer to the rhythmical movements encountered in the limbs in patients with palatal myoclonus.[36] Dubinsky et al.[37] reported that 24 of 296 patients with primary dystonia had dystonic tremor, but that 20 of those patients had focal cervical dystonia with an isolated head-nodding tremor. Only two patients with generalized dystonia had tremor; both were in the arm.

A family history of tremor (and stuttering) is reported to be increased in ITD.[38] Although accompanying essential tremor is recognized in patients with dystonia,[39] it is uncertain how common this occurrence is. Furthermore, linkage studies show that the gene that commonly causes early-onset ITD (DYT1) does not underlie essential tremor.[40,41] Tics are another type of involuntary movement that may be more common in ITD patients and their families than in the general population.[42,43]

In ITD the only neurological abnormalities are dystonic postures and movements. There is no associated loss of postural reflexes, amyotrophy, weakness, spasticity, ataxia, reflex change, abnormality of eye movements, disorder of the retina, dementia, or seizure disorder, except where they may be the result of a concomitant problem such as a complication from a neurosurgical procedure undertaken to correct the dystonia or indicate the presence of some other incidental neurological disease. Because many of the symptomatic dystonias are associated with these neurological findings, the presence of any of these abnormalities in a patient with dystonia immediately suggests that one is dealing with symptomatic dystonia (see Evaluation). However, the absence of such neurological findings does not necessarily exclude the possibility of a symptomatic dystonia, which may present as a pure dystonia.

Epidemiology

The prevalence of ITD is difficult to estimate because of the variation in expression and the tendency for mild cases to go undiagnosed. In one study from Rochester, Minnesota, prevalence was calculated to be 3.4 per 100,000 for generalized dystonia and 29.5 per 100,000 for focal dystonia.[44] There are also ethnic differences in frequency; childhood and adolescent-onset primary dystonia appears to be more common in Jews of Eastern European, or Ashkenazi, ancestry. Based on cases reported in the literature, Zeman and Dyken[45] estimated a disease frequency in American Jews (most had European ancestry) of 2.7 per 100,000, which is about 5 times the frequency of 0.5 per 100,000 that he estimated for the general population. A study of Israeli patients with generalized and segmental primary dystonia found an eightfold higher frequency among Jews of Eastern European ancestry (6.7 per

100,000), compared to that of African and Asian Jews (0.85 per 100,000).[46] More recently, Risch et al.[47] estimated the frequency of early-onset ITD, based on cases diagnosed at Columbia Presbyterian's Movement Disorders Center. Compared to previous studies, they found a higher frequency in Ashkenazi Jews of 20–30 per 100,000; this is about 3 times the frequency they estimate for early-onset dystonia in non-Jews (N Risch, personal communication).

Pathology

There are no consistent morphological abnormalities in ITD, as seen on brain imaging[48] or histological examination.[49] A number of pathological studies have been carried out on patients who died with primary torsion dystonia. When these were reviewed by Zeman,[50] who also added his own cases, he concluded that whereas environmental and inherited etiologies of symptomatic dystonia leave their mark with alterations in the basal ganglia, the hereditary forms of ITD have no tangible pathological abnormalities detectable by means of light microscopy. He felt that the earlier reports of positive findings could be explained as nonspecific alterations or as artifacts resulting from the agonal state prior to death.

Zweig and his colleagues[51] described the histology of the brain stem in four patients with primary torsion dystonia. Two of them started in childhood or adolescence (cases 1 and 2), with case 1 being Jewish and case 2 non-Jewish. Case 1 had numerous neurofibrillary tangles (NFT) in the locus ceruleus, along with mild neuronal loss and extracellular neuromelanin in this nucleus. There were rare NFT in the substantia nigra pars compacta, pedunculopontine nucleus, and dorsal raphe nucleus. Case 2 had no notable abnormality. Cases 3 and 4 had adult-onset cranial-cervical dystonia and cervical dystonia, respectively. Case 3 had remarkable neuronal loss in the substantia nigra pars compacta, dorsal raphe, pedunculopontine nucleus, and locus ceruleus. The pigmented nuclei had extracellular pigment. There was an occasional NFT in the nucleus basalis and infrequent NFT in the substantia nigra. Case 4, like case 2, had no notable abnormality.

The inconsistency of the histology in patients with primary dystonia makes it difficult to interpret the significance of the observations by Zweig and his colleagues.[51] Clearly, there is a great need to have many more cases studied pathologically.

Biochemistry

Hornykiewicz et al.[52] examined the biochemistry of the brain in two patients with childhood-onset generalized dystonia, and Jankovic and Svendsen[53] studied a single case of adult-onset primary cranial segmental dystonia. There were changes in norepinephrine, serotonin, and dopamine levels in various regions of brain. It is not clear which, if any, of these alterations is related to the pathophysiology of dystonia. In a patient with symptomatic dystonia resulting from neuroacanthocytosis, de Yebenes et al.[54] found large increases in norepinephrine in the caudate nucleus, putamen, globus pallidus, and dentate nucleus. Again, it is not clear whether changes in norepinephrine levels are related to dystonia. Many more biochemical studies need to be carried out. In the meantime, fluorodeoxyglucose positron emission tomography (PET) studies have revealed some regional hypometabolism in the frontal cortex and lenticular nucleus.[55,56] PET scans, using a ligand to bind to striatal dopamine D2 receptors, showed a trend to higher uptake in the contralateral striatum in subjects showing lateralization of clinical signs.[57]

In a study of platelet mitochondria, Benecke et al.[58] found a defect in complex I in patients with idiopathic dystonia, most of whom had torticollis and not generalized dystonia.

Genetics

INHERITANCE PATTERN OF EARLY-ONSET ITD

Early reports of ITD described families with affected siblings, parents, second and third degree relatives.[5-8,59-61] Most families had early-onset dystonia, and many were of Eastern European Jewish ancestry. Nevertheless, the genetic basis of dystonia was largely neglected, until the detailed report of Zeman and Dyken in 1967.[45] They reviewed the clinical, pathological, and genetic aspects of 253 cases of *dystonia musculorum deformans*. In this study, patients from 31 families (19 Jewish and 12 non-Jewish) were categorized as familial, and the remaining 105 (50 Jewish and 55 non-Jewish) were considered sporadic. The median age at onset of the affected individuals was 10 years, and more than 90 percent were affected by 21 years of age. The authors concluded that ITD is inherited in both Jewish and non-Jewish populations, as an autosomal-dominant trait with a reduced penetrance of 52 percent. They estimated a higher gene frequency in American Jews (1 in 38,000), compared to that of the general population of the state of Indiana (1 in 200,000); however, they did not propose different inheritance patterns, or the presence of two or more genes, based on this difference in disease frequency.

Three years later Eldridge presented a detailed report of 156 cases representing 96 families (41 families were Ashkenazi Jewish) and came to different conclusions.[62] He proposed that ITD is inherited in an autosomal-recessive fashion in Jews and in an autosomal-dominant fashion in most non-Jewish families. He based his argument of recessive inheritance on three findings: (1) the analysis of sibling risk was consistent with recessive inheritance: (2) The frequency of primary dystonia in Jews is increased over that of non-Jews, and other disorders that are similarly increased in Jews, such as Tay-Sachs, are autosomal-recessive: (3) Clinical differences between Jews and non-Jews were noted. Jews were more likely to have progressive childhood-onset disease with first symptoms in a limb, compared to non-Jews, who had somewhat later onset, less clinical progression, and greater likelihood of initial axial involvement.

Only the first of these points supports directly autosomal-recessive inheritance. This point was first challenged by Korczyn and colleagues.[63] They argued that Eldridge miscalculated the recurrence risk to siblings; also, the consanguinity rate is too low, and there are too many instances of parent and child affected under autosomal-recessive inheritance, unless a very high gene frequency is assumed. Eldridge's third point, that there are clinical differences between non-Jewish and Jewish dystonia cases patients, was also challenged:[64] Burke and colleagues reanalyzed the clinical features in Eldridge's families, as well as those of their own series of families, and found no significant differences in the ages and sites of onset or progression of signs.

Then, in the 1980s, Jewish dystonia families in Israel and the United States were systematically studied, and analyses indicated autosomal-dominant inheritance with reduced penetrance; recessive inheritance was rejected. In the Israeli study, Zilber and colleagues[46] analyzed the families of 47 primary dystonia patients with generalized and segmental dystonia. Analyses of family data were not consistent with an autosomal-recessive pattern: consanguinity was infrequent, the rates of affected parents, offspring, aunts, uncles, and cousins were too high; and the observed rate of affected siblings from presumed heterozygous parents was lower than expected. The authors concluded that primary dystonia is inherited in an autosomal-dominant fashion, with penetrance of 51 percent. In this study the paternal age of isolated cases was increased over that of familial cases, suggesting that some were the result of new mutations.

In the American study, Bressman et al. systematically studied the families of 43 Ashkenazi Jewish probands;[19] this included "blinded" review of videotaped examinations of 90 percent of the living first relatives. The proband group in this study was restricted to patients with onset of ITD before age 28 years, based on the hypothesis that clinical differences between early- and late-onset ITD represent differences in etiologies. However, there were no restrictions in the ages and sites of onset of dystonia in relatives diagnosed as affected. The age adjusted risk to all first degree relatives was 15.5 percent; the risk to second degree relatives was 6.5 percent; and there were no significant sex differences. The risks for parents, offspring, and siblings were similar, as expected for an autosomal dominant disorder. The penetrance was calculated at 30 percent. These results were confirmed in rigorous segregation analysis of the same data.[65] Also, there was no evidence for sporadic cases or new mutations in these families, and the higher frequency of the disorder in Ashkenazim was postulated to be a result of founder mutation and genetic drift.

An interesting finding in this study was the range of clinical features observed in affected relatives. Although relatives had milder disease (only one-half were aware that they had dystonia), most were affected by age 30. There were no relatives with onset of symptoms after age 44, although more than 60 percent of the examined relatives were at least 45 years of age. Also, none had onset in cranial muscles. These findings are consistent with the hypothesis that early- and late-onset ITD have different causes.

These studies demonstrate that early-onset ITD is an autosomal-dominant, not recessive, trait in Jews. Furthermore, Pauls and Korczyn[66] performed complex segregation analysis on Eldridge's previously reported Ashkenazi families. The analysis demonstrates that the trait is inherited in an autosomal-dominant fashion with reduced penetrance.

In almost all studies of early-onset, non-Jewish ITD families the disorder is found to be inherited as an autosomal-dominant trait,[45,60,61,67] with penetrance ranging from nearly complete to about 30 percent. A systematic analysis[68] of 96 non-Jewish British probands with generalized, multifocal, and segmental involvement concluded that approximately 85 percent of cases are inherited as an autosomal-dominant trait, with reduced penetrance of 40 percent; the remaining 15 percent are likely to be nongenetic phenocopies. Increased paternal age of singleton patients was found, and about 14 percent of genetic patients are thought to have new mutations. As in the study of Ashkenazi families, there was variable and often milder expression in affected relatives although, unlike that population, a larger proportion (10–15 percent) of non-Jewish affected family members had late onset (>44 years).

GENETIC LINKAGE STUDIES

Ozelius et al.[69] mapped the first ITD locus (named DYT1) in 1989. They studied a large North American non-Jewish family of French-Canadian ancestry, first reported on by Johnson,[69b] and localized the gene to the 9q32-34 region. Subsequently, Kramer and colleagues found linkage with markers in the same region in 12 Ashkenazi families.[70] Clinical features were similar in the non-Jewish and Jewish families; onset was early in both (average, 14.4 ± 3 and 13.2 ± 1 years, respectively), and symptoms began in a limb (86 percent and 90%, respectively) in almost all. In the study of Kramer, tightest linkage was found with the gene encoding arginosuccinate synthetase (ASS); subsequent multipoint analysis with markers in the 9q region revealed a similar location for the disease genes in both the Jewish and non-Jewish groups,[71] and the same gene is thought to cause dystonia in both. Because the locus for dopamine beta-hydroxylase (DBH) maps to the DYT1 9q region and because this enzyme was implicated in several studies of ITD, this candidate locus was evaluated and excluded soon after DYT1 was localized.[72]

Since the appearance of the initial linkage findings, studies of European,[73] non-Jewish North American,[74] and Ashkenazi[75,76] families confirm that DYT1 is a common cause of early-onset primary dystonia; however, it is not the only gene for ITD.[73,77,78]

In a European study of 27 small families (3 Jewish and 24 non-Jewish), there was evidence for linkage to the chromosomal region containing DYT1, with a combined LOD score of 3.4 at ASS calculated for 24 families. However, tight linkage to ASS was excluded in three non-Jewish families.[73] One of the excluded families was thought to have dopa-responsive dystonia; otherwise, clinical differences between "DYT1" and "non-DYT1" families were not noted.

Evidence implicating DYT1 was also provided in a study of six non-Jewish North American families of European descent.[74] The clinical features of affected members in these six families were similar to each other and similar to those of the non-Jewish and Jewish families first linked to 9q34; age at onset was typically between 6 and 18 years but could occur in the 30s to mid 40s. Symptoms usually started in an arm or leg, and often dystonia spread to involve other limbs and axial muscles. Occasionally, the neck or larynx was affected first, but facial muscles were not commonly involved, and speech was usually normal, except in those treated with thalamotomy. Analyses of haplotypes in these non-Jewish families did not suggest linkage disequilibrium, and it is presumed that most early-onset ITD in the non-Jewish population results from different mutation events in the DYT1 gene.

In two large North American non-Jewish families the DYT1 locus was excluded.[77,78] These families differ clinically from DYT1 families. In one of these non-DYT1 families, symptom onset was later (average 28.4 ± 14.8 years), and most affected family members had first symptoms in the neck or cranial muscles, rather than in a limb. Clinical features in the second "non-DYT1 family" were more similar to those of the typical DYT1 phenotype in that onset was early and that the dystonia began in a limb in many patients. The family differed in that, unlike typical primary dystonia resulting from DYT1, most affected individuals had significant disability because of laryngeal and other cranial muscle involvement.

Although most affected DYT1 gene carriers have early limb-onset dystonia, there is still a wide range of disease severity, and most gene carriers never express the gene. The cause of low penetrance and variable expression is unknown; possible mechanisms include genomic imprinting, anticipation, modifying genes, and environmental factors. Only a few studies have assessed families for these factors. LaBuda et al. analyzed the pedigrees of four previously published series of early-onset or generalized and segmental families for evidence of genomic imprinting or anticipation.[79] They found that the gender of the transmitting parent did not influence site of onset, age of onset, or distribution of dystonia, except that there was maternal transmission in almost all later-onset cases. The data were also consistent with anticipation; however, sampling bias could not be ruled out. A similar trend toward later onset of maternally transmitted dystonia was noted by deLeon in affected Ashkenazi DYT1 gene carriers, but this trend did not reach statistical significance.[80] This same group also assessed Ashkenazi and non-Jewish families with dystonia resulting from DYT1 and found no evidence for anticipation.[81] Intrafamilial correlations of the clinical features, such as age at onset and severity, have also been assessed for evidence of genetic heterogeneity or the presence of modifying genes. A very low correlation for age at onset between 23 first-degree relative pairs was found in one British study of generalized and segmental probands; the authors concluded that there was no evidence of genetic heterogeneity or nonallelic modifying genes; they suggested that ITD was a result of a single gene and that expression may be influenced by environmental factors.[82] The same group found that 16.4 percent of generalized and segmental ITD cases gave a history of trauma exacerbating or precipitating dystonia;[83] the dystonic movements either worsened or began in the same region of the body that was injured. They concluded that peripheral trauma may be a precipitant of dystonia in gene carriers.

LINKAGE DISEQUILIBRIUM OF DYT1 WITH 9q MARKERS IN ASHKENAZI JEWS

Soon after finding linkage of early-onset primary dystonia with 9q markers in Ashkenazi families, it became apparent that these families share a common haplotype of 9q alleles. Very strong allelic association or linkage disequilibrium between the DYT1 gene and a haplotype at the 9q marker loci ABL and ASS was found.[75] For markers that are tightly linked to the disease gene, such an association of linked alleles and the disease gene is consistent with the idea that the disease results largely from a single mutation and that equilibrium has not yet been achieved. The presence of very strong linkage disequilibrium at the relatively large genetic distance of at least a few centiMorgans also suggests that the mutation is recent; Risch et al. have calculated that it first appeared 350 years ago and probably originated in Lithuania or Byelorussia.[47]

A recent study of 174 Ashkenazi individuals affected with both early- and late-onset ITD used additional closely linked microsatellite markers and confirmed that the vast majority of both familial and isolated early-onset ITD cases carry the associated haplotype of 9q markers.[20] This study demonstrated that the clinical features of 1) first symptoms in a limb, (2) involvement of a leg in the course of disease, and (3) early onset discriminate between those who have the associated haplotype from those who do not with about 90 percent accuracy. Conversely, Ashkenazi ITD cases with adult cervical- and cranial-onset ITD very rarely carry the associated haplotype. This implies that a single-founder mutation accounts for most early limb-onset ITD among Ashkenazim, but this mutation event is not responsible for adult cervical- and cranial-onset ITD. The clinical-genetic difference suggests the presence of either different DYT1 mutations or other dystonia genes.

SUMMARY OF GENETICS AND COUNSELING RECOMMENDATIONS

Early-onset ITD is inherited as an autosomal-dominant trait with markedly reduced penetrance of 30–40 percent. Because of this, and also because of the variable expression of dystonia with mild cases being undiagnosed, it is not uncommon for a patient to be the only known person affected in a family.

In most Ashkenazi Jews and in many non-Jews with early limb-onset symptoms, dystonia is a result of mutations in the DYT1 gene on chromosome 9q34. The role of the gene in late-onset and cranial-cervical dystonia is not clear; evidence suggests that DYT1 is not involved in several families with these clinical subtypes, so other dystonia genes are being sought.

In Ashkenazi Jews with early-onset primary dystonia, there is very strong linkage disequilibrium between DYT1 and a haplotype of 9q34 alleles, implying the presence of a founder mutation in this population. As a practical application of this finding, it is possible to perform carrier testing in Ashkenazi families, including those in which only one member is affected with dystonia; diagnosis in an affected person can be confirmed, gene carrier status in an unaffected individual or fetus can be determined, and more accurate counseling can be provided.[84] It is recommended that when DYT1 diagnostic and carrier testing is used, genetic counseling also can be provided. The psychological and social implications of a disorder with autosomal-dominant inheritance that has markedly reduced penetrance and very variable expression are complex. The need for counseling is particu-

larly important for asymptomatic at-risk family members who want carrier testing and in cases of prenatal testing.

In non-Jewish families, carrier testing for the DYT1 gene remains restricted to large families that show linkage to the locus.

Evaluation

Until recently no diagnostic test was available to positively identify cases of ITD; the diagnosis depended on excluding secondary causes. With the finding of linked markers and linkage disequilibrium, it is now possible to diagnose ITD because of the common DYT1 mutation in Ashkenazi Jews (see above). The presence of the DYT1-associated haplotype (at loci D9S62, D9S63 and ASS) in an affected Ashkenazi individual indicates the disorder is a result of the common DYT1 mutation, with greater than 98 percent probability.[47] It is also possible to confirm the diagnosis of ITD resulting from DYT1 in large multiplex non-Jewish families in which linkage to the DYT1 region can be demonstrated.

For the great majority of non-Jewish ITD patients, as well as a minority of Jews with early-onset ITD and most late-onset ITD Jewish patients, the diagnosis of ITD remains one of exclusion. Common causes of symptomatic dystonia at Columbia-Presbyterian Medical Center are listed in Table 30-5, and diagnostic clues that dystonia is secondary are listed in Table 30-6. The investigation of all children and adolescents with uncomplicated "pure" dystonia must include exclusion of Wilson's disease by means of measurement of serum ceruloplasmin, slit-lamp examination for Kayser-Fleischer rings, and using magnetic resonance imaging (MRI). If the history and examination suggest that dystonia is symptomatic, then a more extensive workup is indicated (see Table 30-7).

Dopa-Responsive Dystonia (DRD)

DRD is a "variant" form of childhood-onset dystonia in which dystonia, although usually predominant, is often combined with parkinsonism and hyperreflexia. The disorder is inherited as an autosomal-dominant trait, with an overall reduced penetrance estimated at 30–40 percent.[17,85] There is a female predominance of 2–3:1, and segregation analysis confirms a higher penetrance in women, compared to that

TABLE 30-5 Common Causes of Torsion Dystonia at CPMC

Idiopathic		2431
Tardive dystonia	251	
Birth injury	114	
Psychogenic	82	
Peripheral trauma	68	
Head injury	50	
Stroke	40	
Encephalitis	29	
Miscellaneous	291	
		925
Total	3356	

TABLE 30-6 Clues That Dystonia Is Symptomatic

1. History of possible etiologic factor (e.g., head trauma, peripheral trauma, encephalitis, toxin exposure, drug exposure, perinatal anoxia).
2. Presence of neurological abnormality other than dystonia (e.g., dementia, seizures, ocular abnormalities, ataxia, weakness, spasticity, amyotrophy).
3. Presence of false weakness or nonphysiological sensory exam, or other clues of psychogenic etiology.
4. Onset of rest instead of action dystonia.
5. Early onset of speech involvement.
6. Hemidystonia.
7. Abnormal brain imaging.
8. Abnormal laboratory workup.

TABLE 30-7 Investigation of Patients Suspected as Having Symptomatic (Secondary) Dystonia

Serum ceruloplasmin
Erythrocyte sedimentation rate (ESR)
Antinuclear antibody (ANA)
Blood smear for acanthocytes
Chemistry profile, including uric acid and creatine phosphokinase (CPK)
Serum amino acids
Lysosomal screen
Alpha-fetoprotein
Very long-chain fatty acids
Mitochondrial DNA analysis
Lactate and pyruvate
Urine for amino acids, organic acids, oligosaccharides, and mucopolysaccharide concentrations
Biopsy of skin, muscle, and bone marrow
Ophthalmologic (including slit-lamp) examination
CSF examination
Brain MRI
Electromyography/nerve conduction studies
Electroretinogram
Evoked potential studies

in men. The phenotype in girls and boys, however, is similar, although it is not clear whether the disorder is more severe in one sex.[85,86] The disorder occurs worldwide and the prevalence in both England and Japan has been estimated at 0.5 per million.[17]

The typical clinical picture is that of a child, 4-8 years of age, who develops an abnormal gait that worsens as the day progresses and improves with sleep. The gait is frequently stiff-legged, and there may be plantar flexion or eversion. Dystonia may also involve the trunk, arms and, less commonly, the neck. Parkinsonian features include postural instability, hypomimia, and bradykinesia with progressive slowing, decrementing amplitude, and rigidity as rapid successive or alternating movements are attempted.[10,87] In about 25 percent of cases there is also hyperreflexia, particularly in the legs, and extensor plantar signs; because of the hyperreflexia and also the stiff-legged scissoring gait, children with DRD are not uncommonly misdiagnosed as having spastic diplegic cerebral palsy.[87]

The diagnosis of this condition depends on both the examination findings and a dramatic response to low-dose levodopa therapy. Total daily dosages of as little as 50–200 mg of levodopa (together with a dopa decarboxylase inhibitor) usually result in complete or nearly complete reversal of all signs and symptoms. Furthermore, unlike patients with juvenile Parkinson's disease, with which the disorder may be confused, these patients do not develop fluctuations and maintain an excellent response to levodopa.[87]

The pathogenesis of this condition is thought to involve the synthesis of dopamine. Evidence for this comes from cerebrospinal fluid (CSF), PET, pathological studies and, most recently, DNA analysis of the gene for guanosine triphosphate (GTP) cyclohydrolase 1. Specifically, CSF homovanillic acid (a major metabolite of dopamine) and tetrahydrobiopterin (a cofactor for tyrosine hydroxylase) levels are reduced, suggesting a defect in dopamine production.[88,89] Fluorodopa uptake PET scans, however, are normal, with nearly normal indicating a relatively intact nigrostriatal pathway structurally.[90] These two pieces of evidence are consistent with a functional defect in synthesis, possibly at a level before formation of dopa, e.g., at the level of tyrosine hydroxylation. Confirming the PET studies, which indicate limited structural damage to the nigrostriatal pathway, is a single recent detailed postmortem study.[91] Rajput et al. found a normal num-

ber of nigral dopamine neurons with normal nigral tyrosine hydroxylase activity and protein. There were no inclusion bodies or gliosis, and there was no degeneration in the striatum. The nigral dopamine cells, however, were hypopigmented; there was decreased dopamine in the nigra and striatum, and tyrosine hydroxylase protein and activity was diminished in the striatum.[90] Two possible explanations were posited to explain these findings: (1) disturbed dopamine synthetic capacity or (2) a developmental disturbance with insufficient terminal arborization of dopamine cells. Most recently, strong support for abnormal dopamine synthesis as the underlying cause of DRD has emerged from DNA analyses in DRD patients.

In 1993 Nygaard and colleagues mapped the DRD gene to chromosome 14q,[17] and in 1994 the enzyme GTP cyclohydrolase 1(GTPCH) was mapped to this DRD gene-containing region.[18] GTPCH converts GTP to D-erythro-7,8-dihydroneopterin triphosphate; it is the first step in tetrahydrobiopterin synthesis, and it is the rate-limiting step in this pathway. Thus, GTPCH was considered a candidate gene for DRD. The gene was then assessed in five Japanese DRD cases (four families and one sporadic), and four different point mutations were found in four of the five cases and in no controls. Also, introduction of two of these mutations into a prokaryotic expression system resulted in complete loss of enzyme activity.[18] It is presumed, then, that DRD is caused by insufficient levels of dopamine as a result of low levels of the converting enzyme in heterozygous carriers.

Mutations of GTPCH in DRD have yet to be confirmed by other investigators. Furthermore, there is an autosomal-recessive condition of GTPCH deficiency that produces hyperphenalaninemia and severe neurological dysfunction; heterozygous carriers of this condition do *not* have dystonia. Nevertheless, mutations in this converting enzyme provide a thrifty and cogent explanation for the clinical and laboratory findings in DRD.

References

1. Fahn S (ed): *Movement Disorders 2.* London, Butterworths, 1987, pp 332–358.
2. Fahn S: Concept and classification of dystonia. *Adv Neurol* 50:1–8, 1988.
2a. Redard P. Le torticollis et son traitement. Paris: Carre & Naud, 1898.
3. Oppenheim H: Uber eine eigenartige Krampfkrankheit des kindlichen und jugendlichen Alters (Dysbasia lordotica progressiva, Dystonia musculorum deformans). *Neurol Centrabl* 30:1090–1107, 1911.
4. Fahn S: The varied clinical expressions of dystonia. *Neurol Clin* 2:541–554, 1984.
5. Schwalbe W: *Eine eigentumliche tonische Krampfform mit hysterischen Symptomen. Medicin und chirugie.* Berlin: Universitats-Buchdrukerei von Gustav Schade, 1908.
6. Bernstein S. Ein Fall von Torsionkrampf. *Wien Klin Wochenschr* 25·1567–1571, 1912.
7. Abrahamson I: Presentation of cases of familial dystonia musculorum of Oppenheim. *J Nerv Ment Dis* 51:451–454, 1920.
8. Mankowsky BN, Czerny LI: Zur Frage uber die Hereditat der Torsiodystonie. Moschr Psychiatr Neurol 72:165–179, 1929.
9. Segawa M, Hosaka A, Miyagawa F, et al: Hereditary progressive dystonia with marked diurnal fluctuation. *Adv Neurol* 14:215–233, 1976.
10. Nygaard TG, Marsden CD, Duvoisin RC: Dopa-responsive dystonia. *Adv Neurol* 50:377–384, 1988.
11. Quinn NP, Rothwell JC, Thompson PD, Marsden CD: Hereditary myoclonic dystonia, hereditary torsion dystonia and hereditary essential myoclonus. An area of confusion. *Adv Neurol* 50:391–401, 1988.
12. Dobyns WB, Ozelius LJ, Kramer PL, et al: Rapid-onset dystonia—parkinsonism. *Neurology* 43:2596–2602, 1993.
13. Lee WH, Pascasoi FM, Fuintes FD, Viterbo GH. Torsion dystonia in Panay Philipines. *Adv Neurol* 14:137–151, 1976.
14. Wilhelmsen K, Weeks DE, Nygaard TG, et al: Genetic mapping of "Lubag" (X-linked dystonia-parkinsonism) in a Filipino kindred to the pericentromeric region of the X chromosome. *Ann Neurol* 29:124–131, 1991.
15. Kupke KG, Graeber MB, Miller U: Dystonia-parkinsonism syndrome (XDP) locus-flanking markers in Xq12-q21.1. *Am J Hum Genet* 50:808–815, 1992.
16. Ahmad F, Davis MB, Waddy HM, et al: Evidence for locus heterogeneity in autosomal dominant torsion dystonia. *Genomics* 15:9–12, 1993.
17. Nygaard TG, Wilhelmsen KC, Risch NJ, et al: Linkage mapping of dopa-responsive dystonia (DRD) to chromosome 14q. *Nature Genet* 5:386–391, 1993.
18. Ichinose H, Ohye T, Takahashi E, et al: Hereditary progressive dystonia with marked diurnal fluctuations caused by mutations in the GTP cyclohydrolase 1 gene. *Nature Genet* 8:236–242, 1994.
19. Bressman SB, de Leon D, Brin MF, et al: Idiopathic torsion dystonia among Ashkenazi Jews: Evidence for autosomal dominant inheritance. *Ann Neurol* 26:612–620, 1989.
20. Marsden CD, Harrison MJG, Bundey S. Natural history of idiopathic torsion dystonia. *Adv. Neurol* 14:177–187, 1976.
21. Greene P, Kang UJ, Fahn S. Spread of symptoms in idiopathic torsion dystonia. *Mov Disord* 10:143–152, 1995.
22. Pettigrew LC, Jankovic J: Hemidystonia: A report of 22 patients and a review of the literature. *J Neurol Neurosurg Psychiatry* 48:650–657, 1985.
23. Marsden CD, Obeso JA, Zarranz JJ, Lang AE. The anatomical basis of symptomatic hemidystonia. *Brain* 108:463–483, 1985.
24. Fish DR, Sawyers D, Allen PJ, et al: The effect of sleep on the dyskinetic movements of Parkinson's disease, Gilles de La Tourette syndrome, Huntington's disease, and torsion dystonia. *Arch Neurol* 48:210–214, 1991.
25. Jayne D, Lees AJ, Stern GM. Remission in spasmodic torticollis. *J Neurol Neurosurg Psychiatry* 47:1236–1237, 1984.
26. Friedman A, Fahn S: Spontaneous remissions in spasmodic torticollis. *Neurology* 36:398–400, 1986.
27. Eldridge R, Ince SE, Chernow B, et al: Dystonia in 61-year-old identical twins: Observations over 45 years. *Ann Neurol* 16:356–358, 1984.
28. Chan J, Brin MF, Fahn S: Idiopathic cervical dystonia: Clinical characteristics. *Mov Disord* 6:119–126, 1991.
29. Greene P, Kang U, Fahn S, et al: Double-blind, placebo-controlled trial of botulinum toxin injections for the treatment of spasmodic torticollis. *Neurology* 40:1213–1218, 1990.
30. Burke RE, Fahn S, Marsden CD, et al: Validity and reliability of a rating scale for the primary torsion dystonias. *Neurology* 35:73–77, 1985.
31. Yanagisawa N, Goto A, Narabayashi H: Familial dystonia musculorum deformans and tremor. *J Neurol Sci* 16:125–136, 1972.
32. Jankovic J, Fahn S: Physiologic and pathologic tremors. Diagnosis, mechanism, and management. *Ann Intern Med* 93:460–465, 1980.
33. Yanagisawa N, Goto A: Dystonia musculorum deformans: Analysis with electromyography. *J Neurol Sci* 13:39–65, 1971.
34. Jedynak CP, Bonnet AM, Agid Y: Tremor and idiopathic dystonia. *Mov Disord* 6:230–236, 1991.
35. Herz E: Dystonia. I. Historical review: Analysis of dystonic symptoms and physiologic mechanisms involved. *Arch Neurol Psychiatry* 51:305–318, 1944.
36. Masucci EF, Kurtzke JF, Sorin N: Myorhythmia: widespread movement disorder. Clinicopathological correlations. *Brain* 107:53–79, 1984.
37. Dubinsky RM, Gray CS, Koller WC: Essential tremor and dystonia. *Neurology* 43:2382–2384, 1993.
38. Fletcher NA, Harding AE, Marsden CD: A case-control study of idiopathic torsion dystonia. *Mov Disord* 6:304–309, 1991.
39. Lou JS, Jankovic J: Essential tremor: Clinical correlates in 350 patients. *Neurology* 41:234–238, 1991.
40. Conway D, Bain PG, Warner TT, et al: Linkage analysis with chromosome-9 markers in hereditary essential tremor. *Mov Disord* 8:374–376, 1993.
41. Durr A, Stevanin G, Jedynak CP, et al: Familial essential tremor and idiopathic torsion dystonia are different genetic entities. *Neurology* 43:2212–2214, 1993.
42. Shale HM, Truong DD, Fahn S: Tics in patients with other movement disorders. *Neurology* 36(suppl 1):118, 1986.
43. Stone LA, Jankovic J: The coexistence of tics and dystonia. *Arch Neurol* 48:862–865, 1991.
44. Nutt JG, Muenter MD, Aronson A, et al: Epidemiology of focal and generalized dystonia in Rochester, Minnesota. *Mov Disord* 3:188–194, 1988.
45. Zeman W, Dyken P: Dystonia musculorum deformans: Clinical, genetic and pathoanatomical studies. *Psychiatr Neurol Neurochirio* 77–121, 1967.
46. Zilber N, Korczyn AD, Kahana E, et al: Inheritance of idiopathic torsion dystonia among Jews. *J Med Genet* 21:13–20, 1984.
47. Risch N, de Leon, Bressman SB, et al: Genetic analysis of idiopathic torsion dystonia in Ashkenazi Jews: Evidence for the recent descent of Ashkenazim from a small fournder population. *Nature Genet* 9:152–159, 1995.
48. Rutledge JN, Hilal SK, Silver AJ, et al: Study of movement disorders and brain iron by MR. *AJNR Am J Neuroradiol* 8:397–411, 1987.
49. Zeman W: Dystonia: An overview. *Adv Neurol* 14:91–103, 1976.

50. Zeman W: Pathology of the torsion dystonias (dystonia musculorum deformans). *Neurology* 20(no. 11, part 2):79–88, 1970.

51. Zweig RM, Hedreen JC, Jankel WR, et al: Pathology in brainstem regions of individuals with primary dystonia. *Neurology* 38:702–706, 1988.

52. Hornykiewicz O, Kish SJ, Becker LE, et al: Brain neurotransmitters in dystonia musculorum deformans. *N Engl J Med* 315:347–353, 1986.

53. Jankovic J, Svendsen CN, Bird ED: Brain neurotransmitters in dystonia. *N Engl J Med* 316:278–279, 1987.

54. de Yebenes JG, Brin M, Mena MA, et al: Neurochemical findings in neuroacanthocytosis. *Mov Disord* 3:300–312, 1988.

55. Karbe H, Holthoff VA, Rudolf J, et al: Positron emission tomography demonstrates frontal cortex and basal ganglia hypometabolism in dystonia. *Neurology* 42:1540–1544, 1992.

56. Eidelberg D, Dhawan V, Takikawa S, et al: Regional metabolic covariation in idiopathic torsion dystonia: [18F]flurorodeoxyglucose PET studies. *Mov Disord* 7:297, 1992.

57. Leenders K, Hartvig P, Forsgren L, et al: Striatal [C-11]-N-methyl-spiperone binding in patients with focal dystonia (torticollis) using positron emission tomography. *J Neural Transm Park Dis Dement Sect* 5:79–87, 1993.

58. Benecke R, Strumper P, Weiss H: Electron transfer complex-I defect in idiopathic dystonia. *Ann Neurol* 32:683–686, 1992.

59. Regensburg J. Zur Klinik des hereditaren torsiondystonischen Symptomen komplexen. *Mosch Psychiatr Neurol* 75:323–345, 1930.

60. Zeman W, Kaelbling R, Pasamanick B. Idiopathic dystonia musculorum deformans. I. The hereditary pattern. *Am J Hum Genet* II:188–202, 1959.

61. Johnson, W, Schwartz G, Barbeau A. Studies on dystonia musculorum deformans. *Arch Neurol* 7:301–313, 1962.

62. Eldridge R: The torsion dystonias: Literature review and genetic and clinical studies. *Neurology* 20(no. 11, part 2):1–78, 1970.

63. Korczyn AD, Zilber N, Kahana E, Alter M: Inheritance of torsion dystonia: Reply. *Ann Neurol* 10:204–205, 1981.

64. Burke RE, Brin MF, Fahn S, et al: Analysis of the clinical course of non-Jewish, autosomal dominant torsion dystonia. *Mov Disord* 1:163–178, 1986a.

65. Risch N, Bressmam SB, de Leon D, et al: Segregation analysis of idiopathic torsion dystonia in Ashkenazi Jews suggests autosomal dominant inheritance. *Am J Hum Genet* 46:533–538, 1990.

66. Pauls DL, Korczyn AD: Complex segregation analysis of dystonia pedigrees suggests autosomal dominant inheritance. *Neurology* 40:1107–1110, 1990.

67. Larsson T, Sjogren T: Dystonia musculorum deformans: A genetic and clinical population study of 121 cases. *Acta Neurol Scand, Suppl* 17:1–232, 1966.

68. Fletcher NA, Harding AE, Marsden CD: A genetic study of idiopathic torsion dystonia in the United Kingdom. *Brain* 113:379–395, 1990.

69. Ozelius L, Kramer PL, Moskowitz CB, et al: Human gene for torsion dystonia located on chromosome 9q32-34. *Neuron* 2:1427–1434, 1989.

69b. Johnson W, Schwartz G, Barbeau A: Studies on dystonia musculorum deformans. *Arch Neurol* 7:301–313, 1962.

70. Kramer PL, Ozelius L, de Leon D, et al: Dystonia gene in Ashkenazi Jewish population located on chromosome 9q32-34. *Ann Neurol* 27:114–120, 1990.

71. Kwiatkowski DJ, Ozelius L, Kramer PL, et al: Torsion dystonia genes in two population confined to a small region on chromosome 9q32-34. *Am J Hum Genet* 49:366–371, 1991.

72. Schuback D, Kramer F, Ozelius L, et al: Dopamine beta-hydroxylase gene excluded in four subtypes of hereditary dystonia. *Hum Genet* 87:311–316, 1991.

73. Warner T, Fletcher NA, Davis MB, et al: Linkage analysis in British families with idiopathic torsion dystonia. *Brain* 116:739–744, 1993.

74. Kramer PL, Heiman GA, Gasser T, et al: The DYT1 gene on 9q34 is responsible for most cases of early limb-onset idiopathic torsion dystonia in non-Jews. *Am J Hum Genet* 55:468–475, 1994.

75. Ozelius LJ, Kramer PL, de Leon D, et al: Strong allelic association between the torsion dystonia gene *(DYT1)* and loci on chromosome 9q34 in Ashkenazi Jews. *Am J Hum Genet* 50:619–628, 1992.

76. Bressman SB, de Leon D, Kramer PL, et al: Dystonia in Ashkenazi Jews: Clinical characterization of a founder mutation. *Ann Neurol* 35:771–771, 1994.

77. Bressman SB, Heiman GA, Nygaard TG, et al: A study of idiopathic torsion dystonia in a non-Jewish family: Evidence for genetic heterogeneity. *Neurology* 44:283–287, 1994.

78. Bressman SB, Hunt AL, Heiman G, et al: DYT1 locus is excluded in a non-Jewish family with early onset dystonia. *Mov Disord* 9:626–632, 1994.

79. LaBuda MC, Fletcher NA, Korczyn AD, et al: Genomic imprinting and anticipation in idiopathic torsion dystonia. *Neurology* 43:2040–2043, 1993.

80. deLeon D, Bressman S, Brin MF, et al: Torsion dystonia in Ashkenazi Jew: Is there evidence for an imprinted gene. Mov Disord 7:297, 1992.

81. Almasy L, Bressman S, deLeon D, Risch N: No evidence for anticipation in 9q34-linked idiopathic torsion dystonia. *Am J Gen Epidemiol* 12:326, 1995.

82. Fletcher NA, Harding AE, Marsden CD: Intrafamilial correlation in idiopathic torsion dystonia. *Mov Disord* 6:310–314, 1991.

83. Fletcher NA, Harding AE, Marsden CD: The relationship between trauma and idiopathic torsion dystonia. *J Neurol Neurosurg Psychiatry* 54:713–717, 1991.

84. de Leon D, Brin MF, Murphy P, et al: Genetic counseling for idiopathic torsion dystonia: First use of DNA based carrier detection in Ashkenazic Jews. *Mov Disord* 6:273–274, 1991.

85. Nygaard TG: An analysis of North American families with dopa-responsive dystonia, in Segawa M (ed): *Hereditary Progressive Dystonia with Marked Diurnal Fluctuation.* Carnforth, United Kingdom: Parthenon Publishing, 1993, pp 97–104.

86. Louis E, Lynch T, Bressman SB, et al: Gender differences in dopa-responsive dystonia. *Neurology* 44A 368–369, 1994.

87. Nygaard TG, Marsden CD, Fahn S: Dopa-responsive dystonia: Long-term treatment response and prognosis. *Neurology* 41:174–181, 1991.

88. LeWitt PA, et al. Tetrahydrobiopterin in dystonia: Identification of abnormal metabolism and therapeutic trials. *Neurology* 36:760–764, 1986.

89. Furukawa Y, Nishi K, Kondo T, et al: CSF biopterin levels and clinical features of patients with juvenile parkinsonism. *Adv Neurol* 60:562–567, 1993.

90. Snow BJ, Nygaard TG, Takahashi H, Calne DB: Positron emission tomographic studies of dopa-responsive dystonia and early-onset idiopathic parkinsonism. *Ann Neurol* 34:733–738, 1993.

91. Rajput AH, Gibb WRG, Zhong XH, et al: Dopa-responsive dystonia: Pathologic and biochemical observations in a case. *Ann Neurol* 35:396–462, 1994.

Chapter 31

ADULT-ONSET IDIOPATHIC TORSION DYSTONIAS

EDUARDO S. TOLOSA AND M. J. MARTÍ

CLINICAL FEATURES OF THE IDIOPATHIC ADULT-
    ONSET FOCAL DYSTONIAS (IAOFD)
        Features Common to the Various IAOFD
        Blepharospasm (BSP)
        Oromandibular Distonia (OMD)
        Laryngeal Dystonia (Spasmodic Dysphonia)
        Cervical Dystonia
        Limb Dystonia (LD)
        Other Task-Specific Dystonias
        Other Focal Dystonias
ETIOLOGY
ANATOMIC SUBSTRATE AND PATHOPHYSIOLOGY
    OF THE FOCAL DYSTONIAS
DIFFERENTIAL DIAGNOSIS AND INVESTIGATIONS IN
    PATIENTS WITH FOCAL DYSTONIAS

Dystonia is characterized by involuntary muscular contractions causing twisting movements and abnormal postures. Etiologically dystonia can be classified into primary or idiopathic and secondary or symptomatic. Idiopathic torsion dystonia (ITD) is of unknown cause and is characterized by the development of dystonic movements and postures in the absence of other neurological deficits. Childhood-onset ITD usually involves one lower limb first, with later spread of the dystonia to involve the trunk or other body parts. It is often familial and usually is inherited in an autosomal-dominant pattern with a reduced penetrance. A genetic locus, the DYT1 locus, has been defined on chromosome 9q34 in some Jewish and non-Jewish families and is responsible for susceptibility to generalized torsion dystonia (see Chapter 30).[1] *Some variants of hereditary torsion dystonia can have their onset in early adulthood* (Table 31-1). An X-linked autosomal-recessive dystonia has been shown to occur on the island of Panay in the Philippines. Patients with this variant of ITD develop the initial symptoms in early adulthood, after the age of 20.[2] The disorder may start in the leg, but it may begin with equal or greater frequency in the upper body and generalizes in more than 50 percent of cases. It may also present phenotypically as parkinsonism. A recently reported case presented with adductor laryngeal breathing dystonia.[3] In a Swedish family with ITD of adult onset involving four generations, the disease showed variable expression with focal, multifocal, and generalized forms of dystonia in different family members. In this family, genetic analysis excluded the chromosomal region containing the DYT1 locus as being responsible for dystonia.[4] A new and unique form of hereditary torsion dystonia generally associated with parkinsonism

has been described recently by Dobyns et al.[5] This autosomal-dominant movement disorder, which has been labeled "rapid-onset dystonia-parkinsonism," consists of acute onset over days or weeks of dystonic spasms with parkinsonism. However, dystonia alone is also part of the phenotypic spectrum. Dystonia in patients with this disorder developed between 14 and 45 years of age. DYT1 has been excluded as a candidate gene for rapid-onset dystonia-parkinsonism.

The clinical spectrum of idiopathic dystonia is considerably different when it occurs in adults (Table 31-2). It generally involves the upper body, either the cranial musculature, neck, or arm, and the spasms tend to remain focal or spread only to the adjacent musculature. Idiopathic adult-onset focal dystonias (IAOFD) are sporadic, although, on occasion, more than one member in a family may have a focal dystonia. In Table 31-3 a list of the various IAOFD is depicted.

In the other chapters, childhood onset ITD (Chap. 30) and the symptomatic dystonias (Chap. 33) are covered in detail. In this chapter we cover ITD of adult onset, discussing the clinical manifestations of the various focal dystonias and the current thoughts on the underlying pathophysiology. The IAOFD are much more common than previously recognized. Its *prevalence* has been estimated by Nutt et al.[6] in the population living in Rochester, Minnesota, at 30 per 100,000, compared to generalized ITD at 3.4 per 100,000. Li et al.[7] reported that the prevalence of spasmodic torticollis (ST) in China was 3 per 100,000. A recent study in the Western area of Tottori Prefecture in Japan also encountered a lower prevalence (6.2 per 100,000) for focal dystonias than in Western countries.[8] The reasons for these differences in prevalence are unclear. In any case, these figures are probably underestimates, because patients with focal dystonias may go undiagnosed, and others do not seek medical help. Although the prevalence of generalized ITD is higher among the Ashkenazi Jewish population, this is not the case for IAOFD.[9]

Clinical Features of the Idiopathic Adult-Onset Focal Dystonias (IAOFD)

FEATURES COMMON TO THE VARIOUS IAOFD

Prolonged muscle contractions producing sustained abnormal movements or postures are the clinical hallmark of dystonia. In the IAOFD such spasms are limited to a single body region, with clinical symptoms depending primarily on the group of muscles involved.[10–12]

Characteristics common to the various focal dystonias of adulthood are shown in Table 31-4. IAOFD typically have their onset in the 4th or 5th decades but can also begin much earlier, and they typically affect women more than men (3:1). The onset is generally insidious, with symptoms varying depending on the body region involved and degree of spasm intensity. Dystonias occurring in adult life usually progress during the first few years after the initial manifestations. The time from onset to maximal disability, though, can vary considerably from patient to patient; in some patients, intense disabling spasms develop in just a few days or weeks whereas in others the disorder continues to spread slowly 10–

TABLE 31-1 Clinical Variants of ITD That Can Have Their Onset in Early Adulthood

1. Adult-onset ITD; autosomal-dominant Swedish family (see Ref. 4).
2. X-linked dystonia parkinsonism (see Ref. 2).
3. Rapid-onset dystonia parkinsonism syndrome (see Ref. 5).

TABLE 31-2 Early-Onset versus Late-Onset ITD

Early-Onset
  Onset <age 15
  Frequently starts in one leg
  Commonly becomes generalized with involvement of the trunk
  Usually hereditary
Adult-Onset
  Onset >20
  Focal onset
  Tends to remain focal
  Spreads to neighboring regions (segmental dystonia) in 20% of cases
  Usually sporadic

15 years after onset. Symptoms at onset can be intermittent, appearing only during times of emotional stress or without any apparent reason, but eventually they become steadily present. In about 20–30 percent of patients, dystonia extends to neighboring areas where the spasms are generally mild but can be prominent, with the patient then exhibiting signs of segmental dystonia. Occasionally, progression may skip an adjacent region to involve a more distant one, for example, a patient with blepharospasm (BSP) may later develop writer's cramp (WC) without signs of oromandibular (OMD) or laryngeal dystonia. In most cases dystonia stabilizes after a few years and, eventually, may improve slightly with the passage of time.

Remissions, either partial or complete, can occur in all of the IAOFD, almost always during the first 2–3 years from onset, and are always transient, lasting for days to months. At times symptoms can recur in a different area of the body than was affected originally. Remissions are more common in patients with ST than with other types of IAOFD, and they occur more often in those patients with an earlier age of onset.[10–12,13]

Similar to generalized ITD of childhood, at onset dystonic spasms in IAOFD patients frequently appear during movement (*action dystonia*) and disappear when the affected body part is at rest. With the passage of time, dystonic movements may involve muscles not normally used in a task or movement. In WC, for example, this phenomenon, which is called "*overflow*," produces the characteristic posture of elevation of the elbow and abduction of the shoulder. In some patients dystonia is triggered by actions in other parts of the body, as excessive unwanted concomitants to attempts at voluntary movements (e.g., dystonic movements appearing in the affected arm in a patient with WC when the patient is attempting to write with the healthy hand). Primary idiopathic dystonia often starts as a *task-specific* dystonia. With progression, however, the dystonic movements may appear with other activities. As an example, in patients with limb dysto-

nia, dystonic cramps may occur initially only when writing but later also when using the hands for other tasks such as eating or sawing. In some patients with spasmodic dysphonia, laryngeal spasms occur initially only when the patient is speaking but not when singing or whispering; however, eventually they may be triggered by these actions as well. As the disease progresses, dystonia also may appear even at rest and, if left untreated, may evolve into fixed postures that eventually cause permanent contractures, as can be seen in long-standing untreated cervical dystonia. Although dystonic spasms are usually continuous, the timing and intensity of the movements can be influenced by various factors. Emotional stress and fatigue typically worsen dystonia, whereas rest and relaxation improve the spasms and they disappear during sleep. Some patients notice that certain "sensory tricks" can transiently reduce their dystonia. *This reduction in dystonia by tactile or proprioceptive stimuli* is a feature almost unique to dystonic movements.[14] Touching the back of the head or chin with one or more fingers, for example, allows some patients with torticollis to straighten their head, and gently leaning on the wall when standing may eliminate truncal dystonia transiently.

In addition to prolonged dystonic spasms patients with IAOFD, like those with generalized dystonias, can exhibit other types of involuntary movements. In some patients rapid movements resembling myoclonus occur. Obeso et al.[15] have described *myoclonus* occurring in patients with idiopathic dystonia that occurs irregularly, is seen mostly on voluntary muscle activation, and is superimposed on dystonic muscle spasms. These rapid movements can cause diagnostic confusion in some cases. Rhythmic, tremor-like move-

TABLE 31-3 IAOFD Syndromes

Muscle Groups Involved	Terminology
A. Orbicularis oculi and neighboring facial muscles	Essential BSP, dystonic BSP
B. Peribuccal muscles and platysma	Lower facial dystonia
C. Lower facial, masticatory, pharyngeal, and lingual muscles	OMD syndrome
D. A plus B or A plus C	Meige's syndrome, BSP-OMD syndrome
E. Laryngeal muscles	Laryngeal dystonia, spasmodic dysphonia
F. Cervical muscles	Cervical dystonia, ST
G. Hand, forearm, and arm muscles	Upper LD, WC, TSD, musician's dystonia, athlete's TSD

BSP, blepharospasm; OMD, oromandibular dystonia; ST, spasmodic torticollis; LD, limb dystonia; WC, writer's cramp; TSD, task-specific dystonia.

TABLE 31-4 Clinical Features Common to the Various Adult-Onset Focal Dystonias

Onset generally in 4th to 6th decades

Female predominance

Insidious onset, gradual progression during the first few years

Spread to neighboring regions not uncommon but almost never generalizes

Remissions infrequent but can occur in the early years

Worsened by emotional stress and fatigue

Improved by relaxation and rest

Sensory "tricks" transiently improve dystonic spasms

Tremor is common: focal "dystonic" tremor or essential-like tremor

TABLE 31-5 Eyelid Dysfunction in 17 Patients with Dystonic BSP*

Eyelid Dysfunction	No. of Patients*
Clonic spasms	17 (3)
Dystonic spasms	9 (6)
"Apraxia" of lid opening	11 (3)
Tonic orbicularis contractions	8 (3)
Reflex BSP	6 (2)

*In parentheses is the number of patients in whom the specific type of eyelid dysfunction is the only or the predominant one.

SOURCE: *Modified from Tolosa et al.*[26]

ments are not uncommon in patients with dystonia, especially when the patient attempts to actively resist the involuntary movements. This focal, action-type tremor is generally irregular and slow, and it is called *dystonic tremor.*[16] Occasionally, it may precede the onset of dystonia, as described by Rivest and Marsden,[17] or it may be the only manifestation of the dystonic disorder. Another type of tremor encountered in the idiopathic dystonias, in up to 20 percent of patients in some series, is one that resembles essential tremor and is frequently observed in both hands, even though they may not be affected by dystonic spasms, or in the head. It is a regular tremor, generally of modest amplitude, and has been reported in torticollis, WC, Meige's syndrome, and other focal dystonias.[16,18,19] True essential tremor has been said to occur commonly in patients with idiopathic dystonias, but it is not clear whether this type of postural tremor is a form of essential tremor, or whether it is an expression of some dystonia-related physiological abnormality. The finding that families with essential tremor do not have the DYT1 gene, as determined by means of linkage analysis, indicates that the two disorders are not genetically identical.[20] Mild parkinsonism has been described in some of the IAOFD, such as Meige's syndrome[21] and WC.[19]

BLEPHAROSPASM (BSP)

Patients with BSP have intermittent or sustained bilateral eyelid closure as a result of involuntary contractions of the orbicularis oculi muscles. Mild spasms of the frontalis and the middle and lower facial muscles also occur frequently. When the spasms are limited to the orbital or periorbital muscles, it is frequently called essential or dystonic BSP. The association of BSP with OMD is called cranial dystonia, or Meige's syndrome, because it was the French neurologist Henri Meige who, in 1910, first described in detail this syndrome, calling it "spasm facial median."[21,22] BSP affects women more than men and has its onset in about the 6th decade of life.

Patients with BSP, which may begin in one eye only, complain of eye discomfort, involuntary eye closure, eye narrowing or inability to open the eyes. Common complaints at onset are excessive blinking, eye irritation, burning, and photophobia, similar to symptoms of ocular surface, lid margin, and tear film disorders. BSP patients have variable degrees of difficulty with tasks such as reading, watching television, or driving, and they are frequently disabled, both

occupationally and socially, by the spasms and the resulting functional blindness.[21–25]

Spasms of eye closure are generally aggravated by stress and disappear during sleep. BSP also is worsened by exposure to bright light, and for this reason most patients with BSP wear dark glasses. Other actions that frequently worsen the spasms are looking upward, walking, and reading and, less commonly driving, watching television, or looking downward. Maneuvers or tricks that alleviate some patients include talking, lying down, humming or singing, yawning, laughing, pressure on the eyebrows or the temple, chewing, and opening the mouth.

There are several clinical presentations of BSP (see Ref. 26; Table 31-5). In the dystonic variety, the more common type, the spasms are prolonged, lasting for several seconds or even minutes, and the eyebrows are displaced downward, below the superior orbital rim (Charcot's sign). In the clonic form the repetitive spasms of eye closure (blepharoclonus) are fast and resemble normal blinking. In some patients, as a result of contractions of the pretarsal part of the orbicularis, BSP mimics apraxia of lid opening.[26–29] In these patients the eyes are closed in the absence of overt spasm, and the patient can not initiate or sustain eye opening. Elevation of the eyebrows, as a result of contraction of the frontalis muscles in an effort by the patient to open the eyelids, is common in this form of BSP (Fig. 31-1). Patients with this type of spasm frequently try to open the eyes with their fingers, pulling the lids apart. At times reflex BSP is also present, and such attempts to open the eyes manually are met with increasing resistance by stronger spasms of the orbicularis oculi.[30] Yet in other patients, a persistent narrowing of the palpebral fissure without complete eye closure is observed. The different types of spasms described here can be seen in a given BSP patient but sometimes can occur in isolation.

OROMANDIBULAR DYSTONIA (OMD)

In patients with OMD, spasms occur in the region of the jaw, lower face, and mouth.[31–33] Involvement of the masticatory muscles frequently produces spasms of jaw closure or opening, jaw protrusion, or lateral deviation. Spasms of jaw closure associated with involuntary contractions of the temporalis muscle and the masseters can produce trismus and bruxism. Involuntary contractions of the lower facial muscles result in spasms of lip tightening, involuntary retraction of the corners of the mouth, and lip pursing. Platysmal contrac-

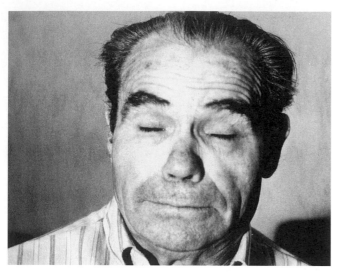

FIGURE 31-1 "Apraxia" of lid opening in patient with BSP. Oribucularis oculi spasms are not clearly evident. The patient tries to open the eyes with vigorous frontalis contraction.

tions are also common. Lingual dystonia is manifested by lateral or upper deviation of the tongue, as well as by tongue protrusion. OMD in isolation is a relatively uncommon form of dystonia, but it is usually very disabling, causing jaw pain, dysarthria, and difficulty chewing and eating. Sensory tricks in OMD include touching the chin, chewing gum, biting on a toothpick, talking, and applying pressure in the submental area. In some patients OMD is triggered by actions such as biting, chewing, or speaking.

In patients with OMD, spasms frequently occur in adjacent regions, and anterocollis, dysphonia, contraction of the nasalis muscles, and BSP are commonly present.

LARYNGEAL DYSTONIA (SPASMODIC DYSHONIA)

Spasmodic dysphonia (SD) occurs between 30 and 50 years of age and, like other IAOFD, affects women more than men. It was originally described by Traube in 1871[34] as "a spastic form of nervous hoarseness" and was wrongly considered to be a psychogenic disorder until recently. Even today, many patients are referred to psychiatrists because the correct diagnosis is not made when the patient presents for treatment. Dystonic spasms in SD occur during speech (action- and task-specific dystonia (TSD)), whereas the muscles and anatomic structures of the larynx are normal during rest. There are two types of SD[35–39]: Adductor SD, which is caused by irregular hyperadduction of the vocal cords, and abductor SD, which is characterized by contraction of the posterior cricoarytenoid muscles during the action of speaking, resulting in inappropriate abduction of the vocal cords. Patients with adductor SD exhibit a choked, strained, staccato, strangled voice quality with abrupt initiation and termination of vocalization, resulting in short breaks in phonation. There is decreased smoothness of speech, which becomes less intelligible. Usually, singing is less affected than speaking, except in severe cases.

Abductor SD is much less frequent. Patients exhibit a breathy, effortful voice, resulting in aphonic whispered seg-

ments of speech.[40] The voice is reduced in loudness, and speech is difficult to understand.

Onset of symptoms in SD is usually gradual, at times following an upper respiratory infection and during either occupational or emotional stress.[41] The initial complaints are increased effort and loss of voice and pitch control, at times only during stress. After 1–2 years of progression, the disease tends to stabilize and become chronic. Maneuvers or tricks that ameliorate SD are usually not as obvious as in other focal dystonias, but some patients report improving transiently when they press their hand on the back of their head[42] or press their hand on their abdomen. Also, speech can improve briefly after a yawn or a sneeze. Laughing, coughing, or crying do not become affected, but in 20–30 percent of patients, dystonia occurs elsewhere, usually in the cranial or cervical region. About 20 percent of patients have an irregular, audible dystonic voice tremor that can, at times, precede the appearance of the dystonic laryngeal spasms.

CERVICAL DYSTONIA

Dystonia of the neck muscles results in a condition characterized by abnormal head and neck posture called cervical dystonia, commonly referred to as spasmodic torticollis (ST). Patients with ST experience jerky movements of the head and intermittent or constant head deviation at rest. Deviation of the head can take any combination of directions: lateral rotation of the head (torticollis), frequently associated with a head tilt, is the most common,[43–45] but there can be lateral torticollis alone, anterocollis, and retrocollis. Frequently, the shoulder is elevated on the side toward which the chin is pointing, and a mild degree of dystonia can be detected commonly in the proximal muscles of the limbs on the same side. Unlike other focal dystonias, the incidence of pain in ST is remarkably high (over two-thirds of the patients) and contributes to disability.[43–45] Pain is most frequent in patients with constant head deviation, and although it is usually localized in the neck, patients can develop secondary cervical radiculopathy (over 30 percent of patients in some series) and experience pain radiating into the arm. Head tremor, considered of a dystonic tremor, and/or hand tremor (essential tremor), occur in about one-third of ST patients.[43,46,47]

Sensory tricks used by torticollis patients to reduce the intensity of spasms include touching of the chin, face, or occiput. One such trick, called "geste antagonistique," consists of correction of head position when a very light touch or pressure is applied to the chin, cheek, or elsewhere in the head contralateral to the direction of the head turn. This trick was used in the past to support a psychogenic basis for ST. Symptoms frequently lessen when the patient lies down in bed, and they worsen when the patient walks and or is under stress. In addition to cervical dystonia, about 20 percent of ST patients exhibit cranial (e.g., BSP) or arm-hand dystonia, which is usually mild.

Reported female to male ratios for idiopathic ST are approximately 2:1. Mean age at onset is between 38 and 42 years, with most cases clustering in the 4th through the 6th decades.[48] Severity of dystonia tends to progress during the first months or years of the illness, and the dystonic spasms can later spread to the oromandibular region or arm and, exceptionally, the leg. Even though ST is mild in some patients, it is usually disabling, interfering with the patients' daily activities and causing frequent pain. In patients with long-standing cervical dystonia contractures may develop and fixed deformities may occur.

Cervical dystonia has been described after neck trauma. Some of these post-traumatic cases differ clinically from the more typical cases of idiopathic cervical dystonia because of the presence of marked limitation of range of motion, absence of geste antagonistique, and lack of improvement after sleep.[49,50]

About 10 percent of patients experience brief spontaneous remission of symptoms, and another 10 percent, mostly with an earlier age at onset, experience a longer period of remission (2–3 years) that occurs usually during the first 5 years of the illness.[51-53]

LIMB DYSTONIA (LD)

LD is characterized by involuntary contractions of limb musculature that result in twisting and repetitive movements or abnormal postures in the extremities. LD can affect the leg or the arm and can be focal, as in WC, or segmental, as when involving the arm and the neck (brachial) or leg and trunk (crural). It is always present in patients with generalized dystonia and in hemidystonia when the upper and the lower extremities on one side are affected.[54,55]

Idiopathic LDs are frequently action dystonias, superimposed on voluntary movements such as writing, using eating utensils, or walking. As the disease progresses, the dystonic postures become more sustained and fixed, even more so when they occur in the legs. When occurring in the arm, distal involvement is more common in the form of wrist flexion, ulnar deviation, and supination. However, elevation, internal rotation, and abduction of the arm can occur also. In some patients the arm pulls behind the patient's back spontaneously.[11]

Many upper LDs are task-specific, that is, they occur exclusively or primarily when the patient performs a specific task. The most frequent task-specific dystonia (TSD) of the arm is WC but, in addition to writing, a large number of dystonia-inducing tasks have been reported in musicians[56,57] (e.g., guitarists, trumpet players) or sportsmen (e.g., golfers, snooker players, dart throwers).[54,58]

Symptoms of WC appear as soon as the pen is picked up or after a few words of writing. It usually presents as a forceful exaggeration of the usual grip of the pen, but in other instances hyperextension of the fingers may prevent the pen from being held in the hand. The wrist can show hyperextension or flexion, or forced supination or pronation. Arm and shoulder involvement can also occur. Writing is jerky, shaky, and laborious, and it may be accompanied by a sensation of tension and discomfort in the forearm. At times, frank pain is associated with writing. Frequently, writing becomes impossible after a few words. Classically, patients with WC can manage to write on a wallboard. Some patients find relief by stabilizing the writing hand by holding it with the contralateral one or by using thicker writing devices.[59-62]

WC is classified as "simple" when dystonia occurs only when writing and as "dystonic" when the spasms appear with other hand tasks, such as using a screwdriver or shaving. WC may evolve from simple to dystonic in about one-third of cases but, generally, the severity of the condition remains relatively unchanged. Extension of dystonia to other adjacent or more distant body regions can occur over months to years after onset of symptoms. In about 25 percent of patients who try to write with the noninvolved hand, bilateral WC develops.[54] As with other dystonias, tremor occurs in about one-third of the cases. It can be a postural symmetrical hand tremor or a tremor triggered by writing. In such cases the differentiation with primary writing tremor, a form of task-specific tremor, can be quite difficult.[63,64]

It is not clear whether extensive writing can cause WC. It is likely that patients who write frequently will recognize their symptoms earlier and will seek early medical attention.[54] WC can be the earliest manifestation of idiopathic generalized torsion dystonia, but it can also represent the presenting complaint of neurological disorders, such as Parkinson's disease or progressive supranuclear palsy.[65-68]

In patients with WC several electrophysiological abnormalities have been found, and these are shared with other TSD (see Ref. 69 for review). Cocontraction of antagonist muscles occurs, such that movement can be undertaken only with the greatest of effort. There is lack of selectivity in attempts to perform independent finger movements, and neural activation may spread ("overflow") to involve muscles not normally used in the task of writing, for example, abduction of the shoulder. Failure to activate the appropriate muscles may also occur. These findings highlight the fact that patients have more problems with voluntary actions than with involuntary muscle spasm.

Dystonia occurring in the lower extremities usually affects distal joints, principally the ankle, with plantar flexion and inversion of the foot. The sole of the foot can also cup and the toes can flex. Initially, foot dystonia occurs only when one is walking, being absent with the limb at rest. Frequently, running, walking in tandem, or walking backwards fails to trigger the abnormal posture. The initial equinovarus posture that occurs when the patient is walking may evolve into a fixed dystonic posture, commonly causing plantar flexion, extension of the knee, and extension, internal rotation and abduction of the hip.

When lower LD occurs in childhood, it usually heralds the onset of early generalized dystonia.[70] When lower LD occurs after the age of 20, it suggests the possibility of focal central nervous system structural disease. Also, when dystonia affects the foot in an adult, the possibility of Parkinson's disease or another parkinsonian syndrome should be considered, because kinesigenic foot dystonia is an early sign of young-onset Parkinson's disease.[66]

OTHER TASK-SPECIFIC DYSTONIAS

In addition to WC, other TSD have been described in milkers, seamstresses, cobblers, shoemakers, musicians, and others whose work involves frequent repetitive movements.[54,71] This population of individuals who repeatedly overuse their limbs is also more predisposed to nerve entrapments and muscle and joints disorders. This may lead to some clinical confusion. Tasks capable of inducing action dystonia almost always require either highly repetitive movements or extreme motor precision. The majority of TSDs involve the upper limb and, rarely, the leg, probably because the use of the lower limb for precise repetitive tasks is unusual. They have been described in knife sharpeners, dancers, tradesmen, cyclists, sewing machine workers, and cello players.

WC is the most common TSD. Telegraphist cramp, found in one study to affect 14 percent of 516 telegraphists,[72] has been progressively disappearing since the introduction of the modern telephone. It is likely that typist's cramp will become more prevalent with the expansion of keyboard-dependent telecommunication. Musicians, with the years of practice and repetition of precise and complicated movements required to achieve professional status, are prone to overuse syndromes, and as many as 15 percent of *professional musicians* may be suffering from overuse syndromes.[56] These focal dystonias are particularly devastating. They can occur in musicians using almost any kind of instrument but are more common in piano players. Newmark and Hochberg[57] evaluated the focal motor syndromes in 57 instrumental musicians and noted three stereotyped afflictions: (a) flexion of 4th and 5th fingers in pianists, (b) flexion of the 3rd finger in guitarists and (c) extension of the 3rd finger in clarinetists. The disabilities in these patients were not progressive. In brass instrumentalists, as well as in double-reed players, musician's dystonia may involve the peribuccal and cervical muscles. Musician's cramps are usually refractory to medical treatment, rest, or physical therapy. Alteration of playing technique may help some patients. The response to botulinum toxin injections is generally insufficient, because for professional musicians, even a marked response to treatment is of no benefit when the abilities needed to play professionally are not maintained.

Athlete's TSD can occur in golfers and other sportsmen, such as tennis players, snooker players, or dart throwers. Golfer's TSD—the "yips"—may affect as many as 28 percent of golfers, more commonly afflicting those who have more cumulative years of golfing.[58] Involuntary movements emerge particularly during putting but are much less evident during chipping or driving.[73] As in patients with other TSD, golfers with the yips use complementary strategies, for example, changing hand preference. About one-fourth of them report that other activities can be similarly affected.

OTHER FOCAL DYSTONIAS

Rarely, isolated dystonia of the pharyngeal muscles occurs causing dysphagia (dystonic dysphagia). Disability in these patients may be severe, and surgical section of the crycopharyngeus muscle may be needed to improve swallowing.[74-76] Patients with dystonic dysphagia frequently have OMD or neck dystonia as well. Isolated lingual dystonia is very rare,[77] but lingual dystonia can certainly be the most prominent manifestation of OMD. Another adult-onset focal dystonia occasionally encountered is *truncal dystonia.* In these patients, continuous or repetitive spasms cause flexion, extension, scoliosis, or torsion of the trunk.[74] As with other focal dystonias, spasms at onset may occur only when walking or standing but, eventually, they can be present even when the patient is lying down. In some patients, spasms are rapid enough

to resemble myoclonus, and this has been referred to as "woodpecker dystonia." Extension to adjacent regions can occur, for example, retrocollis, involvement of proximal limb muscles, or pelvic involvement (so-called copulatory dystonia). Sensory tricks that improve truncal dystonia include gently leaning against the wall when standing, pressing in the back of the neck, or pressing on the hips.

Abdominal wall dystonia (belly dancer's dyskinesia) has recently been described,[78] and Caviness et al.[79] have reported a group of patients with focal or segmental dyskinesias affecting the ears, back, shoulder girdle, abdomen, and pelvic girdle that closely resemble focal dystonias. In these patients the movements were slow, sinuous, semirhythmic, and associated with long-duration bursts of electromyogram (EMG) activity in neurophysiological studies. Peripheral trauma may have played a role in the pathogenesis of the movements in some patients.

Etiology

The cause of adult-onset focal dystonias remains unknown in the majority of cases. Unlike childhood-onset classic ITD, in which current evidence indicates that the mode of inheritance is autosomal-dominant with reduced penetrance in both Jews and non-Jews,[80] the *role of heredity* in adult-onset cases is not well understood. It is not clear to what extent the clinical distinction between early- and late-onset ITD reflects underlying genetic distinctions. A genetic study of ITD in the United Kingdom[81] suggests that in the non-Jewish population a proportion of late-onset cases may be because of the same genetic factors that underlie early onset ITD. On the other hand, findings by Bressman et al.[82] and by Risch et al.[83] suggest that most late-onset ITD in the Ashkenazi Jewish population is etiologically distinct from early-onset ITD.

A role for heredity in adult-onset dystonias is suggested by the observed familial cases of orofacial dystonia, WC, and ST[84,85] and the reports of Meige's syndrome and cervical dystonia in apparently identical twins.[86] Furthermore, several large studies of focal dystonias have reported positive family histories, ranging from 2 to 15 percent of patients.[87] Affected relatives displayed focal and segmental signs but not generalized dystonia. Waddy et al.[88] found that 25 percent of 40 non-Jewish patients with focal dystonia had relatives in whom dystonia could be identified. Most of the secondary cases were not aware of any dystonia. They concluded on the basis of segregation analysis, that focal dystonia is commonly transmitted by an autosomal-dominant gene with reduced penetrance and variable expressivity, and they suggested that a single gene may account for inherited dystonias, regardless of whether they are generalized or focal. Defazio et al. made similar observations in a family study of 29 patients with BSP and craniocervical dystonia.[89] Familial patients were clinically indistinguishable from sporadic ones.

Autoimmune disorders, such as thyroid disease, systemic lupus erythematosus, rheumatoid arthritis, or myasthenia gravis, have been associated with primary dystonia.[25,90] Nivaler et al.,[91] however, could not find anticentral nervous system antibodies in the serum of 11 patients with cranial dystonia, using the direct immunoperoxidase technique; hence, they could not find support for an autoimmune etiology for these disorders. Use of sympathicomimetic drugs, eye color, and focal brain stem and diencephalic lesions have been associated with the focal dystonias only in occasional patients. Therefore, they are not widely accepted as risk factors.

Several studies have indicated that dystonia may be precipitated by *peripheral factors* such as overuse, misuse, or trauma. Fletcher et al.[93] recently showed that peripheral trauma[92] may trigger dystonia in carriers of the idiopathic torsion dystonia gene. A similar phenomenon in isolated BSP is suggested by the finding that up to 12 percent of patients report the occurrence of ocular trauma or lesion before the onset of the movement disorder.[94] Peripheral trauma has also been reported in 5–12 percent of patients with cervical dystonia,[95,96] occurring 3–6 months before the onset of symptoms. Similarly, cases of OMD have occurred soon after facial lacerations and dental work.[97] Laryngitis can precede spasmodic dysphonia.[98] Occasionally, focal LD may be associated with extremity injury, such as electrical injury[99] or with reflex sympathetic dystrophy. Tremor and dystonia are the movement disorders most often associated with reflex sympathetic dystrophy ("causalgia-dystonia syndrome"),[100,101] and it almost always develops after peripheral trauma. In these cases the development of pain may be of importance.

Peripheral factors are also generally accepted to play a role in a variety of occupational or TSDs, such as WC, typist cramp, or the focal dystonias occurring in musicians or sportsmen. A recently described case of OMD occurring in an auctioneer is another example of a focal dystonia that was possibly related to muscle overuse.[102] Inzelberg et al.[103] recently found a highly significant relationship between the motor dominance and the laterality of limb onset in ITD patients, which suggests that the preferred use of a limb may trigger the onset of dystonia.

The exact role of muscle overuse or trauma in the genesis of dystonia remains to be clarified. A recent study by Fletcher et al.[104] does not support the notion that trauma is important in idiopathic dystonia. In their study of 71 patients with ITD and 71 matched controls investigating the role of environmental factors in the development of the disorder, trauma was no more frequent among patients than among control subjects, either in the year preceding the onset of dystonia in the index patients or at any other time. It is unlikely that trauma alone is sufficient for dystonia to develop, because if this were the case, dystonia would be much more common. It has been postulated that trauma may trigger the expression of a previously subclinical or very mild dystonia or trigger dystonia only in patients with preexisting susceptibility, perhaps on a genetic basis.[10,92,105]

It has been suggested that complex movement disorders like dystonia, occurring after a peripheral nerve or spinal nerve root lesion, are generated by reorganization of spinal motor circuitry or by changes in supraspinal somatosensory integration that result in altered basal ganglia function.[105] Some authors believe that there may be a psychogenic basis for many cases of posttraumatic dystonia.[106,107]

Are the adult onset dystonias a focal manifestation of ITD? The concept has been put forward[108,109] that the different IAOFD represent focal manifestations of ITD, with the final distribution of dystonia reflecting the age and site of onset. Several observations support this hypothesis. The clinical manifestations of dystonia in the IAOFD are similar to those encountered in generalized ITD, including the phenomenon of sensory tricks, and focal dystonia can be the presenting feature of generalized ITD. Focal dystonias, for example, BSP, occur in adult members of families with dominantly inherited ITD, suggesting that in these cases the focal dystonias are *formes frustes* of generalized dystonia.[110] Also, similar neurophysiological abnormalities have been found in the IAOFD and the generalized dystonias, and both respond similarly to the same types of drugs.

Whether the IAOFD and generalized ITD are the same disorder, differing only in the extent of the disease, or whether they are distinct and separate entities, however, remains unclear. Genetic studies have shown that dystonia that has its onset in the cranial or cervical regions is rarely associated with the DYT1 gene,[111] suggesting that most cases of focal dystonia not beginning in a limb are distinct from those of generalized dystonia. The DYT1 gene, on the other hand, is present in a high percentage of patients with onset in a limb, suggesting that patients with LD that remains focal are part of the same entity as generalized dystonia.

Anatomic Substrate and Pathophysiology of the Focal Dystonias

Autopsy studies have been performed in 10 patients with presumed idiopathic cranial dystonia. No significant abnormalities were found in four; one had an "incidental" small angioma of the pons; and the other patients had relatively nonspecific abnormalities.[112,113] Mosaic neuronal cell loss and gliosis have been seen in two patients,[114] and three patients have been reported as having cell loss and gliosis of the substantia nigra pars compacta and other brain stem nuclei.[115,116] In two of these patients, there were abundant Lewy bodies present. Lesions in the basal ganglia, thalamus, cerebral cortex, diencephalon, and brain stem have been reported to be associated with some of the focal dystonias.[117,118]

Mostly based on the correlations that exist between the secondary dystonias and lesions of the putamen and thalamus, it is currently believed that the focal dystonias result from an abnormality in the basal ganglia. Static imaging studies have not identified any definite abnormalities in the idiopathic focal dystonias. Dynamic imaging studies, using positron emission tomography (PET), showed hypometabolism in the caudate and lentiform nucleus and in the frontal projection fields of the mediodorsal thalamic nucleus.[119] Hence, functional disturbance in the basal ganglia and their frontal connections is thought to be the underlying cause of the dystonias. In Meige's syndrome relative glucose hypermetabolism of the putamen has been detected.[120] In addition, there are bilateral relative increments in glucose utilization for the thalamus and primary sensorimotor cortices. When the subjects are studied during sleep, the same pattern of hypermetabolism is present, even though no dystonic spasms are occurring.[121] In a recent study cerebral blood flow was measured using $H_2^{15}O$ and PET, at rest and during movement, in a group of six patients with ITD, one of which had isolated WC. Results demonstrated overactivity of the striatum and its frontal association projection areas. Reduced activity in motor executive areas was also detected.[122]

How dysfunction of the basal ganglia results in dystonia is unclear. In dystonia, basal ganglia dysfunction may result in an inability to target inhibition to opposite sets of neurons in the cortex, thus producing excessive motor output, particularly during movement.[10] Ridding et al.[123] have recently reported that ipsilateral corticocortical inhibition is abnormal in patients with WC, which could represent a disturbance in the excitability of local intracortical inhibitory interneurons. In a patient with unilateral focal dystonia resulting from a lesion of the contralateral putamen, Hanjima et al.[124] have detected, using double cortical stimulation techniques, hyperexcitability of the motor cortex ipsilateral to the putaminal lesion with normal excitability of the sensory cortex.

In addition to these alterations in the cortex, many reflex abnormalities have been described in dystonic patients, and these are greatest in muscles affected by dystonia. In cranial, laryngeal, and cervical dystonia blink reflex and masseter inhibitory reflex abnormalities have been clearly documented (Fig. 31-2), suggesting that both excitatory and inhibitory interneuronal pathways in the brainstem are perturbed.[125–127] In many of the focal dystonias, such as ST or spasmodic dysphonia, subclinical abnormalities of the blink reflexes generally occur, suggesting that the clinical abnormalities are not a consequence of the abnormalities observed in these tests. Also, treatment with botulinum toxin markedly improves BSP and ST, but clinical improvement is not accompanied by a concomitant normalization of the blink reflex excitability curve in these patients.[128,129] Another example of abnormal brain stem interneuronal excitability is the finding

of reduced exteroceptive inhibition of the sternocleidomastoid muscle after a supraorbital nerve stimulus.[130] Vestibular abnormalities have also been reported in ST, but they could be secondary to the abnormal head position.[131,132] Reciprocal inhibition has been extensively studied in dystonia. It refers to the active inhibition of activity in antagonist muscles during voluntary contraction of the agonist. In limb dystonia, reciprocal inhibition studied in the flexor and extensor muscles of the forearm is reduced.[133,134] A similar abnormality has been detected in patients with ST and with BSP, even though there was no clinical involvement of forearm muscles. The picture that emerges from all of these physiological studies is that the brain stem and spinal interneuron circuitry are functioning abnormally in patients with focal dystonias, resulting in a change in the tonic control of reflex excitability. An abnormal input from the basal ganglia via cortical or subcortical connections on brainstem and spinal interneurons could result in these static abnormalities. Such changes might produce particular problems during movement, when activity in specific reflex pathways is normally well regulated according to the task being performed.[69]

Differential Diagnosis and Investigations in Patients with Focal Dystonias

The focal dystonias are usually idiopathic, regardless of the location. Occasionally there is a known cause for them. Although the list of such secondary or symptomatic dystonias is quite extensive,[55,135] symptomatic focal dystonias clinically similar to idiopathic ones are not common. Still, the distinction between idiopathic and symptomatic forms is important

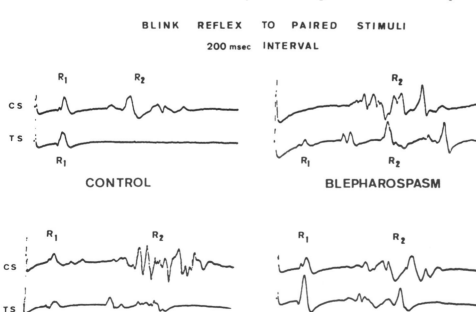

BLINK REFLEX TO PAIRED STIMULI

200 msec INTERVAL

CONTROL

BLEPHAROSPASM

S. TORTICOLLIS

S. DYSPHONIA

0.5 mv
10 msec

FIGURE 31-2 Blink reflexes to pairs of stimuli given at an interstimulus interval of 200 ms in a normal control subject and in patients with focal dystonia. In the normal control subject the conditioning stimulus (CS) completely inhibits the R_2 of the test stimulus (TS). In the patients, on the other hand, a clear R_2 follows the TS already at this short interstimuli interval. Stimuli were delivered at the supraorbital nerve, and the reflex responses (R_1 and R_2) were recorded with surface electrodes from the ipsilateral orbicularis oculi. *(From Tolosa et al.[127] Used with permission.)*

to give patients appropriate prognosis and genetic counseling. Most importantly, adequate treatment of some of the symptomatic dystonias, when appropriately diagnosed, can result in a cure or avoid progression to a more generalized disorder, as could be the case in dystonia associated with Wilson's disease.

The most common cause of symptomatic adult-onset focal dystonia is *tardive dystonia*, induced by chronic neuroleptic administration.[136,137] Cases of tardive dystonia can be identical to those of BSP, OMD, cervical dystonia, spasmodic dysphonia, or idiopathic truncal dystonia and can only be differentiated at times from the idiopathic dystonias by the history of neuroleptic use.[26] Tardive dystonia does not usually lead to WC. Also relatively common in movement disorder clinics are focal dystonias induced by L-dopa in Parkinson's disease[138] and those occurring in the setting of the various *degenerative parkinsonian syndromes*. Kinesigenic foot dystonia can be the presenting manifestation of untreated young-onset Parkinson's disease[139,140] and WC, torticollis, OMD, and BSP have been described as preceding the onset of otherwise typical Parkinson's disease by variable periods of time, from months up to several years (see Ref. 92 for review). LD and BSP can also be the presenting manifestations of progressive supranuclear palsy,[141] and focal dystonia was described as a prominent presenting feature in a group of patients with hereditary or sporadic cerebellar ataxias.[142] When a focal dystonia is the presenting feature of one of these syndromes, when other neurological findings are not yet present, it is usually impossible to differentiate it from one of the "idiopathic" dystonias on clinical grounds.

Focal dystonic spasms similar to the primary ones have been described secondary to focal hemispheric brain pathology and to brain stem/diencephalic lesions in patients with strokes, multiple sclerosis, or hydrocephalus, and we have also seen prominent focal dystonia, either as the initial manifestation or during the course of disorders such as head trauma, kernicterus, delayed-onset dystonia, Hallervorden-Spatz disease, Tourette's syndrome, Huntington's disease, Wilson's disease and acquired nonwilsonian hepatocerebral degeneration and the degenerative cerebellar ataxias, among other disorders.[92,143]

A major portion of the clinical investigations in a patient with adult-onset focal dystonia are directed to uncover a possible cause for the disorder. *Historical features* can be quite useful in ruling out certain etiological factors. A history of exposure to drugs or toxins must be sought diligently. Antidopaminergic drugs, such as the neuroleptics, antiemetics, or some antivertiginous agents, can cause tardive focal dystonias that can be otherwise indistinguishable from idiopathic ones. Toxins such as manganese and methanol can cause similar symptoms, usually after an initial neurological insult. In a number of instances symptomatic dystonia appears months to years after the initial cerebral insult.[144,145] Delayed-onset dystonias can occur in adolescence that are related to birth asphyxia,[146] but this phenomenon can be observed also with central pontine myelinolysis[147] and cyanide intoxication.[148] A history of recent trauma, in the same body region as the focal dystonia, or head trauma, suggests a post-traumatic dystonia.[95,105] Details of the *onset, distribution, and clinical characteristics* of the dystonic spasms is helpful sometimes in diagnosing a symptomatic dystonia. A focal dystonia of abrupt onset suggests a structural nervous system lesion or a psychogenic etiology. Idiopathic dystonias are typically action-induced at onset, followed by overflow dystonia and, eventually, are present at rest. Dystonia at rest, even from the beginning, strongly suggests a secondary dystonia.

In idiopathic dystonia *the only neurological abnormality is the presence of dystonic postures and movements*. Such movements are tremoric at times and exceptionally myoclonic, as described in Clinical Features. There is no associated oculomotor abnormality, ataxia, dementia, seizures, weakness, atrophy, or spasticity. On the contrary, many of the symptomatic dystonias are associated with some of these neurological findings and, therefore, its presence strongly suggests that one is dealing with such a case. The presence of stereotypes (repetitive, patterned, seemingly purposeful but purposeless movements, such as repetitive tongue protrusion ("fly-catching" tongue movements) or the "bon-bon" sign (roving movements of the tongue inside the mouth) in patients with otherwise typical BSP, for example, strongly suggests the diagnosis of tardive dystonia. The absence of such neurological abnormalities, however, does not exclude the possibility of symptomatic dystonia, which may present as pure dystonia. Equally important in the evaluation of a patient with focal dystonia are the findings on general physical examination, which can even be diagnostic of a specific disorder, for example, the presence of a Kayser-Fleischer ring indicates Wilson's disease.

Careful clinical evaluation of the dystonic spasm is always necessary, particularly if the patient is a candidate for botulinum toxin treatment. In some patients diagnosis may not be possible on simple inspection, because dystonia may not be present at all times. In these cases certain clinical maneuvers may bring out the dystonic spasms and allow for a precise diagnosis. Shinning a bright light in front of the patient's eyes or asking the patient to open and close the eyes repeatedly[26] may, for example, trigger BSP. Dystonic tremor, which may be treated successfully with botulinum toxin, may have to be brought out by asking the patient to adopt a certain position, for example, trying to oppose the dystonic spasms. In general an attempt has to be made to find the position with the most severe dystonia, instructing the patient to position the affected body region so as to show maximal abnormality. The patients should always be examined while standing, walking, sitting, and lying down. In patients with LD or cervical dystonia, passive movements of the affected region may help in localizing the contracting muscles and in determining the full range of motion or the presence of contractures.

Palpation of the contracting muscles is also useful in localizing involved muscles and in estimating muscle mass, and it helps in detecting points of tenderness.

Nonorganic *psychogenic dystonia* can be most difficult to diagnose in an adult, but it can occur, particularly in certain subsets of dystonia, such as adult-onset lower LD, paroxysmal dystonia, and adductor laryngeal dystonia. Certain historical or examination features, such as a large number of somatic complaints, abrupt onset, presence of false weakness, or incongruous movements not fitting with typical organic dystonia, provide clues that suggest a psychogenic etiology.[149]

In addition to psychogenic causes, a number of other disorders in which abnormal postures occur but are not associated with underlying inappropriate muscle contraction should be differentiated from dystonia. *Conditions simulating focal dystonia*[55] can be orthopedic (an atlantoaxial subluxation, for example, can lead to an abnormal head posture that mimics torticollis) or neurological (such as posterior fossa tumors, syringomyelia, or extraocular muscle palsies), producing abnormal head or spine postures. Muscle contractures occurring in neurological patients or after orthopedic injuries may also pose difficult diagnostic problems, and infectious, inflammatory, and neoplastic involvement of the soft-tissue structures of the head and neck may simulate cervical dystonia.[150]

In the investigation of patients with adult-onset focal dystonias presumed to be idiopathic, there is little need for laboratory or neuroimaging tests, because a symptomatic cause is almost never found. When the patient is under 40 years of age, investigations for Wilson's disease should be conducted, but older patients with typical focal dystonias require no further workup unless new or atypical features appear on follow-up, particularly when the disorder has been present for several months or longer.

References

1. Kramer PL, DeLeon D, Ozelius L, et al: Dystonia gene in Ashkenazi Jewish population is located on chromosome 9q32-34. *Ann Neurol* 27:114–120, 1990.
2. Lee LV, Kupke KG, Caballar-Gonzaga F, et al: The phenotype of the X-linked dystonia-parkinsonism syndrome—an assessment of 42 cases in the Philippines. *Medicine (Baltimore)* 70:179–187, 1991.
3. Lew MF, Shindo M, Moskowitz CB, et al: Adductor laryngeal breathing dystonia in a patient with Lubag (x-linked dystonia-parkinsonism syndrome). *Mov Disord* 9:318–320, 1994.
4. Holmgren G, Ozelius L, Forsgren L, et al: Adult onset idiopathic torsion dystonia is excluded from the DYT1 region (9q34) in a Swedish family. *J Neurol Neurosurg Psychiatry* 59:178–181, 1995.
5. Dobyns WB, Ozelius LJ, Kramer PL, et al: Rapid-onset dystonia-parkinsonism. *Neurology* 43:2596–2602,1993.
6. Nutt JG, Muenter MD, Aronson A, et al: Epidemiology of focal and generalized dystonia in Rochester, Minnesota. *Mov Disord* 3:188–194, 1988.
7. Li S-C, Schoenberg BS, Wang C-C, et al: A prevalence survey of Parkinson's disease and other movement disorders in the People's Republic of China. *Arch Neurol* 42:655–657, 1985.
8. Nakashima K, Kusumi M, Inoue Y, Takahashi K: Prevalence of focal dystonias in the Western area of Tottori prefecture in Japan. *Mov Disord* 10(4):440–443, 1995.
9. Fahn S: Generalized dystonia, in Tsui JK, Calne DB (eds): *Handbook of Dystonia*. New York: Marcel Dekker, 1995, chap 12, pp 193–211.
10. Jankovic J, Fahn S: Dystonic disorders, in Jankovic J, Tolosa E (eds): *Parkinson's Disease and Movement Disorders*, 2d ed. Baltimore: Williams & Wilkins, 1993, chap 21, pp 337–374.
11. Fahn S: Dystonia, in Jankovic J, Hallett M (eds): *Therapy with Botulinum Toxin*. New York: Marcel Dekker, 1994, chap 12, pp 173–189.
12. Marsden CD: The focal dystonias. *Clin Neuropharmacol* 9(suppl 2):49–60, 1986.
13. Friedman A, Fahn S: Spontaneous remissions in spasmodic torticollis. *Neurology* 36:398–400, 1986.
14. Rothwell JC, Obeso JA, Day BL, Marsden CD: Pathophysiology of dystonias, in Desmedt JE (ed): *Motor Control Mechanisms in Health and Disease,* New York: Raven Press, 1983, pp 851–863.
15. Obeso JA, Rothwell JC, Lang AE, Marsden CD: Myoclonic dystonia. *Neurology* 33:825–830, 1983.
16. Cleeves L, Findley J, Marsden D: Odd tremors, in Marsden D, Fahn S (eds): *Movement Disorders 3*. Oxford, England: Butterworth-Heinemann, 1994, chap 22, pp 434–453.
17. Rivest J, Marsden D: Trunk and head tremor as isolated manifestation of dystonia. *Mov Disord* 5:60–65, 1990.
18. Patterson RM, Little SC: Spasmodic torticollis. *J Nerv Ment Dis* 98:571–599, 1943.
19. Sheehy MP, Marsden CD: Writer's cramp—a focal dystonia. *Brain* 105:461–480, 1982.
20. Conway D, Bain PG, Warner TT, et al: Linkage analysis with chromosome-9 markers in hereditary essential tremor. *Mov Disord* 8:374–376, 1993.
21. Tolosa ES: Clinical features of Meige's disease (idiopathic orofacial dystonia): A report of 17 cases: *Arch Neurol* 38:147–151, 1981.
22. Tolosa ES, Klawans HL: Meige's disease: A clinical form of facial convulsion bilateral and medial. *Arch Neurol* 36:635–637, 1979.
23. Grandas F, Elston JS, Quinn N, Marsden CD: Blepharospasm: A review of 264 patients. *J Neurol Neurosurg Psychiatry* 51:767–772, 1988.
24. Marsden CD: The problem of adult-onset idiopathic torsion dystonia and other isolated dyskinesias in adult life (including blepharospasm, oromandibular dystonia, dystonic writer's cramp and torticollis, or axial dystonia), in Eldridge R, Fahn S (eds): *Dystonia: Advances in Neurology.* New York: Raven Press, 1976, vol. 14, pp 259–276.
25. Jankovic J, Ford J: Blepharospasm and orofacial-cervical dystonia: Clinical and pharmacological findings in 100 patients. *Ann Neurol* 13:402–411, 1983.
26. Tolosa E, Martí MJ: Blepharospasm-oromandibular dystonia syndrome (Meige's syndrome): Clinical aspects, *Adv Neurol* 49:73–84, 1988.
27. Tolosa E, Kulisevsky J, Martí MJ: Apraxia of lid opening in dystonic blepharospasm. IV. International Meeting of the Benign Essential Blepharospasm Research Foundation, Barcelona, Spain, 1986.
28. Tolosa E, Kulisevsky J, Martí MJ: "Apraxia" of lid opening in essential blepharospasm. XXXVIIII Reunión de la American Academy of Neurology, New York, 1987.
29. Elston JS: A new variant of blepharospasm. *J Neurol Neurosurg Psychiatry* 55:369–371, 1992.
30. Obeso JA, Artieda J, Marsden CD: Stretch reflex blepharospasm. *Neurology* 35:1378–1380, 1985.
31. Marsden CD: Blepharospasm-oromandibular dystonia syndrome (Brueghel's syndrome): A variant of adult-onset torsion dystonia? *J Neurol Neurosurg Psychiatry* 39:1204–1209, 1976.
32. Cardosa F, Jankovic J: Oromandibular dystonia, in Ching Tsiu JK, Calne DB (eds): *Handbook of Dystonia.* New York: Marcel Dekker, 1995, chap 11, pp 181–192.
33. Brin MF, Blitzer A, Herman S, Stewart C: Oromandibular dystonia: Treatment of 96 patients with botulinum toxin type A, in Jankovic J, Hallett M (eds): *Therapy with Botulinum Toxin.* New York: Marcel Dekker, 1994, chap 32, pp 429–436.
34. Traube L: Zur Lehre von den Larynxaffectionen beim Ileotyphus, Berlin, Verlag Von August Hirschwald, 1871.
35. Ludlow CL: The spasmodic dysphonias: Speech, movement, and physiological characteristics, in Ching Tsui JK, Calne DB (eds): *Handbook of Dystonia*. New York: Marcel Dekker, 1995, chap 10, pp 159–180.
36. Aronson AE: *Clinical Voice Disorders.* New York: Thieme, 1985.

37. Blitzer A, Brin MF, Fahn S, Lovelace RE: Clinical and laboratory characteristics of focal laryngeal dystonia: Study of 110 cases. *Laryngoscope* 98:636–640, 1988.

38. Rosenfield DB: Spasmodic dysphonia. *Adv Neurol* 49:317–328, 1988.

39. Ludlow CL, Naunton RF, Terada S, Anderson BJ: Successful treatment of selected cases of abductor spasmodic dysphonia using botulinum toxin injection. *Otolaryngol Head Neck Surg* 104:849–855, 1991.

40. Hartman DE, Aronson AE: Clinical investigations of intermittent breathy dysphonia. *J Speech Hear Disord* 46:428–432, 1991.

41. Izdebski K, Dedo HH, Boles L: Spastic dysphonia: A patient profile of 200 cases. *Am J Otolaryngol* 5:7–14, 1984.

42. Aronson AB, Petersen HW, Litin EM: Voice symptomatology in functional dysphonia and aphonia. *J Speech Hear Disord* 29:367–380, 1964.

43. Tsui JKC: Cervical dystonia, in Tsui JKC, Calne DB (eds): *Handbook of Dystonia*. New York: Marcel Dekker, 1995, chap 7, pp 115–127.

44. Jankovic J, Leder S, Warner D, Schwartz K: Cervical dystonia: Clinical findings and associated movement disorders. *Neurology* 41:1088–1091, 1991.

45. Chan J, Brin MF, Fahn S: Idiopathic cervical dystonia: Clinical characteristics. *Mov Disord* 6:119–126, 1991.

46. Couch JR: Dystonia and tremor in spasmodic torticollis. *Adv Neurol* 14:245–258, 1976.

47. Duane DD: Spasmodic torticollis: Clinical and biologic features and their implications for focal dystonia. *Adv Neurol* 50:473–492, 1988.

48. Duane DD: Spasmodic torticollis. *Adv Neurol* 49:135–150, 1988.

49. Truong DD, Dubinsky R, Hermanowicz N, et al: Posttraumatic torticollis. *Arch Neurol* 48(2):221–223, 1991.

50. Schott GD: The relationship of peripheral trauma and pain to dystonia. *J Neurol Neurosurg Psychiatry* 48(7):698–701, 1985.

51. Lowenstein DH, Aminoff MJ: The clinical course of spasmodic torticollis. *Neurology* 38:530–532, 1988.

52. Jahanshahi M, Marion MH, Marsden CD: Natural history of adult-onset idiopathic torticollis. *Arch Neurol* 47:548,1990.

53. Friedman A, Fahn S: Spontaneous remission in spasmodic torticollis. *Neurology* 36(3):398–400, 1986.

54. Uitti RJ, Vingerhoets FJG, Tsui JKC: Limb dystonia, in Tsui JKC, Calne DB (eds): *Handbook of Dystonia*. New York: Marcel Dekker, 1995, chap 9, pp 143.

55. Fahn S, Marsden CD, Calne DB: Classification and investigation of dystonia, in Marsden CD, Fahn S (eds): *Movement Disorders 2*. London: Butterworth, 1987, chap 17, pp 332–358.

56. Lockwood AH: Medical problems in musicians. *N Engl J Med* 320:221–227, 1989.

57. Newmark J, Hochberg FH: Isolated painless manual incoordination in 57 musicians. *J Neurol Neurosurg Psychiatry* 50:291–295, 1987.

58. McDaniel KD, Cummings JL, Shain S: The "yips": A focal dystonia in golfers. *Neurology* 39:192–195, 1989.

59. Sheehy MP, Marden CD: Writer's cramp—a focal dystonia. *Brain* 105:462–480, 1982.

60. Marsden CD, Sheehy MP: Writer's cramp. *Trends Neurosci* 13:148–153, 1990.

61. Sheehy MP, Rothwell JC, Marsden CD: Writer's cramp. *Adv Neurol* 50:457–472, 1988.

62. Ludolph AC, Windgassen K: Klinische Untersuchungen zum Schreibkrampf bei 30 Patienten. *Nervenarzt* 8:462–466, 1992.

63. Rothwell JC, Traub MM, Marsden CD: Primary writing tremor. *J Neurol Neurosurg Psychiatry* 42:1106–1114, 1979.

64. Rosenbaum F, Jankovic J: Focal task-specific tremor and dystonia: Categorization of occupational movement disorders. *Neurology* 38:522–527, 1988.

65. Quinn N, Critchley P, Marsden CD: Young onset Parkinson's disease. *Mov Disord* 2:73–91, 1987.

66. Poewe WH, Lees AJ, Stern GM: Dystonia in Parkinson's disease: Clinical and pharmacological features. *Ann Neurol* 23:73–78, 1988.

67. Rivest J, Quinn N, Marsden CD: Dystonia in Parkinson's disease, multiple system atrophy, and progressive supranuclear palsy. *Neurology* 40:1571–1578, 1990.

68. Rafal RD, Friedman JH: Limb dystonia in progressive supranuclear palsy. *Neurology* 37:1546–1549, 1987.

69. Rothwell JC: The Physiology of dystonia, in Tsui JKC, Calne DB (eds): *Handbook of Dystonia*. New York: Marcel Dekker, 1995, chap 4, pp 59–76.

70. Marsden CD, Harrison MJG, Bundey S: Natural history of idiopathic torsion dystonia, in Eldridge R, Fahn S (eds): *Dystonia*. New York: Raven Press, 1976, pp 177–187.

71. Gowers WR: *A Manual of Diseases of the Nervous System*. London: Churchill, 1888, p 656.

72. Ferguson D: An Australian study of telegraphist's cramp. *Br J Intern Med* 28:280–285,1971.

73. Cohen A. Putting on the agony. *Nurs-Mirror Midwives J* 143(20): 72, 1976.

74. Marsden CD: The focal dystonias. *Clin Neuropharmacol* 9(suppl 2):S49–S60, 1986.

75. Marsden CD: Dystonia: The spectrum of the disease, in Yahr M (ed): *The Basal Ganglia*. New York: Raven Press, 1976, pp 351–367.

76. Marsden CD: Blepharospasm-oromandibular dystonia syndrome (Brueghel's syndrome). *J Neurol Neurosurg Psychiatry* 39:1204 1209, 1976.

77. Robertson-Hoffman DE, Mark MH, Sage JL: Isolated lingual-palatal dystonia. *Mov Disord* 6:177–179, 1991.

78. Iliceto G, Thompson PD, Day BL, et al: Diaphragmatic flutter, the moving umbilicus syndrome, and "belly dancer's" dyskinesia. *Mov Disord* 5:1522, 1990.

79. Caviness JN, Gabellini A, Kneebone CS, et al: Unusual focal dyskinesias: The ears, the shoulders, the back, and the abdomen. *Mov Disord* 9(5):531–538, 1994.

80. Ozelius L, Kramer PL, Moskowitz CB, et al: Human gene for torsion dystonia on chromosome 9q32-34. *Neuron* 2:1427–1434, 1989.

81. Fletcher NA, Harding AE, Marsden CD: A genetic study of idiopathic torsion dystonia in the UK. *Brain* 113:379–395, 1990.

82. Bressman SB, De Leon D, Brin MF, et al: Idiopathic torsion dystonia among Ashkenazi Jews: Evidence for autosomal dominant inheritance. *Ann Neurol* 26:612–620, 1989.

83. Risch NJ, Bressman SB, De Leon D, et al: Segregation analysis of idiopathic torsion dystonia in Ashkenazi Jews suggests autosomal dominant inheritance. *Am J Hum Genet* 46:533–538, 1990.

84. Chan J, Brin MF, Fahn S: Idiopathic cervical dystonia: Clinical characteristics. *Mov Disord* 6:119–126, 1991.

85. De Leon D, Heiman G, Brin MF, et al: Genetic factors in spastic dysphonia. *Neurology* 40(suppl 1):142, 1990.

86. Comella CL, Klawans HL: Meige's syndrome in twins. *Neurology* 38(suppl 1):315, 1988.

87. Kramer PL, Bressman SB, Fahn S, et al: The genetics of dystonia, in Tsui JKC, Calne DB (eds): *Handbook of Dystonia*. New York: Marcel Dekker, 1995, chap 3, pp 43–58.

88. Waddy HM, Fletcher NA, Harding AE, Marsden CD: A genetic study of idiopathic focal dystonias. *Ann Neurol* 29:320–324, 1991.

89. Defazio G, Livrea P, Leon A, Dal Toso R: Antineuronal antibodies in cranial dystonia. *Mov Disord* 6:183–184, 1991.

90. Jankovic J, Patten BM: Blepharospasm and autoimmune diseases. *Mov Disord* 2:159–163, 1987.

91. Nilaver G, Whitling S, Nutt JG: Autoimmune etiology for cranial dystonia. *Mov Disord* 5:179–180, 1990.

92. Tolosa E, Kulisevski J: The pathophysiology of dystonia, in Quinn NP, Jenner PG (eds): *Disorders of Movement. Clinical, Pharmacological and Physiological Aspects.* London: Academic Press, 1989, chap 17, pp 251–262.

93. Fletcher NA, Harding AE, Marsden CD: The relationship between trauma and idiopathic torsion dystonia. *J Neurol Neurosurg Psychiatry* 54:713–717, 1991.

94. Grandas F, Elston J, Quinn N, Marsden CD: Blepharospasm: A review of 264 patients. *J Neurol Neurosurg Psy* 51:767–772, 1988.

95. Jankovic J, Van Der Linden C: Dystonia and tremor induced by peripheral trauma: Predisposing factors. *J Neurol Neurosurg Psychiatry* 51:1512–1519, 1988.

96. Truong DD, Dubinsky R, Hermanowicz N, et al: Posttraumatic torticollis. *Arch Neurol* 48(2):221–223, 1991.

97. Brin MF, Fahn S, Bressman SB, Burke RE: Dystonia precipitated by peripheral trauma. *Neurology* 36(suppl 1):119, 1986.

98. Ludlow CL: The spasmodic dysphonias: Speech, movement, and physiological characteristics, in Tsui JKC, Calne DB (eds): *Handbook of Dystonia.* New York: Marcel Dekker, 1995, chap 10, pp 159–180.

99. Tarsy D, Sudarsky L, Charness ME: Limb dystonia following electrical injury. *Mov Disord* 9(2):230–232, 1994.

100. Schott GD: Induction of involuntary movements by peripheral trauma: An analogy with causalgia. *Lancet* ii:712–715, 1986.

101. Bhatia KP, Bhatt MH, Marsden CD: The causalgia-dystonia syndrome. *Brain* 116:834–851, 1993.

102. Scolding NJ, Smith SM, Sturman S, et al: Auctioneer's jaw: A case of occupational oromandibuar dystonia. *Mov Disord* 10:508–509, 1995.

103. Inzelberg R, Zilber N, Kahana E, Korczyn AD: Laterality of onset in idiopathic torsion dystonia. *Mov Disord* 8(3):327–330, 1993.

104. Fletcher NA, Harding AE, Marsden CD: A case-control study of idiopathic torsion dystonia. *Mov Disord* 6(4):304–309, 1992.

105. Marsden CD. Peripheral movement disorders, in Marsden CD, Fahn S.(eds): *Movement Disordorders 3.* Oxford: Butterworth-Heinemann, 1994, chap 20, pp 406–417.

106. Lang AE, Fahn S: Movement disorders of RSD. *Neurology* 40:1476–1477,1990.

107. Ecker A. Movement disorders of RSD. *Neurology* 40:1477, 1990.

108. Marsden CD: The problem of adult-onset idiopathic torsion dystonia and other isolated dyskinesias in adult life (including blepharospasm, oromandibular dystonia, dystonic writer's cramp, and torticollis, or axial dystonia). *Adv Neurol* 14:259, 1976.

109. Fahn S: Generalized dystonia: Concept and treatment. *Clin Neuropharmacol* 9(suppl 2):S37–S48, 1986.

110. Zeman W, Kaelbling R, Pasamanick B: Idiopathic dystonia musculorum deformans. II. The formes frustes. *Neurology* 10:1068–1075, 1960.

111. Fahn S: Generalized dystonia, in Tsui JKC, Calne DB (eds): *Handbook of Dystonia.* New York: Marcel Dekker, 1995, chap 12, pp 193–212.

112. Garcia-Albea E, Franch O, Muñoz D: Breughel's syndrome: Report of a case with postmortem studies. *J Neurol Neurosurg Psychiatry* 44:437–440, 1981.

113. Jankovic J: Pharmacologic approach to blepharospasm and cranial-cervical dystonia. *Adv Ophtalmol Plast Reconstr Surg* 4:211–217, 1985.

114. Altrocchi PH, Forno LS: Spontaneous oral-facial dyskinesia: Neuropathology of a case. *Neurology* 33:802–805, 1983.

115. Kulisevsky J, Marti MJ, Ferrer I,Tolosa E.: Meige syndrome: Neuropathology of a case. *Mov Disord* 3:170–175, 1988.

116. Zweig RM, Hedreen JC, Jankel WR: Pathology in brainstem regions of individuals with primary dystonia. *Neurology* 38:702–706, 1988.

117. Rothwell JC, Obeso JA: The anatomical and physiological basis of torsion dystonia, in Marsden CD, Fahn S (eds): *Movement Disorders 2.* London: Butterworths, 1987, chap 16, pp 313–331.

118. Jankovic J: Blepharospasm with basal ganglia lesions. *Arch Neurol* 43:866–868, 1986.

119. Karbe H, Holthoff VA, Rudolf J: Positron emission tomography demonstrates frontal cortex and basal ganglia hypometabolism in dystonia. *Neurology* 42:1540–1544, 1992.

120. Fife TD, Hutchinson M, Woods RP, et al: Motor system hypermetabolism in Meige's syndrome. *Neurology* 43(suppl 4):A409–410,1993.

121. Hutchinson M, Fife TD, Woods RP, et al: Glucose metabolism in Meige's syndrome in wakefulness and sleep. *J Cereb Blood Flow Metab* 13(suppl 1):S370, 1993.

122. Ceballos-Baumann O, Passingham RE, Warner T, et al: Overactive prefrontal and underactive motor cortical areas in idiopathic dystonia. *Ann Neurol* 37:363–372, 1995.

123. Ridding MC, Sheean G, Rothwell JC, et al: Changes in the balance between motor cortical excitation and inhibition in focal, task specific dystonia. *J Neurol Neurosurg Psychiatry* 59:493–498, 1995.

124. Hanajima R, Ugawa Y, Masuda N, Kanazawa I: Changes of motor cortical excitability in a patient with unilateral focal dystonia due to a lesion of the contralateral putamen. *Mov Disord* 9(suppl 1):43, 1994.

125. Tolosa ES, Montserrat L: Depressed blink reflex habituation in dystonia blepharospasm. *Neurology* 35:271, 1985.

126. Berardelli A, Rothwell JC, Day BL, Marsden CD: Pathophysiology of blepharospasm and oromandibular dystonia. *Brain* 108:593–608, 1985.

127. Tolosa E, Montserrat L, Bayes A: Blink reflex studies in focal dysonias: Enhanced excitability of brainstem interneurones in cranial dystonia and spasmodic torticollis. *Mov Disord* 3:61–69, 1988.

128. Valls J, Tolosa E, Ribera G: Neurophysiological observation on the effects of botulinum toxin treatment in patients with dystonic blepharospasm. *J Neurol Neurosurg Psychiatry* 54:310–313, 1991.

129. Valls J, Tolosa E., Martí MJ, Allam N: Treatment with botulinum toxin injection does not change brainstem interneuronal excitability in patients with cervical dystonia. *Clin Neuropharmacol* 17(3):229–235, 1994.

130. Carella F, Ciano C, Musicco M, Scaioli V: Exteroceptive reflexes in dystonia: A study of the recovery cycle of the R2 component of the blink reflex and of the exteroceptive suppression of the contracting sternocleidomastoid muscle in blepharospasm and torticollis. *Mov Disord* 9(2):183–187, 1994.

131. Bronstein AM, Rudge P: Vestibular involvement in spasmodic torticollis. *J Neurol Neurosurg Psychiatry* 49:290–295, 1986.

132. Colebatch JG, Di Lazzaro V, Quartarone A, et al: Click-evoked vestibulocollic reflexes in torticollis. *Mov Disord* 10:455–459, 1995.

133. Nakashima K, Rothwell JC, Day BL, et al: Reciprocal inhibition in writer's and other occupational cramps and hemiparesis due to stroke. *Brain* 112:681–697, 1989.

134. Panizza ME, Hallett M, Nilson J: Reciprocal inhibition in patients with hand cramps. *Neurology* 41:553–556, 1991.

135. Calne DB, Lang AE: Secondary dystonia. *Adv Neurol* 50:9–34, 1988.

136. Weiner WJ, Nausieda PA, Glanz RH. Meige syndrome (blepharospasm-oromandibular dystonia) after long term neuroleptic therapy. *Neurology* 31:1555–1556, 1981.

137. Burke RE, Fahn S, Jankovic J, et al: Tardive dystonia: Late onset and persistent dystonia caused by antipsychotic drugs. *Neurology* 32:1335–1346, 1982.

138. Weiner W, Nausieda P: Meige's syndrome during long-term dopaminergic therapy in Parkinson's disease. *Arch Neurol* 39:451–452, 1982.

139. Gershanik OS, Leist A. Juvenile onset Parkinson's disease. *Adv Neurol* 45:213–216, 1986.

140. Poewe WH, Lees AJ, Stern GM: Dystonia in Parkinson's disease: Clinical and pharmacological features. *Ann Neurol* 23:73–79, 1988.

141. Leger JM, Girault JA, Bolgert F : Deux cas de dystonie isolee d'un membre superieur inagurant une maladie de Steele-Richardson-Olszweski. *Rev Neurol (Paris)* 143(2):140–142, 1987.

142. Fletcher NA, Stell R, Harding A, Marsden CD: Degenerative cerebellar ataxia and focal dystonia. *Mov Disord* 3:336–342, 1988.

143. Tolosa E, Kulisevsky J, Fahn S: Meige syndrome: Primary and secondary forms, *Adv Neurol* 50:509–516, 1988.

144. Chu Nai-Shin, Huang Chin-Chang, Lu Chin-Song, Calne DB: Dystonia caused by toxins, in Ching Tsui JK, Calne BC (eds): *Handbook of Dystonia*. New York: Marcel Dekker, 1995, chap 15, pp 241–265.

145. LeWitt PA, Martin SD: Dystonia and hypokinesia with putaminal necrosis after methanol intoxication. *Clin Neuropharmacol* 11:61, 1988.

146. Burke RE, Fahn S, Gold AP: Delayed-onset dystonia in patients with "static" encephalopathy. *J Neurol Neurosurg Psychiatry* 43:789, 1980.

147. Maraganore DM, Folger WN, Swanson JW, Ahlskog JE: Movement disorders as sequelae of central pontine myelinolysis: Report of three cases. *Mov Disord* 7:142–148, 1992.

148. Grandas F, Artieda J, Obeso JA: Clinical and CT scan findings in a case of cyanide intoxication. *Mov Disord* 4:188, 1989.

149. Fahn S, Williams DT: Psychogenic dystonia. *Adv Neurol* 50:431–455, 1988.

150. Lang AE, Weiner WJ: Symptomatic dystonia, in Lang E, Weiner WJ (eds): *Movement Disorders: A Comprehensive Survey*. Mount Kisko, NY: Futura, 1989.

Chapter 32

TREATMENT OF DYSTONIA

JOSEPH JANKOVIC

PHYSICAL AND SUPPORTIVE THERAPY
PHARMACOLOGICAL THERAPY
    Dopaminergic Therapy
    Antidopaminergic Therapy
    Anticholinergic Therapy
    Other Pharmacologic Therapies
BOTULINUM TOXIN
    Blepharospasm
    Oromandibular Dystonia
    Laryngeal Dystonia (Spasmodic Dysphonia)
    Cervical Dystonia
    Writers' Cramps and Other Limb Dystonias
    Other Indications for Botulinum Toxin
SURGICAL TREATMENT OF DYSTONIA
    Thalamotomy
    Peripheral Surgery
SUMMARY

Despite a paucity of knowledge about the cause and pathogenesis of dystonic disorders, the symptomatic treatment of dystonia has markedly improved, particularly since the introduction of botulinum toxin (BTX). In most cases of dystonia, the treatment is merely symptomatic, designed to improve patients posture and function and to relieve associated pain. In rare patients, however, dystonia can be so severe that it can produce not only disabling dystonic movements, sometimes compromising respiration, but also muscle breakdown and life-threatening hyperthermia and myoglobinuria. In such cases of "dystonic storm" proper therapeutic intervention can be life-saving.[1-3]

The assessment of various therapeutic interventions in dystonia is problematic for the following reasons: (1) dystonia and its effects on function are difficult to quantitate, and, therefore, most trials utilize crude clinical rating scales, many of which have not been properly evaluated or validated; (2) dystonia is a syndrome with different etiologies, anatomic distributions, and heterogeneous clinical manifestations producing variable disability; (3) some patients, perhaps up to 15 percent, may have spontaneous, albeit transient, remissions; (4) the vast majority of therapeutic trials in dystonia are not double-blind, placebo-controlled; and (5) most studies, even those that have been otherwise well designed and controlled, have utilized small sample sizes which make the results difficult to interpret, particularly in view of a large placebo effect demonstrated in dystonia. For these and other reasons, the selection of a particular choice of therapy is largely guided by personal clinical experience and by empirical trials (Table 32-1).[4,5] The age of the patient, the anatomic distribution of dystonia, and the potential risk of adverse effects are also important determinants of choice of therapy. The identification of a specific cause of dystonia, such as drug-induced dystonia or Wilson's disease, may lead to a treatment that is targeted to the particular etiology. Therefore, it is prudent to search for identifiable causes of dystonia, particularly when some atypical features are present (see Chaps. 30, 31, and 33).

Physical and Supportive Therapy

Before reviewing pharmacological and surgical therapy of dystonia, it is important to emphasize the role of patient education and supportive care, as these are integral components of a comprehensive approach to patients with dystonia. Physical therapy and well fitted braces are designed primarily to improve posture and to prevent contractures. Although braces are often poorly tolerated, particularly by children, in some cases they may be used as a substitute for a "sensory trick." For example, in some of our patients with cervical dystonia we were able to construct neck-head braces that seem to provide sensory input by touching certain portions of the neck or head in a fashion similar to the patient's own sensory trick, thus enabling the patient to maintain a desirable head position. Various hand devices have been developed in an attempt to help patients who have writer's cramp to use their hands more effectively and comfortably.[6] Some patients find various muscle relaxation techniques and sensory feedback therapy useful adjuncts to medical or surgical treatments.

Pharmacological Therapy

DOPAMINERGIC THERAPY

Pharmacological treatment of dystonia is largely based on empirical, rather than scientific, rationale (Table 32-2). Unlike Parkinson's disease, in which therapy with L-dopa replacement is based on the finding of dopamine depletion in the brains of parkinsonian animals and humans, our knowledge of biochemical alterations in idiopathic dystonia is very limited. One exception is dopa-responsive dystonia (DRD), in which the biochemical and genetic mechanisms have been elucidated by studies of postmortem brains and by molecular DNA and biochemical studies. Decreased neuromelanin in the substantia nigra with otherwise normal nigral cell count and morphology and normal tyrosine hydroxylase immunoreactivity were found in one brain of a patient with classic DRD.[7] There was a marked reduction of dopamine in the substantia nigra and in the striatum. These findings suggested that in DRD the primary abnormality was a defect in dopamine synthesis. This proposal is supported by the finding of a mutation in the GTP cyclohydrolase I gene on chromosome 14q which indirectly regulates the production of tetrahydrobiopterin, a cofactor for tyrosine hydroxylase, the rate-limiting enzyme in the synthesis of dopamine.[8,9]

TABLE 32-1 Treatment of Dystonia

Focal dystonias
  Bleopharospasm
    1. Clonazepam, lorazepam
    2. Botulinum toxin injections
    3. Trihexyphenidyl
    4. Orbicularis oculi myectomy
  Oromandibular dystonia
    1. Baclofen
    2. Trihexyphenidyl
    3. Botulinum toxin injections
  Spasmodic dysphonia
    1. Botulinum toxin injections
    2. Voice and supportive therapy
  Cervical
    1. Trihexyphenidyl
    2. Diazepam, lorazepam, clonazepam
    3. Botulinum toxin injections
    4. Tetrabenazine
    5. Cyclobenzaprine
    6. Carbamazepine
    7. Baclofen (oral)
    8. Peripheral surgical denervation
  Task-specific dystonias (e.g., writer's cramp)
    1. Benztropine, trihexyphenidyl
    2. Botulinum toxin injections
    3. Occupational therapy
Segmental and generalized dystonias
    1. Levodopa (in children to young adults)
    2. Trihexyphenidyl, benztropine
    3. Diazepam, lorazepam, clonazepam
    4. Baclofen (oral, intrathecal)
    5. Carbamazepine
    6. Tetrabenazine (with lithium)
    7. Triple therapy: tetrabenazine, fluphenazine, trihexyphenidyl
    8. Intrathecal baclofen infusion (axial dystonia)
    9. Thalamotomy (in distal dystonia or hemidystonia)

DRD usually presents in childhood with dystonia, mild parkinsonian features, and pseudopyramidal signs (hypertonicity and hyperreflexia) predominantly involving the legs. Many patients have a family history of dystonia or Parkinson's disease. At least half of the patients have diurnal fluctuations with marked progression of their symptoms toward the end of the day and a relief after sleep. Many patients with this form of dystonia are initially misdiagnosed as having "cerebral palsy." Some patients with DRD are not diagnosed until adulthood, and family members of patients with typical DRD may present with adult-onset L-dopa-responsive parkinsonism.[10] The combination of L-dopa-responsive dystonia and parkinsonism, inherited in an autosomal dominant pattern, was also reported in a family characterized by rapidly evolving dystonia (over a period of days to weeks) starting between ages 14 and 45.[11] The take-home message from these reports is that a therapeutic trial of L-dopa should be considered in all patients with childhood-onset dystonia, whether they have classic features of DRD or not.

Most patients with DRD improve dramatically with even small doses of L-dopa (100 mg of L-dopa with 25 mg of decarboxylase inhibitor), but some may require doses of L-dopa as high as 1000 mg per day. In contrast to patients with juvenile Parkinson's disease,[12] DRD patients usually do not develop L-dopa-induced fluctuations or dyskinesias. If no clinically evident improvement is noted after 3 months of therapy, the diagnosis of DRD is probably in error and L-dopa can be discontinued. In addition to L-dopa, patients with DRD also improve with dopamine agonists, with anticholinergic drugs, and with carbamazepine.[13] In contrast to patients with DRD, patients with idiopathic or other types of dystonia rarely improve with dopaminergic therapy.[14]

ANTIDOPAMINERGIC THERAPY

Although used extensively in the past, most clinical trials have produced mixed results with dopamine receptor-blocking drugs. Because of the poor response and the possibility of undesirable side effects, particularly sedation, parkinsonism, and tardive dyskinesia, the use of these drugs in the treatment of dystonia should be discouraged.[15] Dopamine-depleting drugs, however, such as tetrabenazine, have been found useful in some patients with dystonia, particularly in those with tardive dystonia.[16] Tetrabenazine has the advantage over other antidopaminergic drugs that it does not cause tardive dyskinesia. Unfortunately, the drug is not readily available in the United States. It is possible that some of the new atypical neuroleptic drugs will be useful not only as antipsychotics, but also in the treatment of hyperkinetic movement disorders. Clozapine, for example, has been reported to be useful in the treatment of tardive dystonia.[17] The treatment of tardive dystonia and other tardive syndromes is discussed elsewhere in this volume (Chap. 37) and in other reviews.[15]

ANTICHOLINERGIC THERAPY

Anticholinergic medications such as trihexyphenidyl have been found to be most useful in the treatment of generalized and segmental dystonia (Table 32-2).[18] In the experience of Greene et al.,[18] patients with blepharospasm, generalized dystonia, tonic (in contrast to clonic) dystonia, and with onset of dystonia at age younger than 19 years seemed to respond better to anticholinergic drugs than other subgroups, but this difference did not reach statistical significance. Except for short duration of symptoms before onset of therapy, there was no other variable, such as gender or severity, that reliably predicted a favorable response. This therapy is generally well tolerated when the dose is increased slowly. We recommend using a 2-mg preparation of trihexiphenidyl, starting with one-half tablet at bedtime and advancing up to 12 mg/day over the next 4 weeks. Some patients require up to 60–100 mg/day, but at these doses they may experience dose-related drowsiness, confusion, memory difficulty, and hallucinations. In one study of 20 cognitively intact patients with dystonia, only 12 of whom could tolerate 15–74 mg of daily trihexyphenidyl, drug-induced impairments of recall and slowing of mentation were noted particularly in the older patients.[20] Diphenhydramine, an anticholinergic with histamine H_1 antagonist properties, has been reported to have an antidystonic effect in three of five patients.[21] The drug, however, was not effective in 10 other patients with cervical dystonia, and it was associated with sedation and other anti-

TABLE 32-2 Drugs Used in the Treatment of Dystonia

Generic Name	Trade Name	Daily Dosage (mg)	Mechanism of Action
Trihexyphenidyl	Artane	6–10	Anticholinergic
Benztropine	Cogentin	4–15	Anticholinergic
Orphenadrine	Norflex	200–800	Anticholinergic
Clonazepam	Klonopin	1–12	Serotonergic; relaxant
Lorazepam	Ativan	1–16	Relaxant
Diazepam	Valium	10–100	Relaxant
Cyclobenzaprine	Flexeril	20–60	Relaxant
Chlordiazepoxide	Librium	10–100	Relaxant
Baclofen	Lioresal	40–120	Antispastic; GABA agonist; substance P antagonist
Primidone	Mysoline	50–800	Antiepileptic; antitremor
Carbamazepine	Tegretol	600–1600	Antiepileptic
L-dopa/carbidopa	Sinemet (CR)	75/300– 200/2000	Dopamine precursor
Bromocriptine	Parlodel	10–60	Dopamine agonist
Pergolide	Permax	0.5–5	Dopamine agonist
Lithium	Lithobid	600–1800	Antidopaminergic
Tetrabenazine	Nitoman	50–300	Monoamine depleter and blocker
Botulinum A toxin	BOTOX	5–400 units	Blocks Ach release at the neuromuscular junction

cholinergic side effects in most patients. Pyridostigmine and possibly cisapride, peripherally acting anticholinesterase agents, and eye drops of pilocarpine (a muscarinic agonist) often ameliorate at least some of the peripheral side effects such as dry mouth, urinary retention, and blurred vision.

OTHER PHARMACOLOGICAL THERAPIES

Many patients with dystonia require a combination of several medications and treatments (Table 32-2). Benzodiazepines (clonazepam or lorazepam) may provide additional benefit for patients whose response to anticholinergic drugs is unsatisfactory. Clonazepam may be useful in patients with blepharospasm and with myoclonic dystonia. Baclofen may be helpful for oromandibular dystonia, but it is only minimally effective for generalized dystonia. This gamma-aminobutyric (GABA$_b$) autoreceptor agonist has been found to produce substantial and sustained improvement in 29 percent of children at a mean dose of 92 mg/day (range, 40–180).[22] Although initially effective in 28 of 60 (47 percent) of adults with cranial dystonia, only 18 percent continued baclofen at a mean dose of 105 mg/day after a mean of 30.6 months.[23] Narayan et al.[2] first suggested that intrathecal baclofen may be effective in the treatment of dystonia in 1991 in a report of an 18-year-old man with severe cervical and truncal dystonic spasms who was refractory to all forms of oral therapy and to large doses of paraspinal BTX injections. Muscle-paralyzing agents were necessary to relieve these spasms, which compromised his respiration. Within a few hours after the institution of intrathecal baclofen infusion the patient's dystonia markedly improved, and he was able to be discharged from the intensive care unit (ICU) within 1–2 days. The subsequent experience with intrathecal infusions has been quite encouraging, and studies are currently in progress to further evaluate this form of therapy in patients with dystonia.

Peripheral deafferentation with anesthetic was previously reported to improve tremor,[24] but this approach may be also useful in the treatment of focal dystonia.[25] An injection of 5–10 ml of 0.5 percent lidocaine into the target muscle improved focal dystonia for up to 24 hours. This short effect can be extended for up to several weeks if ethanol is simultaneously injected. The observation that blocking muscle spindle afferents reduces dystonia suggests that somatosensory input is important in the pathogenesis of dystonia.[25,26] Local EMG-guided injections of phenol are currently being investigated as a potential treatment of cervical dystonia (J. Massey, personal communication). Chemomyectomy with muscle-necrotizing drugs, such as doxorubicin, has been tried in some patients with blepharospasm and hemifacial spasm,[27] but because of severe local irritation it is doubtful that this approach will be adopted into clinical practice.

Attacks of kinesigenic paroxysmal dystonia may be controlled with anticonvulsants (e.g. carbamezapine, phenytoin). The nonkinesigenic forms of paroxysmal dystonia are less responsive to pharmacological therapy, although clonazepam and acetazolamide may be beneficial. Treatment of paroxysmal dyskinesias is covered in Chapter 38 and in other reviews.[28]

Botulinum Toxin

The introduction of BTX into clinical practice the late 1980s revolutionized treatment of dystonia. The most potent biological toxin, BTX has become a powerful therapeutic tool in the treatment of a variety of neurological, ophthalmologic, and other disorders manifested by abnormal, excessive, or inappropriate muscle contractions.[29–31] In December 1989, after extensive laboratory and clinical testing, the Food and Drug Administration (FDA) approved this biological toxin as a therapeutic agent in patients with strabismus, blepharospasm, and other facial nerve disorders, including hemifacial spasm.

Few therapeutic agents have been better understood in terms of their mechanism of action before their clinical application or have had greater impact on patient's functioning than BTX. The therapeutic value of BTX is due to its ability to cause chemodenervation and to produce local paralysis when injected into a muscle. There are seven immunologically distinct toxins. Type A has been studied most intensely and used most widely, but the clinical applications of other types of toxins, including B and F, are also being explored.[32–34]

BTX-A, currently used most for therapeutic purposes, is harvested from a culture medium after fermentation of a high toxin-producing strain of *Clostridium botulinum* which lyses and liberates the toxin into the culture.[35] The toxin is then extracted, precipitated, purified, and finally crystallized with ammonium sulfate. The crystalline toxin is diluted from milligram to nanogram concentrations, freeze-dried, and dispensed as a white powder in small vials containing 100 mouse units (U) of the toxin. When isolated from bacterial cultures, BTX is noncovalently associated with nontoxic macromolecules, such as hemagglutinin. These nontoxic proteins enhance toxicity by protecting the neurotoxin from proteolytic enzymes in the gut, but they apparently have no effect on the potency of the toxin if injected parenterally.

The therapeutic effects of BTX are thought to be primarily due to its action at the neuromuscular junction. The mechanisms of this primary action are becoming elucidated. The seven antigenically distinct toxins share structurally homologous subunits. Synthesized as single chain polypeptides (molecular weight, 150 kd), these toxin molecules have relatively little potency until they are cleaved by trypsin or bacterial enzymes into a heavy chain (100 K) and light chain (50 K). When linked by a disulfide bond, these dichains exert their paralytic action by preventing the release of acetylcholine (Ach). BTX, therefore, does not affect the synthesis or storage of acetylcholine, but it does interfere with the release from the presynaptic terminal. While the heavy chain of the toxin binds to the presynaptic cholinergic terminal, the light chain acts as a zinc-dependent protease that selectively cleaves proteins that are critical for fusion of the presynaptic vesicle with the presynaptic membrane.[36] Thus, the light chains of BTX-A and E cleave SNAP-25 (synaptosome-associated protein), a protein needed for synaptic vesicle targeting and fusion with the presynaptic membrane.[37] The light chains of BTX-B, D, and F prevent the quantal release of Ach by proteolytically cleaving synaptobrevin-2, also known as VAMP (vesicle-associated membrane protein), an integral protein of the synaptic vesicle membrane.[38] Type C cleaves syntaxin, another plasma membrane-associated protein[39] (Table 32-3).

The primary effect of BTX is to induce paralysis of injected skeletal muscles, especially the most actively contracting muscles. BTX paralyzes not only the extrafusal fibers, but also the intrafusal fibers, thus decreasing the activity of Ib muscle afferents.[40] This may explain the effect of BTX on reciprocal inhibition. In untreated patients with dystonia the

TABLE 32-3 Botulinum Neurotoxins

Neurotoxin	Substrate	Localization
BTX—A, E	SNAP-25	Presynaptic plasma membrane
BTX—B, D, F	VAMP/synaptobrevin	Synaptic vesicle membrane
BTX—C	Syntaxin	Presynaptic plasma membrane

second phase of reciprocal inhibition is usually decreased. BTX "corrects" the abnormal reciprocal inhibition by increasing the second phase, possibly through its effect on the muscle afferents.[41] While the effect on intrafusal fibers may contribute in part to the beneficial action of BTX in patients with dystonia, this is not its main action because BTX is effective in facial dystonia even though the facial muscles do not have spindles.

Measuring variations in fiber diameter and using acetylcholine-esterase staining as indexes of denervation, Borodic et al.[42] showed that BTX diffuses up to 4.5 cm from the site of a single injection (10 U injected in the rabbit longissimus dorsi). Because the size of the denervation field is largely determined by the dose (and volume), multiple-point injections along the affected muscle rather than a single-point injection should, therefore, contain the biological effects of the toxin in the targeted muscle.[43] Blackie and Lees[44] also showed that frequency of dysphagia could be reduced by 50 percent when multiple rather than single injections are used.

It is important to note that the biological activity of BOTOX, distributed by Allergan Pharmaceuticals (originally named Oculinum), is different from the toxin produced in the United Kingdom (UK) or in Japan. The standard unit for measuring potency of BOTOX is derived from a mouse assay: 1 U of BTX is the amount of toxin found to kill 50 percent (LD_{50}) of a group of mice. When administered intravenously or intramuscularly to monkeys, the LD_{50} for the U.S. toxin was estimated to be 40 U/kg, about 3000 U when extracted to a 75-kg man.[45] The dosages used in human therapeutic applications are markedly lower, representing 1–10 percent of this lethal dose. The toxin produced by using anion-exchange chromotography and RNase treatment and supplied by the Vaccine and Research Laboratory, Porton Down, Salisbury (Dysport) in the U.K. has a different potency than BOTOX. One nanogram of the U.K. toxin contains approximately 40 mouse U, whereas 1 ng of the U.S. toxin contains approximately 4 mouse U. The crystallized type A botulinum toxin preparation produced by the Chiba Serum Institute (CS-BOT, Chiba, Japan) has a specific biological activity of 15.2 mouse LD_{50} units/ng.[46] Although the relative potency measured by the number of mouse units per nanogram of the toxin is different for the three preparations (BOTOX = 4 U/ng; Dysport = 40 U/ng; and CS-BOT = 15.2 U/ng); the effective dose for CS-BOT is similar to that of BOTOX. Despite the 10-fold difference in potency per nanogram, it appears that the clinically observable activity of 1 U of BOTOX is roughly equivalent to 2–3 U of the Dysport product. Using quantitative analysis of regional paralysis produced by local injections into the gastrocnemius muscles of mice, Pearce et al.[47] estimated the potency ratio between Dysport and BOTOX to be 4.2:1. In another study, clinical equivalency ratio of 3:1 was determined after titrating dosages of BOTOX in patients previously treated with Dysport.[48]

A small percentage of patients receiving repeated injections develop antibodies against BTX, causing them to be completely resistant to the effects of subsequent BTX injections.[49,50] In one study, 24 of 559 (4.3 percent) patients treated for cervical dystonia developed BTX antibodies.[49] The authors suggested that the true prevalence of antibodies may be more than 7 percent. In addition to patients with BTX antibodies, they studied 8 patients from a cohort of 76 (10.5 percent) who stopped responding to BTX-treatments. These BTX-resistant patients had a shorter interval between injections, more "boosters," and a higher dose at the "nonbooster" injection as compared to nonresistant patients treated during the same period. As a result of this experience clinicians are warned against using booster injections and are encouraged to extend the interval between treatment as long as possible, certainly at least 1 month, and to use the smallest possible doses. In addition to high dosages, we also found that young age is a potential risk factor for the development of immunoresistance to BTX-A.[50] Some of the patients who developed BTX-A antibodies have benefitted from injections by immunologically distinct preparations, such as BTX-F and BTX-B.[32,33,46] The preliminary data suggest that BTX-B provides clinical effects similar to BTX-A, but the benefits of BTX-F seem to last only 1 month. It is likely that future research will result in the development of new and more effective neuromuscular blocking agents that provide therapeutic chemodenervation with long-term benefits and at lower cost.

Despite its proven therapeutic value, there are still many unresolved issues and concerns about BTX. These include lack of standardization of biological activity of the different preparations of BTX, poor understanding of toxin antigenicity, variations in the methods of injection, and inadequate assays for BTX antibodies. Training guidelines for the use of botulinum toxin have been established.[51] Clinicians interested in utilizing BTX chemodenervation in their practice must be aware of these concerns and must exercise proper precautions to minimize the potential risks associated with BTX. Most importantly, they should become thoroughly familiar with the movement disorders they intend to treat and with the anatomy at the injection site. Possible contraindications to the use of BTX include the presence of myasthenia gravis,[52] Eaton-Lambert syndrome, motor neuron disease, aminoglycoside antibiotics, and pregnancy. Besides occasional complications, usually related to local weakness, a major limitation of BTX therapy is its high cost. Several studies analyzing the cost-effectiveness of BTX treatment, however, have demonstrated that the loss of productivity as a result of untreated dystonia and the cost of medications or surgery more than justify the financial expense of BTX treatments.

This review will focus on the use of BTX in the treatment of dystonia. The therapeutic impact of BTX, however, extends to many other disorders including strabismus, spasticity, tremors, tics, achalasia, spastic bladder, and even some cosmetic conditions (Table 32-4).[31] It is likely that the applications of BTX therapy will continue to expand in the future.

TABLE 32-4 Clinical Applications of Botulinum Toxin

Focal dystonia
- Blepharospasm
- Lid "apraxia"
- Oromandibular-facial-lingual dystonia
- Cervical dystonia (torticollis)
- Laryngeal dystonia (spasmodic dysphonia)
- Task-specific dystonia (occupational cramps)
- Other focal dystonias (idiopathic, secondary)

Other involuntary movements
- Voice, head, and limb tremor
- Palatal myoclonus
- Hemifacial spasm
- Tics

Inappropriate contractions
- Strabismus
- Nystagmus
- Myokymia
- Bruxism (TMJ)
- Stuttering
- Painful rigidity
- Muscle contraction headaches
- Lumbosacral strain and back spasms
- Radiculopathy with secondary muscle spasm
- Spasticity
- Spastic bladder
- Achalasia (esophageal, pelvirectal)
- Other spasmic disorders

Other potential applications
- Protective ptosis
- Cosmetic (wrinkles, facial asymmetry)
- Debarking dogs
- Other

BLEPHAROSPASM

The effectiveness of BTX in treating blepharospasm was first demonstrated in a double-blind, placebo-controlled trial in 1987.[53] In a subsequent report of our experience with BTX in 477 patients with various dystonias and hemifacial spasm, Jankovic et al.[54] reviewed the results in 90 patients injected with BTX for blepharospasm. Moderate or marked improvement was noted in 94 percent of the blepharospasm patients. The average latency from the time of the injection to the onset of improvement was 4.2 days, the average duration of maximum benefit was 12.4 weeks, but the total benefit lasted considerably longer, with an average of 15.7 weeks. While 41 percent of all treatment sessions were followed by some side effects (ptosis, blurring of vision or diplopia, tearing, and local hematoma), only 2 percent affected patient's functioning. Complications usually improved spontaneously in less than 2 weeks. These results are consistent with those of other studies.[55] There is no apparent decline in benefit, and the frequency of complications actually decreases after repeat BTX treatments.[56] Reasons for the gradual enhancement in efficacy and reduction in the frequency of complications with repeat treatments include greater experience and improvements in the injection technique. For example, one controlled study showed that an injection into the pretarsal rather than preseptal portion of the orbicularis oculi is associated with significantly lower frequency of ptosis.[57] Ptosis can also be prevented by injecting initially only the lateral and medial portions of the upper lid, thus avoiding the midline levator muscle. We usually initially inject 5 U in each site in the upper lid, 10 U total, and 5 U in the lower lid only laterally (Table 32-5) (Fig. 32-1).

The functional improvement experienced by the vast majority of patients after BTX injection is difficult to express numerically. Many could not work, drive, watch TV, or read prior to the injections. As a result of reduced eyelid and eyebrow spasms, most can now function normally. In addition to the observed functional improvement, there is usually a meaningful amelioration of discomfort and, because of less embarrassment, the patients' self-esteem also frequently improves. BTX injections are now considered by many as the treatment of choice for blepharospasm.[58,59] In addition to idiopathic blepharospasm, BTX injections have been used effectively in the treatment of blepharospasm induced by drugs (e.g., L-dopa in parkinsonian patients or neuroleptics in patients with tardive dystonia), dystonic eyelid and facial tics in patients with Tourette's syndrome, and in patients in whom blepharospasm was associated with "apraxia of eyelid opening."[60,61,62,57]

OROMANDIBULAR DYSTONIA

Oromandibular dystonia is among the most challenging forms of focal dystonia to treat with BTX; it rarely improves with medications, there are no surgical treatments, and BTX therapy can be complicated by swallowing problems. The masseter muscles are usually injected in patients with jaw-closure dystonia, and in patients with jaw-opening dystonia either the submental muscle complex or the lateral pterygoid muscles are injected (Fig. 32-1). In a total of 91 patients treated in 271 visits, the overall improvement was rated as 2.6 (0 = no response to 4 = marked improvement in spasms and

function).[54] A meaningful reduction in the oromandibular-lingual spasms and an improvement in chewing and speech were achieved in more than 70 percent of all patients. The improvement was noted within an average of 5.5 days after injection and lasted 11.5 weeks. Patients with dystonic jaw closure responded better than those with jaw opening dystonia. Temporary swallowing difficulty, noted in less than a third of patients and in only 17 percent of all treatment sessions, was the most frequent complication. BTX injections provide the most effective relief of oromandibular dystonia, and early treatment with BTX may prevent dental and other complications, including the temporomandibular joint (TMJ) syndrome and other oral and dental problems.[63] Oromandi-

TABLE 32-5 Botulinum Toxin: A Dosage Guide

Muscle	Starting Dose (Range) (U/muscle)
Eye brown	10 (5–15)
Upper eyelid	10 (5–15)
Lower lid	5 (2.5–10)
Masseter	50 (25–75)
Sternocleidomastoid (SCM)*	50 (15–75)
Scalenus complex	35 (15–50)
Splenius Capitis	75 (50–150)
Semispinalis Capitis	75 (50–150)
Longissimus Capitis	75 (50–150)
Trapezius	75 (50–100)
Levator scapulae	50 (25–100)
Submental complex	10 (5–25)
Thyroarytenoid**	10 (5–30)
Forearm Flexors	50 (20–75)
Forearm Extensors	15 (10–25)

 * In bilateral injections the dose should be reduced by 50 percent.
** In bilateral injections the dose should be reduced by 75 percent.

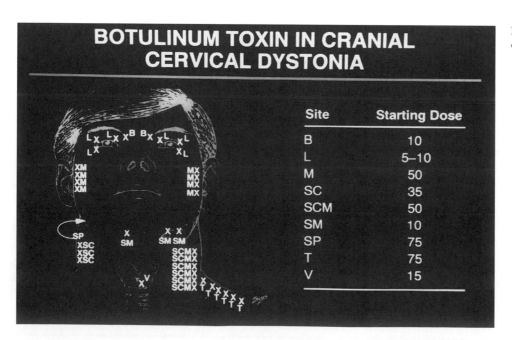

FIGURE 32-1 Botulinum toxin in cranial cervical dystonia.

bular involuntary movements caused by hemimasticatory spasms and other disorders such as Satoyoshi syndrome have been also successfully treated with BTX.[64]

LARYNGEAL DYSTONIA (SPASMODIC DYSPHONIA)

Until the introduction of BTX, the therapy for treating spasmodic dysphonia has been disappointing. The anticholinergic and benzodiazepine drugs only rarely provide meaningful improvement in voice quality. Unilateral transection of the recurrent laryngeal nerve, although effective in most patients, frequently causes unacceptable complications and the voice symptoms often recur.[65] Several studies have established the efficacy and safety of BTX in the treatment of laryngeal dystonia, and this approach is considered by most to be the treatment of choice for spasmodic dysphonia.[54,32,66] Before a patient can be considered a potential candidate for BTX injections, the diagnosis of spasmodic dysphonia must be confirmed by detailed neurological, otolaryngological, and voice assessment and documented by video and voice recordings. There are three approaches currently used in the BTX treatment of spasmodic dysphonia: (1) unilateral EMG-guided injection of 5–30 U;[67] (2) bilateral approach, injecting with EMG-guidance 1.25–4 U in each vocal fold;[66] and (3) an injection via indirect laryngoscopy without EMG.[68] Irrespective of the technique, most investigators report about 75–95 percent improvement in voice symptoms in patients with adductor spasms. One controlled study, however, concluded that unilateral injections "may provide both superior and longer lasting benefits" than bilateral injections.[69] The dosage can be adjusted depending on the severity of glottal spasms and the response to previous injections. Adverse experiences include transient breathy hypophonia, hoarseness, and rare dysphagia with aspiration. Although more complicated and less effective, BTX injections into the posterior cricoarytenoid muscle with the EMG needle placed posterior to the thyroid lamina may be used in the treatment of the abductor form of spasmodic dysphonia.[66] Using a multidisciplinary team approach, consisting of an otolaryngologist experienced in laryngeal injections and a neurologist knowledgeable about motor disorders of speech and voice, BTX injections can provide effective relief for most patients with spasmodic dysphonia.[59,70] BTX may be useful in the treatment of voice tremor and stuttering.[71,72]

CERVICAL DYSTONIA

The goal of therapy of cervical dystonia is not only to improve abnormal posture of the head and associated neck pain, but also to prevent the development of secondary complications such as contractures, cervical radiculopathy, and cervical myelopathy.[73,74] The efficacy and safety of BTX in the treatment of cervical dystonia have been demonstrated in several controlled and open trials.[44,75,54,76,77] In one double-blind, placebo-controlled study of 55 patients with cervical dystonia, 61 percent improved after BTX injection.[75] Open label studies generally report a more dramatic improvement, partly because of a "placebo effect" and, more importantly, because of greater flexibility in selecting the proper dosage and site of injection. Most trials report that about 90 percent of patients

experience improvement in function and control of head-neck movements and in pain. The average latency between injection and the onset of improvement (and muscle atrophy) is 1 week, and the average duration of maximum improvement is 3–4 months. On the average, the injections are repeated every 4–6 months. Patients with long-duration dystonia have been found to respond less well than those treated relatively early, possibly because prolonged dystonia produced contractures.[78] In one study, 28 percent of patients experienced some complication such as swallowing difficulties, neck weakness, and nausea sometime during the course of their treatment (some patients had up to 12 visits in 5 years). Dysphagia, the most common complication, was encountered in 14 percent of all 659 visits, but in only five instances was this problem severe enough to require changing to a soft or liquid diet. Complications are usually related to focal weakness, although distant and systemic subclinical and clinical effects, such as generalized weakness and malaise, rarely occur, possibly as a result of blood distribution or retrograde axonal transport to the spinal motor neurons.[79] Most complications resolve spontaneously, usually within 2 weeks. An injection into one or both sternocleidomastoid muscles was most frequently associated with dysphagia.[80,78,81] One study showed that dosages as small as 20 units administered as a single injection into the sternocleidomastoid muscle completely eliminated muscle activity and could produce neck weakness and dysphagia.[82] In an analysis of patients who received five or more injections we found that the beneficial response was maintained, and the frequency of complications with repeat injections actually declined, presumably as a result of improving skills.[83]

The most important determinants of a favorable response to BTX treatments are a proper selection of the involved muscles and an appropriate dosage (Table 32-6) (Fig. 32-1). EMG may be helpful in some patients with obese necks or in whom the involved muscles are difficult to identify by palpation.[84,85] One study attempted to determine the usefulness of EMG-assisted BTX injections and found that the percentage of patients showing any improvement after BTX was similar whether the injections were assisted by EMG or

TABLE 32-6 Examination of Patients with Cervical Dystonia

1. *Find the most uncompensated position*
   the patient is instructed to allow the head to "draw" into the maximal abnormal posture without resisting the dystonic "pulling" (with eyes open and closed)
   examine while standing, walking, sitting, and writing
2. *Passively move the head*
   to define the dystonic posture
   to localize the contracting muscles
   to determine the full range of motion
   to determine if there are contractures
3. *Palpate contracting muscles*
   to localize the involved muscles
   to estimate the muscle mass
   to find points of tenderness
4. *EMG (needed rarely)*
   to localize involved muscles that cannot be palpated to guide the injection into the muscles that are difficult to access

not.[86] They also noted that "a significantly greater magnitude of improvement" was present in patients treated with EMG-assisted method and that there was "a significantly greater number of patients with marked benefit" in the group randomly assigned to the EMG-assisted method of treatment. Because the majority (70–79 percent) of patients were previously treated with BTX, some may have been experiencing residual effects from previous injection, making the interpretation of the results difficult. Furthermore, the patients who were treated without EMG assistance received a higher dose, indicating more severe dystonia, thus possibly explaining a lesser degree of observed improvement. The general consensus among most BTX users is that EMG is not needed in the vast majority of patients, except in rare instances when the muscles cannot be adequately palpated or the patient does not obtain adequate relief of symptoms with a conventional approach.

WRITERS' CRAMPS AND OTHER LIMB DYSTONIAS

Treatments of writer's cramp with muscle relaxation techniques, physical and occupational therapy, and medical and surgical therapies have been disappointing. Several open[41,87–89] and double-blind controlled[90–92] trials have concluded that BTX injections into selected forearm and hand muscles probably provide the most effective relief in patients with these task-specific occupational dystonias. In some studies fine-wire electrodes were used to localize bursts of muscle activation during the task, and the toxin was injected through a hollow EMG needle into the belly of the most active muscle.[92] Similar beneficial results, however, were obtained in other studies without complex EMG studies.[87] Several lines of evidence support the notion that an intramuscular injection of BTX into the forearm muscles corrects the abnormal reciprocal inhibition.[41]

We studied the effects of BTX in 46 patients with hand dystonia who were injected into forearm muscles in 130 treatment sessions.[88] The average age was 49.4 years, and the dystonic symptoms were present for an average of 8.6 years. After careful examination and palpation of the forearm muscles during writing, the toxin was injected into either the wrist flexors (116 injections) or the wrist extensors (52 injections) (Table 32-5). The average baseline severity of dystonia was 3.5 on a 0–4 (4 = maximum) rating scale. The average peak effect response for all treatment sessions was 2.3 (0 = no response to 4 = maximum benefit). The latency from injection to onset of effect averaged 5.6 days, and the benefit lasted an average of 9.2 weeks. Temporary hand weakness, the chief complication of this treatment, occurred in 54 percent of patients and in 34 percent of all treatment sessions. However, nearly all patients preferred the temporary weakness, which was usually mild, to the disabling writer's cramps. In addition to improving writer's cramps, BTX may provide relief in other task-specific disorders affecting typists, draftsmen, musicians, sportsmen, and other people who depend on skilled movements of their hands.

Other focal distal dystonias, besides those involving the hands, may be amenable to treatment with BTX. Patients with foot dystonia as a manifestation of idiopathic torsion dystonia and patients with parkinsonism who may experi-

ence foot dystonia as an early symptom of their disease, or more commonly as a complication of L-dopa therapy, may benefit from local BTX injections.[93] BTX injections into the foot-toe flexors or extensors may not only alleviate the disability, pain, and discomfort often associated with such dystonia, but may also improve gait. Whether BTX injections will play an important role in the treatment of recurrent painful physiological foot and calf cramps is yet to be determined.

OTHER INDICATIONS FOR BOTULINUM TOXIN

Hemifacial spasm is not considered a form of dystonia, even though it can cause blepharospasm and facial spasms. The chief difference between facial dystonia and hemifacial spasm is that the latter is consistently unilateral. Hemifacial spasm is defined as a neurological disorder manifested by involuntary, recurrent twitches of the eyelids, perinasal, perioral, zygomaticus, platysma, and other muscles of only one side of the face.[94] It is an example of a peripherally induced movement disorder and may be classified as segmental myoclonus in which the muscular contractions result from an irritative lesion of the ipsilateral facial nerve. The condition is not only annoying but also socially embarrassing, and in some patients it causes unilateral blepharospasm that can interfere with vision. Hemifacial spasm is usually due to a compression or irritation of the facial nerve by an aberrant artery or abnormal vasculature around the brain stem. While microvascular decompression of the facial nerve has a high success rate, this surgical treatment is associated with certain risks, such as permanent facial paralysis, deafness, stroke, and death. Therefore, local injections of BTX into involved facial muscles offer a useful alternative to surgical therapy. Nearly all patients improve, the complications are minimal and transient, and the approach can be individualized by injecting only those muscles whose contractions are most disturbing to the patient.[54] In our experience, the average duration of improvement of hemifacial spasm was 5 months, longer than in any of the dystonic disorders. Except for transient facial weakness and ptosis, there are usually no other complications. Along with blepharospasm, the FDA has approved BTX injections also for hemifacial spasm.

Tremor, an oscillatory movement produced by alternating or synchronous contractions of antagonistic muscles, is the commonest movement disorder.[95] While propranolol, primidone, and other antitremor medications are usually satisfactory, when high-amplitude essential tremor significantly impairs activities of daily living, pharmacotherapy alone is not sufficient. In severe cases, neurosurgical treatment (thalamotomy, pallidotomy, or thalamic stimulation) may provide satisfactory relief.

Some form of tremor is present in about half of all dystonic patients.[96] The observation that some patients treated for focal dystonia with BTX noted improvement in their tremor led to trials of BTX specifically for tremor.[96] In a pilot study of 51 patients with disabling tremors of head-neck (42 patients) and hand (10 patients), we noted moderate to marked functional improvement and a reduction in the amplitude of the tremor in 67 percent of patients. The average duration of improvement was 10.5 weeks. Local weakness, lasting up to 3 weeks, occurred after the injection in 60 percent of patients with hand tremor and in 10 percent of those with head-neck tremor. Nearly all patients, however, preferred having mild weakness over disabling tremor. Other open and controlled studies subsequently reported benefit from BTX in patients with hand and head tremor.[97-99]

Motor and phonic tics are usually manifestations of Tourette's syndrome, a familial neurobehavioral disorder. Tics are rarely disabling and they usually improve with antidopaminergic drugs. Some patients, however, have troublesome tics that may cause functional blindness or local discomfort. We have treated 10 patients, 5 with disabling blinking and blepharospasm and 5 with painful dystonic tics involving the neck muscles with BTX injections.[100] All patients noted moderate to marked improvement in the intensity of tics and lessening of the premonitory "tension" that preceded the tics. The improvement lasted 2-20 weeks and, except for transient ptosis in two patients, there were no other complications.

Spasticity, rigidity and *stiff-person syndrome* are examples of hypertonic disorders that may be treated effectively with local injections of BTX.[101-104]

Surgical Treatment of Dystonia

THALAMOTOMY

Improved understanding of the functional anatomy of the basal ganglia and physiological mechanisms underlying movement disorders, coupled with refinements in imaging and surgical techniques, has led to a resurgence of interest in thalamotomy in patients with disabling tremors, dystonia, and other hyperkinetic movement disorders.[105,106] The observation, supported by both physiological and positron emission tomographic (PET) studies, that in dystonia there is a disruption of pallidothalamiccortical projections, provides some rationale for treating dystonia by interrupting the abnormal outflow from the thalamus to the overactive prefrontal motor cortex.[107-109] In a longitudinal study of 17 patients with severe dystonia, eight (47 percent) had a moderate to marked improvement in their abnormal postures and functional disability.[110] Patients with primary and secondary dystonia had a similar response, but 43 percent of the patients with primary dystonia deteriorated during a mean follow-up of 32.9 months, whereas only 30 percent of patients with secondary dystonia deteriorated during a mean follow up of 41.0 months. Neurological complications were observed in 6 of 17 patients (35 percent) immediately after surgery, but deficits (contralateral weakness, dysarthria, and pseudobulbar palsy) persisted in only one subject. Mild weakness contralateral to the surgery was the most common complication, noted in three patients immediately following the procedure. One patient who underwent bilateral procedures had no detectable dysarthria. These results are consistent with other studies that have reported improvement in 34-70 percent of patients with dystonia following thalamotomy.[111-113] While most studies, including ours, concluded that distal dystonia responded more favorably to thalamotomy than axial dystonia, Andrew et al.[111] felt that their patients with axial dystonia, including torticollis, also improved after thal-

amotomy. However, most investigators feel that the best candidates for thalamotomy are those patients who have disabling unilateral dystonia (hemidystonia), unresponsive to medical therapy. Patients with preexisting dysarthria are also good candidates because they have less to lose from thalamotomy-related speech disturbance. Patients with secondary (symptomatic) dystonia seem to respond better than those with idiopathic dystonia. Thalamotomy should not be recommended for patients with facial, laryngeal, and cervical or truncal dystonia. The role of pallidotomy and deep brain stimulation in the treatment of dystonia is currently being evaluated.

PERIPHERAL SURGERY

Peripheral denervation procedures have been used extensively prior to the advent of BTX therapy. In our series of patients with cervical dystonia seen before 1990, 40 of 300 (13 percent) elected to have surgery.[114] While 10 percent of the patients noted worsening after the surgery, 38 percent experienced a noticeable improvement in the ability to control their head position or in reduction of the neck pain.

Three procedures have been used in the treatment of cervical dystonia: (1) extradural selective sectioning of posterior (dorsal) rami (posterior ramisectomy) with or without myotomy; (2) intradural sectioning of anterior cervical roots (anterior cervical rhizotomy); and (3) microvascular decompression of the spinal accessory nerve. Although the first procedure, championed by Bertrand et al.,[115] is considered by many clinicians to be the procedure of choice, no study has compared the different surgical approaches. Bertrand and Molina-Negro[115] reported that 97 of 111 patients (87 percent) had "excellent" or "very good" results. In a smaller series, 5 of 9 patients (56 percent) had moderate benefit which was sustained during up to 21 months of follow-up.[116] The procedure is performed under general anesthesia without a paralyzing agent so that intraoperative nerve root stimulation can be used to identify the innervation to the dystonic muscles. This information, coupled with preoperative EMG, is used to avulse selected nerve roots, usually the branches of the spinal accessory nerve and the posterior rami of C1 through C6. Thorough avulsion of the peripheral branches is felt to be essential in preventing recurrences. Pain seems to improve more than the abnormal posture following the cervical muscle denervation, although some patients complain of "stiff neck" sometimes lasting several months after the surgery. Other complications may include local numbness, neck weakness, and, rarely, dysphagia. The chief disadvantage of anterior rhizotomy compared to posterior primary ramisectomy is that the former procedure causes denervation of both involved and uninvolved muscles, and it cannot be carried out at or below C4 level because of the potential for involvement of the roots to the phrenic nerve leading to paralysis of the diaphragm. The posterior ramisectomy (C2-C6) allows more selective denervation of the involved muscles.

Surgical treatments, such as facial nerve lysis and orbicularis oculi myectomy, once used extensively in the treatment of blepharospasm have been essentially abolished because BTX treatment is usually very effective, and postoperative complications, such as ectropion, exposure keratitis, facial droop, and postoperative swelling and scarring are common. Likewise, recurrent laryngeal nerve section, once used in the treatment of spasmodic dysphonia[65] is used rarely and only when BTX fails to provide satisfactory relief. Another once popular procedure, namely spinal cord stimulation for cervical dystonia, has been shown to be ineffective by a controlled trial.[117]

Continuous intrathecal infusion of baclofen, discussed above, is an established procedure for the treatment of spasticity, but until recently it has not been investigated in the treatment of dystonia.

Summary

Patients with segmental or generalized dystonia beginning in childhood or adolescence should be initially tried on L-dopa/carbidopa, up to 1,000 mg of L-dopa per day. If this therapy is successful, it should be maintained at a lowest possible dose. If ineffective after 3 months, then high-dose anticholinergic (e.g., trihexyphenidyl, benztropine) therapy should be instituted and the dosage increased to the highest tolerated level. If the results are poor, then baclofen, benzodiazepines, carbamazepine, and tetrabenazine should be tried. Some patients may require "triple therapy" consisting of an anticholinergic agent (e.g., trihexyphenidyl), monoamine depleting drug (e.g., tetrabenazine), and a dopamine receptor-blocking drug (e.g., fluphenazine, pimozide, resperidol, or clozapine). Tetrabenazine, alone or with anticholinergic drugs, is particularly useful in the treatment of tardive dystonia. In some patients BTX injections may be helpful to control the most disabling symptom of the segmental or generalized dystonia. In most patients with adult-onset dystonia the distribution is usually focal and, therefore, BTX injections are usually considered the treatment of choice. In some patients this treatment may need to be supplemented by other drugs noted above or by surgical peripheral denervation. Thalamotomy should be reserved only for patients whose symptoms continue to be disabling despite optimal medical therapy. Any form of therapy should, of course, be preceded by a thorough evaluation designed to rule out secondary causes of dystonia. Finally, it is important to emphasize that patient education and counseling are essential components of a comprehensive therapeutic approach to all patients with dystonia.

References

1. Jankovic J, Penn A: Severe dystonia and myoglobinuria. *Neurology* 32:1195–1197, 1982.
2. Narayan RK, Loubser PG, Jankovic J, et al: Intrathecal baclofen for intractable axial dystonia. *Neurology* 41:1141–1142, 1991.
3. Vaamonde J, Narbona J, Weiser R, et al: Dystonic storms: A practical management problem. *Clin Neuropharmacol* 17:344–347, 1994.
4. Jankovic J, Fahn S: Dystonic disorders, in Jankovic J, Tolosa E (eds): *Parkinson's Disease and Movement Disorders,* 2d ed. Baltimore: Williams & Wilkins, 1993, pp 337–374.
5. Greene P: Medical and surgical therapy of idiopathic torsion dystonia, in Kurlan R (ed): *Treatment of Movement Disorders.* Philadelphia: Lippincott, 1995, pp 153–181.
6. Ranawaya R, Lang A: Usefulness of a writing device in writer's cramp. *Neurology* 41:1136–1138, 1991.
7. Rajput AH, Gibb WRG, Zhong XH, et al: DOPA-responsive dystonia—pathological and biochemical observations in a case. *Ann Neurol* 35:396–402, 1994.
8. Ichinose H, Ohye T, Takahi E, et al: Hereditary progressive dystonia with marked diurnal fluctuation caused by mutations in the GTP cyclohydrolase I gene. *Nature Genet* 8:236–242, 1994.
9. Tanaka H, Endo K, Tsuji S, et al: The gene for hereditary progressive dystonia with marked diurnal fluctuation maps to chromosome 14q. *Ann Neurol* 37:405–408, 1995.
10. Harwood G, Hierons R, Fletcher NA, Marsden CD: Lessons from a remarkable family with dopa-responsive dystonia. *J Neurol Neurosurg Psychiatry* 57:460–463, 1994.
11. Dobyns WB, Ozelius LJ, Kramer PL, et al: Rapid-onset dystonia-parkinsonism. *Neurology* 43:2596–2602, 1993.
12. Ishikawa A, Miyatake T: A family with hereditary juvenile dystonia-parkinsonism. *Mov Disord* 10:482–488, 1995.
13. Nygaard TG, Marsden CD, Fahn S: Dopa-responsive dystonia: Long-term treatment response and prognosis. *Neurology* 41:174–181, 1991.
14. Lang AE: Dopamine agonists and antagonists in the treatment of idiopathic dystonia. *Adv Neurol* 50:561–570, 1988.
15. Jankovic J: Tardive syndromes and other drug-induced movement disorders. *Clin Neuropharmacol* 18:197–214, 1995.
16. Jankovic J, Orman J: Tetrabenazine treatment in dystonia, chorea, tics and other dyskinesias. *Neurology* 38:391–394, 1988.
17. Trugman JM, Leadbetter R, Zalis M, et al: Treatment of severe axial tardive dystonia with clozapine: Case report and hypothesis. *Mov Disord* 9:441–446, 1994.
18. Greene P, Shale H, Fahn S: Analysis of open-label trials in torsion dystonia using high dosage of anticholinergics and other drugs. *Mov Disord* 3:46–60, 1988.
19. Jabbari B, Scherokman B, Gunderson CH, et al: Treatment of movement disorders with trihexyphenidyl. *Mov Disord* 4:202–212, 1989.
20. Taylor AE, Lang AE, Saint-Cyr JA, et al: Cognitive processes in idiopathic dystonia treated with high-dose anticholinergic therapy: Implications for treatment strategies. *Clin Neuropharmacol* 14:62–77, 1991.
21. Truong DD, Sandromi P, van der Noort S, Matsumoto RR: Diphenhydramine is effective in the treatment of idiopathic dystonia. *Arch Neurol* 52:405–407, 1995.
22. Greene P: Baclofen in the treatment of dystonia. *Clin Neuropharmacol* 15:276–288, 1992.
23. Fahn S, Henning WA, Bressman S, et al: Long-term usefulness of baclofen in the treatment of essential blepharospasm. *Adv Ophthalmol Plast Reconstr Surg* 4:219–226, 1985.
24. Pozos RS, Iaizo PA: Effects of topical anesthesia on essential tremor. *Electromyogr Clin Neurophysiol* 32:369–372, 1992.
25. Kaji R, Kohara N, Katayama M, et al: Muscle afferent block by intramuscular injection of lidocaine for the treatment of writer's cramp. *Muscle Nerve* 18:234–235, 1995.
26. Hallett M: Is dystonia a sensory disorder? *Ann Neurol* 38:139–140, 1995.
27. Wirtschafter JD: Clinical doxorubicin chemomyectomy: An experimental treatment for benign essential blepharospasm and hemifacial spasm. *Ophthalmology* 98:357–366, 1991.
28. Demirkiran M, Jankovic J: Paroxysmal dyskinesias: Clinical features and classification. *Ann Neurol* 38(4):571–579, 1995.
29. Jankovic J, Brin MF: Therapeutic uses of botulinum toxin. *N Engl J Med* 324:1186–1194, 1991.

30. Clarke CE: Therapeutic potential of botulinum toxin in neurologic disorders. *Q J Med* 82:197–205, 1992.

31. Jankovic J, Hallett M (eds): *Therapy with Botulinum Toxin*. New York: Marcel Dekker, 1994.

32. Ludlow CL, Hallett M, Rhew K, et al: Therapeutic use of type F botulinum toxin. *N Engl J Med* 326:349–350, 1992.

33. Greene P, Fahn S: Treatment of torticollis with injections of botulinum toxin type F in patients with antibodies to botulinum toxin type A. *Mov Disord* 7(suppl 1):134, 1992.

34. Mezaki T, Kaji R, Kohara N, et al: Comparison of therapeutic efficacies of type A and F botulinum toxins for blepharospasm: A double-blind, controlled study. *Neurology* 45:506–508, 1995.

35. Schantz EJ, Johnson EA: Properties and use of botulinum toxin and other mnicrobial neurotoxins in medicine. *Microbiol Rev* 56:80–99, 1992.

36. Blasi J, Chapman ER, Link E, et al: Botulinum neurotoxin A selectively cleaves the synaptic protein SNAP-25. *Nature* 365:160–163, 1993.

37. Sölner T, Whiteheart SW, Brunner M, et al: SNAP receptors implicated in vesicle targeting and fusion. *Nature* 362:318–324, 1993.

38. Schiavo G, Rossetto O, Catsicas S, et al: Identification of the nerve terminal targets of botulinum neurotoxin serotypes A, D, and E. *J Biol Chem* 265:23794–23797, 1993.

39. Huttner W: Snappy exocytoxins. *Nature* 365:104–105, 1993.

40. Filippi GM, Errico P, Samtarelli R, et al: Botulinum A toxin effects on rat jaw muscle spindles. *Acta Otolaryngol (Stockh)* 113:400–404, 1993.

41. Priori A, Berardelli A, Mercuri B, Mafredi M: Physiological effects produced by botulinum toxin treatment of upper limb dystonia: Changes in reciprocal inhibition between forearm muscles. *Brain* 118:801–807, 1995.

42. Borodic GE, Ferrante R, Pearce LB, Smith K: Histologic assessment of dose-related diffusion and muscle fiber response after therapeutic botulinum A toxin injections. *Mov Disord* 9:31–39, 1994.

43. Borodic GE, Pearce LB, Smith K, Joseph M: Botulinum A toxin for spasmodic torticollis: Multiple vs single injection points per muscle. *Head Neck* 14:33–37, 1992.

44. Blackie JD, Lees AJ: Botulinum toxin treatment in spasmodic torticollis. *J Neurol Neurosurg Psychiatry* 53:640–643, 1990.

45. Scott AB, Suzuki D: Systemic toxicity of botulinum toxin by intramuscular injection in the monkey. *Mov Disord* 3:333–335, 1988.

46. Mezaki T, Kaji R, Hamano T, Nagamine T, et al: Optimisation of botulinum treatment for cervical and axial dystonias: Experience with Japanese type A toxin. *J Neurol Neurosurg Psychiatry* 57:1535–1537, 1994.

47. Pearce LB, Borodic GE, Johnson EA, et al: The median paralysis unit: A more pharmacologically relevant unit of biologic activity for botulinum toxin. *J Pharmacol Exp Ther*. In Press.

48. Marion MH, Sheehy MP, Sangla S, et al: A study to compare the clinical efficacy of two different preparations of botulinum toxin in a group of patients with either hemifacial spasm or blepharospasm (abstr.). *Mov Disord* 9(suppl1):51, 1994.

49. Greene P, Fahn S, Diamond B: Development of resistance to botulinum toxin type A in patients with torticollis. *Mov Disord* 9:213–217, 1994.

50. Jankovic J, Schwartz K: Response and immunoresistance to botulinum toxin injections. *Neurology* 45:1743–1746, 1995.

51. American Academy of Neurology: Training guidelines for the use of botulinum toxin for the treatment of neurologic disorders. Report of the Therapeutics and Technology Assessment Subcommittee of the American Academy of Neurology. *Neurology* 44:2401–2403, 1994.

52. Emerson J: Botulinum toxin for spasmodic torticollis in a patient with myasthenia gravis. *Mov Disord* 9:367, 1994.

53. Jankovic J, Orman J: Botulinum A toxin for cranial-cervical dystonia: A double-blind, placebo-controlled study. *Neurology* 37:616–623, 1987.

54. Jankovic J, Schwartz K, Donovan DT: Botulinum toxin treatment of cranial-cervical dystonia, spasmodic dysphonia, other focal dystonias and hemifacial spasm. *J Neurol Neurosurg Psychiatry* 53:633–639, 1990.

55. Elston JS: Botulinum toxin for blepharospasm, in Jankovic J, Hallett M, (eds): *Therapy with Botulinum Toxin*. New York: Marcel Dekker, 1994.

56. Jankovic J, Schwartz K: Longitudinal follow-up of botulinum toxin injections for treatment of blepharospasm and cervical dystonia. *Neurology* 43:834–836, 1993.

57. Jankovic J: Apraxia of eyelid opening. *Mov Disord* 10:686–687, 1995.

58. American Academy of Ophthalmology: Botulinum toxin therapy of eye muscle disorders: Safety and effectiveness. *Ophthalmology* 96(part 2):37–41, 1989.

59. American Academy of Neurology: Assessment: The clinical usefulness of botulinum toxin-A in treating neurologic disorders. Report of the Therapeutics and Technology Assessment Subcommittee of the American Academy of Neurology. *Neurology* 40:1332–1336, 1990.

60. Jankovic J: Botulinum toxin in the treatment of dystonic tics. *Mov Disord* 9:347–349, 1994.

61. Aramideh M, Ongerboer de Visser BW, Koelman JHTM, et al: Motor persistence of orbicularis oculi muscle in eyelid-opening disorders. *Neurology* 45:897–902, 1995.

62. Lepore V, Defazio G, Acquistapance D, et al: Botulinum A toxin for the so-called apraxia of lid opening. *Mov Disord* 10:525–526, 1995.

63. Blitzer A, Brin MF: Laryngeal dystonia: A series with botulinum toxin therapy. *Ann Otol Rhinol Laryngol* 100:85–90, 1991.

64. Merello M, Garcia H, Nogues M, Leiguarda R: Masticatory muscle spasm in non-Japanese patient with Satoyoshi syndrome successfully treated with botulinum toxin. *Mov Disord* 9:104–105, 1994.

65. Dedo HH, Izdebski K: Intermediate results of 306 recurrent laryngeal nerve sections for spastic dysphonia. *Laryngoscope* 93:9–15, 1983.

66. Brin MF, Blitzer A, Stewart C, Fahn S: Treatment of spasmodic dysphonia (laryngeal dystonia) with local injections of botulinum toxin: Review and technical aspects, in Blitzer A, Brin MF, Sasaki CT, Fahn S, Harris KS (eds): *Neurologic Disorders of the Larynx*. New York: Thieme Medical Publishers, 1992, pp 214–228.

67. Jankovic J, Schwartz K: Botulinum toxin injections for cervical dystonia. *Neurology* 41:277–280, 1990.

68. Ford CN, Bless DM, Lowery JD: Indirect laryngoscopic approach for injection of botulinum toxin in spasmodic dysphonia. *Otolaryngol Head Neck Surg* 103:752–758, 1990.

69. Adams SG, Hunt EJ, Charles DA, Lang AE: Unilateral versus bilateral botulinum toxin injections in spasmodic dysphonia: Acoustic and perceptual results. *J Otolaryngol* 22:171–175, 1993.

70. American Academy of Otolaryngology: Position statement on the clinical usefulness of botulinum toxin in the treatment of spasmodic dysphonia. *Arch Otolaryngol Head Neck Surg Bull* 9:8, 1990.

71. Ludlow CL: Treatment of speech and voice disorders with botulinum toxin. *J Am Med Assoc* 264:2671–2675, 1990.

72. Brin MF, Stewart C, Blitzer A, et al: Laryngeal botulinum toxin injections for disabling stuttering in adults. *Neurology* 44:2262–2266, 1994.

73. Treves T, Korczyn AD: Progressive dystonia and paraparesis in cerebral palsy. *Eur Neurol* 25:148–153, 1986.

74. Waterston JA, Swash M, Watkins ES: Idiopathic dystonia and cervical spondylotic myelopathy. *J Neurol Neurosurg Psychiatry* 52:1424–1426, 1989.

75. Greene P, Kang U, Fahn S, et al: Double-blind, placebo controlled trial of botulinum toxin injection for the treatment of spasmodic torticollis. *Neurology* 40:1213–1218, 1990.

76. Poewe W, Schlosky L, Kleedorfer B, et al: Treatment of spasmodic torticollis with local injections of botulinum toxin. *J Neurol* 239:21–25, 1992.

77. Jankovic J, Brin MF, Comella C: *Handbook of Botulinum Toxin Treatment for Cervical Dystonia.* New York: Churchill Livingstone, 1994.

78. Jankovic J, Schwartz KS: Clinical correlates of response to botulinum toxin injections. *Arch Neurol* 48:1253–1256, 1991.

79. Garner CG, Straube A, Witt TN, et al: Time course effects of local injections of botulinum toxin. *Mov Disord* 8:33–37, 1993.

80. Borodic GE, Joseph M, Fay L, et al: Botulinum A toxin for the treatment of spasmodic torticollis: Dysphagia and regional toxin spread. *Head Neck* 12:392–399, 1990.

81. Comella Cl, Tanner CM, DeFoor-Hill L, Smith C: Dysphagia after botulinum toxin injections for spasmodic torticollis. Clinical and radiologic findings. *Neurology* 42:1307–1310, 1992.

82. Buchman AS, Comella CL, Stebbins GT, et al: Determining a dose-effect curve for botulinum toxin in the sternocleidomastoid muscle in cervical dystonia. *Clin Neuropharmacol* 17:188–193, 1994.

83. Jankovic J, Schwartz K: Longitudinal follow-up of botulinum toxin injections for treatment of blepharospasm and cervical dystonia. *Neurology* 43:834–836, 1993.

84. Dubinsky RM, Gray CS, Vetere-Overfield B, Koller WC: Electromyographic guidance of botulinum toxin treatment in cervical dystonia. *Clin Neuropharmacol* 14:262–267, 1991.

85. Gelb DJ, Yoshimura DM, Olney RK, et al: Change in pattern of muscle activity following botulinum toxin injections for torticollis. *Ann Neurol* 29:370–376, 1991.

86. Comella CL, Buchman AS, Tanner CM, et al: Botulinum toxin injection for spasmodic torticollis: Increased magnitude of benefit with electromyographic asssistance. *Neurology* 42:878–882, 1992.

87. Rivest J, Lees AJ, Marsden CD: Writer's cramp: Treatment with botulinum toxin injections. *Mov Disord* 6:55–59, 1990.

88. Jankovic J, Schwartz K: The use of botulinum toxin in the treatment of hand dystonias. *J Hand Surg* 18A:883–887, 1993b.

89. Karp BI, Cole RA, Cohen LG, et al: Long-term botulinum toxin treatment of focal hand dystonia. *Neurology* 44:70–76, 1994.

90. Yoshimura DM, Aminoff MJ, Olney RK. Botulinum toxin therapy for limb dystonias. *Neurology* 42:627–630, 1992.

91. Tsui JKC, Bhatt M, Calne S, Calne DB: Botulinum toxin in treatment of writer's cramp: A double-blind study. *Neurology* 43:183–185, 1993.

92. Cole R, Hallett M, Cohen LG: Double-blind trial of botulinum toxin for treatment of focal hand dystonia. *Mov Disord* 10:466–471, 1995.

93. Pacchetti C, Albani G, Martignoni E, et al: "Off" painful dystonia in Parkinson's disease treated with botulinum toxin. *Mov Disord* 10:333–336, 1995.

94. Digre K, Corbett JJ: Hemifacial spasm: Differential diagnosis, mechanism, and treatment. *Adv Neurol* 49:151–176, 1988.

95. Lou JS, Jankovic J: Essential tremor: Clinical correlates in 350 patients. *Neurology* 41:234–238, 1991.

96. Jankovic J, Schwartz K: Botulinum toxin treatment of tremors. *Neurology* 41:1185–1188, 1991.

97. Trosch RM, Pullman SL: Botulinum toxin A injections for the treatment of hand tremors. *Mov Disord* 9:601–609, 1994.

98. Jankovic J, Schwartz K, Clemence W, et al: A randomized, double-blind, placebo-controlled study to evaluate botulinum toxin type A in essential hand tremor. *Mov Disord* 11:250–256, 1996.

99. Pahwa R, Busenbark K, Swanson-Hyland EF, et al: Botulinum toxin treatment of essential head tremor. *Neurology* 45:822–824, 1995.

100. Jankovic J: Botulinum toxin in the treatment of dystonic tics. *Mov Disord* 9:347–349, 1994.

101. Davis D, Jabbari B: Significant improvement of stiff-person syndrome after paraspinal injection of botulinum toxin A. *Mov Disord* 8:371–373, 1993.

102. Hesse S, Lücke D, Malezic M, et al: Botulinum toxin treatment for lower limb extensor spasticity in chronic hemiparetic patients. *J Neurol Neurosurg Psychiatry* 57:1321–1324, 1994.

103. Tsui JKC, O'Brien C: Clinical trials for spasticity, in Jankovic J, Hallet M (eds): *Therapy with Botulinum Toxin.* New York: Marcel Dekker, 1994, pp 523–534.

104. Grazko M, Polo KB, Jabbari B: Botulinum toxin A for spasticity, muscle spasms, and rigidity. *Neurology* 45:712–717, 1995.

105. Grossman RG, Hamilton WJ: Surgery for movement disorders, in Jankovic J, Tolosa E (eds): *Parkinson's Disease and Movement Disorders,* 2d ed. Baltimore: Williams & Wilkins, 1993, pp 531–548.

106. Jankovic J, Hamilton W, Grossman RG: Thalamic surgery for movement disorders. *Adv Neurol.* In Press.

107. Lenz FA, Martin R, Kwan HC, et al: Thalamic single-unit activity occurring in patients with hemidystonia. *Stereotact Funct Neurosurg* 55:159–62, 1990.

108. Mitchel IJ, Luquin R, Boyce S: Neural mechanisms of dystonia: Evidence from a 2-deoxyglucose uptake study in a primate model of dopamine agonist-induced dystonia. *Mov Disord* 5:49–54, 1990.

109. Ceballos-Baumann AO, Passingham RE, Marsden CD, Brooks DJ: Motor recognization in acquired hemidystonia. *Ann Neurol* 37:746–757, 1995.

110. Cardoso F, Jankovic J, Grossman R, Hamilton W: Outcome after stereotactic thalamotomy for dystonia and hemiballismus. *Neurosurgery* 36:501–508, 1995.

111. Andrew J, Fowler CJ, Harrison MJG: Stereotaxic thalamotomy in 55 cases of dystonia. *Brain* 106:981–1000, 1983.

112. Cooper IS: 20-year followup study of the neurosurgical treatment of dystonia musculorum deformans. *Adv Neurol* 14:423–52, 1976.

113. Tasker RR, Doorly T, Yamashiro K: Thalamotomy in generalized dystonia. *Adv Neurol* 50:615–31, 1988.

114. Jankovic J, Leder S, Warner D, Schwartz K: Cervical dystonia: Clinical findings and associated movement disorders. *Neurology* 41:1088–1091, 1991.

115. Bertrand CM, Molina-Negro P: Selective peripheral denervation in 111 cases of spasmodic torticollis: Rationale and results. *Adv Neurol* 50:637–643, 1987.

116. Davis DH, Ahlskog JE, Litchy WJ, Root LM: Selective peripheral denervation for torticollis: Preliminary results. *Mayo Clin Proc* 66:365–371, 1991.

117. Goetz CG, Penn RD, Tanner CM: Efficacy of cervical cord stimulation in dystonia. *Adv Neurol* 50:645–649, 1988.

Chapter 33

SYMPTOMATIC DYSTONIAS

JUSTO GARCIA DE YÉBENES, ROSARIO SÁNCHEZ
PERNAUTE, and CESAR TABERNERO

DEFINITION OF SECONDARY OR SYMPTOMATIC
  DYSTONIA
SYMPTOMATIC DYSTONIA RELATED TO FOCAL
  BRAIN LESIONS
    Relevant Brain Structures Involved in Dystonia
    Type of Brain Lesion
    Anatomicoclinical Correlation
    Delayed Onset and Independent Progression
DYSTONIA RELATED TO PERIPHERAL INJURY
DYSTONIA IN NEURODEGENERATIVE DISORDERS
    Dystonia In Akinetic-Rigid Syndromes
    Dystonia in Choreic Syndromes
    Dystonia in Other Basal Ganglia Diseases
    Dystonia in Other Neurodegenerations
DYSTONIA IN DISORDERS OF METABOLISM
    Disorders of Lipid Metabolism
    Disorders of Production of Energy
    Disorders of the Metabolism of Organic Acids and
      Amino Acids
    Abnormalities of the Metabolism of Purines
DYSTONIA INDUCED BY PHYSICAL AND CHEMICAL
  AGENTS
THE PSYCHOGENIC DYSTONIAS
PSEUDODYSTONIAS OF ORGANIC ORIGIN

Definition of Secondary or Symptomatic Dystonia

The concept of symptomatic or secondary dystonia, in contrast to the primary or idiopathic dystonias, emerged in the medical literature as a denomination of dystonias of known etiology. Perinatal brain injury was the most representative cause of symptomatic dystonia; more recently, different focal brain lesions, neurodegenerations, metabolic disorders of the nervous system, and drugs and chemicals have been recognized as causes of dystonia. Several genes or gene markers of the formerly considered primary or idiopathic dystonias have been discovered and, in some cases, the mechanism of production is better known in the idiopathic than in the symptomatic dystonias. Therefore, although it is part of a time-revered tradition, the distinction between primary and secondary dystonias caused by different gene defects has lost some of its conceptual background. It is, however, rather useful for the purpose of differential diagnoses to maintain the separation between primary and secondary dystonias. We will include in the group of primary dystonias, and,

therefore, exclude from our discussion, the sporadic cases of unknown origin and the familial cases of autosomal-dominant idiopathic torsion dystonia linked to chromosome 9, myoclonic dystonia of unknown genetic origin, L-dopa-responsive dystonia and parkinsonism related to mutations of the guanosine triphosphate (GTP)-hydrolase gene, and X-linked dystonia and parkinsonism (Table 33-1).

As opposed to primary dystonia, secondary dystonia is considered to be "often accompanied by other neurological deficits,"[1] to "begin suddenly at rest and occur at rest from the onset,"[2] and to be associated with different known hereditary and environmental causes.[3] These differential criteria are relative, because there is a great clinical diversity of secondary dystonias. In this chapter we will discuss the dystonic syndromes secondary to focal, degenerative, metabolic, or chemical insult to the nervous system, as well as the pseudodystonias of organic and psychogenic origin.

The main clinical characteristics of secondary dystonia, as well as the clues for the differential diagnosis, are summarized in Tables 33-2 and 33-3.

Symptomatic Dystonia Related to Focal Brain Lesions

The most frequent cause of dystonia secondary to focal brain lesions is cerebral palsy (Fig. 33-1).[4] With modern neuroimaging techniques it is not uncommon to find focal brain lesions, and frequently perinatal vascular injury is seen in patients with dystonia who are occasionally unaware of perinatal brain damage. Focal brain lesions are responsible for the great majority of cases of hemidystonia.[5-13]

RELEVANT BRAIN STRUCTURES INVOLVED IN DYSTONIA

The identification of the brain structures involved in dystonia is based on neuroimaging and pathology.[5-7] Magnetic resonance imaging (MRI) and positron emission tomography (PET) studies are more sensitive than computed tomography

---

TABLE 33-1 Etiologic Classification of Dystonia

I. Primary Dystonias
  A. Hereditary
    1. Autosomal-dominant idiopathic torsion dystonia linked to chromosome 9
    2. Autosomal-dominant, L-dopa-responsive dystonia related to GTP-hydrolase deficiency.
    3. Autosomal-dominant myoclonic dystonia
    4. X-linked dystonia-parkinsonism
  B. Sporadic idiopathic dystonias
II. Secondary Dystonias
  A. Caused by focal brain lesions
  B. Associated with degeneration of the central nervous system
  C. Resulting from metabolic disorders of the central nervous system
  D. Produced by drugs and chemicals

TABLE 33-2 Differential Diagnosis of Symptomatic Dystonias

Disease	Inheritance	Type of Dystonia	Age at Onset	Clinical Findings	Neuroimaging	Diagnosis
Focal brain lesions	Sporadic	Hemidystonia focal	Children, young adults	Corticospinal & brain-stem signs	Focal lesion	Clinical/MRI
PD	Mostly sporadic	Focal	Adults	Tremor, ARS	Normal (nigral T2 shortening)	Clinical
PSP	Mostly sporadic	Axial	Mature senile	Gaze palsy, ARS	Midbrain tectal atrophy	Clinicopathological
CBD	Sporadic	Limb	Mature senile	Apraxia, myoclonus, alien limb	Asymmetric cerebral atrophy	Clinicopathological
MSA	Sporadic	Axial	Mature senile	ARS, autonomic, cerebellar	OPCA, T2 putaminal hypointensity in SDS and SND	Pathology
Huntington's disease	AD	Generalized	Young adults	Chorea, dementia	Candate and cortical atrophy	Genetic, iT15 CAG expansion
Neuroacantho-cytosis	AR sporadic	Orolingual generalized	Young adults	Chorea, amyotrophy, epilepsy	Caudate atrophy	Acanthocytes
Wilson's disease	AR	Generalized	Children, young adults	Tremor, psychiatric, dysarthria	Putaminal, thalamic dentate, brain stem, T2 high signal	K-F rings, Cu^{2+} levels, ceruloplasmin gene defects of chromosome 13
Hallervorden-Spatz	AR	Multifocal generalized	Children, young adults	Corticospinal, dementia	Pallidal T2 hypointensity ("eye of the tiger" sign)	Pathology
Fahr's syndrome	AD/AR/ sporadic	Generalized hemidystonia	Adults	ARS, corticospinal, ataxia, dementia	Basal ganglia striking calcifications	Imaging (exclusion diagnosis)
Ataxia telangiectasia	AR	Generalized	Children	Ataxia, neuropathy	Cerebellar atrophy	Clinical, low levels IgA
Machado-Joseph	AD	Multifocal generalized	Children, young adults	Ataxia, ophthalmoplegia, amyotrophy	Cerebellar atrophy	Genetic, CAG expansion 14q
Dentatorubropal-lidoluysian at-rophy	AD	Generalized	Adults	Ataxia, dementia, myoclonus	Brain stem, cerebellum A1t signal	genetic, CAG expansion 21p
Intraneuronal inclusion	Sporadic	Focal generalized	Children, young adults	Corticospinal, ataxia, dementia		Pathology (rectal biopsy)
Rett syndrome	Sporadic (females)	Focal	Children	Autism, stereotypia, epilepsy	Brain atrophy	Clinical
GM1 Gangliosidosis, type 3	AR	Generalized	Children, young adults	Ataxia, corticospinal (no dementing)	Basal ganglia lesions	beta-D-galactosidase
GM2 Gangliosidosis	AR	Generalized	Children, young adults	Corticospinal, epilepsy, blindness	T2 high signal in the basal ganglia, severe atrophy	Hexosaminidase
Niemann-Pick type C	AR	Generalized	Children	Dementia, gaze palsy, epilepsy		Defective cholesterol sterification/ sphingomyelinase

TABLE 33-2—*(continued)*

Disease	Inheritance	Type of Dystonia	Age at Onset	Clinical Findings	Neuroimaging	Diagnosis
Metachromatic leukodystrophy	AR	Generalized	Children	Dementia, psychiatric symptoms	White matter, diffuse confluent T2 high signal	Aryl sulphatase A
Ceroid lipofuscinosis Kufs' disease	AR	Focal (cranial) hemidystonia	Children, young adults	Dementia, ataxia, epilepsy	T2 low signal in thalami and striata	Pathology (rectal biopsy)
Leigh's syndrome	AR	Generalized	Children	Hypotonia, ataxia, optic atrophy	Striatal lucencies (T2 basal ganglia hyperintensities)	Pyruvic acid and alanine levels, mtDNA mutations, cytochrome oxidase activity
Glutaric aciduria I	AR	Generalized	Children	Encephalopathic crisis, mental retardation	Frontotemporal atrophy, enlarged Sylvian fissures	Glutaric acid in urine, glutaryl-CoA dehydrogenase
Methylmalonic aciduria	AR	Generalized	Children	Acute encephalopathy	Pallidal T2 hyperintensity	Chromatography of organic acids, Methylmalonic CoA mutase
Homocystinuria	AR	Generalized	Children	Focal deficits, mental retardation	Focal ischemic lesions, sinus thrombosis	AA chromatography
Hartnup disease	AR	Generalized, paroxysmal	Children	Mental retardation, recurrent ataxia, and behavioral alterations	White matter T2 hyperintensity	AA, chromatography
Lesch-Nyhan syndrome	X-linked	Generalized	Children	Mental retardation, self-mutilation		Hypoxanthine guanine phosphoribosyl transferase

ARS, akinetic-rigid syndrome; OPCA, olivopontocerebellar atrophy; SDS, Shy-Drager syndrome; SND, strionigral degeneration; CBD, corticobasal degeneration; AR, autosomal-recessive inheritance; AD, autosomal-dominant inheritance; AA, amino acid; K-F rings, Kayser-Fleisher rings; MRI, magnetic resonance imaging; mtDNA, mitochondrial DNA.

(CT).[9-11] Three regions are most often involved: the basal ganglia, thalamus, and brain stem.[5-7]

The role of the basal ganglia damage in dystonia is firmly established. Putaminal lesions are the most frequent cause of hemidystonia (Fig. 33-2).[5-7,9,13] Even some patients with idiopathic dystonia have a T_2 signal alteration in the putamen in high-field MRI.[14] The caudate nucleus is occasionally involved in limb dystonia. Pallidal lesions with gliosis as a result of kernicterus cause symptomatic dystonia in childhood.[9]

Thalamic lesions are also a cause of secondary dystonia. Limb dystonia may appear after stereotaxic thalamotomy for the treatment of tremor[15] and dystonia.[16] In summary, the appearance of symptomatic dystonia from focal brain lesions suggests that the structural basis of dystonia lies in the basal ganglia-thalamocortical motor circuit, and this has led to the current concept of dystonia as a dysfunction of this loop.

Evidence of brain stem lesions inducing dystonia, namely, cranial dystonia, is supported by neuroimaging, neurophysiological studies, and clinical pathophysiological associations.[17-25] Neuropathological results are not consistent.[26-31] It has not been possible to localize accurately a responsible nucleus or neuronal circuit yet; brain stem projections to and from the basal ganglia are most probably involved.

TYPE OF BRAIN LESION

Dystonia may appear after almost any properly placed focal lesion (i.e., in the basal ganglia, thalamus, or brain stem) (Table 33-4), although the most common cause of dystonia of focal origin is vascular injury. Diffuse brain injuries (anoxia, kernicterus, hydrocephalus, etc.,) may produce a selective involvement of the structures mentioned above (Fig. 33-3). Focal lesions (vascular malformation, tumor, etc.), located away from these regions (basal ganglia, thalami, brain stem), may produce dystonia by indirect mechanisms, which is most probably related to compression or vascular "steal" phenomena. Demyelinating lesions inducing dystonia are most often located at the brain stem level.

Individual features, including age and genetic susceptibility, are distinctly relevant for the different phenotypic expression of similar lesions.[69]

TABLE 33-3 Diagnostic Clues to Secondary Dystonia

Clinical Clues in the Most Common Symptomatic Dystonias	Most Likely Clinical Diagnosis
I. Dystonia in Children	
A. Dystonia associated with focal neurological signs and perinatal brain injury, ectopia lentis, skeletal deformities, mental retardation	Dystonic cerebral palsy, homocystinuria
B. Dystonia after acute encephalopathy associated with macrocephaly, tetraparesis, dysphagia, dysarthria, optic atrophy, hypotonia, tetraparesis, ataxia, dysphagia, dysarthria	Glutaric aciduria, methylmalonic aciduria, Leigh's syndrome
C. Acute dystonia, without any other neurological symptoms	Intake of neuroleptics, antiemetics, catecholamine releasers, antiepileptics, and other drugs and chemicals
D. Fixed congenital focal dystonia	Musculoskeletal deformities
E. Dystonia associated with other neurological deficits, spinocerebellar deficits, tetraparesis, blindness, and seizures	GM1 gangliosidosis
F. Dystonia associated with spasticity, exaggerated startle reaction and seizures, skeletal deformities, mental retardation associated with automutilation, urinary stones, and hyperuricemia	GM2 ganglioisidosis, Niemann-Pick, disease, Lesch-Nyhan's syndrome
II. Dystonia in Youngsters and Adults	
A. Dystonia associated with akinetic-rigid syndromes, foot dystonia, axial dystonia mostly in extension, gaze palsy, dysphagia, dysarthria, gait disturbance, anterocollis, poor response to L-dopa, autonomic disturbances, asymmetric hand dystonia with myoclonus, generalized dystonia with akinetic-rigid syndrome in children and young adults	PD, PSP multiple-system atrophy, CBD, mitochondrial encephalopathy
B. Dystonia associated with chorea and oromandibular dystonia	Neuroacanthocytosis
C. Dystonia associated with ataxia Autosomal-dominant disease with ataxia, dementia, dysarthria, ophthalmoplegia, dystonia and akinetic-rigid syndromes, rhythmic dystonia, and hemidystonia	Machado-Joseph disease, OPCA, drug-induced, focal putaminal lesions

III. MRI Findings	Most Likely Clinical Diagnosis
A. Pattern of atrophy Frontotemporal atrophy with Sylvian enlargement, cerebellar atrophy, caudate atrophy, midbrain atrophy, asymmetric frontoparietal atrophy	Glutaric aciduria, OPCA, Machado-Joseph, ataxia telangiectasia, Huntington's disease, neuroacanthocytosis, PSP, CBD
B. T2 high-intensity signal	
1. Putaminal	Focal vascular lesion, Wilson's, Leigh's, GM2, cyanide
2. Pallidal	Methylmalonic aciduria, carbon monoxide, methyl alcohol
3. White matter	Methachromatic leukodystrophy, homocystinuria, Hartnup disease
C. Low-intensity signal	
1. Putaminal	MSA, Kufs' disease, calcification of the basal ganglia
2. Pallidal	Hallervorden-Spatz disease

Secondary dystonia as a result of basal ganglia and thalamic injuries is much more frequent when the insult takes place in the perinatal period[73] and earlier years of life, rather than in adulthood (Fig. 33-4).[63,66,67,69] An increased vulnerability of the striatum during development, related to different arrangement of matrix/striosomes or to a high level of excitatory neurotransmission at this stage, could be a possible explanation.[74] Age-related differences reflect different grades of neuronal plasticity and different compensatory potential of particular neuronal circuits. The role of genetic susceptibility is well-documented in drug-induced dystonia but unknown in dystonia induced by focal lesions.

ANATOMICOCLINICAL CORRELATION

There is a certain correlation between the topographic localization of the lesion and the pattern of dystonia:

• Putaminal lesion/hemidystonia or limb dystonia
• Thalamic lesion/hand dystonia
• Brain stem lesion/blepharospasm, Meige's syndrome

However, in some cases it is difficult to establish which is the most relevant lesion.[69] Cranial dystonia with putaminal lesions,[28,34,68] and cranial dystonia and hemidystonia with tha-

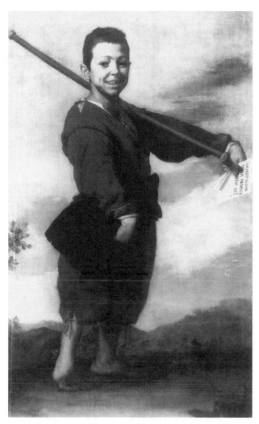

FIGURE 33-1 The limp child. Hemidystonia in cerebral palsy, painted by J. Ribera (1591–1652) in 1642. (*The Louvre, Paris, France.*)

TABLE 33-4 Symptomatic Dystonia as a Result of Focal Lesions of the Nervous System

A. Focal lesions of the basal ganglia, thalamus, and brain stem[5-7]
  1. Vascular:
    a. Infarction[8,9,12,32-37]
    b. Hemorrhage[38,39]
    c. Vascular malformation[40,41]
    d. Arteritis (SLE,[42] primary antiphospholipid syndrome[43])
    e. Migraine[32,44]
  2. Head trauma[45-48]
  3. Tumors and cysts: Astrocytoma,[49] lymphoma,[50] glioma,[51] porencephalic cyst, subarachnoid cyst,[52] metastasis[53]
  4. Infection: *Toxoplasma* (AIDS)[54,55], tuberculoma, viral?[56]
  5. Multiple sclerosis[17,57,58]
  6. Central pontine myelinolysis[25,59,60]
  7. Syringomyelia, cerebellar ectopia[61,62]
B. Diffuse lesions with prominent damage of the basal ganglia, thalamus, or brain stem
  1. Anoxia and energy failure: perinatal asphyxia, cardiac arrest, carbon dioxide, and cyanide intoxication[63 70]
  2. Kernicterus[9]
  3. Hydrocephalus[19]
C. Superficial lesions with unclear effects on the basal ganglia, thalamus, or brain stem
  1. Subdural hematoma[71]
  2. Pachygyria,[72] hemiatrophy

lamic lesions[21,39] are some of the exceptions of this oversimplified scheme. Unilateral diencephalic or brain stem lesions produce bilateral symmetric blepharospasm,[21] although there is one case of a left rostral diencephalic-brain stem lesion with ipsilateral blepharospasm and contralateral hemidystonia.[24]

DELAYED ONSET AND INDEPENDENT PROGRESSION

Some of the most characteristic and intriguing features of dystonia secondary to focal brain lesions are the time delay from injury to the appearance of the movement disorder and its independent progression.

It is unlikely that delayed onset is related to the recovery of an associated corticospinal tract lesion,[9,75] because in many cases dystonia appears without previous hemiparesis. Two alternative pathophysiological mechanisms, *denervation hypersensitivity*[17] and *aberrant sprouting* of the damaged neurons,[63,66] have been proposed.

Dystonia Related to Peripheral Injury

The relationship between peripheral trauma and dystonia is quite controversial. In genetically predisposed individuals, that is, in asymptomatic carriers of the gene for idiopathic torsion dystonia, peripheral trauma may trigger the onset of the dystonia.[46] However, it is not proved that peripheral injury induces dystonia through alteration of the sensory input to the central nervous system or changes of the central processing. Some peculiarities of peripherally induced dystonia[76-81] set it apart from other symptomatic dystonias:

- Short latency of onset (days)
- Present at rest from the start and persists during sleep
- No "geste antagonistique"

FIGURE 33-2 MRI scan showing left perinatal putaminal hemorrhage in a patient with right hemiparesis and right hemidystonia.

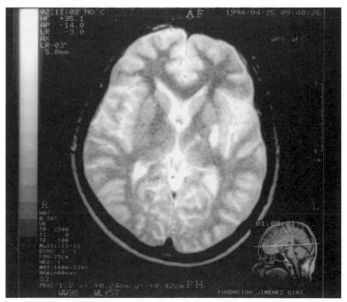

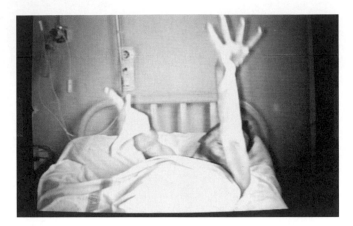

FIGURE 33-3 Generalized dystonia in a patient with AIDS and cerebral toxoplasmosis.

- No overflow
- Fixed postures with limitation of range of motion
- Little response to anticholinergics and botulinum toxin
- Associated causalgia and reflex sympathetic dystrophy

Direct nerve injury or surgery, entrapment neuropathies, and electrical injury have been related to the onset of dystonia. Usually the same region that receives the injury develops the dystonia[81]; hence, local ocular disease is associated with blepharospasm, dental procedures with oromandibular dystonia, whiplash and other neck injuries with cervical dystonia, and limb injury with limb dystonia. In some cases, occupational cramps may be related to repetitive microtraumatisms; hence, they could be considered as a kind of peripherally induced dystonia.

Dystonia in Neurodegenerative Disorders

Dystonia is a common symptom of neurodegenerative disorders, especially those involving the basal ganglia. In most of

FIGURE 33-4 CT scan showing right putaminal infarction in an 8-year-old girl with acute lymphocytic leukemia and left hemidystonia.

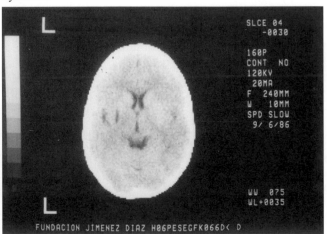

these diseases dystonia is associated with other manifestations of the clinical picture. However, in some instances dystonia may be the unique, most relevant, or first clinical symptom of the neurodegenerative disorder and, therefore, it may be misdiagnosed as idiopathic torsion dystonia.

DYSTONIA IN AKINETIC-RIGID SYNDROMES

PARKINSON'S DISEASE (PD)

Three points deserve discussion regarding dystonia and PD. First, the presence of dystonia in untreated PD; second, the evidence of dystonia and parkinsonism as different phenotypic expression of the same disorders; and third, the appearance of dystonia as a complication of therapy in PD. Dystonia is not uncommon in untreated PD, especially in patients with early onset of clinical symptoms. Adult-onset foot dystonia should raise the possibility of PD.[82,83] The foot is often deviated in equinovarus, with toes 2nd–5th flexed and the great toe dorsiflexed (the so-called striatal toe); this is a typical action dystonia or kinesigenic dystonia, and the deviation worsens with walking. Less frequently, dystonia occurs in the upper extremity in untreated patients with PD, and it is characterized by cubital deviation, metacarpophalangeal flexion, proximal interphalangeal extension, and distal interphalangeal extension. There are some isolated clinical reports of untreated patients suffering blepharospasm, oromandibular dystonia, hemidystonia, writer's cramp, and cervical dystonia,[84,85] and there is a neuropathologically confirmed case of PD with Meige's syndrome.[31] If we consider isolated scoliosis as a symptom of dystonia, then this disorder would be even more frequent in patients with PD.[86] Some authors consider anismus, which is a result of abnormal puborectalis muscle contraction, as a form of dystonia[87] common in PD (see Chap. 13).

The relevance of dystonia in PD has been questioned on the basis that the prevalence of focal dystonia in PD is similar to the expected prevalence of focal dystonia in the same age group.[88]

Dystonia and parkinsonism coexist as different clinical manifestations of the same disease in a number of hereditary conditions, including autosomal-dominant familial parkinsonism,[89] L-dopa-responsive dystonia,[90,91] juvenile parkinsonism,[92,93] early-onset parkinsonism with gliosis of the substantia nigra,[94] and other conditions.

In addition, dystonia occurs in patients under treatment for PD as a complication of the treatment. Off-period dystonia occurs more frequently in the morning (early morning dystonia) after the nocturnal period of L-dopa deprivation or at moments when the patient is akinetic in the interval between two doses of medication (off-period dystonia).

Dystonia also occurs as a side effect of L-dopa treatment at times when the antiparkinsonian effect is present. Peak effect dyskinesia and, more frequently, biphasic dyskinesia are occasionally characterized by repetitive dystonia of the extremities (see Chap. 14).

PROGRESSIVE SUPRANUCLEAR PALSY (PSP)

Oculofaciocervical dystonia[95] is frequent in PSP, which is characterized by akinetic-rigid syndrome, supranuclear gaze palsy, dysphagia, dysarthria, and a variable disturbance of cognitive function. Axial dystonia is characterized by hyperextended neck. Facial expression[96] is related to a tonic-dystonic contraction, making the patients exhibit a "stare." Facial dystonia is often induced by speech. Blepharospasm, often associated with eye lid apraxia, has been described in PSP.[97] Upper limb dystonia, although less typical in PSP, was present in an autopsy-proven patient,[95,98–104] as well as in another pathologically confirmed patient from our group[105] (see Chap. 19).

CORTICOBASAL DEGENERATION (CBD)

Since the original report by Rebeiz et al.,[106] less than 100 clinical patients have been described, and the diagnosis of very few has been confirmed by pathology. The disorder characteristically combines an asymmetric akinetic-rigid syndrome, dystonia, and myoclonus with focal cortical dysfunction. The pathological examination discloses frontoparietal and basal ganglia asymmetrical atrophy and swollen achromatic neurons (see Chap. 45).

Dystonia was present in 83 percent of 36 patients suspected of having CBD, after a mean evolution of 5.2 years.[107] Dystonia began initially in the most affected arm, leading to an adducted and flexed posture with clawed fingers.

MULTIPLE-SYSTEM ATROPHY

Multiple-system atrophy (MSA) is characterized by a varied combination of clinical symptoms derived from the degeneration of several neuronal systems, including the nigrostriatal pathway, striatum, cerebellum, autonomic nervous system, and others. Three subtypes of MSA are currently recognized: striatonigral degeneration, characterized by akinetic-rigid syndrome with poor or short-lasting response to dopaminomimetic agents; Shy-Drager syndrome, characterized by akinetic-rigid syndrome and autonomic failure, and olivopontocerebellar atrophy (OPCA), characterized by ataxia, akinetic-rigid syndrome, different movement disorders, dementia, corticospinal tract signs, and ophthalmoplegia (see Chap. 20).

The frequency of dystonia in MSA is variable. Quinn[88] suggests that around 50 percent of his patients with MSA, as confirmed by pathology, present with anterocollis. Berciano[108] reported the presence of "involuntary movements" in 40 percent of patients with familial and 18 percent of patients with sporadic OPCA. The description of these involuntary movements lacks precise details in most of these patients. Some of them had chorea, probably related to lesions of the subthalamic nucleus; others, including the initial patient described by Menzel,[109] had torticollis. In one case, this torticollis was attributed to atrophy of the vestibuloreticular system.[110]

DYSTONIA IN CHOREIC SYNDROMES

HUNTINGTON'S DISEASE

Dystonia is a frequent clinical symptom in Huntington's disease. In patients with late onset and rapid chorea, dystonia occurs most often as a complication of treatment with neuroleptics. In juvenile patients, motor manifestations are marked

by hypokinesia, rigidity, hypomimia, bradykinesia, and dystonia.[111] In many patients with classical forms, initial rapid chorea disappears with evolution of the illness and is substituted for or accompanied by dystonia (refer to Chap. 35).

NEUROACANTHOCYTOSIS

This unusual disease is inherited in most cases as an autosomal-recessive complex movement disorder. The etiology is unknown, but a membrane defect of protein band 3 is proposed for acanthocytes and striatal neurons.

Clinical manifestations usually start in the 3rd decade as orobuccolinguofacial hyperkinesia, lip smacking, vocalizations, and even orolingual action dystonia leading to lip and tongue automutilation. Thereafter, a generalized chorea develops, often a mixture of chorea and dystonia. In 30 percent of patients there is no cognitive deterioration. About one-half of patients suffer epileptic seizures. Most of them present a motor polyneuropathy with distal amyotrophy and pes cavus. The clinical diagnosis is confirmed by the finding of acanthocytes, usually more than 20 percent of red blood cells, in fresh or saline-incubated blood smears. The neuropathology shows atrophy of the basal ganglia, maximal in caudate nucleus and preferentially affecting small neurons.[112] Neuronal loss also involves the anterior horn of the spinal cord in some cases. The muscle shows denervation and peripheral nerve shows axonal degeneration with demyelination.

Kito et al.[113] described increased noradrenaline in the cerebrospinal fluid and low urinary excretion of dihydroxyphenylacetic acid. De Yebenes et al.[114,115] found moderately decreased striatal levels of dopamine, as well as a great elevation of noradrenaline levels, suggesting that dystonia may be related to disequilibrium of dopamine/noradrenaline neurotransmission in the basal ganglia.

DYSTONIA IN OTHER BASAL GANGLIA DISORDERS

WILSON'S DISEASE

This is an autosomal-recessive systemic disease related to abnormal metabolism of copper and linked to chromosome 13. Tissue damage is a result of copper accumulation. In 217 patients reviewed by Walshe,[116] 43 percent started with hepatic disease and 42 percent with CNS involvement, including two patients with initial psychiatric symptoms. In those patients with neurological onset, tremor in the upper extremities, dysarthria, and dystonia and athetosis were, in that order, the most frequent presenting manifestations. Dystonia also appears during the evolution of the disease, producing bizarre posturing that may affect the four limbs and the trunk (Fig. 33-5). In a clinicoradiological correlation study of 16 symptomatic patients with Wilson's disease, 11 of them, presenting with dystonia, had putaminal lesions in MRI.[117] When considering the differential diagnosis of a patient with dystonia, it is of capital importance to consider and screen for Wilson's disease, because it is a treatable condition in which the reversibility of the clinical symptoms may depend on when definitive therapy is initiated[1] (see also Chap. 46).

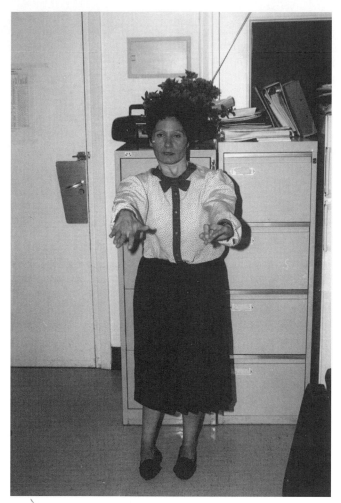

FIGURE 33-5 Generalized dystonia in Wilson's disease.

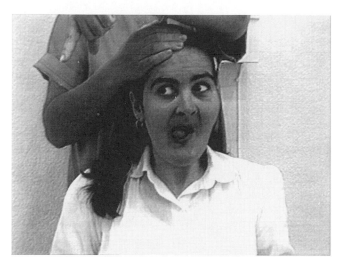

FIGURE 33-6 Orolinguomandibular dystonia in a patient with Hallervorden-Spatz Disease and generalized dystonia.

NEUROAXONAL DYSTROPHY (SEITELBERGER'S DISEASE), INCLUDING HALLERVORDEN-SPATZ DISEASE (HSD)

The pathological marker in this group of related disorders is the neuroaxonal dystrophy or axonal spheroid. Seitelberger[118] classified the primary neuroaxonal dystrophies, including HSD, infantile neuroaxonal dystrophy (INAD), late infantile and juvenile neuroaxonal dystrophy, and neuroaxonal leucodystrophy. Recently, neuroaxonal dystrophy was found in the brain of two siblings presenting with presenile PD.[119]

In INAD the clinical symptoms develop at the end of the 1st year or during the 2nd year of life and are characterized by psychomotor retardation, spasticity and rigidity, loss of vision and hearing, autonomic signs, and death from 3 to 6 years of age. Dystonia may occur with the progression of the disease,[120] especially in cases with long evolution. Pathological involvement is widespread but is most prominent in the posterior spinal horns and the dorsal bulbomedullary nuclei, the pallidum, substantia nigra and other brain stem nuclei, and cerebellar cortex. There is an excess of ferric pigment. Gliosis and long tract degeneration take place.

HSD is an autosomal-recessive disorder that is pathologically characterized by iron deposition in the pallidum and substantia nigra, pars reticularis, and widespread axonal spheroid formation or neuroaxonal dystrophy.[118] The diagnosis must be made by neuropathological examination. Of 64 pathologically confirmed cases, 8 presented with dystonia, and 41 more suffered dystonia during their evolution.[120a] Generalized dystonia was the most frequent presentation, but it could appear as focal or segmental truncal and upper limb dystonia (Fig. 33-6). Dystonia may be associated with tics and other movement disorders in HSD.[121]

CALCIFICATION OF THE BASAL GANGLIA

Calcification of the basal ganglia occurs in a variety of sporadic and hereditary diseases, and it is often associated with different movement disorders, including parkinsonism, chorea, and dystonia. Abnormal parathyroid function is frequently associated with calcification of the basal ganglia, but there are cases without any evidence of biochemical or humoral abnormalities of the metabolism of calcium and phosphorus; these idiopathic cases are often called Fahr's disease. There are reports of familial dystonia as the main manifestation of this disease.[122,123] The patients reported by Caraceni et al.[122] were two brothers with cranial dystonia or limb dystonia; Larsen et al.[123] reported a family with idiopathic calcification of the basal ganglia and autosomal-dominant segmental dystonia.

Two sporadic cases with isolated calcification of the globus pallidus have been described recently.[124] Both patients had cognitive dysfunction, amnesia state, perceptual distortions, complex visual hallucinations, and myoclonus. Patient 1 manifested depression, auditory hallucinations, anxiety, paranoia, and postural tremor; patient 2 manifested multifocal dystonia with dystonic tremor. These cases suggest specific involvement of the pallidal pathways in hallucinations, myoclonus, and dystonia.

PROGRESSIVE PALLIDAL DEGENERATIONS

These rare diseases are be subdivided into four groups according to pathological findings:[125] (a) "pure" pallidal atrophy (PA), (b) "pure" pallidoluysian atrophy (PLA), (c) "extended" forms with nigral, striatal, or dentate nucleus involvement, including pallidoluysionigral atrophy (PLNA), (d) combinations of a–b with thalamic, pyramidal, or spinal motor lesion.

Given the small number of cases, precise clinicopathological correlation has not been possible, but prominent generalized or focal dystonia, together with akinetic-rigid syndromes, is the most common clinical manifestation. Dystonia was described in patients with pure pallidal and pallidoluysian atrophies by van Bogaert.[126] More recently, a patient reported by Wooten et al.[127] had progressive generalized dystonia, dysarthria, and supranuclear gaze palsy. Pathological examination disclosed a pure pallidoluysian atrophy; hence, the authors attributed the symptoms to the damage of the indirect pathway and increased inhibition of internal pallidum.

INTRANEURONAL INCLUSION DISEASE

This is a rare disorder characterized by developmental delay and movement disorders, including dystonia and parkinsonism, with onset from 3 to 30 years of age, most frequently in childhood. The pathological marker is a round autofluorescent eosinophilic inclusion body found in neurons of different regions, more abundant in the basal ganglia but also involving other structures such as the motor neurons, autonomic system, and myenteric plexus. The antemortem diagnosis is possible by means of rectal biopsy.[128]

RETT SYNDROME

This disease characteristically combines psychomotor regression, loss of purposeful use of the hands and stereotypia, ataxia and apraxia of gait, and acquired microcephaly. It only occurs in girls; most of the cases are sporadic; and no diagnostic test is known. Abnormal levels of 5-hydroxyindoleacetic acid and catecholamine metabolites are found in the cerebrospinal fluid. Dystonia is included among the diagnostic criteria.[129] Fitzgerald et al.[130] found that the presence of movement disorders in 32 patients with Rett syndrome was common and increased with age. The disease usually evolves with age from hyperkinetic to hypokinetic patterns. Dystonia, most frequently crural, was present in 59 percent of patients. Bruxism was the most common movement disorder after gait abnormality and stereotyped movements of the hands. Oculogyric crises occurred in 63 percent of cases.

DYSTONIA IN OTHER NEURODEGENERATIONS

MACHADO-JOSEPH DISEASE

This is an autosomal-dominant spinocerebellar degeneration, mainly affecting families descending from ancestors in the Portuguese Islands of the Azores. The clinical manifestations have been classified into different phenotypes. Coutinho and Andrade[131] suggested three clinical subtypes according to the clinical symptoms present in addition to a common ataxic disorder: type I with earliest onset and predominant pyramidal-extrapyramidal signs; type II, the most common, with middle-aged onset and cerebellar plus pyramidal manifestations; and type III of later onset with cerebellar features and distal amyotrophy. Barbeau et al.[132] reviewed 138 patients with this disease and concluded, based on the continuity of

the clinical symptoms in the three subtypes, that this disease was a single clinical entity. The pathological examination usually discloses spinal degeneration affecting anterior horn cells and Clarke's column, and neuronal loss in the dentate nucleus and substantia nigra pars compacta (hence, the name of nigrospinodentatal degeneration).[133] A CAG expansion has been found on chromosome 14q in Japanese cases.[134,134a] Dystonia was present in 20 percent of the 82 patients reported by Gonzalves et al.[135] and involved the hands, feet, face, or neck most commonly, but it was rarely generalized and severe. Dystonia appeared mostly in the younger group. The patient of Lang et al.[136] with double genetic load also had an early onset with generalized dystonia.

The presence of dystonia in Machado-Joseph disease is much more common than in other familial spinocerebellar degenerations. This is attributed to the much more frequent involvement of subthalamopallidal pathways in Machado-Joseph disease, in comparison to other degenerative ataxias.

DYSTONIA IN DENTATORUBROPALLIDOLUYSIAN ATROPHY

In this disease there is degeneration of cerebellar efferent (dentatorubral) and pallidoluysian systems. It is an unusual disease, initially described in Europe by Titica and van Bogaert in 1946,[137] but most of the actual cases are from Japan. The genetic defect has been located on chromosome 21p as an expansion of the trinucleotide CAG.[138,139] Iizuka[140] described three clinical types: an ataxochoreoathetoid, a pseudo-Huntington, and a third type combining myoclonic epilepsy with ataxia. Now that genetic diagnosis is possible, two main clinical groups have been described: adult-onset (at 20 years or older) with ataxia, choreoathetosis, and dementia and juvenile onset (before 20 years) that adds to the previous symptoms a progressive myoclonic epilepsy.[141] Just as it happens in Huntington's disease, paternal transmission correlates with bigger expansions of the repeat and earlier presentation.[142] Dystonia has been described but not as an isolated or prominent manifestation.

ATAXIA TELANGIECTASIA

This is an autosomal-recessive hereditary disorder associated with abnormalities of the DNA repair and clinically characterized by progressive ataxia in childhood, ocular and auricular telangiectasia, increased frequency of respiratory infections resulting from absent or low IgA levels, and increased frequency of malignancies. In most of these patients dystonia is severe, though often not recognized because of the severity of the cerebellar symptoms[143]. After a few years of normal development, affected children develop progressive ataxia of gait, which progressively involves the trunk and upper extremities. Independent gait is progressively more difficult and requires special walkers. Dystonia appears early in the course of the disease[144–148] but usually after the ataxia. Most frequently, it is generalized and further disturbs ambulation (Fig. 33-7). Ocular apraxia, slow saccades, and polyneuropathy may complicate the clinical picture. Severe intellectual deterioration is not typical of this disorder. Telangiectatic lesions appear at about 3–5 years of age and may disappear after several years of progression of disease. Therefore, there may be patients with ataxia telangiectasia with severe dystonia and no prominent telangiectasia in late stages of the

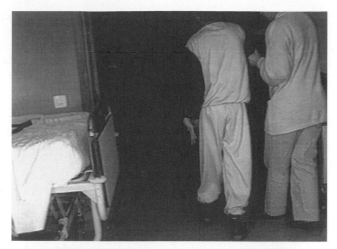

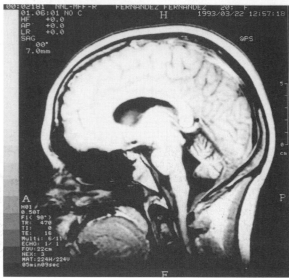

FIGURE 33-7 *Top:* **Generalized dystonia in ataxia telangiectasia.** *Bottom:* **MRI scan showing cerebellar atrophy in ataxia telangiectasia.**

disease. Death occurs as a complication of bronchopulmonary infection or neoplasia, usually a lymphoma.

The pathology of ataxia telangiectasia involves mainly the cerebellar cortex, in which there is a loss of neurons and the pigmented brain stem nuclei, including the substantia nigra and locus ceruleus, which occasionally show Lewy bodies.[149] There is demyelinating neuropathy and loss of fibers in the posterior columns and spinocerebellar tracts.

DYSTONIA IN XERODERMA PIGMENTOSUM

The main manifestations of this entity are dermatological with photosensitivity and skin malignancies, but in some patients neurological manifestations appear with combinations of mental retardation, seizures, spasticity, deafness, ataxia, chorea, dystonia, and axonal sensory neuropathy.[150] There is a defect in DNA repair as in ataxia telangiectasia. The inheritance is autosomal-recessive.

DYSTONIA IN WOLFRAM'S SYNDROME

Although mainly described as an association of diabetes mellitus, diabetes insipidus, optic atrophy, and deafness with autosomal-recessive transmission, it can also be associated with several neurological manifestations. These occur usually later in the course, and consist of ataxia, dizziness, mental and conduct alterations, seizures, tremor and dystonia, areflexia, tonic pupils, and neurogenic bladder.[151]

Dystonia in Disorders of Metabolism

DISORDERS OF LIPID METABOLISM

GM1 GANGLIOSIDOSIS

Dystonia can appear in disorders of lipid metabolism in children and adults. GM1 gangliosidosis is an autosomal-recessive disorder related to a deficiency in beta-galactosidase, leading to intraneuronal storage of GM1 and visceral deposit of compounds with a beta-galactose terminal. GM1 gangliosidosis is clinically characterized by visceromegaly, intellectual impairment, dysmorphism, and a cherry-red spot in the macular region in children. The infantile form, or GM1 type 1, begins at birth or in the first months of life. Affected infants display coarse facial features and skeletal deformities similar to those seen in Hurler's disease. They develop blindness, quadriplegia, and seizures, and they usually die before 2 years of age. Type 2 GM1 begins between 6 and 18 months of age. The course is slower with gait disturbance, mental deterioration, seizures, optic atrophy with a macular cherry-red spot, and late acoustic startle. No marked skeletal deformities are present. Type 3 GM1 gangliosidosis presents from 2 to 27 years of age, with variable manifestations, including a spinocerebellar deficit, dystonia, and myopathy.[152–154]

In adults, GM1 gangliosidosis is characterized by dystonia and early-onset parkinsonism,[153] lack of mental deterioration, and prolonged survival.[155] Atrophy of the head of the caudate nucleus was found in CT scans of two patients,[152,153] and bilateral putaminal lesions on MRI were seen in other patients.[154] Pathological examination of one patient revealed depletion of neurons and intracytoplasmic accumulation of storage material in the basal ganglia, amygdala, and cerebellum.[153] Adult GM1 gangliosidosis occurs with partial deficiencies of beta-galactosidase activity (total lack of activity is associated with the infantile phenotype, partial (from 5 to 15 percent) enzyme activity is associated with adult forms, whereas activity above 15 percent does not produce neurological symptoms.

GM2 GANGLIOSIDOSIS

This disease is a result of intraneuronal accumulation of GM2 ganglioside up to 100–300 times normal values. The cause of the disease is a deficiency in lysosomal hexosaminidase inherited as an autosomal-recessive trait. It is more frequently found among Ashkenazi Jews from eastern Europe.

The symptoms start during infancy. The first symptom is a startle reaction to loud and sudden noises. Quick deterioration of developmental milestones takes place, and few infants reach sitting position. Blindness, spasticity, and convulsions appear, and about 90 percent of these children have a cherry-red spot in one or both maculae. Some children develop macrocephaly related to neuronal storage. Survival after the second year of life is rare.

Diagnosis is made by measuring blood and leukocyte hexosaminidase activity levels. This test shows the heterogeneity of the disease. There are three isoenzymes: A, B, and S, differing in their quaternary structure. Hex A is a trimeric a1 b2; Hex B is a tetrameric b2; and Hex S a dimer a2. There are different mutations of the gene locus. In classic Tay-Sachs, or B variant, Hex A and S are nonfunctional, and normal Hex B is unable to hydrolyze gangliosides. In Sandhoff's disease (O variant), a mutation of the gene coding for B chain on chromosome 5 (5q13) reduces both A and B isoenzymes. In the AB variant, hexosaminidase A and B levels are normal, but the disease is related to a deficit in an activator protein. Individuals with the same enzymatic variants present with similar phenotypes. The parents are heterozygous, and it is possible to perform prenatal diagnosis through chorionic biopsy. There is no effective treatment available, although transplantation of bone marrow and genetic engineering have been attempted.

Most children with classic infantile GM2 gangliosidosis develop an aggressive disease with spastic tetraparesis, seizures, and blindness. Dystonia may appear late in the course of the disease. In juvenile GM2 and in chronic GM2, or adult form, dystonia may appear as the presenting clinical feature[156-159] and, if so, dystonia involves primarily the legs (Fig. 33-8). Some of the juvenile and chronic forms present clinical pictures resembling spinocerebellar degeneration and motor neuron disease.[160]

NIEMANN-PICK DISEASE AND RELATED DISORDERS

This is a heterogeneous group of conditions linked by an accumulation of sphingomyelin in the reticuloendothelial system. Spence and Callahan[161] divided it into group I including former types A and B, with sphingomyelinase deficiency, and group II, including C, D, and E without precise enzymatic deficit.

The main neurological manifestations in Niemann-Pick type A are myoclonic seizures, spasticity, and blindness. Type B disease is also termed visceral or not neuronopathic,

FIGURE 33-8 Foot dystonia in an 8-year-old patient with generalized dystonia resulting from GM2 gangliosidosis.

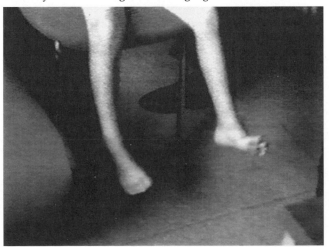

because only occasionally do they develop neurological signs. For types C and D there is no primary metabolic defect identified. Sphingomyelinase activity is normal in most tissues, and only in three-quarters of patients is it decreased in cultured fibroblasts. However, there is a constant defective cholesterol sterification.[162] The initial manifestation is transient neonatal cholestatic icterus, which relapses in 20 percent of patients in the first months of life and leads to death. Surviving patients develop neurological symptoms. Severe cases with onset before 3 years of age suffer a devastating neurological deterioration and may not develop ophthalmoplegia. Patients with later onset present with a very characteristic supranuclear vertical gaze palsy, mental deterioration, gait disorder, cerebellar ataxia, and dystonia. The so-called juvenile dystonic lipidosis may be included in Niemann-Pick type C.[163]

METACHROMATIC LEUKODYSTROPHY

The deficiency of cerebroside sulphatase leads to sulphatide accumulation. Different mutations underlie the late infantile and adult forms, and the juvenile form seems to be related to compound heterozygosity.[164] Rare cases from mutation in an activator protein[165] have also been reported. Juvenile forms present between 4 and 10 years of age with mental deterioration and behavioral disturbances. Nerve conduction velocity may be normal, and a dystonic phenotype has been described.[166]

CEROID LIPOFUSCINOSIS

This group of diseases is marked by the storage of lipopigments, whose nature and production is obscure, in nervous and other tissues. Accumulation takes place in lysosomal-like structures, and the finding of a high concentration of dolichols is supportive of the lysosomal nature of these cytosomes. There is an infantile form, rare outside Finland; a late infantile form; a juvenile form and an adult form, without visual failure and presenting with myoclonic epilepsy, dementia and behavioral disturbances, and extrapyramidal signs, mainly, facial dyskinesias.[167]

PELIZAEUS-MERZBACHER

This disorder has been related to a severe deficiency in myelin-specific lipids caused by a lack of a lipoprotein. Two clinical forms have been described. Type I is X-linked and starts in infancy. Type II is X-linked or autosomal-recessive. The pathology shows a partial-to-total absence of myelinization. In type I, myelin is preserved in the internal capsule and subcortical U fibers. Clinical manifestations include ataxia, nystagmus, and hypotonia, and dystonia occurs later and progresses slowly. In type II there is a severe psychomotor retardation.[168]

DISORDERS OF PRODUCTION OF ENERGY

MITOCHONDRIAL ENCEPHALOMYOPATHIES

Movement disorders, including dystonia, are present in patients with mitochondrial encephalopathies.[169] Truong et al.[170] reviewed 85 patients with mitochondrial myopathies and found that 9 had movement disorders, most frequently myoclonus, but there was generalized dystonia, preceded by mild parkinsonism, in one patient and associated with strokes in another patient.

Generalized dystonia was reported in a patient with suspected mitochondrial myopathy and putaminal hypodensities,[171] and some individuals of a family with patients affected by Leber's hereditary optic neuropathy demonstrated childhood onset dystonia.[172]

SUBACUTE NECROTIZING ENCEPHALOMYELOPATHY OR LEIGH'S DISEASE

Leigh's disease is characterized by intermittent or progressive neurological deterioration after a normal development during the first year of life. Children lose their motor milestones and develop hypotonia, ataxia, corticospinal tract signs, optic atrophy, dystonia, dysphagia, and dysarthria, with relative intellectual preservation. Dystonia is the most common movement disorder in Leigh disease.[173] It may be the principal clinical manifestation in infants,[174] and it is occasionally associated with other movement disorders, including rigidity, tremor, chorea, hypokinesia, myoclonus, and tics. Some patients resemble the primary torsion dystonia phenotype. Neuroradiological studies show basal ganglia lesions, namely, in the putamen, caudate nucleus, substantia nigra, and globus pallidus, in the majority of the patients. MRI is very helpful, because it shows the symmetric lesions of basal ganglia and brain stem in nearly all cases. This pattern of striatal lucencies is consistent with the pathological findings. The pathology of Leigh's disease is characterized by extensive damage of the brain stem and basal ganglia. There is spongiosis of the neuropil and capillary proliferation, but extensive leukoencephalopathy or cortical gray matter damage are uncommon. Leigh's disease is an autosomal-recessive disorder related to abnormalities of the pyruvate kinase complex. The activity of this enzyme in fibroblasts is low, and the blood levels of pyruvate and alanine are usually high. The most common enzymatic defect found in these patients is a reduction of the activity of cytochrome C oxidase. The juvenile forms present with dystonia and movement disorders as protagonistic clinical elements.[175]

Two other disorders related to energy production, Leber's disease and bilateral striatal necrosis, occasionally overlap with Leigh's disease. Therefore, it has been suggested that a variety of energy production disorders, including subacute necrotizing encephalomyelopathy, bilateral striatal necrosis, and Leber's disease, may be grouped under the title of Leigh's syndrome.[176,177] Leber's hereditary optic neuropathy is an X-linked inherited disorder related to different mutations of the mitochondrial genome. Striatal lucencies are present in dystonic patients with Leigh's disease, Leber's hereditary optic neuropathy, and other conditions. In some cases, no biochemical abnormality is found, although some of these may be variants of Leigh's disease. Mutations at point 14459 of the nicotinamide adenine dinucleotide (NADH) dehydrogenase subunit 6 gene are associated with maternally inherited Leber's hereditary optic neuropathy and dystonia.[178] There is a wide variety of clinical presentations, ranging from adult-onset blindness to pediatric dystonia and basal ganglia degeneration in patients with this mutation. Severe nucleotide substitutions are generally new mutations that cause pediatric diseases, such as Leigh's syndrome and dystonia. Mitochondrial DNA rearrangements also cause a variety of phenotypes.[179,180]

DISORDERS OF THE METABOLISM OF ORGANIC ACIDS AND AMINO ACIDS

GLUTARIC ACIDURIA TYPE I

Glutaric aciduria type I (GA-I) is a rare autosomal-recessive disease resulting from a deficiency in glutaryl-CoA dehydrogenase. Homozygous patients have an abnormal degradation of tryptophan, lysine, and hydroxylysine; some of these homozygotes may be clinically asymptomatic. The patients develop their symptoms in infancy. Many of these individuals present with generalized dystonia, which occasionally may appear after recovery from an acute episode of diffuse encephalopathy. Other patients follow a progressive course leading to similar manifestations. Generalized dystonia is the main manifestation, present in 77 percent of 57 patients.[181] Imaging studies show a characteristic frontotemporal atrophy with enlargement of the sylvian fissures.[182] The pathology reveals a severe loss of cells in the basal ganglia, especially in the putamen.[183] The diagnosis is made by measurement of glutaric acid in urine or cerebrospinal fluid. Dietary treatment, with restriction of tryptophan and lysine, reduces the levels of glutaric acid but does not change the course of the disease.[184]

METHYLMALONIC ACIDURIA

This is an autosomal-recessive organic aciduria resulting from abnormal catabolism of methylmalonic acid. During the first years of life patients develop acute neurological symptoms, including generalized dystonia, dysphagia, dysarthria, and different degrees of tetraparesis. These symptoms are considered to be a metabolic stroke involving the globus pallidus and the internal capsule.[185–189] Recent reports of the neurological deficits present in children with different mutations of the methyl-malonyl-CoA mutase gene suggest that there is phenotypic pleomorphism without a consistent pattern of neurological injury and that acidosis and metabolic imbalance are not necessary preconditions for significant neurological morbidity. Analysis of urinary organic acids reveals a massive amount of methylmalonic acid. Some patients obtain relief from dystonic symptoms by taking L-dopa.[188]

FUMARASE DEFICIENCY

This is an inborn error of the tricarboxylic acid cycle characterized by progressive encephalopathy, dystonia, leukopenia, and neutropenia. Elevation of lactate in cerebrospinal fluid and high fumarate excretion in urine provide clues for the investigation of the cytosolic and the mitochondrial fumarase isoenzymes. In two recently reported cases,[190] the analysis of fumarase cDNA demonstrated that both patients were homozygous for a missense mutation, a G-955→C transversion, predicting a Glu-319→Gln substitution. This substitution occurred in a highly conserved region of the fumarase cDNA. Both parents exhibited half the expected fumarase activity in their lymphocytes and were found to be heterozygous for this substitution.

HOMOCYSTINURIA

Homozygous patients for cystathionine beta-synthase deficiency present ectopia lentis, ocular and skeletal deformities, mental retardation, and vascular occlusions that sometimes affect the brain vessels. Dystonia has been described in homocystinuria[191-195] and could be from vascular damage to the basal ganglia. It is also possible that dystonia develops as a metabolic complication[194] through enhanced excitotoxic neurotransmission via stimulation of the glutamate receptors by homocysteic acid or by alteration of the levels of taurine in the basal ganglia.

HARTNUP DISEASE

This disease is characterized by a recurrent personality disorder and cerebellar ataxia, together with a failure to thrive and an intermittent cutaneous rash resembling pellagra. The onset occurs in late infancy and early childhood. Darras et al.[196] described a patient with intermittent focal dystonia. Tamoush et al. report two patients with dystonic features.[197] The biochemical deficit is characterized by a defect in the transport of neutral large amino acids.

ABNORMALITIES OF THE METABOLISM OF PURINES

LESCH-NYHAN SYNDROME

This is an X-linked disorder of the metabolism of purines related to reduced activity of the enzyme hypoxanthine-guanine phosphoribosyltransferase (HGPRT). The clinical features are characterized by normal development up to the age of 6–12 months, followed by developmental delay, mental retardation, spasticity, and a variety of movement disorders (most prominently, dystonia), and automutilation. The patients have high blood levels of uric acid and enhanced urinary elimination of uric acid, which often produces "sandy urine" and urinary stones. Frequent complications of hyperuricemia include gout and tophus. The diagnosis is performed by measurement of the activity of HGPRT in fibroblasts or red blood cells.

HGPRT deficiency may be complete (Lesch-Nyhan syndrome) or partial (Kelley-Seegmiller syndrome). In a recent series[198] of eight patients with complete HGPRT deficiency and four with incomplete enzymatic defect, it was found that the eight patients with Lesch-Nyhan syndrome presented with choreoathetosis, corticospinal motor system dysfunction, mental retardation, and signs of self-mutilation. The patients with Kelley-Seegmiller syndrome were quite heterogeneous: two patients had psychomotor retardation with spasticity; one was mentally retarded with generalized dystonia; and one patient had only gout with no neurological manifestations. A mutation was identified in exon 3 of the gene coding for HGPRT (substitution of guanine with thymine), resulting in the substitution of the normal glycine amino acid by valine (HGPRT Madrid).[199]

Dystonia Induced by Physical and Chemical Agents

Head trauma, which can produce dystonia secondary to focal lesions of the nervous system, and peripheral trauma, which can trigger the development of focal dystonias in individuals at risk, are physical injuries that can produce dystonia. In addition, other physical agents have been reported to induce dystonia. Electrical injuries may produce limb dystonia.[200] Dystonia induced by physical agents has also been described as an occupational disease in users of lasers and in survivors of the Chernobyl nuclear accident.[201,202] The pathogenesis of dystonia in these cases is attributed to radiation-induced lesions of small blood vessels in the brain; the clinical description of these cases is far from clear. Most of these reports are in the Russian literature, and the word "dystonia" is used with different meanings, including disturbances compatible with dystonia and others compatible with autonomic symptoms as well as psychogenic disorders.

Dystonia induced by chemicals is common. Therapeutic agents, with a variety of pharmacological actions, produce dystonia as an acute side effect of the pharmacological treatment or as a persistent, and often permanent, complication. Many of these compounds modify the metabolism of brain monoamines, namely, dopamine (DA), norepinephrine (NE), and serotonin (5-HT). Most frequently, DA stimulating agents, such as L-dopa and DA agonists, induce acute dystonia, especially in patients with akinetic rigid syndromes. Also, there are reports of persistent, and occasionally paroxysmal, dystonia after intake of amphetamine and related compounds.[203,204] DA receptor blockers produce acute and persistent dystonia. Acute dystonic reactions occur frequently with atypical neuroleptics, benzamide derivatives, frequently used as antiemetics in children. These acute dystonic reactions, which occasionally are life-threatening and are always alarming, respond very well to treatment with parenteral anticholinergics (e.g., benzotropine or diphenhydramine).

Persistent dystonia was described in the French literature of the 1950s as a late complication (hence, the name "tardive") of the treatment of schizophrenic patients with chlorpromazine, and it is a frequent complication of long-term neuroleptic treatment (Fig. 33-9). However, the adjective "tardive," meaning "late," may be misleading, because it occasionally occurs very early. Persistent dystonia is very difficult to treat.[205,206] Not infrequently, persistent dystonia is produced by drugs of doubtful indication. Therefore, prevention, early recognition of symptoms, and discontinuation of the offending medication, whenever possible, are the first steps in the treatment of drug-induced dystonia. A list of drugs that produce dystonia is given in Table 33-5. (refer to Chap. 37).

Dystonia may be produced by toxic environmental agents. Manganese toxicity produces dystonia and parkinsonism caused by degeneration of the striatum and pallidum, and it is seen in miners and in patients with chronic liver disease.[276] Dystonia has also been attributed to high copper levels in one patient with cholestatic liver disease.[277] Exogenous toxins, including methanol[278] and cyanide,[279] produce dystonia.

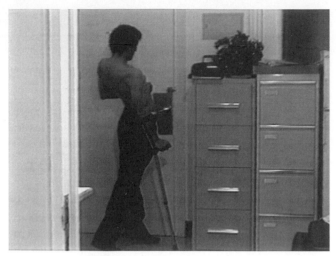

FIGURE 33-9 Generalized persistent dystonia induced by neuroleptics.

Dystonia may be caused by plant derivatives. The best known of these diseases is epidemic ergotism, which is associated with focal and generalized dystonia, epilepsy, stroke, and peripheral ischemia of the limbs (Fig. 33-10).[280,281] Mildeweed sugar cane poisoning produces encephalopathy and dystonia[282] in the developing world.

The Psychogenic Dystonias

Although about 40 percent of patients with dystonia are misdiagnosed as having psychogenic disorders; less than 3 percent of our patients have dystonia of psychogenic etiology. These patients do not belong in a single group but could be subdivided in different subtypes with occasionally imprecise borders. Munchausen's syndrome simulating dystonia[283] is characterized by a chronic factitious disorder consistent with clinical symptoms that are under the patient's voluntary control and that depend on the medical knowledge of the subject. This behavior pretends to ensure to the affected individual a permanent dependence on medical care and may cause unjustified and aggressive, and occasionally risky, medical treatments. Malingering is characterized by consciously simulated illness to obtain social or economic compensation. Hysteria or conversion disorders are characterized by no conscious production of the symptoms. In general, psychogenic dystonia can be differentiated from genuine dystonia by several clinical characteristics, including the presence of associated atypical weakness or sensory complains, fixed postures, and lack of modification of the movement disorder by action or sensory tricks. The pattern of movement changes inconsistently in different situations and in the presence or absence of medical and nursing staff or, at times, when the patient believes he or she is not being observed. There is worsening from stress, improvement by relaxation and psychotherapy, and disappearance by revelation of the nature of the disorder (Table 33-6).

TABLE 33-5 Symptomatic Dystonia to Drugs and Chemicals

I. Chemicals: Therapeutic Agents	TYPE OF DYSTONIA	
	Acute	Persistent
A. Dopamine receptor blockers		
Classic neuroleptics[205-220]	xxx	xx
Clozapine[221-224]	x	
Substituted benzamides[225-233]	xxx	x
Catecholamine depletors[234]	x	
B. Dopamine-stimulating agents		
L-dopa[235-239]	x	x
Dopamine agonists[240-242]	x	
Cocaine[243-245]	x	
Catecholamine releasers[203]	x	x
Ergotamine[246,247]	x	x
Monoamino-oxidase inhibitors[248]	x	
C. Antihistaminics (with DA receptor-blocking properties)		
Thiethylperazine[249]	x	
Prochlorperazine[230]	x	
D. 5-HT-stimulating agents		
Sertraline[250]	x	
Fluoxetine[251-254]	x	
Fluvoxamine[255]	x	
m-CPP[256]	x	
E. Anxiolytics		
Buspirone[257]	x	
Fluspirilene[258-262]	x	
Bromazepam[263]	x	
F. Other		
Carbamazepine[264,265]	x	x
Anesthetics[266-269]	x	
Dilsulfiram[270-272]	x	x
Veralipride[273]	x	
Erythromycin[274]	x	
Flecainide[275]	x	x
Flunarizine and other CA^{2+} blockers	x	x

II. Neurotoxic Chemicals	TYPE OF DYSTONIA	
	Acute	Persistent
A. Minerals		
Manganese[276]		x
Copper[277]		x
B. Organic compounds		
Methyl alcohol[278]		x
Cyanide[279]		x
C. Plant derivatives		
Ergotism[280,281]		x
Mildeweed sugar cane poisoning[282]		x

Pseudodystonias of Organic Origin

These disorders are characterized by abnormal postures or movements related to musculoskeletal deformities or performed to compensate for pain or abnormal function of different elements of the central or peripheral nervous system. These disorders may be confounded with focal or segmental

TABLE 33-6 Clinical Characteristics of Genuine Dystonia, Psychogenic Dystonia, and Pseudodystonia

	Dystonia	Psychogenic Dystonia	Pseudodystonia
Socioeconomic benefit	+ / −	+ + +	+ / −
Atypical symptoms (weakness, sensory complains)	+ / −	+ + +	+ / −
Triggered/worsened by action	+ + +	−	−
Triggered/worsened by stress	+ +	+ + +	+ / −
Fixed dystonia	+	+ + +	+ + +
Improved by sensory tricks or geste antagonistic	+ + +	−	−
Improved by relaxation	+ +	+ + +	−
Abnormal imaging findings	+ / −	−	+ +

−, negative; + / −, questionable; +, positive; + +, very positive; + + +, very characteristic.

dystonias, because they are restricted to a part of the body. The correct diagnosis can be made by taking into consideration the fixed nature of the abnormality, the lack of improvement with sensory tricks, and the absence of aggravation by action. A list of organic disorders simulating dystonias is included in Table 33-7.

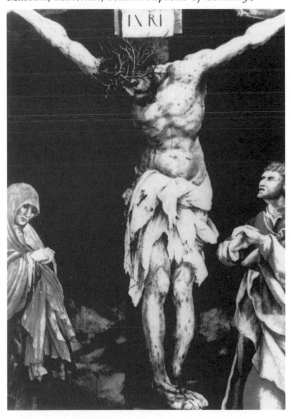

FIGURE 33-10 Foot dystonia in a patient with epidemic ergotism. The painting was done by by M. Grunewald (c 1455–1528), about 1523. The model was probably a patient with epidemic ergotism contacted by Grunewald during his work for the Antonin friars at the Monastery of Issenheim. (*Tauberbischofslein Museum, Karlsruhe, Federal Republic of Germany.*)

TABLE 33-7 Pseudodystonias of Organic Origin

A. Disorders simulating blepharospasm
   Eyelid apraxia
   Palpebral ptosis
B. Disorders simulating oromandibular dystonia
   Trismus
C. Disorders simulating cervical dystonia
   1. Osteoarticular
       Subluxation of the Atlantoaxial articulation
       Klippel-Feil abnormality
       Platybasia and basilar impression
       Cervical hemivertebra
       Damage, absence, or laxity of the cervical ligaments
   2. Muscular
       Congenital or acquired muscle weakness
   3. Neurological
       Diplopia, mainly cranial nerve IV palsy
       Vestibular lesions
       Syringomyelia, syringobulbia
       Tonsillar herniation of any cause, including Arnold-Chiari syndrome
       Posterior fossa tumor or cyst
   4. Remote
       Hiatus hernia
D. Disorders simulating brachial dystonia
   1. Carpal tunnel syndrome and other painful neuropathies
E. Disorders simulating trunk dystonia
   1. Osteoarticular
       Bony abnormalities causing kyphosis, lordosis, or scoliosis
   2. Neuromuscular
       Myopathies or neuropathies
       Stiff-person syndrome
       Opisthotonos
       Muscle cramps
       Compensatory postures due to visceral or anorectal pain
F. Disorders simulating leg dystonia
   1. Osteoarticular
       Asymmetry, bony abnormalities
   2. Neuromuscular
       Spasticity, muscle cramps, restless legs

References

1. Calne DB, Lang AE: Secondary dystonia. *Adv Neurol* 50:9–33, 1988.
2. Jankovic J, Fahn S: Dystonic disorders, in Parkinson's Disease and Movement Disorders. Jankovic J, Tolosa E (eds): Baltimore: Williams & Wilkins, 1993, pp 337–374.
3. Fahn S: Dystonia: Where next?, in Quinn NP, Jenner PG (eds): *Disorders of Movement*. New York: Academic Press, 1989, pp 349–357.
4. Dooling EC, Adams RD: The pathologic anatomy of posthemiplegic athetosis. *Brain* 98:29–48, 1975.
5. Marsden CD, Obeso JA, Zarranz JJ: The anatomical basis of symptomatic dystonia. *Brain* 108:463–483, 1985.
6. Pettigrew LC, Jankovic J: Hemidystonia: A report of 22 cases and a review of the literature. *J Neurol Neurosurg Psychiatry* 48:650–657, 1985.
7. Obeso JA, Giménez-Roldán S: Clinicopathological correlation in symptomatic dystonia. *Adv Neurol* 50:113–122, 1988.
8. Demierre B, Rondot P: Dystonia caused by putamino-capsulo-caudate vascular lesions. *J Neurol Neurosurg Psychiatry* 46:404–409, 1983.
9. Burton K, Farrel K, Li D, Calne DB: Lesions of the putamen and dystonia: Computed tomography and magnetic resonance imaging. *Neurology* 34:962–965, 1984.
10. Perlmutter JS, Raichle ME: Pure hemidystonia with basal ganglion abnormalities on positron emission tomography. *Ann Neurol* 15:228–233, 1984.
11. Quinn N, Bydder G, Leenders N, Marsden CD: Magnetic resonance imaging to detect deep basal ganglia lesions in hemidystonia that are missed by computarized tomography (Letter). *Lancet* Nov 2:1007–1008, 1985.
12. Fross RD, Martin WRW, Li D, et al: Lesions of the putamen: Their relevance to dystonia. *Neurology* 37:1125–1129, 1987.
13. Menkes JH, Curren J: Clinical and MR correlates in children with extrapyramidal cerebral palsy. *AJNR Am J Neuroradiol* 15:451–457, 1994.
14. Schneider S, Feifel E, Ott D, et al: Prolonged MRI T2 times of the lentiform nucleus in idiopathic spasmodic torticollis. *Neurology* 44:846–850, 1994.
15. Krauss JK, Mohadjer M, Nobbe F, Mundinger F: The treatment of post traumatic tremor by stereotactic surgery: Symptomatic and functional outcome in a series of 35 patients. *J Neurosurg* 80:810–819, 1994.
16. Yamashiro K, Tasker RR: Stereotactic thalamotomy for dystonic patients. *Stereotact Funct Neurosurg* 60:81–85, 1993.
17. Jankovic J, Patel SC: Blepharospasm associated with brainstem lesions. *Neurology* 33:1237–1240, 1983.
18. Lang AE, Sharpe JA: Blepharospasm associated with palatal myoclonus (Letter). *Neurology* 34:1522, 1984.
19. Sandyk R, Gillman MA: Blepharospasm associated with communicating hydrocephalus (Letter). *Neurology* 34:1522–1523, 1984.
20. Jankovic J: Blepharospasm associated with palatal myoclonus and communicating hydrocephalus (Letter). *Neurology* 34:1523–1525, 1984.
21. Powers JM: Blepharospasm due to unilateral diencephalon infarction. *Neurology* 35:283–284, 1985.
22. Jankovic J: Blepharospasm with basal ganglia lesions (Letter). *Arch Neurol* 43:866–868, 1986.
23. Day TJ, Lefroy RB, Mastaglia FL: Meige's syndrome and palatal myoclonus associated to brainstem stroke: A common mechanism? *J Neurol Neurosurg Psychiatry* 48:1324–1325, 1986.
24. Leenders KL, Frackowiack RSJ, Quinn N, et al: Ipsilateral blepharospasm and contralateral hemidystonia and parkinsonism in a patient with a unilateral rostral brainstem-thalamic lesion: Structural and functional abnormalities studied with CT, MRI and PET scanning. *Mov Disord* 1:151–158, 1986.
25. Salerno SM, Kurlan R, Joy SE, Shoulson I: Dystonia in central pontine myelinolysis without evidence of extrapontine myelinolysis. *J Neurol Neurosurg Psychiatry* 56:1221–1223, 1993.
26. Garcia-Albea E, Franch O, MuFoz D, Ricoy JR: BrHeghel's syndrome: Report of a case with post-mortem study. *J Neurol Neurosurg Psychiatry* 44:437–440, 1981.
27. Gibb WRG, Lees AJ, Marsden CD: Pathological report of four patients presenting with cranial dystonias. *Mov Disord* 3:211–221, 1988.
28. Altrocchi PH, Forno LS: Spontaneous oral-facial dyskinesia: Neuropathology of a case. *Neurology* 33:802–805, 1983.
29. Zweigg RM, Jankel WR, Whitehouse MF, et al: Brainstem pathology in dystonia. *Neurology* 36(suppl 1):74–75, 1986.
30. Kulisevsky J, Marti MJ, Ferrer I, Tolosa E: Meige syndrome: Neuropathology of a case. *Mov Disord* 3:170–175, 1988.
31. Mark MH, Sage JI, Dickson DW, et al: Meige syndrome in the spectrum of Lewy body disease. *Neurology* 44:1432–1436, 1994.
32. Grimes JD, Hassan MN, Quarrington AM, D'Alton J: Delayed-onset post-hemiplegic dystonia: CT demonstration of basal ganglia pathology. *Neurology* 32:1033–1035, 1982.
33. Russo LS: Focal dystonia and lacunar infarction of the basal ganglia. *Arch Neurol* 40:61–62, 1983.
34. Keane JR, Young JA: Blepharospasm with bilateral basal ganglia infarction. *Arch Neurol* 42:1206–1208, 1985.
35. Giroud M, Dumas R: Dystonie secondaire, un infarctus putamino-capsulo-caud-chez l'enfant. *Rev Neurol (Paris)* 144:375–377, 1988.
36. Picard A, Elghozi D, Schuman-Clacy E, Lacert P: Troubles du langage de type sous-cortical et hemidystonie sequelles d'un infarctus putamino-caude datant de la premiere enfance. *Rev Neurol (Paris)* 145:73–75, 1989.
37. Molho ES, Factor SA: Basal ganglia infarction as a possible cause of cervical dystonia. *Mov Disord* 8:213–216, 1993.
38. Lin JP, Goh W, Brown JK, Steers AJ: Heterogeneity of neurological syndromes in survivors of grade 3 and 4 periventricular haemorrhage. *Childs Nerv Syst* 9:205–214, 1993.
39. Chiang CY, Lu CS: Delayed-onset posthemiplegic dystonia and imitation synkinesia (Letter). *J Neurol Neurosurg Psychiatry* 53(7):623, 1990.
40. Friedman DJ, Jankovic J, Rolak LA: Arteriovenous malformation presenting as hemidystonia. *Neurology* 36:1590–1593, 1986.
41. Lorenzana L, Cabezudo JM, Porras LF, et al: Focal dystonia secondary to cavernous angioma of the basal ganglia: Case report and review of the literature. *Neurosurgery* 31:1108–1112, 1992.
42. Daras M, Georgakopoulos T, Avdelidis D: Late onset post-hemiplegic dystonia in systemic lupus erythematosus. *J Neurol Neurosurg Psychiatry* 51:151–152, 1988.
43. Angelini L, Rumi V, Nardocci N, et al: Hemidystonia symptomatic of primary anti phospholipid syndrome. *Mov Disord* 8:383–386, 1993.
44. Obeso JA, Martinez-Vila E, Delgado G, et al: Delayed onset dystonia following hemiplegic migraine. *Headache* 24:266–268, 1984.
45. Brett EM, Hoare RD, Sweely MP, Marsden CD: Progressive hemidystonia due to focal basal ganglia lesion after mild head trauma. *J Neurol Neurosurg Psychiatry* 44:460, 1981.
46. Fletcher NA, Harding AE, Marsden CD: The relationship between trauma and idiopathic torsion dystonia. *J Neurol Neurosurg Psychiatry* 54:713–717, 1991.
47. Krauss JK, Mohadjer M, Braus DF, et al: Dystonia following head trauma: A report of nine cases and a review of the literature. *Mov Disord* 7:261–272, 1992.

48. Lee MS, Rinne JO, Ceballos-Baumann A, et al: Dystonia after head trauma. *Neurology* 44:1374–1378, 1994.

49. Narbona J, Obeso JA, Luguin R, et al: Hemidystonia secondary to localised basal ganglia tumor. *J Neurol Neurosurg Psychiatry* 47:704–709, 1984.

50. Poewe WH, Kleedorfer B, Willeit J, Gerstenbrand F: Primary CNS lymphoma presenting as a choreic movement disorder followed by segmental dystonia. *Mov Disord* 3:320–325, 1988.

51. Roche S, Godward S, Middleton A, Lane RJ: Dystonic and other movement disorders related to a bifrontal glioma involving the corpus callosum and basal ganglia. *Mov Disord* 8:121–122, 1993.

52. Rosso AL, Mattos JP, Novis SA: A case of periodic sweating associated with a subarachnoid cyst and multifocal dystonia. *Clin Auton Res* 3:299–301, 1993.

53. Krauss JK, Mohadjer M, Nobbe F, Scheremet R: Hemidystonia due to a contralateral parieto-occipital metastasis: Disappearance after removal of the mass lesion. *Neurology* 41:1519–1520, 1991.

54. Nath A, Jankovic J, Pettigrew LC: Movement disorders and AIDS. *Neurology* 37:37–41, 1987.

55. Tolge CF, Factor SA: Focal dystonia secondary to cerebral toxoplasmosis in a patient with acquired immune deficiency syndrome. *Mov Disord* 6:69–72, 1991.

56. Neng T, Yi C, Xiu-Bao Z, Zhi-Jiao Q: Acute infectious torticollis. *Neurology* 33:1344–1346, 1983.

57. Coleman RJ, Quinn NP, Marsden CD: Multiple sclerosis presenting as adult onset dystonia. *Mov Disord* 3:329–332, 1983.

58. Mao C, Gancher ST, Herndon RM: Movement disorders in multiple sclerosis. *Mov Disord* 3:109–116, 1988.

59. Grafton ST, Bahls F, Bell K: Acquired dystonia following central pontine myelinolysis. *Neurology* 37(suppl 1):276, 1987.

60. Maraganore DM, Folger WN, Swanson JW, Ahlskog JE: Movement disorders as sequelae of central pontine myelinolysis: Report of three cases. *Mov Disord* 7:142–148, 1992.

61. Kiwak JK, Deray MJ, Shields WD: Torticollis in three children with syringomyelia and spinal cord tumor. *Neurology* 33:946–948, 1983.

62. Berardelli A, Thompson PD, Day BL, et al: Dystonia of the legs induced by walking or passive movement of the big toe in a patient with syringomyelia and cerebellar ectopia. *Neurology* 36:40–44, 1986.

63. Burke RE, Fahn S, Gold AP: Delayed-onset dystonia in patients with "static" encephalopathy. *J Neurol Neurosurg Psychiatry* 43:789–797, 1982.

64. Hawker K, Lang AE: Hypoxic-ischemic damage of the basal ganglia: Case reports and review of the literature. *Mov Disord* 5:219–225, 1990.

65. Choi IS: Delayed neurologic sequelae in carbon monoxide intoxication. *Arch Neurol* 40:433–435, 1983.

66. Saint Hilaire MH, Burke RE, Bressman SB, et al: Delayed-onset dystonia due to perinatal or early chilhood asphyxia. *Neurology* 41:216–222, 1991.

67. Carella F, Grassi MP, Savoiardo M, et al: Dystonic-parkinsonian syndrome after cyanide poisoning: Clinical and MRI findings. *J Neurol Neurosurg Psychiatry* 51:1345–1348, 1988.

68. Larumbe R, Vaamonde J, Artieda J, et al: Blepharospasm associated with anoxic damage of the basal ganglia during cardiac surgery. *Mov Disord* 8:198–200, 1993.

69. Bhatt MH, Obeso JA, Marsden CD: Time course of post anoxic dystonic syndromes. *Neurology* 43:314–317, 1993.

70. Boylan KB, Chin JH, DeArmond SJ: Progressive dystonia following resuscitation from cardiac arrest. *Neurology* 40:1458–1461, 1990.

71. Eaton JM: Hemidystonia due to subdural hematoma. *Neurology* 38:507, 1988.

72. Leuzzi V, Ricciotti V, Pelliccia A: Hemiplegic dystonia associated with regional cortical dysplasia (pachygyria). *Mov Disord* 8:242–244, 1993.

73. Foley J: Dyskinetic and dystonic cerebral palsy and birth. *Acta Paediatr* 81:57–60, 1992.

74. Giladi N, Burke RE, Kostic V, et al: Hemiparkinsonism-hemiatrophy syndrome: Clinical and neuroradiological features. *Neurology* 40:1731–1734, 1990.

75. Factor SA, Sanchez-Ramos J, Weiner WJ: Delayed-onset dystonia associated with corticospinal tract dysfunction. *Mov Disord* 3(3):201–210, 1988.

76. Schott GD: The relationship of peripheral trauma and pain to dystonia. *J Neurol Neurosurg Psychiatry* 48:698–701, 1985.

77. Jankovic J, Van der Linden C: Dystonia and tremor induced by peripheral trauma: Predisposing factors. *J Neurol Neurosurg Psychiatry* 51:1512–1519, 1988.

78. Truong DD, Dubinsky R, Hermanowicz N, et al: Posttraumatic torticollis. *Arch Neurol* 48:221–223, 1991.

79. Goldman S, Ahlskog JE: Posttraumatic cervical dystonia. *Mayo Clin Proc* 68.443–448, 1993.

80. Foley-Nolan D, Kinirons M, Coughlan RJ, O'Connor P: Post-whiplash dystonia well controlled by transcutaneous electrical nervous stimulation (TENS): Case report. *J Trauma* 30:909–910, 1990.

81. Jankovic J: Post-traumatic movement disorders: Central and peripheral mechanisms. *Neurology* 44:2006–2014, 1994.

82. Lees AJ, Hardie RJ, Stern GM: Kinesigenic foot dystonia as a presenting feature of Parkinson's disease. *J Neurol Neurosurg Psychiatry* 47:885, 1984.

83. Poewe W, Lees AJ, Steiger D, Stern GM: Foot dystonia in Parkinson's disease: Clinical phenomenology and neuropharmacology. *Adv Neurol* 45.357–360, 1986.

84. LeWitt PA, Burns RS, Newman RP: Dystonia in untreated parkinsonism. *Clin Neuropharmacol* 9:293–297, 1986.

85. Katchen M, Duvoisin RC: Parkinsonism following dystonia in three patients. *Mov Disord* 1:151–157, 1986.

86. Grimes JD, Hassan MN, Halle D, Armstrong GWD: Clinical and radiographic features of scoliosis in Parkinson's disease. *Adv Neurol* 45:353–355, 1986.

87. Mathers SE, Kempster PA, Swash M, Lees AJ: Constipation and paradoxical puborectalis contraction in anismus and Parkinson's disease: A dystonic phenomenon? *J Neurol Neurosurg Psychiatry* 51:1503–1507, 1988.

88. Quinn NP: Parkinsonism and dystonia, pseudo-parkinsonism and pseudodystonia. *Adv Neurol* 60:540–543, 1993.

89. Golbe LI, Di Iorio G, Bonavita V, et al: A large kindred with autosomal dominant Parkinson's disease. *Ann Neurol* 27:276–282, 1990.

90. De Yebenes JG, Moskowitz C, Fahn S, Saint-Hilare MH: Long-term treatment with L-dopa in a family with autosomal dominant torsion dystonia. *Adv Neurol* 50:101–111, 1988.

91. Nygaard TG, Trugman JM, de Yebenes JG, Fahn S: DOPA responsive dystonia: The spectrum of clinical manifestations in a large north american family. *Neurology* 40:253–257, 1990.

92. Yokochi M: Nosological concept of juvenile parkinsonism with reference to the dopa-responsive syndrome. *Adv Neurol* 60:548–552, 1993.

93. Bastos Lima A, Levy A, Castro Galdas A, et al: Parkinson's disease before age 30. *Adv Neurol* 60:553–561, 1993.

94. Dwork AJ, Balmaceda C, Fazzini EA, et al: Dominantly inherited, early-onset parkinsonism: Neuropathology of a new form. *Neurology* 43(1):69–74, 1993.

95. Probst A, Dufresne JJ: Paralysie supranucleaire progressive ou dystonie oculo facio cervicale. *Scweitz Arch Neurol Neurochir Psychiatr* 116:107–134, 1975.

96. Constantino A, Bolton CF: The face in progressive supranuclear palsy. *Neurology* 35(suppl 1):161, 1985.

97. Jackson JA, Jankovic J, Ford J: Progressive supranuclear palsy: Clinical features and response to treatment in 16 patients. *Ann Neurol* 13:237–278, 1983.

98. Steele JC, Richardson JC, Olszewsky J: Progressive supranuclear palsy. *Arch Neurol* 10:333–359, 1964.

99. Weimann RL: Heterogeneus degeneration of the central nervous system associated with peripheral neuropathy. *Neurology* 17:507–603, 1967.

100. Steele JC: Progressive supranuclear palsy. *Brain* 95:693–704, 1972.

101. Rafal RD, Friedman JH: Limb dystonia in progressive supranuclear palsy. *Neurology* 37(9):1546–1548, 1987.

102. Kurihara T, Landau WM, Torack RM: Progressive supranuclear palsy with action myoclonus, seizures. *Neurology* 219–223, 1974.

103. Leger JM, Girault JA, Bolgert F: Deux cas de dystonie isole d'un membre superieur inagurant une maladie de Steele Richardson Olszewsky. *Rev Neurol (Paris)* 143:140–142, 1987.

104. Fenelon G, Guillard A, Romanet S, et al: Les signes parkinso-niens du syndrome de Steele-Richardson-Olszewsky. *Rev Neurol Paris* 149(1):69–64, 1993.

105. De Yebenes JG, Sarasa JL, Daniel SE, Lees AJ: Familial progressive supranuclear palsy. In Press.

106. Rebeiz JJ, Kolondy EH, Richardson EP: Corticodentatonigral degeneration with neuronal achromasia. *Arch Neurol* 18:20–33, 1968.

107. Lee MS, Thompson PD, Marsden CD: Corticobasal degeneration: A clinical study of 36 cases. *Brain* 117(5):1183–1196, 1994.

108. Berciano J: Olivopontocerebellar atrophy, in Jancovic J, Tolosa E (eds): *Parkinson's Disease and Movement Disorders*. Baltimore: Williams & Wilkins, 1993, chap 10, pp 163–189.

109. Menzel P: Beitrage zur Kenntnigs der hereditarien ataxie und kleinhinrnatrophie. *Arch Psychiatr Nervenkr* 22:160–190, 1891.

110. Neumann MA: Pontocerebellar atrophy combined with vestibular reticular degeneration. *J Neuropathol Exp Neurol* 36:321–337, 1977.

111. Bruyn GW, Went LN: Huntington's chorea, in Vinken PJ, Bruyn GW, Klawans HL (eds): *Handbook of Clinical Neurology: Extrapyramidal Disorders*. Amsterdam: Elsevier Science Publishers, 1986, vol 5(49), pp 255–266.

112. Rinne JO, Daniels E, Scaravilli F, et al: Neuropathological features of neuroacanthocytosis. *Mov Disord* 9(3):297–304, 1994.

113. Kito S, Itoga E, Hiroshige Y, Matsumoto N: A pedigree of amyotrophic chorea with acanthocytosis. *Arch Neurol* 37:514–517, 1980.

114. de Yebenes JG, Vazquez A, Martinez A, et al: Biochemical findings in symptomatic dystonias. *Adv Neurol* 50:167–175, 1988.

115. de Yebenes JG, Brin MF, Mena MA, et al: Neurochemical findings in neuroacanthocytosis. *Mov Disord* 3(4):300–312, 1988.

116. Walshe JM: Wilson's disease, in Vinken PJ, Bruyn GW, Klawans HL (eds): *Handbook of Clinical Neurology: Extrapyramidal Disorders*. Amsterdam: Elsevier Science Publishers, 1986, vol 5(49), pp 223–238.

117. Magalhaes AC, Caramelli P, Menezes JR, et al: Wilson disease: MRI with clinical correlation. *Neuroradiology* 36:97–100, 1994.

118. Seitelberger F: Neuroaxonal dystrophy: Its relation to aging and neurological diseases, in Vinken PJ, Bruyn GW, Klawans HL (eds): *Handbook of Clinical Neurology: Extrapyramidal Disorders*. Amsterdam: Elsevier Science Publishers, 1986, vol 5(49), pp 391–416.

119. Jankovic J , Kirkpatrick JB, Blomquist KA, et al: Late onset Hallervorden Spatz disease presenting as familial parkinsonism. *Neurology* 35:227–234, 1985.

120. Aicardi J, Castelein P: Infantile neuroaxonal dystrophy. *Brain* 102:727–748, 1979.

120a. Dooling EC, Schoene WC, Richardson EP: Hallervorden Spatz syndrome. *Arch Neurol* 30:70–83, 1974.

121. Nardocci N, Rumi V, Combi ML, et al: Complex tics, stereotypies, and compulsive behavior as clinical presentation of a juvenile progressive dystonia suggestive of Hallervorden Spatz disease. *Mov Disord* 9:369–371, 1994.

122. Caraceni T, Broggi G, Avanzini G: Familial idiopathic basal ganglia calcifications exhibiting "dystonia musculorum deformans." *Eur Neurol* 12:351–359, 1974.

123. Larsen TA, Dunn HG, Jan JE, Calne DB: Dystonia and calcification of the basal ganglia. *Neurology* 35:533–537, 1985.

124. Lauterbach EC, Spears TE, Prewett MJ, et al: Neuropsychiatric disorders, myoclonus, and dystonia in calcification of basal ganglia pathways. *Biol Psychiatry* 35:345–351, 1994.

125. Jellinger K: Pallidal, pallidonigral and pallidoluysionigral degeneration including association with thalamic and dentate degeneration, in Vinken PJ, Bruyn GW, Klawans HL. *Handbook of Clinical Neurology: Extrapyramidal Disorders*. Amsterdam: Elsevier Science Publishers, 1986, vol 5(49), pp 445–464.

126. van Bogaert L: Aspects cliniques et pathologiques des atrophies pallidales et pallido-luysiennes progressives. *J Neurol Neurosurg Psychiatry* 9:125–157, 1946.

127. Wooten GF, Lopes MB, Harris WO, et al: Pallidoluysian atrophy: Dystonia and basal ganglia functional anatomy. *Neurology* 43:1764–1768, 1993.

128. Goutieres F, Mikol J, Aicardi J: Neuronal intranuclear inclusion disease in a child: Diagnoses by rectal biopsy. *Ann Neurol* 27:103–106, 1990.

129. The Rett Syndrome Diagnostic Criteria Study Group: Diagnostic criteria for Rett syndrome. *Ann Neurol* 23:425–428, 1988.

130. Fitzgerald PM, Jankovic J, Percy AK: Rett syndrome and associated movement disorders. *Mov Disord* 5:195–202, 1990.

131. Coutinho P, Andrade C: Autosomal dominant system degeneration in Portuguese families of the Azores islands. *Neurology* 28:703–709, 1978.

132. Barbeau A, Roy M, Cunha L, et al: The natural history of Machado Joseph disease. *Can J Neurol Sci* 11:510–525, 1984.

133. Woods B, Schaumburg H: Nigro-spino-dentatal degeneration with nuclear ophthalmoplegia: A unique and partially treatable clinicopathological entity. *J Neurol Sci* 17:149–166, 1972.

134. Takiyama Y, Oyanagi S, Kawashima S, et al: A clinical and pathological study of a large Japanese family with Machado Joseph disease tightly linked to the DNA markers on chromosome 14q. *Neurology* 44(7):1302–1308, 1994.

134a. Kawaguchi Y, Okamoto T, Taniwaki M, et al. CAG expansions in a novel gene for Machado-Joseph disease at chromosome 14 q 32.1. *Nature Genetics* 8:221–227, 1994.

135. Freire Gonzalves A, Dinis M, Ferro MA, et al: Machado Joseph disease, in Berciano J: *Ataxias y Paraplegias Hereditarias: Aspectos Clinicos y Genticos*. Madrid: Ergon, 1993, chap 11, pp 189–202.

136. Lang AE, Rogaeva EA, Tsuda T, et al: Homozygous inheritance of the Machado Joseph disease gene. *Ann Neurol* 36(3):443–447, 1994.

137. Titica J, Van Bogaert L: Heredodegenerative hemiballismus: A contribution to the question of primary atrophy of the corpus Luysii. *Brain* 69:251–263, 1946.

138. Nagafuchi S, Yanagisawa H, Sato K, et al.: Dentatorubral and pallidoluysian atrophy expansion of an unstable CAG trinucleotide on chromosome 12p. *Nature Genet* 6:14–18, 1994.

139. Koide R, Ikeuchi T, Onodera O, et al: Unstable expansion of CAG repeat in hereditary dentatorubral-pallidoluysian atrophy. *Nature Genet* 6:9–13, 1994.

140. Iizuka R, Hirayama K, Maehara K: Dentato-rubro-pallidoluysian atrophy: A clinico-pathological study. *J Neurol Neurosurg Psychiatry* 47:1288–1298, 1984.

141. Komure O, Sano A, Nishino N, et al: DNA analysis in hereditary

dentatorubral-pallidoluysian atrophy: Correlation between CAG repeat length and phenotipic variation and the molecular basis of anticipation. *Neurology* 45:143–149, 1995.

142. Sano A, Yamamuchi N, Kakimoto Y: Anticipation in hereditary dentatorubral-pallidoluysian atrophy. *Hum Genet* 93:699–702, 1994.

143. Bodesteiner JB, Goldblum RM, Goldman AS: Progressive dystonia masking ataxia telangiectasia. *Arch Neurol* 37:464–465, 1980.

144. Aguilera T, Negrete O: Un caso de ataxia telangiectasia. *Rev Clin Esp* 107:51–54, 1967.

145. Castroviejo P, Rodriguez Costa T, Ojeda Casas A: Ataxia telangiectasia, presentacion de dos casos con agammaglobulinemia. *Rev Clin Esp* 109:439–444, 1968.

146. Garcia Urra D, Campos J, Varela de Seijas E, de Yebenes JG: Movement disorders in ataxia telangiectasia. *Neurology* 39(suppl 1):321, 1989.

147. Garcia Ruiz PJ, Garcia Urra D, Jimenez Jimenez J, et al: Movimientos anormales en ataxia telangiectasia. *Arch Neurobiol* 56:30–33, 1993.

148. Agamanolis DP, Greenstein JI: Ataxia telangiectasia. *J Neuropathol Exp Neurol* 38:475, 1979.

149. Robbins JH, Kraemer KH, Lutzer MA, et al: Xeroderma pigmentosum: An inherited disease with sun sensitivity, multiple cutaneus neoplasm and abnormal DNA repair. *Ann Intern Med* 80:221–248, 1974.

150. Rando TA, Horton JL, Layder BB: Wolfram syndrome: Evidence of a neurodegenerative disease by magnetic resonance imaging. *Neurology* 36:438–440, 1986.

151. Nakano T, Ikeda S, Komdo S, et al: Adult GM1 gangliosidosis: Clinical patterns and rectal biopsy. *Neurology* 35:875–880, 1985.

152. Goldman JE, Katz D, Rapin I, et al: Chronic GM1 gangliosidosis presenting as dystonia: I. Clinical and pathological features. *Ann Neurol* 9:465–475, 1981.

153. Guazzi GC, D'Amore I, Van Hoff F, et al: Type 3 (chronic) GM1 gangliosidosis presenting as infantile choreoathetotic dementia, without epilepsy in three sisters. *Neurology* 38:1124–1127, 1988.

154. Uyama E, Terasaki T, Watanabe S, et al: Type 3 GM1 gangliosidosis: Characteristic MRI findings correlated with dystonia. *Acta Neurol Scand* 86(6):609–615, 1992.

155. Yoshida K, Ikeda S, Kawaguchi K, Yanagisawa N: Adult GM1 gangliosidosis: Immunohistochemical and ultrastructural findings in an autopsy case. *Neurology* 44:2376–2382, 1994.

156. Meek D, Wolfe LS, Andermann E, Andermann F: Juvenile progressive dystonia: A new phenotype of GM2 gangliosidosis. *Ann Neurol* 15:348–352, 1984.

157. Hardie RJ, Morgan Hughes JA: Dystonia in GM2 gangliosidosis (Letter). *Mov Disord* 7:390–391, 1992.

158. Nardocci N, Bertagnolio B, Rumi V, Angelini L: Progressive dystonia symptomatic of juvenile GM2 gangliosidosis [see comments]. *Mov Disord* 7:64–67, 1992.

159. Oates CE, Bosch EP, Hart MN: Movement disorders associated with chronic GM2 gangliosidosis: Case report and review of the literature. *Eur Neurol* 25:154–159, 1986.

160. Johnson WG: The clinical spectrum of hexosaminidase deficiency diseases. *Neurology* 31:1453–1456, 1981.

161. Spence MW, Callahan JW: Sphingomyelin cholesterol lipidoses: The Niemann Pick group of diseases, in Scriver CR, Beaudet Al, Sly WS, Valle D (eds): *The Metabolic Basis of Inherited Disease*, 6th ed. New York: McGraw Hill, 1989, pp 1655–1676.

162. Varier MT, Wenger DA, Comly ME, et al: Niemann Pick disease group C: Clinical variability and diagnosis based on defective cholesterol sterification: A collaborative study of 70 patients. *Clin Genet* 33:311–348, 1988.

163. Martin JJ, Loventhal A, Luteric C, Varier MT: Juvenile dystonic lipidosis (variant of Niemann Pick disease type C). *J Neurol Sci* 66:33–45, 1984.

164. Pollen A, Fluharty AL, Fluharty EB, et al: Molecular basis of different forms of metachromatic leukodystrophy. *N Engl J Med* 324:18–22, 1991.

165. Inui K, Emmett M, Wenger DA: Inmunological evidence for deficiency in an activator protein for sulfatide sulfatase in a variant form of metachromatic leukodystrophy. *Proc Natl Acad Sci U S A* 80:3074–3076, 1983.

166. Lang AE, Clarke JTR, Rosch L, et al: Progressive longstanding "pure" dystonia: A new phenotype of juvenile metachromatic leukodystrophy. *Neurology* 35(suppl 1):194, 1985.

167. Berkovic SF, Carpenter S, Andermann F, et al: "Kufs" disease: A critical reappraisal. *Brain* 111:27–62, 1988.

168. Boulloche J, Aicardi A: Pelizaeus-Merzbacher disease: Clinical and nosological study. *J Child Neurol* 1:233–239, 1986.

169. Harding AE, Shapira A: Mitochondrial disease and movement disorders, in Jankovic J, Tolosa E (eds): *Parkinson's Disease and Movement Disorders*. Baltimore: Williams & Wilkins, 1993, chap 32, pp 569–583.

170. Truong DD, Harding AE, Scaravilli F: Movement disorders in mitochondrial myopathics: A report of nine cases with two autopsy studies. *Mov Disord* 5:109–117, 1990.

171. Bercovic SF, Karpati G, Carpenter S, Lang AE: Progressive dystonia with bilateral putaminal hypodensities. *Arch Neurol* 44:1184–1187, 1987.

172. Novotny EJ, Singh G, Wallace DC, et al: Leber's disease and dystonia: A mitochondrial disease. *Neurology* 36:1053–1060, 1986.

173. Macaya A, Munell F, Burke RE, De Vivo DC: Disorders of movement in Leigh syndrome. *Neuropediatrics* 24(2):60–67, 1993.

174. Munoz-Hiraldo ME, Martinez-Bermejo A, Gutierrez-Molina M, et al: Distonia como manifestacion principal en el sindrome de Leigh del lactante. *Ann Esp Pediatr* 38:348–350, 1993.

175. Whetsell WO, Plaitakis A: Leigh's disease in an adult: Evidence of an "inhibitory factor" in family members. *Ann Neurol* 3:529–524, 1978.

176. Leuzzi V, Bertini F, De Negri AM, et al: Bilateral striatal necrosis, dystonia and optic atrophy in two siblings. *J Neurol Neurosurg Psychiatry* 55:16–19, 1992.

177. Bruyn GW, Bots GTAM, Went LN, Klinkhamer PJJM: Hereditary optic neuropathy: Neuropathological findings. *J Neurol Sci* 113:55–61, 1992.

178. Jun AS, Brown MD, Wallace DC: A mitochondrial DNA mutation at nucleotide pair 14459 of the NADH dehydrogenase subunit 6 gene associated with maternally inherited Leber hereditary optic neuropathy and dystonia. *Proc Natl Acad Sci U S A* 91:6206–6210, 1994.

179. Wallace DC: Mitochondrial DNA mutations in diseases of energy metabolism. *J Bioenerg Biomembr* 26:241–250, 1994.

180. Wallace DC: Mitochondrial DNA sequence variation in human evolution and disease. *Proc Natl Acad Sci U S A* 91:8739–8746, 1994.

181. Kyllerman M, Skjeldal OH, Lundberg M, et al: Dystonia and dyskinesia in glutaric aciduria type I: Clinical heterogeneity and therapeutic considerations. *Mov Disord* 9:22–30, 1994.

182. Voll R, Hoffmann GF, Lipinski CG, et al: Die glutarazidamie/glutarazidurie I als differntialdiagnose der chorea minor. *Klin Padiatr* 205:124–126, 1993.

183. Chow CW, Haan EA, Goodman SI, et al: Neuropathology of glutaric acidemia type I. *Acta Neuropathol (Berl)* 75:590–594, 1988.

184. Lawrence Wolf B, Herberg KP, Hoffmann GF, et al: Entwicklung der Hirnatrophie: Therapie und Therapieuberwachung bei Glutarazidurie Typ 1 (Glutaryl-CoA Dehydrogenase-Mangel) *Klin Padiatr* 205:23–29, 1993.

185. Heindenreich R, Natowicz M, Hainline BE, et al: Acute extrapyramidal syndrome in methylmalonic acidemia: "Metabolic stroke" involving the globus pallidus. *J Pediatr* 113:1022–1027, 1988.

186. Roodhooft AM, Baumgartner ER, Martin JJ, et al: Symmetrical necrosis of the basal ganglia in methylmalonic acidemia. *Eur J Pediar* 149:582–584, 1990.

187. de Sousa C, Piesowicz AT, Brett EM, Leonard JV: Focal changes in the globi pallidi associated with neurological dysfunction in methylmalonic acidemia. *Neuropediatrics* 20:119–201, 1989.

188. Shimoizumi H, Okabe I, Kodama H, Yanagisawa M: Methylmalonic acidemia with bilateral MRI high intensities of the globus pallidus (translated title). *No To Hattatsu.* 25(6):554–557, 1993.

189. Andreula CF, Blasi RD, Carella A: CT and MR studies of methylmalonic acidemia. *AJNR Am J Neuroradiol* 12:410–412, 1991.

190. Bourgeron T, Chretien D, Poggi Bach J, et al: Mutation of the fumarase gene in two siblings with progressive encephalopathy and fumarase deficiency. *J Clin Invest* 93(6):2514–2518, 1994.

191. Hagberg B, Hambraeus L, Bensch K: A case of hompocystinuria with a dystonia neurological syndrome. *Neuropadiatrie* 1:337–343, 1970.

192. Davous P, Rondot P: Homocystinuria and dystonia. *J Neurol Neurosurg Psychiatry* 46:283–286, 1983.

193. Arbour L, Rosenblatt B, Clow C, Wilson GN: Postoperative dystonia in a female patient with homocystinuria. *J Pediatr* 113(5):863–864, 1988.

194. Kempster PA, Brenton DP, Gale AN, Stern GM: Dystonia in homocystinuria. *J Neurol Neurosurg Psychiatry* 51(6):859–862, 1988.

195. Berardelli A, Thompson PD, Zaccagnini M, et al: Two sisters with generalized dystonia associated with homocystinuria. *Mov Disord* 6(2):163–165, 1991.

196. Darras BT, Ampola MG, Dietz WH, Gilmore HE: Intermittent dystonia in Hartnup disease. *Pediatr Neurol* 5:118–120, 1989.

197. Tamoush A, Alpers PH, Feigin RD, et al: Hartnup disease: Clinical, pathological and biochemical observations. *Arch Neurol* 33:797–807, 1976.

198. Jankovic J, Caskey TC, Stout JT, Butler T: Lesch Nyhan syndrome: A study of motor behavior and CSF monoamine turnover. *Ann Neurol* 23:466–469, 1988.

199. Garcia Puig J, Mateos FA, Jimenez ML, et al: Espectro clinico de la deficiencia de hipoxantina-guanina fosforribosiltransferasa: Estudio de 12 pacientes. *Med Clin (Barc)* 14(102):699–700, 1994.

200. Tarsy D, Sudarsky L, Charness ME: Limb dystonia following electric injury. *Mov Disord* 9:230–232, 1994.

201. Panchenko EN, Kazakova SE, Safonova EF: Nervnye narusheniia u likvidatorov avarii na Chernobyl'skoi AES, podvergavshikhsia vozdeistviiu ioniziruiushchego izlucheniia v malykh dozakh. *Vrach Delo* 8:13–16, 1993.

202. Ushkova IN, Koshelev NF: Kliniko-gigigicheskie i eksperimental'nye obosnovaniia nozologii lazernoi bolezni. *Vrach Delo* 2:63–68, 1994.

203. Gay CT, Ryan SG: Paroxysmal kinesigenic dystonia after methylphenidate administration. *J Child Neurol* 9:45–46, 1994.

204. Humphreys A, Tanner AR: Acute dystonic drug reaction or tetanus? An unusual consequence of a 'Whizz' overdose. *Hum Exp Toxicol* 13:311–312, 1994.

205. Burke RE, Fahn S, Jankovic J, et al: Tardive dystonia: Late onset and persistent dystonia caused by antipsychotic drugs. *Neurology* 32:1335–1346, 1982.

206. Gimenez Roldn S, Mateo D, Bartolome P: Tardive dystonia and severe tardive dyskinesia. *Acta Psychiat Scand* 71:488–494, 1985.

207. Owens DG: Extrapyramidal side effects and tolerability of risperidone: A review. *J Clin Psychiatry* 55(suppl):29–35, 1994.

208. Casey DE: Motor and mental aspects of acute extrapyramidal syndromes. *Acta Psychiatr Scand Suppl* 380:14–20, 1994.

209. Khanna R, Damodaran SS, Chakraborty SP: Overflow movements may predict neuroleptic-induced dystonia. *Biol Psychiatry* 35:491–492, 1994.

210. Malhotra AK, Litman RE, Pickar D: Adverse effects of antipsychotic drugs. *Drug Saf* 9:429–436, 1993.

211. Sachdev P: Risk factors for tardive dystonia: A case control comparison with tardive dyskinesia. *Acta Psychiatr Scand* 88:98–103, 1993.

212. Sachdev P: Clinical characteristics of 15 patients with tardive dystonia. *Am J Psychiatry* 150:498–500, 1993.

213. Lauterbach EC: Haloperidol-induced dystonia and parkinsonism on discontinuing metoclopramide: Implications for differential thalamocortical activity. *J Clin Psychopharmacol* 12:442–443, 1992.

214. Meltzer LT, Christoffersen CL, Serpa KA, et al: Lack of involvement of haloperidol-sensitive sigma binding sites in modulation of dopamine neuronal activity and induction of dystonias by antipsychotic drugs. *Neuropharmacology* 31:961–967, 1992.

215. Yassa R, Nastase C, Dupont D, Thibeau M: Tardive dyskinesia in elderly psychiatric patients: A 5-year study. *Am J Psychiatry* 149:1206–1211, 1992.

216. Chiu H, Shum P, Lau J, et al: Prevalence of tardive dyskinesia, tardive dystonia, and respiratory dyskinesia among Chinese psychiatric patients in Hong Kong. *Am J Psychiatry* 149:1081–1085, 1992.

217. Khanna R, Das A, Damodaran SS: Prospective study of neuroleptic-induced dystonia in mania and schizophrenia. *Am J Psychiatry* 149:511–513, 1992.

218. Wojcik JD, Falk WE, Fink JS, et al: A review of 32 cases of tardive dystonia. *Am J Psychiatry* 148:1055–1059, 1991.

219. Matsumoto RR, Hemstreet MK, Lai NL: Drug specificity of pharmacological dystonia. *Pharmacol Biochem Behav* 36:151–155, 1990.

220. Shorten GD, Srithran S, Hendron M: Pseudo-tetanus following trifluoperazine. *Ulster Med J* 59:221–222, 1990.

221. Miller LG, Jankovic J: Neurologic approach to drug-induced movement disorders: A study of 125 patients. *South Med J* 83:525–532, 1990.

222. Dickson R, Williams R, Dalby JT: Dystonic reaction and relapse with clozapine discontinuation and risperidone initiation. *Can J Psychiatry* 39:184, 1994.

223. Thomas P, Lalaux N, Vaiva G, Goudemand M: Dose-dependent stuttering and dystonia in a patient taking clozapine. *Am J Psychiatry* 151:1096, 1994.

224. Kastrup O, Gastpar M, Schwarz M: Acute dystonia due to clozapine. *J Neurol Neurosurg Psychiatry* 57:119, 1994.

225. Cory DA: Adverse reaction to metoclopramide during enteroclysis. *AJR Am J Roentgenol* 163:480, 1994.

226. Ernst M, Gonzalez NM, Campbell M: Acute dystonic reaction with low-dose pimozide. *J Am Acad Child Adolesc Psychiatry* 32:640–642, 1993.

227. Guala A, Mittino D, Ghini T, Quazza G: Le distonie da metoclopramide sono familiari? *Pediatr Med Chir* 14:617–618, 1992.

228. Guala A, Mittino D, Fabbrocini P, Ghini T: Familial metoclopramide-induced dystonic reactions. *Mov Disord* 7:385–386, 1992.

229. Linazasoro G, Marti Masso JF, Olasagasti B: Acute dystonia induced by sulpiride. *Clin Neuropharmacol* 14:463–464, 1991.

230. Factor SA, Matthews MK: Persistent extrapyramidal syndrome with dystonia and rigidity caused by combined metoclopramide and prochlorperazine therapy. *South Med J* 84:626–628, 1991.

231. Bonuccelli U, Nocchiero A, Napolitano A, et al: Domperidone-induced acute dystonia and polycystic ovary syndrome. *Mov Disord* 6:79–81, 1991.

232. Miller LG, Jankovic J: Sulpiride-induced tardive dystonia. *Mov Disord* 5:83–84, 1990.

233. Tait P, Balzer R, Buchanan N: Metoclopramide side effects in children. *Med J Aust* 152:387, 1990.

234. McCann UD, Penetar DM, Belenky G: Acute dystonic reaction in normal humans caused by catecholamine depletion. *Clin Neuropharmacol* 13:565–568, 1990.

235. Zimmerman TR Jr, Sage JI, Lang AE, Mark MH: Severe evening dyskinesias in advanced Parkinson's disease: Clinical description, relation to plasma L-dopa, and treatment. *Mov Disord* 9:173–177, 1994.

236. Marconi R, Lefebvre Caparros D, Bonnet AM, et al: L-dopa-induced dyskinesias in Parkinson's disease phenomenology and pathophysiology. *Mov Disord* 9:2–12, 1994.

237. Bravi D, Mouradian MM, Roberts JW, et al: End-of-dose dystonia in Parkinson's disease. *Neurology* 43:2130–2131, 1993.

238. Rupniak NM, Boyce S, Steventon MJ, et al: Dystonia induced by combined treatment with L-dopa and MK-801 in parkinsonian monkeys. *Ann Neurol* 32:103–105, 1992.

239. Mark MH, Sage JI: L-dopa-associated hemifacial dystonia. *Mov Disord* 6:383, 1991.

240. Leiguarda R, Merello M, Sabe L, Starkstein S: Bromocriptine-induced dystonia in patients with aphasia and hemiparesis. *Neurology* 43:2319–2322, 1993.

241. Peacock L, Lublin H, Gerlach J: The effects of dopamine D1 and D2 receptor agonists and antagonists in monkeys withdrawn from long-term neuroleptic treatment. *Eur J Pharmacol* 186:49–59, 1990.

242. Mitchell IJ, Luquin R, Boyce S, et al: Neural mechanisms of dystonia: Evidence from a 2-deoxyglucose uptake study in a primate model of dopamine agonist-induced dystonia. *Mov Disord* 5:49–54, 1990.

243. Cardoso FE, Jankovic J: Cocaine-related movement disorders. *Mov Disord* 8:175–178, 1993.

244. Hegarty AM, Lipton RB, Merriam AE, Freeman K: Cocaine as a risk factor for acute dystonic reactions. *Neurology* 41:1670–1672, 1991.

245. Farrell PE, Diehl AK: Acute dystonic reaction to crack cocaine. *Ann Emerg Med* 20:322, 1991.

246. Olson WL: Dystonia and reflex sympathetic dystrophy induced by ergotamine. *Mov Disord* 7:188–189, 1992.

247. Merello MJ, Nogues MA, Leiguarda RC, Lopez Saubidet C: Dystonia and reflex sympathetic dystrophy induced by ergotamine. *Mov Disord* 7(2):188–189, 1992.

248. Jarecke CR, Reid PJ: Acute dystonic reaction induced by a monoamine oxidase inhibitor. *J Clin Psychopharmacol* 10:144–145, 1990.

249. Jimenez Jimenez FJ, Vazquez A, Garcia Ruiz P, et al: Chronic hemidystonia following acute dystonic reaction to thiethylperazine. *J Neurol Neurosurg Psychiatry* 54:562, 1991.

250. Shihabuddin L, Rapport D: Sertraline and extrapyramidal side effects. *Am J Psychiatry* 151:288, 1994.

251. Dave M: Fluoxetine-associated dystonia. *Am J Psychiatry* 151:149, 1994.

252. Lock JD, Gwirtsman HE, Targ EF: Possible adverse drug interactions between fluoxetine and other psychotropics. *J Clin Psychopharmacol* 10:383–384, 1990.

253. Reccoppa L, Welch WA, Ware MR: Acute dystonia and fluoxetine. *J Clin Psychiatry* 51:487, 1990.

254. Rio J, Molins A, Viguera ML, Codina A: Distonia aguda por fluoxetina. *Med Clin (Barc)* 99:436–437, 1992.

255. George MS, Trimble MR: Dystonic reaction associated with fluvoxamine. *J Clin Psychopharmacol* 13:220–221, 1993.

256. Adityanjee, Lindenmeyer JP: Precipitation of dystonia by m-CPP in a schizophrenic patient treated with haloperidol. *Am J Psychiatry* 150:837–838, 1993.

257. LeWitt PA, Walters A, Hening W, McHale D: Persistent movement disorders induced by buspirone. *Mov Disord* 8:331–334, 1993.

258. Boylan K: Persistent dystonia associated with buspirone. *Neurology* 40:1904, 1990.

259. Kappler J, Menges C, Ferbert A, Ebel H: Schwere "Spat" dystonie nach "Neuroleptanxiolyse" mit Fluspirilen. *Nervenarzt* 65(1):66–68, 1994.

260. Stones M, Kennie DC, Fulton JD: Dystonic dysphagia associated with fluspirilene. *Br Med J* 301:668–669, 1990.

261. Rittmann M, Steegmanns Schwarz I: Schwere Spatdystonie unter Fluspirilen. *Dtsch Med Wochenschr* 116:1613, 1991.

262. Laux G, Gunreben G: Schwere Spatdystonie unter Fluspirilen. *Dtsch Med Wochenschr* 116:977–980, 1991.

263. Perez Trullen JM, Modrego Pardo PJ, Vazquez Andre M, Lopez Lozano JJ: Bromazepam-induced dystonia. *Biomed Pharmacother* 46:375–376, 1992.

264. Lee JW: Persistent dystonia associated with carbamazepine therapy: A case report. *N Z Med J* 107:360–361, 1994.

265. Soman P, Jain S, Rajsekhar V, et al: Dystonia—A rare manifestation of carbamazepine toxicity. *Postgrad Med J* 70:54–55, 1994.

266. Reddy RV, Moorthy SS, Dierdorf SF, et al: Excitatory effects and electroencephalographic correlation of etomidate, thiopental, methohexital, and propofol. *Anesth Analg* 77:1008–1011, 1993.

267. Lacayo A, Mitra N: Report of a case of phenobarbital-induced dystonia. *Clin Pediatr Phila* 31:252, 1992.

268. Tolarek IH, Ford MJ: Acute dystonia induced by midazolam and abolished by flumazenil. *Br Med J* 300:614, 1990.

269. Mets B: Acute dystonia after alfentanil in untreated Parkinson's disease. *Anesth Analg* 72:557–558, 1991.

270. Riley D: Pallidal and putaminal lesions resulting from disulfiram intoxication. *Mov Disord* 6:166–170, 1991.

271. Riley D: Disulfiram induced dystonia. *Mov Disord* 7:188–192, 1992.

272. Krauss JK, Mohadjer M, Wakhlo Mundinger F: Dystonia and akinesia due to o-AK pallidoputaminal lesions after disulfiram intoxication. *Mov Disord* 6:166–170, 1991.

273. Gabellini AS, Pezzoli A, De Massis P, Sacquegna T: Veralipride-induced tardive dystonia in a patient with bipolar psychosis. *Ital J Neurol Sci* 13:621–623, 1992.

274. Brady W, Hall K: Erythromycin related dystonic reaction. *Am J Emerg Med* 10:616, 1992.

275. Miller LG, Jankovic J: Persistent dystonia possibly induced by flecainide. *Mov Disord* 7:62–63, 1992.

276. Barbeau A, Inoue N, Cloutier T: Role of manganese in dystonia. *Adv Neurol* 14:339–352, 1976.

277. Danks DM: Copper-induced dystonia secondary to cholestatic liver disease. *Lancet* 335:410, 1990.

278. Ross. Methanol induced dystonia. *Can J Neurol Sci* 97:155–162, 1990.

279. Valenzuela R, Court J, Godoy J: Delayed cyanide induced dystonia. *J Neurol Neurosurg Psychiatry* 55:198–199, 1992.

280. De Yebenes JG, de Yebenes PG: La distonia en la pintura de Matias Grunewald: El ergotismo epidemico en la baja Edad Media. *Arch Neurobiol* 54:37–40, 1991.

281. Quinn NP: Dystonia in epidemic ergotism. *Neurology* 33:1267, 1983.

282. Spencer PS, Ludolph AC, Kisby GE: Neurologic diseases associated with use of plant components with toxic potential. *Environ Res* 62:106–113, 1993.

283. Batshaw ML, Wachtel RC, Deckel AW, et al: Munchausen's syndrome simulating torsion dystonia. *N Engl J Med* 312:1437–1439, 1985.

Chapter 34

GENETICS AND MOLECULAR BIOLOGY OF HUNTINGTON'S DISEASE

JAMES F. GUSELLA and MARCY E. MacDONALD

HISTORY AND EPIDEMIOLOGY
GENETIC LINKAGE APPROACH
GENETIC AND PHYSICAL MAPPING OF THE HD
  REGION
MINIMIZING THE CANDIDATE REGION WITH
  HISTORICAL RECOMBINATIONS
IDENTIFICATION OF THE HD DEFECT
CHARACTERISTICS OF THE CAG REPEAT
CLINICAL CORRELATES OF CAG REPEAT LENGTH
STRUCTURE AND EXPRESSION OF THE HD GENE
MECHANISM OF ACTION OF THE HD DEFECT
COMPARISON TO MOVEMENT DISORDERS
CLINICAL CONSEQUENCES: DIAGNOSIS AND
  PROSPECTS FOR THERAPY

History and Epidemiology

In 1872, George Huntington described a unique ailment involving characteristic involuntary movements that begin insidiously, usually in middle age, and progress gradually until the victim is consumed by full-blown chorea.[1] His description was based on his observations of families with the disorder in his clinical practice as a family physician in East Hampton, on Long Island, New York. As members of the same families had been cared for by his father and grandfather, who were also physicians, Huntington was attuned to the inherited nature of the peculiar disorder. He described frequent transmission of the defect from either an affected mother or an affected father to offspring, with no skipping of generations. Huntington also noted that "if by any chance these children go through life without it, the thread is broken and the children and great-grandchildren of the original shakers may rest assured that they are free from the disease." This pattern of transmission was recognized as the result of a Mendelian autosomal-dominant defect by Osler in 1908.[2] Indeed, Vessie[3] later traced many of the Long Island families to immigrants from Bures, England, who landed in New England in 1649, confirming Huntington's description of this hereditary chorea as "an heirloom from generations away back in the dim past." George Huntington's accurate, lucid, and succinct description of this nightmarish affliction led to its appellation of Huntington's chorea, subsequently changed to Huntington's disease (HD), as its manifestations are not limited to loss of motor control.

Although Huntington believed that the disorder existed only in eastern Long Island, it is now known to be widespread throughout the world. The prevalence is highest in populations of western European ancestry, in which 4–7 persons/100,000 are affected.[4] However, the actual disease gene frequency is 2.5–3 times higher, as HD typically has its onset only in midlife, and at any given time, two-thirds of gene carriers have yet to become symptomatic. The prevalence is relatively consistent across Europe and in other regions of the world that have populations of western European descent, with the exception of Finland, where a significantly lower rate reflects this population's restricted genetic origin. HD is also seen in Africans and Asians, although with a much lower prevalence.

Many of the early studies of HD concentrated on its familial nature, documenting large kindreds in which the defect was passed from generation to generation. HD, as an autosomal-dominant disorder, is transmitted equally from males and females, and both sexes have a 50:50 chance of inheriting the defect. The disease gene is highly penetrant, but onset is variable, ranging from early childhood to late in life. As most cases manifest in middle age, the HD gene is often passed on to children before the parent is aware of the disorder. The rare cases of juvenile onset (<15 years of age) are usually inherited from an affected father.[5,6] HD is untreatable, and its victims are condemned to slow, inexorable progression of their disease that ends in death 10–20 years after onset.

Genetic Linkage Approach

The high penetrance, late onset, and characteristic clinical manifestations, which combine to produce large identifiable disease families (Fig. 34-1), made this disorder the ideal candidate for pioneering a novel strategy that emerged in the early 1980s for establishing the chromosomal location of a genetic defect.[7] This approach relied on merging the tenets of Mendelian inheritance with the power of recombinant DNA technology, using naturally occurring variations in DNA sequence as highly informative genetic markers to search for genetic linkage with the disease gene. The goal was to discover a polymorphic DNA marker that cosegregates with the disorder in families and thereby infers the presence of the disease gene in the same chromosomal vicinity. It would then be possible to identify the genetic defect on the basis of its chromosomal location, without any additional knowledge of its biochemical nature.

Previous genetic linkage studies of HD had used a limited panel of expressed polymorphic systems, blood group antigens, and serum enzymes that permitted only 15 percent of the autosomal genome to be searched.[8] The concept of DNA markers offered a potential route to making the remaining 85 percent of the genome accessible to examination, but only a handful of DNA markers had been described. These were restriction fragment-length polymorphisms, or RFLPs, detected by using single-copy human DNA clones to probe genomic DNA blots for variations in restriction fragment size that reflected differences in the primary DNA sequence. As RFLP markers were generated, they were tested for genetic linkage to HD in two large pedigrees, one of American

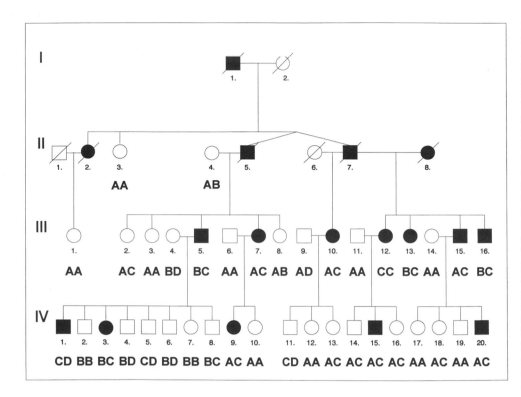

FIGURE 34-1 An idealized HD pedigree showing cosegregation of *D4S10* with the disorder. An imaginary four generation (I–IV) HD pedigree is shown with genotypes for the *D4S10* marker (4 alleles: A, B, C, D) shown under the symbol for each living family member. In each generation, the family members are numbered sequentially. Circles and squares denote females and males, respectively. Slashed symbols indicate deceased individuals. Filled symbols represent those individuals clinically diagnosed with HD. Individuals II-5 and II-7 are monozygotic twins. The disorder is segregating in this pedigree with the C allele of *D4S10*. As this marker displays 4 percent recombination with HD, all individuals who inherit the C allele from their affected parent have a 96 percent chance of also having inherited the HD defect. Individual II-8 is an HD-affected individual who married into the pedigree and, with II-7, produced progeny at risk of having two copies of the HD defect.

and one of Venezuelan origin. In 1983, success came quickly, as one of the initial 13 RFLP markers tested revealed strong genetic linkage to the disorder[9] (e.g., see Fig. 34-1). This marker, *D4S10*, consisting of two *Hind III* polymorphisms detected by an anonymous DNA probe, G8, placed HD on the short arm of chromosome 4 (Fig. 34-2). There were no crossovers between the marker and HD, either in a large section of the Venezuela pedigree or in the independent American HD family with 14 affected members, producing odds of greater than 100 million:1 in favor of genetic linkage. This was the first example of mapping a genetic defect to a human chromosome using only genetic linkage to a DNA polymorphism, without any prior clue to the disease gene's location. This approach has been replicated subsequently in a host of different disorders and has become increasingly sophisticated as newer and more informative markers have been elaborated, and the human genetic map has become increasingly detailed. The success of the linkage strategy, and the opportunities that it created for isolating disease genes via their chromosomal location, provided a major impetus for undertaking the Human Genome Initiative to map and sequence the human genome.

Genetic and Physical Mapping of the HD Region

The anonymous DNA marker, *D4S10*, genetically linked to HD, was initially assigned to chromosome 4 by hybridization of the G8 probe to a panel of human X mouse somatic cell

hybrid lines that had segregated various human chromosomes.[9] The marker was then regionally assigned to the terminal cytogenetic band of the chromosome 4 short arm, because it was hemizygous (present in a single copy) in patients with Wolf-Hirschhorn syndrome, a congenital anomaly caused by heterozygous deletion on 4p.[10] Several groups later confirmed this assignment by in situ hybridization to metaphase chromosomes.[11–13] Genotyping of *HD* families revealed that the HD gene is located on chromosome 4 in all of the families tested, yielding no evidence of other genes that can cause the clinical symptoms of HD (nonallelic heterogeneity).[14] These same investigations made HD the first genetic disorder in man established to be completely dominant. Several individuals who were homozygous for the HD defect, having inherited a disease allele from both parents, were found to be clinically indistinguishable from typical heterozygous HD gene carriers.[15,16] This surprising result indicated that in HD heterozygotes, the remaining normal allele does not act to delay the disease process or to alter its manifestation, and two doses of the defective gene are not significantly more damaging than a single dose.

The position of the *HD* defect relative to the cytogenetic map could be determined only indirectly, by linkage analysis with *D4S10* and other surrounding DNA markers. HD and *D4S10* displayed 4 percent recombination, placing the disease gene within about 4×10^6 base pair (bp) of DNA either centromeric or telomeric to the DNA marker (Fig. 34-2). DNA markers were identified centromeric to *D4S10* in 4p16, using Wolf-Hirschhorn patients with different extents of 4p16 deletion. When the highly polymorphic 4p16.1 marker *RAF1P1* (then know as *RAF2*) was typed in the same *HD* kindreds

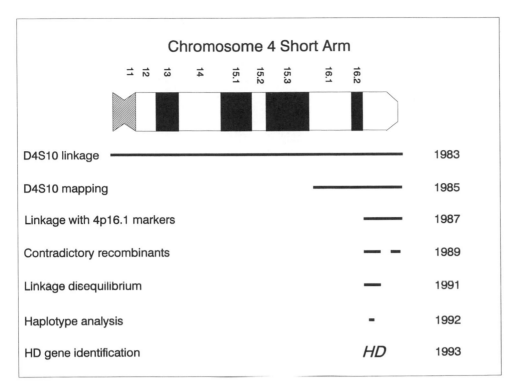

Chromosome 4 Short Arm

D4S10 linkage	1983
D4S10 mapping	1985
Linkage with 4p16.1 markers	1987
Contradictory recombinants	1989
Linkage disequilibrium	1991
Haplotype analysis	1992
HD gene identification *HD*	1993

FIGURE 34-2 Progressive narrowing of the HD gene search. In 1983, genetic linkage with *D4S10* assigned the HD gene to chromosome 4. The horizontal lines below the schematic diagram of the chromosome 4 short arm depict the chronology of the HD search (1983–1993), as the candidate region was progressively narrowed using the techniques listed and described in the text.

as *D4S10*, it revealed additional crossovers, indicating that the disease gene must be located telomeric to both DNA markers.[17] This assigned the HD gene to the 4p16.3 subband, between *D4S10* and the short-arm telomere, a segment corresponding to about 0.2 percent of the genome, or 6 million bp of DNA (Fig. 34-2).

The chromosomal localization of the HD gene, and, subsequently, many other genetic defects created the need to improve standard mapping methods and to develop new techniques to clone genes based on their map location, without a knowledge of the protein defect involved. As with the DNA marker linkage approach, the search for the *HD* gene also acted as the proving ground for several of these technologies. The initial stages of more detailed mapping in 4p16.3 were aided by the construction of regional somatic cell hybrid panels that permitted rapid assignment and ordering of new DNA probes to several regions of 4p16.[18,19] These hybrid panels acted as a backbone on which more sophisticated approaches, such as radiation hybrid mapping[20,21] and pulsed-field gel electrophoresis,[22] could be appended. Numerous novel sources of DNA probes, including phage libraries of flow-sorted chromosome 4 DNA, chromosome 4-enriched somatic cell hybrid genomic libraries, chromosome "jumping" libraries, Not I "linking" clones, P1 clones, yeast artificial chromosome clones, combined with pulsed-field gel electrophoresis, and somatic cell hybrid mapping eventually produced a physical map that spanned 5×10^6 bp in 4p16.3[23–25] (Fig. 34-2).

Because the HD gene had been assigned to 4p16.3, using only genetic linkage techniques, and because there was no physical rearrangement of the region associated with the disorder, the only means of locating the defect on the physical map was to construct a parallel genetic map by tracking the

inheritance of informative DNA markers through normal and HD pedigrees. Although RFLP markers, like *D4S10*, were used initially, successive generations of newer, more informative markers were added to the map as they emerged. First, variable number of tandem repeat markers (VNTR), detected like RFLPs by DNA blotting but displaying many different potential restriction fragment sizes as a result of variation in the copy number and, therefore, length, of a repeated DNA motif located between two restriction sites were found to be particularly frequent in telomeric regions like 4p16.[26,27] Later, the advent of the polymerase chain reaction (PCR) permitted the easy use of simple-sequence repeats (SSRs), di-, tri-, and tetranucleotide repeat, varying in repeat unit number, as highly informative multi-allele polymorphisms.[28,29] The genetic map of 4p16.3 was anchored to the physical map by DNA sites common to both, revealing that the 5×10^6 bp of DNA between *D4S10* and *D4S90* in 4p16.3 spanned 6 percent recombination.[30–32] However, there was a striking difference between the apparent distance between markers suggested by the genetic map and their actual physical separation on the physical map. Markers located within a 300 to 400-kb genetic "hot spot" immediately telomeric to *D4S10* revealed far more recombination than expected, such that this small physical interval accounted for more than one-half of the genetic distance of the entire 4p16.3 genetic map.[31] The remaining segment between *D4S125* and the telomere spans at least 4 Mb of physical distance but shows only 2.6 percent recombination.

In the absence of a physical benchmark, such as a deletion or translocation, to precisely position the disease gene within the linked segment, genetic crossovers between 4p16.3 DNA markers and the disease gene in HD families remained the only potential route to defining the DNA segment containing the defect. The success of this strategy depends on unequivocal diagnosis of the disorder in affected individuals, on accurate DNA typing, and on the frequency of double, as opposed to single, crossovers on HD chromosomes. HD was readily mapped beyond the "hot spot" of increased recombination telomeric to D4S10, as most crossovers with the defect occurred within this interval. However, the position of the disease gene in the remaining 3.5 × 10⁶ of the physical map was not so easily discerned, as several genetic events in well-defined HD pedigrees yielded contradictory implications concerning its location.[30,33] Initially, a few diagnosed individuals in well-defined HD pedigrees were found to possess only marker alleles characteristic of the affected parent's normal chromosome. These events, in which no evidence of marker-marker crossover was seen, suggested that *HD* must be located in the telomeric 100-kb segment of the chromosome, beyond all informative DNA markers then available. However, several other HD cases were subsequently discovered that predicted a location closer to D4S10, as markers in the terminal 1.5 × 10⁶ bp of the chromosome showed crossover with HD, whereas markers in the 2.5 × 10⁶ bp telomeric to D4S10 did not. Thus, the two classes of apparent recombination events implied mutually exclusive locations for the defect (Fig. 34-2).

One explanation for this genetic conundrum was the possibility of double recombination in the latter cases, with the chromosome switching back to the *HD* version telomeric to the final marker (D4S142) in the terminal 100 kb predicted by former events. This scenario led to the isolation of the entire segment between D4S142 and the telomere of an HD chromosome as a yeast artificial chromosome (YAC).[34] Analysis of this DNA was complicated by the presence of subtelomeric repeat sequences and by sequence similarities to acrocentric chromosomes.[35] No evidence was found for a double crossover or for the presence of genes that could cause HD. Mounting evidence (see below) gradually favored the internal region of 4p16.3 as the site of the HD gene, but an explanation for the apparent crossovers that predicted this telomeric location had to await the identification of the genetic defect. Pulsed-field gel mapping initially produced a long-range physical map spanning the 2.5 × 10⁶ bp of this internal region, which was subsequently isolated as overlapping clone sets, first of YACs and later of cosmids.[22–25]

Minimizing the Candidate Region with Historical Recombinations

With genetic recombination having failed to provide a single, unequivocal site for the HD gene, innovative genetic strategies were required to progress with the search. The observation that some markers in the internal 4p16.3 segment displayed allele association with HD implicated this region as the site of the defect and provided the opportunity for a more powerful approach to localizing it.[36,37] Certain alleles for D4S95 and D4S98 RFLPs were more frequently represented on *HD* chromosomes than expected from their frequency on normal chromosomes. This was presumed to be a result of the presence of these alleles on the original chromo-

some 4 that underwent an HD mutation, with an insufficient number of subsequent generations to return the markers to their equilibrium frequencies. A comprehensive analysis of 4p16.3 DNA markers revealed the patterns of allele association to be quite complex.[38] Markers with evident allele association were interspersed on the physical map with sites that showed no association with *HD*. This supported the view that the current pool of *HD* chromosomes reflects more than one independent *HD* mutation or primordial chromosome. It also suggested that if HD chromosomes could be grouped based on their mutational ancestry, the identification of a minimum cluster of shared marker alleles of 4p16.3 might pinpoint the location of the genetic defect.

The implementation of this novel approach was feasible because of the emergence of VNTR and SSR markers with a sufficiently large array of alleles to discriminate many potential primordial haplotypes.[39] Haplotype analysis unearthed evidence for a multitude of independent HD mutations, with 78 *HD* chromosomes exhibiting 26 different haplotypes within the region of maximal linkage disequilibrium, around D4S127 and D4S95. The most frequent *HD* haplotype accounted for about one-third of *HD* chromosomes, and the initial assessment of decay in strength of linkage disequilibrium within this class of chromosomes predicted a most likely location for *HD* in the 500-kb region between D4S180 and D4S182 (Figs. 34-2 and 34-3).

Identification of the HD Defect

A set of overlapping cosmid clones between D4S180 and D4S182 acted as the source of genomic DNA for exon amplification, a novel approach for identifying candidate genes that takes advantage of the splicing signals bordering exons to permit rapid and efficient isolation of the small proportion of genomic DNA that codes for proteins. This strategy identified a number of candidate genes[40–42]: *ADD1*, encoding alpha-adducin, a protein that participates in organizing the actin-spectrin cytoskeletal lattice; IT10C3, a probable small-molecule transporter with similarity to the tetracycline efflux proteins of *Escherichia coli*; GPRK2L, a G protein-coupled receptor kinase; and several anonymous genes with no similarity to previously described sequences (Fig. 34-3). Scanning of the full coding sequence of the first three candidates revealed no evidence of abnormalities or sequence differences specific to HD. Similarly, examination of the genomic segment spanned by each of these genes failed to disclose any alteration on disease chromosomes, with the exception of one report that mistakenly interpreted a rare Alu repeat sequence insertion within an intron of *ADD1* in two individuals as causative of HD.[43] This change was relegated to the status of a rare polymorphism by the discovery of the actual HD defect that had emerged from investigation of IT15, one of the anonymous candidate genes.[44]

Continued haplotype analysis with markers in the D4S180–D4S182 interval, particularly a codon deletion polymorphism in the very long IT15 transcript, refined the size of the candidate region as additional HD chromosomes, previously thought to be unrelated, were exposed to belong to the most common haplotype class, based on sharing of a

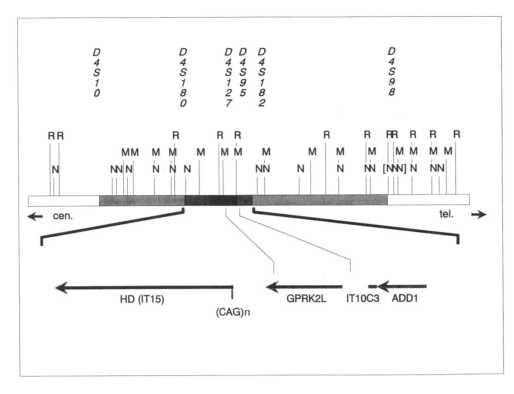

FIGURE 34-3 Isolation of HD candidate gene from the region of haplotype sharing. The long-range restriction enzyme map of ~3 × 10⁶ bp of the central portion of 4p16.3 is shown, with the progressively narrowing candidate region denoted by increasing intensity of shading. The unshaded region was eliminated by recombination events in HD families, placing the defect within the region between the DNA markers *D4S10* and *D4S98*. Initial haplotype analysis placed the defect in the 500-kb segment between DNA markers *D4S180* and *D4S182*. Candidate genes from this region are depicted below the map. Detailed haplotype analysis eventually narrowed the search to the interval of darkest shading, targeting the search to the 5′ end of the IT15 gene. This proved to contain the HD defect as an unstable, expanded CAG trinucleotide repeat ((CAG)n). R, NruI site; M, M1uI site; N, NotI site; cen., centromeric direction; tel., telomeric direction.

small segment of 150 kb immediately centromeric to *D4S95* (Fig. 34-3). This finding, which represented the ultimate distillation of the genetic approach, targeted the search for the defect to the extreme 5′ end of IT15. The culmination of the location cloning strategy came in 1993 with the discovery of an expanded, unstable trinucleotide repeat with the sequence CAG as the cause of HD (Fig. 34-4).[45]

Characteristics of the CAG Repeat

The IT15 CAG repeat on normal chromosomes is polymorphic, ranging from 6 to 34 units (Fig. 34-5) and is inherited in a Mendelian fashion.[46,47] Adjacent to the CAG trinucleotide stretch is a segment of consecutive CCG codons that is also polymorphic, varying from 6 to 12 repeat units.[48] The CCG alleles are also inherited in a Mendelian fashion but show strong linkage disequilibrium in HD, as more than 90 percent of disease chromosomes have 7 CCG units.[49] The CAG repeat of disease chromosomes is expanded, ranging from 37 to more than 100 units (Fig. 34-5). By contrast with the normal CAG alleles and with the CCG repeat, the HD CAG alleles do not show Mendelian inheritance. Rather, they change in length, becoming either shorter or longer, when passed to progeny from either a male or a female parent (Fig. 34-6). In most cases, the magnitude of the changes is small (<6 repeat units), with a bias toward repeat length increases, but fathers sometimes transmit alleles with larger expansions, up to a doubling or more in the number of CAG units.[46] The different allele sizes among progeny of an HD gene carrier are reflected in similar variation in DNA prepared from sperm, although the normal alleles in these individuals remain identical in somatic and sperm DNA.[50] It has not yet been established at what stage in spermatogenesis this HD-specific vari-

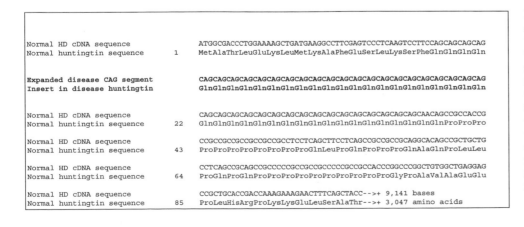

FIGURE 34-4 The N-terminal sequence of huntingtin encoded by the 5′ end of the HD gene. The huntingtin cDNA 5′ coding sequence for a normal allele is shown above the amino acids (1–96) specified by each codon. This normal allele produces a huntingtin protein with 22 consecutive glutamine (Gln) residues. The effect of the HD mutation is shown as an inserted sequence of an additional 21 CAG repeats, encoding 21 Gln residues.

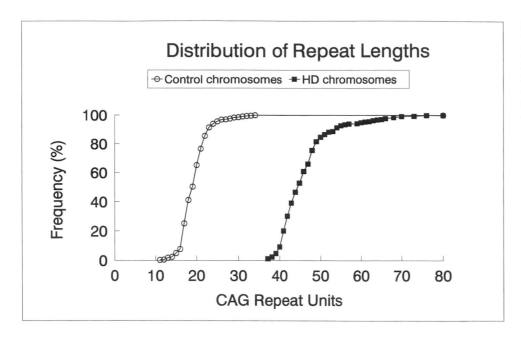

FIGURE 34-5 The cumulative distribution of CAG repeat lengths on HD and normal chromosomes. The frequency of CAG allele sizes on normal (circles) and disease (squares) chromosomes determined in Ref. 92 is depicted as a cumulative distribution for each.

ation occurs, what biological parameters (e.g., parental age, disease status, etc.) may affect it, whether all HD alleles of a given CAG length are equally unstable, and whether the degree of instability can be altered by the surrounding haplotype. Similar CAG repeat variation, albeit of reduced magnitude, is expected to occur in HD oogenesis but has not yet been demonstrated directly.

By contrast with gametic variation, the expanded HD CAG repeat exhibits very limited somatic alteration for most repeat lengths.[50–53] For example, several pairs of identical twins have been shown to possess repeats of identical length. For the very longest HD alleles (>60 CAG units), somatic changes

may be more frequent, but these do not correlate with neuropathology. Surprisingly, decreases in the number of CAG units in these cases may be most pronounced in the cerebellum, although this region is relatively insensitive to the pathological effects of the mutation.

Clinical Correlates of CAG Repeat Length

After the cloning of the HD gene, a plethora of reports analyzed the CAG repeat in cohorts of individuals with a clinical diagnosis of HD.[47] In all studies, the vast majority of patients

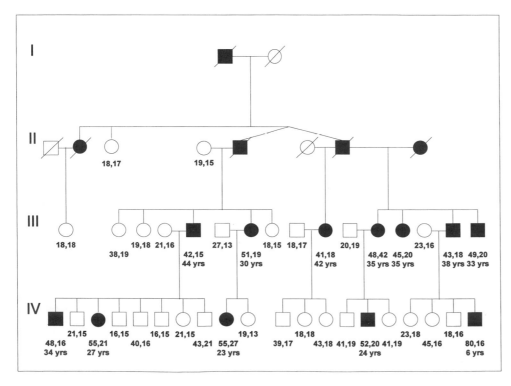

FIGURE 34-6 CAG repeat lengths and age of onset in the idealized HD pedigree. The same pedigree shown in Figure 34-1 is displayed with CAG repeat length for both alleles (larger allele shown first by convention) under each symbol. For those individuals who are symptomatic, age of onset (in years) is also shown. Of the four progeny who were potential HD homozygotes, only the eldest possesses two HD alleles with CAG repeat lengths of 48 and 42, respectively. Juvenile onset has occurred in the youngest member of the pedigree in generation IV, because of an HD allele with 80 CAG units, whereas the eldest member of generation III remains asymptomatic with an HD allele of 38 CAG repeats.

possessed a CAG repeat in the expanded size range, attesting to the universality of this mutational mechanism of HD in many races, nationalities, and ethnic groups. In some studies, a number of HD-diagnosed individuals did not possess an expanded CAG allele, but careful analysis of one such data set showed that the majority of these can be explained as sample mix-ups, lab errors, or erroneous diagnoses based on atypical features.[54] The latter category is well-established to exist, based on the absence of HD-like neuropathology in a small percentage of postmortem brains from individuals with a clinical diagnosis of HD.

As almost all cases of HD are familial, the disorder has traditionally been viewed as having a very low rate of new mutation. Support for this notion came in the failure of the few sporadic cases to meet stringent criteria for new mutation status, including absence of disease in elderly parents, proof of paternity, and disease transmission. The linkage disequilibrium approach used in the search for the *HD* gene provided the first evidence that new mutations to HD do occur, as the many different 4p16.3 haplotypes on HD chromosomes indicated independent origins for some chromosomes.[39] Identification of the HD CAG repeat has provided a direct genetic test of whether sporadic cases of HD-like symptoms are a result of new mutations. Indeed, sporadic cases with classic HD symptoms display an expanded CAG repeat in the HD size range.[45,55,56] Interestingly, their unaffected relatives who have the same chromosome possess a CAG repeat that is intermediate between the size ranges associated with normal and HD chromosomes. Several cases of HD new mutation have occurred on a chromosome bearing the major HD haplotype, that shared by one-third of HD chromosomes. This indicates that many of the HD families with this major haplotype may share a common ancestor who was not in fact affected with the disorder. Chromosomes with intermediate

alleles on this and other haplotype backgrounds thus represent a reservoir from which new sporadic HD cases may arise.

The complement of the clinical HD studies is the analysis of postmortem brain tissue, in which HD neuropathology has been documented. In a study of 310 brains assessed for HD neuropathology, using the grading system of Vonsattel et al.,[57] only three were found not to have an expanded CAG repeat.[58] Examination of the clinical records in these three cases revealed numerous features atypical of HD, suggesting a distinct disorder. Consequently, use of a combination of clinical and neuropathological criteria to assign a diagnosis of HD yields a collection of cases that all display an expanded CAG allele. If another type of mutation, either at the HD locus or elsewhere in the genome, can cause the same constellation of clinical and neuropathological features typically associated with HD, then it is quite rare.

Before the identification of the HD defect, family studies had established that inheritance of the HD defect invariably produced the disorder but with significant variation in clinical presentation. The most dramatic example is the manifestation of HD in juveniles in some cases of paternal transmission of the defect. The nature of the HD mutation has explained much of this variation, including the effect of paternal inheritance, as there is a strong inverse correlation between CAG repeat length and age at onset of neurological symptoms (Fig. 34-7) in all populations examined.[47] The increased magnitude of size changes in spermatogenesis dictates that paternal transmissions are the major source of the long CAG repeats that underlie juvenile onset.

The assessment of neurological onset and, to an even greater degree, psychiatric onset, has been viewed as prone to considerable subjective error. However, inverse correlations of CAG repeat length with age at onset of both neuro-

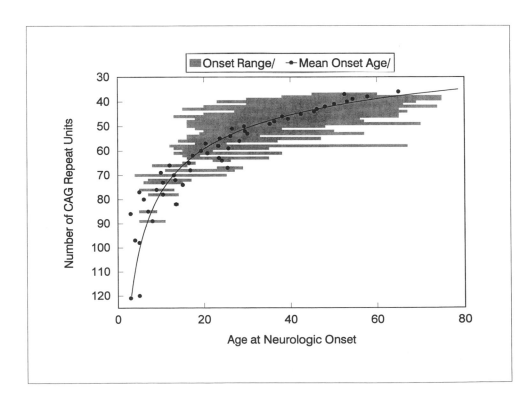

FIGURE 34-7 Inverse correlation between onset age and CAG repeat length. Published age at onset data for 1070 HD patients was used to calculate the average age at onset associated with any given repeat length. This mean age at onset (filled circles) and the associated range of onset ages (shaded bars) are plotted against CAG repeat length with curve fitting by power regression. A highly significant inverse correlation ($r = -.87$, $p < .00001$) between age at onset of neurological symptoms and CAG repeat length occurs across all HD alleles. However, in the adult-onset age group, there is a very wide range of possible ages of onset associated with any given repeat length, precluding its use in predicting the timing of the disorder in individual cases.

logical and psychiatric symptoms and with the objective parameter, age at death, are evident even when clinical data is contributed by many independent reporting physicians from different areas.[58] About one-half of the variation in age at onset and death is explained by CAG repeat length, as there can be significant differences between individual patients with identical HD alleles, presumably because of modifying factors, such as interacting genes, environmental influences, or stochastic events. The question as to whether rate of progression also varies with repeat length remains open, as studies comparing CAG repeat with functional decline have been in conflict.[59,60]

Structure and Expression of the HD Gene

The HD CAG repeat is located in exon 1 of a 67-exon gene, 17 codons downstream from the initiator ATG.[44] The gene is transcribed in a telomere-to-centromere orientation and encodes a protein of more than 3140 amino acids named huntingtin.[45] The CAG repeat produces a polymorphic segment of consecutive glutamine residues, adjacent to a set of proline residues encoded by the CCG repeat. Huntingtin's function is not known. Its sequence is not related to other proteins but shows a high degree of evolutionary conservation relative to mouse, rat, and puffer fish homologs.[61–64] The latter is 73 percent identical to human huntingtin, with the homology segregated into numerous patches likely to represent regions most critical for function. Interestingly, the most evolutionarily divergent segment is the polyglutamine-polyproline stretch, encoded by the adjacent CAG and CCG repeats. The normal human gene encodes 12–36 glutamines whereas the rat, mouse, and puffer fish genes encode 8, 7, and 4 glutamines. The human glutamine segment is followed by a region of 42 amino acids that includes 29 prolines. The corresponding regions of rat and mouse huntingtins have 28 and 27 prolines of 36 and 35 residues, respectively, while puffer fish huntingtin has only 2 prolines out of 4 residues. These comparisons suggest that the long polyglutamine and polyproline segments are not essential for huntingtin's normal function.

Huntingtin is expressed widely in both neural and nonneural (e.g., kidney, liver, lymphoblast, lung, heart, etc.) tissues based on studies of both mRNA and protein, suggesting that its normal function is not confined to cells in the areas of HD neuropathology.[65–73] Antisera against the N-terminal peptide encoded 5' to the CAG stretch have provided direct evidence that the CAG repeat is translated, as they react with the same large ~350-kd Western blot band detected by antisera raised against C-terminal regions.[69,71–73] The size change caused by the expanded CAG of the disease allele permits normal and HD isoforms of huntingtin to be distinguished by sodium dodecyl sulfate (SDS)-polyacrylamide gel electrophoresis. Cell fractionation experiments have indicated that huntingtin is a cytoplasmic protein and that this gross localization is not altered in HD cells.[72] Similar cytoplasmic localization has also been revealed in immunohistochemical analyses of rat, monkey, and human brain tissues, in which the pattern of huntingtin expression does not parallel the regions of HD neuropathology.[69,70,73] In both normal and HD neurons, huntingtin reactivity is seen in cell bodies, dendrites, axons, and terminals but not in nuclei. Thus, the neuronal target cells that succumb to the effects of the HD defect represent only a small subset of the neural and nonneural cell populations that express the mutant protein.

Mechanism of Action of the HD Defect

The mechanism by which the expanded HD CAG repeat produces the characteristic HD neuropathology is not known. It ultimately causes HD symptoms through the premature death of selected adult neurons, exemplified by the progressive loss of medium-sized spiny neurons along the posteroanterior, dorsoventral, and mediolateral axes of the caudate loss. However, it is not clear how many biochemical steps reside between the initial trigger, the expanded CAG repeat, and the final stages of neuronal demise. The cell death could be a proximal consequence of the presence of an expanded CAG repeat in adult neurons, or it could be a relatively late by-product of a change early in development that produces a compromised tissue structure susceptible to premature neuronal cell loss.

Whatever the stage at which the mutation acts, there are several conceivable biochemical mechanisms that could be involved, a few of which have been effectively eliminated by recent experimentation. The expanded CAG repeat does not drastically alter transcription, as huntingtin mRNA is expressed at comparable levels from the disease and normal alleles.[44,74] Similarly, the ability to distinguish HD and normal huntingtin based on electrophoretic mobility has revealed that the defect does not prevent translation of the mRNA. Thus, the lack of transcriptional and translational effects suggests that the HD defect acts through the altered structure of huntingtin and its extended polyglutamine segment.

The lengthened polyglutamine stretch does not cause HD by elimination of huntingtin's activity, as there is direct genetic evidence in both man and mouse that disruption of this gene does not produce disease symptoms. In humans, individuals with an HD gene translocation that eliminates 50 percent of huntingtin production do not develop HD.[44] Similarly, mice with one copy of the HD gene homolog (*Hdh*) inactivated by targeted mutagenesis show no abnormality.[75] Interestingly, transgenic mice expressing a novel truncated version of murine huntingtin's NH_2-terminus display pathology in the subthalamic nucleus and develop behavioral anxieties, suggesting that abnormal versions of huntingtin can have neuronal consequences.[76] However, homozygosity for complete inactivation of the mouse gene results in early embryonic death, before development of the nervous system, which is in sharp contrast with the adult-onset neuropathology in humans. The mouse experiments establish that huntingtin activity is essential for normal development. Thus, the existence of adult individuals homozygous for an expanded CAG allele indicates that the HD mutation does not remove huntingtin's normal activity.

The most probable mechanism of HD pathogenesis is a "gain of function," in which the lengthened polyglutamine segment confers a new property on the protein. This "gain of function" could act through huntingtin's normal physiological role if it elevated, rather than inhibited, huntingtin's normal activity. Alternatively, the novel property could leave huntingtin's normal activity intact while also promoting a new interaction of huntingtin or one of its breakdown products with a biochemical pathway unrelated to huntingtin's normal physiological role. This new interaction would then constitute huntingtin's "gain of function," although it could produce either activation or inactivation of the target pathway.

Ultimately, any model of the CAG repeat's mode of action must explain the complete dominance of the defect, the specificity of cell loss, and the correlation between repeat length and disease severity. In the gain of function model, dominance is expected, as the normal protein would not likely interfere with the action of HD huntingtin's added property. However, complete dominance is expected only when the effect of the new property already exceeds a critical effective threshold with a single dose of the disease gene. Specificity of the cell loss would be achieved if the novel property were effective only in particular cells because of peculiarities in their metabolism, such as restricted expression of a target-interacting protein. Increasing functional effectiveness of the interaction with lengthening of the polyglutamine stretch would then explain the correlation with disease severity. Thus, the gain of function model is an attractive working hypothesis that suggests several lines of investigation, with primary focus on discerning the cascade of events triggered by HD huntingtin's altered structure, rather than on defining normal huntingtin's physiological role.

Comparison to Movement Disorders

Several other neurodegenerative disorders (Fig. 34-8) are also caused by expanded trinucleotide repeats and show striking genetic similarities with HD. In each case, a normally polymorphic CAG repeat is expanded and unstable on disease chromosomes. The CAG repeat is located within the coding sequence of the respective gene, predicting an altered protein with an extended stretch of consecutive glutamine residues.

In Kennedy's disease, or spinal bulbar muscular atrophy (SBMA), expansion of CAG alters the primary structure of the androgen receptor, encoded at Xq11.2-q12.[77–79] The result of this mutation in males is a progressive loss of anterior horn cells in the spinal cord with consequent progressive muscular weakness, sometimes in association with mental retardation and androgen insensitivity. Although variable endocrine abnormalities, presumably related to reduced androgen receptor function, may include gynecomastia and testicular atrophy before the onset of muscle weakness, there is no abnormal development of the genitalia. By contrast, inactivating mutations in the androgen receptor gene do not mimic SBMA but rather produce testicular feminization. Thus, the expanded CAG repeat does not appear to cause degeneration of the anterior horn cells by simply causing androgen insensitivity.

Spinocerebellar ataxia type 1 (SCA1) is a progressive cerebellar ataxia resulting from neuronal loss in the cerebellum, including both Purkinje cells and dentate nucleus neurons in the inferior olive and in cranial nerve nuclei III, IV, IX, X, and XII. Additional clinical symptoms include muscle atrophy, decreased deep tendon reflexes, and loss of proprioception, although cognitive function remains relatively intact. SCA1 is inherited in an autosomal-dominant fashion because of an expanded CAG repeat on 6p, located in the first third of the coding sequence of ataxin-1, a protein of unknown function.[80,81] This 87-kd protein is widely expressed in the cytoplasm of nonneuronal tissues, in the nuclei of neurons from various brain regions, and in both cytoplasm and nuclei of cerebellar Purkinje cells. Unlike HD, SBMA, and other CAG expansion disorders, the larger *SCA1* normal alleles do not encode a pure CAG stretch, as the repeat is interrupted by CAT codons not found in the expanded CAG segment of the disease allele.

Machado-Joseph disease (MJD), another genetic ataxia, was originally described in a Portuguese family from the

FIGURE 34-8 Neurodegenerative disorders caused by translated expanded CAG trinucleotide repeats.

Disorder	Chromosome	Gene and Product	Repeat	Location	Number of Repeat Units
Kennedy's disease (spinal bulbar muscular atrophy)	Xq11.2-q12	*AR* androgen receptor	CAG	coding	normal 11 to 33 affected 40 to 62
Huntington's disease	4p16.3	*HD* huntingtin	CAG	coding	normal 11 to 34 affected 37 to 121
Spinocerebellar ataxia 1	6p24	*SCA1* ataxin-1	CAG	coding	normal 19 to 36 affected 40 to 81
Dentatorubropallido-luysian atrophy, Haw River syndrome	12p	*DRPLA* atrophin	CAG	coding	normal 8 to 35 affected 49 to 79
Machado-Joseph disease, Spinocerebellar ataxia 3	14q32.1	*MJD, SCA3* MJD1a protein	CAG	coding	normal 12 to 40 affected 67 to 82

Azores and was subsequently identified as one of the most frequently inherited spinocerebellar degenerative disorders in many populations. MJD shows progressive degeneration of the spinocerebellar tracts, but unlike SCA1, displays relative sparing of the inferior olive and cerebellar cortex. In addition to cerebellar ataxia, the manifestations of MJD include pyramidal and extrapyramidal signs, external ophthalmoplegia, facial and lingual fasciculation, and bulging eyes. It is inherited as an autosomal-dominant disorder caused by an expanded CAG repeat in a novel gene encoded at 14q32.1.[82] Recently, it has been shown that the clinically similar spinocerebellar ataxia type 3, previously thought to be a genetically distinct disorder, is also caused by expansion of this same CAG repeat on chromosome 14.[83]

Dentatorubral-pallidoluysian atrophy (DRPLA) is a rare degenerative disorder characterized by neuronal loss in both dentatofugal and pallidofugal systems that causes both ataxia and choreoathetosis, along with myoclonus, epilepsy, and dementia.[84] The defect in DRPLA, which is also inherited as an autosomal-dominant disorder, is located in the coding sequence of a novel gene on chromosome 12p that produces a 190-kd cytoplasmic protein of unknown function.[85] Expansion of the same CAG stretch is also the underlying defect in Haw River syndrome, a DRPLA-like disorder described in a single African-American family in North Carolina.[86]

Each of these other CAG repeat disorders displays normal alleles that are polymorphic and expanded alleles that are unstable, each within a respective size range comparable to the normal and disease alleles in HD. CAG instability appears in each case to be most important in gametogenesis, although somatic changes in the size of the expanded alleles have been observed. The CAG repeat length of disease alleles is typically correlated in an inverse manner with age at onset of symptoms, and like HD, the most severe cases emanate from paternal transmissions, as the magnitude of allelic length increases tends to be greatest in spermatogenesis. In each disorder, the defect produces an elongated stretch of polyglutamine in the corresponding protein that makes the disease version electrophoretically distinguishable from its normal counterpart. In all cases, the primary feature of pathogenesis is progressive neurodegeneration, although a different constellation of neurons in different locations within the central nervous system is affected in each of the different disorders. These similarities suggest that the ultimate mechanism of neuronal toxicity may be similar in each case, but that the susceptibility of individual types of neurons can be modified by the protein context in which the expanded polyglutamine segment is presented, resulting in different patterns of neuropathology. Thus, as a similar gain of function may be acting in HD and in these other neurodegenerative disorders, delineating the mechanism of neuronal death in any one might have positive implications for developing therapies in all of them.

Clinical Consequences: Diagnosis and Prospects for Therapy

The major impact of molecular biology on clinical care of HD has been the capacity to perform predictive testing, determining whether asymptomatic individuals born "at risk" because of a parent with HD have, in fact, inherited the defect. The discovery of DNA markers for HD in 1983 made it possible to perform presymptomatic or prenatal diagnostic testing for some interested individuals. However, the test was cumbersome and prone to various forms of inaccuracy, as it required tracing genetically linked markers through several related family members, at least one of whom was clinically affected. Thus, it was only applicable to at-risk individuals for whom several family members were able and willing to donate their DNA. This newfound ability to predict the future presence of a devastating, untreatable neurological disorder in a currently unaffected individual raised numerous ethical dilemmas that were debated at length. Pilot testing programs began cautiously, with a heavy emphasis on counseling both before and after delivery of the test result.[87–89] A high level of psychological and emotional support was built in because of the potentially calamitous consequences of a positive test result in a disorder with psychiatric disturbances and the lack of a precedent for determining ability to cope with such information. This experience led to the establishment of formal guidelines sanctioned by the International Huntington Association (IHA) and by the World Federation of Neurology (WFN) to ensure ethical administration of predictive testing.[90] This precedent has become an increasingly important guide, as genetic defects have been found in numerous other late-onset human disorders, including the other CAG repeat diseases referred to above.

The discovery of the nature of the genetic defect in HD has revolutionized the technical aspects of predictive testing, providing an inexpensive method that can be applied to any at-risk individual, without the critical need for DNA from relatives. CAG repeat measurement can also be applied to prenatal testing for confirmation of a clinical diagnosis of HD and for differential diagnosis in difficult cases (Fig. 34-9). Although direct assay of CAG length is more accurate and more widely applicable than the former linkage test, the essential nature of the information being obtained remains the same. Thus, the IHA-WFN guidelines remain in force, revised to take into account the nature of direct testing.[91]

Despite the improvement in the testing procedure, there remain complicating factors that must be considered in applying CAG repeat measurement to disease prediction. Normal and HD chromosomes may differ by as few as three repeat units. Moreover, chromosomes from unaffected members of the rare "new mutation" families can possess intermediate alleles closer to HD size or even overlapping with the lower end of the HD size range.[45,55,56] It is not clear whether these individuals are truly "normal" or will develop HD when they have a sufficiently long life. Indeed, there may be no precise border between chromosomes that cause HD and those that do not, as modifying factors become paramount in determining onset for alleles low in the HD range. Thus, intermediate alleles represent a dilemma for predictive testing of at-risk individuals. They also pose a problem in assessing the potential risk of transmitting HD, as the degree to which individual intermediate alleles are prone to expansion is not clear.

A second consideration in using the CAG assay for predictive testing derives from the linkage studies aimed at delineating the HD candidate region. As noted above, several

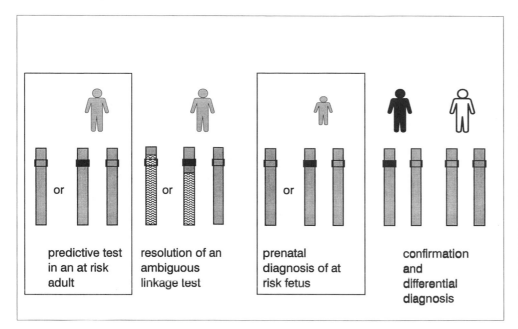

FIGURE 34-9 Applications of molecular diagnosis. A schematic diagram is shown to illustrate the clinical uses of direct measurement of CAG repeats. An expanded CAG repeat is depicted by a black box on one chromosome. The normal allele is denoted by an unfilled box. CAG repeat measurement distinguishes between normal and HD chromosomes in predictive testing of "at-risk" individuals, including those who have received an ambiguous result from the HD linkage test because of recombination between the markers and the disease gene. CAG repeat length can also provide prenatal diagnosis in at-risk pregnancies and is of value in confirming or refuting the clinical diagnosis of HD in atypical or difficult cases.

clinically diagnosed individuals in different HD pedigrees yielded marker genotypes characteristic of the normal chromosome from the corresponding affected parent, confusing the localization of the defect by predicting a second candidate region.[30,33] Discovery of the HD CAG mutation permitted resolution of this genetic conundrum. Despite the presence of expanded trinucleotide repeats in all other affected members of these HD families, the exceptional individuals had only normal alleles. Thus, these individuals appear to have another movement disorder mistakenly diagnosed as HD because of an extensive family history. Such cases can be expected to occur at a low frequency in families undergoing presymptomatic testing. Thus, the fact that a negative HD test does not exclude the future occurrence of another movement disorder should be conveyed to at-risk individuals.

Finally, the strong inverse correlation between age at onset and CAG repeat length raises special problems in delivering the results of the HD CAG test.[92] Every HD test that yields an allele in the established disease range can be considered diagnostic of the future onset of the disorder. However, despite the precision with which the number of CAG units can be measured, the CAG length cannot be considered an accurate predictor of age at onset in any individual case, because the range of ages at onset observed for any particular repeat length is far too extensive to make such predictions meaningful. Effective communication of the dubious prognostic value of CAG length for each at-risk individual represents another significant challenge for genetic counselors dealing with this disorder.

Although delivery of the HD predictive test has become more practical and experience with its associated genetic counseling has grown, many at-risk individuals choose not to undergo testing. Despite its reduced cost, increased accuracy, and wider applicability, the CAG repeat test shares the major drawback of the linkage test: Nothing can be done to prevent the disease in those found to carry the defective gene. Without an effective treatment, the predictive test is a mixed blessing.

Over the past 15 years, molecular biology has brought us to identification of HD's primary defect, but it has yet to define its biochemical mechanism. This mechanism appears likely to involve a "gain of function," i.e., a new property conferred upon the huntingtin protein by the expanded glutamine segment. This property may or may not be related to huntingtin's normal activity. The gain-of-function model for the mechanism of pathogenesis suggests that development of a therapy will require interfering with a novel property of mutant huntingtin, rather than simply replacing lost activity of this protein. However, delineation of the cascade of events that leads from the expanded polyglutamine segment to eventual cell death may reveal numerous potential targets for intervention. For example, toxicity of the mutant protein (or a breakdown product thereof) would be a novel property, as it is not a feature of the normal protein. Therefore, toxicity would constitute a gain-of-function whose ultimate mechanism of action is to inhibit another cellular process and whose effects could presumably be reversed by replacing the inhibited activity. Alternatively, it would also be a gain-of-function if huntingtin's normal activity were augmented by mutation, thus producing "too much of a good thing." Unlike the toxicity model, this gain of function must necessarily act through huntingtin's normal pathway. However, these scenarios are only two of many possible gain-of-function effects that could be proposed as the mechanism whereby the expanded HD CAG repeat causes specific neuronal cell loss. Hopefully, the understanding of the HD's biochemical mechanism that will eventually emerge from continued molecular analysis will reveal a mechanism that is amenable to intervention.

References

1. Huntington G: On chorea. *Med Surg Report* 26:317, 1872.
2. Osler W: Historical note on hereditary chorea, in Browning W (ed): *Neurographs.* Brooklyn, NY: Albert C. Huntington Publishing, 1908, vol 1, pp 113–116.

3. Vessie PR: On the transmission of Huntington's chorea for 300 years: The Bures family group. *J Nerv Ment Dis* 76:553, 1932.

4. Harper PS: The epidemiology of Huntington's disease. *Hum Genet* 89:365, 1992.

5. Merritt AD, Conneally PM, Rahman NF, Drew AL: Juvenile Huntington's chorea, in Barbeau A, Brunette TR (eds): *Progress in Neurogenetics*. Amsterdam: Excerpta Medica Foundation, 1969, pp 645–650.

6. Bird ED, Caro AJ, Pilling JB: A sex related factor in the inheritance of Huntington's chorea. *Ann Hum Genet* 37:255, 1974.

7. Gusella JF: DNA polymorphism and human disease. *Ann Rev Biochem* 55:831, 1986.

8. Pericak-Vance MA, Conneally PM, Merritt AD, et al: Genetic linkage studies in Huntington disease. *Cytogenet Cell Genet* 22:640, 1978.

9. Gusella JF, Wexler NS, Conneally PM, et al: A polymorphic DNA marker genetically linked to Huntington's disease. *Nature* 306:234, 1983.

10. Gusella JF, Tanzi RE, Bader PI, et al: Deletion of Huntington's disease-linked G8 (*D4S10*) locus in Wolf-Hirschhorn syndrome. *Nature* 318:75, 1985.

11. Zabel BU, Naylor SL, Sakaguchi AY, Gusella JF: Mapping of the DNA locus *D4S10* and the linked Huntington's disease gene to 4p16-p15. *Cytogenet Cell Genet* 42:187, 1986.

12. Wang HS, Greenberg CR, Hewitt J, et al: Subregional assignment of the linked marker G8 (D4S10) for Huntington's disease to chromosome 4p16.1–16.3. *Am J Hum Genet* 39:392, 1986.

13. Landegent JE, Jansen IN, De Wal N, et al: Fine mapping of the Huntington disease linked *D4S20* locus by non-radioactive in situ hybridization. *Hum Genet* 73:354, 1986.

14. Conneally PM, Haines JL, Tanzi RE, et al: Huntington disease: No evidence for locus heterogeneity. *Genomics* 5:304, 1989.

15. Wexler NS, Young AB, Tanzi RE, et al: Homozygotes for Huntington's disease. *Nature* 326:194, 1987.

16. Myers RH, Leavitt J, Farrer LA, et al: Homozygote for Huntington's disease. *Am J Hum Genet* 45:615, 1989.

17. Gilliam TC, Tanzi RE, Haines JL, et al: Localization of the Huntington's disease gene to a small segment of chromosome 4 flanked by D4S10 and the telomere. *Cell* 50:565, 1987.

18. Smith B, Skarecky D, Bengtsson U, et al: Isolation of DNA markers in the direction of the Huntington disease gene from the G8 locus. *Am J Hum Genet* 42:335, 1988.

19. MacDonald ME, Anderson MA, Gilliam TC, et al: A somatic cell hybrid panel for localizing DNA segments near the Huntington's disease gene. *Genomics* 1:29, 1987.

20. Doucette-Stamm LA, Riba L, Handelin B, et al: Generation and characterization of irradiation hybrids of human chromosome 4. *Somat Cell Mol Genet* 17:471, 1991.

21. Altherr MR, Plummer S, Bates GP, et al: Radiation hybrid map spanning the Huntington disease gene region of chromosome 4. *Genomics* 13:1040, 1992.

22. Bucan M, Zimmer M, Whaley WL, et al: Physical maps of 4p16.3, the area expected to contain the Huntington's disease mutation. *Genomics* 6:1, 1990.

23. Bates GP, MacDonald ME, Baxendale S, et al: Defined physical limits of the Huntington disease gene candidate region. *Am J Hum Genet* 49:7, 1991.

24. Bates GP, Valdes J, Hummerich H, et al: Characterisation of a YAC contig spanning the Huntington's disease gene candidate region. *Nature Genet* 1:180, 1992.

25. Baxendale S, MacDonald ME, Mott R, et al: Construction of cosmid contigs and high resolution restriction maps of a 2 megabase region containing the Huntington's disease gene. *Nature Genet* 4:181, 1993.

26. Wasmuth JJ, Hewitt J, Smith B, et al: A highly polymorphic locus very tightly linked to the Huntington's disease. *Nature* 332:73, 1988.

27. MacDonald ME, Cheng SV, Zimmer M, et al: Clustering of multi-allele DNA markers near the Huntington's disease gene. *J Clin Invest* 84:1013, 1989.

28. Taylor SAM, Barnes GT, MacDonald ME, Gusella JF: A dinucleotide repeat polymorphism at the *D4S127* locus. *Hum Mol Genet* 1:147, 1992.

29. Tagle DA, Blanchard-McQuate L, Valdes J, et al: Dinucleotide repeat polymorphism in the Huntington's disease region at the *D4S182* locus. *Hum Mol Genet* 2:489, 1993.

30. MacDonald ME, Haines JL, Zimmer M, et al: Recombination events suggest possible locations for the Huntington's disease gene. *Neuron* 3:183, 1989.

31. Allitto BA, MacDonald ME, Bucan M, et al: Increased recombination adjacent to the Huntington's disease-linked D4S10 marker. *Genomics* 9:104, 1991.

32. Youngman S, Sarafarazi M, Bucan M, et al: A new DNA marker [*D4S90*] is terminally located on the short arm of chromosome 4 close to the Huntington's disease gene. *Genomics* 5:802, 1989.

33. Robbins C, Theilmann J, Youngman S, et al: Evidence from family studies that the gene causing Huntington disease is telomeric to *D4S95* and *D4S90*. *Am J Hum Genet* 44:422, 1989.

34. Bates GP, MacDonald ME, Baxendale S, et al: A YAC telomere clone spanning a possible location of the Huntington's disease gene. *Am J Hum Genet* 46:762, 1990.

35. Youngman S, Bates GP, Williams S, et al: The telomeric 60 Kb of chromosome arm 4p is homologous to telomeric regions on 13p, 15p, 21p and 22p. *Genomics* 14:350, 1992.

36. Snell RG, Lazarou L, Youngman S, et al: Linkage disequilibrium in Huntington's disease: An improved localization for the gene. *J Med Genet* 26:673, 1989.

37. Theilmann J, Kanani S, Shiang R, et al: Non-random association between alleles detected at *D4S95* and *D4S98* and the Huntington's disease gene. *J Med Genet* 26:676, 1989.

38. MacDonald ME, Lin C, Srinidhi L, et al: Complex patterns of linkage disequilibrium in the Huntington disease region. *Am J Hum Genet* 49:723, 1991.

39. MacDonald ME, Novelletto A, Lin C, et al: The Huntington's disease candidate region exhibits many different haplotypes. *Nature Genet* 1:99, 1992.

40. Taylor SAM, Snell RG, Buckler A, et al: Cloning of the alpha-adducin gene from the Huntington's disease candidate region of chromosome 4 by exon amplification. *Nature Genet* 2:223, 1992.

41. Duyao MP, Taylor SAM, Buckler AJ, et al: A gene from the Huntington's disease candidate region with similarity to a super-family of transporter proteins. *Hum Mol Genet* 2:673, 1993.

42. Ambrose C, James M, Barnes G, et al: A novel G protein-coupled receptor kinase cloned from 4p16.3. *Hum Mol Genet* 1:697, 1992.

43. Goldberg PY, Rommens JM, Andrew SE, et al: Identification of an Alu retrotransposition event in close proximity to a strong candidate gene for Huntington's disease. *Nature* 362:370, 1993.

44. Ambrose CM, Duyao MP, Barnes G, et al: Structure and expression of the Huntington's disease gene: Evidence against simple inactivation due to an expanded CAG repeat. *Somat Cell Molec Genet* 20:27, 1994.

45. Huntington's Disease Collaborative Research Group: A novel gene containing a trinucleotide repeat that is expanded and unstable on Huntington's disease chromosomes. *Cell* 72:971, 1993.

46. Gusella JF, MacDonald ME: Huntington's disease. *Semin Cell Biol* 6:21, 1995.

47. Gusella JF, MacDonald ME: Huntington's disease: CAG genetics expands neurobiology. *Curr Opin Neurobiol* 5:656, 1995.

48. Rubinsztein DC, Barton DE, Davison BCC, Ferguson-Smith MA: Analysis of the Huntington gene reveals a trinucleotide-length polymorphism in the region of the gene that contains two CCG-rich stretches and a correlation between decreased age of onset

of Huntington's disease and CAG repeat number. *Hum Mol Genet* 2:1713, 1993.

49. Andrew SE, Goldberg YP, Theilmann J, et al: A CCG repeat polymorphism adjacent to the CAG repeat in the Huntington disease gene: Implications for diagnostic accuracy and predictive testing. *Hum Mol Genet* 3:65, 1994.

50. MacDonald ME, Barnes G, Srinidhi J, et al: Gametic but not somatic instability of CAG repeat length in Huntington's disease. *J Med Genet* 30:982, 1993.

51. De Rooij KE, De Konig Gans PA, et al: Somatic expansion of the (CAG)n repeat in Huntington disease brains. *Hum Genet* 95:270, 1995.

52. Zuhlke C, Riess O, Bockel B, et al: Mitotic stability and meiotic variability of the (CAG)n repeat in the Huntington disease gene. *Hum Mol Genet* 2:2063, 1993.

53. Telenius H, Kremer B, Goldberg YP, et al: Somatic and gonadal mosaicism of the Huntington disease gene CAG repeat in brain and sperm [published erratum appears in Nature Genet 7:113, 1994]. *Nature Genet* 6:409, 1994.

54. Andrew SE, Goldberg YP, Kremer B, et al: Huntington disease without CAG expansion: Phenocopies or errors in assignment? *Am J Hum Genet* 54:852, 1994.

55. Myers RH, MacDonald ME, Koroshetz WJ, et al: De novo expansion of a (CAG)n repeat in sporadic Huntington's disease. *Nature Genet* 5:168, 1993.

56. Goldberg YP, Kremer B, Andrew SE, et al: Molecular analysis of new mutations for Huntington's disease: Intermediate alleles and sex of origin effects. *Nature Genet* 5:174, 1993.

57. Vonsattel JP, Myers RH, Stevens TJ, et al: Neuropathologic classification of Huntington's disease. *J Neuropathol Exp Neurol* 44:559, 1985.

58. Persichetti F, Srinidhi J, Kanaley L, et al: Huntington's disease CAG trinucleotide repeats in pathologically confirmed post-mortem brains. *Neurobiol Dis* 1:159, 1994.

59. Kieburtz K, MacDonald M, Shih C, et al: Trinucleotide repeat length and progression of illness in Huntington's disease. *J Med Genet* 31:872, 1994.

60. Illarioshkin SN, Igarashi S, Onodera O, et al: Trinucleotide repeat length and rate of progression of Huntington's disease. *Ann Neurol* 36:630, 1994.

61. Barnes GT, Duyao MP, Ambrose CM, et al: Mouse Huntington's disease gene homolog (Hdh). *Somat Cell Mol Genet* 20:87, 1994.

62. Lin B, Nasir J, MacDonald H, et al: Sequence of the murine Huntington disease gene: Evidence for conservation, alternate splicing and polymorphism in a triplet (CCG) repeat [corrected] [published erratum appears in Hum Mol Genet 3:530, 1994]. *Hum Mol Genet* 3:85, 1994.

63. Schmitt I, Baechner D, Megow D, et al: Expression of the Huntington disease gene in rodents: Cloning the rat homologue and evidence for down regulation in non-neuronal tissues during development. *Hum Mol Genet* 4:1173, 1995.

64. Baxendale S, Abdulla S, Elgar G, et al: Comparative sequence analysis of the human and pufferfish Huntington's disease genes. *Nature Genet* 10:67, 1995.

65. Li SH, Schilling G, Young WS III, et al: Huntington's disease gene (IT15) is widely expressed in human and rat tissues. *Neuron* 11:985, 1993.

66. Strong TV, Tagle DA, Valdes JM, et al: Widespread expression of the human and rat Huntington's disease gene in brain and nonneural tissues. *Nature Genet* 5:259, 1993.

67. Landwehrmeyer GB, McNeil SM, Dure LS IV, et al: Huntington's disease gene: Regional and cellular expression in brain of normal and affected individuals. *Ann Neurol* 37:218, 1995.

68. Hoogeveen AT, Willemsen R, Meyer N, et al: Characterization and localization of the Huntington disease gene product. *Hum Mol Genet* 2:2069, 1993.

69. Sharp AH, Loev SJ, Schilling G, et al: Widespread expression of Huntington's disease gene (IT15) protein product. *Neuron* 14:1065, 1995.

70. DiFiglia M, Sapp E, Chase K, et al: Huntingtin is a cytoplasmic protein associated with vesicles in human and rat brain neurons. *Neuron* 14:1075, 1995.

71. Jou YS, Myers RM: Evidence from antibody studies that the CAG repeat in the Huntington disease gene is expressed in the protein. *Hum Mol Genet* 4:465, 1995.

72. Persichetti F, Ambrose CM, Ge P, et al: Normal and expanded Huntington's disease alleles produce distinguishable proteins due to translation across the CAG repeat. *Mol Med* 1:374, 1995.

73. Trottier Y, Devys D, Imbert G, et al: Cellular localization of the Huntington's disease protein and discrimination of the normal and mutated form. *Nature Genet* 10:104, 1995.

74. Stine OC, Li SH, Pleasant N, et al: Expression of the mutant allele of IT-15 (the HD gene) in striatum and cortex of Huntington's disease patients. *Hum Mol Genet* 4:15, 1995.

75. Duyao MP, Auerbach AB, Ryan A, et al: Homozygous inactivation of the mouse Hdh gene does not produce a Huntington's disease-like phenotype. *Science* 269:407, 1995.

76. Nasir J, Floresco JB, O'Kusky JR, et al: Targeted disruption of the Huntington's disease gene results in embryonic lethality and behavioral and morphological changes in heterozygotes. *Cell* 81:811, 1995.

77. LaSpada AR, Wilson EM, Lubahn DB, et al: Androgen receptor gene mutations in X-linked spinal and bulbar muscular atrophy. *Nature* 352:77, 1991.

78. Biancalana V, Serville F, Pommier J, et al: Moderate instability of the trinucleotide repeat in spino-bulbar muscular atrophy. *Hum Mol Genet* 1:255, 1992.

79. LaSpada AR, Roling DB, Harding AE, et al: Meiotic stability and genotype-phenotype correlation of the trinucleotide repeat in X-linked spinal and bulbar muscular atrophy. *Nature Genet* 2:301, 1992.

80. Zoghbi HY, Orr HT: Spinocerebellar ataxia type 1. *Semin Cell Biol* 6:29, 1995.

81. Servadio A, Koshy B, Armstrong D, et al: Expression of the ataxin-1 protein in tissues from normal and spinocerebellar ataxia type 1 individuals. *Nature Genet* 10:94, 1995.

82. Kawaguchi Y, Okamoto T, Taniwaki M, et al: CAG expansions in a novel gene for Machado-Joseph disease at chromosome 14q32.1. *Nature Genet* 8:221, 1994.

83. Schöls L, Menezes Saecker-Vieira AM, Schöls S, et al: Trinucleotide expansion within the MJD1 gene presents clinically as spinocerebellar ataxia and occurs most frequently in German SCA patients. *Hum Mol Genet* 4:1001, 1995.

84. Ikeuchi T, Onodera O, Oyake M, et al: Dentatorubral-pallidoluysian atrophy (DRPLA): Close correlation of CAG repeat expansions with the wide spectrum of clinical presentations and prominent anticipation. *Semin Cell Biol* 6:37, 1995.

85. Yazawa I, Nukina N, Hashida H, et al: Abnormal gene product identified in hereditary dentorubral-pallidoluysian atrophy (DRPLA) brain. *Nature Genet* 10:99, 1995.

86. Burke JR, Wingfield MS, Lewis KE, et al: The Haw River syndrome: Dentatorubropallidoluysian atrophy (DRPLA) in a African-American family. *Nature Genet* 7:521, 1994.

87. Meissen GJ, Myers RH, Mastromauro CA, et al: Predictive testing for Huntington's disease with use of a linked DNA marker. *N Engl J Med* 318:535, 1988.

88. Brandt J, Quaid KA, Folstein SE, et al: Presymptomatic diagnosis of delayed-onset disease with linked DNA markers: The experience in Huntington's disease. *J Am Med Assoc* 261:3108, 1989.

89. Wiggins S, Whyte P, Huggins M, et al: The psychological consequences of predictive testing for Huntington's disease. *N Engl J Med* 327:1401, 1992.

90. World Federation of Neurology Research Group on Huntington's Disease: Ethical issues policy statement on Huntington's disease molecular genetics predictive test. *J Med Genet* 27:34, 1990.

91. International Huntington Association and World Federation of Neurology Research Group on Huntington's Chorea: Guidelines for the molecular genetics predictive test in Huntington's disease. *Neurology* 44:1533, 1994.

92. Duyao M, Ambrose C, Myers R, et al: Trinucleotide repeat length instability and age of onset in Huntington's disease. *Nature Genet* 4:387, 1993.

Chapter 35

CLINICAL FEATURES AND TREATMENT OF HUNTINGTON'S DISEASE

FREDERICK J. MARSHALL and IRA SHOULSON

EPIDEMIOLOGY
NATURAL HISTORY
CLINICAL FEATURES
    Movement Disorder
    Cognitive Disorder
    Behavioral Disorder
    Progressive Functional Decline
DIAGNOSIS
    Positive Family History
    Negative or Absent Family History
    Imaging Studies
    Electrophysiological Studies
    Genetic Testing
TREATMENT
    Symptomatic Intervention
    Experimental Therapeutics

Huntington's disease (HD) is an autosomal-dominant neurodegenerative disorder characterized clinically by abnormal movements, intellectual decline, behavioral disturbances, and relentless functional deterioration. Gene carriers typically manifest illness in adulthood after normal birth and development. George Huntington first described the cardinal features of "hereditary chorea" in 1872, culling from his own clinical experience and that of his father and grandfather, who preceded him in the rural practice of medicine on Long Island.[1]

A cooperative investigative effort over the past 2 decades has culminated in the characterization of the HD gene (IT15), located near the telomere of the short arm of chromosome 4.[2] The mutant gene contains an excessive number of trinucleotide CAG repeats that code for a polyglutamine stretch in the 348-kd protein product, often referred to as *huntingtin*. The protein product is widely expressed in both neuronal and non-neuronal tissues.[3–5] Deletions within the region of chromosome 4 encompassing IT15, such as occur in Wolf-Hirschhorn syndrome, do not give rise to the HD phenotype, suggesting that the expanded gene codes for a protein resulting in an abnormal "gain of function."[6] Although concerted efforts are underway to develop a transgenic animal model of HD, neurobiological research has focused on the pathogenetic role of free-radical and excitotoxic mechanisms operating in the context of cellular bioenergetic defects.[7] Current research on the genetics and pathophysiology of HD is reviewed in detail elsewhere in this volume (Chap. 34 and Chap. 36). In this chapter, we focus on the clinical features and treatment of HD.

Epidemiology

HD occurs with a worldwide prevalence of approximately 5–10 per 100,000 population.[8] Northern and Southern European, as well as Indian and Central Asian populations, are similarly affected.[9] Some areas have a low frequency of HD, notably Japan (0.1 per 100,000)[10] and Finland (0.5 per 100,00).[11] The highest known concentration of HD is in the state of Zulia, in Venezuela, where a single large family, now numbering more than 10,000 individuals, is thought to be descended from a progenitor who lived on the shores of Lake Maracaibo approximately 200 years ago.[12]

In the United States, approximately 25,000 individuals have clinical features of HD, with an additional 125,000 people at risk of developing HD.[8,13] Although analysis of restriction fragment length polymorphisms (RFLP) to determine carrier status became available by the mid-1980s,[14] and direct testing for CAG repeat length has been conducted since 1993,[2] the vast majority of asymptomatic at-risk individuals have not been tested.[15] In the past 2 decades, nondirective and supportive genetic counseling appears to have lowered the frequency of the HD gene.[16,17]

Natural History

The age at onset of symptoms and the initial clinical manifestations of illness vary widely. The majority of patients have onset of symptoms normally distributed around a mean age of 39 years.[18] Juvenile HD, as defined by onset of illness before age 20, accounts for about 5–10 percent of all affected patients.[19,20] Rigidity, dystonia, and bradykinesia are the predominant motor features in juvenile-onset patients, in whom paternal inheritance of the HD gene is more common than in the more typical adult-onset form.[18,21,22]

It is difficult to date the onset of illness precisely, and there is typically a delay of months to years between symptom onset and diagnosis. Patients from the Venezuelan family who were examined annually often showed subtle "soft" neurological signs as much as 5 years or more before manifest illness could be diagnosed.[12,23]

Duration of illness also varies considerably around a mean of about 19 years. Most patients survive for 10–25 years after onset of illness.[20] Although juvenile-onset HD may be a risk factor for rapid progression,[24] Roos et al. found no relationship between duration of illness and age at onset in a retrospective study of 1106 patients, although male patients with affected fathers progressed the fastest.[25]

An inverse relationship between CAG repeat length and age at onset of HD has been reported and confirmed.[26–30] This relationship accounts for about 50 percent of the variance in age at onset. A strong correlation persists between very high CAG repeat lengths and juvenile presentation. However, for the majority of gene carriers with CAG repeat lengths ranging from 37 to 52, age at onset varies considerably from 15 to 75 years of age. Therefore, CAG repeat length by itself is not an accurate or sufficient predictor of HD onset.[26] Interestingly, the correlation between the degree of CAG expansion and the natural $\log_n$ of age at onset appears stronger, suggesting a higher-order relationship between symptom onset and CAG length[31] (Fig. 35-1).

The relationship between CAG repeat length and clinical progression of illness remains unsettled. Several studies have failed to show a link between CAG repeat length and the mode of presentation or pace of deterioration in HD.[32–34] Others have reported a strong relationship between CAG repeat length and selected clinical outcomes.[35] Differences in study design and the definitions of illness onset and duration may account for the discrepant findings.

As HD advances, patients experience progressive debility and weight loss. Heightened immobility and dysphagia often lead to aspiration pneumonia, a common cause of death. Among 395 affected patients in a Danish study, pneumonia and cardiovascular disease were the most common primary causes of death.[36]

Clinical Features

MOVEMENT DISORDER

CHOREA
The term *chorea* derives from the Greek verb meaning "to dance." Chorea is reminiscent of the continuous, irregular, and fleeting movements of a marionette. In less dramatic forms, chorea may pass for fidgetiness. These movements eventually occur throughout the body, including respiratory, pharyngeal, and laryngeal musculature. Patients may incorporate involuntary choreiform movements into apparently purposeful gestures, a phenomenon referred to as parakinesia. In some patients, chorea may appear as severe uncontrollable flailing of the extremities, or ballism, interfering with the patient's ability to feed, sit in a chair, or sleep in a bed.

Although conspicuous and of cosmetic concern, chorea is not disabling per se. Individuals with relatively severe chorea may be able to function, ambulate, and care for themselves surprisingly well. Bradykinesia, rigidity, dystonia, and postural instability more commonly impair function.

DYSTONIA AND PARKINSONISM
As HD progresses, chorea often gives way to axial posturing (dystonia) and parkinsonian features of bradykinesia, rigidity, and postural instability.[12,37,38] Mild dystonia in combination with chorea gives the writhing appearance of choreoathetosis. Sustained dystonic posturing affecting the neck, trunk, or limbs may result in contractures, immobility, and skin breakdown. Bradykinesia and dystonia, with or without significant rigidity, are often heralding features of juvenile-onset HD.[38]

Progressive postural instability occurs in both juvenile-onset and advanced adult-onset HD. Severe chorea, dystonia, rigidity, postural sway, and disruption of central vestibular reflexes contribute to the progressive balance problems attending HD.[39]

In the terminal stages of illness, patients may become akinetic and rigid, with little or no evidence of chorea. Pyramidal tract signs, such as spasticity, clonus, and extensor plantar responses, may appear.

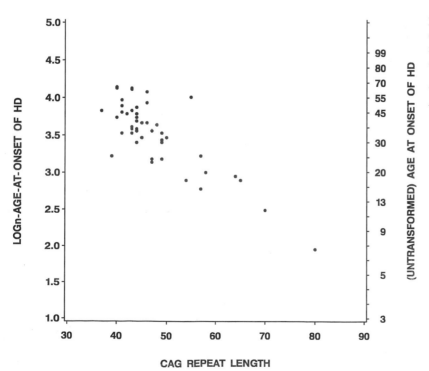

FIGURE 35-1 Relationship between $\log_n$-age-at-onset or untransformed-age-at-onset and CAG repeat length in 50 patients with HD. For $\log_n$-age-at-onset versus CAG repeat length, $r = -.82$, $p < .0001$. For untransformed-age-at-onset versus CAG repeat length, $r = -.69$, $p < .001$. *Adapted from Kieburtz et al.*[31]

DYSARTHRIA AND DYSPHAGIA

Deterioration in communication abilities and swallowing also characterizes the advanced stages of illness. Initially, speech may be hypophonic, with irregular rate, rhythm, and pitch in the setting of impaired respiratory coordination. HD patients show variability of utterance duration and/or voice-onset-time in tests of acoustic speech signals.[40] As articulation disturbances progress from understandable to unintelligible, the ability to sustain voluntary tongue protrusion is lost.

EYE MOVEMENT ABNORMALITIES

Disordered ocular motility is one of the earliest motor signs of HD.[41,42] Voluntary initiation of ocular saccades becomes slowed and uncoordinated. Patients find it more difficult to suppress head movements and often blink in order to break fixation and generate a saccadic burst.[43] Smooth pursuit movements are frequently disrupted by saccadic intrusions and impersistence. Initiation of internally generated saccades is more difficult than initiation of externally triggered ones, suggesting a relative sparing of parietosuperior collicular pathways in the setting of extensive damage to frontostriatal circuits.[44] Opticokinetic nystagmus is impaired both vertically and horizontally, although vertical movements are generally affected earlier.[45] Despite the prominence of oculomotor impairment, quantitative oculomotor assessment does not appear to be sufficiently sensitive or specific to distinguish accurately between asymptomatic gene carriers and nongene carriers at risk for HD.[46]

OTHER HYPERKINESIAS

Patients with HD may manifest other movement disorders, such as tics and involuntary vocalizations resembling Tourette syndrome.[47,48] Some individuals may exhibit myoclonus as a dominant feature of their movement disorder.[49–51]

COGNITIVE DISORDER

The cognitive and psychiatric features of HD are perhaps the earliest and most important indicators of functional decline.[52] The dementia of HD has been characterized as "subcortical" because of the prominence of bradyphrenia—slowed thinking—and because of attentional and sequencing impairments in the absence of cortical deficits such as aphasia, agnosia, and apraxia.[53,54] Executive function—the ability to plan, sequence, and carry out complex tasks—is thought to be selectively lost, perhaps related to damage to frontostriatal circuits.[55,56]

Paulsen and co-workers have emphasized that the memory impairment in "cortical dementias" typically involves deficits of both recognition and recall, whereas recognition is generally spared in patients with subcortical dementia. They found that Alzheimer patients performed poorly on tests of memory function, regardless of the severity of dementia, whereas Huntington patients performed poorly on tests of initiation (e.g., the double alternating movement task of the Mattis Dementia Rating Scale).[57] These observations are consistent with the findings of other investigators.[58–61] Registration and immediate memory recall are relatively spared in HD patients, whereas retrieval of recent and remote memories is impaired.[62–64]

Neuropsychological tests that appear to be sensitive indicators of disease progression include the Symbol Digit Modalities Test,[65] the Verbal Fluency Subtest of the Multilingual Aphasia Examination,[66] and the Stroop Interference Test.[67] These tests are part of the Unified Huntington's Disease Rating Scale (UHDRS), a battery of motor, cognitive, behavioral, and functional assessments used primarily as a clinical research tool.[68] The Trail Making Test-Part B, designed to assess executive functions, may also be useful in characterizing the progressive dementia of HD.[69]

Several investigators have examined the cognitive profile of asymptomatic persons at risk for HD.[70,71] Foroud and co-workers administered the Wechsler Adult Intelligence Scale–Revised (WAIS-R) to 394 at-risk individuals who denied symptoms referable to HD. After cognitive testing was complete, CAG repeat length measures revealed that gene carriers generally scored lower on all portions of the WAIS-R than noncarriers. There was an inverse correlation between CAG repeat length in gene carriers and scores on the WAIS-R.[70] These findings suggest that subtle intellectual impairment may antedate overt signs or symptoms of illness.

Cognitive decline is characteristic of HD, but the pace of progression among patients varies considerably.[72,73] Some individuals may remain cognitively intact despite many years of motor impairment. Insight and central language function generally remain preserved, even in the advanced stages of illness.[54,74]

BEHAVIORAL DISORDER

AFFECTIVE ILLNESS

Affective illness is a common presentation for HD[75] and occurs in as many as 30–50 percent of patients during the course of the illness.[76–78] Depressed patients experience enduring feelings of sadness, worthlessness, or guilt. Anhedonia—the loss of pleasure in activities—is commonly associated with poor concentration, decreased libido, hypersomnia, and psychomotor retardation. Affective disorder may be more prevalent in some families, particularly in those with a relatively late age at onset.[79] Only 10 percent of depressed HD patients experience episodic bouts of mania and agitation characteristic of bipolar disorder.[80]

SUICIDE

George Huntington was aware of the risk of suicide in HD. He noted that "the tendency to insanity, and sometimes that form of insanity which leads to suicide, is marked. I know of several instances of suicide of people suffering from this form of chorea, or who belonged to families in which the disease existed."[1] Suicide is influenced not only by the severity of the affective disorder but also by the degree of functional capacity retained, the level of insight remaining, and the extent of social supports available. Identified risk factors (many of which are inter-related) include childlessness, depression, single marital status, living alone, and other suicides in the family.[81] An increased rate of suicide has also been reported in those at risk for HD.[82–84] In a retrospective study, suicide was nearly as common in 282 asymptomatic siblings (5.3 percent) as it was in 395 HD patients (5.6 percent).[36]

PSYCHOSIS

The lifetime prevalence of psychosis in HD has been estimated at about 10 percent.[85] Impaired reality testing may occur at any time in the course of the illness, and patients may display psychotic features long before they manifest motor signs. When HD presents as an isolated thought disorder in a young person, it may be misdiagnosed as schizophrenia.[85]

Apathy is a common manifestation of affective illness in HD. Extreme social withdrawal may also represent an underlying thought disorder. Other psychotic features include paranoid delusions (typically, of spousal infidelity), thought broadcasting (the feeling that one's thoughts are immediately accessible to others), thought insertion (the feeling that others' thoughts are forcing their way into one's mind), and hallucinations, most commonly auditory or visual.[85]

SEXUAL DISORDERS

George Huntington commented on hypersexuality in his patients,[1] although hyposexuality is more common in HD.[86] HD patients may rarely develop paraphilias in the form of misdirected sexual feelings or behaviors.[86]

OBSESSIVE-COMPULSIVE SYMPTOMS

Current theories implicate the basal ganglia and frontal lobes in obsessive-compulsive disorders,[87] and compulsive handwashing and other ritualistic behaviors may occur in HD patients who have no other affective illness.[88]

PERSONALITY AND BEHAVIOR CHANGES

Personality changes occur commonly in HD patients, often beginning years before the onset of cognitive or motor manifestations.[78] Irritability, apathy, or anxiety may be the first signs of personality change.[89] Conduct disorder and antisocial personality disorder occur in about 5 percent of patients with HD, but their presence in at-risk teens does not accurately predict gene carrier status.[79,85] Although the prevalence of alcohol abuse in HD is similar to that in the population at large, alcohol and other substance abuse no doubt contribute to the social disruption and turmoil in many HD families.[90]

In general, psychiatric illness among individuals at-risk for HD does not predict gene carrier status. The risk of developing major depressive disorder increases when HD patients begin to show motor manifestations of the illness.[91] However, no differences in the incidence of depression, psychosis, or behavioral disorders reliably distinguish between asymptomatic gene-positive and gene-negative individuals. Major psychiatric illness is common in at-risk individuals, regardless of gene carrier status, suggesting that childhood and adolescent environments, as well as the HD gene, predispose a patient to behavioral disturbances.[92]

SLEEP DISORDERS

HD patients frequently experience daytime hypersomnolence and nocturnal insomnia. Increased latency to nocturnal sleep onset, frequent awakenings, and decreased slow-wave sleep on polysomnography have been correlated with severity of motor impairment, duration of illness, and extent of caudate atrophy as shown by computed tomography.[93] Underlying affective illness remains a major and remediable cause of sleep disruption in HD.

PROGRESSIVE FUNCTIONAL DECLINE

As motor, cognitive, and behavioral problems come to the surface, accustomed functions become compromised. A number of rating scales provide quantitative assessments of the functional impact of HD.[24,94,95] The total functional capacity (TFC) score derived from the HD Functional Capacity Scale[94] (Tables 35-1 and 35-2) has been validated against radiographic measures of disease progression, including computed tomography (CT) and magnetic resonance (MR) measures of striatal volume, as well as fluorodeoxyglucose positron emission tomography (PET) measures of striatal metabolism.[55,56,96,97] Reliability has been demonstrated among a variety of health professionals.[98] A prospective evaluation of 129 HD patients by a single examiner demonstrated an overall TFC decline of 0.63 ± 0.75 (mean $\pm$ SD) units per year.[99] The pace of functional decline was not reliably predicted by age at onset, body weight, gender of affected parent, or neuroleptic use.[99] Furthermore, no association between CAG repeat length and the rate of functional deterioration has been found among patients followed prospectively by a single examiner who was kept unaware of CAG repeat length.[31]

The Unified Huntington's Disease Rating Scale (UHDRS) includes standardized assessments of motor, cognitive, and behavioral performance, as well as the TFC and other functional measures of illness.[68] The UHDRS appears to be a reliable and internally consistent tool in assessing the progression of illness and the impact of therapeutic interventions.[68,100,101]

Diagnosis

POSITIVE FAMILY HISTORY

Diagnosis is relatively straightforward when a characteristic movement disorder occurs in the setting of a clear-cut family history of HD. The failure to obtain a complete and accurate family history is the most common cause of misdiagnosis in patients who present primarily with psychiatric features.[89]

There are other heritable neurological disorders that may present with chorea, progress inexorably, and involve cognitive and behavioral changes.[102] Dentatorubropallidoluysian atrophy (DRPLA) is an autosomal-dominant disorder, phenotypically similar to HD, which results from CAG repeat expansion in a gene located on chromosome 12.[103] Ataxia is a prominent presenting feature of DRPLA, with oculomotor abnormalities, chorea, and dementia developing as the disease progresses.[104,105] Genetic testing is available for both HD and DRPLA and may be helpful when clinical features alone are insufficient to establish the diagnosis.

Neuroacanthocytosis may present in adulthood with progressive dementia and chorea accompanied by seizures, orolingual dystonia with self-mutilation, progressive muscle wasting, elevated creatine kinase, and peripheral neuropathy. Neuroacanthocytosis can occur in dominant, recessive, or sporadic patterns. The diagnosis may be confirmed by the presence of acanthocytes on peripheral blood smear.[106,107]

TABLE 35-1 Criteria for Quantified Staging of Functional Capacities in HD

A. Engagement in occupation
  3 = *Usual level*—Full-time salaried employment, actual or potential (e.g., job offer or qualified), with normal work expectations and satisfactory performance.
  2 = *Lower level*—Full- or part-time salaried employment, actual or potential, with a lower-than-usual work expectation (relative to patient's training and education) but with satisfactory performance.
  1 = *Marginal level*—Part-time voluntary or salaried employment, actual or potential, with lower expectation and less-than-satisfactory work performance.
  0 = *Unable*—Totally unable to engage in voluntary or salaried employment.
B. Capacity to handle financial affairs
  3 = *Full*—Normal capacity to handle personal and family finances (income tax, balancing checkbook, paying bills, budgeting, shopping).
  2 = *Requires slight assistance*—Mildly impaired ability to handle financial affairs, such that accustomed routine responsiblities require some organization and assistance from family member or financial advisor.
  1 = *Requires major assistance*—Moderately impaired ability to handle financial affairs, such that patient comprehends the nature and purpose of routine financial procedures and is competent to handle funds but requires major assistance in the performance of these tasks.
  0 = *Unable*—Patient is unable to comprehend the financial process and is totally unable to perform task-related routine financial procedures.
C. Capacity to manage domestic responsibilities
  2 = *Full*—No impairment in performance of routine domestic tasks (cleaning, laundering, dishwashing, table setting, recipes, lawn care, answering mail, civic responsibilities).
  1 = *Impaired*—Moderate impairment in performance of routine domestic tasks, such that patient requires some assistance in carrying out these tasks.
  0 = *Unable*—Marked impairment in function and marginal performance; requires major assistance.
D. Capacity to perform activities of daily living
  3 = *Full*—Complete independence in eating, dressing, and bathing.
  2 = *Mildly impaired*—Somewhat labored peformance: in eating (avoids certain foods that cause chewing and swallowing problems), in dressing (difficulty in fine tasks only, e.g., buttoning or tying shoes), in bathing (difficulty in fine performance only, e.g., brushing teeth); requires only slight assistance.
  1 = *Moderately impaired*—Substantial difficulty in eating (swallows only liquid or soft foods and requires considerable assistance), in dressing (performs only gross dressing activities and requires assistance with everything else), in bathing (performs only gross bathing tasks; otherwise, requires assistance).
  0 = *Severely impaired*—Requires total care in activities of daily living.
E. Care can be provided at:
  2 = *Home*—Patient living at home and family readily able to meet care needs.
  1 = *Home or extended care facility*—Patient may be living at home, but care needs would be better provided at an extended care facility.
  0 = *Total care facility only*—Patient requires full-time, skilled nursing care.

SOURCE: *From Shoulson et al.[98] Used with permission.*

NEGATIVE OR ABSENT FAMILY HISTORY

When characteristic abnormalities of movement, cognition, and behavior occur in the absence of a family history of progressive neurodegenerative disease, a broader differential diagnosis should be considered (see Chap. 38). Identification of the mutation causing HD has made definitive diagnosis possible in the absence of a family history. In a study of apparently sporadic cases, 25 of 28 patients with signs and symptoms typical of HD showed expanded CAG repeats on chromosome 4, whereas only 5 of 16 patients with atypical clinical features (e.g., static illness, history of cerebrovascular disease, or Sydenham's chorea) tested positive for the expansion.[108,109]

There are several reasons why a patient with confirmed HD might not have a positive family history of this highly penetrant disease. Nonpaternity or ancestral death before manifestation of the disease may obscure the history. Alternatively, expansion of an unstable intermediate CAG length paternal allele into the HD range (>36 CAG repeats) may occur during spermatogenesis, giving rise to an affected individual whose father was unaffected.[110] Goldberg and colleagues have explored the genetic risk to siblings of sporadic cases, identifying a family with "pseudo-recessive" Huntington's disease on the basis of this type of expansion.[111] The frequency of *de novo* HD mutations remains exceedingly low.[112]

IMAGING STUDIES

Although a number of imaging methods have been used in the investigation of patients with HD, no single technique has emerged as necessary or sufficient for diagnosis.[96,113,114]

CT AND MRI
CT studies have demonstrated that measurement of the bicaudate diameter (the shortest linear distance between the heads of the caudate nuclei) is a simple and reliable marker of disease[113] and that progressive caudate atrophy parallels the deterioration of functional capacity.[55,56] Loss of putaminal volume may be detected by MRI in the early stages of illness and possibly antedate caudate atropy.[114] Studies in at-risk individuals who have undergone CAG testing suggest that volumetric MRI evidence of atrophy in the basal ganglia may appear before the clinical onset of illness.[115]

PET
PET studies using several ligands have attempted to detect metabolic changes that accompany the onset and progression of HD. Reduced fluorodeoxyglucose caudate metabolism

TABLE 35-2 Relationships of Stage of Illness to TFC Scores in HD

Stage	Corresponding TFC Score
I	11–13
II	7–11
III	3–6
IV	1–2
V	0

SOURCE: *Adapted from Shoulson et al.[98]*

correlates with functional capacity and bradykinesia/rigidity, whereas putamen hypometabolism correlates with chorea, oculomotor abnormalities, and fine motor coordination.[97] It remains unclear as to whether PET can reliably detect abnormalities in presymptomatic gene carriers.[116,117]

HD patients have a significantly decreased number and density of striatal dopamine D1 receptors as measured by the radiolabeled dopamine D1 receptor ligand [^{11}C]SCH-23390.[118] However, binding of the dopamine D2 receptor ligand 11C-labeled raclopride appears to correlate better with behavioral recovery in animal models of striatal transplantation.[119]

PROTON MR SPECTROSCOPY

The ability to assess *in vivo* chemical concentrations in a defined volume of brain tissue has become feasible, using MR spectroscopy.[120] Patients with HD have elevated levels of lactate in cortex and basal ganglia, raising the possibility that *in vivo* assessment of lactate might prove useful as a biological marker of disease progression. The biological impact of experimental therapeutic interventions might also be followed using these techniques.[121]

ELECTROPHYSIOLOGICAL STUDIES

Several investigators have reported the variable loss of frontal somatosensory evoked potentials in HD, but these findings are nonspecific and are frequently encountered in other disorders of the basal ganglia.[122–124]

GENETIC TESTING

An international study has evaluated the sensitivity and specificity of CAG repeat analysis in patients who were diagnosed with HD on the basis of characteristic clinical features. Of the 1007 clinically diagnosed patients, 995 had expanded CAG repeats (sensitivity, 98.8 percent). None of the 113 patients with other neuropsychiatric illnesses showed repeat expansion (specificity, 100 percent).[125] Therefore, clinical assessment of symptomatic individuals remains a very accurate means of diagnosis.

The ethical, psychological, and social implications of presymptomatic testing for HD have received wide attention.[126–128] A recent study of participation in the a predictive testing program revealed no differences between nonparticipants and participants with regard to gender, average age, stability of relationship, or level of education. Nonparticipants tended to have learned of their at-risk status during adolescence, whereas participants had done so in adulthood.[129] The World Federation of Neurology-International Huntington Association Research Group on Huntington's Chorea has recently published guidelines for predictive testing that emphasize the importance of confidentiality, informed consent, and multidisciplinary supportive counseling both before and after reporting of test results. The guidelines stress that predictive testing should not be performed on minors.[130]

Treatment

SYMPTOMATIC INTERVENTION

George Huntington said of HD in 1872:

> I have never known a recovery or even an amelioration of symptoms in this form of chorea; when once it begins it clings to the bitter end. No treatment seems to be of any avail, and indeed nowadays its end is so well known to the sufferer and his friends, that medical advice is seldom sought. It seems at least to be one of the incurables.

Despite the therapeutic nihilism so prevalent since HD was first described, several interventions may appreciably improve the quality of life for patients and their families. Although pharmacotherapies are available for the amelioration of some of the motor and psychiatric manifestations of HD, the provision of clear and accurate information and psychosocial support measures remains central to the care of HD patients and families.

Psychosocial support aimed at the family and the patient should ensure the availability of compassionate care providers, psychological and genetic counseling and referral, and access to social and legal services, including concrete assistance with long-term planning, facilitation of disability reviews, and support groups. Several clinical support and research organizations may be of help to the patient, family, and clinicians in their efforts to ease the burden of illness (see Table 35-3 and Appendix). Awareness of active research into the cause and treatment of HD is an important component of comprehensive care.

TREATING THE MOVEMENT DISORDER

There is no evidence that treatment of chorea or other hyperkinetic manifestations of HD results in functional improvement.[131] More often than not, antichoreic therapies are ineffective, and their long-term use is attended by a variety of untoward side effects. Occasionally, patients with disabling chorea may benefit temporarily from antichoreic pharmacotherapy to facilitate self-care. Reduction of heightened dopaminergic activity by use of dopamine receptor antagonists (e.g., phenothiazines, butyrophenones, thioxanthines)[131–133] or dopamine-depleting agents (e.g., reserpine and tetrabenazine)[134–136] may suppress chorea in the short term. Use of these neuroleptic agents commonly exacerbates bradykinesia and rigidity and may also lead to further functional decline from drug-induced sedation, apathy, akathisia, depression, dysarthria, or dysphagia. When chorea is sufficiently disabling, neuroleptic agents should be initiated, using the smallest effective dosage. Because the severity of chorea tends to diminish over time as HD progresses, continued use of dopamine antagonists or dopamine depletors requires frequent reassessment. The routine use of neuroleptics in juvenile-onset illness or in patients with advanced illness should be avoided.

The antichoreic effect of neuroleptics is thought to be mediated primarily by their blockade of D2 receptors on neurons projecting to the lateral globus pallidus via the indirect path-

TABLE 35-3 Huntington's Disease Organizations

HUNTINGTON'S DISEASE SOCIETY OF AMERICA 140 West 22nd St., 6th Floor New York, NY 10011-2420 Phone: (212) 242-1968; (800) 345-HDSA Fax: (212) 243-2443	HUNTINGTON SOCIETY OF CANADA 13 Water Street North, Suite 3 PO Box 1269 Cambridge, Ontario N1R 7G6 CANADA Phone: (519) 622-1002 Fax: (519) 622-7370
FOUNDATION FOR THE CARE AND CURE OF HUNTINGTON'S DISEASE, INC. PO Box 1084 82681 Overseas Highway Islamorada, FL 33036 Phone: (305) 664-5044 Fax: (305) 664-8524	HEREDITARY DISEASE FOUNDATION 1427 7th St., Suite 2 Santa Monica, CA 90401 Phone: (310) 458-4183 Fax: (310) 458-3937
INTERNATIONAL HUNTINGTON ASSOCIATION c/o Gerritt Dommerholt Callunahof 8 7217 ST Harfsen NETHERLANDS Phone: 31-573-43-1595	

way of basal ganglia transmission (see Chap. 36). The selective D4 receptor antagonist, clozapine, has been found to exert antichoreic effects in a small open-label study,[137] but controlled trials have not been done.

HD patients with predominant features of bradykinesia and rigidity may benefit from treatment with L-dopa or directly acting dopamine agonists,[138] but caution should be used with such agents because they can exacerbate chorea and dystonia and provoke hallucinations and psychosis. There are no effective pharmacotherapies for treating the disabling dystonic features of HD.

TREATMENT OF THE PSYCHIATRIC AND BEHAVIORAL DISORDER

Depression represents the single most remediable feature of HD.[76,85] The relative efficacies of various tricyclic compounds, monoamine oxidase inhibitors, and selective serotonin reuptake inhibitors have not been established. In patients for whom sedation is a concern, antidepressants with minimal anticholinergic effects (e.g., nortriptyline, desipramine) may be useful. Alternatively, if agitation and irritability predominate, using agents with more anticholinergic effects (e.g., amitriptyline, imipramine) may be appropriate. Fluoxetine may be beneficial as a first-line therapy for depression or as an alternative if tricyclics have failed. A controlled trial of fluoxetine in nondepressed HD patients did not show functional benefits.[139] Other serotonin reuptake inhibitors (e.g., sertraline, paroxitine, venlafaxine) have not been examined systematically in HD.

Rarely, depressed patients may not respond to adequate trials of tricyclics or serotonin reuptake inhibitors. Monoamine oxidase inhibitors such as phenelzine or tranylcypromine may be useful, but these agents can induce untoward effects on blood pressure when foods high in tyramine or other interacting medications are not restricted. Electroconvulsive therapy (ECT) may be effective in treating selected patients with HD who suffer from depression that is otherwise unresponsive to pharmacotherapeutic interventions.[140]

HD patients with bipolar affective illness may benefit from supervised trials of carbamazepine, valproate, or lithium, but there are no studies that have examined this problem systematically.[38]

Frank psychosis with agitation and behavioral aggression usually requires antipsychotic neuroleptic medications for short-term and often long-term treatment. When required, fluphenazine, haloperidol, thioridazine, or other antipsychotics should be used in the lowest possible dosage, with attention to the risks of a patient developing extrapyramidal side effects. Clozapine's possible use for treatment of psychosis in HD has been advocated,[141] but no controlled studies have been reported.

The novel tricyclic compound, clomipramine, as well as other inhibitors of serotonin reuptake already mentioned, may be useful in treating patients with compulsive behaviors or obsessive preoccupations.

EXPERIMENTAL THERAPEUTICS

REPLACEMENT STRATEGIES

Given the complexity of neurochemical changes in HD (see Chap. 36, Neuropathology and Pathophysiology of Huntington's Disease), it appears extremely unlikely that replacing neurotransmitter loss (as L-dopa restores dopamine for Parkinson's disease) will be a successful treatment strategy for HD.[52] The loss of gamma-aminobutyric acid (GABA)-ergic neurons in the striatum has prompted several unsuccessful pharmacological efforts to increase GABA activity.[142,143] Increasing cholinergic activity has also proved to be of little benefit.[144] Attempts to reduce the increased concentration of somatostatin in the HD basal ganglia using cysteamine have not produced clinical benefits.[145] Although there is a decrease in the number of cannabinoid receptors in HD,[146] there was no difference between placebo and cannabidiol (a nonpsychotropic constituent of cannabis that stimulates cannabinoid receptors) in a 6-week, double-blind, crossover trial of efficacy and safety for the treatment of chorea.[147]

NEUROPROTECTIVE STRATEGIES

A number of strategies are being aimed at slowing the progression of HD based on the emerging knowledge of pathogenesis. Premature neuronal dysfunction and death in HD are thought to be mediated by glutamate-triggered influx of calcium ions into neurons, leading to the formation of membrane-damaging free radicals in the setting of underlying bioenergetic defects (see Chap. 36).

The notion that retarding glutamatergic neurotransmission may slow cell death and thereby slow clinical decline has been reviewed extensively.[148,149] Baclofen (an inhibitor of presynaptic corticostriatal glutamate release) failed to slow functional decline in 60 patients with early signs of HD who were followed for up to 42 months in a randomized, placebo-controlled trial.[150] Dextromethorphan, a weak, noncompetitive *N*-methyl-D-aspartate (NMDA) receptor ion-channel blocker showed no short-term benefits in an open-label trial involving 11 patients.[151] A controlled trial of lamotrigine, another agent that retards glutamate release, is currently in progress. Remacemide, a noncompetitive NMDA receptor antagonist that blocks the ion channel, has been found to be well-tolerated in a placebo-controlled trial of 31 HD patients treated for up to 5 weeks.[100] Modest antichoreic effects attributable to remacemide were also observed.[152]

Strategies designed to buttress mitochondrial energy metabolism have a neuroprotective rationale in the experimental therapeutics of HD. Under normal resting potentials, the NMDA ion channel is blocked by magnesium, preventing glutamate from inducing a toxic influx of calcium into the cell. Because this channel is voltage-gated, conditions that depolarize the cell—such as defects in mitochondrial energy metabolism—may result in displacement of magnesium, thereby promoting influx of calcium, even in the setting of normal glutamate concentrations and activity.[7] Ubiquinone (coenzyme Q10), an intermediary in the mitochondrial electron transport chain, has been examined in a 6-month, open-label trial and has been found to be well tolerated at dosages of up to 1200 mg daily.[101] Ubiquinone has also been shown to lower occipital lactate levels in patients with HD, as measured by proton MR spectroscopy.[153] Controlled clinical trials of ubiquinone in HD have not yet been undertaken. A controlled trial of L-acetylcarnitine, another mitochondrial-buttressing agent, failed to show symptomatic benefits in 10 HD patients.[154]

Free-radical scavengers warrant investigation in light of the putative role of free radical generation in the terminal events of the neurodegenerative cascade.[155] A 24-week, placebo-controlled crossover trial of vitamin E in 10 patients with HD showed no benefit.[156] A 12-month, double-blinded, placebo-controlled trial in 73 HD patients failed to show consistent benefit, although patients in the earlier stages of illness responded more favorably.[157] Studies of other free-radical scavengers are under way.

Based on the contention that the primary degenerative process in HD is linked to intrinsic striatal vulnerabilities, implantation of normal fetal striatal tissue is under investigation as a possible method of intervention for HD.[158] This approach is also supported by preliminary findings suggesting short-term benefits of fetal nigral transplantation for Parkinson's disease.[159] Two case reports of transplantation in HD patients leave many important questions—such as graft site, graft number, and appropriate fetal age—unanswered.[160,161] At present, this approach should be considered highly experimental.

Identification of the gene responsible for HD and current efforts to develop transgenic animal models has buoyed the prospects for gene therapy strategies aimed at replacing or repairing the primary mutation.

To date, the early experimental therapeutics of HD has little to show in tangible terms. Rapidly increasing knowledge of etiology and pathogenesis, however, has expanded the options for rational therapeutic interventions and the prospects for substantive benefits for persons affected by, and at risk for, HD.

Acknowledgments

This work was supported by Training Grant NS-07338 from the National Institute of Neurological Disorders and Stroke.

References

1. Huntington G: On chorea. *Med Surg Report* 26:320, 1872.
2. The Huntington's Disease Collaborative Research Group: A novel gene containing a trinucleotide repeat that is expanded and unstable on Huntington's disease chromosomes. *Cell* 72:971–983, 1993.
3. Sharp AH, Loev SJ, Schilling G, et al: Widespread expression of Huntington's disease gene (IT15) protein product. *Neuron* 4:1065–74, 1995.
4. Strong TV, Tagle DA, Valdes JM, et al: Widespread expression of the human and rat Huntington's disease gene in brain and nonneural tissues. *Nature Genet* 5:259–65, 1993.
5. Li SH, Schilling G, Young WS, et al: Huntington's disease gene (IT15) is widely expressed in human and rat tissues. *Neuron* 1:985–93, 1993.
6. Albin RL, Tagle DA: Genetics and molecular biology of Huntington's disease. *Trends Neurosci* 8:11–14, 1995.
7. Albin RL, Greenamyre JT: Alternative excitotoxic hypotheses. *Neurology* 42:733–738, 1992.
8. Conneally PM: Huntington's disease: Genetics and epidemiology. *Am J Hum Genet* 36:506–526, 1984.
9. Harper PS: The epidemiology of Huntington's disease. *Hum Genet* 89:365–376, 1992.
10. Narabayashi H: Huntington's chorea in Japan: Review of the literature. *Adv Neurol* 1:253–259, 1973.
11. Palo J, Somer H, Ikonen EM: Low prevalence of Huntington's disease in Finland. *Lancet* 2(8562):805–806, 1987.
12. Penney JB, Young AB, Shoulson I, et al: Huntington's disease in Venezuela: 7-year follow-up on symptomatic and asymptomatic individuals. *Mov Disord* 5:93–99, 1990.
13. Tanner CM, Goldman SM: Epidemiology of movement disorders. *Curr Opin in Neurol* 7:325–332, 1994.

14. Gusella JF, Wexler NS, Conneally PM, et al: A polymorphic DNA marker linked to Huntington's disease. *Nature* 306:234–238, 1983.

15. Quaid KA, Morris M: Reluctance to undergo predictive testing: The case of Huntington's disease. *Am J Med Genet* 45:41–45, 1993.

16. Harper PS, Tyler A, Smith S, et al: Decline in the predicted incidence of Huntington's chorea associated with systematic genetic counseling and family support. *Lancet* ii:411–413, 1981.

17. Carter CO, Evans KA, Baraitser M: Effect of genetic counseling on the prevalence of Huntington's chorea. *Br Med J* 286:281–283, 1983.

18. Riley DE, Lang A: Movement disorders, in Bradley WG, Daroff RB, Fenichel GM, Marsden CD (eds): *Neurology in Clinical Practice: The Neurological Disorders*. Boston: Butterworth-Heinemann, 1991, vol 2, chap 76, pp 1563–1601.

19. Adams P, Falek A, Arnold J: Huntington's disease in Georgia: Age at onset. *Am J Hum Genet* 43:695–704, 1988.

20. Oliver JE: Huntington's chorea in Northamptonshire. *Br J Psychiatry* 116:241–253, 1970.

21. Bruyn GW: Huntington's chorea: Historical clinical and laboratory synopsis, in Vinken PJ, Bruyn GW (eds): *Handbook of Clinical Neurology*. Amsterdam: North Holland, 1968, vol 16, pp 298–378.

22. Merrit AD, Conneally PM, Rahman NF, Drew AL: Juvenile Huntington's chorea, in Barbeau A, Brunette JR (eds): *Progress in Neurogenetics 1*. Amsterdam: Excerpta Medica, 1969, pp 645–650.

23. Young AB, Shoulson I, Penney JB, et al: Huntington's disease in Venezuela: Neurologic features and functional decline. *Neurology* 36:244–249, 1986.

24. Myers RH, Sax DS, Koroshetz WJ, et al: Factors associated with slow progression in Huntington's disease. *Arch Neurol* 48:800–804, 1991.

25. Roos RA, Hermans J, Vegter-van der Vlis M, et al: Duration of illness in Huntington's disease is not related to age at onset. *J Neurol Neurosurg Psychiatry* 56:98–100, 1993.

26. Duyao M, Ambrose C, Myers R, et al: Trinucleotide repeat length instability and age of onset in Huntington's disease. *Nature Genet* 4:387–392, 1993.

27. Stine OC, Pleasant N, Franz ML, et al: Correlation between the onset age of Huntington's disease and length of the trinucleotide repeat in IT-15. *Hum Mol Genet* 2:1547–1549, 1993.

28. Craufurd D, Dodge A: Mutation size and age at onset in Huntington's disease. *J Med Genet* 30:1008–1011, 1993.

29. Simpson SA, Davidson MJ, Barron LH: Huntington's disease in Grampian region: Correlation of the CAG repeat number and the age of onset of the disease. *J Med Genet* 30:1014–1017, 1993.

30. Andrew SE, Goldberg YP, Kremer B, et al: The relationship between trinucleotide (CAG) repeat length and clinical features of Huntington's disease. *Nature Genet* 4:398–403, 1993.

31. Kieburtz K, MacDonald M, Shih C, et al: Trinucleotide repeat length and progression of illness in Huntington's disease. *J Med Genet* 31:872–874, 1994.

32. Ashizawa T, Wong LJ, Richards CS, et al: CAG repeat size and clinical presentation in Huntington's disease. *Neurology* 44:1137–1143, 1994.

33. Claes S, Van Zand K, Legius E, et al: Correlations between triplet repeat expansion and clinical features in Huntington's disease. *Arch Neurol* 52:749–753, 1995.

34. Marshall FJ, Kieburtz K, MacDonald M, et al: Lack of correlation between CAG-repeat length and rate of motor decline in Huntington disease, in Cassiman JJ (ed): *Proceedings of the 16th International Meeting of the World Federation of Neurology Research Group on Huntington's Disease,* July 15–18, 1995. Leuven, Belgium, University of Leuven, 1995, p 19.

35. Illarioshkin SN, Igarashi S, Onodera O, et al: Trinucleotide

repeat length and rate of progression of Huntington's disease. *Ann Neurol* 36:360–365, 1994.

36. Sorensen SA, Fenger K: Causes of death in patients with Huntington's disease and in unaffected first degree relatives. *J Med Genet* 29:911–914, 1992.

37. Kremer B, Weber B, Hayden MR: New insights into the clinical features, pathogenesis and molecular genetics of Huntington's disease. *Brain Pathol* 2:321–335, 1992.

38. Shoulson I: Care of patients and families with Huntington's disease, in Marsden CD, Fahn S (eds): *Movement Disorders*. London: Butterworth, 1982, pp 277–290.

39. Tian JR, Herman SJ, Zee DS, Folstein SE: Postural control in Huntington's disease (HD). *Acta Otolaryngol* Suppl (Stockh) 481:333–336, 1991.

40. Hertrich I, Ackermann H: Acoustic analysis of speech timing in Huntington's disease. *Brain Lang* 47:182–196, 1994.

41. Leigh RJ, Newman SA, Folstein SE, Lasker AG: Abnormal ocular motor control in Huntington's disease. *Neurology* 33:1268–1275, 1983.

42. Collewijn H, Went LN, Tomminga EP, Vegter-van de Vlis M: Oculomotor defects in patients with Huntington's disease and their offspring. *J Neurol Sci* 86:307–320, 1988.

43. Lasker AG, Zee DA, Hain TC, et al: Saccades in Huntington's disease: Initiation defects and distractability. *Neurology* 37:364–370, 1987.

44. Tian JR, Zee DS, Lasker AG, Folstein SE: Saccades in Huntington's disease: Predictive tracking and interaction between release of fixation and initiation of saccades. *Neurology* 41:875–881, 1991.

45. Rubin AJ, King WM, Reinbold KA, Shoulson I: Quantitative longitudinal assessment of saccades in Huntington's disease. *J Clin Neuroophthalmol* 13:59–66, 1993.

46. Rothlind JC, Brandt J, Zee D, et al: Unimpaired verbal memory and oculomotor control in asymptomatic adults with the genetic marker for Huntington's disease. *Arch Neurol* 50:799–802, 1993.

47. Jankovic J, Ashizawa T: Tourettism associated with Huntington's disease. *Mov Disord* 10:103–105, 1995.

48. Kerbeshian J, Burd L, Leech C, Rorabaugh A: Huntington disease and childhood onset Tourette syndrome. *Am J Med Genet* 39:1–3, 1991.

49. Thompson PD, Bhatia KP, Brown P, et al: Cortical myoclonus in Huntington's disease. *Mov Disord* 9:633–641, 1994.

50. Carella F, Scaioli V, Ciano C, et al: Adult onset myoclonic Huntington's disease. *Mov Disord* 8:201–205, 1993.

51. Vogul CM, Drury I, Terry LC, Young AB: Myoclonus in adult Huntington's disease. *Ann Neurol* 29:213–215, 1991.

52. Feigin A, Kieburtz K, Shoulson I: Treatment of Huntington's disease and other choreic disorders, in Kurlan R (ed): *Treatment of Movement Disorders*. Philadelphia: Lippincott, 1995, pp 337–364.

53. Kennedy JS, Kenny JT: Cognitive disorders associated with psychiatric illnesses, in Thal LJ, Moos WJ, Gamzu ER (eds): *Cognitive Disorders*. New York: Marcel Dekker, 1992, p 138.

54. Shoulson I: Huntington's disease: cognitive and psychiatric features. *Neuropsychiatr Neuropsychol Behav Neurol* 3:15–22, 1990.

55. Bamford KA, Caine ED, Kido DK, et al: Clinical-pathological correlation in Huntington's disease: A neuropsychological and computed tomography study. *Neurology* 39:796–801, 1989.

56. Bamford KA, Caine ED, Kido DK, et al: A prospective evaluation of cognitive decline in early Huntington's disease: Functional and radiographic correlates. *Neurology* 45:1867–1873, 1995.

57. Paulsen JS, Butters N, Sadek JR, et al: Distinct cognitive profiles of cortical and subcortical dementia in advanced illness. *Neurology* 45:951–956, 1995.

58. Lange KW, Sahakian BJ, Quinn NP, et al: Comparison of executive and visuospatial memory function in Huntington's disease and dementia of Alzheimer type matched for degree of dementia. *J Neurol Neurosurg Psychiatry* 58:598–606, 1995.

59. Rosser AE, Hodges JR: The dementia rating scale in Alzheimer's disease, Huntington's disease and progressive supranuclear palsy. *J Neurol* 241:531–536, 1994.

60. Mohr E, Brouwers P, Claus JJ, et al: Visuospatial cognition in Huntington's disease. *Mov Disord* 6:127–132, 1991.

61. Brandt J, Folstein SE, Folstein MF: Differential cognitive impairment in Alzheimer's and Huntington's disease. *Ann Neurol* 23:555–561, 1988.

62. Aminoff MJ, Marshall J, Smith EM, Wyke MA: Pattern of intellectual impairment in Huntington's chorea. *Psychol Med* 5:169–172, 1975.

63. Caine ED, Ebert MH, Weingartner H: An outline for the analysis of dementia: The memory disorder of Huntington's disease. *Neurology* 27:1087–1092-1977.

64. Brandt J: Access to knowledge in dementia of Huntington's disease. *Dev Neuropsychol* 1:335–348, 1985.

65. Smith A: *Symbol Digit Modalities Test Manual*. Los Angeles: Western Psychological Services, 1973.

66. Benton AL, Hamsher K: *Multilingual Aphasia Examination Manual*. Iowa City, Iowa: University of Iowa, 1978.

67. Stroop JR: Studies of interference in serial verbal reactions. *J Exp Psychol* 18:643–662, 1935.

68. Huntington Study Group: Unified Huntington's Disease Rating Scale: Reliability and consistency. *Mov Disord.* 11:136–142, 1996.

69. Lezak MD: *Neuropsychological Assessment*. New York: Oxford University Press, 1983.

70. Foroud T, Siemers E, Kleindorfer D, et al: Cognitive scores in carriers of Huntington's disease gene compared to noncarriers. *Ann Neurol* 37:657–664, 1995.

71. Diamond R, White RF, Myers RH, et al: Evidence of presymptomatic cognitive decline in Huntington's disease. *J Clin Exp Neuropsychol* 14:961–975, 1992.

72. MacMillan JC, Morrison PJ, Nevin NC, et al: Identification of an expanded CAG repeat in the Huntington's disease gene (IT15) in a family reported to have benign hereditary chorea. *J Med Genet* 30:1012–1013, 1993.

73. Britton JW, Uitti RJ, Ahlskog JE, et al: Hereditary late-onset chorea without dementia: Genetic evidence for substantial phenotypic variation in Huntington's disease. *Neurology* 45:443–447, 1995.

74. Caine ED, Hunt RD, Weingartner H, Ebert MH: Huntington's dementia: Clinical and neuropsychological features. *Arch Gen Psychiatry* 35:377–384, 1978.

75. Di Maio L, Squitieri F, Napolitano G, et al: Onset symptoms in 510 patients with Huntington's disease. *J Med Genet* 30:289–292, 1993.

76. Caine ED, Shoulson I: Psychiatric syndromes in Huntington's disease. *Am J Psychiatry* 140:728–733, 1983.

77. Folstein SE, Folstein MF: Psychiatric features of Huntington's dsease: recent approaches and findings. *Psychiatr Dev* 2:193–205, 1983.

78. Shiwach R: Psychopathology in Huntington's disease patients. *Acta Psychiatr Scand* 90:241–246, 1994.

79. Folstein SE: The psychopathology of Huntington's disease, in McHugh RR, McKurick VA (eds): *Genes, Brain and Behavior*. New York: Raven Press, 1991.

80. Folstein SE, Chase GA, Wahl WE, et al: Huntington's disease in Maryland: Clinical aspects of racial variation. *Am J Hum Genet* 41:168–171, 1987.

81. Lipe H, Schultz A, Bird TD: Risk factors for suicide in Huntington's disease: a retrospective case controlled study. *Am J Med Genet* 48:231–233, 1993.

82. Schoenfeld M, Myers RH, Cupples LA, et al: Increased rate of suicide among patients with Huntington's disease. *J Neurol Neurosurg Psychiatry* 47:1283–1287, 1984.

83. Farrer LA: Suicide and attempted suicide in Huntington's disease: Implications for preclinical tests of persons at risk. *Am J Med Genet* 24:305–311, 1986.

84. Wong MT, Chang PC, Yu YL, et al: Psychosocial impact of Huntington's disease on Hong Kong Chinese families. *Acta Psychiatr Scand* 90:16–18, 1994.

85. Folstein SE: *Huntington's Disease: A Disorder of Families*. Baltimore: Johns Hopkins University Press, 1989.

86. Fedoroff JP, Peyser C, Franz ML, Folstein SE: Sexual disorders in Huntington's disease. *J Neuropsychiatr Clin Neurosci* 6:147–153, 1994.

87. Luxenberg JS, Swedo SE, Flament MF, et al: Neuroanatomical abnormalities in obsessive-compulsive disorder detected with quantitative X-ray computed tomography. *Am J Psychiatry* 145:1089–1093, 1988.

88. Cummings JL, Cunningham K: Obsessive-compulsive disorder in Huntington's disease. *Biol Psychiatry* 31:263–270, 1992.

89. Pflanz S, Besson JA, Ebmeier KP, Simpson S: The clinical manifestation of mental disorder in Huntington's disease: A retrospective case record study of disease progression. *Acta Psychiat Scand* 83:53–60, 1991.

90. King M: Alcohol abuse and Huntington's disease. *Psychol Med* 15:815–819, 1985.

91. Watt DC, Seller A: A clinico-genetic study of psychiatric disorder in Huntington's chorea. *Psychol Med* 23(suppl 1):1–46, 1993.

92. Shiwach RS, Norbury CG: A controlled psychiatric study of individuals at risk for Huntington's disease. *Br J Psychiatry* 165:500–505, 1994.

93. Wiegand M, Moller AA, Lauer CJ, et al: Nocturnal sleep in Huntington's disease. *J Neurol* 238:203–208, 1991.

94. Shoulson I, Fahn S: Huntington's disease: Clinical care and evaluation. *Neurology* 29:1–3, 1979.

95. Blysma FW, Rothlind J, Hall MR, et al: Assessment of adaptive functioning in Huntington's disease. *Mov Dis* 8:183–190, 1993.

96. Kido DK, Shoulson I, Manzione JV, Harnish PP: Measurements of caudate and putamen atrophy in patients with Huntington's disease. *Neuroradiology* 33 (suppl 1):604–606, 1991.

97. Young AB, Penney JB, Starosta-Rubenstein S, et al: PET scan investigations of Huntington's disease: Cerebral metabolic correlates of neurological features and functional decline. *Ann Neurol* 20:296–303, 1986.

98. Shoulson I, Kurlan R, Rubin AJ, et al: Assessment of functional capacity in neurodegenerative movement disorders: Hunting-ton's disease as a prototype, in Munsat TL (ed): *Quantification of Neurological Deficit*. Boston: Butterworth, 1989, pp 271–283.

99. Feigin A, Kieburtz K, Bordwell K, et al: Functional decline in Huntington's disease. *Mov Disord* 10(suppl 2):211–214, 1995.

100. Kieburtz K, Feigin A, Como P, et al: A controlled trial of the glutamate antagonist remacemide hydrochloride in Huntington's disease. *Soc Neurosci Abstr* 20:1256, 1994.

101. Feigin A, Kieburtz K, Como P, et al: An open-label trial of coenzyme Q10 (CoQ) in Huntington's disease (HD). *Neurology* 44(suppl 2):A398–A399, 1994.

102. Greenamyre JT, Shoulson I: Huntington's disease, in Calne D (ed): *Neurodegenerative Diseases*. Philadelphia: WB Saunders, 1994, pp 684–704.

103. Koide R, Ikeuchi T, Onodera O, et al: Unstable expansion of CAG repeat in hereditary dentatorubral-pallidoluysian atrophy (DRPLA). *Nat Genet* 6:9–13, 1994.

104. Warner TT, Lennox GG, Janota I, Harding AE: Autosomal-dominant dentatorubropallidoluysian atrophy in the United Kingdom. *Mov Disord* 9:289–296, 1994.

105. Iazuka R, Hirayama K, Machara K: Denatato-rubro-pallido-

luysian atrophy: A clinico-pathological study. *J Neurol Neurosurg Psychiatry* 47:1288–1298, 1984.

106. Hardie RJ, Pullon HWH, Harding AE, et al: Neuroacanthocytosis: A clinical heamatological and pathological study of 19 cases. *Brain* 114:13–49, 1991.

107. Rinne JO, Daniel SE, Scaravilli F, et al: The neuropathological features of neuroacanthyocytosis. *Mov Disord* 9:297–304, 1994.

108. Bateman D, Boughey AM, Scaravilli F, et al: A follow-up study of isolated cases of suspected Huntington's disease. *Ann Neurol* 31:2983–2987, 1992.

109. David MB, Bateman D, Quinn NP, et al: Mutation analysis in patients with possible but apparently sporadic Huntington's disease. *Lancet* 344(8924):714–717, 1994.

110. MacDonald ME, Barnes G, Srinidhi J, et al: Gametic but not somatic instability of CAG repeat length in Huntington's disease. *J Med Genet* 30:982–986, 1993.

111. Goldberg YP, Andrew SE, Theilmann J, et al: Familial predisposition to recurrent mutations causing Huntington's disease: Genetic risk to sibs of sporadic cases. *J Med Genet* 30:987–990, 1993.

112. Vogel F, Motulsky AG: *Human Genetics. Problems and Approaches.* Berlin, Springer-Verlag, 1986, p 419.

113. Stober T, Wussow W, Schimrigk K: Bi-caudate diameter—the most specific and simple CT parameter in the diagnosis of Huntington's disease. *Neuroradiology* 26:25–28, 1984.

114. Harris GJ, Pearlson GD, Peyser CE, et al: Putamen volume reduction on magnetic resonance imaging exceeds caudate changes in mild Huntington's disease. *Ann Neurol* 31:69–75, 1992.

115. Aylward EH, Brandt J, Codori AM, et al: Reduced basal ganglia volume associated with the gene for Huntington's disease in asymptomatic at-risk persons. *Neurology* 44:823–828, 1994.

116. Kuwert T, Lange HW, Boecker H, et al: Striatal glucose consumption in chorea-free subjects at risk of Huntington's disease. *J Neurol* 241:31–36, 1993.

117. Grafton ST, Mazziotta JC, Pahl JJ, St. et al: Serial changes of cerebral glucose metabolism and caudate size in persons at risk of Huntington's disease. *Arch Neurol* 49:1161–1167, 1992.

118. Sedval G, Karlsson P, Lundin A, et al: Dopamine D1 receptor number—a sensitive PET marker for early brain degeneration in Huntington's disease. *Eur Arch Psychiatry Clin Neurosci* 243:249–255, 1994.

119. Dunnett SE, Fricker RA, Torres EM, et al: Correlation between anatomical reconstruction, PET imaging and behavioral recovery in striatal grafts derived from embryos of different donor ages, in Cassiman JJ (ed): *Proceedings of the 16th International Meeting of the World Federation of Neurology Research Group on Huntington's Disease,* July 15–18, 1995. Leuven, Belgium, University of Leuven, 1995, pp 40–41.

120. Kauppinen RA, Williams SR, Busza AL, van Bruggen N: Applications of magnetic resonance spectroscopy and diffusion weighted imaging to the study of brain biochemistry and pathology. *Trends Neursci* 16:88–95, 1993.

121. Jenkins BG, Koroshetz WJ, Beal MF, Rosen BR: Evidence for impairment of energy metabolism in vivo in Huntington's disease. *Neurology* 43(suppl 14):A334, 1993.

122. Topper R, Schwarz M, Podoll K, et al: Absence of frontal somatosensory evoked potentials in Huntington's disease. *Brain* 116:87–101, 1993.

123. Yamada T, Rodnitzky RL, Kameyama S, et al: Alternation of SEP topography in Huntington's patients and their relatives at risk. *Electroencephalogr Clin Neurophysiol* 80:251–261, 1991.

124. Kuwert T, Noth J, Scholz D, et al: Comparison of somatosensory evoked potentials with striatal glucose consumption measured by positron emission tomography in the early diagnosis of Huntington's disease. *Mov Disord* 8:98–106, 1993.

125. Kremer B, Goldberg P, Andrew SE, et al: A worldwide study of the Huntington's disease mutation: The sensitivity and specificity of measuring CAG repeats. *N Engl J Med* 330:1401–1406, 1994.

126. Terrenoire G: Huntington's disease and the ethics of genetic prediction. *J Med Ethics* 18:79–95, 1992.

127. Hayden MR, Bloch M, Wiggens S: Psychological effects of predictive testing for Huntington's disease. *Adv Neurol* 65:201–210, 1995.

128. Tibben A, Duivenvoorden HJ, Niermeijer MF, et al: Psychological effects of presymptomatic DNA testing for Huntington's disease in the Dutch program. *Psychosom Med* 56:526–532, 1994.

129. van der Steenstraten IM, Tibben A, Roos RA, et al: Predictive testing for Huntington's disease: Nonparticipants compared with participants in the Dutch program. *Am J Med Genet* 55:618–625, 1994.

130. World Federation of Neurology and International Huntington Association Research Group on Huntington's Chorea: Guidelines for the molecular genetics predictive test in Huntington's disease. *Neurology* 44:1533–1536, 1994.

131. Shoulson I: Huntington's disease: Functional capacities in patients treated with neuroleptic and antidepressant drugs. *Neurology* 31:1333–1335, 1981.

132. Girotti F, Carella F, Scigliano G, et al: Effect of neuroleptic treatment of involuntary movements and motor performances in Huntington's disease. *J Neurol Neurosurg Psychiatry* 47:848–852, 1984.

133. Barr AN, Fischer JH, Koller WC, et al: Serum haloperidol concentration and choreiform movements in Huntington's disease. *Neurology* 38:84–88, 1988.

134. Kempinski WH, Boniface WR, Morgan PP, et al: Reserpine in Huntington's chorea. *Neurology* 10:38–42, 1960.

135. Jankovic J, Orman J: Tetrabenazine therapy of dystonia, chorea, tics and other dyskinesias. *Neurology* 38:391–394, 1988.

136. Friedman JH: A case of progressive hemichorea responsive to high-dose reserpine. *J Clin Psychiatry* 47:149–150, 1986.

137. Bonuccelli U, Ceravolo R, Maremmani C, et al: Clozapine in Huntington's chorea. *Neurology* 44:821–823, 1994.

138. Jongen PJ, Renier WO, Gabreels FJ: Seven cases of Huntington's disease in childhood and L-dopa-induced improvement in the hypokinetic-rigid form. *Clin Neurol Neurosurg* 82:251–261, 1980.

139. Como PG, Rubin AF, O'Brien CF, et al: A controlled trial of fluoxetine in non-depressed patients with Huntington's disease. *Neurology* 43(suppl 4):A334, 1993.

140. Ranen NG, Peyser CE, Folstein SE: ECT as a treatment for depression in Huntington's disease. *J Neuropsychiatr Clin Neurosci* 6:154–159, 1994.

141. Sajotovic M, Verbanac P, Ramirez LF, Meltzer HY: Clozapine treatment of psychiatric symptoms resistant to neuroleptic treatment in patients with Huntington's chorea. *Neurology* 41:156, 1991.

142. Shoulson I, Goldblatt D, Charlton M, Joynt RJ: Huntington's disease: Treatment with muscimol, a GABA-mimetic drug. *Ann Neurol* 4:279–284, 1978.

143. Manyam N, Hare T, Katz L: Effect if isoniazid on CSF and plasma GABA levels in Huntington's disease. *Life Sci* 26:1303–1308, 1980.

144. Nutt JG, Rosin A, Chase TN: Treatment of Huntington's disease with a cholinergic agonist. *Neurology* 28:1061–1064, 1978.

145. Schults C, Steardo L, Barone P, et al: Huntington's disease: Effect of cysteamine, a somatostatin-depleting agent. *Neurology* 36:1099–1102, 1986.

146. Glass M, Faull RL, Dragunow M: Loss of cannabinoid receptors in the substantia nigra in Huntington's disease. *Neuroscience* 56:523–527, 1993.

147. Consroe P, Laguna J, Allender J, et al: Controlled clinical trial of cannabidiol in Huntington's disease. *Pharmacol Biochem Behav* 40:701–708, 1991.

148. Greenamyre JT: The role of glutamate in neurotransmission and neurologic disease. *Arch Neurol* 43:1058–1063, 1986.

149. Shoulson I: Huntington's disease: Anti-neurotoxic therapeutic strategies, in Fuxe K, Roberts R, Schwarcz R (eds): *Excitotoxins.* London: MacMillan, 1983, pp 343–353.

150. Shoulson I, Odoroff C, Oakes D, et al: A controlled clinical trial of baclofen in Huntington's disease. *Ann Neurol* 25:252–259, 1989.

151. Walker FO, Hunt VP: An open label trial of dextromethorphan in Huntington's disease. *Clin Neuropharmacol* 12:322–330, 1989.

152. Kieburtz K, McDermott M, Marshall FJ, et al: Evaluation of the glutamate antagonist remacemide hydrochloride in Huntington's disease. *Neurology* 45(suppl 4):A254, 1995.

153. Koroshetz WJ, Jenkins B, Rosen B, Beal MF: Ubiquinone lowers occipital lactate levels in patients with Huntington's disease. *Neurology* 43(suppl 4):A334, 1993.

154. Goetz CG, Tanner CM, Cohen JA, et al: L-acetyl carnitine in Huntington's disease: Double blind placebo controlled crossover study of drug effects on movement disorders and dementia. *Mov Disord* 5:263–264, 1990.

155. Coyle JT, Puttfarken P: Oxidative stress, glutamate and neurodegenerative disorders. *Science* 262:689–700, 1993.

156. Caro AJ, Caro S: Vitamin E treatment of Huntington's chorea. *Br Med J* 1(6106):153, 1978.

157. Peyser CE, Folstein M, Chase GA, et al: Trial of d-alpha tocopherol in Huntington's disease. *Am J Psychiatry.* 152:1771–1775, 1995.

158. Schumacher JM, Hantraye P, Brownell AL, et al: A primate model of Huntington's disease: Functional neural transplantation and CT-guided stereotactic procedures. *Cell Transplant* 1:313–322, 1992.

159. Freeman TB, Olanow CW, Hauser RA, et al: Bilateral fetal nigral transplantation into the postcommissural putamen in Parkinson's disease. *Ann Neurol* 38:379–388, 1995.

160. Sramka M, Rattaj M, Molina H, et al: Stereotactic technique and pathophysiological mechanisms of neurotransplantation in Huntington's chorea. *Stereotact Funct Neurosurg* 58:79–83, 1992.

161. Madrazo I, Cuevas C, Castrejon H, et al: The first homotopic fetal homograft of the striatum in the treatment of Huntington's disease. *Gac Med Mex* 129:109–117, 1993.

Chapter 36

NEUROPATHOLOGY AND PATHOPHYSIOLOGY OF HUNTINGTON'S DISEASE

STEVEN M. HERSCH and ROBERT J. FERRANTE

NEUROPATHOLOGY
    Striatum
    Globus Pallidus
    Substantia Nigra
    Diencephalon
    Cerebral Cortex
    Cerebellum and Brain Stem
PATHOPHYSIOLOGY
    Role of Excitatory Amino Acids
    Role of Cellular Metabolism
MOLECULAR NEUROPATHOLOGY
    Huntingtin Transcription
    Role of Mutant Huntingtin Protein

Huntington's disease (HD) is a neurodegenerative disorder related to a mutation occurring in the coding region of the IT15 gene on chromosome 4. The average age of onset is about 40 years of age; however, the range is extremely broad, with pediatric and late-life onsets not infrequent. The genetic mutation consists of expansion of a polymorphic trinucleotide (CAG) repeat, near the 5' end of the gene, that normally ranges from about 17–30 copies. Individuals with more than 37 repeats develop HD, with the largest numbers (greater than 60) correlating with juvenile onset of HD. Genetic anticipation occurs such that the affected offspring of males have an increased probability of developing the disease at an earlier age than their fathers. The IT15 gene codes for a normal protein, named huntingtin, which is of unknown function. In individuals heterozygous for HD, both normal protein and protein containing an expanded polyglutamine tract, transcribed by the CAG expansion, are expressed. The relationship between this abnormal protein and neuropathology is just beginning to be explored. The clinical expression of HD is characteristic and consists of progressively disordered movement, behavior, and cognition. The specific symptoms and progression of HD can be related to its neuropathology, which is characterized by relatively selective loss of specific neuronal populations in a variety of brain regions. Basal ganglia pathology has been the most thoroughly characterized and has been central to the development of animal models and hypotheses about the circuitry involved in chorea and about potential mechanisms of neuronal death in HD. Pathology in other brain regions has not been studied as extensively but is more widespread than the customary focus on basal ganglia might suggest and undoubtedly contributes to disease phenotype. Pathology outside the brain has neither been identified nor completely excluded. This review will focus on research occurring in the last 2 decades, during which new methods in quantitative anatomy, immunocytochemistry, biochemistry, and molecular biology have emerged and provided an explosion of new knowledge and ideas about HD.

Neuropathology

STRIATUM

GROSS AND HISTOLOGICAL PATHOLOGY
The most striking neuropathology in HD occurs within the neostriatum, in which there is gross atrophy of the caudate nucleus and putamen, accompanied by marked neuronal loss and astrogliosis (Fig. 36-1).[1,2] The striatal astrogliosis appears to reflect relative astrocyte survival in a shrinking striatum,[3] rather than a primary or reactive astrocytosis. The extent of gross striatal pathology, neuronal loss, and gliosis provides a basis for grading the severity of HD pathology (grades 0–4),[4] which also correlates to the extent of clinical disability (Fig. 36-2). Grade 0 cases have a strong clinical and familial history suggesting HD but no detectable histological neuropathology at autopsy. In grade 1 cases, neuropathological changes can be detected microscopically with as much as 50 percent depletion of striatal neurons but without gross atrophy. In more severe grades (2–4), gross atrophy, neuronal depletion, and gliosis are progressively more pronounced, and pallidal pathology becomes evident. In the most severe grade (4), more than 90 percent of striatal neurons are lost, and microscopy predominantly reveals astrocytes. There is a dorsal-to-ventral, anterior-to-posterior, and medial-to-lateral progression of neuronal death, with the dorsomedial striatum affected earliest and relative sparing of the ventral striatum and nucleus accumbens.[4,5]

SELECTIVE NEURONAL LOSS AND PRESERVATION
Quantitative microscopic studies demonstrating relative preservation of large striatal neurons and severe loss of medium sized striatal neurons provided early evidence for selective neuronal degeneration in the neostriatum.[3,6] Since then, extensive biochemical, tissue binding, and immunocytochemical studies of HD brain tissue have demonstrated marked disparities, with loss versus preservation of a variety of neurochemical substances within the basal ganglia, suggesting that the destructive process is not equally expressed in all striatal neurons and that there is a selective pattern of neuronal vulnerability.

Medium spiny neurons are inhibitory projection neurons that use gamma-aminobutyric acid (GABA) as their primary neurotransmitter, and they comprise more than 80 percent of all striatal neurons. Reductions in GABA, its synthetic enzyme glutamic acid decarboxylase (GAD), and its degradative enzyme GABA-transaminase in the neostriatum were among the earliest neurochemical changes detected in HD

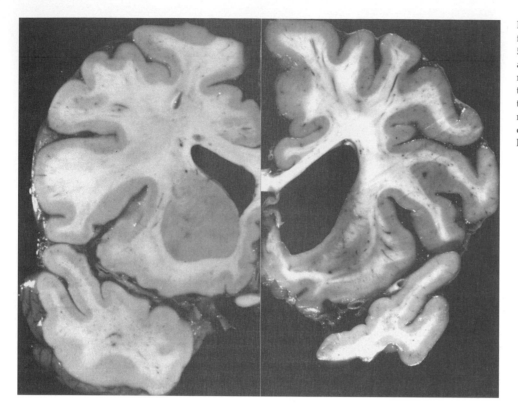

FIGURE 36-1 Photomicrographs of fixed cerebral hemispheres from a 58-year-old female with HD *(right)* and an age-matched normal specimen *(left)* at a coronal level through the rostral striatum. Note the marked atrophy of the caudate nucleus and putamen, along with cortical atrophy and white matter loss in HD.

and could be correlated with loss of medium spiny neurons.[7–11] Medium spiny neurons have further been shown to be depleted in HD based on the loss of substance P,[12] enkephalin,[12] calcineurin,[13] calbindin,[14,15] adenosine receptors,[16] and dopamine receptors[17,18] (Fig. 36-3). Medium spiny neurons can be divided into two populations based upon both connectional and neurochemical differences. One subpopulation expresses D1 dopamine receptors and the cotransmitter substance P, and projects primarily to the internal segment of the globus pallidus (GPi) and the substantia nigra pars reticulata. The other population expresses the D2 dopamine receptor and enkephalin and projects primarily to the

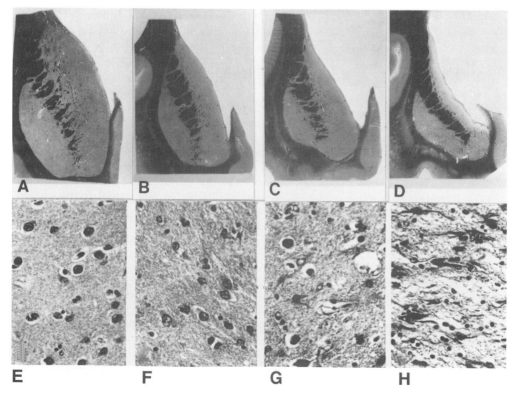

FIGURE 36-2 Coronal sections through the level of the caudate nucleus and putamen, demonstrating the grades of severity of striatal involvement. A normal specimen is represented in *A*. No gross striatal atrophy is observed in grades 0 and 1. In grade 2 *(B)*, there is striatal atrophy, but the caudate nucleus remains convex. In grade 3 *(C)*, striatal atrophy is more severe, with the caudate nucleus flat. In grade 4 *(D)*, striatal atrophy is most severe with the medial surface concave. Concomitant with the severity of gross atrophy observed in grades 2, 3, and 4, progressive neuronal loss and astrogliosis occur within the caudate nucleus and putamen in *F*, *G*, and *H*, respectively. There is a dorsoventral gradient of cell death, with the dorsal striatum most severely involved.

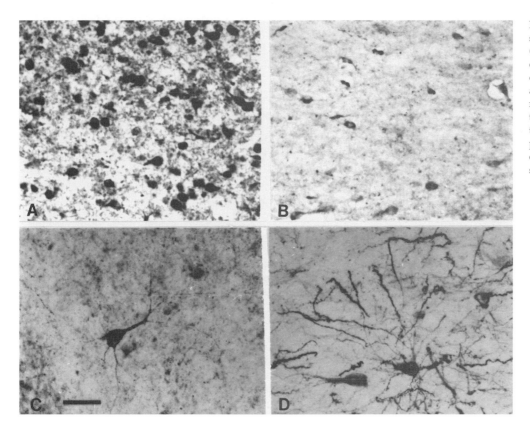

FIGURE 36-3 Calbindin-positive spiny striatal neurons in normal (*A* and *C*) and Huntington's disease (HD) (*B* and *D*) caudate nucleus. The number of immunoreactive neurons is significantly reduced in HD. Degenerative alterations of this neuronal population, as demonstrated in Golgi preparations (see Fig. 36-5), are observed in *D*. There is a distal shift in dendritic staining in HD.

external segment of the globus pallidus (GPe).[19] All of these markers of striatal projection neurons and their axonal projections are progressively lost in HD, correlating with the loss of medium spiny neurons.[12,13,17,20–25]

Although both populations of medium spiny neurons are lost, there is evidence that, particularly in the early stages of HD, striatal neurons projecting to the GPe are preferentially lost in comparison to striatal neurons projecting to the GPi.[26–28] It has been suggested that this differential loss of striatal projections leads to imbalanced activity in the so-called direct and indirect pathways, causing chorea.[29–31] More specifically, the release of the GPe from inhibitory striatal input is hypothesized to result in excessive inhibition of the subthalamic nucleus which, in turn, causes decreased activation of the GPi and reduced inhibition of the thalamus, leading to increased cortical excitation and chorea. Consistent with this hypothesis, bicuculline blockade of the GABAergic input to the GPe causes chorea in primates.[32] Furthermore, more equal loss of neurons projecting to both GPi and GPe may be associated with the occurrence of the rigid-akinetic variant of HD,[33] which usually occurs in juveniles. This model has been very useful but is probably oversimplified, because it does not account for such findings as increased thalamic levels of GABA,[28] for simultaneous pathology in other parts of the circuit, or for the finding that the D1 dopamine receptor is reduced more than D2 in the striatum and in the termination zones of striatal afferents.[17,18] This latter finding is contrary to what would be predicted, based on the changes in substance P and enkephalin.

In addition to medium spiny neurons, there are a variety of interneurons in the striatum, expressing other neuroactive substances. Those interneurons that have been studied appear resistant to the neurodegeneration that occurs in HD (Fig. 36-4). These include several types of large- and medium-sized aspiny or sparsely spiny neurons, including one type that expresses somatostatin and neuropeptide Y and can be visualized by the reduced form of NADP (NADPH)-diaphorase histochemistry,[34] a type of substance P expressing neuron,[35] and large cholinergic interneurons.[36] There is a striking persistence of somatostatin and neuropeptide Y[37,38] and of the somatostatin/neuropeptide Y/NADPH-diaphorase neurons that express them in both caudate nucleus and putamen in HD.[33,39–41] The density of these neurons is actually increased four- to fivefold, reflecting the combined effects of both neuronal sparing and tissue shrinkage. The preservation of large cholinergic interneurons likely accounts for the increased ratio of large to small neurons seen in morphometric studies[3,6] of the striatum in HD and also for the preservation of acetylcholinesterase activity.[42] Levels of choline acetyltransferase, the synthetic enzyme for acetylcholine, by contrast, are progressively reduced.[9,36] This may be a result of loss of local postsynaptic targets for cholinergic neurons, most of which are spiny dendrites,[43] and of subsequent reduction in their axons and in acetylcholine synthesis. The preservation of classes of neurons has been invaluable experimentally, providing a means for determining whether animal models of HD reproduce the selective vulnerability that occurs in human HD.

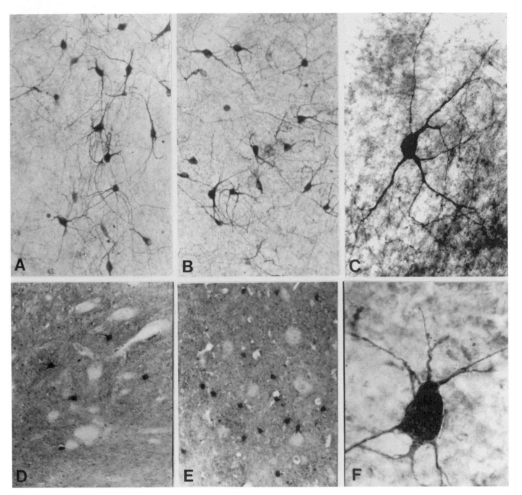

FIGURE 36-4 Photomicrographs of aspiny striatal neuron populations, which are relatively spared in HD. Medium-sized NADPH-diaphorase striatal neurons are represented in *A–C,* with normal staining found in *A* and preservation in an HD case demonstrated in *B*. Large acetylcholinesterase striatal neurons are demonstarted in *D–F*. *D* demonstrates the normal density of these neurons, while *E* demonstrates that their numbers increase in HD as a result of survival in a shrinking striatum. The density of both neuronal types is significantly increased in HD.

NEURONAL REMODELING

Alterations in the dendritic structure of several types of neurons vulnerable in HD have suggested that both proliferative and degenerative alterations occur for some time before cell death finally ensues. Whether these alterations reflect a primary abnormality in the regulation of dendritic architecture or a secondary compensation and decompensation for altered striatal circuitry is unknown. Early morphological alterations of spiny striatal neurons have been described using Golgi and calbindin immunocytochemical methods (Fig. 36-5).[44,45] Proliferative changes, found primarily in moderate grades of HD, include prominent recurving of distal dendritic segments, short-segment branching along the length of dendrites, and increased numbers and size of dendritic spines. Degenerative alterations, found primarily in more severe cases, consist of truncated dendritic arbors, focal dendritic swelling, and marked spine loss. The relative extent to which enkephalin and substance P subsets develop proliferative changes is not known. It is also not known whether such alterations also occur in striatal interneurons that are spared in HD. These newly formed dendritic arbors and increased numbers of dendritic spines may form functional connections and represent a plastic increase in postsynaptic surfaces in compensation for lost neurons. It has been sug-

gested that the resulting increase in synapses could facilitate neuronal excitability and exacerbate excitotoxic cell, death.[45]

STRIOSOME AND MATRIX PATHOLOGY

The striatum is also composed of chemically and connectionally heterogeneous compartments termed patches or striosomes and matrix.[19,46] Striosomes consist of discrete areas distributed throughout the striatum in which opiate receptors, substance P, met-enkephalin, and cholecystokinin are concentrated. The intervening matrix is enriched in somatostatin, neuropeptide Y, NADPH-diaphorase, calbindin, choline acetyltransferase, acetylcholinesterase, and cytochrome oxidase. Although the striosome-matrix compartments, as determined by acetylcholinesterase[47,48] or by calbindin immunocytochemistry,[15,49] persist in the striatum in HD, the total area of the matrix is reduced whereas the total area of striosomes is unchanged (Fig. 36-6). These findings are consistent with the preferential loss of striatal D1 receptors[17,18] but would be unexpected when striatal neurons projecting to the GPe are preferentially lost. Because both types of projection neurons are actually admixed in the striatum,[50] patterns of connectivity may not relate quite exactly to striosome/matrix organization.

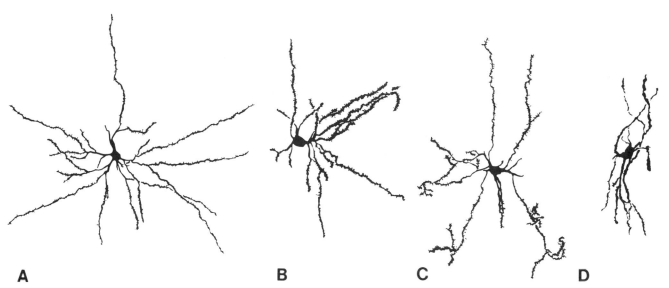

A **B** **C** **D**

FIGURE 36-5 Camera lucida drawings of representative spiny striatal neurons in normal *(A)*, moderate grades of HD *(B and C)*, and severe grades of HD *(D)*. Normal spiny neurons have 3–7 primary dendrites that centrifugally radiate from the soma. In moderate grades of HD, the dysmorphic alterations are proliferative. There is an increase in spine density with short-segment branching and terminal dendritic curving. In severe grades of HD, the changes are degenerative, consisting of truncated dendritic arbors, focal swellings, and marked spine loss.

GLOBUS PALLIDUS

Pallidal atrophy and gliosis have long been recognized to occur in HD[4,51]; however, its extent is probably underappreciated. In a standard-setting quantitative study,[3] Lange and his colleagues determined that both the GPe and GPi can lose more than 50 percent of volume and more than 40 percent of neurons while glia increase both in concentration and in absolute number (Fig. 36-7). These authors felt that pallidal degeneration is more likely a result of primary degeneration of pallidal neurons than of a transneuronal consequence of striatal atrophy. As they also pointed out, pallidal degeneration and loss of pallidal projections has not been sufficiently

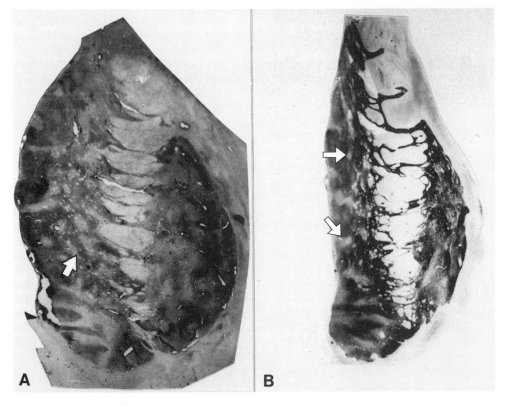

A **B**

FIGURE 36-6 Acetylcholinesterase staining in the striatum in normal *(A)* and severe HD *(B)*. The intensity of staining is heterogeneous, with lighter-stained areas *(arrows)* referred to as patches and the intervening more intensely stained area referred to as the matrix. There is a significant reduction in the matrix compartment, in comparison to that of the total area of patch compartments in HD.

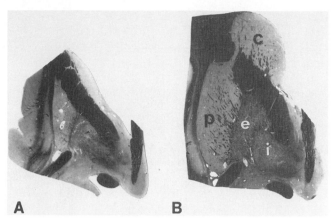

FIGURE 36-7 Coronal sections through the globus pallidus in HD *(A)* and a normal age-matched specimen *(B)* stained for myelin. The caudate nucleus (c) is reduced to a thin ribbon, whereas the putamen (p) and GPi(i) and GPe(e) of the pallidum are severely atrophic in HD.

considered in models attempting to explain chorea. Most recent studies concerned with pallidal pathology in HD have focused more on striatopallidal afferents than on pallidal neurons or their projections. Inhibitory striatal afferents project differentially to the GPi and GPe and coat pallidal dendrites with terminals. Striatopallidal neurons expressing substance P project primarily to the GPi whereas those expressing enkephalin project primarily to the GPe.[19] As discussed above, there has been some evidence of preferential loss of GPe afferents in choreatic HD, based primarily on the differential loss of substance P and enkephalin immunoreactivity.[26–28] Whether these results were in any way affected by pallidal neuron loss is unknown.

SUBSTANTIA NIGRA

Loss of striatonigral fibers, as well as nigral neurons, has previously been reported to occur in HD.[2,52,53] There have

been two recent quantitative studies of nigral pathology in HD, using distinct methods that may explain the differences in their results.[54,55] Both studies found substantial atrophy and gliosis of both the pars compacta (SNc) and pars reticulata (SNr), with a loss in cross-sectional area of as much as 40 percent (Fig. 36-8). Ferrante and his colleagues observed that the SNr, however, had a greater area loss than the SNc. Both studies also reported that nonpigmented neurons were reduced in both nigral zones and by as much as 45 percent. Oyanagi and colleagues found that pigmented neurons were reduced by about 50 percent medially and laterally but were preserved centrally, whereas Ferrante and colleagues found pigmented neurons to be relatively spared with an increase in number resulting from their preservation in a shrinking SNc. The loss of nonpigmented cells may be quite relevant to the development of motor symptoms, because these neurons are the source of nigral afferents to the thalamus, superior colliculus, and brain stem. The relative preservation of pigmented neurons is consistent with preservation of dopaminergic nigrostriatal projections.[56] The topography of nigral atrophy did not correlate with the dorsomedial to ventrolateral pattern of striatal atrophy,[54] suggesting that nigral cell loss cannot be fully explained by loss of striatonigral afferents. However, the possibility of transneuronal degeneration remains, because striatal excitotoxic lesions in rodents can cause subsequent neuronal degeneration in the SNr.[57] Interestingly, because the neuronal loss can be prevented by administration of a specific GABA agonist, neuronal death may be related to the loss of inhibitory GABAergic input

DIENCEPHALON

THALAMUS
There is very limited mention in any literature of thalamic pathology in HD, although its presence has been acknowledged. The only specific study was performed by Dom and his colleagues,[58] who examined the ventrolateral thalamus in seven cases of HD. Because the basal ganglia outflow

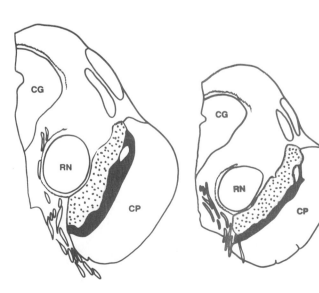

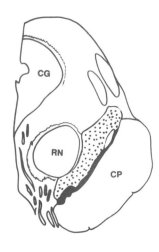

CONTROL   **HD GRADE 3**   **HD GRADE 4**

FIGURE 36-8 Sections through the substantia nigra at the level of the red nucleus (RN) and third nerve in normal control and grade 3 and 4 HD. The total area of the substantia nigra, pars compacta (stippled area), and pars reticulata (solid black area) are significantly reduced in HD, with the substantia nigra pars reticulata most severely involved and pars compacta relatively spared.

directed to the frontal cortex is relayed by the ventrolateral thalamus, pathology in this nucleus may be quite relevant to the movement disorders occurring in HD. These investigators found that 50 percent of small neurons disappeared, whereas large neurons were not altered. If these small thalamic neurons are inhibitory interneurons, their loss could be related to thalamic disinhibition. Increased levels of thalamic GABA in HD,[28] however, are not consistent with this hypothesis, unless it can somehow be viewed as a compensatory upregulation of GABA. Clearly, further study of thalamic neuropathology is needed to clarify its contribution to HD symptoms.

SUBTHALAMUS

The subthalamus is an extremely interesting nucleus in regard to HD. Subthalamic strokes have long been known to cause ballistic involuntary movements that are very similar to those of chorea. The subthalamus is also postulated to be excessively inhibited in HD, leading to alterations in pallido-thalamic excitation, as previously outlined, that may be the basis for chorea. Furthermore, the subthalamus gives rise to one of the few excitatory pathways in the basal ganglia and thus may be relevant in excitotoxic cell death (see Pathophysiology). Nevertheless, little has been added to knowledge of subthalamic pathology in HD since the morphometric study by Lange and his colleagues, who found that subthalamic volume and neuron number are reduced by about 25 percent.[3] Studies examining how neurotransmitters and receptors are altered in the subthalamus have not been performed but may help elucidate its role in the pathogenesis of chorea.

HYPOTHALAMUS

Hypothalamic pathology has been postulated to be related to the cachexia and autonomic disturbance that occurs in HD patients. Bruyn noted significant neuronal loss and gliosis in the supraoptic nucleus and lateral hypothalamic nucleus.[51] In the only quantitative studies of hypothalamic pathology, Kremer[59,60] found up to a 90 percent neuronal loss in the lateral tuberal nucleus, which was worse in patients developing motor symptoms at an early age. The percentage of astrocytes did not change, whereas oligodendrocytes were reduced by 40 percent. It was further postulated that the high levels of glutamate receptors normally present in the lateral tuberal nucleus renders these neurons selectively susceptible to excitotoxic cell death.[61] Although little is known about the normal function of the lateral tuberal nucleus, the possibility that its degeneration underlies the catabolic state that frequently occurs in HD patients is intriguing. Furthermore, because cell loss is so severe, this nucleus may have value in experimental investigations of cell death and neuroprotection in HD.

CEREBRAL CORTEX

Cortical atrophy has long been recognized as occurring in HD.[62,63] Its extent, clinical significance, and relationship to striatal degeneration, however, remain incompletely characterized. Particularly, the relative roles of the cerebral cortex and basal ganglia in psychiatric, behavioral, and cognitive symptoms of HD is poorly understood, although there should be little doubt that cortical degeneration is at least involved in personality change, dementia, and spasticity. If cortical atrophy contributes significantly to these symptoms, as seems likely from its extent, this may be a crucial area for further research. Because the entire cerebral cortex projects to the striatum and much of the frontal lobe receives the outflow of striatal-pallidal-thalamocortical circuits,[64,65] cortical and basal ganglia pathology may not be very separable clinically. Most studies related to potential medical and surgical therapies have focused on the striatum; however, when treatments preserve the striatum but not the cortex, many of the worst symptoms of the disease might still occur. Thus, understanding whether cortical degeneration is a primary process or a secondary retrograde phenomenon related to loss of a major cortical afferent target, the neostriatum, and whether cortical and striatal cell death occur by similar cellular mechanisms, may be of great importance.

GROSS AND REGIONAL PATHOLOGY

Generalized cortical atrophy is frequently apparent at autopsy (Fig. 36-1) and accounts for the majority of the 15–30 percent loss in brain weight that occurs in HD.[66,67] Gross and regional cortical atrophy has been studied planimetrically by several investigators. Lange[66] reported an overall cortical shrinkage of 15 percent in five cases of HD and noted that atrophy occurred the least in frontal regions and the most in occipital association areas (30 percent). De la Monte and her colleagues[67] studied 30 HD brains and demonstrated a 20–30 percent overall reduction in the cross-sectional area of cerebral cortex, accompanied by a 29–34 percent reduction in subcortical white matter. Thinning of the cortical gray matter ranged only from 9–16 percent, perhaps explaining why obvious cortical pathology is easily missed when one is examining individual sections. The severity of atrophy occurring in the cortex, as well as in the striatum and thalamus, correlated with the clinical progression of the disease.[4,67] With increasing pathological grades of HD, brain weight declined, ventricular volume increased, cerebral atrophy increased, and the cortical ribbon thinned. Depression and dementia corresponded to the extent of both cortical and basal ganglia atrophy. It is not clear to what extent any cortical areas undergo more atrophy than others; however, pronounced degenerative changes occur in medial postcentral cortex, occipital isocortex (areas 18 and 19), prepyriform cortex, cingulate cortex,[66] primary motor cortex,[68] dorsolateral prefrontal cortex (areas 8, 9, 10, and 46),[69–71] and perihippocampal allocortex.[72]

LAMINAR AND CELLULAR PATHOLOGY

The laminar pattern of cerebral cortical degeneration in HD has been studied qualitatively, with varying results. McCaughey[73] described diffuse degeneration through layers III, V, and VI with some patchy involvement of IV. In four pediatric cases,[74] cortical degeneration appeared panlaminar. Forno and Jose[52] observed layer III to be the most severely affected in a series of adults. Roizin and Kaufman[75] found that the middle layers of cortex were most affected in some cases whereas the deeper layers were most affected in others. Bruyn et al.[2] later reported that layers III and V and, sometimes, IV had the most neuronal loss.

Quantitative studies have been performed more recently in a variety frontal and prefrontal areas, using varying methods.[68–71] The most consistent findings have been loss of volume and neurons in layers III, V, and VI. The concentration of neurons in these layers may not change,[69,70,71] however, indicating that cortical neuronal loss is proportional to cortical volume loss. Astrocyte and oligodendrocyte numbers and concentration increase dramatically, especially in layers III–VI (Fig. 36-9). These increases likely indicate glial survival in a shrinking cortex and not reactive gliosis, because cortical glial fibrillary acidic protein (GFAP) staining does not increase.[76] The size of cortical neurons also declines in HD, suggesting selective loss or shrinkage of larger pyramidal cells (Fig. 36-9). Although there have been differing interpretations of this data, cortical cell loss is clearly not confined to neurons projecting to the striatum, which consist of a limited population of medium-sized pyramidal cells located deep in layer III and superficially in layer V. Thus, retrograde degeneration of corticostriatal neurons cannot readily account for cortical atrophy. These studies also suggest that there is relative sparing of cortical interneurons, which typically are small neurons. Further evidence for this includes data indicating that substance P-expressing interneurons are spared,[77] and that cortical concentrations of GABA, somatostatin, neuropeptide Y, cholecystokinin, and vasoactive intestinal polypeptide (VIP), which are expressed by interneurons, are all elevated in HD.[78–80] Cerebral cortical pyramidal cells have also been shown, by means of Golgi staining, to develop increased numbers of dendrites and dendritic spines whereas others appear to have degenerative changes,[81] suggesting that proliferative and degenerative changes occur in these neurons before cell death.

NEUROCHEMISTRY

Neurochemical alterations in the cerebral cortex in HD have also been identified, although findings have been inconsistent. Two laboratories[11,82] have found that glutamate, the putative neurotransmitter of pyramidal cells, and GABA, a marker for inhibitory cortical interneurons, are reduced in the cerebral cortex. In contrast, Storey et al. showed glutamate and aspartate to increase in most areas of cortex that they examined.[80] Unlike the striatum, N-methyl-D-aspartate (NMDA) receptor binding is unchanged in cortex, whereas oc-amino-3-hydroxy-5-methyl-4-isoxazole-propionic acid (AMPA) and kainate receptor binding is reduced in layer VI.[83] Such studies may offer evidence of selective vulnerability of distinct neuronal types; however, biochemical changes can be difficult to interpret without a detailed understanding of the underlying anatomic changes. For example, glutamate could be reduced from loss of neurons, loss of glutamatergic afferents, or alteration of glutamate metabolism in the absence of degenerative change. Understanding how the expression of glutamate receptors is altered in the cortex in HD may help explain altered cortical levels of glutamate. Whether cortical alterations in glutamate or glutamate receptors plays a role in excitotoxic cell death in the striatum, via corticostriatal projections, is an interesting question, about which there is little information.

CEREBELLUM AND BRAIN STEM

Reports of cerebellar involvement in HD have been variable, with cerebellar atrophy being reported in some pediatric and adult cases.[84–87] At a cellular level, Purkinje cell loss has been the primary consistent finding;[2] however, thinning of the

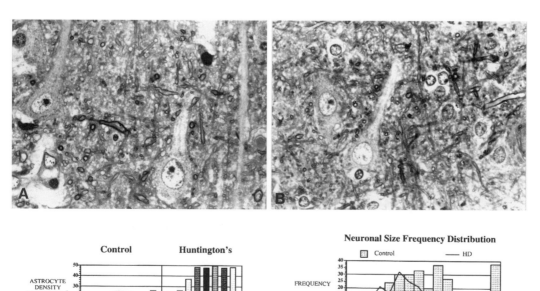

FIGURE 36-9 Toluidine blue-stained 2μm sections from control *(A)* and HD *(B)* primary motor cortex. Normal-appearing pyramidal cells are visible in each. The HD case, however, contains many more astrocytes, as well as nuclear ghosts from degenerated neurons. Quantitative data *(C)* demonstrate that the density of astrocytes is more than doubled in layers III–VI. Measurement of nuclear diameters demonstrates that surviving neurons are smaller than control neurons and that the largest neurons seem to have disappeared.

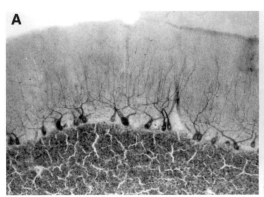 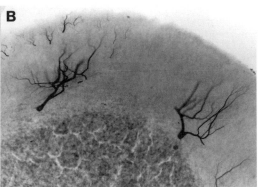

FIGURE 36-10 Immunocyto-chemistry in control (*A*) and HD cerebellum (*B*), using antihuntingtin antibodies. Purkinje cell drop-out is evident in the HD case (*B*), as is remodeling of the dendritic trees of those that survive.

granule cell layer has also been observed and has been taken to indicate loss of this cell type as well.[87] One quantitative study[88] examined Purkinje cell loss in 17 HD cases of unknown grade. More than one-half had a reduction in Purkinje cell density greater than 50 percent. With huntingtin immunocytochemistry, we have also noted severe loss of Purkinje cells in advanced grades of HD (Fig. 36-10). In addition, proliferative and degenerative changes are visible in Purkinje cells. Dentate cell loss and gliosis and involvement of cerebellar efferent and afferent pathways have also been noted.[2,87] The clinical significance of cerebellar atrophy is difficult to gauge, as involuntary movements and dystonia may obscure the cardinal signs of cerebellar dysfunction. Nevertheless, contributions to gait ataxia, postural instability, dysrhythmic voluntary movements, altered speech cadence, and disordered eye movements are all possible.

Brain stem alterations in HD have received almost no attention in the last 2 decades, so there is little to add to the review[2] of Bruyn et al. from 1979, in which severe degeneration of the superior and inferior olivary, lateral vestibular, dorsal vagal, and hypoglossal nuclei was noted. Additional significant regions of neuropathology from the earlier literature include the red nucleus, the basis pontis, and the spinal cord.[1,2,52,73,85]

Pathophysiology

ROLE OF EXCITATORY AMINO ACIDS

The initial observation suggesting that excitotoxicity may play a role in HD was made by the McGeers[89] and Coyle and Schwarcz.[90] Both sets of investigators showed that injections of the glutamate agonist kainic acid produced axon-sparing lesions of the striatum resembling HD. This model was refined by the use of selective NMDA agonists, such as quinolinic acid,[71–93] which cause medium spiny neurons to degenerate (astrogliosis) but are sparing of NADPH-diaphorase and cholinergic interneurons. Chronic lesions result in significantly increased striatal atrophy, more closely replicating the neuropathology of HD.[94,95] Furthermore, in the monkey, quinolinic acid excitotoxic lesions lead to hyperkinesis and dopamine agonist-induced chorea.[80] The close match of these models with HD neuropathology strongly suggests an excitotoxic

mechanism of cell death. Selective depletion of NMDA receptors in the putamen in HD suggested that neurons expressing this glutamate receptor are selectively vulnerable.[96] However, alterations in other types of glutamate receptors also occur.[97,98] Because increased glutamate levels, abnormal functioning of glutamate receptor function, or the significant presence of endogenous excitotoxins have not been demonstrated in the striatum in HD, a basis for why excitotoxicity should occur has been elusive. Nevertheless, the evidence for excitotoxic cell death has been compelling enough to justify medication trials with glutamate antagonists.

ROLE OF CELLULAR METABOLISM

A novel hypothesis explaining the pattern of degeneration in HD has recently evolved that suggests that impaired energy metabolism may be involved in the degenerative process.[99–102] Several studies have suggested that altered energy metabolism occurs in HD. Cytochrome oxidase (complex IV) activity is reduced in striatum; complex I activity is reduced in platelets[103]; complex II/III activity is reduced in the caudate nucleus.[104] Increased lactate has been demonstrated in HD cortex and striatum *in vivo* by means of MR spectroscopy.[105] These studies in HD suggest that metabolic dysfunction does occur, but is it a secondary marker of degeneration or is it related to the pathopysiology of neuronal death? Experimentally, energy (adenosine triphosphatase) depletion can produce partial membrane depolarization and removal of the voltage-dependent magnesium block of the NMDA-linked calcium channel.[106] The open calcium channel could then permit normal amounts of glutamate to produce a heightened NMDA receptor response which, in turn, could cause excitotoxic cell death. Animal studies show that striatal injection of mitochondrial toxins, such as the succinic dehydrogenase inhibitors 3-nitropropionic acid (3-NP) and malonic acid, produces selective neuronal loss identical to that produced by NMDA agonists and identical to the neuropathological pattern in HD, as well as analogous motor symptoms (Fig. 36-11 and Table 36-1).[107–109] Importantly, mitochondrial toxin-induced striatal pathology is dramatically reduced by NMDA receptor blockade, as well as by antioxidants and free radical scavengers.[110–111] This further strengthens the hypothesis of a metabolic defect underlying selective

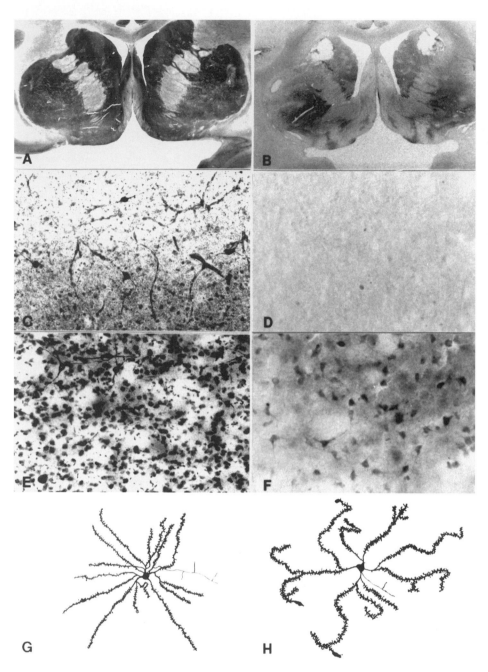

FIGURE 36-11 Histopathological alterations observed in a 3-nitropropionic acid-treated primate. Gross lesions are found in the dorsal aspect of the caudate nucleus and putamen in Nissl- and calbindin-stained sections through the striatum (*A* and *B*), respectively. There is a dorsoventral gradient of neuronal loss, with the dorsal striatum more severely involved. Only aspiny NADPH-diaphorase neurons persist in the dorsal striatum (*C*), with few spiny calbindin neurons (*D*). All neuronal populations are better preserved in the ventral striatum (*E* and *F*). Similar dysmorphic alterations, as observed in HD, are found in treated animals (*H*) in comparison to controls (*G*). From Brouillet et al.[109] *Used with permission.*

excitotoxicity[106,112] and provides a rationale for treating HD with glutamate antagonists combined with protectants against oxygen-free radical activity.

Molecular Neuropathology

HUNTINGTIN TRANSCRIPTION

At what level does the HD mutation act? Huntingtin mRNA is normally distributed in diverse tissues in humans and rats and is expressed predominantly in neurons within the brain.[113–115] All neurons appear to express huntingtin, and there is no apparent correlation within particular types of neurons between levels of mRNA and their vulnerability to

cell death. Because mRNA for both the normal and mutant alleles is produced by individuals with HD and because known "knockout" mutations affecting one HD allele do not cause the HD phenotype,[116–118] simple gene inactivation is unlikely to underlie disease pathogenesis. Because mRNA for the mutant allele is expressed in HD brain in amounts similar to that of the normal allele,[114,119] an alteration in transcription is also unlikely to be pathogenic. The remaining possibilities are that the genetic mutation affects ribosomal translation or that it acts at the protein level to alter the normal function of huntingtin. RNA binding proteins, which are tissue-specific and have been demonstrated to interact with the huntingtin CAG repeat,[120] could affect translation and also the intracellular localization of huntingtin mRNA.

TABLE 36-1 Comparison of HD and 3-NP Striatal Lesions

Huntington's Disease	3-NP Striatal Lesions
Young-adult onset	Vulnerability in young adult animals
Striatal vulnerability	Striatal vulnerability
Dorsal-ventral gradient	Dorsal-ventral gradient
Movement disorder	Movement disorder
Chorea	Dystonia in rats, chorea in primates
Loss of spiny projection neurons	Loss of spiny projection neurons
Sparing of NADPH-diaphorase neurons	Sparing of NADPH-diaphorase neurons
Dendritic changes in spiny neurons	Dendritic changes in spiny neurons
Sparing of striatal afferents	Sparing of striatal afferents

Other translational effects are possible. Because inactivation of one allele does not cause HD, however, it would be difficult for a translational block to account for disease pathogenesis. Thus, it remains more likely that HD is the result of a protein level effect, rather than an alteration in translation. Nevertheless, levels of mutant protein have not yet been fully measured in HD brain tissue.

ROLE OF MUTANT HUNTINGTIN PROTEIN

Because huntingtin is an unknown protein, it has not yet been possible to elucidate how its mutation could cause the disease, or whether it can be linked specifically to excitotoxicity or to an energetic defect. The approach currently being taken is to study huntingtin, using specific antibodies raised against it.[122–126] The preliminary results of most investigators have been generally consistent. Huntingtin is found primarily in soluble fractions, and its relative levels in various tissues and brain areas correspond to the levels of its mRNA. Both normal and mutant proteins are expressed in cell lines and tissues from HD patients (Fig 36-12). It is not yet clear whether the mutation alters the levels of mutant huntingtin in brain, although decreased levels have been reported in lymphoblasts from individuals with HD.[122] Immunocytochemistry (Fig. 36-13) indicates that huntingtin is located in neurons throughout the brain, with high levels evident in

cortical pyramidal cells, cerebellar Purkinje cells, and large striatal interneurons, among others. Striatal medium spiny neurons are also well labeled, whereas medium-sized neurons in other brain regions may be quite variable. There are significant levels of huntingtin in the striatum, with heterogeneous expression evident both in medium spiny neurons and in interneurons. It has not yet been determined whether the heterogeneity of huntingtin expression corresponds to the differential vulnerabilty of neurons to degeneration. Subcellular localization of huntingtin is consistent with a cytosolic protein primarily found in somatodendritic regions but with some presence in axons as well (Fig. 36-14). Huntingtin appears to particularly associate with dendritic microtubules, although some is also associated with synaptic vesicles in axon terminals. Localization studies would argue against a direct role in synaptic transmission, because little is found, either pre- or post-synaptically. Similarly, a direct role in oxidative metabolism seems unlikely, because huntingtin is not found within mitochondria. There are many cellular processes, however, that bear less directly on synaptic transmission and metabolism that may be affected by the HD mutation and still be an upstream cause of excitotoxicity. Based on limited sequence homology with transcription factors,[127] it has been suggested that huntingtin binds protein factors along DNA strands.[128] This possibility is unlikely, however, because huntingtin protein has not been found in cell nuclei (Fig. 36-14). A suggestion that has not yet been investigated is that proteins with expanded polyglutamine tracts could serve as substrates for transglutaminases and become cross-linked to lysine donors, leading to aggregation of the protein within the cell.[129] Huntingtin also contains a polyproline sequence, which could bind to the SH3 domains of a variety of molecules, including tyrosine kinases involved in signal transduction and cell growth[130] and cytoskeleton-related molecules[130] that regulate cytoskeleton integrity or serve to target specific proteins or organelles to particular regions of the cytoskeleton.[131] Dysfunction in these pathways could conceivably provide a metabolic burden or impair the cytoskeletal anchoring or transport of mitochondria, vesicles, ribosomes, or other organelles and molecules, causing a cellular defect that renders neurons susceptible to excitotoxicity. Another possibility, not yet explored, is that huntingtin catabolism is impaired, causing altered levels, toxic or dysfunctional breakdown products, or impairment of cellular cata-

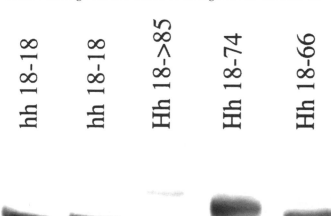

FIGURE 36-12 Western blot, using monoclonal antihuntingtin antibodies of lymphoblast lysates from control (hh) patients, heterozygote HD patients (Hh), and a homozygote HD patient (HH). The numbers correspond to the number of CAG repeats contained in each huntingtin allele. A single band is detected in control and homozygote cases, because the alleles have identical numbers of repeats; however, the homozygote is at a higher molecular weight. Two bands are visible in each of the heterozygote cases, corresponding to the differing molecular weights of normal and mutant huntingtin. This immunoblot demonstrates that both normal and mutant forms of huntingtin are expressed in tissue from HD patients. *From Gutekunst et al.*[122] *Used with permission.*

hh 18-18 hh 18-18 Hh 18->85 Hh 18-74 Hh 18-66 HH 45-45

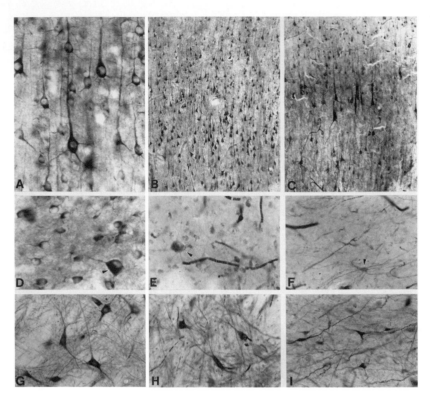

FIGURE 36-13 Immunocytochemistry using monoclonal antihuntingtin antibodies in sections from monkey (first column), from human controls (middle column), and from human HD cases (last column). The first row is from frontal cortex (*A–C*), the second row is from caudate nucleus (*D–F*), and the third row is from globus pallidus (*G–I*). As a result of optimal fixation, the monkey tissue is better stained and permits better resolution of cellular detail. In each region, neurons are well-stained, glia are unstained, nuclei are not labeled, and most label is somatodendritic, with some additional staining of axons and more diffuse staining of the neuropil. In cerebral cortex (*A–C*), pyramidal cells are most prominently stained. In normal monkey (*D*) and human (*E*) caudate nucleus, medium-sized neurons and large interneurons (arrows) are visible. In HD (*F*), only one neuron (arrow) is visible that appears to be an aspiny interneuron. GPe and GPi neurons are also well-stained in monkey (*G*) and human (*H*), although they appear shrunken in HD (*I*). (Several of these micrographs were *from Gutekunst et al.*[122] and were *used with permission.*)

FIGURE 36-14 Electron microscopic immunocytochemistry of huntingtin in monkey, using the diffusible reaction product, DAB (*A, C, E, G*) and also immunogold (*B, D, F, H*), which permits much higher spatial resolution. DAB reaction product is visible in the perikaryon of a cortical pyramidal cell (center) but not in an adjacent astrocyte (bottom right) or oligodendrocyte (top left). All nuclei are unlabeled. At a higher magnification, immunogold particles are primarily free in the cytoplasm and are not associated with endoplasmic reticulum or Golgi apparatus, suggesting that the protein is synthesized by free ribosomes. A Purkinje cell dendrite (*C*), in longitudinal section, is filled with reaction product that coats all its organelles but appears to associate particularly with its microtubules. Immunogold labeling of another Purkinje cell dendrite (*D*) shows many immunogold particles contacting microtubules. A DAB-labeled dendritic spine (*E*) from the putamen is diffusely filled with reaction product that also appears to label the postsynaptic density; however, with immunogold labeling (*F*), *neither plasma membrane nor postsynaptic density labeling is seen.* Axon terminals from the cerebellum (*G*) and cerebral cortex (*H*) are also shown. DAB coats the membrane, synaptic vesicles, and presynaptic density. In contrast, immunogold particles appear to associate primarily with synaptic vesicles but not with the presynaptic density or membrane. (Several of these micrographs were reproduced *from Gutekunst et al.*[122] and were *used with permission.*)

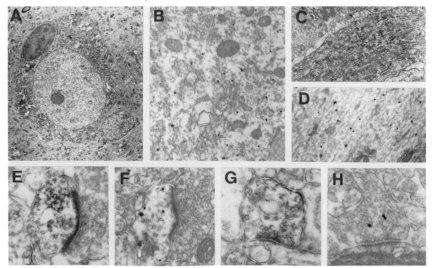

bolic machinery. Elucidating the normal function of huntingtin and the effects of its mutation on its own function and on other cellular processes holds great promise for understanding the pathogenesis of HD and perhaps for novel treatments.

References

1. Bruyn GW: Huntington's chorea: Historical, clinical and laboratory synopsis, in Vinken PJ, Bruyn GW (eds): *Handbook of Clinical Neurology*. New York: John Wiley & Sons, 1968, pp 298–378.
2. Bruyn G, Bots G, Dom R: Huntington's chorea: Current neuropathological status. *Adv Neurol* 1:83–93, 1979.
3. Lange H, Thorner G, Hopf A, Schroder K: Morphometric studies of the neuropathological changes in choreatic diseases. *J Neurol Sci* 28:401–425, 1976.
4. Vonsattel J-P, Myers RH, Stevens TJ, et al: Neuropathological classification of Huntington's disease. *J Neuropathol Exp Neurol* 44:559–577, 1985.
5. Roos R, Pruyt JFM, de Vries J, Bots GTHAM: Neuronal distribution in the putamen in Huntington's disease. *J Neurol Neurosurg Psychiatry* 48:422–425, 1985.
6. Dom R, Baro F, Brucher JM: A cytometric study of the putamen in different types of Huntington's chorea. *Adv Neurol* 1:369–385, 1973.
7. Perry TL, Hansen S, Kloster M: Huntington's chorea: Deficiency of gamma-aminobutyric acid in brain. *N Engl J Med* 288:337–342, 1973.
8. Bird ED, Iversen LL: Huntington's chorea. Post-mortem measurement of glutamic acid decarboxylase, choline acetyltransferase and dopamine in basal ganglia. *Brain* 97:457–472, 1974.
9. Spokes EGS: Neurochemical alterations in Huntington's chorea: A study of post mortem brain tissue. *Brain* 103:179 210, 1980.
10. Carter CJ: Reduced GABA transaminase activity in the Huntington's disease putamen. *Neurosci Lett* 48:339–342, 1984.
11. Reynolds GP, Pearson SJ: Decreased glutamic acid and increased 5-hydroxytryptamine in Huntington's disease brain. *Neurosci Lett* 78:233–238, 1987.
12. Marshall P, Landis D, Zalneraitis E: Immunocytochemical studies of substance P and leucine-enkephalin in Huntington's disease. *Brain Res* 289:11–26, 1983.
13. Goto S, Hirano A, Rojas CRR: An immunohistochemical investigation of the human neostriatum in Huntington's disease. *Ann Neurol* 25:298–304, 1989.
14. Ferrante R, Kowall N, Richardson E Jr: Immunocytochemical localization of calcium binding protein in normal and Huntington's disease striatum. *J Neuropathol Exp Neurol* 47:352, 1988.
15. Seto-Ohshima A, Emson PC, Lawson E, et al: Loss of matrix calcium-binding protein-containing neurons in Huntington's disease. *Lancet* 1:1252–1255, 1988.
16. Martinez-Mir MI, Probst A, Palacios JM: Adenosine A2 receptors: Selective localization in the human basal ganglia and alterations with disease. *Neuroscience* 42:697–706, 1991.
17. Joyce JN, Lexow N, Bird E, Winokur A: Organization of dopamine D1 and D2 receptors in human striatum: Receptor autoradiographic studies in Huntington's disease and schizophrenia. *Synapse* 2:546–557, 1988.
18. Richfield EK, OBrien CF, Eskin T, Shoulson I: Heterogeneous dopamine receptor changes in early and late Huntington's disease. *Neurosci Lett* 132:121–126, 1991.
19. Gerfen C: The neostriatal mosaic: Multiple levels of compartmental organization in the basal ganglia. *Ann Rev Neurosci* 15:285–320, 1992.
20. Kanazawa I, Bird E, O'Connell R, Powell D: Evidence for the decrease in substance P content of substantia nigra in Huntington's chorea. *Brain Res* 120:387–392, 1977.
21. Gale JS, Bird ED, Spokes EG, et al: Human brain substance P: Distribution in controls and Huntington's chorea. *Neurochem* 30:633–634, 1978.
22. Emson PC, Arrequi A, Clement-Jones V, et al: Regional distribution of met-enkephalin and substance P immunoreactivity in normal human brain and in Huntington's disease. *Brain Res* 199:147–160, 1980.
23. Grafe MR, Forno LS, Eng LF: Immunocytochemical studies of substance P and met-enkephalin in the basal ganglia and substantia nigra in Huntington's, Parkinson's and Alzheimer's diseases. *J Neuropathol Exp Neurol* 44:47–59, 1985.
24. Waters CM, Peck R, Rossor M, et al: Immunocytochemical studies on the basal ganglia and substantia nigra in Parkinson's disease and Huntington's chorea. *Neuroscience* 25:419–438, 1988.
25. Beal MF, Ellison DW, Mazurek MF, et al: A detailed examination of substance P in pathologically graded cases of Huntington's disease. *J Neurol Sci* 84:51–61, 1988.
26. Reiner A, Albin RL, Anderson KD, et al: Differential loss of striatal projection neurons in Huntington disease. *Proc Natl Acad Sci U S A* 85:5733–5737, 1988.
27. Albin RL, Young AB, Penny JB, et al: Abnormalities of striatal projection neurons and N-methyl-D-aspartate receptors in presymptomatic Huntington's disease. *N Engl J Med* 322:1293–1298, 1990.
28. Storey E, Beal M: Neurochemical substrates of rigidity and chorea in Huntington's disease. *Brain* 116:1201–1222, 1993.
29. Crossman A: Primate models of dyskinesia: The experimental approach to the study of basal ganglia-related involuntary movement disorders. *Neuroscience* 21:1–40, 1987.
30. Albin R, Young A, Penney J: The functional anatomy of basal ganglia disorders. *Trends Neurosci* 12:366–375, 1989.
31. DeLong M: Primate models of movement disorders of basal ganglia origin. *Trends Neurosci* 13:281–285, 1990.
32. Crossman A, Mitchell I, Sambrook M, Jackson A: Chorea and myoclonus in the monkey induced by gamma-aminobutyric acid antagonism in the lentiform complex. *Brain* 111:1211–1233, 1988.
33. Albin RL, Reiner A, Anderson KD, et al: Striatal and nigral neuron subpopulations in rigid Huntington's disease: Implications for the functional anatomy of chorea and rigidity-akinesia. *Ann Neurol* 27:357–365, 1990.
34. Kowall N, Ferrante R, Martin J: Patterns of cell loss in Huntington's disease. *Trends Neurosci* 10:24–29, 1987.
35. Ferrante R, Kowall N, Martin J, Richardson E Jr: Substance P-containing striatal neurons in Huntington's disease. *Exp Neurol* 46:375, 1987.
36. Ferrante RJ, Beal MF, Kowall NW, et al: Sparing of acetylcholinesterase-containing striatal neurons in Huntington's disease. *Brain Res* 411:162–166, 1987.
37. Beal MF, Mazurek MF, Ellison DW, et al: Somatostatin and neuropeptide Y concentrations in pathologically graded cases of Huntington's disease. *Ann Neurol* 23:562–569, 1988.
38. Aronin N, Cooper PE, Lorenz LJ, et al: Somatostatin is increased in the basal ganglia in Huntington's disease. *Ann Neurol* 13:519–526, 1983.
39. Ferrante RJ, Kowall NW, Beal MF, et al: Morphologic and histochemical characteristics of a spared subset of striatal neurons in Huntington's disease. *J Neuropathol Exp Neurol* 46:12–27, 1987.
40. Ferrante RJ, Kowall NW, Beal MF, et al: Selective sparing of a class of striatal neurons in Huntington's disease. *Science* 230:561–563, 1985.
41. Dawbarn D, Quidt MED, Emson PC: Survival of basal ganglia neuropeptide Y-somatostatin neurones in Huntington's disease. *Brain Res* 340:251–260, 1985.

42. McGeer P, McGeer E: Enzymes associated with the metabolism of catecholamines, acetylcholine and GABA in human controls and patients with Parkinson's disease and Huntington's chorea. *J Neurochem* 26:65–76, 1976.

43. Hersch SM, Gutekunst C-A, Rees HD, et al: Distribution of m1-4 muscarinic receptor proteins in the rat striatum: Light and electron microscopic immunocytochemistry using subtype specific antibodies. *J Neurosci* 14:3351–3363, 1994.

44. Graveland GA, Williams RS, Difiglia M: Evidence for degenerative and regenerative changes in neostriatal spiny neurons in Huntington's disease. *Science* 227:770–773, 1985.

45. Ferrante RJ, Kowall NW, Richardson EPJ: Proliferative and degenerative changes in striatal spiny neurons in Huntington's disease: A combined study using the section-Golgi method and calbindin D28k immunocytochemistry. *J Neurosci* 11:3877–3887, 1991.

46. Graybiel A: Neurotransmitters and neuromodulators in the basal ganglia. *Trends Neurosci* 13:244–254, 1990.

47. Ferrante RJ, Kowall NW, Richardson EP, Jr., et al: Topography of enkephalin, substance P and acetylcholinesterase staining in Huntington's disease striatum. *Neurosci Lett* 71:283–288, 1986.

48. Ferrante RJ, Kowall NW: Tyrosine hydroxylase-like immunoreactivity is distributed in the matrix compartment of normal human and Huntington's disease striatum. *Brain Res* 416:141–146, 1987.

49. Kiyama H, Seto-Ohshima A, Emson PC: Calbindin D28K as a marker for the degeneration of the striatonigral pathway in Huntington's disease. *Brain Res* 525:209–214, 1990.

50. Hersch SM, Ciliax BJ, Gutekunst C-A, et al: Electron microscopic analysis of D1 and D2 dopamine receptor proteins in the dorsal striatum and their synaptic relationships with motor corticostriatal afferents. *J Neurosci* 15:5222–5237, 1995.

51. Bruyn G: Neuropathological changes in Huntington's chorea. *Adv Neurol* 1:399–403, 1973.

52. Forno LS, Jose C: Huntington's chorea: A pathological study. *Adv Neurol* 1:453–470, 1973.

53. Bugiani O, Tabaton M, Cammarata S: Huntington's disease: Survival of large striatal neurons in the rigid variant. *Ann Neurol* 15:154–156, 1984.

54. Oyanagi K, Takeda S, Takahasi H, et al: A quantitative investigation of the substantia nigra in Huntington's disease. *Ann Neurol* 26:13–9, 1989.

55. Ferrante R, Kowall N, Richardson EJ: Neuronal and neuropil loss in the substantia nigra in Huntington's disease. *J Neuropathol Exp Neurol* 48:380, 1989.

56. Beal M, Martin J: Neuropeptides in neurological disease. *Ann Neurol* 20:547–565, 1986.

57. Saji M, Reis D: Delayed transneuronal death of substantia nigra neurons prevented by gamma-aminobutyric acid. *Science* 235:66–69, 1987.

58. Dom R, Malfroid M, Baro F: Neuropathology of Huntington's chorea. Studies of the ventrobasal complex of the thalamus. *Neurology* 26:64–68, 1976.

59. Kremer HP, Roos RA, Dingjan GM, et al: Atrophy of the hypothalamic lateral tuberal nucleus in Huntington's disease. *J Neuropathol Exp Neurol* 49:371–382, 1990.

60. Kremer HP, Roos RA, Dingjan GM, et al: The hypothalamic lateral tuberal nucleus and the characteristics of neuronal loss in Huntington's disease. *Neurosci Lett* 132:101–104, 1991.

61. Kremer B, Tallaksen GSJ, Albin RL: AMPA and NMDA binding sites in the hypothalamic lateral tuberal nucleus: Implications for Huntington's disease. *Neurology* 43:1593–1595, 1993.

62. Alzheimer A: Über die anatomische grunglage der Huntingtonschen chorea und der choreatischen bewegungen überhaupt. *Neurol Zentral* 30:891–892, 1911.

63. Hallervorden J: Huntingtonsche chorea (chorea chronica progressiva herditaria), in Lubarsch O, et al (eds): *Handbuch der Speziellen Pathologischen Anatomie und Histologie*. Berlin: Springer-Verlag, 1957, pp 793–822.

64. Alexander GE, Delong MR, Strick PL: Parallel organization of functionally segregated circuits linking basal ganglia and cortex. *Annu Rev Neurosci* 9:357–381, 1986.

65. Alexander GE, Crutcher MD, DeLong MR: Basal ganglia-thalamocortical circuits: Parallel substrates for motor, oculomotor, 'prefrontal' and 'limbic' functions. *Prog Brain Res* 85:119–146, 1990.

66. Lange HW: Quantitative changes of telencephalon, diencephalon, and mesencephalon in Huntington's chorea, postencephalic, and idiopathic Parkinson's disease. *Verh Anat Ges* 75:923–925, 1981.

67. de la Monte S, Vonsattel J-P, Richardson EPJ: Morphometric demonstration of atrophic changes in the cerebral cortex, white matter, and neostriatum in Huntington's disease. *J Neuropathol Exp Neurol* 47:516–525, 1988.

68. Hersch SM, Rosenfeld V, Gutekunst C-A, et al: A quantitative laminar analysis of cerebral cortical degeneration in Huntington's disease. *Soc Neurosci Abstr* 17:1449, 1991.

69. Sotrel A, Paskevich PA, Kiely DK, et al: Morphometric analysis of the prefrontal cortex in Huntington's disease. *Neurology* 41:1117–1123, 1991.

70. Hedreen JC, Peyser CE, Folstein SE, Ross CA: Neuronal loss in layers V and VI of cerebral cortex in Huntington's disease. *Neurosci Lett* 133:257–261, 1991.

71. Rajkowska G, Selemon L, Goldman-Rakic P: Morphometric evidence for prefrontal cellular atrophy in advanced Huntington's disease. *Soc Neurosci Abstr* 19:838, 1993.

72. Braak H, Braak E: Allocortical involvement in Huntington's disease. *Neuropathol Appl Neurobiol* 18:539–547, 1992.

73. McCaughey W: The pathologic spectrum of Huntington's chorea. *J Nerv Ment Dis* 133:91–103, 1961.

74. Byers RK, Gilles FH, Fung C: Huntington's disease in children. Neuropathologic study of four cases. *Neurology* 23:561–569, 1973.

75. Roizin L, Kaufman MA: Neuropathologic observations in Huntington's chorea, in Zimmerman HM (ed): *Progress in Neuropathology*. New York: Grune & Stratton, 1976, pp 447–488.

76. Zalneraitis EL, Landis DMA, Richardson EPJ, Selkoe DJ: A comparison of astrocytic structure in cerebral cortex and striatum in Huntington's disease (abstr.). *Neurology* 31:151, 1981.

77. Cudkowicz M, Kowall NW: Degeneration of pyramidal projection neurons in Huntington's disease cortex. *Ann Neurol* 27:200–204, 1990.

78. Beal MF, Swartz KJ, Finn SF, et al: Amino acid and neuropeptide neurotransmitters in Huntington's disease cerebellum. *Brain Res* 454:393–396, 1988.

79. Mazurek MF, Beal MF, Knowlton SF, et al: Elevated concentrations of cholecystokinin and vasoactive intestinal peptide in Huntington's disease postmortem cerebral cortex. *Neurology* 39(suppl 1):203, 1989.

80. Storey E, Kowall NW, Finn SF, et al: The cortical lesion of Huntington's disease: Further neurochemical characterization, and reproduction of some of the histological and neurochemical features by N-methyl-D-aspartate lesions of rat cortex. *Ann Neurol* 32:526–534, 1992.

81. Sotrel A, Williams R, Kaufmann W, Myers R: Evidence for neuronal degeneration and dendritic plasticity in cortical pyramidal neurons of Huntington's disease: A quantitative Golgi study. *Neurology* 43:2088–2096, 1993.

82. Ellison DW, Beal MF, Mazurek MF, et al: Amino acid neurotransmitter abnormalities in Huntington's disease and in the quinolinic acid animal model of Huntington's disease. *Brain* 110:1657–1673, 1987.

83. Wagster MV, Hedreen JC, Peyser CE, et al: Selective loss of [³H] kainic acid and [³H] AMPA binding in layer VI of frontal cortex in Huntington's disease. *Exp Neurol* 127:70–75, 1994.

84. Markham C, Knox J: Observations on Huntington's chorea in childhood. *J Pediatr* 67:46–57, 1965.

85. Jervis G: Huntington's chorea in childhood. *Arch Neurol* 9:50–63, 1963.

86. Byers R, Gilles F, Fung C: Huntington's disease in children: Neuropathologic study of four cases. *Neurology* 23:561–569, 1973.

87. Rodda R: Cerebellar atrophy in Huntington's disease. *J Neurol Sci* 50:147–157, 1981.

88. Jeste DV, Barban L, Parisi J: Reduced Purkinje cell density in Huntington's disease. *Exp Neurol* 85:78–86, 1984.

89. McGeer E, McGeer P: Duplication of biochemical changes of Huntington's chorea by intrastriatal injections of glutamic and kainic acids. *Nature* 263:517–519, 1976.

90. Coyle J, Schwarcz R: Lesions of striatal neurons with kainic acid provides a model for Huntington's chorea. *Nature* 263:244–246, 1976.

91. Beal MF Kowall NW, Ellison DW, et al: Replication of the neurochemical characteristics of Huntington's disease by quinolinic acid. *Nature* 321:168–171, 1986.

92. Beal MF, Kowall NW, Ferrante RJ, Cipolloni PB: Quinolinic acid striatal lesions in primates as a model of Huntington's disease. *Ann Neurol* 26:137, 1989.

93. Ferrante RJ, Kowall NW, Cipolloni PB, et al: Excitotoxin lesions in primates as a model for Huntington's disease: histopathologic and neurochemical characterization. *Exp Neurol* 119:46–71, 1993.

94. Beal M, Ferrante R, Swartz K, Kowall N: Chronic quinolinic acid lesions in rats closely resemble Huntington's disease. *J Neurosci* 11:1649–1659, 1991.

95. Bazzett TJ, Becker JB, Kaatz KW, Albin RL: Chronic intrastriatal dialytic administration of quinolinic acid produces selective neural degeneration. *Exp Neurol* 120:177–185, 1993.

96. Young AB, Greenamyre JT, Hollingsworth Z, et al: NMDA receptor losses in putamen from patients with Huntington's disease. *Science* 241:981–983, 1988.

97. Dure LS, Young AB, Penney JB: Excitatory amino acid binding sites in the caudate nucleus and frontal cortex of Huntington's disease. *Ann Neurol* 30:785–793, 1991.

98. Gutekunst C-A, Hersch SM, Wimpey T, et al: Western blot analysis of glutamate receptor subunits in Huntington's disease. *Soc Neurosci* 19:410, 1993.

99. Beal MF, Hyman BT, Koroshetz W: Do defects in mitochondrial energy metabolism underlie the pathology of neurodegenerative diseases? Trends Neurosci 16:125–31, 1993.

100. Beal MF: Does impairment of energy metabolism result in excitotoxic neuronal death in neurodegenerative illnesses? Ann Neurol 31:119–130, 1992.

101. Albin R, Greenamyre J: Alternative excitotoxic hypotheses. *Neurology* 42:733–738, 1992.

102. Beal MF: *Mitochondrial Dysfunction and Oxidative Damage in Neurodegenerative Diseases.* Austin, TX: RG Landes Company, 1995.

103. Parker WD Jr, Boyson SJ, Luder AS, Parks JK: Evidence for a defect in NADH:Ubiquinone oxidoreductase (complex 1) in Huntington's disease. *Neurology* 40:1231–1234, 1990.

104. Brennan W, Bird E, Aprille J: Regional mitochondrial respiratory activity in Huntington's disease brain. *J Neurochem* 44:1948–1950, 1985.

105. Jenkins B, Koroshetz W, Beal M, Rosen B: Localized proton-NMR spectroscopy in patients with Huntington's disease (HD) demonstrates abnormal lactate levels in occipital cortex: Evidence for compromised metabolism in HD. *Neurology* 42:223–229, 1992.

106. Novelli A, Reilly J, Lysko P, Henneberry R: Glutamate becomes neurotoxic via the N-methyl-D-aspartate receptor when intracellular energy levels are reduced. *Brain Res* 451:205–212, 1988.

107. Greene J, Porter R, Eller R, Greenamyre J: Inhibition of succinate dehydrogenase by malonic acid produces an 'excitotoxic' lesion in rat striatum. *J Neurochem* 61:1151–1154, 1993.

108. Beal MF, Brouillet E, Jenkins BG, et al: Neurochemical and histologic characterization of striatal excitotoxic lesions produced by the mitochondrial toxin 3-nitropropionic acid. *J Neurosci* 13:4181–4192, 1993.

109. Brouillet E, Hantraye P, Ferrante RJ, et al: Chronic mitochondrial energy impairment produces selective striatal degeneration and abnormal choreiform movements in primates. *Proc Natl Acad Sci U S A* 92:7105–7109, 1995.

110. Greene J, Greenamyre J: Characterization of the excitotoxic potential of the reversible succinate dehydrogenase inhibitor malonate. *J Neurochem* 64:430–436, 1995.

111. Beal MF, Henshaw DR, Jenkins BG, et al: Coenzyme Q₁₀ and nicotinamide block striatal lesions produced by the mitochondrial toxin malonate. *Ann. Neurol* 36(6):882–888, 1994.

112. Henshaw R, Jenkins BG, Schulz JB, et al: Malonate produces striatal lesions by indirect NMDA receptor activation. *Brain Res* 647:161–166, 1994.

113. Huntington's Disease Collaborative Research Group: A novel gene containing a trinucleotide repeat that is expanded and unstable on Huntington's disease chromosomes. *Cell* 72:971–983, 1993.

114. Li S-H, Schilling G, Young WS, III, et al: Hungtington's disease gene (IT15) is widely expressed in human and rat tissues. *Neuron* 11:985–993, 1993.

115. Strong T, Tagle DA, Valdes JM, et al: Widespread expression of the human and rat Huntington's disease gene in brain and nonneural tissues. *Nature Genet* 5:259–265, 1993.

116. Ambrose CM, Duyao MP, Barnes G, et al: Structure and expression of the Huntington's disease gene: evidence against simple inactivation due to an expanded CAG repeat. *Somat Cell Mol Genet* 20:27–38, 1994.

117. Duyao MP, Auerbach AB, Ryan A, et al: Inactivation of the mouse Huntington's disease gene homolog Hdh. *Science* 269:407–410, 1995.

118. Nasir J, Floresco SB, O'Kulsky JR, et al: Targeted disruption of the Huntington's disease gene results in embryonic lethality and behavioral and morphological changes in heterozygotes. *Cell* 81:811–823, 1995.

119. Landwehrmeyer GB, McNeil SM, Dure LS, IV, et al: Huntington's disease gene: regional and cellular expression in brain of normal and affected individuals. *Ann Neurol* 37:218–230, 1995.

120. Eberwine J, McLaughlin B: Striatal RNA-binding proteins interact with huntingtin mRNA, in MA Ariano, DJ Surmeier (eds): *Molecular and Cellular Mechanisms of Neostriatal function.* Austin, TX: RG Landes Company, 1995, pp 143–149.

121. Feng Y, Zhang F, Lokey LK, et al: Translational suppression by trinucleotide repeat expansion at FMR1. *Science* 268:731–734, 1995.

122. Gutekunst C-A, Levey AL, Heilman CJ, et al: Localization of huntingtin in rat, monkey and human tissues with anti-fusion protein antibodies. *Proc Natl Acad Sci U S A* 92:8710–8714, 1995.

123. Hoogeveen AT, Willemsen R, Meyer N, et al: Characterization and localization of the Huntington disease gene product. *Hum Mol Genet* 2:2069–2073, 1993.

124. Sharp AH, Loev SJ, Schilling G, et al: Widespread expression of Huntington's disease gene (IT15) protein product. *Neuron* 14:1065–1074, 1995.

125. DiFiglia M, Sapp E, Chase K, et al: Huntingtin is a cytoplasmic protein associated with vesicles in human and rat brain neurons. *Neuron* 14:1075–1081, 1995.

126. Trottier Y, Devys D, Imbert G, et al: Cellular localization of the Huntington's disease protein and discrimination of the normal and mutated form. *Nature Genet* 10:104–110, 1995.

127. Gerber H-P, Seipel K, Georgiev D, et al: Transcriptional activation modulated by homopolymeric glutamine and proline stretches. *Science* 263:808–811, 1994.

128. Perutz M, Johnson T, Suzuki M, Finch J: Glutamine repeats as polar zippers: Their possible role in inherited neurodegenerative diseases. *Proc Natl Acad Sci U S A* 91:5355–5358, 1994.

129. Green H: Human genetic disease due to codon reiteration: Relationship to an evolutionary mechanism (letter to the editor). *Cell* 74:955–956, 1993.

130. Seedorf K, Kostka G, Lammers R, et al: Dynamin binds to SH3 domains of phospholipase C gamma and GRB-2. *J Biol Chem* 269:16009–16014, 1994.

131. Bar-Sagi D, Rotin D, Batzer A, et al: SH3 domains direct cellular localization of signaling molecules. *Cell* 74:83–91, 1993.

Chapter 37

TARDIVE DYSKINESIA

CHRISTOPHER G. GOETZ

PHENOMENOLOGY
EPIDEMIOLOGY AND NATURAL HISTORY
PATHOPHYSIOLOGY
NEUROIMAGING AND NEUROPATHOLOGY
PREVENTION AND TREATMENT: GENERAL
    CONSIDERATIONS
        Conservative Use of Neuroleptics
        Choice of Neuroleptics
        Treatment with Other Drugs
TREATMENT OF SPECIFIC FORMS OF TARDIVE
    DYSKINESIA
        Choreic/Stereotypic Movements
        Dystonic Movements
        Tardive Akathisia
FUTURE PERSPECTIVES

The term "tardive dyskinesia" (TD) applies only to abnormal involuntary movements resulting from chronic treatment with agents that block central dopamine receptors (Table 37-1). In most instances, these drugs are antipsychotic neuroleptic (NL) agents. Nonetheless, other dopaminergic receptor blockers, such as metoclopramide, are associated with the same disorder.[1] Schoenecker associated oral-facial dyskinesia with chlorpromazine treatment in 1957, yet 3 decades later, a cause-and-effect relationship between NL therapy and involuntary movements was still questioned.[2,3] The controversy persisted in part because NLs are most commonly used to treat psychosis and agitated senile depression; mannerisms resembling the movements of TD can occur spontaneously in some persons with psychosis and in normal elderly patients.[4]

Nonetheless, the unequivocal occurrence of involuntary movements after chronic NL therapy in nonpsychotic young adults without another cause for movement disorders[5] leaves no doubt that TD does occur. The 1980 American Psychiatric Association Task Force provided a useful definition of TD as "an abnormal involuntary movement, not including tremor, resulting from treatment with a neuroleptic drug for 3 months in persons with no other identifiable cause for movement disorder."[6] New descriptions add the possibility that tremor might need to be included as a form of TD. This discussion focuses on four topics: phenomenology, epidemiology and natural history, pathophysiology, and treatment of TD.

Phenomenology

A variety of movements occur in TD. Most common are rapid unsustained movements variously described as choreic or stereotypic.[7,8] The former term refers to movements that are unpredictable and flow from one body region to another, whereas stereotypies are reproducible and regular, remaining generally restricted in their anatomic distribution. Controversy exists currently as to which term is best-suited for most rapid TD movements, and the author has personally seen instances of both, sometimes in the same patient. Any body area may be affected, but the mouth is commonly involved, producing lip-smacking, tongue protrusion, or grimacing. In addition to facial movements, rapid movements of the fingers, hands, or the more proximal arm; nodding or head bobbing; pelvic rocking motions; fine movements of the toes; or a nonrhythmic motion of both legs may develop. TD may involve the trunk and diaphragm, sometimes leading to speech disorders[9,10] or even respiratory distress,[11,12] which may, rarely, be life-threatening.[13,14]

Dystonic movements also occur in TD, either alone or in combination with choreic or stereotypic movements. Dystonic movements are sustained abnormal postures of a body part or parts, induced or increased with use of the affected part, often with superimposed spasm. Although axial dystonia was first reported as a sequel of chronic NL treatment in 1962,[15] the term "tardive dystonia" was only recently applied to a series of NL-treated patients,[16] most of whom suffered from axial dystonias.

"Tardive akathisia" is an unpleasant sensation of internal restlessness that is partially relieved by volitional movements occurring in a patient who has received chronic NLs. These movements typically involve the lower extremities.[17] Tardive akathisia is phenomenologically indistinguishable from acute or subacute akathisia, but these latter entities occur when a patient's normal dose is increased, and akathisia occurs within days or weeks. Tardive akathisia occurs after chronic exposure to NLs and a steady or decreasing drug dosage.

Tics and myoclonic movements are also within the potential repertoire of TD, as well as "tardive tremor."[8,18,19] This latter movement disorder is a parkinsonian tremor that develops in the context of a constant or decreasing dose of NL. Importantly, it does not refer to parkinsonism or mouth tremor (rabbit syndrome) seen with starting NL medication or with a recent increase in NL dose. As a group, tardive movements often represent combinations of various movement disorders, so that dystonia and chorea, myoclonus and stereotypy, or dystonia and myoclonus occur together, rather than as isolated phenomena. When a physician encounters a patient with such mixed disorders, drug-induced dyskinesia and, specifically, TD should be carefully considered.

Epidemiology and Natural History

Despite methodological differences, recent reviews have shown a striking consistency in prevalence estimates of TD.[20] Jeste and Wyatt[21] reviewed 37 studies and, using a weighted-mean methodology, found a prevalence of 17.6 percent. Kane and Smith[22] reviewed 56 studies and found a prevalence of 20 percent. Although more recent estimates (1981–1986) have been higher, with an average prevalence of 30 percent, overall, the average prevalence of TD is 15–20 percent.[23]

Another condition termed spontaneous dyskinesia resembles TD but occurs independently of NL treatment. To esti-

TABLE 37-1 Drugs Associated with Tardive Dyskinesia

- Antipsychotic agents (e.g., neuroleptic drugs)
- Antidepressants with dopamine receptor blockade (e.g., amoxapine)
- Antinausea medications with dopamine receptor blockade (e.g., metoclopramide)

mate the true prevalence of TD, the frequency of this movement disorder should be subtracted from those for TD. The prevalence of spontaneous dyskinesia ranges from 0 to 53 percent.[24] Based on a series of 18 studies carried out between 1966 and 1983, Casey and Gerlach[25] calculated the prevalence rate of TD to be 19.8 percent and that of spontaneous dyskinesia as 5.9 percent. The net difference of 13.9 may, therefore, be a better estimate of the prevalence of TD.

Gardos and Cole estimate that the risk for a schizophrenic inpatient developing TD during 1 year of continuous NL exposure is 4–5 percent.[26] Cumulative incidence of TD is approximately 10 percent after 2 years, 15 percent after 3 years, and 19 percent after 4 years. This linear increase over the first years of NL exposure argues against the idea of a period of maximal risk. Incidence estimates in other prospective studies range from 3–7 percent, with an average of approximately 5 percent.[27]

The above data do not take into account several putative risk factors related to either the patient or to the NL treatment. The most consistently observed risk factors are age and gender. Several studies have shown that the prevalence of TD is higher in women,[28,1] particularly when they are elderly.[29] Patients with affective disorders appear to be more susceptible to TD than patients with schizophrenia.[30,31] Crane first suggested that TD was more likely to develop in patients with NL-induced parkinsonism,[32] but this issue has been debated. Likewise, early studies suggested an association between TD and prior brain injury, electroconvulsive therapy (ECT), and lobotomy, but more recent studies have been less conclusive.[33]

Treatment-related variables, such as type of NL used, dose, duration of treatment, and concurrent drug treatment have additionally been studied as putative risk factors for TD. Early reports suggested that piperazine phenothiazines were most likely to result in TD,[34] but subsequent studies[35] have not confirmed this observation. Several studies[36] found that depot fluphenazine increased the prevalence of TD. Dose and duration of NL exposure have not been established as definite risk factors, but recent studies suggest that high dose[37] and high cumulative dose[38] are risk factors for eventual TD. Other drug exposure, including antiparkinson agents like anticholinergics, has not been consistently related to an increased risk of TD.[20]

Whereas most of the risk factors appear to relate to TD regardless of phenomenological form, for tardive dystonia, special risk factor analyses have been performed with the use of case-control methodology. In one study, tardive dystonia was more likely in patients with a prior history of acute NL-induced dystonia.[39]

When NLs can be discontinued, the signs of TD resolve spontaneously in some patients,[6] transiently worsen in oth-

ers, and persist in some. Predicting which symptomatic patients have "reversible," rather than "persistent" dyskinesias, is at present impossible.[7] Approximately one-third of patients with TD on NLs remit within 3 months of discontinuation.[40] Resolution of movements can occur as long as 5 years after NL withdrawal.[28,41] Some studies suggest that discontinuation shortly after the onset of dyskinesias makes remission more likely, and that remissions are less likely in persons over the age of 60.[42]

In patients who remain on NLs, there is little difference in overall prevalence over a 10-year period. In 63 patients examined at baseline and 5 and 10 years later, most TD patients continued to have involuntary movements at all time points. Some patients (15 percent) however, remitted completely despite continued therapy.[43]

Pathophysiology

The pathophysiology of TD remains unknown, but interaction between dopamine, acetylcholine, gamma-aminobutyric acid (GABA), and glutamate systems may be important. In 1973, Klawans[44] proposed that the hyperkinetic movements of TD reflected a relative overactivity of striatal dopaminergic systems and that a reciprocal antagonism existed between striatal cholinergic and dopaminergic systems. He suggested that TD was related to denervation hypersensitivity of striatal dopamine receptors, resulting from "chemical denervation" by a NL. This behavior was suggested to lead to increased numbers and affinity of D2 receptors.

Despite its usefulness, this hypothesis met with several problems. For example, in laboratory studies, NL-induced receptor changes occur within days,[45] whereas movements in TD typically develop after months or years. Second, only about 15–20 percent of NL-exposed individuals develop TD,[20] whereas the NL-related increases in receptor density and sensitivity observed in animals were essentially a universal phenomenon.[46] In animals, NL-induced changes in motor behavior rarely persisted after drug withdrawal.[46] Finally, attempts to identify receptor changes specifically associated with TD in humans were uniformly inconclusive.

Gunne and Haggstrom[47] proposed that an abnormality of GABA-related striatal neurons caused TD. They observed changes in the GABA-synthesizing enzyme glutamic acid decarboxylase (GAD) in animals treated with NLs and noted similar changes in humans with TD.[48,49] Although they suggested that neuroleptics specifically injured GABAergic neurons, others have not replicated these findings.[50] Even when GABA changes occur, these changes could reflect increased dopaminergic activity and, thereby, be only a secondary phenomenon.

New interest focuses on the glutamate system and theories of excitotoxins. Basal ganglia function is mediated in part by cortical glutaminergic afferents, which innervate two putaminal GABAergic neuronal populations.[51] Anatomic, physiological, and pharmacological studies suggest that these neuronal populations form specific parallel efferent pathways that function with peptide co-transmitters.[52] These peptide-specific pathways have been termed "direct" and "indirect" by DeLong, and the "indirect" system[53] has been shown to be dysfunctional in some hyperkinetic disorders. In the "indirect" basal ganglia-thalamocortical circuit, somatotopically organized input from specific cortical areas facilitates striatal GABA/enkephalin (and, possibly, neurotensin) neurons. These putaminal neurons contain D2 receptors and are inhibited by nigral dopamine input. They inhibit a second population of GABAergic neurons in the external portion of the globus pallidus. The pallidal GABAergic neurons, in turn, inhibit excitatory glutaminergic outflow from the subthalamic nucleus to GABA/substance-P (and, possibly, dynorphin) neurons in the internal portion of the globus pallidus. These GABA/substance-P/dynorphin cells inhibit thalamic outflow. A parallel "direct" system involves putaminal GABA/substance-P neurons and does not include subthalamic nucleus. Studies using 2-deoxyglucose autoradiography in primates suggest that chronic neuroleptics lead to underactivity of the pathway from the subthalamic nucleus to the medial pallidal segment and substantia nigra (pars reticulata), leading ultimately to facilitation of thalamic outflow.[54]

Dysfunction of "indirect" striatal outflow may be consistent with the dopaminergic hypothesis of TD and other forms of chorea.[55] A drug-induced overactivity of dopaminergic function, perhaps via NL-induced changes in D2 receptors, could cause excessive inhibition of subthalamic nucleus neurons and functional disinhibition of pallidothalamic outflow. Indirectly, blockade of dopamine receptors and resultant striatal changes can thereby alter expression of peptide co-transmitters. Haloperidol is known to cause alterations of concentrations of several peptide neurotransmitters, including enkephalins and neurotensin, although the clinical significance of such changes is unknown. The unusual temporal course of TD, becoming evident after prolonged exposure and persisting long after drug withdrawal, could in part reflect alterations of these peptide systems. A neurotransmitter system under greater current scrutiny is the cholinergic interneuron pathway in the striatum. Miller and Chouinard[56] reviewed clinical and laboratory evidence to suggest that primary attention to this cell population should not be overshadowed by studies of the dopaminergic system.

Neuroimaging and Neuropathology

Magnetic resonance studies have not revealed differences in size or configuration of basal ganglia or other structures in TD subjects.[57] In a study of eight patients with TD, using positron emission tomography, D2 receptor density was not greater than that in age-matched controls.[58] TD is not associated with a characteristic pathological finding. In some reports, the brains are normal,[59] whereas other reports show inferior olive damage, substantia nigra or nigrostriatal degeneration, or swelling of large neurons of the caudate.[7] In two studies comparing the brains of TD patients to those of controls with similar psychiatric and treatment histories, nonspecific abnormalities were more common in TD.[60,61] Postmortem neurochemical studies found alterations in dopamine concentrations and receptor binding in the brains of persons with schizophrenia, but no specific change correlated with TD.[62]

Prevention and Treatment: General Considerations

CONSERVATIVE USE OF NEUROLEPTICS

TD has no universally effective therapy, and, therefore, prevention of its development must be the cornerstone of therapy (Table 37-2). The first tenet of prevention is to use neuroleptics only when necessary. The American Psychiatric Association[6] published useful guidelines. Indications for the short-term use of NLs (for 6 months or less) included the management of acute psychosis, preoperative medication, control of nausea, and treatment of primary neurological disorders, such as Huntington's disease and Gilles de la Tourette's syndrome. Treatment for longer than 6 months was recommended for psychotic patients with objective evidence of continuing psychosis, recurrent psychosis with NL withdrawal, disabling neurological illnesses requiring chronic treatment, and demonstrated responsiveness to therapy. The continued need for chronic NL treatment should be regularly reassessed. NLs should be discontinued when their efficacy is uncertain and should not be used when other agents can be substituted.

Although never evaluated in a clinical trial, simple precautions, such as using the lowest effective NL dose and regularly reevaluating the need for treatment, make intuitive sense.

CHOICE OF NEUROLEPTICS

For decades pharmacologists have searched for a specific antipsychotic drug that acts only on receptors mediating psychosis, without any dopamine-blocking effects elsewhere. This goal has not been achieved, but several "atypical" NLs, most notably, clozapine, have relatively greater effects on limbic than on striatal dopamine neurons and appear to be less associated with TD.[62] Sokoloff and colleagues,[63] using molecular genetic techniques, proposed that a third dopamine receptor (D3) distributed primarily in anterior, limbic, striatal regions may be important. "Typical" NLs have much stronger affinities for D2 than for D3 receptors, whereas "atypical" NLs have only a slightly greater preference for D2 than for D3 receptors.[64] If D3 receptors primarily mediate behavior, rather than motor function, specific D3 antagonists should have minimal motor-adverse effects. Although a specific D3 antagonist is not yet available, use of agents with high D3 affinity, such as clozapine, sulpiride, and

TABLE 37-2 Treatment of Tardive Dyskinesia

Phenomenology	Recommended Treatment
Stereotypies, chorea, tics	Reserpine, Tetrabenazine, baclofen, benzodiazepines
Dystonia	Reserpine, Tetrabenazine, anticholinergics, botulinum toxin
Akathisia	Reserpine, Tetrabenazine, propranolol, opioids

thioridazine, may lower the relative risk of TD, compared to other NLs. With clozapine, frequent blood counts are necessary to monitor for the possibility of aplastic anemia. It is important to recognize that atypical NLs too can cause TD and that no NL is entirely safe.

When a patient is receiving an NL and develops early signs of TD, ideally, the drug should be stopped immediately. Unfortunately, withdrawal of NL agents is impossible in the case of many psychotic patients or in patients with disorders such as severe Gilles de la Tourette's syndrome, in which NLs play a specific therapeutic role. In these cases, the behavioral benefit of continuing NLs must be weighed against the relative neurological risk of TD. Specific data on this question are unclear. In many patients, the movement disorder may not progressively worsen, despite continued therapy.[6] It is well established that TD symptoms will diminish when the NL dose is increased, because higher medication doses increase the blockade of striatal dopamine receptors. The use of the pathogenetic agent, however, for the treatment of TD is advised only in life-threatening situations in which all other treatments have failed.

TREATMENT WITH OTHER DRUGS

Because many patients do not have spontaneous remissions of TD, and because severe psychosis precludes NL discontinuation in others, a variety of therapeutic agents have been studied in TD. Evaluations of all therapeutic regimens are confounded by the inability to distinguish spontaneous remission from treatment-related resolution; by the wide variation in age, sex, duration, and severity of movements; by the lack of universal diagnostic techniques; and by the absence of a single standardized rating scale. Also, some studies have treated only patients receiving concurrent NLs; others have treated those no longer taking NLs; and others have mixed the two groups.

Treatment of Specific Forms of Tardive Dyskinesia

The movements of TD are generally choreic/stereotypic or dystonic, and drug treatment protocols have primarily focused attention on one or the other. Because many TD patients have a combination of movement types, the treating physician may need to weigh the relative impact of medications on each component of the movement disorder in a patient. Some treatments ameliorate one type of movement disorder while aggravating another.

CHOREIC/STEREOTYPIC MOVEMENTS

TREATMENTS INVOLVING THE DOPAMINE SYSTEM
The dopamine-depleting agents reserpine and tetrabenazine are the treatment of choice for the choreic or stereotypic movements of typical TD.[65] Reserpine depletes presynaptic stores of biogenic amines and is not believed to cause TD. Tetrabenazine, an experimental agent in the United States, also depletes presynaptic stores of biogenic amines but, in addition, blocks postsynaptic dopamine receptors. Because of this latter action,[65] it could theoretically cause TD. Both drugs control the movements of TD in the majority of patients and, in some cases, treatment is followed by complete remission of TD.[66] The major side effects of these agents are orthostatic hypotension, depression, and parkinsonism. Orthostatic hypotension occurs most commonly in older patients and may be avoided or minimized through the gradual introduction of the drug, beginning with 0.125–0.25 mg daily and increasing by 0.124–0.25 mg weekly, while monitoring blood pressure. Depression occurs commonly after prolonged (months to years), continuous therapy and generally requires drug discontinuation. Concurrent or latent depression can be severely exacerbated by reserpine. The full therapeutic response to a given dose of these agents is not apparent for several weeks, and doses as high as 6 mg/day of reserpine may be necessary. Sometimes, an NL will be needed for short-term control of TD during the few weeks when reserpine is being introduced.[67]

Low doses of dopamine agonists designed to activate presynaptic autoreceptors and thereby decrease dopamine release have not been consistently successful.[68] "Desensitizing" dopamine receptors by using increasing doses of L-dopa has not proved regularly beneficial.[69] The monoamine oxidase B inhibitor, selegiline, with putative antioxidant properties, along with its dopaminergic facilitation, was tried in a placebo-controlled sample of TD patients, but drug-treated patients fared worse than those receiving placebo.[70] Calcium-channel blocking agents, usually used in cardiac patients, have been suggested to have dopamine-blocking properties, but in one placebo-controlled study, diltiazem had no efficacy in treated TD.[71] Other studies have suggested that nifedipine and verapamil may be more effective,[72] but better placebo-controlled and blinded protocols are needed to evaluate this drug class.

In severely disabled patients, particularly those with respiratory or oropharyngeal dyskinesias, withdrawal of the NL agent may be potentially life-threatening. In such severe cases, a return to NL medication may be the only feasible therapy. On the other hand, reserpine may be added to a stable dose of the NL and increased until the movements abate. When movements decrease, the NL may be slowly withdrawn to keep the dose of the causative agent at its very lowest level. Novel or atypical NLs, such as clozapine, have been tried at high doses in treating TD, but side effects in the elderly (primarily, sedation) preclude its general use.[73] In low doses (50–250 mg/day), clozapine has no significant effect on TD.[74]

TREATMENTS INVOLVING THE GABA SYSTEM
Based on observations that programide coadminstration with chronic haloperidol can reduce vacuous chewing movements in experimental animals,[75] agents with effects on the GABA system have been tried in TD. The magnitude of benefit achieved with agents that are designed to augment GABA function is generally less than that with drugs affecting dopamine systems. However, the therapeutic index is generally greater, so that a short trial with a GABAergic agent is often indicated in mild or moderate TD, before attempting treatment with dopamine-depleting agents. Respiratory depres-

sion may accompany an overdose with this class of drugs, and the respiratory depressant effect may be additive with other central nervous system (CNS) depressants, including ethanol. The physician must carefully consider suicide risk and concurrent medications when prescribing these agents.

Small studies have suggested that baclofen,[76] sodium valproate,[77] and gamma-vinyl GABA[78] produce mild improvement in TD, but the effects were inconsistent, short-lasting, or limited by side effects. Of these, baclofen, starting at 5 or 10 mg daily and increasing in 5- to 10-mg/day increments, up to a maximum daily dose of 60–80 mg/day in three or four doses, is most likely to be beneficial. In patients receiving concurrent NLs, baclofen may aggravate drug-induced parkinsonism. Sedation is a common adverse effect, and ataxia, confusion, and auditory or visual hallucinations may rarely occur. Abrupt discontinuation should be avoided, because anxiety or hallucinations may occur. Coma, respiratory depression, and seizures may follow severe overdosage.

Benzodiazepines may potentiate central GABA transmission and are mildly beneficial in TD, especially clonazepam and diazepam.[79] Sedation, a common dose-limiting side effect of clonazepam, can be minimized by gradual drug introduction, beginning with 0.5 mg daily and increasing in 0.5 to 1 mg/week increments. Tolerance for the antidyskinetic effect is common after months of therapy, but Thaker et al.[79] found gradual withdrawal, followed by a 2-week drug-free period, to be associated with renewed efficacy when the drug was reintroduced.

ANTIOXIDANT AND OTHER PHARMACOLOGICAL STRATEGIES

A recent focus for studying the pathophysiology of several movement disorders is membrane damage caused by free radical formation.[80,81] The antioxidant vitamin, tocopherol, a free radical scavenger, was found to be useful in several short trials of TD,[82,83] but not in all.[84] Because the doses used (400–1,200 IU/day) are not associated with adverse effects, tocopherol could become an important therapeutic agent if further trials replicate these results. At present, a 2- or 3-week trial of tocopherol in mildly to moderately affected patients could be attempted before other therapeutic regimens, because there is no risk of treatment-related adverse effects. Higher doses have also been studied with positive effects, but coagulation status and cholesterol levels need to be monitored.[85,86] The effect is not a result of changes in NL drug levels.[86] Whereas most studies are short term, one has shown maintained improvement for as long as 36 weeks.[87]

In uncontrolled studies of small numbers of patients, a large number of other agents have been reported to have minimal benefit on TD, including propranolol,[88] clonidine,[89] tryptophan,[90] cyproheptadine,[91] opiates,[92,93] manganese and niacin,[94] and GM1 ganglioside.[95] Lithium was beneficial in several studies[96], but not in others.[97] Agents affecting the cholinergic system have not had a consistent benefit.[7] Buspirone has been used in an open-label trial with statistically significant improvement.[98] With the new interest in neuropeptides, ceruletide has been examined with clinical improvement. The putative advantage to such therapy is its once weekly administration.[99]

Finally, ECT was reported both to ameliorate TD[100] and to increase its occurrence.[101] Because others have noted that mood fluctuations alter the expression of TD,[101,102] these observations may relate to ECT effects on mood more than movement disorders.

DYSTONIC MOVEMENTS

Some drugs are useful for dystonic, as well as choreic/stereotypic, TD.[16] As with patients with unusual TD, those with tardive dystonia are helped by dopamine-depleting agents, such as reserpine and tetrabenazine.[103] Clonazepam[79] and ECT[102] have been reported to be beneficial in a few patients.

In contrast, however, centrally active anticholinergic drugs (muscarinic receptor blockers) are a major therapeutic tool in tardive dystonia,[16] whereas in typical choreic/stereotypic TD, movements worsen when an anticholinergic is given.[45] In patients with both dystonia and typical TD, use of anticholinergics may improve dystonia but worsen other signs. In such cases, the physician should analyze which movements are causing the most pronounced disability. In most instances, other than cosmetic, dystonic movements are more disabling than choreic/stereotypic.

A new treatment, primarily designed for idiopathic dystonia but recently applied to other dystonic syndromes, is botulinum toxin injection. This biological toxin, when injected directly into overactive muscles, weakens them by decreasing acetylcholine release at the neuromuscular junction. For patients whose tardive dystonia affects primarily one body region, this treatment could be considered.[104] In patients with combined tardive dystonia and choreic tardive dyskinesia movements, botulinum toxin can abate dystonia, whereas other medications focus on dyskinesias.[105]

In setting an order for medication trials in tardive dystonia, clonazepam or baclofen may be selected first when the dystonia is painful. A trial of anticholinergic agents may be useful in those without prominent choreic or stereotypic movements. Dopamine-depleting agents may be tried as a more aggressive treatment in patients without depression. In persons with extreme disability, as is often the case in those with predominantly axial dystonias, NL agents may be necessary. In this case, careful explanation of the potential for the treatment to aggravate the tardive disorder is recommended. Botulinum toxin is usually an adjunct medication, supplementing other drugs, and is used to focus specific attention to one or two prominently involved body areas.

TARDIVE AKATHISIA

Tardive akathisia is phenomenologically indistinguishable from subacute akathisia accompanying NL treatment and, hence, in patients requiring continued use of NL agents, making a distinction between the two is particularly problematic. Dopamine-depleting agents are useful in tardive akathisia, in doses similar to those used in typical TD.[17] In a few persons, agents useful in treating subacute akathisia, such as propranolol (60 mg daily)[106] and opiates (propoxyphene up to 100 mg daily or codeine up to 60 mg daily) may be helpful.[107] In contrast to subacute akathisia, anticholinergic agents are not helpful in tardive akathisia.

Future Perspectives

The development of functional MR scanning and PET technology may provide clearer evidence of the pathophysiological changes that occur with the introduction of NL drugs in humans and the progressive, long-term consequences of their use. The appreciation of receptor subtypes for the dopaminergic system provides solid evidence that TD occurs when striatal dopaminergic receptors are blocked, and such studies support the concept that TD may be avoided by selective antagonists that avoid striatal dopaminergic receptor antagonism. More complete understanding of neurotransmitter systems other than the dopaminergic system promises direct clinical impact for treatment and prevention, especially as related to the GABAergic pathways. Finally, new discoveries on oxidative metabolism in the central nervous system and the role of such chemical reactions in neurodegenerative and neurotoxic syndromes may lead to significant treatment breakthroughs that do not necessarily relate to specific neurotransmitters systems but rather to general chemical reactions affecting neuronal and glial function.

References

1. Sewell DD, Jeste DV: Metoclopramide-associated tardive dyskinesia: An analysis of 67 cases. *Arch Fam Med* 1(2):271–278, 1992.
2. Schoenecker VM: Ein eigentümliches syndrom in oralen Bereich bei Megphen Applikation. *Nervenarzt* 28:35–43, 1957.
3. Waddington JL: Tardive dyskinesia: A critical re-evaluation of the causal role of neuroleptics and of the dopamine receptor supersensitivity hypothesis, in Callaghan N, Galvin R (eds): *Recent Researches in Neurology.* London: Pitman, 1984, pp 34–48.
4. Marsden CD, Tarsy D, Baldessarini RJ: Spontaneous and drug-induced movement disorders in psychotic patients, in Benson DF, Blumer D (eds): *Psychiatric Aspects of Neurologic Disease.* New York: Grune & Stratton, 1975, pp 219–265.
5. Klawans HL, Bergen D, Bruyn GW, Paulson GW: Neuroleptic-induced tardive dyskinesia in nonpsychotic patients. *Arch Neurol* 30:338–339, 1974.
6. Baldessarini RJ, Cole JO, Davis JM, et al: Tardive dyskinesia: Summary of a Task Force Report of the American Psychiatric Association. *Am J Psychiatry* 137:1163–1172, 1980.
7. Tanner CM: Drug-induced movement disorders (tardive dyskinesia and dopa-induced dyskinesia), in Vinken PJ, Bruyn GW, Klawans HL (eds). *Handbook of Clinical Neurology.* Amsterdam: Elsevier Science Publishers, 1986, pp 185–212.
8. Stacy M, Jankovic J: Tardive dyskinesia. *Curr Opin Neurol Neurosurg* 4:343–349, 1991.
9. Feve A, Angelard B, Benelon G, et al: Postneuroleptic laryngeal dyskinesias: A cause of upper airway obstructive syndrome improved by local injections of botulinum toxin. *Mov Disord* 7(1):217–219, 1993.
10. Gerratt BR, Goetz CG, Fisher HB: Speech abnormalities in tardive dyskinesia. *Arch Neurol* 41:273–276, 1984.
11. Weiner WJ, Goetz CG, Nausieda PA, Klawans HL: Respiratory dyskinesias: Extrapyramidal dysfunction and dyspnea. *Am J Intern Med* 88:327–331, 1978.
12. Wilcos PG, Bassett A, Jones B, Fleetham JA: Respiratory arrhythmias in patients with tardive dyskinesia. *Chest* 105(1):203–207, 1994.
13. Casey DE, Rabins P: Tardive dyskinesias as a life-threatening illness. *Am J Psychiatry* 135:486–488, 1978.
14. Feve A, Angelard B, Fenelon G, et al: Postneuroleptic laryngeal dyskinesias: A cause of upper airway obstructive syndrome improved by local injections of botulinum toxin. *Mov Disord* 8(2):217–219, 1993.
15. Druckman R, Seelinger D, Thulin B: Chronic involuntary movements induced by phenothiazines. *J Nerv Ment Dis* 135:69–76, 1962.
16. Burke RE, Fahn S, Jankovic J, et al: Tardive dystonia: Late-onset and persistent dystonia caused by anti-psychotic drugs. *Neurology* 32:1335–1346, 1982.
17. Christiansen E, Moller JE, Faurbye A: Neurological investigation of 28 brains from patients with dyskinesia. *Acta Psychiatr Scand* 46:14–23, 1970.
18. Stacy M, Jankovic J: Tardive tremor. *Mov Disord* 7(1):75–57, 1992.
19. Adler LA, Peselow E, Duncan E, et al: Vitamin E in tardive dyskinesia: Time course of effect after placebo substitution. *Psychopharmacol Bull* 39(3):371–374, 1993.
20. Khot V, Egan MF, Hyde TM, Wyatt J: Neuroleptics and classic tardive dyskinesia, in Lang AE, Weiner, WJ (eds): *Drug-Induced Movement Disorders.* Mt. Kisco, NY: Futura Publishing Company, 1982, pp 121–166.
21. Jeste DV, Wyatt RJ: *Understanding and Treating Tardive Dyskinesia.* New York: Guilford Press, 1982.
22. Kane JM, Smith JM: Tardive dyskinesia. *Arch Gen Psychiatry* 39:473–481, 1982.
23. Baldessarini RJ, Cole JO, Davis JM, et al: *Tardive Dyskinesia: A Task Force Report.* Washington, DC: American Psychiatric Association, 1980.
24. Casey DE, Hansen TE: Spontaneous dyskinesia, in Jeste DV, Wyatt RJ (eds): *Neuropsychiatric Movement Disorders.* Washington DC: American Psychiatric Press, 1984, pp 68–95.
25. Casey DE, Gerlach J: Tardive dyskinesia. *Acta Psychiatr Scand* 77:369–378, 1988.
26. Gardos G, Cole JO: Overview: Public health issues in tardive dyskinesia. *Am J Psychiatry* 137:776–781, 1980.
27. Chouinard G, Annable L, Ross-Chouinard A, Mercier P: A 5-year prospective longitudinal study of tardive dyskinesia: Factors predicting appearance of new cases. *J Clin Psychopharmacol* 8(suppl):21–26, 1988.
28. Jeste DV, Wyatt RJ: *Understanding and Treating Tardive Dyskinesia.* New York: Guilford Press, 1982.
29. Smith JM, Oswald WT, Kucharski LT, Waterman LJ: Tardive dyskinesia: Age and sex differences in hospitalized schizophrenics. *Psychopharmacology* 58:207–211, 1978.
30. Gardos G, Casey D (eds): *Tardive Dyskinesia and Affective Disorders.* Washington DC: American Psychiatric Press, 1983.
31. Yassa R, Nastase C, Dupont D, Thibeau M: Tardive dyskinesia in elderly psychiatric patients: A 5-year study. *Am J Psychiatry* 149(9):1206–1211, 1992.
32. Crane GE: Persistent dyskinesia. *Br J Psychiatry* 122:395–405, 1973.
33. Gupta S, Egan MF, Hyde TM: An unusual presentation of tardive dyskinesia with prominent involvement of the pectoral musculature. *Biol Psychiatry* 33(4):291–292, 1993.
34. Gershanik OS: Drug-induced movement disorders. *Curr Opin Neurol Neurosurg* 6(3):369–376, 1993.
35. Klawans HL, Goetz CG, Perlik S: Tardive dyskinesia: Review and update. *Am J Psychiatry* 137:900–908, 1980.
36. Gardos G, Cole JO, LaBrie RA: Drug variables in the etiology of tardive dyskinesia: Application of discriminant function analysis, in Fahn WE, Smith RC, Davis JM, Domino EF (eds): *Tardive Dyskinesia: Research and Treatment.* New York: SP Medical and Scientific Books, 1980, pp 291–296.

37. Morgenstern H, Glazer WM: Identifying risk factors for tardive dyskinesia among long-term outpatients maintained with neuroleptic medications: Results of the Yale Tardive Dyskinesia Study. *Arch Gen Psychiatry* 50(9):723–733, 1993.

38. Cavallaro R, Regazzetti MG, Mundo E, et al: Tardive dyskinesia outcomes: Clinical and pharmacologic correlates of remission and persistence. *Neuropsychopharmacology* 8(3):233–239, May 1993.

39. Sachdev P: Risk factors for tardive dystonia: A case-control comparison with tardive dyskinesia. *Acta Psychiatr Scand* 88(2):98–103, 1993.

40. Jeste DV, Jeste SD, Wyatt RJ: Reversible tardive dyskinesia: Implications for therapeutic strategy and prevention of tardive dyskinesia. *Mod Probl Pharmacopsychiatry* 21:34–48, 1983.

41. Klawans HL, Tanner CM: The reversibility of permanent tardive dyskinesia. *Neurology* 33(suppl 2):163, 1983.

42. Quitkin F, Rifkin A, Gochfeld L, Klein DF: Tardive dyskinesia: Are first signs reversible? *Am J Psychiatry* 134:84–87, 1977.

43. Gardos G, Casey DE, Cole HO, et al: Ten-year outcome of tardive dyskinesia. *Am J Psychiatry* 151(6):836–841, 1994.

44. Klawans HL: *The Pharmacology of Extrapyramidal Movement Disorders.* Basel, Switzerland: Karger, 1973.

45. Klawans HL, Rubovits R: The effect of cholinergic and anticholinergic agents on tardive dyskinesias. *J Neurol Neurosurg Psychiatry* 37:941–947, 1974.

46. Goetz CG, Klawans HL: Controversies in animal models of tardive dyskinesia, in Marsden CD, Fahn S (eds): *Movement Disorders.* Boston: Butterworth Scientific, 1982, pp 263–276.

47. Gunne LM, Haggstrom JE: Pathophysiology of tardive dyskinesia. *Psychopharmacology* suppl 232:191–193, 1985.

48. Gunne LM, Haggstrom JE, Sjoquist B: Association with persistent neuroleptic-induced dyskinesia of regional changes in brain: GABA synthesis. *Nature* 309:347–349, 1984.

49. Andersson U, Haggstrom JE, Levin ED, et al: Reduced glutamate decarboxylase activity in the subthalamic nucleus in patients with tardive dyskinesia. *Mov Disord* 4:37–46, 1989.

50. Mithani S, Atmada S, Baimbridge KG, Fubuger HC: Neuroleptic-induced oral dyskinesias: Effects of progabide and lack of correlation with regional changes in glutamic acid decarboxylase and choline acetyl transferase activities. *Psychopharmacology* 93:94–100, 1987.

51. Alexander GE, Crutcher MD: Functional architecture of basal ganglia circuits: Neural substrates of parallel processing. *Tr in Neurosci* 13:266–271, 1990.

52. Graybiel AM: Neurotransmitters and neuromodulators in the basal ganglia. *Tr in Neurosci* 13:244–254, 1990.

53. DeLong MR: Primate model of movement disorders of basal ganglia origin. *Tr in Neurosci* 13:281–285, 1990.

54. Feve A, Angelard B, Fenelon G, et al: Neuroleptic-induced tardive dyskinesia in the Cebus monkey. *Mov Disord* 7(1):32–37, 1990.

55. Reiner A, Albin RL, Anderson KD, et al: Differential loss of striatal projection neurons in Huntington disease. *Proc Natl Acad Sci U S A* 85:5733–5737, 1988.

56. Miller R, Chouinard G: Loss of striatal cholinergic neurons as a basis for tardive and L-dopa-induced dyskinesias, neuroleptic-induced supersensitivity psychosis and refractory schizophrenia. *Biol Psychiatry* 34(10):713–738, 1993.

57. Abad V, Ovsiew F: Treatment of persistent myoclonic tardive dystonia with verapamil. *Br J Psychiatry* 162:554–556, 1993.

58. Blin J, Baron JC, Cambon H, et al: PET study. *J Neurol Neurosurg Psychiatry* 52:1248–1252, 1989.

59. Hunter R, Blackwood W, Smith MC: Neuropathological findings in three cases of persistent dyskinesias following phenothiazines. *J Neurol Sci* 7:263–273, 1968.

60. Christiansen E, Moller JE, Faurbye A: Neurological investigation of 28 brains from patients with dyskinesia. *Acta Psychiatr Scand* 46:14–23, 1970.

61. Jellinger K: Neuropathologic findings after neuroleptic long-term therapy. *Neurotoxicology,* 71:25–42, 1977.

62. Lieberman J, Johns C, Cooper T, et al: Clozapine pharmacology and tardive dyskinesia. *Psychopharmacology* 99:S54–S59, 1989.

63. Sokoloff P, Giros B, Mrtres MP, et al: Molecular cloning and characterization of a novel dopamine receptor (D3) as a target for neuroleptics. *Nature* 347:146–151, 1990.

64. Strange PG: Interesting times for dopamine receptors. *Tr in Neurosci* 14:43–45, 1991.

65. Jankovic J, Orman J: Tetrabenazine therapy of dystonia, chorea, tics and other dyskinesias. *Neurology* 38:391–394, 1988.

66. Lang AE, Marsden CD: Alphamethylparatyrosine and tetrabenazine in movement disorders. *Clin Neuropharmacol* 5:375–387, 1982.

67. Stacy M, Cardosa F, Jankovic J: Tardive stereotypy and other movement disorders in tardive dyskinesias. *Neurology* 43(5):937–941, 1993.

68. Tamminga CA, Chase TN: Bromocriptine and CF 25-396 in the treatment of tardive dyskinesia. *Arch Neurol* 37:204–205, 1980.

69. Alpert M, Friedhoff A: Clinical application of receptor modification treatment, in Fann WE, Smith RC, Davis JM, Domino EF (eds): *Tardive dyskinesia: Research and Treatment.* New York: Spectrum, 1980, pp 471–474.

70. Goff DC, Renshaw PF, Sarid-Segal O, et al: A placebo-controlled trial of selegiline (L-deprenyl) in the treatment of tardive dyskinesia. *Biol Psychiatry* 33(10):700–706, 1993.

71. Loonen AJ, Verwey HA, Roels PR, et al: Is diltiazem effective in treating the symptoms of (tardive) dyskinesia in chronic psychiatric inpatients? A negative, double-blind, placebo-controlled trial. *J Clin Psychopharmacology* 12(1):39–42, 1992.

72. Cates M, Lusk K, Wells BG: Are calcium-channel blockers effective in the treatment of tardive dyskinesia? *Ann Pharmacother* 27(2):191–196, 1993.

73. Simpson CM, Lee JH, Shrivastava RK: Clozapine and tardive dyskinesia. *Psychopharmacologia* 56:75–80, 1978.

74. Gerlach J, Simmelsgaard H: Tardive dyskinesia during and following treatment with haloperidol, biperiden, thioridizine, and clozapine. *Psychopharmacologia* 59:105–112, 1978.

75. Kaneda H, Shirakawa O, Dale J, et al: Co-administration of progabid inhibits haloperidol-induced oral dyskinesias in rats. *Eur J Pharmacol* 212(1):43–49, 1992.

76. Stewart RM, Rollins J, Beckham B, Roffman M: Baclofen in tardive dyskinesia patients maintained on neuroleptics. *Clin Neuropharmacol* 5:365–373, 1982.

77. Nair NPV, Lal S, Schwartz G, Tharundayil JX: Effects of sodium valproate and baclofen in tardive dyskinesia: Clinical and neuroendocrine studies. *Adv Biochem Psychopharmacol* 24:437–441, 1980.

78. Tell GP, Schecter PJ, Koch-Weser J, et al: Effects of gamma vinyl GABA (letter). *N Engl J Med* 305:581–582, 1981.

79. Thaker GK, Nguyen JA, Strauss ME, et al: Clonazepam treatment of tardive dyskinesia: A practical GABA mimetic strategy. *Am J Psychiatry* 147:445–451, 1990.

80. Lohr JB, Kuczenski R, Bracha HS, et al: Increased indices of free radical activity in the cerebrospinal fluid of patients with tardive dyskinesia. *Biol Psychiatry* 28:535–539, 1990.

81. Cadet JL: Movement disorders: Therapeutic role of vitamin E (Review). *Toxicol Ind Health* 9(1-2):337–347, 1993.

82. Elkashef AM, Ruskin PE, Bacher N, Barrett D: Vitamin E and the treatment of tardive dyskinesia. *Am J Psychiatry* 147:505–506, 1990.

83. Dabiri LM, Pasta D, Darby JK, Mosbacher D: Effectiveness of vitamin E for treatment of long-term tardive dyskinesia. *Am J Psychiatry* 151(6):925–926, 1994 June.

84. Shriqui CL, Bradwejn J, Annable L, Jones BD: Vitamin E in the treatment of tardive dyskinesia: A double-blind placebo-controlled study. *Am J Psychiatry* 149(3):391–393, 1992.

85. Adler LA, Peselow E, Rotrosen J, et al: Vitamin E treatment of tardive dyskinesia. *Am J Psychiatry* 150(9):1405–1407, 1993.

86. Egan MF, Hyde TM, Albers GW, et al: Treatment of tardive dyskinesia with vitamin E. *Am J Psychiatry* 149(6):773–777, 1992.

87. Adler LA, Peselow E, Duncan E, et al: Vitamin E in tardive dyskinesia: Time course of effect after placebo substitution. *Psychopharmacol Bull* 29(3):371–374, 1993.

88. Bacher NM, Lewis HA: Low dose propranolol in tardive dyskinesia. *Am J Psychiatry* 137:495–497, 1980.

89. Freedman R, Bell J, Kirch D: Clonidine therapy for coexisting psychosis and tardive dyskinesia. *Am J Psychiatry* 137:629–630, 1980.

90. Prange AJ Jr, Wilson IC, Morris CE: Preliminary experience with tryptophan and lithium in the treatment of tardive dyskinesia. *Psychopharmacol Bull* 9:36–37, 1973.

91. Gardos G, Cole JO: Pilot study of cyproheptadine (Periactin) in tardive dyskinesia. *Psychopharmacol Bull* 14:18–20, 1978.

92. Bjorndal N, Casey DE, Gerlach J: Enkephalin, morphine, and naloxone in tardive dyskinesia. *Psychopharmacology (Berl)* 69:133–136, 1980.

93. Stoessl AJ, Polanski E, Frydryszak H: The opiate antagonist naloxone suppresses a rodent model of tardive dyskinesia. *Mov Disord* 8(4):44–452, 1993.

94. Kunin RA: Manganese and niacin in the treatment of drug-induced dyskinesia. *J Orthomol Psychiatry* 5:4–27, 1976.

95. Peselow ED, Irons S, Rotrosen J, et al: GMI ganglioside as a potential treatment in tardive dyskinesia. *Psychopharmacology* 25:277–280, 1989.

96. Reda FA, Scanlan JM, Kemp K, Escobar JI: Treatment of tardive dyskinesia with lithium carbonate. *N Engl J Med* 137:84–87, 1983.

97. Simpson GM, Branchez MH, Lee HJ: Lithium in tardive dyskinesia. *Pharmakopsychiatr Neuropsychopharmakol* 9:76–80, 1976.

98. Moss LE, Neppe VM, Drevets WC: Buspiron in the treatment of tardive dyskinesia. *J Clin Psychopharmacol* 13(3):204–209, 1993.

99. Kojima T, Yamauchi T, Miyasaka M, et al: Treatment of tardive dyskinesia with ceruletide: A double-blind, controlled study. *Psychiatry Res* 43(2):129–136, 1992.

100. Price TRP, Levin R: Effects of electroconvulsive therapy on tardive dyskinesia. *Am J Psychiatry* 135:991–993, 1978.

101. Unrbrand L, Faurbye A: Reversible and irreversible dyskinesia after treatment with perphenazine, chlorpromazine, reserpine and ECT therapy. *Psychopharmacologia* 1:408–418, 1960.

102. Adityanjee SK, Jayaswal SK, Chan TM, Subramaniam M: Temporary remission of tardive dystonia following electroconvulsive therapy. *Br J Psychiatry* 156:433–435, 1990.

103. Kang JU, Burke RE, Fahn S: Natural history and treatment of tardive dystonia. *Mov Disord* 1:193–208, 1986.

104. Jankovic J, Brin MF: Therapeutic uses of botulinum toxin. *N Engl J Med* 324:1186–1194, 1991.

105. Stip E, Faughnan M, Desjardin I, Labrecque R: Botulinum toxin in a case of severe tardive dyskinesia mixed with dystonia. *Br J Psychiatry* 161:867–868, 1992.

106. Fleischhacker WW, Roth SD, Kane JM: The pharmacologic treatment of neuroleptic-induced akathisia. *J Clin Psychopharmacol* 10:12–21, 1990.

107. Burke RE, Kang UJ, Jankovic J, et al: Tardive akathisia: An analysis of clinical features and response to open therapeutic trials. *Mov Disord* 4:157–175, 1989.

Chapter 38

OTHER CHOREATIC DISORDERS

MARGERY H. MARK

CHOREA
IMMUNE SYSTEM, HORMONES, AND CHOREA
    Sydenham's Chorea
    Chorea Gravidarum
    Systemic Lupus Erythematosus and Antiphospholipid
      Antibody Syndrome
    Pathophysiology: Immune-mediated Mechanism
HEREDITARY CHOREAS: NEUROACANTHOCYTOSIS
HEREDITARY CHOREAS: BENIGN HEREDITARY
   CHOREA
HEREDITARY CHOREAS:
   DENTATORUBROPALLIDOLUYSIAN ATROPHY
SENILE CHOREA
VASCULAR CHOREA, HEMICHOREA, AND
   HEMIBALLISMUS
OTHER NEUROLOGICAL AND SYSTEMIC DISEASES
    Hyperthyroidism
    Polycythemia Vera
    Metabolic Disorders
    Multiple Sclerosis
    Postpump Chorea
OTHER CAUSES
    Drugs, Toxins, Infections, Neoplasms, and
      Degenerative Disorders
PAROXYSMAL DYSKINESIAS
PAINFUL LEGS AND MOVING TOES
SUMMARY

Chorea

Chorea (Greek for "dance") consists of irregular, unpredictable, brief movements that flow from one body part to another in a nonstereotyped fashion. They may be incorporated, especially in milder cases, into more purposeful movements. They may consist of small twitches or larger jerks of any body part. Choreiform movements rarely occur in isolation; rather, they may often be seen in a spectrum with slower, distal, writhing, sinuous movements called *athetosis* and described as *choreoathetosis*. In many disorders in which chorea is a feature, it is not uncommon to see other movement disorders as well, particularly dystonia. The opposite side of speed and amplitude from athetoid movements are *ballistic* movements, which are usually seen unilaterally as *hemiballism*, although bilateral (*paraballism* or *biballism*) may be encountered. Ballistic movements, the most extreme type of movement disorder, are large amplitude, usually proximal flinging of a limb or body part. Although some investigators separate these disorders, others (including this author) consider ballism to be a severe form of chorea and, in fact, many cases of resolving ballistic movements taper down to chorea.[1]

The prototypic choreic disorder is *Huntington's disease* (HD), discussed in detail in the preceding chapters. The phenomenology of chorea in other disorders, both primary and secondary, is essentially the same as in HD; likewise, theories of the pathophysiology of the choreas, for the most part, are very similar. Similarly, Wilson's disease (Chap. 46), tardive dyskinesia (Chap. 37), and treated Parkinson's disease (Chap. 14) may also demonstrate chorea; the reader is referred to those chapters for more details. In this chapter, we will focus on several clinical entities in which chorea plays a significant role. Other related movement disorders will also be discussed.

Immune System, Hormones, and Chorea

It has long been recognized that several seemingly unrelated conditions have been uncommonly associated with chorea: rheumatic fever, systemic lupus erythematosus (SLE), and pregnancy (and its flip side, use of oral contraceptives). The pathophysiology of chorea in these conditions may be similar and will be explored below.

SYDENHAM'S CHOREA

In 1686, Thomas Sydenham described the clinical syndrome that now bears his name.[2] Originally called St. Vitus' dance, as well as chorea minor, acute chorea, and rheumatic chorea, *Sydenham's chorea* (SC) not uncommonly follows rheumatic fever in children and adolescents. Antecedent infection with group A streptococcus is usual, although many patients do not give a history of strep infection and, as the chorea may occur 6 months or more after infection, antistreptolysin and antistreptococcal antibodies may not be elevated. Adequate antibiotic therapy in the United States has dramatically reduced the occurrence of rheumatic fever, and thus of SC,[3] although it may still be found. It may be seen more often in children from developing countries who lack routine antibiotic care. In fact, a recent series from Turkey showed that acute rheumatic fever is not only still very prevalent in that country but also remains a significant cause of morbidity and revealed that 20 percent of patients (45/228) admitted to hospital with rheumatic fever had chorea.[4] Another series of admissions to one hospital in Chile from 1976 to 1989 demonstrated that 16 percent of attacks of acute rheumatic fever (70/438 in 402 patients) presented with SC.[5]

The clinical syndrome of SC, in addition to the chorea, is characterized by a semiacute illness involving muscular weakness, hypotonia, dysarthria, and behavioral abnormalities. The most common of the behavioral problems is obsessive-compulsive symptomatology, with 82 percent of individuals affected in one series; nearly one-half of these children met criteria for frank obsessive-compulsive disorder.[6,7] They also demonstrated increased emotional lability, motoric hyperactivity, irritability, distractibility, and age-regressed behavior. Behavioral symptoms may begin several days to weeks before onset of chorea and wax and wane with motor signs.[6] The chorea is usually bilateral, but may be unilateral in about 20 percent of patients. It may begin either abruptly or insidiously, worsen over 2–4 weeks, and usually resolves spontaneously in 3–6 months, although some patients may have residual chorea. Recurrences may occur in about 20 percent of patients, usually within about 2 years.[3,8] The vast majority of patients are between 5 and 15 years old at first occurrence, and girls are affected about twice as frequently as boys, especially in the peripubescent ages, suggesting a role for sex hormones in this disorder.[9]

The electroencephalogram (EEG) is often abnormal, with slowing, particularly irregular occipital slowing.[10,11] Recent neuroimaging studies may shed some light on the pathophysiology (discussed below). Magnetic resonance imaging (MRI) in two cases revealed increased signal on T_2-weighted images in the striatum and globus pallidus, with resolution of signal intensity on clinical improvement.[12,13] A recent analysis of MRI of 24 subjects with SC demonstrated increased size of caudate, putamen, and globus pallidus,[14] suggesting an inflammatory process. Functional neuroimaging, evaluating regional cerebral glucose metabolism using ^{18}F-fluoro-deoxy-glucose and positron emission tomography (FDG-PET), in SC differs from HD and other hereditary choreas. In HD, there is striatal hypometabolism[15]; but in SC, there is demonstrated increased glucose metabolism in bilateral striatum in two girls with Sydenham's and contralaterally in an elderly woman with hemichorea as a residual to adolescent-onset Sydenham's[16,17]; the abnormality on PET was reversible in the girls after clinical improvement.

The chorea in SC responds to dopaminergic blockers (pimozide may be less sedating than haloperidol)[18] or depleters[19] but, as it tends to be self-limited, treatment should be restricted to those in whom the chorea is so severe as to interfere with function. Valproate may also be helpful.[16,20] Corticosteroids, intravenous immunoglobulin, and plasmapheresis may also play a role in the treatment of SC.[11] Antibiotic therapy with penicillin to prevent cardiac dysfunction may be indicated as well.

CHOREA GRAVIDARUM

Pregnancy is another nonneurological condition that may, rarely, present with chorea as *chorea gravidarum* (CG); it is more frequently seen in women with a prior history of SC, or the chorea may be secondary to other conditions (e.g., SLE[21]). It is far less common than when first reviewed in 1932,[22] and morbidity and maternal and fetal mortality have continued to drop with each subsequent decade.[23,24] In the original reports, approximately 60 percent of women with CG had an antecedent episode of chorea in childhood, almost certainly SC. CG may also herald HD[25] or SLE.[26] It usually resolves without sequelae after delivery. In a single report of a fatal case,[27] neuronal loss and astrocytosis in the striatum, especially the caudate, were found. Although this pathology was nonspecific for CG, it suggests that the chorea has a structural basis in some cases.

Similarly, chorea may occur with the use of estrogens. Chorea after oral contraceptive use has been reported.[28–31] An interesting recent report[32] describes recurrent chorea in a 61-year-old woman after the use of a topical vaginal cream that contained conjugated estrogen. She had chorea gravidarum when she was younger. As estrogen may affect dopa-

mine receptor sensitivity by upregulating receptors in experimental animals, these reports suggest a role for hormone-induced chorea, especially in the setting of previously damaged basal ganglia.[9,28,33] As with CG, chorea with oral contraceptive use may be the presenting symptom of SLE.[34]

SYSTEMIC LUPUS ERYTHEMATOSUS AND ANTIPHOSPHOLIPID ANTIBODY SYNDROME

Of the other systemic disorders that cause chorea, SLE is the most common, although only about 2 percent of SLE patients have chorea.[35] As with SLE in general, it tends to occur primarily in girls and women, and it occurs more commonly in those with younger onset of their SLE. Chorea may be the sole neurological manifestation preceding the diagnosis of SLE in nearly one-quarter of those afflicted.[36] The chorea may last from days to years; it may be episodic and recurrent. It is often unilateral, although it may be generalized. Other neurological manifestations of SLE include stroke, transient ischemic attacks, seizures, migraine, psychosis, and dementia. Diagnosis of SLE is important because of treatment aimed at the more serious and life-threatening complications of the disease. Treatment of the chorea, as in other disorders, may occasionally require antidopaminergics. Steroids and antithrombotic agents, such as aspirin and warfarin, have also been found to be effective.[37]

A relatively new disorder, *primary antiphospholipid antibody syndrome* (PAPS), has also been associated with chorea.[38] These patients do not fit criteria for SLE. Clinically, PAPS is also associated with, among other things, stroke, transient cerebral ischemia, migraines, recurrent spontaneous abortions, venous thrombosis, cardiac valvular dysfunction, and thrombocytopenia.[39–42] The hallmark is the presence of antiphospholipid antibodies (aPL), consisting of false-positive Venereal Disease Research Laboratories (VDRL) test, anticardiolipin antibody, and lupus anticoagulant, all of which are also associated with (and were first described in) SLE. These antibodies, both IgG and IgM, inhibit coagulation by interfering with phospholipid-dependent coagulation tests and prolong activated partial thromboplastin time *in vitro* but are paradoxically associated with thrombosis rather than bleeding.[43]

PATHOPHYSIOLOGY: IMMUNE-MEDIATED MECHANISM

Most interesting is the occurrence of chorea in SC, CG, SLE, PAPS, or without such associations in the presence of aPL.[44] Although thrombotic vascular occlusion is implicated in some cases,[45,46] the current theory of the pathophysiology of chorea in all these disorders in immunological. Many cases of chorea have now been reported with the presence of aPL in SLE[46,47] and PAPS.[48] Interestingly, there are now also cases of SC (or rheumatic fever)[49] and CG and/or oral contraceptive use[50,51] with evidence of aPL, and there are others with isolated aPL[52,53] who do not meet criteria for either SLE or PAPS. There are further cases with combination of SC, SLE, and aPL with chorea.[54]

As with SC, increased striatal to cortical FDG metabolism measured with PET was found in SLE patients,[55] and in a woman with alternating hemichorea with PAPS, evidence was found on PET for contralateral striatal hypermetabolism.[56] These findings, along with similar results in SC,[16,17] suggest that hypermetabolism in these disorders reflects an autoimmune process, with antibodies directly affecting basal ganglia neurons.[44,56] This hypothesis is supported by the work of Husby et al.,[57] who showed that antibodies from both serum and spinal fluid from SC patients cross-reacted with antigens in the cytoplasm of caudate and subthalamic nucleus neurons. Streptococcal antigens have also been shown to cross-react to neuronal epitopes,[58,59] as well as to cardiolipin,[58] further supporting the hypothesis of cross-reactive, antibody-mediated inflammation or hypermetabolic dysfunction in these conditions.

Hereditary Choreas: Neuroacanthocytosis

Neuroacanthocytosis (NA) is an uncommon familial disorder, recognized since the mid-1960s, that has also been called choreoacanthocytosis, familial amyotrophic chorea, amyotrophic chorea with acanthocytes, and Levine-Critchley syndrome.[60–66] The more general nomenclature is more appropriate, given the wide variety of neurological abnormalities involved. NA is characterized by acanthocytosis, normal beta-lipoproteins, and multiple movement disorders. Chorea is the most prominent finding, but dystonia (especially lingual action dystonia), motor and vocal tics, and parkinsonism all occur and may occur in the same individual. Lingual-labial dyskinesias may be so severe as to cause self-mutilation. An axonal sensorimotor polyneuropathy, mostly affecting the distal portion of nerves,[67] is common, along with attendant amyotrophy and, consequently, elevated creatine phosphokinase (CPK). Decreased or absent reflexes, dysarthria, and dysphagia also occur. Generalized seizures occur in more than one-half the cases. Cognitive impairment, on the other hand, has been less commonly reported, but mild frontal lobe dysfunction probably exists in at least one-half of affected individuals.[68–70] Onset is usually in the 20s to 30s, and death occurs, on average, in about 9 years.[69] It is most likely an autosomal-recessive disorder,[71] but autosomal dominance and X-linked inheritance have been proposed[70]; association of some cases with the McLeod phenotype (a weak expression of Kell blood group antigens), which is X-linked, has raised the issue of whether some patients with apparent NA and McLeod's syndrome have the same disease.[72–74] Treatment is symptomatic; the chorea may respond to reduction of dopaminergic transmission (although concomitant parkinsonism may worsen), and seizures should be treated with appropriate anticonvulsants.

Pathologically, the findings in the central nervous system are principally confined to the basal ganglia. The caudate and putamen are primarily affected, with neuronal loss and gliosis. The globus pallidus is almost as severely involved. Cortex, subthalamic nucleus, cerebellum, pons, and medulla are generally spared.[69] In cases with prominent parkinsonism, reduced neuronal density in the substantia nigra, primarily in the ventrolateral region, has been reported.[75] The pathology of the peripheral nerves reveals a distal axonal neuropathy.[67,76] In a study of the neurochemical findings in the brains of patients with NA, the main abnormality was depletion of dopamine and its metabolites, particularly in the striatum; there were also increases in norepinephrine in putamen and globus pallidus and marked reduction in substance P in striatum and substantia nigra.[77]

Functional neuroimaging with PET in patients with NA has demonstrated striatal hypometabolism with FDG,[78,79] which is similar to findings in HD.[15] Brooks et al. evaluated the presynaptic and postsynaptic dopaminergic system in NA.[80] They found ^{18}F-fluorodopa (^{18}F-dopa) uptake to be normal in caudate and anterior putamen but significantly reduced (in the range of patients with Parkinson's disease) in the posterior putamen. Using ^{11}C-labeled raclopride to evaluate the integrity of striatal D2 receptors, they found reduction in both caudate and putamen to cerebellum uptake ratios, reflecting a 65 percent (caudate) and 53 percent (putamen) loss of D2 receptor binding sites. Their findings indicate a loss of nigrostriatal dopaminergic projections and of D2-receptor neurons and are consistent with a clinical picture of both chorea and parkinsonism in NA.

The erythrocyte abnormalities in NA have been a subject of scrutiny, and some feel that the red cell membrane dysfunction may hold the key to understanding the pathophysiology of this disorder. Although acanthocytes define the disorder, they are variably seen in this disease, and they may be absent in an occasional patient.[76] They are also frequently seen, or can be induced, in obligate heterozygotes.[81] The red blood cells of patients with NA can be induced to form spiny or rounded projections by dilution in normal saline, in vitro aging, or contact with glass.[82] Interestingly, echinocytic transformation is completely reversible by incubation with chlorpromazine. NA erythrocytes also have abnormal membrane-bound fatty acid structures, with increases in palmitic (C16:0) and docosahexaenoic (C22:6) acids and reduction in stearic acid (C18:0).[83] Bosman and coworkers[84,85] have demonstrated abnormal erythrocyte band 3 structure and sulfate flux measurements, indicating that anion transport activity is reduced in the erythrocytes of patients with definite NA and with likely NA but without acanthocytes. Their plasma also showed distinct antibrain immunoreactivity; measuring sulfate transport and plasma antibrain immunoreactivity may be useful in cementing a diagnosis in a disorder with a variable phenotype.

Hereditary Choreas: Benign Hereditary Chorea

Benign hereditary chorea (BHC), also called hereditary nonprogressive chorea, is another rare disorder. It is primarily symmetric and distal, with onset in childhood and little if any progression beyond adolescence, which may help differentiate it from HD.[86,87] Few other neurological abnormalities are present, with the occasional exception of ataxia, dysarthria, pyramidal tract signs, and postural/action tremor.[88] Although cognitive processes are generally normal, intellectual impairment has been reported in one family.[89] Occasionally, the chorea has been found to be progressive.[90,91] In another sibship in which the basic disorder was compatible with a diagnosis of BHC, monocular horizontal nystagmus (beginning in infancy and remitting in childhood, along with the chorea) and peripheral cataracts were also found. It is questioned whether this is a form of BHC or another familial illness.[92] Functional neuroimaging has not been helpful in differentiating this form of chorea from others. Striatal FDG metabolism was found to be decreased in one study[93] and normal in another.[94]

BHC appears to be autosomal-dominant, although rare reports of autosomal-recessive and X-linkage are extant.[95] The suggestion has also been made that BHC and HD may represent allelic forms of the same disorder. It is very likely that some families may, in fact, have HD, as in some of the cases with progressive chorea. Recently, one family was reported to have the expanded CAG repeat in the HD gene, suggesting that some families with so-called "benign" chorea may, in fact, be a phenotypic variant of HD.[96] Genetic testing should be performed in these families to rule out HD. The genetics of BHC should ultimately be able to define the disease.

Hereditary Choreas: Dentatorubropallidoluysian Atrophy

An extremely rare autosomal-dominant disorder, *dentatorubropallidoluysian atrophy* (DRPLA) is characterized by its distinctive pathology with extensive cell loss and gliosis in (as its name implies) the dentate nucleus, the red nucleus, the external globus pallidus, and the subthalamic nucleus.[97] DRPLA has a variable phenotypic picture, including chorea, myoclonus, epilepsy, cerebellar ataxia, and dementia, and comprising both juvenile and adult onset. Three clinical subtypes have been proposed: Type I, ataxochoreoathetoid type; Type II, the pseudo-Huntington type; Type III, the myoclonic-epileptic type.[98] Warner et al.,[97] however, suggest that, as phenotypic variation is the rule, rather than the exception, in autosomal-dominant inherited diseases (as in the hereditary ataxias and the probably mislabeled olivopontocerebellar atrophies[99]), the clinical subclassification is inappropriate and misleading.

The molecular genetic defect of DPRLA has recently been determined. It is, like HD, a trinucleotide repeat of CAG on chromosome 12p.[100–103] Anticipation is a feature of this disorder, as it is in HD, and accounts for the differences in juvenile and adult onset.[100] The molecular genetics of this disorder become key information in defining syndromes, as in the case of a kindred with the so-called Haw River syndrome,[104] which underwent molecular reevaluation; expanded DRPLA alleles were discovered in this family.[105]

Senile Chorea

Senile chorea is an insidiously developing generalized choreic disorder, primarily involving the limbs and occurring in individuals more than 60 years old with normal mentation, no family history, and no other apparent etiology. It is another unusual and controversial entity, with opinion divided as to whether it is a single disorder or a syndrome with multiple etiologies.[106] Few pathological reports exist; a very early study by Alcock[107] described atrophy and cell loss in both the caudate and putamen to a lesser degree than that seen in HD, whereas a more recent case examined by Friedman and Ambler demonstrated primarily putaminal cell loss and gliosis but with caudate sparing.[106]

Some authors have considered senile chorea to be a variant of late-onset HD. A study by Shinotoh et al.,[108] in which they measured CAG trinucleotide repeat expansion in the HD gene in four patients with senile chorea, demonstrated normal repeat lengths, supporting the notion that senile chorea is a separate and distinct nosological entity.

Vascular Chorea, Hemichorea, and Hemiballismus

Both generalized chorea and, more commonly, hemichorea and hemiballismus may occur as a result of vascular disease. Classically, hemiballismus was considered a result of a lesion of the subthalamic nucleus[109–111]; it is now known that a variety of lesions in the basal ganglia (and in corticostriatal pathways as well) that interrupt both afferent and efferent subthalamopallidal pathways, detected both at autopsy and with modern neuroimaging, may cause persistent or paroxysmal choreic or ballistic movements, and vascular insults in many areas, including caudate, putamen, thalamus, and corona radiata, have been reported.[45,112–126] Vascular etiologies include ischemia, infarction, hemorrhage, and vascular malformations (arteriovenous malformations,[127,128] venous angiomas,[129] and cavernous angiomas[130,131]). Both *hyperglycemia* and *hypoglycemia* may produce hemichorea/hemiballism, generalized chorea, and paroxysmal chorea, presumably also on a vascular basis.[132–141] We will consider the generation of all of these types of movements to be interchangeable. In fact, early authors, including Martin and Alcock,[110] argued that hemiballism was really just an intense, more violent form of hemichorea and that ballistic movements generally were more proximal than choreiform movements. More recent evidence shows that experimental chorea and ballism from different lesions may result in the same reduction in subthalamopallidal activity,[142,143] and may also be produced by the same lesion as well,[144,145] further supporting the notion that they result from a common neural mechanism.

Clinically, in the majority of patients with chorea or ballism of vascular etiology, the onset is abrupt. The face is usually spared. Most patients recover spontaneously within 2–4 weeks, although some do continue to have choreic movement of long duration. In the interim, when the movement interferes with function, patients may respond very well to neuroleptics (low-dose haloperidol) or to dopamine depleters, in the short term. Nevertheless, as many of these patients may be elderly, they may be more susceptible to the side effects of these drugs, such as parkinsonism and tardive dyskinesia. A safer (from the perspective of extrapyramidal adverse effects) and, possibly, an equally effective therapeutic choice is clozapine.[146] Unlike SC, the response to valproate in vascular hemichorea-hemiballism is variable.[147–149]

As mentioned above, neuroimaging (computed tomography (CT) and, especially, MRI) are particularly helpful in localizing an anatomic lesion. PET, however, has not shown specific abnormalities. In one study of hemichorea, the contralateral striatum had decreased glucose metabolism, and striatal ^{18}F-dopa uptake was normal.[150]

Other Neurological and Systemic Diseases

HYPERTHYROIDISM

Chorea secondary to *hyperthyroidism*, an eminently treatable disorder, is rare but may affect about 2 percent of individuals with hyperthyroidism,[151] although this may be an overestimation. It may be clinically indistinguishable from the chorea of other etiologies and may be bilateral or unilateral, persistent[152–158] or paroxysmal.[159,160] Hyperthyroidism is generally reversible with normalization of thyroid hormone levels but may also respond (while still in the hyperthyroid state) to dopaminergic blocking agents.[161] The pathophysiology of hyperthyroid chorea is not understood, but theories include altered function, rather than altered structure, of the striatum.[1] In view of the seriousness of the disease and the ease of evaluation and treatment, a thyroid screen should be checked in adults who develop chorea, including paroxysmal choreic movements, of otherwise undetermined cause.

POLYCYTHEMIA VERA

Polycythemia vera, a hematologic disorder that is more prevalent in men, can rarely be the cause of chorea; interestingly, when it occurs (in less than 1 percent of cases), it is more common in women (again, invoking a suspicion of hormonal influence?) and may be the presenting sign of polycythemia in about two-thirds of patients.[162] Patients may also demonstrate facial erythrosis or splenomegaly.[163] Onset is usually after age 50, and the chorea is generally bilateral and symmetric. It responds to treatment with both reduction of hyperviscosity and antidopaminergics.[164–166] Pathophysiologically, the hyperviscosity may lead to reduced cerebral blood flow with resultant localized ischemia, and the results may be similar to those in other vascular choreas. As with hyperthyroidism, presentation of chorea in later adulthood should trigger a hematologic workup.

METABOLIC DISORDERS

Other *metabolic* causes of chorea, in addition to the aforementioned hyperglycemia,[132–136,139–141] hypoglycemia,[137–139] and hyperthyroidism,[151–161] include hyponatremia,[167] hypernatremia,[168] hypocalcemia,[169] hypomagnesemia,[170] hypoparathyroidism,[171–174] hyperparathyroidism,[175] and hepatic encephalopathy (acquired hepatocerebral degeneration).[176–180] Rapid correction of hyponatremia with resultant central pontine myelinolysis has also been reported to be associated with chorea.[181,182]

MULTIPLE SCLEROSIS

Although it too is rare, movement disorders have been reported as a complication of *multiple sclerosis*. Paroxysmal dyskinesias may be the most common presentation and may include choreic movements.[183] Persistent chorea (bilateral or hemichorea) and hemiballism have also been noted to be an infrequent accompaniment with multiple sclerosis.[184–188] Demyelinating plaques in the basal ganglia have occasionally been seen.[184,188]

POSTPUMP CHOREA

A little-known entity outside of pediatric cardiovascular services, *postpump chorea* not infrequently accompanies cardiopulmonary bypass surgery with deep hypothermia for congenital heart disease in children. It was first recognized in 1960[189] and described fully the following year by Bergouignan et al.[190] There have been a number of other reports since then, with the incidence of chorea within 2 weeks of surgery varying from 1.2 to 18 percent, depending on the center studied.[191–199] Children range from a few months to 3 years old at the time they undergo surgery. They undergo deep hypothermia, and there is an association with circulatory arrest. The chorea may resolve within a few months,[194,197] or it may persist (the longest follow-up of a child with irreversible chorea is >10 years).[197] Most patients with postpump chorea syndrome develop other neurological abnormalities, including seizures (postoperative and occasionally persistent) and developmental delay and cognitive deficits.[193,195,197] The persistent chorea does not respond well to most treatment modalites.[197] Most reports of CT and MRI scans have been normal or show diffuse cerebral atrophy, but a single study with FDG-PET demonstrated hypometabolism in the left frontal lobe.[197] Interestingly, a single-photon emission computed tomographic (SPECT) evaluation of another child showed nonspecific hypoperfusion of frontal lobe and cerebellum; this child had an unremarkable CT and MRI as well.[198]

The pathophysiology of this intriguing disorder is, not surprisingly, unknown. Hypoxic-ischemic damage and thromboembolic infarction in the basal ganglia circuitry have been proposed, especially as their occurrence is not uncommon in the setting of cardiac bypass surgery.[197] Medlock and colleagues concluded that the absence of structural lesions in the basal ganglia after prolonged chorea suggested a biochemical or microembolic etiology.[197] Another study, by Curless et al.,[199] of three children with postpump chorea found that none had significant intraoperative hypoxemia or hypotension but that all three had hypocapnia and respiratory alkalosis during the rewarming period; those researchers hypothesize that hypocapnia-induced cerebral vasoconstriction may contribute to ischemic damage in critical focal brain areas. In a recent neuropathological examination of two patients, Kupsky and co-workers[200] demonstrated selective neuronal loss and gliosis of the external globus pallidus; areas of the brain usually susceptible to hypoxic-ischemic necrosis were spared. This finding correlates with the older evidence that the globus pallidus bears the brunt of the damage in children who die after cardiac surgery.[189] One other theory proposed for the mechanism of injury here is based on auto-immunity[197]; as with the situation in rheumatic disease,[57] could there be antibodies directed against the basal ganglia in these children? In a slightly different but related story,[201] a child with congenital heart disease received a heart transplant, with deep hypothermia and circulatory arrest, at age 12. Four weeks later, she developed generalized chorea that responded dramatically to corticosteroids, which makes an autoimmune mechanism a reasonable hypothesis. It is unclear as to whether there is a connection between this patient's cardiac transplantation and the chorea that developed after bypass surgery. There are no reports of specific aPL being evaluated in any of these cases, which may shed more light on the situation.

Other Causes

DRUGS, TOXINS, INFECTIONS, NEOPLASMS, AND DEGENERATIVE DISORDERS

A plethora of case reports exist describing the association of chorea with drugs, degenerative disorders, medical conditions, and a variety of other situations. In some instances, there is only a single report that documents the connection. Previous authors have compiled extensive lists[1,202,203]; Table 38-1 serves to amend and to expand those before its compilation with more recent references (previously mentioned in text, as well as Refs.[204–254]). (Accordingly, only those new references will be noted; all others are to be understood as referred

to the lists of Weiner and Lang,[1] Duvoisin,[202] or Shoulson.[203]) As with other conditions, treatment of the underlying disease process should be the primary goal in correcting the cause of the chorea.

Paroxysmal Dyskinesias

Paroxysmal dyskinesias are movement disorders occurring as "attacks" without loss of consciousness, with recovery between attacks. Many of the etiologic factors already discussed as the causes of choreic and/or ballistic movements can result in paroxysmal chorea, as well as persistent movements. Nonepileptic causes of symptomatic paroxysmal chorea include vascular causes,[126,128] hypoglycemia,[138] hyperglycemia,[141] hyperthyroidism,[159,160] hypoparathyroidism,[171,172] and multiple sclerosis.[183]

There are two major primary forms of paroxysmal dyskinesias, *paroxysmal kinesigenic choreoathetosis* (PKC) and *paroxysmal dystonic choreoathetosis* (PDC), and an *intermediate form* of paroxysmal choreoathetosis between PKC and PDC.[1] None are particularly good terms, as the movements may not necessarily be choreoathetotic, but they are ingrained in the literature. They may be primarily dystonic syndromes, in fact, but will be described briefly here.

PKC is precipitated by sudden movements, particularly after the patient is coming out of a rest position, and by focal movements, stress, excitement, or hyperventilation. Abnormal involuntary movements may span the spectrum of dystonic to choreic to ballistic, but dystonic movements probably

---

TABLE 38-1 Conditions Associated with Chorea and Ballism

Drugs	Calcium-channel blockers
Neuroleptics, dopamine receptor blockers	Cinnarizine
Phenothiazines (e.g., chlorpromazine)	Flunarizine
Butyrophenones (e.g., haloperidol)	Verapamil[212]
Thioxanthines (e.g., thiothixene)	Other drugs
Benzamides (e.g., metoclopramide)	Alcohol (intoxication and withdrawal)
Antiparkinson agents	Amoxapine
L-dopa	Baclofen[213]
Dopamine agonists (bromocriptine, pergolide)	Cyclizine
Amantadine	Cyclosporine[214]
Anticholinergics (including atropine)[204,205]	Cyproheptadine,[215] other antihistamines
Anticonvulsants	Diazepam-pentobarbital withdrawal[216]
Phenytoin[206]	Diazoxide
Carbamazepine	Digoxin[217]
Phenobarbital	Isoniazid
Ethosuximide	Lithium[212,218,219]
Valproate[207]	Methyldopa
Stimulants	Pentamidine[220]
Methamphetamine,[208] other amphetamines[209]	Ranitidine, cimetidine[221]
Methylphenidate	Reserpine
Cocaine, crack cocaine ("crack dancing")[210]	Triazolam
Caffeine	Tricyclic antidepressants[222]
Pemoline	**Hereditary/Degenerative Disorders**
Aminophylline	Alzheimer's disease[223]
Theophylline[211]	Amino acid disorders (glutaric acidemia/aciduria type I,[224]
Steroids	propionic acidemia,[225] cystinuria, homocystinuria,
Anabolic steroids	phenylketonuria, Hartnup disease,
Conjugated topical estrogens[32]	argininosuccinicaciduria)
Oral contraceptives	Ataxia-telangiectasia[226]
Opiates	Benign hereditary chorea[87,91,94]
Methadone	

TABLE 38-1—(*continued*)

Hereditary/Degenerative Disorders
  Carbohydrate metabolism (galactosemia,
    mucopolysaccharidoses, mucolipidoses, pyruvate
    dehydrogenase deficiency)
  Dentatorubropallidoluysian atrophy[97,100–105]
  Familial striatal necrosis
  Gilles de la Tourette syndrome
  Hallervorden-Spatz disease
  Hereditary spinocerebellar ataxias, including Machado-Joseph
    disease
  Huntington's disease
  Idiopathic basal ganglia calcinosis
  Leigh's disease
  Lesch-Nyhan syndrome
  Lipidoses (GM$_1$ and GM$_2$ gangliosidosis, sphingolipidosis,
    Gaucher's disease, globoid cell leukodystrophy,
    metachromatic leukodystrophy, ceroid
    lipofuscinosis)
  Mitochondrial encephalomyopathy[227,228]
  Multiple-system atrophy[229]
  Myoclonus epilepsy
  Neuroacanthocytosis[66–71,75–85]
  Paroxysmal dystonic choreoathetosis
  Paroxysmal kinesigenic choreoathetosis
  Pelizaeus-Merzbacher disease
  Pick's disease
  Progressive supranuclear palsy[230]
  Sea-blue histiocytosis
  Sturge-Weber syndrome
  Sulfite-oxidase deficiency
  Tuberous sclerosis[231]
  Wilson's disease
  Xeroderma pigmentosum
Autoimmune/Collagen Vascular
  Systemic lupus erythematosus[39,55]
  Primary antiphospholipid syndrome[39–42,56]
  Rheumatoid arthritis
  Behçet's disease
  Henoch-Schönlein syndrome
  Periarteritis nodosa
  Churg-Straus syndrome[232]
Autoimmune Parainfectious
  Sydenham's chorea (poststreptococcal)[6,7,11–14,16,17]
  Other infections: Pertussis, varicella, diphtheria
  Serum sickness reaction to tetanus toxoid
Infectious Disease, including Prions-Related
  Scarlet fever (streptococcal)
  Bacterial endocarditis
  Typhoid fever
  Legionnaire's disease
  Lyme disease
  Neurosyphilis[233]
  Mycoplasma pneumoniae encephalitis[234]
  Encephalitis lethargica (von Economo's encephalitis)
  Viral meningoencephalitis[235] (mumps, measles, varicella,
    influenza)
  Postvaccinial
  Infectious mononucleosis
  Herpes simplex encephalitis relapse[236,237]
  Creutzfeldt-Jakob disease[222]
  Subacute sclerosing panencephalitis
  Cysticercosis[238]

  Human immunodeficiency virus-related
  Toxoplasmosis[239–241]
Other Systemic
  Acute intermittent porphyria
  Polycythemia vera[164–166]
  Sarcoidosis
  Sickle cell anemia
  Transitional myeloproliferative disease
Metabolic
  Hypoglycemia[137,139] and hyperglycemia[133–136,139–141]
  Hyponatremia and hypernatremia (and central pontine
    myelinolysis[181,182])
  Hypocalcemia
  Hypomagnesemia
  Hepatic failure, acquired hepatocerebral degeneration[180]
  Renal failure
Endocrine
  Hyperthyroidism[154–158,160]
  Hypoparathyroidism,[173] pseudohypoparathyroidism, and
    hyperparathyroidism
  Chorea gravidarum
  Addison's disease
Nutritional
  Beriberi (thiamine deficiency)
  Wernicke's encephalopathy[242]
  Pellagra (niacin deficiency)
  B$_{12}$ deficiency in infants
Toxins
  Carbon monoxide[243]
  Manganese[244]
  Mercury
  Organophosphate poisoning[245]
  Thallium
  Toluene (glue-sniffing)
Neoplastic
  Primary brain tumor
  Metastatic brain tumor
  Primary central nervous system (CNS) lymphoma[246,247]
  Acute lymphoblastic leukemia (with lupus anticoagulant)[248]
  Paraneoplastic[249]
Cerebrovascular
  Basal ganglia, subcortical infarcts[119–121,124,136]
  Basal ganglia, subcortical ischemia[123]
  Basal ganglia, thalamic hemorrhage[118,122]
  Epidural hematoma
  Subdural hematoma
  Moyamoya disease[250–252]
  Vascular malformations (arteriovenous malformations,[127,128]
    venous angioma,[129] cavernous angioma[130,131])
Other Neurological and Miscellaneous Disorders
  Head trauma
  Migraine
  Multiple sclerosis[183,188]
  Orobuccolingual dyskinesias of aging
  Poststatus epilepticus[253]
  Senile chorea[106,108]
  Cerebral palsy
  Infantile chorea in bronchopulmonary dysplasia[254]
  Kernicterus
  Physiological chorea of infancy
  Postpump chorea[192–201]

New additions or updated references only are noted. More than one category may apply to a single condition (e.g., Autoimmune and Endocrine for chorea gravidarum, Autoimmune and Neoplastic for acute lymphoblastic leukemia with antiphospholipid antibodies), and some are difficult to classify (e.g., post-pump chorea), but each item will only be listed once.

SOURCE: Adapted from Weiner and Lang,[1] and Duvoisin,[202] and Shoulson.[203]

predominate; they may be bilateral or unilateral. They usually begin in youth and diminish with age. Attacks may be frequent (100/day) or rare (2/year). Consciousness is spared. The attacks usually do not last longer than 2 minutes, and never more than 5 minutes. There is often a prodromal sensation of tightness or tingling, and it may warn the individual to allow avoidance of the attacks. Although the EEG is normal, patients respond well to low doses of phenytoin or other anticonvulsants. PKC, as well as PDC and the intermediate form, may be familial.[1]

PDC has similarities to PKC but differs in that onset age is younger (infancy) and the duration of the attacks is longer (up to hours). The movements are mostly dystonic, but may be choreic as well. The diseases also differ in terms of their precipitating events: in PDC, alcohol and caffeine are the precipitants, as well as stress or excitement. Frequency is also less than in PKC, and treatment differs. Anticonvulsants do not usually help. In PDC, oxazepam is the treatment of choice. Also effective are clonazepam, acetazolamide, and low-dose haloperidol.[1]

Painful Legs and Moving Toes

Although it is not a true choreic disorder, we include the uncommon entity *painful legs and moving toes* in this chapter. First described in 1971,[255] this condition appears to be a peripherally derived movement disorder. The syndrome consists of pain in the affected limb associated with spontaneous, involuntary, wriggling movements of the toes. The movements may be bilateral or unilateral, continuous or intermittent, occasionally stopping completely for a number of minutes.[255-260] Rarely, the upper limbs may be involved instead of the legs and toes (*painful arms and moving fingers*).[261,262] The disability involved results largely from the pain and rarely from digit movement. Unfortunately, all treatment modalities, both for hyperkinetic movements and for pain, have been fruitless, with the occasional exception of those used for sympathetic block. Painful legs and moving toes frequently occurs in individuals with a history of lumbosacral disease, including spinal nerve root injury, peripheral trauma, or peripheral neuropathy, suggesting a peripheral origin for the disorder, but with postulated central nervous system alterations in segmental motor pathways.[263] The severe and unrelenting pain makes the diagnosis clear, despite the disorder's rarity. There also exists a variant, *painless legs and moving toes,* in which the characteristics of the movements are the same, but pain is absent.[263,264] In these patients, the digit movements may be bothersome, and partial relief may be attained by means of injection of botulinum toxin into the toe extensor and flexor muscles, (MH Mark, personal observations).

Summary

Chorea is a rare manifestation of some very common diseases (vascular disease, hyperthyroidism), as well as a common finding in very rare disorders (neuroacanthocytosis, benign hereditary chorea). Choreiform movements should alert the physician that any one of a legion of conditions may be responsible, and a thorough physical examination with appropriate laboratory tests is in order. The pathophysiology of chorea is still not understood, but both animal studies and careful observation of clinical phenomena are bringing us closer to elucidating the elusive puzzle of the choreas.

References

1. Weiner WJ, Lang AE: *Movement Disorders—A Comprehensive Survey.* Mount Kisco, NY: Futura Publishing Company, 1989.
2. Sydenham T: *The Entire Works of Thomas Sydenham.* London: Sydenham Society, 1848–1850.
3. Nausieda PA, Grossman BJ, Koller WC, et al: Sydenham's chorea: An update. *Neurology* 30:331–334, 1980.
4. Karademir S, Demirceken F, Atalay S, et al: Acute rheumatic fever in children in the Ankara area in 1990–1992 and comparison with a previous study in 1980–1989. *Acta Paediatr* 83:862–865, 1994.
5. Figueroa F, Berrios X, Gutierrez M, et al: Anticardiolipin antibodies in acute rheumatic fever. *J Rheumatol* 19:1175–1180, 1992.
6. Swedo SE, Leonard HL, Schapiro MB, et al: Sydenham's chorea: Physical and psychological symptoms of St Vitus dance. *Pediatrics* 91:706–713, 1993.
7. Swedo SE, Leonard HL: Childhood movement disorders and obsessive compulsive disorder. *J Clin Psychiatry* 55(suppl):32–37, 1994.
8. Bird MT, Palkes H, Prensky AL: A follow up study of Sydenham's chorea. *Neurology* 26:601–606, 1976.
9. Schipper HM: Sex hormones in stroke, chorea, and anticonvulsant therapy. *Semin Neurol* 8:181–186, 1988.
10. Ch'ien LT, Economides AN, Lemmi H: Sydenham's chorea and seizures: Clinical and electroencephalographic studies. *Arch Neurol* 35:382–385, 1978.
11. Swedo SE: Sydenham's chorea: A model for childhood autoimmune neuropsychiatric disorders. *J Am Med Assoc* 272:1788–1791, 1994.
12. Kienzle GD, Breger RK, Chun RW, et al: Sydenham chorea: MR manifestations in two cases. *AJR Am J Neuroradiol* 12:73–76, 1991.
13. Traill Z, Pike M, Byrne J: Sydenham's chorea: A case showing reversible striatal abnormalities on CT and MRI. *Dev Med Child Neurol* 37:270–273, 1995.
14. Giedd JN, Rapoport JL, Kruesi MJP, et al: Sydenham's chorea: Magnetic resonance imaging of the basal ganglia. *Neurology* 45:2199–2202, 1995.
15. Grafton ST, Mazziotta JC, Pahl JJ, et al: Serial changes of cerebral glucose metabolism and caudate size in persons at risk for Huntington's disease. *Arch Neurol* 49:1161–1167, 1992.
16. Goldman S, Amrom D, Szliwowski HB, et al: Reversible striatal hypermetabolism in a case of Sydenham's chorea. *Mov Disord* 8:355–358, 1993.
17. Weindl A, Kuwert T, Leenders KL, et al: Increased striatal glucose consumption in Sydenham's chorea. *Mov Disord* 8:437–444, 1993.
18. Shannon KM, Fenichel GM. Pimozide treatment of Sydenham's chorea. *Neurology* 40:186, 1990.
19. Jankovic J, Orman J. Tetrabenazine therapy of dystonia, chorea, tics, and other dyskinesias. *Neurology* 38:391–394, 1988.
20. Daoud AS, Zaki M, Shakir R, al-Saleh Q: Effectiveness of sodium valproate in the treatment of Sydenham's chorea. *Neurology* 40:1140–1141, 1990.
21. Wolf RE, McBeath JG: Chorea gravidarum in systemic lupus erythematosus. *J Rheumatol* 12:992–993, 1985.

22. Willson P, Preece AA: Chorea gravidarum: A statistical study of 951 collected cases, 846 from the literature and 105 previously unreported. *Arch Intern Med* 49:471–533, 1932.

23. Beresford OD, Graham AM: Chorea gravidarum. *J Obstet Gynaecol Br Emp* 57:616–625, 1950.

24. Lewis BV, Parsons M: Chorea gravidarum. *Lancet* 1:284–288, 1966.

25. Bolt JM: Abortion and Huntington's chorea. *Br Med J* 1:840, 1968.

26. Donaldson IM, Espiner EA: Disseminated lupus erythematosus presenting as chorea gravidarum. *Arch Neurol* 25:240–244, 1971.

27. Ishikawa K, Kim RC, Givelber H, Collins GH: Chorea gravidarum: Report of a fatal case with neuropathological observations. *Arch Neurol* 37:429–432, 1980.

28. Nausieda PA, Koller WC, Weiner WJ, Klawans HL: Chorea induced by oral contraceptives. *Neurology* 29:1605–1609, 1979.

29. Galimberti D: Chorea induced by the use of oral contraceptives: Report of a case and review of the literature. *Ital J Neurol Sci* 8:383–386, 1987.

30. Leys D, Destee A, Petit H, Warot P: Chorea associated with oral contraception. *J Neurol* 235:46–48, 1987.

31. Driesen JJ, Wolters EC: Oral contraceptive induced paraballism. *Clin Neurol Neurosurg* 89:49–51, 1987.

32. Caviness JN, Muenter MD: An unusual cause of recurrent chorea. *Mov Disord* 6:355–357, 1991.

33. Hruska RE, Silbergeld EK: Increased dopamine receptor sensitivity after estrogen treatment using the rat rotation model. *Science* 208:1466–1468, 1980.

34. Iskander MK, Khan M: Chorea as the initial presentation of oral contraceptive related systemic lupus erythematosus. *J Rheumatol* 16:850–851, 1989.

35. Gibson T, Myers AR: Nervous system involvement in systemic lupus erythematosus. *Ann Rheum Dis* 35:398–406, 1976.

36. Bruyn GW, Padberg G: Chorea and systemic lupus erythematosus. *Eur Neurol* 23:278–290, 1984.

37. Feigin A, Kieburtz K, Shoulson I: Treatment of Huntington's disease and other choreic disorders, in Kurlan R (ed): *Treatment of Movement Disorders*. Philadelphia: JB Lippincott, pp 337–364, 1995.

38. Hughes GRV: Thrombosis, abortion, cerebral disease and the lupus anticoagulant. *Br Med J* 287:1088–1089, 1983.

39. Asherson RA, Khamashta MA, Gil A, et al: Cerebrovascular disease and antiphospholipid antibodies in systemic lupus erythematosus, lupus-like disease, and the primary antiphospholipid syndrome. *Am J Med* 86:391–399, 1989.

40. Asherson RA, Khamashta MA, Ordi-Ros J, et al: The "primary" antiphospholipid syndrome: Major clinical and serological features. *Medicine* 68:366–374, 1989.

41. Levine SR, Welch KM: The spectrum of neurologic disease associated with antiphospholipid antibodies: Lupus anticoagulants and anticardiolipin antibodies. *Arch Neurol* 44:876–883, 1987.

42. Levine SR, Deegan MJ, Futrell N, Welch KMA: Cerebrovascular and neurologic disease associated with antiphospholipid antibodies: 48 cases. *Neurology* 40:1181–1189, 1990.

43. Boey ML, Colaco CB, Gharavi AE, et al: Thrombosis in SLE: Striking association with the presence of circulating "lupus" anticoagulant. *Br Med J* 287:1021–1023, 1983.

44. Bouchez B, Arnott G, Hatron PY, et al: Chorée et lupus erythemateux disséminé avec anticoagulant circulant. Trois cas. *Rev Neurol (Paris)* 141:571–577, 1985.

45. Kirk A, Harding SR: Cardioembolic caudate infarction as a cause of hemichorea in lupus anticoagulant syndrome. *Can J Neurol Sci* 20:162–164, 1993.

46. Asherson RA, Derksen RH, Harris EN, et al: Chorea in systemic lupus erythematosus and "lupus-like" disease: Association with antiphospholipid antibodies. *Sem Arthritis Rheum* 16:253–259, 1987.

47. Khamashta MA, Gil A, Anciones B, et al: Chorea in systemic lupus erythematosus: Association with antiphospholipid antibodies. *Ann Rheum Dis* 47:681–683, 1988.

48. Vlachoyiannopoulos PG, Dimou G, Siamopoulou-Mavridou A: Chorea as a manifestation of the antiphospholipid syndrome in childhood. *Clin Exp Rheumatol* 9:303–305, 1991.

49. de la Fuente Fernandez R: Rheumatic chorea and lupus anticoagulant. *J Neurol Neurosurg Psychiatry* 57:1545, 1994.

50. Lubbe WF, Walker EB: Chorea gravidarum associated with circulating lupus anticoagulant: Successful outcome of pregnancy with prednisone and aspirin therapy: Case report. *Br J Obstet Gynaecol* 90:487–490, 1983.

51. Omdal R, Roalso S: Chorea gravidarum and chorea associated with oral contraceptives—diseases due to antiphospholipid antibodies? *Acta Neurol Scand* 86:219–220, 1992.

52. Okseter K, Sirnes K: Chorea and lupus anticoagulant: A case report. *Acta Neurol Scand* 78:206–209, 1988.

53. Shimomura T, Takahashi S, Takahashi S: Chorea associated with antiphospholipid antibodies. *Clin Neurol* 32:989–993, 1992.

54. Besbas N, Damarguc I, Ozen S, et al: Association of antiphospholipid antibodies with systemic lupus erythematosus in a child presenting with chorea: A case report. *Eur J Pediatr* 153:891–893, 1994.

55. Guttman M, Lang AE, Garnett ES, et al: Regional cerebral glucose metabolism in SLE chorea: Further evidence that striatal hypometabolism is not a correlate of chorea. *Mov Disord* 2:201–210, 1987.

56. Furie R, Ishikawa T, Dhawan V, Eidelberg D: Alternating hemichorea in primary antiphospholipid syndrome: Evidence for contralateral striatal hypermetabolism. *Neurology* 44:2197–2199, 1994.

57. Hushy G, van de Rijn I, Zabriskie JB, et al: Antibodies reacting with cytoplasm of subthalamic and caudate nuclei neurons in chorea and acute rheumatic fever. *J Exp Med* 144:1094–1110, 1976.

58. Cunningham MW, Swerlick RA: Polyspecificity of antistreptococcal murine monoclonal antibodies and their implications in autoimmunity. *J Exp Med* 164:998–1012, 1986.

59. Bronze MS, Dale JB: Epitopes of streptococcal M proteins that evoke antibodies that cross-react with human brain. *J Immunol* 151:2820–2828, 1993.

60. Levine IM, Estes JW, Looney JM: Hereditary neurological disease with acanthocytosis. *Arch Neurol* 19:403–409, 1968.

61. Critchley EMR, Clark DB, Wikler A: Acanthocytosis and neurological disorder without abetalipoproteinemia. *Arch Neurol* 18:134–140, 1968.

62. Kito S, Itoga E, Hiroshige Y, et al: A pedigree of amyotrophic chorea with acanthocytosis. *Arch Neurol* 37:514–517, 1980.

63. Sakai T, Mawatari S, Iwashita H, et al: Choreoacanthocytosis: Clues to clinical diagnosis. *Arch Neurol* 38:335–338, 1981.

64. Sotaniemi KA: Chorea-acanthocytosis. Neurological disease with acanthocytosis. *Acta Neurol Scand* 68:53–56, 1983.

65. Sakai T, Iwashita H, Goto I, Kakugawa M: Neuroacanthocytosis syndrome and choreoacanthocytosis (Levine-Critchley syndrome). *Neurology* 35:1679, 1985.

66. Hardie RJ: Acanthocytosis and neurological impairment—a review. *Q J Med* 71:291–306, 1989.

67. Vita G, Serra S, Dattola R, et al: Peripheral neuropathy in amyotrophic chorea-acanthocytosis. *Ann Neurol* 26:583–587, 1989.

68. Delecluse F, Deleval J, Gerard J-M, et al: Frontal impairment and hypoperfusion in neuroacanthocytosis. *Arch Neurol* 48:232–234, 1991.

69. Rinne JO, Daniel SE, Scaravilli F, et al: The neuropathological features of neuroacanthocytosis. *Mov Disord* 9:297–304, 1994.

70. Hardie RJ, Pullon HWH, Harding AE, et al: Neuroacanthocytosis—a clinical, haematological and pathological study of 19 cases. *Brain* 114:13–49, 1991.

71. Vance JM, Pericak-Vance MA, Bowman MH, et al: Chorea-acanthocytosis: A report of three new families and implications for genetic counselling. *Am J Med Genet* 28:403–410, 1987.

72. Witt TN, Danek A, Reiter M, et al: McLeod syndrome: A distinct form of neuroacanthocytosis—report of 2 cases and literature review with emphasis on neuromuscular manifestations. *J Neurol* 239:302–306, 1992.

73. Takashima H, Sakai T, Iwashita H, et al: A family of McLeod syndrome, masquerading as chorea-acanthocytosis. *J Neurol Sci* 124:56–60, 1994.

74. Malandrini A, Fabrizi GM, Truschi F, et al: Atypical McLeod syndrome manifested as X-linked chorea-acanthocytosis, neuromyopathy and dilated cardiomyopathy: Report of a family. *J Neurol Sci* 124:89–94, 1994.

75. Rinne JO, Daniel SE, Scaravilli F, et al: Nigral degeneration in neuroacanthocytosis. *Neurology* 44:1629–1632, 1994.

76. Malandrini A, Fabrizi GM, Palmeri S, et al: Choreo-acanthocytosis-like phenotype without acanthocytes: Clinicopathological case report: A contribution to the knowledge of the functional pathology of the caudate nucleus. *Acta Neuropathol* 86:651–658, 1993.

77. de Yebenes JG, Brin MF, Mena MA, et al: Neurochemical findings in neuroacanthocytosis. *Mov Disord* 3:300–312, 1988.

78. Dubinsky RM, Hallett M, Levey R, Di Chiro G: Regional brain glucose metabolism in neuroacanthocytosis. *Neurology* 39:1253–1255, 1989.

79. Hosokawa S, Ichiya Y, Kuwabara Y, et al: Positron emission tomography in cases of chorea with different underlying diseases. *J Neurol Neurosurg Psychiatry* 50;1284–1287, 1987.

80. Brooks DJ, Ibanez V, Playford ED, et al: Presynaptic and postsynaptic striatal dopaminergic function in neuroacanthocytosis: A positron emission tomographic study. *Ann Neurol* 30:166–171, 1991.

81. Brin MF, Bressman SB, Fahn S, et al: Chorea-acanthocytosis: Clinical and laboratory features in five cases (abstr.) *Neurology* 35(suppl 1):110, 1985.

82. Feinberg TE, Cianci CD, Morrow JS, et al: Diagnostic tests for choreoacanthocytosis. *Neurology* 41:1000–1006, 1991.

83. Sakai T, Antoku Y, Iwashita H, et al: Chorea-acanthocytosis: Abnormal composition of covalently bound fatty acids of erythrocyte membrane proteins. *Ann Neurol* 29:664–669, 1991.

84. Kay MM, Goodman J, Lawrence C, Bosman G: Membrane channel protein abnormalities and autoantibodies in neurological disease. *Brain Res Bull* 24:105–111, 1990.

85. Bosman GJ, Bartholmeus IG, De Grip WJ, Horstink MW: Erythrocyte anion transporter and antibrain immunoreactivity in chorea-acanthocytosis: A contribution to etiology, genetics, and diagnosis. *Brain Res Bull* 33:523–528, 1994.

86. Haerer AF, Currier RD, Jackson JF: Hereditary nonprogressive chorea of early onset. N Engl J Med 276:1220–1224, 1967.

87. Wheeler PG, Weaver DD, Dobyns WB: Benign hereditary chorea. *Pediatr Neurol* 9:337–340, 1993.

88. Pincus JH, Chutorian A: Familial benign chorea with intention tremor: A clinical entity. *J Pediatr* 70:724–729, 1967.

89. Leli DA, Furlow TW, Falgout JC: Benign familial chorea: An association with intellectual impairment. *J Neurol Neurosurg Psychiatry* 47:471–474, 1984.

90. Behan PO, Bone I: Hereditary chorea without dementia. *J Neurol Neurosurg Psychiatry* 40:687–691, 1977.

91. Schady W, Meara RJ: Hereditary progressive chorea without dementia. *J Neurol Neurosurg Psychiatry* 51:295–297, 1988.

92. Wheeler PG, Dobyns WB, Plager DA, Ellis FD: Familial remitting chorea, nystagmus, cataracts. *Am J Med Genet* 47:1215–1217, 1993.

93. Suchowersky O, Hayden MR, Martin WRW, et al: Cerebral metabolism of glucose in benign hereditary chorea. *Mov Disord* 1:33–45, 1986.

94. Kuwert T, Lange HW, Langen KJ, et al: Normal striatal glucose consumption in two patients with benign hereditary chorea as measured by positron emission tomography. *J Neurol* 237:80–84, 1990.

95. Bruyn GW, Myrianthopoulos NC: Chronic juvenile hereditary chorea, in Vinken PH, Bruyn GW, Klawans HL (eds): *Handbook of Clinical Neurology.* Amsterdam: Elsevier Science Publishers, 49:335–348, 1986.

96. MacMillan JC, Morrison PJ, Nevin NC, et al: Identification of an expanded CAG repeat in the Huntington's disease gene (IT15) in a family reported to have benign hereditary chorea. *J Med Genet* 30:1012–1013, 1993.

97. Warner TT, Lennox GG, Janota I, Harding AE: Autosomal-dominant dentatorubropallidoluysian atrophy in the United Kingdom. *Mov Disord* 9:289–296, 1994.

98. Iizuka R, Hirayama K, Machara K: Dentato-rubro-pallido-luysian atrophy: A clinico-pathological study. *J Neurol Neurosurg Psychiatry* 47:1288–1298, 1984.

99. Mark MH, Sage JI: Olivopontocerebellar atrophy, in Stern MB, Koller WC (eds): *Parkinsonian Syndromes.* New York: Marcel Dekker, pp. 43–67, 1993.

100. Potter NT, Meyer MA, Zimmerman AW, et al: Molecular and clinical findings in a family with dentatorubral-pallidoluysian atrophy. *Ann Neurol* 37:273–277, 1995.

101. Koide R, Ikeuchi T, Onodera O, et al: Unstable expansion of CAG repeat in hereditary dentatorubral-pallidoluysian atrophy (DRPLA). *Nature Genet* 6:9–13, 1994.

102. Nagafuchi S, Yanagisawa H, Sato K, et al: Dentatorubral and pallidoluysian atrophy expansion of an unstable CAG trinucleotide on chromosome 12p. *Nature Genet* 6:14–18, 1994.

103. Nagafuchi S, Yanagisawa H, Ohsaki E, et al: Structure and expression of the gene responsible for the triplet repeat disorder, dentatorubral and pallidoluysian atrophy (DRPLA). *Nature Genet* 8:177–182, 1994.

104. Farmer TW, Wingfield MS, Lynch SA, et al: Ataxia, chorea, seizures, and dementia. Pathologic features of a newly defined familial disorder. *Arch Neurol* 46:774–779, 1989.

105. Burke JR, Wingfield MS, Lewis KE, et al: The Haw River syndrome: Dentatorubropallidoluysian atrophy (DRPLA) in an African-American family. *Nature Genet* 7:521–524, 1994.

106. Friedman JH, Ambler M: A case of senile chorea. *Mov Disord* 5:251–253, 1990.

107. Alcock NS: A note on the pathology of senile chorea (nonhereditary). *Brain* 59:376–387, 1936.

108. Shinotoh H, Calne DB, Snow B, et al: Normal CAG repeat length in the Huntington's disease gene in senile chorea. *Neurology* 44:2183–2184, 1994.

109. Jakob A: *Die extrapyramidalen Enkrankungen.* Berlin: Springer-Verlag, 1923.

110. Martin JP, Alcock NS: Hemichorea associated with a lesion of the Corpus Luysii. *Brain* 504–516, 1934.

111. Melamed E, Korn-Lubetzki I, Reches A, Siew F: Hemiballismus: Detection of focal hemorrhage in subthalamic nucleus by CT scan. *Ann Neurol* 4:582, 1978.

112. Martin JP: Hemichorea (hemiballismus) without lesions in the corpus Luysii. *Brain* 80:1–10, 1957.

113. Kase CS, Maulsby GO, deJuan E, Mohr JP: Hemichorea-hemiballism and lacunar infarction of the basal ganglia. *Neurology* 31:452–455, 1981.

114. Folstein S, Abbott M, Moses R, et al: A phenocopy of Huntington's disease: Lacunar infarcts of the corpus striatum. *Johns Hopkins Med J* 148:104–113, 1981.

115. Saris S: Chorea caused by caudate infarction. *Arch Neurol* 40:590–591, 1983.

116. Tabaton M, Mancardi G, Loeb C: Generalized chorea due to bilateral small, deep cerebral infarcts. *Neurology* 35:588–589, 1985.

117. Sethi KD, Nichols FT, Yaghmai F: Generalized chorea due to basal ganglia lacunar infarcts. *Mov Disord* 2:61–66, 1987.

118. Altafullah I, Pascual-Leone A, Duvall K, et al: Putaminal hemorrhage accompanied by hemichorea-hemiballism. *Stroke* 21:1093–1094, 1990.

119. Defebvre L, Destee A, Cassim F, et al: Vermersch E. Transient hemiballism and striatal infarction. *Stroke* 21:967–968, 1990.

120. Destee A, Muller JP, Vermersch P, et al: Hemiballismus, hemichorea, striatal infarction. *Rev Neurol (Paris)* 146:150–152, 1990.

121. Bhatia KP, Lera G, Luthert PJ, Marsden CD: Vascular chorea: Case report with pathology. *Mov Disord* 9:447–450, 1994.

122. Freilich RJ, Chambers BR: Choreoathetosis and thalamic haemorrhage. *Clin Exp Neurol* 25:115–120, 1988.

123. Fukui T, Hasegawa Y, Seriyama S, et al: Hemiballism-hemichorea induced by subcortical ischemia. *Can J Neurol Sci* 20:324–328, 1993.

124. Barinagarrementeria F, Vega F, DelBrutto OH: Acute hemichorea due to infarction in the corona radiata. *J Neurol* 236:371–372, 1989.

125. Vidakovic A, Dragasevic N, Kostic VS: Hemiballism: Report of 25 cases. *J Neurol Neurosurg Psychiatry* 57:945–949, 1994.

126. Calzetti S, Moretti G, Gemignani F, et al: Transient hemiballismus and subclavian steal syndrome. *Acta Neurol Belg* 80:329–335, 1980.

127. Tamaoka A, Sakuta M, Yamada H: Hemichorea-hemiballism caused by arteriovenous malformations in the putamen. *J Neurol* 234:124–125, 1987.

128. Shintani S, Shiozawa Z, Tsunoda S, Shiigai T: Paroxysmal choreoathetosis precipitated by movement, sound and photic stimulation in a case of artero-venous malformation in the parietal lobe. *Clin Neurol Neurosurg* 93.237–239, 1991.

129. Vincent FM: Hyperglycemia-induced hemichoreoathetosis: The presenting manifestation of a vascular malformation of the lenticular nucleus. *Neurosurgery* 18:787–790, 1986.

130. Carpay HA, Arts WF, Kloet A, et al: Hemichorea reversible after operation in a boy with cavernous angioma in the head of the caudate nucleus. *J Neurol Neurosurg Psychiatry* 57:1547–1548, 1994.

131. Carella F, Caraceni T, Girotti F: Hemichorea due to a cavernous angioma of the caudate. Case report of an aged patient. *Ital J Neurol Sci* 13:783–785, 1992.

132. Linazasoro G, Urtasun M, Poza JJ, et al: Generalized chorea induced by nonketotic hyperglycemia. *Mov Disord* 8:119–120, 1993.

133. Lin JJ, Chang MK: Hemiballism-hemichorea and non-ketotic hyperglycaemia. *J Neurol Neurosurg Psychiatry* 57:748–750, 1994.

134. Nakagawa T, Mitani K, Nagura H, et al: Chorea-ballism associated with nonketotic hyperglycemia and presenting with bilateral hyperintensity of the putamen on MR T1-weighted images—a case report. *Clin Neurol* 34:52–55, 1994.

135. Shimomura T, Nozaki Y, Tamura K: Hemichorea-hemiballism associated with nonketotic hyperglycemia and presenting with unilateral hyperintensity of the putamen on MRI T₁-weighted images—a case report. *Brain Nerve* 47:557–561, 1995.

136. Broderick JP, Hagen T, Brott T, Tomsick T: Hyperglycemia and hemorrhagic transformation of cerebral infarcts. *Stroke* 26:484–487, 1995.

137. Hefter H, Mayer P, Benecke R: Persistent chorea after recurrent hypoglycemia. *Eur Neurol* 33:244–247, 1993.

138. Newman RP, Kinkel WR: Paroxysmal choreoathetosis due to hypoglycemia. *Arch Neurol* 41:341–342, 1984.

139. Sethi KD, Allen M, Sethi RK, McCord JW: Chorea in hypoglycemia and hyperglycemia (abstr.) *Neurology* 40(suppl 1):337, 1990.

140. Stone LA, Armstrong RM: An unusual presentation of diabetes: Hyperglycemia inducing hemiballismus (abstr.) *Ann Neurol* 26:164, 1989.

141. Haan J, Kremer HPH, Padberg G: Paroxysmal choreoathetosis as presenting symptom of diabetes mellitus. *J Neurol Neurosurg Psychiatry* 52:133, 1989.

142. Crossman AR, Sambrook MA, Jackson A: Experimental hemichorea/hemiballismus: Studies on the intracerebral site of action in a drug-induced dyskinesia. *Brain* 107:579–596, 1984.

143. Mitchell IJ, Jackson A, Sambrook MA, Crossman AR: Common neurological mechanism in experimental chorea and hemiballismus in the monkey: Evidence from 2-deoxyglucose autoradiography. *Brain Res* 339:346–350, 1985.

144. Mitchell IJ, Jackson A, Sambrook MA, Crossman AR: The role of the subthalamic nucleus in experimental chorea: Evidence from 2-deoxyglucose metabolic mapping and horseradish peroxidase tracing studies. *Brain* 112:1533–1548, 1989.

145. Crossman AR, Mitchell IJ, Sambrook MA, Jackson A: Chorea and myoclonus in the monkey induced by gamma-aminobutyric acid antagonism in the lentiform complex. The site of drug action and a hypothesis for the neural mechanisms of chorea. *Brain* 111:1211–1233, 1988.

146. Bashir K, Manyam BV: Clozapine for the control of hemiballismus. *Clin Neuropharmacol* 17:477–480, 1994.

147. Chandra V, Wharton S, Spunt AL: Amelioration of hemiballismus with sodium valproate. *Ann Neurol* 12:407, 1982.

148. Dewey RB Jr, Jankovic J: Hemiballism-hemichorea: Clinical and pharmacologic findings in 21 patients. *Arch Neurol* 46:862–867, 1989.

149. Sethi KD, Patel BP: Inconsistent response to divalproex sodium in hemichorea-hemiballism. *Neurology* 40:1630–1631, 1990.

150. Otsuka M, Ichiya Y, Kuwabara Y, et al: Cerebral glucose metabolism and ¹⁸F-dopa uptake by PET in cases of chorea with or without dementia. *J Neurol Sci* 115:153–157, 1993.

151. Logothetic J: Neurologic and muscular manifestations of hyperthyroidism. *Arch Neurol* 5:533–544, 1961.

152. Fidler SM, O'Rourke RA, Buchsbaum HM: Choreoathetosis as a manifestation of thyrotoxicosis. *Neurology* 21:55–57, 1971.

153. Delwaide PJ, Schoenen J: Hyperthyroidism as a cause of persistent choreic movements. *Acta Neurol Scand* 58:309–312, 1978.

154. Shahar E, Shapiro MS, Shenkman L: Hyperthyroid-induced chorea: Case report and review of the literature. *Israel J Med Sci* 24:264–266, 1988.

155. Ahronheim JC: Hyperthyroid chorea in an elderly woman associated with sole elevation of T3. *J Am Geriatr Soc* 36:242–244, 1988.

156. Lucantoni C, Grottoli S, Moretti A: Chorea due to hyperthyroidism in old age: A case report. *Acta Neurol Scand* 16:129–133, 1994.

157. Baba M, Terada A, Hishida R, et al: Persistent hemichorea associated with thyrotoxicosis. *Intern Med* 31:1144–1146, 1992.

158. Pozzan GB, Battistella PA, Rigon F, et al: Hyperthyroid-induced chorea in an adolescent girl. *Brain Dev* 14:126–127, 1992.

159. Fischbeck KH, Layzer RB: Paroxysmal choreoathetosis associated with thyrotoxicosis. *Ann Neurol* 6:453–454, 1979.

160. Drake ME Jr: Paroxysmal kinesigenic choreoathetosis in hyperthyroidism. *Postgrad Med J* 63:1089–1090, 1987.

161. Klawans HL, Shenker DM, Weiner WJ: Observations on the dopaminergic nature of hyperthyroid chorea. *Adv Neurol* 1:543–549, 1973.

162. Bruyn GW, Padberg G: Chorea and polycythemia. *Eur Neurol* 23:26–33, 1984.

163. Mas JL, Guergen B, Bouche P, et al: Chorea and polycythaemia. *J Neurol* 232:168–171, 1985.

164. Rigon G, Baratti M, Quaini F, Calzetti S: Polycythemia chorea: Description of a clinical case. *Minerva Med* 78:1325–1329, 1987.

165. Cohen AM, Gelvan A, Yarmolovsky A, Djaldetti M: Chorea in polycythemia vera: A rare presentation of hyperviscosity. *Blut* 58:47–48, 1989.

166. Chamouard JM, Smagghe A, Malalanirina BH, et al: Chorea disclosing polycythemia and renal adenocarcinoma. *Rev Neurol (Paris)* 148:380–382, 1992.

167. Tang WY, Gill DS,Chuan PS: Chorea, a manifestation of hyponatremia? *Singapore Med J* 22:92–93, 1981.

168. Sparacio RR, Anziska B, Schutta HS: Hypernatremia and chorea. *Neurology* 26:46–50, 1976.

169. Howdle PD, Bone I, Losowsky MS: Hypocalcemic chorea secondary to malabsorption. *Postgrad Med J* 55:560–563, 1979.

170. Greenhouse AH: On chorea, lupus erythematosus, and cerebral vasculitis. *Arch Intern Med* 117:389–393, 1966.

171. Tabee-Zadeh MJ, Frame B, Kapphahn K: Kinesiogenic choreoathetosis and idiopathic hypoparathyroidism. *N Engl J Med* 286:762–763, 1972.

172. Soffer D, Licht A, Yaar I, Abramsky O: Paroxysmal choreoathetosis as a presenting symptom in idiopathic hypoparathyroidism. *J Neurol Neurosurg Psychiatry* 40:692–694, 1977.

173. Kashihara K, Yabuki S: Unilateral choreic movements in idiopathic hypoparathyroidism. *Brain Nerve* 44:477–480, 1992.

174. Salti I, Paris A, Tannir N, Khouri K: Rapid correction by 1-alpha-hydroxycholecalciferol of hemichorea in surgical hypoparathyroidism. *J Neurol Neurosurg Psychiatry* 45:89–90, 1982.

175. Rizzo GN, Olanow CW, Roses AD: Chorea in hyperparathyroidism: Report of a case. *AMB* 27:155–156, 1981.

176. Hurwitz LJ, Montgomery AD: Persistent choreoathetotic movements in liver disease. *Arch Neurol* 13:421–426, 1965.

177. Toghill PJ, Johnston AW, Smith JF: Choreoathetosis in portosystemic encephalopathy. *J Neurol Neurosurg Psychiatry* 30:358–363, 1967.

178. Gerard JM, Vanderhaeghen JJ, Telerman-Toppet N, Coers C: Choreo-athetosis with hepato-cerebral degeneration in a patient with a portocaval shunt. *Acta Neurol Belg* 73:100–109, 1973.

179. Spitaleri DL, Vitolo S, Fasanaro AM, Valiani R: Choreoathetosis: Uncommon manifestation during chronic liver disease with portocaval shunt. *Riv Neurol* 53:293–299, 1983.

180. Yokota T, Tsuchiya K, Umetani K, et al: Choreoathetoid movements associated with a spleno-renal shunt. *J Neurol* 235:487–488, 1988.

181. Tison FX, Ferrer X, Julien J: Delayed onset movement disorders as a complication of central pontine myelinolysis. *Mov Disord* 6:171–173, 1991.

182. Tsutada T, Hayashi H, Kitano S, et al: A case report of central pontine and extrapontine myelinolysis which occurred during pregnancy and was accompanied by choreic movement. *Clin Neurol* 29:1294–1297, 1989.

183. Roos RA, Wintzen AR, Vielvoye G, Polder TW: Paroxysmal kinesigenic choreoathetosis as presenting symptom of multiple sclerosis. *J Neurol Neurosurg Psychiatry* 154:657–658, 1991.

184. Mouren P, Tatassian A, Toga M, et al: Etude critique du syndrome hemiballique. *Encephale* 55:212–274, 1966.

185. Sarkari NBS: Involuntary movements in multiple sclerosis. *Br Med J* 2:738–740, 1968.

186. Bachman DS, Lao-Velez C, Estanol B: Dystonia and choreoathetosis in multiple sclerosis. *Arch Neurol* 33:590, 1976.

187. Taff I, Sabato UC, Lehrer G: Choreoathetosis in multiple sclerosis. *Clin Neurol Neurosurg* 87:41–43, 1985.

188. Mao C-C, Gancher ST, Herndon RM: Movement disorders in multiple sclerosis. *Mov Disord* 3:109–116, 1988.

189. Bjork VO, Hultquist G: Brain damage in children after deep hypothermia for open-heart surgery. *Thorax* 15:284–291, 1960.

190. Bergouignan M, Fontan F, Trarieux M, Julien J: Syndromes choreiformes de l'enfant au décours d'interventions cardiochirurgicales sous hypothermie profonde. *Rev Neurol (Paris)* 105:48–60, 1961.

191. Brunberg JA, Doty DB, Reilly EL: Choreoathetosis in infants following cardiac surgery with deep hypothermia and circulatory arrest. *J Pediatr* 84:232–235, 1974.

192. Robinson RO, Samuels M, Pohl KRE: Choreic syndrome after cardiac surgery. *Arch Dis Child* 63:1466–1469, 1988.

193. DeLeon S, Ilbawi M, Arcilla R, et al: Choreoathetosis after deep hypothermia without circulatory arrest. *Ann Thorac Surg* 50:714–719, 1990.

194. Barratt-Boyes BG: Choreoathetosis as a complication of cardiopulmonary bypass. *Ann Thorac Surg* 50:693–694, 1990.

195. Wical BS, Tomasi LG: A distinctive neurological syndrome after profound hypothermia. *Pediatr Neurol* 6:202–205, 1990.

196. Wong PC, Barlow CF, Hickey PR, et al: Factors associated with choreoathetosis after cardiopulmonary bypass in children with congenital heart disease. *Circulation* 86:118–126, 1992.

197. Medlock MD, Cruse RS, Winek SJ, et al: A 10-year experience with postpump chorea. *Ann Neurol* 34:820–826, 1993.

198. Yoshii S, Mohri N, Suzuki S, et al: Postoperative choreoathetosis in a case of tetralogy of Fallot. *J Jpn Assoc Thorac Surg* 43:109–112, 1995.

199. Curless RG, Katz DA, Perryman RA, et al: Choreoathetosis after surgery for congenital heart disease. *J Pediatr* 124:737–739, 1994.

200. Kupsky WJ, Drozd MA, Barlow CF: Selective injury of the globus pallidus in children with post-cardiac surgery choreic syndrome. *Dev Med Child Neurol* 37:135–144, 1995.

201. Blunt SB, Brooks DJ, Kennard C: Steroid-responsive chorea in childhood following cardiac transplantation. *Mov Disord* 9:112–114, 1994.

202. Duvoisin RC: Chorea. *Semin Neurol* 2:351–358, 1982.

203. Shoulson I: On chorea. *Clin Neuropharmacol* 9(suppl 2):S85–S99, 1986.

204. Nomoto M, Thompson PD, Sheehy MP, et al: Anticholinergic-induced chorea in the treatment of focal dystonia. *Mov Disord* 2:53–56, 1987.

205. Matsumoto K, Nogaki H, Morimatsu M: A case of choreoathetoid movements induced by anticholinergic drugs, trihexyphenidyl HCl and dosulepin HCl. *Jpn J Geriatr* 29:686–689, 1992.

206. Harrison MB, Lyons GR, Landow ER: Phenytoin and dyskinesias: A report of two cases and review of the literature. *Mov Disord* 8:19–27, 1993.

207. Lancman ME, Asconape JJ, Penry JK: Choreiform movements associated with the use of valproate. *Arch Neurol* 51:702–704, 1994.

208. Sperling LS, Horowitz JL: Methamphetamine-induced choreoathetosis and rhabdomyolysis. *Ann Intern Med* 121:986, 1994.

209. Rhee KJ, Albertson TE, Douglas JC: Choreoathetoid disorder associated with amphetamine-like drugs. *Am J Emerg Med* 6:131–133, 1988.

210. Daras M, Koppel BS, Atos-Radzion E: Cocaine-induced choreoathetoid movements ('crack dancing'). *Neurology* 44:751–752, 1994.

211. Stuart AM, Worley LM, Spillane J: Choreiform movements observed in an 8-year-old child following use of an oral theophylline preparation. *Clin Pediatr* 31:692–694, 1992.

212. Helmuth D, Ljaljevic Z, Ramirez L, Meltzer HY: Choreoathetosis induced by verapamil and lithium treatment. *J Clin Psychopharmacol* 9:454–455, 1989.

213. Crystal HA: Baclofen therapy may be associated with chorea in Alzheimer's disease. *Ann Neurol* 28:839, 1990.

214. Combarros O, Fabrega E, Polo JM, Berciano J: Cyclosporine-induced chorea after liver transplantation for Wilson's disease. *Ann Neurol* 33:108–109, 1993.

215. Samie MR, Ashton AK: Choreoathetosis induced by cyproheptadine. *Mov Disord* 4:81–84, 1989.

216. Patrick SJ, Snelling LK, Ment LR: Infantile chorea following abrupt withdrawal of diazepam and pentobarbital therapy. *J Toxicol Clin Toxicol* 31:127–132, 1993.

217. Mulder LJ, van der Mast RC, Meerwaldt JD: Generalised chorea due to digoxin toxicity. *Br Med J Clin Res Ed* 296:1262, 1988.

218. Matsis PP, Fisher RA, Tasman-Jones C: Acute lithium toxicity—chorea, hypercalcemia and hyperamylasemia. *Aust N Z J Med* 19:718–720, 1989.

219. Reed SM, Wise MG, Timmerman I: Choreoathetosis: A sign of lithium toxicity. *J Neuropsychiatry Clin Neurosci* 1:57–60, 1989.

220. Sweeney BJ, Edgecombe J, Churchill DR, et al: Choreoathetosis/ballismus associated with pentamidine-induced hypoglycemia in a patient with the acquired immunodeficiency syndrome. *Arch Neurol* 51:723–725, 1994.

221. Lehmann AB: Reversible chorea due to ranitidine and cimetidine. *Lancet* 8603:158, 1988.

222. Clarke CE, Bamford JM, House A: Dyskinesia in Creutzfeld-Jakob disease precipitated by antidepressant therapy. *Mov Disord* 7:86–87, 1992.

223. Fukutani Y, Nakamura I, Kobayashi K, et al: A case of familial juvenile Alzheimer's disease with apallic state at the relatively early stage and various neurological features—a clinicopathological study. *Clin Neurol* 29:633–638, 1989.

224. Voll R, Hoffmann GF, Lipinski CG, et al: Glutaric acidemia/glutaric aciduria I as differential chorea minor diagnosis. *Klin Padiatrie* 205:124–126, 1993.

225. Sethi KD, Ray R, Roesel RA, et al: Adult-onset chorea and dementia with propionic acidemia. *Neurology* 39:1343–1345, 1989.

226. Friedman JH, Weitberg A: Ataxia without telangiectasia. *Mov Disord* 8:223–226, 1993.

227. Nelson I, Hanna MG, Alsanjari N, et al: A new mitochondrial DNA mutation associated with progressive dementia and chorea: A clinical, pathological, and molecular genetic study. *Ann Neurol* 37:400–403, 1995.

228. Truong DD, Harding AE, Scaravilli F, et al: Movement disorders in mitochondrial myopathies: A study of nine cases with two autopsy studies. *Mov Disord* 5:109–117, 1990.

229. Steiger MJ, Pires M, Scaravilli F, et al: Hemiballism and chorea in a patient with parkinsonism due to a multisystem degeneration. *Mov Disord* 7:71–77, 1992.

230. Colosimo C, Rossi P, Elia M, et al: Transient alternating hemichorea as presenting sign of progressive supranuclear palsy. *Ital J Neurol Sci* 1991;12:99–101, 1991.

231. Wright RA, Pollock M, Donaldson IM: Chorea and tuberous sclerosis. *Mov Disord* 7:87–89, 1992.

232. Kok J, Bosscray A, Brion JP, et al: Chorea in a child with Churg-Straus syndrome. *Stroke* 24:1263–1264, 1993.

233. Jones AL, Bouchier IA: A patient with neurosyphilis presenting as chorea. *Scot Med J.* 38:82–84, 1993.

234. Beskind DL, Keim SM: Choreoathetotic movement disorder in a boy with Mycoplasma pneumoniae encephalitis. *Ann Emerg Med* 23:1375–1378, 1994.

235. Krauss JK, Mohadjer M, Nobbe F: Mundinger F. Bilateral ballismus in children. *Child Nerv Syst* 7:342–346, 1991.

236. Gascon GG, al-Jarallah AA, Okamoto E, et al: Chorea as a presentation of herpes simplex encephalitis relapse. *Brain Dev* 15:178–181, 1993.

237. Wang HS, Kuo MF, Huang SC, Chou ML: Choreoathetosis as an initial sign of relapsing of herpes simplex encephalitis. *Pediatr Neurol* 11:341–345, 1994.

238. Bhigjee AI, Kemp T, Cosnett JE: Cerebral cysticercosis presenting with hemichorea. *J Neurol Neurosurg Psychiatry* 50:1561–1562, 1987.

239. Sanchez-Ramos JR, Factor SA, Weiner WJ, Marquez J: Hemichorea-hemiballismus associated with acquired immune deficiency syndrome and cerebral toxoplasmosis. *Mov Disord* 4:266–273, 1989.

240. Pestre P, Milandre L, Farnarier P, Gallais H: Hemichorea in acquired immunodeficiency syndrome. Toxoplasmosis abscess in the striatum. *Rev Neurol (Paris)* 147:833–837, 1991.

241. Nath A, Hobson DE, Russell A: Movement disorders with cerebral toxoplasmosis and AIDS. *Mov Disord* 8:107–112, 1993.

242. Moodley R, Seebaran AR, Rajput MC: Dystonia and choreoathetosis in Wernicke's encephalopathy: A case report. *S Afr Med J* 75:543–544, 1989.

243. Meucci G, Rossi G, Mazzoni M: A case of transient choreoathetosis with amnesic syndrome after acute carbon monoxide poisoning. *Ital J Neurol Sci* 10:513–517, 1989.

244. de Krom MC, Boreas AM, Hardy EL: Manganese poisoning due to use of Chien Pu Wan tablets. *Ned Tijdschr Geneeskd* 138:2010–2012, 1994.

245. Joubert J, Joubert PH: Chorea and psychiatric changes in organophsophate poisoning. A report of 2 further cases. *S Afr Med J* 74:32–34, 1988.

246. Poewe WH, Kleedorfer B, Willeit J, Gerstenbrand F: Primary CNS lymphoma presenting as a choreic movement disorder followed by segmental dystonia. *Mov Disord* 3:320–325, 1988.

247. Sakai M, Hashizume Y, Yamamoto H, Kawakami A: An autopsy case of primary cerebral malignant lymphoma initiated with choreoathetosis. *Clin Neurol* 30:849–854, 1990.

248. Schiff DE, Ortega JA: Chorea, eosinophilia, and lupus anticoagulant associated with acute lymphoblastic leukemia. *Pediatr Neurol* 8:466–468, 1992.

249. Albin RL, Bromberg MB, Penney JB, Knapp R: Chorea and dystonia: A remote effect of carcinoma. *Mov Disord* 3:162–169, 1988.

250. Watanabe K, Negoro T, Machara M, et al: Moyamoya disease presenting with chorea. *Pediatr Neurol* 6:40–42, 1990.

251. Pavlakis SG, Schneider S, Black K, Gould RJ: Steroid-responsive chorea in moyamoya disease. *Mov Disord* 6:347–349, 1991.

252. Takanashi J, Sugita K, Honda A, Niimi II. Moyamoya syndrome in a patient with Down's syndrome presenting with chorea. *Pediatr Neurol* 9:396–398, 1993.

253. Fowler WE, Kriel RL, Krach LE: Movement disorders after status epilepticus and other brain injuries. *Pediatr Neurol* 8:281–284, 1992.

254. Hadders-Algra M, Bos AF, Martijn A, Prechtl HF: Infantile chorea in an infant with severe bronchopulmonary dysplasia: An EMG study. *Dev Med Child Neurol* 36:177–182, 1994.

255. Spillane JD, Nathan PW, Kelly RE, Marsden CD: Painful legs and moving toes. *Brain* 94:541–556, 1971.

256. Nathan PW: Painful legs and moving toes: Evidence on the site of the lesion. *J Neurol Neurosurg Psychiatry* 41:934–939, 1978.

257. Schott GD: Painful legs and moving toes: The role of trauma. *J Neurol Neurosurg Psychiatry* 44:344–346, 1981.

258. Barrett RE, Singh N, Fahn S: The syndrome of painful legs and moving toes. *Neurology* 31(suppl 1):79, 1981.

259. Wulff CH: Painful legs and moving toes: A report of 3 cases with neurophysiologic studies. *Acta Neurol Scand* 66:283–287, 1982.

260. Schoenen J, Gonce M, Delwaide PJ: Painful legs and moving toes: A syndrome with different pathophysiologic mechanisms. *Neurology* 34:1108–1112, 1984.

261. Funakawa I, Muno Y, Takayanagi T: Painful hand and moving fingers. *J Neurol* 234:342–343, 1987.

262. Verhagen WIM, Horstink WMIM, Notermans SLH: Painful arm and moving fingers. *J Neurol Neurosurg Psychiatry* 48:384–385, 1985.

263. Dressler D, Thompson PD, Gledhill RF, Marsden CD: The syndrome of painful leg and moving toes. *Mov Disord* 9:13–21, 1994.

264. Walters AS, Hening WA, Shah SK, Chokroverty S: Painless legs and moving toes: A syndrome related to painful legs and moving toes? *Mov Disord* 8:377–379, 1993.

CLASSIFICATION, CLINICAL FEATURES, AND TREATMENT OF MYOCLONUS

JOSÉ A. OBESO

DIFFERENTIATION FROM OTHER MOVEMENT
   DISORDERS
CLINICAL PRESENTATION
   Reflex Myoclonus
   Action Myoclonus
   Negative Myoclonus
   Spontaneous Myoclonus
   Rhythmic Myoclonus
NEUROPHYSIOLOGICAL ORIGIN
   Cortical Myoclonus
   Subcortical Myoclonus
   Spinal Myoclonus
ETIOLOGY
   Etiologic Classification
   Major Diagnostic Categories
TREATMENT
   Multifocal Action Myoclonus
   Focal Myoclonus of Cortical Origin

Myoclonus is a brief muscle jerk caused by neuronal discharges. A sudden and short-lasting interruption of ongoing voluntary muscle contraction may produce a postural pause clinically very similar to myoclonus, hence the recently applied term "negative myoclonus." Both forms often share the same etiology, coincide in the same patients, and can even affect the same muscle group.[1]

Myoclonus can be classified from various points of view (Table 39-1). The major categories are (1) clinical presentation; (2) neurophysiological origin; and (3) etiology. Myoclonus may occur spontaneously, may be triggered by external stimulation ("reflex") or may be induced during voluntary muscle activation ("action"). According to its distribution, myoclonus may be focal, segmental, generalized, or multifocal. The timing of myoclonus can be rhythmic or irregular.

A myoclonic jerk consists of a single muscle discharge but can be repetitive, giving rise to a salvo of muscle activity (Fig. 39-1). The latter is particularly frequent in action myoclonus and interferes severely with the execution of even the most simple motor tasks. For this reason, action myoclonus (both positive and negative types) may be considered as the movement disorder that produces the greatest interference with voluntary movements.

Differentiation from Other Movement Disorders

Myoclonus must be differentiated from other dyskinesias, such as tics, chorea, postural tremor, dystonia, and hemifacial spasm.[2]

Tics, as present in Gilles de la Tourette's syndrome, are frequently as brief as myoclonus. The main elements to distinguish between these two categories of muscle jerks include the following: (1) Myoclonus usually interferes notably with voluntary movement and is aggravated by action, whereas tics almost never disrupt motor acts. (2) Tics can be voluntarily suppressed and myoclonus cannot. (3) A high proportion of patients will feel a somesthetic sensation preceding the tic or an internal urgency to produce the movement. Myoclonus is not accompanied by any special sensation. (4) Most forms of myoclonus stop during sleep whereas tics often persist.

Chorea is a flowing combination of irregular muscle activity. Some of the movements of chorea may look "myoclonic" if taken in isolation, but it is the unpredictable concatenation of different patterns of movement which typifies chorea.

Postural and action tremor, when very severe, may be associated with sudden changes in the amplitude and rhythmicity of the muscle activity, giving rise to a false impression of a myoclonic jerk. This problem is easily resolved, when in doubt, by electromyographic (EMG) recording.[3] Slow resting tremor or myorrhythmia is difficult to distinguish clinically from rhythmical segmental myoclonus. True myoclonus, even when repetitive and rhythmical, must have a sudden and shock-like onset and end.

Dystonia consists of prolonged muscle spasms, which are longer than those of myoclonus and produce twisting, repetitive movements and abnormal postures.[4] Similarly, the muscle activity of hemifacial spasm lasts longer and provokes sustained, tonic contractions. However, such differentiation might not be so easy in early stages, when only clonic twitching of either the upper or lower facial musculature is present. In such instances, EMG studies are needed to clarify the diagnosis.

It should be kept in mind that myoclonus may coincide with other involuntary movement disorders in the same patients. For instance, some families with essential tremor and myoclonus have been described;[5] myoclonus and dystonia are combined in inherited myoclonic dystonia[6] (Fig. 39-2), and both action and reflex myoclonic jerks may be present in patients with Huntington's chorea.[7] These and other combinations also illustrate the point that the major motor manifestation of a given nosological entity does not imply that other movement disorders cannot be present in such diseases and syndromes. For example, not all the abnormal movements of Gilles de la Tourette's syndrome are tics, nor is chorea the only movement disorder present in Huntington's disease.

TABLE 39-1 Classification of Myoclonus

Clinical
   Presentation:
      Spontaneous
      Action
      Reflex
   Distribution:
      Generalized
      Multifocal
      Segmental
      Focal
Neurophysiological origin
   Cortical
   Subcortical (brainstem)
   Spinal
Etiology
   Physiological
   Essential
   Symptomatic
      Associated with epilepsy
      Associated with other causes

Clinical Presentation

REFLEX MYOCLONUS

Somesthetic, visual, and auditory stimuli, independently and in combination, may trigger myoclonic jerking. Such myoclonus is focal or generalized in distribution. Pinpricking the limbs distally (wrist and palmar surface of the upper limbs and the soles of the feet), as well as flicking the fingers and toes are probably the most sensitive clinical methods of evoking reflex myoclonus limited to a body area.[8] In some instances the jerks are so sensitive to somesthetic stimuli that focal myoclonus may become self-perpetuated and simulate spontaneous myoclonus as in epilepsia partialis continua or even look like a tremor.

Generalized reflex myoclonus to somesthetic stimulation is more commonly obtained by touching or tapping the face, particularly the mentalis zone (J A Obeso, personal observations).[9] Visually triggered reflex myoclonus may be evoked

clinically by a threatening stimulus but more often requires flash stimulation.[10] Auditory stimulation is not a frequent cause of myoclonus, except in children. Both visually and auditorily evoked myoclonus are always generalized. Generalized reflex myoclonus induced by unexpected sounds has to be distinguished from *hyperekplexia*, which is a pathological exaggeration of the startle response (see below).

ACTION MYOCLONUS

This occurs during active muscular contraction and affects both posturally acting muscles and prime movers. Action myoclonus may be focal or segmental, but the most common distribution is multifocal or generalized. This form is undoubtedly the one which produces the greatest disability. This is usually due to the concatenation of several brief EMG discharges (Fig. 39-1), which forces the limbs and trunk to move in unintended directions. The abnormal neuronal activity provoking action myoclonus probably arises from the same areas as those subserving normal motor control mechanisms. Thus, action myoclonus interferes with, prevents, and disrupts very gross voluntary movements to a much greater extent than other movement disorders such as dystonia and tics.

NEGATIVE MYOCLONUS

Negative myoclonus is by definition only present during active muscular contraction and in fact is almost always combined with positive action myoclonus. There are two major clinical presentations: asterixis and postural lapses.[1] Asterixis is the most common and best characterized form of negative myoclonus. It consists of a silence of EMG discharges for a short period of time (50–200 ms), thus producing a brief loss of antigravitational activity and postural control (Fig. 39-2, *arrow*). Asterixis is usually multifocal in distribution but may affect a muscle group in isolation. Recently, Shibasaki et al.[11] have described reflex negative myoclonus limited to muscles of one limb. Postural lapses consist of a long-duration EMG silence (200–500 ms), usually occu-

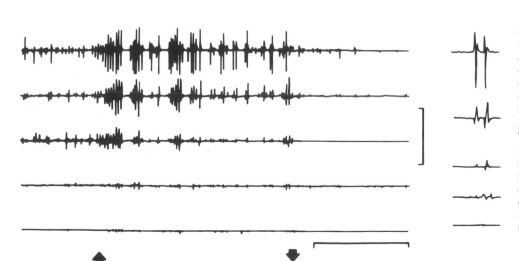

FIGURE 39-1 EMG recording from several muscles in the right arm of a patient with action myoclonus (Ramsay Hunt syndrome). From *top* to *bottom* are deltoid, biceps, triceps, finger extensors, and finger flexors. The horizontal scale bar indicates 2 s. The insert on the right shows the EMG discharges in more detail. Scale bar = 100 ms. The salvo of repetitive myoclonic discharges associated with silent periods is clearly seen in the proximal arm muscles. (*From Obeso et al.*[8] *Used with permission.*)

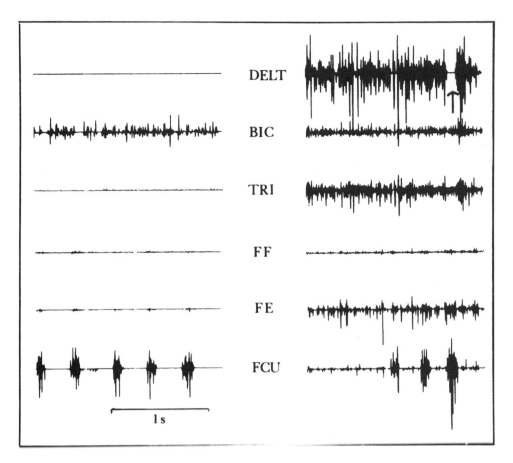

FIGURE 39-2 EMG recording from the right arm of a patient with myoclonic dystonia. On the *left*, spontaneous myoclonic activity is present in flexor carpi ulnaris (FCU) at rest. On the *right*, exaggerated EMG activity is seen in proximal arm muscles (deltoid, biceps, triceps) while the myoclonus persists in FCU. A brief negative myoclonus (asterixis) is indicated by the arrow in deltoid EMG (DELT). BIC, biceps; TRI, triceps. *(From Obeso et al.[17] Used with permission.)*

pying axial and proximal muscles of the lower limbs, with a tendency for repetitive appearance over a few seconds.[1] In patients with severe myoclonic encephalopathies, such as postanoxic myoclonus, these postural lapses may follow a myoclonic discharge and may actually lead to greater functional disability than the myoclonus.

SPONTANEOUS MYOCLONUS

Spontaneous myoclonus may be focal, multifocal, or generalized and have several presentations. It may be sporadic and occur unpredictably or coincide with specific moments, such as in normal people with nocturnal myoclonus or in patients with early morning myoclonic epilepsy. In other instances, it may be almost continuously present, as in patients with metabolic encephalopathies or Creutzfeldt-Jakob disease.

RHYTHMIC MYOCLONUS

This is almost always spontaneous in presentation, with a focal or segmental distribution. The myoclonic discharge may persist during sleep and is little affected by sensory stimulation. The frequency is variable but usually slow (1–4 Hz). The two most common types are palatal and spinal myoclonus.

It is important to realize that different patterns are often combined in the same subject. For instance, reflex and action myoclonus may coincide and affect the same body region(s);

multifocal spontaneous myoclonus, as seen in metabolic encephalopathies, is very commonly aggravated during action, and focal myoclonus may spread to become generalized.

Neurophysiological Origin

This topic is thoroughly covered in Chap. 40, but it will be briefly addressed here because it is important to understand some clinical and therapeutic aspects.

Electrophysiological analysis of myoclonus is mainly aimed at identifying the site of the discharges producing the jerks and the pathophysiological mechanisms involved in their origin. It should be noted that the origin of the discharges producing myoclonus does not necessarily coincide with the topography of the lesion(s) and that on many occasions, the pathological basis cannot be determined.

Myoclonus can be divided into three major pathophysiological categories.

CORTICAL MYOCLONUS

Cortical myoclonus results from abnormal activity arising in the sensorimotor cortex and spreading down via the corticospinal pathway. The EMG discharge is of short duration (usually 10–50 ms), and the somatosensory evoked potentials (SEPs) are increased in amplitude (20–50 μV) and frequently associated with a reflex muscle response (C-wave) that follows the cortical potential by a short latency of 15–20 ms for the forearm muscles.[8] Back-averaging the EEG activity preceding the jerks reveals a biphasic potential over the contralateral sensorimotor cortex preceding the muscle discharge by some 20 ms in the arm and 35 ms in the leg (see Chap. 40).

SUBCORTICAL MYOCLONUS

Subcortical myoclonus indicates that the neuronal discharge originates in structures between the cortex and the spinal cord. The most common type is "reticular reflex myoclonus," characterized by generalized jerks, with predominant involvement of proximal limb and axial muscles provoked by sensory stimulation. Electromyographic recording of the spreading of the jerk through different muscles is necessary to determine the brain stem origin (see Chap. 40).

SPINAL MYOCLONUS

Spinal myoclonus is secondary to abnormal neuronal discharge originating in the spinal cord. It is frequently rhythmical and only exceptionally stimuli-sensitive. A newly described form is propiospinal myoclonus,[12] in which spontaneous and stimuli-sensitive (tapping) jerks involve mainly the trunk and abdominal muscles. The EMG discharges consist of repetitive bursts with a frequency of 1–7 Hz.

Etiology

Myoclonus may occur in the setting of a wide variety of conditions. Indeed, a list of all causes of myoclonus could be almost as long as the index of a neurology textbook. However, in many instances myoclonus is a nonspecific manifestation and is accompanied by many other neurological signs. In such cases, myoclonus is not a key clinical indicator.

The etiologic classification of myoclonus, as originally outlined by Marsden et al.,[13] is briefly summarized below; more detailed attention is given to those conditions in which myoclonus is a major complaint or the main clinical sign leading to a correct diagnosis.

ETIOLOGIC CLASSIFICATION

PHYSIOLOGICAL MYOCLONUS
This occurs in normal people in special circumstances and does not indicate an underlying abnormality. Nocturnal myoclonus of the legs is probably the most common type.

ESSENTIAL MYOCLONUS
This occurs in individuals in whom myoclonus is the only or most important neurological manifestation and the course is not progressive. It is now recognized that most cases are familial and frequently associated with dystonia (see below).

MYOCLONIC EPILEPSIES
Idiopathic epilepsy without any other neurological problem may have myoclonus as a major clinical expression. This includes entities such as benign myoclonus of infancy, myoclonic absences, juvenile myoclonic epilepsy of Janz, and photosensitive epileptic myoclonus. In such instances, the jerks are usually generalized and occur spontaneously, are frequently facilitated by lack of sleep, alcohol, etc., and may be triggered by visual stimuli.

Myoclonus may also be present in patients with generalized tonic-clonic epilepsy in the setting of a progressive encephalopathy (progressive myoclonic epilepsy), which will be discussed in detail below.

SECONDARY MYOCLONUS
As indicated above, any process causing central nervous system (CNS) damage or dysfunction may be associated with myoclonus. However, the list of conditions in which myoclonus is the only or major clinical manifestation is much less extensive. This includes anoxia (Lance-Adams syndrome), trauma, bismuth intoxication, and some metabolic problems such as renal failure, hyponatremia, hypokalemia, etc., which may show myoclonus as an initial sign. More rarely, a late-onset degenerative disease such as progressive supranuclear palsy, olivopontocerebellar atrophy, or Huntington's disease may have action myoclonus as a major feature. Reflex myoclonus is a common feature of corticobasal degeneration and olivopontocerebellar atrophy and may be a prominent feature in some rare families with Huntington's disease. Focal lesion of the CNS may produce focal or segmental myoclonus (see below).

The list of drugs causing myoclonus is fairly long. Thus, the possibility of drug abuse should always be considered in any patient with a myoclonic encephalopathy of unknown origin.

MAJOR DIAGNOSTIC CATEGORIES

The principal clinical presentations and the most common etiologies of myoclonus as a movement disorder will be discussed in this section. Myoclonus in patients with epilepsy (i.e. myoclonic absences, juvenile myoclonic epilepsy, etc.) as the major clinical problem is not included here.

CAUSES OF SEVERE MULTIFOCAL OR GENERALIZED MYOCLONUS
This section deals with conditions in which myoclonus may be overt and a predominant clinical problem. The jerks usually have a multifocal distribution and appear spontaneously, but they may be aggravated by action and be stimulus sensitive.

Essential Myoclonus
In this condition the jerks are usually multifocal, extremely brief (hence the term "lightning"), and aggravated by action. The amplitude and intensity of the jerks are variable. In some patients the jerks are large and almost continuous, provoking severe disability, but in others the amplitude is so small that they interfere only minimally with routine motor acts. Essential myoclonus is a heterogenous disorder, which may be sporadic but more often has a genetic basis (hereditary essential myoclonus). In familial cases, inheritance is autosomal dominant with variable penetrance and expression, on-

set occurs in the first two decades of life, severity may be variable within the same family, and all routine laboratory tests and neuroimaging studies are normal.

While the existence of patients with myoclonus as the only manifestation must be admitted,[6] recent observations indicate that essential myoclonus very often occurs in combination with dystonic postures and movements and shows an extreme sensitivity to alcohol ("alcohol-sensitive myoclonic dystonia"). Interestingly, none of the drugs commonly effective in other types of myoclonus has been capable of mimicking the dramatic antimyoclonic effect of alcohol.[14]

The association of myoclonus and dystonia has been the subject of considerable debate and confusion.[15] The term "myoclonic dystonia" was actually used a long time ago by Davidenkow[16] and refers to the association of two movement disorders, namely, brief (<100 ms) myoclonic jerking and long-lasting (>500 ms) dystonic spasms, usually in different muscle groups (Fig. 39-2). This combination may occur in a low proportion of patients with idiopathic torsion dystonia[15,17] and also in other clinical settings, such as after trauma and anoxia, or as part of the tardive dyskinesia syndrome. However, the most common, albeit infrequent, presentation is that of "hereditary myoclonic dystonia with dramatic response to alcohol."[15] Several families have been described in recent years.[6] The disease is autosomal dominant, of early onset (<10 years), and has a relatively stereotyped clinical picture, characterized by predominance of dystonia in the neck and shoulder muscles and very brief myoclonic jerking in the arms and hands. Legs are rarely or minimally involved. The response to small amounts of alcohol is very impressive, with eradication of both myoclonus and dystonia. It is now clear that within the same family the presence and intensity of either myoclonus or dystonia are variable,[6,18] explaining the difficulties and uncertainties in understanding and accepting the existence of hereditary myoclonic dystonia as an entity. Clearly, genetic studies in the near future will resolve definitively the remaining unknowns.

Hereditary essential myoclonus may also be associated with postural tremor. For instance, in 15 family members reported by Korten et al.,[19] 8 had myoclonus alone, 4 showed myoclonus and tremor, and 3 had tremor only. Alcohol also has a striking effect on tremor in such families. It should be realized that sporadic cases with positive response to alcohol have been reported in individuals with progressive myoclonic epilepsy, progressive myoclonic ataxia, postanoxic myoclonus,[6] and dystonia.[20] The sensitivity to alcohol is probably relatively unspecific and specific to hereditary essential myoclonus with or without dystonia.

A variant form of essential myoclonus consists of families with generalized myoclonus in whom the jerks occurred predominantly at the onset of rapid movement and the EMG showed alternating activity in antagonist muscles, mimicking the triphasic pattern of a normal "ballistic" movement[21] (refer to Chap. 40).

Progressive Myoclonic Encephalopathies (PMEs)

In patients with a progressive myoclonic encephalopathy, the features of myoclonus are not distinctive enough to enable the correct identification of the different entities under this title. The key to a correct diagnosis and understanding of the nosology of the progressive myoclonic encephalopathies is the predominant clinical signs associated with myoclonus.

PME WITH EPILEPSY AND DEMENTIA   The major clinical features consist of action and stimuli-sensitive multifocal and generalized myoclonus, tonic-clonic seizures which are difficult to control, and progressive dementia. Age of onset is usually in the first two decades of life, but patients with late onset are occasionally encountered. Other possible signs are ataxia, spasticity, or visual defects, etc. In this setting the diagnoses to consider are Lafora's disease, myoclonic epilepsy with ragged-red fibers (MERRF), lipofuscinosis (Kufs' disease), and sialidosis. In Japan, dentatorubralpallidoluysian atrophy is relatively common and probably the most common cause of the syndrome, which is now well defined as a mitochondrial DNA mutation.

Electrophysiological analysis of the myoclonus frequently indicates a cortical origin, but this finding is not sufficiently specific to enable a definitive diagnosis to be reached. Equally, neuroimaging studies may be abnormal but are not specific.

Lafora's disease has a mean age of onset of 14 years (ranging from 5 to 20) and consists of a rapidly progressing dementia, frequent grand mal seizures which are relatively difficult to control, and visual hallucinations. The disease is inherited by autosomal recessive transmission. Visual evoked potentials may be extremely increased in amplitude (>70 μV). Definitive diagnosis is established by skin and muscle biopsy which shows the characteristic inclusions ("Lafora bodies"). The disease has a fatal evolution in less than 10 years from diagnosis, although more slowly evolving cases have been described.

MERRF is typically suspected in patients with a maternal inheritance pattern and a clinical picture dominated by myoclonus, epilepsy, ataxia, and dementia, associated with other problems such as deafness, myocardiopathy, diabetes, hypertension, and short stature.[22] However, there is tremendous phenotypic variation, and extremely mild forms without dementia and epilepsy (see below) have been reported. MERRF is a typical example of a respiratory chain/oxidative phosphorylation disease, most patients showing a 8234 type of mitochondrial RNA mutation.[23] Final diagnosis is achieved by molecular biology techniques.

Neuronal storage diseases are the most frequent cause of PME in children.[24] Tay-Sachs disease (hexosaminidase A deficiency), Sandhoff's disease (hexosaminidase A and B deficiency), infantile neuropathic Gaucher's disease, and the sialidoses are the most common diagnostic entities.[24] Common to all is the generalized, stimuli-sensitive myoclonus and prominent photosensitivity. In the cherry-red-spot myoclonus syndrome (sialidosis type I), somatosensory evoked potentials are giant, but the visual evoked potentials are decreased in amplitude,[24] a rare combination which may have diagnostic value. In adults, Kufs' disease and sialidosis have been described but are indeed very rare causes of PME.

PME WITH EPILEPSY AND WITHOUT OR WITH ONLY MINOR COGNITIVE DEFECT   This group is made up of patients with a slowly progressing disease with the combination of action myoclonus, epilepsy, and ataxia, in whom no evidence of mitochondrial or any other abnormality is found.[25] Proper recognition of these patients has been marred by several factors, the least of which is semantic. Thus, such patients have been labeled as Unverricht-Lundborg's disease, Baltic myoclonus, and Ramsay-Hunt syndrome. In fact, various types of neurodegenerations, most of which have cerebellar involvement in common, constitute the underlying pathology of the disease process in most cases.[26] Two major clinical subgroups are now recognized: (1) progressive myoclonic epilepsy (PME) and (2) progressive myoclonic ataxia (PMA).

The major cause of PME is Unverritch-Lundborg's disease, which may have associated dementia but more often has minimal or absent cognitive changes. The disease has a worldwide spread and is probably a genetically determined neurodegeneration. In most patients, symptoms begin in the first decade of life. Evolution is slow, with a marked variation within the same family as to the degree of progression and disability.[27] Action and stimuli-sensitive multifocal myoclonus is a major problem. Generalized tonic-clonic seizures may be difficult to control in some cases.[27] Ataxia may be present but usually to a minor degree. Cortical somatosensory evoked potentials are of large amplitude, photosensitivity is frequent, and the EEG is abnormal. Back-averaging the EEG activity preceding the myoclonus will often show a cortical potential antedating the jerks by a few milliseconds (i.e., 15–20 ms for the upper limb). Magnetic resonance imaging/computed tomography (MRI/CT) brain scans are normal or show mild atrophy. In a few cases, atrophy of the cerebellum out of proportion with that present supratentorially can be encountered.[25] All diagnostic tests used to assess the above-mentioned causes of PME with dementia are normal.

PMA is characterized by action myoclonus with multifocal and occasionally generalized distribution, variable presence of stimuli-induced myoclonus, and ataxia. The latter affects mainly gait in the early stage of evolution but evolves towards a widespread cerebellar syndrome. Clinical assessment of the ataxia is hampered by action myoclonus.[2] It is only after proper drug control of the myoclonus that cerebellar signs may be properly evaluated. Epilepsy is absent or mild and almost always well controlled with the drugs used to treat the myoclonus.[25,26] Dementia is certainly not a feature of PMA, but changes in mood and depression are relatively common as disability increases due to disease progression. Many cases are sporadic, but familial forms have also been described.[2] Age at onset varies widely from the first to the seventh decade of life.

A cortical origin for the myoclonus is demonstrated in about 70 percent of cases. It should be noted that drug treatment of the myoclonus (see below) at the time of neurophysiological analysis reduces the likelihood of recording abnormal cortical potentials. The term Ramsay-Hunt syndrome (RHS) may be more properly used in this group of patients. Mitochondrial disease, MERRF in particular, may have a milder course and show the clinical picture of PMA, including late onset and absent cognitive deficit,[28] but the notion that mitochondrial respiratory chain diseases are the most common etiology of progressive myoclonic syndromes with epilepsy or ataxia is erroneous. In fact, most patients

have a neurodegeneration with variable pathological basis. This includes pure spinocerebellar degeneration, spinocerebellar plus dentatorubral degeneration, olivopontocerebellar atrophy (OPCA), and dentatorubropallidoluysian atrophy.[2,26] A deficit of vitamin E (tocopherol) secondary to malabsorption is also a cause of RHS. Recently Bhatia et al.[29] described four patients with sporadic celiac disease coursing without overt malabsorption or malnutrional symptoms with the typical clinical picture of PMA: action and stimuli-sensitive myoclonus, mild ataxia, and infrequent generalized seizures. The myoclonus has all of the electrophysiological characteristics of cortical myoclonus. Stressing a point we had made in earlier writings,[8,10] the pathology of one case revealed Purkinje cell loss in the cerebellum but indemnity of the cortex, thus indicating that cortical myoclonus obeys a disinhibition mechanism.

Particularly interesting is the recent description[30] of a 70-year-old patient from Japan with a spinocerebellear syndrome in whom a mutation was found in the gene coding for the alpha-tocopherol transfer protein, giving rise to the intriguing possibiity of a similar or related defect in patients with RHS or PMA.

PME WITH DEMENTIA AND WITHOUT EPILEPSY   Three neurodegenerative diseases are important to consider in this section: Alzheimer's disease (AD), corticobasal degeneration (CBD), and Huntington's disease (HD).

Alzheimer's disease may have spontaneous and action-induced generalized myoclonus as a prominent and early sign. This form frequently courses clinically with the triad of myoclonus, dementia, and parkinsonism and is a frequent cause of diagnostic confusion. More typically, however, the jerks in AD consist of small amplitude, irregular twitching of the hand muscles, producing a pseudotremulous appearance called "polyminimyoclonus."[31] A slow frontal cortical potential has been recorded preceding these small amplitude jerks.[31]

Corticobasal degeneration (see Chap. 45) is a progressive disorder of asymmetric onset, beginning in the 60s and 70s and mainly characterized by limb apraxia, alien limb phenomenon, slowness and rigidity, cortical sensory defects, dysarthria and aphasia, hand dystonia, and stimuli-sensitive myoclonus. The evolution of CBD is slowly progressive. Most patients become bedridden over a period of 5–8 years. Severe cognitive deficit does not occur in the majority of patients, but in about 30 percent it appears late in the evolution.[32]

The myoclonus of CBD is highly characteristic and a very frequent feature,[32] although nonexclusive of this condition. The affected limb, particularly the forearm and hand muscles, shows what appears to be spontaneous, irregular, and practically continuous jerking, aggravated by any attempt to move voluntarily. Careful observation indicates that the apparently spontaneous jerks are actually due to background ongoing muscle activity.[8] Thus, the myoclonic limb will stop moving when complete relaxation is achieved. The most notorious semiological feature of the myoclonus in CBD is the exquisite sensitivity to sensory stimuli such as light touching, stretching, or even air-puffing the affected hand.[8] These will cause a salvo of muscle jerking that will continue indefinitely unless the explorer can obtain full relaxation of the limb. The extreme tendency for the affected limb to move continuously very often leads to the movement disorder being regarded as tremor, which in addition to the clumsiness and rigidity provokes an early diagnosis of Parkinson's disease that is wrong.

The features of myoclonus in CBD strongly suggest a cortical origin,[33] but the neurophysiological findings are not totally typical. SEPs are not enlarged, and back-averaging frequently fails to detect a potential preceding the jerks.

In Huntington's disease, action myoclonus is a rare manifestation, but a few patients with genetic and autopsy-proven studies have been described in whom multifocal action myoclonus was the primary manifestation. In one such family,[34] electrophysiological studies showed large SEPs and reflex muscle responses typical of cortical myoclonus, and visual stimulation elicited an EEG pattern consistent with visual reflex myoclonus.[10]

Other causes of severe myoclonus associated with cognitive deficit are viral or prion related encephalopathies, particularly Creutzfeldt-Jakob disease (CJD), herpes simplex, and subacute sclerosing panencephalitis (SSPE). The myoclonus in CJD is spontaneous, symmetrical, and generalized. The typical EEG triphasic waves are always associated with the spontaneous myoclonus.

In patients with a subacute myoclonic encephalopathy of unknown cause accompanied by cognitive deficit associated or not with other neurological problems (ataxia, seizures, etc.), the diagnostic possibilities include metabolic derangements (renal and liver failure, hyperglycemia, hypokalemia, hyponatremia, etc.), toxic agents (bismuth, methyl bromide, heavy metals), and drugs (antidepressants, antibiotics, phenytoin, cocaine, amphetamine, etc).

Static Myoclonic Encephalopathies

Action and spontaneous, multifocal, and/or generalized myoclonus may be extremely disabling in patients who have suffered severe anoxia or head trauma. Posthypoxic myoclonus was described by Lance and Adams in 1963,[35] and it received much attention after the discovery of its dramatic sensitivity to treatment with 5-hydroxytryptophan (5-HTP). However, a high proportion of patients show additional neurological deficits (i.e., ataxia, speech difficulties, memory loss, etc.), which reduce the chances of adequate therapeutic control. In their original article, Lance and Adams also described in detail the existence of long EMG silences following the myoclonic jerks. They recognized the importance of these silent periods as being responsible for the postural lapses (negative myoclonus) often seen in posthypoxic myoclonus.

In children with a history of perinatal hypoxia, Obeso et al.[36] described "oscillatory myoclonus" associated with spasticity in the legs, limb dystonia, and dysarthria. The jerks consisted of sudden bursts of myoclonic activity, lasting for a few seconds (1–3 s) and greatly interfering with voluntary motor commands. Recording the muscle activity during such jerking bouts revealed reciprocal activation of antagonist muscles, a very unusual EMG finding in patients with myoclonus of any type and origin.[2] The recent observation of a new case suggests that the seemingly myoclonic bursts may actually be action tremor, explaining the EMG findings.

CAUSES OF FOCAL MYOCLONUS

This section describes conditions characterized by focal or segmental myoclonus which may be spontaneous and rhythmical, may occur in response to sensory stimulation, and/or may occur during action.

Focal Myoclonus of the Limbs

A "jerking limb" may occur in a wide variety of clinical settings. Lesions located along the neuraxis, including the sensorimotor cerebral cortex, thalamus, mesencephalon, and spinal cord, may be associated with focal myoclonus. However, the major causes to consider here are those affecting the cortex or the spinal cord.

CORTICAL MYOCLONUS   In general, cortical myoclonus must be used as a neurophysiological concept and not as a clinical entity. This is so because there are many conditions which course with myoclonus of cortical origin but in which no pathological abnormality at the cortical level is found (for example, see the description of celiac disease in Ref. 29). In this section, cortical myoclonus is used to refer to focal myoclonus associated with a lesion or dysfunction of the cerebral cortex.

In cortical myoclonus the jerks are restricted to a few muscles with predominant activation of distal and flexor muscles. The most common presentation is during action and provoked by somesthetic stimulation. Stretching the fingers, delicate stimulation such as touching the hand or foot with a feather, and pinpricking the wrist are all very effective in triggering a salvo of focal myoclonic jerking. In many patients the reflex myoclonus is modality-specific, and only one of the above stimuli is capable of eliciting the myoclonus. The condition most likely to be associated with cortical reflex myoclonus of one hand is CBD.[8,32,33]

Spontaneous and rhythmical presentation is the main characteristic of epilepsia partialis continua (EPC), which may also be stimuli-sensitive and aggravated by action.[8] The causes of EPC include tumors, arteriovenous (A-V) malformations, focal encephalitis of Kozhevnikov, abcess, stroke, and disorders of neuronal migration. In a proportion of patients with EPC secondary to ischemia or tumors, the lesion is located subcortically.

Focal stimuli-sensitive myoclonus elicited by stimulation of any of the four limbs is very common in multiple system atrophy with predominant OPCA.[37] However, the presence of reflex myoclonus may well pass unnoticed unless actively investigated. The best type of stimulus consists of pinpricking the palmar surface of the wrist and the metacarpal region of the index finger while the examiner extends the fingers and wrist. The rate of stimulation must be low (<1/s) to avoid habituation. Small jerks will be seen or felt in the forearm and intrinsic hand muscles. Occasionally, the same stimuli will induce a generalized jerk. SEPs are enhanced in amplitude and usually associated with a reflex muscle discharge, thus having the characteristics of cortical reflex myoclonus. Flash stimulation is also accompanied by reflex jerks in about 50 percent of patients with OPCA.[37] In contrast with the common photomyoclonic response more frequently found in patients with epilepsy, visual reflex myoclonus in OPCA is induced by low frequency (<10Hz) flash stimulation, each stimulus being accompanied by a cortical spike which antedates a myoclonic jerk.[10] The origin of the abnormal discharge is in the premotor and motor cortex.

The sensitivity to visual stimulus is blocked by L-dopa and dopamine agonists.[10] Because many patients with OPCA also have parkinsonian features, care must be taken to stop medication for at least 12 hours before conducting the electrophysiological evaluation.

SPINAL MYOCLONUS Spinal myoclonus is a typical, albeit rare, cause of focal and usually rhythmical myoclonus. The most frequent clinical presentation consists of spontaneous, repetitive jerks of one limb, sometimes spreading to adjacent neck and trunk muscles. The frequency of the myoclonus is very variable, from 10 to 50/min. In many reported cases the myoclonus persists during sleep. The most common etiologies are cervical myelopathy (including posttraumatic), tumors, multiple sclerosis, and infections.[38] A rather similar presentation may be observed in patients with evidence of peripheral nerve damage (nerve, plexus, and root) with or without accompanying sympathetic changes (Sudeck's atrophy).

Palatal Myoclonus

This is the classic example of focal or segmental rhythmic jerking. A few years ago, however, analysis of this movement disorder by experts in the field led to the conclusion that palatal "myoclonus" is actually a form of tremor and should not be included under the category of myoclonus.[39] Nevertheless, the term "palatal myoclonus" remains in general use in most clinical quarters and deserves a brief summary in this chapter.

Palatal movements occur unilaterally or bilaterally, at 0.5–3 Hz, and are frequently associated with synchronous movements of the tongue, face, larynx, neck, and even arm muscles. Hypertrophic degeneration of the inferior olive is the pathological basis of this disorder,[40] but interruption or lesions of the connections between the dentate nucleus and the inferior olives via the red nucleus (Guillain-Mollaret triangle) may also induce the tremor.[40] Two distinct clinical forms can be distinguished:[41] essential palatal tremor (EPT) and symptomatic palatal tremor (SPT). EPT is characterized, in addition to the palatal movements, by ear clicking in phase with the tremor and no history of neurological disorders. Patients with SPT have clinical evidence of cerebellar and brain stem dysfunction, but ear clicking is not a feature.[41] EPT ceases almost completely during sleep, but SPT is only slightly reduced.[41] The most common causes of SPT are trauma, multiple sclerosis, stroke, and degenerative diseases.[42]

Facial Myoclonus

Twitching of some facial muscles may occur in normal people when tired and after excessive tobacco and alcohol consumption, in hemifacial spasm, and following focal brain stem lesions. In most instances, the EMG pattern is that of myokymia or spasms rather than truly myoclonic. Rhythmic slow movements of the orbicularis oris sometimes spreading to the adjacent musculature leads one to consider Whipple's disease.

Authentic facial myoclonus without involvement of any other body part is actually rare. The most common condition associated with it is EPC.

Axial Myoclonus

Segmental and rhythmical myoclonus of the neck and trunk may rarely arise as a consequence of brain stem lesions, Arnold-Chiari malformation, and upper cervical cord damage.[38] Vela et al.[42] recently described an exceptional patient with focal myoclonic jerking of the neck as the initial sign of SSPE.

Nonrhythmic, repetitive axial flexion, and more rarely extension jerks, occurring spontaneously but aggravated by action and sensitive to stretching, are the major features of "propiospinal myoclonus."[9] The EMG shows irregular, brief bursts at a variable frequency of 1–7 Hz. Detailed neurophysiological analysis (refer to Chap. 40) is necessary to confirm the spinal origin of this uncommon presentation.

GENERALIZED, STIMULI-SENSITIVE MYOCLONUS
In a small proportion of all patients with myoclonus, the main problem consists in whole body jerks triggered by sensory stimuli (sound, touching, stretching, or visual threatening). This clinical presentation may correspond to three different mechanisms: (1) reticular reflex myoclonus; (2) hyperekplexia; and (3) psychogenic (also refer to Chap. 40).

Reticular reflex myoclonus (RRM) is a pathophysiological term describing the origin of myoclonus in the brain stem reticular formation. Anoxia, uremia, liver failure, drugs, and brain stem encephalitis are the major causes of RRM.

Hyperekplexia is the pathological manifestation of startle.[43] Clinical differences from RRM are that the latter may also occur during action whereas hyperekplexia is always stimuli-induced. Tonic spasms following stimulation may be present in hyperekplexia but are not associated with RRM. Otherwise, precise differentiation of the two conditions require electrophysiological assessment. Hyperekplexia may be symptomatic or inherited as an autosomal dominant condition. The latter has been defined as a mutation in the alpha-1 subunit of the glycine receptor.

Normal people may, for a variety of reasons, jump and jerk in response to external stimulation mimicking myoclonus and startle.[44] Clinical hints to the diagnosis are the acute onset, variability in the stimuli triggering the jerks, and variable recruitment of the muscles.[44] In such cases, the onset of the EMG discharge is always within the range of normal reaction time.[44]

Treatment

Myoclonus is a very disabling movement disorder because it utilizes the same motor control mechanisms that are necessary for normal voluntary movements. The treatment of myoclonus is largely empirical, because there has been little progress in understanding its biochemical basis. In this section the therapeutic possibilities are discussed in accordance with the major clinical presentations, as described above, and the pathophysiological origin of myoclonus regardless of the etiology.

MULTIFOCAL ACTION MYOCLONUS

This is the most incapacitating form and the one requiring the major therapeutic effort. In around 70 percent of patients with action myoclonus, electrophysiological assessment indicates a cortical origin. This is a very important feature to consider when addressing the pharmacological approach. The initiation of drug treatments in action myoclonus occurred in the 1970s when 5-HTP, the precursor of serotonin, was given to a French patient with postanoxic action myoclonus[45] in whom a large number of drugs had been tried without success and a thalamotomy had also been performed with no benefit. Administration of 5-HTP with carbidopa to prevent peripheral decarboxylation produced a dramatic improvement in the patient. This result led to a number of studies on posthypoxic action myoclonus, which confirmed the therapeutic action of 5-HTP plus carbidopa (100–300/25 mg/day). It was found that the CSF concentration of the major serotonin metabolite, 5-hydroxyindolacetic acid (5-HIAA), was lowered in most of these patients.[46,47] Physiological analysis revealed that patients with postanoxic myoclonus with an excellent response to 5-HTP had reticular reflex myoclonus, whereas those with a moderate or no response had cortical reflex myoclonus.[47] The failure to control equally well all cases with 5-HTP and the associated side effects (nausea, vomiting, diarrhea, hypotension and gastrointestinal bleeding) led to the examination of other alternative drugs. Clonazepam, sodium valproate, and fluoxetine were found useful.[48] In later years, several patients with action myoclonus have been physiologically and pharmacologically studied, and a general picture of the treatment of severe action myoclonus has emerged.

The major factor recognized as a predictor of the drug responsiveness is the neurophysiological origin. Cortical myoclonus responds exceedingly well to piracetam (8–20 g/day), clonazepam (2–15 mg/day), sodium valproate (1200–3000 mg/day), and primidone (500–1000 mg/day).[49] In the majority of patients with severe, highly disabling action myoclonus, these drugs have to be given in combination to achieve adequate control.[49,50] This is thought to be due to the various mechanisms implicated in the pathophysiology of cortical myoclonus.[8,49] Clonazepam is the most efficient antimyoclonic drug, but piracetam is the first drug to be used because of its excellent tolerance up to 24 g/day.[50,51] All of these drugs are believed to act by increasing gamma-aminobutyric acid (GABA) activity in the cortex, but direct evidence of their mechanism of action against cortical myoclonus is still lacking. Surprisingly, the initial experience with other recently acquired anticonvulsant drugs such as vigabatrin and gabapentin has not been positive. Milacemide, a prodrug of glycine, was tried without benefit in a few patients with myoclonus, but neurophysiological assessment was not reported.[52]

In two patients with progressive myoclonic ataxia and cortical myoclonus, the addition of acetozalamide to the combination discussed above led to better control of the jerks.[53]

The degree of symptomatic control achieved in patients with action myoclonus of cortical origin is usually very striking at the beginning of treatment, but the long-term treatment response pattern is variable. This depends on several factors, the most important of which is the underlying disease. Patients with a static encephalopathy, e.g., posthypoxia, in whom myoclonus is the only or major clinical problem, achieve a very long-lasting and adequate control. On the other hand, patients with progressive illness, e.g., MERFF, sialidosis, neurodegenerations, etc, are very difficult to control for any length of time. An important practical point in the management of such cases is the ease with which generalized seizures may occur when manipulating the drug regimen. Thus, when a given drug treatment is judged inefficient, its withdrawal must be achieved very carefully and slowly.

The above discussion relates to the treatment of action myoclonus understood to be a positive muscle discharge. However, in most patients the jerks are actually a combination of positive and negative (EMG silence) myoclonus.[1] The latter is as incapacitating as the former. However, there has not been any study specifically analyzing the effect of antimyoclonic drugs against negative myoclonus. In many patients, the postural lapses that affect the trunk and proximal leg muscles are the most difficult feature to keep under control.[49,50]

Patients with action myoclonus originating in the brain stem (reticular reflex myoclonus) are much less frequent. Clonazepam is the drug of choice. Fluoxetine (10–20 mg/day) and 5-HTP may produce additional benefit.

FOCAL MYOCLONUS OF CORTICAL ORIGIN

This myoclonus also responds very well to the drugs discussed above.[8] The only exception is CBD, but this is a very special pathophysiological type of cortical myoclonus and a rapidly evolving disease.[33,34] In extremely severe cases of cortical myoclonus producing epilepsia partialis continua, surgery may be considered after rigorous assessment.

Spinal myoclonus has no specific drug treatment. The best therapeutic approach is to treat the causative condition whenever this is possible. Drugs used with some benefit include clonazepam, carbamazepine, and tetrabenazine. Palatal myoclonus may respond to 5-HTP, trihexyphenidyl (up to 60 mg/day), carbamazepine, and piracetam.

Nocturnal myoclonus, usually involving the legs but occasionally the whole body, may require treatment when very frequent and so severe as to interfere with falling asleep. Clonazepam at a relatively low dose (1–3 mg, bed time) is very effective for controlling this problem.

References

1. Obeso JA, Artieda J, Burleigh A: Clinical aspects of negative myoclonus. *Adv Neurol* 67:1–8, 1996.
2. Obeso JA, Artieda J, Marsden CD: Different clinical presentations of myoclonus in Jankovic J, Tolosa E (eds): *Parkinson's Disease and Movement Disorders,* 2nd edition. Baltimore: Williams and Wilkins, chap 19, pp 315–328, 1993.
3. Obeso JA, Narbona J: Post-traumatic tremor and myoclonic jerking. *J Neurol Neurosurg Psychiatry* 46:788, 1983.

4. Rothwell JC, Obeso JA: The anatomical and physiological basis of torsion dystonia in Marsden CD and Fahn S (eds): *Movement Disorders-2*. London: Butterworth, chap 16, pp 313–331, 1987.
5. Mahloudji M, Pikely RT: Hereditary essential myoclonus. *Brain* 90:669–674, 1967.
6. Quinn NP: Essential myoclonus and myoclonic dystonia—a review. *Mov Disord*. 11:119–124, 1996.
7. Vogel CM, Drury I, Terry LC, Young AB. Myoclonus in adult Huntington's disease. *Ann Neurol* 29:213–215, 1991.
8. Obeso JA, Rothwell JC, Marsden CD: The spectrum of cortical myoclonus—from focal reflex jerks to spontaneous motor epilepsy. *Brain* 108:193–224, 1985.
9. Brown P, Thompson PD, Rothwell JC, et al: Axial myoclonus of propiospinal origin. *Brain* 114:197–214, 1991.
10. Artieda J, Obeso JA: The pathophysiology and pharmacology of photic cortical reflex myoclonus. *Ann Neurol* 34:175–184, 1993.
11. Shibasaki H, Ikeda A, Nagamine T, et al: Cortical reflex negative myoclonus. *Brain* 117:477–486, 1994.
12. Brown P, Rothwell JC, Thompson PD, Marsden CD. Propiospinal myoclonus: "Pattern" generators in humans. *Mov Disord* 9:571–576, 1994.
13. Marsden CD, Hallett M, Fahn S: The nosology and patho-physiology of myoclonus, in *Movement Disorders-1*. London: Butterworth, 1982, chap 13, pp 196–248.
14. Artieda J, Luquin MR, Vaamonde J, et al: Generalized reflex myoclonus in a patient with alcohol-sensitive spontaneous myoclonus and an abnormal gait pattern. *Mov Disord* 5:85–88, 1990.
15. Kurlan R, Berh J, Medved L, Shoulson I: Myoclonus and dystonia: A family study. *Adv Neur* 50:385-389, 1988.
16. Davidenkow F: Auf hereditar-abiotrophischer Grundlage akut auf tretende, regressierende und episodische Erkrankungen des Nervensystems und Bemerkungen über die familäre subakute, myoklonische Dystonie. *Z Neurol Psychiatry* 104:596–622, 1926.
17. Obeso JA, Rothwell JC, Lang AE, Marsden CD: Myoclonic dystonia. *Neurology* 33:825–830, 1983.
18. Fahn S, Sjaastad O. Hereditary essential myoclonus in a large Norwegian family. *Mov Disord* 6:237–247, 1991.
19. Korten JJ, Notermans SLH, Frenken CWGM, et al: Familial essential myoclonus. *Brain* 97:131–138, 1974.
20. Gudin M, Vaamonde J, Rodriguez M, et al: Alcohol-sensitive dystonia. *Mov Disord* 8:122–123, 1993.
21. Hallett M, Chadwick D, Marsden CD: Ballistic movement overflow myoclonus: A form of essential myoclonus. *Brain* 110:299-312, 1977.
22. DiMauro S, Moraes CT: Mitochondrial encephalomyopathies. *Arch Neurol* 50:1197-1208.
23. Jackson MJ, Schaefer JA, Johnson MA et al: Presentation and clinical investigation of mitochondrial respiratory chain disease. A study of 51 patients. *Brain* 118:339–358, 1995.
24. Rapin I: Myoclonus in neuronal storage and Lafora disease. *Adv Neurol* 43:65–86, 1986.
25. Marsden CD, Harding A, Obeso JA, Lu CS: Progressive myoclonic ataxia (the Ramsay Hunt syndrome). *Arch of Neurol* 47:1121–1125, 1990.
26. Marsden CD, Obeso JA: The Ramsay Hunt syndrome is a useful clinical entity. *Mov Disord* 4:6–12, 1989.
27. Berkovic SF, Andermann F, Carpenter S, Wolfe SL: Progressive myoclonus epilepsies: Specific causes and diagnosis. *N Engl J Med* 315:296–305, 1986.
28. Vaamonde J, Muruzabal J, Tuñon T, et al: Abnormal muscle and skin mitochondria in a family with myoclonus, ataxia and deafness (May and White syndrome). *J Neurol Neurosurg Psychiatry* 55:128–132, 1992.
29. Bhatia KP, Brown P, Gregory R, et al: Progressive myoclonic ataxia associated with coeliac disease. *Brain* 118:1087--1093, 1995.
30. Gotoda T, Arita M, Hiroyuki A, et al: Adult-onset spino-cerebellar dysfunction caused by a mutation in the gene for the alpha-tocopherol-transfer protein. *N Engl J Med* 333:1313–1318, 1995.
31. Wilkins DE, Hallett M, Berardelli A, et al: Physiological analysis of the myoclonus of Alzheimer's disease. *Neurology* 34:898–903, 1984.
32. Rinne JO, Lee MS, Thompson PD, Marsden CD: Corticobasal degeneration: A clinical study of 36 cases. *Brain* 117:1183–1196, 1994.
33. Thompson PD, Day BL, Rothwell JC, et al: The myoclonus in corticobasal degeneration: Evidence for two forms of cortical reflex myoclonus. *Brain* 117:1197–1208, 1995.
34. Thompson PD, Bhatia KP, Brown P, et al: Cortical myoclonus in Huntington's disease. *Mov Disord* 9:633–641, 1994.
35. Lance JW, Adams RD: The syndrome of intention or action myoclonus as a sequel to hypoxic encephalopathy. *Brain* 86:111–136, 1963.
36. Obeso JA, Lang AE, Rothwell JC, Marsden CD: Post-anoxic symptomatic oscillatory myoclonus. *Neurology* 33:240–243, 1983.
37. Rodriguez M, Artieda J, Zubieta JL, Obeso JA: Reflex myoclonous in olivopontocerebellar atrophy. *J Neurol. Neurosurg Psychiatry* 57:316–319, 1994.
38. Jankovic J, Pardo R: Segmental myoclonus: Clinical and pharmacological study. *Arch Neurol* 43:1025–1031, 1986.
39. Hallett M, Shibasaki H, Obeso JA: Criteria for visual identification of myoclonus. *Mov Disord*. In Press.
40. Lapresle J: Palatal myoclonus. *Adv Neurol* 43:265–274, 1986.
41. Deuschl G, Toro C, Valls-Solé J, et al: Symptomatic and essential palatal tremor. *Brain* 117:775–788, 1994.
42. Vela L, Felgueroso B, Villar ME, et al: Panaencefalitis esclerosante subaguda del adulto con mioclonias segmentarias como sintoma inicial. *Neurologia* 10:470, 1995.
43. Brown P, Rothwell JC, Thompson PD, et al: The hyperekplexias and their relationship to a normal startle reflex. *Brain* 114:1903–1928, 1991.
44. Thompson PD, Colebatch JG, Rothwell JC, et al: Voluntary stimulus sensitive jerks and jumps mimicking myoclonus or pathological startle syndrome. *Mov Dis* 7:257–262, 1992.
45. Lhermitte F, Oeterfalvi M, Marteau R, et al: Analyse pharmacologique d'un cas de myoclonus d'intention et d'action postanoxique. *Rev Neurol (Paris)* 124:21–31, 1971.
46. Van Woert MH, Sethy VH: Therapy of intention myoclonus with l-5-hydroxytryptophan and a peripheral decarboxylase inhibitor, MK 486. *Neurology* 25:135–140, 1975.
47. Chadwick D, Hallett M, Harris R, et al: Clinical, biochemical and physiological features distinguishing myoclonus responsive to 5-hydroxytryptophan, tryptophan with a monoamine oxidase inhibitor and clonazepam. *Brain* 100:455–487, 1977.
48. Fahn S: Posthypoxic action myoclonus: Literature review update. *Adv Neurol* 43:157–169, 1986.
49. Obeso JA, Artieda J, Rothwell JC, et al: The treatment of severe action myoclonus. *Brain* 112:765–777, 1989.
50. Obeso JA, Artieda J, Quinn NP, et al: Piracetam in the treatment of different types of myoclonus. *Clin Neuropharmacol* 11:529–536, 1988.
51. Brown P, Steiger MJ, Thompson PD, et al: Effectiveness of piracetam in cortical myoclonus. *Mov Disord* 8:63–68, 1993.
52. Gordon Forrest M, Diaz-Olivo R, Hunt AL, Fahn S: Therapeutic trial of milacemide in patients with myoclonus and other intractable movement disorders. *Mov Disord* 8:484–488, 1993.
53. Vaamonde J, Legarda I, Jimenez-Jimenez J, Obeso JA: Acetazolamide improves action myoclonus in Ramsay Hunt syndrome. *Clin Neuropharmacol* 15:392–396, 1992.

Chapter 40

PATHOPHYSIOLOGY OF MYOCLONIC DISORDERS

CAMILO TORO and MARK HALLETT

PHYSIOLOGICAL CLASSIFICATION OF MYOCLONUS
    Epileptic Myoclonus
    Nonepileptic Myoclonus
ELECTROPHYSIOLOGICAL EVALUATION OF
MYOCLONUS
    Polygraphic EMG Studies
    Routine Electroencephalography
    EEG Back-Averaging
    SEPs
    Reflex Studies
    Transcranial Magnetic Stimulation (TMS)
NEGATIVE MYOCLONUS

The electrophysiological study of myoclonic movements has interested clinical electrophysiologists, epileptologists, movement disorders specialists, and sleep medicine specialists. As early as 1935, Gibbs et al.[1] had described patients with spike-and-wave discharges in the electroencephalogram (EEG) with muscle jerking at the same rate of the EEG spikes. Grinker et al.[2] are credited with the first description of polyspike discharges in the EEG, with close association to myoclonic jerking in patients with progressive myoclonic epilepsy. In 1946, Dawson produced a detailed description of the relationship between EEG spikes and muscle jerks in patients with myoclonus, reporting also, in some of his patients, the possibility of inducing myoclonic jerks by tendon tapping.[3] One year later, Dawson himself demonstrated not only the first recording of somatosensory evoked potentials (SEPs) from the scalp in humans[4] but also showed that SEPs in patients with myoclonus could be grossly exaggerated in amplitude.[5]

Electrophysiological studies aid in making the diagnosis and provide insight into the pathophysiology of myoclonus.[6-11] From a clinical perspective, myoclonus refers to quick muscle jerks, either irregular or rhythmic, and almost always arising from the central nervous system. This definition itself is quite nonspecific and is of little value in establishing a precise etiologic diagnosis or understanding the basic pathophysiological mechanisms of the disorder. Myoclonus can be focal, involving only a few adjacent muscles; generalized, involving many or most of the muscles in the body; or multifocal, involving many muscles but in different jerks.[8] Myoclonus can be spontaneous, can be activated or accentuated by voluntary movement (action myoclonus), and can be activated or accentuated by sensory stimulation (reflex myoclonus).[8,9,11-13] In the differential diagnosis of myoclonus, the principal features that favor myoclonus are the quickness and fragmentary nature of the movement and the absence of voluntary influence.[12] Some simple tics look identical to myoclonus and cannot be visually distinguished. Another disorder that could be confused with myoclonus is tremor, because some forms of myoclonus are rhythmic.[14] Conversely, some tremors, despite a regular frequency, have a variable amplitude of the EMG and present an irregular appearance that is not unlike that of myoclonus.[12]

Perhaps the only electrophysiological finding that can be generalized across the broad clinical definition of myoclonus is that myoclonus arises from abnormal muscle activation in the form of short (50–300 ms) electromyogram (EMG) bursts (positive myoclonus).[6,7] Less often, myoclonus is the result of brief interruptions of ongoing tonic EMG (negative myoclonus).[15,16] In both instances this abnormal EMG activity leads to a brief displacement of the involved body segment and/or disruption of posture. These features alone may aid in differentiating myoclonus from fragments of other movement disorders with more complex and lengthy patterns of muscle coactivation, such as chorea and dystonia.[6,7] Additional electrophysiological assessment can aid in deciding whether the movement disorder is indeed myoclonus, and, if so, which physiological type.[8]

Physiological Classification of Myoclonus

There are several useful schemes for classifying myoclonus.[8] For the purposes of therapy, it is valuable to consider both an etiologic classification and a physiological classification. The etiologic and physiological classifications of myoclonus often do not coincide. An etiologic classification of myoclonus provides guidance for treatment of the underlying metabolic, infectious, or toxic derangement, and it has clear implications in the prognosis and counseling of relatives of afflicted individuals. The physiological classification of myoclonus searches for the site and mechanism of origin of the symptoms, the precipitating factors, and the pathways of spread. Myoclonic disorders, with strikingly different etiologic, genetic, and prognostic implications, may fall into the same physiological group, sharing relatively homogeneous electrophysiological properties that usually point to common physiological derangement.[8-11,14] These findings, in turn, may aid the selection of the most appropriate symptomatic therapy and may serve as a quantitative tool for evaluating efficacy and mechanisms of action of antimyoclonic medications.[17-19]

Halliday[20] can be credited with the first comprehensive attempt to classify the myoclonias, based on their electrophysiological correlates. He divided myoclonus into three main groups: *pyramidal, extrapyramidal,* and *segmental. Pyramidal* myoclonus encompassed those myoclonic disorders characterized by a brief burst of EMG activity associated with an EEG correlate. Because of the short latency between the EEG event and the EMG burst (15–40 ms), he proposed an origin in the cortex propagated via the pyramidal tract. In *extrapyramidal* myoclonus, Halliday included those myoclonic movements in which the EEG events were less obvious and the EMG bursts were of longer duration. He considered the movements seen in subacute sclerosing panencephalitis (SSPE) as prototypical of this group. The loose association between EEG and EMG and the long and variable length of EMG bursts suggested to Halliday an extrapyramidal site of origin. *Segmental* myoclonus was used by Halliday to denote myoclonus, often symmetrical and rhythmic, confined to discrete brain stem segments or spinal cord myotomes and arising from brain stem or spinal cord damage as a result of trauma, infection, or neoplasm.

We now classify myoclonus in two broad groups (Table 40-1). By defining epileptic myoclonus as myoclonus that is a fragment of epilepsy, myoclonus can be divided into *epileptic* and *nonepileptic* types.[21,22] The physiological characteristics of epileptic myoclonus are (1) EMG burst length of 10–50 ms, (2) synchronous antagonist activity, and (3) an EEG correlate. Nonepileptic myoclonus shows (1) EMG burst lengths of 50–300 ms, (2) synchronous or asynchronous antagonist activity, and (3) no EEG correlate. The classification of myoclonus into epileptic and nonepileptic groups has a value beyond simple taxonomic curiosity. Response to anticonvulsant agents and other antimyoclonic medications, such as piracetam, appears to be closely linked to the physiological features of the myoclonus.[17,18]

The terms cortical and subcortical myoclonus are used to classify myoclonus according to the location in the nervous system of the presumed generator of the myoclonus.[8] Cortical and subcortical myoclonus can be used almost interchangeably with epileptic and nonepileptic myoclonus, respectively. Reticular reflex myoclonus, classified as epileptic myoclonus, is the only form of myoclonus at odds with the overlap in the two classification schemes. Reticular reflex myoclonus originates from abnormal paroxysmal discharges in the brain stem reticular formation and thus has a subcortical origin.

EPILEPTIC MYOCLONUS

Cortical reflex myoclonus is a fragment of focal or partial epilepsy.[21] Each myoclonic jerk involves only a few adjacent muscles, but larger jerks with more muscles involved can be seen. The disorder is commonly multifocal and is accentuated by action and sensory stimulation. The EEG reveals a focal positive-negative event over the sensorimotor cortex contralateral to the jerk preceding both spontaneous and reflex-induced myoclonic jerks. With stimulus sensitivity, C-reflexes are seen and are correlated with giant SEPs. The EEG

event associated with reflex jerks is a giant P1-N2 component of the SEP[19,21-24] (Fig. 40-1). Often, the P1-N2 has exactly the same topography as the positive-negative event preceding the spontaneous myoclonus, but at times there are some differences.[9,19,23,24] A final feature is that if the cranial nerve muscles are active, then the timing of onset of activation is from above downward; that is, the masseter (5th cranial nerve) is active before the orbicularis oculi (7th cranial nerve), which is itself active before the sternocleidomastoid (11th cranial nerve).[21]

Reticular reflex myoclonus is a fragment of a type of generalized epilepsy.[25] These jerks are usually generalized with predominance that is proximal more than distal and flexor more than extensor. Voluntary action and sensory stimulation increase the jerking. This disorder has the following features: (1) There are brief generalized EMG bursts, lasting 10–30 ms and triggered by sensory stimulation, such as touch or muscle stretch, or by action. (2) The EEG correlates, when present, are not time-locked to the muscle activation. (3) The pattern of EMG activation in cranial nerve muscles is with the sternocleidomastoid muscle activated first and the other cranial nerve muscles activated in reverse numerical order. It is as if the front of activation originates in proximity to the motor nucleus of the eleventh cranial nerve and travels bidirectionally along the neuroaxis.[25] Reticular reflex myoclonus can be seen in patients with postanoxic myoclonus and in other toxic-metabolic encephalopathies associated with myoclonus, such as uremia.[26] In cats, urea infusions give rise to this form of myoclonus. Depth electrode recordings in these animals have defined the origin of the abnormal discharge in the nucleus reticularis gigantocellularis.[27]

TABLE 40-1 Physiological Classification of Myoclonus

Epileptic myoclonus
  Cortical reflex myoclonus
  Reticular reflex myoclonus
  Primary generalized epileptic myoclonus
  Photic cortical reflex myoclonus
Nonepileptic myoclonus
  Normal physiological phenomena (e.g., hypnic jerk)
  Essential myoclonus
  Palatal myoclonus (tremor)
  Spinal myoclonus, including propriospinal myoclonus
  Peripheral myoclonus
  Exaggerated startle
  Nocturnal myoclonus (e.g., periodic movements in sleep)
  Psychogenic myoclonus

FIGURE 40-1 Giant SEPs in a patient with cortical sensory-reflex myoclonus. Taps to the fingers on the left hand (indicated by the vertical dashed line) give rise to a giant SEP response, which is larger over the contralateral central regions (C4). A reflex EMG response (C-reflex) in the left abductor pollicis brevis muscle (LAPB) is elicited after most of the taps. The onset of the reflex response, indicated by the arrow, has a latency of 42 ms.

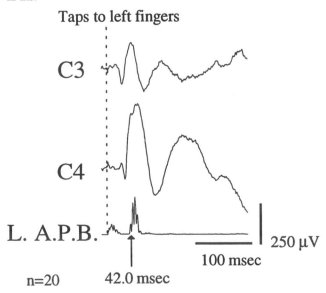

Both cortical and reticular reflex myoclonus may be seen in the same patient.[21,28] Clinically, there will be both multifocal and generalized jerks, and physiological analysis will reveal features of both disorders.

Primary generalized epileptic myoclonus is a fragment of primary generalized epilepsy.[22] The most common clinical manifestation is small, focal jerks, often involving only the fingers; thus, the myoclonus is sometimes called minipolymyoclonus.[29] The term minipolymyoclonus was originally coined to refer to small jerks seen in patients with motor neuron disease. Minipolymyoclonus of central origin and minipolymyoclonus of peripheral origin have a similar clinical appearance and are probably most easily separated by the company they keep, epilepsy and muscle denervation, respectively. A second clinical presentation of primary generalized epileptic myoclonus consists of generalized, synchronized whole-body jerks not unlike those seen with reticular reflex myoclonus.[29] The EEG correlate is a slow, bilateral frontocentrally predominant negativity similar to the wave of a primary generalized paroxysm.

Recent detailed studies of photic cortical reflex myoclonus show that it has an origin in a hyperexcitable motor cortex and is driven by an occipital response of normal appearance.[30] There is a remarkable similarity in these findings and those of the myoclonus in the photosensitive Papio papio baboon.[31,32] Intermittent light stimulation in the photosensitive baboon gives rise to frontocentral paroxysmal discharges. The surface-positive component of the cortical discharge precedes activation of the orbicularis oculi by 4 ms, the masseter by 7 ms, the biceps by 8 ms, and the paraspinal muscles by 24 ms. These results are consistent with a pyramidal tract route of spread. Unit recordings indicate areas 4 and 6 of the cortex with the highest levels of activity.[33] Recordings from subcortical structures show that their involvement is always secondary to the cortical activation. A failure of intracortical recurrent inhibition seems responsible, at least in part, for these findings.[32]

NONEPILEPTIC MYOCLONUS

Some myoclonic movements reflect normal physiological phenomena. One such phenomenon is the hypnic jerk experienced by all people at one time or another.[8]

Essential myoclonus is a term that is used for those patients whose sole neurological abnormality is myoclonus and who specifically do not have seizures, dementia, or ataxia.[8] The EEG and other laboratory investigations should be normal. Familial cases as well as sporadic cases are seen. Ballistic movement overflow myoclonus is one type of essential myoclonus that has been seen as an autosomal-dominant disorder.[8] The myoclonus is generalized, appears to occur a little at rest, and is clearly increased by action. The EMG is characterized by the ballistic "triphasic" EMG pattern with alternating activity in antagonist muscles (although more tonic EMG patterns might also be seen).[34]

Palatal myoclonus, now preferentially called palatal tremor, is the prototypical rhythmic focal myoclonic disorder.[35–38] Palatal tremor has now been shown to consist of two separate disorders: essential palatal tremor (EPT), which manifests an ear click, and symptomatic palatal tremor (SPT),

which is associated with cerebellar disturbances.[36–38] The palatal movements are consistent with activation of the tensor veli palatini muscle in EPT and of the levator veli palatini muscle in SPT.[38] Palatal movements, unilaterally or bilaterally, occur at 1.5–3 Hz and, in SPT, may be accompanied by synchronous movements of adjacent muscles, such as the external ocular muscles, tongue, larynx, face, neck, diaphragm, or even limb muscles. During sleep, EPT stops, whereas SPT continues, with only slight variations in the tremor rate. The palatal tremor cycle exerts remote effects on the tonic EMG activity of the upper and lower extremities only in patients with SPT. In SPT, cerebellar dysfunction ipsilateral to the palatal tremor may be a result in part of abnormal function of the contralateral hypertrophic inferior olive, but the pathophysiological basis of EPT remains unknown.[36–38] Focal movements of tongue or neck can occur without palatal movement and have been called bulbar myoclonus or branchial myoclonus.[35]

Spinal myoclonus is more commonly rhythmic than arrhythmic.[8,20] Involved regions can be one limb, one limb and adjacent trunk, or both legs. Lesions of the spinal cord giving rise to focal movements include infection, degenerative disease, tumor, cervical myelopathy, and demyelinating disease, and it may follow spinal anesthesia or the introduction of contrast media into the cerebrospinal fluid (CSF). Unlike palatal myoclonus, spinal myoclonus is only rarely idiopathic. Spinal myoclonus usually occurs spontaneously and may persist during sleep.

A new form of spinal myoclonus, propriospinal myoclonus, has been recently recognized.[39,40] This is clinically characterized by axial jerks that are nonrhythmic and that lead to symmetric flexion of neck, trunk, hips, and knees. Jerks can be spontaneous or stimulus-induced. By EMG studies, the myoclonus starts in the midthoracic region and propagates slowly, about 5 m/s, both rostrally and caudally.

Peripheral myoclonus has been reported, but it is not clear that this is always distinct from fasciculation or myokymia. Peripheral myoclonus is recognized by signs of acute or chronic denervation in the involved muscles. Cases have been reported with lesions of nerve, brachial plexus, and nerve root.[7,8]

Exaggerated startle is being increasingly recognized clinically as a form of myoclonus.[41–43] It is normal to have a quick muscular response to a surprise stimulus; this is the startle response. It can be considered exaggerated because it is too large a response or too complex but, most commonly, it is exaggerated because it appears when it is not expected. A startle would not be expected when the stimulus is not a surprise, and normal human beings adapt fairly quickly to low-intensity or repeated stimuli. There has been considerable confusion in the literature as to which myoclonic phenomena are truly exaggerated startle reflexes. One source of confusion, for example, is stimulus-sensitive myoclonus, which might be difficult to distinguish purely on clinical grounds from exaggerated startle. Creutzfeldt-Jakob disease is commonly said to be characterized by an exaggerated startle, but the stimulus-induced response is a myoclonic jerk.[8,42]

The normal parameters of the audiogenic startle response have been well-characterized and enable proper recognition.[43,44] There is a bilaterally symmetric pattern with an invariable blink; other craniocervical muscles almost always are activated, but recruitment in the limbs is variable (Fig. 40-2). Onset latencies of EMG activity are 20–40 ms in the orbicularis oculi, 35–80 ms in masseter and sternocleidomastoid, 50–100 ms in biceps brachii, 100–125 ms in hamstrings and quadriceps, and 130–140 ms in tibialis anterior. The latency of the response in abductor pollicis brevis is much delayed, compared to what would be expected from the latency of the response in the biceps.[41,43] There is synchronous activation of antagonist muscles with an EMG burst duration of 50–400 ms, shortening with habituation. The response significantly habituates within a few trials.

Recent studies have shown that hyperekplexia or startle disease is characterized by a truly exaggerated startle.[41–43] Startle epilepsy is a disorder consisting of epilepsy after a startle. The interesting syndrome known by many names, including *jumping* or *latah,* appears also to be initiated with a startle, but its physiology has never been investigated in detail.

Nocturnal myoclonus includes several different phenomena, including the hypnic jerk, periodic movements in sleep, and excessive fragmentary myoclonus in non-rapid eye movement (NREM) sleep. Myoclonus associated with epilepsy, intention myoclonus associated with semivolitional

FIGURE 40-2 **Polygraphic average of 20 trials of rectified EMG reflex responses to stimulation of the right median nerve in a patient with cortical reflex myoclonus. In this patient, focal stimulation often resulted in generalized body twitches. The latency of activation of the different muscles is consistent with a rostrocaudal pattern of activation with muscles innervated by the highest cranial nerves activating first. R, right; L, left; APB, abductor pollicis brevis muscle; SCM, sternocleidomastoid muscle; Orb. Oc, orbicularis oculi. Activation of the L. APB follows activation of the R. APB by about 15 ms. This difference probably represents a delay related to transcallosal spread of the activation from the left to the right hemisphere.**

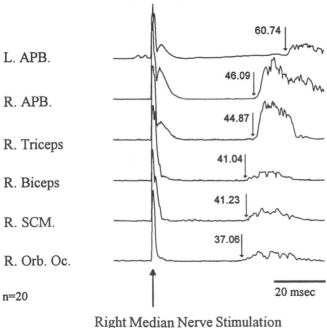

L. APB.

60.74

R. APB.

46.09

R. Triceps

44.87

R. Biceps

41.04

R. SCM.

41.23

R. Orb. Oc.

37.06

n=20

20 msec

Right Median Nerve Stimulation

movements, and segmental myoclonus also occur in sleep but are not primarily nocturnal.[8] Periodic movements of sleep are characterized by a pattern that is unmistakable. EMG bursts of tonic type, lasting 500–2000 ms (really out of the myoclonus range), come every 10–30 s, and are most prominent in the tibialis anterior muscles. The two sides of the body can be activated independently, simultaneously, or even alternately. They occur in NREM sleep but can occur also in drowsiness, when the patient can be fully conscious of their occurrence.[45]

Myoclonus can also be psychogenic. Monday and Jankovic[46] reported on the clinical features of 18 such patients. The myoclonus was present for 1–110 months; it was segmental in ten, generalized in seven, and focal in one patient. Stress precipitated or exacerbated the myoclonic movements in 15 patients; 14 had a definite increase in myoclonic activity during periods of anxiety. The following findings helped to establish the psychogenic nature of the myoclonus: (1) clinical features incongruous with "organic" myoclonus, (2) evidence of underlying psychopathology, (3) an improvement with distraction or placebo, and (4) the presence of incongruous sensory loss or false weakness. More than one-half of all patients with adequate follow-up improved after gaining insight into the psychogenic mechanisms of their movement disorder. Physiological investigation in such cases is lacking. One single case report of a patient with a paroxysmal psychogenic movement disorder showed evidence of a "readiness" potential in relation to movement.[47]

Electrophysiological Evaluation of Myoclonus

POLYGRAPHIC EMG STUDIES

Because EMG is a direct measure of alpha motor neuron activity, it provides information about the central nervous system command that generates the movement. Numerous muscles act on each joint, and it is usually necessary to record from at least two muscles with antagonist actions. EMG is mainly used for the purpose of timing information and in most cases can be collected from surface electrodes.[6]

Inspection of the EMG signal of an involuntary movement reveals, first, whether the movement is regular (usually a tremor) or irregular. Irregular EMG activity will sometimes clinically appear rhythmic if it is rapid. The duration of the EMG burst correlating with an involuntary movement can be measured; specific ranges of duration are associated with different types of movements. Specification of duration in the range from 30 to 300 ms merely by clinical inspection is virtually impossible as a result of the relative slowness of the mechanical events, compared to that of the electrical events. Antagonist muscle relationships also can be specified as synchronous or asynchronous (reciprocal). In a tremor, asynchronous activity is described as alternating. It is important to keep in mind that some disorders of the peripheral nervous system can also give rise to involuntary movements. These include fasciculations, tetany, myokymia, and neuromyotonic discharges and, generally, they can be recognized with needle EMG.[7]

The polygraphic study of the EMG activity alone can provide useful information in classifying and understanding the pathophysiology of myoclonus. EMG bursts of brief duration (50 ms or less) are almost exclusively seen in epileptic myoclonus. Discharges approaching 150 ms are typical of nonepileptic myoclonus. Rapid movements with EMG bursts lasting between 150 and 300 ms are often seen as fragments of other movement disorders, such as dystonia. The time relation of activation of different muscles involved in a generalized twitch also provides information on the type of myoclonus. A rostrocaudal "wave" of activation, beginning with the uppermost motor cranial nerves and progressing in a descending fashion along the neuroaxis with a conduction velocity appropriate for the pyramidal tract is typical of epileptic myoclonus originating in the cortex.[21] A pattern of activation initiating with the sternocleidomastoid muscle and progressing with the activation of both rostrally and caudally innervated muscles is typical for reticular reflex myoclonus. Proximal muscles are most often involved in nonepileptic myoclonus. Synchronous activation of distal antagonist muscles is usually the rule in epileptic myoclonus.

The latency differences between homologous muscles in the upper and lower extremities and among muscles innervated by different segments along the neuroaxis may also provide insight into intracortical and transcallosal spread of activation[48] (Fig. 40-3).

ROUTINE ELECTROENCEPHALOGRAPHY

The most common encounter of the neurologist with the electrophysiology of myoclonus occurs in the setting of studies involving a routine EEG, using additional EMG monitoring leads. A similar procedure is routinely used in polygraphic sleep recordings when sleep-related movement disorders are suspected. The presence of well-defined spike, spike-wave, or polyspike discharges in close association with the bursts of EMG activation may indicate an epileptic mechanism. Other encephalopathies not necessarily regarded as epileptic in nature may also show EEG events time-locked to myoclonus, as is the case in Creutzfelt-Jakob disease.[49] In some patients, despite an obvious epileptic disorder, the routine EEG may not reveal a distinct abnormality associated with myoclonic movements. Many patients with epilepsia partialis continua may not have a distinct EEG-EMG correlation.[11,50,51] This may be related in part to the specific three-dimensional arrangement of the involved cortical ribbon generating tangential dipoles or to involvement of a relatively small area of cortical area lacking the "critical mass" necessary to project an abnormality to the scalp with an amplitude discernible from the background EEG signal. Under these circumstances, back-averaging of EEG to the EMG burst may help identify the location and characteristics of EEG abnormalities related to the movements.

The EEG itself is also of value in the diagnosis and follow-up of patients with metabolic or degenerative forms of myoclonic disorders.[10,52] Occipital and rolandic spikes, as well as paroxysms of generalized spikes and polyspikes, are often seen in the setting of the syndrome of progressive myoclonic epilepsy.[10] Progressive deterioration of background rhythms parallels disease progression.[10,52]

Nose Taps

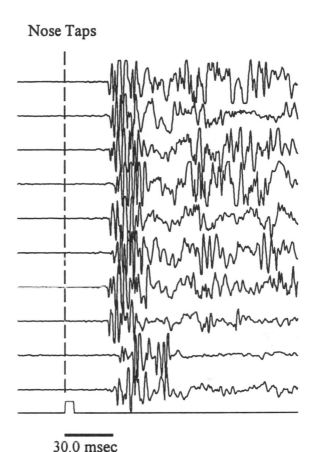

30.0 msec

FIGURE 40-3 Sample of 10 reflex EMG responses from the cervical paraspinal muscles to rhythmic nose taps (0.25 Hz) in a patient with acquired startle after a brain stem encephalitis. The responses did not show the normal expected habituation with repeated stimuli and were clinically associated with brief head retraction. The time of the stimulus is indicated by the vertical dashed line. A brief burst of activity at a latency of 30 ms was followed by a more sustained EMG activation of variable degree.

EEG BACK-AVERAGING

Averaging of EEG activity time-locked to the onset of myoclonic EMG bursts, known as EEG back-averaging or "jerk-locked" averaging, is used to establish the presence, location, and characteristics of cortical activity that is correlated (time-locked) to the onset of the positive myoclonic event.[8,9,11,21] A similar averaging procedure but one that is time-locked to the onset of EMG silent periods can be applied to the study of negative myoclonus (silent period-locked averaging).[16,53,54] These techniques can be performed "on-line," using most conventional evoked potential equipment driving the triggering of an averager with a threshold trigger set to fire at myoclonic EMG burst onset. The sampled EEG epochs should include at least 100 ms of data before EMG onset. The exact number of averaged epochs may vary, depending on the signal-to-noise ratio. Most laboratories studying myoclonus electrophysiologically record the EEG and EMG data using magnetic or digital media and conduct the analysis "off-line." This offers the advantage of *post hoc* sorting of different myoclonic events and better control of artifact rejection. Multiple scalp and EMG leads are desirable. The use of back-averaging may not be necessary with patients whose clear-cut spikes time-locked to myoclonic EMG burst can be seen in the raw EEG. Even in this situation, however, back-averaging may provide more detailed information on the topography and components of the epileptiform paroxysms that best correlate with the myoclonic movements.[7]

A cortical participation in the genesis of myoclonus is indicated by the presence of a reproducible EEG potential that precedes the onset of the myoclonic EMG activity. The prototypical finding is the presence of a myoclonus-related cortical spike.[9,11,21] This is usually a positive-negative, biphasic sharp EEG potential time-locked to the myoclonus. In most cases, the spike is located over the central region contralateral to the upper extremity muscle used to drive the averaging when the myoclonus is focal or multifocal. The early positive peak of the spike precedes the EMG onset in upper extremity muscles by about 15–25 ms and for the lower extremity by about 40 ms[9] (Fig. 40-4). These latencies are compatible with the corticospinal conduction times for the hand and foot muscles, respectively. Other patterns of myoclonus-related EEG activity have been described. Those include monophasic and triphasic EEG potentials or even more complex sets of wavelets time-locked to the myoclonus.[14]

The discharge is maximal over the vertex when myoclonus is recorded from the lower extremities, in keeping with the homuncular organization of the motor cortex. When the myoclonic movements are generalized or bilaterally synchronous, the EEG discharge is widespread with a vertex maximum.[14] In some patients with cortical myoclonus, the initial cortical discharge, spontaneous or reflex, spreads to adjacent motor cortical areas or to homologous areas in the other hemisphere. A high degree of spread characterizes those subjects with a tendency to experience generalized myoclonic twitches and frequent seizures.[48]

SEPs

Since Dawson's initial observations in 1947,[5] it is well-known that a subgroup of patients with myoclonus have a grossly enhanced SEP amplitude.[9,19,23] "Giant" SEPs is the term generally used to describe this abnormality in patients with cortical myoclonus.[9] Giant SEPs deviate from normal SEPs not only in their amplitude but also in the distortion of the waveform components (Fig. 40-5). The waveform morphology in giant SEPs is usually "simplified" into three large amplitude peaks. Naming the waveforms according to their polarity and sequence (N1, P1, N2, etc.), rather than according to the more conventional terminology (N20, P25/P30, N35, etc.) is favored by some authors.[19] When labeled by its polarity, the N1 component is usually normal in amplitude and has a latency comparable to that of the N20 component of regular SEPs. In contrast, the P1 and N2 components are enlarged in magnitude and usually are delayed, when compared to those of normal SEPs.[9,19] A N1/P1 or a P1/N2 amplitude greater than 10 μV and measured at the contralateral central region in ear-referenced recordings is considered a giant response.[9] In many patients, giant SEPs resemble typical spike-wave paroxysms (Figs. 40-1 and 40-5). Giant SEPs are

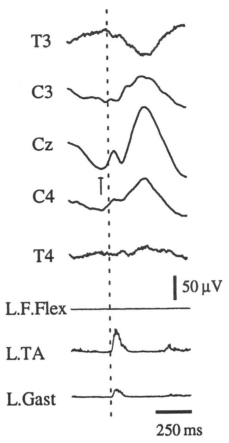

FIGURE 40-4 Back-averaging of the EEG activity in a patient with epilepsia partialis continua manifested as irregular twitching of the left leg. The routine EEG showed widespread spike-slow wave activity involving the right hemisphere. Averaging of 100 EEG epochs aligned to the onset EMG burst from the left tibialis anterior muscle (L. TA) shows a focal surface positive potential over the vertex area (indicated by the arrow) with a latency of 40 ms preceding the EMG twitches. Activation of the left gastrocnemius muscle (L. Gast.) shows a synchronous burst to that of the L.TA muscle. L.F. Flex, left finger flexors.

often associated with a reflex myoclonic jerk at a latency of approximately 45 ms in hand muscles after median nerve stimulation (C-reflex).[9,19,55,56] The concomitant presence of these two is the hallmark of sensory-reflex cortical myoclonus. The striking resemblance in latency and morphology of the giant SEP-C-reflex complex to the myoclonus-related cortical spike suggests that both originate from common cortical mechanisms.[9,19,21]

The generator of the giant SEP resides in or in close proximity to the central sulcus.[23,24,57,58] Because the subcortical components and the first cortical component (N1) are usually normal in amplitude, it can be suggested that an abnormality in intracortical inhibition after the arrival of the first volley of thalamocortical activity might be responsible for the abnormal activation of surrounding cortex which, in turn, leads to enlargement of both the giant SEP responses and activation of descending motor outputs leading to the C-reflex.[9,19]

The use of paired somatosensory stimuli at variable intervals has been used to trace the excitability cycle of the sensori-

Electrode C4

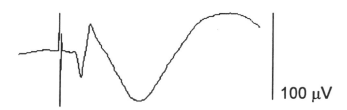

Lafora Body Myoclonus

100 µV

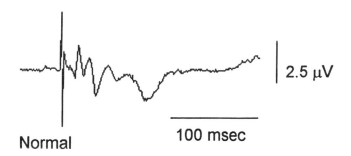

2.5 µV

Normal

100 msec

L. Median Nerve Stimulation

FIGURE 40-5 Differences in the morphology and amplitude of SEPs to median nerve stimulation in a patient with progressive myoclonic epilepsy secondary to Lafora body disease (*top*) and in a normal individual (*bottom*). The waveform morphology in patients with epileptic cortical myoclonus is often of large amplitude, "simplified" in morphology and reminiscent of an epileptiform spike-wave paroxysm.

motor cortex in cortical myoclonus.[59,60] Patients with cortical myoclonus tend to show a "triphasic" cycle of initial depression of cortical excitability, followed within 20–80 ms by a period of increased excitability and a subsequent period of depression with recovery of the baseline excitability after 300 ms.[60] There is evidence suggesting that this cycle may be heavily weighted towards inhibition in patients presenting with epileptic negative myoclonus.[61]

REFLEX STUDIES

In some patients with myoclonus, certain types of stimulation will produce a reflex response that is not present in normal subjects. This was named the C-reflex by Sutton and Mayer,[55] who thought it was the result of an abnormal cortically mediated reflex. The latency of the C-reflex in upper extremity muscles is approximately 36–50 ms after the stimulus given to the hand and 60–70 ms when the reflex is elicited and recorded in lower extremities. These latencies are about twice those of the first cortical component of the SEPs (18–25 ms in upper limb and 30–35 ms in lower limb)[9] (Fig. 40-1). In

cases of cortical reflex myoclonus, the C-reflex is the result of abnormal activity in a cortical loop. This loop would involve fast-conducting tracts up to the sensory cortex, using the posterior column, lemniscal, and thalamocortical pathways. The events in the cortex that lead to large SEPs may in parallel activate the motor cortex via corticocortical connections generating a rapid descending discharge to the anterior horn motor neurons. In rare patients, the reflex may only occur in response to cutaneous stimuli whereas in others it occurs in response only to passive stretch.[55,56] A direct relationship is most often seen between the amplitude of the giant SEP and the presence of a reflex myoclonic jerk.[19] These two events, however, appear to be differentially affected by pharmacological interventions such as lisuride or clonazepam.[19]

Care should be exerted not to confuse the C-reflex with normal reflex EMG responses. For example, electrical stimulation of a mixed nerve gives rise to an F-wave. In normal individuals, some degree of voluntary activation of the recorded muscle results in several responses after the direct muscle response.[62] There are also late responses after stimulation of a cutaneous nerve when the recorded muscle is not at rest. One of these responses, the E2 response, is mediated via a long-loop pathway. The use of the reflex responses to differentiate different types of myoclonus has been demonstrated by Chen et al.[63] They studied the responses to cutaneous stimulation in patients with Parkinson's disease and other akinetic-rigid syndromes. In patients with myoclonus in the setting of Parkinson's disease or multiple-system atrophy, there was facilitation of the E2 component of the response. In patients with cortical-basal ganglionic degeneration, there was a response at a shorter latency than E2.[63,64] The pathways for these responses are not completely clear, but they do differ, and the physiological test can be used clinically for differential diagnosis.[63–65]

TRANSCRANIAL MAGNETIC STIMULATION (TMS)

Motor thresholds to magnetic stimulation are low in those myoclonic patients with a tendency to experience generalized twitches and seizures and are high, even higher than in normal subjects, in those with only focal twitches.[66] Cortical excitability is also enhanced in cortical myoclonus when TMS is presented with a concomitant somatosensory stimulus.[67] After TMS there is a brief period of cortical inhibition in which the cortex is relatively refractory to a second stimulus. In normal subjects this phenomenon relies on intact intracortical inhibition. The recovery of cortical excitability can be probed with the use of pairs of cortical stimuli.[66] Patients with cortical myoclonus and the tendency to have generalized and multifocal twitches and frequent seizures exhibit a deficient intra- and transcortical inhibition to paired stimuli[66] and a tendency for spread of their cortical EEG discharges.[48]

Negative Myoclonus

Asterixis, a form of negative myoclonus, was the name given to brief postural lapses associated with cessation of tonic

EMG activity. Asterixis was first described by Adams and Foley[67] in patients with hepatic encephalopathy, but it is known now to represent a nonspecific neurological finding associated with multiple forms of toxic and metabolic encephalophathies. Asterixis has been reported to arise from subcortical and brain stem lesions,[15] but physiological studies in these cases are lacking. EEG abnormalities similar to those of epileptic cortical myoclonus can also present in the setting of negative myoclonus. In fact, positive and negative myoclonus often coexist. The classification scheme and the electrophysiological methods proposed for positive myoclonus can all be identically applied to negative myoclonus.

Ugawa et al.[53,68] have evaluated the EEG correlates of asterixis, using the silent period-locked averaging technique in patients with well-defined postural lapses associated with EMG silent periods. The silent periods in these patients were classified in two forms. In form, type I silent periods were associated with a complete cessation of background EMG activity, lasting for 50–100 ms. The second form, type II, was characterized by a primarily negative event that was associated with a brief and discrete but definite burst of EMG activity that occurred before the silence. Only type II silent periods were preceded by well-defined EEG discharges. The discharges were localized to the contralateral central regions and preceded the event by 20–30 ms. Similar findings have been reported in other patients.[16,53]

Epileptiform discharges preceding negative myoclonus have been reported in children with epilepsy.[69–71] The presenting symptoms in these patients were tremulousness or postural lapses of tonically activated muscles and rare convulsions. The EEG showed focal epileptiform discharges on average 30–50 ms before the onset of the EMG silence. It remains undetermined as to when the EEG discharge of positive and negative myoclonus is consistently different. Giant SEPs are variably present in patients with negative myoclonus. The recovery curve of SEP amplitude to paired somatosensory stimuli in patients with epileptic negative myoclonus shows a more prominent inhibition, compared to that of patients with positive myoclonus.[61]

The C-reflex elicited by electrical stimulation of the median nerve is sometimes present in patients with negative myoclonus. Rare patients may show negative myoclonus in response to sensory stimulation (sensory-reflex asterixis)[16,61] (Fig. 40-6).

It can be postulated that epileptic negative and positive myoclonus are parts of the same phenomenon. During the abnormal cortical discharge, positive and negative influences on motor activity are generated. These influences may differ in their time of maximal expression, threshold for clinical manifestation, their time course, pathways of spread, their sensitivity to medications, and sensitivity to different physiological states such as sleep-wake cycles and fatigue.[16]

Negative myoclonus of subcortical origin may have a completely different pathophysiology. Type I silent periods, without an EEG correlate, may originate primarily from subcortical structures. The high coexistence of type I and type II silent periods in the same patient population may indicate that important cortical-subcortical interactions are operative in the genesis of negative myoclonus.[16]

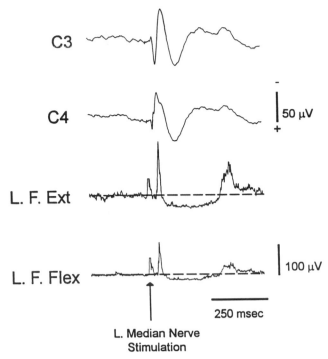

FIGURE 40-6 SEP and averaged rectified EMG responses in a patient with sensory-reflex asterixis recorded while the patient's hands were held against gravity. There is a giant SEP in response to left median nerve stimulation. Associated with each stimulus, there is a brief reflex EMG activation (C-reflex), followed by a period of EMG suppression clinically associated with a postural lapse (asterixis) lasting about 250 ms. L.F. Ext, left finger extensors; L.F. Flex, left finger flexors.

References

1. Gibbs FA, Davis H, Lennox WG: The electro-encephalogram in epilepsy and in conditions of impaired conciousness. *Arch Neurol Psychiatry* 34:1133–1148, 1935.
2. Grinker RR, Serota H, Stein SI: Myoclonic epilepsy. *Arch Neurol Psychiatry* 40:968–980, 1938.
3. Dawson GD: The relation between the electroencephalogram and muscle action potentials in certain convulsive states. *J Neurol Neurosurg Psychiatry* 9:5–22, 1946.
4. Dawson GD: Cerebral responses to electrical stimulation of peripheral nerve in man. *J Neurol Neurosurg Psychiatry* 10:134–140, 1947.
5. Dawson GD: Investigations on a patient subject to myoclonic seizures after sensory stimulation. *J Neurol Neurosurg Psychiatry* 10:141–162, 1947.
6. Hallett M: Analysis of abnormal voluntary and involuntary movements with surface electromyography, in Desmedt JE (ed): *Motor Control Mechanisms in Health and Disease.* New York: Raven Press, 1983, pp 907–914.
7. Hallett M: Electrophysiologic evaluation of movement disorders, in Aminoff MJ (ed): *Electrodiagnosis in Clinical Neurology*, 3d ed. New York: Churchill Livingstone, 1992, pp 403–419.
8. Marsden CD, Hallett M, Fahn S: The nosology and pathophysiology of myoclonus, in Marsden CD, Fahn S (eds): Neurology 2: *Movement Disorders.* London: Butterworths Scientific, 1982, pp 196–248.

9. Shibasaki H, Yamashita Y, Kuroiwa Y: Electroencephalographic studies of myoclonus: Myoclonus-related cortical spikes in progressive myoclonic epilepsy. *Brain* 108:225–240, 1978.

10. So N, Berkovic S, Andermann F, et al: Myoclonus epilepsy and ragged red fibres (MERRF). 2. Electrophysiological studies and comparison with other progressive myoclonus epilepsies. *Brain* 112:1261–1276, 1989.

11. Obeso JA, Rothwell JC, Marsden CD: The spectrum of cortical myoclonus. *Brain* 108:193–224, 1985.

12. Hallett M, Obeso J, Shibasaki H: Visual recognition of myoclonus. *Mov Disord.* In Press.

13. Lance JW, Adams RD: The syndrome of intention or action myoclonus as a sequel to hypoxic encephalopathy. *Brain* 86:111–136, 1963.

14. Toro C, Pascual-Leone A, Deuschl G, et al: Cortical tremor: A common manifestation of cortical myoclonus. *Neurology* 43:2346–2353, 1993.

15. Shahani BT, Young RR: Asterixis—a disorder of the neural mechanisms underlying sustained muscle contraction, in Shahani M (ed): *The Motor System: Neurophysiological and Muscle Mechanisms.* Amsterdam: Elsevier, 1976, pp 301–306.

16. Toro C, Hallett M, Rothwell JC, et al: Physiology of negative myoclonus, in Fahn S, Hallett M, Luders HO, Marsden CD (eds): *Negative Motor Phenomena.* New York: Raven Press, 1995, pp 211–217.

17. Brown P, Steiger MJ, Thompson, PD et al: Effectiveness of piracetam in cortical myoclonus. *Mov Disord* 8:63–68, 1993.

18. Chadwick D, Hallett M, Harris R, et al: Clinical, biochemical and physiologic features distinguishing myoclonus responsive to 5-hydroxytryptophan, tryptophan with monoamine oxidase inhibitor and clonazepam. *Brain* 100:455–487, 1977.

19. Rothwell JC, Obeso JA, Marsden CD: On the significance of giant somatosensory evoked potentials in cortical myoclonus. *J Neurol Neurosurg Psychiatry* 47:33–42, 1984.

20. Halliday AM: The electrophysiological study of myoclonus in man. *Brain* 90:241–284, 1967.

21. Hallett M, Chadwick D, Marsden CD: Cortical reflex myoclonus. *Neurology* 29:1107–1125, 1979.

22. Hallett M: Myoclonus: Relation to epilepsy. *Epilepsia* 26(suppl):s67–s77, 1985.

23. Shibasaki H, Yamashita Y, Neshigi R, et al: Pathogenesis of giant somatosensory evoked potentials in progressive myoclonic epilepsy. *Brain* 108:225–240, 1985.

24. Shibasaki H, Kakigi R, Ikeda A: Scalp topography of giant SEP and pre- myoclonus spike in cortical reflex myoclonus. *Electroencephalogr Clin Neurophysiol* 81:31–37, 1991.

25. Hallett M, Chadwick D, Adam J, Marsden CD: Reticular reflex myoclonus: A physiological type of human post-hypoxic myoclonus. *J Neurol Neurosurg Psychiatry* 40:253–264, 1977.

26. Chadwick D, French AT: Uraemic myoclonus: An example of reticular reflex myoclonus? *J Neurol Neurosurg Psychiatry* 42:52–55, 1979.

27. Zuckerman EG, Glasser GH: Urea-induced myoclonic seizures. *Arch Neurol* 27:14–28, 1972.

28. Thompson PD, Maertens de Noordhout A, Day BL, et al: Clinical and electrophysiological observations in post-anoxic myoclonus, in Crossman AR, Sambrook MA (eds): *Current Problems in Neurology 9: Neuronal Mechanisms in Disorders of Movement.* London: John Libbey, 1989, pp 375–381.

29. Wilkins DE, Hallett M, Erba G: Primary generalized epileptic myoclonus: A frequent manifestation of minipolymyoclonus of central origin. *J Neurol Neurosurg Psychiatry* 48:506–516, 1985.

30. Artieda J, Obeso JA: The pathophysiology and pharmacology of photic cortical reflex myoclonus. *Ann Neurol* 34:175–184, 1993.

31. Brailowsky S: Myoclonus in Papio papio. *Mov Disord* 6:98–104, 1991.

32. Naquet R, Meldrum BS: Myoclonus induced by intermittent light stimulation in the baboon: Neurophysiological and neuropharmacological approaches. *Adv Neurol* 43:611–627, 1986.

33. Fischer-Williams M, Poncet M, Riche D, Naquet R: Light induced epilepsy in the baboon Papio papio: Cortical and depth recordings. *Electroencephalogr Clin Neurophysiol* 25:557–569, 1968.

34. Hallett M, Chadwick D, Marsden CD: Ballistic movement overflow myoclonus. *Brain* 100:299–312, 1977.

35. Dubinsky RM, Hallett M: Palatal myoclonus and facial involvement in other types of myoclonus. *Adv Neurol* 49:263–278, 1988.

36. Deuschl G, Mischke G, Schenck E, et al: Symptomatic and essential rhythmic palatal myoclonus. *Brain* 113:1645–1672, 1990.

37. Deuschl G, Toro C, Valls-Sole J, et al: Symptomatic and essential palatal tremor. 1. Clinical, physiological, and MRI analysis. *Brain* 117:775–788, 1994.

38. Deuschl G, Toro C, Hallett M: Symptomatic and essential palatal tremor. 2. Differences in palatal movements. *Mov Disord* 9:676–678, 1994.

39. Brown P, Thompson PD, Rothwell JC, et al: Axial myoclonus of propriospinal origin. *Brain* 114:197–214, 1991.

40. Chokroverty S, Walters A, Zimmerman T, Picone M: Propriospinal myoclonus: A neurophysiologic analysis. *Neurology* 42:1591–1595, 1992.

41. Brown P, Rothwell JC, Thompson PD, et al: The hyperekplexias and their relationship to the normal startle reflex. *Brain* 114:1903–1928, 1991.

42. Thompson PD, Colebatch JG, Brown P, et al: Voluntary stimulus-sensitive jerks and jumps mimicking myoclonus or pathological startle syndromes. *Mov Disord* 7:257–262, 1992.

43. Matsumoto J, Fuhr P, Nigro M, Hallett M: Physiological abnormalities in hereditary hyperekplexia. *Ann Neurol* 32:41–50, 1992.

44. Wilkins DE, Hallett M, Wess MM: Audiogenic startle reflex of man and its relationship to startle syndromes: A review. *Brain* 109:561–573, 1986.

45. Hening WA, Walters AS, Chokroverty S: Movement disorders and sleep, in Chokroverty S (ed): *Movement Disorders.* Great Neck, NY: PMA Publishing Corp, 1990, pp 127–157.

46. Monday K, Jankovic J: Psychogenic myoclonus. *Neurology* 43:349–352, 1993.

47. Toro C, Torres F: Electrophysiological correlates of a paroxysmal movement disorder. *Ann Neurol* 20:731–734, 1986.

48. Brown P, Day BL, Rothwell JC, et al: Interhemispheric and intrahemispheric spread of cerebral cortical myoclonic activity and its relevance to epilepsy. *Brain* 114:2333–2352, 1991.

49. Shibasaki H, Motomura S, Yamashita Y, et al: Periodic synchronous discharge and myoclonus in Creutzfeldt-Jacob disease: Diagnostic application of jerk-locked averaging method. *Ann Neurol* 9:150–156, 1981.

50. Kugelberg E, Widen L: Epilepsia partialis continua. *Electroencephalogr Clin Neurophysiol* 6:503–506, 1954.

51. Thomas JE, Reagan TJ, Klass DW: Epilepsia partialis continua: A review of 32 cases. *Arch Neurol* 34:266–275, 1977.

52. Reese K, Toro C, Malow B, Sato S: Progression of the EEG in Lafora-body disease. *Am J EEG Tech* 33:229–235, 1993.

53. Ugawa Y, Shimpo T, Mannen T: Physiological analysis of asterixis: Silent period locked averaging. *J Neurol Neurosurg Psychiatry* 52:89–93, 1989.

54. Artieda J, Muruzabal J, Larumbe R, et al: Cortical mechanisms mediating asterixis. *Mov Disord* 7:209–216, 1992.

55. Sutton GG, Mayer RF: Focal reflex myoclonus. *J Neurol Neurosurg Psychiatry* 37:207–217, 1974.

56. Sutton GG: Receptors in focal reflex myoclonus. *J Neurol Neurosurg Psychiatry* 38:505–507, 1975.

57. Cowan JMA, Rothwell JC, Wise RJS, Marsden CD: Electrophysiological and positron emission studies in a patient with cortical myoclonus, epilepsia partialis continua and motor epilepsy. *J Neurol Neurosurg Psychiatry* 49:796–807, 1986.

58. Kakigi R, Shibasaki H: Generator mechanisms of giant somatosensory evoked potentials in cortical reflex myoclonus. *Brain* 110:1359–1373, 1987.

59. Shibasaki H, Neshige R, Hashiba Y: Cortical excitability after myoclonus: Jerk-locked somatosensory evoked potentials. *Neurology* 35:36–41, 1985.

60. Ugawa Y, Gemba K, Shimpo T, Mannen T: Somatosensory evoked potential recovery (SEP-R) in myoclonic patients. *Electroencephalogr Clin Neurophysiol* 80:21–25, 1991.

61. Shibasaki H, Ikeda A, Nagamine T, et al: Cortical reflex negative myoclonus. *Brain* 117:477–486, 1994.

62. Deuschl G, Lücking CH: Physiological and clinical application of hand muscle reflexes, in Rossini PM, Mauguiere F (eds): *New Trends and Advanced Techniques in Clinical Neurophysiology*. Amsterdam: Elsevier, 1990, pp 84–101.

63. Chen R, Ashby P, Lang AE: Stimulus-sensitive myoclonus in akinetic-rigid syndromes. *Brain* 115:1875–1888, 1992.

64. Thomson PD, Day BL, Rothwell JC, et al: The myoclonus in corticobasal degeneration: Evidence for two forms of cortical reflex myoclonus. *Brain* 117:1197–1207, 1994.

65. Brunt ER, van Weerden TW, Pruim J, Lakke JW: Unique myoclonic pattern in corticobasal degeneration. *Mov Disord* 10:132–142, 1995.

66. Reutens DC, Puce A, Berkovic SF: Cortical hyperexcitability in progressive myoclonic epilepsy: A study with transcranial magnetic stimulation. *Neurology* 43:186–192, 1993.

67. Adams RD, Foley JM: The neurological changes in the more common types of severe liver disease. *Trans Neurol Assoc* 74:217–219, 1949.

68. Ugawa Y, Genba K, Shimpo T, Mannen T: Onset and offset of electromyographic (EMG) silence in asterixis. *J Neurol Neurosurg Psychiatry* 53:260–262, 1990.

69. Cirignotta F, Lugaresi E: Partial motor epilepsy with "negative myoclonus." *Epilepsia* 32:54–58, 1991.

70. Guerrini R, Dravet C, Genton P, et al: Epileptic negative myoclonus. *Neurology* 43:1078–1083, 1993.

71. Takanori Y, Tsukagoshi H: Cortical activity-associated negative myoclonus. *J Neurol Sci* 111:77–81, 1992.

Chapter 41

PATHOPHYSIOLOGY AND DIFFERENTIAL DIAGNOSIS OF TICS

JORGE L. JUNCOS and ALAN FREEMAN

CLINICAL SPECTRUM
PATHOPHYSIOLOGY
DIFFERENTIAL DIAGNOSIS
    Phenomenology
    Etiologies
TREATMENT

A tic is a brief, rapid, repetitive, and seemingly purposeless stereotyped action that may involve a single muscle or multiple muscle groups. Its hyperkinetic properties may make it difficult to distinguish from other fast "jerky" movements, such as chorea and myoclonus. The most common and best-studied disorder characterized by tics is Tourette's syndrome (TS), which is discussed in more detail in Chap. 42. This chapter will focus on what is known about the phenomenology, pathophysiology, and differential diagnosis of tics.

Clinical Spectrum

Tics typically present in childhood or adolescence and may be transient or last a lifetime. With aging most tics tend to reach a stable plateau or disappear altogether.[1,2] Traditionally, tics are divided into motor or vocal, depending on the affected muscle group, and into simple or complex, depending on the intricacy of their phenomenology (Table 41-1). Tics have a wide spectrum of severity, ranging from the barely detectable and easily rationalized "nervous habits" to the complex, emotionally laden, sometimes offensive utterances found in a minority of patients with TS.

Phenomenologically, motor tics may be fast or clonic (blinking, nose twitching, head jerking) or more sustained and dystonic.[3] Dystonic motor tics are relatively slow, compared to clonic tics. They are characterized by sustained twisting, pulling, or squeezing movements, producing a briefly maintained body posture. Examples include painless oculogyric eye movements, blepharospasm, and brief dystonic neck movements.[4,5] Clonic tics respond to selected dopamine blockers and other therapies, as discussed in Chap. 42. In our experience dystonic tics may be more difficult to control with conventional pharmacotherapy. A recent report suggests that some of these painful dystonic tics refractory to pharmacotherapy may respond to local injections of botulinum toxin.[6] Tics may be aggravated by psychostimulants and other drugs that cause excitation or anxiety (see below).

Tics can be associated with brief focal sensory experiences which may precede, accompany or follow the movements or vocalization.[7] These sensory experiences or premonitory urges have been termed "sensory tics" and commonly affect the face, head, and neck areas, with the limbs less often involved. In TS these urges may be present in 41–92 percent of patients.[8,9] In the authors' experience, these premonitory phenomena are occasionally reported by other patients with tics, such as those with cranial dystonia ("Meige's syndrome"). These uncomfortable sensations are temporarily relieved by an associated motor tic affecting the same or a nearby body region. If sensory tics indeed affect such a large proportion of individuals with tics, it is unclear whether the sensory experience is an independent entity or just a subjective component of the more readily recognized motor or vocal tic.

Are tics voluntary or involuntary? Motor tics have traditionally been interpreted as involuntary, because they are not associated with the negative premotor electroencephalographic potential (Bereitschaftspotential) normally associated with voluntary movement.[10] However, more recently it has been reported that not all voluntary movements are necessarily preceded by these potentials.[11] Furthermore, when patients are asked directly, many of them report that the tics are under "voluntary control."[12] More specifically, motor tics that occur in response to premonitory urges are interpreted by patients as a voluntary act to relieve the often-uncomfortable sensation.[12] The term "unvoluntary" was recently coined in an effort to reconcile this dichotomy that underlies the terms voluntary and involuntary when referring to tics.[13] Unvoluntary refers to an "automatic movement performed without conscious effort" such as scratching in response to an itch.[13]

In contrast to motor and vocal tics, sensory tics are interpreted by patients as involuntary.[9] More complex sensations or affects associated with tics have been referred to as "complex sensory tics."[3] It is unclear, however, whether these complex phenomena are themselves related to the more involved comorbid conditions associated with tic disorders, such as obsessions and compulsions (see Chap. 42). For instance, Karp and Hallett recently described a patient whose tics were associated with out-of-body sensations that were relieved by intentional movements, or tics, directed at the object in question.[14] These "phantom tics" may represent a continuum with obsession and compulsions that are common in primary tic disorders (see Chap. 42). Previous authors have used the term "impulsion" to refer to similar actions that fall between the spectrum of compulsions and tics.[15]

Finally, motor tics, although conspicuous, are seldom the most disabling feature of a chronic tic disorder. Vocal tics can be more socially incapacitating than motor tics, especially the complex utterances and the coprolalia seen in TS. Sensory tics are highly variable but can be distressing, particularly when they present as pain syndromes.[8] In our experience they are less responsive than the above tics to dopamine blockers and other therapies. Furthermore, in TS, comorbid entities such as obsessions, compulsions, learning disabilities, attention deficit disorder (ADD), and its associated behaviors, when present, are more disabling than the tics themselves. Much like stressors from any source, poor control of these comorbid entities will aggravate the tics.

TABLE 41-1 Classification of Tic Phenomenology

	Motor	Vocal	Sensory
Simple	Frequent blinking	Sniffing	Burning sensations
	Blepharospasm	Grunting	Tightness
	Grimacing	Throat clearing	Muscle tension
	Pouting	Barking	Tingling
	Jaw opening	Growling	Itching
	Head jerking	Coughing	Impulsions
	Shoulder shrugging	Moaning	
	Fist clenching	Humming	
Complex	Head twisting or shaking	Panting	Inner tension
	Spitting	Belching	Pain syndromes
	Hitting (self, others)	Stuttering	Premonitory
	Jumping, kicking	Echolalia	Exertional
	Squatting	Coprolalia	2° to tic suppression
	Pelvic/abdominal thrusting	Palilalia	"Phantom tics"

Pathophysiology

The neurobiological substrate of tics is unknown but is thought to involve abnormalities in corticostriatothalamic circuits modulated by ascending monoaminergic pathways.[16] Evidence for this has been obtained in part from autopsies in neurological conditions in which tics are a secondary manifestation. For instance, tics have been described as late sequelae of encephalitis lethargica (i.e., postencephalitic parkinsonism), in which there is extensive pathological involvement of the ascending monoaminergic pathways, the midbrain tegmentum, and the periaqueductal gray.[17,18] Presumably, the resulting dopaminergic denervation of basal ganglia leads to "postsynaptic dopamine hypersensitivity," which can lead to tics when combined with the extensive midbrain pathology found in postencephalitic parkinsonism.[18]

Striatal regions forming part of the above circuits, such as the caudate and putamen, are thought to be involved in the generation of motor tics. Vocal tics may involve nonmotor circuits such as those projecting to the prefrontal and limbic cortices.[19,20] Unlike the striatum that receives dopaminergic innervation from the pars compacta of the substantia nigra, these nonmotor circuits receive dopaminergic projections from the ventral tegmental area of the midbrain.[20] The cortical projection regions of these circuits include the prefrontal cortex, the cingulate gyrus, the entorhinal cortex, the olfactory tubercle, the amygdala, and selected regions of the midbrain tegmentum. Experiments in primates indicate that manipulations of the cingulate gyrus and other limbic forebrain regions can lead to changes in vocalization that depend on the nature of the perturbation and the testing conditions.[21,22] The cingulate gyrus is of particular interest in that it connects cortical and limbic structures involved in vocalization.[21] Other limbic structures have also been associated with obsessions and compulsions, in primary tic disorders and postencephlitic parkinsonism.[18]

Morphometic neuroanatomic studies of these structures, using high-resolution magnetic resonance imaging (MRI) with volumetric analysis, support the view that there are basal ganglia abnormalities in TS.[23,24] The studies indicate that children and adults with TS have reduced volumes in the region of the left lenticular nucleus (globus pallidus and putamen), compared to those of age-matched controls.[23,24] Because the left hemisphere is typically larger than the right, TS subjects also exhibited significant attenuation in the normal interhemispheric asymmetries seen in controls. In one study this lack of asymmetry was particularly striking in individuals with comorbid TS and ADD.[24,25]

Positron emission tomography (PET), using ^{18}F-fluorodeoxyglucose studies, suggest that in TS there is *decreased* metabolic activity in subcortical regions, including basal ganglia and limbic cortices, and *increased* normalized metabolic activity in overlying cortex.[26] These regions are connected by the motor/limbic-striatal-thalamic circuitry described above.[20] Areas that exhibit decreased metabolic rates include the orbital, frontal, and superior insular cortices, the mesial temporal regions, and the striatum. Regions exhibiting increased metabolic rate include the premotor regions (lateral premotor and supplementary motor areas), the rolandic cortices, and the postrolandic sensory association areas.[26] More importantly, it seems that the functional metabolic relationship between these regions is altered in TS, compared to that of controls.

Much like the morphometric studies discussed above, these altered relationships gravitate around the ventral striatum, including the globus pallidus. In TS, striatal metabolic changes are positively coupled to the metabolic rates in overlying cortical regions.[26] In normal subjects, this relationship is negatively correlated, that is, if the metabolic activity in the ventral striatum *increases*, it is expected to *decrease* that in the corresponding target cortical regions. This has led to speculation that, in TS, there is functional cortical-subcortical "short circuiting" between these regions, leading to failure of "gating mechanisms" responsible for the coupling of motor and limbic cortical regions through the ventral striatum.[26] Clinically, this may lead to inability to suppress activity generated somewhere within the motor/limbic-striatal-thalamic circuitry. Depending on where in the circuitry this activity originates, the patient may present with inability to control motor impulses (tics, compulsions), failure to control sensory overload (ADD), or intrusive thoughts and impulsions (OCD). Using auditory and visual startle responses as a model of sensori-motor "gating" by striatal outflow, animal experiments have produced evidence that indirectly support this hypothesis.[27] Startle responses are profoundly affected by dopaminergic transmission in the basal ganglia, thereby tying this model to what is known about the pharmacology of tics and TS (see below).

Key questions for which there are still only speculative answers are: Where in the supposedly abnormal motor/limbic-striatal-thalamic circuits is the abnormal activity generated? What sustains, and at the same time makes so variable, the clinical course of TS? These questions force us again to examine the key role that the ventral striatum may play in transforming motivation into action by serving as an interface between the above motor circuits, the limbic system, and the hypothalamus.[28] However, if tics are viewed as involuntary (or "unvoluntary," as discussed above) phenomena, then theories regarding motivation, decision making, and action would be only limited value in explaining tics.

Gedye has proposed a theory that incorporates the involuntary quality of tics.[29] He theorized that "abnormal discharges in the frontal lobes" mediate the numerous phenomena that constitute TS.[29] He suggests that the phenomenology of tics is similar to that of the motor and vocal manifestations of frontal lobe seizures. Frontal cortical dysfunction resulting from abnormal electrical activity may help to explain the neuropsychological abnormalities described in some cases of TS (e.g., inattention, difficulties with planning, sequencing, and with shifting mental sets).[29] He tries to dispel skepticism regarding this theory by pointing out that: (a) frontal lobe epileptiform discharges are often missed on surface electroencephalograpy (EEG). (b) Frontal seizures are not necessarily associated with loss of consciousness. (c) Frontal seizures are less responsive to anticonvulsants than the more common seizures originating from other brain regions. Presumably, this would explain the lack of response of tics to anticonvulsants. The authors' view is that this theory is weakened by several observations. Although patients with frontal seizures do not necessarily *lose* consciousness during an event, they frequently exhibit subtle and not-so-subtle alterations of consciousness not seen in TS. Although anticonvulsants have been used to treat several aspects of TS, they are typically not very effective at treating the tics.[3]

Detailed electrophysiological studies also fail to support the above theory. The contribution of electrophysiological studies to the understanding of the involuntary ("unvoluntary") nature or tics was discussed above. Beyond this they provide little insight into the pathogenesis of tics. A number of electroencephalographic studies have failed to document consistent abnormalities in subjects with TS.[30,31] Bergen et al. reported a 34 percent incidence of nonspecific EEG abnormalities in a random selection of 38 TS patients, most of which could be attributed to coexisting signs of neurological dysfunction (so-called "soft neurologic signs").[30] Only two patients exhibited electroencephalographic epileptiform activity, but none reported seizures.[30] Neufeld et al. examined quantitative EEGs in 48 consecutive patients with TS and concluded that "there was no significant difference between TS patients and matched controls".[31] Krumholz et al. exam-

ined the EEG (n = 40) and the visual, brain stem, and auditory evoked responses (n = 17) in TS and found no "diagnostic or therapeutic value to justify their routine use in this syndrome."[32]

Polysomnographic contributions to the study of TS are limited, even though insomnia and other sleep related complaints are not uncommon in TS.[33] In selected cases, polysomnographic studies have shown a higher percentage of stage III/IV sleep and decreased rapid eye movement (REM) sleep in patients with TS, compared to that of controls.[33] Although these findings fail to explain the frequent sleep disruption in TS, they suggest that disordered arousal may be playing a role in TS. Two tantalizing studies suggest that disorders of arousal such as somnambulism and night terrors, are more common in TS than in controls.[34,35] It can be speculated that disordered arousal may be the sleep cycle equivalent of the "gating" abnormalities postulated above. This hypothesis predicts that, just as tics do not disappear during sleep, TS patients are more likely than controls to "be driven" by urges associated with dreaming, for instance, sleep walking or somnambulism. In the case of night terrors the subject is unable to suppress the energy typically generated by nightmares and, as a result, is awakened in a panic. The mechanisms for these intrusions into normal sleep have yet to be defined.

Based in part on the above findings and on speculations regarding the neural circuitry involved in tic disorders, several neurosurgical procedures have been proposed for the treatment of TS.[36] These include stereotactic coagulation of the rostral intralaminar and medial thalamic nuclei, lesions of the cerebellar dentate nucleus, and frontal lobotomies.[36] These procedures have remained unpopular because of their limited and inconsistent results and their considerable morbidity. Leckman et al. recently reported a case in which bilateral anterior cingulotomies was followed by bilateral infrathalamic lesions for the treatment of severe TS. The patient's tics and obsessive compulsive symptoms improved. However, the patient developed marked dysarthria, dysphasia, and a lasting parkinsonian syndrome.[37] Limbic leukotomies and isolated lesions of the cingulate gyrus carry much less morbidity than the above combined procedures and may be effective in the treatment of OCD and selected cases of TS.[36,38]

Dysfunction of central dopaminergic pathways is suspected as playing a role in the pathophysiology of tic disorders, in particular TS.[16,39] This suspicion is based on indirect clinical and pharmacological evidence discussed in detail in the TS chapter (Chap. 42). An alternative hypothesis is that tics may result in part from dysfunction in cerebral cholinergic systems.[40,41] According to this hypothesis, evidence for central dopaminergic "hyperfunction" in tic disorders could be interpreted instead as indirect evidence of cerebral cholinergic "hypofunction." In experimental animals, dopamine and acetylcholine play complementary and often reciprocal roles.[42] In man, clinical evidence suggests dopaminergic transmission can be enhanced by cholinergic antagonists.[42] Examples of this include the response of hypodopaminergic states like neuroleptic-induced extrapyramidal syndromes and Parkinson's disease to cholinergic antagonists. Conversely, cholinergic agonists may alleviate hyperdopaminergic states, such as tics and chorea.[43]

Indirect evidence for abnormal cholinergic transmission in TS has been obtained through a series of pharmacological experiments. For instance, oral anticholinergic agents have a definite but variable effect on tics.[44] Most studies support the view that augmentation of central cholinergic transmission relieves tics and possibly other symptoms of TS.[40,41,44] Accordingly, several purported cholinomimetics have been investigated as possible alternatives to the standard dopamine-blocking strategies in TS.[43] The results have been limited by the agents used which, like choline and lecithin, are poorly tolerated and poorly penetrate the central nervous system (CNS).[41,45] Further work on this hypothesis will have to await the availability of new cholinergic agents with better therapeutic profiles that are now being tested for Alzheimer's disease.

Serotonin is another potentially important neurotransmitter in the pathogenesis of tic disorders and, in particular, TS. Most of its relevance to TS appears to be in its relationship to OCD symptomatology, for which serotonin reuptake blockers (SSRIs) have proven moderately effective.[43,46,47] This is discussed in more detail in Chapter 42. It has been our experience, however, that the SSRIs, which are normally tolerated in OCD patients without TS, not infrequently aggravate tics, limiting their use in some patients with TS.

Differential Diagnosis

The clinical features of tics have been extensively studied in primary tic disorders such as TS but not in other conditions in which tics are a secondary manifestation. For the purposes of this chapter we will discuss primary and secondary tics together because, phenomenologically, there is no evidence that there are significant differences between them.

PHENOMENOLOGY

Tics can be differentiated from hyperkinesias by their suppressibility, by their tendency to persist during sleep, and by the associated premonitory symptoms mentioned above (see Table 41-2). Unlike tics, and perhaps chorea, other movement disorders are seldom suppressible or perceived by patients as "voluntary." In particular, motor or vocal tics occurring in response to a premonitory urge are often viewed by patients as voluntary. Note that voluntary control may be difficult to assess in children. Table 41-2 also illustrates other aspects of the history and the physical exam that may help differentiate tics from other movement disorders.

Other features that help differentiate tics from hyperkinesias are their variability and course. For instance, over the course of primary tic disorders the severity of tics typically waxes and wanes, with predictable crises during adolescence. Tics may temporarily "disappear" or, more likely, become barely noticeable for extended periods, only to recur unprovoked, or triggered by nonspecific stressors. The character of the tics can also change from time to time, more typically, over the course of years. For example, excessive blinking or grimacing in childhood may transform into intermittent nose flaring and grunting in adolescense or into neck jerking in adulthood. Compounding this intrinsic variability are the profound effects that stress, stimulants, and other drugs can have on tics. Sensitivity to drugs, unfortunately,

TABLE 41-2 Response of Patients with Selected Movement Disorders to Questions Regarding Subjective Perception and Other Maneuvers*

	Subjective Perception	Premonitory Urges	Distraction	Suppression	Effect of Selected Movements
Tics	Vol or Invol	Yes	↓	+ + +	Usually ↓
Myoclonus	Invol	No	0 or ↑	0	Commonly ↑
Chorea	Invol	No	0 or ↑	±	Variable
Akathitic movements	Vol	Yes	↓	+ +	↓
Orofacial tardive dyskinesia	Invol	No	↑	+ +	Commonly ↑
Drug-induced dyskinesia	Invol	No	↑	+ +	Commonly ↑
Psychogenic movements	Invol	±Yes**	↓	±	Usually ↓**
Tremors	Invol	No	0 or ↑	In PD + +, in others 0	±↑
Dystonia	Invol	No	0 or ↑	±	Commonly ↑

*This important information should be elicited in the course of the history. "Vol" and "Invol" refer to the patients' interpretation of the activity as voluntary or not. The direction of the arrow refers to an increase or a decrease in movement; the thickness of the arrow is an arbitrary representation of the intensity of this change. 0, no change; ±, variable change; +, + +, + + +, mild, moderate, or marked suppressibility, respectively.
**This is highly variable from patient to patient.

SOURCE: Modified from Lang AE: Clinical phenomenology of tic disorders: Selected aspects. *Adv Neurol* 58:27, 1992.

does not help differentiate tics from any other movement disorders.

Dyskinesias (hyperkinesias) that may be difficult to differentiate from tics include myoclonus, chorea, akathisia, tardive dyskinesia, L-dopa-induced dyskinesia, the nonspecific movements (stereotypies) encountered in psychotic patients, and psychogenic movement disorders. Dystonic tics can be differentiated from dystonia by the company they keep; that is, they seldom occur in the absence of clonic or tonic tics. Compared to other tics, dystonic tics are more commonly associated with uncomfortable sensations that are relieved by movements.[4,8] Unlike myoclonus, a patient with tics would not be expected to loose motor control while executing a task such as holding a glass.

Chorea and tics are hard to differentiate phenomenologically, because both are quick, involuntary movements. However, chorea is less suppressible and is not associated with premonitory urges. Chorea, unlike tics, consists of a dance-like flow of "irregularly irregular" finger, limb, trunk, or facial movements that ebb or cease during sleep. L-dopa-induced dyskinesia occurs in association with the treatment of Parkinson's disease. Tics are seldom mistaken for tremors, which are, in contrast to tics, regular and oscillatory in nature. Tardive dyskinesia can be distinguished from tics by drug history and a typical pattern of predominant orobuccolingual involvement. Interestingly, in TS, tardive dyskinesia in response to chronic neuroleptic therapy appears to be exceedingly rare.

Other movements superficially resembling tics include mannerisms, disorders of excessive startle, and hyperekplexia. Mannerisms are physiological tics or patterned, sequential movements that are commonly outgrown during childhood. Although they appear in normal children, they are more commonly associated with mental subnormality.

ETIOLOGIES

PRIMARY TIC DISORDER

In tic disorders, the terms primary and secondary are again arbitrary, because we are uncertain of their pathophysiology and mechanisms. *Transient tic disorder*, by definition, lasts more than 1 month but less than 1 year. This diagnosis is made retrospectively, because there is no way to predict the course of tics when they first appear. The age of onset is always in childhood or early adolescence. For a tic to qualify as a *chronic motor tic disorder*, it must be present for more than 1 year. This entity presents in childhood and is frequently encountered in an individual from a family with TS; hence, it may be a variant of TS. *TS* is discussed in chapter 42. Adult onset tic disorders are rare and are frequently associated with other neurological disorders (discussed below).

SECONDARY TIC DISORDERS

Secondary tics are associated with a variety of neurological disorders. The tics themselves may be indistinguishable from those in TS, but the neurological signs associated with these conditions are not features of TS. Table 41-3 lists most medical and neurological conditions in which tics have been described. A detailed description of each one is beyond the scope of this chapter, but many are discussed elsewhere in this book.

Infections and parainfectious processes, including selected viral encephalitides and Sydenham's chorea, may be associated with tic-like movements.[17,48,49] This tic-like activity is often missed clinically due to coexisting choreiform movements. Tics associated with viral encephalitis may be missed due to the otherwise critical state of the patient. Tics may also be secondary to hypertensive or lacunar states or systemic vasculitidies involving the basal ganglia.[49] When these disorders are complicated by hyperkinesias, typically the choreatic movement tends to obscure the tics. These entities should be sought in individuals with tics and systemic symptoms, and when appropriate, in individuals presenting with tics above age twenty-one, the arbitrary upper age of onset of primary tic disorders.

Neuroacanthocytosis is a rare inherited neurodegenerative syndrome characterized by acanthocytosis in the peripheral blood smear and progressive neurological dysfunction. Associated neurological findings not encountered in primary tic disorders include: orofacial dyskinesia, chorea, lip and tongue biting, hypertonia, and hyporeflexia. Spitz and Jankovic recently described a neuroacanthotic syndrome in which tics are the predominant movement disorder.[50]

Hyperekplexias represent a group of disorders of unknown etiology that can superficially mimic tics. Clinical manifestations consist of an exaggerated startle response sometimes accompanied by congenital hypertonia and prominent nocturnal myoclonus.[51] Clusters of familial cases have been described in the literature under the rubrics of "Jumping Frenchman of Maine" and "Latah," with the latter cases being limited to certain Malaysian and Indonesian cultures.[49] Symptoms usually present in childhood and persist into adulthood, yet the course of the illness is relatively benign. Typically, the patients have a tendency to drop things or fall in response to a startling stimulus.

Hyperekplexia can be differentiated from tics by the following: it causes loss of postural tone, cannot be supressed, is stimulus sensitive, and is devoid of vocalizations. Hyperekplexia can be treated with clonazepam or methysergide[52,53]; anticonvulsants, such as phenobarbital, are of only partial or inconsistent benefit. Recently, a mutation in the alpha-1 subunit of inhibitory glycine receptor was described in one of the familial pedigrees.[54] There is now evidence that abnormalities in spinal reciprocal inhibitory mechanisms modulated by glycine receptors may be abnormal in patients with hereditary hyperekplexia.[55]

More unusual causes of secondary tics include trauma,[56,57] cerebral malaria,[58] and carbon monoxide poisoning.[59]

DRUG-INDUCED TICS

Drugs capable of inducing or aggravating tics include stimulants (methylphenidate, dexedrine, pemoline, decongestants, and illicit substances such as amphetamine, cocaine, or their derivatives)[60]; anticonvulsants[61–63]; L-dopa; tricyclic antidepressants; and birth control pills.[34] Neuroleptics can paradoxically aggravate tics when they provoke motor restlessness or akathisia.[64] Except for tardive (neuroleptic-induced) tics, most cases of drug-induced tic disorders are readily reversible when the offending agent is withdrawn. In cases where

TABLE 41-3 Etiologies of Tic and Tic-Like Disorders

Primary	Toxic-metabolic
Acute transient tic of childhood	• Carbon monoxide poisoning
Chronic motor tic disorder*	• Hypoglycemia
Gilles de la Tourette's syndrome*	Drug-induced
Adult onset tic disorder	• Neuroleptics (tardive tics)
Senile tic disorder	• Stimulants
Secondary	• Anticonvulsants
Hereditary	• L-dopa (in parkinsonism)
• Chromosomal abnormalities	*Infectious*
Down syndrome	• Sydenham's chorea
Fragile X, others (e.g., XXY)	• Encephalitis
• Huntington's disease	• Postencephalitic parkinsonism
• Dystonia (e.g., Meige's syndrome)	• Creutzfeldt-Jakob disease
• Hyperekplexias (see text)	• Rubella syndrome
Developmental	Habitual Body Manipulations**
• Autistic syndromes	• Finger sucking
Rett syndrome	• Nail biting, trichtilomania***
• Static encephalopathy (anoxic, etc.)	• Eye rubbing, ear touching
• Pervasive developmental delay	• Genital manipulation
Degenerative	• Nose picking
• Neuroacanthocytosis	Stereotypies****
• Progressive supranuclear palsy	• Head nodding or banging
Psychiatric	• Body rocking
• Schizophrenia	• Arm jerking
• Obsessive-compulsive disorder	

*Discussed in Chap. 42. Chronic motor tic disorder is now considered part of the clinical spectrum of Gilles de la Tourette's syndrome.

**May be nonspecifically associated with emotional disturbance.

***May be seen in obsessive compulsive disorders.

****Most commonly seen with pervasive developmental delay and mental retardation.

SOURCE: Modified from Lees AJ, Tolosa E: Tics, in Jankovic J, Tolosa E (eds): *Parkinson's Disease and Movement Disorders*. Baltimore: Urban & Schwarzenberg, 1988.

the tic problem persists longer than a few weeks, the suspicion has been that the drug may have unmasked an underlying primary tic disorder.

Carbamazepine-induced tics constitute an idiosyncratic reaction that can occur at therapeutic blood levels and without signs of toxicity.[61] Neuroleptics can produce transient tics when abruptly withdrawn ("emergence" hyperkinesis), or chronic tics secondary to long-term neuroleptic exposure, i.e., "tardive tics."[64] L-dopa-induced tics have been reported with the treatment of Parkinson's disease but are an exceedingly rare complication of this disorder.

Treatment

Pharmacological and nonpharmacological management of tics is covered with the treatment of Tourette's syndrome in Chap. 42.

Acknowledgment

Supported in part by a research grant from the Comstock family to JLJ.

References

1. Erenberg G, Cruse RP, Rothner AD: The natural history of Tourette's syndrome: A follow-up study. *Ann Neurol* 22:383–385, 1987.
2. Goetz CG, Tanner CM, Stebbin GT, et al: Adult tics in Gilles de la Tourette's syndrome: Description and risk factors. *Neurology* 42:784–788, 1992.
3. Jankovic J: The neurology of tics, in Marsden CD, Fahn S (eds.): *Movement Disorders*. London: Butterworth, 1987, chap 19, pp 383–405.
4. Jankovic J, Stone L: Dystonic tics in patients with Tourette's syndrome. *Mov Disord* 6:248–252, 1991.
5. Stone LA, Jankovic J: The coexistence of tics and dystonia. *Arch Neurol* 48:862–865, 1991.
6. Jankovic J: Botulinum toxin in the treatment of tics associated with Tourette's syndrome. *Neurology* 43(suppl 2):A310, 1993.
7. Bliss J: Sensory experiences of Gilles de la Tourette's syndrome. *Arch Gen Psychiatry* 37:1343–1347, 1980.
8. Kurlan R, Lichter D, Hewitt D: Sensory tics in Tourette's syndrome. *Neurology* 39:731–734, 1989.
9. Leckman JF, Walker DE, Cohen DJ: Premonitory urges in Tourette's syndrome. *Am J Psychiatry* 150:98–102, 1993.
10. Obeso JA, Rothwell JC, Marsden CD: Simple tics in Gilles de la Tourette's syndrome are not prefaced by a normal premovement EEG potential. *J Neurol Neurosurg Psychiatry* 14:735–738, 1981.
11. Papa SM, Artieda J, Obeso JA: Cortical activity preceding self-initiated and externally triggered voluntary movement. *Mov Disord* 6:217–224, 1991.

12. Lang A: Patient perception of tics and other movement disorders. *Neurology* 41:223–238, 1991.

13. Fahn S: Motor and vocal tics, in Kurlan R (ed): *Handbook of Tourette's Syndrome and Related Tic and Behavioral Disorders.* New York: Marcel Dekker, 1993, pp 3–16.

14. Karp BI, Hallett M: Extracorporeal "phantom tics" in Tourette's syndrome. *Neurology* 46:38–40, 1996.

15. Green RC, Pitman RK: Tourette's syndrome and obsessive-compulsive disorder: Clinical relationships, in Jenike MA, Baer L, Minichiello WE (eds): *Obsessive Compulsive Disorders: Theory and Management,* 2d ed. Chicago: Yearbook Medical Publishers, 1990, chap 5, pp 61–75.

16. Singer HS: Neurobiological issues in Tourette's syndrome. *Br Dev* 16:353–364, 1994.

17. Sacks OW: Acquired Tourettism in adult life. *Adv Neurol* 35:89–92, 1982.

18. Devinsky O: Neuroanatomy of Gilles de la Tourette's syndrome: Possible midbrain involvement. *Arch Neurol* 40:508–514, 1983.

19. Alexander GE, DeLong MR, Strick PL: Parallel organization of functionally segregated circuits linking basal ganglia and cortex. *Annu Rev Neurosci* 9:357–381, 1986.

20. Alexander GE, Crutcher MD, DeLong MR: Basal ganglia-thalamocortical circuits: Parallel substrates for motor, oculomotor, "prefrontal" and "limbic" functions. *Prog Brain Res* 85:119–145, 1990.

21. Muller-Preus P, Jurgens U: Projections from the "cingular" vocalization area in the squirrel monkey. *Brain Res* 103:29–43, 1976.

22. Baleydier C, Mauguierre F: The duality of the cingulate gyrus in monkey. *Brain* 103:525–554, 1980.

23. Peterson B, Riddle MA, Cohen DJ, et al: Reduced basal ganglia volumes in Tourette's syndrome using three-dimensional reconstruction techniques from magnetic resonance images. *Neurology* 43:941–948, 1993.

24. Singer HS, Reiss AL, Brown JE, et al: Volumetric MRI changes in basal ganglia of children with Tourette's syndrome. *Neurology* 43:950–956, 1993.

25. Witelson SF: Clinical neurology as data for basic neuroscience: Tourette's syndrome and the human motor system. *Neurology* 43:859–861, 1993.

26. Stoetter B, Braun AR, Randolph C, et al: Functional neuroanatomy of Tourette's syndrome limbic-motor interactions studied with FDG PET. *Adv Neurol* 58:213–226, 1992.

27. Swerdlow NB, Caine SB, Geyer MA: Regionally selective effects of intracerebral dopamine infusion on sensorimotor gating of the startle reflex in rats. *Psychopharmacology* 108:189–195, 1992.

28. Mogenson GJ, Jones DL, Chi YY: From motivation to action: Functional interface between the limbic system and the motor system. *Prog Neurobiol* 14:69–97, 1980.

29. Gedye A: Tourette's syndrome attributed to frontal lobe dysfunction: Numerous etiologies involved. *J Clin Psychol* 47(2):233–252, 1991.

30. Bergen D, Tanner C, Wilson R: The electroencephalogram in Tourette's syndrome. *Ann Neurol* 11:382–385, 1982.

31. Neufeld MY, Berger Y, Chapman J, Korcyzn A: Routine and quantitative EEG analysis in Gilles de la Tourette's syndrome. *Neurology* 40:1837–1839, 1990.

32. Krumholz A, Singer HS, Niedermeyer E, et al: Electrophysiological studies in Tourette's syndrome. *Ann Neurol* 14:638–641, 1983.

33. Glaze DG, Frost JD, Jankovic J: Sleep in Gilles de la Tourette's syndrome. *Neurology* 33:586–592, 1983.

34. Gabor B, Matthewes WS, Ferrari M: Disorders of arousal in Gilles de la Tourette's syndrome. *Neurology* 34:815–817, 1984.

35. Bock RD, Goldberger L: Tonic, phasic, and cortical arousal in Gilles de la Tourette's syndrome. *J Neurol Neurosurg Psychiatry* 48:535–544, 1985.

36. Robertson M, Doran M, Trimble M, Lees AJ: The treatment of Gilles de la Tourette's syndrome by limbic leucotomy. *J Neurol Neurosurg Psychiatry* 53:691–694, 1990.

37. Leckman JF, de Lotbinière, Marek K, et al: Severe disturbances in speech, swallowing, and gait following stereotactic infrathalamic lesions in Gilles de la Tourette's syndrome. *Neurology* 43:890–893, 1993.

38. Kurlan R, Kersun J, Ballantine HT Jr., Caine ED: Neurosurgical treatment of severe obsessive-compulsive disorder associated with Tourette's syndrome. *Mov Disord* 5(2):152–155, 1990.

39. Messiha FS: Biochemical pharmacology of Gilles de la Tourette's syndrome. *Neurosci Biobehav Rev* 12:295–305, 1988.

40. Barbeau A: Cholinergic treatment in Tourette's syndrome. *N Engl J Med* 302:1310–1311, 1980.

41. Sandyk R: Cholinergic mechanisms in Gilles de la Tourette's syndrome: *Int J Neurosci* 81:95–100, 1995.

42. Guyenet PG, Agid Y, Javoy F, et al: Effects of dopaminergic receptor agonists and antagonists on the activity of the neostriatal cholinergic system. *Brain Res* 84:227–244, 1975.

43. Jankovic J, Rohaidy H: Motor, behavioral, and pharmacologic findings in Tourette's syndrome. *Can J Neurol Sci* 14:541–546, 1987.

44. Tanner CM, Goetz CG, Klawans HL: Cholinergic mechanisms in Tourette's syndrome. *Neurology* 32:1315–1317, 1982.

45. Polinsky RJ, Ebert MH, Caine ED, et al: Cholinergic treatment in the Tourette's syndrome. *N Engl J Med* 302:1310, 1980.

46. Comings DE: *Tourette's Syndrome and Human Behavior.* Duarte, CA: Hope Press, 1990, chaps 59–63, pp 417–462.

47. Charney DS, Goodman WK, Price LH, et al: Serotonin function in obsessive-compulsive disorder. *Arch Gen Psychiatry* 45:177–185, 1988.

48. Northam RS, Singer HS: Postencephalitic acquired Tourette-like syndrome in a child. *Neurology* 41:592–593, 1991.

49. Lees AJ: *Tics and Related Disorders.* London: Churchill Livingstone, 1985, pp 80–81.

50. Spitz MC, Jankovic J, Killian JM: Familial tic disorder, parkinsonism, motor neuron disease, and acanthocytosis: A new syndrome. *Neurology* 35:366–370, 1985.

51. Kurczynski TW: Hyperekplexia. *Arch Neurol* 40:246–248, 1983.

52. Andermann F, Keene DL, Andermann E, Quesney LF: Startle disease or hyperekplexia: Further delineation of the syndrome. *Brain* 103:985–997, 1980.

53. Saenz-Lope E, Herranz-Tanarro FJ, Masdeu JC, Chacón-Pena JR: Hyperplexia: A syndrome of pathologic startle responses. *Ann Neurol* 15:36–41, 1984.

54. Milani N, Dalpra L, del Prete A, et al: A novel mutation (GIn266—His) in the alpha 1 subunit of the inhibitory glycine-receptor gene (GLRA1) in hereditary hyperekplexia (letter). *Am J Hum Genet* 58(2):420–422, 1996.

55. Floeter MK, Andermann F, Andermann E, et al: Physiological studies of spinal inhibitory pathways in patients with hereditary hyperekplexia. *Neurology* 46:766–772, 1996.

56. Fahn S: A case of post-traumatic tic syndrome. *Adv Neurol* 35:349–350, 1982.

57. Gaul JJ: Posttraumatic tic disorder. *Mov Disord* 9(1):121, 1994.

58. Davis TME, Knezevick W: Multiple tics following cerebral malaria. *Med J Aust* 160:307–308, 1994.

59. Pulst SM, Walshe TM, Romero JA: Carbon monoxide poisoning with features of Gilles de la Tourette's syndrome. *Arch Neurol* 40:443–444, 1983.

60. Pasqual-Leone A, Dhuna A: Cocaine-associated multifacial tics. *Neurology* 40:999–1000, 1990.

61. Robertson PL, Garofalo AG, Silverstein FS, Komarynski MA: Carbamazepine-induced tics. *Epilepsia* 34(5):965–968, 1993.

62. Howrie DL, Crumrine PK: Phenytoin-induced movement disorder associated with intravenous administration for status epilepticus. *Clin Pediatr* 24(8):467–469, 1985.

63. Burd L, Kerbeshian J, Fisher W, Gascon G: Anticonvulsant medications: An iatrogenic cause of tic disorders. *Can J Psychiatry* 31:419–423, 1986.

64. Klawans HL, Nausieda PA, Goetz CC, et al: Tourette-like symptoms following chronic neuroleptic therapy. *Adv Neurol* 35:415–418, 1982.

Chapter 42

TOURETTE'S SYNDROME
ROGER M. KURLAN

CLINICAL FEATURES
    Tic Disorders
    Behavioral Features
NATURAL COURSE
EPIDEMIOLOGY
DIFFERENTIAL DIAGNOSIS
    Distinguishing Tics from Other Movement Disorders
    Primary and Secondary Tic Disorders
ETIOLOGY/PATHOGENESIS
    Genetics
    Neurobiology
THERAPY
    Treatment of Tics
    Treatment of ADHD
    Treatment of OCD
    Nonmedication Therapies

In his now famous publication of 1885 where he described the illness that bears his name, George Gilles de la Tourette reported nine patients with motor and vocal tics, some of whom had echophenomena and coprolalia. Since that time, Gilles de la Tourette's syndrome (TS) has been generally viewed as a rare, severe, and disabling condition with bizarre symptoms and an unknown etiology. However, notions concerning TS and related disorders have undergone a dramatic evolution in recent years[1] and will serve as the focus for this chapter.

Clinical Features

The fourth (1994) edition of the Diagnostic and Statistical Manual of Psychiatry (DSM-IV) lists the following diagnostic criteria for TS:[2]

1. Both multiple motor and one or more vocal tics have been present at some time during the illness, although not necessarily concurrently.
2. The tics occur many times a day (usually in bouts) nearly every day or intermittently throughout a period of more than one year, and during this period there was never a tic-free period of more than three consecutive months.
3. The disturbance causes marked distress or significant impairment in social, occupational, or other important areas of functioning.
4. The onset is before age 18 years.
5. The disturbance is not due to the direct physiological effects of a substance (e.g., stimulants) or a general medical condition (e.g., Huntington's disease or post-viral encephalitis).

The formulation of such criteria, however, fails to convey the very heterogeneous clinical characteristics of the condition. The clinical manifestations of TS can best be viewed as a spectrum that includes both tics and associated behavioral features (Table 42-1).

TIC DISORDERS

Tics are recurrent, nonrhythmic, stereotyped movements (motor tics) or sounds produced by moving air through the nose, mouth, or throat (vocal tics).[3] In contrast to most other types of involuntary movements, tics are not constantly present (except when extremely severe) and occur out of a background of normal motor activity. Motor and vocal tics may take a variety of forms and can be divided conceptually into simple and complex types. *Simple motor tics* are sudden, brief, isolated movements such as an eye blink, a shoulder shrug, or a head jerk. Although most simple motor tics are fast and abrupt, some may appear as slower, sustained, tonic movements (e.g., neck twisting, abdominal or buttock tightening) that resemble dystonia and are therefore termed "dystonic tics."[4] *Complex motor tics* consist of more coordinated and complicated movements that may appear purposeful, as if performing a voluntary motor act. Examples include touching, smelling, jumping, copropraxia (obscene gestures), and echopraxia (mimicking movements performed by others). Motor tics usually recur in the same part of the body, and multiple body regions can be involved. Over time, tics often recede from one body part and evolve elsewhere.

Simple vocal tics include a variety of inarticulate noises and sounds, such as throat clearing, sniffling, and grunting. *Complex vocal tics* have linguistic meaning and consist of full or truncated words, such as echolalia (repeating the words of others), palilalia (repeating the individual's own words), and coprolalia (obscene words). Although coprolalia has perhaps been the symptom most responsible for the public notoriety of TS, the presence of this symptom is certainly not required for diagnosis. It is now clear that this symptom may be mild and transient and occurs in only a minority of cases. Some patients experience the obscene words only internally in thought (mental coprolalia).

Tics may manifest themselves by virtually any body movement or noise. Thus, the tic disorder of TS represents a wide spectrum of involuntary movements and noises, some of which may appear quite bizarre (e.g., throwing objects, pulling down pants) and be misinterpreted as manifestations of psychological illness.

The patient often experiences an irresistible urge to tic. This urge can usually be suppressed temporarily, but at the expense of a build-up of psychic tension that can be relieved only by the production of a tic.

Recent attention has focused on sensory symptoms that may occur in TS. "Sensory tics" are patterns of uncomfortable somatic sensations, such as pressure, tickling, or warmth that are localized to specific body regions, such as face, shoulder, or neck.[5,6] Patients attempt to relieve the uncomfortable sensations with movements often interpreted as voluntary, usually tonic tightening or stretching of muscles indicative of a dystonic tic. Relief is temporary, however, and the movements are repeated. Some patients produce vocalizations that

TABLE 42-1 Clinical Heterogeneity of Tourette's Syndrome

The tic disorder
  Tic types
    Simple motor tics
    Simple vocal tics
    Complex motor tics
    Complex vocal tics
    Tic variants
      Dystonic tics
      Sensory tics
  Tic disorder syndromes
    Tourette's syndrome
    Chronic tic disorder (motor or vocal)
    Transient tic disorder
  Tic severity
The behavioral disorder
  Obsessive-compulsive behavior
  Attention deficit hyperactivity disorder
  Other behavioral disturbances

are responses to a sensory stimulus in the larynx or throat. Sensory tics, reported by about 40 percent of surveyed TS patients, may be the most prominent feature of illness for some patients and are often misdiagnosed.

The motor and vocal tics of TS characteristically follow a waxing and waning pattern, such that there are periods lasting days or weeks during which tics worsen followed by other periods during which tics are less severe. The tics also characteristically occur in "waves," with a certain combination of tic types being present, only to eventually resolve and be replaced by another group of tics.

BEHAVIORAL FEATURES

Although chronic, multiple motor and vocal tics are usually the most prominent clinical features of TS and represent the signs on which the diagnosis of the disorder is currently based, tics may also be accompanied by a variety of behavioral disturbances. Studies have demonstrated a high incidence of obsessive-compulsive behavior (OCB), generally about 50 percent, in TS patients.[7–9] Common examples of such symptoms include compulsive checking, counting, and perfectionism, and obsessive worries or fears. About half of patients with TS will also show evidence of attention deficit hyperactivity disorder (ADHD), manifested by inattention, distractibility, impulsivity, and hyperactivity.[10] TS has been reported to have a close clinical association with a variety of other behavioral disturbances, including conduct disorder, panic attacks, phobias, depression, mania, anxiety disorders, stuttering, obesity, and alcoholism.[11] At present, however, the full spectrum of the TS behavioral disorder has not been accurately delineated and remains an area of controversy.[12–14]

A number of distinctive personality traits, such as argumentativeness, defensiveness, negativism, and impulsiveness, are seen commonly among TS patients. It is unclear whether these behavioral traits are specific for TS, reflect associated behavioral disorders (e.g., ADHD), or result from the peculiar social and emotional difficulties associated with living with the illness. Disturbed interpersonal relationships

with parents, siblings, peers, teachers, and others may underlie some of the observed problems.

Self-injurious behavior occurs occasionally in patients with TS.[15] This type of behavior has been linked to high levels of obsessionality and hostility. Other socially inappropriate behavior may accompany TS, such as verbalizing insults and other derogatory remarks or destroying personal property.[16] Such behavior may have a substantial functional impact on patients with TS and may contribute to social difficulties and isolation.

It is not uncommon to encounter difficulties with reading, writing, and arithmetic, including specific learning disabilities, in children with TS.[17] Patients with TS usually have normal intelligence, as their IQ distribution parallels that of the general population.[18]

Natural Course

The onset of tics occurs between the ages of 2 and 15 years in most cases, with the mean age of onset being 7 years.[19] The initial tics usually occur in the upper body, commonly involving the eyes (e.g., blinking) or other parts of the face. Vocal tics represent the initial manifestation of illness for a minority of patients.

Over the short term, tics characteristically change in type and wax and wane in severity. The longer-term, lifelong course of the TS tic disorder has been investigated in several studies. Erenberg et al. found that 73 percent of adult TS subjects reported that over a period of years their tics had either lessened considerably or almost disappeared.[20] Bruun followed 136 TS patients from 5 to 15 years and found that tic severity lessened over time with 59 percent rated mild-moderate initially and 91 percent rated so at follow-up.[21] Over time, 28 percent no longer required medications, and 52 percent reported spontaneous improvement. Shapiro and Shapiro observed that 5–8 percent of TS patients recover completely and permanently in adolescence; tics become less severe in 35 percent of cases during adolescence and less severe in "most patients" in adulthood.[22] Thus, many patients with TS experience an improvement or resolution of tics after adolescence.

Although the natural course of the tic disorder in TS has received considerable attention, little investigative work has focused on the behavioral components. Comings and Comings have suggested that for many children with TS, symptoms of ADHD antedate the appearance of tics by an average of 2.5 years.[23] Park and colleagues found it unusual for ADHD or obsessive-compulsive disorder (OCD) to be absent at the time of initial diagnosis of TS and then to appear later on, with only 4–6 percent of patients following this course.[24] On the other hand, disruptive behaviors (20 percent) and school problems (13 percent) more likely appeared over time.

Epidemiology

There is a 3:1 male predominance among patients with TS.[19] However, if one considers OCD to be an alternative clinical expression of the condition (see below), the gender ratio is nearly equal.[25] The disorder has been identified in all races and appears to be uniformly distributed across socioeconomic classes.[19] The clinical features appear to be uniform among different cultural groups, except that coprolalia is particularly uncommon in Japanese patients.[19]

Traditionally, TS has been viewed as a rare disorder. However, recent evidence suggests that it is much more common than generally appreciated. An accurate lifetime prevalence rate for TS has not been established. Past estimates, ranging from 0.03–1.6 percent,[26] have been based largely on case series of patients referred for medical evaluation or on data obtained from questionnaires without direct clinical examinations. For example, in estimating the prevalence of TS in North Dakota adults and children, Burd and colleagues included only subjects on a state-wide list of medical diagnoses.[27,28] The epidemiological survey of TS conducted by Caine et al. in Monroe County, New York, involved only children referred by school and health personnel following an extensive informational campaign in the local news media.[29] Several lines of recent evidence suggest that these approaches are likely to be inaccurate and lead to gross underestimates of disease prevalence. Systematic analysis of large TS kindreds using a family study method in which all available members are directly interviewed and examined indicates that most cases of TS are mild and do not come to medical attention and that the disorder is often unrecognized and misdiagnosed by physicians.[26,30] Furthermore, studies of the prevalence of TS have been restricted to an analysis of the tic disorder, and mounting evidence (see below) indicates that behavioral disorders, including OCD and ADHD, may be the only clinical manifestations of illness for some individuals.[8,25] Thus, the prevalence of the disorder may be much higher than current estimates, particularly if behavioral manifestations are included. Although his conclusions have been challenged,[12,14] Comings has estimated that if one accepts TS as a broadly based behavioral disorder, up to 1 in 100 individuals may manifest one or more clinical aspects of the TS genetic trait, making it one of the most common neurobehavioral disorders affecting man.[11]

Further support for a high prevalence of tic disorders comes from epidemiological surveys of school-age children which have identified tic rates ranging from 4 to 50 percent.[31-33] Two recent epidemiological studies found that nearly one-third of school-age children who required special educational programs had evidence of a tic disorder.[34,35] Although such studies have identified a high rate of tics during the course of childhood development, the authors have not examined the clinical characteristics of tics (e.g., presence of motor and vocal types, duration of at least 1 year) that are necessary to determine whether or not they satisfy criteria for TS. For most subjects identified with tics in these community-based surveys, the severity of tics observed has generally been quite mild.

Taken together, current evidence suggests that TS and related tic disorders are quite common in the general childhood population. For the most part, they appear to represent mild, nondisabling conditions which do not lead to medical attention or therapy, although they do appear to be linked to childhood school problems. It remains unclear whether all cases of chronic motor and vocal tics represent TS. The recent DSM edition has added the diagnostic criteria for TS that tics must cause marked distress or a significant impairment in daily functioning (see above). It has not been established, however, that such functional criteria are truly valid for making diagnostic distinctions.

Differential Diagnosis

DISTINGUISHING TICS FROM OTHER MOVEMENT DISORDERS[3]

Simple motor tics may resemble the rapid muscle jerks of myoclonus. However, even when most tics are simple jerks, more complex forms of motor tics or more sustained dystonic tics may also be present, allowing one to establish the diagnosis by association with these other forms of motor tics. Moreover, simple motor tics tend to have a less random, more predictable body distribution and a wider range of amplitude and forcefulness when compared with myoclonus. The characteristic voluntary suppressibility of tics and the tendency of myoclonus to increase with intentional acts may also help distinguish between the conditions. It is important to recognize, however, that voluntary suppressibility is a feature that is not specific for tics but can be seen to at least some degree in virtually all hyperkinetic movement disorders (see also Chap. 41).

Repetitive eye blinking and forceful eye closures from tics and from blepharospasm, a form of focal cranial dystonia, can usually be differentiated by the presence of other tics or dystonic movements at other sites. In addition, whereas tics typically begin in childhood, blepharospasm is predominantly a disorder with onset in later adult life. Dystonic tics may be differentiated from torsion dystonia in that the latter is a continual movement that can result in a sustained abnormal posture, while dystonic tics usually cause an abnormal posture that is present for only a short period of time. The presence of more typical jerk-like tics in other body regions would favor the notion that the sustained contractions could be dystonic tics rather than torsion dystonia. In addition, dystonic tics are often preceded by localized uncomfortable sensations (sensory tics) which may be relieved by the movement.[5] Such sensory experiences are typically absent in torsion dystonia.

It may be difficult to distinguish complex motor tics and compulsions. In contrast to tics, compulsions are closely associated with obsessions, are often performed in response to an obsessive thought pattern, and may be performed according to certain rules (rituals), such as a specified number of times, in a specified order, or at a particular time of day (e.g., bedtime rituals). In addition, compulsive rituals may be performed with the thought of preventing discomfort or a future dreaded event. The repetitive complex motor acts, known as stereotypies, of patients with mental retardation, psychosis, autism, or congenital blindness or deafness, may also be difficult to distinguish from motor tics. The correct diagnosis of tics is usually made by excluding conditions known to be associated with stereotypies or by identifying associated simple motor or vocal tics (see also Chap. 41 and Table 41-3).

Response to drug therapy (see below) may be helpful for differential diagnosis as well. For example, whereas tics usually predictably respond to dopamine antagonist drugs, compulsions do not. Rather, antidepressant drugs that selectively inhibit serotonin reuptake (e.g., fluoxetine, clomipramine) may be quite effective for compulsions.

PRIMARY AND SECONDARY TIC DISORDERS

A variety of primary tic disorders are now recognized, and TS can be considered to represent one member of a family of tic disorders.[1] Chronic motor tic disorders and chronic vocal tic disorders differ from TS in that motor or vocal tics, but not both, are present. Transient tic disorders differs from the others by having a duration of less than 1 year. Chronic motor and vocal tic disorders and transient tic disorders are now generally viewed as clinical variants of TS.[36,37]

It is now generally believed that the primary tic disorders occur on a hereditary basis.[38] Occasional cases of acute or chronic tics may represent phenocopies of the genetic disorder, and examples include chronic neuroleptic exposure (tardive TS),[39] viral encephalitis,[40] head trauma,[41] and carbon monoxide intoxication[42] (Table 42-2). Tics may also occur in a number of neurological disorders, including Huntington's disease, Parkinson's disease, progressive supranuclear palsy, neuroacanthocytosis, Meige's syndrome (cranial dystonia), and startle disorders. The excessive startle syndromes may be associated with echolalia, coprolalia, and echopraxia. For these secondary tic disorders, tics are usually combined with other disorders of movement (e.g., with chorea in Huntington's disease and neuroacanthocytosis).[43] In our experience, it is common to find a clinical syndrome resembling TS, including tics, OCB, inattention, and impulsivity in children with an array of developmental disorders that are often difficult to characterize. The Tourette-like features are often associated with developmental delays (motor, cognitive, social/emotional), learning disabilities, other involuntary movements (dystonia, chorea, stereotypies), and other movement disturbances (clumsiness, stuttering). We have observed this

TABLE 42-2 Secondary Tic Disorders

Inherited
  Huntington's disease
  Neuroacanthocytosis
  Torsion dystonia
  Chromosomal abnormalities
  Other
Acquired
  Drugs: neuroleptics (tardive tics), stimulants, anticonvulsants, L-dopa
  Trauma
  Infectious: encephalitis, Creutzfeldt-Jakob disease, Sydenham's chorea
  Developmental: static encephalopathy, mental retardation, autism, pervasive developmental disorder
  Stroke
  Degenerative: Parkinson's disease, progressive supranuclear palsy
  Toxic: carbon monoxide

constellation of symptoms in children with pervasive developmental disorders, fetal-alcohol syndrome, intrauterine exposure to illicit drugs, and other perinatal insults, and we suspect that it reflects a disruption of normal basal ganglia developmental processes which can occur from a variety of causes.

Etiology/Pathogenesis

GENETICS

Although Gilles de la Tourette himself stated that the disorder was hereditary in nature, for many years the etiology of TS was ascribed to psychogenic causes, and the importance of genetic factors was overlooked. It was not until the late 1970s that investigators demonstrated a familial concentration for TS and found that susceptibility to the illness is transmitted vertically from generation to generation, indicating a genetic trait.[44] Studies of monozygotic twins have confirmed a genetic influence.[45] Single major-locus, polygenic, and multifactorial patterns of transmission within families have been proposed.[38,45] The most widely held notion of transmission pattern derives from segregation analysis of 30 families affected by TS which indicates that the disorder is inherited in an autosomal-dominant pattern with incomplete and sex-specific penetrances (affected males are more common that affected females) and variable clinical expression which includes TS, chronic tic disorder, and obsessive-compulsive disorder (OCD).[25] When OCD is considered an alternative expression of the putative TS gene, penetrance estimates for females rise from 56 percent (when only TS or chronic tic disorder is considered) to 70 percent.[25] Other family studies have supported the notion that OCD is an alternative expression of the TS trait.[45]

Thus, current evidence suggests that the TS genetic trait can be expressed by a behavioral disorder alone, even in the absence of tics. This notion appears to be well-supported for OCD, particularly in females. Recent data also suggest that ADHD, at least in some families, is another possible behavioral variant of TS.[10,46] However, it remains undetermined whether any other psychopathological condition represents an alternative expression of the disorder as well. An observed association between TS and other psychopathology may simply be secondary to ascertainment bias, in that individuals with both problems may be more likely to be referred for medical evaluation. Furthermore, patients may experience behavioral disorders (e.g., depression or anxiety) as a consequence of living with the illness.

A recent report by Kurlan and colleagues indicates that the true hereditary transmission pattern for TS remains to be fully clarified.[47] The authors found a high frequency of bilineal (from maternal *and* paternal sides) transmission of TS in studied families. In addition, the frequency of bilineal transmission appeared to be related to the proband's severity of TS in that the frequency of both parents being affected was higher in families in which the proband's symptoms were most severe. These findings indicate that bilineal transmission and possible homozygosity or polygenic influences are common in TS and suggest that these genetic phenomena might play a role in determining severity of illness.

NEUROBIOLOGY

While genetic factors are now recognized as most important for the development of TS and related tic disorders, investigators continue to search for underlying neuroanatomic and neurochemical disturbances that may be manifestations of the gene defect and involved in the pathogenesis of the disorder. Several lines of evidence support the notion that striatal dopamine receptor supersensitivity at least partly underlies the tic disorder: (1) dopamine receptor antagonists are the most effective drugs for suppressing tics; (2) tics may be exacerbated by dopaminergic medications such as amphetamines; (3) reduced levels of the dopamine metabolite homovanillic acid have been identified in the cerebrospinal fluid of patients with TS[48]; and (4) the phenomenon of tardive tics follows chronic dopamine antagonist therapy.[39] The reported absence of staining for dynorphin in the globus pallidus of a postmortem brain from a patient with TS[49] and clinical observations that drugs affecting the endogenous opioid system may influence the symptoms of TS[50–52] have focused attention on the role of this neurochemical system in the pathogenesis of the disorder. Another study of postmortem TS brains revealed reduced concentrations of adenosine 3', 5'-monophosphate (cyclic AMP) in the cerebral cortex and suggests a possible dysfunction of secondary neurochemical messengers.[53] Other authors have suggested that sex hormone influences on brain development and function may be important in the pathogenesis of TS.[54,55] Two recent studies involving cerebral magnetic resonance imaging have revealed that the basal ganglia in patients with TS do not have the volumetric asymmetry (left greater than right) seen in normal controls (see also Chap. 41).

Therapy

The management of patients with TS can be both challenging and rewarding. The initial step is to identify the clinical features that are interfering most with daily activities and direct initial therapy at this "target" symptom (Table 42-3). The target symptom is not always tics—it may be ADHD, OCD, or other behavior problems (e.g., depression or anxiety).

TREATMENT OF TICS

Most patients with mild tics who have made a good adaptation in their lives can avoid the use of any medications. Educating patients, family members, peers, and school personnel regarding the nature of TS, restructuring the educational environment, and supportive counseling are measures that may be sufficient to avoid drug therapy. Pharmacotherapy should be considered once it is determined that the tics are functionally disabling and not remediable to psychosocial interventions. The goal in treating tics is generally to achieve "satisfactory" suppression or control rather than to attempt to make the patient completely free of tics. For the patient

TABLE 42-3 Pharmacological Treatment of Tourette's Syndrome

Tics
  Neuroleptics (haloperidol, pimozide, fluphenazine, others)
  Clonidine (oral, transdermal)
  Tetrabenazine
  Clonazepam
  Calcium-channel antagonists
  Botulinum toxin (dystonic tics)
Attention deficit hyperactivity disorder
  Clonidine
  Stimulants
  Deprenyl
  Tricyclic antidepressants
Obsessive-compulsive behavior
  Serotonin reuptake inhibitors (clomipramine, fluoxetine, others)

with mild or moderate tics, treatment is usually initiated with clonidine (Catapres). Brand name Catapres is recommended because of concerns about variable bioavailability for generic clonidine products. This drug is initiated at 0.05 mg at bedtime, and the dosage is increased by 0.05 mg every few days until satisfactory control of tics is achieved or unacceptable side effects are encountered. Most patients respond to 1 tablet (0.1 mg) 3 times per day (before and after school and at bedtime for children), but the maintenance dose should be the lowest one that gives satisfactory suppression of tics. Due to a short duration of action, particularly in children, 4 times daily dosing may be required. When necessary, higher doses of Catapres can be used, letting adverse effects be the dose-limiting factor. Transdermal Catapres is a good alternative dosing form, particularly for children who cannot swallow pills.

If Catapres alone is insufficient, one can add a neuroleptic (if partial relief with Catapres was observed) or replace Catapres with a neuroleptic (if no benefit was perceived). If Catapres is to be discontinued, the drug should be tapered by 0.05 mg every few days in order to avoid potential withdrawal phenomena, usually tachycardia and hypertension. Haloperidol (Haldol) remains one of the most commonly prescribed neuroleptics for treating tics. The drug is initiated at 0.25 mg at bedtime, increasing as necessary; most patients have a favorable response to 2 mg/day or less, given at bedtime. If haloperidol is unsuccessful or produces unacceptable side effects, one can then switch to pimozide (Orap), fluphenazine (Prolixin), or another neuroleptic.

For patients with very severe tics that are extremely problematic, one can initiate therapy with a neuroleptic rather than clonidine. Local intramuscular injections of botulinum toxin have been used to treat patients with painful dystonic tics.[56] Other medications that have been reported to improve tics include tetrabenazine, clonazepam, and calcium channel antagonists.

TREATMENT OF ADHD

When ADHD is the target symptom, Catapres is a useful starting medication. If symptoms are not adequately controlled, one can switch to a stimulant, such as methylphenidate (Ritalin) or pemoline (Cylert). Although treatment with stimulants may exacerbate tics in some patients, the occasional worsening of tics may be tolerable when these medications are effective in improving attentional abilities and alleviating hyperactivity.[57] If tics are significantly worsened by stimulant therapy, clonidine or a neuroleptic can be added. Recent, preliminary studies suggest that the selective monoamine oxidase-B (MAO-B) inhibitor deprenyl shows evidence of improving both ADHD and tics in children with both disorders.[58,59] Tricyclic antidepressants can be considered for the treatment of ADHD, but recent cases of sudden death in children treated with desipramine have raised concerns about the safety of this class of medications.

TREATMENT OF OCD

Recently introduced antidepressant drugs that inhibit serotonin reuptake, including fluoxetine (Prozac), clomipramine (Anafranil), and others may be effective for the treatment of OCD associated with TS.[60,61] Clinicians should be aware that the combined use of a serotonin reuptake inhibitor with deprenyl is not recommended due to potential serious interactions. Psychosurgical approaches have been used for occasional patients severely disabled by OCD who had inadequate responses to medications.[62,63]

NONMEDICATION THERAPIES

One of the most important aspects of treating TS is educating the patient and family members about tic disorders, ADHD, OCD, and other behavioral disturbances. A variety of educational brochures, videotapes, and other materials are available from the Tourette Syndrome Association (4240 Bell Boulevard, Bayside, NY 11361). A local TS support group may be of great benefit to patients and family members. Individual, group, or family counseling may be helpful in facilitating a healthy adaptation to the illness. Specific psychoeducational assessments and therapy are often needed for children with school problems.

References

1. Kurlan R: Tourette's syndrome: Current concepts. *Neurology* 39:1625–1630, 1989.
2. American Psychiatric Association: *Diagnostic and Statistical Manual of Mental Disorders,* 4th ed. Washington DC: American Psychiatric Association, 1994.
3. The Tourette Syndrome Classification Study Group: Definitions and classification of tic disorders. *Arch Neurol* 50:1013–1016, 1993.
4. Jankovic J, Stone L: Dystonic tics in patients with Tourette's syndrome. *Mov Disord* 6:248–252, 1991.
5. Kurlan R, Lichter D, Hewitt D: Sensory tics in Tourette's syndrome. *Neurology* 39:731–734, 1989.
6. Scahill LD, Leckman JF, Marek KL: Sensory phenomena in Tourette's syndrome. *Adv Neurol* 65:273–280, 1995.
7. Frankel M, Cummings JL, Robertson MM, et al: Obsessions and compulsions in Gilles de la Tourette's syndrome. *Neurology* 36:378–382, 1986.
8. Pauls DL, Towbin KE, Leckman JF, et al: Gilles de la Tourette's syndrome and obsessive-compulsive disorder: Evidence supporting a genetic relationship. *Arch Gen Psychiatry* 43:1180–1182, 1986.
9. Como PG: Obsessive-compulsive disorder in Tourette's syndrome. *Adv Neurol* 65:281–291, 1995.
10. Comings DE, Comings BG: Tourette's syndrome and attention deficit disorder with hyperactivity: Are they genetically related? *J Am Acad Child Psychiatry* 23:138–146, 1984.
11. Comings DE: A controlled study of Tourette's syndrome. VII. Summary: A common genetic disorder causing disinhibition of the limbic system. *Am J Hum Genet* 41:839–866, 1987.
12. Cohen DJ: Gilles de la Tourette's syndrome and attention deficit disorder with hyperactivity: Evidence against a genetic relationship. *Arch Gen Psychiatry* 43:1177–1179, 1986.
13. Pauls DL, Cohen DJ, Kidd KK, Leckman JR: Tourette's syndrome and neuropsychiatric disorders: Is there a genetic relationship? (Letter). *Am J Hum Genet* 43:206–209, 1988.
14. Kurlan R: What is the spectrum of Tourette's syndrome? *Curr Opin Neurol Neurosurg* 1:294–298, 1988.
15. Robertson MM, Yakeley JW: Obsessive-compulsive disorder and self-injurious behavior. In Kurlan R (ed): *Handbook of Tourette's Syndrome and Related Tic and Behavioral Disorders.* New York: Marcel Dekker, 1983, pp 45–87.
16. Kurlan R, Daragjati C, Como PG, et al: Non-obscene, complex, socially inappropriate behavior in Tourette's syndrome. *Neurology* 1995; 4(suppl 4):A253.
17. Walkup JT, Scahill LD, Riddle MA: Disruptive behavior, hyperactivity, and learning disabilities in Tourette's syndrome. *Adv Neurol* 65:259–272, 1995.
18. Como PG: Neuropsychological testing, in Kurlan R (ed): *Handbook of Tourette's Syndrome and Related Tic and Behavioral Disorders.* New York: Marcel Dekker, 1993, pp 221–239.
19. Shapiro AK, Shapiro ES, Young JG, Feinberg TE (eds): *Gilles de la Tourette Syndrome,* 2d ed. New York: Raven Press, 1988, pp 61–193.
20. Erenberg G, Cruse RP, Rothner AD: The natural history of Tourette syndrome: A follow-up study. *Ann Neurol* 22:383–385, 1987.
21. Bruun RD: The natural history of Tourette's syndrome. In Cohen DJ, Bruun RD, Leckman (eds): *Tourette's Syndrome and Tic Disorders: Clinical Understanding and Treatment.* New York: John Wiley & Sons, 1988, pp 21–39.
22. Shapiro ES, Shapiro AK: Gilles de la Tourette syndrome and tic disorders. *Harvard Medical School Mental Health Letter,* May 1989, p 5.
23. Comings DE, Comings BG: Tourette syndrome: Clinical and psychological aspects of 250 cases. *Am J Hum Genet* 37:435–450, 1985.
24. Park S, Como PG, Cui L, Kurlan R: The early course of the Tourette's syndrome clinical spectrum. *Neurology* 43:1712–1715, 1993.
25. Pauls DL, Leckman JF: The inheritance of Gilles de la Tourette's syndrome and associated behaviors: Evidence for autosomal dominant transmission. *N Engl J Med* 315:993–997, 1986.
26. Kurlan R, Behr J, Medved L, et al: Severity of Tourette's syndrome in one large kindred: Implication for determination of disease prevalence rate. *Arch Neurol* 44:268–269, 1987.
27. Burd L, Kerbeshian J, Wikenheiser M, et al: Prevalence of Gilles de la Tourette's syndrome in North Dakota adults. *Am J Psychiatry* 143:787–788, 1986.
28. Burd L, Kerbeshian J, Wikenheiser M, Fisher W: A prevalence study of Gilles de la Tourette syndrome in North Dakota school-age children. *J Am Acad Child Psychiatry* 4:552–555, 1986.
29. Caine ED, McBride MC, Chiverton P, et al: Tourette's syndrome in Monroe County school children. *Neurology* 38:472–475, 1988.
30. McMahon WM, Leppert M, Filloux F, et al: Tourette symptoms in 161 related family members. *Adv Neurol* 58:159–165, 1992.
31. Kellmer Pringle ML, Butler NR, Davie R: 1st report of national child development study, in: *11,000 Seven-Year-Olds.* National Bureau for Co-operation in Child Care, London, 1967, p 185.

32. MacFarlane JW, Honzik MP, Allen L: *Behavior Problems in Normal Children*. University of California Publications in Child Development, 1954.

33. Lapouse R, Monk M: Behavior deviations in a representative sample of children: Variation by sex, age, race, social class and family size. *Am J Orthopsychiatry* 34:436–446, 1964.

34. Comings DE, Himes JA, Comings BG: An epidemiologic study of Tourette's syndrome in a single school district. *J Clin Psychiatry* 51:463–469, 1990.

35. Kurlan R, Whitmore D, Irvine C, et al: Tourette's syndrome in a special education population: A pilot study involving a single school district. *Neurology* 44:699–702, 1994.

36. Golden GS: Tics and Tourette's syndrome: A continuum of symptoms? *Ann Neurol* 4:145–148, 1978.

37. Kurlan R, Behr J, Medved L, Como P: Transient tic disorder and the clinical spectrum of Tourette's syndrome. *Arch Neurol* 45:1200–1201, 1988.

38. Pauls DL: The inheritance pattern, in Kurlan R (ed): *Handbook of Tourette's Syndrome and Related Tic and Behavioral Disorders*. New York: Marcel Dekker, 1993, pp 307–315.

39. Klawans HL, Falk DK, Nausieda PA, Weiner WJ: Gilles de la Tourette's syndrome after long-term chlorpromazine therapy. *Neurology* 28:1064–1068, 1978.

40. Sacks OW: Acquired tourettism in adult life, in Friedhoff AJ, Chase TN (eds): *Gilles de la Tourette's Syndrome*. New York: Raven Press, 1982, pp 89–92.

41. Fahn S: A case of post-traumatic tic syndrome, in Friedhoff AJ, Chase TN (eds): *Gilles de la Tourette's Syndrome*. New York: Raven Press, 1982, pp 349–350.

42. Pulst SM, Walshe TM, Romero JA: Carbon monoxide poisoning with features of Gilles de la Tourette's syndrome. *Arch Neurol* 40:443–444, 1983.

43. Jankovic J: Tics in other neurological disorders. In Kurlan R (ed): *Handbook of Tourette's Syndrome and Related Tic and Behavioral Disorders*. New York: Marcel Dekker 1993, pp 167–182.

44. Price RA, Kidd KK, Cohen DJ, et al: A twin study of Tourette's syndrome. *Arch Gen Psychiatry* 42:815–820, 1985.

45. Pauls DL: Issues in genetic linkage studies of Tourette syndrome: Phenotypic spectrum and genetic model parameters. *Adv Neurol* 58:151–157, 1992.

46. Knell ER, Comings DE: Tourette's syndrome and attention-deficit hyperactivity disorder: Evidence for a genetic relationship. *J Clin Psychiatry* 54:331–337, 1993.

47. Kurlan R, Eapen V, Stern J, et al: Bilineal transmission in Tourette's syndrome families. *Neurology* 44:2336–2342, 1994.

48. Singer HS, Butler IJ, Tune LE, et al: Dopaminergic dysfunction in Tourette's syndrome. *Ann Neurol* 12:361–366, 1982.

49. Haber SN, Kowell NW, Vonsattel JP, et al: Gilles de la Tourette's syndrome: A postmortem neuropathological and immunohistochemical study. *J Neurol Sci* 75:225–241, 1986.

50. Gilman MA, Sandyk R: The endogenous opioid system in Gilles de la Tourette's syndrome. *Med Hypotheses* 19:371–378, 1986.

51. Lichter D, Majumdar L, Kurlan R: Opiate withdrawal unmasks Tourette's syndrome. *Clin Neuropharmacol* 11:559–564, 1988.

52. Kurlan R, Majumdar L, Deeley C, et al: A controlled trial of propoxyphene and naltrexone in Tourette's syndrome. *Ann Neurol* 30:19–23, 1991.

53. Singer HS, Hahn I-H, Krowiak E, et al: Tourette's syndrome: A neurochemical analysis of postmortem cortical brain tissue. *Ann Neurol* 27:443–446, 1990.

54. Kurlan R: The pathogenesis of Tourette's syndrome: A possible role for hormonal and excitatory neurotransmitter influences in brain development. *Arch Neurol* 49:874–876, 1992.

55. Peterson BS, Leckman JF, Scahill L, et al: Steroid hormones and CNS sexual dimorphisms modulate symptom expression in Tourette's syndrome. *Psychoneuroendocrinology* 17:553–563, 1993.

56. Jankovic J: Botulinum toxin in the treatment of tics associated with Tourette's syndrome (abstr.). *Neurology* 1993; 43(suppl 2):A310.

57. Robertson MM, Eapen V: Pharmacologic controversy of CNS stimulants in Gilles de la Tourette's syndrome. *Clin Neuropharmacol* 15:408–425, 1992.

58. Jankovic J: Deprenyl in attention deficit associated with Tourette's syndrome. *Arch Neurol* 50:286 288, 1993.

59. Feigin A, Kurlan R, McDermott M, et al: A double-blind, placebo-controlled, cross-over study of deprenyl in children with Tourette's syndrome (TS) and attention-deficit hyperactivity disorder (ADHD) (abstr.). *Neurology* 45(suppl 4):A254–A255, 1995.

60. Como PG, Kurlan R: An open-label trial of fluoxetine for obsessive-compulsive disorder in Gilles de la Tourette's syndrome. *Neurology* 41:872, 1991.

61. Kurlan R, Como PG, Deeley C, et al: A pilot controlled study of fluoxetine for obsessive-compulsive symptoms in children with Tourette's syndrome. *Clin Neuropharmacol* 16:167, 1993.

62. Kurlan R, Kersun J, Ballentine HT Jr, et al: Neurosurgical treatment of severe obsessive-compulsive disorder associated with Tourette's syndrome. *Mov Disord* 5:152, 1990.

63. Robertson M, Doran M, Trimble M, et al: The treatment of Gilles de la Tourette Syndrome by limbic leucotomy. *J Neurol Neurosurg Psychiatry* 53:691, 1990.

Chapter 43

CLINICAL FEATURES AND TREATMENT OF CEREBELLAR DISORDERS

SID GILMAN

FUNCTIONS OF THE CEREBELLUM
    Control of Posture and Movement
    Motor Learning
    Cognitive Functions
    Cerebellar Abnormalities in Autism and
      Schizophrenia
CLINICALLY RELEVANT CEREBELLAR ANATOMY
CLINICAL SIGNS OF CEREBELLAR DISORDERS
    Abnormalities of Stance and Gait
    Titubation
    Rotated or Tilted Postures of the Head
    Disturbances of Extraocular Movements
    Decomposition of Movement
    Dysmetria
    Dysdiadochokinesis and Dysrhythmokinesis
    Ataxia
    Check and Rebound
    Tremor
    Ataxia Dysarthria
    Abnormalities of Muscle Tone
TREATMENT OF CEREBELLAR DISORDERS

Functions of the Cerebellum

CONTROL OF POSTURE AND MOVEMENT

Studies in experimental animals beginning early in the last century demonstrated that the key role of the cerebellum is in the control of motor function.[1,2] This view was buttressed by observations in patients with disorders of cerebellar structure and function dating to the turn of the century.[3,4] These observations demonstrated that lesions of the cerebellum disturb posture and gait and the smoothly integrated coordination of movements, both simple and compound. Disturbed cerebellar function disrupts movements requiring an accurate estimate of the goal in time and space. Lesions of the cerebellum delay the initiation of movement and lead to clumsiness of movement; however, these lesions do not prevent the execution of movement. With cerebellar injury, muscles that normally act together lose their capacity to do so. Movements then deteriorate into incomplete or inaccurate forms, producing errors of force, velocity, and timing. Muscle strength may be diminished somewhat, but is not lost. Essentially all movements coordinated by the somatic musculature are affected, including extraocular movements and speech. Cerebellar lesions alone do not disrupt sensation in the body (except for weight discrimination) (see Chap. 44).

MOTOR LEARNING

Recent studies revealed that the cerebellum participates in motor tasks by learning new movements and by adapting already learned movements to a new task. Evidence for this comes from theoretical considerations[5-7]; anatomic observations in animals[8,9]; physiological studies in animals[10-16]; observations with positron emission tomography in normal humans[17-24]; and clinical/physiological testing of humans with cerebellar lesions.[25-30] Taken together, these observations indicate that the initial learning of skilled motor acts begins consciously under the control of the cerebral cortex. From the very start of the learning situation, the cerebellum participates in the control of the task and, as learning proceeds, the cerebellum assumes increasing responsibility until it gains essentially complete control of the task. The cerebellum comes to recognize the context requiring the movement, links together each component of the movement, and automatically triggers the movement upon presentation of the appropriate stimulus in the correct context. Through the cerebellum, the nervous system controls the sequence of many complex movements automatically, without the need for conscious awareness of the planning, execution, and termination required. Thus, movements programmed by the cerebellum can combine muscular actions, prevent movement errors, and develop complex movement sequences involving both single joints and multiple joints.

COGNITIVE FUNCTIONS

The observation that memory and intellect remain preserved in humans with large volumes of cerebellar tissue destroyed[4] led to the conclusion that the cerebellum is not involved in cognitive functions. Recently, however, growing evidence has been adduced linking the cerebellum to at least certain aspects of cognition. The initial interest in this idea came from the observation that in phylogenetic development the lateral cerebellum and the cognitively important structures of the forebrain developed phylogenetically in parallel.[31-33] Recent anatomic studies have begun to demonstrate linkages of the cerebellum with the motor association areas of the cerebral cortex that participate in motor planning, including premotor cortex, primary and secondary frontal eye fields, and areas 44, 45, and 46.[34-37] These motor association areas are thought to include regions important in the motor components of speech in humans (areas 44 and 45 of Brodmann). The motor association areas receive projections from regions of the brain associated with perception and awareness. Studies in both experimental animals utilizing single neuronal unit recordings and in humans with positron emission tomography have shown that these areas become active with anticipation of a movement or rehearsal of a movement, even without actual performance of the movement.[18] Moreover, both the left frontal lobe of the cerebrum and the right cerebellar hemisphere become active when human subjects are required to generate a word in an association task.[38] With repetition of the same task to the point of familiarity, frontal activity declines and cerebellar activity decreases,[39] suggesting that the cerebellum becomes responsible for execution of the task. Support for the idea that the cerebellum functions in this fashion came from the demonstration of impaired word production in an association task after a vascular insult of the right cerebellar hemisphere in one report[40] and agrammatic speech after a similar lesion in another.[41] Observations in patients with cerebellar degenerations and focal lesions suggest other high-level functions for the cerebellum, including cognitive planning,[42] associative learning,[43] classical conditioning,[44] instrumental learning,[45] and voluntary shifts of selective attention between sensory modalities.[46,47] Synaptic plasticity has been cited as a mechanism accounting for motor and cognitive learning in the cerebellum.[48]

CEREBELLAR ABNORMALITIES IN AUTISM AND SCHIZOPHRENIA

Anatomic abnormalities have been found in the cerebellum of patients with autism, a developmental disorder that results in severe deficits of language, social, and cognitive function.[49–52] Similar evidence has linked cerebellar abnormalities with schizophrenia.[53] Neither of these observations has been sufficiently consistent to establish a cause and effect relationship.

Clinically Relevant Cerebellar Anatomy

The cerebellum consists of a central longitudinal structure, the vermis, and two hemispheres.[54] A zone between the vermis and the lateral part of the hemisphere on each side is called the paravermis. The cerebellar cortex is divided by fissures into three major lobes: the anterior, posterior, and flocculonodular. The primary fissure separates the anterior and posterior lobes, and the postnodular fissure divides the posterior and flocculonodular lobes. Additional shallow fissures subdivide the anterior and posterior lobes into a series of transverse lobules (also see Fig. 44-6).

Comparative anatomic studies led to the division of the cerebellum into the archicerebellum (flocculonodular lobe), paleocerebellum (the vermis of the anterior lobe and the pyramis, uvula, and paraflocculus), and neocerebellum (the lateral parts of the cerebellum, including most of the hemi-

spheres and the middle portion of the vermis)[55] (Table 43-1). These divisions correspond moderately well to the sites of afferent projections to the cerebellum.[55] Vestibular fibers project densely into the flocculonodular lobe (the archicerebellum), and correspondingly the term "vestibulocerebellum" has been applied to this lobe. The major projections from the spinal cord[56] terminate in the vermis (the paleocerebellum), leading to the designation "spinocerebellum" for this region. The projections from the pons, which are derived principally from the cerebral cortex, terminate in the cerebellar hemispheres, and the term "pontocerebellum" is used for the hemispheres. This system of nomenclature has been useful, but it provides only approximate localization because the locations of the termination sites describe only partially the regions activated physiologically.[54,57–59]

Clinically, the organization of the cerebellum is best viewed as a series of sagittal zones,[54] including: (1) a vermal zone containing cerebellar cortical efferent neurons projecting to the fastigial nucleus; (2) an intermediate (paravermal) zone with cerebellar cortical efferents projecting to the interposed nuclei; and (3) a lateral zone, including the most lateral region of the anterior lobe and the lateral portion of the hemispheres, which contain cerebellar cortical efferents projecting to the lateral (dentate) nucleus (Table 43-2 and Fig. 44-7). Many additional sagittal zones have been identified,[60,61] but are not helpful clinically. Additional anatomic sites important clinically for eye movement abnormalities are regions receiving major inputs from the vestibular nuclei, including the dorsal vermis and fastigial nucleus, the flocculus and paraflocculus, and the nodulus.[62]

The midline zone of the cerebellum contains major afferents originating in the spinal cord and the brain stem reticular and vestibular nuclei and major efferents projecting via the fastigial nucleus to vestibulospinal and reticulospinal neurons. These connections are concerned with posture, locomotion, the position of the head in relation to the trunk, and the control of extraocular movements.[54] Correspondingly, the clinical signs resulting from midline cerebellar disease consist of disordered stance and gait,[63] truncal titubation,[54] rotated postures of the head,[64] and disturbances of extraocular movements[62] (Table 43-3). Some authors consider disorders of the flocculus, nodules, and uvula as a separate group, comprising the "vestibulocerebellum."[65–67] In the past, dysarthria has been considered a sign of midline cerebellar disease, but this disorder may be linked to several sites in the cerebellum, including the hemispheres.[40,41,68]

TABLE 43-1 Anatomic and Phylogenetic Organization of the Cerebellum

Structure	Phylogenetic Designation	Afferent Projections	Current Designation
Flocculonodular lobe	Archicerebellum	Vestibular receptors and nuclei	Vestibulocerebellum
Vermis of anterior lobe, pyramis, uvula, paraflocculus	Paleocerebellum	Spinal cord	Spinocerebellum
Cerebellar hemispheres, middle portions of vermis	Neocerebellum	Pons	Pontocerebellum

TABLE 43-2 Sagittal Organization of the Cerebellum

Zone	Principal Afferent Projections	Associated Deep Cerebellar Nuclei	Efferent Projections of Cerebellar Nuclei
Vermal	Spinal cord, reticular and vestibular nuclei	Fastigial	Vestibulospinal tract, reticulospinal tract
Intermediate (paravermal)	Spinal cord, brain stem, cerebral cortex	Interposed	Red nucleus, thalamus
Lateral	Pons, cerebral cortex	Dentate	Thalamus, cerebral cortex

The intermediate zone of the cerebellum is comprised of the paravermal region of the cerebellar cortex and the interposed nuclei on each side. Major afferents to this zone arise in many structures, including the spinal cord, brain stem, and cerebral cortex, with cerebral cortical projections mediated through synapses in the brain stem. Similarly, efferent projections reach both rostral and caudal regions of the nervous system. Diseases strictly limited to the intermediate zone appear to be rare, and consequently the clinical disorders from injury to this zone have been linked with those due to disease of the midline zone or the lateral zone.

The lateral zone includes the cerebellar hemisphere and the dentate nucleus of each side. This zone receives afferent projections heavily from the cerebral cortex through relay nuclei in the pons and brain stem reticular nuclei. The lateral zone sends projections to brain stem and thalamic structures that make connections with both forebrain and spinal levels of the nervous system. The abnormalities resulting from lesions of the lateral zone are related chiefly to voluntary movements and consist of abnormalities of stance and gait, disturbances of extraocular movements, decomposition of movement, dysmetria, dysdiadochokinesis, dysrhythmokinesis, ataxia, impaired check, excessive rebound, kinetic and static tremor, dysarthria, and hypotonia[54] (Table 43-3).

Clinical Signs of Cerebellar Disorders

Clinical signs of cerebellar disease commonly result from disease processes directly involving the cerebellum; however, similar signs can result from disorders of structures separate from the cerebellum. These structures include the

TABLE 43-3 Principal Clinical Signs Linked to the Sagittal Organization of the Cerebellum

Zone	Clinical Signs
Vermal	Abnormal stance and gait; truncal titubation; rotated postures of the head; disturbances of extraocular movements
Lateral	Abnormal stance and gait, disturbances of extraocular movements, decomposition of movement, dysmetria, dysdiadochokinesis, dysrhythmokinesis, ataxia, impaired check, excessive rebound, kinetic and static tremor, dysarthria, hypotonia

spinal cord, usually from involvement of the spinocerebellar pathways, the pons, midbrain, and thalamus,[69–71] the internal capsule,[72,73] and even the parietal cortex.[74]

ABNORMALITIES OF STANCE AND GAIT

The most common clinical signs of cerebellar disease are abnormalities of standing and walking.[64] With disease restricted to the midline zone, these abnormalities usually appear with minimal disturbances in the coordinated movements of the limbs when tested separately. With disease of the lateral zone, difficulty in standing and walking accompanies cerebellar movement disorders of the other limbs. The patient with a cerebellar gait disorder usually stands on a wide base and may develop a severe truncal tremor. As the patient walks, truncal instability may result in falls to the right, left, forward, or backward,[4] and coordination of postural control with voluntary movement is difficult.[75] Walking is performed with a series of steps irregularly placed, some too far forward, some inadequately far forward, and some too far to the sides. The legs are often lifted excessively during ambulation. Gait deficits can be enhanced by various maneuvers, including walking in tandem (heel to toe) or walking on the heels, the toes, or backward. The side toward which a patient falls, swerves, drifts, or leans does not necessarily indicate the side of the cerebellar lesion. Ataxia of gait with unimpaired limb coordination otherwise occurs with injury to the anterior superior portion of the cerebellar vermis and frequently results from nutritional and alcoholic damage to the nervous system.[76] Lesions of the flocculonodular lobe are also associated with disorders of stance and gait, often in association with multidirectional nystagmus and head rotation.[54]

TITUBATION

This is a rhythmic tremor of the body or head, consisting of a rocking motion forward and backward, from side to side, or in a rotatory movement, and usually occurring several times per second. The patient may have an associated distal static tremor of the fingers and wrist.

ROTATED OR TILTED POSTURES OF THE HEAD

Abnormal postures of the head can be associated with disease of the vermis or the flocculonodular lobule. The direction of head tilt does not have localizing significance with respect to the side of the cerebellar pathology.[54]

DISTURBANCES OF EXTRAOCULAR MOVEMENTS

Based upon experimental work in animals and correlations with neurological disorders in humans, three principal sites in the cerebellum are associated with distinctive disorders of extraocular movement.[62,77] The sites are: (1) the dorsal vermis and underlying fastigial nucleus; (2) the flocculus and paraflocculus; and (3) the nodulus. Lesions of the dorsal vermis and fastigial nucleus result in saccadic dysmetria, typically with hypermetric movements and at times with macrosaccadic oscillations. Saccadic lateropulsion[78] and deficits of pursuit can also occur. Lesions of the flocculus and paraflocculus cause gaze-evoked nystagmus, rebound nystagmus, and downbeat nystagmus; impaired smooth tracking; glissadic, postsaccadic drift; and disturbances in adjusting the gain of the vestibulo-ocular reflex.[79–81] Lesions of the nodulus lead to an increase in the duration of the vestibular response, which is manifested clinically by periodic alternating nystagmus.

In addition to the disturbances of extraocular movements associated with the three sites described above, many other disorders are described with cerebellar diseases, but are not as yet associated with specific known sites. These disturbances include square-wave jerks, divergent nystagmus, centripetal nystagmus, primary position upbeating nystagmus, increased responsiveness of the cervico-ocular reflex, and pendular oscillations.[62]

DECOMPOSITION OF MOVEMENT

Disease in the lateral zone of the cerebellum results in abnormalities of both simple and compound movements.[54,82,83] Simple movements consist of changes of posture or movements restricted to one joint or plane and can be slow or rapid. Compound movements involve a change of posture at two or more joints. The lateral zone of the cerebellum participates in many aspects of the control of both types of movements.[84–87]

Cerebellar lesions impair the control of simple movements, both slow[88–90] and rapid.[4,86,91] Muscular contractions under both isotonic and isometric conditions are affected,[92,93] and the execution of serial movements is impaired.[94] Self-terminated simple movements are abnormal after cerebellar lesions in that movement initiation is delayed[83] and braking is abnormal.[95] Ballistic movements are carried out abnormally after cerebellar lesions.[96] Injury to the cerebellar hemispheres results in deterioration of compound arm movements with decomposition into their constituent parts. This leads to errors of direction, delay in the initiation of one portion of the compound movement, and an excessive trajectory with movement.[97,98] Dysfunction of the lateral zone of the cerebellum also influences long latency stretch reflexes.[99–101] The disorders of movement with cerebellar disease result from a variety of abnormalities, including disturbances in the central commands that initiate movements and in the regulation of sensory feedback.[93,102]

DYSMETRIA

This is a disturbance of the trajectory or placement of a body part during active movements. Hypometria refers to a trajectory in which the body part falls short of its goal, and hypermetria indicates a trajectory in which the body part extends beyond its goal. Dysmetria is a common finding in patients with cerebellar disorders and can be detected by increasing the inertial load of the moving limb in patients with cerebellar lesions without otherwise clinically apparent dysmetria.[103]

DYSDIADOCHOKINESIS AND DYSRHYTHMOKINESIS

Dysdiadochokinesis is a manifestation of cerebellar disease seen with alternating or fine repetitive movements. When the patient taps one hand with the other, rapidly placing the palmar and dorsal surfaces alternately upward, deficits appear in the rate of alternation and in the completeness of the sequence. The patient cannot produce rhythmic movements, and the hand is supinated or pronated incompletely. Opposing each finger in rapid succession against the thumb of the same hand reveals finer deficits in coordination. Alternate tapping of the heel and toe on the floor also demonstrates deficits in movements of the feet. Dysrhythmokinesis is a disorder of the rhythm of rapidly alternating movements and can be demonstrated when patients attempt to tap out a rhythm such as three rapid beats followed by one delayed beat. The rhythm is abnormal and irregular with cerebellar lesions.

ATAXIA

The term "ataxia" is used to describe multiple problems with movement, including delay in movement initiation, disorders of movement termination (dysmetria), disturbances of velocity and acceleration, and difficulty applying constant force.[104] These abnormalities result in decomposition of movement so that errors occur in the sequence and speed of the component parts of a movement. The result is a lack of speed and skill in acts requiring the smoothly coordinated activity of several muscles. Another term for the abnormalities of movement with cerebellar disease is asynergia or dyssynergia. These terms indicate that the patient is unable to perform the various components of a movement at the right time in the appropriate space.

CHECK AND REBOUND

Impaired check and excessive rebound are related signs of cerebellar injury. To examine for abnormal check, the examiner asks the patient to maintain the limbs extended forward in space while the examiner taps the wrists strongly enough to displace the arms. The patient keeps the eyes shut and the hands pronated. A small displacement should result in a rapid, accurate return to the original position in a normal subject. With injury to the cerebellum, a light tap to the wrist results in a large displacement of the affected limb followed by an overshoot beyond the original position. Return to the original position is achieved by oscillation of the arm around its initial position. Wide excursion of the affected limb, which is termed excessive rebound, results from impaired check. Excessive rebound results in overshoot beyond the original position. Impaired check can also be assessed by forcefully pulling on the patient's forearm while the patient flexes the elbow. On releasing the forearm abruptly, the examiner will evoke an unchecked contraction of the arm, and patients will strike their chest with their hand or wrist. The basic phenomenon underlying impaired check and rebound is the inability to stop abruptly an ongoing movement.

TREMOR

Cerebellar dysfunction results in static and kinetic tremors.[54,82,105,106] The term "intention tremor" is a widely used but ambiguous term, usually referring to the tremor that occurs with limb movement. The term "kinetic tremor" is preferable. Static tremor can be demonstrated by observing a patient with arms extended parallel to the floor and hands open. Often this position can be sustained steadily for several seconds, but then a rhythmic oscillation occurs, generated at the shoulder. Recent studies suggest that static tremor is driven by stretch-evoked peripheral feedback to the cerebal cortex.[105,107] A kinetic tremor, usually affecting the proximal musculature exclusively in cerebellar disease, can be brought out by having the patient perform the finger-to-nose and heel-to-shin tests.

ATAXIC DYSARTHRIA

Patients with disease restricted to the cerebellum develop an ataxia of speech characterized by imprecise consonants, excessive and equalized stress patterns, irregular articulatory breakdowns, distorted vowels, prolonged phonemes, prolonged intervals, and slowness of rate, as well as excessive loudness variations, pitch breaks, and voice tremor.[108,109] Cerebellar disease alone does not lead to strained, strangled speech, which appears to result from corticobulbar disease.[110]

Recently, transient loss of speech termed 'cerebellar mutism' was described in children after posterior fossa surgery.[111–116] The disorder occurs following manipulation at surgery of structures in the posterior fossa, including the cerebellum and the dorsal brain stem. Currently this disorder is thought to result from an interaction of trauma to the brain stem and cerebellum coupled with hydrocephalus.[115]

ABNORMALITIES OF MUSCLE TONE

Hypotonia (decreased resistance to passive muscular extension) can result from lateral cerebellar lesions, usually acutely after cerebellar injury, with decreased abnormality over time.[4] Associated pendular deep tendon reflexes may be seen. Tonic stretch reflexes induced by muscle vibration[117] are abnormal in patients with cerebellar disorder and appear to be related to clinical hypotonia. Hypotonia has been found in monkeys after complete cerebellectomy,[118] in the ipsilateral limbs after unilateral cerebellar ablation,[118] and after lesions of the cerebellar nuclei.[119] Hypotonia is most marked in the extensor muscles of monkeys with cerebellar lesions but decreases with time and is replaced by tonic flexion of the affected limbs.[54] Hypotonia does not appear in cats and dogs after cerebellar ablation; these animals develop marked extensor rigidity with opisthotonos. The extensor rigidity of

dogs and cats with cerebellar ablation is termed "alpha rigidity" because it persists after sectioning of the dorsal roots, which abolishes decerebrate gamma rigidity.[54]

The cerebellum manipulates the linkage of alpha and gamma motoneurons in the performance of movements. Inactivation of the cerebellar cortex in the cat by cooling results in a decrease in the excitability of muscle spindle afferents.[54] In the decerebellate monkey, muscle spindle primary afferents are defective in function, showing raised thresholds and depressed static and dynamic sensitivities.[118] Muscle spindle secondary afferents, however, show essentially normal responses. Hypotonia appears to be related to the muscle spindle abnormalities. Cerebellectomy in the cat reduces muscle spindle sensitivity to static extension and a variety of natural external inputs,[120] with greater abnormalities affecting afferents with high rather than low conduction velocity,[121] along with low baseline rates of alpha motoneuron firing.[122] The reason for this is that cerebellar lesions result in defective gamma motoneuron regulation of muscle spindle output.[54] Thus, alpha motoneurons having synaptic connection with spindle receptors innervated by afferent fibers of high conduction velocity receive a falsely low indication of static muscle length. The decrease of fusimotor activity leading to abnormalities in muscle spindle function is an important factor in the pathogenesis of cerebellar hypotonia. Although the decrease of fusimotor activity after cerebellar lesions results from abnormal function of a long reflex loop through the precentral cortex,[123,124] vestibulospinal and reticulospinal pathways also appear to be involved because lesions of the fastigial nucleus markedly decrease muscle spindle activity.[125]

Treatment of Cerebellar Disorders

Medical treatment of the symptoms of cerebellar disorders is limited at best. Despite the appearance periodically of enthusiastic claims for therapeutic benefits from administration of isoniazid, physostigmine, L-5-hydroxytryptophan, thyrotropin-releasing hormone, vitamin E, amantadine, and propranolol, most clinicians have found these medications to have limited results or no benefit. I have found administration of clonazepam 1.5–5 mg daily in divided doses to have limited benefit in some patients. I usually begin treatment with one-half of a 0.5 mg tablet at bedtime and then gradually escalate the dose over many weeks, depending upon patient tolerance of the side effects, which include drowsiness, lethargy, and worsening of ataxia. The key to treatment of cerebellar disorders is an accurate diagnosis so that the appropriate therapeutic intervention can be made.

Disorders of cerebellar function can arise from degenerative, demyelinative, neoplastic, paraneoplastic, vascular, and infectious diseases, and from drug effects, heavy metal intoxications, malformations, inherited metabolic diseases, and endocrinopathies.[54] Table 43-4 provides a summary of the common disorders affecting cerebellar function, the laboratory tests helpful in the diagnosis, and the specific treatments available. Recent publications provide lists of the inherited ataxias of infancy, childhood, and adulthood, the pattern of inheritance, the appropriate laboratory tests, and the specific treatment available.[126,127]

TABLE 43-4 Differential Diagnosis and Treatment of Cerebellar Disorders

Disorders	Laboratory Tests	Specific Treatment
Disease		
Degenerative (OPCA, MSA, FA, alcoholic cerebellar degeneration)	MRI; CT; PET	None for OPCA and FA, thiamine and proper nutrition for alcoholic cerebellar degeneration
Demyelinative	MRI, CSF evaluation, evoked potential studies	Immunosuppressive therapy
Neoplasm (primary or secondary, von Hippel-Lindau syndrome)	MRI, angiogram, CBC, x-rays, bone marrow, bone scan	Surgery, chemotherapy, radiation therapy
Paraneoplastic	Search for primary neoplasm (ovarian, lung, breast, uterine, sarcomatous neoplasms in adults, neuroblastoma in children)	Surgery, chemotherapy, radiation therapy of the primary neoplasm
Vascular (AVM, infarction, hemorrhage)	MRI, CT, angiogram	Surgical and medical management
Infections		
Abscess	MRI, CT, angiogram	Surgery, antibiotics
Creutzfeldt-Jakob disease	EEG	None
Acute cerebellar ataxia in children	CSF evaluation, viral studies, search for neuroblastoma	None
Drug effects		
Anticonvulsants (phenytoin, valproate, carbamazepine, clonazepam, phenobarbital)	Serum anticonvulsant drug levels	Decrease anticonvulsant drug intake
Psychotropic medications (neuroleptic, antidepressant)	Serum levels if available	Decrease psychotropic medication intake
Lithium	Serum level of lithium	Decrease lithium intake
Heavy metals		
Thallium	Urinalysis for thallium, nerve conduction velocity	Chelating agents, hemodialysis
Lead (children)	Serum and urine levels of lead	Chelating agents, hemodialysis
Malformations (Dandy-Walker, Arnold-Chiari)	MRI, angiogram, myelogram, skull and spine films	Surgery
Inherited ataxias	Specific serum, tissue and urine tests	Correction of metabolic defect
Endocrinopathy (myxedema)	T3, T4, TSH	Thyroid replacement medication

OPCA, olivopontocerebellar atrophy; MSA, multiple system atrophy; FA, Friedreich's ataxia; MRI, magnetic resonance imaging; CT, computed tomographic scanning; CSF, cerebrospinal fluid; CBC, complete blood count; AVM, arteriovenous malformation; EEG, electroencephalogram; T3, T4, TSH, specific serum tests of thyroid function.

References

1. Fluorens P: *Recherches Expérimentales sur les Propriétés et les Fonctions du Système Nerveux dans les Animaux Vertébrés.* Paris: Crevot, 1824.
2. Luciani L: Il Cervelletto: *Nuovi Studi di Fisiologia Normale e Pathologica.* Florence: LeMonnier, 1891.
3. André-Thomas: *Le Cervelet: Etude Anatomique, Clinique, et Physiologique.* Paris: Steinheil, 1897.
4. Holmes G: The Croonian lectures on the clinical symptoms of cerebellar disease and their interpretation. *Lancet* i:1177–1182, 1231–1237; ii:59–65, 111–115, 1922.
5. Brindley GS: The use made by the cerebellum of the information that it receives from the sense organs. *Int Brain Res Org Bull* 3:80, 1964.
6. Marr D: A theory of cerebellar cortex. *J Physiol (Lond)* 202:437–470, 1969.
7. Albus JS: A theory of cerebellar function. *Math Biosci* 10:25–61, 1971.
8. Brand S, Dahl A-L, Mugnaini E: The length of parallel fibers in the cat cerebellar cortex: An experimental light and electron microscopic study. *Exp Brain Res* 26:39–58, 1976.
9. Mugnaini E: The length of cerebellar parallel fibers in chicken and rhesus monkey. *J Comp Neurol* 220:7–15, 1983.

10. Ito M, Shiida N, Yagi N, Yamamoto M: The cerebellar modification of rabbit's horizontal vestibulo-ocular reflex induced by sustained head rotation combined with visual stimulation. *Proc Jpn Acad* 50:85–89, 1974.

11. Robinson DA: Adaptive gain control of the vestibulo-ocular reflex by the cerebellum. *J Neurophysiol* 39:954–969, 1976.

12. Yeo CH, Hardiman MJ, Glickstein M: Discrete lesions of the cerebellar cortex abolish classically conditioned nictitating membrane response of the rabbit. *Behav Brain Res* 13:261–266.

13. Thach WT, Goodkin HP, Keating JG: The cerebellum and the adaptive coordination of movement. *Ann Rev Neurosci* 15:403–442, 1992.

14. Thompson RF: The neurobiology of learning and memory. *Science* 233:941–947, 1986.

15. Thompson RF: Neural mechanisms of classical conditioning in mammals. *Philos Trans R Soc Lond Biol* 329:161–170, 1990.

16. Thompson RF, Krupa DJ: Origin of memory traces in the mammalian brain. *Ann Rev Neurosci* 17:519–549, 1994.

17. Roland PE: Metabolic mapping of sensorimotor integration in the human brain, in Bock G, O'Connor M, Marsh J (eds): *Motor Areas of the Cerebral Cortex*, Ciba Foundation Symposium #132. Chichester, UK: John Wiley & Sons, 1987, pp 251–268.

18. Roland PE, Eriksson L, Widen L, Stone-Elander S: Changes in regional cerebral oxidative metabolism induced by tactile learning and recognition in man. *Eur J Neurosci* 1:3–17, 1988.

19. Seitz RJ, Roland PE, Bohm C, et al: Motor learning in man: A positron emission tomography study. *Neuroreport* 1:57–66, 1990.

20. Haier RJ, Siegel BV Jr, MacLachlan A, et al: Regional glucose metabolic changes after learning a complex visuospatial motor task: A positron emission tomography study. *Brain Res* 570:134–143, 1991.

21. Mazziotta JC, Grafton ST, Woods RC: The human motor system studied with PET measurements of cerebral blood flow: Topography and motor learning, in Lassen NA, Ingvar DH, Raichle ME, Friberg L (eds): *Brain Work and Mental Activity*, Alfred Benzen Symposium 31. Copenhagen: Munksgaard, 1991, pp 280–290.

22. Friston KJ, Frith CD, Passingham RE, et al: Motor practice and neurophysiological adaptation in the cerebellum: A positron emission tomography study. *Proc R Soc Lond [Biol]* 248:223–228, 1992.

23. Grafton ST, Mazziotta JC, Presty S, et al: Functional anatomy of human procedural learning determined with regional cerebral blood flow and PET. *J Neurosci* 12:2542–2548, 1992.

24. Jenkins IH, Brooks DJ, Nixon PD, et al: Motor sequence learning: A study with positron emission tomography. *J Neurosci* 14:3775–3790, 1994.

25. Horak FB, Diener HC: Cerebellar control of postural scaling and central set in stance. *J Neurophysiol* 72:479–93, 1994.

26. Horak FB: Comparison of cerebellar and vestibular loss on scaling of postural responses, in Brandt T, Paulus W, Bles W, et al. (eds): *Disorders of Posture and Gait*. Stuttgart, Germany: Georg Thieme Verlag, 1990, pp 370–373.

27. Gautier GM, Hofferer J-M, Hoyt WF, Stark L: Visual-motor adaptation: Quantitative demonstration in patients with posterior fossa involvement. *Arch Neurol* 36:155–160, 1979.

28. Baizer JS, Glickstein M: Role of cerebellum in prism adaptation. *J Physiol* 23:34–35, 1974.

29. Weiner MJ, Hallett M, Funkenstein HH: Adaptation to lateral displacement of vision in patients with lesions of the central nervous system. *Neurology* 33:766–772, 1983.

30. Sanes JN, Dimitrov B, Hallett M: Motor learning in patients with cerebellar dysfunction. *Brain* 113:103–120, 1990.

31. Leiner HC, Leiner AL, Dow RS: Does the cerebellum contribute to mental skills? *Behav Neurosci* 100:443–453, 1986.

32. Leiner HC, Leiner Al, Dow RS: Cerebro-cerebellar learning loops in apes and humans. *Ital J Neurol Sci* 8:425–436, 1987.

33. Leiner HC, Leiner AL, Dow RS: The human cerebro-cerebellar system: Its computing, cognitive, and language skills. *Behav Brain Res* 44:113–128, 1991.

34. Schell GR, Strick PL: The origin of thalamic inputs to the arcuate premotor and supplementary motor areas. *J Neurosci* 4:539–560, 1983.

35. Orioli PJ, Strick PL: Cerebellar connections with the motor cortex and the arcuate premotor area: An analysis employing retrograde transneuronal transport of WGA-HRP. *J Comp Neurol* 288:612–626.

36. Yamamoto T, Yoshida K, Yoshikawa H, et al: The medial dorsal nucleus is one of the thalamic relays of the cerebellocerebral responses to the frontal association cortex in the monkey: Horseradish peroxidase and fluorescent dye double staining study. *Brain Res* 579:315–320, 1992.

37. Middleton FA, Strick PL: Anatomic evidence for cerebellar and basal ganglia involvement in higher cognitive functions. *Science* 266:458–461, 1994.

38. Petersen SE, Fox PT, Posner MI, et al: Positron emission tomographic studies of the processing of single words. *J Cog Neurosci* 1:153–170, 1989.

39. Raichle ME, Fiez JA, Videen TO, et al: Practice-related changes in human brain functional anatomy during nonmotor learning. *Cereb Cortex* 4:8–26, 1994.

40. Fiez JA, Petersen SE, Cheney MK, Raichle ME: Impaired nonmotor learning and error detection associated with cerebellar damage. *Brain* 115:155–178, 1992.

41. Silveri MC, Leggio MG, Molinari M: The cerebellum contributes to linguistic production: A case of agrammatic speech following a right cerebellar lesion. *Neurology* 44:2047–2050, 1994.

42. Grafman J, Litvan I, Massaquoi S, et al: Cognitive planning deficit in patients with cerebellar atrophy. *Neurology* 42:1493–1496, 1992.

43. Bracke-Tolkmitt R, Linden A, Canavan AGM, et al: The cerebellum contributes to mental skills. *Behav Neurosci* 103:442–446, 1989.

44. Topka H, Valls-Solé J, Massaquoi SG, Hallett M: Deficit in classical conditioning in patients with cerebellar degeneration. *Brain* 116:961–969, 1993.

45. Lalonde R: Cerebellar contributions to instrumental learning. *Neurosci Biobehav Rev* 18:161–170, 1994.

46. Akshoomoff NA, Courchesne E: A new role for the cerebellum in cognitive operations. *Behav Neurosci* 106:731–738, 1992.

47. Akshoomoff NA, Courchesne E: ERP evidence for a shifting attention deficit in patients with damage to the cerebellum. *J Cog Neurosci* 6:388–399, 1994.

48. Ito M: Synaptic plasticity in the cerebellar cortex and its role in motor learning. *Can J Neurol Sci* 20:S70–S74, 1993.

49. Courchesne E, Yeung-Courchesne R, Press GA, et al: Hypoplasia of cerebellar vermal lobules VI and VII in autism. *N Engl J Med* 318:1349–1354, 1988.

50. Murakami JW, Courchesne E, Press GA, et al: Reduced cerebellar hemisphere size and its relationship to vermal hypoplasia in autism. *Arch Neurol* 46:689–694, 1989.

51. Holroyd S, Reiss AL, Bryan RN: Autistic features in Joubert syndrome: A genetic disorder with agenesis of the cerebellar vermis. *Biol Psychiatry* 29:287–294, 1991.

52. Ciesielski KT, Knight JE: Cerebellar abnormality in autism: A nonspecific effect of early brain damage? *Acta Neurobiol Exp* 54:151–154, 1994.

53. Weinberger D, Kleinman J, Luchins D, et al: Cerebellar pathology in schizophrenia: A controlled post-mortem study. *Am J Psychiatry* 137:359–361, 1980.

54. Gilman S, Bloedel JR, Lechtenberg R: *Disorders of the Cerebellum.* Philadelphia: FA Davis, 1981.

55. Brodal A: *Neurological Anatomy in Relation to Clinical Medicine,* 3rd ed. New York: Oxford University Press, 1981.

56. Kitamura T, Yamada J: Spinocerebellar tract neurons with axons passing through the inferior or superior cerebellar peduncles. *Brain Behav Evol* 34:133–142, 1989.

57. Brodal A, Brodal P: Observations on the secondary vestibulocerebellar projections in the macaque monkey. *Exp Brain Res* 58:62–74, 1985.

58. Suzuki DA, Keller EL: The role of the posterior vermis of monkey cerebellum in smooth-pursuit eye movement control. I. Eye and head movement-related activity. *J Neurophysiol* 59:1–18, 1988.

59. Suzuki DA, Keller EL: The role of the posterior vermis of monkey cerebellum in smooth-pursuit eye movement control. II. Target velocity-related Purkinje cell activity. *J Neurophysiol* 59:19–40, 1988.

60. Voogd J: The importance of fibre connections in the comparative anatomy of the mammalian cerebellum, in Llinas R (ed): *Neurobiology of Cerebellar Evolution and Development.* Chicago: American Medical Association, 1969.

61. Voogd J: The olivocerebellar projection in the cat. *Exp Brain Res* suppl. 6:134, 1982.

62. Leigh RJ, Zee DS: *The Neurology of Eye Movements,* 2d ed. Philadelphia: FA Davis, 1991.

63. Maurice-Williams RS: Mechanisms of production of gait unsteadiness by tumors of the posterior fossa. *J Neurol Neurosurg Psychiatry* 38:143–148, 1975.

64. Amici R, Avanzini G, Pacini L: Cerebellar tumors, in *Monographs in Neural Sciences.* Basel, Switzerland: Karger, 1976, vol 4.

65. Dichgans J: Clinical symptoms of cerebellar dysfunction and their topodiagnostical significance. *Hum Neurobiol* 2:269–279, 1984.

66. Dichgans J, Diener H-C: Clinical evidence for functional compartmentalization of the cerebellum, in Bloedel JR, Dichgans J, Precht W (eds): *Cerebellar Functions.* Berlin: Springer-Verlag, 1984.

67. Dichgans J, Diener H-C: Different forms of postural ataxia in patients with cerebellar diseases, in Bles W, Brandt T (eds): *Disorders of Posture and Gait,* Amsterdam: Elsevier, 1986.

68. Lechtenberg R, Gilman S: Speech disorders in cerebellar disease. *Ann Neurol* 3:285–290, 1978.

69. Melo TP, Bogousslavsky J: Hemiataxia-hypesthesia: A thalamic stroke syndrome. *J Neurol Neurosurg Psychiatry* 55:581–584, 1992.

70. Melo TP, Bogousslavsky J, Moulin T, et al: Thalamic ataxia. *J Neurol* 239:331–337, 1992.

71. Solomon DH, Barohn RJ, Bazan C, Grissom J: The thalamic ataxia syndrome. *Neurology* 44:810–814, 1994.

72. Fisher CM, Cole M: Homolateral ataxia and crural paresis—a vascular syndrome. *J Neurol Neurosurg Psychiatry* 28:45–55, 1965.

73. Giroud M, Creisson E, Fayolle H, et al: Homolateral ataxia and crural paresis: A crossed cerebral-cerebellar diaschisis. *J Neurol Neurosurg Psychiatry* 57:221–222, 1994.

74. Yagnik PM, Dhaduk V, Huen L: Parietal ataxic hemiparesis. *Eur Neurol* 28:164–166, 1988.

75. Diener H-C, Dichgans J, Guschlbauer B, et al: The coordination of posture and voluntary movement in patients with cerebellar dysfunction. *Mov Disord* 7:14–22, 1992.

76. Victor M, Adams RD, Collins GC: *The Wernicke-Korsakoff Syndrome and Related Neurologic Disorders Due to Alcoholism and Malnutrition,* 2d ed. Philadelphia: FA Davis, 1989.

77. Lewis RF, Zee DS: Ocular motor disorders associated with cerebellar lesions: Pathophysiology and topical localization. *Rev Neurol (Paris)* 149:665–677, 1993.

78. Helmchen C, Straube A, Büttner U: Saccadic lateropulsion in Wallenberg's syndrome may be caused by a functional lesion of the fastigial nucleus. *J Neurol* 241:421–426, 1994.

79. Waterson JA, Barnes GR, Grealy MA: A quantitative study of eye and head movements during smooth pursuit in patients with cerebellar disease. *Brain* 115:1343–1358, 1992.

80. Grant MP, Leigh RJ, Seidman SH, et al: Comparison of predictable smooth ocular and combined eye-head tracking behaviour in patients with lesions affecting the brainstem and cerebellum. *Brain* 115:1323–1342, 1992.

81. Vahedi K, Rivaud S, Amarenco P, Pierrot-Deseilligny C: Horizontal eye movement disorders after posterior vermis infarctions. *J Neurol Neurosurg Psychiatry* 58:91–94, 1995.

82. Flament D, Hore J: Movement and electromyographic disorders associated with cerebellar dysmetria. *J Neurophysiol* 55:1221–1233, 1986.

83. Hallett M, Shahani BT, Young RR: EMG analysis of patients with cerebellar deficits. *J Neurol Neurosurg Psychiatry* 38:1163–1169, 1975.

84. Brown SH, Hefter H, Mertens M, Freund H-J: Disturbances in human arm movement trajectory due to mild cerebellar dysfunction. *J Neurol Neurosurg Psychiatry* 53:306–313, 1990.

85. Morrice B-L, Becker WJ, Hoffer JA, Lee RG: Manual tracking performance in patients with cerebellar incoordination: Effects of mechanical loading. *Can J Neurol Sci* 17:275–285, 1990.

86. Becker WJ, Kunesch E, Freund H-J: Coordination of a multi-joint movement in normal humans and in patients with cerebellar dysfunction. *Can J Neurol Sci* 17:264–274, 1990.

87. Thach WT, Perry JG, Kane SA, Goodkin HP: Cerebellar nuclei: Rapid alternating movement, motor somatotopy, and a mechanism for the control of motor synergy. *Rev Neurol (Paris)* 149:607–628, 1993.

88. Beppu H, Suda M, Tanaka R: Analysis of cerebellar motor disorders by visually guided elbow tracking movements. *Brain* 107:787–809, 1984.

89. Hermsdörfer J, Wessel K, Mai N, Marquardt C: Perturbation of precision grip in Friedreich's ataxia and late-onset cerebellar ataxia. *Mov Disord* 9:650–654, 1994.

90. Müller F, Dichgans J: Dyscoordination of pinch and lift forces during grasp in patients with cerebellar lesions. *Exp Brain Res* 101:485–492, 1994.

91. Bonnefoi-Kyriacou B, Trouche E, Legallet E, Viallet F: Planning and execution of pointing movements in cerebellar patients. *Mov Disord* 10:171–178, 1995.

92. Mai N, Bolsinger P, Avarello M, et al: Control of isometric finger force in patients with cerebellar disease. *Brain* 111:973–998, 1988.

93. Flament D, Hore J: Comparison of cerebellar intention tremor under isotonic and isometric conditions. *Brain Res* 439:179–186, 1988.

94. Inhoff AW, Diener H-C, Rafal RD, Ivry R: The role of cerebellar structures in the execution of serial movements. *Brain* 112:565–581, 1989.

95. Vilis T, Hore J: Central neural mechanisms contributing to cerebellar tremor produced by limb perturbations. *J Neurophysiol* 43:279–291, 1980.

96. Spidalieri G, Busby L, Lamarre Y: Fast ballistic arm movements triggered by visual, auditory, and somesthetic stimuli in the monkey. II. Effects of unilateral dentate lesion on discharge of precentral cortical neurons and reaction time. *J Neurophysiol* 50:1359–1379, 1983.

97. Brooks VB, Thach WT: Cerebellar control of posture and movement, in Brooks VB (ed): *Handbook of Physiology. Neurophysiology: Motor Control.* Bethesda, MD: American Physiological Society, 1981, sect 1, vol 2, part 2.

98. Miall RC, Weir DJ, Stein JF: Visuo-motor tracking during reversible inactivation of the cerebellum. *Exp. Brain Res* 65:455–464, 1987.

99. Diener H-C, Dichgans J: Long loop reflexes and posture, in Bles W, Brandt T (eds): *Disorders of Posture and Gait.* Amsterdam: Elsevier, 1986.

100. Diener H-C, Dichgans J, Bacher M, Guschlbauer B: Characteristic alterations of long-loop 'reflexes' in patients with Friedreich's disease and late atrophy of the cerebellar anterior lobe. *J Neurol Neurosurg Psychiatry* 47:679–685, 1984.

101. Tokuda T, Tako K, Hayashi R, Yanagisawa N: Disturbed modulation of the stretch reflex gain during standing in cerebellar ataxia. *EEG Clin Neurophysiol* 81:421–426, 1991.

102. Grill SE, Hallett M, Marcus C, McShane L: Disturbances of kinaesthesia in patients with cerebellar disorders. *Brain* 117:1433–1447, 1994.

103. Manto M, Godaux E, Jacquy J: Detection of silent cerebellar lesions by increasing the inertial load of the moving hand. *Ann Neurol* 37:344–350, 1995.

104. Diener H-C, Dichgans J: Pathophysiology of cerebellar ataxia. *Mov Disord* 7:95–109, 1992.

105. Hore J, Flament D: Evidence that a disordered servo-like mechanism contributes to tremor in movements during cerebellar dysfunction. *J Neurophysiol* 56:123–136, 1986.

106. Cole JD, Philip HI, Sedgwick EM: Stability and tremor in the fingers associated with cerebellar hemisphere and cerebellar tract lesions in man. *J Neurol Neurosurg Psychiatry* 51:1558–1568, 1988.

107. Flament D, Vilis T, Hore J: Dependence of cerebellar tremor on proprioceptive but not visual feedback. *Exp Neurol* 84:314–325, 1984.

108. Kluin KJ, Gilman S, Markel DS, et al: Speech disorders in olivopontocerebellar atrophy correlate with positron emission tomography findings. *Ann Neurol* 23:547–554, 1988.

109. Ackermann H, Ziegler W: Cerebellar voice tremor: An acoustic analysis. *J Neurol Neurosurg Psychiatry* 54:74–76, 1991.

110. Gilman S, Kluin K: Perceptual analysis of speech disorders in Friedreich disease and olivopontocerebellar atrophy, in Bloedel JR, Dichgans J, Precht W (eds): *Cerebellar Functions.* Berlin: Springer-Verlag, 1984.

111. Ammirati M, Mirzai S, Samii M: Transient mutism following removal of a cerebellar tumor. *Child Nerv Syst* 5:12–14, 1989.

112. Dietze DD, Mickle JP: Cerebellar mutism after posterior fossa surgery. *Pediatr Neurosurg* 16:25–31, 1990.

113. Ferrante L, Mastronardi L, Acqui M, Fortuna A: Mutism after posterior fossa surgery in children. *J Neurosurg* 72:959–963, 1990.

114. Catsman-Berrevoets CE, van Dongen HR, Zwetsloot CP: Transient loss of speech followed by dysarthria after removal of posterior fossa tumour. *Dev Med Child Neurol* 34:1102–1117, 1992.

115. van Dongen HR, Catsman-Berrevoets CE, van Mourik M: The syndrome of 'cerebellar' mutism and subsequent dysarthria. *Neurology* 44:2040–2046, 1994.

116. Cole M: The foreign policy of the cerebellum. *Neurology* 44:2001–2005, 1994.

117. Lance JW, Degail P, Nielson PD: Tonic and phasic spinal cord mechanisms in man. *J Neurol Neurosurg Psychiatry* 29:535–544,1966.

118. Gilman S: The mechanism of cerebellar hypotonia: An experimental study in the monkey. *Brain* 92:621–638, 1969.

119. Growdon JH, Chambers WW, Liu CN: An experimental study of cerebellar dyskinesia in the rhesus monkey. *Brain* 90:603–632, 1967.

120. Gilman S, McDonald WI: Cerebellar facilitation of muscle spindle activity. *J Neurophysiol* 30:1495–1512, 1967.

121. Gilman S, McDonald WI: Relation of afferent fiber conduction velocity to reactivity of muscle spindle receptors after cerebellectomy. *J Neurophysiol* 30:1513–1522, 1967.

122. Gilman S, Ebel HC: Fusimotor neuron responses to natural stimuli as a function of prestimulus fusimotor activity in decerebellate cats. *Brain Res* 21:367–384, 1970.

123. Gilman S, Marco LA, Ebel HC: Effects of medullary pryamidotomy in the monkey. II. Abnormalities of muscle spindle afferent responses. *Brain* 94:515–530, 1971.

124. Gilman S, Lieberman JS, Marco LA: Spinal mechanism underlying the effects of unilateral ablation of areas 4 and 6 in monkeys. *Brain* 97:49–64, 1974.

125. Kornhauser D, Bromberg MB, Gilman S: Effects of lesions of fastigial nucleus on static and dynamic responses of muscle spindle primary afferents in the cat. *J Neurophysiol* 47:977–986,1982.

126. Gilman S: Inherited ataxia, in Johnson RT (ed): *Current Therapy in Neurologic Disease,* 2d ed. Toronto: Marcel Decker, 1987, pp 224–232.

127. Hurko O: Hereditary cerebellar ataxia, in Johnson RT, Griffin JW (eds): *Current Therapy in Neurologic Disease,* 4th ed. St. Louis: Marcel Decker, 1993, pp 254–261.

Chapter 44 _____

PATHOPHYSIOLOGY OF CEREBELLAR DISORDERS

DARRY S. JOHNSON and ERWIN B. MONTGOMERY, JR.

MECHANISMS UNDERLYING CEREBELLAR
  SYMPTOMS AND SIGNS
    Dysmetria
    Tremor
    Dysdiadochokinesia
    Dysarthria
    Hypotonia
    Nystagmus
    Ataxia/Gait Disturbance
    Decomposition of Movement
    Is There a Common Fundamental Underlying
      Mechanism?
    Mechanisms of Dysmetria
    Cerebellar Effects on the Alpha Motor System
    Cerebellar Effects on the Gamma Motor System
    Is It Alpha or Gamma?
THREE THEORIES REGARDING CEREBELLAR
  MOVEMENT STRATEGY
    Cerebellum as a Servocontroller or Feedback-based
      Mechanism
    Cerebellum as a Feedforward Generator
    Concept of Efferent Copy: A Hybrid of Two Theories
    Which Is It—Feedback, Feedforward, or Efference
      Copy?
ORGANIZATION OF THE CEREBELLUM
    Macroscopic View
    Microscopic View
CEREBELLAR SYNDROMES
    Vermal Syndrome
    Paravermal Syndrome
    Lateral Zone
    Nystagmus
    Dysarthria
MECHANISMS OF DYSFUNCTION
THE CEREBELLUM AND LEARNING
SUMMARY

The concept of the cerebellum as being responsible only for the smooth coordination of motor acts has undergone a dramatic transformation since the work of the Italian neurophysiologist, Luigi Luciani, who in the latter part of the nineteenth century described the effects of ablation experiments in dogs.[1,2] Later, in 1917, Gordon Holmes produced what may still be considered the gold standard description of cerebellar signs and symptoms in soldiers with gunshot and shrapnel wounds during World War I[3] (Fig. 44-1). Since the descriptions of Holmes much has been discovered about cerebellar physiology via such techniques as selective abla-

tion, electrical stimulation, reversible cooling, and functional imaging with single-photon emission computed tomography (SPECT) and positron emission tomography (PET). However, there remains much to be discovered. The objective of this chapter is to summarize what has been learned to date in regard to cerebellar pathophysiology and to give the clinician a useful background of information on which to base decisions when treating a patient with cerebellar disease.

The diverse signs of cerebellar pathology will first be presented briefly to identify a common underlying mechanism or set of mechanisms. Then hypotheses regarding the pathophysiology of the common underlying mechanism(s) will be described, based on anatomy and physiology. Three fundamental theories of cerebellar physiology will be presented.

The macroscopic and microscopic anatomy and the physiology of the cerebellum then will be described. This will lead to a discussion of clear, definable cerebellar syndromes that are special cases of the common underlying mechanism(s) that differ based on body representation in the cerebellum, as defined by input and output connections. Finally, research as it relates to learning and the potential role of the cerebellum in cognitive and language processes will be explored.

Mechanisms Underlying Cerebellar Symptoms and Signs

DYSMETRIA

Dysmetria is one of the cardinal signs of cerebellar disease. Holmes, in 1917, described dysmetria in terms of abnormal range and force of movement.[3] The movement either falls short or goes past the intended target. The sign of past pointing is an example of dysmetria, in which the hand goes beyond the target. Hypometria is a premature arrest of movement, whereas hypermetria is a result of excessive range of movement. Dysmetria is best seen in the finger-to-nose test, or in the case of the lower extremity, great toe-to-examiner's finger test, provided that the patient has movement only at the hip. During these tests the arm (or foot) typically overshoots or undershoots the target, manifesting an erratic trajectory (Fig. 44-2).

There are at least two possible mechanisms underlying dysmetria. First, dysmetria may result from an error in programming the precise patterns of muscle activity that initiate and execute a movement. It is a "disturbance of the trajectory or placement of a body part during active movements."[4] It often takes longer than normal to initiate and to stop voluntary movements, and there is a lack of uniform velocity.[5]

Alternatively, a second mechanism may be a failure to stop the movement. This could be because of a delay and slowness in arresting muscle contraction[6] or because the body part in movement is literally too floppy (meaning decreased resistance to passive movement) as a result of decreased muscle tone. Stopping the movement uses passive and active elements. The elastic properties of the limb resist movement and may help in stopping a movement. Normal braking or stopping mechanisms must consider passive resistance and may be inappropriate in the face of decreased muscle tone (Fig. 44-3).

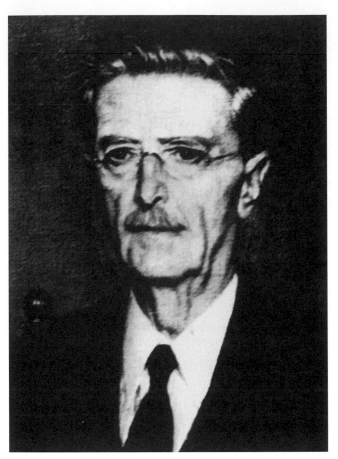

FIGURE 44-1 Gordon Holmes provided the classic description of symptoms and signs resulting from lesions of the cerebellum. *(From McHenry: Garrison's History of Neurology. Springfield, IL: Charles C Thomas, 1969. Used with permission.)*

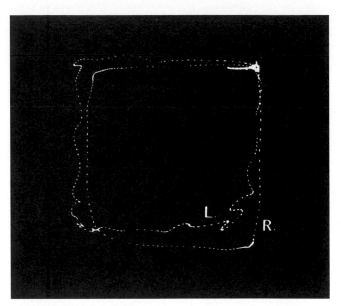

FIGURE 44-2 The patient has a lesion of the left cerebellar hemisphere. The patient is asked to outline the square end of a room with the normal (*right*) and affected (*left*) forefingers. Holmes secured a light to the end of the forefingers, and subsequent recordings were made; each flash of light represents 0.04 s of finger movement. *(From Holmes.*[7] *Used with permission.)*

TREMOR

A tremor is a rhythmic, involuntary, oscillatory movement. Although tremors can be classified in numerous ways, perhaps the best way is to characterize them by their relationship to rest, movement, and maintenance of a particular posture. Rest tremor, also known as static tremor, is the typical slow, coarse tremor, such as is seen, for example, in patients with parkinsonism and related disorders of the basal ganglia. It typically has a frequency of 4–6 Hz. Postural tremor, or tension tremor, is that seen when a limb is maintained in a position against gravity, as when outstretched. One example is the physiological tremor seen when the hands are held outstretched with a frequency of about 8–12 Hz. This tremor is accentuated with such stressors as fear, anxiety, or fatigue. Subsets of this type of tremor include benign essential tremor (idiopathic) or familial tremor (autosomal dominant). The toxic tremor resulting from thyrotoxicosis, uremia, drug toxins (such as bronchodilators, tricyclic antidepressants, and lithium), carbon monoxide poisoning, heavy metal poisoning (mercury, arsenic, or lead) or from withdrawal from alcohol

FIGURE 44-3 Cerebellar dysmetria and associated patterns of movement abnormalities. *A.* Delay of initiation and termination of movement. The delay may be 0.1–0.2 s of both start and stop. *B.* Abnormal change of direction as evidenced by increased oscillations during attempt to trace a square. (See original work from Holmes.) *C.* Irregular velocity when attempting to touch objects sequentially. *D.* Lack of synergy between muscles upon attempting to touch the nose with the tip of a finger, an example of dysmetria. *(From Pearlman et al: Neurological Pathophysiology, 3rd ed. New York: Oxford University Press, 1984. Used with permission.)*

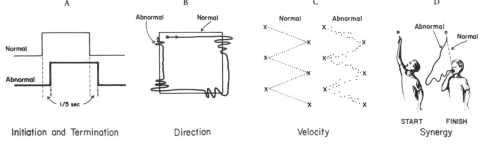

A Initiation and Termination   B Direction   C Velocity   D Synergy

or sedative drugs is another type of postural tremor. The third tremor type, known as intention, action, motor, or (preferably) kinetic, occurs during activity. It is this type of tremor that is most frequently associated with disorders of the cerebellum.

Holmes described the tremor seen in patients with cerebellar injuries as irregular oscillations in the intended direction that result from failure of uniform deceleration, complicated by secondary or correcting jerks when the object has not been accurately reached in the first attempt.[7] Holmes also said that "the tremulousness usually increases towards its completion when accuracy is most essential."[3] He described a static tremor as well; titubation (shaking of the head and trunk) increases when one is fatigued, and the body as a whole tends to sway with standing. This static tremor tends to be coarse. He observed slow displacements by gravity and quicker voluntary jerks back toward the original position. Many recent authors, however, have indicated that static tremor that accompanies posture maintenance rarely occurs and has poor localizing value.[5,6]

Gilman et al.[4] emphasize, as do other authors, that the term "intention tremor" is a poor one and has often been misused. They prefer the term kinetic tremor. Also, it is pointed out that kinetic tremor tends to involve primarily proximal limb muscles, in contradistinction to distal tremor, as seen in patients with parkinsonism.

Kinetic tremor can be seen by having the patient do finger-to-nose testing, as well as heel-to-knee testing. Tremor appears when movement is initiated, during the course of the movement, or when the limb approaches the target. The amplitude of the tremor is especially prominent as the target is approached. Static tremor is demonstrated by having the patient extend the arms parallel to the floor with hands open. After several seconds the arms will begin to oscillate rhythmically at the shoulder. This can also be demonstrated in the lower limb by asking the patient to extend one leg and hold the great toe close to, but not touching, the examiner's index finger. This posture, in a few seconds, will produce oscillations at the hip joint.[4]

DYSDIADOCHOKINESIA

First described by Babinski in 1902, dysdiadochokinesia is a disturbance in the patient's ability to perform rapid alternating movements. This is most easily demonstrated in the clinical setting by having the patient perform rapid supination/pronation of the forearms on a table top or on his or her lap[8] (Fig. 44-4). Holmes said that this was a very persistent sign, unlike that of hypotonia, which will be described shortly.[3,7] In 1929 Wertham described a related abnormality, arrhythmokinesis, which is a disturbance in tapping out a definite rhythmic pattern; the two sides are then compared.[9]

DYSARTHRIA

Holmes described the speech pattern of patients with cerebellar disease as "slow, drawling, and monotonous, but at the same time (it) tends to be staccato and scanning."[3] The dysarthric speech of a patient with cerebellar disease typically

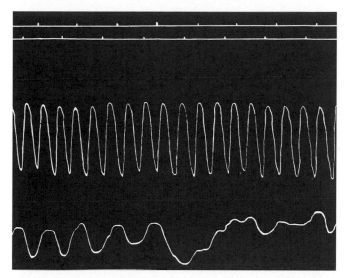

FIGURE 44-4 These tracings are of rapid alternating movements of the affected arm (*below*) and the unaffected arm (*above*). Note the slower velocity and smaller amplitude of the affected arm; notice how it becomes more irregular as the arm becomes almost locked in supination. This is dysdiadochokinesis. (*From Holmes.[7] Used with permission.*)

has a sing-song character. Syllables can be explosive intermittently and at incorrect points of emphasis. This type of speech has also been described as having a nasal character. Production can be labored with excessive facial grimacing. Zentay described the speech by way of four components: (1) ataxic speech (interference of articulation, respiration, and phonation); (2) adiadochokinesis of speech (slowness of speech); (3) explosive-hesitant speech; and (4) scanning speech (stretching of the syllables, which are sharply cut off from one another).[10] Comprehension and grammar remain intact.

In the work by Amici et al. in studying over 250 patients with cerebellar tumors, the authors described the speech as "scanning and explosive against a background of monotony," quoted from Lhermitte in 1958.[6] Brown et al. studied 30 patients with cerebellar ataxia without other neurological disturbances.[11] They analyzed the speech patterns of these patients and characterized ataxic dysarthria on the basis of 10 "deviant dimensions." Of the 10 dimensions they discovered that excess and equal stress were prominent, that is, a prosodic disorder of speech in which magnified vocal emphasis is issued to normally unstressed words and syllables. The second dimension that was specific for cerebellar disease was irregular articulatory breakdown, which is recognized by sudden, intermittent telescoping (running together) of one or more syllables.

HYPOTONIA

Luciani, in 1891, defined hypotonia as a decreased resistance to passive limb manipulation.[1] Muscles tend to be flaccid on the involved side. The muscle mass has a reduced consistency on palpation with decreased resistance to passive movement.

These muscles have a greater-than-normal range of motion. Dow and Moruzzi also define hypotonia as a loss or diminution of muscle tone or a decreased resistance to passive movement.[8] Limbs on the affected side show greater range of motion than normal when shaken passively; this tends to occur acutely after cerebellar injury and usually resolves within 1 week to 10 days. It is less apparent and less easy to detect in chronic cerebellar disease[7] (Fig. 44-5).

Holmes believed that static tremor and rebound are also manifestations of hypotonia. He defined tone as "the constant slight tension characteristic of healthy muscle, which offers a steadily maintained resistance to stretching." It is usually more easily demonstrated in the arm than in the leg. It is more pronounced proximally, with muscles that are more involved with determination of postures. The pendular knee jerk sometimes seen is evidence of diminished postural tone. He also observed that the ipsilateral shoulder often drooped, with the arm hanging fully extended by the side. Holmes viewed hypotonia as one of the fundamental or essential signs resulting from cerebellar disease.[3,7]

NYSTAGMUS

Perhaps the most insightful statement made concerning eye movements associated with cerebellar disease was made by Miller in 1988, when he said that "many patients with cerebellar disease also have involvement of the brainstem as well. Thus, it is often unwarranted to attribute associated ocular motor abnormalities to cerebellar dysfunction."[12] This, for the majority of cases, seems to be intuitive. Mass lesions of the cerebellum usually compress the adjoining brain stem. The most commonly encountered lesions involving the cerebellum, such as those produced by stroke, multiple sclerosis,

FIGURE 44-5 This is an extreme example of the hypotonia that can be seen following an acute cerebellar injury. In this case, the left cerebellar hemisphere has been injured, leading to the dramatic decrease in tone of the left wrist. (The photo was taken 1 week after the lesion occurred.) *(From Holmes.[3] Used with permission.)*

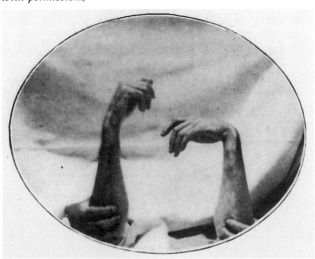

or the spinocerebellar degenerations, commonly affect the brain stem as well.

Even so, years of clinical and experimental work have shown some ocular motor signs to be associated with cerebellar disease. These include: (1) different types of nystagmus, such as gaze-evoked, rebound, downbeat, or positional; (2) skew deviation; (3) saccadic dysmetria; (4) impairments in smooth pursuit, optokinetic nystagmus, or fixation suppression of caloric-induce nystagmus; (5) fixation abnormalities; (6) postsaccadic drift (glissades); and (7) increased gain in the vestibulo-ocular (VOR) reflex.[12]

ATAXIA/GAIT DISTURBANCE

Patients with ataxia resulting from cerebellar disease walk with a wide base and tend to stagger, as if intoxicated. Their gait may be stiff-legged because of disturbed postural reflexes.[8] It has been described as "drunken reeling." Patients walk with their legs apart, trunk swaying, with a tendency to "barge" to one or both sides.[6] They generally fall to the side of the lesion when only one cerebellar hemisphere is affected.

Another type of ataxia that must be differentiated from that which is a result of cerebellar lesions is caused by disrupted proprioceptive pathways. Disturbances can be either in the periphery in sensory nerves, sensory roots, in dorsal columns in the spinal cord, in the parietal cortex (Brodman areas 3, 1, 2, and 5), or in the occipital cortex.[13,14] This ataxia is known as sensory ataxia, and often it is indistinguishable from ataxia of cerebellar origin. The characteristics that delineate sensory ataxia from that resulting from cerebellar disease include absence of other cerebellar signs, such as nystagmus or dysarthria. With dorsal column involvement, vibratory and position sense are commonly impaired as well, leading to Romberg's sign. This sign is usually absent in cerebellar disease.[14]

Sensory ataxias tend to worsen when the patient is denied visual feedback, as would occur with closing the eyes or walking in the dark. Cerebellar ataxia does not significantly worsen when the subject is denied visual feedback. Consequently, Romberg's sign defined as worsening ataxia with the eyes closed is indicative of a sensory ataxia and is not a result of cerebellar disease.[14]

Another form of ataxia primarily affecting gait arises from lesions in the frontal lobe and is known as Bruns' ataxia.[14] Before the discovery of neuroimaging, neurosurgeons knew that if they did not find a lesion in the cerebellum during a suboccipital exploration, they would then have to look in the contralateral frontal lobe.[15,16]

Ataxias can be associated also with lesions of the internal capsule, and the middle and superior cerebellar peduncles (input and output pathways to and from the cerebellum, respectively). One theory as to why such diverse noncerebellar lesions cause symptoms virtually identical to those associated with direct cerebellar lesions is that these noncerebellar lesions still produce cerebellar dysfunction. Lesions of input systems, such as the frontopontocerebellar pathways in the internal capsule, the pontocerebellar fibers in the middle cerebellar peduncle, or the sensory system, result in failure to provide the cerebellum with information necessary for the normal successful programming of movement.[13]

DECOMPOSITION OF MOVEMENT

Holmes described a sign of cerebellar disease called decomposition of movement, in which complex movements are broken down into their elemental components.[3] He also used the term asynergia,[2] meaning the inability to perform all the different movements necessary to accomplish an act smoothly. Holmes explained that when the cerebellum is diseased, patients will perform each element of the sequenced movement as a functionally separate entity, rather than in one smooth, fluid motion.

IS THERE A COMMON FUNDAMENTAL UNDERLYING MECHANISM?

Some of the classical symptoms and signs of cerebellar dysfunction can be considered special cases of other, more fundamental symptoms and signs. For example, kinetic tremor can be considered a special case of dysmetria. Ataxia may be seen as a combination of kinetic tremor and dysmetria, particularly when it occurs in the context of walking or balance. The dysarthric speech could also be considered a form of dysmetria in which articulatory targets are under- or overshot, leading to abnormal intonations and inflections.

One argument that kinetic tremor is a special case of dysmetria is that it does not occur unless there is an initial error in the original movement. Subsequent correcting movements are dysmetric also, leading to another error requiring further correcting movements that also are dysmetric. These dysmetric correcting movements are most likely to occur toward the end of the movement. These oscillating movements at the end explain why kinetic tremor is sometimes described as terminal tremor. Vilis and Hore showed that monkeys whose dentate nucleus of the cerebellum is rendered inactive by cooling will not have tremor during movements unless there is an error. In the case of these experiments, error was introduced into the movements by injecting a brief resistance. In the normal monkey, such perturbations produced a rapid oscillation (or tremor) that dampened quickly. When the dentate nucleus was cooled, the tremor was slower and of much longer duration.[17]

It is possible that dysdiadochokinesia also may be a special case of dysmetria. In this case, the dysmetria of the component sequential movements may have an additive effect, thereby easily disrupting rapidly alternating movements. Alternatively, rapidly alternating movements may be physiologically distinct types of movements, thereby having their own unique pathophysiology.

It is possible that decomposition of movement is a learned response used to simplify the movement task. Breaking down complex synergistic movements reduces the degrees of freedom, thereby reducing the possibilities of error. This may be analogous to patients with ataxic gait that learn to walk with a wide-based gait to provide a better base of support, thereby reducing the risk of a fall.

It is unclear as to how dysmetria can explain static or positional tremor and nystagmus. It could be argued that maintenance of limb or eye position is an active process requiring continuous corrections. Dysmetria affecting these corrections could result in an inability to maintain position and errors in attempting to return to the intended position. These repetitive errors and corrections then lead to oscillation that appears as tremor and nystagmus. Clearly, dysmetria can not explain hypotonia.

MECHANISMS OF DYSMETRIA

Dysmetria appears to be a fundamental abnormality associated with cerebellar dysfunction. Most of the symptoms and signs of cerebellar disease can be interpreted as special cases of dysmetria. The question now becomes: What is the nature of dysmetria? There are several possibilities that relate to abnormalities manifested either through the alpha motor system or the gamma motor system. The alpha motor system is that which drives the limb musculature directly. The gamma motor system may drive the musculature indirectly by first affecting the muscle spindle fibers. This changes the excitability of the muscle spindle that reflexively, through muscle spindle afferents, drives the alpha motor neurons.

CEREBELLAR EFFECTS ON THE ALPHA MOTOR SYSTEM

Ultimately, the alpha motor system must be activated either directly or indirectly. The alpha motor system must precisely control the activations of individual muscles and must closely coordinate activities in muscles synergistic and antagonistic to the intended movement. Normal movement requires the precise control of muscles that facilitate the movement (agonist muscles) and of those that oppose the movement (antagonist muscles). The precise control of these muscles includes what muscles are affected and the timing of those effects.

The control mechanisms are complex. For example, the antagonist muscles that oppose the intended movement are often activated during movement. Although this seems counterintuitive, activation of the antagonist muscles is necessary to brake the movement so that it does not overshoot. An abnormality in muscle selection and timing of activation leads to abnormal movements. Actual movements have separate components, each of which have to be precisely controlled. Mechanisms that initiate a movement are separate from those that control the final trajectory of the movement.[18]

Even within a single muscle there is a complex pattern of activation. Rapid movements are associated with a triphasic pattern of muscle activation. There is an initial agonist burst of electromyographic activity (EMG), followed by a pause during which there is a burst of EMG in the antagonist muscle. This is then followed by a third burst of EMG, this time occurring in the agonist. The first burst of EMG is thought to control movement initiation and is used to overcome the initial inertial load that would resist movement. The second burst, occurring in the antagonist, acts as a brake on the initial burst so that the movement does not overshoot. The third and final burst, in the agonist, brings the movement to the final target.[19]

EMG studies in nonhuman primates have confirmed that lateral cerebellar lesions (affecting the lateral cerebellar hemisphere and/or the dentate nucleus) produce prolonged agonist and delayed antagonist onset during muscle contraction,[20] which could readily lead to dysmetria. Also, with flexion, as compared to that of controls, acceleration had smaller magnitude, and deceleration had larger magnitude. The disorder in acceleration showed agonist EMG activity that was less abrupt in onset, smaller in magnitude, and longer in duration. The authors concluded that the normal function of the cerebellum is needed for the generation of agonist and antagonist muscle activity that is of both the correct timing and magnitude to control the dynamic phase of arm movements.[20]

EMG studies in humans with cerebellar disease, compared to those with normal subjects, confirmed the conclusions of this work, suggesting that the cerebellum plays an important role in the timing mechanisms of agonist and antagonist contraction.[21-23] It was shown that the EMG abnormalities associated with clinical dysmetria consisted of delayed and prolonged agonist activity, as well as delayed onset of antagonist activity. One example of such a study involved 20 patients with cerebellar deficits.[21] This study, examining the EMG of fast elbow flexion, showed that biceps, triceps, or the activities of both were prolonged during elbow flexion. When triceps (antagonist) activity was prolonged, the developing movement was prematurely halted, correlating with the clinical finding of hypometria, or the undershooting of the target.

In regard to dysdiadochokinesia, a majority of patients with cerebellar lesions had antagonistic muscle activity that either ceased too late or not at all. Normally, the antagonistic activity decreases during the 50 ms or so before the initiation of biceps activity, and it always ends before that point.[21] The clinical sign of rebound may be a result of failure to reduce activity in the tonically active agonist muscle. To test for rebound, a patient is asked to keep his arms in an outstretched position in front of him, pronated and with eyes closed. The examiner than displaces one arm at a time by strongly tapping the wrist. The normal outstretched arm will return promptly to its original position, whereas the affected limb will overshoot its original position because of a larger displacement. The affected limb returns to the approximate original position through a series of oscillations. Holmes initially thought that rebound was caused by hypotonia, but the evidence suggests that it results from a failure or delay in the correct termination of muscle activity.

Hallett et al.[21] concluded that the cerebellum plays a role in the organization of the relationship between agonists and antagonists in successive movements. The distortion of the initial part of the motor pattern was a consistent finding in their EMG analysis. They surmised, then, that the deficit must be in the supraspinal segment, even before the program reaching the anterior horn cells. This is consistent with the view that the cerebellum normally contributes to the generation of the agonist burst that initiates learned movements.

Recordings of changes in neuronal activities in nonhuman primates performing limb movement tasks have shown that the neurons in the lateral cerebellum become active before those of the motor cortex.[24] This suggests that the lateral cerebellum is involved in motor programming that encodes the precise patterns and timing of synergistic and antagonist muscle activities. Now this program is relayed to the motor cortex for execution. Lesions of the lateral cerebellum then could cause abnormal motor programs that incorrectly drive the motor cortex neurons necessary for movement. Evidence supporting this comes from the work of Meyer-Lohmann et al. in 1977, who showed that activity changes in movement-related motor cortex neurons are delayed by 50–150 ms during cerebellar dentate cooling.[25] These observations correlate with prolongation of the reaction times in patients or experimental animals with cerebellar lesions.[20,22,23]

In light of this, Hore and Vilis, in 1984, used torque pulse perturbation experiments with monkeys, in which the monkeys moved a lever. As they did so, a force was added that either moved the lever toward the target or opposed the movement. The researchers showed that training and practice allows skilled movements to be done that are predictive or anticipatory.[26] Cooling of the dentate severely impaired the ability of the monkey to predict accurate movement range and force, resulting in overshoot and, hence, dysmetria. The evidence showed that the early antagonist response is preprogrammed and is likely formed to act as a braking response to prevent overshoot of the initial agonist burst. Even Holmes, in his early works, stated that delayed antagonist onset is largely responsible for dysmetria.[3,7]

This concept of inappropriate timing can be used to help explain the sign of dysdiadochokinesia, which is basically an inability of the patient to time the onset and offset of agonist and antagonist muscles accurately. Tremor is likewise related; it is postulated that the intention tremor seen in cerebellar disease involves an error in this braking system. Because the patient is unable to predict when braking should be initiated, the patient depends on external cues, or afferent input, in order to engage the antagonist. This explains the worsening seen as the target is approached, and it can be postulated to be a result of the patient trying to correct the movement by relying on external cues. This closed loop causes delays in the system, leading to the oscillations of intention tremor.[17]

Relating nystagmus or saccadic dysmetria to limb dysmetria seems to break down, though. Although numerous studies already mentioned have shown that limb dysmetria is associated with increased reaction times, reversible cooling of cerebellar nuclei (fastigial, interpositus, or dentate) in monkeys had no effect on the reaction time (initiation) of saccades, lending evidence to the theory that the cerebellum is involved instead in *terminating* saccadic eye movements.[27]

The complexity of motor programs generated in the cerebellum may vary according to the complexity of the intended movement. Quantitative differences in task complexity could translate into qualitative differences in underlying physiology. In other words, simpler task programming may not be as dependent on cerebellar function as more complex tasks. Sternberg et al., in 1978, have shown experimentally that the reaction time to start the first movement of a sequence of movements increases in direct proportion with the length of the sequence to be completed.[28] The hypothesis is that a plan, or abstract copy of the motor program (the response sequence) is devised before the actual movement and is sent to a "motor buffer." Then, during actual movement, the intended motor sequence is transcribed from the buffer to define the exact pattern of muscle activation. This pattern specifies the spaciotemporal pattern of movement. As the number of component responses rises, so too will the time needed to interpret the motor buffer and to organize the sequences of motor output into their proper order. In the normal setting, then, this results in an increased latency to initiate the first response component in the planned motor sequence.

There is evidence in both animal and human studies that the cerebellum appears to be involved in the programming of such a complex practiced movement before movement onset, so that the sequence will be performed as a single fluid unit. Robertson and Grimm, in 1975 in their studies of dentate recordings in monkeys, showed that some dentate neurons fire before movement that involves a sequenced (not just a simple) response.[29]

Human subjects with moderate cerebellar deficiency have been studied as well in this regard. They were tested, along with controls, in executing a single-, two-, or three-keypress command in a certain sequence.[30] In patients with cerebellar disease there were negligible or no effects of sequence length on response time, whereas normal control subjects showed the expected increase in response onset time with an increase in sequence length. This observation suggests that patients with cerebellar disease are slow in their reaction times and cannot modify those times according to the complexity of the required task. A breakdown of the sequence into functional independent elements was also noted, correlating with Holmes' "decomposition of movement."[3,7] The authors concluded that the translation of a programmed sequence of responses into action involves cerebellar structures that schedule a sequence of ordered responses before movement onset. In other words, cerebellar disease interferes with the correct timing of a sequence of movements before movement onset.

The notion of precise timing of events in the motor program is very important. There is evidence that the cerebellum participates in the perception of timing as well. In the study done by Ivry and Keele,[31] two tasks were examined: (1) a production task of rhythmic tapping and (2) a perception task of testing the patient's perceptual acuity of comparable temporal intervals. Of patients diagnosed with parkinsonism, cortical disease (lesions affecting the posterior regions of the frontal lobe), peripheral neuropathy, or cerebellar disease, only those patients with cerebellar disease displayed a deficit in both the production and perception of timing tasks. This study not only demonstrated a deficit in the production task of finger tapping but also revealed a severe impairment in the cerebellar patients' ability to perceive time intervals.[31]

These results offered evidence for the theory that cerebellar integrity is critical for the operation of an internal timing process, which was first proposed by Braitenberg in 1967.[32] The authors used this evidence to support their belief that the cerebellum performs the operation of computing the timing requirements of a motor program.

CEREBELLAR EFFECTS ON THE GAMMA MOTOR SYSTEM

The descriptions above clearly demonstrate that the timing and patterns of muscle activity are abnormal in patients with cerebellar pathology. Because the muscles are driven directly by alpha motor neurons, the activities of these neurons must also be abnormal in cerebellar disease. The question then becomes: Is the abnormality of the alpha motor system a direct or indirect consequence of cerebellar disease? The links from the cerebellum through the motor cortex to the alpha motor system at least provide a pathway for a direct effect of the cerebellum on the alpha motor system. However, what is anatomically possible may not be physiologically relevant.

The gamma motor system has an effect on the alpha motor system through a servocontroller reflex mechanism involving the muscle spindles. If the cerebellum were to have an effect on the gamma motor system that affects the function of the muscle spindles, it could be another means by which the cerebellum affects movement. To this extent, it has been theorized that this association extends to the skeletal muscle level, involving alpha-gamma coactivation, that is, the process that acts to maintain muscle spindle sensitivity during muscle contraction. This produces appropriate tone and, hence, hypothetically, smooth and coordinated movements. Thus the cerebellum acts as the "head ganglion of the proprioceptive system," as Sherrington stated earlier in this century.[33]

To better understand how the cerebellum can influence muscle tone via its effects on the gamma motor system, it is necessary first to summarize the basic structures of skeletal muscle involved. The two types of nerve fibers that innervate skeletal muscle are the alpha motor neurons and the gamma motor neurons, both arising from the anterior horn cells in the spinal cord. The alpha motor neurons are fibers large in diameter (9–20 μm) that innervate extrafusal muscle fibers, which produce muscle tension, contraction, and movement. Gamma motor neurons average 5 μm in diameter and innervate the small, specialized intrafusal muscle fibers, which are contained within muscle spindles, constituting approximately 30 percent of the motor nerve fibers.[34] (For a more in-depth review, see the work of Granit[35] and Kandel et al.[36])

Two receptors in skeletal muscle exist that are necessary for motor control. Muscle spindles respond to stretch and signal changes in muscle length. The sensory input from the spindles is used by the brain to determine the relative attitudes (positions) of the limb portion in question. This system is extremely sensitive to very small changes in length and may be used by the brain to compensate and to correct for disturbances in movement. This sensitivity of Ia afferent discharge (from the muscle spindles) to small changes in velocity relies upon the coactivation of alpha-gamma motor neurons.[35] According to Granit, this coactivation *may* be important, because the responses by the spinal cord to changes of muscle length are made more symmetrical by the summed action of muscle spindles and extrafusal fibers.

The intrafusal fibers are specialized muscle fibers that make up part of the muscle spindle. Gamma motor neurons innervate the contractile polar regions of these fibers. The gamma motor neurons that innervate the muscle spindles are also known as the fusimotor system. Gamma motor neurons regulate and modulate spindle afferent discharge according to the following scheme: activation of a gamma efferent leads to shortening and contraction of the polar regions of the intrafusal fibers. This stretches the noncontractile region, leading to increased sensitivity and firing of the sensory endings.[34-36]

To better understand how the cerebellum relates to muscle tone, one must understand the ascending and descending pathways that affect the gamma motor system. Information from muscle spindles from the legs and trunk is transmitted via the dorsal spinocerebellar tract, keeping the cerebellum updated regarding evolving movement in terms of tension, position, force, and rate of movement. The cuneocerebellar tract subserves the upper extremity in the same manner. These tracts enter the cerebellum through the inferior cerebellar peduncle, ending on the same side as their origin. The ventral spinocerebellar tract, however, conveys different information. These tracts are mainly concerned with the information from segmental interneurons that synthesize input from the periphery and mainly from descending commands through the corticospinal and rubrospinal tracts.[3,7] These tracts enter the cerebellum through the superior cerebellar peduncle, terminating mostly in the ipsilateral medial and intermediate zones. The function of this pathway is to keep the cerebellum updated regarding the ongoing execution of movement and regulation of muscle tone.

The two main descending systems that exert influence on the gamma motor neuron system include the vestibulospinal tract that is concerned with extensors and the rubrospinal tract that is concerned with flexors. The cerebellum sends information to both origins of these tracts, namely, the lateral vestibular nucleus (for the vestibulospinal tract) and the red nucleus (for the rubrospinal tract). These descending systems connect in parallel ways with both alpha and gamma motor neurons, lending evidence to the concept of coactivation.

Gilman, in 1969, showed that cerebellar ablation (specifically of the interpositus and fastigial nucleus) in the monkey led to hypotonia, defined as decreased resistance to passive limb manipulation.[37] By deactivating cerebellar influence, stretch responses of muscle spindle afferents are decreased, possibly by decreasing the tonic facilitation of fusimotor activity. This decrease of spindle primary afferent input would then be expected to affect homonymous alpha motor neurons, in turn decreasing their facilitatory drive, hence, leading to a decrease of tonic extrafusal motor activity. He proposed that this may be the cause of cerebellar dysmetria. In summary, he concluded that a decrease in fusimotor activity, leading to abnormalities in muscle spindle function, is an important factor in the pathogenesis of cerebellar hypotonia.[37]

IS IT ALPHA OR GAMMA?

More recent data conflict somewhat with Gilman's hypothesis, however. Experiments in deafferented primates abolish the influence of the gamma motor system. Liu and Chambers, in 1971, proved that monkeys with lesioned cerebellar nuclei and that were deafferented by dorsal rhizotomy showed marked cerebellar ataxia in contradistinction to those monkeys that were deafferented only.[38] Gilman et al., in 1976, found that cerebellar ablation in deafferented monkeys resulted in a worse motor performance.[39] This led Flament and Hore, in 1986, to suggest that cerebellar movement deficits are a result of disordered central commands, rather than of primarily to the influence of the gamma motor system.[20] Holmes himself postulated that hypermetria was related to

decreased tone of the antagonist,[3,7] whereas other authors showed that instead of decreased tone, prolonged, or delayed, antagonistic tone during movements accounted for the dysmetria.[20,23] Thus, the theory[37] that dysmetria is caused by decreased fusimotor activity to antagonist muscle does not explain the disorders seen involving the antagonistic muscles in these studies.

Three Theories Regarding Cerebellar Movement Strategy

CEREBELLUM AS A SERVOCONTROLLER OR FEEDBACK-BASED MECHANISM

The cerebellum is involved in the timing of movement in two ways: in a feedback control function and in a feedforward control function.[40] Regarding the former, it is proposed that the cerebellum is in charge of an instant-by-instant fine tuning of the cerebral cortex's ongoing motor output. In 1967, John C. Eccles proposed that the cerebellum is involved in the ongoing correction of movement, postulating a dynamic feedback loop control of movement.[41] He described the notion that with perturbations of evolving movements, changes occurred in peripheral receptors that signaled new information into the cerebellum. This then led to corrections by the cerebellar efferent discharges via descending pathways. In this model, meaningful feedback could only occur when there was some change or evolution in the continuing movement.[43] In regard to pyramidal tract efferent flow, Eccles stated that "it is incessantly subject to revision by the continuous feedback of information to the cerebellum with the further integration of its output."[43] The underlying theme to this theory is the ongoing correction of movement.

CEREBELLUM AS A FEEDFORWARD GENERATOR

The feed-forward control function proposes that the cerebellum, before actual movement initiation, sends to the motor cortex a preprogrammed sequence of movements. Hence, a defect in this function would clinically be discerned as difficulty with starting, conducting, and stopping muscular contractions (i.e., dysdiadochokinesia or dysmetria). Clinical evidence for this dates back to the observations of Holmes,[3,7] who noted that the initiation of movement was delayed in patients with lateral cerebellar damage; movements were slow to start and slow to relax. He believed, then, that this slowness in movement initiation was not a result of muscle tone disturbance but rather "a delay in initiating corticospinal innervation."[7] Walshe, in 1927, concurred, stating that in humans the cerebellum's essential function was in the generation of movement.[44]

Evarts and Thach, in 1969, postulated that this indeed was the case, that the lateral part of the cerebellum influenced motor output by means of a feedforward mechanism.[4,7] Ito, in 1970, agreed, especially for learned movements.[40] He viewed the cerebellum as providing an internal substitute for the external world. This, then, eliminated the requirement for peripheral sensory input, speeding the rate at which a movement could be implemented via preprogramming. Ito expanded this concept,[46] in which he proposes that as a movement is learned during repeated practice, the slower, feedback mechanisms are used. Gradually, as the movement is learned, it becomes more automatic, eventually being done "without much thought." It is this function that is thought to be subserved by the lateral, or dentate, cerebellum. This process uses the feedforward mechanism.[46]

The work of Thach, in 1975,[24] and of Sasaki and Gemba, in 1984,[47] showed that lateral cerebellar output precedes motor cortex activity in movement production. Thach, in 1970, showed that dentate activity precedes EMG changes when monkeys make self-initiated movements, and that the dentate activity preceded motor cortex response.[48] Thus, it is postulated that the output of the lateral cerebellum is concerned with and precedes intended movement.

Other evidence for this stems from the work of Allen and Tsukahara,[49] who theorize that the dentate is well-suited for the preprogramming of movements, given its enormous size in humans, being 10 times larger than the interpositus nuclei. They point out that rapid and ballistic-type movements, such as a boxer striking an adversary or a piano player rapidly striking the keys, must be served by preprogrammed movements, as there would be no time for peripheral feedback to sufficiently update the movement, once begun. Allen and Tsukahara comment that the more rapid the intended movement, the more the pyramidal tract needs a preprogrammed sequence to produce a good result.[49]

CONCEPT OF EFFERENT COPY: A HYBRID OF TWO THEORIES

This is defined as a process in which a system (the cerebellum) is provided with some sort of a model of an intended movement from the motor cortex before the actual execution of the movement.[26] In this model, the cerebellum can compare the program for the intended movement to its knowledge of the state of the organisms. When there is an error, a feedback-corrective program can be relayed back to the motor cortex. Thus, the motor program from the motor cortex is amended before the movement is accomplished. Eccles has noted that "the cerebrum cannot begin instituting any action without the cerebellum immediately knowing about it."[50] Neuroanatomically, this theory fits with the known connections. Neural activity projects from the motor cortex to both spinal motor neurons and to cerebellum via collaterals through the pontine nuclei.

The efference copy hypothesis has several tenants. First, for rapid correction of any sudden perturbations in the environment, the efference copy must be compared with the actual afferent signal. Second, the efference copy must use a delay device, or predictive capability, because the afferent signal is changing constantly. Third, the efference copy is formed simultaneously as the movement command is sent. Fourth, the cerebellum can formulate subsequent components of the cerebrum's response—this must be based on prior experience or learning. The cerebellum must be given the neural signals for the efference copy before receiving the afferent signals to allow for correction, hence, the need for a delay device. It has been proposed that each cortical command is transformed by the cerebellum into the next of a sequence of command components. Therefore, the particular preprogrammed response evolves on the basis of transformation set up in the cerebellum according to prior experience.

WHICH IS IT—FEEDBACK, FEEDFORWARD, OR EFFERENCE COPY?

Much more research will be needed to definitively answer this question. However, there is some indirect evidence to suggest that all of the above may be operative. Different mechanisms may be used by different regions of the cerebellum. Both the feedback and efferent copy models depend on sensory information received from the body. The lateral cerebellum receives little direct sensory input from the periphery.[51] Therefore, the lateral cerebellum is least likely to use a feedback or an efferent copy mechanism. Yet, the most likely area of the cerebellum to produce ataxia and tremor when lesioned is the lateral cerebellum.[4,8] Changes in neuronal activity associated with movement generation occur in dentate neurons before those in the motor cortex. This would be consistent with a feedforward mechanism.

The interpositus nucleus (globose and emboliform in humans) receives input from both the motor cortex and periphery. Neuronal activity in the interpositus nucleus associated with movement initiation occurs almost simultaneously with those of the motor cortex. These observations are consistent with the interpositus nuclei operating by means of efferent copy mechanisms.

The fastigial nucleus receives most of its input from the periphery, and little of the output goes to the motor cortex. Neuronal activity in this structure occurs usually after the onset of movement. These observations would be consistent with the fastigial nucleus operating in a feedback manner.

Organization of the Cerebellum

MACROSCOPIC VIEW

Located in the posterior fossa, the cerebellum is a derivative of the metencephalon, or pons. It is attached to the dorsum of the pons by three sets of paired peduncles that transmit afferent and efferent signals. The cerebellum is separated from the cerebrum by the tentorium cerebelli. Grossly, the cerebellum is composed of the cortex (made up of folia), the internal white matter or medullary substance, four paired deep nuclei, and three paired peduncles. Folia represent a series of (mostly) transversely oriented cortical ridges or folds. When sectioned sagittally, the white matter of the cerebellum gives the appearance of tree-like branching, thus called the arbor vitae (tree of life). On the surface of the arbor vitae rests each folium (which is Latin for leaf.[52,53]

Anatomists have observed that the cerebellar cortex contains five deeper clefts than the folia, running in a transverse manner and separating the groups of folia into 10 named lobules and 3 named lobes (Fig. 44-6). The deepest of all the cerebellar fissures, the primary fissure, separates the anterior lobe (made up of lobules I through V) from the posterior lobe (made up of lobules VI through IX). The third lobe, the flocculonodular lobe, corresponds to lobule X and is sepa-

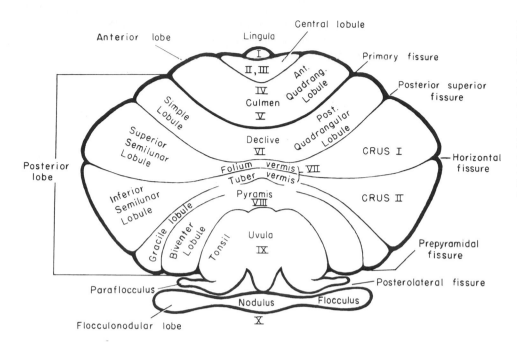

Central lobule

Anterior lobe

Lingula

Primary fissure

Posterior superior fissure

Horizontal fissure

Posterior lobe

CRUS I

CRUS II

Prepyramidal fissure

Posterolateral fissure

Paraflocculus

Flocculus

Nodulus

Flocculonodular lobe

I

II, III

IV

V

VI

VII

VIII

IX

X

Culmen

Simple Lobule

Ant. Quadrang. Lobule

Post. Quadrangular Lobule

Superior Semilunar Lobule

Declive

Folium vermis

Tuber vermis

Inferior Semilunar Lobule

Pyramis

Gracile lobule

Biventer Lobule

Tonsil

Uvula

FIGURE 44-6 Classic neuroanatomic description of the fissures and lobules of the cerebellum. The anterior lobe, or paleocerebellum, is located rostral to the primary fissure. The posterior lobe, or neocerebellum, lies between the primary and posterolateral fissures. The flocculonodular lobe, or archicerebellum, lies caudal to the posterolateral fissure. Lobules are labeled with roman numerals. *(From Carpenter.[53] Used with permission.)*

rated from the posterior lobe by the posterolateral fissure. In the sagittal plane, a midline vermis and two cerebellar hemispheres are present.

The embryologic divisions of the cerebellum consist of three sections. The archicerebellum is made up of the nodulus and the paired flocculi. Phylogenetically, it is the oldest division and is related to the vestibular system. The paleocerebellum corresponds to the anterior lobe, or spinocerebellum, located rostral to the primary fissure, the deepest in the cerebellum. It receives information regarding stretch receptors by way of the spinocerebellar tracts and is primarily involved with muscle tone regulation. The third portion is the neocerebellum, which is the largest and newest part of the cerebellum, and is the most prominent in primates.[54] It corresponds anatomically to the posterior lobe. Classically, it is thought to be involved primarily with coordinating movement of ipsilateral limbs.

The cells of the four paired deep cerebellar nuclei lie within the medullary substance of the cerebellum proper. From medial to lateral these nuclei are the fastigial, globose, emboliform, and dentate. The globose and emboliform nuclei are known collectively as the interpositus nucleus, with the emboliform situated more anteriorly than the globose. Output from cells of these nuclei is excitatory, in contradistinction to the output of the cerebellar cortex via the Purkinje cells, which is entirely inhibitory.

The archicerebellum, made up of the flocculonodular lobe, is often considered separate and distinct from the remainder of the cerebellum. It is thought to be an outgrowth of the vestibular nuclei. The cerebellar cortex of this lobe does not project to any of the deep cerebellar nuclei. It projects to the vestibular nuclei in the brain stem. The flocculonodular lobe has a different embryological origin, compared to the remainder of the cerebellum.[55]

AFFERENT CONNECTIONS TO THE CEREBELLUM

All afferent information that goes into the cerebellum, whether motor or sensory, courses through one of the three paired peduncles. Information then proceeds through the deep white medullary substance, ultimately to terminate in the cerebellar cortex. Collateral information is sent to appropriate deep cerebellar nuclei. As mentioned before, information from muscle spindles is transmitted to the cerebellum through spinocerebellar tracts. Vestibular end organ information is also relayed, as is information from joint proprioceptors. Afferents from the cerebral cortex are relayed via the corticopontocerebellar complex (which will ultimately enter the cerebellar cortex as mossy fibers), and the inferior olivary complex (which will ultimately enter the cerebellar cortex as climbing fibers). The primary projections from the cerebral cortex that form the corticopontocerebellar tracts include the premotor cortex and supplementary motor area (Brodman's area 6), the primary motor cortex (area 4), and the primary sensory cortex (areas 1, 2, and 3). It is of interest to note that the number of fibers involved in input from the cerebral cortex is on the order of 20 million, as compared to that of the pyramidal tract, made up of only 1 million or so fibers.[54] In fact, the ratio of afferent to efferent connections is approximately 40:1,[53] leading theorists to surmise that the cerebellum is involved with higher cognitive functions.[54,56,57] This will be dealt with in a later section.

The three paired cerebellar peduncles include the superior, middle, and inferior, all uniting to attach the cerebellum to the dorsum of the pons. Afferent connections to the cerebellum via the inferior peduncle include a relay to the fastigial nucleus from fibers of the vestibular nucleus. A structure known as the restiform body is entirely concerned with afferent information, whereas a juxtarestiform body contains both afferent and efferent information. In addition to fibers from the vestibular nucleus, fibers from the posterior spinocerebellar tract, accessory cuneate nucleus, olivocerebellar tract (from the contralateral inferior olive), and reticular formation in the brain stem are also relayed by way of the inferior peduncle to cerebellar cortex.[52,53,55]

The middle cerebellar peduncle, or brachium pontis, contains the massive bundle of crossed corticopontocerebellar fibers; the vermis receives both ipsilateral and contralateral fibers. These end as mossy fibers, which will be expanded on when the cerebellar cortex circuitry is discussed. Thus, the middle cerebellar peduncle conveys only afferent information. The main afferent fibers carried in the superior cerebellar peduncle are those from the ventral spinocerebellar tract, ending mainly in ipsilateral medial and intermediate cerebellar zones.[52,53,55]

EFFERENT CONNECTIONS FROM THE CEREBELLUM

The efferent output of the cerebellum goes by way of both the superior cerebellar peduncle and the fastigial nucleus fibers in the inferior peduncle. The superior cerebellar peduncle is composed of fibers from the dentate and interpositus nuclei. These fibers enter the brain stem and divide into an ascending and descending branch. Fibers in the ascending branch cross the midline in the tegmentum at the junction of the pons and midbrain and ascend to the contralateral red nucleus. Some fibers, predominantly from the interpositus nuclei, synapse on neurons in the magnocellular division of the red nucleus. Most of the fibers continue on to the thalamus, specifically to the ventral lateral pars caudalis and ventral posterolateral pars oralis nuclei. From there, the fibers proceed to the primary motor cortex (area 4). This fiber tract bundle is known as the dentatorubrothalamic tract, also called the brachium conjunctivum. The descending division of the superior cerebellar peduncle travels to the reticular nuclei and the inferior olive. Some of these fibers project back to the contralateral cerebellar cortex and nuclei.[52,53,55]

The fastigial efferent fibers are both crossed and uncrossed. The crossed fibers from the fastigial nucleus travel in the uncinate fasciculus, arching around the superior cerebellar peduncle, projecting bilaterally and symmetrically to both lateral and inferior vestibular nuclei, as well as to upper cervical cord motor neurons. A small number of fibers also ascend in the superior cerebellar peduncle to reach the ventral lateral and ventral posterolateral thalamus. Similarly, the uncrossed, smaller juxtarestiform body projects to the vestibular nuclei, as well as to lower brain stem structures.[52,53,55]

The modern functional organization is quite different from the anatomic organization described above. The functional organization is divided into zones based on behavioral observation in ablation experiments[59–61] and anatomic connectivity (Fig. 44-7). This organization was based largely on the work of Jansen and Brodal in 1940.[58] Their general concept stated that the cerebellar cortex is anatomically organized into longitudinal corticonuclear zones. As in most of the central nervous system, there is a gradient between the three zones. That is to say, sharp borders do not exist but rather blend and overlap. As stated by Evarts and Thach, "localization is more-or-less rather that all-or-none."[45]

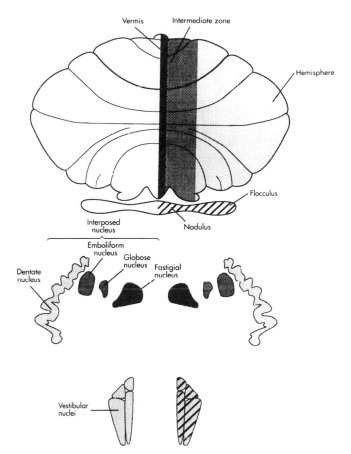

FIGURE 44-7 This shows that the cerebellar cortex is divided into three longitudinal zones with its subsequent projections to the four paired cerebellar nuclei. *(From Nolte.*[52] *Used with permission.)*

The midline, or vermal, zone is made up of the cerebellar cortex of the vermis and the unpaired fastigial nucleus. The cerebellar cortex in this region projects primarily to the fastigial nuclei. This part of the cerebellum receives input primarily from the periphery, in contrast to the lateral zone, which receives very little input directly from the periphery. The outputs of the vermal zone project directly to brain stem structures or to the spinal cord, with very little going directly to the thalamus and cerebral cortex. The lateral cerebellum, in contrast, sends most of its output to the cerebral cortex via the thalamus.[53] The fastigial nucleus and its efferent target, the vestibular nuclei, are involved in limb extension to maintain posture. The human cerebellar stimulation and ablation studies of Nashold and Slaughter, in 1969, confirmed this. Nuchal and truncal postural mechanisms are under fastigial control as well[62] (Fig. 44-8).

The cerebellar cortex has a somatotopic arrangement, as well as a functional zone arrangement. It does, however, appear to be less discrete and less acutely outlined than that of the cerebral cortex homunculus.[8] From numerous animal experiments, most notably, those performed by Chambers and Sprague in 1955, the head and truncal regions occupy the vermis of the anterior lobe with the representation of the limbs extending into the paravermal zone.[60,61] Ablations of

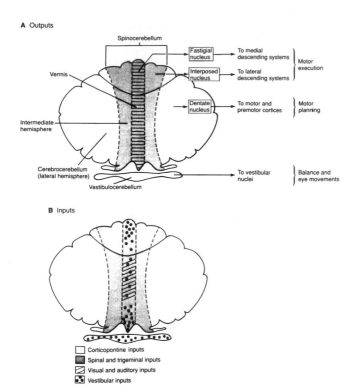

FIGURE 44-8 Schematic representation of the outputs (*A*) and inputs (*B*) of the cerebellum. *(From Kandel et al.[36] Used with permission.)*

the vermal region in experimental animals produce abnormalities of gait and posture. In humans, lesions of this region most often produce gait and truncal ataxia without producing symptoms in the extremities during volitional movement. Consequently, the vermal region of the cerebellum is thought to be concerned primarily with modifying muscle tone and controlling posture, locomotion, and whole-body equilibrium.

The lateral zone, made up of the dentate nucleus and its overlying cerebellar cortex, is involved with the coordination of ipsilateral somatic motor activity and preprogramming of learned volitional movements. The dentate is the largest cerebellar nucleus in man; it relays chiefly the efferent outflow from the lateral hemispheric area of the cerebellum, exerting its influence on tone and movement of ipsilateral limbs. Nashold and Slaughter, in 1969, showed that stimulation within the lateral interpositus nucleus or dentate nucleus results in facilitation of ipsilateral flexor tone.[62]

The paravermal zone is comprised of the interpositus nucleus and the overlying cerebellar cortex, which projects to the interpositus nucleus. The interpositus receives input from the motor cortex, as well as from the periphery. The interpositus nucleus projects to both the cerebral cortex and to the brain stem. Lesions of the interpositus in experimental animals show postural defects in the ipsilateral limbs, as well as difficulties with locomotion and the righting postural response.[60] Animal experiments suggest that the interpositus nucleus and its efferent target, the red nucleus, are concerned more with flexor mechanisms.[60,63] Consequently, the paravermal zone of the cerebellum is thought to facilitate ipsilateral flexor muscle tone via the rubrospinal tract.

Evarts and Thach, in 1969, stated that almost all of the cerebellar cortex receives at least some input from the cerebral cortex.[45] Somatotopic projections from sensory and motor areas of the cerebral cortex have been mapped to medial and intermediate zones of the cerebellar cortex. In the intermediate zone, both motor and sensory areas of the cerebral cortex project to the contralateral anterior lobe in the sagittal dimension as well, so that the head is oriented posteriorly in the simplex, the legs are represented anteriorly in the centralis, and the arms are in between, in the culmen[64] (Fig. 44-9). Even auditory and visual receiving areas project to the medial simplex, folium, and tuber, overlapping the two head regions from cerebral cortex (corresponding to the lobules, as diagrammed in Fig. 44-6).

These different zones also differ in the timing of the neuronal activity changes associated with the generation of movement. Neurons in the dentate nucleus tend to become active before those of the motor cortex.[24] Neurons in the interpositus become active later, at approximately the same time as those of the motor cortex.[65] Neurons in the fastigial nucleus change activity latest and usually after the movement has been initiated.[66]

THE FLOCCULONODULAR LOBE

As previously mentioned, the flocculonodular lobe is phylogenetically the oldest, most primitive portion of the cerebellum and arises from the vestibular nuclei. As such, it retains both afferent and efferent connections with the vestibular apparatus. The tract that carries such information is the juxtarestiform body. It conveys both afferent signals via direct and secondary vestibulocerebellar tracts and efferent signals via cerebellovestibular tracts. This vast amount of information comes and goes through the inferior cerebellar peduncle.

FIGURE 44-9 Homunculus of the cerebellum of the macaque. Note the two different representations of the somatotopic map, bilateral in paramedian lobules and ipsilateral in the anterior lobe. *(From Pearlman et al: Neurological Pathophysiology, 3rd ed. New York: Oxford University Press, 1984. Used with permission.)*

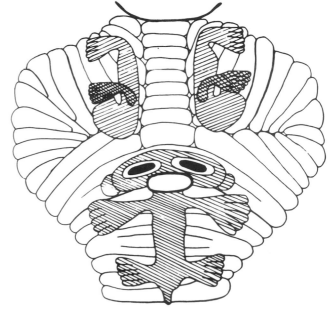

The flocculonodular syndrome is caused by lesions of the nodulus, flocculus, and uvula. The hallmarks seen are poor equilibrium, both during standing and walking, nystagmus, and, sometimes, a rotated posture of the head.[8] Dow and Moruzzi stated that "when the body as a whole is at rest, individual movements, especially of the hand, can be carried out without evidence of locomotor disturbance; the heel-to-knee test can be performed without tremor, etc. Only when the body is propelled through space are difficulties encountered."[8] The basic mechanism of dysfunction is believed to result from the patient being unable to access vestibular information needed to coordinate movements of either the body or the eyes. This will be covered in greater detail shortly.

MICROSCOPIC VIEW

To better understand how lesions in certain zones of the cerebellum produce the signs described above, it is essential to have a clear understanding of the circuitry involved, both in cerebellar cortical function and cerebrocerebellar loops and spinocerebellar loops. Much of this has been described elegantly in the text by Eccles et al.[67] A brief description is given here.

CEREBELLAR CORTEX CIRCUITRY

The cerebellar cortex is divided into three layers (Fig. 44-10). From the outside toward the medullary white matter, these layers are the molecular, Purkinje, and granular layers. These cortical layers contain five types of neurons, and they are distributed in a laminar manner. The focal point of the cere-

bellar cortex is logically the Purkinje cell, from which the entire output of the cerebellum originates. Thus, the Purkinje cell is the final common output pathway.[40] It is the only neuron whose soma is in the Purkinje layer. The majority of its fibers project to the deep cerebellar nuclei, exerting inhibitory synaptic action. A few Purkinje cell axons synapse directly on vestibular nuclei. These come from the flocculonodular lobe. Finally, Purkinje cells send recurrent collaterals back to adjacent Purkinje cells, as well as to another type of cerebellar cortical cell, the Golgi type II neuron, which will be described shortly. The following discussion will focus on the relationship of the other neuron types to the Purkinje cell.

Purkinje cells receive input from two sources of fibers, mossy and climbing, both of which exert excitatory action. The climbing fibers originate from the inferior olivary complex and make monosynaptic connections with Purkinje cells. Each Purkinje cell receives afferent information from a single climbing fiber, but multiple synaptic connections are made. This is perhaps one of the strongest excitatory synapses found in the central nervous system (CNS). Mossy fibers are the primary afferent input into the cerebellar cortex, originating from spinocerebellar, pontocerebellar, and vestibulocerebellar systems. Mossy fibers do not make direct synapses on Purkinje cells but rather synapse on granule and Golgi cells. The cell bodies of the granule cells are located in the granular layer, whereas its axons ascend through the Purkinje layer to the molecular layer, where they bifurcate into parallel fibers, so named because these axons run parallel to each other and to the long axis of the folia. These axons run for 1–2 mm in both directions, synapsing on Purkinje cells. Each

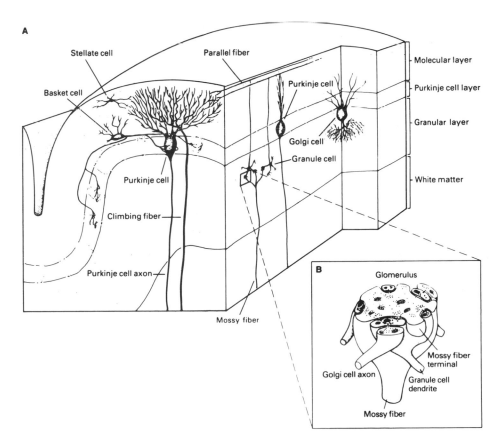

FIGURE 44-10 Diagram of the three layers of the cerebellar cortex. *A.* This shows the transverse and longitudinal planes of a single cerebellar folium, with the five types of neurons. *B.* Detailed drawing of a glomerulus, a clear space in the granular layer where terminals of mossy fibers synapse with Golgi cell axons and granule cell axons. *(From Kandel et al.[36] Used with permission.)*

parallel fiber will make synaptic connection with thousands of Purkinje cells, but only a few synapses will be made with each individual Purkinje cell (in contrast to the numerous connections made by climbing fibers). Each Purkinje cell, in turn, receives synapses from thousands of parallel axons.

Granule cells also send processes to stellate and basket cells, located in the molecular layer, as well as to those parts of the Golgi II neuron dendrites that penetrate the molecular layer. The postsynaptic action of granule cells, and thus of parallel fibers, is excitatory, although it is not as strong as that exhibited by climbing fibers.

As mentioned earlier, parallel fibers synapse on stellate and basket cells. These are cerebellar cortical interneurons located in the molecular layer (some authors define these as the outer and inner stellate cells, respectively). Both cells produce inhibitory input to the Purkinje cell, although basket cell inhibition is much stronger, owing to its synapse directly onto the Purkinje cell body. Its axons form tangential fibers that synapse on Purkinje cell dendrites, thus producing a web, or basket, of inhibitory synapses. The stellate cells, on the other hand, send their axons to synapse on the distal dendrites of the Purkinje cell.

The fifth cerebellar cortical neuron is known as the Golgi cell, located in the granular layer. It receives mossy fiber synapses and climbing fiber synapses on dendrites in the granular layer. The Golgi cell also receives excitatory synapses from parallel fibers onto its dendrites that travel up to the molecular layer. The Golgi cell's main mode of action is the inhibition of up to 10,000 granule cells.[68] This serves to sharpen the input via mossy fibers by suppressing all weak excitatory actions on granule cells.

As mentioned previously, the entire output from the cerebellar cortex is via the Purkinje cell discharges.[40] They exert inhibitory synaptic action on their target neurons, the deep cerebellar nuclei. Eccles calls this sculpturing, in that the cerebellar nuclei also receive constant excitatory discharges from axon collaterals of mossy and climbing fibers.[42] Thus the cerebellar nuclei, which are in a state of background excitation from mossy and climbing collateral input, are subjected to changing inhibitory input from the cerebellar cortex via Purkinje cells.

CEREBELLAR CORTEX STRUCTURE AND DYSMETRIA

One of the fundamental abnormalities associated with cerebellar dysfunction is dysmetria. Analysis of the muscle activities associated with movement strongly suggests that the major cause of dysmetria is the proper timing of activities in muscle synergistic and antagonistic to the intended movement. This suggests that a major function of the intact cerebellum is to provide for the precise timing of muscle activities by developing a motor program that is executed through the motor cortex. In order to do so, the cerebellum must integrate information from wide sources throughout the brain. It must then transmit a motor program to a small part of the brain, namely, the motor cortex.

At least in simple reaction time tasks, the amount of time used in developing a motor program is small, compared to the amount of time it takes muscle activities to execute a particular movement. Thus, the challenge of the cerebellum is to convert information widely distributed spatially over a short duration of time into a spatially narrow output information of a longer time duration that is consistent with the time required for movement execution. The cerebellar cortex circuitry may be uniquely suited to just such a purpose.

Braitenberg proposed, in 1967, that the parallel fibers of the cerebellar cortex act as a delay line with the ability to transform spatial into temporal patterns.[32] The temporal pattern can be created as a sequence over time of Purkinje cell discharges. The regular spatial organization of flattened Purkinje cell dendrite trees oriented transversely to the direction of the parallel fibers ensures that one Purkinje cell was excited at one time. An action potential running down the parallel fiber would excite one Purkinje cell at a time. Purkinje cells most proximal to the origin of the parallel fiber would be excited earlier whereas more distal Purkinje cells would discharge later. The small caliber of the parallel fiber carries a slower conduction velocity, which further contributes to spreading out Purkinje cell responses over time. Ultimately, this sequencing of Purkinje cell activity is translated to a sequence of activity in specific muscles appropriate for the initiation and execution of movement.

Cerebellar Syndromes

Are there clear definable syndromes related to differences in anatomy and physiology? How do the basic mechanisms described above produce these syndromes when applied to specific regions of the cerebellum? What is the relation to the input and output connections of the cerebellum?

The concept of cerebellar syndromes has been dichotomized differently in the literature. Authors have discussed it both on the basis of classic anatomy and on the basis of functional zones, as described earlier. There is considerable overlap, because some of the descriptions ascribed to the lobe approach of classical anatomy correlate with the modern longitudinal organizations based on zones. For example, much of the anterior lobe of the cerebellum corresponds to the paravermal zone. Therefore, descriptions of symptoms and signs previously ascribed to the paleocerebellar syndromes are very similar to those described with lesions of the paravermal zone. In addition, much of the neocerebellum is correlated with the lateral zone. Descriptions of the neocerebellar syndromes then share significant similarities to the lesions of the lateral zone. With time, there should be less reference to paleo-, neo-, and archicerebellar syndromes that will be replaced by vermal, paravermal, and lateral syndromes.

Much of what is known about the cerebellar syndromes stems from animal ablation studies, begun by Luciani in 1891, when he studied the effects in dogs.[1,2] Chambers and Sprague helped to define the concept of functional zones in their ablation studies in cats.[60,61] Other authors have added important data in primate studies.[8,59,69]

The effects in man were analyzed with great insight by the work of Gordon Holmes, describing the signs and symptoms in soldiers who suffered gunshot and shrapnel wounds (mostly to the lateral cerebellum) in World War I.[3,7] Later, effects of surgical manipulation were noted.[62] The accumulated evidence amassed from these and other studies allows for the categorization of cerebellar syndromes (Table 44-1).

VERMAL SYNDROME

The midline of the cerebellum, consisting of the vermis of the cortex and fastigial nucleus, regulates posture, locomotion, tone, and equilibrium of the entire body.[60,61] An ataxic, titubating gait (a stumbling, staggering gait with shaking of the head and trunk), oscillations of the head and neck, and frequent falling have been observed in ablation studies in primates.[8] No tremor of the limbs and no change in reflexes or tone are seen. This part of the cerebellum is relatively independent from the rest of the cerebrum, lacking substantial cerebral cortical input.[45] It does, however, have close connections with the vestibular system, both sensory and motor components. Thus, it is involved in the automatic (and autonomous) regulation of whole body position, i.e., posture.[49] It has been called "a closed loop system that regulates the segmental reflexes important in postural fixation or truncal movement."[4]

As noted earlier in the section regarding nystagmus, this section of the cerebellum is involved in phasic eye and head movements as well. In addition to the ocular motor aberrancies produced with lesions in this area, humans with lesions of the cerebellar vermis will tend to have a wide-based, ataxic gait, reeling and staggering as if drunk. When the lesion is in one cerebellar hemisphere, patients may tend to fall to the side of the lesion, but this is secondary to defective control of the affected leg, not weakness. Balance in hemispheric (lateral) lesions is often surprisingly well maintained in distinction to vermal lesions. Victor et al., in 1959, showed a clinical correlation with the somatotopic map,[70,71] namely, that the marked and disproportionate gait disturbance in alcoholic cerebellar degeneration is related to the earliest and most marked degeneration in the most ante-

rior folia of the vermis, associated with control of the lower extremities.[72] In this condition, marked ataxia during standing and ambulation is observed, as well as dysmetric heel-to-shin maneuver of the legs. The arms are relatively spared, however. Patients walk with a staggering, wide-based gait. Also noted are exaggerated positive supporting reactions, seen as well in dog ablation models. Some authors believe that gait ataxia is the only sign that can be ascribed to anterior lobe lesions in man, but that in order to use gait ataxia as a sign indicating involvement of the anterior vermis, there must be few or no signs of involvement of the posterior vermis or neocerebellum.[5] Lesions restricted to the neocerebellum produce no equilibrium disturbances or primary gait ataxia. Dow and Moruzzi pointed out that with the patient lying in bed, the movement abnormalities so easily seen during ambulation could not be appreciated with volitional movements of the lower extremities.[8]

Another interesting phenomenon that has been described is the evanescent character of the signs seen. Isolated unilateral lesions in the fastigial nucleus of the monkey produced equilibrium disturbances with a staggering gait and falling to the side of the lesion, whereas bilateral lesions produced the same but more pronounced errors in coordination of gait and in equilibrium.[8] However, these lasted only briefly and became attenuated and subsequently resolved in as little as 2 weeks. In regard to human clinical relevance, this "extraordinary capacity for compensation" may be the reason why isolated lesions restricted to cerebellar parenchyma that are slow growing, such as some tumors, can become quite substantial in size before any deficit in cerebellar function is appreciated.[8]

PARAVERMAL SYNDROME

There does not seem to be a discrete intermediate cerebellar syndrome in humans, because of the unlikelihood of lesions

TABLE 44-1 Categories of Cerebellar Syndromes

Properties	Vermal Zone	Paravermal Zone	Lateral Zone
Deep cerebellar nuclei	Fastigial	Interpositus (globose and emboliform)	Dentate
Afferents	Mostly from periphery and brain stem, little from cerebral cortex	From periphery, brain stem, and cerebral cortex (particularly motor cortex)	Mostly from the cerebral cortex, little from the periphery
Efferents	Mostly to brain stem and spinal cord, little to the cerebral cortex	Both to brain stem and cerebral cortex	Mostly to cerebral cortex, but also to brain stem
Timing of changes in neuronal activity	After activity changes in the motor cortex and after movement	After activity changes in the motor cortex and just before movement onset	Before activity changes the motor cortex and before movement
Putative functions	Affects control of posture and balance	May be involved in on-line modification of the motor program such as efferent copy mechanisms	Develops programs for volitional movement, particularly for the limb
Clinical symptomatology	Gait and truncal ataxia that may spare volitional movement of the extremities, also called "axial ataxia"	No distinguishing symptoms or signs as lesions usually not restricted to this area	Produces ataxia and tremor, particularly of the extremities during volitional movement, called "appendicular ataxia"

restricted to this area. The anterior portion of the nucleus interpositus projects to the magnocellular portion of the red nucleus, whereas the posterior portion primarily innervates the vestibular complex and secondarily projects to the red nucleus. This intermediate portion of the cerebellum is believed to regulate the spatially organized and skilled movements of ipsilateral limbs, as well as the posture and tone associated with them, according to the ablation experiments done in cats by Chambers and Sprague.[60,61] Recent studies of movement-related mossy fiber discharges in nonhuman primates reveal that the intermediate cerebellum receives information regarding velocity, position, and direction of movement from individual forelimb muscles. In turn, these interpositus neurons incorporate this information and help coordinate movement of the whole limb, with an emphasis on hand and finger joint manipulation.[73] The term "spinocerebellum" is roughly analogous to this area, as it receives somatotopic afferent projections from the spinal cord through the spinocerebellar tracts. The dorsal part of the spinocerebellar tract relays information about peripheral sensory events, providing the cerebellum with evolving movement information. The ventral spinocerebellar tract relays information from segmental interneurons that integrate both peripheral and descending information, a sort of internal feedback loop.[36] This feedback informs the cerebellum of the effect of its output to the red nucleus and ultimately to the spinal cord, therefore involving it in the constant update of intended movement.[45]

LATERAL ZONE

In animal ablation studies lesions in the lateral zone, or neocerebellum, produce no lasting changes in postural tone or in deep tendon reflexes.[60,61] Tremor was mainly attributed to dentate nucleus lesioning. It was Gordon Holmes, however, who brought the classic signs of lateral cerebellar deficiency to light in human subjects. His description has been called "the clearest which has ever been presented."[8] As mentioned previously, the lateral cerebellum is concerned chiefly with the timing of movement. Lesions are manifested by the signs of dysmetria, tremor, dysdiadochokinesia, hypotonia, and decomposition of movement. Lesions restricted to the lateral cerebellum in humans produce no equilibrium or balance disturbances or primary gait disorders.

Patients studied with lateral cerebellar lesions have shown in experimental situations that the lateral regions of the cerebellum are needed for accurate timing. Medial regions are mainly involved in implementation and execution of motor responses or ongoing regulation of movement.[74] This agrees with the hypothesis that lateral cerebellar regions contribute to movement planning and that the more medial zones contribute to movement execution, correction, and regulation.

NYSTAGMUS

Before describing the eye findings in cerebellar disease, definitions of different types of eye movements will be provided to serve as a basis for the discussion. Nystagmus is a rhythmic back and forth oscillation of the eyes. Pendular nystagmus has smooth, equal velocity in both directions of gaze whereas jerk nystagmus is characterized by a slow drift, followed by a quick corrective phase in the opposite direction. Saccades are rapid eye movements, bringing the fovea to bear almost immediately on the target. They quickly change visual fixation. Pursuit refers to slow eye movements. Convergence refers to slow movements that bring both eyes onto a close target. The VOR is seen when eye deviation or nystagmus occurs in response to vestibular system stimulation by caloric testing (irrigation of the ears with either warm or cold water) or by angular acceleration or deceleration. (Caloric stimulation with cold water causes nystagmus with the fast component to the opposite side, whereas warm water produces nystagmus with the fast component to the same side in a normally functioning brain.) The VOR is largely responsible for image stabilization during movements of the head and eyes.

In regard to nystagmus, the first report to document ocular motor abnormalities was published in 1973, when Westheimer and Blair described findings in monkeys after total cerebellectomy.[75] These included defects in holding eccentric positions of gaze, smooth pursuit, convergence, and optokinetic nystagmus. It was reported soon thereafter that hemicerebellectomy produced the same defects on the ipsilateral side of the lesion.[76] A persistent saccadic dysmetria is also seen after complete cerebellectomy in the monkey.[77] Their report and others[78] revealed that the dorsal cerebellar vermis, paravermis, and fastigial nuclei are necessary for proper placement of saccades. These lesions of the cerebellar vermis also tend to affect the magnitude of ipsilateral saccades.[83] Selhorst et al., in 1976, revealed similar findings in humans with cerebellar lesions and reported that lesions of the dorsal vermis and underlying fastigial nucleus lead to abnormally large saccades or hypermetria of saccades.[80,81] It is postulated that the cerebellar vermis acts as a calibrator organ by constantly adjusting the gain of the direct visual motor pathway, without actually being in the direct loop. With a cerebellar lesion (vermian lesion), this control is lost, and the gain subsequently increases, leading to overshoot of saccades or dysmetria of saccades. In fact, the authors propose that "saccadic overshoot dysmetria is a specific ocular motor sign occurring only in patients with cerebellar disease."[80]

Lesions of the deep cerebellar nuclei have been shown to cause saccadic oscillations, defined as horizontal clusters of saccades that reverberate about the intended fixation point and take the fovea off the target.[81] At the bedside, patients will often report a blurring of vision as they attempt to fixate on the intended target because of inability to keep the visual image on the fovea. Another proposed function, then, of this part of the cerebellum is to provide long-term adaptation functions that correlate eye movements correctly to the visual stimulus or target, thereby correcting for ocular motor dysmetria and ensuring accuracy of saccades.[12]

In addition to the vermis and fastigial nuclei, the flocculus and paraflocculus are important in coordinating eye movement. Ablation studies of this part of the cerebellum in monkeys has led to impaired smooth pursuit, whether the head is still or moving.[82] Furthermore, rebound nystagmus, downbeat nystagmus, and horizontal gaze-evoked nystagmus were shown to result from such ablations. These observations are evidence that the flocculus is important in preventing retinal slip and in stabilizing gaze holding.[77] In regard to the VOR, Ito showed that the flocculus monitors the gain of the VOR to provide visual stability during movements of the head. The flocculus does so by direct connections to the vestibular nuclei.[83] This allows for compensation of head movement by allowing the eyes to move appropriately, thereby reducing blur to a minimum. When a lesion occurs affecting the flocculus, the gain of the VOR is increased, as the flocculus normally has inhibitory control of the VOR, leading to retinal slip and image destabilization.

Kornhuber, in 1973, categorized the eye findings in cerebellar pathology differently.[84] He dichotomized the aberrant eye movements on the basis of cortical versus nuclear disease. In cerebellar cortex disease, he found that dysmetria of saccadic eye movements usually occurs, with preservation of smooth pursuit. The dysmetria is usually of the hypometric form, in which the patient initiates eye movement in the correct direction but fails to reach the target, resulting in many smaller saccades, rather than in one single large movement. The anatomic location for production of voluntary saccades lies in the middle part of the vermis around the primary fissure. A lesion in this area then leads to ipsilateral hypometria of saccades. With unilateral lesioning of the cerebellar cortex in this area, unilateral dysmetria is encountered. He found the best examples of cerebellar dysmetria of saccades to result from subacute cerebellar cortical atrophy. He then looked at the literature regarding cerebellar eye movements in relation to cerebellar nuclear lesions and found that the nucleus interpositus is responsible for active eye holding. Nashold and Slaughter, in their lesion studies in humans, found that coagulation of the nucleus interpositus and medial dentate led to ipsilateral gaze paralysis. Pure lesioning of the dentate nucleus, taking care to spare the interpositus nucleus, caused no oculomotor deficits.[85] Kornhuber concluded that the cerebellar cortex functions to preprogram saccadic (discontinuous) eye movements, whereas the nucleus interpositus functions to govern the continuous hold command. (He was quick to point out, however, that the commands for voluntary saccades do not originate in the cerebellum but rather in the forebrain.)[84]

Thus, the cerebellum plays an integral role in maintaining both adequate visual fixation and stabilization during eye movements. Saccadic overshoot dysmetria is considered to be consistent with a lesion in the vermis, whereas retinal slip is found with flocculus lesions. Other categories of nystagmus are not as specific, owing to the degree of complexity and integration of the structures involved. The distinct message is that one type of nystagmus, saccadic overshoot dysmetria, appears to be specific to the cerebellum.

DYSARTHRIA

Speech disturbances are most often seen in patients with bilateral or diffuse cerebellar lesions, although it has been shown pathologically that the midportion of the vermis and adjacent paravermian regions are likely to produce such dysfunction.[5,72] In contrast, the work of Amici et al. found that the cerebellar dysarthric pattern was more common in lesions of the lateral and intermediate cerebellar zones in their group of approximately 250 patients.[6] The classic work by Dow and Moruzzi, in 1958, although not greatly expanded on, also localized the ataxic dysarthria to the lateral zones as well.[8]

A most intriguing twist to the dysarthria story came in 1978, when Lechtenberg and Gilman published their results of patients with dysarthria and focal cerebellar disease.[86] They found a surprising correlation between dysarthria and focal left cerebellar hemisphere disease; in fact, 22 of 31 patients with dysarthria had mainly or exclusively left cerebellar hemisphere disease, whereas only two patients had vermal disease. Like Amici et al., they found no correlation between lesions of the vermis and ataxic dysarthria.[6] This report is not as clear-cut as it seems, however, because of the patient population studied. Most of the lesions were tumors, producing mass effect and most likely affecting other nearby structures. This, then, opens a new insight into cerebellar physiology. Could it be that the contralateral connections with the nondominant right cerebral hemisphere help to explain the qualities of cerebellar speech? The evidence seems to point in that direction.

Grammar, per se, is not affected in cerebellar speech disorders. Rather, it is prosody and intonation that are affected. It has been proposed that the right hemisphere is concerned with the perception of harmony and melody.[87] This holds true, except for professional musicians.[88] This cerebrocerebellar link seems to be a plausible reason as to why predominantly left cerebellar hemisphere lesions are involved in dysarthric speech. Certainly, more work needs to be done to better elucidate the anatomic substrate for the entity known as ataxic dysarthria.

Mechanisms of Dysfunction

Typically, when cerebellar symptomatology is evident in a patient, it is because of ischemia, stroke, demyelination, tumor, mass effect, degeneration, or other such pathology. These lesions may involve the cerebellar parenchyma directly or may disrupt any one or more of the numerous inputs to or outputs from the cerebellum (nuclei, tracts, etc.), leading to a disconnection syndrome. Another possibility exists, however, whereby a remote area of pathology leads to secondary cerebellar dysfunction. One example is known as crossed cerebellar diaschisis; examples of this phenomenon have already been described.[13–16]

Originally defined by von Monakow in the early part of this century, diaschisis is a potentially reversible functional hypometabolism. The first description relating the cerebellum with the cerebrum in terms of this concept was provided by Baron et al., in 1980, who presented cases in which there was a matched decrease in cerebral blood flow and oxygen metabolism in the cerebellar hemisphere contralateral to a cerebral infarct, ipsilateral to clinical symptoms (typically, hemiparesis).[89] Of interest is the finding that the diaschisis appears to be reversible, in that the phenomenon was not observed for more than 2 months after cerebral infarct. Another study of 55 patients with a single infarct in the distribution of the internal carotid artery revealed crossed cerebellar diaschisis in 58 percent of the patients.[90] Two processes may be suggested by this finding, according to the authors: That transient hypometabolism could indeed represent true diaschisis or that persistent contralateral cerebellar degeneration may represent corticopontocerebellar transsynaptic degeneration. That the association of cerebellar hypometabolism was more prominent with involvement of the cortex or the internal capsule lends support to the latter hypothesis.

Cerebellar glucose metabolism has also been studied in relation to patients with aphasia.[91] Of 37 patients with aphasia resulting from left cerebral infarcts or hemorrhages, 21 were found to have contralateral cerebellar hypometabolism; interestingly, all of the patients with Broca's aphasia (8 of 37) were found to have decreased right cerebellar glucose metabolic rates. The significance of this finding may not be fully appreciated; suffice it to say that this, and other studies, revealing contralateral cerebellar hypometabolism in PET studies highlight the importance of the association of cortex, cerebellum, and the connections in between for motor, and perhaps, language system integrity.

The Cerebellum and Learning

Marr, in an eloquent dissertation regarding the theory of motor programming in 1969, proposed that the cerebellum actually learns to perform motor skills.[92] The tenet basic to his theory is that the afferent input via the mossy fibers are transformed into a language that is stored; he called this the "codon representation of an input." He goes on to propose that during learning, the cerebral cortex organizes the movement, causing the appropriate olivary cells to fire in a specified sequence. This, in turn, causes the Purkinje cells to fire in a correctly sequenced manner for that particular movement. Then, the next time a similar command appears, the activity of the mossy fibers stimulates the Purkinje cell, now "familiar" with the desired movement. This would constitute a learned response. He proposed that the function of the climbing fiber input was to modify the response of Purkinje neurons to mossy fiber input by increasing the effectiveness of the mossy fiber synapses on the Purkinje cells.[92] During execution of a learned movement, the mossy fibers are responsible for the initiation of the various basic movements. It is, therefore, essential that during learning, the Purkinje cell is associated with the desired movement, or context of movement, immediately before performing the organism's elemental movement.

Some background information about input to the Purkinje cell is justified before proceeding. Each Purkinje cell receives two types of excitatory input, each of which generates different action potentials. The multiple parallel fiber inputs from granule cells cause simple spikes, whereas the single climbing fiber input produces complex spikes. (Recall that each granule cell collects input from many mossy fibers.) The simple spike corresponds to the short-latency cerebellar evoked potential of 2–6 ms, whereas the complex spike is the long latency response of 12–25 ms.[93]

In work by Gilbert and Thach, in 1977,[94] monkeys were trained to hold onto a movable handle and to keep that handle in a particular location by using wrist flexors or exten-

sors; a motor was applied that could easily change the load that the monkeys were accustomed to moving at random times. The monkeys were trained for many months to move a fixed load. It was found that the control response (no load increase) generated random simple spikes with intermittent complex spikes. When load was suddenly increased, the number of complex spikes increased, and after practice at this new load the number of complex spikes returned to control values. On the other hand, there was a marked decrease in the frequency of *simple* spike discharges, both during the initial load increase and after practice, after the complex spikes had returned to baseline values.

The study showed that the activity of the climbing fiber is modulated during motor learning, which suggests that the modulation might serve to reduce the strength of the mossy fiber input to the Purkinje cells. This would then lead to a decrease in Purkinje cell firing, and, because of this disinhibition, lead ultimately to an increased output of the deep cerebellar nuclei. The authors contend that the results of their experiment support the theories of cerebellar learning, which propose that complex spike frequency changes should occur during learning.[94] The initial increase of complex spike firing, followed by the decrease in firing rate, corresponded to the time period needed to relearn the task with a new load. In regard to the simple spike data, it is proposed that there could be a decrease in strength of the parallel fiber synapses on Purkinje cells when the climbing fibers are active during learning. This agrees with the hypothesis put forward by Albus in 1971; he believed that climbing fibers can decrease mossy fiber activity via what he termed "heterosynaptic inhibition."[57] He said that this was needed and designed to correct any discrepancy between the intended movement and the actual movement produced.

It is hypothesized that the strength of parallel fiber excitation of Purkinje cells is magnified after climbing fiber excitation of Purkinje cells.[67,68] The importance of climbing fiber discharge during the learning phase may relate to Hebbian learning.[95] This concept holds that the discharge of the climbing fiber ensures to reinforce the effect of other afferents to the Purkinje cell. This may change the way the Purkinje cell will respond to the inputs in the future and not require continued simultaneous activity in the climbing fiber. This long-lasting change in Purkinje response to the other inputs would constitute learning.

While the work of Gilbert and Thach showed indirect evidence that the cerebellum is involved in motor learning, direct evidence for the same came from the work of Robinson with the VOR, in which he showed that when the flocculus is lesioned, the gain of the reflex is no longer modifiable.[96]

The cerebellum has also been implicated in connection with classical conditioning. Experiments in rabbits use the nictitating membrane response (NMR), in which a puff of air to the eye (unconditioned stimulus) provokes a blink (unconditioned response). This unconditioned stimulus is then paired with the conditioned stimuli of white noise and light. The NMR then occurs in response to the conditioned stimulus with the unconditioned stimuli. Lesions of the ipsilateral dentate-interpositus nuclei terminate the classically conditioned response.[97] These authors also stated that rabbits or cats can preserve this response after all brain tissue superior to the thalamus has been removed; it was then surmised that some structure below the thalamus must be necessary to preserve the response.

Yeo et al., in 1985, were more selective in their lesion experiments and discovered that it is the anterior division of the interpositus nucleus, as well as its afferent connection with lobule VI (lobulus simplex), that abolishes the NMR conditioning and also prevents relearning of the response.[98,99] In other words, the rabbit loses the ability to learn the conditioned response on the ipsilateral side of the lesion, even though the eye still blinks in response to the puff of air. If the rabbit had learned the conditioned response before a cerebellar lesion in the regions was noted, the conditioned response vanishes on the ipsilateral side, whereas the conditioned response on the contralateral side remains intact. Two recent reports have extended these observations to human subjects with damaged cerebellar circuitry, implying that the cerebellum is essential for the classically conditioned somatic response.[100,101]

There is evidence that in the course of the evolution of humans, the dentate nucleus has undergone a marked expansion that seems to parallel the growth of the cerebral cortex in the frontal lobes. There appears to be a newly evolved part of the dentate that is macrogyric and located ventrolaterally (called the neodentate), whereas the older, microgyric part is located dorsomedially.[54] It has been argued that the increased size of the dentate paralleling the increased size of the frontal cortex is evidence for the dentate influencing the frontal cortex. In humans it has also been shown that the primary target of the neodentate is the frontal lobe, motor areas 4 and 6, as well as projections to the inferior prefrontal cortex (areas 44 and 45, Broca's area), and area 8, the superior prefrontal cortex.[54] These authors go on to state that, in addition to functioning as the purely motor aspect of word articulation, Broca's prefrontal area and the surrounding prefrontal areas subserve the function of word finding, a cognitive process. Thus, by virtue of the neodentate's connection to Broca's prefrontal area, the neodentate also may be involved with cognitive processing.

The authors further expand their theory by postulating that a neural loop exists in which motor commands from association areas of the cortex not only travel to the cerebellum via pontine pathways but also send a copy of the commands through the red nucleus and then the inferior olive. The latter then sends its climbing fibers into the cerebellar cortex and to the neodentate[54] (Fig. 44-11). Ito proposes a similar neural loop.[102] In this fashion the cerebellum receives a copy of the motor command that can be regarded as a motor simulation, or motor imagery. In this way the cerebellum participates in a feedforward control in which the actual motor command is compared with prior memories from earlier training, improving its output. Leiner et al. further postulate that the input to the red nucleus, in addition to providing motor command information, can also allow the neodentate to participate in language functions as well.[54] It is unproven that the dentate is involved in the cognitive process of word finding, as well as in the motor process of word articulation.

Several recent studies using neuroimaging have given us new insights regarding the role of the cerebellum in higher functioning, particularly language. In a study by Petersen

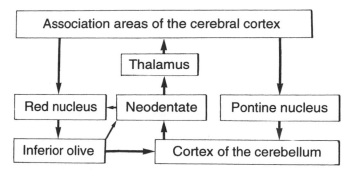

FIGURE 44-11 Diagram of the neural loop showing the connections between the cerebellum and cerebral cortex as postulated by Leiner, Leiner, and Dow[54] (see text). (*From Leiner et al.[54] Used with permission.*)

and Fiez in 1993, normal human subjects were required to generate a cognitive association between words.[103] They were presented a noun and were asked to think (not speak) of a verb associated with that noun (for instance, "dog" and "bark"). During this rule-based word generation task, using PET, it was found that the right lateral-inferior portion of the cerebellum was activated. This was anatomically distinct from the paramedian cerebellar activation that occurred during motor tasks, including speech (Fig. 44-12 and Fig. 44-13, respectively). Another study, using single-photon emission computed tomography (SPECT), required 17 normal human subjects to count silently and to imagine certain movement sequences via motor imagery, both purely cognitive tasks. Again, the inferior lateral part of the cerebellum was markedly activated during both cognitive tasks, supporting the notion that temporally organized planning of future motor acts depends on the integrity of the lateral inferior cerebellum. This is not identical to those parts of the cerebellum

FIGURE 44-12 Sagittal slices through averaged subtraction images are shown of subjects asked to think of a verb associated with a noun utilizing PET technology. Note the activation in several prefrontal regions, (*A*), the anterior cingulate (*B*), and in the contralateral cerebellar hemisphere (*C*). Note the difference between this and the paramedian activation of the cerebellum during motor tasks. (*From Peterson et al.[103] Used with permission.*)

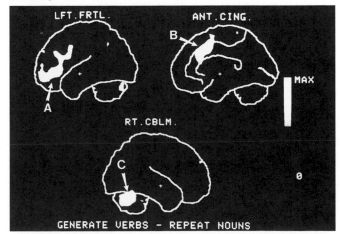

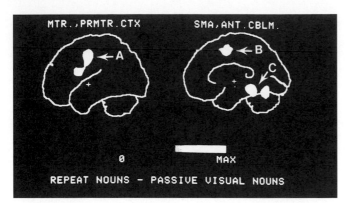

FIGURE 44-13 Sagittal slices through averaged subtraction images are displayed of subjects asked to repeat nouns aloud that were visually presented. Note the activation in the left motor (*upper*) and premotor (*lower*) cortex (*A*). The image on the *right* shows supplementary motor cortex activation (*upper, B*) and midline cerebellum activation (*lower, C*). Notice the difference in the areas of cerebellar activation between this task and the verb generation task. (*From Petersen et al.[103] Used with permission.*)

that are activated during actual voluntary motor movement, namely, the superior part of the vermis[104] (Fig. 44-14).

A third line of evidence for cerebellar cognitive processing, obtained by way of neuroimaging, is from the recent work of Kim et al.[103] In this study humans were imaged in a 4-Tesla magnetic resonance imaging (MRI) device while performing two tasks. The first task involved a visually guided task, moving pegs from one end of a pegboard to another. The other task involved solving a puzzle, a sort of brain teaser requiring cognitive processing (Fig. 44-15). During attempts to solve the puzzle a dramatic bilateral activation was seen in the dentate nucleus in all seven participants, with an intensity three to four times greater than that seen during the visually guided movement of pegs (Figs. 44-16 and 44-17). Again, the conclusion was reached that the dentate is involved in cognitive processing and that the specific regions responsible are distinct from those activated during eye and limb movement control.

A different approach was used by Middleton and Strick, in 1994, when they examined the retrograde transneuronal transport of herpes simplex virus type I (HSV-1).[106] The HSV-1 was injected into area 46, the dorsolateral prefrontal cortex,

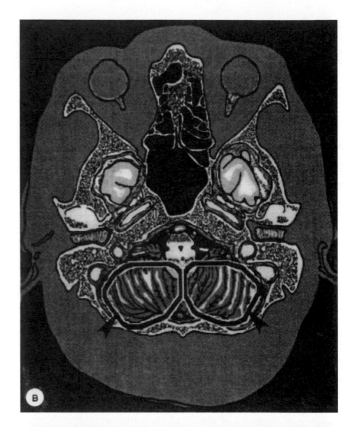

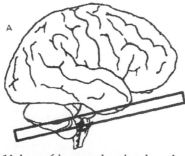

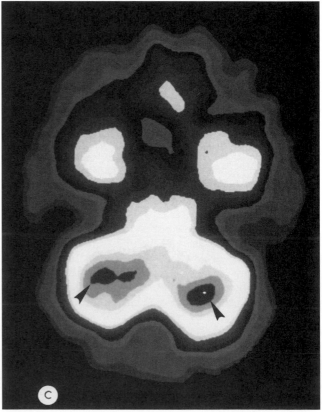

FIGURE 44-14 Area of increased regional cerebral blood flow (rCBF) during mental imagery. *A.* Lateral view of the brain; the boxed area is that corresponding to the orbitomeatal line. *B.* Anatomic model of the area of interest, 1 cm below the orbitomeatal line, where the thick black lines encircle the area affected. *C.* An actual SPECT rCBF recording, where the higher ⁹⁹ᵐTc-HMPAO (rCBF) levels are indicated by the darkened "bulls-eye"-shaped areas within each cerebellar hemisphere (lateral cerebellum). (*From Ryding et al.[104] Used with permission.*)

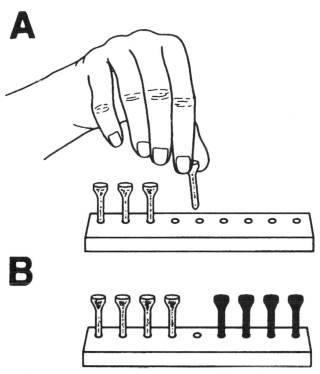

A

B

FIGURE 44-15 Sketch of the tasks performed in the work by Kim et al.[105] (see text). *A.* For the visually guided task, pegs were moved one at a time from one end of the pegboard to another. *B.* The brain teaser task involved moving the four pegs of each color from one end to the other. Three rules existed: Only one peg could be moved at a time; a peg could only be moved forward, never backward; and a peg could be moved to an adjacent open space or could jump an adjacent peg of a different color. *(From Kim et al.[105] Used with permission.)*

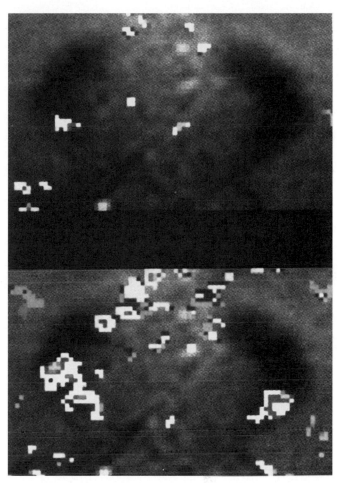

FIGURE 44-16 Functional maps of dentate nucleus during activation for one patient during the visually guided task (*top*) and during the brain teaser task (*bottom*). The dentate nuclei are the dark crescent-shaped areas with decreased signal intensity. Note the dramatic increase in dentate activation during the brain teaser task as opposed to the visually guided movement task. (See Fig. 44-17 for structure identification). *(From Kim et al.[105] Used with permission.)*

which is known to be involved in spatial working memory and in planning the order and timing of future behavior. Retrograde transneuronal transport of the virus was noted to occur in many neurons of the dentate nucleus, mostly contralateral to the injection site and mostly in the ventral portion, concentrated there primarily in the middle third of the dentate. The authors pointed out that this region of the dentate differs considerably from more dorsal nucleus regions, which have been labeled in other experiments from motor and premotor areas, and from more caudal nucleus regions, which have been labeled from frontal eye fields. The results provide evidence that the dorsolateral prefrontal cortex is one of the targets of dentate nucleus output, separate from those with connections to cerebral cortex motor areas.[106]

It is proposed, then, that based on the preceding evidence that the region of the neodentate may be involved in cognitive planning, practice-related learning, error detection, learning arbitrary associations between words, judging time intervals, and cognitive processing in three-dimensional space.[54] This area of cerebellar research is currently a hotbed of activity and, as more is uncovered about how the cerebellum processes information, the effects of cerebellar disease on higher cognitive functions may be more recognized. The current evidence favors a direct link (see the review by Schmahmann in Ref. 107).

FIGURE 44-17 Line drawing corresponding to the functional maps of dentate nucleus (see Fig. 44-16).

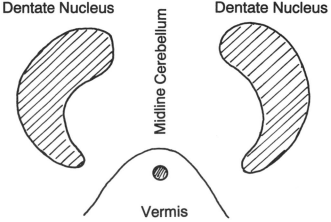

Dentate Nucleus   **Dentate Nucleus**

Midline Cerebellum

Vermis

Summary

The functions of the cerebellum and the pathophysiology of the symptoms and signs of cerebellar dysfunction have become more understood and, at the same time, more complex. Analysis of kinematics and EMG behaviors disordered by cerebellar disease point to a set of fundamental mechanisms. Chief of these mechanisms is abnormalities in the timing of activity in muscles synergistic and antagonistic to the intended movements. The abnormalities of muscle activations lead to dysmetria. Most of the classical symptoms and signs of cerebellar disease can be considered special cases of dysmetria. Hypotonia is another fundamental abnormality, but its contributions to the classical symptoms and signs of cerebellar disease is unclear and only incidental.

Although there may be only a few fundamental mechanisms underlying the symptoms and signs of cerebellar disease, the manifestations of this mechanism differ according to the region of the cerebellum affected. Thus, there is a regional differentiation. Initially, syndromes defined by a specific constellation of symptoms and signs were defined by the classical lobar anatomic descriptions. Newer concepts of functional organization are now based on longitudinal zones. These zones are consistent with the anatomic connections between the deep cerebellar nuclei and the cerebellar cortex projecting to the nuclei. This longitudinal organization is also consistent with efferent and afferent connections to and from the cerebellum and the timing of activity changes relative to movement generation. These concepts have heuristic value in increasing the understanding of how cerebellar disorders present clinically. These concepts aid in differential diagnosis.

Until recently, the primary, if not only, role of the cerebellum has been related to the control of movement. Recent studies have now shown a possible role of the cerebellum, particularly the dentate nucleus, in cognitive functions including, but not limited to, language. Although the clinical syndromes typically identified today do not include symptoms and signs of cognitive dysfunction, better understanding of these functions, as well as better testing instruments, may clearly identify abnormalities in these domains.

Although much has been learned about the function and dysfunction of the cerebellum, much more remains to be done. Compared to our understanding of the basal ganglia, less is known about the cerebellum. Consequently, the development of therapeutics for cerebellar diseases has lagged far behind those for basal ganglia diseases. Yet, cerebellar disorders are a common and important source of disability and suffering. Hopefully, scientists and clinicians will have an opportunity in the future to narrow this gap of knowledge.

References

1. Luciani L: *Il Cervelletto: Nuori Studi de Fisiologia Normale e Patologica.* Florence: Le Monnier, 1891.
2. Luciani L: *Muscular and Nervous System,* translated by FA Welby. London: MacMillan, 1915, vol 3.
3. Holmes G: The symptoms of acute cerebellar injuries due to gunshot injuries. *Brain* 40:461–535, 1917.
4. Gilman S, Bloedel JR, Lechtenberg R: *Disorders of the Cerebellum.* Philadelphia: F.A. Davis, 1981.
5. Nyberg-Hansen R, Horn J: Functional aspects of cerebellar signs in clinical neurology. *Acta Neurol Scand Suppl* 51:219–245, 1972.
6. Amici R, Avanzini G, Pacini L: Cerebellar tumors: Clinical analysis and physiopathologic correlations, in *Monographs in Neural Science.* Basel, Switzerland: Karger, 1976, vol 4.
7. Holmes G: The cerebellum of man. *Brain* 62:1–30, 1939.
8. Dow RS, Moruzzi G: *The Physiology and Pathology of the Cerebellum.* Minneapolis: The University of Minneapolis Press, 1958.
9. Wertham FI: A new sign of cerebellar disease. *J Nerv Ment Dis* 69:486–493, 1929.
10. Zentay PJ: Motor disorders of the central nervous system and their significance for speech: Cerebral and cerebellar dysarthrias (part I). *Laryngoscope* 47:147–156, 1937.
11. Brown JR, Darley FL, Aronson AE: Ataxic dysarthria. *Int J Neurol* 7:302–318, 1970.
12. Miller NR: *Walsh and Hoyt's Clinical Neuro-Ophthalmology,* 4th ed. Baltimore: Williams & Wilkins, 1988, pp 618–746.
13. Montgomery EBM Jr: Signs and symptoms from a cerebral lesion that suggest cerebellar dysfunction. *Arch Neurol* 40:422–423, 1983.
14. Garcin R: The ataxias: Disturbances of nervous function, in Vinken PJ, Bruyn GW (eds): *Handbook of Clinical Neurology.* Amsterdam, North-Holland Publishing Co, 1969, vol 1, pp 309–355.
15. Grant FC: Cerebellar symptoms produced by supratentorial tumors. *AMA Arch Neurol* 20:292–308, 1928.
16. Frazier CH: Tumor involving the frontal lobe alone. *AMA Arch Neurol* 35:525–571, 1936.
17. Vilis T, Hore J: Central neural mechanisms contributing to cerebellar tremor produced by limb perturbations. *J Neurophysiol* 43:279–291, 1980.
18. Montgomery EBM Jr, Gorman DS, Nuessen J: Motor initiation versus execution in normal and Parkinson's disease subjects. *Neurology* 41:1469–1475, 1991.
19. Hallett M, Shahani BT, Young RR: EMG analysis of stereotyped voluntary movements in man. *J Neurol Neurosurg Psychiatry* 38:1154–1162, 1975.
20. Flament D, Hore J: Movement and electromyographic disorders associated with cerebellar dysmetria. *J Neurophysiol* 55:1221–1233, 1986.
21. Hallett M, Shahani BT, Young RR: EMG analysis of patients with cerebellar deficits. *J Neurol Neurosurg Psychiatry* 38:1163–1169, 1975.
22. Hore J, Wild B, Diener HC: Cerebellar dysmetria at the elbow, wrist, and fingers. *J Neurophysiol* 65:563–571, 1991.
23. Hallett M, Berardelli A, Matheson J, et al: Physiological analysis of simple rapid movements in patients with cerebellar deficits. *J Neurol Neurosurg Psychiatry* 53:124–133, 1991.
24. Thach WT: Timing of activity in cerebellar dentate nucleus and cerebral motor cortex during prompt volitional movement. *Brain Res* 88:233–241, 1975.
25. Meyer-Lohmann J, Hore J, Brooks VB: Cerebellar participation in generation of prompt arm movements. *J Neurophysiol* 40:1038–1050, 1977.
26. Hore J, Vilis T: A cerebellar-dependent efference copy mechanism for generating appropriate muscle responses to limb perturbations, in Bloedel JR, Dichgans J, Precht W (eds): *Cerebellar Functions.* Berlin: Springer-Verlag, 1984, pp 24–35.
27. Vilis T, Hore J: Characteristics of saccadic dysmetria in monkeys during reversible lesions of medical cerebellar nuclei. *J Neurophysiol* 46:828–838, 1981.
28. Sternberg S, Monsell S, Knoll RL, Wright CE: The latency and duration of rapid movement sequences: Comparison of speech and typewriting, in Stelmach GE (ed): *Information Processing in*

Motor Control and Learning. New York: Academic Press, 1978, pp 117–152.

29. Robertson LT, Grimm RJ: Responses of primate dentate neurons to different trajectories of the limb. *Exp Brain Res* 23:447–462, 1975.

30. Inhoff AW, Diener HC, Rafal RD, Ivry R: The role of cerebellar structures in the execution of serial movements. *Brain* 112:565–581, 1989.

31. Ivry RB, Keele SW: Timing functions of the cerebellum. *J Cogn Neurosci* 1:136–152, 1989.

32. Braitenberg V: Is the cerebellar cortex a biological clock in the millisecond range? *Prog Brain Res* 25:334–346, 1967.

33. Sherrington CS: *The Integrative Action of the Nervous System.* New York: Charles Scribner's Sons, 1906.

34. Guyton AC: *Textbook of Medical Physiology.* Philadelphia: WB Saunders, 1986.

35. Granit R: *The Basis of Motor Control.* London: Academic Press, 1970.

36. Kandel ER, Schwartz JH, Jessell TM (eds): *Principles of Neural Science.* Norwalk, CT: Appleton & Lange, 1991.

37. Gilman S: The mechanism of cerebellar hypotonia. *Brain* 92:621–638, 1969.

38. Liu CN, Chambers WW: A study of cerebellar dyskinesia in the bilaterally deafferented forelimbs of the monkey (Macaca mulatta and Macaca speciosa). *ACTA Neurobiol Exp* 31:263–289, 1971.

39. Gilman S, Carr D, Hollenberg J: Kinematic effects of deafferentation and cerebellar ablation. *Brain* 99:311–330, 1976.

40. Ito M: Neurophysiological aspects of the cerebellar motor control system. *Int J Neurol* 7:162–176, 1970.

41. Eccles JC: Circuits in the cerebellar control of movement. *Proc Natl Acad Sci U S A* 58:336–343, 1967.

42. Eccles JC: The role of the cerebellum in controlling movement, in Downman CBB (ed): *Modern Trends in Physiology.* London: Butterworth, 1972, vol 1, pp 86–111.

43. Eccles JC, Sabah NH, Schmidt RF, Taborikova H: Mode of operation of the cerebellum in the dynamic loop control of movement. *Brain Res* 40:73–80, 1972.

44. Walshe FMR: The significance of the voluntary element in the genesis of cerebellar ataxy. *Brain* 50:377–385, 1927.

45. Evarts EV, Thach WT: Motor mechanisms of the CNS: Cerebrocerebellar interrelations. *Annu Rev Physiol* 31:451–498, 1969.

46. Ito M: A new physiological concept on cerebellum. *Rev Neurol (Paris)* 146:564–569, 1990.

47. Sasaki K, Gemba H: Compensatory motor function of the somatosensory cortex for dysfunction of the motor cortex following cerebellar hemispherectomy in the monkey. *Exp Brain Res* 56:532–538, 1984.

48. Thach WT: Discharge of cerebellar neurons related to two maintained postures and two prompt movements: I. Nuclear cell output (and) II. Purkinje cell output and input. *J Neurophysiol* 33:527–546, 1970.

49. Allen GI, Tsukahara N: Cerebrocerebellar communication systems. *Physiol Rev* 54:957–1006, 1974.

50. Eccles JC: *The Understanding of the Brain.* New York: McGraw Hill, 1977, pp 106–145.

51. Allen GI, Gilbert PFC, Yin TCT: Convergence of cerebral inputs onto dentate neurons in monkey. *Exp Brain Res* 32:151–170, 1978.

52. Nolte J: *The Human Brain.* St. Louis: Mosby-Year Book, 1993, pp 337–359.

53. Carpenter MB: *Core Text of Neuroanatomy.* Baltimore: Williams & Wilkins, 1991, pp 224–249.

54. Leiner HC, Leiner AL, Dow RS: Cognitive and language functions of the human cerebellum. *Trends Neurosci* 16:444–447, 1993.

55. DeMyer W: *Neuroanatomy.* New York: John Wiley & Sons, 1988, pp 187–206.

56. Marr, D: A theory of cerebellar cortex. *J Physiol* 202:437–470, 1969.

57. Albus JS: A theory of cerebellar function. *Math Biosci* 10:25–61, 1971.

58. Jansen J, Brodal, A: Experimental studies on the intrinsic fibers of the cerebellum. II: The cortico-nuclear projection. *J Comp Neurol* 73:267–321, 1940.

59. Carrea RME, Mettler FA: Physiologic consequences following extensive removals of the cerebellar cortex and deep cerebellar nuclei and effect of secondary cerebral ablations in the primate. *J Comp Neurol* 87:169–288, 1947.

60. Chambers WW, Sprague JM: Functional localization in the cerebellum. I: Organization in longitudinal cortico-nuclear zones and their contribution to the control of posture, both extrapyramidal and pyramidal. *J Comp Neurol* 103:105–129, 1955.

61. Chambers WW, Sprague JM: Functional localization in the cerebellum. II: Somatotopic organization in cortex and nuclei. *AMA Arch Neurol Psychiatry* 74:653–680, 1955.

62. Nashold BS Jr, Slaughter DG: Effects of stimulating or destroying the deep cerebellar regions in man. *J Neurosurg* 31:172–186, 1969.

63. Dow RS: Some aspects of cerebellar physiology. *J Neurosurg* 18:512–530, 1961.

64. Snider RS: The cerebellum. *Sci Am* 199:84–90, 1958.

65. Thach W: Correlation of neural discharge with pattern and force of muscular activity, joint position, and direction of the intended movement in motor cortex and cerebellum. *J Neurophysiol* 41:654–676, 1978.

66. Bava A, Grimm R, Rushmer D: Fastigial unit activity during voluntary movement in primates. *Brain Res* 288:371–374, 1983.

67. Eccles JC, Ito M, Szentagothai J: *The Cerebellum as a Neuronal Machine.* New York: Springer-Verlag, 1967.

68. Eccles JC: The cerebellum as a computer: Patterns in space and time. *J Physiol* 229:1–32, 1973.

69. Botterell EH, Fulton JF: Functional localization in the cerebellum of primates. III: Lesions of hemispheres (neocerebellum). *J Comp Neurol* 69:63–87, 1938.

70. Adrian ED: Afferent areas in the cerebellum connected with the limbs. *Brain* 66:289–315, 1943.

71. Snider RS, Eldred E: Cerebro-cerebellar relationships in the monkey. *J Neurophysiol* 15:27–40, 1952.

72. Victor M, Adams RD, Mancall EL: A restricted form of cerebellar cortical degeneration occurring in alcohol patients. *AMA Arch Neurol* 1:579–688, 1959.

73. van Kan PLE, Gibson AR, Houk JC: Movement-related inputs to intermediate cerebellum of the monkey. *J Neurophysiol* 69:74–94, 1993.

74. Ivry RB, Keele SW, Diener HC: Dissociation of the lateral and medial cerebellum in movement timing and movement execution. *Exp Brain Res* 73:167–180, 1988.

75. Westheimer G, Blair SM: Oculomotor defects in cerebellectomized monkeys. *Invest Ophthalmol* 12:618–621, 1973.

76. Westheimer G, Blair SM: Functional organization of primate oculomotor system revealed by cerebellectomy. *Exp Brain Res* 21:463–472, 1974.

77. Optican LM, Robinson DA: Cerebellar-dependent adaptive control of primate saccadic system. *J Neurophysiol* 44:1058–1076, 1980.

78. Ritchie L: Effects of cerebellar lesions on saccadic eye movements. *J Neurophysiol* 39:1246–1256, 1976.

79. Aschoff JC, Cohen B: Changes in saccadic eye movements produced by cerebellar cortical lesions. *Exp Neurol* 32:123–133, 1971.

80. Selhorst JB, Stark L, Ochs AL, Hoyt WF: Disorders in cerebellar ocular motor control. I. Saccadic overshoot dysmetria: An oculographic, control system and clinico-anatomical analysis. *Brain* 99:497–508, 1976.

81. Selhorst JB, Stark L, Ochs AL, Hoyt WF: Disorders in cerebellar ocular motor control. II. Macrosaccadic oscillation: An oculographic, control system and clinico-anatomical analysis. *Brain* 99:509–522, 1976.

82. Zee DS, Yamazaki A, Butler PH, Gucer G: Effects of ablation of flocculus and paraflocculus on eye movements in primate. *J Neurophysiol* 46:878–899, 1981.

83. Ito M: Neural design of the cerebellar motor control system. *Brain Res* 40:81–84, 1972.

84. Kornhuber HH: Cerebellar control of eye movements. *Adv Otorhinolaryngol* 19:241–253, 1973.

85. Nashold BS Jr, Slaughter G, Gills JP: Ocular reactions in man from deep cerebellar stimulation and lesions. *Arch Ophthalmol* 81:538–543, 1969.

86. Lechtenberg R, Gilman S: Speech disorders in cerebellar disease. *Ann Neurol* 3:285–290, 1978.

87. Shankweiler D: Effects of temporal lobe lesions on recognition of dichotically presented melodies. *J Comp Physiol Psychol* 62:115–119, 1966.

88. Bever TG, Chiariello RJ: Cerebral dominance in musicians. *Science* 185:537–539, 1974.

89. Baron JC, Bousser MG, Comar D, Castaigne P: "Crossed cerebellar diaschisis" in human supratentorial brain infarction. *Trans Am Neurol Assoc* 105:459–461, 1980.

90. Pantano P, Baron JC, Samson Y, et al: Crossed cerebellar diaschisis: Further studies. *Brain* 109:677–694, 1986.

91. Metter EJ, Kempler D, Jackson CA, et al: Cerebellar glucose metabolism in chronic aphasia. *Neurology* 37:1599–1606, 1987.

92. Marr D: A theory of cerebellar cortex. *J Physiol* 202:437–470, 1969.

93. Granit R, Phillips CG: Excitatory and inhibitory processes acting upon individual Purkinje cells of the cerebellum in cats. *J Physiol* 133:520–547, 1956.

94. Gilbert PFC, Thach WT: Purkinje cell activity during motor learning. *Brain Res* 128:309–328, 1977.

95. Hebb DO: *The Organization of Behavior*. New York: John Wiley & Sons, 1949.

96. Robinson DA: Adaptive gain control of vertibuloocular reflex by the cerebellum. *J Neurophysiol* 39:954–969, 1976.

97. McCormick DA, Thompson RF: Cerebellum: Essential involvement in the classically conditioned eyelid response. *Science* 223:296–299, 1984.

98. Yeo CH, Hardiman MJ, Glickstein M: Classical conditioning of the nictitating membrane response of the rabbit. II: Lesions of the cerebellar cortex. *Exp Brain Res* 60:99–113, 1985.

99. Yeo CH, Hardiman MJ, Glickstein M: Classical conditioning of the nictitating membrane response of the rabbit. III: Connections of cerebellar lobule HVI. *Exp Brain Res* 60:114–126, 1985.

100. Lye RH, O'Boyle DJ, Ramsden RT, Schady W: Effects of a unilateral cerebellar lesion on the acquisition of eyeblink conditioning in man. *J Physiol* 403:58P, 1988.

101. Solomon PR, Stowe GT, Pendlebury WW: Disrupted eyelid conditioning in a patient with damage to cerebellar afferents. *Behav Neurosci* 103:898–902, 1989.

102. Ito M: *The Cerebellum and Neural Control*. New York: Raven Press, 1984.

103. Petersen SE, Fiez JA: The processing of single words studied with positron emission tomography. *Ann Rev Neurosci* 16:509–530, 1993.

104. Ryding E, Decety J, Sjoholm H, et al: Motor imagery activates the cerebellum regionally. A SPECT rCBF study with ^{99m}Tc-HMPAO. *Cogn Brain Res* 1:94–99, 1993.

105. Kim SG, Ugurbil K, Strick PL: Activation of a cerebellar output nucleus during cognitive processing. *Science* 265:949–951, 1994.

106. Middleton FA, Strick PL: Anatomical evidence for cerebellar and basal ganglia involvement in higher cognitive function. *Science* 266:458–461, 1994.

107. Schmahmann JD: An emerging concept: The cerebellar contribution to higher function. *Arch Neurol* 48:1178–1187, 1991.

Chapter 45

CORTICOBASAL DEGENERATION

RAY L. WATTS, RANDALL P. BREWER, JULIE A. SCHNEIDER
and SUZANNE S. MIRRA

SYNOPSIS OF THREE EARLY PATIENTS
CLINICAL FEATURES
LABORATORY AND IMAGING STUDIES
NEUROPATHOLOGY
    Cortical Degeneration
    Achromatic Neurons
    Subcortical Degeneration
    Tau-Associated Changes
    Tau Cytopathology in CBD and Other Disorders
    Neuropathological Criteria for the Diagnosis of CBD
    Neuropathological Heterogeneity and Overlap
    Relationship among CBD, Pick's Disease, and PSP
DIFFERENTIAL DIAGNOSIS
THERAPY
FUTURE DIRECTIONS

Interest in corticobasal degeneration (CBD) has expanded exponentially in recent years and, as a result, our understanding of this disorder continues to evolve. This is largely a result of the recognition of its clinical and neuropathological features, as well as the further characterization of CBD, using modern clinical and laboratory approaches. Yet, many questions remain unresolved: Is CBD a movement disorder or a cognitive disorder, or both in some situations? Is CBD a distinctive nosological entity or a syndrome? Are there molecular and neuropathological changes unique to CBD? What is the relationship between CBD and other neurodegenerative disorders that cause abnormalities of movement and cognition, such as progressive supranuclear palsy (PSP), multisystem atrophy, Pick's disease, Alzheimer's disease (AD), Parkinson's disease (PD) with dementia, diffuse Lewy body disease, etc.? Although we cannot answer most of these questions, in this chapter we will describe our current understanding of CBD and its place in the spectrum of neurodegenerative *movement disorders,* based on our experience and work of others over the last decade. However, before we embark on a formal delineation of current concepts, a brief review of the original three cases is warranted.

Synopsis of Three Early Patients

Rebeiz et al.[1,2] described three patients with a unique pattern of progressive motor impairment in later adult life. The disorder was characterized by slow, awkward voluntary limb movements accompanied by tremor and dystonic posturing. In all three patients, dysfunction began and remained most prominent in the left limbs; stiffness, lack of dexterity, and

"numbness" or "deadness" were the initial symptoms. The gradual progression included gait impairment, with particular difficulty initiating steps, marked limb rigidity, loss of dexterity, impaired position and other sensory function of the left limbs, as well as interference with attempted movements from involuntary synkinesia of the contralateral limbs. Although motor impairment progressed, intellectual function was said to remain relatively intact. Motor disability progressed, and the illness terminated in death 6–8 years after the onset of neurological disease.

The pathological findings in all three patients were distinctive, with an unusual pattern of frontoparietal neuronal loss. The asymmetrical presentation of signs and symptoms correlated with asymmetrical atrophy in the contralateral frontal and parietal cortex in two of the three patients. The atrophic cortex showed extensive neuronal loss, with associated gliosis. Some of the pyramidal neurons, in the third and fifth layers, were swollen, with an eosinophilic hyaline appearance. The swollen neurons often had eccentric nuclei and, occasionally, displayed cytoplasmic vacuoles. The neurons were often devoid of Nissl substance, thus prompting the use of the term "achromatic."

These striking pathological findings were not accompanied by features typical of other neurodegenerative conditions, such as Pick bodies, senile plaques, or Lewy bodies. The topography of neuronal loss in the cortex coincided with sites of the distribution of the achromatic neurons, mostly in the frontal, Rolandic, and parietal regions. Although neuronal loss and gliosis were also observed elsewhere in cerebral cortex, the hippocampal formation, occipital cortex, and inferior and medial temporal cortex were spared. Considerable loss of pigmented neurons in the substantia nigra was observed in the three patients. The medial portion of the subthalamic nucleus also showed gliosis and swollen neurons. In two patients, there were similar neuronal changes in the dentate and roof nuclei of the cerebellum; the cerebellar cortex, however, was spared. Evidence of secondary corticospinal tract degeneration was present in two of the three patients. In each case, the general autopsy, including examination of the circulatory system, as well as other organ systems, gave no clues concerning the pathogenesis of the intriguing neuropathological findings. With this historical backdrop, we will now address current knowledge of clinical features, laboratory studies, and neuropathological findings of CBD.

Clinical Features

CBD makes its appearance in mid- to late adult life, with symptoms usually beginning after age 60. Typically, onset is insidious. Both sexes seem to be equally affected by CBD,[3–5] although in our retrospective study of *neuropathologically* diagnosed CBD, we encountered an inexplicable predominance of women (10 of 11 patients).[6] The occurrence appears to be sporadic because, with the possible exception of case 2 of Rebeiz et al.,[2] family histories of affected patients are usually negative for any type of similar disorder. No other risk factors, such as exposure to toxic or infectious agents, have been identified thus far.

The core clinical picture of CBD in our experience consists of an asymmetric extrapyramidal syndrome of the akinetic-rigid type, with or without tremor, beginning insidiously on one side[7-9] (Table 45-1). Rinne et al.[3] analyzed the clinical features of 36 cases (6 with pathological confirmation). Of the 36 patients, 20 presented with symptoms related to a jerky, stiff, or clumsy upper extremity. Of the 36 patients, 10 began with the symptom of difficulty walking (stiffness, jerking, or clumsiness of a leg or "unsteadiness" without leg complaints). Other less common presentations include combined arm and leg involvement, dysphasia, dysarthria, and orofacial dyspraxia.[10,11] The symptoms gradually extend to the contralateral limbs within one to several years of onset. Postural instability, loss of facial expression, speech impairment, and other signs of midline or generalized motor impairment of extrapyramidal type also develop within one or more years.

Signs of cortical dysfunction are usually evident within 1 to 3 years of onset, with apraxia and cortical sensory loss especially prominent. In our recent series of 11 neuropathologically confirmed CBD cases,[6] 7 of the 11 patients presented with unilateral limb dysfunction. The remaining four patients had less typical presentations, including memory loss, behavioral changes, and difficulties with speech or gait. All 11 patients eventually developed extrapyramidal signs, as well as cortical features, most commonly apraxia.

Leiguarda et al.[12] studied 10 patients with suspected CBD and found that ideomotor apraxia occurred most frequently. Combined ideomotor and ideational apraxia correlated with global cognitive impairment. Many patients exhibit the "alien hand/limb" phenomenon, and this feature may be striking.[13] Rosenfield et al.[11] presented two patients (one with pathologi-

cal confirmation) with speech apraxia as a presenting sign in the evolution of the classical clinical syndrome.

A very important early *clinical clue* suggesting that one is confronted with a "Parkinson-plus" disorder, instead of idiopathic PD, is the *lack of beneficial response to L-dopa therapy*. Other clinical features commonly seen are: (1) an irregular, jerky action/postural tremor, (2) myoclonus, (3) corticospinal signs (hyperreflexia and Babinski sign(s)), (4) supranuclear gaze abnormalities, (5) choreoathetotic involuntary movements, (6) blepharospasm, and (7) frontal release signs (Table 45-1). The tremor differs from the typical rest or postural tremor seen with PD; it is a more rapid (6–8 Hz), irregular, jerky action/postural tremor; myoclonus is often superimposed in advanced stages.

The myoclonus is focal, at least initially, and tends to be present to a greater extent in the most affected limb(s). Myoclonus, like tremor, is best seen during action or maintenance of a posture; it is also stimulus-sensitive in many cases.[14,15] The myoclonus of CBD appears most often as a late manifestation, frequently superseding the action tremor. Eventually, most patients exhibit signs of corticospinal dysfunction, with extensor plantar responses and hyperreflexia. The differentiation of spasticity from rigidity in these patients is clinically very difficult, but the loss of voluntary movement is almost certainly related in part to degeneration of primary and secondary motor cortical regions that contribute to the corticospinal tracts.

Eye movement abnormalities are common in CBD. In the early stages of the disease, smooth-pursuit eye movements may be slow and exhibit saccadic breakdown, but the range of movement is generally full (except for upgaze in elderly patients). As the illness progresses, patients gradually lose the ability to make rapid saccades to verbal command, with retained spontaneous saccades and optokinetic-nystagmus.[16] Oculocephalic reflexes are preserved and are even accentuated as eye movement abnormalities worsen, indicating the supranuclear nature of the gaze palsy.[17] Distinctive differences between the ocular motility disorder in clinically diagnosed CBD, PSP, striatonigral degeneration (SND), and PD have been described.[18] Horizontal saccadic latencies were significantly increased in the CBD group, compared to those of the PSP group. Vertical saccadic paralysis was not observed, interestingly, in the PD, SND, or CBD groups, but it was present in 9 of 10 patients in the PSP group.

Spontaneous onset of choreoathetotic involuntary movements involving the limb and facial muscles may be seen, as well as blepharospasm and other focal dystonias. In fairly advanced stages, frontal "release" signs (grasp, glabellar, and exaggerated facial and palmomental reflexes) may become prominent. Speech becomes slow and monotonous, and paraphasic errors and dysphasia may evolve. In the most advanced stages, patients may become anarthric.

Although many cases show little, if any, cognitive dysfunction, varying degrees of intellectual, memory, and language impairment may develop; cognitive impairment may be the presenting or even sole feature in some cases.[6,19] In our own series of 11 cases of neuropathologically confirmed CBD,[6] all patients eventually developed cognitive deficits; the onset, nature, and severity of the impairment, however, varied widely. Cognitive disturbances preceded or accompanied the

TABLE 45-1 Clinical Features of CBD

Major
  Akinetic-rigid parkinsonian syndrome (loss of dexterity, slowness of movement, increased muscle tone, postural/gait disturbance, hypomimia, hypophonic dysarthria)
  Cortical signs (apraxia-limb, orobuccolingual, oculomotor; cortical sensory disturbance—astereognosis, decreased graphesthesia, double simultaneous tactile extinction; dysphasia—especially paraphasic errors; extensor plantar responses and other corticospinal tract signs)
  Dystonia (especially flexion dystonia of upper limb(s), distal greater than proximal)
  Action/postural tremor (rapid, irregular, jerky)
  Myoclonus
  "Alien hand/limb" phenomenon
Minor
  Choreoathetic involuntary movements
  Supranuclear-gaze abnormalities (saccades affected more than smooth pursuit)
  Intellectual impairment/dementia (cognition may be remarkably well preserved until late in the course)
  Frontal "release" signs (grasps, brisk facial, and palmomental reflexes)
  Cerebellar signs
  Blepharospasm

SOURCE: *From Watts et al.[7] Used with permission.*

onset of the movement disorder in four patients; an additional three patients developed memory loss, progressing to more global dementia, within 2–3 years of the onset of neurological symptoms. Another patient displayed mild early memory impairment and, in three individuals, dementia was a late feature.

The neuropsychological profile of CBD has received little attention until recently.[20,21] Interestingly, patients with clinically diagnosed CBD show marked similarity to patients with PSP (dysexecutive syndrome), but with substantially more impairment of dynamic motor execution and praxis. In a study comparing clinically diagnosed CBD with clinically diagnosed AD with extrapyramidal features,[21] CBD patients displayed better performance on tests of immediate recall and attention, whereas they performed significantly worse on tests of praxis and digit span.

As voluntary limb movement becomes progressively slower and clumsier, many patients develop a characteristic dystonic posture with the hand and forearm flexed and the arm adducted, asymmetrically, in earlier stages. The illness generally progresses to a state of bilateral rigid immobility after 5–7 years, and a patient usually dies from aspiration pneumonia and sepsis.

In summary, based on current evidence, CBD appears to be a distinctive nosological entity. When fully developed and observed over time, the *motoric presentation* is sufficiently characteristic to allow correct diagnosis during life with a relatively high accuracy. Additional studies, summarized below, including laboratory studies, computed tomography (CT) and magnetic resonance imaging (MRI), electrophysiology, positron emission tomography (PET) and cerebrospinal fluid (CSF) neurotransmitter studies, although not diagnostic, can provide supportive data. The ultimate confirmation, however, still depends on the neuropathological findings in concert with the clinical picture, and the full scope of clinical presentation is still being defined.

Laboratory and Imaging Studies

Routine laboratory studies of blood, urine, and CSF are normal, including copper and ceruloplasmin levels. Heavy metal toxic screens of urine have been negative. Watts et al.[22] found that cerebrospinal fluid levels of somatostatin were significantly decreased in all three patients assayed, two of whom had autopsy confirmation of CBD.

Radiographic evaluation with brain CT scans and MRI may be normal in the early stages, but as the disease progresses a pattern of asymmetric frontoparietal cortical atrophy (greatest contralateral to the most severely affected limbs; see Fig. 45-1) or bilateral cortical atrophy evolves. As the atrophy becomes more prominent, abnormal signal attenuation is seen in the underlying subcortical white matter (Fig. 45-1A). Serial evaluation of CT or MRI scans over time at 6- to 12-month intervals is generally more useful than one isolated scan. A recent review by Savoiardo et al.[23] addresses the role of MRI in various parkinsonian syndromes.

Electrophysiological studies can be useful in the evaluation of patients with CBD. *Electroencephalography (EEG)* is usually normal when symptoms first emerge, but as the disease pro-

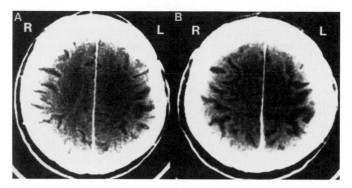

FIGURE 45-1 Cranial CT images from the autopsied case of Watts et al. in 1985, in the fifth year of the patient's illness. There is asymmetrical (left greater than right) frontoparietal cortical atrophy, which is most prominent in the perirolandic regions. Note the attenuation of subcortical white matter underlying the central sulcus in *A*.

gresses the EEG may reveal asymmetric slowing (most prominent over the cerebral hemisphere contralateral to the most affected limbs). When correlated with asymmetric radiographic changes in a similar distribution and a typical clinical picture of CBD, this laboratory finding further supports the diagnosis. In late stages, the EEG usually shows bilateral slowing, so the time reference of the EEG in the evaluation of an individual patient can be very important. *Electrophysiological tremor/movement studies*, using accelerometric and electromyographic (EMG) recording techniques, indicate that the tremor present with CBD clearly differs from the classic parkinsonian "rest" or postural tremor. It is more rapid (typically, 6–8 Hz) and is most evident during action, and the amplitude may vary, giving it a more irregular appearance. *Myoclonus* may be recorded using similar techniques of examination, and provocative maneuvers, such as action of a limb, startle, or tactile stimulation, help to bring it out. Thompson et al.[15,24] and Carella et al.[25] found that myoclonus was not preceded by a cortical discharge and reported that central motor conduction was normal. Results of *evoked potential (EP) studies* have been mixed. *Somatosensory EP* (SSEP) studies may yield poorly formed or absent thalamocortical potentials, and latencies have been normal or minimally prolonged. We and other groups[24–26] have not found enlargement of the secondary component of the SSEP cortical potential, which can be seen with cortical reflex myoclonus or epilepsia partialis continua. Pattern shift *visual EP* studies have been normal in most patients, but one of our pathologically confirmed cases had prolonged P100 latencies bilaterally. *Brain stem auditory EP* studies have been normal in our experience. Routine *EMG/nerve conduction studies* have turned up occasional focal or generalized neuropathies in a few patients, but no clear-cut pattern has emerged, and these are usually subclinical or do not contribute significantly to overall disability.

PET and single-photon emission computed tomography (SPECT) findings in CBD patients have been reported from several institutions.[6,22,27–35] Two general approaches have been taken, and these have given similar patterns of results in different centers: (1) studies of cerebral metabolism (oxygen or glucose) and blood flow, and (2) assessment of nigrostriatal dopaminergic system function. Several groups have found abnormalities of cerebral metabolism with a corresponding reduction of cerebral blood flow (CBF): (1) decreased oxygen metabolism in the frontoparietal[22,27,34] and medial frontal, parietal,[35] and temporal cortical regions,[5,29] most prominently in the cerebral hemisphere contralateral to the most affected limbs and (2) decreased glucose metabolism (fluorodeoxyglucose, FDG) in the parietal cortex and thalamus, in an asymmetric distribution with the greatest decrease contralateral to the most affected limbs (as with oxygen metabolism and CBF).[30–32] Dysfunction of the nigrostriatal dopaminergic system has been demonstrated by: (a) decreased ^{18}F-dopa uptake in the striatum (F-dopa PET)[5,16,28,29] and (b) reduced postsynaptic striatal D2 receptor binding of [[123m]I]-iodobenzamide (IBZM) on SPECT scanning.[35] The general patterns of these *in vivo* metabolic abnormalities conform to the known pattern of neuronal degeneration in CBD, indicating that PET and/or SPECT studies may help differentiate this disorder from other types of "Parkinson-plus" or motor system degeneration syndromes. This matter has been reviewed by Brooks.[36] Recently, SPECT labeling of the dopamine transporter by [2β-carboxymethoxy 3β(4-iodophenyl)-tropane [^{123}I]β-CIT has demonstrated symmetric striatal reduction in clinically diagnosed CBD, multiple-system atrophy (MSA), and PSP, compared with asymmetric reductions in PD.[37] The number of cases of CBD studied by functional imaging is still small, indicating the need for further correlative studies with neuropathological confirmation.

Neuropathology

CORTICAL DEGENERATION

Frontal-parietal cortical degeneration, often asymmetrical and predominantly involving perirolandic cortex (Figs. 45-2 and 45-3), is a characteristic feature of CBD. Asymmetrical cortical degeneration at autopsy is observed in more than 80 percent of CBD cases, in our experience, and this asymmetry almost always correlates with the laterality of the clinical manifestations. In about two-thirds of cases, the atrophy is predominantly perirolandic; less commonly, more rostral frontal cortex is involved and tends to be associated with more atypical clinical presentations.[6] Cingulate and insular cortex exhibit variable involvement. As in the original reports described earlier in this chapter, temporal cortex is usually spared (except in cases exhibiting concomitant AD pathology or other processes involving temporal lobe, e.g., hippocampal sclerosis). Occipital cortex is generally unremarkable.

Corresponding microscopic examination reveals neuronal loss and gliosis in cortical regions with grossly apparent atrophy. When the changes are mild, however, they may only be appreciated microscopically. Thus, in brains derived from individuals suspected of having CBD or other unusual movement disorders, the pathologist should consider taking sections when feasible from bilateral perirolandic cortex. Changes in the white matter consisting of loss of myelin and axons may be severe, particularly in regions underlying extensively involved cortex. Associated hydrocephalus ex

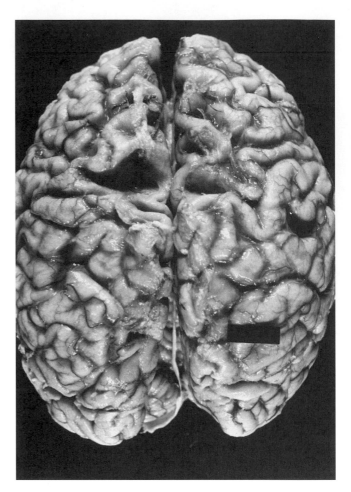

FIGURE 45-2 The convexity of the brain of a 75-year-old man with CBD exhibits striking asymmetric perirolandic cortical atrophy, which is greater on the left, where the sulcus is gaping. *(From Watts et al.[7] Used with permission.)*

vacuo and attenuation of the corpus callosum result from the loss of tissue (Fig. 45-3).

ACHROMATIC NEURONS

Ballooned or achromatic neurons are another characteristic feature of CBD. They most commonly occur in the deeper layers of degenerated frontoparietal cortex but may be observed in other cortical and subcortical regions. (Fig. 45-4). Indeed, when one considers ballooned neurons to be requisite for the neuropathological diagnosis of CBD (see below), then, by definition, they will be seen in virtually every case. Although ballooned neurons are readily stained using a hematoxylin & eosin (H&E) preparation or neurofilament immunohistochemistry, in some cases with extensive neuronal loss and gliosis in cortex they may be difficult to detect, and multiple sections of involved cortex may be needed to ascertain their presence.

SUBCORTICAL DEGENERATION

Degeneration of the substantia nigra, in our experience, is almost uniformly severe (Fig. 45-5). Involvement of other

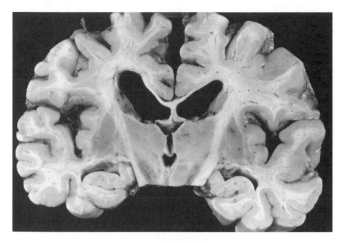

FIGURE 45-3 Coronal section through the cerebrum reveals asymmetric cortical atrophy (L > R) with thinning of the corpus callosum, loss of cerebral white matter, and resulting dilatation of the lateral ventricles (hydrocephalus ex vacuo). Note, too, the asymmetric narrowing predominantly involving the left posterior limb of the internal capsule and left cerebral peduncle. (*From Watts et al.*[7] *Used with permission.*)

subcortical nuclei, however, varies widely from patient to patient in severity and topography. Basal ganglia, thalamus, periaqueductal gray matter, colliculi, oculomotor complex, red nucleus, dentate nucleus, and inferior olivary nuclei exhibit variable neuronal loss and gliosis.

TAU-ASSOCIATED CHANGES

A spectrum of silver and tau-immunopositive structures are commonly encountered in CBD. Neurofibrillary tangles (NFT) are frequently identified on silver stains such as Gall-

FIGURE 45-4 Cytoskeletal pathology in corticobasal degeneration. *a*, ballooned neuron, perirolandic cortex; *b*, glial inclusion, white matter; *c*, neuropil threads, perirolandic cortex; *d*, globose-type tangle, globus pallidus; *e*, globular tangle or Pick-like inclusion, basis pontis; *f*, thread-like tangle, subthalamic nucleus. Stains used were as follows: H&E (*a*); tau immunostain (*b* and *c*); modified Bielschowsky silver stain (*d–f*); Magnifications: 450× (*a*); 730× (*b*); 440× (*c*); 730× (*d*); 600× (*e* and *f*). (*From Schneider et al.*[6] *Used with permission.*)

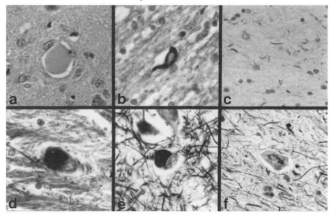

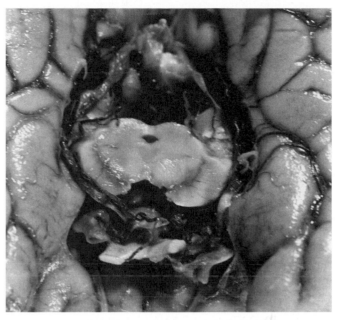

FIGURE 45-5 Pallor of the substantia nigra is seen, along with reduction in size of the left cerebral peduncle, as a result of degeneration of subcortical white matter. (*From Watts et al.*[7] *Used with permission.*)

yas preparation and tau immunohistochemistry within neurons of cortex; subcortical nuclei, for example, basal ganglia and subthalamic nucleus; and brain stem nuclei, for example, oculomotor complex and inferior olives. While the distribution of the NFT in CBD is reminiscent of that of PSP, the appearance of the NFT generally differs. The NFT of PSP are typically globose in conformation, whereas those in CBD vary from thread-like cytoplasmic strands occasionally encircling the nucleus to more confluent irregular globules resembling Pick bodies. However, some of these distinctions are subtle ones and, in fact, NFTs show a spectrum of occasionally overlapping morphologies in PSP, Pick's disease, and CBD, as illustrated by Feany and colleagues.[38]

In virtually all CBD cases, neuropil threads, grains, and glial and neuronal inclusions are observed on silver stains and tau immunohistochemistry. These changes are usually most marked in the degenerated cortex, underlying white matter, basal ganglia, internal capsule, and basis pontis. Neuropil threads are particularly prominent in the deeper layers of cortex and the immediate subjacent white matter and their frequency may parallel white matter degeneration on H&E stain. Tau-positive argyrophilic structures described as "astrocytic plaques" by Ksiezak-Reding et al.[39] and believed to be characteristic of CBD are identified in many CBD cases (Fig. 45-6), although they have also been observed in PSP (see Ref. 40; SS Mirra, personal observations).

TAU CYTOPATHOLOGY IN CBD AND OTHER DISORDERS

The presence of widespread tau-positive inclusions in CBD[4,38–44] suggests a relationship between CBD and other neurodegenerative disorders exhibiting tau-associated cyto-

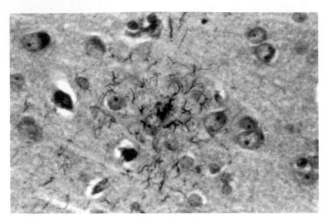

FIGURE 45-6 "Astrocytic plaque" seen on tau immunostain. Magnification: 450×.

pathology, for example, Pick's disease, PSP, and AD. Ultrastructural and molecular studies have revealed both distinctions and similarities of tau-associated changes among these disorders. PSP classically exhibits 15–18-nm tau-positive, ubiquitin-negative straight filaments with occasional paired helical filaments (PHF) similar to AD, Pick's disease shows 10- to 15-nm straight filaments and 24-nm-wide PHF-like filaments with 130- to 160-nm intervals and a 12-nm minimum width; AD shows PHFs with 80-nm intervals, and 10-nm minimum and 20-nm maximum widths. Wakabayashi[45] demonstrated 15-nm-wide tau-positive, ubiquitin-negative straight tubules in CBD, whereas Ksiezak-Reding et al.[39] described 13- to 28-nm-wide twisted filaments with a periodicity of 169–202 nm, rather than straight tubules in CBD inclusions. Although the inclusions in all three disorders are composed of phosphorylated tau, biochemical studies suggest differences in the tau polypeptides. In CBD and PSP, two major tau polypeptides of molecular weight 64 and 69 kd were identified, whereas in AD three major polypeptides with molecular weights of 60, 64, and 68 kd were found.[39]

NEUROPATHOLOGICAL CRITERIA FOR THE DIAGNOSIS OF CBD

In a series of two reports emanating from an NIH consensus conference, investigators have sought to establish and validate neuropathological criteria for the diagnosis of PSP and related disorders, including Pick's disease and postencephalitic parkinsonism.[46,47] Briefly, the diagnostic neuropathology criteria for CBD, as proposed by Litvan and colleagues,[47] included: circumscribed or lobar atrophy in parietal or frontoparietal areas; tau-positive cortical neurons; swollen and achromatic neurons, basophilic inclusions, numerous neuropil threads, and severe neuronal loss in substantia nigra, basal ganglia, or dentatorubrothalamic tract; gliosis and spongiosis in subcortical white matter; and a clinical history compatible with CBD. Thus, the authors did not rely on neuropathological markers alone to diagnose these disorders; clinical features were also included.[47] However, they exclude cases with large or multiple infarcts, Lewy bodies, AD diagnostic changes, silver-positive oligodendroglial inclusions (usually seen in MSAs), Pick bodies, and prion-

reactive protein-positive amyloid plaques. Thus, these exclusion criteria would eliminate cases with coexisting PD, AD, or certain other pathologies. Our experience with overlap among neurodegenerative disorders such as PSP and CBD,[6,48] as well as that of others discussed below, suggests that a substantial proportion of otherwise typical CBD cases would be excluded on the basis of these criteria.

We base neuropathological diagnosis of CBD on the presence of asymmetrical frontoparietal neuronal loss and gliosis, cortical ballooned neurons, nigral degeneration, and variable involvement of subcortical nuclei, such as basal ganglia. However, we believe that it is the compendium of neuropathological findings, often in concert with clinical features, that allows the diagnosis of CBD. Taken alone, each of the neuropathological findings is nonspecific. Ballooned neurons, for example, are found in a wide spectrum of disorders.[49] They occur in Pick's disease, Creutzfeldt-Jakob disease,[50] PSP,[51] ALS,[52] and AD.[49] Nor are the tau-positive inclusions or other changes specific for CBD as discussed above. Asymmetric cortical degeneration of CBD occurs in other neurodegenerative disorders, for example, Pick's disease, frontal lobe dementia, and ALS with frontal lobe dementia, although the distribution of changes usually differs from that of CBD. Indeed, some would designate all neurodegenerative disorders with focal or asymmetric cortical degeneration as "asymmetric cortical degenerative syndromes" or "Pick complex."[53]

NEUROPATHOLOGICAL HETEROGENEITY AND OVERLAP

Neuropathologists and clinicians are increasingly aware of the overlap and heterogeneity encountered among neurodegenerative diseases such as AD, PD, and PSP. Extrapyramidal signs are common in patients with AD, and PD patients may develop dementia. We have found striking neuropathological and clinical overlap and heterogeneity in 20 cases of neuropathologically diagnosed PSP.[48] Twelve of these cases showed concomitant pathological changes of AD, PD, or both disorders; those with PD exhibited cortical and subcortical Lewy bodies. Two cases evidenced neuropathological features of both PSP and CBD, and one of these also displayed hippocampal, amygdala, and entorhinal sclerosis. Still another case exhibited combined features of PSP, AD, and pontocerebellar degeneration at autopsy.

We have encountered similar neuropathological and clinical overlap in a series of 11 patients of neuropathologically confirmed CBD.[6] Only 5 of the 11 patients (45 percent) showed "pure" CBD pathology. The remaining six patients manifested overlapping neuropathological features of one or more disorders, including AD, PSP, PD, and hippocampal sclerosis. Interestingly, these six patients all exhibited memory loss early in the course of their illness. Others, too, have observed overlap between CBD and other disorders.[17,38,54,55]

RELATIONSHIP AMONG CBD, PICK'S DISEASE, AND PSP

There is substantial neuropathological overlap between Pick's disease and CBD. Ballooned neurons, variable degeneration of the substantia nigra and basal ganglia, and tau-positive inclusions occur in both disorders. However, Pick bodies, a characteristic feature of Pick disease, are rarely observed in CBD. Although both disorders exhibit asymmetrical cortical atrophy, the temporal cortex, as well as the hippocampus, are usually involved in Pick's disease but are relatively spared in CBD. CBD and Pick's disease can also have overlapping clinical features, and CBD patients may manifest behavioral changes and language disturbances. So called "parietal Pick's disease" has been reported as a potential mimicker of CBD.[56] The full relationship between these two disorders awaits further clarification.

We and others[6,38,48,54] have observed pathological overlap between CBD and PSP. As discussed above, there is similarity in the distribution and appearance of neurofibrillary pathology. In addition, we have also observed grumose degeneration of the dentate nucleus in two CBD patients. Grumose degeneration, an eosinophilic granular change in the dentate nucleus attributed to clusters of distended axon terminals,[57] occurs most commonly in PSP but has occasionally been observed in other neurodegenerative diseases.[58–62]

Links between these three disorders may occur at a molecular level as well. The apolipoprotein E e4 allele is recognized as a major risk factor for familial and sporadic AD.[63,64] However, Schneider et al.[65] also observed an increased frequency of the apoE e4 allele in CBD, Pick's disease, and PSP, compared to that of control populations. Although others have not observed this trend in PSP,[66] another group has recently reported an increased e4 allele frequency in Pick's disease.[67] Studies of ApoE genotype in larger numbers of cases of CBD and other neurodegenerative disorders, and further investigation of its relationship to tau-associated cytoskeletal pathology, are warranted.

Differential Diagnosis

The pattern of motoric deficits presented by CBD is sufficiently distinctive such that, when fully developed, the syndrome generally would not be misdiagnosed as PD. However, this is the most common misdiagnosis early in the course. The best early clues that allow one to distinguish this disorder from idiopathic PD are (1) the lack of beneficial response to L-dopa or dopamine agonists and (2) signs of cortical dysfunction, most notably, apraxia and/or cortical sensory impairment.

The differential diagnosis of the motoric presentation of CBD consists of the nosologically distinct extrapyramidal syndromes associated with basal ganglionic and cortical degeneration that present as a "Parkinson-plus" syndrome.[68] Disorders with similar presentations include PSP[69–71] (see Chap. 19), striatonigral degeneration[72,73] (see Chap. 20), MSA (including olivopontocerebellar atrophy)[73,74] (see Chap. 20), diffuse Lewy Body disease[76,77] (see Chap. 24), atypical variants of Pick's disease,[55,56,78–80] PD with dementia, AD with extrapyramidal features,[81,82] the parkinsonism-dementia-amyotrophic lateral sclerosis complex,[83,84] Wilson's disease[85] (see Chap. 46), Huntington's disease (especially the rigid form usually seen in juveniles)[86] (see Chap. 35), variants of

Azorean disease,[87–90] familial progressive basal ganglia, corticobulbar, and corticospinal systems degeneration[91–96] (see Chap. 24), late-onset Hallervorden-Spatz disease[97,98] (see Chap. 25), and adult neuronal ceroid lipofuscinosis,[97,99] all of which typically differ in several clinical and pathological respects. Some cases of CBD, however, may show overlapping clinical and pathological features with other disorders.[6,19,53,100]

PSP classically presents with prominent axial rigidity, postural instability, and eye movement abnormalities. Several cases of "atypical" PSP have been reported, with clinical features similar to those of CBD.[70,71] Atypical features such as asymmetric onset, oculomotor impairment that is only mild, focal dystonia, and involuntary limb elevation resembling the "alien limb phenomenon" are the most frequent characteristics shared by both disorders.

Asymmetric cortical degenerations,[101,102] Pick's disease,[56,101,102] AD,[81,82] and primary progressive aphasia[53,103–106] may present with features resembling early CBD, such as focal myoclonus, apraxia, "alien limb phenomenon," and asymmetric rigidity. These syndromes, in general, lack the prominent and progressive extrapyramidal dysfunction characteristic of the typical motoric presentation CBD. However, there may be significant overlap of these disorders with CBD, the full delineation of which awaits further careful clinical, pathological, and molecular studies.

Table 45-2 summarizes the differential clinical features which are helpful in the evaluation of patients with combined parkinsonism and cerebral cortical-cognitive dysfunction.

Therapy

Pharmacotherapy has generally been of limited benefit, and this can best be ascribed to the multisystem degenerative nature and predominance of cortical involvement in CBD. There is little or no beneficial response to L-dopa/carbidopa or dopamine agonists (bromocriptine, pergolide); indeed, this is a characteristic feature. Clonazepam has been the most beneficial agent for action tremor and myoclonus. Baclofen may improve rigidity and tremor also but to a lesser degree. Anticholinergics have not been beneficial, and they have been tolerated poorly. Dopamine antagonists, such as haloperidol, have been used sparingly and have not been helpful. Propranolol may benefit the action tremor early in the course in some, but later its effectiveness wanes, particularly as the tremor becomes myoclonic. Trials of ethanol, physostigmine, methysergide, diphenhydramine, and clonidine have produced no improvement.

In some instances stereotaxic thalamotomy or pallidotomy is indicated for relief of severe painful dystonia involving the extremities. Other aspects of patient care, not involving pharmacotherapy, can be of special importance for these patients. *Physiotherapy* is very helpful for maintenance of mobility and prevention of contractures. Pain related to dystonic posturing can be lessened by maintenance of good range of motion and, occasionally, splinting can be helpful. *Occupational therapy* can help patients maintain some degree of functional independence by providing specially made devices such as eating utensils with large handles. *Speech therapy*

TABLE 45-2 Differential Clinical Features in Patients Presenting with Parkinsonism and Cognitive Dysfunction*

	Disorders Presenting with Parkinsonism and Subsequent Cognitive Decline	
Diagnosis	Principal Clinical Features	Features Suggesting Another Disorder or Concurrent Pathology
CBD	Apraxia, cortical sensory loss, unilateral or asymmetric rigidity and dystonia, action tremor superseded by focal myoclonus, alien limb behavior, rapid course, lack of response to L-dopa therapy	Prominent ocular impairment, axial-rigidity or dystonia out of proportion to limb involvement, rest tremor, autonomic failure, aphasia, early or severe dementia
MSA	Symmetric rigidity (less commonly asymmetric); lack of rest tremor; cerebellar and autonomic dysfunction; choreoathetosis; rapid course; lack of or suboptimal response to L-dopa therapy	Early and prominent ocular impairment, apraxia, cortical sensory loss
PSP	Supranuclear ophthalmoplegia (especially vertical), axial dystonia in extension, early gait impairment and postural instability, dysarthria and pseudobulbar palsy, frontal lobe-type dementia (dysexecutive syndrome), lack of or suboptimal response to L-dopa therapy	Lack of or minimal ocular impairment, asymmetric rigidity, prominent dementia early in course, alien limb-type behavior, apraxia, cortical sensory loss
PD with dementia	Rest tremor, bradykinesia, asymmetric rigidity, gait impairment, memory loss, dementia, L-dopa responsiveness	Symmetric rigidity, lack of rest tremor, axial dystonia, early ocular impairment, early myoclonus, apraxia, cortical sensory loss, lack of or suboptimal response to L-dopa therapy

	Disorders Presenting with Dementia and Subsequent Extrapyramidal Dysfunction	
Diagnosis	Principal Clinical Features	Features Suggesting Another Disorder or Concurrent Pathology
AD with extrapyramidal dysfunction	Early cognitive impairment (especially memory loss), cortical dysfunction (visuospatial, language, praxis), mild bradykinesia and rigidity, protracted progressive course	Parkinsonism before memory loss, progressive frontal lobe dysfunction, aphasia or apraxia without significant memory loss, early gait impairment, axial rigidity, ophthalmoplegia, alien limb-type behavior
DLBD	Early cognitive dysfunction (especially with fluctuating features), L-dopa-induced psychosis, mild parkinsonism (initially)	Isolated cortical dysfunction (memory loss, aphasia, apraxia, cortical sensory loss, frontal lobe dementia), axial rigidity and dystonia, ophthalmoplegia
Pick's disease	Prominent frontal lobe dementia with personality changes (disinhibition or apathy), aphasia, memory loss	Progressive aphasia or apraxia without dementia, prominent extrapyramidal features, rest tremor, L-dopa responsiveness, ophthalmoplegia
CJD	Rapid course of dementia, personality changes, myoclonus; upper motor neuron, cerebellar and/or extrapyramidal signs	Protracted course, isolated parkinsonism or cortical dysfunction (apraxia, cortical sensory loss), rest tremor, L-dopa responsiveness

DLBD, diffuse Lewy body disease; CJD, Creutzfeldt-Jakob disease.

*Significant overlap exists between many neurodegenerative disorders. These guidelines help to clinically differentiate some of the disorders with combined cognitive and extrapyramidal dysfunction; many pathologically proven variants have been described. This overlap underscores the need to consider a thorough evaluation in patients presenting with movement disorders.[107] There is ongoing debate regarding the nosology of PD with dementia, DLBD, and AD with extrapyramidal dysfunction.

may offer practical hints and exercises to optimize speech function and guard against aspiration secondary to swallowing difficulty. Over time, most patients develop severe dysphagia and require percutaneous feeding gastrostomy tube placement. This assists with maintenance of nutrition with a reduced risk of aspiration. The decision to place a gastrostomy in a patient with a chronically progressive neurodegenerative disease must be handled on an individual basis. Good home care assistance can help prolong the time a patient can remain at home before requiring nursing home placement.

Despite all therapeutic efforts, the illness is relentlessly progressive, leading to rigid immobility within 3–5 years and death within 5–10 years.

Future Directions

Identification of disease-specific biological markers to improve diagnostic accuracy, the development of better therapeutic strategies, and the elucidation of the cellular and molecular abnormalities associated with CBD are much needed to further our knowledge of the disorder and improve the care of our patients.

Acknowledgments

We are indebted to the many neurologists and other physicians who have referred patients and collaborated over the years: At Massachusetts General Hospital, Robert R. Young, John H. Growdon, M. Flint Beal, E.P. Richardson, Jr., Roger Williams, C. Miller Fisher, Raymond D. Adams; at Emory University, Alan Freeman, Donal Costigan, Charles Epstein, Robert F. Kibler, Steven Hersch, and Allan Levey; at Duke University, Albert Heyman and James Villier (Charlotte); in Virginia, Jon D. Dorman and Della C. Williams. We are grateful to Lisa Taylor and Selena Nelson for assistance in manuscript preparation. This work was supported in part by the Emory University Parkinson Research Fund, the Sartain Lanier Family Foundation, the Mary Louise Morris Brown Foundation, the Francis Hollis Brain Foundation, and the American Parkinson Disease Association. Suzanne S. Mirra's work is supported by Veterans Affairs Merit Award and National Institutes of Health Grant AG10130.

References

1. Rebeiz JJ, Kolodny EH, Richardson EP: Corticodentatonigral degeneration with neuronal achromasia: A progressive disorder of late adult life. *Trans Am Neurol Assoc* 92:23–26, 1967.

2. Rebeiz JJ, Kolodny EH, Richardson EP: Corticodentatonigral degeneration with neuronal achromasia. *Arch Neurol* 18:20–33, 1968.

3. Rinne JO, Lee MS, Thompson PD, Marsden CD: Corticobasal degeneration: A clinical study of 36 cases. *Brain* 117:1183–1196, 1994.

4. Feany MB, Dickson DW: Widespread cytoskeletal pathology characterizes corticobasal degeneration. *Am J Pathol* 146:1388–1396, 1995.

5. Sawle GV, Brooks DJ, Marsden CD, Frackowiak RS: Corticobasal degeneration: A unique pattern of regional cortical oxygen hypometabolism and striatal fluorodopa uptake demonstrated by positron emission tomography. *Brain* 114:541–556, 1991.

6. Schneider JA, Watts RL, Gearing M, et al: Corticobasal degeneration: Neuropathological and clinical heterogeneity. Neurology. In Press.

7. Watts RL, Mirra SS, Richardson EP: Corticobasal ganglionic degeneration, in Marsden CD, Fahn S (eds): *Movement Disorders 3.* London: Butterworth, 1994, pp 282–299.

8. Case Records of the Massachusetts General Hospital (Case 38-1985) (Case of corticonigral degeneration with neuronal achromasia). *N Engl J Med* 313:739–748, 1985.

9. Greene PE, Fahn S, Lang AE, et al: Progressive unilateral rigidity, bradykinesia, tremulousness, and apraxia, leading to fixed postural deformity of the involved limb. *Mov Disord* 5:(4)341–351, 1990.

10. Lang AE: Corticobasal ganglionic degeneration presenting with "progressive loss of speech output and orofacial dyspraxia." *J Neurol Neurosurg Psychiatry* 55:1101, 1992.

11. Rosenfield DB, Bogatka CJ, Viswanath NS, et al: Speech apraxia in corticobasal ganglionic degeneration. *Ann Neurol* 30:296–297, 1991.

12. Leiguarda R, Lees AJ, Merello M, et al: The nature of apraxia in corticobasal degeneration. *J Neurol Neurosurg Psychiatry* 57:455–459, 1994.

13. Doody RS, Jankovic J: The alien hand and related signs. *J Neurol Neurosurg Psychiatry* 55:806–810, 1992.

14. Chen R, Ashby P, Lang AE: Stimulus sensitive myoclonus in akinetic-rigid syndromes. *Brain* 115:1875–1888, 1992.

15. Thompson PD, Day BL, Rothwell JC, et al: The myoclonus of corticobasal degeneration: Evidence of two forms of corticobasal reflex myoclonus. *Brain* 117:1197–1207, 1994.

16. Riley DE, Lang AE, Lewis A, et al: Cortical-basal ganglionic degeneration. *Neurology* 40:1203–1212, 1990.

17. Gibb WRG, Luthert PJ, Marsden CD: Corticobasal degeneration. *Brain* 112:1171–1192, 1989.

18. Vidailhet M, Rivaud S, Gouider-Khouja N, et al: Eye movements in parkinsonian syndromes. *Ann Neurol* 35:420–426, 1994.

19. Lerner A, Friedland R, Riley D, et al: Dementia with pathological findings of corticobasal ganglionic degeneration. *Ann Neurol* 32:271, 1992.

20. Pillon B, Blin J, Vidailhet M, et al: The neuropsychological pattern of corticobasal degeneration: Comparison with progressive supranuclear palsy and Alzheimer's disease. *Neurology* 45:1477–1483, 1995.

21. Massman PJ, Kreiter KT, Jankovic J, Doody RS: Neuropsychological distinction between corticobasal ganglionic degeneration and Alzheimer's disease with extrapyramidal signs. *Neurology* (suppl 2) 44:194–195, 1994.

22. Watts RL, William RS, Growdon JH, et al: Corticobasal ganglionic degeneration. *Neurology* 35(suppl 1):178, 1995.

23. Savoiardo M, Girotti F, Strada L, Ciceri E: Magnetic resonance imaging in progressive supranuclear palsy and other parkinsonian disorders. *J Neural Transm Park Dir Dement Sect* 42:93–110, 1994.

24. Thompson PD, Day BL, Rothwell JC, Marsden CD: Clinical and electrophysiological findings in corticobasal degeneration. *Mov Disord* 5(1):43, 1990.

25. Carella F, Scaioli V, Franceschetti S, et al: Focal reflex myoclonus in corticobasal degeneration. *Funct Neurol* 6:165–170, 1991.

26. Brunt ERP, van Weerden TW, Pruim J, Lakke JWPF: Unique myoclonic pattern in corticobasal degeneration. *Mov Disord* 10(2):132–142, 1995.

27. Watts RL, Mirra SS, Young RR, et al: Corticobasal ganglionic degeneration (CBD) with neuronal achromasia: Clinicopathological study of two cases. *Neurology* 39(suppl 1):140, 1989.

28. Riley DE, Lang AE: Corticobasal ganglionic degeneration (CBD): Further observations on six additional cases. *Neurology* 38(suppl 1):360, 1988.

29. Sawle GV, Brooks DJ, Thompson PD, et al: PET studies on the dopaminergic system and regional cortical metabolism in corticobasal degeneration. *Neurology* 39(suppl 1):163, 1989.

30. Eidelberg D, Moeller JR, Sidtis JJ, et al: (1989) Corticodentatonigral degeneration: Metabolic asymmetries studied with 18F-fluorodeoxyglucose and positron emission tomography. *Neurology* 39(suppl 1):164, 1989.

31. Eidelberg D, Dhawan V, Moeller JR, et al: The metabolic landscape of corticobasal ganglionic degeneration: Regional asymmetries studied with positron emission tomography. *J Neurol Neurosurg Psychiatry* 54:856–862, 1991.

32. Blin J, Vidailhet M, Bonnet AM, et al: PET study in corticobasal degeneration. *Mov Disord* 5(suppl 1):19, 1990.

33. Blin J, Vidailhet MJ, Pillon B, et al: Corticobasal degeneration: Decreased and asymmetrical glucose consumption as studied with PET. *Mov Disord* 7(4):348–354, 1992.

34. Markus HS, Lees AJ, Lennox G, et al: Patterns of regional cerebral blood flow in corticobasal degeneration studied using HMPAO SPECT: Comparison with Parkinson's disease and normal controls. *Mov Disord* 10(2):179–187, 1995.

35. Frisoni GB, Pizzolato G, Zanetti O, et al: Corticobasal degeneration: Neuropsychological assessment and dopamine D2 receptor SPECT analysis. *Eur Neurol* 35(1):50–54, 1995.

36. Brooks DJ: PET studies on the early and differential diagnosis of Parkinson's disease. *Neurology* 43(6):S6–16, 1993.

37. Marek K, Seibyl J, Fussell B, et al: Dopamine transporter imaging in Parkinson disease and Parkinson plus syndromes. *Mov Disord* 10(5):3, 1995.

38. Feany MB, Mattiace LA, Dickson DW: Neuropathologic overlap of progressive supranuclear palsy, Pick's disease, and corticobasal degeneration. *J Neuropathol Exp Neurol* 55:53–67, 1996.

39. Ksiezak-Reding H, Morgan K, Mattiace LA, et al: Ultrastructure and biochemical composition of paired helical filaments in corticobasal degeneration. *Am J Pathol* 145:1496–1508, 1994.

40. Nishimura T, Ikeda K, Akiyama H, et al: Immunohistochemical investigation of tau-positive structures in the cerebral cortex of patients with progressive supranuclear palsy. *Neurosci Lett* 201:123–126, 1995.

41. Mori H, Nishimura M, Namba Y, Oda T: Corticobasal degeneration: A disease with widespread appearance of abnormal tau and neurofibrillary tangles, and its relation to progressive supranuclear palsy. *Acta Neuropathol (Berl)* 87:545–553, 1994.

42. Horoupian DS, Chu PL: Unusual case of corticobasal degeneration with tau/Gallyas-positive neuronal and glial tangles. *Acta Neuropathol (Berl)* 88:592–598, 1994.

43. Uchihara T, Mitani K, Mori H, et al: Abnormal cytoskeletal pathology peculiar to corticobasal degeneration is different from that of Alzheimer's disease or progressive supranuclear palsy. *Acta Neuropathol (Berl)* 88:379–383, 1994.

44. Feany MB, Ksiezak-Reding H, Liu WK, et al: Epitope expression and hyperphosphorylation of tau protein in corticobasal degeneration: Differentiation from progressive supranuclear palsy. *Acta Neuropathol (Berl)* 90:37–43, 1995.

45. Wakabayashi K, Oyanagi K, Mahifuchi T, et al: Corticobasal degeneration: Etiopathological significance of the cytoskeletal alterations. *Acta Neuropathol (Berl)* 87:545–553, 1994.

46. Hauw JJ, Daniel SE, Dickson D, et al: Preliminary NINDS neuropathologic criteria for Steele-Richardson-Olszewski syndrome (progressive supranuclear palsy). *Neurology* 44:2015–2019, 1994.

47. Litvan I, Hauw JJ, Bartko JJ, et al: Validity and reliability of the preliminary NINDS neuropathologic criteria for progressive supranuclear palsy and related disorders. *J Neuropathol Exp Neurol* 55:97–105, 1996.

48. Gearing M, Olson DA, Watts RL, Mirra SS: Progressive supranuclear palsy: Neuropathologic and clinical heterogeneity. *Neurology* 44:1015–1024, 1994.

49. Dickson DW, Yen S-H, Suzuki KI, et al: Ballooned neurons in select neurodegenerative diseases contain phosphorylated neurofilament epitopes. *Acta Neuropathol (Berl)* 71:216–223, 1986.

50. Nakazato Y, Hirato J, Ishida Y, et al: Swollen cortical neurons in Creutzfeldt-Jakob disease contain a phosphorylated neurofilament epitope. *J Neuropathol Exp Neurol* 49:197–205, 1990.

51. Mackenzie IRA, Hudson LP: Achromatic neurons in the cortex of progressive supranuclear palsy. *Acta Neuropathol (Berl)* 90:615–619, 1995.

52. Manetto V, Sternberger NH, Perry G, et al: Phosphorylation of neurofilaments is altered in amyotrophic lateral sclerosis. *J Neuropathol Exp Neurol* 47:642–653, 1988.

53. Kertesz A, Hudson L, Mackenzie IRA, Munoz DG: The pathology and nosology of primary progressive aphasia. *Neurology* 44:2065–2072, 1994.

54. Ikeda K, Akiyama H, Haga C, et al: Argyrophilic thread-like structure in corticobasal degeneration and supranuclear palsy. *Neurosci Lett* 174:157–159, 1994.

55. Jendroska K, Rossor MN, Mathias CJ, Daniel SE: Morphological overlap between corticobasal degeneration and Pick's disease: A clinicopathological report. *Mov Disord* 10:111–114, 1995.

56. Lang AE, Bergeron C, Pollanen MS, Ashby P: Parietal Pick's disease mimicking cortical-basal ganglionic degeneration. *Neurology* 44:1436–1440, 1994.

57. Mizusawa H, Yen S-H, Hirano A, Llena JF: Pathology of the dentate nucleus in progressive supranuclear palsy: A histological, immunohistochemical and ultrastructural study. *Acta Neuropathol (Berl)* 78:419–428, 1989.

58. Yamashita S, Iwamoto H, Hara M, et al: Sisters with early onset hereditary dentatorubral-pallidoluysian atrophy of childhood-DNA analysis and clinicopathological findings (title translated from Japanese). *No To Hattatsu* 27:473–479, 1995.

59. Kogure T, Oda T, Katoh Y: Autopsy cases of hereditary ataxia pathologically diagnosed as the Japanese type of Joseph disease-cliniconeuropathological findings (title translated from Japanese). *Seishin Shinkeigaku Zasshi* 92:161–183, 1990.

60. Iwabuchi K, Nagatomo H, Tanabe T, et al: An autopsied case of type 2 Machado-Joseph's disease or spino-pontine degeneration (title translated from Japanese). *No To Shinkei* 45:733–740, 1993.

61. Hayashi M, Itoh M, Kabasawa Y, et al: A neuropathologic study of a case of the Prader-Willi syndrome with an interstitial deletion of the proximal long arm of chromosome 15. *Brain Dev* 14:58–62, 1992.

62. Hattori H, Tanaka S, Kondoh H, et al: A case of juvenile Alzheimer's disease with various neurological features such as myoclonus, showing grumose degeneration in the dentate nucleus (title translated from Japanese). *Rinsho Shinkeigaku* 30:647–653, 1990.

63. Strittmatter WJ, Saunders AM, Schmechel D, et al: Apolipoprotein E: High avidity binding to beta-amyloid and increased frequency of type 4 allele in late onset familial Alzheimer's disease. *Proc Natl Acad Sci USA* 90:1977–1981, 1993.

64. Corder EH, Saunders AM, Strittmatter WJ, et al: Gene dose of apolipoprotein E type 4 allele and the risk of Alzheimer's disease in late onset families. *Science* 261:921–923, 1993.

65. Schneider JA, Gearing M, Robbins RS, et al: Apolipoprotein E genotype in diverse neurodegenerative disorders. *Ann Neurol* 30:296–297, 1995.

66. Tabaton M, Rolleri M, Masturzo P, et al: Apolipoprotein E epsilon 4 allele frequency is not increased in progressive supranuclear palsy. *Neurology* 45:1764–1765, 1995.

67. Farrer LA, Abraham CR, Volicer L, et al: Allele e4 of apolipoprotein E shows a dose effect on age at onset of Pick disease. *Exp Neurol* 136:162–170, 1995.

68. Stacy M, Jankovic J: Differential diagnosis of Parkinson's disease and the parkinsonism plus syndromes. *Neurol Clin* 10:341–359, 1992.

69. Steele JC, Richardson JC, Olszewski J: Progressive supranuclear palsy. *Arch Neurol* 10:333–358, 1964.

70. Barclay CL, Bergeron C, Lang AE: Arm levitation in progressive supranuclear palsy. *Mov Disord* 10:15–16, 1995.

71. Case Records of the Massachusetts General Hospital: Weekly Clinicopathological exercises: A 75-year-old man with right sided rigidity, dysarthria, and abnormal gait. *N Engl J Med* 329:1560–1567, 1993. (Published erratum appears in *N Engl J Med* 330:448, 1994.

72. Adams RD, Van Bogaert L, Vander Eecken H: Striatonigral degeneration. *J Neuropathol Exp Neurol* 23:584–608, 1964.

73. Takei Y, Mirra SS: Striatonigral degeneration: A form of multiple system atrophy with clinical parkinsonism. *Prog Neuropathol* 2:217–251, 1973.

74. Spokes EGS, Bannister R, Oppenheimer DR: Multiple system atrophy with autonomic failure. *J Neurol Sci* 43:59–82, 1979.

75. Quinn N: Multiple system atrophy, in Marsden CD, Fahn S (eds): *Movement Disorders 3*. London: Butterworth, 1994, pp 262–281.

76. Kosaka K: Dementia and neuropathology in Lewy body disease. *Adv Neurol* 60:456–463, 1993.

77. Burkhardt CR, Filey CM, Kleinschmidt-DeMasters BK, et al: Diffuse Lewy body disease and dementia. *Neurology* 38:1520–1528, 1988.

78. Akelaitis AJ: Atrophy of basal ganglia in Pick's disease: A clinicopathologic study. *Arch Neurol Psychiatry* 51:27–34, 1944.

79. Tissot R, Constantinidis J, Richard J: *La Maladie de Pick*. Paris: Paul Masson, 1975.

80. Cole M, Wright D, Banker BQ: Familial aphasia due to Pick's disease. *Ann Neurol* 6:158, 1979.

81. Wojcieszek J, Lang AE, Jankovic J, et al: Rapidly progressive aphasia, apraxia, dementia, myoclonus and parkinsonism. *Mov Disord* 9:358–366, 1994.

82. Ball JA, Lantos PL, Jackson M, et al: Alien hand sign in association with Alzheimer's histopathology. *J Neurol Neurosurg Psychiatry* 56(9):1020–1023, 1993.

83. Hirano A, Kurland LT, Krooth RS, et al: Parkinsonism-dementia complex: An endemic disease on the Island of Guam. I. Clinical features. *Brain* 84:642–661, 1961.

84. Hirano A, Malamud M, Kurland LT: Parkinsonism-dementia complex on the Island of Guam. II. Pathological features. *Brain* 84:662–679, 1961.

85. Wilson SAK: Lenticular degeneration. *Brain* 34:295–321, 1912.

86. Bruyn GW: The Westphal variant and juvenile type of Huntington's chorea, in Barbeau A, Brunette JR (eds): *Progress in Neurogenetics*. Amsterdam: Excerpta Medica Foundation, 1967, pp 666–673.

87. Woods BT, Schaumburg HH: Nigrospinodentatal degeneration with nuclear ophthalmoplegia, in Vinken PJ, Bruyn GW (eds): *Handbook of Clinical Neurology*. Amsterdam: North-Holland Publishing Co, 1975, vol 22, pp 157–176.

88. Nakano KK, Dawson DM, Spence A: Machado disease: A hereditary ataxia in Portuguese emigrants to Massachusetts. *Neurology* 22: 49–55, 1972.

89. Romanul FCA, Fowler HL, Radvany J, et al: Azorean disease of the nervous system. *N Engl J Med* 296:1505–1508, 1977.

90. Sachdev HS, Forno LS, Kane CA: Joseph disease: A multisystem degenerative disorder of the nervous system. *Neurology* 32:192–195, 1982.

91. Boustany RM, Tyler KL, Kolodny EH, Adams RD: A new familial progressive degeneration of the basal ganglia, cortocobulbar, and corticospinal systems. *Neurology* 34(suppl 1):149, 1984.

92. Jendroska K, Hoffman O, Schelosky L, et al: Absence of disease related prion protein in neurodegenerative disorders presenting with Parkinson's syndrome. *J Neurol Neurosurg Psychiatry* 57(10):1249–1251, 1994.

93. Morin P, Lechevalier B, Bianco C: Atrophie cerebelleuse et lesions pallido-luyso-nigriques avec corps de Lewy. *Rev Neurol (Paris)* 136:381–390, 1980.

94. Brown P, Rodgers-Johnson P, Cathala F, et al: Creutzfeldt-Jakob disease of long duration: Clinicopathological characteristics, transmissibility and differential diagnosis. *Ann Neurol* 16:295–304, 1984.

95. Dorfman LJ, Forno LS: Paravicoplastic encephalomyelitis. *Acta Neurol Scand* 48:556–574, 1992.

96. Giladi N, Fahn S: Hemiparkinsonism-hemiatrophy syndrome may mimic early stage cortical-basal ganglionic degeneration. *Mov Disord* 7:384–385, 1992.

97. Jankovic J, Kirkpatrick JB, Blonquist KA, et al: Late onset Halloverden-Spatz disease presenting as familial parkinsonism. *Neurology* 35:227–234, 1985.

98. Kritchevsky N, Hansen LA, Deteresa R, et al: Slowly progressive ideomotor apraxia: A presentation of adult onset Halloverden-Spatz disease. *Neurology* 39(suppl):237, 1989.

99. Martin JJ: Adult type of neuronal ceroid lipofuscinosis. *Dev Neurosci* 13:331–338, 1991.

100. Paulus W, Selim M: Corticonigral degeneration with neuronal achromasia and basal neurofibrillary tangles. *Acta Neuropathol (Berl)* 81:89–94, 1990.

101. Caselli RJ, Jack CR Jr, Peterson RC, et al: Asymmetric cortical degeneration syndrome: Clinical and radiologic correlation. *Neurology* 42:1462–1468, 1992.

102. Caselli RJ, Jack CR Jr: Asymmetric cortical degeneration syndromes: A proposed clinical classification. *Arch Neurol* 49:770–780, 1992.

103. Mesulam MM: Slowly progressive aphasia without dementia. *Ann Neurol* 11:592–598, 1982.

104. Morris JC, Cole M, Banker BQ, Wright D: Hereditary dysphasia dementia and the Pick-Alzheimer spectrum. *Ann Neurol* 16:455–466, 1984.

105. Goulding PJ, Northen B, Snowden JS, et al: Progressive aphasia with right sided extrapyramidal signs: Another manifestation with localized cerebral atrophy. *J Neurol Neurosurg Psychiatry* 52:128–130, 1989.

106. Lippa CF, Cohen R, Smith TW, Drachman DA: Primary progressive aphasia with focal neuronal achromasia. *Neurology* 41:882–886, 1991.

107. Pillon B, Dubois B, Agid Y: Testing cognition may contribute to the diagnosis of movement disorders. *Neurology* 46:329–334, 1996.

Chapter 46

WILSON'S DISEASE

RONALD F. PFEIFFER

EPIDEMIOLOGY
GENETICS
PATHOPHYSIOLOGY
CLINICAL FEATURES
    Hepatic Manifestations
    Neurological Manifestations
    Psychiatric Manifestations
    Ophthalmologic Manifestations
    Musculoskeletal Manifestations
    Other Manifestations
DIAGNOSIS
TREATMENT
    Dietary Therapy
    Inhibition of Intestinal Copper Absorption
    Copper Chelation Therapy
    Liver Transplantation
    Treatment Guidelines
SUMMARY

In 1912 Wilson penned, as his doctoral thesis, his now classic treatise describing the clinical and pathological features of the disease he labeled progressive hepatolenticular degeneration.[1] He was not, however, the first to describe the illness that now bears his name. Case descriptions of what likely was Wilson's disease (WD) were published by Frerichs in 1860,[2] Westphal in 1885,[3] Gowers in 1888,[4] Ormerod in 1890,[5] Homen in 1892,[6] and Strümpell in 1898,[7] but it was Wilson who accurately and exhaustingly detailed the characteristics of this illness and distilled this information into a coherent clinical picture.

After Wilson's description, our present-day understanding of WD has evolved and matured as a result of contributions from many individuals. Kayser, in 1902,[8] and Fleischer, in 1903[9] and 1912,[10] first described the rings of corneal pigmentation that are now so firmly linked with WD. Although Rumpel first described increased hepatic copper content in WD in 1913,[11] it was not until 1948, when Mandelbrote et al.[12] noted increased urinary excretion of copper and Cumings[13] documented copper deposits in both liver and brain, that WD was finally recognized as a disturbance of copper metabolism. Ceruloplasmin deficiency was subsequently documented by Scheinberg in 1952.[14] The past 4 decades have been marked by dramatic advances in our ability to treat WD, and the past several years have witnessed the unfolding of the search for the WD gene.

Epidemiology

Although not recognized by Wilson himself—he noted it to be familial but believed that a toxin was the likely cause—

WD was identified as a hereditary process by Hall in 1921.[15] It is an autosomal-recessive inherited disease. Estimates of prevalence vary widely, but WD is, by all accounts, a rare disorder. A prevalence figure of 30 cases per million is most frequently quoted,[16,17] but other lower estimates have been published.[18–20] A birth incidence rate of 17 per million was reported in Ireland by Reilly for the years 1950–1969.[20] In northern Europe, calculations of WD gene frequency range from 0.34 to 0.53, whereas, in locales with higher rates of consanguinity, such as Japan, Israel, and Sardinia, gene frequencies are higher.[20]

Genetics

In 1985 Frydman and colleagues suggested that the WD gene was located on chromosome 13.[21] The subsequent search for the gene location eventually was focused on the 13q14.3 region between D13S59 and D13S31.[22–25] In 1993 Bull and colleagues and Yamaguchi and colleagues suggested that WD is the result of a defect in a gene, which Bull labeled as Wc1, that encodes a copper transporting P-type adenosine triphosphatase (ATPase) that is expressed in liver and kidney.[26,27] Moreover, they noted that the Wc1 gene was very similar to the gene for Menkes' disease, another disorder of copper metabolism.

Pathophysiology

Our understanding of the pathophysiological processes that characterize WD has expanded considerably beyond the seminal recognition in the 1940s of copper excess in the liver and copper deposition in other tissues. The exact molecular defect responsible for these events, however, has remained enigmatic as of the date of this writing although, with the rapidly unfolding events in the realm of molecular genetics, it is entirely possible that this statement will be outdated by the time this reaches press.

As a vital component of enzyme systems such as cytochrome C oxidase, dopamine beta-hydroxylase, superoxide dismutase, and tyrosinase, copper is an essential element for cellular functioning.[28] However, outside of these enzyme systems, free copper is an extremely toxic substance that can produce irreversible cellular damage and death. To protect against such cellular damage, elegant systems have evolved that bind the copper molecule so that it can be safely absorbed, correct amounts can be delivered to the required sites, and excess copper can be eliminated from the body. When these delivery systems malfunction, dysfunction and damage can result, either from too much or too little copper.

Menkes' disease is an x-linked recessive disorder in which intestinal copper absorption is impaired, with consequent copper deficiency in body tissues, including liver and brain. Ceruloplasmin is also reduced. WD is a disease of copper toxicity. The problem is not one of excessive absorption of copper but rather, it is a consequence of faulty transport and elimination of this element.

First isolated in 1948, ceruloplasmin is α globulin that binds and transports six copper molecules.[29] There are actually multiple forms of ceruloplasmin, with molecular weights varying from 115,000 to 200,000.[30] Although ceruloplasmin is characteristically decreased in WD, this is not absolute, and WD is not merely a disease of ceruloplasmin deficiency. In fact, 5–15 percent of individuals with WD may have normal or only slightly reduced ceruloplasmin, whereas 10–20 percent of heterozygotes who are clinically asymptomatic may have reduced ceruloplasmin.[31] It is also unclear what role ceruloplasmin deficiency actually plays in the production of symptoms in WD. Symptom severity clearly does not correlate with magnitude of ceruloplasmin deficiency,[32] nor does correction of the deficiency with exogenous ceruloplasmin administration correct the clinical picture.[33] It is not clear as to whether the reduction of ceruloplasmin in WD is a result of reduced production or accelerated degradation of the compound. It has been suggested that there may be reduced transcription of the ceruloplasmin gene or reduced translation of ceruloplasmin mRNA in WD,[34,35] but this is speculation.

Ceruloplasmin deficiency is not unique to WD. As noted above, ceruloplasmin deficiency is also characteristic of Menkes' disease. A hereditary ceruloplasmin deficiency with only modest hepatic copper accumulation, but dramatic iron deposition in liver, pancreas, and brain has recently been described.[36] Transient ceruloplasmin deficiency may also occur in a variety of conditions, including protein-losing enteropathy, nephrotic syndrome, hepatic failure, sprue, as well as in other situations in which both protein and total calorie intake are deficient.[31,37]

The recognition that ceruloplasmin deficiency is not the primary explanation for the copper deposition in tissues in WD has led investigators to focus on copper elimination as the potential etiopathological mechanism. The primary route of elimination of copper is the gastrointestinal tract.[38] Copper is also excreted in the urine, but this is only a secondary route, which has been emphasized in the past because of the ease in measuring copper elimination via this route. It has now been recognized that impairment of gastrointestinal (GI) elimination of copper stands at the root of the copper accumulation in WD.[17,39] Copper is routinely secreted in saliva, gastric juice, and bile, but the copper in the saliva and gastric juice is subsequently reabsorbed more distally in the gut, leaving biliary excretion of copper as the primary source of copper elimination.[39,40] It is a defect in biliary excretion of copper that is the hallmark of WD.[17,39] This defect in biliary excretion of copper results in slow, but steady, accumulation of copper in the body.[41] Initially, the copper is stored in the liver, but eventually the storage capacity of the liver is exceeded, and unbound copper spills out of the liver and finds its way to other organs and tissues, where it also begins to accumulate. As the excess copper escapes from the liver, urinary copper excretion markedly increases but is not able to fully compensate for the defect in biliary excretion. This results in a positive copper balance with consequent relentless deposition of copper in other tissues.

With the identification of the WD gene (Wc1) as encoding for a copper transporting ATPase, it has been suggested that both impaired incorporation of copper into ceruloplasmin in the liver and reduced copper excretion from liver into bile could be accounted for by an abnormal ATPase that is not able to maintain the copper in the correct redox state.[26] Other hypotheses have also been proposed.

Clinical Features

Although the fundamental pathogenetic defect in WD has its source in the hepatobiliary system, the consequences of the defect play themselves out in multiple organs and systems. This multisystem involvement lends itself to an extremely diverse clinical picture which, at times, presents a formidable challenge for even the most astute clinician.

HEPATIC MANIFESTATIONS

Hepatic symptoms or signs of hepatic dysfunction are the most frequent mode of clinical presentation of WD, representing the initial feature in more than 50 percent of cases.[42] This percentage is even higher in Asian populations,[43] although the reason for this difference is not clear. The average age of onset of hepatic symptoms is 11.4 years.[44] It is rare for WD to become clinically apparent before age 6. "Hepatic" presentation beyond age 40, although unusual, has been documented.[45] Thus, WD should still be considered in the differential diagnosis of individuals in their 40s and even 50s who present with hepatic dysfunction.

Hepatic dysfunction in WD can follow one of several routes in its evolution. It can present with asymptomatic enlargement of both liver and spleen. Liver function tests may, however, be elevated, and spider angiomata may appear.

Acute transient hepatitis is a second, more common mode of presentation. This occurs in 25 percent of individuals and is typically characterized by jaundice, anorexia, and easy fatigability with a reduced sense of energy.[17] Although this may be all too easily passed off as a viral-induced hepatitis or infectious mononucleosis, especially when family history is silent, the concomitant presence of a hemolytic anemia should serve as an important portent of the presence of WD.[17] Other abnormalities that may also be clues to a diagnosis of WD in this setting include elevated unconjugated bilirubin[46] and reduced uric acid.

Acute fulminant hepatitis, with rapidly progressive liver failure, encephalopathy, and coagulopathy, is yet another potential mode of hepatic presentation of WD.[47] The mortality rate with this presentation is extremely high.[48] A severe Coombs'-negative hemolytic anemia, presumably from destruction of erythrocytes by the suddenly released hepatic copper, may occur.[49] Relatively low aminotransferase levels and low alkaline phosphatase levels may also be noted.[50]

Chronic active hepatitis occurs in 10–30 percent of individuals with WD.[51,52] One diagnostically treacherous aspect of this presentation of WD is the potential for the serum ceruloplasmin, as an acute-phase reactant, to become "elevated" into the low normal range.[51]

The most common hepatic manifestation of WD is the development of progressive cirrhosis with a postnecrotic picture.[53] Individuals typically develop slowly progressive hepatic failure with splenomegaly (often without hepatomegaly), ascites, esophageal varices, and encephalopathy. There are no specific identifying characteristics of the cirrhosis;

thus a high index of suspicion remains a necessity in the evaluation of young (and even middle-aged) individuals with progressive liver failure.

NEUROLOGICAL MANIFESTATIONS

Left untreated, most individuals with WD will eventually develop symptoms or signs of neurological dysfunction. In 40–50 percent of individuals neurological symptoms are actually the initially recognized clinical feature.[42] As might be suspected from the pathophysiological basis of WD, the average age at which neurological features appear is significantly later than the average age of onset of hepatic WD manifestations—18.9 years versus 11.4 years—although neurological symptoms have been reported as early as age 6.[44,53] Although it is uncommon, delayed appearance of neurological symptoms beyond age 50 can also occur.[54]

Tremor is the most frequent neurological presenting feature in WD, occurring in approximately 50 percent of individuals.[55] The tremor may be resting, postural, or kinetic in character. Asymmetry is the rule. The tremor may be fine or coarse, proximal or distal. A proximal component of tremor in the arms can endow the tremor with a "wing-beating" appearance. Head titubation may also be present. An unusual presentation of tremor in WD is isolated tongue tremor.[56,57]

Dysarthria is another common feature of neurological WD, eventually developing in the vast majority of patients. Two broad categories of dysarthria have been described.[37] A hypokinetic dysarthria resulting from extrapyramidal dysfunction, particularly dystonia, affecting the tongue, face, and pharynx, commonly occurs. Speech can be severely compromised. The dysarthria can become so severe, the patient becomes virtually mute. Drooling, another common feature of WD, is also the result of this dystonic involvement, as is the "risus sardonicus," or fixed grimace-smile, seen in some individuals with WD. An unusual "whispering dysphonia" has also been described in WD,[58] as has a very unusual laugh in which most of the sound is generated with inspiration.[59] The second type of dysarthria observed in WD is a cerebellar-type characterized by scanning, explosive speech. This type of dysarthria is a result of cerebellar and brain stem involvement.

Cerebellar dysfunction, which initially gave rise to the term "pseudosclerotic" as a type of WD, is seen in approximately 25 percent of WD patients with neurological dysfunction.[60] In addition to the scanning speech described above, individuals may display impaired coordination and kinetic (intention) tremor as part of the clinical picture.

Although dystonia, which in addition to facial and pharyngeal muscles can also involve the limbs and trunk, is seen quite frequently in WD, chorea is uncommon. Tics or myoclonus are very unusual.

Gait abnormalities are another hallmark of WD. As with dysarthria, both extrapyramidal and cerebellar patterns of impairment have been described. An individual with WD may display a parkinsonian gait, a wide-based ataxic gait, or a combination of the two.

Seizures have been reported in up to 6 percent of patients with WD, especially in younger individuals.[61] The combination of seizures and psychiatric disturbances may indicate the presence of frontal white matter lesions.[62] Pseudobulbar

emotional lability,[63] muscle cramps, and even priapism[64] have been reported in WD. Headache can be the presenting neurological symptom, according to some investigators, in approximately 10 percent of individuals.[17]

Neither upper motor neuron (weakness, spasticity, hyperreflexia, Babinski responses) nor lower motor neuron signs (hyporeflexia) are often seen in WD. Sensory loss, sphincter dysfunction, and autonomic disturbances are also unusual.[17]

Historically, WD has been segregated into two types, the classic (dystonic) WD and the pseudosclerotic (Westphal) forms.[65] Classic WD is characterized primarily by extrapyramidal dysfunction, especially dystonia, whereas the pseudosclerotic form presents with kinetic (intention) tremor and dysarthria of the cerebellar type. The term pseudosclerotic derives from its superficial resemblance to multiple sclerosis. A more recent categorization of WD has used three subgroups: pseudoparkinsonian, pseudosclerosis, and dyskinesia.[66] Although this most recent categorization includes some anatomic specificity, these attempts at classification are of limited practical value, because considerable variability and overlap exist.

PSYCHIATRIC MANIFESTATIONS

The psychiatric features of WD are often underappreciated and underdiagnosed. Most reports indicate that psychiatric symptoms are the presenting clinical feature in approximately 20 percent of individuals with WD.[67] However, percentages ranging from 10 to 51 percent have been reported.[68] Up to 20 percent of individuals with WD will be referred to a psychiatrist for evaluation before a diagnosis of WD is made.[69]

Most individuals with WD will experience psychiatric symptomatology at some point during the course of their illness. Reported figures range from 30 to 100 percent.[70] Not surprisingly, psychiatric manifestations of WD are most commonly seen in persons who also display neurological dysfunction. Because of these facts, Yarze and colleagues caution that WD should be considered and excluded in any young person who develops otherwise-unexplained psychiatric dysfunction, especially when signs of associated neurological dysfunction are also present.[50]

As with the neurological picture of WD, there is no archetypal psychiatric WD presentation. Akil and Brewer have divided the psychiatric symptoms of WD into five categories: behavioral/personality abnormalities, affective disorders, cognitive impairment, psychosis, and an "others" category.[71] Subtle changes in personality and behavior may develop, including emotional lability, impulsiveness, childishness, aggressiveness, recklessness, and disinhibition.[72] Self-injurious behavior may occur.[73] More severe psychiatric features may also develop. Depression is reported in 20–30 percent of persons with WD and is probably significantly underdiagnosed.[71] As with some other neurodegenerative disorders, there is controversy as to whether depression in WD is reactive or endogenous. Mania may also occur.

Although clear-cut dementia is uncommon in WD, it may occur in advanced situations in which structural central nervous system (CNS) damage has occurred. Formal IQ testing can demonstrate reductions of 12–35 points in individuals with WD, but the explanation for this is not clear.[74] It has been suggested that cognitive impairment in WD is a result of subclinical hepatic encephalopathy,[75] but this assessment is controversial.[71] It should also be remembered that the appearance of an individual with WD, with dysarthria, drooling, impaired coordination, and bradykinesia, may be mistakenly perceived as indicative of cognitive impairment when, in fact, intellect is unaffected.

Psychosis, although unusual in WD, may occur and be characterized by paranoid thinking, delusional thoughts, hallucinations, and even catatonia.[70,73,76] These psychiatric symptoms often respond poorly to conventional psychiatric medical management, and it may be difficult to differentiate adverse effects of psychiatric medications from developing neurological symptoms of WD itself.[59]

A variety of other psychiatric difficulties may also appear in the setting of WD. Anxiety may be a troublesome problem.[77] Sexual preoccupation and decreased sexual inhibition have been described in WD by several investigators.[17,77] Deterioration in work or academic performance may also occur, although not necessarily correlating with impairment of cognitive function. Anorexia nervosa has been described in an individual with WD.[68]

Psychiatric symptoms often improve with appropriate treatment of WD, but improvement often is delayed into the 6- to 18-month time frame. Permanent psychiatric dysfunction may persist, despite adequate treatment.

OPHTHALMOLOGIC MANIFESTATIONS

As noted earlier, Kayser's initial description of the pigmented corneal rings that now bear his name was published in 1902, fully 10 years before Wilson's clinical compilation. Kayser's patient was felt at the time to be suffering from multiple sclerosis.[8] Fleischer described similar ocular changes in 1903, and in 1912 connected the corneal pigmented rings with the neurological picture of "pseudosclerosis."[9,10]

Kayser-Fleischer rings (KFRs) are formed by the deposition of copper in Descemet's membrane. The excess copper is actually deposited throughout the cornea, but it is only in Descemet's membrane that sulfur-copper complexes are formed, producing the visible copper deposits.[78,79] They are almost always bilateral, but unilateral KFRs have been described.[80] Vision is not obstructed or impaired by the KFRs. Their color is quite variable and can range from gold to brown to green. Because of their color composition, fully developed KFRs are often quite readily seen in blue eyes but can be very difficult to discern when the iris is brown. The visible KFR pigment appears first in the periphery of the cornea at the limbus and spreads centrally. In some individuals a clear area between the pigment and the corneoscleral junction may be present.[81] The superior aspect of the cornea is involved initially, followed by the inferior aspect and then, finally, the medial and lateral aspects of the cornea fill in. A KFR is depicted in Fig. 46-1. An excellent color photograph of KFRs was recently provided by Finelli.[82]

There are two important caveats to remember with regard to the identification of KFRs. Because the first appearance of a KFR is superiorly, it is important to lift the eyelid when examining the patient so that the entire cornea is exposed and inspected.[83] Furthermore, in many individuals, espe-

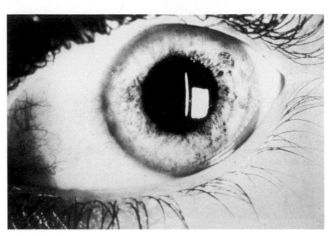

FIGURE 46-1 Kayser-Fleischer ring in an individual with Wilson's disease. See Plate 9. (*Courtesy of Rowen Zetterman.*)

cially those with brown eyes, or when the KFR is not "mature," it may be impossible to see the KFR under routine ophthalmoscopic exam, and slit-lamp examination by an experienced ophthalmologist is necessary.

Corneal pigment deposition can occur in conditions other than WD. Copper-containing corneal rings indistinguishable from KFRs on slit-lamp examination have been described in a variety of hepatic conditions, including primary biliary cirrhosis,[81,84] chronic active hepatitis,[85] possible partial biliary atresia,[85] cirrhosis, and chronic cholestatic jaundice.[86] Intraocular copper-containing foreign bodies, or "grinders," can stain the iris and cornea (chalcosis) and mimic KFRs.[78] Copper sulfate-containing ophthalmic solutions, used to treat trachoma, can also stain the cornea.[87] In some individuals with multiple myeloma,[88,89] and in others with pulmonary carcinoma,[90] marked elevations of gamma globulin and copper have led to corneal ring formation but in a central rather than peripheral pattern.

In several other situations corneal staining unrelated to copper deposition can occur. Arcus senilis is usually easily distinguishable from KFRs by its whitish color, even though its location coincides with KFR "territory." However, if an individual has superimposed carotenemia, the arcus senilis may assume a yellowish tint or cast and can be mistaken for KFRs.[91] Corneal heme staining after cataract removal may also transiently mimic KFRs.[85]

KFRs are virtually always present, at least under slit-lamp examination, in individuals with WD who have developed neurological dysfunction but may not have yet developed in asymptomatic (preclinical) persons or in those with only hepatic symptoms. There are case reports of absence of KFRs in WD patients with neurological symptoms, although this must be exceedingly rare.[54]

Another ocular manifestation of WD is the sunflower cataract, which was first described by Siemerling and Oloff in 1922.[92] The sunflower cataract is much less common than the KFR, occurring in only 17 percent of untreated individuals.[78] It consists of copper deposits in the lens that have a green, gold, brown, or grey coloration and a sunburst or sunflowerlike appearance, with a central powder-like disc and radiating petal-like spokes.[78,93] The sunflower cataract usually does not interfere with vision and, typically, can only be seen during slit-lamp examination.

Other ophthalmologic abnormalities may also be seen in WD. Eye movement abnormalities,[94] white retinal spot formation,[95] and night blindness[96] all have been described in WD, but it is not clear whether as part of the WD or simply a coincidence. Difficulty with gaze fixation has been reported in WD,[97] as has eyelid-opening apraxia.[98] Noteworthy for their absence in WD are nystagmus and cranial nerve palsies.[78]

MUSCULOSKELETAL MANIFESTATIONS

Joint and bone involvement is an under-recognized component of WD. It has been reported with especially high frequency in Asian populations;[43] in fact, the term "osteomuscular type" has been used to describe individuals with skeletal involvement and additional muscle weakness and wasting.[43,99] This higher frequency of musculoskeletal manifestations has been noted in Chinese,[100,101] Japanese,[102] and Indian[99] populations.

Osteoporosis, characterized by radiographic evidence of decreased bone density, may develop in two-thirds of individuals with WD.[103] Osteomalacia, rickets, and localized bone demineralization all may occur.[50] These boney changes may lead to frequent, and even spontaneous, fractures.

Joint involvement, especially the knees, can lead to joint hypermobility or, alternatively, to pain and stiffness, suggesting premature osteoarthrosis.[103,104] Periarticular and intraarticular calcifications can also develop.[50]

Radiological evidence of spinal abnormalities is reported in 20–33 percent of persons with WD.[103,105] Both vertebral body abnormalities and narrowing of the intervertebral disk space are described. Destruction of intervertebral discs and adjacent vertebral bodies severe enough to be mistaken for pyogenic or tuberculous discitis was reported in an individual with WD by Hu, who suggested the possibility of Charcot's disease of the spine because of a subclinical neurological defect of sensation.[106]

The mechanism of bone and joint damage in WD is not clear. With the use of x-ray microprobe spectrometry, synovial copper and iron deposition have been documented in WD.[107] Tissue destruction, mediated by oxygen-derived free radicals, may be responsible for the cartilage and synovial damage.[107]

OTHER MANIFESTATIONS

Hemolytic anemia may be the initial manifestation of WD in 10–15 percent of cases.[50,108,109] As noted earlier, it may also develop in the setting of transient hepatitis and may itself be transient in this setting.[17,110] Severe hemolytic anemia can occur during acute fulminant hepatic failure in WD.[50] Any young person with an otherwise-unexplained nonspherocytic, Coombs-negative hemolytic anemia should be investigated for possible WD. The hemolysis is probably a result of free copper-induced oxidative injury to erythrocytes.[108,111,112]

Renal involvement may also be a part of WD. Excessive amounts of copper in the urine induce renal tubular dysfunction which, in turn, can produce hypercalciuria and hyperphosphaturia with consequent nephrocalcinosis.[113] In fact, hypercalciuria and nephrocalcinosis may be the presenting features of WD.[114] Aminoaciduria and reduction of serum uric acid may also be seen in WD.[53,115]

Wilson mentioned the presence of hyperpigmentation of the legs and a dark complexion in his description of WD.[1] Skin changes seem to develop with particular frequency in Chinese WD patients,[43] with anterior lower leg hyperpigmentation noted in 60 percent in one series.[116] These changes can be misinterpreted as Addison's disease by the unwary. Bluish discoloration of the lunulae of the nails[28,117] and acanthosis nigricans[118] have also been reported.

Menstrual irregularity,[41,119] delayed puberty,[120] and gynecomastia all have been reported in WD, as have congestive heart failure, cardiac arrhythmia, glucose intolerance, and parathyroid insufficiency.[50]

Diagnosis

McIntyre has aptly stated that "the most important single factor in early diagnosis (of WD) is *suspicion* of the disease."[110] When the diagnosis is not considered, it will not be made. WD should be considered and excluded in any young person who develops unexplained neurological dysfunction, especially if the basal ganglia or cerebellum are involved. Moreover, because of its protean manifestations, similar consideration of WD is important in young individuals presenting with hepatic, psychiatric, and even other symptoms. The definition of "young" is relative but certainly should include individuals up to the age of 40 and probably to age 60.

There presently (this may change with molecular genetic advances and recognition of the WD gene) is no fail-safe diagnostic test for WD. Certain identification of WD can only be reached with judicious use of a combination of studies, which may include determination of hepatic copper content, serum ceruloplasmin, 24-hour urinary copper, and slit-lamp examination for KFRs. Additional studies, such as determination of the rate of incorporation of radiocopper into ceruloplasmin, neuroimaging studies, neurophysiological studies, serum free copper, and even cerebrospinal fluid (CSF) copper levels, may be useful. It is not necessary to obtain each of these studies in every patient.

It is important to perform the necessary studies in laboratories where the procedures are run frequently and the reported values are reliable. Care must be taken in collecting samples for analysis. Urine collections should always be in copper-free jugs supplied by the laboratory. Scheinberg and Sternlieb also stress that precautions must be taken performing liver biopsy to avoid specimen contamination by the biopsy needle.[17]

Determination of hepatic copper content via liver biopsy is the single most sensitive and accurate test for WD. Hepatic copper content will be elevated in virtually all individuals with WD, even those who are clinically asymptomatic. Because copper is not uniformly distributed in the liver, however, it is possible for a sampling error to give a falsely low copper level when a sufficiently sized biopsy (1–2 cm of tissue) is not obtained.[121] Hepatic copper elevation in WD is typically quite striking, generally greater than 250 μg/g dry tissue, compared to the normal values of 15–55 μg/g. Hepatic copper elevation is not, by itself, pathognomonic for WD and can occur in obstructive liver diseases, such as primary biliary cirrhosis, biliary atresia, extrahepatic biliary obstruction, primary sclerosing cholangitis, intrahepatic cholestasis of childhood, Indian childhood cirrhosis, and chronic active hepatitis.[122-126] Deceptively low hepatic copper levels may also be found in individuals with WD when the biopsy is performed just as copper is being mobilized from the liver and released into the general circulation. In this situation the hepatic copper content is still elevated, but levels in the range of "only" 100 μg/g may be recorded.[127] Although measurement of hepatic copper content is the most sensitive and accurate diagnostic study for WD, the invasiveness and small, but definite, risk of complication from the procedure dictate that this study be used only when simpler approaches have not yielded a definitive diagnosis.

Slit-lamp examination by an experienced ophthalmologist to look for KFRs is a vital part of the diagnostic evaluation for suspected WD. The presence of KFRs, although not absolutely specific for WD, is strong supportive evidence of the diagnosis in an individual with neurological or psychiatric features suggesting WD. It has been stated that the absence of KFRs in an individual with CNS symptoms or signs excludes the diagnosis of WD.[17] Exceptions to this "doctrine," however, have been reported, and individuals with neurological WD but no KFRs described.[54,128,129] Of course, in persons with only hepatic symptoms (where copper has not yet been released systemically) or in asymptomatic individuals, KFRs are typically absent.

As a screening test for WD, assay of serum ceruloplasmin is both simple and practical and should be performed on every individual in whom the diagnosis of WD is being considered. However, because ceruloplasmin may fall within or only slightly below the normal range in 5–15 percent of persons with WD,[17] it should not be the sole screening measure used. Moreover, in addition to falling into the subnormal range in 10–20 percent of WD heterozygotes[17] (who do not develop WD and do not require any WD treatment), serum ceruloplasmin may also be reduced in a number of other conditions, as mentioned earlier. Because it is an acute-phase reactant, ceruloplasmin may increase in pregnancy, during estrogen administration, with infection or inflammation (including hepatitis),[31] and it is, therefore, possible for ceruloplasmin to actually transiently reach normal or near-normal levels in persons with WD who also develop these conditions.[51] However, Yarze and colleagues believe that a serum ceruloplasmin level greater than 30 mg/dL virtually excludes the possibility of WD[50] whereas Snow suggests a level of 40 as the exclusion mark.[121]

As noted earlier, urinary copper excretion rises dramatically in symptomatic WD, even though the increase never is sufficient to establish a negative copper balance. Urinary copper levels in symptomatic WD typically exceed 100 μg/day, but in asymptomatic individuals, where copper is still accumulating in the liver, urinary copper may still be in the normal range. Obstructive liver disease, such as primary biliary cirrhosis, can also produce elevation of urinary copper.[126,130] Despite these drawbacks, 24-h urinary copper determination remains a useful and relatively simple screening test for WD that effectively complements ceruloplasmin determination. As a screening tool, the 24-h character of the test may cause some practical difficulties for the patient in urine storage and transport to the laboratory, especially for individuals who have to travel long distances to their clinic visit, but the information obtained makes the test worth the trouble.

Routine serum copper levels, which measure total serum copper, are frequently obtained as a screening test for WD but are actually of little real value. Total serum copper is usually reduced in WD simply as a reflection of reduced ceruloplasmin and provides no additional useful diagnostic information.[50,127,131] Determination of nonceruloplasmin (free) serum copper, however, directly measures the unbound (actually loosely albumin-complexed), and thus potentially toxic, copper in the blood.[50] This is typically elevated in symptomatic WD and is useful as another diagnostic test.[132]

Measurement of the incorporation of radioactive copper into ceruloplasmin may also be of value in selected situations in the diagnostic evaluation of suspected WD. In the normal individual there is an initial rise in serum ^{64}Cu after its oral administration as it enters the blood and is complexed with albumin and amino acids. Serum ^{64}Cu levels then drop as the copper is cleared by the liver, only to show a secondary rise, peaking at 48 h as the ^{64}Cu is incorporated into newly synthesized ceruloplasmin by the liver and released into the circulation. This secondary rise in ^{64}Cu does not occur in WD, even in those WD patients with normal or near-normal ceruloplasmin levels. Thus, this study can be useful in identifying such "covert" WD individuals.[133]

CSF copper levels have been measured in WD and found to be elevated in persons with neurological symptoms.[134] Levels have also been noted to decline in concert with symptomatic neurological improvement, suggesting that CSF copper levels may be the most accurate reflection of the brain copper load.[135] However, this method of copper monitoring is not performed on a routine clinical basis, and such use would require extensive additional validation.

Neuroimaging studies frequently demonstrate abnormalities in WD. The changes are not specific for WD but may consist of very suggestive patterns of abnormality. As might be expected, magnetic resonance imaging (MRI) is a more sensitive indicator of brain involvement in WD than is computed tomography (CT). Recent reports, in fact, have demonstrated MRI abnormalities in 100 percent of individuals with WD who have neurological dysfunction.[136,137] The basal ganglia are the most consistently involved brain area, with the brain stem and thalamus also frequently affected.[138,139] Increased signal intensity on T_2-weighted images is the characteristic abnormality; sometimes, an area of increased signal intensity surrounds an area of decreased intensity.[139] It has been suggested that either edema or demyelination may account for the increased signal intensity whereas either iron or copper deposition (both are paramagnetic substances) may produce the area of reduced signal intensity.[139] Certain abnormalities, such as the "face of the panda" midbrain sign[140] and the "bright claustrum" sign,[141] have been suggested to be characteristic of WD but are not consistently present.

Positron emission tomography (PET) scanning, both with [18F]deoxyglucose[142–144] and with [18F]dopa,[145] typically demonstrates abnormalities in WD. However, this modality is not currently in routine clinical use and is not part of the standard evaluation of suspected WD. Evoked potentials of various types may be abnormal in many patients with WD but are nonspecific and of no clear-cut diagnostic value.[146]

Practical guidelines to follow suggest that in individuals presenting with hepatic disease, liver biopsy for hepatic copper content is usually necessary to confirm diagnosis, because KFRs may not yet have formed, and ceruloplasmin and urinary copper levels are not invariably abnormal. In individuals with neurological symptoms a liver biopsy is usually not necessary. The presence of KFRs on slit-lamp examination, coupled with reduced ceruloplasmin and increased urinary copper excretion, virtually confirms the diagnosis in the presence of neurological symptoms. There may be instances, such as when KFRs are present but ceruloplasmin is not markedly reduced, that liver biopsy is still necessary. When a liver biopsy cannot be performed or when its results are inconclusive, a radiocopper incorporation study may be useful.

Treatment

Treatment strategies in WD center on restoring and maintaining appropriate copper balance within body tissues. With the possible exception of liver transplantation, treatment of WD is palliative rather than curative; the underlying defect that produces WD is not corrected, and treatment must be continued for the individual's lifetime, although the specific type of treatment or mix of treatment modalities may change with time and circumstances.

Treatment of WD can be stratified into four primary approaches: dietary therapy, therapy to reduce copper absorption, therapy to increase copper chelation and elimination, and liver transplantation.

DIETARY THERAPY

Limitation of dietary copper intake seems like a prudent and sensible maneuver in treating WD, but it has not been shown to be of significant benefit in most instances.[147] Nevertheless, foods particularly high in copper content, such as shellfish, liver, nuts, chocolate, and mushrooms, should probably be avoided by individuals with WD.[127,147,148]

In contrast to the usual ineffectiveness of dietary therapy in WD, however, Brewer and colleagues have reported two anecdotal descriptions of individuals in which a strict lactovegetarian diet seemed to control WD adequately without other therapy.[149] They postulated that in the lactovegetarian diet the bioavailability of copper was sufficiently reduced by fiber and phytate to stabilize copper balance.

Copper content in the primary drinking source of an individual with WD should be measured and, if it proves to be unacceptably high, distilled water should be used instead.[147,148] It should also be remembered that domestic water softeners increase the copper content of water.[50] Copper content in any vitamin/mineral preparations the patient might be taking should also be considered.

INHIBITION OF INTESTINAL COPPER ABSORPTION

POTASSIUM
Potassium iodide or potassium sulfide has been advocated in the past as a means of decreasing dietary copper absorption by interacting with copper to form insoluble copper iodide or sulfide.[150] However, this approach is of no proven practical value and is not typically used in treating WD.

ZINC
Zinc, administered as either acetate[148,151] or sulfate salt,[152] provides another mechanism to limit gastrointestinal copper absorption in WD. The effect of zinc is mediated through the cysteine-rich 61-amino acid protein, metallothionein, which is present in many body tissues including brain, liver, and intestinal cells (enterocytes).[153,154] The primary role of metallothionein in the body is probably as a zinc-binding ligand and, as such, it is important for zinc homeostasis and transport.[154] Metallothionein has a high affinity for zinc but an even higher affinity for copper.[155] When given on an empty stomach, supplementary oral zinc administration induces metallothionein formation in the intestinal cells. The increased metallothionein then binds zinc and limits zinc absorption[156] but is also capable of binding dietary copper.[157] The bound copper, like the bound zinc, is then trapped and stored within the intestinal mucosal cells until the cells are eventually sloughed and excreted in the feces.[148,156] By means of the same mechanism the reabsorption of copper secreted into the GI tract via saliva and gastric juices is also blocked.[156] The net result of these actions is induction of a small, but real, negative copper balance.

The role of zinc administration in the treatment of WD is still not completely settled. It is generally very well tolerated, and this low toxicity makes it very appealing as primary therapy of WD in the presymptomatic individual.[148,158] Its role in the treatment of the symptomatic patient is less clear. The effect of zinc administration on copper absorption does not appear for 1–2 weeks, because the induction of metallothionein is rather slow. Moreover, the negative copper balance induced by zinc is relatively small. These characteristics may make zinc monotherapy unsuitable as initial therapy in the individual with WD who is already experiencing neurological symptoms,[159] although it actually has been successfully used in this manner.[160] Brewer and colleagues strongly advocate switching to zinc as "maintenance" therapy after initial therapy with other more potent agents in neurologically symptomatic individuals and have reported extensive favorable experience with zinc in this role.[159,161] This management approach receives support from some investigators, but others are less enthusiastic and recommend that zinc therapy be confined to those unable to tolerate penicillamine or trientine.[50,162] A dosage regimen of 50 mg elemental zinc three times daily is generally used.

Although zinc is almost always well-tolerated, adverse effects may occur. Gastric irritation,[163] typically with the morning dose, is more frequent with zinc sulfate than with zinc acetate.[148] It has been suggested that administering zinc with a small amount of luncheon meat may limit the gastric discomfort while minimizing any effect on efficiency.[159] Sideroblastic anemia resulting from impaired iron utilization has been reported with zinc therapy.[164] Zinc can lower high-density lipoprotein (HDL) cholesterol in men by approximately 20 percent and total cholesterol in both men and women by about 10 percent.[159,165] Serum amylase and lipase may increase early in the course of zinc therapy, later returning to normal.[166] The same phenomenon may be noted with alkaline phosphatase.[166]

Brewer and colleagues have suggested the potential for interaction between zinc and penicillamine when they are used concurrently; their studies have shown increased urinary copper excretion but an offsetting reduction in fecal copper excretion when penicillamine is added to zinc therapy.[167] Whether neurological deterioration can occur as a direct result of initiating zinc therapy, as can occur with penicillamine, is a subject of dispute.[168,169]

TETRATHIOMOLYBDATE

Ammonium tetrathiomolybdate (TM), the most recently developed treatment for WD,[170,171] actually is capable of reducing the copper load in WD by working at two distinct sites.[172] It, like zinc, is able to limit gastrointestinal absorption of copper, but it does so by an entirely different mechanism of action. In the gut lumen TM forms a tripartite complex with copper and albumin; the complexed copper cannot be absorbed by the intestinal mucosal cells and is excreted in the feces.[172] Both food-derived copper and endogenously secreted copper are complexed by the TM. Unlike zinc, the negative copper balance produced by TM is present immediately, because metallothionein induction is not necessary.

When TM is given without food, it is readily absorbed into the bloodstream. Once absorbed, it forms the same tripartite complex with albumin and unbound (free) copper in the blood, which renders the copper unavailable for cellular uptake and, therefore, nontoxic.[172] Thus, TM can reduce the copper load systemically, in addition to its action in the gut lumen.

In initial studies TM has been administered in a regimen of six doses daily—3 with meals and three inbetween meals—to promote copper complex formation both in the gut and in the blood. In this regimen the mealtime doses of TM were 20 mg, whereas the intermeal dosage was titrated progressively upward until nonceruloplasmin (free) plasma copper and plasma molybdenum levels (converted to micromoles) were equivalent, a process termed "closing the plasma copper molybdenum gap" by Brewer and colleagues.[172] This generally required a between-meals dose of 20–60 mg.

When administered as the initial therapy to individuals with neurologically symptomatic WD in the fashion described above, Brewer and colleagues noted an immediate and significant reduction in plasma-free copper[172] (more specifically, in the percentage of trichloroacetic acid-soluble plasma copper). In no instance did initial deterioration in neurological function, as can occur with penicillamine therapy, develop. After 8 weeks of TM therapy all patients were switched to zinc therapy for long-term management; TM was not used as maintenance therapy.

Although TM is generally very well-tolerated, reversible bone marrow depression has been reported.[163] Brewer attributes this to impaired erythropoiesis resulting from copper depletion in the bone marrow (R Pfeiffer, personal communication). In rats, TM has also been shown to damage epiphyses in growing bone,[173] leading Walshe to suggest that TM not be used for more than short courses in children or adolescents with unfused epiphyses.[163]

Although experience with TM in the treatment of WD is currently still quite limited, it appears to be a very promising, although still experimental, treatment modality. With the proposed regimen of six doses daily, however, patient compliance may be an issue.

COPPER CHELATION THERAPY

PENICILLAMINE

Penicillamine (dimethylcysteine) is a metabolic product of penicillin that avidly chelates copper; the resulting complexed copper is excreted in the urine. Since its introduction into usage in WD by Walshe,[174] penicillamine has become the mainstay of WD treatment. Although it has been accepted that penicillamine produces its primary effect by copper chelation and cupriuresis, additional actions, including induction of metallothionein, have also been suggested.[50]

Penicillamine should always be given on an empty stomach. The traditionally recommended initial dosage is 1–2 g daily, but some have advocated a less aggressive induction, such as 250 mg daily, with subsequent upward titration based on the amount of urinary copper excretion, aiming for 1–3 mg daily.[147,148] Shoulson and colleagues have suggested that penicillamine doses exceeding 750 mg daily are seldom necessary.[147] Concomitant administration of pyridoxine (25 mg daily) has also been recommended by some researchers because of an antipyridoxine effect of penicillamine,[50,175] but others believe that penicillamine-induced pyridoxine deficiency only occurs in special circumstances, such as pregnancy, during a growth spurt, or with dietary deficiency.[163,176]

One troublesome aspect of penicillamine is its propensity to produce initial deterioration in neurological function as treatment is begun. The frequency with which this occurs is not entirely clear, but Walshe and Yealland[163] noted it in 22 percent of patients (30 of 137) that they treated, and Brewer et al. noted it[177] in 52 percent (13 of 25) in a retrospective survey. More ominously, Brewer adds that 50 percent of those in whom neurological deterioration occurs on initiation of penicillamine therapy do not fully recover to their baseline level of functioning.[177] Emergence of neurological dysfunction in previously neurologically asymptomatic individuals has also been described after initiation of penicillamine therapy.[178,179] The reason for this neurological deterioration is uncertain. Mobilization of copper from the liver with subsequent redistribution to the brain has been suggested,[177] but studies of CSF copper levels during this deterioration do not support this hypothesis.[135] It is this potential for initial neurological deterioration that has led some investigators to propose the "gentler" initiation of penicillamine therapy described above and others to advocate induction of therapy with zinc or TM.

Improvement in function may begin within 2 weeks of initiating penicillamine therapy but, more typically, it is delayed for 2–3 months.[180] With continued therapy, gradual improvement may continue for up to 1–2 years.[148] Improvement in virtually all facets of clinical dysfunction may occur. Tremor and cerebellar signs seem to improve more readily than dystonia, whereas the fixed smile and dysarthria may show no improvement at all. KFRs recede gradually in a sequence inverse to their appearance.[83] Sunflower cataracts also clear, often more rapidly than KFRs.[78,93] Psychiatric symptoms improve with penicillamine therapy, although not as fully or as consistently as neurological symptoms and signs.[37,71] The same is true of psychometric testing.[181] Neuroimaging abnormalities, both CT[182] and MRI,[136,137,183] may improve after penicillamine.

A variety of other problems may also attend penicillamine therapy. Acute sensitivity reactions may develop in 20–30 percent of individuals on penicillamine in conventional doses.[184,185] Consisting of skin rash, fever, eosinophilia, thrombocytopenia, leukopenia, and lymphadenopathy, these reactions typically develop within 2 weeks of initiation of treatment. Even in the face of a severe reaction, however, it is not always necessary to abandon penicillamine therapy permanently. It should be discontinued until the rash clears. Often, it is then possible to carefully reinstitute therapy, beginning with much lower doses. Chan and Baker[186] outline a protocol for penicillamine desensitization in which the rash and fever are first allowed to improve after discontinuation of penicillamine. Prednisone (30 mg daily) is then started 2 days before reinstitution of penicillamine at a reduced dosage of 125 mg daily. Penicillamine is then increased by 125 mg at 3-day intervals to reach a dose of 500 mg daily. Subsequently, prednisone is gradually tapered and discontinued over a 1-month period whereas penicillamine is increased further by 250 mg at 3- to 5-day intervals to a dose of 1.0 g daily. Kher and colleagues[187] report successful reintroduction of penicillamine by resorting to an initial dosage of 1 mg/kg/day in a child who developed recrudescence of the allergic reaction when penicillamine was reintroduced at a dose of 250 mg daily. Despite these measures, 5–20 percent of individuals are ultimately unable to tolerate penicillamine at all.[148] Agranulocytosis induced by penicillamine can be fatal.[188]

With chronic penicillamine administration a variety of other adverse effects may occur. Nephrotic syndrome,[189] Goodpasture's syndrome,[190] a lupus-like syndrome,[191] a myasthenia-like syndrome,[192] acute polyarthritis,[103] thrombocytopenia,[17] and retinal hemorrhages[193] all have been reported. Loss of the sense of taste may also develop with penicillamine therapy; a favorable response of this dysgeusia to zinc administration has been demonstrated.[147,194] Optic neuritis was a rare complication of D,L-penicillamine administration but does not occur with D-penicillamine alone.[17,195] Serum IgA deficiency has also occurred with penicillamine therapy.[196] Adverse reactions to penicillamine may still develop after prolonged therapy; Walshe and Yealland report that lupus has developed after 30 years of therapy.[163]

Dermatologic problems also may develop with chronic penicillamine treatment. Penicillamine dermatopathy is characterized by brownish skin discoloration, which develops as a consequence of recurrent subcutaneous bleeding during incidental trauma.[197] The bleeding is attributed to penicillamine-induced inhibition of collagen and elastin cross-linking.[198] Penicillamine can also produce impairment of wound healing,[199] which has led to the recommendation that penicillamine dosage should be reduced to 250–500 mg daily during perioperative periods.[17] Elastosis perforans serpiginosa,[200,201] pemphigus,[202] and aphthous stomatitis[203] are other reported penicillamine-induced dermatologic processes.

TRIENTINE

Triethylene tetramine dihydrochloride, or trientine, is a copper chelation agent with a mechanism of action similar to that of penicillamine.[204–207] Trientine appears to be somewhat less potent than penicillamine and, thus, does not induce as vigorous "decoppering," which may make it less likely to provoke the initial neurological deterioration that penicillamine can invoke.

As with penicillamine, trientine should be taken on an empty stomach, and a typical daily dosage is 750–2000 mg, given in three divided doses.[50] Experience with trientine has been much less extensive than with penicillamine, but trientine appears to be a less toxic compound.[17] Lupus nephritis[206] and sideroblastic anemia[208] both have been reported with trientine.

Trientine has primarily been used as an alternative copper chelation therapy when penicillamine has not been tolerated. It has not been widely used as a first-line agent in the treatment of WD.

BRITISH ANTILEWISITE (BAL)

Dimercaprol, or British anti-Lewisite (BAL), was the initial copper-chelating agent used in the treatment of WD[209,210] but has now been virtually abandoned because of the necessity to administer it parenterally and because of its proclivity to produce a plethora of adverse effects, such as headache, nausea, dizziness, and pain at the injection site. Scheinberg and Sternlieb[211] still reserve a place for BAL in individuals with severe WD who do not improve with penicillamine, trientine, or both used in combination. In such individuals they advocate up to four courses of BAL injections, with each course consisting of five injections on the weekdays of 4 successive weeks. They report significant improvement in approximately 33 percent of individuals thus treated and maintenance of the improvement with subsequent chronic penicillamine or trientine therapy. Brewer, however, hotly disputes both the theory and clinical data behind this recommendation and suggests that BAL be relegated to the "historical scrapheap" of WD management.[212]

LIVER TRANSPLANTATION

The most dreaded complication of WD is the development of fulminant hepatic failure. Wilsonian fulminant hepatic failure primarily occurs in children and young adults, more frequently in females than in males.[17,213] It is characterized by relatively modest transaminase and alkaline phosphatase elevations and by a nonimmune hemolytic anemia.[213,214]

When treatment of Wilsonian fulminant hepatic failure is confined to medical management, the mortality rate is virtually 100 percent.[213–215] Because of this ghastly statistic, orthotopic liver transplantation (OLT) has been used with increasing frequency in this desperate situation. Chronic, severe hepatic insufficiency unresponsive to medical measures is also seen as an appropriate indication for OLT.[213]

Schilsky et al. have reviewed the experience with OLT in the treatment of WD at 15 transplant centers in the United States and 3 in Europe.[213] Data on 55 patients were reviewed. The survival rate at 1 year was 79 percent. Similar survival rates have been noted by other investigators.[214,216] In addition to correction of hepatic dysfunction, improvement has been observed in the neurological, psychiatric, and ophthalmologic features of WD after OLT.[213] Because the transplanted liver is free of the genetic defect responsible for WD, copper metabolism normalizes after OLT, and continued chelation or another WD therapy is generally not necessary.[213,214] Although OLT may thus be viewed as curative therapy, it carries with it significant morbidity and mortality. Moreover, transplanted individuals still retain the genetic abnormality in other body tissues and will pass on the trait to all children.

Because of the success of OLT in treating WD patients with hepatic failure, the question as to whether individuals with stable hepatic function but severe neurological dysfunction not responding to medical therapy should also be considered for OLT has been raised. There has been at least one case report of OLT performed in this situation,[217] but most investigators view such a treatment approach as experimental and not as the current standard of therapy.

TREATMENT GUIDELINES

In the individual with WD who is still asymptomatic (presymptomatic) some, but not all, investigators recommend that therapy be initiated and maintained with zinc alone. Still others view zinc therapy as an unproven modality and continue to recommend primary treatment with penicillamine.

In the individual who has hepatic, but not neurologic, symptoms introduction of both a chelating agent and zinc may be ideal. Pencillamine is the standard chelating agent in this situation, although trientine has its advocates.

In the individual who has developed neurological dysfunction, penicillamine remains the standard therapy for initial management. When tetrathiomolybdate becomes available and experience with it grows, it may become an acceptable, or even preferred, treatment alternative. Zinc is recommended by some investigators for maintenance therapy after initial decoppering, but still others prefer maintenance with penicillamine. Trientine remains an alternative chelating agent for those individuals unable to tolerate penicillamine, but is not usually employed as a first-line drug.

For the individual with fulminant or chronic hepatic failure, liver transplantation may be the only viable treatment option.

Summary

In the more than 8 decades since Wilson's seminal description, our understanding of and ability to effectively treat WD has dramatically advanced. Nevertheless, because of its protean clinical features WD remains a tremendous diagnostic and therapeutic challenge to the clinician. The palliative nature of WD therapy dictates constant vigilance on the part of the treating physician to ensure ongoing patient compliance and to watch closely for treatment complications. The reward, however, of prompt diagnosis and attentive therapy can be an asymptomatic and healthy individual faced with an otherwise fatal disease.

Acknowledgments

The excellent secretarial assistance of Mary Reed and Helen Ham in manuscript preparation is deeply appreciated.

References

1. Wilson SAK: Progressive lenticular degeneration: A familial nervous disease associated with cirrhosis of the liver. *Brain* 34:295–507, 1912.
2. Frerichs FT: *A Clinical Treatise on Diseases of the Liver.* London: The New Sydenham Society, 1860, vol 2, pp 60–62.
3. Westphal C: Über eine dem Bilde der cerebrospinalen grauen Degeneration ähnliche Erkrankung des centralen Nervensystems ohne anatomischen Befund, nebst einigen Bermerkungen über paradoxe Contraction. *Arch Psychiatr Nervenkrank* 14:87–134, 1883.
4. Gowers W: *A Manual of Diseases of the Nervous System.* London: J & A Churchill, 1888.
5. Ormerod JA: Cirrhosis of the liver in a boy, with obscure and fatal nervous symptoms. *St Bart Hosp Rep* XXVI:57, 1890.
6. Homen EA: Eine Eigenthümliche bei drei Geschwistern auftretende typische Krankheit unter der Form einer progressiven Dementia, in Verbindung mit ausgedehnten gefässveränderungen (wohl lues hereditaria tarda). *Arch Psychiatr* XXIV:191–228, 1892.
7. Strümpell A: Über die Westphal'sche Pseudosklerose und über diffuse Hirnsklerose, inbesondere bei Kindern. *Dtsch Z Nervenheilk* 12:115–149, 1898.
8. Kayser B: Über einen Fall von angeborener grünlicher Verfärbung der Kornea. *Klin Monatsbl Augenheilkd* 40:22–25, 1902.
9. Fleischer B: Zwei weitere Falle von grünlicher Verfärbung der Kornea. *Klin Monatsbl Augenheilkd* 41:489–491, 1903.
10. Fleischer B: Über eine der "Pseudosklerose" nahestehende, bisher unbekannte Krankheit (gekennzeichnet durch tremor, psychische storungen, braunliche Pigmentierung bestimmter gewebe, insbesondere auch der Hornhautperipherie, Lebercirrhose). *Dtsch Z Nervenheilkd* 44:179–201, 1912.
11. Rumpel A: Über das Wesen und die Bedeutung der Leberveränderungen und der Pigmentierunen bei den damit verbundenen Fällen von Pseudosklerose, zugleich ein Beitrag zur Lehre von der Pseudosklerose (Westphal-Strümpell). *Dtsch Z Nervenheilkd* 49:54–73, 1913.
12. Mandelbrote BM, Stanier MW, Thompson RHS, Thruston MN: Studies on copper metabolism in demyelinating diseases of the central nervous system. *Brain* 71:212–228, 1948.
13. Cumings JN: The copper and iron content of brain and liver in the normal and in hepato-lenticular degeneration. *Brain* 71:410–415, 1948.
14. Scheinberg IH, Giblin D: Deficiency of ceruloplasmin in patients with hepatolenticular degeneration (Wilson's disease). *Science* 116:484–485, 1952.
15. Hall HC: *La Dégénérescence Hépato-lenticulaire: Maladie de Wilson-Pseudosclérose.* Paris: Paul Masson, 1921.

16. Saito T: An assessment of efficiency in potential screening for Wilson's disease. *J Epidemiol Community Health* 35:274–280, 1981.

17. Scheinberg IH, Sternlieb I: *Wilson's Disease*. Philadelphia: WB Saunders, 1984.

18. Bachmann H, Lossner J, Gruss B, Rucholtz U: Die epidemiologie der Wilsonschen erkrankung in der DDR und die derzeitige problematik einer populations genetischen bearbeitung. *Psychiatr Neurol Med Psychol Leipzig* 31:393–400, 1979.

19. Przuntek H, Hofmann E: Epidemiologische untersuchung zum morbus Wilson in der Bundesrepublik Deutschland. *Nervenarzt* 58:150–157, 1987.

20. Reilly M, Daly L, Hutchinson M: An epidemiological study of Wilson's disease in the Republic of Ireland. *J Neurol Neurosurg Psychiatry* 56:298–300, 1993.

21. Frydman M, Bonné-Tamir B, Farrer LA, et al: Assignment of the gene for Wilson's disease to chromosome 13. *Proc Natl Acad Sci U S A* 82:1819–1821, 1985.

22. Kooy RF, Van der Veen AY, Verlind E, et al: Physical localization of the chromosomal marker D13S31 places the Wilson disease locus at the junction of bands q14.3 and q21.1 of chromosome 13. *Hum Genet* 91:504–506, 1993.

23. Thomas GR, Roberts EA, Rosales TO, et al: Allelic association and linkage studies in Wilson disease. *Hum Molec Genet* 2:1401–1405, 1993.

24. Stewart EA, White A, Tomfohrde J, et al: Polymorphic microsatellites and Wilson disease (WD). *Am J Hum Genet* 53:864–873, 1993.

25. Bowcock AM, Tomfohrde J, Weissenbach J, et al: Refining the position of Wilson disease by linkage dysequilibrium with polymorphic microsatellites. *Am J Hum Genet* 54:79–87, 1994.

26. Bull PC, Thomas GR, Rommens JM, et al: The Wilson disease gene is a putative copper transporting P-type ATPase similar to the Menkes gene. *Nature Genet* 5:327–337, 1993.

27. Yamaguchi Y, Heiny ME, Gitlin JD: Isolation and characterization of a human liver cDNA as a candidate gene for Wilson disease. *Biochem Biophys Res Commun* 197:271–277, 1993.

28. Patten BM: Wilson's disease. In Jankovic J, Tolosa E, (eds): *Parkinson's Disease and Movement Disorders*. Baltimore: Urban & Schwarzenberg, 1988, pp 179–190.

29. Holmberg CG, Laurell CB: Investigations in serum copper. II. Isolation of the copper containing protein and a description of some of its properties. *Acta Chem Scand* 2:550–556, 1948.

30. Sato M, Schilsky ML, Stockert RJ, et al: Detection of multiple forms of human ceruloplasmin: A novel Mr 200,000 form. *J Biol Chem* 265:2533–2537, 1990.

31. Gibbs K, Walshe JM: A study of the ceruloplasmin concentrations found in 75 patients with Wilson's disease, their kinships and various control groups. *Q J Med* 48:447–463, 1979.

32. Cartwright GE, Markowitz H, Shields GS, Wintrobe MM: Studies on copper metabolism. XXIX. A critical analysis of serum copper and ceruloplasmin concentrations in normal subjects, patients with Wilson's disease and relatives of patients with Wilson's disease. *Am J Med* 28:555–563, 1960.

33. Scheinberg IH, Sternlieb I: Environmental treatment of a hereditary illness: Wilson's disease. *Ann Intern Med* 53:1151–1161, 1960.

34. Neifakh SA, Vakharlovskii VG, Gaitskhoki VS, et al: Ekspressiia gena, tseruloplazmina pri bolezni Vil'sona-Konovalova. *Vestn Akad Med Nauk SSR* 1:53–63, 1982.

35. Czaja MJ, Weiner FR, Schwarzenberg SJ, et al: Molecular studies of ceruloplasmin deficiency in Wilson's disease. *J Clin Invest* 80:1200–1204, 1987.

36. Morita H, Ikeda S, Yamamoto K, et al: Hereditary ceruloplasmin deficiency with hemosiderosis: A clinicopathological study of a Japanese family. *Ann Neurol* 37:646–656, 1995.

37. Weiner WJ, Lang AE: *Movement Disorders: A Comprehensive Survey*. Mt Kisco, NY: Futura Publishing Co, 1989, pp 257–291.

38. van Berge Henegouwen GP, Tangedahl TN, Hofmann AF, et al: Biliary secretion of copper in healthy man. *Gastroenterology* 72:1228–1231, 1977.

39. O'Reilly S, Weber PM, Oswald M, Shipley L: Abnormalities of the physiology of copper in Wilson's disease. *Arch Neurol* 25:28–32, 1971.

40. Owen CA Jr: Absorption and excretion of Cu^{64}-labelled copper by the rat. *Am J Physiol* 207:1203–1206, 1964.

41. Scheinberg IH, Sternlieb I: Wilson's disease. *Annu Rev Med* 16:119–134, 1965.

42. Walshe JM: Wilson's disease: The presenting symptoms. *Arch Dis Child* 37:253–256, 1962.

43. Chu N-S, Hung T-P: Geographic variations in Wilson's disease. *J Neurol Sci* 117:1–7, 1993.

44. Walshe JM: Wilson's disease (HLD), in Vinken PJ, Bruyn GW (eds): *Handbook of Clinical Neurology*. Amsterdam: North-Holland Publishing Co, 1976, vol 27, pp 379–414.

45. Bellary SV, VanThiel DH: Wilson's disease: A diagnosis made in two individuals greater than 40 years of age. *J Okla State Med Assoc* 86:441–444, 1993.

46. Black M, Billing BH: Hepatic bilirubin UDP-glucuronyl transferase activity in liver disease and Gilbert's syndrome. *N Engl J Med* 280:1266–1271, 1969.

47. O'Donnell JG, Watson ID, Fell GS, et al: Wilson's disease presenting as acute fulminant hepatic failure. *Scott Med J* 35:118–119, 1990.

48. Mowat AP: Orthotopic liver transplantation in liver-based metabolic disorders. *Eur J Pediatr* 151(suppl 1):S32–S38, 1992.

49. Roche-Sicot J, Benhamou J-P: Acute intravascular hemolysis and acute liver failure associated as a first manifestation of Wilson's disease. *Ann Intern Med* 86:301–303, 1977.

50. Yarze JC, Martin P, Munoz SJ, Friedman LS: Wilson's disease: Current status. *Am J Med* 92:643–654, 1992.

51. Sternlieb I, Scheinberg IH: Chronic hepatitis as a first manifestation of Wilson's disease. *Ann Intern Med* 76:59–64, 1972.

52. Scott J, Gollan JL, Samourian S, Sherlock S: Wilson's disease presenting as chronic active hepatitis. *Gastroenterology* 74:645–651, 1978.

53. Strickland GT, Leu ML: Wilson's disease: Clinical and laboratory manifestations in 40 patients. *Medicine* 54:113–137, 1975.

54. Ross E, Jacobson IM, Dienstag JL, Martin JB: Late onset Wilson's disease with neurologic involvement in the absence of Kayser-Fleischer rings. *Ann Neurol* 17:411–413, 1985.

55. Walshe JM: Wilson's disease, in Vinken PJ, Bruyn GW, Klawans HL (eds): *Handbook of Clinical Neurology*. New York: American Elsevier, 1986, vol 49, pp 223–238.

56. Topaloglu H, Renda Y: Tongue dyskinesia in Wilson disease. *Brain Dev* 14:128, 1992.

57. Topaloglu H, Gucuyener K, Orkun C, Renda Y: Tremor of tongue and dysarthria as the sole manifestation of Wilson disease. *Clin Neurol Neurosurg* 92:295–296, 1990.

58. Parker N: Hereditary whispering dysphonia. *J Neurol Neurosurg Pscyhiatry* 48:218–224, 1985.

59. Cartwright GE: Diagnosis of treatable Wilson's disease. *N Engl J Med* 298:1347–1350, 1978.

60. Walshe JM, Yealland M: Wilson's disease: The problem of delayed diagnosis. *J Neurol Neurosurg Pscyhiatry* 55:692–696, 1992.

61. Dening TR, Berrios GE, Walshe JM: Wilson disease and epilepsy. *Brain* 111:129–1155, 1988.

62. Huang C-C, Chu N-S: Psychosis and epileptic seizures in Wilson's disease with predominantly white matter lesions in the frontal lobe. *Parkinsonism Relat Disord* 1:53–58, 1995.

63. Mingazzini G: Über das Zwangsweinen und -lachen. *Klin Wochenschr (Wien)* 41:998–1002, 1928.

64. Nair KR, Pillai PG: Trunkal myoclonus with spontaneous priapism and seminal ejaculation in Wilson's disease. *J Neurol Neurosurg Pscyhiatry* 53:174, 1990.

65. Denny-Brown D: Hepatolenticular degeneration (Wilson's disease): Two different components. *N Engl J Med* 270:1149–1156, 1964.

66. Oder W, Prayer L, Grimm G, et al: Wilson's disease: Evidence of subgroups derived from clinical findings and brain lesions. *Neurology* 43:120–124, 1993.

67. Medalia A, Scheinberg IH: Psychopathology in patients with Wilson's disease. *Am J Psychiatry* 146:662–664, 1989.

68. Gwirtsman HE, Prager J, Henkin R: Case report of anorexia nervosa associated with Wilson's disease. *Int J Eating Disord* 13:241–244, 1993.

69. Dening TR, Berrios GE: Wilson's disease: Psychiatric symptoms in 195 cases. *Arch Gen Psychiatry* 46:1126–1134, 1989.

70. Scheinberg IH, Sternlieb I, Richman J. Psychiatric manifestations in patients with Wilson's disease, in Bergsma D, Scheinberg IH, Sternlieb I (eds): *Wilson's Disease: Birth Defects,* Original Article Series. New York: The National Foundation-March of Dimes, 1968, vol 4, pp 85–87.

71. Akil M, Brewer GJ: Psychiatric and behavioral abnormalities in Wilson's disease. *Adv Neurol* 65:71–178, 1995.

72. Walshe JM: Missed Wilson's disease. *Lancet* 2:405–406, 1975.

73. Dening TR: Psychiatric aspects of Wilson's disease. *Br J Psychiatry* 147:677–682, 1985.

74. Knehr CA, Bearn AG: Psychological impairment in Wilson's disease. *J Nerv Ment Dis* 124:251–255, 1956.

75. Tarter RE, Switala J, Carra J, et al: Neuropsychological impairment associated with hepatolenticular degeneration (Wilson's disease) in the absense of overt encephalopathy. *Int J Neurosci* 37:67–71, 1987.

76. Davis EJ, Borde M: Wilson's disease and catatonia. *Br J Psychiatry* 162:256–259, 1993.

77. Akil M, Schwartz JA Dutchak D, et al: The psychiatric presentations of Wilson's disease. *J Neuropsychiatry Clin Neurosci* 3:377–382, 1991.

78. Wiebers DO, Hollenhorst RW, Goldstein NP: The ophthalmologic manifestations of Wilson's disease. *Mayo Clin Proc* 52:409–416, 1977.

79. Johnson RD, Campbell RJ: Wilson's disease: Electron microscopic, x-ray energy spectroscopic and atomic absorption spectroscopic studies of corneal copper deposition and distribution. *Lab Invest* 46:546–569, 1982.

80. Innes JR, Strachan IM, Triger DR: Unilateral Kayser-Fleischer ring. *Br J Ophthalmol* 70:469–470, 1979.

81. Tauber J, Steinert RF: Pseudo-Kayser-Fleischer ring of the cornea associated with non-Wilsonian liver disease: A case report and literature review. *Cornea* 12:74–77, 1993.

82. Finelli PF: Kayser-Fleischer ring: Hepatolenticular degeneration (Wilson's disease). *Neurology* 45:1261–1262, 1995.

83. Sussman W, Scheinberg IH: Disappearance of Kayser-Fleischer rings. Effects of penicillamine. *Arch Ophthalmol* 82:738–741, 1969.

84. Fleming CR, Dickson ER, Wahner HW, et al: Pigmented corneal rings in non-Wilsonian liver disease. *Ann Intern Med* 86:285–288, 1977.

85. Frommer D, Morris J, Sherlock S, et al: Kayser-Fleischer-like rings in patients without Wilson's disease. *Gastroenterology* 72:1331–1335, 1977.

86. Kaplinsky C, Sternlieb I, Javitt N, Rotem Y: Familial cholestatic cirrhosis associated with Kayser-Fleischer rings. *Pediatrics* 65:782–788, 1980.

87. Stephenson S: Cases illustrating an unusual form of corneal opacity due to the long-continued application of copper sulphate to the palpebral conjunctiva. *Trans Ophthalmol Soc UK* 23:25–27, 1902.

88. Goodman SI, Rodgerson DO, Kaufman J: Hypercupremia in a patient with multiple myeloma. *J Lab Clin Med* 70:57–62, 1967.

89. Lewis RA, Falls HF, Troyer DO: Ocular manifestations of hyercupremia associated with multiple myeloma. *Arch Ophthalmol* 93:1050–1053, 1995.

90. Martin NF, Kincaid MC, Stark WJ, et al: Ocular copper deposition associated with pulmonary carcinoma, IgG monoclonal gammopathy and hypercupremia: A clinicopathologic correlation. *Ophthalmology* 90:110–116, 1983.

91. Giorgio AJ, Cartwright GE, Wintrobe MM: Pseudo-Kayser-Fleischer rings. *Arch Intern Med* 113:817–818, 1964.

92. Siemerling E, Oloff H: Pseudosklerose (Westphal-Strümpell) mit Cornealring (Kayser Fleischer) und doppelseitiger Scheinkatarakt, die nur bei seitlicher Beleuchtung sichtbar ist und die der nach Verletzung durch Kupfersplitter entstehenden Kataract ähnlich ist. *Klin Wochenschr* 1:1087–1089, 1922.

93. Cairns JE, Williams HP, Walshe JM: "Sunflower cataract" in Wilson's disease. *Br Med J* 3:95–96, 1969

94. Goldberg MF, von Noorden GK: Ophthalmologic findings in Wilson's hepatolenticular degeneration: With emphasis on ocular motility. *Arch Ophthalmol* 75:162–170, 1966.

95. Pillat A: Changes in the eyegrounds in Wilson's disease (pseudosclerosis). *Am J Ophthalmol* 16:1–6, 1933.

96. Walsh FB, Hoyt WF: *Clinical Neuroophthalmology,* 3rd ed. Baltimore: Williams & Wilkins, 1969, vol 2, p 1140.

97. Lennox G, Jones R: Gaze distractibility in Wilson's disease. *Ann Neurol* 25:415–417, 1989.

98. Keane JR: Lid-opening apraxia in Wilson's disease. *J Clin Neuroophhthalmol* 8:31–33, 1988.

99. Dastur DK, Manghani DK, Wadia NH: Wilson's disease in India. I. Geographic, genetic, and clinical aspects in 16 families. *Neurology* 18:21–31, 1968.

100. Tu JB: A genetic, biochemical and clinical study of Wilson's disease among Chinese in Taiwan. *Acta Paediatr Sin* 4:81–104, 1963.

101. Xu XH, Yang BX, Feng YK: Wilson's disease (hepatolenticular degeneration): Clinical analysis of 80 cases. *Chin Med J* 94:673–678, 1981.

102. Saito T: Presenting symptoms and natural history of Wilson's disease. *Eur J Pediatr* 146:261–265, 1987.

103. Golding DN, Walshe JM: Arthropathy of Wilson's disease: Study of clinical and radiological features in 32 patients. *Ann Rheum Dis* 36:99–111, 1977.

104. Feller E, Schumacher HR: Osteoarticular changes in Wilson's disease. *Arthritis Rheum* 15:259–266, 1972.

105. Mindelzun R, Elkin M, Scheinberg IH, Sternlieb I: Skeletal changes in Wilson's disease: A radiological study. *Radiology* 94:127–132, 1970.

106. Hu R: Severe spinal degeneration in Wilson's disease. *Spine* 19:372–375, 1994.

107. Kramer U, Weinberger A, Yarom R, et al: Synovial copper deposition as a possible explanation of arthropathy in Wilson's disease. *Bull Hosp Jt Dis* 52:46–49, 1993.

108. McIntyre N, Clink HM, Levi AJ, et al: Hemolytic anemia in Wilson's disease. *N Engl J Med* 276:439–444, 1967.

109. Sternlieb I: Wilson's disease: Indications for liver transplants. *Hepatology* 4:15S–17S, 1984.

110. McIntyre N: Neurological Wilson's disease. *Q J Med* 86:349–350, 1993.

111. Meyer RJ, Zalusky R: The mechanisms of hemolysis in Wilson's disease: Study of a case and review of the literature. *Mt Sinai J Med* 44:530–538, 1977.

112. Forman SJ, Kumar KS, Redeker AG, Hochstein P: Hemolytic anemia in Wilson disease: Clinical findings and biochemical mechanisms. *Am J Hematol* 9:269–275, 1980.

113. Wiebers DO, Wilson DM, McLeod RA, Goldstein NP: Renal stones in Wilson's disease. *Am J Med* 67:249–254, 1979.

114. Hoppe B, Neuhaus T, Superti-Furga A, et al: Hypercalciuria and nephrocalcinosis, a feature of Wilson's disease. *Nephron* 65:460–462, 1993.

115. Diess A, Lynch RE, Lee GR, Cartwright GE: Long-term therapy of Wilson's disease. *Ann Intern Med* 75:57–65, 1971.

116. Leu ML, Strickland GT, Wang CC, Chen TSM: Skin pigmentation in Wilson's disease. *J Am Med Assoc* 211:1542–1543, 1970.

117. Bearn AG, McKusick VA: Azure lunulae: An unusual change in the fingernails in two patients with hepatolenticular degeneration (Wilson's disease). *J Am Med Assoc* 166:904–906, 1958.

118. Ezzo JA, Rowley JF, Finnegin JV: Hepatolenticular degeneration associated with acanthosis nigricans. *Arch Intern Med* 100:827–832, 1957.

119. Lau JY, Lai CL, Wu PC, et al: Wilson's disease: 35 years' experience. *Q J Med* 75:597–605, 1990.

120. Sternlieb I, Scheinberg IH: Wilson's disease, in Wright R, Alberti KGM, Karran S, et al (eds): *Liver and Biliary Disease*. London: Bailliere Tindall, 1985, pp 949–961.

121. Snow B: Laboratory diagnosis and monitoring of Wilson's disease, in *Neurological Aspects of Wilson's Disease*, American Academy of Neurology Course 411. 1995, pp 25–30.

122. Smallwood RA, Williams HA, Rosenauer VM: Liver copper levels in liver disease: Studies using neutron activation analysis. *Lancet* 2:1310–1313, 1968.

123. Benson GD: Hepatic copper accumulation in primary biliary cirrhosis. *Yale J Biol Med* 52:83–88, 1979.

124. Evans J, Newman S, Sherlock S: Liver copper levels in intrahepatic cholestasis of childhood. *Gastroenterology* 75:875–878, 1978.

125. Tanner MS, Portmann B, Mowat AP, et al: Increased hepatic copper concentration in Indian childhood cirrhosis. *Lancet* 1:1203–1205, 1979.

126. LaRusso NF, Summerskill WH, McCall JT: Abnormalities of chemical tests for copper metabolism in chronic active liver disease: Differentiation from Wilson's disease. *Gastroenterology* 70:653–655, 1976.

127. Sternlieb I, Giblin DR, Scheinberg IH: Wilson's disease, in Marsden CD, Fahn S (eds): *Movement Disorders*. London: Butterworth, 1987, vol 2, pp 288–302.

128. Willeit J, Kiechl SG: Wilson's disease with neurologic impairment but no Kayser-Fleischer rings. *Lancet* 337:1426, 1991.

129. Oder W, Grimm G, Kollegger H, et al: Neurological and neuropsychiatric spectrum of Wilson's disease: A prospective study of 45 cases. *J Neurol* 238:281–287, 1991.

130. Frommer DJ: Urinary copper excretion and hepatic copper concentrations in liver disease. *Digestion* 21:169–178. 1981.

131. Cumings JN: Trace metals in the brain and in Wilson's disease. *J Clin Pathol* 21:1–7, 1968.

132. Stremmel W, Meyerrose K-W, Niederau C, et al: Wilson disease: Clinical presentation, treatment, and survival. *Ann Intern Med* 115:720–726, 1991.

133. Sternlieb I, Scheinberg IH: The role of radiocopper in the diagnosis of Wilson's disease. *Gastroenterology* 77:138–142, 1979.

134. Weisner B, Hartard C, Dieu C: CSF copper concentration: A new parameter for diagnosis and monitoring therapy of Wilson's disease with cerebral manifestation. *J Neurol Sci* 79:229–237, 1987.

135. Hartard C, Weisner B, Dieu C, Kunze K: Wilson's disease with cerebral manifestations: Monitoring therapy by CSF copper concentration. *J Neurol* 241:101–107, 1993.

136. Thuomas KA, Aquilonius SM, Bergstrom K, Westermark K: Magnetic resonance imaging of the brain in Wilson's disease. *Neuroradiology* 35:134–141, 1993.

137. Roh JK, Lee TG, Wie BA, et al: Initial and follow-up brain MRI findings and correlation with the clinical course in Wilson's disease. *Neurology* 44:1064–1068, 1994.

138. Selwa LM, Vanderzant CW, Brunberg JA, et al: Correlation of evoked potential and MRI findings in Wilson's disease. *Neurology* 43:2059–2064, 1993.

139. Magalhaes ACA, Caramelli P, Menezes JR, et al: Wilson's disease: MRI with clinical correlation. *Neuroradiology* 36:97–100, 1994.

140. Hitoshi S, Iwata M, Yoshikawa K: Midbrain pathology of Wilson's disease: MRI analysis of three cases. *J Neurol Neurosurg Pscyhiatry* 54:624–626, 1991.

141. Sener RN: The claustrum on MRI: Normal anatomy, and the bright claustrum as a new sign in Wilson's disease. *Pediatr Radiol* 23:594–596, 1993.

142. Hawkins RA, Mazziotta JC, Phelps ME: Wilson's disease studied with FDG and positron emission tomography. *Neurology* 37:1707–1711, 1987.

143. Kuwert T, Hefter H, Scholz D, et al: Regional cerebral glucose consumption measured by positron emission tomography in patients with Wilson's disease. *Eur J Nucl Med* 19:96–101, 1992.

144. Hefter H, Kuwert T, Herzog H, et al: Relationship between striatal glucose consumption and copper excretion in patients with Wilson's disease treated with D-penicillamine. *J Neurol* 241:49–53, 1993.

145. Snow BJ, Bhatt MH, Martin WRW, et al: The nigrostriatal dopaminergic pathway in Wilson's disease studied with position emission tomography. *J Neurol Neurosurg Pscyhiatry* 54:12–17, 1991.

146. Grimm G, Madl C, Katzenschlager R, et al: Detailed evaluation of evoked potentials in Wilson's disease. *Electroencephalogr Clin Neurophysiol* 82:119–124, 1992.

147. Shoulson I, Goldblatt D, Plassche W, Wilson G: Some therapeutic observations in Wilson's disease. *Adv Neurol* 37:239–246, 1983.

148. Brewer GJ, Yuzbasiyan-Gurkan V. Wilson's disease, in Klawans HL, Goetz CG, Tanner CM (eds): *Textbook of Clinical Neuropharmacology and Therapeutics*. New York: Raven Press, 1992, pp 191–205.

149. Brewer GJ, Yuzbasiyan-Gurkan V, Dick R, et al: Does a vegetarian diet control Wilson's disease? *J Am Coll Nutr* 12:527–530, 1993.

150. Barbeau A: Treatment of Wilson's disease, in Barbeau A (ed): *Disorders of Movement*. Philadelphia: JB Lippincott, 1981, pp 209–220.

151. Brewer GJ, Yuzbasiyan-Gurkan V, Young AB: Treatment of Wilson's disease. *Semin Neurol* 7:209–220, 1987.

152. Hoogenraad TU, Van Hattum J, Van den Hamer CJA: Management of Wilson's disease with zinc sulphate: Experience in a series of 27 patients. *J Neurol Sci* 77:137–146, 1987.

153. Ebadi M, Paliwal VK, Takahashi T, Iversen PL: Zinc metallothionein in mammalian brain. *UCLA Symp Mol Cell Biol* 98:257–267, 1989.

154. Ebadi M: Metallothionein and other zinc-binding proteins in brain. *Methods Enzymol* 205:363–387, 1991.

155. Day FA, Panemangalore M, Brady FO: In vivo and ex vivo effects of copper on rat liver metallothionein. *Proc Soc Exp Biol Med* 168:306–310, 1981.

156. Brewer GJ, Hill GM, Prasad AS, et al: Oral zinc therapy for Wilson's disease. *Ann Intern Med* 99:314–320, 1983.

157. Hall AC, Young BW, Bremner I: Intestinal metallothionein and the mutual antagonism between copper and zinc in the rat. *J Inorg Biochem* 11:57–66, 1979.

158. Brewer GJ, Yuzbasiyan-Gurkan V, Lee DY, Appelman H: Treatment of Wilson's disease with zinc. VI. Initial treatment studies. *J Lab Clin Med* 114:633–638, 1989.

159. Brewer GJ, Yuzbasiyan-Gurkan V, Lee D-Y: Molecular genetics and zinc-copper interactions in human Wilson's disease and

canine copper toxicosis, in Prasad AS (ed): *Essential and Toxic Trace Elements in Human Health and Disease: An Update.* New York: Wiley-Liss, 1992, pp 129–145.

160. Rossaro L, Sturniolo GC, Giacon G, et al: Zinc therapy in Wilson's disease: Observations in five patients. *Am J Gastroenterol* 85:665–668, 1990.

161. Brewer GJ, Yuzbasiyan-Gurkan V: Wilson's disease. *Medicine* 71:139–164, 1992.

162. Lipsky MA, Gollan JL: Treatment of Wilson's disease: In D-penicillamine we trust—what about zinc? *Hepatology* 7:593–595, 1987.

163. Walshe JM, Yealland M: Chelation treatment of neurological Wilson's disease. *Q J Med* 86:197–204, 1993.

164. Simon SR, Branda RF, Tindle BH, Burns SL: Copper deficiency and sideroblastic anaemia associated with zinc ingestion. *Am J Hematol* 28:181–183, 1988.

165. Hooper PL, Visconti L, Garry PJ, Johnson GE: Zinc lowers high-density lipoprotein-cholesterol levels. *J Am Med Assoc* 244:1960–1961, 1980.

166. Yuzbasiyan-Gurkan V, Brewer GJ, Abrams GD, et al: Treatment of Wilson's disease with zinc: V. Changes in serum levels of lipase, amylase and alkaline phosphatase in Wilson's disease patients. *J Lab Clin Med* 114:520–526, 1989.

167. Brewer GJ, Yuzbasiyan-Gurkan V, Johnson V, et al: Treatment of Wilson's disease with zinc: XI. Interaction with other anticopper agents. *J Am Coll Nutr* 12:26–30, 1993.

168. Hoogenraad TU: Dangers of interrupting decoppering treatment in Wilson's disease. *Arch Neurol* 51:972–973, 1994.

169. Lang CJG: In reply. *Arch Neurol* 5:973, 1994.

170. Walshe JM: Wilson's disease: Yesterday, today and tomorrow. *Mov Disord* 3:10–29, 1988.

171. Brewer GJ, Dick RD, Yuzbasiyan-Gurkan V, et al: Initial therapy of patients with Wilson's disease with tetrathiomolybdate. *Arch Neurol* 48:42–47, 1991.

172. Brewer GJ, Dick RD, Johnson V, et al: Treatment of Wilson's disease with ammonium tetrathiomolybdate. I. Initial therapy in 17 neurologically affected patients. *Arch Neurol* 51:545–554, 1994.

173. Spence JA, Suttle NF, Wenham G, et al: A sequential study of the skeletal abnormalities which develop in rats given a small dietary supplement of ammonium tetrathiomolybdate. *J Comp Pathol* 90:139–153, 1980.

174. Walshe JM: Penicillamine: A new oral therapy for Wilson's disease. *Am J Med* 21:487–495, 1956.

175. Marsden CD: Wilson's disease. *Q J Med* 248:959–966, 1987.

176. Gibbs KR, Walshe JM: Interruption of the tryptophan-nicotinic acid pathway by penicillamine-induced pyridoxine deficiency in patients with Wilson's disease and in experimental animals. *Ann NY Acad Sci* 111:158–169, 1969.

177. Brewer GH, Terry CA, Aisen AM, Hill GM: Worsening of neurological syndrome in patients with Wilson's disease with initial penicillamine therapy. *Arch Neurol* 44:490–494, 1987.

178. Glass JD, Reich SG, DeLong MR: Wilson's disease: Development of neurological disease after beginning penicillamine therapy. *Arch Neurol* 47:595–596, 1990.

179. Brewer GJ, Turkay A, Yuzbasiyan-Gurkan V: Development of neurologic symptoms in a patient with asymptomatic Wilson's disease treated with penicillamine. *Arch Neurol* 51:304–305, 1994.

180. Deiss A: Treatment of Wilson's disease. *Ann Intern Med* 99:398–399, 1983.

181. Goldstein NP, Ewert JC, Randall RV, Gross JB: Psychiatric aspects of Wilson's disease (hepatolenticular degeneration): Results of psychometric tests during long-term therapy. *Am J Psychiatry* 124:1555–1561, 1968.

182. Williams FJB, Walshe JM: Wilson's disease. An analysis of the cranial computerized tomographic appearances found in pa-

tients and the changes in response to treatment with chelating agents. *Brain* 104:735–752, 1981.

183. Nazer H, Brismar J, Al-Kawi MZ, et al: Magnetic resonance imaging of the brain in Wilson's disease. *Neuroradiology* 35:130–133, 1993.

184. Sternlieb I, Scheinberg IH: Penicillamine therapy in hepatolenticular degeneration. *J Am Med Assoc* 189:748–754, 1964.

185. Haggstrom GC, Hirschowitz BI, Flint A: Long-term penicillamine therapy for Wilson's disease. *South Med J* 73:530–531, 1980.

186. Chan C-Y, Baker AL: Penicillamine hypersensitivity: Successful desensitization of a patient with severe hepatic Wilson's disease. *Am J Gastroenterol* 89:442–443, 1994.

187. Kher A, Bharucha BA, Kumta NB: Wilson's disease: Initial worsening of neurologic syndrome with penicillamine therapy. *Indian Pediatrics* 29:927–928, 1992.

188. Corcos JM, Soler-Bechera J, Mayer K, et al: Neutrophilic agranulocytosis during administration of penicillamine. *J Am Med Assoc* 189:265–268, 1964.

189. Hirschman SZ, Isselbacher KJ: The nephrotic syndrome as a complication of penicillamine therapy of hepatolenticular degeneration (Wilson's disease). *Ann Intern Med* 62:1297–1300, 1965.

190. Sternlieb I, Bennett B, Scheinberg IH: D-penicillamine induced Goodpasture's syndrome in Wilson's disease. *Ann Intern Med* 82:673–675, 1975.

191. Walshe JM: Penicillamine and the SLE syndrome. *J Rheumatol* 8(suppl 7):155–160, 1981.

192. Czlonkowska A: Myasthenia syndrome during penicillamine treatment. *Br Med J* 2:726–727, 1975.

193. Bigger JF: Retinal hemorrhages during penicillamine therapy of cystinuria. *Am J Ophthalmol* 66:954–955, 1968.

194. Henkin RI, Keiser HR, Jaffe IA, et al: Decreased taste sensitivity after D-Penicillamine reversed by copper administration. *Lancet* 2:1268–1271, 1967.

195. Tu J, Blackwell RQ, Lee PF: DL-Penicillamine as a cause of optic axial neuritis. *J Am Med Assoc* 185:83–86, 1963.

196. Proesman W, Jaeken J, Eckels R: D-Penicillamine induced IgA deficiency in Wilson's disease. *Lancet* 2:804–805, 1976.

197. Sternlieb I, Fisher M, Scheinberg IH: Penicillamine-induced skin lesions. *J Rheumatol* 8(suppl 7):149–154, 1981.

198. Nimni ME: Mechanism of inhibition of collagen cross-linking by penicillamine. *Proc R Soc Med* 70(suppl 3):65–72, 1977.

199. Morris JJ, Seifter E, Rettura G, et al: Effect of penicillamine upon wound healing. *J Surg Res* 9:143–149, 1969.

200. Kirsch N, Hukill PB: Elastosis perforans serpiginosa by penicillamine. Electron microscopic observations. *Arch Dermatol* 113:630–635, 1977.

201 Pass F, Goldfischer S, Sternlieb I, Scheinberg IH: Elastosis perforans serpiginosa after penicillamine therapy for Wilson's disease. *Arch Dermatol* 108:713–715, 1973.

202. Eisenberg E, Ballow M, Wolfe SH, et al: Pemphigus-like mucosal lesions: A side effect of penicillamine therapy. *Oral Surg Oral Med Oral Pathol* 51:409–414, 1981.

203. Bennett RA, Harbilas E: Wilson's disease with aseptic meningitis and penicillamine-related cheilosis. *Arch Intern Med* 120:374–376, 1967.

204. Walshe JM: The management of penicillamine nephropathy in Wilson's disease: A new chelating agent. *Lancet* 2:1401–1402, 1969.

205. Walshe JM: Assessment of the treatment of Wilson's disease with triethylene tetramine 2HCL (Trien 2HCl), in Sarkar B (ed): *Biological Aspects of Metal Related Diseases.* New York: Raven Press, 1983, pp 243–261.

206. Walshe JM: Treatment of Wilson's disease with trientine (triethylene tetramine) dihydrochloride. *Lancet* 1:643–647, 1982.

207. Walshe JM: Copper chelation in patients with Wilson's disease: A comparison of penicillamine and triethylene tetramine hydrochloride. *Q J Med* 42:441–452, 1973.

208. Condamine L, Hermine O, Alvin P, et al: Acquired sideroblastic anaemia during treatment of Wilson's disease with triethylene tetramine dihydrochloride. *Brit J Hematol* 83:166–168, 1993.

209. Denny-Brown D, Porter H: The effect of BAL (2,3 dimercaptopropanol) on hepato-lenticular degeneration (Wilson's disease). *N Engl J Med* 245:917–925, 1951.

210. Cumings JN: The effects of BAL in hepatolenticular degeneration. *Brain* 74:10–22, 1951.

211. Scheinberg IH, Sternlieb I: Treatment of the neurologic manifestations of Wilson's disease. *Arch Neurol* 52:339–340, 1995.

212. Brewer GJ: In reply. *Arch Neurol* 52:340, 1995

213. Schilsky ML, Scheinberg IH, Sternlieb I: Liver transplantation for Wilson's disease: Indications and outcome. *Hepatology* 19:583–587, 1994.

214. Rela M, Heaton ND, Vougas V, et al: Orthotopic liver transplantation for hepatic complications of Wilson's disease. *Br J Surg* 80:909–911, 1993.

215. Shafer DF, Shaw BW Jr: Fulminant hepatic failure and orthotopic liver transplantation. *Semin Liver Dis* 9:189–194, 1989.

216. Chen CL, Kuo YC: Metabolic effects of liver transplantation in Wilson's disease. *Transplant Proc* 25:2944–2947, 1993.

217. Mason AL, Marsh W, Alpers DH: Intractable neurological Wilson's disease treated with orthotopic liver transplantation. *Dig Dis Sci* 38:1746–1750, 1993.

Chapter 47

STIFF-PERSON SYNDROME

OSCAR S. GERSHANIK

HISTORICAL BACKGROUND
CLINICAL ASPECTS
    Physical Examination
    Laboratory Examination
    Electromyography (EMG)
    Muscle Biopsy
    Imaging Studies
ASSOCIATED CONDITIONS
DIAGNOSIS
DIFFERENTIAL DIAGNOSIS
PATHOPHYSIOLOGY AND PATHOGENESIS
    Pathology
    Physiology
    Biochemistry and Pharmacology
    Immunology
    Etiology and Pathogenesis
TREATMENT

The stiff-person syndrome (SPS) is a rare neurological disorder of unknown cause, characterized by severe and incapacitating axial and proximal limb rigidity as a result of continuous motor unit activity. Rigidity is often enhanced by anxiety, sudden movements, or external stimuli, causing intermittent painful muscle spasms. The disease follows a progressive, unremitting course, resulting in pronounced disability, when left untreated.

Historical Background

This unusual syndrome was first described by Moersch and Woltman in 1956.[1] The authors coined the term "Stiff-man syndrome" in reporting on 14 patients with clinical features of progressive fluctuating muscular rigidity and spasms. Their first patient, a 49-year-old man, initially complained of a feeling of tightness of the neck musculature that was of variable occurrence. Over a period of 4 years this disorder progressively affected the muscles of the shoulders, back, abdomen, and thighs, causing the muscles to appear stiff and "board-like." Continuous muscle contraction, causing pronounced stiffness of the axial and limb muscles, forced the patient to walk in a peculiar way that was both slow and awkward. Voluntary movement or passive displacement of the limbs triggered prolonged and painful muscle spasms. When severe enough, the spasms caused postural instability and falls. In the words of the authors, the patient would fall like a "wooden man." The additional 13 patients in the original report were similar in all respects.

The clinical features of this previously unreported condition were described in detail in Moersch and Woltman's study. No other signs of central or peripheral nervous system involvement were present in their 14 patients. The only additional clinical abnormality found in 4 of the 14 original patients was diabetes mellitus. Of their 14 patients, 5 underwent electromyographic studies, revealing motor unit activity resembling "that which accompanies contraction of voluntary muscle." In their 1967 review on the subject, Gordon et al.[2] summarized the electromyographic findings reported in the literature until then as "one of persistent tonic contraction reflected in constant firing even at rest." No attempt at relaxation could alter the continuous motor unit discharges, according to these authors. Their observations provided the electrophysiological substrate of muscle stiffness in these patients.

Since the publication of Moersch and Woltman's description of the syndrome, more than 100 cases have been reported from different regions of the world. The first successful attempt at treatment of this condition was that of Howard in 1963[3] with the use of diazepam to reduce stiffness and spasms.

A major breakthrough in the understanding of the pathogenesis of SPS came through the work of Solimena and co-workers in 1988,[4] who reported the presence of antibodies against glutamic acid decarboxylase (GAD), an enzyme involved in the synthesis of gamma-aminobutyric acid (GABA) in a patient with SPS, diabetes mellitus, and evidence of additional immunological involvement. Since then, SPS has been postulated to be an immunologic disorder.

Gordon et al.[2] and, later, Lorish et al.[5] defined the clinical criteria necessary for the diagnosis of SPS. These criteria have been widely accepted and are currently used for the identification of cases of SPS.

Numerous attempts at therapeutic intervention followed Howard's observation of clinical improvement with diazepam in patients with SPS. Benzodiazepines and baclofen have been recognized as the drugs of choice,[6] although reports of improvement with other drugs, such as sodium valproate, tizanidine, steroids, and with nonpharmacological treatments, such as plasmapheresis, have been published in recent years.[6]

Clinical Aspects

The disease is sporadic, affecting individuals of both sexes in variable proportions. In their analysis of 34 "valid" cases, Gordon et al.[2] found a 2 to 1 male/female preponderance; this ratio, however, is not maintained in subsequent cases in the more recent literature.[5,7] Although the age at onset varies considerably, the majority of those afflicted are adults ranging from 29 to 59 years of age. Both older and younger cases have been occasionally reported (extreme range, 7–71 years).[8–10] Although families with "congenital" SPS have been described, doubts have been raised concerning their identity with sporadic SPS of later onset.[6,11,12] Mean age at onset in the original Mayo Clinic series was 45.5 ± 9.3 years.[5]

Symptoms usually start slowly and insidiously; patients often complaining of episodic aching and tightness of the axial musculature (neck, paraspinal, and abdominal muscles). Muscle tightness, stiffness, and rigidity become constant within several weeks or months. Involvement is usually symmetrical, spreading on to include proximal muscle groups in all four limbs.[5,6] Sparing of distal muscles of the limbs and facial musculature is usually the rule in these patients, although involvement of the cranial musculature has been reported occasionally (e.g., difficulty swallowing, dysphagia, changes in facial expression, pursing of the lips, etc.).[2] Stiffness as a result of involvement of antagonistic muscles causes significant restriction of voluntary movements. Patients are almost unable to bend over and find walking extremely difficult. They adopt a typical hyperlordotic lumbar posture causing folding of the skin in that region; the neck is held in a somewhat extended position; and there is marked limitation of back and hip movement. Of importance is the fact that lumbar hyperlordosis persists even when patients are lying down on their back. This peculiar pattern of stiffness "has prompted patients and physicians to use such descriptions as 'stiff as a board' and 'he walks like a wooden man' or 'looks like a tin soldier'," as it was colorfully reported by Lorish et al.[5] in their 1989 update on SPS. The rigidity or stiffness may fluctuate in intensity from hour to hour or from day to day, usually disappearing during sleep. Activities of daily living become severely impaired in these patients, as they find it extremely difficult to dress by themselves; even leaning forward to tie their shoelaces or put on their socks is difficult. When severe rigidity of the cervical spine is present, patients must discontinue driving as they are limited in their capacity to rotate their head to look back or to the side.[5]

An additional incapacitating symptom is the occurrence of intermittent severe spasms in affected muscles.[1,2,5] Spasms are precipitated by a wide range of triggering factors. A sudden noise, an unexpected movement, a simple touch, or just being gently nudged may often be the cause of severe spasmodic contraction of the affected muscles. Passive stretching of the muscles will also cause spasms. Emotional stimuli, as well as stress or fatigue may prompt a paroxysm. Spasms are short lasting (minutes) and gradually disappear if the triggering stimulus is removed. Muscle spasms are often associated with pain. Painful sensation has been variably reported in the literature; either as an acute, sharp, or excruciating pain or, more often, as a dull, cramping feeling of fatigue.[1,2,5] Patients experiencing a bout of spasms present a distressful picture, as they "appear to be in a shock-like state associated with sweating, tachycardia and restlessness."[2] An increase in blood pressure has been documented during these crises.[10] Spasms are a compounding factor of motor disability in these patients, as they frequently are the cause of sudden falls. Anecdotal reports abound in the literature: patients complaining of spasmodic fits triggered by the ringing of the phone; being awakened in the middle of the night by a soft nudge by a spouse; or falling out of a chair while attempting to sit down.[5] The magnitude and intensity of the spasms is quite variable. In a few reported cases they became severe enough to cause the fracture of long bones.[2]

In a recent analysis of clinical and laboratory findings in SPS patients, Meinck et al.[13] extended the repertoire of symptoms in this disorder, adding three new and distinct clinical features to those previously described. Of their eight patients, five reported an "aura"-like feeling preceding spontaneous spasmodic attacks. In the majority of their cases, spasmodic jerks adopted a stereotyped motor pattern, consisting of brief opisthotonos, stiffening of the slightly abducted legs and inversion of the plantarflexed feet. In addition, their patients reported a feeling of paroxysmal fear invading them whenever they crossed an open space unaided. Moreover, even the thought of doing it would precipitate it.

The illness follows a variable course with a duration ranging from 6 to 28 years measured from onset of symptoms to either death or last follow-up visit.[5] In the majority of cases the disease slowly and steadily progresses over time. There are, however, some cases in whom stabilization is achieved through medication. Lorish et al.[5] reported on the follow-up of 13 patients seen at the Mayo Clinic during the period from 1955 to 1985. These patients had a disease duration ranging from 1 to 28 years. All 13 cases were under treatment with variable doses of diazepam, and the great majority remained independently mobile despite the long duration of the disease in some of them. The rate of progression of the disease and the final outcome will depend in part on the conditions usually associated with this disorder (e.g., diabetes, malignancy, etc.). Unexpected sudden death has been reported in SPS cases.[14] Two patients carrying a diagnosis of SPS experienced sudden death, apparently secondary to autonomic instability. Of these two cases, however, one had atypical clinical signs and inflammatory changes in the basal ganglia, brain stem, and spinal cord, which is more suggestive of encephalomyelitis.[15,16] Severe autonomic symptomatology may be precipitated in SPS patients by sudden withdrawal of medication. This contingency should always be entertained when making changes in medication in SPS patients.

PHYSICAL EXAMINATION

Neurological examination is usually noncontributory, except for those findings related to muscle rigidity. Palpatory examination of the affected muscles will reveal a "tight, rock-hard, boardlike quality." Postural changes have been described in detail in the preceding paragraphs. Gait is slow and cautious to avoid precipitation of spasms and falls. Cognitive function, cranial nerves, muscle strength, sensory function, and coordination are all normal; deep-tendon reflexes have often been found to be increased, without further evidence of pyramidal tract involvement. Some investigators have reported mild atrophy and weakness in the advanced stages of the disease. Studies of respiratory function may reveal, in some cases, a restrictive pattern resulting from involvement of the thoracic musculature.[1,2,5,6]

LABORATORY EXAMINATION

Routine laboratory examinations are usually within normal limits, except in those patients in whom insulin-dependent diabetes mellitus (IDDM), thyroid disorders, malignancy, or other associated conditions are present (see Associated Conditions).[1,2,5–7] Creatinuria is a rare finding in these patients and is most probably linked to disuse atrophy.[2] Immunological determinations reveal the presence of antibodies directed against gamma-aminobutyric acid (GABAergic) neurons, more specifically, to GAD in a large proportion of SPS patients;[4,7,17,18] autoantibodies directed against other cellular systems also are found frequently in these patients.[7,17] Oligoclonal IgG banding, both in serum and cerebrospinal fluid (CSF), may be found in some cases.[4,7,17,19–21] Elevated CSF IgG has been reported in isolated cases.[22] The presence of significant CSF abnormalities is, on the contrary, the rule in encephalomyelitis (see Differential Diagnosis).[15,16] Certain human lymphocyte antigen (HLA) phenotypes appear to be more frequent than others in cases of SPS.[7,23–25] All of the above point in the direction of an immunological disorder as the underlying cause of SPS (see Pathophysiology and Pathogenesis).

ELECTROMYOGRAPHY (EMG)

The presence of continuous motor unit activity at rest and its persistence, despite attempts at relaxation, is a constant finding in SPS patients. There are no abnormalities in the morphology of motor units; peripheral nerve motor and sensory conduction velocities are normal, and no signs of denervation, such as fasciculations, fibrillations, and positive sharp waves, can be found. No evidence of grouping of rhythmic discharges or atypical high-frequency bursts are usually found. Electromyographic (EMG) recordings show this pattern of continuous motor unit activity to be more prominent in paraspinal muscles (thoracolumbar and rectus abdominis), as well as in proximal arm and leg muscles. Involvement of both agonist and antagonist muscle groups is common. Peripheral stimulation (gentle touching or stroking of the skin) of the muscles explored is followed by marked enhancement of motor unit activity, either continuous or intermittent (spasms) (Fig. 47-1). The abnormal EMG activity is absent during sleep. Peripheral nerve or spinal nerve root block, spinal anesthesia and general anesthesia, or intravenous injection of diazepam can also abolish this pattern of motor unit activity.[2,5,6,26]

MUSCLE BIOPSY

Histological study of muscle is usually noncontributory. Most studies performed have reported normal findings in muscle biopsy specimens. In some cases, nonspecific findings, such as minimal atrophy, slight fibrosis, occasional degeneration, and regeneration of muscle fibers with associated sprouting of nerve terminals, edema, perivascular infiltration, and proliferation of connective tissue, have been described.[2] The majority of authors are in agreement in the interpretation of these findings as secondary to prolonged ischemia linked to intense muscular contraction.[2]

IMAGING STUDIES

Plain x-ray films of the spine may reveal signs of spondylosis and ossification of spinal ligaments.[1] Although these findings have been reported in SPS patients, they probably represent common, nonspecific phenomena, equally present in the general population.[2] Cortical atrophy on computed tomography and white matter lesions on magnetic resonance imaging (MRI) have been reported in isolated cases of SPS, although

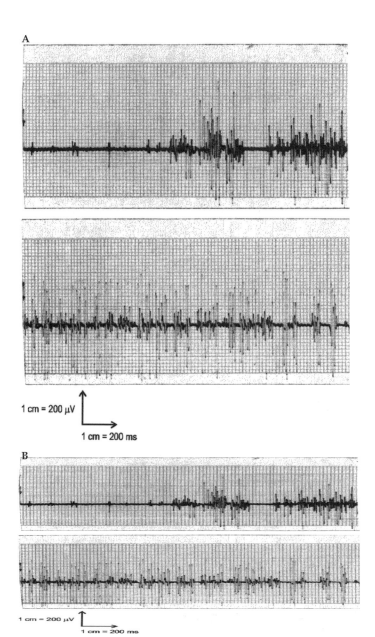

FIGURE 47-1 *A.* Simultaneous EMG recording of antagonist muscles of the upper extremity (biceps and triceps brachialis), showing bursts of motor unit discharges at rest. *B.* EMG recording of biceps brachialis, showing intermittent bursts of motor unit discharges after a mechanical stimulus (light tapping).

their relevance to this condition has not been discussed.[6,19,22] It is indeed possible that the above-mentioned abnormalities would correspond to underlying encephalomyelitis. Progressive encephalomyelitis with rigidity (PEWR) is often misdiagnosed as SPS (see Differential Diagnosis).

Associated Conditions

A number of medical conditions are commonly associated with SPS and are useful in validating its diagnosis, as well as in providing clues concerning the pathogenesis of this disorder.

In Blum and Jankovic's review of reported cases until 1991,[7] of 84 patients fulfilling Gordon's criteria for SPS, 18 percent had definite clinical evidence of one or more organ-specific autoimmune diseases. These included pernicious anemia, vitiligo, myasthenia gravis, hypothyroidism, hyperthyroidism, and Hashimoto's thyroiditis.

Of special importance is the relationship of SPS and IDDM, not only because of the frequent association of these two conditions but also because the reason for their simultaneous occurrence may have a bearing on the pathogenesis of SPS.[7] It should be noted that 4 of the original 14 patients reported on in Moersch and Woltman's study,[1] and 8 of 13 patients in an update from Lorish et al.'s[5] made on SPS and published in 1989 had diabetes. The type of diabetes was not mentioned in these two reports. It is currently accepted that diabetes is present in one-third to two-thirds of patients with SPS. A review of the literature[7] by Blum and Jankovic found that in 8 percent of the published cases IDDM was present, whereas 13 additional patients had diabetes but without further characterization of its type. According to these authors the frequency of IDDM in SPS patients is, therefore, more than 30 times that of the general population (0.25 percent). These findings are of relevance in the light of the current hypothesis on the pathogenesis of IDDM. It is presently accepted that an abnormal immune response directed against pancreatic islet cells is triggered by an exogenous agent, possibly a virus, causing the development of IDDM in genetically predisposed individuals.[7] A similar mechanism may be involved in the pathogenesis of SPS (see Pathophysiology and Pathogenesis).

Nocturnal myoclonus and epilepsy have also been reported in association with SPS. In their 1978 publication, Martinelli et al.[27] calculated, from a review of the literature, that the prevalence of epilepsy in SPS cases was close to 10 percent. They concluded that this figure was much higher than the prevalence of epilepsy in the general population, supporting the concept that this association was not by chance. However, this assertion has been contested by others, justifying the higher prevalence of epilepsy in SPS patients as a withdrawal phenomenon in individuals under diazepam therapy for extended periods.[28] In addition to nocturnal myoclonus, other types of myoclonic jerks have been reported in patients diagnosed as having SPS. Leigh et al.[29] published the clinical and electrophysiological findings in a 38-year-old patient with reflex myoclonus and muscle rigidity. The authors coined the term "Jerking-stiff-man syndrome" in view of the prominent jerking with similar characteristics to reticular reflex myoclonus that was present in their patient. Although the patient had many of the clinical features necessary for the diagnosis of SPS, the presence of clinical and radiological signs of brain stem and cerebellar involvement would be more in favor of either encephalomyelitis or of an atypical form of sporadic cerebellar system degeneration. An additional case reported by Alberca et al.[30] shares many of the clinical features described in the previous patient, although no evidence of structural involvement of the CNS was found.

Diagnosis

Gordon et al.[2] were the first to establish a set of criteria for the diagnosis of SPS. They were based on the analysis of the original 14 cases of Moersch and Woltman and subsequent reports from the world literature. Their criteria included clinical and neurophysiological findings, as well as a number of supportive tests. Clinical criteria were subdivided into six "key features" as follows:

1. *Prodrome* ("episodic aching and tightness of the axial musculature");
2. *Progression* ("symmetrical, continuous stiffness characterized by tight, stone-hard, board-like muscles spreads to involve most of the limb, trunk and neck musculature");
3. *Painful spasms and precipitating factors* ("Superimposed upon this persistent rigidity of muscles, sudden stimuli often precipitate paroxysms of muscle spasm of such intensity as to lead, although not invariably, to excruciating pain");
4. *Sleep* ("In this state rigidity is abolished . . . .");
5. *Neurologic findings* ("Normal motor and sensory examinations are the rule, except for the difficulty in active movement and the board-hard muscles referred to under 'Progression.' ");
6. *Intellect* ("Invariably intellect has been found intact . . . .")

According to the criteria of Gordon et al. the EMG "defines the peculiar state of voluntary muscle in stiff-man syndrome as one of persistent tonic contraction reflected in constant firing even 'at rest.'" Additional supportive tests included: (1) a response to myoneural blocking agents; (2) the effect of chemical block of peripheral motor fibers, and (3) a response to general anesthesia. Furthermore, the beneficial effect of diazepam on muscle stiffness was included as a final supportive criterion.

More recently, Thompson[6] modified and expanded the criteria for diagnosis proposed by Gordon et al.[2] and Lorish et al.[5] (Table 47-1).

Differential Diagnosis

Any patient presenting with muscle stiffness, rigidity and cramps, or muscle spasms may, at one time or another, be considered as a possible case of SPS. Moreover, there are several conditions with clinical features resembling SPS but with demonstrable central nervous system (CNS) pathology that have been reported in the literature as atypical cases of this disorder. The list of conditions is long and includes disorders of muscle contraction of both central and peripheral origin (Table 47-2). Dealing with each of these disorders exceeds the scope of this chapter (for a review, see Refs. 6 and 26).

Strict adherence to the criteria carefully delineated by Gordon et al.,[2] Lorish et al.,[5] and, more recently, Thompson[6] will help in identifying cases of SPS, differentiating them from the conditions listed in Table 47-2.

TABLE 47-1 Criteria for the Diagnosis of the Stiff-Man Syndrome

Clinical
   Gradual onset of aching and tightness of axial muscles
   Slow progression; stiffness spreads from axial muscles to limbs
      (legs > arms)
   Persistent contraction of thoracolumbar, paraspinal, and
      abdominal muscles
   Abnormal hyperlordotic posture of lumbar spine
   Board-like rigidity of abdominal muscles
   Rigidity abolished by sleep
   Stimulus-sensitive painful muscle spasms
   No other abnormal neurological signs
   Intellect normal
   Cranial muscles rarely (if ever) involved
Neurophysiological
   Continuous motor unit activity
   EMG activity abolished by sleep, peripheral nerve block, spinal
      or general anesthesia
   Normal peripheral nerve conduction
   Normal motor unit morphology
Other observations that may be helpful but are of uncertain
      diagnostic specificity
   Autoantibodies directed against GABAergic neurons, in
      particular to GAD
   Association with autoimmune endocrine disease

Some of the disorders included in Table 47-2 deserve special consideration because of the difficulties they may present in the differential diagnosis with SPS.

PEWR with painful spasms is a rare, usually paraneoplastic disorder featuring, in addition to the cardinal symptoms of SPS, evidence of brain stem and spinal cord involvement.[15,16,31] The latter may manifest in terms of cranial nerve signs, segmental and long-tract spinal cord symptomatology. Myoclonus and opsoclonus have also been reported in this disorder. Imaging studies may reveal cortical, brain stem, and cerebellar atrophy and, sometimes, hyperintense signals in the white matter on MRI examination. Abnormal findings in the CSF are frequent (lymphocytic pleocytosis, elevated protein levels, increased immunoglobulins, and oligoclonal IgG bands). In a single patient, diagnosed as having PEWR on the basis of a few atypical features (pattern of distribution of rigidity, loss of tendon jerks, nuclear and supranuclear gaze palsies, and reticular reflex myoclonus) GAD autoantibodies were detected.[32] However, no confirmation of an inflammatory process within the CNS was available. Results of biopsy or postmortem examination in PEWR cases show an inflammatory process, with perivascular lymphocitic infiltration, gliosis, and severe neuronal loss, involving mainly the lower brain stem and spinal cord (encephalomyelitis). In some cases there is more widespread involvement, including brain cortical regions (hippocampus) and subcortical gray nuclei (basal ganglia). The most striking pathological changes are usually restricted to the central gray zones of the spinal cord containing inhibitory interneurons. The disease follows a relentless course, ending in death in a few months or years. This condition has been reported either as an isolated illness or, more frequently, as being associated with malignancy (oat cell carcinoma of the lung, Hodgkin's disease).[33,34]

The question of SPS as a paraneoplastic autoimmune disorder in isolated cases has been raised in several publications. Three women with breast cancer, presenting with clinical features fullfilling the criteria necessary for the diagnosis of

TABLE 47-2 Differential Diagnosis of Stiff-Person Syndrome

| | PERIPHERAL | |
CENTRAL	Nerve	Muscle
Encephalitis (including brain stem, spinal cord: "Progressive encephalomyelitis with rigidity")	Myokimia, neuromyotonia, and pseudomyotonia	Myotonic syndromes (channelopathies)
Dystonia	Idiopathic	Myotonic dystrophy
Idiopathic	Isaacs syndrome (continuous muscle fiber activity)	Myotonia congenita
Symptomatic	Associated with neuropathy	Paramyotonia
Akinetic-rigid syndromes	Hereditary	Myopathies
Parkinson's disease	Inflammatory	Metabolic
Multiple system atrophy	Toxic	Inflammatory
Progressive supranuclear palsy	Radiation	Endocrine
Drug-induced parkinsonism	Paraneoplastic	Congenital
Toxic parkinsonism (MPTP, carbon monoxide, manganese)	Schwartz-Jampel syndrome	Contracture
Neuroleptic malignant syndrome	Tetanus	Arthritis
Myelopathies (infectious, trauma, ischemia, hemorrhage, spondylosis)	Cramps	Ankylosing spondylitis
Spinal cord tumor		Volkmann's ischemic contracture
Spinal cord AVM		
Toxins (tetanus, strychnine, etc.)		
Motor neuron disease (primary lateral sclerosis, amyotrophic lateral sclerosis)		
Psychiatric illness (hysteria, malingering)		

MPTP, 1-methyl-4-phenyl-1,2,3,6-tetrahydropyridine; AVM, arteriovenous malformation.

SPS, were recently reported.[35] These patients had none of the conditions frequently associated with SPS (IDDM and other immunological disorders), and no GAD autoantibodies were detected. Extensive immunologic screening detected the presence of a humoral autoimmune response against a neuronal protein of 128 kd. This antigen was found to be concentrated at synapses, and its distribution outside the nervous system was highly restricted. Similar to GAD, the 128-kd antigen is localized in the cytoplasmic compartment and is not a membrane surface protein. In a follow-up study, this 128-kd antigen has been identified as the synaptic vesicle-associated protein amphiphysin.[36] Both GAD and amphiphysin are concentrated in nerve terminals, associated with the cytoplasmic surface of synaptic vesicles. This finding suggests a possible link between the mechanism of autoimmunity in SPS and some paraneoplastic cases. It is also worth noting that 40 percent of SPS cases lack autoantibodies directed against GAD and that not all patients suffer from IDDM as an associated condition.

Therefore, it is possible that SPS may be, in fact, a heterogeneous disorder in which different pathogenetic mechanisms, including a paraneoplastic immune response with or without inflammatory changes (PEWR), play a role.[32,33,37]

Pathophysiology and Pathogenesis

PATHOLOGY

Postmortem examination of the CNS, including the spinal cord in patients with SPS, has not yielded evidence of any significant abnormality.[1,2,5,6,8] The only exception was a case reported by Nakamura et al.,[38] showing involvement of the anterior columns of the spinal cord. No consistent macroscopic or microscopic changes have been found in the few remaining cases that underwent autopsy. The lack of pathological correlates to the marked derangement of motor unit activity and muscle contraction appears to indicate that SPS is a functional rather than a structural disorder.

PHYSIOLOGY

All evidence suggests a central origin for spasms, rigidity, and continuous motor unit activity. This is sustantiated by their disappearance with sleep, peripheral nerve block, general anesthesia, and systemic administration of diazepam.[1,2,5] Several hypotheses have been proposed to explain this enhancement of spinal motor neuron activity, including increased primary excitability of alpha motoneurons, a disorder of presynaptic inhibition of Ia terminals in the spinal cord, increased fusimotor activity, defective Renshaw cell function, and abnormalities in the suprasegmental descending pathways controlling spinal interneuronal systems. Several authors have addressed these hypotheses using different investigative techniques.

Monosynaptic stretch reflexes and F-waves are normal in SPS patients.[39] In addition, assessment of the ratio of the maximal H-reflex to M-wave size in the soleus muscle has failed to reveal any abnormality, excluding a primary enhancement of alpha motor neuron excitability.[39]

Evaluation of the recovery curve of the soleus H-reflex after a conditioning stimulus in patients with SPS yielded normal results, thus ruling out the Ia afferent system as the source of abnormal inputs to the motor neurons of the spinal cord.[27,40]

Although there is no conclusive evidence for or against the presence of increased gamma motoneuron (fusimotor) activity, most authors consider it unlikely in view of the normal tendon reflexes and peculiar pattern of distribution of muscle rigidity.[2,39]

Involvement of the recurrent inhibitory loop mediated by Renshaw cells has also been ruled out as the silent period after a supramaximal peripheral nerve stimulus was found to be normal in SPS patients.[39–42]

Evidence in favor of a disorder of presynaptic inhibition of Ia terminals in the spinal cord is based on the lack of depression in amplitude of the soleus H-reflex conditioned by tonic vibration applied to the Achilles tendon in SPS cases.[40]

Another consistent abnormal finding in SPS patients is the presence of a widespread enhancement of exteroceptive reflexes, probably a result of a disorder of descending pathways controlling segmental interneuronal systems.[39,43] The responses to exteroceptive stimuli have been found to be grossly exaggerated, with abnormally short transmission times and the presence of abnormal excitatory reflex phases in face, arm, and leg muscles. Both somatosensory and acoustic stimuli are the most effective in evoking an abnormal reflex response. The presence of an abnormally exaggerated blink reflex has also been noted in SPS cases.[39] A more prominent and persistent response of the acoustic startle reflex has been found in SPS patients, in comparison to that of controls.[44] Most nonnociceptive reflexes have been found to behave abnormally, showing a low stimulation threshold, lacking habituation phenomena, and exhibiting cocontraction, suggesting nonspecific disturbances of the polysynaptic system.[27,39]

BIOCHEMISTRY AND PHARMACOLOGY

The existence of a disorder involving suprasegmental influences on inhibitory interneuronal systems at the spinal cord level is supported by a number of biochemical and pharmacological studies.

An increase in the severity of spasms induced by catecholamine precursors such as L-dopa or reuptake inhibitors such as clorimipramine has been reported.[9,39,43,45] On the contrary, opposite effects were observed with the use of drugs reducing aminergic activity within the CNS, such as clonidine and tizanidine,[39] or drugs such as diazepam and baclofen that probably act by enhancing GABAergic transmission.[46] In addition, diazepam may also act indirectly through inhibition of catecholaminergic transmission.[9,39] These findings suggest an imbalance between noradrenergic and GABAergic neurotransmitter systems descending from the brain stem to the spinal cord.[9,39] The detection of reduced levels of GABA in the CSF of SPS patients lends further support to this hypothesis.[7]

Neither physostigmine, a cholinergic drug, glycine, a putative inhibitory neurotransmitter at the spinal cord level, nor milacemide, a glycine precursor, produce any modification in the clinical status of SPS patients.[9,46,47] These observations lend little support to theories proposing a defective synaptic transmission, either at the cholinergic synapse of recurrent axons of alpha motoneurons involving Renshaw cells or at the proposed glycinergic synapse between axons of spinal cord interneurons and cell bodies of alpha motoneurons.

The hypothesis of an imbalance between a descending excitatory catecholamine neuronal system and a GABAergic counterpart with net inhibitory effects on alpha motoneurons was further bolstered by findings of increased 3-methoxy-4-hydroxyphenylglycol (MHPG) excretion in a patient with SPS.[48] MHPG is the major metabolite of brain norepinephrine. Pharmacological manipulations in this patient showed a direct correlation between clinical status and levels of MHPG in the urine, suggesting the presence of an overactive catecholamine system as one of the underlying mechanisms of rigidity and spasms.[9,39,48] However, a subsequent report failed to confirm these findings.[41]

Although, on the basis of the therapeutic response to drugs, most authors agree on the possibility of such an imbalance, there is as yet no firm evidence to substantiate it.

IMMUNOLOGY

Young, in 1966,[49] was the first to advance the hypothesis of an autoimmune mechanism in the pathogenesis of SPS, based on the findings of pernicious anemia and possible Hashimoto's thyroiditis in a patient with this disorder. The coexistence of diseases of autoimmune origin in patients with SPS is a consistent finding, suggesting a possible common pathogenetic mechanism. As mentioned before, in Blum and Jankovic's review of 84 published cases, including 2 of their own, 18 percent had clinical evidence of one or more autoimmune diseases.[7]

A compelling argument in favor of the autoimmune origin of SPS came through the work of Solimena et al.[4] These authors detected the presence of autoantibodies against several nonneuronal tissues in the serum of a patient with SPS, epilepsy, and IDDM, carrying an autoimmunity predisposing HLA phenotype. These included complement-fixing islet cell antibodies, gastric parietal cell antibodies, and thyroglobulin and thyroid microsomal antibodies. In addition, both the serum and the CSF of the patient contained antibodies to mammalian CNS antigens. Antibodies were detected through immunocytochemistry and Western blot analysis. The cellular and subcellular distribution of immunoreactivity was identical to that of GAD, an enzyme involved in the synthesis of GABA. GAD is concentrated in GABAergic nerve terminals and, outside the CNS, in pancreatic beta cells. Cross-immunoreactivity was found in this patient. An important additional piece of evidence in support of the hypothesis of an autoimmune process directed against the CNS was the finding of elevated levels of IgG, with an oligoclonal pattern, in the CSF of the patient.

In a subsequent publication, Solimena et al.[17] reported on the results of a systematic immunological study of patients with SPS. They studied the serum of 32 patients with an established diagnosis of SPS; in 24 patients the CSF was also available. Control serum samples of 218 individuals were used, including 16 healthy subjects, 111 patients with varied neurologic disorders, 74 with IDDM, 20 with other organ-specific autoimmune disorders, and 3 with systemic autoimmune disease. The techniques used in the study included immunocytochemical assays to detect autoantibodies against GABAergic neurons, standard laboratory procedures to detect different organ-specific autoantibodies (islet cell, gastric parietal cell, thyroglobulin, and thyroid microsomal-fraction antibodies), immunoblotting, immunoprecipitation, and isoelectric focusing and silver staining of serum and CSF to detect oligoclonal IgG bands. Sixty percent of the sera of SPS patients tested were positive for autoantibodies against GABAergic neurons, whereas 50 percent of the CSF samples were also positive. Twenty-seven percent of the CSF samples tested revealed the presence of oligoclonal IgG bands, including two patients negative for GABAergic neuron autoantibodies. In all patients who tested positive for GABAergic neuron antibodies there was cross-immunoreactivity directed against pancreatic beta cells. Other organ-specific autoantibodies that were positive in the same patient group included: gastric parietal cell antibodies (15/19), thyroid microsomal-fraction antibodies (9/19), and thyroglobulin antibodies (4/15). In the control population, only four patients (1.8 percent) tested positive for GABAergic neuron autoantibodies. A Western blot assay was performed to investigate whether GAD was the autoantigen responsible for the positive immunoreactivity against brain and pancreas. A band comigrating with GAD was detected in the large majority of serum and CSF samples that were positive for autoantibodies against GABAergic neurons, confirming GAD as the antigen responsible for the autoimmune response.

More recent studies have attempted to characterize the immunological response both in SPS and IDDM better. GAD, the major autoantigen in both disorders, is present in two isoforms, GAD-65 and GAD-67, which have different molecular weights and are the product of two different genes.[50] The majority of SPS patients carry autoantibodies that react with the smaller isoform and specifically identify a dominant autoreactive target region (epitope) in the antigen.[51] The pattern of reactivity is somewhat different in IDDM, suggesting differences in epitope recognition in these two disorders.[52] These findings may indicate that during the development of these diseases, the autoantigen is presented to the immune system through separate pathogenetic mechanisms.[53] Depending on the method of detection used, autoantibodies against the larger GAD-67 isoform and to an 80-kd antigen can also be identified in SPS cases.[50,54] In a recent report Johnstone and Nussey[21] detected the presence of autoantibodies reacting against the large isoform of human GAD (GAD-67), using recombinant techniques, providing direct evidence for a clonally restricted response to GAD in SPS patients. These findings confirm previous observations suggesting immunological heterogeneity in SPS.[55] They also underline the need to perform different immunological techniques to identify the specific antigen involved in the production of anti-GABAergic autoantibodies in SPS cases.

The possibility of a genetically determined susceptibility to the development of SPS has been discussed by different authors. Several studies have reported on the detection of specific HLA haplotypes frequently linked to this disorder.

The original patient of Solimena et al. with autoantibodies to GAD was found to have the B44 and DR-3/4 antigens as major haplotypes. In the same year, Williams and coworkers[23] found that four of their five SPS patients, all suffering from autoimmune endocrinopathies, also typed to the B44 antigen, which is in linkage dysequilibrium with DR-4. HLA DR3 and DR4 are the alleles most commonly associated with IDDM in whites. Subsequently, Blum and Jankovic[7] speculated on the possibility that the specific organization of HLA-determined immunoregulatory molecules, apparently involved in the development of IDDM, possibly constitute the pathogenetic mechanism of autoimmunity to GABAergic cells in the CNS. The demonstration of HLA phenotypes common to both IDDM and SPS would lend further support to this hypothesis. In a more recent study on the genetics of susceptibility and resistance to IDDM in SPS, Pugliese et al.[24] found that, as in IDDM, SPS was associated with the allele DQB1*0201. In addition, the presence or absence of the related allele DQB1*0602 will, in turn, confer either a protective or predisposing factor for the development of IDDM in SPS patients.[25] These findings are, according to the authors, further evidence of the importance of the HLA genetic background in the development of SPS and related autoimmune disorders.

ETIOLOGY AND PATHOGENESIS

Although as yet there is no definitive answer concerning the etiology and pathogenesis of SPS, all of the available evidence already discussed in previous paragraphs suggests that an autoimmune mechanism is responsible for its development. An unknown noxious stimulus will trigger the cascade of events leading to the exposure of intracellular GAD to the immune system, causing the production of autoantibodies against this enzyme and GABA-containing neurons. This, in turn, will lead to a selective impairment of GABAergic transmission in suprasegmental systems influencing the inhibitory activity of spinal interneurons. The resulting imbalance between excitatory and inhibitory influences at the segmental level will be the cause of the enhancement of spinal motor neuron activity.

Treatment

Benzodiazepines have become the cornerstone of treatment of SPS, ever since Howard[3] first reported dramatic improvement of muscle spasms with diazepam in three patients with this disorder. The rationale behind Howard's approach was that, because diazepam blocked strychnine convulsions in mice and spinal reflexes in cats, he speculated that this drug would supress the constant discharges originating in the motor neurons of the spinal cord that were believed to be the cause of rigidity and stiffness in individuals affected with this syndrome. His patients were treated with up to 60 mg/day of diazepam in four divided doses, achieving significant functional improvement. Moreover, with the use of this drug, in addition to symptomatic benefit there were modifications in the EMG at rest. Unfortunately, the dose of diazepam usually needed to produce functional improvement is often associated with untoward side effects, mainly, profound se-

dation.[5,6] The dose range of diazepam presently used is between 10 and 100 mg daily in most cases. With this treatment regimen, patients tend to stabilize and maintain some degree of functional capacity.[5] However, most patients experience their symptoms on a continual basis, and some cases continue to deteriorate. Other benzodiazepines, such as clonazepam, have also been used in doses of 4–6 mg/day (1 mg of clonazepam is equivalent to 4–5 mg of diazepam), with apparent benefit in a few selected cases.[56] The second drug of choice, according to several authors is baclofen, administered in doses of up to 100 mg/day in order to achieve maximum benefit.[41,46,57] A relative absence or unavailability of GABA, a putative inhibitory neurotransmitter at the level of the gamma motor neuron system in the spinal cord, had been proposed by Gordon[2] as the underlying mechanism for rigidity in SPS. The beneficial effects of baclofen would derive from its properties as a GABA analogue (GABA-B receptor agonist).[46,58] As with diazepam, the main side effect observed with this drug is sedation. The administration of intrathecal baclofen through an infusion pump has been recently proposed.[58] The rationale behind this approach is to provide sufficiently high concentrations of the drug to the spinal cord receptors without the systemic side effects usually seen with oral administration. Only a few patients have been treated with this method of drug delivery, and the results so far have been variable.[59] Special attention should be paid to the adequate operation of the drug delivery system, as pump malfunctioning has been responsible for severe autonomic complications in one case of SPS.[60]

The standard treatment regimen in clinical practice today is a combination of diazepam and baclofen in lower doses than those used when each drug is given alone.[6] Furthermore, the best strategy is to gradually titrate the dosage of both drugs so as to minimize the sedative effects of these drugs. The best results are obtained in the control of spontaneous and stimulus-sensitive muscle spasms, whereas axial rigidity, abnormal posturing, and limitations of mobility respond less well. Valproic acid has also been advocated, and anecdotal reports of marked benefit in some cases can be found in the literature.[61] As an anticonvulsant, valproic acid is thought to augment GABAergic transmission, and perhaps its beneficial effect could be attributed to its ability to compensate for a deficiency of GABA at the spinal cord level. Several other drugs, including tizanidine, carbamazepine, sodium dantrolene, phenytoin, phenobarbital, cyclobenzaprine, mephenesin, L-dopa, 5-hydroxytryptophan, glycine, biperiden, dipropylacetate, gamma-hydroxybutyric acid, and milacemide, have also been tried with inconsistent or detrimental results.[7,9,39,47,62]

Plasmapheresis became an obvious choice after reports of the presence of antibodies reacting against GAD in both serum and CSF of patients with SPS and additional evidence of immunological involvement. The few cases undergoing this treatment obtained variable results. Two patients reported in separate papers had an excellent response to plasmapheresis; improvement was observed at variable times during the course of treatment in these two cases.[63,64] In one of them, clinical response was evident immediately after the second exchange, whereas subjective improvement lagged behind. Return to almost normal was reported by the patient almost 2 weeks after the end of plasmapheresis. Parallel to the reduction of rigidity and spasms there were signs of improvement in EMG studies, and the areas of evoked exteroceptive reflex responses were dramatically reduced. In one of the cases, antibody levels remained unchanged, whereas in the other GAD-like immunoreactivity fell from 1:1280 to 1:80 during plasmapheresis. In contrast, in the two additional patients reported on by Harding et al.,[20] the results were disappointing, although the immunological markers in these patients were similar to the previous ones. Plasmapheresis remains a promising therapeutic strategy, although controlled studies on the efficacy of this intervention have not been conducted yet.

The benefits of steroid treatment and immunosupressive drugs have been reported on an anecdotal basis.[20,65,66] Most patients appear to require a daily dose of 30–60 mg of prednisone to achieve noticeable improvement; however, reappearance of symptoms develops whenever the steroid dosage is tapered.[66] The use of high-dose, long-term steroids in the treatment of a chronic disorder, frequently associated with IDDM, does not seem convenient.

Two recent publications have reported on the beneficial effects of intravenous immunoglobulin (IVIG) in the treatment of SPS.[67,68] A total of six patients showed significant subjective and functional improvement after treatment with IVIG, lending additional support to the hypothesis of an immune origin of SPS. As with other immune disorders, IVIG therapy could be effective through either neutralization of autoantibodies or downregulation of antibody production.

An anecdotal report on the benefits of paraspinal injection of botulinum toxin A in a patient with SPS has been published recently.[69] Significant reduction of rigidity at the paraspinal and thigh muscles, improvement of ambulation, and cessation of pain were obtained with the use of this medication.

In summary, present-day strategies for the treatment of SPS can be divided into two separate categories. The first category includes drugs known to interact with the pharmacological mechanisms underlying the production of muscle rigidity (diazepam, baclofen, valproic acid, clonidine, tizanidine, etc.), and the benefit derived from their use is purely symptomatic. On the other hand, the use of plasmapheresis, steroids, and other immunomodulating agents (immunosupressive drugs, IVIG) represent an attempt to modify or control the immunologic factors potentially involved in the pathogenesis of SPS.

References

1. Moersch FP, Woltman HW: Progressive fluctuating muscular rigidity and spasm ("stiff-man" syndrome): Report of a case and some observations in 13 other cases. *Mayo Clin Proc* 31:421–427, 1956.

2. Gordon EE, Januszko DM, Kaufman L: A critical survey of stiff-man syndrome. *Am J Med* 42:582–599, 1967.

3. Howard FM: A new and effective drug in the treatment of stiff-man syndrome: Preliminary report. *Mayo Clin Proc* 38:203–212, 1963.

4. Solimena M, Folli F, Denis-Donini S, et al: Autoantibodies to glutamic acid decarboxylase in a patient with stiff-man syn-drome, epilepsy, and type I diabetes mellitus. *N Engl J Med* 318:1012–1020, 1988.

5. Lorish TR, Thorsteinsson G, Howard FM: Stiff-man syndrome updated. *Mayo Clin Proc* 64:629–636, 1989.

6. Thompson PD: Stiff people, in Marsden CD, Fahn S (eds): *Movement Disorders 3.* Oxford, England: Butterworth-Heinemann, 1994, chap 19, pp 373–405.

7. Blum P, Jankovic J: Stiff-person syndrome: An autoimmune disease. *Mov Disord* 6:12–20, 1991.

8. Trethowan WH, Allsop JL, Turner B: The stiff-man syndrome. *Arch Neurol* 3:114–122, 1960.

9. Isaacs H: Stiff-man syndrome in a black girl. *J Neurol Neurosurg Psychiatry* 42:988–994, 1979.

10. Kugelmass N: Stiff-man syndrome in a child. *N Y State J Med* 61:2483–2487, 1961.

11. Klein R, Haddow JE, De Luca C: Familial congenital disorder resembling the stiff-man syndrome. *Am J Dis Child* 124:730–731, 1972.

12. Sander JE, Layzer RB, Goldsobel AB: Congenital stiff-man syndrome. *Ann Neurol* 8:195–197, 1979.

13. Meinck HM, Ricker K, Hulser PJ, et al: Stiff man syndrome: Clinical and laboratory findings in eight patients. *J Neurol* 241:157–166, 1994.

14. Schwartzman MJ, Mitsumoto H, Chou SM, et al: Sudden death in stiff-man syndrome with autonomic instability. *Ann Neurol* 26:166, 1989.

15. Kasperek S, Zebrowski S: Stiff-man syndrome and encephalomyelitis. *Arch Neurol* 24:22–31, 1971.

16. Whiteley AM, Swash M, Urich H: Progressive encephalomyelitis with rigidity. *Brain* 99:27–42, 1976.

17. Solimena M, Folli F, Morello F, et al: Autoantibodies to GABA-ergic neurones and pancreatic beta cells in stiff-man syndrome. *N Engl J Med* 322:1555–1560, 1990.

18. Baekkeskov S, Aanstoot H-J, Christgau S, et al: Identification of the 64K autoantigen in insulin dependent diabetes mellitus as the GABA-synthesizing enzyme glutamic acid decarboxylase. *Nature* 347:151–156, 1990.

19. Meinck HM, Ricker K: Long-standing "stiff-man" syndrome: A particular form of disseminated inflammatory CNS disease? *J Neurol Neurosurg Psychiatry* 50:1556–1557, 1987.

20. Harding AE, Thompson PD, Kocen RS, et al: Plasma exchange and immunosuppression in the stiff-man syndrome. *Lancet* ii:915, 1989.

21. Johnstone AP, Nussey SS: Direct evidence for limited clonality of antibodies to glutamic acid decarboxylase (GAD) in stiff-man syndrome using baculovirus expressed GAD. *J Neurol Neurosurg Psychiatry* 57:659, 1994.

22. Maida E, Reisner T, Summer K, Sandor-Eggerth H: Stiff-man syndrome with abnormalities in CSF and computerized tomography findings. *Arch Neurol* 37:182–183, 1980.

23. Williams AC, Nutt JG, Hare T: Autoimmunity in stiff-man syndrome. *Lancet* ii:22, 1988.

24. Pugliese A, Gianani R, Eisenbarth GS, et al: Genetics of susceptibility and resistance to insulin-dependent diabetes in stiff-man syndrome. *Lancet* 344:1027–1028, 1994.

25. Pugliese A, Solimena M, Awdeh ZL, et al: Association of HLA-DQB1*0201 with stiff-man syndrome. *J Clin Endocrinol Metab* 77:1550–1553, 1993.

26. Auger RG: AAEM minimonograph #44: Diseases associated with excess motor unit activity. *Muscle Nerve* 17:1250–1263, 1994.

27. Martinelli P, Pazzaglia P, Montagna P, et al: Stiff-man syndrome associated with nocturnal myoclonus and epilepsy. *J Neurol Neurosurg Psychiatry* 41:458–462, 1978.

28. Meinck HM: Exteroceptive reflex abnormalities in stiff-man syndrome. *J Neurol Neurosurg Psychiatry* 48:92–93, 1985.

29. Leigh PN, Rothwell JC, Traub M, Marsden CD: A patient with reflex myoclonus and muscle rigidity: "Jerking stiff-man syndrome." *J Neurol Neurosurg Psychiatry* 43:1125–1131, 1980.
30. Alberca R, Romero M, Chaparro J: Jerking stiff-man syndrome. *J Neurol Neurosurg Psychiatry* 45:1159–1160, 1982.
31. McCombe PA, Chalk JB, Searle JW, et al: Progressive encephalomyelitis with rigidity: A case report with magnetic resonance imaging findings. *J Neurol Neurosurg Psychiatry* 52:1429–1431, 1989.
32. Burn DJ, Ball J, Lees AJ, et al: A case of progressive encephalomyelitis with rigidity and positive antiglutamic acid dehydrogenase antibodies. *J Neurol Neurosurg Psychiatry* 54:449–451, 1991.
33. Bateman DE, Weller RO, Kennedy P: Stiff-man syndrome. *J Neurol Neurosurg Psychiatry* 53:695–696, 1990.
34. Ferari P, Fedeico M. Grimaldi LME, Silingardi V: Stiff man syndrome in a patient with Hodgkin's disease: An unusual paraneoplastic syndrome. *Haematologica* 75:570–572, 1990.
35. Folli F, Solimena M, Cofiell R, et al: Autoantibodies to a 128-kd synaptic protein in three women with the stiff-man syndrome and breast cancer. *N Engl J Med* 328:546–551, 1993.
36. De Camilli P, Thomas A, Cofiell R, et al: The synaptic vesicle-associated protein amphiphysin is the 128-kD autoantigen of stiff-man syndrome with breast cancer. *J Exp Med* 178:2219–2223, 1993.
37. Piccolo G, Cosi V: Stiff-man syndrome, dysimmune disorder and cancer. *Ann Neurol* 25:105, 1989.
38. Nakamura N, Fujiya S, Yahara O, et al: Stiff-man syndrome with spinal cord lesion. *Clin Neuropathol* 5:40–46, 1986.
39. Meinck HM, Ricker K, Conrad B: The stiff-man syndrome: New pathophysiological aspects from abnormal exteroceptive reflexes and the response to clomipramine, clonidine and tizanidine. *J Neurol Neurosurg Psychiatry* 47:280–287, 1984.
40. Rossi B, Massetani R, Guidi M, et al: Electrophysiological findings in a case of stiff-man syndrome. *Electromyogr Clin Neurophysiol* 28:137–140, 1988.
41. Mamoli B, Heiss WD, Maida E, Podreka I: Electrophysiological studies on the stiff-man syndrome. *J Neurol* 217:111–121, 1977.
42. Boiardi A, Crenna P, Negri S, Merati B: Neurological and pharmacological evaluation of a case of stiff-man syndrome. *J Neurol* 223:127–133, 1980.
43. Meinck HM, Conrad B: Neuropharmacological investigations in the stiff-man syndrome. *J Neurol* 233:340–347, 1986.
44. Matsumoto JY, Caviness JN, McEvoy KM: The acoustic startle reflex in stiff-man syndrome. *Neurology* 44:1952–1955, 1994.
45. Guilleminault C, Sigwald J, Castaigne P: Sleep studies and therapeutic trial with L-dopa in a case of stiff-man syndrome. *Eur Neurol* 10:89–96, 1973.
46. Miller F, Korsvik H: Baclofen in the treatment of stiff-man syndrome. *Ann Neurol* 9:511 512, 1981.
47. Brown P, Thompson PD, Rothwell JC, et al: A therapeutic trial of milacemide in myoclonus and the stiff person syndrome. *Mov Disord* 6:73–75, 1991.
48. Schmidt RT, Stahl SM, Spehlmann R: A pharmacologic study of the stiff-man syndrome. *Neurology* 25:622–626, 1975.
49. Young W: The stiff-man syndrome. *Br J Clin Pract* 20:507–510, 1966.
50. Butler MH, Solimena M, Dirkx R Jr, et al: Identification of a dominant epitope of glutamic acid decarboxylase (GAD-65) recognized by autoantibodies in stiff-man syndrome. *J Exp Med* 178:2097–2106, 1993.
51. Li L, Hagopian WA, Brashear HR, et al: Identification of autoantibody epitopes of glutamic acid decarboxylase in stiff-man syndrome patients. *J Immunol* 152:930–934, 1994.
52. Kim J, Namchuk M, Bugawan T, et al: Higher autoantibody levels and recognition of a linear NH2-terminal epitope in the autoantigen GAD65, distinguish stiff-man syndrome from insulin-dependent diabetes mellitus. *J Exp Med* 180:595–606, 1994.
53. Bjork E, Velloso LA, Kampe O, Karlsson FA: GAD autoantibodies in IDDM, stiff-man syndrome, and autoimmune polyendocrine syndrome type I recognize different epitopes. *Diabetes* 43:161–165, 1994.
54. Darnell RB, Victor J, Rubin M, et al: A novel antineuronal antibody in stiff-man syndrome. *Neurology* 43:114–120, 1993.
55. Gorin F, Baldwin B, Tait R, et al: Stiff-man syndrome: A disorder with autoantigenic heterogeneity. *Ann Neurol* 28:711–714, 1990.
56. Westblom U: Stiff-man syndrome and clonazepam. *J Am Med Assoc* 237:1930, 1977.
57. Whelan JL: Baclofen in the treatment of the "stiff-man" syndrome. *Arch Neurol* 37:600–601, 1980.
58. Penn RD, Mangieri EA: Stiff-man syndrome treated with intrathecal baclofen. *Neurology* 43:2412, 1993.
59. Ford B, Fahn S: Intrathecal baclofen. *Neurology* 44:1367–1368, 1994.
60. Meinck HM, Tronnier V, Rieke K, et al: Intrathecal baclofen treatment for stiff-man syndrome: Pump failure may be fatal. *Neurology* 44:2209–2210, 1994.
61. Spehlmann R, Norcross K, Rasmus SC, Schlageter NL: Improvement of stiff-man syndrome and sodium valproate. *Neurology* 31:1162–1163, 1981.
62. Gordon MF, Diaz Olivo R, Hunt AL, Fahn S: Therapeutic trial of milacemide in patients with myoclonus and other intractable movement disorders. *Mov Disord* 8:484–488, 1993.
63. Brashear HR, Phillips LH: Autoantibodies to GABAergic neurones and response to plasmapheresis in stiff-man syndrome. *Neurology* 41:1588–1592, 1991.
64. Vicari AM, Folli F, Pozza G, et al: Plasmapheresis in the treatment of stiff-man syndrome. *N Engl J Med* 320:1499, 1989.
65. George TM, Burke JM, Sobotak PA, et al: Resolution of stiff-man syndrome with cortisol replacement in a patient with deficiencies of ACTH, growth hormone, and prolactin. *N Engl J Med* 310:1511–1513, 1984.
66. Piccolo G, Cosi V, Zandrini C, Moglia A: Steroid-responsive and dependent stiff-man syndrome: A clinical and electrophysiological study of two cases. *Ital J Neurol Sci* 9:559–566, 1988.
67. Amato AA, Cornman EW, Kissel JT: Treatment of stiff-man syndrome with intravenous immunoglobulin. *Neurology* 44:1652–1654, 1994.
68. Karlson EW, Sudarsky L, Ruderman E, et al: Treatment of stiff-man syndrome with intravenous immune globulin. *Arthritis Rheum* 37:915–918, 1994.
69. Davis D, Jabbari B: Significant improvement of stiff-person syndrome after paraspinal injection of botulinum toxin A. *Mov Disord* 8:371–373, 1993.

Chapter 48

GAIT AND BALANCE DISORDERS

JOHN G. NUTT and FAY B. HORAK

COMPONENTS OF AMBULATION
    Posture or Balance Tasks
    Gait or Locomotor Tasks
OVERVIEW OF SYSTEMS REQUIRED FOR BALANCE
  AND GAIT AND THEIR ANATOMIC SUBSTRATES
SENSORY SYSTEMS
    Vestibular Disorders
    Somatosensory Disorders
    Visual Disorders
ORIENTATION
    Subcortical Lesions
    Posterior Parietal Lesions and Sensory Neglect
FORCE PRODUCTION
SCALING OF FORCE
    Parkinsonism
    Hyperkinetic Movement Disorders
    Cerebellar Disorders
    Spasticity
BALANCE AND LOCOMOTOR SYNERGIES
    Brain Stem Lesions
    Frontal Lesions
    Freezing
DEPLOYMENT OF STRATEGIES (COGNITIVE)
    Dementia
    Impaired Attention
    Fear of Falling Gaits
    Cautious Gait
SUMMARY

Balance and gait disorders are a common cause of perplexity for the clinician. Hemiplegic, ataxic, waddling, and parkinsonian gaits are readily recognized, but the cause of many patients' slowness, unsteadiness, and falls do not fit these classical gait patterns. Some of this difficulty for the clinician is because there is no general scheme for considering balance and gait disorders nor a clear pathophysiological basis for a differential as exists for other neurological syndromes. For example, disordered communication may arise from dysarthria, receptive and expressive aphasia, alexia, etc., and the clinical signs can be interpreted in terms of dysfunction in particular areas of the brain. The same is not true of balance and gait disorders. The terminology for balance and gait abnormalities is confusing, poorly defined, and never related to an overall scheme for gait dysfunction. Senile, apractic, marché à petits pas, and frontal ataxia are common examples of confusing and ill-defined clinical entities. The physiological basis of various abnormal gaits or disequilibrium syndromes is rarely considered. Finally, there is only a vague concept of the anatomic substrates essential for balance and gait.

This chapter will develop a scheme for approaching human balance and gait disorders. Balance and gait are intertwined. Balance is a prerequisite for walking, and many so-called gait disorders are, in reality, balance disorders. However, balance and gait are, to some extent, separable and independent functions. We use a system approach for the categorization and attempt to relate system dysfunction to various neural structures.[1] We acknowledge at the outset that some of our scheme is hypothetical; the clinical, physiological, and pathological data are insufficient to allow confident categorization. One function of this chapter is to stimulate clinicians and scientists to consider these problems.

Components of Ambulation

Walking may be considered the result of successful execution of several balance and locomotion tasks (Table 48-1).

POSTURAL OR BALANCE TASKS

Balance tasks get the body in an upright position and keep it upright during voluntary activities, including ambulation. This requires orienting the body segments with respect to each other, the environment, and gravity and generating forces to maintain equilibrium during voluntary movements and externally induced perturbations. These tasks may be clinically divided into four categories.

1. Switching (transitioning between) postures: changing from a lying to a sitting position or a sitting to standing position.
2. Standing (antigravity support) maintains stationary, upright stance. This is not simply a static balancing of the body above the feet (base of support) because the body is constantly moving. Therefore, postural control systems are necessary to constrain the sway such that it stays within the limits of the base of support.
3. Anticipatory adjustments are the postural changes that precede voluntary movements including stepping. These are feedforward processes that anticipate the changes in posture necessary to support voluntary movement. They are not dependent upon sensory input resulting from the movement itself.
4. Reactive postural responses protect against unexpected external perturbations. These are sensory-triggered or feedback-controlled postural responses that result from unexpected displacement of the body by forces arising in the environment or by voluntary movements.

GAIT OR LOCOMOTOR TASKS

Locomotion produces the repetitive limb and trunk movements that progressively propel the person through space. In addition to the rhythmical movements causing progression, locomotion requires stability in an upright position and adaptability to the changing environment and to ongoing voluntary activities. Upright postural stability during ambulation is produced by the balance tasks described above. The other tasks are:

1. Initiate and arrest stepping.
2. Alter stepping patterns for turns, for different speeds, and for various support surfaces.
3. Avoid obstacles.

   Both balance and locomotor tasks must be adapted to changing constraints of the support surface, body, environment, and ongoing voluntary tasks. Effective and efficient execution of each of the above tasks depends upon the integrity of the physiological systems underlying their control. Dysfunction in any physiological system will result in compensatory strategies for accomplishing the basic balance and locomotor tasks to achieve task goals.

Overview of Systems Required for Balance and Gait and Their Anatomic Substrates

Gait and balance dysfunction can be categorized into systems by six questions (Table 48-2).

1. Do patients have the correct information about their bodies and the environment to ambulate? This requires accurate information from vestibular, visual, and somatosensory systems.
2. Can patients process and integrate sensory information to form an internal representation of the body in space and gravitational field? Sensory information is converted into egocentric (body-oriented) and exocentric (world-oriented) spatial maps in posterior parietal cortical areas, premotor areas, putamen, frontal eye fields, and superior colliculus.[2]
3. Can patients produce adequate force to execute balance and locomotor tasks? Force generation depends upon motor nerves, muscle, and skeletal systems.
4. Can patients scale forces accurately and appropriately? Patients must be able to modify the force exerted in proportion to the balance and locomotor requirements for a given situation. Scaling depends upon the basal ganglia, cerebellum, and corticospinal system.
5. Do patients have accessible balance and locomotor synergies? Synergies are groups of muscles activated in a specific temporal/spatial order to produce a coordinated movement. Fundamental locomotor and equilibrium syn-

TABLE 48-1 Components of Stable Ambulation

Balance tasks
  1. Transitions
  2. Stance
  3. Anticipatory
  4. Reactive
Locomotor tasks
  1. Initiate and arrest stepping
  2. Alter steps (speed, turns, obstacles)
  3. Integrate voluntary tasks
Adapt to changing constraints of:
  Environment
  Body

TABLE 48-2 Anatomic Correlates of Balance and Gait Disorders

Sensory
  Vestibular
  Proprioceptive
  Visual
  Multisensory
Perception/Orientation
  Vestibular
  Vestibulocerebellum
  Parietal
  Premotor
Force Production
  Musculoskeletal
  Motor nerves or motoneurons
Scaling of Force
  Basal ganglia
  Cerebellum
  Corticospinal
Synergy Organization and Access
  Spinal cord
  Brain stem
  Motor cortex
Cognitive
  Frontal lobe

ergies are in the spinal cord and brainstem. They appear to be accessed through subcortical and frontal lobe structures.
6. Do patients appropriately deploy balance and locomotor synergies? Attention, judgment, and learning mediated by cortical areas are required to deploy synergies that are appropriate for constraints imposed by the person's physical condition and the environment.

Sensory Systems

Sensory disturbances of gait and balance are caused by inadequate or erroneous knowledge of body position, environment, and gravity (Table 48-3). The consequences of deprivation or distortion of the sensory input are delays, inappropriate gain, and improper selection of synergies for balance. Balance or gait are normal except when the individual is in an environment in which they are dependent upon the deficient sense(s). In this setting, inappropriate synergies may be selected or timing may be wrong. These balance and gait disturbances will be associated with evidence of loss of vestibular, proprioceptive, or visual input.

VESTIBULAR DISORDERS

Balance and gait disorders associated with vestibular lesions are related to the roles of the vestibular system in sensing and perceiving self-motion, orienting to a vertical position, controlling the center of body mass, and stabilizing the head in space. The type of balance and gait deficits related to abnormal vestibular information depends on the location, extent, and type of vestibular lesion as well as on central compensation for the lesion. Functionally, two very different balance disorder syndromes are associated with vestibular

TABLE 48-3 Clinical and Pathological Features of System Dysfunction

Syndrome	History	Signs	Balance and Gait	Lesions
SENSORY				
Vestibular	Dizziness—worse with head motion Disorientation—environmentally specific Visual vertigo Blurred vision with head movement Falls in dark and/or on uneven surfaces	Spontaneous or positional vertigo and/or nystagmus Abnormal subjective vertical Gaze instability	Ataxia with head motion En bloc gait Excessive or absent hip sway Asymmetry of posture and gait Inability to stand on one foot or tandem Ataxia in presence of visual motion Fall while standing on foam with eyes closed	Labyrinth Eighth cranial nerve Vestibular nuclei Central vestibular pathways Vestibulocerebellum
Somatosensory	Tripping Ankle injuries Difficulty walking in dark	Paresthesia Reduced somatosensation Reduced ankle DTRs	Delayed postural responses High stepping, slapping feet Visual dependence Reduced limits of stability	Peripheral nerves Posterior columns of spinal cord
Vision	Fear of falling Impaired vision Double vision	Reduced visual acuity Visual field loss Abnormal extraocular movements	Haptic cues improve stability Trips over obstacles Cautious gait Tilted posture	Retina Optic nerve Extraocular muscles Central visual pathways
ORIENTATION	Falls in complex environments Spatial disorientation Hemineglect Difficulty transferring Trips over obstacles	Intact sensation Body alignment abnormal Poor subjective vertical Ocular tilt Difficulty manipulating objects	Unstable in sensory conflict conditions Asymmetrical alignment Falls without corrective efforts Inappropriate stability limits May be unable to stand	Midbrain Thalamus Parietal cortex
FORCE PRODUCTION	Weakness Slowness Pain Fatigue	Weakness Decrease ROM Limb and joint deformity Abnormal postural alignment	Limp Waddling gait Foot drop Decrease posture response magnitude	Bones Joints Muscles Motor nerves Motor neurons
SCALING OF FORCE	Clumsiness Slowness Falls	Dysmetria Slowness Abnormal tone Involuntary movements	Abnormal magnitude of postural responses Hypermetric: Falls opposite of direction pushed Hypometric: Falls in direction pushed Narrow range gait velocities Excessive sway to perturbation Sway in stance may be larger or smaller than normal	Basal ganglia Cerebellum Corticospinal tracts
ORGANIZATION AND ACCESS TO SYNERGIES	Unable to stand/sit independently Knees/hips buckle Uncoordinated	Brain stem/frontal lobe signs	Freezing gait Excessive joint motion Poorly coordinated legs, arms, head in gait	Frontal cortex Midbrain Deep white matter
COGNITIVE	Careless falls Impulsiveness Instability during cognitive tasking Fear of falling	Dementia Inattention Reckless, poor judgment Excessive anxiety about falls	Failure to adapt to changing constraints Decreased balance with distracting tasks	Diffuse cortical involvement

disorders; one is caused from chronic loss of vestibular information and the other from present, but distorted, vestibular information produced by acute vestibular disorders, fluctuating function, or mechanical pathology in the inner ear resulting in abnormal sensory signals.[3,4] Well-compensated loss of vestibular function produces balance and gait problems when patients are in environments in which there is inadequate visual and somatosensory information for orientation in space. In contrast, distortion of vestibular information may affect interpretation of visual and somatosensory information such that balance is impaired in many sensory environments, and often imbalance is accompanied by perceptions of vertigo and disorientation.[5] Although the basic coordination, latency, and scaling of balance and gait synergies are normal in vestibular patients, head-trunk coordination is abnormal, and the selection of balance synergies is limited.[6]

LOSS OF VESTIBULAR FUNCTION

Vestibular hair cell and eighth nerve fiber degeneration that occurs gradually with aging or neurotoxicity are not associated with dizziness, so patients may not recognize their balance instability until they find themselves in an environment in which vestibular information is critical for postural orientation. For example, patients may suddenly fall or feel totally disoriented in space when they attempt to walk at night on a sandy beach. Because of the redundancy of vestibular, vision, and somatosensory information for postural orientation in most environments, even patients with complete, bilateral absence of vestibular function may have normal gait and stance on normal, firm surfaces, even with eyes closed. This is particularly true for vestibular loss occurring early in life.

Profound loss of vestibular function in adults is usually associated with en bloc gait in which there is lack of normal counterrotation among the head, trunk, and legs to reduce excessive head accelerations during locomotion.[7] Gait ataxia can be provoked in patients with vestibular loss by requiring head movements or whole-body turns while walking.[8,9] Profound loss of vestibular function is also associated with inability to stand on one foot, even with eyes open, or to stand or walk on narrow beams or in tandem. This inability to balance on narrow surfaces is thought to result from an inability to coordinate rapid, large postural movements of the head and trunk required in these tasks.[10]

Unilateral loss of vestibular function results in asymmetrical posture and gait. After acute loss of vestibular function on one side, patients tend to lean their heads and body toward that side, but this asymmetry gradually resolves as the patient compensates over a period of several weeks.[11] Subtle asymmetries in stabilization of the head and trunk may persist, however. For example, patients may not be stable when their center of body mass is shifted to the side of the vestibular lesion in sitting and standing. One test for this asymmetry is the Fukuda walking in place test, in which patients attempt to step in place with eyes closed.[12] Patients with unilateral loss may rotate toward the side of the lesion in the acute phase, and this rotation gradually lessens as they compensate for the loss. After compensation, patients with complete unilateral loss of vestibular function may be able to balance on a compliant surface with eyes closed, suggesting that vestibular information from one side is adequate for stability.[13]

DISTORTED VESTIBULAR FUNCTION

Mechanical or electrolytic disruption of labyrinthine fluid dynamics, such as fistulas, cupulolithiasis, or hydrops (Ménière's disease), can result in abnormal vestibular information to the nervous system regarding head motion. Abnormally activated vestibular receptors may signal self-motion to the nervous system when no actual motion exists. As a consequence, patients may activate large balance reactions in circumstances when no postural response is called for, causing instability or falls. Distorted vestibular function may result in the perception of the body spinning or rocking or of the room spinning or tilting. These abnormal perceptions may be caused by particular head positions or motions, depending on the specific pathophysiology. During severe attacks of vertigo, patients may be completely unable to stand, even if they are supported. Prolonged vestibular distortions are usually compensated for by central suppression of vestibular information, or the disease may progress to permanent loss of receptors, at which point patients exhibit a vestibular loss balance and gait pattern.

Patients with uncompensated, distorted vestibular function often become overly reliant on visual cues for balance and may have dizziness and instability in response to environmental visual motion or when visual information is unreliable for postural orientation.[14,15] Patients with visual motion sensitivity appear to interpret environmental motion as self-motion and show postural unsteadiness in these environments. Such patients commonly report balance difficulties on busy streets when they are surrounded by vehicular and pedestrian traffic. Many of these patients are stable with eyes closed, even when surface somatosensory cues are altered, suggesting that they have adequate vestibular information for postural orientation.[14,15]

Some patients with vestibular disorders become overly reliant on somatosensory cues for balance and thus become unstable on surfaces that do not yield reliable information regarding body sway.[16] For instance, these patients are unstable on compliant surfaces such as foam, soft soil, and sand. They may be reluctant to lift their feet to walk, resulting in shuffling. They often touch walls, furniture, and companions to aid spatial orientation.

Patients with distorted vestibular function may show excessive hip and trunk motions while maintaining equilibrium, resulting in very large head accelerations.[17] These large trunk motions can be observed in response to perturbations of stance, during gait with voluntary head motions, and when asked to stop walking suddenly.

Thus, in contrast to patients with loss of vestibular function, patients with distorted vestibular function often use visual or somatosensory information abnormally for postural orientation and show excessive, instead of reduced, head and trunk motion.

SOMATOSENSORY DISORDERS

Absent, delayed, or disordered peripheral sensory information from cutaneous and deep pressure sensors in the soles of the feet and from proprioceptive and joint receptors in the feet, legs, and trunk can have distinctive effects on balance and gait. Somatosensory loss from the feet alone does not result in increased sway in stance or in changes in the latency of postural responses.[10] In contrast, somatosensory loss that includes loss of proprioceptive information from the leg muscles, such as from diabetic peripheral neuropathy, results in increased anterior/posterior sway in stance and significant delays in automatic postural responses.[18,19] The postural synergies are intact, however, suggesting a slowing in triggering synergies.

Somatosensory loss from demyelination of central sensory pathways in multiple sclerosis results in even longer delays in postural responses. The delays are highly correlated with spinal sensory conduction from evoked potentials.[1] Abnormal, delayed somatosensory conduction may be more destabilizing than complete loss of somatosensory information from the lower extremities. Neuropathy patients with partial sensory loss showed more deficits scaling the magnitude of their responses to increasing postural disturbances than patients with almost total sensory loss.[19]

Patients with significant loss of sensory information in the feet may move their center of body mass with large trunk motions as if they are standing across narrow beams, a situation in which force at the ankles is ineffective for maintaining balance.[10] Thus, somatosensory loss appears to result in altered perceptions of limits of stability. This is apparent from very small shifts of center of mass when the patient is asked to lean forward or backward as far as they can without moving their feet.

Somatosensory loss results in great dependence on vision for orientation as revealed by great unsteadiness in stance and gait with eyes closed. This, of course, is the basis of the Romberg sign, initially described as a sign of tabes dorsalis and posterior column dysfunction. Patients with severe loss of somatosensation are even more unstable with eyes closed than patients with complete vestibular loss, suggesting that somatosensation is more critical for stance than is vestibular sense.

The ataxic gait in patients with loss of somatosensation, especially in spinal pathways, is distinctive for slapping of the feet, high stepping, and excessive lateral body motion. When the loss of somatosensation is from cerebral lesions such as strokes, patients may not bear weight fully on the affected limb, even when strength is normal.

VISUAL DISORDERS

Loss of visual information from pathology in the cornea, retina, optic nerve, or central visual pathways leaves a patient dependent on somatosensory and vestibular information for postural orientation. Static visual references are used to align the trunk and head to a vertical orientation. Visual motion information is used to determine self-motion with reference to the environment. Peripheral visual flow information is particularly critical for postural stability, although motion in the central visual field may also affect postural sway.[20,21] Aging often is associated with degeneration of the peripheral retina and central visual pathways. The resulting visual impairments, loss of sensitivity to moving objects, reduced con-

trast sensitivity, night blindness, and impaired eye movements affect postural stability. Distorted vision, rather than visual loss, caused by diplopia, cataracts, new bifocals, etc., limit the use of vision for obstacle avoidance and orientation in space.

Vision is not critical for stability in stance and gait as evidenced by the small increase in body sway when the eyes are closed.[15] When somatosensory information is reduced, however, such as when the surface is compliant or a patient has somatosensory loss, the sway induced by eye closure or by environmental visual motion is significantly greater.[22] Vision is critical for obstacle avoidance during gait. Visual information about upcoming obstacles is used to alter the locomotor pattern in an anticipatory manner during gait.[23] When one eye is patched, subjects tend to step over obstacles with the leg on the side of the unpatched eye, suggesting that vision is used not only to judge the dimensions and distance of the obstacle but also to monitor the progress of the stepping leg to ensure toe clearance.

Disorders of eye movements can have dramatic effects on balance and posture. When gaze stabilization during head movement is abnormal, such as occurs with oscillopsia, burred vision disrupts use of vision for orientation and motion perception. Paresis of extraocular muscles can result in tilted and shifted perception of vertical orientation accompanied by disturbances of gait and grasping, abnormalities that are ameliorated by eye closure.[24] Sometimes abnormalities of eye positions, such as ocular torsion, reflect lesions in central vestibular brainstem pathways that affect perception of vertical and spatial orientation.[25]

Orientation

In disorders of orientation, patients have no significant disruption of primary sensation but appear to be unaware of orientation of the body in space and in the gravitational field or to misinterpret sensory information (Table 48-3). Patients exhibit distorted perception of egocentric space (neglect of body parts) and exoceptive space (visual and sensory neglect or abnormal subjective verticality). Inappropriate balance and gait synergies may be selected because of faulty interpretation of position of body in space. Patients do not complain of dizziness or vertigo but may complain of unexplained falls.

The pathophysiological explanation for these syndromes may be disturbances in any sensory-motor area containing spatial maps. This includes the posterior parietal cortex, putamen, ventral premotor cortex, superior colliculus, and frontal eye fields.[2]

SUBCORTICAL LESIONS

Infarcts and hemorrhages of the midbrain tegmentum, thalamus, and basal ganglia have been associated with orientation problems and with falls. Lesions in the vicinity of the interstitial nucleus of Cajal cause the ocular tilt reaction consisting of lateral head tilt opposite to the side of the lesion, skew deviation with ipsilateral eye higher, bilateral ocular torsion, and deviation of subjective visual vertical orientation.[26] This body alignment abnormality is generally not associated with impaired balance.[26] Posterolateral thalamic infarctions produce abnormalities in subjective visual vertical orientation and, in a few patients, is associated with postural instability.[26]

At this point categorization of subcortical lesions into our classification runs into difficulty. Many cases to be described below have not been studied in sufficient detail to allow definitive assignment to the categories of orientation, scaling, or absent synergies. That is, the clinical evidence is inadequate to decide if the patients had: (1) abnormal sensory orientation; (2) normal but hypometric synergies; or (3) absent or disrupted synergies. The patients described below are assigned to orientation because they seemed to have intact synergies for other motor acts but appeared oblivious to orientation within the earth's gravitational field. More detailed studies of these types of patients may revise these tentative assignments.

Bilateral lesions of the interstitial nucleus of Cajal in cats cause a hyperextension of the neck that may be analogous to the nuchal dystonia of progressive supranuclear palsy (PSP).[27] Furthermore, these lesions produce visual motor behavior in the cats that is reminiscent of the visual equilibrium problems experienced by people with PSP.[27] The interstitial nucleus of Cajal may be involved pathologically in cases of PSP.[27] Thus, the striking disequilibrium of PSP may be due to disturbances of orientation.

Severe postural instability can result from acute infarcts and hemorrhages of the dorsal and posterior regions of the thalamus (thalamic astasia)[28] or of the putamen.[29] Patients with these lesions appear to be unaware of their orientation in the gravitational field and often fall with no corrective efforts.[28,29] Similarly, a unilateral infarct in the vicinity of the left dorsomedial red nucleus caused a patient to lean her head and trunk to the right while sitting or standing and to fall to the right without protective reactions.[30]

POSTERIOR PARIETAL LESIONS AND SENSORY NEGLECT

Lesions of the posterior parietal lobe can present with profoundly complex abnormalities in behavior including apraxia, agnosia, abnormal body scheme, and hemineglect, often with the preservation of sensation and strength. Although most studies of the effect of lesions in the sensory association areas of parietal cortex investigate use of the arm and hand in reaching, similar deficits in use of the legs and trunk for balance and gait are likely to be present.[31] Because the parietal cortex receives information regarding position and movement of the body in space to control operation of the limbs, ambulation activities requiring knowledge of egocentric space and immediate extrapersonal space could also be affected by posterior parietal lesions.[32–34] Likely deficits include abnormal orientation of the body to vertical, difficulty negotiating in space, difficulty transferring from one position to another, and difficulty adjusting leg positions and movements to overcome obstacles.

Recently, the posterior parietal cortex has been associated with the "dorsal stream" of the central visual pathways.[35] There is mounting evidence that the dorsal visual stream that projects to posterior parietal cortex is specialized for control of movement or action, whereas the ventral visual stream that projects to inferotemporal cortex is specialized for visual perception. Patients with damage of the posterior parietal cortex show deficits called "optic ataxia" consisting of problems with shaping hand posture and orienting the arm for manipulation of objects, although they have no difficulty describing the features of the object they are manipulating.[36] We would predict that patients with these lesions would also show difficulty in automatically using vision for avoiding obstacles during ambulation (lifting the swing leg the correct amount to go over, bending the trunk to go under, and changing stride to go around obstacles), although they would be able to describe the relevant features of the obstacles.[37,38] A patient with a lesion localized to the ventral visual stream was shown to have the same type of severe deficits in the perception and description of obstacles for gait as he or she had in the perception and description of objects for grasping but had no problem using vision to automatically step over obstacles or to manipulate objects for grasping.[37] The weak co-occurrence of optic ataxia and hemispatial neglect and their different lesion sites indicate a dissociation between these two syndromes.[36] More studies on the specific balance and gait deficits associated with posterior parietal lesions are needed.

Force Production

This category of balance and gait abnormalities is related to biomechanical constraints imposed by the musculoskeletal system and can be thought of in terms of springs, levers, and hinges. Equilibrium and locomotor synergies are normal insofar as abnormal muscles, bones, and joints allow. Disordered balance and gait can easily be attributed to weakness from muscle or motor nerve disorders, to joint problems such as arthritis, to connective tissue, and to bone abnormalities. Patients can generally adapt to these problems when the remainder of the nervous system is intact. In fact, patients often ambulate surprisingly well with marked weakness or skeletal deformity. When biomechanical constraints are combined with dysfunction in other systems, balance and gait can be severely compromised. For example, arthritis in the feet and ankles that poses no threat to postural and gait stability in young individuals with intact nervous systems becomes a major risk factor for falls in the elderly in whom other neurological deficits often exist.[39]

The syndromes produced by failure of force production and by skeletal and connective tissue disorders are well described in texts and include: (1) waddling gait of proximal muscle weakness; (2) steppage or equine gait (foot drop) of distal muscle weakness; (3) limps from arthritis or pain of hip, knee, and ankle joints; and (4) stiff, careful gait of painful spine disorders. These will not be discussed further in this chapter.

Scaling of Force

Scaling abnormalities of balance and gait are characterized by hyper- or hypometric synergies and by overflow (activation of muscles not necessary for execution of the synergy).

Synergies are intact, but execution is faulty because of inappropriate modification of force, despite an adequate biomechanical system. These disorders are associated with signs of cerebellar, basal ganglia, or corticospinal dysfunction. The clinician must differentiate absent balance responses of sensory or orientation dysfunction from hypometric responses secondary to scaling disorders. Scaling force magnitude is dependent on both feedforward (predictive preprograming) and feedback.[40]

The characteristics of parkinsonian, choreic, dystonic, ataxic, and spastic gaits are familiar to clinicians and well-described in textbooks so only the evidence that they are failures of scaling will be discussed.

PARKINSONISM

Abnormalities of postural responses are such an important and integral part of the parkinsonism syndrome that disturbed postural responses are included as one of the four features defining the syndrome (the others being tremor, rigidity, and bradykinesia). The clinically apparent postural abnormalities include stooped posture, shuffling gait, freezing, propulsion, retropulsion, drifting of postural alignment to the side or backwards during sitting and standing, and falls. Clinically, many patients do not appear to have any postural responses in some settings, falling like a toppling tree. The prominent postural abnormalities in parkinsonism led Martin to deduce that the basal ganglia must be the origin of many postural responses,[41] a view still popular, as evidenced by the tendency to include postural disturbances as a key component of the syndrome. However, many studies of patients with Parkinson's disease, using platforms that can measure surface forces and simultaneously record electromyogram (EMG) activity of leg and trunk muscles, reveal that even patients that clinically appear to have no postural responses do, indeed, have a response that is normal in latency and temporal organization. It is, however, of low magnitude and not sufficient to be effective.[42] The postural responses in Parkinson's disease are also inflexible; they do not adapt to changed conditions as readily as do those of normal subjects.[42] Thus, the evidence from physiological studies is that the postural responses are retained, but their execution is defective. The studies, demonstrating hypometric responses in severely affected patients with seemingly absent responses, do point out the difficulty with understanding postural disturbances in patients without some objective measures of postural responses.

The recognition of parkinsonism as a cause of a balance and gait disorder is based on the presence of the typical postural and locomotor difficulties accompanied by other signs of parkinsonism. A similar gait pattern but without other parkinsonian signs and unresponsive to L-dopa (sometimes termed lower body parkinsonism) can be produced by vascular disease.[43,44]

The gait and postural abnormalities of parkinsonism are partially responsive to L-dopa. Background postural tone is reduced, and self-initiated muscle force is increased.[45] The hypometric automatic postural responses of parkinsonian patients recorded in the lab or evaluated by physical examination in the clinic may or may not improve after L-dopa.[45,46]

HYPERKINETIC MOVEMENT DISORDERS

Chorea and dystonia may markedly impact gait and balance but, from clinical observation, it appears that the equilibrium and locomotor synergies are preserved in most patients.[41] As with parkinsonism, there appears to be defective execution of balance and locomotor strategies caused by superimposed or incorporated involuntary movements of chorea or the overflow of muscle activation in dystonia. Huntington's disease may be complicated because there may be components of parkinsonism and of frontal lobe dysfunction, so that all postural problems cannot be attributed to chorea alone.[41,47]

CEREBELLAR DISORDERS

Cerebellar dysfunction generally results in increased sway in quiet stance. With flocculonodular (vestibulocerebellum) lesions, there is a slow (less than 1 Hz) sway in all directions; with anterior lobe (spinocerebellum) lesions, the sway is faster (3 Hz) and is in an anterior-posterior direction.[48] Lesions restricted to the cerebellar hemispheres (paleocerebellum) do not produce abnormalities of balance or gait, although limb movements may be dysmetric (see also Chaps. 43 and 44).

The automatic postural responses in patients with cerebellar disease are of normal latency but are hypermetric, such that patients fall in a direction opposite to the one in which they were perturbed.[49] The ataxic gait can result from these abnormalities in balance, as well as from dysmetria of the legs. The widened base that is characteristic of cerebellar disorders may partly result from the increased sway and from the inability of the patient to exactly predict where the dysmetric limb will make contact with the support surface. Uncertainty about where the feet will make contact with the support surface appears to be a common cause of widened base. A widened base may also be seen in normal individuals standing on a moving support surface, such as a pitching ship deck, or in patients who do not know where their limbs are in space, such as those with sensory ataxia. The cerebellum does not appear to be the origin of postural responses, because the latency and timing of balance synergies are normal, although the magnitude of the responses is too large.[49] Patients with cerebellar lesions have particular difficulty scaling the magnitude of postural responses based on prediction from prior experience.[49]

SPASTICITY

Spasticity of spinal or cerebral origin produces a stiff, slow gait. The majority of forward movement of a spastic leg seems to come from the hip, and because of weakness of dorsiflexors of the ankle and increased tone in the leg, circumduction of the leg is necessary to prevent catching the toe during the swing phase of a step. When there is adequate strength, spasticity rarely prohibits ambulation, although it may make it precarious. These characteristic changes in gait are generally readily recognized in the clinic. The clinician may be surprised by discrepancies between the signs of spasticity elicited when the patient is supine and the degree of spasticity apparent when the patient walks. Presumably, this reflects a loss of specificity in synergies such that there is overflow and involvement of muscles not normally incorporated into the synergy, or alternatively, it is a compensatory mechanism for weak and ineffective synergies.

In subjects with spastic legs, the EMG patterns of automatic postural responses,[50] anticipatory postural adjustments,[51] and gait[52,53] are basically preserved, although there is less force (scaling deficit), delays in distal muscle activation, and cocontraction. The pattern in spastic cerebral palsy may be more complex,[54] but the uncertainty about the extent of the lesion in these patients, as well as the effect of lesions in the immature brain, makes interpretation more problematic. Overall, the conclusion is that pure corticospinal tract dysfunction mainly affects execution of balance and gait synergies by altering scaling of synergies, although there are other physiological abnormalities present as well.

The cortical motor areas are important in adjusting and adapting the locomotor pattern to the demands of the task and the environment. Walking straight ahead may be generated from spinal and brainstem regions, but the adaptation of the pattern to uneven surfaces, steps, and so forth (skilled walking) requires cortical input.[55]

Balance and Locomotor Synergies

Locomotor synergies exist in the spinal cord in vertebrates,[56] including man.[57,58] These locomotor synergies are engaged by brainstem and subcortical centers to produce walking, trotting, or running.[55,59,60] Balance and posture tasks appear to be brainstem synergies, as evidenced by the ability of selective stimulation to alter postural tone[60,61] and the ability of decerebrate cats to stand. Disruption of these "basic" equilibrium and locomotor synergies is a rare cause of balance and gait disturbances in humans, because most spinal cord and brainstem lesions cause so much dysfunction that there are multiple causes for balance and gait difficulties without invoking disruption of synergies. However, rare brainstem lesions appear to selectively disrupt balance synergies, as discussed below.

The brainstem locomotor and postural equilibrium centers, such as the pedunculopontine nucleus, receive input from frontal cortex[62] and from basal ganglia.[59] It may be that frontal areas are necessary for normal access to spinal and brainstem postural and locomotor synergies; frontal lesions or lesions interrupting the connections between frontal cortical areas and brainstem will make the synergies unavailable, as though they were absent or totally disrupted. Several observations are consistent with the hypothesis that the frontal regions are important in recruiting postural synergies for voluntary movement, including walking. Electrical stimulation and seizures of human frontal cortex, particularly in the region of the supplementary motor cortex, elicit complex movements that include tonic proximal muscle movements that could be postural.[63,64] Flexion of a forelimb of the cat, elicited by electrical stimulation of motor cortex, is preceded by postural adjustments to allow the animal to maintain balance when the limb is flexed.[65] Anticipatory postural adjustments are impaired by mesial frontal lesions (includes SMA) in humans.[66,67] Frontal lesions in monkeys cause a postural asymmetry and forced circling.[68]

These observations suggest that balance and gait disorders could arise from: (1) disruption of spinal and brainstem synergies and (2) access to these synergies by frontal motor areas and, perhaps, basal ganglia. The practical difficulty with this classification is differentiating the inappropriate postural and locomotor synergies resulting from deranged orientation from disruption of the synergies themselves or from loss of access to synergies.

BRAINSTEM LESIONS

There are a paucity of reports of brainstem lesions causing dissolution of balance and locomotor synergies that cannot be explained by other sensory or motor abnormalities. A small infarct in the region of the pontomesencephalic junction and the pedunculopontine nucleus produced a gait characterized by poor equilibrium and irregular steps reminiscent of "gait apraxia."[69] Bilateral infrathalamic stereotactic lesions in the vicinity of the superior border of the red nuclei produced axial rigidity, bradykinesia, marked disequilibrium (fell with turns and sudden movements), and a wide-based, slow, unsteady gait.[70] We encountered six patients with apparent brainstem lesions (no brain imaging was obtained) and markedly impaired balance that could not be explained by proprioceptive sensory loss, cerebellar deficits, or weakness.[71] It is likely that brainstem lesions (particularly midbrain) may produce disequilibrium and locomotor difficulties more commonly than clinically appreciated, with the instability and falling instead incorrectly attributed to cerebellar dysfunction.

FRONTAL LESIONS

Hydrocephalus, multiple lacunar infarcts, and large frontal lesions can be associated with marked disequilibrium that is not explained by weakness or sensory loss. The patients may have difficulty arising, failing to bring their feet under them as they try to stand and in trying to push themselves up from a chair without even placing their feet on the ground. Helped to an erect position, the patients do not bring their weight over their feet and, instead, push backward with seeming disregard for their support base. Stepping may be bizarre, with feet crossing and with no coordination between trunk and feet. Difficulty initiating gait (freezing, to be discussed below) may or may not be present. This clinical phenomenon was first reported by Bruns[72] and is sometimes termed Bruns' or frontal ataxia. Frontal ataxia is often assumed to be an ataxia similar to that produced by cerebellar lesions. However, Bruns' description of the cases suggests severe disequilibrium with signs generally not seen with cerebellar dysfunction, such as retropulsion and crossing the legs when attempting to walk. Subsequent descriptions of balance and gait abnormalities associated with frontal lesions considered them to be an apraxia of gait.[73-78] By the case descriptions in the reports, the disability was dominated by disequilibrium and would better be termed apraxia of balance, if apraxia is correct at all. Deep white matter lesions may produce severe disequilibrium as well, presumably by disrupting subcortical-frontal connections.[43]

FREEZING

Freezing is the inability to initiate gait and the interruption of gait by distraction, passing through doorways, and turning.[79] Freezing is reduced by tricks that help the affected person focus on walking, such as targets on the floor on which to step, counting out loud, marching to music, and walking straight forward in an uncluttered walking space.[79] Freezing may be a relatively isolated sign without marked problems with balance or other motor function,[71,80] or it may be associated with impaired balance and other motor dysfunction.[71,81]

Freezing is a widely recognized sign of parkinsonism[79] but also occurs in other brain disorders that do not include parkinsonism as part of the clinical picture. These other disorders generally affect the frontal lobes or the deep white matter. The same array of lesions causing disequilibrium—hydrocephalus, frontal mass lesions, and deep white matter lesions—have been most commonly incriminated.[44,71,77,80,82]

Patients who exhibit freezing may have virtually normal gait when they get underway, so the problem appears to be access to brainstem locomotor centers, not loss of walking programs or an apraxia. The observation that locomotion can be induced in animals by stimulation of subthalamic and midbrain locomotor regions[55,83] suggests that some form of excitatory drive to locomotor centers is sufficient to elicit coordinated locomotion. Lesions producing freezing are in the basal ganglia, which have connections to the pedunculopontine nucleus (a possible midbrain locomotor center),[59] in frontal lobes that project heavily to midbrain[62,84] and in deep white matter that might interrupt connections between frontal lobes and brainstem locomotor nuclei. The situations that induce freezing and the tricks that aid freezing may be interpreted as factors that interfere or assist with concentration and voluntary control of walking by cortical motor areas.

Deployment of Strategies (Cognitive)

Gait patterns are often considered fixed; abnormal gaits are thought of as neurological signs that are as immutable as Babinski signs. However, consider how a normal person's gait will appropriately change depending upon whether the surface is flat pavement, a rough uneven surface, a slippery surface such as ice or upon footwear (shoes versus thongs versus skis versus stilts). Likewise, postural synergies are adapted to the situation. The postural response to a perturbation when standing at the end of a low diving board will depend on whether the pool is filled with water and how the person is attired (formally or in a swimming suit)! Thus, to be effective, equilibrium and gait are adapted to the situation through awareness of the body and environment, as well as by using insight, judgment, and past experience.

Balance and locomotor synergies must be adapted to the limitations imposed by the person's physical capabilities, the environment, and ongoing voluntary activity. This adaptation is dependent upon sensory information, experience, and learning. It requires: (1) attention to physical limitations imposed by body and tasks; (2) attention to environmental setting; (3) judgment; and (4) ability to direct attention as appropriate to ensure effective locomotion and stability.

DEMENTIA

Many epidemiological studies of falls in the elderly identify dementia as one risk factor for falls.[85,86] A portion of this propensity to fall may be explained by abnormalities identified in physiological studies of balance and gait. The basic postural balance synergies are intact[87] (FB Horak, unpublished observations), but the patients exhibit more sway in standing[88] and walking.[89] They have difficulty maintaining their equilibrium in novel situations[87] (FB Horak, unpublished observations) and do not adapt or learn to balance in complex situations (FB Horak, unpublished observations). The gait is slower in patients with dementia[87,89] and is more disrupted by distractors such as performing a word fluency test during walking (RM Camicioli, unpublished observations).

Other reasons might be postulated for falls in demented patients. Some falls appear to be a result of poor insight; the patients attempt do things that are not reasonable for their physical capabilities. Demented patients do not attend to their environment as well as age-matched controls do. This inattention may be the cause of impaired obstacle clearance while walking.[87]

In conclusion, demented patients may have normal balance synergies but do not use them effectively because of impaired attention and insight and an inability to profit from experience. It is probable that when dementia is combined with other problems with balance and gait, the chance of falls will markedly increase because the patient will be unable to adapt to the disabilities.

IMPAIRED ATTENTION

The effect of attention on balance and gait has not been investigated, but the attentional demands of balance and locomotion have been studied. Attentional demands have been measured by the reaction time to auditory cues while subjects were balancing and walking. As the difficulty of maintaining balance increased, the reaction time also increased, indicating that more attention was required for the balance task.[90,91] Walking increased attentional demands,[91] as did using a walker.[92] Although it has not been proven, one can postulate that inattention or distraction may impede balance or walking. It also may be that the increased risk of falling associated with psychotropic drug use[85] is partially related to effects on attention and not solely to alterations in vestibular or motor function.

The converse of these observations is that some patients with severely compromised balance and gait do not fall because they are very attentive to their safety. Attentional capacity may be a critical factor in the security of gait. The slow, short-stepped gait with en block turns seen in many elderly patients (cautious gait or so-called, "senile gait") may be an appropriate adaptation of gait to a person's perceived capacity to maintain balance.[93,94] That is, the cautious gait may indicate that cognitive aspects of balance and locomotion are intact!

Above, we have discussed attention or inattention in a global sense. There is another form of inattention that must be considered, hemi-inattention or motor neglect.[95,96] Lesions in the frontal and parietal lobes, as well as in the thalamus, may reduce the use of the contralateral limbs despite normal strength and coordination and no evidence of sensory neglect.[95-97] Motor neglect could account for the thalamic, basal ganglia, and midbrain astasia discussed in the section on orientation, but because there was no mention in the case reports of motor neglect during other motor tasks we think this is less likely than an orientation deficit.

FEAR OF FALLING GAITS

A post-fall syndrome consists of the sudden inability to walk without support of objects or the assistance of another person occurring after a fall in which there is no evidence of neurological or orthopedic abnormality to explain the inability to walk.[98,99] With assistance, many of these patients may walk normally. This inability to walk appears to be the result of excessive fear, a perceived insecurity of balance that does not match the person's physical capacity. It might thus be termed the "overcautious" gait.

CAUTIOUS GAIT

The cautious gait needs to be considered under this category but not as a pathological gait. The proper response to postural insecurity is to adopt more conservative balance and gait patterns. The gait pattern often referred to as "senile" and characterized by slowing, shorter steps, and en bloc turns is an appropriate response to perceived risk of falls in the anterior and, posterior directions. A normal person assumes this gait pattern on a slippery surface. Widening of the base of support is an appropriate response to uncertainty as to where the feet will make contact with the support surface, and there is a risk of falls laterally. A normal person widens the base on a pitching ship deck. The perceived risk of falls may arise from within (impairment of balance and gait systems) or from without (the environment).

Summary

Balance and gait disorders can be related to disturbances in six different systems. The balance and gait patterns that the clinician observes is a result of the dysfunction and the compensatory adaptations made for the dysfunction. The adaptation can simultaneously occur at a wiring level (sprouting of axons and establishment of new connections), a reorganization of existing neural function (for example, using visual, rather than somatosensory information, for balance) and modification of behavior (voluntary adaptation). Recognizing the balance and gait patterns characteristic of dysfunction in each system will guide the diagnostic evaluation of patients and specific treatment. Recognizing the interaction of the systems and the adaptations used for dysfunction will suggest methods that promote adaptation.

References

1. Pratt C, Horak F, Herndon R: Differential effects of somatosensory and motor system deficits on postural dyscontrol in multiple sclerosis, in Woollacott M, Horak FB (eds): *Posture and Gait: Control Mechanisms.* Eugene, OR: University of Oregon Press, 1992, pp 118–121.

2. Gross CG, Graziano MSA: Multiple representations of space in the brain. *Neuroscientist* 1:43–50, 1995.

3. Black FO: Peripheral vestibular disorders. In: Harker LA, ed. *Otolaryngology—Head and Neck Surgery.* Vol. IV. *Ear and Skull Base,* 1986, pp 3293–3311.

4. Horak FB, Shupert CL: Role of the vestibular system in postural control, in Herdman SJ, Whitney SL, Borello-France DF (eds): *Vestibular Rehabilitation.* Philadelphia: FA Davis, 1994, pp 22–46.

5. Shumway-Cook A, Horak FB, Yardley L, Bronstein AM: Rehabilitation of balance disorders in the patient with vestibular pathology, in Bronstein A, Brandt T, Woollacott M (eds): *Aspects of Balance and Related Gait Disorders.* Kent, England: Edward Arnold Publishers, 1995 pp 211–235.

6. Horak FB, Shupert CL, Dietz V, Horstmann G: Vestibular and somatosensory contributions to responses to head and body displacements. *Exp Brain Res* 100:93–106, 1994.

7. Pozzo T, Berthoz A, Lefort L, Vitte E: Head stabilization during various locomotor tasks in humans. II. Patients with bilateral peripheral vestibular deficits. *Exp Brain Res* 82:97–106, 1990.

8. Shumway-Cook A, Horak FB: Vestibular rehabilitation: An exercise approach to managing symptoms of vestibular dysfunction. *Semin Hear* 10:196–208, 1989.

9. Shumway-Cook A, Horak FB: Rehabilitation strategies for patients with vestibular deficits. *Neurol Clin N Am* 8:441–457, 1990.

10. Horak FB, Nashner LM, Diener HC: Postural strategies associated with somatosensory and vestibular loss. *Exp Brain Res* 82:167–177, 1990.

11. Takemori S, Ida M, Umezu H: Vestibular training after sudden loss of vestibular functions. *Otorhinolaryngol* 47:76, 1985.

12. Fukuda R: The stepping test: Two phases of the labyrinthine reflex. *Acta Otolaryngol (Stockh)* 50:95, 1959.

13. Black F, Peterka RJ, Shupert C, Nashner L: Effects of unilateral loss of vestibular function on the vestibulo-ocular reflex and postural control. *Ann Oto Rhinol Laryngol* 98:884–889, 1989.

14. Black FO, Wall C, Nashner LM: Effect of visual and support surface orientation references upon postural control in vestibular deficient subjects. *Acta Otolaryngol (Stockh)* 95:199–210, 1983.

15. Nashner LM, Black FO, Wall CI: Adaptation to altered support and visual conditions during stance: Patients with vestibular deficits. *J Neurophysiol* 2:536–544, 1982.

16. Horak FB, Mirka A, Shupert CL: The role of peripheral vestibular disorders in postural dyscontrol in the elderly, in Woollacot M, Shumway-Cook A (eds): *The Development of Posture and Gait across the Lifespan.* Columbia, SC: Univ. of South Carolina Press, 1989, pp 253–279.

17. Shupert CL, Horak FB, Black FO: Hip sway associated with vestibulopathy. *J Vestibular Res* 4:231–244, 1994.

18. Diener HC, Dichgans J, Guschlbauer B, Langenbach P: The significance of proprioception on postural stabilization as assessed by ischemia. *Brain Res* 296:103–109, 1984.

19. Inglis JT, Horak FB, Shupert CL, Jones-Rycewicz C: The importance of somatosensory information in triggering and scaling automatic postural responses in humans. *Exp Brain Res* 101:159–164, 1994.

20. Leibowitz HW, Johnson CA, Isabelle E: Peripheral motion detection and refractive error. *Science* 177:1207–1208, 1972.

21. Stoffregen TA: Flow structure versus retinal location in the optical control of stance. *J Exp Psychol Hum Percept Perform* 11:554–565, 1985.

22. Peterka RJ, Benolken MS: Role of somatosensory and vestibular cues in attenuating visually-induced human postural sway, in Woollacott M, Horak F (eds): *Posture and Gait: Control Mechanisms.* Eugene, OR: University of Oregon Press, 1992, pp 272–275.

23. Patla AE, Prentice SD, Robinson C, Neufeld J: Visual control of locomotion: Strategies for changing direction and for going over obstacles. *J Exp Psychol Hum Percept Perform* 17:603–634, 1991.

24. Grusser OJ: Multimodal structure of the extrapersonal space, in Hein A, Jeannerod M (eds): *Spatially Oriented Behavior*. New York: Springer-Verlag, 1983, pp 327–352.

25. Brandt TH, Esser J, Buchele W, Krafczk S: Visuo-spinal ataxia caused by disorders of eye movements, in Roucoux A, Crommelinck M (eds): *Physiological and Pathological Aspects of Eye Movements*. The Hague: Dr. W Junk, 1982, pp 425–430.

26. Dieterich M, Brandt T: Thalamic infarctions: Differential effects on vestibular function in the roll plane (35 patients). *Neurology* 43:1732–1740, 1993.

27. Fukushima-Kudo J, Fukushima K, Tashiro K: Rigidity and dorsiflexion of the neck in progressive supranuclear palsy and the interstitial nucleus of Cajal. *J Neurol Neurosurg Psychiatry* 50:1197–1203, 1987.

28. Masdeu JC, Gorelick PB: Thalamic astasia: Inability to stand after unilateral thalamic lesions. *Ann Neurol* 23:596–603, 1988.

29. Labadie EL, Awerbuch GI, Hamilton RH, Rapesak SZ: Falling and postural deficits due to acute unilateral basal ganglia lesions. *Arch Neurol* 45:492–496, 1989.

30. Felice KJ, Keilson GR, Schwartz WJ: Rubral gait ataxia. *Neurology* 40:1004–1005, 1990.

31. Heilman KM, Watson RT: The neglect syndrome—a unilateral defect of the orienting response, in Harnad S, Doty RW, Goldstein L, (eds): *Lateralization in the Nervous System*. New York: Academic Press, 1977.

32. Karnath HO, Fetter M: Ocular space exploration in the dark and its relation to subjective and objective body orientation in neglect patients with parietal lesions. *Neuropsychologia* 33:371–377, 1995.

33. Karnath HO: Subjective body orientation in neglect and the interactive contribution of neck muscle proprioception and vestibular stimulation. *Brain* 117:1001–1012, 1994.

34. Mountcastle VB, Lynch JC, Georgopoulos A, et al: Posterior parietal association cortex of the monkey: Command functions for operation within extra-personal space. *J Neurophysiol* 38:871–908, 1975.

35. Goodale MA: Visual pathways supporting perception and action in the primate cerebral cortex. *Curr Opin Neurobiol* 3:578–585, 1993.

36. Perenin MT, Vighetto A: Optic ataxia: A specific disorder in visuomotor coordination, in Perenin MT, Vighetto A (eds): *Spatially Oriented Behavior*. New York: Springer-Verlag, 1983, pp 305–326.

37. Patla AE: Neurobiomechanical basis for the control of human locomotion, in Bronstein A, Brandt T, Woollacott M (eds): *Aspects of Balance and Related Gait Disorders*. Kent, England: Edward Arnold, 1995, pp 19–40.

38. Patla AE, Rietdyk S: Visual control of limb trajectory over obstacles during locomotion: Effect of obstacle height and width. *Gait Posture* 1:45–60, 1993.

39. Tinetti ME, Williams TF, Mayewski R: Fall risk index for elderly patients based on number of chronic disabilities. *Am J Med* 80:429–434, 1986.

40. Horak FB, Diener HC, Nashner LM: Influence of central set on human postural responses. *J Neurophysiol* 62:841–853, 1989.

41. Martin JP: *The Basal Ganglia and Posture*. Philadelphia: JB Lippincott, 1967, p 1.

42. Horak FB, Nutt JG, Nashner LM: Postural inflexibility in parkinsonian subjects. *J Neurol Sci* 111:46–58, 1992.

43. Thompson PD, Marsden CD: Gait disorder of subcortical arteriosclerotic encephalopathy: Binswanger's disease. *Mov Disord* 2:1–8, 1987.

44. Fitzgerald PM, Jankovic J: Lower body parkinsonism: Evidence for vascular etiology. *Mov Disord* 4:249–260, 1989.

45. Horak FB, Frank J, Nutt J: Effect of dopamine on postural control in parkinsonian subjects: Scaling, set and tone. *J Neurophysiol* 75:2380–2396, 1996.

46. Johnson MT, Mendez A, Kipnis AN, et al: Acute effects of L-dopa on wrist movements in Parkinson's disease: Kinematics, volitional EMG modulation and reflex amplitude modulation. *Brain* 117:1409–1422, 1994.

47. Tian J, Herdman SJ, Zee DS, Folstein SE: Postural stability in patients with Huntington's disease. *Neurology* 42:1232–1238, 1992.

48. Diener HC, Dichgans J, Bacher M, Gompf B: Quantification of postural sway in normals and patients with cerebellar disease. *Electroencephalogr Clin Neurophysiol* 57:134–142, 1984.

49. Horak FC, Diener HC: Cerebellar control of postural scaling and central set in stance. *J Neurophysiol* 72:479–493, 1994.

50. Berger W, Horstmann G, Dietz V: Spastic paresis: Impaired spinal reflexes and intact motor programs. *J Neurol Neurosurg Psychiatry* 51:568–571, 1988.

51. Horak FB, Esselman P, Anderson ME, Lynch MK: The effects of movement velocity, mass displaced, and task certainty on associated postural adjustments made by normal and hemiplegic individuals. *J Neurol Neurosurg Psychiatry* 47:1020–1028, 1984.

52. Dietz V, Quintern J, Berger W: Electrophysiological studies of gait in spasticity and rigidity: Evidence that altered mechanical properties of muscle contribute to hypertonia. *Brain* 104:431–449, 1981.

53. Berger W, Horstmann G, Dietz V: Tension development and muscle activation in the leg during gait in spastic hemiparesis: The independence of muscle hypertonia and exaggerated stretch reflexes. *J Neurol Neurosurg Psychiatry* 47:1029–1033, 1984.

54. Nashner LM, Shumway-Cook A, Marin O: Stance posture control in select groups of children with cerebral palsy: Deficits in sensory organization and muscular coordination. *Exp Brain Res* 49:393–409, 1983.

55. Armstrong DM: Supraspinal control of locomotion. *J Physiol* 405:1–37, 1988.

56. Grillner S, Wallen P: Central pattern generators for locomotion with special reference to vertebrates. *Annu Rev Neurosci* 8:233–261, 1985.

57. Calancie B, Needham-Shropshire B, Jacobs P, et al: Involuntary stepping after chronic spinal cord injury: Evidence for a central rhythm generator for locomotion in man. *Brain* 117:1143–1159, 1994.

58. Dietz V, Colombo G, Jensen L: Locomotor activity in spinal man. *Lancet* 344:1260–1263, 1994.

59. Garcia-Rill E: The basal ganglia and the locomotor regions. *Brain Res Brain Res Rev* 11:47–63, 1986.

60. Mori S, Sakamoto T, Ohta Y, et al: Site-specific postural and locomotor changes evoked in awake, freely moving intact cats by stimulating the brainstem. *Brain Res* 505:66–74, 1989.

61. Mori S: Contribution of postural muscle tone to full expression of posture and locomotor movements: Multi-faceted analyses of its setting brainstem-spinal cord mechanisms in the cat. *Jpn J Physiol* 39:785–809, 1989.

62. Kuypers HGJM, Lawrence DG: Cortical projections to the red nucleus and the brainstem in the rhesus monkey. *Brain Res* 4:151–188, 1967.

63. Salanova V, Morris HH, Van Ness P, et al: Frontal lobe seizures: Electroclinical syndromes. *Epilepsia* 36:16–24, 1995.

64. Penfield W, Welch K: The supplementary motor area of the cerebral cortex: A clinical and experimental study. *Arch Neurol Psychiatry* 66:289–317, 1951.

65. Gahery Y, Nieoullon A: Postural and kinetic coordination following cortical stimuli which induce flexion movements in the cat's limbs. *Brain Res* 149:25–37, 1978.

66. Gurfinkel VS, El'ner AM: Contribution of the frontal lobe secondary motor area to organization of postural components in human voluntary movement. *Neirofiziologiya* 20:7–15, 1988.

67. Viallet F, Massion J, Massarino R, Khalil R: Coordination between posture and movement in a bimanual load lifting task: Putative

role of a medial frontal region including the supplementary motor area. *Exp Brain Res* 88:674–684, 1992.

68. Kennard MA, Ectors L: Forced circling in monkeys following lesions of the frontal lobes. *J Neurophysiol* 1:45–51, 1938.

69. Masdeu JC, Alampur U, Cavaliere R, Tavoulareas G: Astasia and gait failure with damage of the pontomesencephalic locomotor region. *Ann Neurol* 35:619–621, 1994.

70. Leckman JF, de Lotbiniere AJ, Marek K, et al: Severe disturbances in speech, swallowing, and gait following stereotactic infrathalamic lesions in Gilles de la Tourette's syndrome. *Neurology* 43:890–894, 1993.

71. Nutt JG, Marsden CD, Thompson PD: Human walking and higher level gait disorders, particularly in the elderly. *Neurology* 43:268–279, 1993.

72. Bruns L: Uber sturungen des gleichgewichtes bei stirnhirntumoren. *Dtsch Med Wochenschr* 18:138–140, 1892.

73. Gerstmann J, Schilder P: Uber eine besondere gangstorung bei stirnhirner kranting. *Wien Med Schr* 76:97–107, 1926.

74. van Bogaert L, Martin P: Sur deux signes du syndrome de desequilibration frontale: L'apraxie de la marche et l'antonie statique. *Encephale* 24:11–18, 1929.

75. Bell A: Apraxia in corpus callosum lesions. *J Neurol Psychopathol* 15:137–146, 1934.

76. Denny-Brown D: The nature of apraxia. *J Nerv Ment Dis* 126:9–31, 1958.

77. Meyer JS, Barron DW: Apraxia of gait: A clinicophysiological study. *Brain* 83:261–284, 1960.

78. Petrovici K: Apraxia of gait and of trunk movements. *J Neurol Sci* 7:229–243, 1968.

79. Stern GM, Lander CM, Lees AJ: Akinetic freezing and trick movements in Parkinson's disease. *J Neural Transm Suppl* 16:137–141, 1980.

80. Atchison PR, Thompson PD, Frackowiak RSJ, Marsden CD: The syndrome of gait initiation failure: A report of six cases. *Mov Disord* 8:285–292, 1993.

81. Achiron A, Ziv I, Goren M, et al: Primary progressive freezing gait. *Mov Disord* 8:293–297, 1993.

82. Messert B, Baker NH: Symptoms of progressive spastic ataxia and apraxia associated with occult hydrocephalus. *Neurology* 16:440–452, 1966.

83. Eidelberg E, Walden JG, Nguyen LH: Locomotor control in Macaque monkeys. *Brain* 104:647–663, 1981.

84. Kuypers HGJM: Anatomy of the descending pathways, in Brooks VB (ed): *Handbook of Physiology. The Nervous System: Motor Control.* Bethesda, MD: American Physiological Society, 1981, sect 1, part 1, vol 2, pp 597–666.

85. Tinetti ME, Speechley M, Ginter SF: Risk factors for falls among elderly persons living in the community. *N Engl J Med* 319:1701–1707, 1988.

86. Salgado R, Lord SR, Packer J, Ehrlich F: Factors associated with falling in elderly hospital patients. *Gerontology* 40:325–331, 1994.

87. Alexander NB, Mollo JM, Giordani B, et al: Maintenance of balance, gait patterns, and obstacle clearance in Alzheimer's disease. *Neurology* 45:908–914, 1995.

88. Sharma JC, MacLennan WJ: Causes of ataxia in patients attending a falls laboratory. *Age Ageing* 17:94–102, 1988.

89. Visser H: Gait and balance in senile dementia of Alzheimer's type. *Age Ageing* 12:296–301, 1983.

90. Teasdale N, Bard K, LaRue J, Fleury M: Cognitive demands of posture control. *Exp Aging Res* 19:1–13, 1993.

91. Lajoie Y, Teasdale N, Bard C, Fleury M: Attentional demands for static and dynamic equilibrium. *Exp Brain Res* 97:139–144, 1993.

92. Wright DL, Kemp TL: The dual-task methodology and assessing the attentional demands of ambulation with walking devices. *Phys Ther* 72:306–315, 1992.

93. Elble RJ, Sienko-Thomas S, Higgins C, Colliver J: Stride-dependent changes in gait of older people. *J Neurol* 238:1–5, 1991.

94. Elble RJ, Hughes L, Higgins C: The syndrome of senile gait. *J Neurol* 239:71–75, 1992.

95. Laplane D, Degos JD: Motor neglect. *J Neurol Neurosurg Psychiatry* 46:152–158, 1983.

96. Valenstein E, Heilman KM: Unilateral hypokinesia and motor extinction. *Neurology* 31:445–448, 1981.

97. von Giesen H, Schlaug G, Steinmetz H, et al: Cerebral network underlying unilateral motor neglect: Evidence from positron emission tomography. *J Neurol Sci* 125:29–38, 1994.

98. Marks I: Space "phobia" a pseudo-agoraphobic syndrome. *J Neurol Neurosurg Psychiatry* 44:387–391, 1981.

99. Murphy J, Isaacs B: The post-fall syndrome: A study of 36 elderly patients. *Gerontology* 82:265–270, 1982.

Chapter 49

MOVEMENT DISORDERS IN CHILDHOOD

GEORGE W. PAULSON and CARSON R. REIDER

"NORMAL" MOVEMENT PHENOMENA DURING
  DEVELOPMENT
DYSKINETIC MOVEMENTS
  Tics
  Tremor
  Dystonic Phenomena
  Chorea
  Myoclonus
JUVENILE PARKINSON'S DISEASE
ATAXIA AND SPASTICITY
PAROXYSMAL MOVEMENT DISORDERS
MISCELLANEOUS DISORDERS
PSYCHOLOGICAL PROBLEMS ASSOCIATED WITH
  MOVEMENT DISORDERS

A discussion of movement disorders, whether those seen in children or in adults, can use multiple classifications. Conditions that affect the cortex or anterior horn cells may logically be excluded, as can cerebellar disorders, but in neurological practice, and most particularly in childhood, the appearance of a disorder of movement may be associated with disorders throughout many areas of the nervous system (Table 49-1). "Movement disorders" could be limited to presumed extrapyramidal disorders. Several alternative classifications for movement disorders are reflected in this volume; these include descriptive labels, specific diseases, genetic classification, degenerative or infectious disorders, etc. Ideally, the abnormalities that cause movement disorders would be described precisely on the basis of the underlying neuropathology, but even in forms of common dystonia, often no clearly reflective neuropathology exists. The traditional reliance on clinical diagnosis and the paucity of objective diagnostic tests contribute significantly to the lack of consistency in classification. In some conditions, dystonia again, for example, a topographical listing, such as generalized, segmental, or focal, can be used. Classification of dystonias could also be made according to age of onset, presumed etiology, clinical features, or even severity.[1] For decades, the tendency was to classify movement disorders as hypokinetic or hyperkinetic, with the unspoken hypothesis of a loss of intrinsic homeostasis reflecting too much, too little, or too rapidly changing conditions within the nervous system. Conditions such as juvenile Parkinson's disease (PD)[2] or Huntington's disease (HD)[3] actually display aspects of both hypokinesia and hyperkinesia. The dyskinesias also can be subdivided into cho-

rea, dystonia, tremor, tic, and myoclonus. However, then, where does ataxia fit in?

This chapter is less than rigid in format, is mixed in classification, and cannot be encyclopedic. It will include comments on normal phenomena, with distinction of the normal and the less severe from the more severe disorders, with an attempt to separate relatively stable from relatively progressive disorders. In addition to this chapter, there are several fine texts on pediatric neurology, including the works by Swaiman[4] and by Volpe.[5]

"Normal" Movement Phenomena During Development

Fundamental work over several decades done by Prechtl[6] and others[7] has confirmed an evolution of fetal movements from those more generalized to those more discrete as birth approaches. Massive truncal flexion movements, and later limb flexion movements, become more delicate as the fetus develops patterns turning "toward" or turning "away." Eventually, more precise limb and finger movements appear, even before birth ensues. Shortly after a child's birth, parents can be fascinated by the movements of their newborn and, to an anxious new parent, normal movements may be interpreted as anything from seizures to quiet sleep.

Newborns may not initially perform coordinated sucking movements and may manifest a mixture of tongue thrust, sucking, turning toward and turning away. The gentle and attentive parent leads the child beyond inappropriate movements toward coordinative function. On the infant's face there is a play of apparent but inappropriate emotional responses during the first several months, appearances that can shift rapidly from what appears to be a smile into what is a grimace or an admixture of both a wince and a smile. The play of expression seems fickle, random, and unrelated to the external world. The new parent who studies the child may notice pursed lips, fine myoclonic jerks around the face, and inchoate mouth twitches. During sleep, sucking movements of the lips and fluttering of the eyelids can be observed. Multiple motor reflections of the paradoxical sleep phenomena of the newborn also may be seen. Shortly after birth, coarse jerking movements of the arms, or portions of an exaggerated or partial Moro response, are joined by more delicate movements of the fingers.

Development of motor function is not smooth during the first year. A new skill appears, seems lost for a few weeks, and then returns in a more predictable form. At times, for example, when a 6-month-old child is attempting to sit, there will be an inappropriately rigid posture and limb extension, as the child falls to one side, followed by a delayed look of consternation or an outright cry. It is possible to observe a mixture of numerous reflex responses, including the "fencing response," "parachute" response, or "placing" response, or even the residual bilateral Moro reflex, joined to an apparently voluntary motion.

Jitteriness is frequently seen during the neonatal period. Although sometimes attributable to hypocalcemia, hypogly-

TABLE 49-1 A Classification of Movement Disorders

Primary
  Genetic
    Essential tremor
    Familial nonprogressive chorea
    Huntington's disease
    Inherited ataxias
    Torsion dystonias
    Wilson's disease
  Idiopathic
    Blepharospasm
    Gilles de la Tourette's syndrome
    Parkinson's disease
    Dystonia
Secondary
  Birth injury
    Double athetosis
  Head injury
  Metabolic
    Asterixis
    Kernicterus
  Vascular
    Hemiballism
  Inflammatory
    Chorea secondary to SLE
  Hormonal
    Hyperthyroidism
    Hypothyroidism
    Hypoparathyrodism
    Pseudohypoparathyroidism
    Pseudopseudohypoparathyroidism
  Neoplastic
    Tumor in basal ganglia or skull base
  Infection
    Sydenham's chorea
    Postviral
  Drugs (neuroleptics, antipsychotics)
    Action dystonia
    Parkinsonism
    Akathisia
    Tardive dyskinesia/dystonia
  Toxic
    Metallic
      Parkinsonism (manganese)
    Nonmetallic
      Parkinsonism (carbon dioxide, MPTP)
Psychogenic
  Abasia astasia
  Myoclonus
  Tremor

SLE, systemic lupus erythematosus; MPTP, 1-methyl-4-phenyl-1,2,3,6-tetra-hydropyridine.
SOURCE: Modified from Manyan BV: Rehabilitation of parkinsonism, other movement disorders and ataxia, in Good DC, Couch JR (eds): *Handbook of Rehabilitation*. New York: Marcel Dekker, 1994.

cemia, or encephalopathy, jitteriness has also been observed in a significant percentage of healthy neonates. Extreme jitteriness should always raise the suspicion of drug withdrawal or hypothermia. After infancy the phenomenon usually disappears, but continuance of jitteriness may warrant

follow-up to rule out a seizure disorder. The long-term significance (i.e., the relation to essential tremor) remains unclear. Some normal babies, age 3–8 months, develop a form of benign myoclonus with repetitive flexor spasms that do not bear the ominous prognosis of infantile spasms.[8]

Walking during the first several years appears to be, and indeed is, ataxic. Not uncommonly, a child appears to favor one leg over the other, or the toes may turn out more on one foot than on the other. Most of these initial asymmetries gradually develop into a fully coordinated gait. As emphasized by Butler,[9] apparently abnormal movement patterns can often be benign as well as transient. Motor development may not be solely related also to maturation of the cerebral cortex but related to feedback mechanisms, as well as dependent on various structural developments, for example, bone growth, muscle mass, etc. The process is complex, not smooth, but for most, it is wonderfully hopeful and healthful.

Repetitive touching, stroking, gentle gesturing, or tics may be seen in the early years of life. For example, a normal child may repetitively touch one eyelid with no apparent cause or may tug at an earlobe, even when there is not an infection. By age 5, inconsistent tics or mannerisms seem almost universal but only infrequently evolve into Tourette's syndrome. A gender difference does exist. Boys not only are more often clumsy and act more aggressively but also may be more inclined to stutter and to manifest more tics, as well as to display facial grimacing during speech. One of ten children has obvious isolated tics, with a peak in frequency at age 7, and although most such tics disappear they may recur in old age.[10] Just as facial mannerisms and tics can be observed in a bus or on a roadside in adults,[11] so, too, children often have idiosyncratic mannerisms. Up until age 12 or 13, some patterned movements continue to be performed with difficulty. For example, it may be hard to spread the fingers selectively and, until the teen years, there may be overflow phenomena, such as curling in of the fingers when the child walks on the outside of the foot.

All of the delays, even in the development of the subtle motor phenomena, may be enhanced in the child who is retarded. Many of the early measurements of development actually measure motor development, because cognitive function will be less accessible to testing. Those children with mental retardation or blindness may use a gait that is perhaps best described as graceless. Overt physical handicaps can accentuate any abnormal movement pattern.

Any normal child, even after age 2, can occasionally manifest head banging, but in children that are blind or sensory deprived, rocking or repetitive hand and head movements are almost universal. Once called "blindisms," these repetitive movements or "stereotypies" can be seen in the severely retarded child and are accentuated during times of boredom or anxiety.[12]

For decades there has been discussion of "minimal neurological deficit," "minimal brain damage," or "attention deficit disorder" with potential linkage of the difficulties in learning or in sustained attention with putative neurological problems. This usually first becomes a consideration as school begins but may remain a problem until puberty or beyond.[13] The lay, as well as the medical, literature abounds with discussions of difficulties in fine manipulation, coordination problems, subtle choreiform movements, or hypotonia in such children. Just as motor deficits are used to measure developmental milestones, so too have these presumed and yet subtle abnormalities been linked with troublesome or obsessive-compulsive behavior, hyperactivity, or problems in concentration. Classical neurology has contributed relatively little in this potential area of research, and it is possible that most practicing neurologists feel uncomfortable in declaring such children as either neurologically normal or abnormal. It is certainly clear that many superficially "abnormal" movements in children are transient, do not necessarily indicate the presence of a progressive disorder and do not necessarily imply long-term disability. Nevertheless, childhood autism and schizophrenia have been reported to be related to hypotonia and repetitive stereotyped movements,[14] and severe hypotonia always raises the issue of organic encephalopathy.

Even when there is obvious clumsiness, a clear difference between normal and abnormal phenomena can be difficult to identify. Some children seem congenitally maladroit[15] but are otherwise entirely normal. Every child discovers there are other children who can run faster and can throw with more apparently instinctive skills. Unfortunately, many normal children discover themselves near the end of the line when there is selection for group athletics, are slower to learn how to color "within the lines," or are less able to disentangle the shape of letters when they learn to write. Just as most parents can be patient with overt masturbation, thumb suck ing, or enuresis, so, too, many of the subtle deficits in motor performance deserve little formal attention. It is not necessarily true that the dyslexic child is also clumsy, nor that the clumsy child is also "brain damaged."

Generally speaking, most developmental disorders do not require specific imaging or extensive laboratory tests, and for most children development offers great promise, because time often produces significant amelioration. Premature labeling of apparent movement disorders can have profound and long-lasting effects on the child's self-esteem and capabilities.

Dyskinetic Movements

The principal dyskinesias include tics, tremor, athetosis, dystonia, and chorea. Children exhibit almost all of the principal types of dyskinesia seen in adults.[16] Distinction between these movements may be difficult in children, and the incidence of associated diseases is different. The definitions are not different than in the adult and are provided elsewhere in this book. In addition to the major classification categories listed above, myoclonus and ataxia are features of some of the movement disorders of childhood. Many movement disorders in childhood are also combined with spasticity.

TICS

Tics may be transient or permanent, innocent or progressive, familial or sporadic[17] (Table 49-2). Most tics last for only weeks or months, but motor tics can be chronic. The usual

TABLE 49-2 Etiological Classification of Childhood Tics

Idiopathic
  Acute transient tics
  Persistent simple or multiple tics of childhood that clear before
    adulthood
  Chronic simple or multiple motor tics that persist
  Gilles de la Tourette's syndrome
Secondary tics
  Postencephalitic
  Sydenham's chorea
  Head trauma
  Carbon monoxide poisoning
  Poststroke
  Neuroacanthocytosis
  Drugs: carbamazepine, L-dopa, neuroleptics, phenobarbital,
    phenytoin, stimulants
  Mental retardation syndromes, including chromosomal
    abnormalities
  Other

SOURCE: Modified from Lockman LA: Movement disorders, in Swaiman KF, Wright FS (ed): *The Practice of Pediatric Neurology.* St. Louis: CV Mosby, 1982.

fear is that tics represent a feature of the Gilles de la Tourette syndrome (TS)[18] (see also Chaps. 41 and 42). The motor tics in TS vary but often include facial grimacing and limb jerking. In contrast to simple persistent motor tics, which may remain very stereotyped, the motor tics in TS vary with time and circumstances and are multiple. As many as 50 percent of children with TS also have behavioral disorders or an obsessive-compulsive disorder,[19] and some have extensive somatic complaints.[20] TS is far from rare in a pediatric or neurological practice. It has been claimed,[21] but not truly proven, that stimulant medications used for presumed attention deficit disorders may elicit or worsen TS. The cause of TS remains uncertain, but TS can certainly be familial. In some families TS is autosomal-dominant with variable penetrance.[22]

Management of the patient with TS usually requires medication, time, and counseling. The physician may choose to emphasize nonpharmaceutical measures, such as biofeedback and support of the school and family, because the efficacy of current pharmacotherapy is limited. Medications used for symptomatic relief include haloperidol, imipramine, pimozide, and clonidine. It is wise to emphasize that medications do not erase TS, that all drugs have side effects, and that for many children with mild-to-moderate TS, medication is not required. The condition will often, but not always, extend into adulthood. Sporadic facial contractions, as well as compulsive disorders, interestingly, have been noted in schizophrenia,[23] but TS is not characterized by the major features of schizophrenia.

TREMOR

One common tremor in childhood is that related to nonspecific cerebral inflammation or secondary to fever. Another is the mixed type of tremor linked with cerebral palsy. Any person, adult or child, who exerts maximum strength, who is fatigued, or who is anxious, may display a transient tremor (Table 49-3).

TABLE 49-3 Some Varieties of Tremor

	Postural	Intention	Task Specific	Hysterical
Physiological		Ataxic syndromes	Primary writing	Conversion
Essential			Vocal	symptom
Cerebellar			Orthostatic	
Peripheral neuropathy				
Wilson's disease				
Posttraumatic				
Nonspecific (i.e., weakness, fatigue, infection, etc.)				

SOURCE: Modified from Hallett M: Differential diagnosis of tremor, in Vinken PJ, Bruyn GW, Klawans HL (eds): *Handbook of Clinical Neurology.* Amsterdam: Elsevier, 1986, vol 49, no. 5.

"Benign" essential tremor (ET) is also common in childhood[24] and may be the most common persistent tremor (see also Chap. 27). ET may markedly increase with anxiety, and in both children and adults is often attributed to "nerves." The characteristics of ET in the child are similar to those of ET in adulthood,[25] but the tremor in some children may actually improve in young adulthood and then reappear in later years. Children who have had postinfectious polyneuropathy may be left with residual tremor, and some patients with variants of both hereditary and nonhereditary neuropathy may manifest tremor early in the course of the disorder. Some children with cerebral palsy or with residua of brain injury manifest a nonspecific tremor, which is often postural and worse with action. It is wise to consider hyperthyroidism in any child who develops a new disorder that is characterized by tremor, but imaging—as with most movement disorders—is rarely useful for the child with tremor. Tremor can be a conspicuous feature of several of the inherited conditions, such as Wilson's disease, but dystonic phenomena are also present in the children with Wilson's disease. ET is characterized, in most instances, by tremor with no other neurological handicap.

Brief shuddering attacks can be seen in infancy or early childhood and, usually, pass with time. Although, as mentioned earlier, some normal or premature newborns may be jittery,[26] this can occur after a pregnancy during which drugs or alcohol had been used. Although seizures may be associated with such withdrawal phenomena in children, the overall prognosis, even in these children, is usually good. Seizures can be distinguished from jitteriness in a newborn, in that when the child is jittery there is no ocular component, and the movement is tremorous, not clonic. Passive movements will stop jitter, and in jitterness there are no autonomic changes.[27] Some true seizures in such children can, of course, appear to represent facial automatisms or a movement disorder.[28,29]

DYSTONIC PHENOMENA

It is an unusual child that has not had sore muscles and a stiff or "wry" neck at one time or another but, fortunately, children are less likely to actually injure the vertebral bodies and compress the spinal cord than the elderly. A stiff neck may be related to a throat infection. When chronic neck

spasticity is seen in a child, it usually represents a variant of cerebral palsy. Torticollis can be a transient problem in the newborn, particularly if caused by a hematoma in the sternocleidomastoid muscle. This form of torticollis is treatable by means of physical therapy with gentle repetitive stretching of the muscle. Cases of a benign and self-limited form of paroxysmal torticollis in children have been reported.[30]

More persistent torticollis can be a manifestation of a treatable disorder, such as familial L-dopa-responsive dystonia, a condition that is rare and usually occurs in more than one family member.[31,32] L-dopa-responsive dystonia may be seen with a diurnal variation and may worsen in late afternoon (see also Chap. 30).

Unfortunately, as reviewed in Chap. 30 in this volume, more severe and less treatable progressive generalized dystonia may also begin in childhood and is often misidentified, particularly when there is no other affected family member. Such idiopathic dystonia is often slowly progressive and can represent an inherited disorder[33] (Tables 49-4 and 49-5).

The diagnosis of dystonia, at least until genetic testing is more generally applicable, continues to rest on clinical symptomatology. Mental retardation is not a consistent associated feature, but it is rare for a child and family not to suffer severe secondary emotional stress when dystonia appears. Trials of numerous drugs, such as trihexyphenidyl, baclofen, and even L-dopa, are appropriate but for many will offer only limited symptomatic benefit. Neurosurgical procedures such as thalamotomy or implantation of a baclofen pump[34] can occasionally be useful (see also Chap. 32).

Children are particularly vulnerable to the acute dystonic reaction caused by phenothiazines and similar medications.[35-37] Only one or two doses of a dopamine-blocking antiemetic might trigger a profound acute dystonic phenomenon, a reaction that is frightening and may appear to the uninitiated as life-threatening. These episodes are now usually quickly identified in emergency rooms and are easily treated with antihistamines, anticholinergics, or sedatives. It is interesting to speculate as to why acute dystonia is more common in the young, although tardive dyskinesia is more common in the elderly than in children. In Wilson's disease, when CNS manifestations are present early in life the peculiar plastic rigidity of this disorder is readily apparent, but when symptoms of the disease first appear in a patient's 20s or 30s,

TABLE 49-4 A Classification of Dystonia

By cause
  Idiopathic
    Sporadic
    Familial
      Autosomal-dominant
      Autosomal-recessive
      X-linked recessive
  Symptomatic
    Hereditary neurological disorders
    Environmental
      Cerebral, focal cerebral vascular, or cervical cord injury
      Head trauma
      Encephalitis and postinfectious
      Multiple sclerosis
      Brain tumor
By age of onset
  Childhood (0–12 yr)
  Adolescent (13–20 yr)
  Adult (≥21 yr)
By distribution
  Focal
    Eyelids (blepharospasm)
    Mouth (oromandibular dystonia)
    Larynx (dystonic adductor dysphonia)
    Neck (torticollis)
    Arm (writer's cramp)
  Segmental
    Cranial
    Axial
    Brachial
    Crural
  Multifocal
  Hemidystonia
  Generalized
Psychogenic

SOURCE: Modified from Fahn S, Marsden CD, Calne DB: Classification and investigation of dystonia, in Fahn S, Marsden CD (eds): *Movement Disorders 2*. London: Butterworths, 1987.

TABLE 49-5 Differential Diagnosis of Dystonia

Congenital and developmental	Benign dystonia of infancy
	Cerebral palsy (dystonic form)
	Dyspeptic dystonia with hiatus hernia
Degenerative disorders of unknown cause	Ataxia-telangiectasia
	Dystonia musculorum deformans
	Focal dystonias
	Hallervorden-Spatz disease
	Hemidystonia
	Idiopathic torsion dystonia
	Leber's disease (variant)
	Myoclonic dystonia (paroxysmal)
	L-dopa responsive dystonia
	Subacute necrotizing encephalomyelopathy
	Dystonia-parkinsonian syndrome
Metabolic conditions	Gangliosidosis
	Phenylketonuria
	Triosephosphate isomerase deficiency
	Wilson's disease
Infectious disease	Viral encephalitis
Medication reaction	Bethanechol
	Butyrophenones
	Carbamazepine
	Phenothiazines
	Reserpine
	Tetrabenazine
Sleep abnormalities	Paroxysmal sleep dystonia
Psychogenic	Munchausen syndrome simulating dystonia or psychogenic dystonia

SOURCE: Modified from Swaiman KF: *Pediatric Neurology: Principles and Practice*, 2d ed. St. Louis: CV Mosby, 1994.

a characteristic and even pathognomonic flapping tremor is more likely. Similarly, in the childhood form of Huntington's disease (HD), rigidity and relatively little chorea may occur, whereas patients with the more common later onset of HD manifest obvious chorea with minimal rigidity and bradykinesia until later in the course.

There are numerous inherited causes of severe dystonia. These include young onset PD, and rare conditions such as Hallervorden-Spatz disease.[66] In the latter the extrapyramidal features are linked with dementia, and some patients exhibit a distinctive pattern on MRI ("tigereye"). There can also be acquired dystonias secondary to tumor, trauma, metabolic disorders, etc. Sandifer's syndrome is an apparent movement disorder related to gastroesophageal reflux.[67,68] The stomach contents bathe the esophagus, and with regurgitation the patient suddenly flexes forward and appears to have an almost choreoathetotic movement. The movement can include torticollis, extension, or rotation of the neck, as related to intake of meals. Rarely, apneic episodes occur. The bizarre movements can be cured when the reflux is treated.

CHOREA

Chorea can be seen with childhood HD, but the classic childhood chorea is Sydenham's[38] (see also Chaps. 35 and 38). This presumably postinfectious disorder usually follows group A beta hemolytic streptococcal pharyngitis. The process reflects individual vulnerability, as well as a postinfectious response. As is so often the case with other movement disorders of childhood, Sydenham's chorea overlaps with psychiatric disturbances. The chorea may not even be identified initially, because the patient is considered "simply" restless, aggressive, or hyperemotional. Anatomic areas affected in Sydenham's chorea include the caudate and subthalamus, but the process does not spare the cortex or cranial nerve nuclei.[39] It seems probable that Sydenham's chorea relates to an autoimmune response, which may account for the fact that some acutely ill patients seem to respond to a brief course of steroids.

The clinical course tends to be insidious with fatigue, clumsiness, and abnormal movements involving the face and limbs. As noted in the last century, the movement is even more abrupt and unpredictable than that of chorea associated with HD.[40] Although the chorea is usually generalized, hemichorea can also be seen. As many as one-half of the patients with Sydenham's chorea who are seen by neurologists will not present with other signs of rheumatic fever. Nevertheless, preventive measures, including long-term antibiotic prophylaxis, are recommended, and adequate sedation or tranquilization is necessary in the short term to protect the child. Chorea paralytica or mollis, older labels for extremely severe cases, may be associated with profound disability but fortunately this, as well as the other forms of Sydenham's chorea, are not only treatable but are relatively preventable.

HD in childhood presents a slightly different concatenation of symptoms than the adult form, with rigidity, easily observed slowing of eye movements from loss of rapid saccadic eye movements and, occasionally, seizures as early features.[41] HD in childhood can present as difficulty in school, even before there are clinical signs relating to the movement disorder. The patient may appear to be primarily clumsy, rather than either rigid or choreiform, on initial evaluation. Reflexes are usually brisk, and the patient may have trouble keeping the tongue protruded.

The identification of the gene on chromosome 4 has led to definitive testing for HD (see also Chap. 34). This has not eliminated ethical issues: Does one test the asymptomatic child who is unable to give informed consent for a test that may indicate a disease in which overt diagnosis can change the child's social potential, and for which there is no current cure? When, however, the cause for a potentially severe disorder in childhood is obscure and diagnosis is necessary for medical management, DNA testing can clarify issues of care. Computed tomography, magnetic resonance imaging, etc., are not required when DNA testing is definitive. Management consists of symptomatic therapy and counseling. Carbamazepine may be useful for mood swings, and some patients benefit from antidepressants or from a trial of haloperidol for temporary suppression of the chorea.

Benign familial chorea[42] is even less common than HD and is benign particularly in the sense that mental deterioration is not apparent. As with HD, the condition is usually considered to be an autosomal-dominant one, with more limited penetrance than is true of HD. Also, in contrast to HD, benign familial chorea may not worsen with time, and abnormal movements usually begin in childhood. Some patients manifest conspicuous jerking along with the chorea, and for such patients clonazepam or haloperidol may be helpful.

Chorea can result from bilirubin encephalopathy, a condition that has now become infrequent, because the modern approach to Rh disease of the newborn is so successful.[43] Nevertheless, kernicterus can still occur in low-birth weight or premature infants. The children with chronic bilirubin encephalopathy may develop athetosis or chorea only some months after the insult. The delay in development of athetosis may reflect a phenomena similar to that of the child who is hypotonic at birth and who then later becomes spastic. A spectrum of extrapyramidal deficits may be noted in children with kernicterus, and the auditory system is often affected. Athetosis is a relatively nonspecific response to many disorders, but, traditionally, bilirubin abnormalities, hypoxia, and genetics have been key causal factors.[44,45] There are also a host of even more obscure causes for childhood chorea, athetosis, or dystonia[46–49] (Table 49-6).

TABLE 49-6 Differential Diagnosis of Chorea

Congenital	*Traumatic*	*Genetic*
Cerebral palsy	Burns in children	Ataxia-telangiectasia
		Bassen-Kornweig disease
Neoplastic	*Toxic*	Benign familial chorea of early onset
Brain tumors	Carbon monoxide	Dystonia musculorum deformans
	Isoniazide	Fabry's disease
Metabolic-endocrinologic	Lithium	Familial microencephaly with curvilinear bodies
Addison's disease	Mercury	Familial microencephaly, retardation, and chorea
Beriberi	Oral contraceptives	Familial paroxysmal choreoathetosis
Cerebral lipidosis	Phenothiazine	Friedreich's ataxia
Hypocalcemia	Reserpine	Glutaric aciduria
Hypoglycemia	Scopolamine	Huntington's disease
Hypomagnesemia		Incontinentia pigmenti
Hypernatremia	*Infectious*	Lesch-Nyhan syndrome
Hypoparathyroidism	Diphtheria	Phenylketonuria
Kernicterus	Encephalitis	Porphyria
Phenylketonuria	Neurosyphilis	Sturge-Weber syndrome
Polycythemia	Pertussis	Wilson's disease
Porphyria	Poststreptococcal (Sydenham)	
Pregnancy	Typhoid fever	*Unknown and miscellaneous*
Thyrotoxicosis		Hyperkinetic syndrome
Vitamin B$_{12}$	*Vascular*	Intranuclear hyaline inclusion disease
deficiency	Anaphylactoid purpura (Henoch-Schonlein	Nevus lateralis
Wilson's disease	purpura)	Parietal chorea
	Cerebral infarction	
Degenerative	Lupus erythematosus	
(of unknown cause)	Posthemiplegic chorea	
Canavan spongy		
degeneration		

SOURCE: Modified from Swaiman KF: *Pediatric Neurology: Principles and Practice*, 2d ed. St. Louis: CV Mosby, 1994.

Chorea can be seen with multiple-system illnesses, such as lupus erythematosus, or even as a result of hyperthyroidism. There are numerous reports of chorea related to large doses of anticonvulsants or other toxins. Chorea can be one feature of numerous degenerative disorders, and it may be a feature of encephalopathy resulting from viral illnesses. Neuroacanthocytosis may present with chorea, but other neurological deficits, including peripheral neuropathy or facial tics, may be more obvious.[50,51] Recent reports emphasize vaccination as one additional cause for chorea,[52] but traditionally the reaction to the varicella virus is more commonly manifested as cerebellar ataxia or opsoclonus.

MYOCLONUS

Myoclonus in childhood is commonly observed by parents and can be an entirely benign phenomenon.[53] When, however, myoclonus is the harbinger of infantile spasms or other seizure phenomena it is far from innocent. Whenever myoclonus is present, it is reasonable to search for a seizure disorder, because progressive myoclonic phenomena linked with seizures can be particularly ominous for the child's future. Multiple epileptic syndromes manifest seizures with myoclonus, and the same is true of the numerous metabolic disorders of childhood. Many children have myoclonic jerks when they sleep, or as part of a parasomnia or sleep disorder, with or without night terrors. For the infant with generalized myoclonus, particularly when it is linked with "dancing eyes," neuroblastoma must be a consideration.

Many degenerative disorders are associated with myoclonus, particularly when the gray matter is involved (Table 49-7). Some children with degenerative disorders and myoclonus will have evoked responses that are intense, and, even-

TABLE 49-7 Classification of Myoclonus

Segmental

Type:	*Etiology:*
Brain stem	Vascular
Eye	Infectious
Palate	Demyelinating
Jaw	Neoplastic
Face and tongue	Traumatic
Spinal	Unknown
Neck	
Truncal or extremity	

Generalized myoclonus (cortical, subcortical, or brain stem involvement)

Acute or subacute
Encephalomyelitis
Toxic (tetanus, other infections, strychnine, other toxins)
Anoxic
Metabolic (uremia, hepatic insufficiency, other)
Degenerative

Chronic
Progressive myoclonus epilepsy (Lafora body epilepsy, lipidoses, system degeneration, or Ramsay Hunt syndrome)
Nonprogressive intermittent myoclonus with epilepsy
Essential myoclonus (paramyoclonus multiplex)
Nocturnal myoclonus

SOURCE: Modified from Swaiman KF: *Pediatric Neurology: Principles and Practices*, 2d ed. St. Louis: CV Mosby, 1994.

tually, do clearly manifest a seizure disorder. Paramyoclonus multiplex and nonepileptic jerking in the mornings on awakening may be difficult to distinguish from the myoclonic epilepsy of Janz.[54,55] Epileptic facial automatisms, jerks, or movements can present as a movement disorder. Although there are many nonepileptic paroxsymal events in childhood,[56] any child with sudden severe myoclonus or paroxysmal changes, e.g., a drop attack, warrants an electroencephalogram (EEG) as an initial step in discovery and treatment of a seizure disorder. Some of the recurrent events that are nonepileptic (including paroxysmal vertigo, shuddering attacks, breath-holding spells, syncope, etc.) can be diagnostically confusing. Worsening myoclonus may suggest a metabolic, hereditary, or infectious process and, as in all neurological illness, attention must be directed to sorting the benign from the serious (see also Chaps. 39 and 40).

There are a series of paroxysmal choreoathetotic phenomena that manifest as unusual responsiveness to stimulation, which is similar to the original description of the Mount Reback syndrome,[58] which is more prominent in childhood than in the later years of life. The startle syndromes[59,60] include a range from exaggerated normal startle to profound incapacity with any abrupt movement or sound. "Hyperekplexia" can be a familial disorder[61] and may be associated with echolalia, clumsiness, sudden jerky movements or even with acute prostration triggered by sound or startle.

Juvenile Parkinson's Disease

Patients with juvenile or early-onset parkinsonism may be considered as dystonic initially; however, in most cases, after conditions such as Wilson's disease have been ruled out, the diagnosis of parkinsonism is obvious, although always troublesome in the very young.[57] Clinical features are similar to those of adult PD, and treatment options are the same. There may be a predominance of rigidity, postural tremor, and dystonic features, and the response to medication may be very intense, with an initial brisk improvement followed after some years by severe fluctuations. Dementia is less common in the young, and hereditary patterns may be more common than in the more usual cases of idiopathic PD. (See also Chaps. 13, 14, and 26.)

Ataxia and Spasticity

Ataxia can be secondary to damage of various types to the cerebellar pathways,[62] including the classic Friedreich's ataxia, as so well-described in the review by Manyan.[63] In addition to the ataxia seen with Friedreich's disease there are usually associated physical findings that include evidence of posterior column dysfunction, diabetes, or cardiac dysfunction that make the diagnosis of Friedreich's disease relatively easy. The cerebellar degenerative diseases are numerous and controversial in classification, but they are closer to the threshold of definitive nosological distinction (see Chaps. 20 and 43).

Ataxia may be familial and periodic, consisting of paroxysmal episodes of ataxia combined with nystagmus. Some children complain of intermittent and almost inexplicable vertigo, and a few of these patients manifest subtle neurological deficits, even between episodes. Acetazolamide can eliminate the episodic ataxia for occasional patients.

Numerous inherited and degenerative disorders may present as ataxic syndromes, and they are well reviewed in standard pediatric neurology texts[4] (Tables 49-8 and 49-9).

Many disorders affecting the neuromuscular system initially can be misinterpreted as a movement disorder, for example, the patient with muscular dystrophy who has a waddling gait but does not appear overtly weak. It may be difficult with such a child to be certain early in the course of the disease whether or not the child is normal. Some normal infants scoot on their buttocks, rather than ever crawl and, yet, may walk at the proper time. Failure or a fear to ambulate in the young child can be an indication of significant dysfunction, including underlying imbalance.

Mirror movements, that is, overflow of movements into one hand when the other hand is being used, can be normal in a child.[64,65] The hemiplegic child is more likely to have associated mirror movements in the hemiplegic limb than the adult with hemiplegia. Nevertheless, mirror movements, which are often benign even when familial, may also be associated with platybasia and similar disorders of the upper cervical spine or cord.

The term "cerebral palsy" (CP) includes multiple disorders with multiple causes, with the implication that CP represents a static process that began before or around the time of birth (usually, perinatal hypoxia). The most common manifestations of CP include spasticity that is reflected in gait or choreathetosis (secondary to basal ganglia lesions). There may be eyes crossed as well as legs crossed, as pointed out a century ago, and mild athetosis or tremor may be linked with spasticity. Facial expression may be less vivacious, and may appear more "extrapyramidal," than for a normal child. Although spasticity, often worse in the legs, is the most common motor handicap, followed in frequency by choreathetosis and dystonia, a small subgroup of those with CP will be predominantly ataxic. In patients with CP there can be an associated mental retardation or a seizure disorder.

Spasticity can result from overt postnatal brain or cord trauma, and in either this posttraumatic state or the more usual CP, the condition may be stable or slowly improve during the years after the insult. Sometimes, when the insult has been exceptionally severe in childhood, after decades the process can retrogress, and the patient may actually slowly worsen. Whether or not this represents something like the "postpolio syndrome" is unknown. Such deterioration in CP or posttraumatic states usually occurs only when the spasticity and injuries have been extremely severe. In addition to the limb spasticity after head injury, there is often difficulty with hand coordination, and the motivational deficit so common in the adult with head injury may also be noted in the child with brain injury.

Congenital or familial difficulties can be relatively stable, but when they represent a rare but severe dominant disorder, such as HD, or a profound recessive disorder, such as Wilson's disease, the process can be progressive. Ataxia is common in almost all of the degenerative disorders of childhood, and it can be linked with behavioral changes and with loss of developmental milestones. Although most developmental disorders do not require an extensive workup, as was stated above, progressive disorders must be defined as fully as possible. Child abuse, malnutrition, or parental neglect can also produce apparent clumsiness in a child with partial failure to develop both physically and mentally. The different inherited metabolic disorders, although commonly causing generalized ataxia, can also lead to relatively specific or even unique neurological patterns, as in Wilson's disease, Lesch-Nyhan disease, glutaric acid deficiency, Leigh's syndrome, etc.

Some postinfectious conditions are not permanent and will tend to improve. For example, the cerebellar ataxia seen after chicken pox or similar viral disorders generally has a good prognosis, and the opsoclonus and other bizarre eye movement abnormalities of encephalitis are usually transient.

Paroxysmal Movement Disorders

For most movement disorders, the pattern of abnormality tends to remain similar during much of the day, unless medication or stress produces a shift from hypokinetic to hyperkinetic phenomena. There are, however, a series of movement disorders in which paroxysmal and abrupt shifts are the major characteristic. These conditions consist of involuntary

TABLE 49-9 Causes of Chronic or Progressive Ataxia

Hereditary
  Autosomal-dominant inheritance (including Machado-Joseph disease, olivopontocerebellar degeneration, Ramsay Hunt syndrome)
  Autosomal-recessive of mt DNA inheritance (including abetalipoproteinemia and hypobetalipoproteinemia, ataxia-ocular motor apraxia, ataxia-telangiectasia, ataxia with episodic dystonia, Friedreich's ataxia, juvenile gangliosidosis and lipidosis, Marinesco-Sjogren syndrome, pyruvate dysmetabolism, Refsum's disease, respiratory chain disorders, sea-blue histiocytosis)
  X-linked inheritance (including adrenoleukodystrophy)
Congenital malformations (including basilar impression, cerebellar aplasias, Chiari malformation)
Brain tumors

mt DNA, mitochondrial DNA

TABLE 49-8 Causes of Acute or Recurrent Ataxia

Conversion reaction, "pseudoataxia"
Migraine and benign paroxysmal vertigo
Genetic disorders (including dominant recurrent ataxia, Hartnup's disease, maple syrup urine and other metabolic disorders, paroxysmal ataxia and myokymia)
Vascular disorders (including cerebellar hemorrhage, Kawasaki's disease, lupus erythematosus)
Encephalitis
Presumed postinfectious or immune disorder (acute postinfectious cerebellitis, Miller Fisher's syndrome, myoclonic encephalopathy, neuroblastoma, multiple sclerosis)
Brain tumor
Trauma
Drug ingestion

jerks, twitches, or flinging movements without any associated loss of consciousness. At times the movements occur with absolutely no premonition, but for some patients an aura occurs. In this group of disorders the patients are conscious, and when they fall they are quite aware that they are falling. It may be very difficult to distinguish some of these movements from a seizure. As a rule when the patient has a loss of consciousness, seizures should be strongly considered. Classic drop attacks in childhood may be associated with EEG phenomena similar to those seen with absence attacks, and the EEG phenomena may be so brief and the episodes so infrequent that they are missed during a routine EEG.

Acquired forms of paroxysmal movement disorders that are not genetic include multiple sclerosis, which is uncommon in childhood but does occur. The paroxysmal disorders of multiple sclerosis include tetanic spasms of the limbs or trunk. The attacks tend to be brief, and although they are usually dystonic they may appear choreoathetotic in pattern. As a group the patients with multiple sclerosis are most likely to have flexor spasms of the limbs, and these usually respond to anticonvulsants. Paroxysmal episodes can occasionally occur in endocrine disorders.

Paroxysmal dystonic choreoathetosis has become the common label for the disease that afflicts patients who manifest brief dystonic episodes.[69] The spells last only a few seconds, or for up to 5 minutes. Attacks can be precipitated by movement, but there can be overlap between these and similar conditions that are associated with sudden dystonic movements in response to abrupt sounds. Paroxysmal dystonic choreoathetosis tends to be inherited, and, in some families, it is inherited as an autosomal-dominant disorder.

Paroxysmal kinesiogenic choreoathetosis has had many other names.[70,71] In this condition the abnormal movement follows a brisk or sudden event, such as hitting a ball, attempting to run, etc. The episodes are brief and consist of more sudden and overt twisting than is true of dystonia, and the spells may occur several times a day. Occasionally, these patients have a sense of "tightness" before the episode. As a rule this paroxysmal condition begins in childhood, and a dominant inheritance may be present, although in some families a recessive pattern has been suggested. For all of these paroxysmal conditions and startle syndromes, there should be trials of anticonvulsant medications, but these may not be successful.

Miscellaneous Disorders

The neurology of movement disorders includes numerous miscellaneous disorders of unknown etiology.

Stereotypy has been considered a habit pattern or ritualistic behavior. As many as 10 percent of normal infants develop repetitive phenomena such as head banging, head rolling, or rocking, but this usually passes after the first several years. When head banging occurs, it is distressing for parents. More common in boys, as is true of many of the aggressive behavioral phenomena, the explanation for childhood head banging remains unclear.

Normal children, as normal adults, may display finger gestures or movements of various kinds, some of which have cultural meanings and some of which seem purely random. In Rett syndrome, seen in girls, repetitive hand-wringing movements may occur, along with progressive mental retardation and seizures.[72] Stereotyped posturing in response to numerous stimuli has been reported in children with basal ganglia diseases. Episodic hyperextension of the head or flexion during sleep or just before sleep may be entirely normal, but severe spasms in childhood can raise the possibility of tetanus, a seizure disorder, or hypocalcemia and other metabolic disorders.

The relationship between generalized hyperactivity and movement disorders is not entirely clear. Many children with chronic brain damage are indeed hyperactive, and this may be associated with distractibility and impulsivity. Akathisia consists of pathological restlessness and is typically seen with the extrapyramidal disorders. Most feel an irresistible need to move and manifest overt restlessness. They may also complain of insomnia. Restless leg syndrome, which has been linked to pregnancy, genetics, anemia,[73,74] and extrapyramidal disease, can be noted in adolescence (see also Chap. 51). It is possible that some of the children, who were once told they had "growing pains," had a variant of restless leg syndrome.

Numerous periodic movements in sleep have been reported and consist particularly of flexion or extension of the hip or knee. These seem to be quite common in childhood, although their incidence has been inadequately documented. Bruxism is characteristically seen in otherwise-normal children, and, folk wisdom notwithstanding, it is not usually associated with parasites or undue daytime anxiety. Bruxism can be familial. The amount of pressure against the surface of the teeth is immense, and other than wear and tear of the teeth and occasional pain in the temporal or masseter muscles, bruxism is usually harmless.

Psychological Problems Associated with Movement Disorders

Far more common than misidentification of movement disorders are their psychological consequences. The detection and diagnosis of primarily psychogenic movement disorders, as with the psychogenic gait disturbance of astasia-abasia or psychogenic myoclonus, can be difficult and uncertainty may lead to unnecessary medication (see also Chap. 52). The majority of patients with psychogenic movement disorders do not appear overtly disturbed emotionally, as is true for many children with psychogenic seizures. Nonetheless, psychiatric counseling and intervention should usually be sought, even though it may be relatively fruitless. Most patients have access to a video record, and prolonged video and electroencephalographic monitoring may be helpful in the diagnosis of psychogenic phenomena, but there is no substitute for evaluation by an experienced clinician.

Movement disorders not only produce physical handicaps but also may lead to persistent and lifelong disability secondary to embarrassment and social withdrawal. Secondary problem behaviors can limit the child's activities of daily living, school performance, and social interaction. Stress may exacerbate the abnormal movements. Severe emotional stress may even be increased by sincere efforts at rehabilitation, leading to adverse secondary consequences that limit the efficacy of physical therapy and similar measures. Management is far from simple and requires sustained effort by patient, family, and therapists.

The child with a movement disorder is often of normal intelligence, but some have attention deficit disorder or another neurobehavioral dysfunction. For example, children of average intelligence with Tourette's syndrome may continue to suffer from attentional problems into adulthood. Children with fine motor disabilities and coordination difficulties who also have lower initial IQs, school achievement, and developmental test scores appear to show an increase in troublesome behavior, hyperactivity, and decreased ability to concentrate. Children with Wilson's disease may suffer not only from major psychiatric complications and clumsiness but also from a disability in memory. Symptomatic patients with Wilson's disease exhibit greater psychological difficulties than those who carry the gene but are yet asymptomatic.[75]

Because motor impairment can significantly confound school performance, a child may appear below average, although his or her intelligence is not. An inappropriate but common response is to educate the child with a movement disorder among the mentally subnormal. When problems are left unaddressed, such individuals may suffer from, at best, psychological trauma that can have profound implications for self-esteem and future success. Learning problems may continue during adolescence, even as neurological signs diminish. Nevertheless, puberty tends to offer a normalizing effect in many adolescents, with only the most severe cases persisting. Adolescents with a history of hypotonia or coordination problems often eventually demonstrate behavior and cognitive skills comparable to those of their normal peers.[76,77]

It is the responsibility of the physician to help educate teachers and school personnel, as well as family members, regarding the significance of dystonia or other movement disorders. Behavioral therapy, physical therapy with active parental participation, and a carefully structured educational program for the child can be valuable adjuncts to medical treatment. In the absence of a cure, successful management of a child with a movement abnormality begins with correct diagnosis and should include a comprehensive treatment plan. Specialists in health care other than neurology, but such as psychiatry, social work, or rehabilitation, offer hope, adjustment, and practical advice to the child and parent. The medical therapist may seek resolution without medications, using a team approach and avoiding the potential complications of drug therapy.

The impact of the movement disorder on the patient is not determined solely by the diagnostic label or limited to physical, behavioral, and mental impairments. The extent of physical and occupational disability and the social handicap may be the most important determinants of the impact of the underlying biological impairment.[78] Disability thus refers to the effect of the impairment on an individual's capabilities, for example, on walking, writing, and talking, as well as to the effects of primary or secondary behavioral changes resulting from the disorder. Complete diagnosis implies both a neurological label and a determination of disability.

A child's ability to overcome or adjust to disabilities depends, in part, on the child's and the family's personal resources, and the extent of disability may not necessarily be identical with the degree of physical impairment. The level of ultimate disability also results partly from the societal response, especially from peers, to the child's handicap. Failure to meet perceived norms can produce impediments to functional independence and lead to ultimate discrimination. Limitations of our present medical interventions necessitates awareness from all relevant therapists of the potential for help from multiple, and often nonmedical, sources. The medical counselor is, of course, often limited because of lack of certainty in prognosis, as with dystonias, or is limited by the absence of therapy, as with HD. Nevertheless, the child and the family can be comforted and helped greatly by a careful neurological assessment and team approach to treatment. Because so often diagnosis, therapy, and prognosis are all uncertain on a patient's first visit, an active and planned follow-up often becomes the best diagnostic test. In the process the physician often becomes friend and counselor to the family, and the rewards to all, including to the physician, can be immeasurable.

References

1. Jankovic J, Fahn S: Dystonic disorders, in Jankovic J, Tolosa E (eds): *Parkinson's Disease and Movement Disorders*, 2d ed. Baltimore: Williams & Wilkins, 1993, pp 337–374.
2. Narabayaski H, Yokochi M, Iizuka R, Nagatsu T: Juvenile parkinsonism, in Vinken PJ, Bruyn GW, Klawans HL (eds): *Handbook of Clinical Neurology: Extrapyramidal Disorders*. New York: Elsevier, 1986, vol 5(49), 1986, pp 153–165.
3. Paulson GW: Diagnosis of Huntington's disease. *Adv Neurol* 23:177–184, 1979.
4. Swaiman KF: *Pediatric Neurology: Principles and Practice*, 2nd ed. St. Louis: Mosby-Year Book, 1994.
5. Volpe JJ: *Neurology of the Newborn*, 3d ed. Philadelphia: WB Saunders, 1994.
6. Prechtl HFR: *Continuity of Neurological Functions from Prenatal to Postnatal Life*. Oxford, England: Spastics International Medical, 1984.
7. Volpe JJ: *Neurology of the Newborn*, 3d ed. Philadelphia: WB Saunders, 1994.
8. Resnick TJ, Moshi SL, Perotta L, et al: Benign neonatal sleep myoclonus: Relationship to sleep states. *Arch Neurol* 43:266–268, 1986.
9. Butler IJ: Movement disorders of children. *Pediatr Clin North Am* 39(4):727–742, 1992.
10. Lees AJ, Tolosa E: Tics, in Jankovic J, Tolosa E (eds): *Parkinson's Disease and Movement Disorders*, 2d ed. Baltimore: Williams & Wilkins, 1993, pp 329–335.
11. Lees AJ: Facial mannerisms and tics. *Adv Neurol* 49:255–261, 1988.
12. Pranzatelli MR: Miscellaneous movement disorders of childhood. *Pediatr Ann* 22:65–68, 1993.
13. Soorani-Lunsing RJ, Hadders-Algra M, Huisjes HJ, Touwen BC: Neurobehavioral relationships after the onset of puberty. *Dev Med Child Neurol* 36(4):334–343, 1994.
14. Bender L: Childhood schizophrenia: Clinical study of 100 schizophrenic children. *Am J Orthopsychiatry* 17:40, 1947.
15. Ford F: *Diseases of the Nervous System in Infancy, Childhood and Adolescence*, 6th ed. Springfield, IL: Charles C Thomas, 1973.

16. Pranzatelli MR: An approach to movement disorders of childhood. *Pediatr Ann* 22:13–16, 1993.

17. Jankovic J: The neurology of tics, in Marsden CD, Fahn S. (eds): *Movement Disorders 2*. London: Butterworth, 1987, pp 383–405.

18. Singer HS, Walkup JT: Tourette's syndrome and other tic disorders: Diagnosis, pathophysiology, and treatment. *Medicine* 70(1):15–32, 1991.

19. Swedo SE, Leonard HL: Childhood movement disorders and obsessive compulsive disorder. *J Clin Psychiatry* 55(suppl):32–37, 1994.

20. Frank MS, Sieg KG, Gaffney GR: Somatic complaints in childhood tic disorders. *Psychosomatics* 32(4):396–399, 1991.

21. Goetz CG: Tics: Gilles de la Tourette's syndrome, in Vinken PJ, Bruyn GW, Klawans HL(eds): *Handbook of Clinical Neurology*. Amsterdam: Elsevier, 1986, vol 5(49), pp 627–639.

22. Pauls DL, Leckman JF: The inheritance of Gille de la Tourette's syndrome and associated behavior: Evidence for autosomal dominant transmission. *N Engl J Med* 315:993–997, 1986.

23. Rodgers D, Hymas N: Sporadic facial stereotypies in patients with schizophrenia and compulsive disorders. *Adv Neurol* 49:383–394, 1988.

24. Paulson GW: Benign essential tremor in childhood. *Clin Pediatr* 15:67–70, 1976.

25. Findley LJ: Tremors: Differential diagnosis and pharmacology, in Jankovic J and Tolosa E.(eds): *Parkinson's Disease and Movement Disorders*, 2nd ed. Baltimore: Williams & Wilkins, 1993, pp 293–313.

26. Shuper A, Zalzberg J, Weitz R, Mimouni M: Jitteriness beyond the neonatal period: A benign pattern of movement in infancy. *J Child Neurol* 6(3):243–245, 1991.

27. Volpe JJ: *Neurology of the Newborn*, 3rd ed. Philadelphia: WB Saunders, 1994.

28. Mizrahi EM: Epileptic facial automatisms and head movements. *Adv Neurol* 49:274–287, 1988.

29. Lance JW: Sporadic and familial forms of tonic seizures. *J Neurol Neurosurg Psychiatry* 26:51–59, 1963.

30. Snyder CH: Paroxysmal torticollis in infancy. *Am J Dis Child* 117:458, 1969.

31. Boyd K, Patterson V: Dopa responsive dystonia: A treatable condition misdiagnosed as cerebral palsy. *Br Med J* 298:1019–1020, 1989.

32. Nygaard TG, Marsden CD, Fahn S: Dopa responsive dystonia: Long term treatment response and prognosis. *Neurology* 41:174–181, 1991.

33. Rowland LP: The first decade of molecular genetics in neurology: Changing clinical thought and practice. *Ann Neurol* 32(2):207–214, 1992.

34. Greene PE, Fahn S: Baclofen in the treatment of idiopathic dystonia in children. *Mov Disord* 7(1):48–52, 1992.

35. Swett C: Drug induced dystonia. *Am J Psychol* 123:532–534, 1975.

36. Lang AE: Miscellaneous drug induced movement disorders, in Lang AE, Weiner WJ (eds): *Drug Induced Movement Disorders*. Mt. Kisco, New York: Futura, 1992, pp 339–381.

37. Tolosa E, Alom J, Marti MJ: Drug induced dyskinesias, in Jankovic J, Tolosa E (eds): *Parkinson's Disease and Movement Disorders*, 2nd ed. Baltimore: Williams & Wilkins, 1993, pp 375–397.

38. Brett EM: Some syndromes of involuntary movements, in *Pediatric Neurology*, 2nd ed. New York: Churchill-Livingstone, 1991, pp 271–283.

39. Nausieda PA: Sydenham's chorea, chorea gravidarum and contraceptive-induced chorea, in Vinken PJ, Bruyn GW, Klawans HL (eds): *Handbook of Clinical Neurology*. Amsterdam: Elsevier, 1986, vol 5(49), pp 359–367.

40. Paulson GW. William Osler's views on chorea. *Adv Neurol* 1:41–44, 1973.

41. Bird M, Paulson G: The rigid form of Huntington's chorea. *Neurology* 21:271–276, 1971.

42. Bruyn GW, Myrianthopoulos NC: Chronic juvenile hereditary chorea (benign hereditary chorea of early onset), in Vinken PJ, Bruyn GW, Klawans HL (eds): *Handbook of Clinical Neurology*. Amsterdam: Elsevier, 1986, vol 5(49), pp 335–348.

43. Salam-Adams M, Adams RD: Acquired hepatocerebral syndromes, in Vinken PJ, Bruyn GW, Klawans HL (eds): *Handbook of Clinical Neurology*. Amsterdam: Elsevier, 1986, vol 5(49), pp 213–221.

44. Salam-Adams M, Adams RD: Athetotic syndromes, in Vinken PJ, Bruyn GW, Klawans HL (eds): *Handbook of Clinical Neurology*. Amsterdam: Elsevier, 1986, vol 5(49), pp 381–389.

45. Spiegel EA, Baird HW: Athetotic syndrome, in Vinken PJ, Bruyn GW (eds): *Handbook of Clinical Neurology: Diseases of Basal Ganglia*. Amsterdam: North-Holland, 1968, vol 6, pp 440–475.

46. Seitelberger F: Neuroaxonal dystrophy: Its relation to aging and neurological diseases, in Vinken PJ, Bruyn GW, Klawans HL (eds): *Handbook of Clinical Neurology*. Amsterdam: Elsevier, 1986, vol 5(49), pp 391–415.

47. Lowenthal A: Striopallidodentate calcifications, in Vinken PJ, Bruyn GW, Klawans HL (eds): *Handbook of Clinical Neurology*. Amsterdam, Elsevier, pp 417–436, 1986.

48. Iizuka R, Hirayama K: Dentato-rubro-pallido-luysian atrophy, in Vinken PJ, Bruyn GW, Klawans HL(eds): *Handbook of Clinical Neurology*. Amsterdam: Elsevier, 1986, vol 5(49), pp 437–443.

49. Jellinger K: Exogenous lesions of the pallidum, in Vinken PJ, Bruyn GW, Klawans HL(eds): *Handbook of Clinical Neurology*. Amsterdam: Elsevier, 1986, vol 5(49), pp 465–491.

50. Bruyn GW. Chorea-acanthocytosis, in Vinken PJ, Bruyn GW, Klawans HL(eds): *Handbook of Clinical Neurology*. Amsterdam: Elsevier, 1986, vol 5(49), pp 327–334.

51. Spitz MC, Jankovic J, Killian JM: Familial tic disorder, parkinsonism, motor neuron disease, and acanthocytosis: A new syndrome. *Neurology* 35:366–370, 1985.

52. Plesner AM: Gait disturbances after measles, mumps, and rubella vaccine. *Lancet* 345:316, 1995.

53. Lombroso CT, Fejerman N: Benign myoclonus of early infancy. *Ann Neurol* 1:38–43, 1977.

54. Delgado-Escueta AV, Eenrile-Bacsal F: Juvenile myoclonus of Janz. *Neurology* 34:285, 1984.

55. Murphy JV, Dehkharghani F: Diagnosis of childhood seizure disorders. *Epilepsia* 35(suppl 2):S7–17, 1994.

56. Golden GS: Nonepileptic paroxysmal events in childhood. *Pediatr Clin North Am* 39(4):715–725, 1992.

57. Gershanik OS: Early onset parkinsonism, in Jankovic J, Tolosa E (eds): *Parkinson's Disease and Movement Disorders*, 2nd ed. Baltimore: Williams & Wilkins, 1993, pp 235–252.

58. Mount LA, Reback S. Familial paroxysmal choreoathetosis: Preliminary report on a hitherto undescribed clinical syndrome. *Arch Neurol* 44:841–846, 1990.

59. Marsden CD, Fahn S: Problems in the dyskinesias, in Marsden CD, Fahn S (eds): *Movement Disorders 2*. Boston: Butterworth, 1987, pp 311–312.

60. Andermann F, Andermann E: Excessive startle syndrome: Startle disease, jumping and startle epilepsy. *Adv Neurol* 43:321–338, 1986.

61. Tijssen MA, Shiang R, Van Deutekom J, et al: Molecular genetic reevaluation of the Dutch hyperekplexia family. *Arch Neurol* 52:578–582, 1995.

62. Lechtenberg R: Ataxia and other cerebellar syndromes, in Jankovic J, Tolosa E(eds): *Parkinson's Disease and Movement Disorders*, 2nd ed. Baltimore: Williams & Wilkins, 1993, pp 419–431.

63. Manyan BV: Friedreich's disease, in deJong JMBV (ed): *Handbook of Clinical Neurology: Hereditary Neuropathies and Spinocerebellar Atrophies*. New York: Elsevier, 1991, vol 16(60), pp 299–333.

64. Rasmussen P: Persistent mirror movements: A clinical study of 17 children, adolescents and young adults. *Dev Med Child Neurol* 35(8):699–707, 1993.

65. Cohen LG, Meer J, Tarkka I, et al: Congenital mirror movements. Abnormal organization of motor pathways in two patients. *Brain* (114):381–403, 1991.

66. Paulson GW, Dadmehr N: Hallervorden-Spatz disease, in Rosenberg RN, Prusiner SB, Mauro S, Barchi RL (eds): *The Molecular and Genetic Basis of Neurological Disease*. Newton, MA, Butterworth-Heinimann, 1992, pp 343–348.

67. Kinsbourne, M: Hiatus hernia with contortions of the neck. *Lancet* 1:1058–1061, 1964.

68. Menkes JH, Ament ME: Neurologic disorders of gastroesophageal function, *Adv Neurol* 49:409–416, 1988.

69. Lance JW: Familial paroxysmal dystonic choreoathetosis and its differential from related syndromes. *Ann Neurol* 2:285–293, 1977.

70. Plant GT: Focal paroxysmal kinesiogenic choreoathetosis. *J Neurol Neurosurg Psychiatry* 46:345–348, 1983.

71. Buruma OJS, Roos RAC: Paroxysmal choreoathetosis, in Vinken PJ, Bruyn GW (eds): *Handbook of Clinical Neurology*. Amsterdam: New-Holland Publishing Co, 1986, vol 5(49), pp 344–355.

72. Hagberg B, Aicardi J, Dias K, et al: A progressive syndrome of autism, dementia, ataxia and loss of purposeful hand use in girls: Rett's syndrome. Report of 35 cases. *Ann Neurol* 14:471–479, 1983.

73. Ekbom KA: Restless leg syndrome. *Neurology* 10:868–873, 1960.

74. Lugaresi E, Cirignotta F, Coccagna G, Montagna P: Nocturnal myoclonus and restless leg syndrome. *Adv Neurol* 43:295, 1986.

75. Medalia A, Galynker I, Scheinberg IH: The interaction of motor, memory, and emotional dysfunction in Wilson's disease. *Biol Psychiatry* 31(8):823–826, 1992.

76. Kalverborg AF: Neurobehavioral study in pre-school children, in *Clinics in Developmental Medicine*, No. 54. London: Spastics International Medical Publications, 1975.

77. Soorani-Lunsing RJ, Huisier HJ, Touwen BCL: Minor neurological dysfunction after the onset of puberty: association with specific prenatal events. *Early Hum Dev* 33:71–80, 1993.

78. World Health Organization: *International Classification of Impairment, Distribution and Handicaps: A Manual of Classification Relating to the Consequences of Disease*. Geneva: World Health Organization, 1980.

Chapter 50

MOVEMENT DISORDERS AND AGING

ALI H. RAJPUT

DISTINCTION BETWEEN NORMAL AGING AND
  MOVEMENT DISORDERS
    Akinesia/Hypokinesia/Bradykinesia and Old Age
    Tone Changes and Old Age
    Hyperkinetic Disorders and Old Age
    Station, Posture, Postural Reflexes, and Old Age
    Gait Abnormality and Old Age
    Gait Apraxia
    Ophthalmoplegia in the Elderly and in Movement
      Disorders
    Primitive Reflexes in Movement Disorders and the
      Elderly
CONSIDERATION OF MOVEMENT DISORDERS THAT
  ARE CONCENTRATED IN OLD AGE
    Parkinsonism in the Elderly
    Drug-Induced Parkinsonism
    Essential Tremor in the Elderly
    Stroke and Movement Disorders
    Orofacial Dyskinesias in the Elderly
MOVEMENT DISORDERS ASSOCIATED WITH OTHER
  NEURODEGENERATIVE DISEASES IN THE ELDERLY
SPECIAL CONSIDERATION OF MOVEMENT
  DISORDERS MANAGEMENT IN THE ELDERLY

There is no uniformly agreed upon definition of old age. For the purpose of this chapter, the usual retirement age of 65 years will be used as the start of old age.[1-4] The proportion of elderly in the general population has been steadily rising in Western countries for several decades.[5] The prevalence of aging-related disorders in the population has, therefore, been increasing. Several movement disorders (MD) are concentrated in old age, and some features of normal aging resemble MD.

Posture and gait, to a large extent, depend on normal vestibular, visual, proprioceptive, postural sway adjustment and motor functions. With advancing age there is decline in vestibular,[6] visual,[7,8] and proprioceptive[9] functions. The postural sway increases[10,11] and the muscle mass decreases progressively[12] in old age. Old age is also associated with slowed speed of motor activity, reduced vibration sensation in feet, reduced ankle jerks,[9] memory decline,[9,13] reduced vertical gaze,[13] and emergence of primitive reflexes.[13,14] Together, these anatomic and physiological changes lead to alteration in station, posture, gait, postural reflexes, motor functions, and extraocular movements—all well-known features in some movement disorders.

The elderly are liable to suffer from other systemic diseases,[5] from malnutrition,[15] and to take multiple prescription drugs.[1,5,16-18] The frequency and the severity of drug side ef-

fects, including MD,[19-29] increase with advancing age.[5,30] When compared with those of young adults, the drug adverse effects occur twice as frequently in patients 60 years and older, and those over age 80 years have a 25% risk of intoxication with some drugs.[5]

Several common MD are concentrated in the elderly,[2,3,19,31-33] and there is an increased concentration of other neurological illnesses, such as Alzheimer's disease and stroke, which may simulate or be associated with movement abnormalities in the elderly.[34-38]

The appropriate chapters in this volume will cover MD in greater detail. This chapter will concentrate on age-related changes that resemble MD and those aspects of MD that require special considerations in the old age.

Distinction Between Normal Aging and Movement Disorders

The MD can be broadly classified into (a) hypokinetic and (b) hyperkinetic disorders. These two clinical features, tremor (hyperkinesia) and bradykinesia (hypokinesia), typically coexist in Parkinson's syndrome (PS). Motor slowing; abnormalities of posture, gait, and extraocular movements; and the presence of primitive reflexes that are characteristic of some MD, are also part of normal aging. Because there are no biological markers to distinguish between age-related findings and MD, their significance in the elderly is based on careful clinical assessment.[13,14,39-44]

AKINESIA/HYPOKINESIA/BRADYKINESIA AND OLD AGE

The akinesia/hypokinesia/bradykinesia complex, usually referred to as bradykinesia, is characterized by slowed movement initiation, small amplitude of movement, and reduced motor velocity.[45] Bradykinesia is a common feature in PS.[24,45,46] Slowed motor performance is also a part of normal aging.[9,47] Clinical assessment is the main tool used to differentiate normal slowing down from MD-related bradykinesia. Table 50-1 is a summary of clinical features that are helpful in distinguishing age-related slowing from hypokinetic MD and some other disorders that produce motor slowing.

Focal pain producing pathology and mechanical restriction at a joint lead to reduced focal movement and, therefore, may be mistaken for bradykinesia. Careful examination of the suspected joint and testing for bradykinesia at an unaffected joint will help ascertain the nature of the problem. Detailed assessment of sensory functions, tone, muscle strength, and reflexes, as noted in Table 50-1, are valuable adjuncts used to distinguish hypokinetic MD from other neurological diseases and from normal age-related slowing. Age-related slowing is symmetrical and generalized whereas hypokinesia from MD is often asymmetrical.

TONE CHANGES AND OLD AGE

Testing for tone is dependent on a patient's ability to comprehend, follow instructions, and cooperate. In normal elderly persons, there is no change in the muscle tone. In cognitive and in language-impaired elderly persons, there may be an

TABLE 50-1 Normal Aging and Hypokinetic Disorders

	Normal Aging-Related Slowing	Focal Pathology Emulating Slowing	Movement Disorder (PS, dystonia)-Related Slowing	Other NS Pathology (central or peripheral)-Causing Slowing
Symmetry of findings	Symmetrical	Asymmetrical	Often asymmetrical	Frequently asymmetrical
Focal examination	Normal	Abnormal	Normal	Normal
Tone	Normal	Normal (if pain and joint movement restriction discounted). Testing at unaffected joint helpful to identify normal tone.	Increased (rigidity or dystonia)	May have paratonia Spasticity when there is corticospinal involvement Decreased when there is lower motor neuron pathology
Sensory function	Normal (except vibration reduction in feet)	As in normal aging	As in normal aging	May be impaired, depending on nature of lesion
Reflexes	Normal symmetrical (ankle jerks may be hypoactive), plantars flexor	As in normal aging	As in normal aging	Hyperactive with extensor plantar or hypoactive, depending on site of lesion. Frequently asymmetrical.
Strength	Normal	Normal, but patient unable to fully exert because of pain or joint restriction	Normal in PS (if repeatedly tested), may appear reduced in dystonia	Reduced or inconsistent

PS, Parkinson's syndrome; NS, nervous system

apparent increase in tone known as paratonia (gegenhalten).[42] Paratonia is characterized either by progressively increasing resistance to an attempted passive movement in any direction *or* an irregular unpredictable opposition to passive movement and may be mistaken for cogwheel rigidity.[13,21,42] Making this distinction is possible in most cases upon careful clinical assessment (Table 50-2).

The two main forms of increased resistance to passive movements in MD are rigidity and dystonia. Rigidity is characterized by sustained resistance through the range of passive movement, is of equal severity in opposite directions at a joint, that is, flexor and extensor movement would have comparable resistance,[48] and is reproducible. Cogwheel rigidity is characteristic of PS patients who also manifest tremor. Based on personal experience, the author submits that cogwheel rigidity can also be detected when there is no visible tremor.

Dystonia is characterized by cocontraction of agonist and antagonist muscles. The force of muscle contraction is, however, unequal in the opposing groups of muscles, thus resulting in dystonic movement or dystonic posture. Although the resistance to passive movement is increased in all directions, the degree of hypertonicity depends on the direction of attempted movement. The resistance is more pronounced when the passive movement counteracts the dystonic posture than when the movement is attempted in the same direction as that of the dystonic movement or posture. A passive movement away from the sustained dystonic posture may be interrupted by irregular jerks, indicating dystonic tremor.

Increased tone is also a feature of corticospinal tract dysfunction known as spasticity. It is characterized by a velocity-dependent "catch" which is followed by a release without further increase in resistance through the remainder of the movement, that is, the clasp knife phenomenon. By contrast,

in rigidity the increased tone is evident through the entire range of movement (i.e., "plastic"). In mild corticospinal dysfunction the tone abnormality may not be easily distinguishable from rigidity. One helpful maneuver is to let an extended knee of the patient suddenly drop over the examiner's arm and observe the flexion pattern at the knee joint as the leg drops downward. Spastic leg manifests as one extensor "catch," which is followed by the heel rapidly falling downward. The rigid leg, by contrast, falls slowly at a relatively steady velocity until the movement is completed.

The tendon reflexes are, for all practical purposes, normal in MD, except that they may be difficult to elicit when optimal positioning is prevented by dystonia. In some extrapyramidal disease patients there is spontaneous or gait-related dystonic extension of the big toe on the affected side. When the plantar reflex is attempted, that toe will either flex or its extended position will become less pronounced. Such toe abnormality is known as striatal toe.[49] The presence of hyperreflexia and extensor-plantar response support spasticity.

Any joint movement that produces pain will be involuntarily guarded and may, therefore, be mistaken as rigidity. Mechanical restriction to movement can also simulate hypertonicity. Examination of the affected joint for pain and range of movement and tone assessment at a nonaffected joint will help clarify this situation.

Cogwheeling phenomenon, which is characterized by *rhythmic* interruption of attempted passive movement,[48,50] is seen in patients with medium-to-large amplitude tremor. The cogwheel rigidity in PS typically lacks the rhythmicity that is characteristic of the cogwheeling phenomenon. Rhythmic *resistance* to passive movement, which is detected only with reinforcement, that is, voluntary motor activity at a distant, noncontiguous part of body, is known as Froment's sign. It may be detected in a variety of disorders in which

TABLE 50-2 Muscle Tone Changes in Normal Elderly, Movement Disorders, and Selected Conditions

	Normal Elderly	(a) Rigidity and (b) Dystonia	Spasticity (Mild)	Paratonia (Gegenhalten)	Cogwheeling Phenomenon (Froment's Sign)
Characteristic	Equal and normal resistance in all directions of movement	(a) Resistance sustained and equal in opposite directions of movement; reproducible (b) Increased tone different when passive movement is with rather than when against dystonic posture	Increased tone, velocity-dependent catch: "clasp-knife"	Irregular, unpredictable, intermittently increased tone or progressively greater resistance on attempted movement	*Rhythmic* interruption of passive movement coinciding with tremor; rhythmic resistance to passive movement seen only on reinforcement in tremor-producing conditions (Froments sign)
Symmetry	Symmetrical	Usually asymmetrical	Frequently asymmetrical	Usually symmetrical	May be symmetrical or asymmetrical, depending on tremor location
Reflexes	Normal; reduced at ankles and plantars flexor	Normal (may be difficult to elicit when there is pronounced dystonia)—striatal toe	Exaggerated and extensor plantar response	Usually normal	Normal
Tremor	Absent	Frequently part of PD	Absent	Absent	Prominent feature
Reinforcement Related Tone Increase	No significant change; minimal when there is any and is symmetrical	Usually asymmetrical increase	May increase slightly asymmetrically	Unpredictable change	Rhythmic symmetrical increase (Froment's sign)

tremor is the prominent feature, for example, essential tremor (ET) and Parkinson's disease (PD).[48] Table 50-2 is a summary of tone changes in normal elderly, major MD, and selected other conditions.

HYPERKINETIC DISORDERS AND OLD AGE

The most common hyperkinetic disorder in adults is tremor.[43,51-53] Rautakorpi et al.[53] noted tremor in 25 percent of the general population over 40 years of age in Finland. The most common tremor-associated MD in adults are ET and PS[51]—both of which are concentrated in old age.[19,31-33,51,53,54] For other illnesses, the elderly take a large number of drugs, including tricyclics, monoamine oxidase inhibitors, antihistamines, valproate, anticholinergics, corticosteroids, calcium-channel blockers, amiodarone, lithium, sympatheticomimetic drugs, drugs for asthma, such as isoproterenol, terbutaline, methylxanthines (theophylline), each of that may produce tremor.[1,44,55,56] Nutritional disorders, other systemic illnesses, and metabolic diseases, such as hyperthyroidism, which accentuate physiological tremor or produce pathological tremor are also more common in old age.[15,44,53,56] In those patients more than 65 years of age, the prevalence of tremor is, therefore, greater than the 25 percent reported in the population over more than 40 years old.[53] The high prevalence rate of tremor in old age has sometimes been erroneously interpreted as an indication that tremor is part of normal aging. There is no evidence that old age by itself leads to tremor production.[13,44,46,47,50,57,58] All tremors are pathological or are enhanced physiological manifestations of drugs or other stresses.

STATION, POSTURE, POSTURAL REFLEXES, AND OLD AGE

The manner or attitude of standing is known as "station," and the position of the whole body and its different parts indicates the posture. As noted above, visual,[7,8] vestibular,[6] and proprioceptive functions[9] decline, and the normal postural sway in the standing position increases[10,11] with aging. Dizziness, characterized by a sensation of instability, is a common symptom in the elderly.[6,59,60] By 65 years of age 30 percent and by 80 years of age approximately 66 percent of the general population have experienced dizziness at some time or another.[60] In general, the sensation of stability in the standing position declines with old age. Because of that, the normal elderly have a slightly widened base when standing or walking[9] (see also Chap. 48).

Posture in the elderly is slightly flexed at the neck and trunk in the standing position, with the knees and elbows remaining straight. Flexed neck, trunk, hips, knees, and elbows are features of PS, except in PSP, in which the posture is unduly erect. Advanced PS patients have difficulty maintaining an erect posture for more than several seconds, whereas normal elderly can do that easily.

The ability to regain balance in response to spontaneous body sway or after active perturbation depends on the integrity of postural reflexes. Maki et al.[10] noted that both the spontaneous and the induced sway are exaggerated in the normal elderly. In old age there is significantly increased sway velocity, both with eyes open and closed,[11] that is most pronounced in those who fear falling.[11] Duncan et al.[61] noted that elderly with poor balance have impairment of at least two of the three related processes regulating balance—sensory, effector, and central processing—and concluded that a cumulative, rather than a single, deficit is the basis of impaired mobility.[61]

Postural stability is clinically tested as follows. The patient, while standing with eyes open and feet comfortably apart, is asked to resist the examiner's pull. He or she is instructed to take one step, when necessary, to regain balance in response to the pull and is assured that the examiner will prevent falling. Depending on the size of the patient and the force of the pull, any individual may be displaced. The examiner first applies a *modest* forward pull.[40,41,62] This is then followed by a similar backward pull.[40,41,62] When the patient takes one or two steps, the postural reflexes are considered normal. When three to four steps are taken the posture is considered to be minimally abnormal, and more than four steps indicate definitely impaired postural reflexes.[40,41,62] When in response to pull the patient makes no effort to regain balance and would fall like a solid object when not prevented, it indicates even more pronounced impairment of postural reflexes.

Loss of postural reflexes is part of normal aging,[41,42,63] and the prevalence of this finding increases with advancing age. Between 80 and 89 years of age, the postural reflexes are impaired in 70 percent of the elderly.[41] Loss of postural reflexes is a well-known feature of PS and is used to classify the severity of disability. A Hoehn and Yahr stage III or higher rating[62,64] is characterized by impairment of postural reflexes. Duncan and Wilson noted bradykinesia in 37 percent of normal elderly community residents and in 76 percent of day hospital cases.[47] Thus, when the two features—bradykinesia and loss of postural reflexes—were used as the minimum requirement for the diagnosis of PS,[65] a large number of normal elderly would be diagnosed erroneously and treated unnecessarily.[24,41,42,63,66,67] Therefore, it is recommended that the diagnosis of PS be made when two of three—bradykinesia, rigidity, and tremor—are present.[24,42,66,67] Rest tremor is perhaps the most reliable sign for the diagnosis of PS in the elderly. Impaired postural reflexes should only be used as an adjunct to other PS features when one is making a PS diagnosis in an elderly individual.[41,42]

GAIT ABNORMALITY AND OLD AGE

The gait in normal elderly is slightly wide based and has short, slow strides, but the heel strike and the arm swing are normal and symmetrical.[9,42] The stride velocity declines by 10–20 percent by the 80 years of age.[40,68] Those who have an excessively slow or abnormal pattern of ambulation are classified as having a gait disorder (see also Chap. 48). It is estimated that 15 percent of those 60 years and older have a gait abnormality.[40] In addition to identifiable causes, for

example, arthritis, motor weakness, coordination difficulty, PS, etc., between 10 and 20 percent of the elderly with gait abnormality, that is approximately 2.25 percent of those 60 years of age and older, have no identifiable cause.[40,69]

Parkinson's syndrome is the most common MD associated with gait abnormality in old age. Flexed posture, *narrow base*, slow short shuffling steps, reduced arm-swing, and impaired postural reflexes are typical of PS[42,64]—the exception being PSP. The PSP cases have an unduly erect posture, narrow or broad base, and their feet are lifted high, striking the ground flat, giving their gait a mechanical (robotic) quality. Unlike PD, the parkinsonian features in PSP are usually symmetrical.[70–72]

GAIT APRAXIA

In gait apraxia (GA) walking difficulty cannot be attributed to mechanical, motor, sensory, coordination, visual, or vestibular dysfunction.[42,73–75] These patients have normal lower limb functions when tested in the sitting or lying position.[73] The GA patient can tap normally, can make a circle or simple drawings in the air or on the floor, and can emulate complex actions like riding a bicycle, in the supine position.[41,42,46,69,73,74] On the other hand, the leg functions in the weight-bearing position, such as would be necessary for walking, are impaired.[74,75] The posture is erect, and gait is typically broad-based with short, shuffling, hesitating steps, as if the patient were "glued" to the floor.[69,75,76] The gait in the GA cases has some features resembling a parkinsonian abnormality. However, unlike PD, the GA patients cannot copy steps or improve with visual guiding lines—features well-known in PD.[76] The arm swing, which is reduced in PS, is usually unaffected in GA and the leg function dissociation between supine and standing positions, a prominent feature of GA, is not seen in PS. Similarly, the normal upper limb function, but marked walking related leg dysfunction, characteristic of GA, is not part of PD. In PD some functional impairment is seen in both the upper and lower limb on the same side. Nearly all PD patients benefit from L-dopa (LD),[24,77] but GA patients do not. Most GA patients have frontal lobe disease or normal pressure hydrocephalus.[42,73–75]

Table 50-3 highlights a comparison of gait in the normal elderly, gait apraxia, and PS.

Another less clearly understood gait abnormality resembling PD is known as senile gait.[78] It is characterized by stooped posture; *broad-base*, reduced arm-swing; stiff turns; and a tendency to fall.[78] These patients do not manifest other major parkinsonian features, such as rest tremor,[57,58,79] upper limb bradykinesia or rigidity and, unlike PD, they do not improve on L-dopa or other antiparkinsonian drugs.[78]

OPHTHALMOPLEGIA IN THE ELDERLY AND IN MOVEMENT DISORDERS

Vertical gaze palsy, the characteristic manifestation of PSP,[70–72] is also noted in rare cases of multiple-system atrophy,[80] PD,[81] Whipple's disease,[82] and other rare diseases. Limitation of vertical gaze is also seen in some normal elderly.[13] Jenkyn et al.[13] contend that an upward-gaze deviation of 5 mm or less and a downward gaze deviation of 7 mm or less from the midposition should be regarded as abnormal. Based

TABLE 50-3 Posture and Gait in Normal Elderly, Parkinson's Disease, and Gait Apraxia

Clinical Features	Normal Elderly	Parkinson's Disease	Gait Apraxia
Base (distance between feet)	Slightly wider than at younger age	Narrow	Broad
Symmetry of abnormality	Symmetrical	Usually asymmetrical	Symmetrical
Functions in the involved lower limb	Normal and symmetrical	Impaired, regardless of weight bearing or not (no dissociation)	Impaired only when weight bearing, but normal when not weight bearing (dissociation pronounced and early)
Upper limb motor function	Normal	Impaired on the involved side	Unimpaired
Arm swing	Normal	Reduced on involved side	Normal on both sides
Posture	Erect	Generalized flexion—neck, trunk, hip, knee, elbow	As in normal elderly
Postural reflexes	May be normal or impaired	Impaired in moderately advanced disease	Impaired early
Foot tapping in sitting or lying position	Normal	Affected side slow and progressively slowed	As in normal elderly
Gait abnormality	Uncommon, increases with age	Late manifestation	Major problems—early manifestation
Stripes on the floor for visual guidance	No change in gait	Improved gait	No improvement in gait
Tremor	Absent	Frequently seen; typically, at rest	As in normal elderly
Dementia	Absent	In about one-third of cases	Common but not invariable
Reflexes	Normal (may be reduced at ankles)	As in normal (may have striatal toe)	May be brisk; may have Babinski sign
Grasp reflex	Normal	Usually negative	Usually positive
Bladder function	Normal	Normal or hypertonic or hypotonic bladder	Incontinence common
L-dopa response	None	Improvement	None

on a study of more than 2000 normal volunteers between 50 and 93 years of age, they[13] observed that in the 8th decade of life, upward gaze was impaired in 29 percent and downward gaze in 34 percent. The diagnostic significance of gaze palsy should, therefore, be interpreted in conjunction with other clinical features.[80]

PRIMITIVE REFLEXES IN MOVEMENT DISORDERS AND THE ELDERLY

A sustained glabellar reflex and a positive snout reflex are common features in PD. Jenkyn et al.[13] noted that 37 percent of normal elderly in the 8th decade had a persistent glabellar

reflex, and 26 percent had a positive snout reflex. Koller et al.[14] concluded that the frequency of positive snout reflex correlates with increasing age. The presence of primitive reflexes is, therefore, a soft clinical sign that, when considered with other findings, strengthens the diagnosis but in isolation has limited significance in the diagnosis of PS.

In summary, the distinction between normal elderly and those with MD may be difficult, as several features of MD are also present in normal elderly. In this regard tremor in general, and rest tremor in particular, is not a part of normal aging and strongly indicates an MD. Because diagnosis of MD is based on clinical assessment, the global clinical picture should be considered as distinguishing between normal aging and MD. In the event of doubt, a short therapeutic trial of L-dopa or another agent is justifiable to arrive at the correct diagnosis.

Consideration of Movement Disorders That Are Concentrated in Old Age

The common movement disorders concentrated in old age include parkinsonism, essential tremor, MD resulting from stroke, drug-induced MD, and orofacial dyskinesias.

PARKINSONISM IN THE ELDERLY

The onset of PS before 40 years is rare.[83] In a large series of PS, the mean onset age was in the early 60s.[83,84] The incidence and prevalence rates of PS rise sharply after 60 years of age.[19,32,33,64,83,85–88] In a door-to-door survey, the prevalence ratio of PD in elderly 75 years and older was seven times higher than that in the 40- to 64-year-old group.[33] This chapter will focus on those aspects of PS pertinent to the elderly.

Parkinsonism in the elderly can be divided into two subgroups: (1) onset at an early age, with the patient surviving to old age; and (2) parkinsonism first manifesting in old age.[89]

When the disease begins at a younger age, the patient is likely to have received antiparkinsonian drugs, including L-dopa for several years before reaching old age. Most such cases would, therefore, manifest chronic L-dopa side effects, including dyskinesias, wearing-off, on-off fluctuations, and freezing episodes[77,90] (see also Chaps. 13 and 14). When PS starts in old age, the distinction from normal aging may be difficult, as some features of PS are also seen in normal elderly. As noted above, a sizable portion of normal elderly have motor slowing, primitive reflexes, vertical-gaze palsy, and impaired postural reflexes.[13,14,40–42,46] Based on a survey of 92 elderly community residents with no neurological disease, Duncan and Wilson[47] concluded that nearly one-half of subjects had one manifestation (excluding postural instability) of PS. In a similar survey of day hospital patients, they detected that nearly everyone had at least one clinical feature of PS.[47] The normal elderly may, therefore, be mistaken as PS and treated unnecessarily with drugs, which can produce side effects and financial hardship. On the other hand, PS features may be mistaken as part of normal aging and the individual deprived of appropriate treatment. Careful population surveys indicate that between 35 and 41 percent of PS cases are undiagnosed and, hence, untreated.[33,91] In a Saskatchewan survey of patients 65 years and older, we detected that 50 percent of PS cases were undiagnosed in the community[2] and 25 percent in the institutionalized population.[3] Missed diagnosis deprives these patients of the opportunity to live an optimal quality of life. A 60-year-old woman, a patient of mine, illustrates that point. She had slowed down and could no longer live alone safely. Her seven children (including a nurse) attributed that to old age and arranged admission to a private care home. While there, she deteriorated further, as she was unable to get out of bed and feed herself. Neurological examination after hospitalization revealed stage IV Hoehn and Yahr[64] akinetic-rigid PS. On LD she improved remarkably, regaining full functional independence.

In 1958 Kurland[88] estimated a 1 percent prevalence rate of PD in patients 60 years of age and older and 2.6 percent in patiens 85 years and older. More recently, we have observed a PD prevalence rate of 3 percent in the community[2] and 6 percent in institutionalized patiens 65 years and older in a Saskatchewan population.[3] The proportion of the North American population over age 65 and over age 85 has increased substantially since 1958. Because the prevalence rate of PD increases with advancing age, it is reasonable to assume that in the contemporary general population the prevalence rate is greater than 1 percent and is probably closer to 3 percent.[2,3] Akinetic-rigid PS cases are most likely to remain undiagnosed, however, even those elderly who have classical PS features, including tremor, and advanced disability may be unrecognized.

Tremor is the most common first manifestation of PS, ranging from 41[92] to 70.5 percent[64] in different studies. In autopsy-verified cases, we noted that tremor alone was the first manifestation in 49 percent.[93] In 41 percent of PS cases the initial tremor was restricted to the upper limbs.[93] By contrast, only 3 percent of cases first manifested as lower limb tremor.[93] Other PS features, in conjunction with tremor, were the first manifestations in 53 percent of cases.[93] The akinetic-rigid PS onset cases are prone to developing gait abnormalities early[93,94] and are classified as postural instability and gait difficulty (PIGD) variant.[93–95] Other, less dramatic, presentations include: upper or lower limb functional decline; handwriting deterioration; foot dragging when tired; difficulty with fine tasks, such as doing buttons or piano playing; loss of self-confidence; feeling of stiffness; declined "coordination"; a sense of leg control loss; lack of energy; fatigue; general physical slowing[93] and frozen shoulder.[96]

Because rest tremor (RT) is not a feature of normal aging, it is the most reliable single distinction between normal aging and parkinsonism.[44,46,79,93,97,98] Isolated lower limb RT has even higher diagnostic value.[93,97] On fluorodopa position emission tomography (PET) scanning, isolated RT cases have the same profile as PD cases.[98]

The most common PS variant is the Lewy body (LB) substantia nigra (SN) pathology type,[19,24,65,99] also known as idiopathic Parkinson's disease (PD).[99] It is distinguished from other PS variants by lack of history of a preceding insult and by associated clinical features.[22,24,42,65] Most other variants may not manifest tremor whereas nearly all PD cases have RT at some point.[79] Akinetic-rigid symmetrical onset and presence of autonomic, corticospinal, or cerebellar dysfunction favor a diagnosis of multiple-system atrophy (MSA).[24,46,57,100] Symmetrical neurological findings, vertical-gaze palsy, absence of tremor, early gait and balance abnormalities, and erect posture favor a PSP diagnosis.[24,70–72] Clinical features in PS depend on the anatomic site of the lesion, rather than on the pathological process involved.[24,58,93,101,102] Like PD, other diseases focused on the SN lead to all the major parkinsonian features, and they respond to LD.[24,77,101,102] Such entities include cases who may or may not have identifiable inclusions.[24,101] Collectively, the SN-centered pathology group of PS can be clinically distinguished from that of other variants in 85 percent of cases.[24] Nearly all PD cases improve on LD,[77] although isolated LD-nonresponsive PD cases have been reported.[103,104] About one-third of the cases of other PS variants also improve on LD, although the benefit in those is of shorter duration (usually, less than 3 years[77]) In suspected PS cases, a trial on LD is, therefore, justifiable. When Sinemet (LD/carbidopa) and Symmetrel (amantadine) are initiated simultaneously, the improvement is seen sooner than on Sinemet alone. A positive response, although helpful, is not diagnostic of PD.

The elderly PS patients have a more rapid functional decline than the younger cases.[92,95,105,106] However, late-onset age by itself does not shorten survival, when compared with age- and sex-matched population.[84,107,108] The PIGD onset mode has been reported as being more common in old age,[94] but one autopsy confirmed study revealed no difference in onset age between PIGD and tremor patients.[93] Whereas 74 percent of the tremor-onset cases had LB disease, only 27 percent of PIGD cases had the same pathology.[93] The PIGD cases had more widespread pathology, which accounted for the rapid progression of disability and reduced survival.[93] The accelerated disability in the elderly PS patients may also reflect additional functional decline related to the aging process or concurrent senile gait[78] or gait apraxia.[73]

Compared to early-onset PS cases, dementia is nearly 10 times more frequent when onset is in old age.[105,109,110] A larger proportion of elderly PS cases are, therefore, demented. At any point, nearly one-third of PD cases have dementia,[111–114] and new dementia cases emerge three to five times more commonly in patients with PD, as compared to those that develop in age-matched normal controls during 5 years of follow-up.[109,112,114–116] Demented cases more frequently experience psychiatric and other adverse effects on antiparkinsonian drugs,[89,105,107,108,117] thus making symptomatic control difficult. Demented PS cases also have a significantly reduced life expectancy.[84,105,107,108,115,116,118]

It has been suggested that elderly PD cases are resistant to developing LD-induced dyskinesias. However, in a carefully conducted study comparing early onset (mean age, 38 years) and late onset (mean age, 73 years) patients on comparable LD doses, there was no difference in the duration of LD exposure before dyskinesia onset.[92] Several of our elderly cases have developed dyskinesias early and on a small dose of LD. Thus, the elderly PS patients are not unduly resistant to dyskinesia.

DRUG-INDUCED PARKINSONISM

Drug-induced parkinsonism (DIP) has been well-known since the 1960s.[22,25,26] There are very few reports on incidence and prevalence of DIP in the general population. In a community survey of PS between 1967 and 1979, the DIP incidence was second only to PD.[19] In the nursing-home population over 65 years of age, we noted a 3 percent prevalence of DIP.[3] Use of multiple drugs is common in the elderly.[1] In a study of 100 consecutively hospitalized elderly, we noted an average of 5.15 drugs per patient, and 3 percent of patients were receiving 12 or more drugs,[1] including drugs well-known as causing DIP. Another reason for exaggerated frequency of DIP in old age[22,23,27,89] is the age-related striatal dopamine (DA) deficiency.[23,119,120] In more than 90 percent of cases, the DIP emerges within 90 days of neuroleptic initiation.[22] Although akinesia and rigidity may be prominent features in these patients, DIP is clinically indistinguishable

from PD.[24,28,29,89] Some DIP patients may have associated tardive dyskinesias. Theoretically, the DIP should be symmetrical; however, that is not always the case.[22,24] One reason is that some DIP cases have an underlying PD pathology, and dopaminergic stress precipitates asymmetrical PS.[23] The PS manifestations, which are entirely a result of drug-induced DA depletion or receptor block, improve when the offending agent is discontinued.[29] When there is preclinical PD pathology, the drug-induced clinical features may continue or worsen slowly after the drug is discontinued.[28,29] Careful drug history in the elderly PS cases is vital, as discontinuing an unnecessary drug may be the only treatment required. The time for full recovery after discontinuing neuroleptics may be as long as 6 months.

The best symptomatic drugs for DIP are the anticholinergics. Because only a small proportion of neuroleptic-treated patients develop DIP,[19,22,25,27] prophylactic use of anticholinergics, which the elderly tolerate poorly, is not justifiable.[27] Amantadine or LD may be beneficial in some DIP cases.[27,28] When the antipsychotic agents cannot be withdrawn safely in DIP, they should be replaced with atypical antipsychotic agents—clozapine or risperidone.[22]

ESSENTIAL TREMOR IN THE ELDERLY

The ET onset age ranges from childhood to old age,[31,54,55] but the incidence and prevalence rates increase markedly in old age[31,51,53,54,121,122] (see also Chap. 27). One-quarter of the Finnish population over 40 years of age had tremor.[53] Of the 25 percent with tremor, the majority (55 percent) of the population studied had ET.[53] We found nearly similar prevalence rates of ET—14 percent in the community[2] and 10 percent in the institutionalized[3] populations 65 years of age and older in Saskatchewan, Canada.

The tremor frequency in ET varies from 4 to 12 Hz, and there is an inverse relation between the frequency and tremor amplitudes.[123,124] With advancing age the tremor involves wider body areas, the amplitude increases,[123] and the frequency decreases in most ET cases.[55,120,125] Functional disability in ET is mainly related to tremor amplitude which, as noted above, increases in old age.[120,123] Therefore, the tremor-related dysfunction is more common in the elderly, as compared to that in younger ET patients.[120]

Because life expectancy in ET is normal[31] and tremor is the only clinical abnormality in most cases, it was once known as "benign essential tremor." When we consider the psychological and functional handicap related to tremor, even at a young age there is a significant handicap.[31,122,126,127] In one sickness profile study dealing with patients' own assessment of emotional behavior, work, communication, home management, recreation, and pastime, the ET cases, compared to controls were significantly handicapped in nearly every category.[127] In childhood they are often embarrassed by the tremor and may be ridiculed by other children. These patients frequently experience anxiety that may lead to depression and, in rare cases, to suicide attempts.[120,127,128] These patients may, therefore, have to settle for lesser social and employment opportunities than their abilities and qualifications warrant.[31,120,122,126–129] In old age, the exaggerated tremor makes these patients self-conscious, resulting in self-imposed social isolation. The functional disability is usually a result of the upper limb action tremor, including impaired writing, drinking from a cup, feeding, manipulating fine objects, etc.[31,122,126,127,129] Head and voice tremor each may also interfere significantly in the everyday lives of elderly ET cases. One elderly patient had such pronounced head tremor that he could not get a haircut at a barber shop. He needed to consume several alcoholic drinks before the head tremor would sufficiently subside and a family member could give him a haircut. I have also seen several other ET patients in whom the voice tremor presented the main handicap in their daily life.

In addition to the action tremor, in old age some ET patients may develop rest tremor (RT) without evidence of bradykinesia or rigidity.[120] In an autopsy study, one-third of ET cases had developed RT later in age.[120] Each of these cases had upper limb tremor of more than 10 years' duration, and each was over 60 years of age when the RT emerged.[120] The ET patients who first manifested the disease in old age may simultaneously develop RT, in addition to the typical action tremor. However, RT alone is not a manifestation of ET.[57,58,97] ET patients who have RT are sometimes labeled as senile tremor patients.[44,55] That label is not justifiable, as there is no other clinical difference and the pathological findings in these cases are similar to those for other ET patients.[120,128] Leg RT alone at the onset without head or upper action tremor is against the ET diagnosis.[97] The PET scan pattern in these patients is similar to parkinsonism.[98] The reason for the emergence of RT is unknown; however, it has been postulated that an age-related decline in the striatal DA level[119] contributes to the emergence of RT.[120]

Several clinical studies have reported an increased risk of PS in ET cases,[130-132] but others found no such association.[31,54,133,134] In our autopsy series of nine ET cases—the largest series in the world—in which the PS diagnosis was made when rest tremor, bradykinesia, and rigidity were observed, 3 (33 percent) patients had PS.[120,128] Two of those patients had DIP, and one had basal ganglia ischemic lesions.[120,128] None of these cases had LB pathology.[120,128] In addition to our study, there are only six other ET autopsy cases that have been reported since 1919, when the link between SN atrophy, LB inclusions, and PD was first established.[120] None of those six had LB pathology.[120,128] The elderly ET patients, like other elderly individuals, are predisposed to DIP.[22,27,28] Thus, PS in general is more common in ET, but the risk of PD (LB disease) in these patients is not different from the general population.[120,128]

Cogwheeling phenomena in ET cases may be mistaken for cogwheel rigidity,[48,50,135,136] and RT, as noted above, is a natural evolution in some ET cases.[120,128] Considering that the distinction between the natural evolution of ET and superimposed PS may be difficult,[120] the additional diagnosis of PS is justifiable only when there has been a distinct change in the classical ET profile and when bradykinesia, rigidity, and RT are unequivocally detected.[120,128] Asymmetry of bradykinesia and rigidity, especially when more pronounced on the side least affected by tremor, is a valuable clue for making the additional diagnosis of PS in ET cases. Piano playing finger movements and rapid hand tapping, contrasted to pronation/supination movements, are better indicators of bradykinesia

in ET cases. The distinction between cogwheeling and cogwheel rigidity is outlined in Table 50-2. An alcoholic beverage temporarily relieves symptoms in most, but not all, ET cases.[129,137] However, this effect is not specific for ET, as other tremor variants may also improve with alcohol.[129] With time the benefit of alcohol declines, requiring larger quantities or producing no relief of tremor. Based on self-made observations that alcohol alleviates tremor, some ET patients come to rely on that and progressively consume larger quantities,[31,128,129,138] eventually developing alcohol-related complications.[31]

STROKE AND MOVEMENT DISORDERS

Stroke is a common disorder in old age,[38] and some stroke patients may have abnormal movements, for example, hemiballismus, dystonia, and PS.

HEMIBALLISMUS

Hemiballismus (HB) is characterized by proximal large amplitude, irregular, flinging unilateral limb movements. Rarely, the ballistic movements involve only one limb[139-141]—monoballismus—or both sides, known as paraballismus or biballismus.[141-144] In one study of 25 patients, 19 had HB, 5 monoballismus, and 2 biballismus.[141] In only 2 of these 25 (8 percent) cases, the clinical picture was that of pure ballismus. Most cases had additional abnormalities such as dystonia or chorea.[141] In 72 percent of cases the HB was a result of ischemia, followed by hemorrhage in 8 percent.[141] The main site of pathology in HB is the subthalamic nucleus (STN). The lesion, however, may not be restricted to the STN, or that nucleus may be unaffected. A lesion of the caudate, putamen, or thalamus, alone or in conjunction with an STN lesion, can also produce hemiballismus.[141,145-147] A neuroimaging study[141] of 22 ballismus patients revealed that only 1 (4 percent) had a lesion restricted to the STN, and in five (23 percent) there were STN plus other basal ganglia, pons, or midbrain lesions. In six (27 percent) cases the lesion was restricted to other basal ganglia or the thalamus, without STN involvement, and in three (14 percent) cases there were parietal and/or temporal cortex lesions. In seven (32 percent) cases no neuroimaging abnormality could be identified.[141]

In rare cases, multiple basal ganglia lacunar infarcts may produce generalized chorea.[148]

The onset in HB is usually sudden but, in some cases, it evolves over several days to weeks.[141] With time the ballistic movements become less violent and acquire a choreic quality.[149,150] When STN stroke is the basis of HB, usually there is a spontaneous recovery. Symptomatic control of ballistic movements can be achieved with haloperidol or other neuroleptics within several days.[141,143] Valproate and sulpiride are also useful drugs in some cases.[146,151]

DYSTONIA

In the elderly, focal and hemidystonia (HD) may result from a basal ganglia stroke[152,153] (see also Chap. 33). In one study of 22 hemidystonia patients, 36 percent of cases of all ages, and nearly all those over age 65 years of age had HD consequent to stroke.[152] Another study of 28 cases noted that 15 (56 percent) of the posthemiplegic dystonia cases were caused by stroke.[153] HD in patients 50 years of age and older is almost always secondary to stroke.[153] When there is only one discrete lesion as the basis of HD, it may be localized to the lentiform nucleus, head of the caudate, or the posterolateral thalamus,[153] but most HD cases have larger lesions or multiple sites of pathology. The contralateral putamen is the most common site involved in HD.[152–154] As noted above, a putamen, globus pallidus, caudate (head), or thalamus (posterolateral) lesion in isolation, or in different combinations with other sites, can produce contralateral focal or hemidystonia.[152–154] The onset of HD after stroke may be delayed for several weeks to years,[152,153] but in rare cases, depending on the site of pathology, dystonia may emerge within several days. In most cases HD emerges as the severity of motor weakness declines.

The other forms of dystonia, blepharospasm and Meige's syndrome,[155] although common in old age, are not related to stroke.

STROKE AND PS

Parkinsonism secondary to stroke is very rare. Chang et al.[156] studied ischemia as a basis of parkinson-like syndrome. Bradykinesia, rigidity, and gait disturbance were common manifestations, but these patients did not have tremor, and none improved on LD.[156] Ischemic lesions in the basal ganglia, frontal lobe, or deep subcortical white matter were responsible for this parkinson-like clinical picture.[156] Parkinsonism secondary to SN infarction is very rare. These cases can have all the clinical characteristics of PD, including improvement on LD.[102] (See also Chap. 25.)

OROFACIAL DYSKINESIAS IN THE ELDERLY

Chronic neuroleptic-treated patients are prone to developing tardive dyskinesia (TD), the frequency of which rises with advancing age.[155,157–159] TD patients have oral-buccal-lingual-masticatory, cervical, truncal, or extremity stereotyped movements in different combinations. Orofacial dyskinesias are also reported in elderly who have never used neuroleptics.[159–161] Wide variation in the prevalence rate of drug-induced and spontaneous orofacial dyskinesias (SOFD) has been reported.[155] One community-based survey of individuals 71 years of age and older, reported only 0.22 percent prevalence of TD.[162] Khot and Wyatt[163] reviewed nine TD studies conducted in psychiatric patient populations. The cumulative TD prevalence rate was approximately 20 percent in all ages but increased markedly in patients after age 40. Most of the TD cases had a history of neuroleptic usage.[163]

The existence of SOFD has been questioned by some experts.[164,165] Sweet et al.[164] studied 45 patients over 60 years of age at a psychiatric hospital and detected neuroleptic-induced dyskinesias in 21 percent but noted no instance of SOFD. Based on a survey of institutionalized elderly, a study by Ticehurst[165] concluded that the case of the presumed SOFD patients represents an incomplete history of neuroleptic usage. On the other hand, Chiu et al.[160] noted a 26 percent prevalence of neuroleptic-induced TD and a 2.4 percent prevalence of SOFD in a psychogeriatric clinic population. Klawans and Barr[159] noted SOFD in 0.8 percent in patients between 50 and 59 years of age, in 6 percent of those between

60 and 69 years old, and in 7.8 percent of those between 70 and 79 years old, in the general population who had neither a neurological illness nor were receiving neuroleptics. Waddington and Youssef[161] reported four elderly schizophrenics with SOFD who had never received neuroleptics. On balance, the current evidence favors the hypothesis that rare elderly individuals suffer from orofacial dyskinesias of unknown etiology.

The pathogenesis of orofacial dyskinesia is unknown. It has been suggested that dental extraction and ill-fitting dentures may be contributory factors.[159,166–168] Sandyk and Kay[169] studied the role of edentulousness in neuroleptic-induced dyskinesias in 131 psychiatric patients. Dyskinesias of the tongue, face, or extremities did not correlate with edentulous status.[169] Edentulous patients, on the other hand, were more liable to developing cervical and truncal dyskinesias.[169]

Movement Disorders Associated with Other Neurodegenerative Diseases in the Elderly

The most common neurodegenerative disorder in the elderly population is Alzheimer's disease (AD).[4,34,35] Several forms of abnormal movements have been reported in AD cases, with the most common being Parkinsonism.[170–174] There is considerable evidence that PS is significantly more common in AD than expected in matched general population, and its frequency increases with the progression of AD. Kischka et al[175] conducted electrophysiological tests on AD patients and controls. Movement time (bradykinesia) and muscle tone (rigidity) were significantly increased in AD patients, compared to normal controls, thus indicating that preclinical PS features are common in AD. A 3-year follow-up of AD cases noted a progressively more common emergence of bradykinesia.[174] Bradykinesia was noted initially in 39 percent of untreated cases and in 72 percent 3 years later. The presence of rigidity also increased from 11 percent in untreated to 61 percent in AD cases at the end of 3 years.[174] However, tremor was not evident in the early or the late AD cases.[174] Nearly every AD patient treated with neuroleptics developed bradykinesia, rigidity, or orofacial dyskinesias when followed for a long time.[174] Although tremor is rarely reported in AD-associated PS, one study of untreated community residents with mild AD noted RT in 10 percent of cases.[172] Unlike PD, none of these cases improved on LD.[172] Bennett et al.[173] studied a 235-bed nursing home patient population and noted some parkinsonian features in a large proportion of the AD cases, some of whom improved on antiparkinsonian drugs.[173] Personal experience indicates that some AD cases manifest tremor[24] and those with AD + PD improve on LD.[117] Morris et al.[170] longitudinally studied 44 AD and 58 controls, none of whom had PS at entry point. At the end of a 66-month follow-up, based on the presence of two of these three factors—bradykinesia, rigidity, and rest tremor—PS was detected in 16 (37 percent) patients. Six (14 percent) of those were on neuroleptics, and 10 (23 percent) evolved into PS spontaneously. By contrast, over the same interval only three

(5 percent) of the 58 controls developed PS.[170] Thus, the spontaneous emergence of new PS in AD cases over 66 months was nearly 5 times that expected in the general population of the same age.

The reasons for PS manifestations in AD include neuroleptic usage,[170] concomitant PD,[117] diffuse LB disease,[176,177] LB variant of AD,[37] and extranigral pathology.[170] Like AD, PD is concentrated in the elderly;[19,32,33] therefore, the two diseases may coexist.[117] When the PD features are later followed by AD, the initial clinical picture is indistinguishable from that of PD.[117] As the AD evolves in such cases, RT becomes less prominent, and an irregular small amplitude kinetic tremor emerges. Although there is motor function improvement on LD, in the sequentially evolving cases psychiatric side effects are a common and early problem.[117] In those who manifest PD and AD simultaneously, the typical parkinsonian RT is less evident, and the response to LD is poor.[117] The AD cases who develop extrapyramidal features early have a rapid progression of disability.[170,174,178]

Myoclonus may be a feature in some AD patients[178,179] and rare AD cases may have prominent chorea, thus resembling Huntington's disease.[180]

Parkinsonism, chorea, and myoclonus in different combinations are also seen in Jakob-Creuzfeldt disease.[181] Corticobasal degeneration patients typically present as action tremor, unilateral dystonia, and apraxia and later develop stimulus-sensitive myoclonus[182–184] (see also Chap. 45). In rare Pick's disease patients the clinical picture is indistinguishable from that of corticobasal degeneration.[185–187]

Special Consideration of Movement Disorders Management in the Elderly

The elderly are prone to having other systemic disorders[5] and consume large numbers of drugs.[1,5,188] Altered drug metabolism[16–18,189] predisposes them to drug toxicity and drug side effects.[1,5] Drug-induced MD are more likely in the elderly than in the younger subjects. Therefore, when considering the diagnosis and management of MD, taking a careful history of drug intake is necessary. The elderly are liable to having prostate hypertrophy, glaucoma, age-related memory deficit, cardiac dysrhythmias, leg edema, etc., which are contraindications to the use of commonly prescribed drugs for movement disorders—anticholinergics, beta-adrenergic blockers, dopamine precursors, dopamine agonists, amantadine, etc. Wherever possible, the first choice in treatment of drug-induced MD is to discontinue the offending agent.

The major goals of treatment in elderly retired individuals are self-sufficiency for personal, physical, and social needs and physical safety. Job performance is not a significant consideration in this age group. The expected survival in the elderly is naturally shortened. Therefore, drugs that may slow down the disease[190] need not be used as the first line of PD treatment in those over 75 years of age. When one drug is sufficient to control the symptoms, additional drugs should be avoided, as they increase the risk of side effects. Nonmedical supports such as physiotherapy, occupational therapy, home care, home safety measures, proper diet, and judicious physical and social activity are important adjuncts. Many elderly individuals suffering from MD are liable to isolate themselves socially. Nonprofit disease-specific organizations are highly valuable in providing social support and interaction among those suffering from similar disease (see Appendix). Surgical procedures to treat movement disorders should be used only after careful consideration and then very cautiously, especially in the elderly with a MD.

References

1. Desai T, Rajput AH, Desai HB: Uuse and abuse of drugs in the elderly. *Prog Neuropsychopharmacol Biol Psychiatry* 14:779–784, 1990.

2. Moghal S, Rajput AH, D'Arcy C, Rajput R: Prevalence of movement disorders in elderly community residents. *Neuroepidemiology* 13:175–178, 1994.

3. Moghal S, Rajput AH, Meleth R, et al: Prevalence of movement disorders in institutionalized elderly. *Neuroepidemiology* 14:297–300, 1995.

4. Canadian Study of Health and Aging Working Group: Canadian Study of Health and Aging: Study methods and prevalence of dementia. *Can Med Assoc J* 150(6):899–913, 1994.

5. Rowe JW: Aging and geriatric medicine, in Wyngaarden JB, Smith LH (eds): *Cecil Textbook of Medicine*. Philadelphia: WB Saunders, 1988, pp 21–27.

6. Parker SW: Dizziness in the elderl, in Albert ML, Knoefel JE (eds): *Clinical Neurology of Aging*, 2d ed. New York: Oxford University Press, 1994, pp 569–579.

7. Matjucha ICA, Katz B: Neuro-ophthalmology of aging, in Albert ML, Knoefel JE (eds): *Clinical Neurology of Aging*, 2d ed. New York: Oxford University Press, 1994, pp 447.

8. Kline D, Sekuler R, Dismukes K: Social issues, human needs, and opportunities for research on the effects of age on vision: An over-view, in Sekuler R, Kline D, Dismukes K (eds): *Aging and Human Visual Function*. New York: Alan R. Liss, 1982, pp 3–6.

9. Drachman DA, Long RR, Swearer JM: Neurological evaluation of the elderly patient, in Albert ML, Knoefel JE (eds): *Clinical Neurology of Aging*, 2d ed. New York: Oxford University Press, 1994, pp 159–180.

10. Maki BE, Holliday PJ, Fernie GR: Aging and postural control: A comparison of spontaneous- and induced-sway balance tests. *J Am Geriatr Soc* 38(1):1–9, 1990.

11. Baloh RW, Fife TD, Zerling L, Socotch T: Comparison of static and dynamic posturography in young and older normal people. *J Am Geriatr Soc* 42(4):405–412, 1994.

12. Lexell J, Taylor CC, Sjostrom M: What is the cause of the ageing atrophy? Total number, size and proportion of different fiber types studied in whole vastus lateralis muscle for 15- to 83-year-old men. *J Neurol Sci* 84:275–294, 1988.

13. Jenkyn LR, Reeves AG, Warren T, et al: Neurological signs in senescence. *Arch Neurol* 42:1154–1157, 1985.

14. Koller WC, Glatt S, Wilson RS, Fox JH: Primitive reflexes and cognitive function in the elderly. *Ann Neurol* 12:302–304, 1982.

15. Duckett S, Schoedler S: Nutritional disorders and alcoholism, in Duckett S (ed): *The Pathology of the Aging Human Nervous System*. Philadelphia: Lea & Febiger, 1991, pp 200–209.

16. Benet LZ, Sheiner LB: Pharmacokinetics: The dynamics of drug absorption, distribution, and elimination, in Gilman AG, Goodman LS, Rall TW, Murad F (eds): *The Pharmacological Basis of Therapeutics*, 7th ed. New York: MacMillan Publishing Company, 1985, pp 3–34.

17. Ross EM, Gilman AG: Pharmacodynamics: Mechanisms of drug action and the relationship between drug concentraton and effect, in Gilman AG, Goodman LS, Rall TW, Murad F (eds): *The Pharmacological Basis of Therapeutics,* 7th ed. New York: Mac-Millan Publishing Company, 1985, pp 35–48.

18. Blaschke TF, Nies AS, Mamelok RD: Principles of therapeutics, in Gilman AG, Goodman LS, Rall TW, Murad F (eds): *The Pharmacological Basis of Therapeutics,* 7th ed. New York: MacMillan Publishing Company, 1985, pp 49–65.

19. Rajput AH, Offord KP, Beard CM, Kurland LT: Epidemiology of parkinsonism: Incidence, classification, and mortality. *Ann Neurol* 16:278–282, 1984.

20. Lang AE: Lithium and parkinsonism. *Ann Neurol* 15:214, 1984.

21. Klawans HL: Abnormal movements in the elderly. *Sandorama* 15–18, 1981.

22. Friedman JH: Drug-induced parkinsonism, in Lang AE, Weiner WJ (eds): *Drug-Induced Movement Disorders.* Mount Kisco, NY: Futura Publishing Co, 1992, pp 41–83.

23. Rajput AH, Rozdilsky B, Hornykiewicz O, et al: Reversible drug-induced parkinsonism: Clinicopathologic study of two cases. *Arch Neurol* 39:644–646, 1982.

24. Rajput AH, Rozdilsky B, Rajput Alex H: Accuracy of clinical diagnosis in parkinsonism—a prospective study. *Can J Neurol Sci* 18:275–278, 1991.

25. Ayd FJ: A survey of drug-induced extrapyramidal reaction. *J Am Med Assoc* 175:1054–1060, 1961.

26. Delay J, Deniker P: Drug-induced extrapyramidal syndromes, in Vinken PJ, Bruyn GW (eds): *Handbook of Clinical Neurology,* 6th ed. New York: Elsevier-North Holland, 1968, pp 248–266.

27. Rajput AH: Drug induced parkinsonism in the elderly. *Geriatr Med Today* 3:99–107, 1984.

28. Hardie RJ, Lees AJ: Neuroleptic-induced Parkinson's syndrome: Clinical features and results of treatment with l-dopa. *J Neurol Neurosurg Psychiatry* 51:850–854, 1988.

29. Burn DJ, Brooks DJ: Nigral dysfunction in drug-induced parkinsonism: An ^{18}F-dopa PET study. *Neurology* 43:552–556, 1993.

30. Gordon M, Preiksaitis HG: Drugs and the aging brain, in Duckett S (ed): *The Pathology of the Aging Human Nervous System.* Philadelphia: Lea & Febiger, 1991, pp 443–448.

31. Rajput AH, Offord KP, Beard CM, Kurland LT: Essential tremor in Rochester, Minnesota: A 45-year study. *J Neurol Neurosurg Psychiatry* 47:466–470, 1984.

32. Bharucha NE, Bharucha EP, Bharucha AE, et al: Prevalence of Parkinson's disease in the Parsi Community of Bombay, India. *Arch Neurol* 45:1321–1323, 1988.

33. Schoenberg BS, Anderson DW, Haerer AF: Prevalence of Parkinson's disease in the biracial population of Copiah County, Mississippi. *Neurology* 35(6):841–845, 1985.

34. Schoenberg BS, Kokmen E, Okazaki H: Alzheimer's disease and other dementing illnesses in a defined United States population: Incidence rates and clinical features. *Ann Neurol* 22:724–729, 1987.

35. Terry RD, Katzman R: Senile dementia of the Alzheimer type. *Ann Neurol* 14:497–506, 1983.

36. Boller F, Mizutani T, Roessmann U, et al: Parkinson's disease, dementia, and Alzheimer's disease: Clinicopathological Correlations. *Ann Neurol* 7:329–335, 1980.

37. Hansen L, Salmon D, Galasko D, et al: The Lewy body variant of Alzheimer's disease: A clinical and pathological entity. *Neurology* 40:1–8, 1990.

38. Babikian VL, Kase CS, Wolf PA: Cerebrovascular disease in the elderly, in Albert ML, Knoefel JE (eds): *Clinical Neurology of Aging,* 2d ed. New York: Oxford University Press, 1994, pp 548–568.

39. Sudarsky L: Gait disturbances in the elderly, in Albert ML, Knoefel JE (eds): *Clinical Neurology of Aging,* 2d ed. New York: Oxford University Press, 1994, pp 483–492.

40. Sudarsky L: Geriatrics: Gait disorders in the elderly. *N Engl J Med* 322:1441–1446, 1990.

41. Weiner WJ, Nora LM, Glantz RH: Elderly inpatients: Postural reflex impairment. *Neurology* 34:945–947, 1984.

42. Rajput AH: Parkinsonism, aging and gait apraxia, in Stern MB, Koller WC (eds): *Parkinsonian Syndromes.* New York: Marcel Dekker, 1993, pp 511–532.

43. Jankovic J, Fahn S: Physiologic and pathologic tremors: Diagnosis, mechanism, and management. *Ann Intern Med* 93:460–465, 1980.

44. Kelly J, Taggart HMcA, McCullagh P: Normal and abnormal tremor in the elderly, in Findley LJ, Koller WC (eds): *Handbook of Tremor disorders.* New York: Marcel Dekker, 1995, pp 351–370.

45. Marsden CD: Slowness of movement in Parkinson's disease. *Mov Disord* 1989;4(suppl l):S26–S37.

46. Rajput AH: Clinical features and natural history of Parkinson's disease (special consideration of aging), in Calne DB (ed): *Neurodegenerative Diseases.* Philadelphia: WB Saunders, 1994, pp 555–571.

47. Duncan G, Wilson JA: Normal elderly have some signs of PS. *Lancet* 1989;1392.

48. Findley LJ, Koller WC: Definitions and behavioral classifications, in Koller WC, Findley LJ (eds): *Handbook of Tremor Disorders.* New York: Marcel Dekker, 1995, pp 1–5.

49. Duvoisin RG: The differential diagnosis of parkinsonism, in Stern GM, ed. *Parkinson's Disease.* Baltimore: John Hopkins University Press, 1990, pp 431–466.

50. Findley LJ, Gresty MA, Halmagyi GM: Tremor and cogwheel phenomena and clonus in Parkinson's disease. *J Neurol Neurosurg Psychiatry* 44:534–546, 1981.

51. Rautakorpi I, Takala J, Marttila RJ, et al: Essential tremor in a Finnish population. *Acta Neurol Scand* 66:58–67, 1982.

52. Findley LJ, Gresty MA: Tremor. *Br J Hosp Med* 16–32, 1981.

53. Rautakorpi I, Marttila RJ, Takala J, Rinne UK: Occurrences and causes of tremors. *Neuroepidemiology* 1:209–215, 1982.

54. Haerer AF, Anderson DW, Schoenberg BS: Prevalence of essential tremor: Results from the Copiah County study. *Arch Neurol* 39:750–751, 1982.

55. Koller WC, Hubble JP, Busenbark KL: Essential tremor, in Calne DB (ed): *Neurodegenerative Diseases.* Philadelphia: WB Saunders, 1994, pp 717–742.

56. LeWitt PA: Tremor induced or enhanced by pharmacological means, in Findley LJ, Koller WC (eds): *Handbook of Tremor Disorders.* New York: Marcel Dekker, 1995, pp 473–481.

57. Rajput AH: Clinical features of tremor in extrapyramidal syndromes, in Findley LJ, Koller WC (eds): *Handbook of Tremor Disorders.* New York: Marcel Dekker, 1994, pp 275–291.

58. Rajput AH, Rozdilsky B, Ang L: Site(s) of lesion and resting tremor. *Ann Neurol* 28(2):296–297, 1990.

59. Koch H, Smith MC: Office-based ambulatory care for patients 75 years old and over. *National Ambulatory Medical Care Survey, 1980 and 1981.* Hyattsville, MD: National Center for Health Statistics, Public Health Service, 1985.

60. Luxon LM. A bit dizzy. *Br J Hosp Med* 32:315, 1984.

61. Duncan PW, Chandler J, Studenski S, et al: How do physiological components of balance affect mobility in elderly men? *Arch Phys Med Rehabil* 74(12):1343–1349, 1993.

62. Fahn S, Elton RL: UPDRS Development Committee: Unified Parkinson's disease rating scale, in Fahn S, Marsden CD, Calne D, Goldstein M (eds): *Recent Developments in Parkinson's Disease,* 2d ed. Florham Park, NJ: Macmillan Healthcare Information, 1987, pp 153–305.

63. Tinetti ME, Speechley M, Ginter SF: Risk factors for falls among elderly persons living in the community. *N Engl J Med* 319:1701–1707, 1988.

64. Hoehn MM, Yahr MD. Parkinsonism: Onset, progression, and mortality. *Neurology* 17:427–442, 1967.

65. Hughes AJ, Daniel SE, Kilford L, Lees AJ: Accuracy of clinical diagnosis of idiopathic Parkinson's disease: A clinico-pathological study of 100 cases. *J Neurol Neurosurg Psychiatry* 55:181–184, 1992.

66. Rajput AH: Diagnosis of PD (letter) *Neurology* 43:1629–1630, 1993.

67. Rajput AH: Accuracy of clinical diagnosis of idiopathic Parkinson's disease. *J Neurol Neurosurg Psychiatry* 56:938–939, 1993.

68. Winter DA, Patla AE, Frank JS, Walt SE: Biomechanical walking pattern changes in the fit and healthy elderly. *Phys Ther* 70(6):340–347, 1990.

69. Sudarsky L, Ronthal M: Gait disorders among elderly patients. A survey study of 50 patients. *Arch Neurol* 40:740–743, 1983.

70. Rajput AH, Chornell G, Rozdilsky B: Progressive external ophthalmoplegia with parkinsonism and dementia treatment with L-dopa. *Can J Ophthalmol* 7:368–374, 1972.

71. Steele JC, Richardson JC, Olszewski J: Progressive supranuclear palsy. *Arch Neurol* 10:333–359, 1964.

72. Jackson JA, Jankovic J, Ford J: Progressive supranuclear palsy: Clinical features and response to treatment in 16 patients. *Ann Neurol* 13:273–278, 1983.

73. Sudarsky L, Simon S: Gait disorder in late-life hydrocephalus. *Arch Neurol* 44:263–267, 1987.

74. Estanol BV: Gait apraxia in communicating hydrocephalus. *J Neurol Neurosurg Psychiatry* 44:305–308, 1981.

75. Fisher CM: Hydrocephalus as a cause of disturbances of gait in the elderly. *Neurology* 32:1358–1363, 1982.

76. Forssberg H, Johnels B, Steg G: Is parkinsonian gait caused by a regression to an immature walking pattern? *Adv Neurol.* 40:375–379, 1984.

77. Rajput AH, Rozdilsky B, Rajput Alex, Ang L: L-dopa efficacy and pathological basis of Parkinson syndrome. *Clin Neuropharmacol* 13(6):553–558, 1990.

78. Koller W, Wilson R, Glatt S, et al: Senile gait: Correlation with computed tomographic scan. *Ann Neurol* 13:343–344, 1983.

79. Rajput AH, Rozdilsky B, Ang L: Occurrence of resting tremor in Parkinson's disease. *Neurology* 41:1298–1299, 1991.

80. Jankovic J, Rajput AH, Golbe LI, Goodman JC: What is it? Case 1, 1993: Parkinsonism, dysautonomia, and ophthalmoparesis. *Mov Disord* 8(4):525–532, 1993.

81. Stewart BJ, Rajput AH, Ravindran J: Ophthalmoplegia in parkinsonism (abstr). *Can J Neurol Sci* 21:S27, 1994.

82. Simpson DA, Wishnow R, Gargulinski RB, Pawlak AM: Oculo-facial-skeletal myorhythmia in central nervous system Whipple's disease: Additional case and review of the literature. *Mov Disord* 10(2):195–200, 1995.

83. Rajput AH: Frequency and cause of Parkinson's disease. *Can J Neurol Sci* 19:103–107, 1992.

84. Rajput AH, Uitti Ryan J, Rajput Alex H, Basran P: Life expectancy in parkinsonism today (abstr.). *Mov Disord* 1990;5(suppl 1):13.

85. Nobrega FT, Glattre E, Kurland LT, Okazaki H: Comments on the epidemiology of parkinsonism including prevalence and incidence statistics for Rochester, Minnesota, 1935–1966, in Barbeau A, Brunette JR (eds): *Progress in Neurogenetics.* Amsterdam: Excerpta Medica, 1967, pp 474–485.

86. Schoenberg BS: Environmental risk factors for Parkinson's disease: The epidemiologic evidence. *Can J Neurol Sci* 14:407–413, 1987.

87. Marttila RJ: Epidemiology, in Koller WC (ed): *Handbook of Parkinson's Disease.* New York: Marcel Dekker, 1987, pp 35–50.

88. Kurland LT: Epidemiology: Incidence, geographic distribution and genetic considerations, in Fields WS (ed): *Pathogenesis and Treatment of Parkinsonism.* Springfield, IL: Charles C Thomas, 1958, pp 5–43.

89. Rajput AH: Parkinson's disease in the elderly. MEDICINE North America 1:101–106, 1986.

90. Rajput AH, Stern W, Laverty WH: Chronic low dose therapy in Parkinson's disease: An argument for delaying L-dopa therapy. *Neurology* 34(8):991–996, 1984.

91. Morgante L, Rocca WA, Di rosa AE, et al: Prevalence of Parkinson's disease and other types of parkinsonism: A door-to-door survey in three Sicilian municipalities. *Neurology* 42:1901–1907, 1992.

92. Gibb WR, Lees AJ: A comparison of clinical and pathological features of young- and old-onset Parkinson's disease. *Neurology* 38:1402–1406, 1988.

93. Rajput AH, Pahwa R, Pahwa P, Rajput Alex: Prognostic significance of the onset mode in parkinsonism. *Neurology* 43:829–830, 1993.

94. Zetusky WJ, Jankovic J, Pirozzolo FJ: The heterogeneity of Parkinson's disease: Clinical and prognostic implications. *Neurology* 35:522–526, 1985.

95. Jankovic J, McDermott M, Carter J, et al: Variable expression of Parkinson's disease: A base-line analysis of the DATATOP cohort. *Neurology* 40:1529–1534, 1990.

96. Riley D, Lang AE, Blair RDG, et al: Frozen shoulder and other shoulder disturbances in Parkinson's disease. *J Neurol Neurosurg Psychiatry* 52:63–66, 1989.

97. Rajput AH, Rozdilsky B, Rajput Alex H: Essential leg tremor. *Neurology* 40:1909, 1909.

98. Brooks DJ, Playford ED, Ibanez V, et al: Isolated tremor and disruption of the nigrostriatal dopaminergic system: An 18F-dopa PET study. *Neurology* 42:1554–1560, 1992.

99. Duvoisin R, Golbe LI: Toward a definition of Parkinson's disease. *Neurology* 39:746, 1989.

100. Rajput AH, Kazi KH, Rozdilsky B: Striatonigral degeneration response to L-dopa therapy. *J Neurol Sci* 16:331–341, 1972.

101. Rajput AH, Uitti RJ, Sudhakar S, Rozdilsky B: Parkinsonism and neurofibrillary tangle pathology in pigmented nuclei. *Ann Neurol* 25:602–606, 1989.

102. Murrow RW, Schweiger GD, Kepes JJ, Koller WC: Parkinsonism due to a basal ganglia lacunar state: Clinicopathologic correlation. *Neurology* 40:897–900, 1990.

103. Mark MH, Sage JI, Dickson DW, et al: L-dopa-nonresponsive Lewy body parkinsonism: Clinicopathologic study of two cases. *Neurology* 42:1323–1327, 1992.

104. Sage JI, Miller DC, Golbe LI, et al: Clinically atypical expression of pathologically typical Lewy-Body parkinsonism. *Clin Neuropharmacol* 13(1):36–47, 1991.

105. Hietanen M, Teravainen H: The effect of age of disease onset on neuropsychological performance in Parkinson's disease. *J Neurol Neurosurg Psychiatry* 51:244–249, 1988.

106. Goetz CG, Tanner CM, Stebbins GT, Buchman AS: Risk factors for progression in Parkinson's disease. *Neurology* 38:1841–1844, 1988.

107. Uitti RJ, Rajput AH, Offord KP: Parkinsonism survival in the L-dopa era. *Neurology* 41(suppl 1):190, 1991.

108. Rajput AH, Uitti RJ, Rajput Alex H, Basran P. Parkinsonism-onset and mortality update (abstr.). *Can J Neurol Sci* 16(2):241, 1989.

109. Mayeux R, Stern Y, Rosenstein R, et al: An estimate of the prevalence of dementia in idiopathic Parkinson's disease. *Arch Neurol* 45:260–262, 1988.

110. Mayeux R, Chen J, Mirabello E, et al: An estimate of the incidence of dementia in idiopathic Parkinson's disease. *Neurology* 40:1513–1517, 1990.

111. Marttila RJ, Rinne UK: Dementia in Parkinson's disease. *Acta Neurol Scand* 54:431–441, 1976.

112. Rajput AH: Prevalence of dementia in Parkinson's disease, in Huber SJ, Cummings JL (eds): *Parkinson's Disease. Neurobehavioral Aspects.* New York: Oxford University Press, 1992, pp 119–131.

113. Rajput AH, Rozdilsky B: Parkinsonism and dementia: Effects of L-dopa. *Lancet* 1:1084, 1975.

114. Rajput AH, Offord KP, Beard CM, Kurland LT: A case control study of smoking habits, dementia and other illnesses in idiopathic Parkinson's disease. *Neurology* 37:226–232, 1987.

115. Marder K, Leung D, Tang M, et al: Are demented patients with Parkinson's disease accurately reflected in prevalence surveys? A survival analysis. *Neurology* 41:1240–1243, 1991.

116. Mindham RHS, Ahmed SWA, Clough CG: A controlled study of dementia in Parkinson's disease. *J Neurol Neurosurg Psychiatry* 45:969–974, 1982.

117. Rajput AH, Rozdilsky B, Rajput A: Alzheimer's disease and idiopathic Parkinson's disease coexistence. *J Geriatr Psychiatry Neurol* 6:170–176, 1993.

118. Marder K, Mirabello E, Chen J, et al: Death rates among demented and nondemented patients with Parkinson's disease. *Ann Neurol* 28(2):295, 1990.

119. Kish SJ, Shannak K, Rajput A, et al: Aging produces a specific pattern of striatal dopamine loss: Implications for the etiology of idiopathic Parkinson's disease. *J Neurochem* 58:642–648, 1992.

120. Rajput AH, Rozdilsky B, Ang L, Rajput A: Significance of Parkinsonian manifestations in essential tremor. *Can J Neurol Sci* 20:114–117, 1993.

121. Salemi G, Savettieri G, Rocca WA, et al: Prevalence of essential tremor: A door-to-door survey in Terrasini, Sicily. *Neurology* 44(1):61–64, 1994.

122. Bain PG, Findley LJ, Thompson PD, et al: A study of hereditary essential tremor. *Brain* 117:805–824, 1994.

123. Elble RJ: Physiologic and essential tremor. *Neurology* 36:225–231, 1986.

124. Stiles RN: Frequency and displacement amplitude relations for normal hand tremor. *J Appl Physiol* 40(1):44–54, 1976.

125. Calzetti S, Baratti M, Findley LJ: Frequency/amplitude characteristic of postural tremor of the hands in a population of patients with bilateral essential tremor: Implications for the classification and mechanism of essential tremor. *J Neurol Neurosurg Psychiatry* 50:561–567, 1987.

126. Rajput AH: Essential tremor that is not "benign" (abstr.). *Trans Can Congr Neurol* 55:151, 1976.

127. Busenbark KL, Nash J, Nash S, et al: Is essential tremor benign? *Neurology* 41:1982–1983, 1991.

128. Rajput AH: Pathological and neurochemical basis of essential tremor, in Findley LJ, Koller WC (eds): *Handbook of Movement Disorders.* New York: Marcel Dekker, 1994, pp 233–244.

129. Rajput AH, Jamieson H, Hirsch S, Quraishi A: Relative efficacy of alcohol and propranolol in action tremor. *Can J Neurol Sci* 2:31–35, 1975.

130. Geraghty JJ, Jankovic J, Zetusky WJ: Association between essential tremor and Parkinson's disease. *Ann Neurol* 17:329–333, 1985.

131. Barbeau A, Roy M: Familial subsets in idiopathic Parkinson's disease. *Can J Neurol Sci* 11:144–150, 1984.

132. Hornabrook RW, Nagurney JT: Essential tremor in Papua, New Guinea. *Brain* 99:659–672, 1976.

133. Cleeves L, Findley LJ, Koller W: Lack of association between essential tremor and Parkinson's disease. *Ann Neurol* 24:23–26, 1988.

134. Marttila RJ, Rautakorpi I, Rinne UK: The relation of essential tremor to Parkinson's disease. *J Neurol Neurosurg Psychiatry* 47:734–735, 1984.

135. Findley LJ, Gresty MA: Tremor and rhythmical involuntary movements in Parkinson's disease, in Findley LJ, Capildeo R (eds): *Movement Disorders: Tremor.* London: The Scientific and Medical Division of The MacMillan Press, 1984, pp 295–304.

136. Salisachs P, Findley LJ: Problems in the differential diagnosis of essential tremor, in Findley LJ, Capildeo R (eds): *Movement Disorders: Tremor.* London: MacMillan Press, 1984, pp 219–224.

137. Koller WC, Biary N: Effect of alcohol on tremors: Comparison with propranolol. *Neurology* 34:221–222, 1984.

138. Rajput AH, Rozdilsky B, Ang L, Rajput A: Clinicopathological observations in essential tremor: Report of 6 cases. *Neurology* 41:1422–1424, 1991.

139. Maruyama T, Hasimoto T, Miyasaka M, Yanagisawa N: A case of thalamo-subthalamic hemorrhage presenting monoballism in the contralateral lower extremity. *Rinsho Shinkeigaku* 32(9):1022–1027, 1992.

140. Ikeda M, Tsukagoshi H: Monochorea caused by a striatal lesion. *Eur Neurol* 31(4):257–258, 1991.

141. Vidakovic A, Dragasevic N, Kostic VS: Hemiballism: Report of 25 cases. *J Neurol Neurosurg Psychiatry* 57(8):945–949, 1994.

142. Nicolai A, Lazzarino LG: Paraballism associated with anterior opercular syndrome: A case report. *Clin Neurol Neurosurg* 96(2):145–147, 1994.

143. Caparros-Lefebvre D, Deleume JF, Bradaik N, Petit H: Biballism caused by bilateral infarction in the substantia nigra. *Mov Disord* 9(1):108–110, 1994.

144. Lodder J, Baard WC: Paraballism caused by bilateral hemorrhagic infarction in basal ganglia. *Neurology* 31:484–486, 1981.

145. Lazzarino LG, Nicolai A: Hemichorea-hemiballism and anosognosia following a contralateral infarction of the caudate nucleus and anterior limb of the internal capsule. *Riv Neurol* 61(1):9–11, 1991.

146. Hanaoka Y, Ohi T, Matsukura S: A case of hemiballism successfully treated by sulpiride, caused by lesions of the striatum. *Rinsho Shinkeigaku* 30(7):774–776, 1990.

147. Konagaya M, Nakamuro T, Sugata T, et al: MRI study of hemiballism. *Rinsho Shinkeigaku* 30(1):17–23, 1990.

148. Sethi KD, Nichols FT, Yaghmai F: Generalized chorea due to basal ganglia lacunar infarcts. *Mov Disord* 2(1):61–66, 1987.

149. Hyland HH, Forman DM: Prognosis in hemiballismus. *Neurology* 7:381–391, 1957.

150. Pappenheim E: Therapeutic response in hemiballismus. *Ann Neurol* 6:139, 1979.

151. Lenton RJ, Copti M, Smith RG: Hemiballismus treated with sodium valproate. *Br Med J* 283:17–18, 1981.

152. Pettigrew LC, Jankovic J: Hemidystonia: A report of 22 patients and a review of the literature. *J Neurol Neurosurg Psychiatry* 48:650–657, 1985.

153. Marsden CD, Obeso JA, Zarranz JJ, Lang AE: The anatomical basis of symptomatic hemidystonia. *Brain* 108:463–483, 1985.

154. Fross RD, Martin WRW, Li D, et al: Lesions of the putamen: Their relevance to dystonia. *Neurology* 37:1125–1129, 1987.

155. Comella CL, Klawans HL: Nonparkinsonian movement disorders in the elderly, in Albert ML, Knoefel JE (eds): *Clinical Neurology of Aging,* 2d ed. New York: Oxford University Press, 1994, pp 502–520.

156. Chang CM, Yu UL, Ng HK, et al: Vascular pseudoparkinsonism. *Acta Neurol Scand* 86(6):588–592, 1991.

157. Schwartz M, Silver H, Tal I, Sharf B: Tardive dyskinesia in northern Israel: Preliminary study. *Eur Neurol* 33(3):264–266, 1993.

158. Casey DE: Tardive dyskinesia. *West J Med* 153(5):535–541, 1990.

159. Klawans HL, Barr A: Prevalence of spontaneous lingual-facial-buccal dyskinesias in the elderly. *Neurology* 32:558–559, 1982.

160. Chiu HF, Wing YK, Kwong PK, et al: Prevalence of tardive dyskinesia in samples of elderly people in Hong Kong. *Acta Psychiatr Scand* 87(4):266–268, 1993.

161. Waddington JL, Youssef HA: The lifetime outcome and involuntary movements of schizophrenia never treated with neuroleptic drugs: Four rare cases in Ireland. *Br J Psychiatry* 156:106–108, 1990.

162. Green BH, Dewey ME, Copeland JR, et al: Prospective data on the prevalence of abnormal involuntary movements among elderly people living in the community. *Acta Psychiatr Scand* 87(6):418–421, 1993.

163. Khot V, Wyatt RJ: Not all that moves is tardive dyskinesia. *Am J Psychiatry* 148(5):661–666, 1991.

164. Sweet RA, Mulsant BH, Rifai AH, Zubenko GS: Dyskinesia and neuroleptic exposure in elderly psychiatric inpatients. *J Geriatr Psychiatry Neurol* 5(3):156–161, 1992.

165. Ticehurst SB: Is spontaneous orofacial dysinesia an artefact due to incomplete drug history? *J Geriatr Psychiatry Neurol* 3(4):208–211, 1990.

166. Klawans HL, Bergen D, Bruyn GW, Paulson GW: Neuroleptic-induced tardive dyskinesias in nonpsychotic patients. *Arch Neurol* 30:338–339, 1974.

167. Koller WC: Edentulous Orodyskinesia. *Ann Neurol* 13:97–99, 1983.

168. Kai S, Kai H, Tashiro H: Tardive dyskinesia affected by occlusal treatment—a case report. *Cranio* 12(3):199–203, 1994.

169. Sandyk R, Kay SR: Edentulousness and neuroleptic-induced neck and trunk dyskinesia. *Funct Neurol* 5(4):361–363, 1990.

170. Morris JC, Drazner M, Fulling K, et al: Clinical and pathological aspects of parkinsonism in Alzheimer's disease. *Arch Neurol* 46:651–657, 1989.

171. Molsa PK, Marttila RJ, Rinne UK: Extrapyramidal signs in Alzheimer's disease. *Neurology* 34:1114–1116, 1984.

172. Tyrrell PJ, Rossor MN: Extrapyramidal signs in dementia of Alzheimer type. *Lancet* 1989;October 14:920.

173. Bennett RG, Greenough WB, Gloth FM III, et al: Extrapyramidal signs in dementia of Alzheimer type. *Lancet* 1989;December 9:1392.

174. Soininen H, Laulumaa V, Helkala EL, et al: Extrapyramidal signs in Alzheimer's disease: A 3-year follow-up study. *J Neural Transm Park Dis Dement Sect* 4(2):107–119, 1992.

175. Kischka U, Mandir AS, Ghika J, Growdon JH: Electrophysiologic detection of extrapyramidal motor signs in Alzheimer's disease. *Neurology* 43:500–505, 1993.

176. Crystal HA, Dickson DW, Lizardi JE, et al: Antemortem diagnosis of diffuse Lewy body disease. *Neurology* 40:1523–1528, 1990.

177. Dickson DW, Ruan D, Crystal H, et al: Hippocampal degeneration differentiates diffuse Lewy body disease (DLBD) from Alzheimer's disease: Light and electron microscopic immunocytochemistry of CA2-3 neurites specific to DLBD. *Neurology* 41:1402–1409, 1991.

178. Chui HC, Teng EL, Henderson VW, Moy AC: Clinical subtypes of dementia of the Alzheimer type. *Neurology* 35:1544–1550, 1985.

179. Mayeux R, Stern Y, Spanton S: Heterogeneity in dementia of the Alzheimer type: Evidence of subgroups. *Neurology* 35:453–461, 1985.

180. Ravindran J, Stewart BJ, Siemens P, et al: Chorea as a presenting feature of Alzheimer's disease (abstr.). *Can J Neurol Sci* 21:S67, 1994.

181. Weiner WJ, Lang AE: Other akinetic-rigid and related syndromes, in Weiner WJ, Lang AE (eds): *Movement Disorders: A Comprehensive Survey*. Mount Kisco, NY: Futura Publishing, 1989, pp 117–219.

182. Watts RL, Mirra SM, Richardson EP: Cortical basal ganglionic degeneration, in Marsden CD, Fahn S (eds): *Movement Disorders 3*. Oxford, England: Butterworth-Heineman, 1994, pp 282–299.

183. Lang AE, Riley DE, Bergeron C: Cortical-basal ganglionic degeneration, in Calne DB (ed): *Neurogenerative Diseases*. Philadelphia: WB Saunders, 1994, pp 877–894.

184. Brunt ER, van Weerden TW, Pruim J, Lakke JWPF: Unique myoclonic pattern in corticobasal degeneration. *Mov Disord* 10(2):132–142, 1995.

185. Lang AE, Bergeron C, Pollanen MS, Ashby P: Parietal Pick's disease mimicking cortical-basal ganglionic degeneration. *Neurology* 44:1436–1440, 1994.

186. Kertesz A, Hudson L, Mackenzie IRA, Munoz DG: The pathology and nosology of primary progressive aphasia. *Neurology* 44:2065–2072, 1994.

187. Jendroska K, Rossor MN, Mathias CJ, Daniel SE: Morphological overlap between corticobasal degeneration and Pick's disease: A Clinicopathological report. *Mov Disord* 10(1):111–114, 1995.

188. McKim WA, Mishara BL: Prescription and over-the-counter drugs, in Hines L, Turner J, Kee L, et al (eds): *Drugs and Aging*. Toronto: Butterworth, 1987, pp 17–40.

189. McKim WA, Mishara BL: Age-related changes in absorption, distribution, excretion and sensitivity to drugs, in Hines L, Turner J, Kee L, et al (eds): *Drugs and Aging*. Toronto: Butterworth, 1987, pp 7–15.

190. The Parkinson Study Group: Effect of deprenyl on the progression of disability in early Parkinson's disease. *N Engl J Med* 321:1364–1371, 1989.

Chapter 51

MOVEMENT DISORDERS SPECIFIC TO SLEEP AND THE NOCTURNAL MANIFESTATIONS OF WAKING MOVEMENT DISORDERS

DAVID B. RYE and DONALD L. BLIWISE

NORMAL MOVEMENT IN SLEEP
MOVEMENT DISORDERS SPECIFIC TO SLEEP
    Periodic Leg Movements in Sleep/Restless Legs
       Syndrome
    Rapid Eye Movement Sleep Behavior Disorder
OTHER MOVEMENT DISORDERS SPECIFIC TO SLEEP
    Fragmentary NREM Myoclonus
    Nocturnal Paroxysmal Dystonia
    Head Banging (Jactatio Capitis Nocturna) and Body
       Rocking
    Bruxism
    Sleeptalking (Somniloquy)
    Sleepwalking (Somnambulism)
    Night Terrors (Pavor Nocturnus)
    Nocturnal Eating
SLEEP IN WAKING MOVEMENT DISORDERS
    Sleep in Parkinson's Disease
    Sleep in Other Waking Movement Disorders
    Treatment of Disturbed Sleep in Waking Movement
       Disorders
MECHANISMS CONTRIBUTING TO DISTURBED SLEEP
  IN WAKING MOVEMENT DISORDERS
    Etiologic Factors Related to Disrupted Sleep in
       Parkinson's Disease
    Role of Dopamine in Behavioral State Control
    Significance of the Ascending Reticular Activating
       System to Behavioral State Control
    Role of the Basal Ganglia in Behavioral State Control

In this chapter we will review nonepileptiform movement disorders in sleep. The disorders reviewed below encompass an extraordinarily wide range of movements and behaviors. For ease of presentation, we have divided this review into movement disorders known to be specific to sleep versus those movement disorders characteristic of wakefulness that may be modulated by sleep. Additionally, we will focus on practical guidelines for treatment that are, in part, driven by anatomic and physiological considerations of movement in sleep, using Parkinson's disease (PD) as the prototypical dis-order. The similarity of the sleep-related manifestations of many of these disorders and their assumed common underlying pathophysiology lead to treatment considerations that are parallel, despite heterogeneity of waking clinical disease. In fact, it is our belief that the various states of sleep may represent an exquisitely sensitive window on the functional anatomy and pharmacology of the basal ganglia and related structures, which may enhance our knowledge of the mechanisms underlying these conditions.

Much of our knowledge of sleep and movement disorders derives from studies on small groups of patients, including many individual patient reports. There are sparingly few comprehensive studies which: (1) evaluate the natural history of disordered sleep in various movement disorders; (2) control adequately for all variables that may confound clinical presentation, including aging, dementia, and affective state; and (3) evaluate response to treatment in a placebo-controlled fashion. This is not surprising, given the existence of multiple interacting variables that hinder identification of homogeneous patient populations. Moreover, complex combinations of pathology in brain regions such as the basal forebrain, raphe nuclei, locus ceruleus, and pedunculopontine nucleus occur in many movement disorders and would be expected to contribute appreciably to the manifestations of most of the conditions discussed below.

Normal Movement in Sleep

In order to define abnormal quantities or qualities of nocturnal movement, it is first necessary to establish the parameters of what constitutes normal movement during sleep. In some cases (e.g., nocturnal paroxysmal dystonia (NPD) or rapid eye movement sleep behavior disorder (RBD)), the pattern and amplitude of movement is clearly abnormal. Conversely, in other cases, either by virtue of the widespread prevalence of a condition (e.g., periodic leg movements in sleep ([PLMs])) or its transient expression during development (e.g., somnambulism), defining the limits of normality may be problematic. Undoubtedly, some of the complexity stems from the varying sensitivities of the techniques used to detect movements; that is, can they be documented videographically or do they require more sophisticated detection methods, such as accelerometers (e.g., actigraphy), surface, or even needle electromyography? Muscle activity recorded from surface electrodes, as is used in most polysomnographic studies, for example, may reveal some information regarding individual motor units when those units are not deeply distributed but, in other situations involving higher threshold force or when the muscle group of interest is further from skin, such surface electromyography (EMGs) may be insufficient.[1] Additionally, determining whether movement in sleep is focal or is a manifestation of a more complex pattern of movement adds another dimension of complexity. Polysomnographic studies often rely on surface EMG recordings of only several muscle groups (mentalis, anterior tibialis), which may show somewhat different patterns of activation relative to other muscles. Using actigraphic measures, for example, Van Hilten et al.[2] recently have shown that the upper limbs consistently reflect more movement during sleep relative to body trunk.

Although most skeletal muscles show reduced tonic activity during sleep,[3,4] it has long been known that the body of the sleeper is far from still throughout the night. Seminal studies from the first part of this century by Kleitman et al.[4] and Johnson et al.,[5] using primitive techniques, confirmed that the average sleeper exhibits from 40 to 50 movements during a night of sleep. Later work, using video time-lapse photography, confirmed these findings.[6] Gardner and Grossman[7] have maintained that gross body movements represent the end points of afferent stimulation as the sleeper adjusts position to maintain comfort. For example, a hard bed surface has been associated with a larger number of body movements relative to a more comfortable bed.[8] Generally, however, the characteristic number of such gross body movements during sleep has been demonstrated to be a relatively stable individual trait[9] that predicts change in sleep state,[10] decreases during postsleep deprivation recovery sleep,[11] and is often preceded by autonomic activation.[12]

In contrast to these gross body movements are brief twitches of distal limb muscles also known to occur during sleep. These were originally described in humans by De Lisi[13] and have been associated with both sleep onset ('hypnic jerks' or 'sleep starts')[14] and REM sleep, as recorded both in the finger,[15] in the leg,[16] and in the mimetic muscles.[17,18] Middle ear muscle activity has been investigated extensively during sleep and has been shown to relate at above chance levels with motor activity in the face, neck, and extremities.[19,20] Brief isolated twitches in rapid eye movement (REM) sleep have also been described in normal animals, including the cat[21] and baboon.[22] In humans, they have been likened to fasciculations and are without pathological significance.[23] Fasciculations in patients with lower motor neuron disease appear unaffected by sleep.[24]

Although limb jerks and twitches can be seen in normal sleepers, an increasingly large body of evidence suggests that waking movement disorders in general and disorders of the basal ganglia specifically may be characterized by excessive amounts of such activity within sleep.[25–27] Parkinsonian patients undergoing long-term L-dopa therapy are known to demonstrate myoclonic-like limb activity.[28] Such activation of motor systems during sleep in basal ganglia disorders may be distinguished from the normal activity during sleep described above because of its duration, frequency, and/or widespread distribution across muscle groups. A more complete description of these movements, as well as potential mechanisms underlying their occurrence, will be explored in greater detail below.

Movement Disorders Specific to Sleep

In recent years, the development of the multidisciplinary field of sleep disorders has led clinicians and researchers to examine movement patterns during sleep. In this section we will briefly review many of the movement disorders confined to sleep or, in some cases, those exacerbated by sleep. The enormous range and rich panoply of movements observed in otherwise neurologically normal individuals challenges the assumption that human sleep is a period of virtual quiescence.

PERIODIC LEG MOVEMENTS IN SLEEP/RESTLESS LEGS SYNDROME

Originally coined 'nocturnal myoclonus' by Symonds in 1953, periodic leg movements during sleep (PLMs) are repetitive, stereotypic, nonepileptiform movements of the lower limbs unique to sleep. The conventional definition requires that each movement lasts between 0.5 and 5.0 s, with a frequency of 1 every 20–40 s.[29] PLMs seldom occur in the upper limbs.[30–33] Movements typically consist of uni- or bilateral ankle dorsiflexion that occurs in clusters and can be followed by arousal on the EEG as manifested by K-complexes, bursts of alpha activity or lightening of sleep stages. They are most common in light (stages 1 and 2) non-REM (NREM) sleep, when compared to deep (stages 3 and 4) NREM and REM-sleep.[34] PLMs are clearly more prevalent in the aged population[35] without demonstrating a gender proclivity. Although PLMs are frequently associated with brief arousals from sleep that result in sleep fragmentation and, sometimes, profound excessive daytime sleepiness (EDS), the patient suffering with PLMs is just as likely to complain of insomnia.[36–38] Because the prevalence of PLMs approaches 50 percent of the geriatric population,[36,37] they may represent a common end point of many different medical conditions. For example, folate or iron deficiency and renal failure have been associated with PLMs, and a history of prior alcohol use may be a contributing factor.[39] Other etiologic factors potentially important in modulating PLMs include lumbosacral narrowing[40] and limb position.[41]

The underlying neurophysiological mechanisms for PLMs remain enigmatic. Nerve conductions[33,42] and sensory evoked potentials[43] are normal in patients with PLMs, suggesting that a primary afferent sensory disturbance is not at play. Cinematography has shown that PLMs resemble a Babinski response; however, during wakefulness this pathological response is generally absent.[44,45] Others have implicated brain stem dysfunction in noting a long latency component of the blink reflex.[43,46] The remarkably constant 20- to 40-s periodicity of leg movements mimics and even coincides with alterations in blood pressure,[47,48] respiration, intraventricular pressure, pulse frequency and electroencephalogram (EEG) arousal, suggesting the presence of an underlying central nervous system pacemaker. Neuropharmacological hypotheses regarding the pathophysiological basis of PLMs derive in part from the observed therapeutic benefits of dopaminomimetics and opioids.[49] A recent study[50] has suggested that impaired dopaminergic neurotransmission underlying PLMs reflects a decreased density of D2 receptors in the basal ganglia. It is premature, however, to rule out other potential substrates as contributors to the pathophysiology of PLMs, because dopaminergic and opioid systems interact outside of the basal ganglia in the brain stem and spinal cord.

The restless legs syndrome (RLS) is a nosological entity distinct from PLMs that was first described by Ekbom.[51–53] A great majority of patients with RLS, however, also experience PLMs, and because associated risk factors and treatment strategies are common to both conditions, they are commonly discussed together. The RLS manifests as irresistible leg movements accompanied by paresthesias that occur upon rest, most commonly just before or upon retiring to bed.

These paresthesias are perceived variably as 'pins and needles,' a 'crawling sensation,' and even as a deep-seated 'fullness' in the calves. Because vigorous leg movements or walking bring some relief, sleep onset is markedly delayed. Symptoms may also occur after awakenings that are spontaneous or possibly precipitated by PLMs and, therefore, interfere with sleep continuity as well. Taking a careful family history often reveals the presence of RLS, because it is frequently hereditary.[54] Medical conditions associated with RLS are the same as those discussed above for PLMs and, as is the case for PLMS, gender proclivity is ambiguous, and the syndrome increases in prevalence with age.[52] Analysis of EEG immediately before leg movements has shown no evidence of cortical Bereitschafts potential,[53] unlike voluntary movements in the same patients. RLS is to be distinguished from nocturnal leg cramps (systremma), which are thought to reflect muscle spasms secondary to excessive muscular fatigue and salt loss and are typically treated with quinine or skeletal muscle relaxants more or less successfully.[55,56] Some patients with RLS have been reported to experience leg cramps as well.[57]

TREATMENT

Because PLMs/RLS are associated with a variety of other conditions, including myelopathies, neuropathies, anemia, uremia, and narcolepsy, as well as others,[49] these entities should be carefully screened for and properly treated, when present. Treatment strategies for RLS are generally the same as those for PLMs. Nonpharmacological approaches include encouraging abstinence from caffeine, an agent that reportedly worsens RLS but not PLMs.[58] Alcohol and a variety of antidepressants make the condition more severe and should also be avoided if possible. It has been our clinical impression that antidepressants with potent 5-hydroxytryptamine (5-HT) reuptake blocking activity demonstrate a proclivity to increase PLMs. There are presently three well-established treatments for PLMs/RLS: dopaminomimetics, benzodiazepines, and opioid agonists. The therapeutic benefit observed with L-dopa and bromocriptine on PLMs, in fact, is part of a series of findings that supports the hypothesis that a deficit in central dopaminergic transmission,[49] possibly at the level of the D2-receptor,[50] underlies their pathophysiology. Opioids are also potent suppressors of PLMs,[59,60] whereas benzodiazepines improve sleep continuity only by decreasing arousals without decreasing the number of PLMs.[49,61] In the patient with PLMs, we suggest beginning treatment with an oral dose of 25/100 carbidopa/L-dopa 30–60 minutes before bedtime and doubling this dose if a satisfactory benefit is not observed. Alternatively, the dopamine agonist bromocriptine (1.25–3.75 mg qhs or 7.5 mg in divided doses) can be tried. When these approaches are unsatisfactory or result in 'rebound' leg movements in the early morning, we will discontinue dopaminomimetics and substitute clonazepam (0.5–2.0 mg), temazepam (15–30 mg) or triazolam (0.125–0.375 mg) at least 1 h before bedtime. We reserve the use of oxycodone (5–15 mg) or propoxyphene (65–100 mg) for patients who are refractory to the above approaches in order to avoid the development of tolerance and dependence to opioids. We have also noted beneficial effects with other

opioids, including codeine and methadone. Several other treatments have been proposed for PLMs, but few of them have been systematically evaluated and, therefore, have not gained widespread acceptance, including tegretol, baclofen, and clonidine.[49] Recent successes have also been reported with valproate,[62] and we and other investigators have also had some limited success with gabapentin (200–1200 mg qhs).[62a]

RAPID EYE MOVEMENT SLEEP BEHAVIOR DISORDER

In the mid-1980s, Schenck et al. described patients (predominantly older males in their 50s and 60s) with purposeful nocturnal motor activity, often violent in nature, that resembled dream enactment.[63] The patients typically demonstrated full dream recall and a history of self-injurious behavior that originated from REM sleep unaccompanied by epileptiform activity. Shouting and other loud vocalizations were common. Many of the patients had been mislabeled as having a long-standing psychiatric disorder. This condition, now termed rapid eye movement behavior disorder (RBD), is defined as a condition ". . . characterized by the intermittent loss of REM sleep electromyographic atonia and by the appearance of elaborate motor activity associated with dream mentation."[64] The novel concept resulting from the recognition of RBD is that certain electrophysiologically defined measures (EEG, electro-ocylogram [EOG], EMG) that define states of consciousness (e.g., waking, NREM sleep, REM sleep) can be dissociated from each other in certain disease states. Studies from the 1970s and early 1980s had originally demonstrated that lesions of the dorsolateral pontine tegmental field in cats[65,66] produced behavioral dissociation, with suspension of normal REM atonia, so that the animals appeared to be literally acting out their dreams. A number of studies had already suggested that a wide range of pharmacological agents in humans could be associated with some loss of REM atonia, including tricyclic antidepressants, monoamine oxidase inhibitors, and alcohol.[67–70] More recently, RBD-like syndromes have been related to use of selective 5-HT reuptake inhibitors.[71]

That RBD-like behavior frequently precedes the overt waking manifestations of PD,[26,72,73] as well as multiple-system atrophy,[74] underscores the importance of a thorough sleep history when evaluating patients with neurological complaints. Of the patients originally diagnosed with idiopathic RBD by Schenck et al., 38 percent eventually developed PD.[73] History should carefully consider other conditions that may precipitate RBD, such as abstinence from alcohol, benzodiazepine withdrawal, or chronic use of some psychotropic medications.[72] Differentiating RBD from panic attacks or nocturnal terrors can be more problematic. The later, however, arise from stage 2 at the transition to stage 3 and from stage 3/4 sleep, respectively.[75] Nocturnal motor behavior with lack of dream recall, abrupt arousal accompanied by diffuse autonomic symptoms, and amnesia for the event suggests the diagnosis of panic attacks. Although nocturnal terrors also manifest with extreme autonomic activation and retrograde amnesia, motor behaviors are usually more pronounced and marked by confusion and violence on attempted arousal.[75]

In RBD, on the other hand, dreams are frequently recalled and described as vivid, unpleasant, or action-filled. Polysomnography reveals heightened periodic and aperiodic movements in NREM sleep in both upper and lower limbs (in ~50 percent of patients), as well as heightened phasic and/or tonic REM-EMG activity during REM-sleep epochs not accompanied by dream enactment behavior. Elevated amounts of stages 3 and 4 NREM sleep have been noted as well. Clinicopathological studies of idiopathic human RBD are not yet available; however, magnetic resonance imaging studies indicate that symptoms may result from lesions involving the pontine tegmentum.[76] Patients with known brain stem degeneration,[77] as well as narcoleptics, also frequently demonstrate such motor dyscontrol.[78] In Mahowald and Schenck's[72] patient series, slightly more than one-third of RBD patients also had known central nervous system disorders, with the remainder considered idiopathic. The midbrain-pontine junction figures prominently in the pathophysiology of RBD and, given its position as a route by which the basal ganglia may modulate REM-sleep atonia, may account for how PD may manifest as RBD (see below; Fig. 51-6).

TREATMENT

The treatment of choice for RBD is clonazepam (0.5–2.0 mg qhs), which is reported to be effective in 75–90 percent of patients.[72]

Other Movement Disorders Specific to Sleep

FRAGMENTARY NREM MYOCLONUS

Broughton et al.[79] have reported on brief (150 ms) bursts of potentials of 50–250 μV amplitude occurring in seemingly random fashion throughout NREM sleep. Unlike PLMS, which are confined to the lower limbs,[33] these potentials are less prolonged and occur in widespread fashion in various limbs bilaterally and in different muscle groups. In most cases visible movements are not noted. Among sleep apnea patients, the presence of such surface EMG activity is not systematically accompanied by oxygen desaturation. Based on the data of Broughton et al., the most parsimonious interpretation is that fragmentary myoclonus represents an incidental finding made in patients diagnosed with other primary sleep disorders (e.g., sleep apnea, narcolepsy, insomnia). Nonetheless, Broughton et al. concluded that such fragmentary myoclonus may be associated with excessive daytime sleepiness (EDS) in some cases.

NOCTURNAL PAROXYSMAL DYSTONIA

This condition, which consists of paroxysmal motor attacks during NREM, but not REM sleep, is characterized by normal interictal EEG activity during both sleep and wakefulness.[80] During an episode, which may last for 20–60 s, spike waves, often prominent in frontal regions, may be observed[81]; however, most patients have been described without any paroxysmal EEG activity.[82] Behaviorally, patients may show dystonic posturing or hyperextension; on some occasions,

vocalizations are also noted.[83] In other patients, semipurposeful arm activity or even sexual automatisms may be seen. Thus, NPD patients share some characteristic features with RBD; however, the episodes in NPD clearly evolve from NREM (typically stage 4) sleep. Data suggest that the modal interval between attacks is 10–40 s,[83] which has led some researchers to speculate that the condition parallels the periodic waxing and waning of EEG activation in NREM sleep (cyclic alternating pattern) described in normals.[84] These fluctuations in corticosubcortical arousability could exert a modulating effect on the motor attacks.

HEAD BANGING (JACTATIO CAPITIS NOCTURNA) AND BODY ROCKING

These movement disorders may occur during NREM[85] or REM sleep,[86,87] with more than 600 distinct movements observed on a given night. Head movements are typically anteroposterior. Occasionally headrolling, consisting of lateral movements, may also occur. Body rocking occurs with the sleeper often on his or her knees in bed with anteroposterior thrusting of the entire body into the pillow. These conditions are most typically seen in infants where, at the age of 9 months, a prevalence of 60 percent has been reported[88]; they are much less frequent in older children and adults. Spontaneous presentations in adults have been noted; one report implied that head banging may have resulted from closed-head injury.[89] Other variants may exist as well. A case of repetitive, nocturnal tongue biting in a 2-year-old child, occurring in slow-wave sleep and not associated with epileptiform activity in waking or sleep, was reported by Tuxhorn and Hoppe.[90]

BRUXISM

Excessively high masseter electromyogram activity during sleep, particularly when associated with tooth wear, temporomandibular joint pain, or destruction of dental restorations, is labeled bruxism. Bruxism has been variously described as occurring in both NREM and REM sleep.[91–93] There is some suggestion that bruxing in REM may lead to greater mouth damage, because a greater masticatory force is generated when antigravity muscles are overcome by REM related atonia.[94] Of note is that 75–85 percent of bruxing events co-occur with more generalized body movements, typically, in the anterior tibialis.[95] There is also some evidence that bruxism, more than any other movement disorder of sleep, is associated with acute psychological stress.[96,97] Alcohol has been reported to increase bruxism,[98] and several types of medications, including serotonin reuptake inhibitors[99] and long-term phenothiazine usage,[100] have been suggested to predispose for bruxism. Animal studies indicate that dopamine agonists can increase its occurrence,[101] whereas in humans, bruxism has been attributed to long-term use of L-dopa.[102]

SLEEPTALKING (SOMNILOQUY)

This phenomenon has been investigated extensively by Arkin,[103] who reported that episodes may arise from both NREM and REM sleep and have varying levels of complexity and semantic structure. There was little relationship to psychopathology. MacNeilage[104] reported that episodes of sleeptalking were preceded by an average of 10 s of muscle activity, as recorded in the genioglossus and other oral/buccal muscles. Additionally, individuals who characteristically talked in their sleep showed a greater abundance of such activity, even during periods without vocalization. Vocalizations during sleep are also common during RBD and night terrors.

SLEEPWALKING (SOMNAMBULISM)

Classic sleepwalking (somnambulism) was described polysomnographically in the 1960s,[105] and appeared to occur largely in stage 4 sleep and not uncommonly in children. More recent reports have confirmed these findings.[106] Because the condition derives out of slow-wave sleep and often involves incomplete awakening, some have considered the condition as a disorder of arousal.[107] It is distinguished from complex partial seizures by a normal EEG during both waking and sleep. The subject remains amnestic during and after the event and, unlike the case of the complex, purposeful movements of RBD, the sleeper's movements are awkward and gangly. Somnambulism is common in children, with a prevalence as high as 39–48 percent in 4 to 6 year olds noted in some epidemiological studies.[108] It is thought to be of little psychopathological consequence in childhood, although adults who sleepwalk have been reported to have schizoid tendencies.[109] Childhood trauma or posttraumatic stress disorder are risk factors. At all ages, the sleepwalker should be considered potentially dangerous to self and others. Adult sleepwalkers have been shown to have higher amounts of stages 3 and 4 sleep and have more spontaneously occurring disruptions of these stages as well.[110] There appears to be a hereditary component. Somnambulism should be differentiated from the phenomenon of sundowning in geriatric patients.[111]

NIGHT TERRORS (PAVOR NOCTURNUS)

Often occurring with somnambulism with arousals from stage 4 sleep,[112] night terrors are characterized by dramatic awakenings, accompanied by extraordinarily loud vocalizations, screaming, and a heightened affective state. Tachycardia, tachypnea, sweating, and enlarged pupils have been described.[113] As is the case with somnambulism, this condition is usually seen in children, rather than in adults, and may represent a transiently normal developmental event. More serious psychopathology may be implicated in adults.[114] Retrograde amnesia usually exists, although the sleeper may have a vague recollection of frightening experiences. Some potential overlap with RBD may exist.

NOCTURNAL EATING

Of apparent similarity to RBD is a syndrome involving excessive nighttime food consumption in patients without a comorbid eating disorder diagnosis in the waking state. Schenck et al.[115] and others[116,117] have described a dissociated state involving complex, purposeful motor behavior, specifically limited to eating, in several series of patients. Patients are usually amnestic for the experiences, which are identified by the patients by containers, etc., and other food remnants in the morning. Those few cases documented in the laboratory suggest that the awakenings may occur out of NREM, rather than REM sleep.[117]

TREATMENT OF OTHER MOVEMENT DISORDERS SPECIFIC TO SLEEP

Historical or polysomnographic identification of the specific form of nocturnal movement disorder will dictate the course of treatment. Once the proper diagnosis is established, the vast majority are treatable by either behavioral or pharmacological means. Because their etiologies are likely to be diverse, however, the proposed treatments are legion and usually lack validated objective results. The physician should first attempt to rule out any associated condition and/or medication that may account for nocturnal movements or parasomnic behaviors. Antidepressant medications, for example, may worsen fragmentary non-REM myoclonus, whereas cardiac antiarrhythmic agents and some antidepressants may exacerbate nocturnal terrors.[118,119] Before pharmacological interventions, the physician should always council the patient and family on proper sleep hygiene, including: (1) avoidance of sleep deprivation; (2) maintenance of a strict sleep-wake schedule; and (3) avoidance of alcoholic and caffeinated beverages, as well as nicotine, secondary to their tendencies to worsen sleep fragmentation.

Fragmentary non-REM sleep myoclonus is a disorder that may be associated with marked EDS.[79,120] Treatment typically includes clonazepam (0.5–2.0 mg) at bedtime, although it should be noted that there is insufficient information on the etiology and treatment of this specific disorder. NPD responds remarkably well to carbamazepine (200–400 mg) at bedtime. Rare successes have also been reported with phenytoin (5 mg/kg) and phenobarbital (100–150 mg) at bedtime. There is no clear consensus on the treatment of head banging/body rocking. In severe cases with self-injurious behavior, the judicious use of clonazepam (0.5–2.0 mg) at bedtime seems warranted. In milder cases, behavioral modification that involves audio masking with a metronome may be of benefit. Overpracticing of rhythmic behavior in a rocking chair or more vigorous rhythmic exercises before retiring may be of additional benefit, and self-hypnosis has also been reported to be successful.[121] There are no established direct treatments of bruxism.[96] Most measures are aimed at limiting the morbidity associated with bruxism and include the use of mouth guards and nonsteroidal anti-inflammatory agents. Given the observations that dopaminergic agonists may worsen bruxism,[101,102] it would be interesting to establish whether there is a role for dopamine antagonists in treatment. Muscle relaxation, biofeedback, and psychotherapy may be of some benefit, but their effectiveness has not been further defined.[96]

Sleeptalking, sleepwalking, night terrors, and nocturnal binge eating comprise a group of parasomnias that frequently coexist.[122] One of the most important aspects of the treatment of these disorders is ruling out coexistent depression or other psychopathology, particularly in the elderly patient. A medication history is also important, because these parasomnias may be associated with long-term benzodiazepine use or withdrawal, as well as cardiac anti-arrhythmic agents. A wide variety of stimuli, such as PLMs, apnea, and gastroesophageal reflux, may also present with complaints of parasomnic behavior, presumably secondary to their precipitating nocturnal arousals. Polysomnography, therefore, is frequently indicated to consider these etiologies that demand distinct treatment strategies. Nocturnal seizures less commonly present with complaints simulating one of these parasomnias or head banging/body rocking. Video monitoring and polysomnography with EEG montages that are more elaborate than those typically used in routine studies are, therefore, only occasionally required for proper diagnosis.

Sleeptalking, when present without other associated parasomnic behaviors, is of unknown significance and has no known treatment. Sleepwalking may respond to psychotherapy[123] and/or hypnosis.[106,124] Symptomatic treatment with clonazepam (0.5–2.0 mg qhs) is effective in about one-half of cases. Night terrors frequently respond to diazepam or alprazolam alone or in combination with a tricyclic antidepressant, such as nortryptiline. In the elderly patient in whom benzodiazepines may induce confusion or disorientation, trazodone (25–150 mg), carbamazepine (200–300 mg), or valproate (125–500 mg) at bedtime may be of some benefit. The mainstays of treatment for nocturnal binge eating include L-dopa/carbidopa alone or in combination with clonazepam.[116,125] Favorable response to L-dopa is thought, in part, to be related to the frequent coexistence of PLMs in these patients, so that treatments with opioids may also be indicated.[125] Favorable responses to 5-HT reuptake inhibitors, representing a smaller subset of patients, have also been reported.[116,125]

Sleep in Waking Movement Disorders

SLEEP IN PARKINSON'S DISEASE

Disorders of sleep in patients with PD have long been recognized; however, their pathophysiological basis remains ill-defined, and universal treatment strategies have not been established. Reasons for these deficiencies are many, and they include the pathological heterogeneity of PD and coincident factors such as medication use, aging, dementia, and mood disturbances, each of which are known to independently affect sleep parameters. The sleep of PD patients is profoundly disturbed, even relative to other neurodegenerative conditions. One survey placed the prevalence of sleep disturbance in PD at 98 percent.[126] Polysomnographic studies of PD patients, extending back into the 1960s, consistently demonstrate poor sleep efficiency, decreases in stages 3 and 4 sleep, and marked sleep fragmentation.[127–132] The sleep stage-specific EEG may also change in PD, with sleep spindles being reduced during slow-wave sleep[130,133,134] and alpha activity intruding into REM sleep.[127] Changes in REM sleep have been more variable across studies and appear highly dependent on dose and length of L-dopa, or bromocriptine treatment and individual patient differences.[128,129,135,136] Therefore, although L-dopa is known to suppress REM sleep in normal adult volunteers,[137] potent REM-sleep suppression,[138,139] increased REM sleep amounts,[128,130] and elevated REM density[138,139] have all been reported in PD. REM sleep rebound effects have been suggested as underlying the hallucinations experienced by many PD patients subsequent to

years of pharmacotherapy.[140–145] Comella et al.,[146] however, recently suggested that unique pathology may underlie these hallucinations, because these patients have more profoundly disturbed sleep when controlling for medication effects. Absence of customary REM atonia and/or excessive limb movement during sleep have long been appreciated,[127,132,147] and were first documented systematically in PD by Askenasky[148] and in other basal ganglia diseases by Mano.[149] More recently, the London[150] and Mayo Clinic[26,151] groups have also focused on such activity. The sleep of PD patients can also be characterized by the occurrence of intense dream-like motor and verbal behavior during REM sleep that is typically violent and potentially injurious.[26,72–74,77,151,152] To summarize the results of these and other studies[153–156]:

1. Sleep can be punctuated by parkinsonian tremor (Figs. 51-1 and 51-2), although tremor may be preceded by microawakenings; and during REM, isolated muscle contractions frequently predominate (Fig. 51-3).
2. Non-REM *and* REM sleep are characterized by large numbers of isolated *and* periodic limb movements (PLMs) (Fig. 51-4).
3. Stages 3 and 4 of non-REM sleep are least likely to manifest movements.
4. Nocturnal movements are likely in both upper and lower extremities.
5. Nocturnal movements are likely in both flexor and extensor muscles.
6. Nocturnal movements are generally best controlled when waking motor symptomatology is best treated, although movement may persist even in the presence of antiparkinsonian medication in advanced patients.
7. RBD can accompany and even precede waking signs of PD, as well as other degenerative conditions affecting the basal ganglia and/or brain stem.

In summary, difficulty with sleep maintenance (i.e., sleep fragmentation) is the earliest and most frequent sleep disorder recognized in PD. Despite the widely held belief that involuntary movements associated with disease of the extrapyramidal motor system disappear during sleep, motor dyscontrol in sleep, either in the form of tremor (Figs. 51-1 and 51-2), isolated movements (Fig. 51-3), PLMS (Fig. 51-4), increased REM sleep EMG activity (Fig. 51-3), or RBD frequently accompany PD and other neurodegenerative diseases affecting the basal ganglia.[157] The prevalence of nocturnal motor dyscontrol is difficult to establish, because most published data derive from polysomnographic studies carried out at referral centers, thereby selecting for patients with disturbed sleep. The degree to which nocturnal movements contribute to sleep fragmentation, and whether these are disease-specific or treatment-related phenomena, remain controversial issues that are still to be resolved. Many clinicians, for example, consider nocturnal movements severe enough to awaken the patient as evidenced below, in excerpts from Parkinson's *Essay on the Shaking Palsy*:

In this stage, the sleep becomes much disturbed. The tremulous motion of the limbs occur during sleep, and augment until they awaken the patient, and frequently with much agitation and

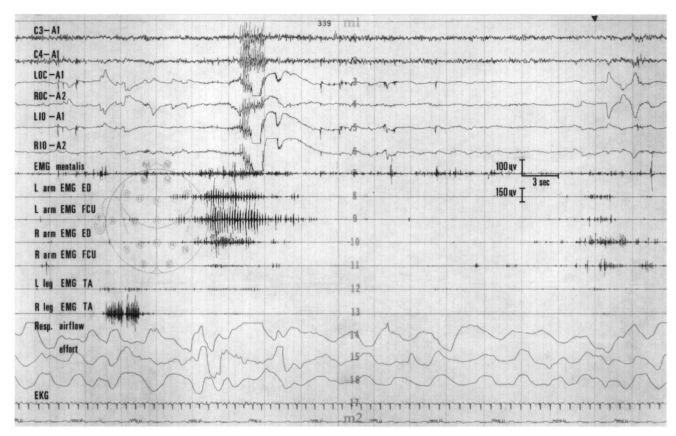

FIGURE 51-1 Polysomnographic recording of an episode of tremor intruding on an epoch of REM sleep in a patient with PD. Also note the increased level of tonic activity in the chin EMG (EMG mentalis). R, right; L, left; ED, extensor digitorum; FCU, flexor carpi ulnaris; TA, tibialis anterior.

alarm. . . . As the debility increases and the influence of the will over the muscles fades away, the tremulous agitation becomes more vehement. It now seldom leaves him for a moment; but even when exhausted nature seizes a small portion of sleep, the motion becomes so violent as not only to shake the bed-hangings, but even the floor and sashes of the room. (James Parkinson (1755–1824). From: *James Parkinson (1755–1824)*, edited by Macdonald Critchley. London: Macmillan & Co., 1955.)

Other investigators argue that awakenings almost always precede nocturnal movement in support of the contention that movement disorders disappear in sleep.[150,158] In our own experience with PD patients, referred for evaluation from a large movement disorders clinic, it has become commonplace to record movement preceding awakenings, although it is difficult to be certain whether a direct causal relationship exists.

The daytime consequences of sleep fragmentation, whatever the underlying pathophysiology, have not been established, although patients and their spouses frequently volunteer that activities of daily living are improved when sleep is undisturbed.[159] One might suspect EDS to be a direct consequence of disturbed sleep in PD, but this issue has only been addressed with questionnaire-based surveys, and the results paint a conflicting picture. Although one study suggests that EDS and 'dozing,' but not napping, are more frequent in PD patients than in elderly controls,[160] another argues that

subjective 'fatigue' related to exertion, but not EDS, is more common in PD.[161] Quantitative assessments of EDS or arousal with the mean sleep latency test (MSLT) or maintenance of wakefulness test (MWT), respectively, would be most useful in establishing the clinical relevance of these subjective complaints. Our own and other's[158,162] experiences with PD patients suggests a wide range of daytime sleep latencies between and within subjects that likely reflects not only the degree of sleep fragmentation but also a complex interplay between the effects of medication, the 'on-off' phenomena (Fig. 51-5) and, potentially, the degree of pathology in brain regions critical for maintaining arousal (see below). Because sleep and levels of arousal have generally accepted benefits on the mobility in parkinsonism,[146,159,163,164] investigations into the precise nature and prevalence of the disturbed sleep of PD seem warranted.

Suprisingly little attention has been directed toward relating sleep disruption to the cognitive disabilities of PD. Sleep loss in humans, for example, impairs cognitive performance in a manner imitating frontal lobe dysfunction,[165,166] a commonly observed and studied disorder in PD patients that has been attributed to dopamine depletion (see Chap. 2). Dependence on REM sleep for overnight learning of a visuospatial task[167] also suggests that reductions of REM sleep that are intrinsic to PD or that result from L-dopa administration might contribute to the visuospatial abnormalities experi-

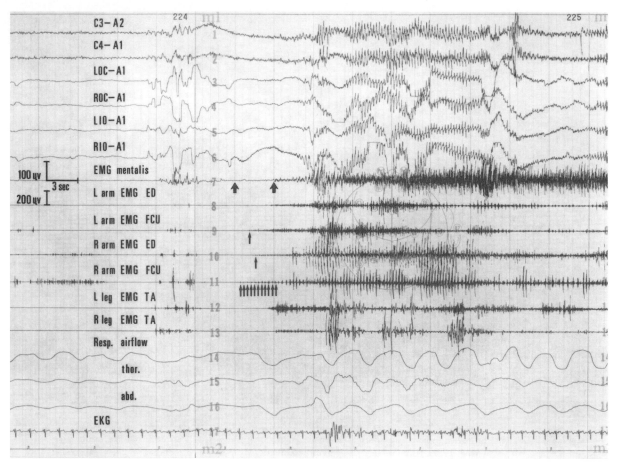

FIGURE 51-2 Polysomnographic recording of an episode of tremor intruding on REM sleep with subsequent arousal in a patient with PD. Multiple small arrows denote tremor that begins in the right flexor carpi ulnaris (FCU), coincident with the development of tonic activity in the right extensor digitorum (ED) and left flexor carpi ulnaris (small arrows). During this 3-second epoch there is no change in chin muscle activity, as detected by the mentalis EMG (two broad arrows) or in the cortical EEG. Arousal from REM sleep, therefore, clearly occurs after these EMG changes. Abbreviations are as designated in Fig. 52-1.

enced by PD patients.[168] Ascribing cognitive deficits in PD to insufficient sleep is problematic because: (1) each may be a secondary phenomena reflecting dopamine depletion, and (2) they may reflect extranigral pathology in brain regions known to affect behavioral state (see below). Although correlations can be made between cognitive deficits and EDS or hypoarousal in markedly sleep-deprived normals,[169,170] the MSLT or MWT have never been systematically applied to a population of PD patients. The potential contributions of EDS and hypoarousal to deficits of cognition, attention, or motivation in PD, therefore, remain obscure. Impaired attentional and mnemonic functions circumvested within the terms 'bradyphrenia' or 'subcortical dementia,' are therefore most frequently ascribed to nigral or extranigral pathology in PD (see Chap. 18).[168,171] A better understanding of the pathophysiology underlying the disturbed sleep of PD patients, and its contribution to daytime sleepiness and hypoarousal might yield novel insights into the treatment of cognitive disabilities in PD patients.

TREATMENT

Clinicians treating patients with PD and other neurodegenerative diseases of the basal ganglia should always carefully inquire about sleep quality, since disturbed sleep can presage the development of further more troublesome sleep disorders.[143] When sleep disturbances in patients with PD occur, their management is highly individualized. Askenasy and Yahr,[156] however, demonstrated that appropriate management of waking motor symptoms generally reduces nocturnal movement and improves sleep efficiency. Although amelioration of waking motor symptoms is always the desired outcome, that anywhere from 74 to 98 percent of medicated PD patients complain of sleep disturbances[126,143] suggests that suboptimal management may well be the rule, rather than the exception. Because a typical pattern of disordered sleep has not been clearly delineated and etiology is generally unknown, no clear-cut algorithms exist for approaching the treatment of PD patients with disordered sleep. Specific treatments need to be customized to com-

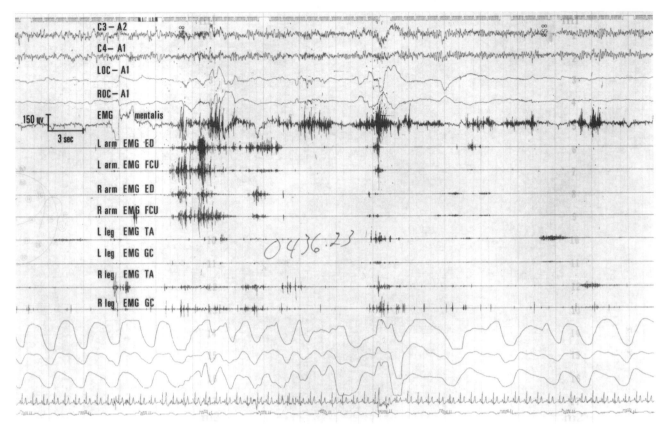

FIGURE 51-3 Polysomnographic recording of intermittent phasic muscle activity during REM sleep in a patient with PD. It is not unusual to detect similar phasic muscle activity coincident with other phasic events of REM sleep (e.g., eye movements) in normals. Note, however, the occurrence of heightened phasic and tonic muscle activity in the chin (EMG mentalis) that occurs independent of eye movements in the parkinsonian patient. REM sleep appears to persist despite these EMG changes. Abbreviations as for Fig. 51-1; GC, gastrocnemius.

plaints only after an adequate sleep history and review of polysomnographic findings, as discussed in detail below, have been completed. History should not rely on subjective reports of sleep alone, since reliability of personal assessments is well-known to be poor secondary to sleep state misperception. Information from a caregiver and preferably a bed partner is a sine qua non to guide treatment decisions, as is historical information on the timing of medications and nocturnal symptoms, as well as the relationship of symptoms to any changes in medication. Whenever historical evidence exists for nocturnal motor behavior, abnormal respiratory patterns, or EDS, polysomnography should be performed. Before pharmacological interventions, the physician should always counsel the patient and family on proper sleep hygiene, which includes, but is not restricted to, avoidance of alcoholic beverages, nicotine, and caffeine.[172]

SLEEP ONSET INSOMNIA

Sleep onset insomnia appears to be no greater a problem in the PD patient than in the general aged population, based on questionnaire data.[126,145,160,161] In most instances, sleep-onset problems can be related to anxiety or to agitated depression, which should then be the focus of treatment. Additional contributors to sleep-onset insomnia in small subpopulations

of PD patients include RLS and akathisia, which are discussed in more detail below.

When treatment with L-dopa is instituted, some patients may experience sleep-onset insomnia that typically resolves with time.[158] Sleep-onset insomnia, at the outset of L-dopa therapy, is best treated by administering medications earlier and waiting patiently. When insomnia is severe enough to produce a significant and persistent phase delay in sleep onset, the use of fairly rapidly absorbed and/or short-acting benzodiazepines, such as temazepam (15–30 mg), alprazolam (0.125–0.25 mg), estazolam (1–2 mg) or triazolam (0.125–0.25 mg), seems warranted. In our own experience, we have been most satisfied with triazolam, with the comment that it should be used with caution in elderly and demented patients. Our own repeated attempts to treat advanced patients with zolpidem (5–10 mg), a very rapidly absorbed and short-acting benzodiazepine-like medication, as well as other sedative-hypnotics (chloral hydrate, pentobarbital) have met with limited success.

SLEEP MAINTENANCE INSOMNIA

Sleep maintenance insomnia, i.e., sleep fragmentation, is the most common nocturnal complaint in PD patients. It is of primary importance to first rule out, by history, other comor-

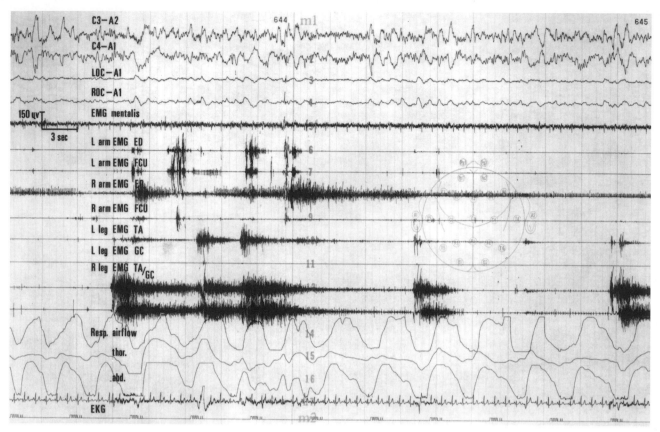

FIGURE 51-4 Polysomnographic recording of periodic leg movements during stage 2 non-REM sleep in a PD patient. Note the periodic cocontraction of the right tibialis anterior (TA) and gastrocnemius (GC) indicative of PLMs. In the parkinsonian patient this is more likely to occur coincident with, as well as independent of, activity in several other upper and lower extremity muscle groups. Arousal from sleep clearly does not accompany these EMG changes.

bid conditions that might present as a complaint of sleep maintenance insomnia. For example, poor sleep characterized by early morning awakenings can signal the appearance of depression, the use of alcohol as a sedative, or the natural effect of aging in phase advancing the wake-sleep cycle. Having ruled out these possibilities, the clinician should recognize that the complaint of sleep fragmentation in PD manifests polysomographically as a continuum from unexplained spontaneous awakenings to awakenings associated with quite specific nocturnal motor disturbances. Each of the latter conditions can be associated with either under- or over-treatment of the daytime symptoms of PD or represent side effects of adjunct medications and, therefore, require very different treatment strategies.

Clinical experience dictates that early in the course of treatment with L-dopa, daytime administration improves motor symptoms and may not disrupt sleep. Frequent awakenings, for the most part unassociated with movements, are treated with sedating antidepressants, such as trazodone, nefazodone, nortriptyline, amitriptyline, or clomipramine. Some caution should be exercised in prescribing antidepressants, because they may precipitate confusion/hallucinosis,[158] worsen PD,[173] or worsen PLMs (see below). Because the later two side effects appear related to serotoninergic mechanisms, the antidepressants listed above are presented in order of

preference, based on their increasing potencies in blocking 5-HT reuptake.[174]

As PD progresses and/or L-dopa use becomes long-term, patients may experience 'off' phenomena during the night. These patients, usually advanced in their disease, typically relate a history of marked interdose motor fluctuations during the day. Not only dyskinesia but also immobility with subsequent inability to rise to use the bathroom may be troubling for the patient at night.[126] In this instance, historical documentation frequently uncovers the presence of nocturnal movements, severe akinesia, and/or prolonged awakenings that occur *later* in the night. This situation should be carefully distinguished, preferably by polysomnography, from nocturnal movements *early* in the night, which is more suggestive for nocturnal myoclonus secondary to over-treatment or PLMs. Treatment for PD patients with distinct nocturnal motor disabilities such as tremor, dyskinesias, akinesia, and prolonged awakenings should begin with dosing L-dopa closer to bedtime, particularly in sustained-release form, because this is felt to diminish sleep fragmentation by nocturnal movements.[175,176] Alternatively, selegiline and bromocriptine have been shown to improve sleep in patients with PD, even when L-dopa has minimal effect.[139,158] High evening doses, however, might increase sleep latency and disrupt sleep in the first half of the night, despite improving sleep continuity in the second half of the night.[129,130] When polysomnograhpically documented nocturnal movements persist, we complement treatment with benzodiazepines, which are known to markedly reduce phasic sleep events and small and large body movements.[177] We prefer the use of triazolam (0.125–0.25 mg qhs) in nondemented patients because of its documented benefit for elderly patients with PLMs, sleep fragmentation, and daytime sleepiness.[178]

Frequently encountered in our practice has been the worsening of nocturnal myoclonus and PLMs with antidepressants, particularly 5-HT reuptake inhibitors, which is an infrequently recognized side effect but is commonly accepted among sleep clinicians.[94,144,179,180] This phenomenon is consistent with reports of benefits from methysergide, a serotonin antagonist, in alleviating the nocturnal myoclonus of PD (see below).[16,28,144] Treatment options include discontinuation of antidepressant medication or its substitution with an antidepressant, whose potency in blocking 5-HT reuptake is less. We have also observed worsening of PLMs in PD, secondary to the inadvertent prescription of metaclopromide for the gastrointestinal symptoms of PD that presumably reflects its dopamine antagonist action.

FRAGMENTARY NOCTURNAL MYOCLONUS

The chronic administration of L-dopa can lead to the development of fragmentary nocturnal myoclonus during slow-wave sleep.[28,144] Historical data that may suggest the presence of nocturnal myoclonus include the complaint of troubling daytime dyskinesias related to L-dopa dosing[28] or that of exaggerated *axial* myoclonus at sleep onset that may precipitate abrupt arousals from sleep. This phenomenon is thought to reflect L-dopa-induced upregulation of serotoninergic neurotransmission, because it is alleviated by methysergide (2 mg), a serotoninergic antagonist, and by discontinuing L-dopa but not by altering anticholinergic medications.[28] Treatment options include a reduction in nighttime dosing of dopamine agonists, addition of a benzodiazepine, such as temazepam, clonazepam, or triazolam and, possibly, a trial with methysergide (2 mg) shortly before bedtime.

PERIODIC LEG MOVEMENTS OF SLEEP

PLMs are an entity distinct from fragmentary nocturnal myoclonus, although their presence early in non-REM sleep disrupts sleep in a similar manner. They can be differentiated clinically from myoclonus, because they are more often unilateral and prolonged, spaced at very regular intervals, and characterized by a flexor withdrawal type movement typically restricted to the lower extremities. Although a careful history from a spouse or bed partner may, therefore, distinguish between these two entities, polysomnography is sometimes required and warranted since treatment modalities are distinct. It is unclear whether PLMs are more prevalent in PD patients, given their relatively high prevalence rates in the general population over the age of 65.[37,52] However, that neurophysiological abnormalities delineated in patients with PLMs but not suffering from PD[43,46] approximate those seen in PD patients,[181,182] suggests a common pathophysiology. The therapeutic benefits observed with L-dopa and bromocriptine on PLMs, in fact, support the hypothesis that a deficit in central dopaminergic transmission,[49] possibly at the level of the D2 receptor,[50] underlies their pathophysiology. In treating PD patients with coexistent PLMs, we follow the strategies outlined above for PLMs in the nonparkinsonian population. Given the decreased capacity of the pathologically effected substantia nigra (SN) to synthesize dopamine from L-dopa, trials with the dopamine agonist bromocriptine (1.25–3.75 mg qhs or 7.5 mg in divided doses) or selegiline (2.5–5.0 mg) seem particularly warranted. When dopaminomimetics are unsatisfactory, aggravate insomnia, produce troubling nocturnal myoclonus, or result in 'rebound' leg movements in the early morning,[49] we will substitute oxycodone (5–15 mg) or propoxyphene (65–100 mg) at bedtime for the dopaminomimetics. We reserve the use of benzodiazepines for patients that are refractory to these approaches to avoid problems associated with the development of tolerance and possible worsening of coexistent depression.

RLS

Several investigators have failed to note the coincidence of RLS in patients with PD[158,162]; however, in our experience the two frequently coexist. The reason for this apparent discrepancy may be a definitional one, because the distinction between PLMs and RLS is a somewhat artificial one. Suspected RLS in a PD patient should be very carefully differentiated from akathisia, which is also encountered in the PD patient population.

AKATHISIA

Nocturnal akathisia is a reported problem in a small subgroup of PD patients and should be carefully differentiated from RLS. Akathisia is not associated with prominent paresthesias, and symptoms are not typically relieved by movements or pacing, unlike those of RLS. Moreover, there is no polysomnographically documented hallmark that has yet been defined in the PD patient experiencing akathisia. Akathisia is frequently described by the PD patient as a vague sensation of an 'inner restlessness.' Moreover, akathisia is thought to be precipitated by L-dopa,[183,184] whereas it would be expected to suppress the symptoms of RLS. While one report suggests that akathisia more commonly occurs in PD patients with bradykinesia and 'stiffness,'[183] another notes that it is unrelated to motor or mental state or time of day.[184] Successful treatments include alterations in the timing or dosage of L-dopa[183] and bedtime dosing of clozapine, which has the added benefit of reducing nighttime tremor.[184] Successful treatment of akathisia has also been reported, using fluoxetine alone or together with amitriptyline in one depressed PD patient.[185]

REM SLEEP BEHAVIOR DISORDER

RBD is another example of nocturnal motor dyscontrol that can manifest in patients with PD and other neurodegenerative conditions.[72,77,152] This entity is more frequently encountered in the male PD patient (~90 percent), as is the case with 'idiopathic' RBD. The treatment of choice for RBD is clonazepam (0.5–2.0 mg qhs), which is effective in 75–90 percent of cases, although it is unclear whether PD patients exhibiting RBD represent a unique subpopulation. Dopaminomimetics and/or antidepressants, which block dopamine reuptake (e.g., buproprion and sertraline) theoretically, may prove to be a useful alternative or adjunct medications in the PD patient with RBD.

OTHER PARASOMNIAS

Parasomnia is a term that includes a variety of complex sleep-related behavioral phenomena in addition to RBD. In PD patients, these include sleeptalking, sleepwalking (i.e., somnambulism), altered dream content, nocturnal hallucinations, nocturnal terrors, and panic disorder. Difficulties in differentiating between parasomnias on the basis of history and the lack of specific polysomnographic features in PD has precluded accurate delineation of their pathophysiology and treatment. Because many of these parasomnias have been reported as prodromes to the development of full-blown RBD,[72] they may describe a continuum reflecting a common pathophysiology. The sleep of patients experiencing nocturnal terrors, however, lacks any distinct alterations in sleep architecture,[158] whereas that of patients with nocturnal hallucinations is markedly fragmented and approximates that seen in RBD.[146] Although panic disorder could theoretically manifest nocturnally in PD, it is rarely encountered and typically occurs during the 'off' phase in depressed PD patients taking L-dopa but not direct agonists.[186] Most studies attribute parasomnias in PD to the long-term effects of L-dopa treatment.[141–143,158,162] Pathological differences between individual PD patients are as likely to contribute to parasomnias, because nocturnal hallucinations[146] and nocturnal wandering/disruptive behavior[187] in PD can be unrelated to medication type or dose. A greater prevalence of parasomnia type behaviors in the subpopulation of PD patients with dementia further supports this contention.[162] There is little information on the treatment of patients with nocturnal terrors or panic attacks, particularly those with coexistent PD. Instruction on proper sleep hygiene, and sedating antidepressants, alone or together with an anxiolytic such as alprazolam, are the mainstays of treatment. The parasomnia condition most familiar to the clinician treating PD patients is that of nocturnal hallucinations/delirium, where preexisting sleep complaints are more common,[143] sleep deprivation markedly aggravates the severity of symptoms,[188] and sleep efficiency, total REM-sleep time, and percentage are significantly reduced.[146] Other than reducing the dosage of dopaminomimetics, the mainstays of treatment include clozapine (6.25–50 mg qhs)[189,190] or risperidone (0.5–2.0 mg qhs).[191,192] The nature of their beneficial effects in the PD population has not been defined; however, it might be expected to reflect the tendency of the atypical neuroleptics to enhance sedation, improve sleep continuity, reduce gross body movements, and enhance REM sleep.[193–196] Sedating antidepressants such as amitriptyline or trazodone may be of additional added benefit. Ondansteron, a 5-HT$_3$ receptor antagonist, may also be effective and safe in relieving hallucinosis in the PD patient,[197] but the precise mechanism of benefit and how this medication affects sleep are unknown.

SLEEP APNEA

Central or obstructive sleep apnea, hypoventilation, and irregular patterns of respiration likely contribute to sleep fragmentation in a small subpopulation of PD patients, however, few detailed studies have been reported.[198,199] With the possible exception of multisystems atrophy (MSA), encompassing the Shy-Drager syndrome and olivopontocerebellar degeneration (OPCD), nocturnal respiratory disturbances probably are no more likely to occur in PD or other movement disorders, given their high prevalence in the normal adult population.[162,200] Increased tone or dyskinesias in the upper airway muscles, caused by either the disease itself or medications,[201] can predispose the PD patient to obstructive apneas. Dyscoordination of respiratory muscle activity and abnormalities in respiratory drive have also been observed that might contribute to nocturnal respiratory disturbances.[202–204] The severity of respiratory abnormalities is greater in patients with coincident autonomic dysfunction,[199] so that EDS is more regularly present in patients with Shy-Drager and OPCD. Obstructive and central sleep apnea, respirations with variable amplitude and arrhythmic respiration are commonly observed in such patients.[205–209] Although in PD it is generally felt that respiratory disturbances correlate with the severity of rigidity and tremor, they do not typically improve with administration of L-dopa.[162] Treatment of the sleep-related respiratory disturbances in PD and other neurodegenerative conditions is, therefore, similar to that when these problems are encountered in the normal adult population. For obstructive and central sleep apnea, treatment with continuous positive airway pressure (CPAP) offers the best chance of success and can be used effectively by most patients. In patients who cannot tolerate CPAP, we first explore the use of bilevel positive airway pressure before adding adjunct medications such as sedative antidepressants or the extremely short-acting sedative/hypnotic zolpidem (5–10 mg qhs). The use of Breathe-Right® nasal strips to decrease intranasal airflow resistance has also increased compliance with CPAP or bilevel positive airway pressure in our hands. One anecdotal report notes successful treatment of central sleep apnea in OPCD using trazadone (50 mg qhs).[210]

EXCESSIVE DAYTIME SLEEPINESS

Whether EDS is more prevalent in the PD patient population is an issue of considerable controversy (see above). The clinician treating PD patients, however, will nonetheless commonly encounter this complaint, which is likely to have numerous underlying pathophysiologies. In one subpopulation of patients, who more frequently exhibit comorbid dementia,[158,162] EDS can represent an acute effect of L-dopa administration, possibly as a result of its action on D2-like receptors in the ventral tegmental area (VTA) (see below). In a second population, who frequently exhibit the 'on-off' phenomenon, EDS appears to reflect an alteration in intrinsic circadian rhythms. These patients tend to sleep poorly at night and disperse sleep into multiple brief daytime naps (see Fig. 51-5). A reduction of the patients' homeostatic drive to sleep nocturnally, therefore, indirectly contributes to many nocturnal, and, subsequently daytime symptoms. In other PD patients, EDS may be the consequence of sleep that is disrupted by any one of a number of causes already discussed or simply reflect pathology to brain regions known to be involved in attention and arousal (see below). There is little hard evidence, however, that convincingly demonstrates the existence of EDS in the PD patient population, let alone its prevalence and pathophysiology.

In approaching the treatment of EDS in the PD patient, the clinician should first differentiate as to whether EDS is related temporally to L-dopa administration. In the case of medication-related EDS, two approaches have been used. The first is concomitant use of amphetamines such as pemoline, methylphenidate, or dextroamphetamine, which enhance arousal and improve motor performance in PD but whose value is limited secondary to the development of tolerance.[158,211,212] Selegiline (15–30 mg/day) may have similar beneficial effects, reflecting either its inhibition of monoamine oxidase inhibitor-B (MAO-B) or metabolism into amphetamine and metamphetamine, especially at higher doses. Although the use of selegiline in treating the EDS in PD has not been systematically explored, it improves memory and learning of word associations in PD patients independent of effects on depression and other cognitive tasks,[213,214] increases theta EEG frequency bands over delta activity[215] and is useful in treating the EDS accompanying other disorders such as narcolepsy.[216–218] The use of bromocriptine has not been found to be effective in alleviating EDS in PD or narcolepsy, likely because this direct dopamine agonist acts primarily at D2 and not D1 receptors (see below). The second, less satisfactory solution to treating the medication-related EDS of PD is alternate-day dosing of L-dopa, which may precipitate sudden freeze attacks and akinesia.[158,162] When EDS is unrelated to timing of medication, one should next consider a circadian disruption, sleep fragmentation, or pathological involvement of brain stem arousal centers as central to its etiology. Intrinsic disruption of the circadian timing system is frequently encountered, coincidentally, with the 'on-off' phenomenon and treatment should be aimed at maximizing 'on' periods, possibly by using the slow-release formulation of L-dopa at night.[175,176] Sleep fragmentation manifests in many forms as discussed above and, ideally, should be defined with polysomnography so that directed treatments can be instituted. Finally, when EDS unrelated to timing of medication cannot

be attributed to either a circadian factor or sleep fragmentation, treatment with amphetamines or 'activating' antidepressants seems appropriate where these agents presumably compensate for the pathological involvement of brain stem nuclei involved in attention and arousal.

SLEEP IN OTHER WAKING MOVEMENT DISORDERS

HUNTINGTON'S DISEASE

Polysomnographic studies of Huntington's disease (HD) have demonstrated some disturbance of sleep architecture, including reduced sleep efficiency, prolonged sleep latency, and reduced slow-wave sleep.[219] Early studies claimed an absence of REM sleep in HD,[220] but this has not been confirmed by others.[219,221] Increased density of sleep spindles (12–14 Hz) activity has been noted in the stage 2 sleep of HD patients.

Dyskinesias have been reported to occur in sleep in HD,[149] with lowest frequency during slow-wave sleep (stages 3 and 4). REM sleep, by contrast, appeared to be a time of relative activation of the chorea. Fish et al.[150] reported that HD patients showed a larger number of movements across the entire sleep period relative to PD patients, although they contended that such apparent sleep-related movements were preceded by several seconds of EEG arousal before the movement itself. PLMS are sometimes noted in the sleep of HD patients.

PROGRESSIVE SUPRANUCLEAR PALSY (PSP)

The sleep of patients with PSP is characterized by a near absence of REM sleep.[222,223] This decrease may reflect selective cell loss within the pedunculopontine nucleus. Additionally, sleep efficiency and sleep fragmentation indicate severe sleep disturbance and have been correlated with extent of dementia,[???] although body movement in these patients appears to be no more severe than in age-matched controls.

TORSION DYSTONIA

There is a general consensus that the elevated muscle tonus, seen in many conditions characterized by dystonia, decreases in sleep.[149,224,225] Hemifacial spasm has been shown to be decreased during sleep, as well.[226] REM atonia is generally unchanged in both primary and secondary dystonia.[227]

Although Fish et al.[150] also contend that sleep-related movements during sleep, in both primary and secondary torsion dystonia, emerge only after brief awakenings, other investigators have noted that muscle tension in the affected sternocleidomastoid in spasmodic torticollis can appear as a specific sleep-related event.[228,229] Emser et al.[229] even suggested a temporal linkage of such EMG activity with vertex sharp waves during stage 1 sleep. Mano et al.[149] also concluded that the long-lasting EMG discharges corresponding to the waking clinical dystonic condition can "... appear in any sleep stage with the same EMG characteristics as in wakefulness."

FIGURE 51-5 Multiple sleep latencies (SL) in a patient with PD demonstrate extreme variability across time of day and are likely to reflect complex interrelationships among circadian factors, medications, and 'on-off' status. Note sleep latencies of 2 minutes at 9:00 A.M. and 3:00 P.M. (1500) while the patient was 'on,' versus no sleep (i.e., sleep latencies of 20 minutes) during 'off' periods or peak-dose dyskinesias (star). Arrowheads indicate times of dosing of one-half tablet of controlled-release carbi-dopa/L-dopa 50/200 (Sinemet-CR).

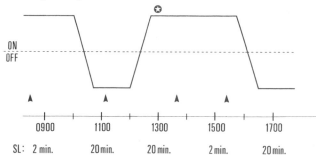

Segawa et al.[225] and others[230] have described diurnal variation in a juvenile form of dystonia, with symptoms greatly improved during and immediately subsequent to sleep. REM sleep deprivation has been shown to aggravate movement during sleep in these patients, and administration of L-dopa increased the number and frequency of movements in sleep.[225]

CREUTZFELDT-JAKOB DISEASE
In Creutzfeldt-Jakob disease, generalized paroxysmal spike activity precludes normal identification of NREM sleep stages. REM sleep is typically difficult to discern.[231] Diffuse myoclonus is seen in all limbs and is apparent throughout sleep and wakefulness.

OLIVOPONTOCEREBELLAR ATROPHY (OPCA)
Shimizu et al.[77] reported that patients with OPCA demonstrated RBD-like behaviors with awakening from REM sleep characterized by dream-enactment behavior. Of note, however, were patients with late cerebellar cortical atrophy without brain stem involvement, who did not show such behavior.

HEMIFACIAL SPASM/BLEPHAROSPASM
Movements associated with blepharospasm and hemifacial spasm can occur at night and interfere with sleep continuity. Several studies have demonstrated that these movements decrease in amplitude and frequency through sleep stages, with the lowest values seen in REM sleep.[226,232]

HEMIBALLISMUS
A small number of cases have been reported in the literature.[149] Results are similar to those seen in HD, in that movements are decreased in NREM sleep but continue to be detectable.

TOURETTE'S SYNDROME (TS)
Clinical data indicate that sleep disturbance is present in 62 percent (69/112) of TS patients, with tics during sleep reported in about one-third of these patients and somnambulism and bruxism reported in a lower percentage of these.[233] Sandyk and Bamford[234] have suggested that decreases in tic frequency during sleep may be a useful indicator of improvement in waking clinical state in these patients.

Early polysomnographic studies of TS patients did not report on movement during sleep[235] but did note normalization of sleep architecture after haloperidol administration. Some studies have reported reduced REM sleep percentages or slow-wave sleep in these patients,[235] but these results may reflect the fact that the subjects in these studies were not drug-naive.[236] Among 34 patients studied polysomnographically, motor activity was reported to be present in 23,[233] although quantified polysomnographic data were not presented. Numerous other studies have confirmed the persistence of polysomnographically defined movement during sleep in TS.[237–239] Movements were reported to decrease from wakefulness to sleep, although they reoccurred during the sleep period. As was the case for many movement disorders studied by Fish et al.,[150] these authors contend that most of the sleep-related movements in TS, although technically occurring during the "sleep period," actually represent events that are preceded by brief microawakenings or by lightening of sleep stages to stage 1. Movements were rare, according to these authors, during stages 2, 3, 4, or REM.

Glaze et al.[236] noted "unusual" behavior episodes in TS which originated from stage 4 sleep and consisted of high-amplitude delta activity accompanied by disorientation, confusion, or combativeness. Unlike typical episodes of night terrors or somnambulism, there was no evidence of elevated heart rate or breathing rate during these episodes.

PALATAL MYOCLONUS
Chokroverty and Barron[240] first noted persistence of palatal myoclonus in sleep in patients with brain stem infarcts. Later, Kayed et al.[241] reported several cases of palatal myoclonus in patients without infarcts, which clearly persisted in sleep. Although rates of movement typically declined from high rates during wakefulness (120–200/min) to rates as low as 80/min, the data of Kayed et al. conclusively indicated continued presence of palatal myoclonus during EEG defined sleep. Of particular interest was that in REM sleep, the amplitude of the movements showed considerable clustering with two to four high-amplitude movements alternating with lower-amplitude movements. This did not appear related to bursting of eye movements. Yokota et al.[242] reported that palatal myoclonus was exacerbated in REM sleep.

TREATMENT OF DISTURBED SLEEP IN WAKING MOVEMENT DISORDERS
The nature and prevalence of disturbed sleep across the spectrum of waking movement disorders is complex, and their pathophysiologies are poorly defined. It is not, therefore, surprising that scientifically validated objective results documenting specific treatments of disturbed sleep in each waking movement disorder do not exist. Nonetheless, it has been our impression that effective treatment of the core symptoms of the underlying waking movement disorder will typically result in a corresponding improvement in any associated sleep disturbances. Difficulties with sleep onset and sleep maintenance seem to be the most frequent complaints encountered in patients with waking movement disorders. As detailed above for patients with PD, sleep maintenance problems can respond favorably to sedating antidepressants or the judicious use of benzodiazepines (e.g., clonazepam). Clozapine and risperidone in low doses seem particularly useful in PSP. As is the case with the PD patient, we have also noted the worsening of nocturnal movements in many patients receiving tricyclic antidepressants and potent 5-HT reuptake inhibitors, although the prevalence of this complication is unclear. When sleep complaints persist after the successful treatment of the core waking motor disturbance and/or the simple approaches outlined here, a re-evaluation of the patient for a possible underlying sleep disorder should be performed that includes polysomnography.

Mechanisms Contributing to Disturbed Sleep in Waking Movement Disorders

As reviewed in earlier chapters (see Chaps. 5–7 and 9), the neural and pharmacological substrates underlying the pathophysiology of waking movement disorders lie primarily in the basal ganglia. It is unclear, however, how this knowledge can be extrapolated to account for the sleep disturbances manifested in these disorders. What follows is a discussion of several neural and pharmacological factors that represent a framework from which the pathophysiology behind sleep disturbances in waking movement disorders and more rational treatment strategies can be derived. Because most of our knowledge concerning waking movement disorders derives from PD, we will focus this discussion around PD. It should be recognized that sleep disruption in other waking movement disorders and movement disorders specific to sleep may involve similar substrates.

The neural and pharmacological substrates underlying the disturbed sleep of PD remain poorly defined. Dopamine, 5-HT, norepinephrine, and acetylcholine play critical roles in wake-sleep regulation and might be suspected to be primary contributors to the disturbed sleep of PD, given their depletion in PD (see Chap. 18).[243] An alternative neurobiological model considers the sleep disturbances of PD to be secondary in character; i.e., directly related to impaired motor functions. It has been suggested, for example, that nocturnal motor dyscontrol in PD is mediated by the same neuroanatomic and neurochemical substrates responsible for bradykinesia/akinesia, tremor, rigidity, and other waking disturbances in PD.[148,153,156] Before presenting what is known about the role of dopamine and other neurotransmitters in behavioral state control, and the role of the basal ganglia in modulating behavioral state and nocturnal movement, we will briefly review the potential contributions of medications, aging, depression, and dementia to the disturbed sleep of PD.

ETIOLOGIC FACTORS RELATED TO DISRUPTED SLEEP IN PARKINSON'S DISEASE

Questionnaire and polysomnographic studies in PD patients indicate that medication effects alone cannot account for the problems with their sleep.[146,157,187] Therefore, the intrinsic pathology in PD itself is likely to be a major contributor to disturbed sleep, because early and/or untreated PD patients clearly have disturbed sleep,[128,130] and sleep deteriorates with severity of disease.[134,136,229] Other studies have associated the disturbed sleep of PD with comorbid conditions such as age[161,244] or depression,[245–249] but none have addressed dementia. Preservation of a decreased REM sleep latency in depressed PD patients is consistent with models of diminished serotonergic tone in depression and might have a biological basis in the pathology of the serotonergic raphe nuclei in PD.[250] Some questionnaire data suggest that depressed PD patients have markedly worse sleep relative to nondepressed patients,[247,248] although not all studies agree.[249] Quality of sleep (i.e., total sleep time and sleep efficiency) in depressed PD patients might not be as severely affected by parkinsonian medications.[245,246] Surprisingly, few studies have discrimi-

nated between sleep disturbances in subtypes of PD patients (e.g., tremor versus rigid/bradykinetic). Traczynska-Kubin et al.[132] implied that REM sleep was higher in their 3 tremorous patients relative to their 10 bradykinetic patients, whereas Askenasy and Yahr[154] divided their 10 patients into four groups but provided little additional data. Mouret[127] reported less disturbed sleep architecture in patients experiencing blepharospasm versus those with excessive muscle activity in REM. Phenomenologically based questionnaires suggest that factors such as difficulty in turning over in bed, nocturia, and pain frequently contribute to disturbed sleep in PD.[126,161,251] In summary, a mutual underlying pathophysiology that correlates specific sleep disturbances in PD with specific daytime symptoms has not been firmly established. Such information would be critical to the clinician, for example, in establishing an index of suspicion for nocturnal disruptions and how they might best be treated. A careful longitudinal study addressing the natural history of disturbed sleep in PD is clearly needed, as well as a determination of the intrinsic physiological dysfunction specific to sleep, because both are likely to have important therapeutic implications for PD, as well as other movement disorders.

ROLE OF DOPAMINE IN BEHAVIORAL STATE CONTROL

Dopamine, like other biogenic amines, has long been suspected to have important effects on the behavioral state.[252–255] A parsimonious explanation for wake-sleep-related alterations in PD might, therefore, relate directly to the pathological involvement of dopaminergic neurons, which is the hallmark of the disease[256,257] (see Chaps. 11 and 18). The cellular and pharmacological substrates mediating dopamine's role in behavioral state control, however, are ill-defined and, therefore, preclude simple pathophysiological associations in PD. A principal problem associated with ascribing specific wake-sleep effects to dopamine has been the inability to distinguish its role from that of norepinephrine, because pharmacological manipulations effect both transmitters. Systemic alpha-methyltyrosine[258] or intracisternal 6-hydroxydopamine,[259] for example, decrease behavioral and EEG waking activity and/or increase REM-sleep percentages, and this effect has been attributed to norepinephrine depletion.[252] Nonetheless, drugs that potentiate dopaminergic transmission, either acting as agonists primarily at D1 receptors, as precursors (e.g., L-dopa), catecholamine releasers (e.g., reserpine), catecholamine reuptake inhibitors (e.g., amphetamines) or irreversible inhibitors of transmitter breakdown (e.g., selegiline), all produce behavioral arousal and EEG desynchronization and enhance wakefulness at the expense of slow-wave and REM-sleep.[137,255,260,261–263] These findings have, in fact, motivated treatments of the EDS and inappropriate REM-sleep expression in narcolepsy with L-dopa[264,265] and selegiline.[216–218] Low-doses of apomorphine or L-dopa, conversely, produce sedation that is antagonized by nonsedating doses of neuroleptics, suggesting presynaptic inhibition through D2-like autoreceptors in the ventral tegmental area (VTA).[266–268] Blockade of dopaminergic transmission (D1 and/or D2 receptor antagonism at unknown postsynaptic sites) with classical neuroleptics[269] or with the atypical neuroleptic clozapine also induce sedation[193,194] and can markedly augment REM sleep.[195,196] Sleepiness and hypoarousal in individual parkinsonian patients may, therefore, reflect dopamine depletion or be related to the effects of dopaminomimetics on the VTA.

As reviewed by Bjorklund and Lindvall,[270] the mesencephalic dopamine system provides a striking example of how a small number of neurons can exert widespread and global control of brain function, as might be expected for neurons involved in behavioral state control. The evidence supporting a direct role for these specific cell groups in modulating wakefulness and sleep, however, is incomplete and yields a conflicting picture. Although single-cell activity in the VTA[271,272] and the SN[273,274] exhibit little variation across the wake-sleep cycle, manipulations that deplete dopamine originating in these cell groups produce varied effects on behavioral state. In hemiparkinsonian patients, there are no discernible EEG correlates that identify the affected hemisphere.[275] Electrolytic lesions of the SN-pars compacta (SN-pc) also lack an EEG correlate but do decrease 'behavioral arousal'.[276] Larger excitotoxic lesions of the ventral mesopontine reticular formation, including the SN-pc, produce a wake-sleep disruption remarkably similar to that seen in PD.[277] Conversely, smaller lesions primarily involving the VTA cause hyperactivity and either loss of attentive immobile behavior[278] or disturbance of organized behavior,[279,280] with little effect on sleep. More selective destruction of the dopaminergic nigrostriatal system with the neurotoxin 1-methyl-4-phenyl-1,2,3,6-tetrahydropyridine (MPTP) selectively suppresses REM sleep acutely. During the recovery period, however, REM sleep re-emerges in parallel with the resolution of parkinsonian symptoms.[281] Interpretative difficulties with all of these studies preclude a definition of a precise role for dopamine or the VTA/SN complex in the control of behavioral state. To a great degree, this difficulty reflects previous inabilities to distinguish between different types of catecholamine neurons and pathways that are necessary to precisely map the central dopamine systems.[270] The recent development of specific antibodies to the dopamine transporter[282] and several of the five genetically-defined dopamine receptor subtypes[283] should soon help define the cellular and subcellular loci at which dopamine might affect behavioral state (see Chap. 7). Dopamine innervation of the thalamus and locus ceruleus, which have not received widespread attention,[270,284] but might be expected to influence behavioral state, for example, should become more clearly delineated. Dopaminergic neurons in the diencephalon and their innervation of the posterior pituitary, hypothalamus, and spinal cord might also be implicated in behavioral state control, either directly or indirectly (e.g., by influencing PLMS); however, they are rarely pathologically involved in idiopathic PD.[285,286]

In addition to the potential direct role of the mesotelencephalic dopamine system in modulating behavioral state, some attention has been directed to the inverse relationship, i.e., how behavioral state may modulate the nigrostriatal pathway. Tyrosine hydroxylase activity in the striatum, for example, undergoes diurnal modulation,[287] despite the fact that neuronal firing rates of dopaminergic neurons in the VTA and SN show no diurnal nor sleep stage-specific modulation. Plasticity in the nigrostriatal system, governed by

behavioral state, is also suggested by the downregulation of striatal dopamine receptor number and increased receptor affinity with REM sleep deprivation[288] and during hibernation.[289] In light of the known REM sleep-suppressant effects of L-dopa and decreased REM sleep in PD, these findings may be relevant to the morning/daytime motor fluctuations encountered in PD.[155,159–161,290] The reported lack of diurnal responsiveness to subcutaneous injections of apomorphine, however, argues that at least the proposed dopamine receptor changes during sleep are not clinically relevant.[291]

In summary, despite significant experimental evidence supporting a direct role for dopamine and/or the SN/VTA complex in modulating behavioral state, a coherent synthesis has not yet emerged.

SIGNIFICANCE OF THE ASCENDING RETICULAR ACTIVATING SYSTEM TO BEHAVIORAL STATE CONTROL

In addition to degeneration of the nigrostriatal and mesocortical dopaminergic pathways, neurotransmitter specific systems constituting the ascending reticular activating system (ARAS) are involved by the neuropathology of PD. Cell loss in the ARAS ranges from 30–90 percent and has been proposed to underlie many of the functional deficits observed in PD, particularly akinesia, depression, and dementia.[243,292] Neuronal degeneration has been described in the serotoninergic dorsal and median raphe, noradrenergic locus ceruleus, and cholinergic pedunculopontine tegmental nucleus.[241,293–295] Pathological involvement of some of these same structures in PSP,[293,296] torsion dystonia,[297] and HD[298] may also be relevant to the pathological sleep observed in these diseases. Pathological involvement of the forebrain cholinergic magnocelullar basal nucleus and its widespread connections to the cerebral cortex also occurs in some cases of PD (see Chap. 18) and might be expected to contribute to some of the observed behavioral state related alterations. The significance of pathological involvement of the ARAS to the etiology and treatment of state-specific disorders in PD is limited. Review of experimental studies of the effects of lesioning or stimulating these structures, and their wake-sleep-specific neural activity, however, is of some heuristic value in attempting to appreciate potential contributions of their pathology to the disturbed wake-sleep observed in PD (Table 51-1). More detailed discussions of most of this information can be found in excellent reviews by Saper[299] and Szymusiak.[300] A great deal remains to be learned concerning the interactions of these diffusely projecting systems with one another[301,302] and with the SN[303–306] before their role in wake-sleep behavior can be assessed definitively.

ROLE OF THE BASAL GANGLIA IN BEHAVIORAL STATE CONTROL

Considerable evidence suggests that the basal ganglia influence sleep. Although there are several plausible substrates that might mediate this effect, our present understanding of the contribution of the basal ganglia to normal and pathological sleep is limited. According to current concepts, the basal ganglia may be viewed as components of a family of segre-

TABLE 51-1 Summary of Some Behavioral, Physiological, and Pharmacological Data Pointing to Proposed Roles in Sleep/Wake Control for Brain Stem Nuclei Comprising the Ascending Reticular Activating System

Nucleus	Transmitter	Effects of Lesions on Sleep/Wake	Proposed Role in Sleep/Wake	Neural Activity (Hz)			References
				Quiet W	SWS	REM	
SN	Dopamine	None (?)	Sedation (D2) Arousal (D1)	3–4	3–4	3–4	272, 273, 359, see text
Dorsal raphe	Serotonin	Insomnia	↑SWS ↓REM sleep	2–3	1–2	0	252, 360–362
Median raphe	Serotonin	(?)	(?)	11	6	0–16	363–365
Locus Ceruleus	Norepinephrine	↓W ↑SWS ↓REM sleep(?)	Arousal (e.g., sustained attention) ↓REM sleep	3–4	1–2	0	276, 366–368
PPN	Acetylcholine	↓W ↑SWS ↓REM sleep ↓Phasic REM	REM sleep effector(↑) Arousal/attention	20	13	30	350, 370–371

Degeneration in nondopaminergic nuclei of the ARAS ranges from 30–90 percent in PD[743] and is likely to contribute significantly to the observed behavioral state-related disorders in PD and other neurodegenerative diseases. Pathology in the raphe, for example, might be expected to contribute to insomnia whereas cell loss in the locus ceruleus and PPN might account for deficits in arousal/attention and decrements in REM sleep known to accompany PD. Significant interconnections between each of these nuclei and the SN and individual differences in their pathological involvement likely accounts for the wide variety of sleep/wake alterations observed in PD. W, wakefulness; SWS, slow-wave sleep; REM sleep, REM sleep.

gated, cortical-subcortical reentrant pathways centered upon thalamocortical relationships (see Chap. 5). An extensive literature invokes basal ganglia-thalamocortical circuits in modulating sleep, particularly sleep spindling,[307] but a unifying picture has not emerged. Cortical synchronization and somnolence, followed by increased REM sleep, after the withdrawal of low-frequency caudate stimulation in rats, monkey, and man[308,309] has been attributed to inhibition of the ARAS.[310,311] Furthermore, REM sleep is enhanced after bilateral caudate ablation in rats.[312] Dopamine infusions into the caudate produce frontal sleep spindling and somnolence that are antagonized by acetylcholine.[313] Also intriguing are the reductions of REM sleep reported in animals and schizophrenics after frontal lobotomy/leukotomy.[314–317] Bilateral thalamotomy in animals and PD results in marked insomnia.[317–319] In summary, lesions and stimulation of individual components of basal ganglia-thalamocortical circuits clearly influence sleep, but the neural and pharmacological bases are poorly understood.

Functional models of the basal ganglia focus themselves, therefore, on an accounting of many aspects of normal and pathological *waking* movement.[320,321] The emphasis of these models on basal ganglia-thalamocortical circuitry largely ignores two pathways through which the basal ganglia might have important effects on sleep. First, the thalamic reticular nucleus, whose inhibition of thalamocortical activity is critical for entering slow-wave sleep,[322] is innervated by the external segment of the globus pallidus (GPe)[323] and substantia nigra pars reticulata (SNr).[324] Second, the pedunculopontine tegmental nucleus (PPN), located at the junction of the midbrain and pons and considered critical in REM sleep generation, is in a midbrain extrapyramidal area (MEA/PPN) (Fig. 51-6),[325–328] and is innervated by the internal segment of the globus pallidus (GPi) via collaterals of the pallidothalamic pathway in subprimates,[329–332] monkey,[332–336] and human.[336] The MEA/PPN and the subceruleal region, with which they merge imperceptibly, contain neurons character-

ized as either "REM-on" or "REM-off"[337] and project to ventromedullary reticulospinal neurons of the "bulbospinal inhibitory zone" (BIZ) of Magoun and Rhines (Fig. 51-6).[337–341] The BIZ contains neurons that display REM sleep-specific increases in discharge rates and that are necessary for maintaining REM atonia via active, glycine-mediated inhibition of motor neurons.[342–344] The influence of basal ganglia on brain stem/reticulospinal pathways originating from the MEA/PPN/subceruleal region has also been inferred on the basis of accentuated blink reflexes[345–347] and acoustic facilitation of spinal reflexes in PD patients.[181,182] Similar reflex pathway abnormalities in patients with PLMs, but not suffering from PD, suggest modulation of PLMs by the same neuropharmacological substrates.[43,46] In summary, a well-substantiated multisynaptic route exists by which the basal ganglia might modulate brain stem circuits, particularly those involved in modulating REM atonia.[336]

The functional role and behavioral relevance of this multisynaptic pathway between the basal ganglia and lower neural axis remains ill defined. The GABA-ergic output of the GPi to cholinergic PPN neurons has been proposed to play an active role in generating pontogeniculate-occipital (PGO)-waves that herald the onset of REM sleep and presumably correlate with dream imagery.[326,348] The MEA/PPN/subceruleal region and its afferent control by output from the GPi may also play an important role in modulating motor activity in REM-sleep. In both cats and humans, for example, lesions of the MEA/PPN/subceruleal region or interruption of their descending output tract (i.e., the central tegmental or reticulotegmental tracts) to the BIZ eliminate REM atonia[337,343,349] or result in RBD.[72,76,77] The occurrence of RBD in PD, therefore, suggests a disruption of midbrain-pontine neural circuits manifesting as insufficient motor inhibition in REM sleep. The pathophysiological basis of RBD may lie in degeneration of the PPN itself, because this nucleus is involved in the primary pathology of PD in *some* cases[293,294]; however, recent studies suggest that such pathology might result in *decreased*

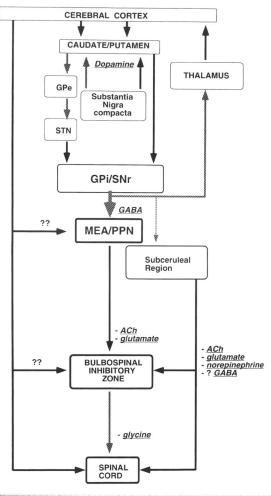

FIGURE 51-6 Schematic representation of established pathways through which the basal ganglia can influence lower motor centers and thereby motor activity during sleep. The MEA and PPN are key structures in the midbrain that can relay basal ganglia influences to the BIZ in the medulla. The MEA/PPN region receives descending inhibitory GABAergic pathways from the GPi and SNr. Descending pathways from the MEA and PPN that use glutamate and acetylcholine (Ach), respectively, are largely responsible for the REM sleep-related increase in BIZ neural activity. Because this increased neural activity is necessary to maintain REM atonia, any decrements in the glutamatergic or cholinergic influences on the BIZ will, therefore, result in loss of REM atonia and, possibly, RBD. We hypothesize that such decrements occur in PD secondary to heightened neural discharge in the GPi (i.e., excessive inhibition) and/or loss of PPN neurons (i.e., absent source of excitation), thereby accounting for the loss of REM atonia and RBD that sometimes accompany PD. Because the pathophysiological basis of many waking movement disorders and movement disorders specific to sleep are thought to lie in the basal ganglia, these brain stem pathways may also represent the substrates mediating many additional motor disturbances in sleep. GPe, external pallidum; STN, subthalamic nucleus.

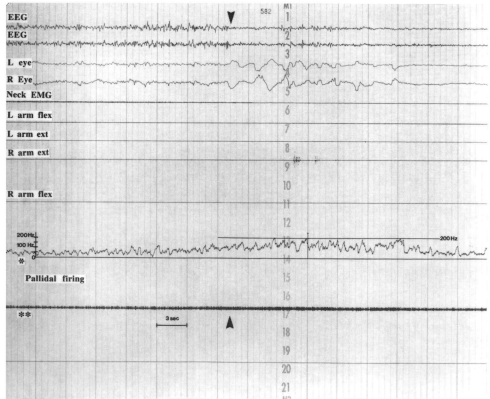

FIGURE 51-7 Neural discharge in the primate GPi increases at transitions to REM sleep, as well as during phasic events of REM sleep consistent with a role for the basal ganglia in modulating behavioral state. This figure demonstrates increasing single-unit activity in the GPi, preceding and at the transition (arrowheads) from stage 2 non-REM sleep to REM sleep. During quiet wakefulness or slow-wave sleep, GPi firing rates average 35–45 Hz. During 12–15 s before definable REM sleep, however, GPi unit discharge slowly escalates to approximately 150 Hz. Periodic bursts of 200-Hz discharge appear to coincide with phasic events of REM sleep (e.g., eye movements). In quiet REM sleep (e.g., to the extreme right hand side of this figure, where phasic eye and/or muscle activity is absent), GPi discharge decreases to waking levels.

The single unit illustrated here was located in the sensorimotor portion of the GPi and exhibited responsiveness in wakefulness to limb movement. The recording paradigm allowed uninterrupted monitoring of this same unit for 3 continuous hours of sleep, over which an identical discharge pattern was observed in two additional transitions to REM sleep. *, single-unit activity in the GPi, expressed as a 200-ms moving average of frequency of firing. Ordinate divisions in increments of 50 Hz. **, single-unit activity in the GPi, recorded as acceptance pulse indicating time-discriminated spikes.

phasic activity in REM sleep.[350] Therefore, the neural basis underlying REM-related myoclonus and RBD in PD more likely reflects abnormalities in the afferent input to the MEA/PPN/subceruleal region from the GPi. We hypothesize that much of the GABAergic basal ganglia output targets glutamatergic neurons that, in turn, are important modulators of BIZ reticulospinal neurons whose excitation is necessary for maintaining REM atonia.[336] Phasic neural activity in nuclei implicated in waking movement, in fact, coincides with EMG activity during eye movement episodes of REM sleep; for example, in the GPi[351] (Fig. 51-7), reticulospinal neurons,[352] red nucleus,[353] and pyramidal cells in the motor cortex,[354] suggesting their possible roles in overcoming the somatic motoneuron inhibition of REM sleep. Lesion and microstimulation studies of the red nucleus and motor cortex, however, indicate that they are not responsible for REM-related myoclonus.[353,355,356] Pallidotomy in PD improves waking motor function[357] (see Chaps. 6 and 16) and also decreases REM-related EMG activity (DB Rye and D Bliwise, personal observations),[157] suggesting that heightened tonic waking discharge of the parkinsonian GPi[358] is further enhanced in REM-sleep. Such an enhancement might be expected to produce excessive myoclonic activity, either indirectly by excessively inhibiting glutamatergic pathways from the MEA to the BIZ that are necessary for maintaining atonia or alternatively by directly enhancing phasic discharges in cholinergic PPN neurons. Investigation of the sleep-stage specific changes of the GPi and MEA/PPN/subceruleal region in the normal and parkinsonian condition are critical to furthering our understanding of the pathophysiological basis of disturbed sleep, particularly nocturnal movements occurring de novo or as part of diseases of the basal ganglia, in PD and other movement disorders.

Acknowledgments

The authors would like to extend their greatest appreciation to Ms. Katy Hair for her excellent secretarial support in preparing this work. We would also like to acknowledge Dr. Dainis Irbe for his assistance in performing and scoring polysomnographic records from a variety of movement disorder patients, as well as Dr. Robert Turner for his critical help in recording sleep/wake-specific neuronal discharge in the primate globus pallidus. Supported in part by a Cotzias fellowship from the American Parkinson Disease Association to DBR and NIH grants NS-35345 and AG-10643 to DLB.

References

1. Fujimoto T, Nishizono H: Muscle contractile properties by surface electrodes compared with those by needle electrodes. *Electroencephalogr Clin Neurophysiol* 89:247–251, 1993.
2. van Hilten J, Middelkoop H, Kuiper S, et al: Where to record motor activity: An evaluation of commonly used sites of placement for activity monitors. *Electroencephalogr Clin Neurophysiol* 89:359–362, 1993.
3. Jacobson A, Kales A, Lehmann D, Hoedemaker F: Muscle tonus in human subjects during sleep and dreaming. *Exp Neurol* 10:418–424, 1964.
4. Kleitman N, Cooperman N, Mullin F: Studies on the physiology of sleep. IX. Motility and body temperature during sleep. *Am J Physiol* 105:574–584, 1933.
5. Johnson H, Swan T, Weigand G: In what positions do healthy people sleep? *J Am Med Assoc* 94:2058–2062, 1930.
6. Hobson J, Spagna T, Malenka R: Ethology of sleep studied with time-lapse photography: Postural immobility and sleep-cycle phase in humans. *Science* 204:251–253, 1978.
7. Gardner JR, Grossman W: Normal motor patterns in sleep in man, in *Advances in Sleep Research*. New York: Spectrum Publications, 1975, pp 67–107.
8. Suckling E, Koenig E, Hoffman B, Brooks C: The physiological effects of sleeping on hard or soft beds. *Hum Biol* 29:274–288, 1957.
9. Moses J, Lubin A, Naitoh P, Johnson L: Methodology: Reliability of sleep measures. *Psychophysiology* 9:78–82, 1972.
10. Muzet A, Naitoh P, Townsend R, Johnson L: Body movements during sleep as a predictor of stage change. *Psychon Sci* 29(1):7–10, 1972.
11. Naitoh P, Muzet A, Johnson L, Moses J: Body movements during sleep after sleep loss. *Psychophysiology* 10(4):363–368, 1973.
12. Townsend R, Johnson L, Naitoh P: Heart rate preceding motility in sleep. *Psychophysiology* 12:217–219, 1975.
13. De Lisi L: Su di un fenomeno motorio constate del sonno normale: Le mioclonie ipniche fisiologiche. *Riv Pat Nerv Ment* 39:481–496, 1932.
14. Oswald I: Sudden bodily jerks on falling asleep. *Brain* 82:92–103, 1959.
15. Stoyva J: Finger electromyographic activity during sleep: Its relation to dreaming in deaf and normal subjects. *J Abnorm Psychol* 70(5):343–349, 1965.
16. Askenasy J, Yahr M, Davidovitch S: Isolated phasic discharges in anterior tibial muscle: A stable feature of paradoxical sleep. *J Clin Neurophysiol* 5(2):175–181, 1988.
17. Chokroverty S: Phasic tongue movements in human rapid-eye-movement sleep. *Neurology* 30:665–668, 1980.
18. Bliwise D, Coleman R, Bergmann B, et al: Facial muscle tonus during REM and NREM Sleep. *Psychophysiology* 11:447–508, 1974.
19. Slegel D, Benson K, VP Zarcone J, Schubert E: Middle-ear muscle activity (MEMA) and its association with motor activity in the extremities and head in sleep. *Sleep* 14(5):454–459, 1991.
20. Pessah M, Roffwarg H: Spontaneous middle ear muscle activity in man: A rapid eye movement sleep phenomenon. *Science* 178(62):773–776, 1972.
21. Gassel M, Marchiafava P, Pompeiano O: Phasic changes in muscular activity during desynchronized sleep in unrestrained cats. *Arch Ital Biol* 102:449–470, 1964.
22. Cepeda C, Naquet R: Physiological sleep myoclonus in baboons. *Electroencephalogr Clin Neurophysiol* 60:158–162, 1985.
23. Montagna P, Liguori R, Zucconi M, et al: Physiological hypnic myoclonus. *Electroencephalogr Clin Neurophysiol* 70:172–175, 1988.
24. Montagna P, Liguiori R, Zucconi M, et al: Fasciculations during wakefulness and sleep. *Acta Neurol Scand* 76:152–154, 1987.
25. van Hilten B, Hoff J, Middelkoop H, et al: Sleep disruption in Parkinson's disease: Assessment by continuous activity monitoring. *Arch Neurol* 51:922–928, 1994.
26. Silber M, Dexter D, Ahlskog J, et al: Abnormal REM sleep motor activity in untreated Parkinson's disease (abstr.). *Sleep Res* 22:274, 1993.
27. Laihinen A, Alihanka J, Raitasuo S, Rinne U: Sleep movements and associated autonomic nervous activities in patients with Parkinson's disease. *Acta Neurol Scand* 76:64–68, 1987.
28. Klawans H, Goetz C, Bergen D: L-dopa-induced myoclonus. *Arch Neurol* 32:331–334, 1975.
29. Bliwise D, Keenan S, Burnburg D, et al: Inter-rater reliability for scoring periodic leg movements in sleep. *Sleep* 14:249–251, 1991.
30. Askenasy, JJM, Yahr MD: Different laws govern motor activity in sleep than in wakefulness. *J Neural Trans* 79:103–111, 1990.

31. Askensay JJM, Yahr MD, Davidovitch S: Isolated phasic discharges in anterior tibial muscle: a stable feature of paradoxical sleep. *J Clin Neurophys* 5:175–181, 1988.

32. Coleman RM: Periodic movements in sleep (nocturnal myoclonus) and restless legs syndrome, in Guilleminault C. (ed): *Sleeping and Waking Disorders: Indications and Techniques.* Menlo Park, CA: Addison-Wesley, 1982, pp 265–295.

33. Bliwise D, Ingham R, Date E, Dement W: Nerve conduction and creatinine clearance in aged subjects with periodic movements in sleep. *J Gerontol Med Sci* 44:M164–M167, 1989.

34. Pollmächer T, Schulz H: Periodic leg movements (PLM): Their relationship to sleep stages. *Sleep* 16(6):572–577, 1993.

35. Bliwise D: Sleep in normal aging and dementia. *Sleep* 16:40–81, 1993.

36. Bliwise D, Petta D, Seidel W, Dement W: Periodic leg movements during sleep in the elderly. *Arch Gerontol Geriatr* 4:273–281, 1985.

37. Ancoli-Israel S, Kripke D, Klauber M, et al: Periodic limb movements in sleep in community dwelling elderly. *Sleep* 14:496–500, 1991.

38. Kales A, Bixler E, Soldatos C, et al: Biopsychobehavioral correlates of insomnia, part 1: Role of sleep apnea and nocturnal myoclonus. *Pschosomatics* 23:589–600, 1982.

39. Aldrich M, Shipley J: Alcohol use and periodic limb movements of sleep. *Alcohol Clin Exp Res* 17(1):192–196, 1993.

40. Shafor R: Prevalence of abnormal lumbo-sacral spine imaging in patients with insomnia associated restless legs, periodic movements in sleep. *Sleep Res* 20:396, 1991.

41. Dzvonik M, Kripke D, Klauber M, Ancoli-Israel S: Body position changes and periodic movements in sleep. *Sleep* 9(4):484–491, 1986.

42. Smith R, Gouin P, Minkley P, et al: Periodic limb movement disorder is associated with normal motor conduction latencies when studied by central magnetic stimulation—successful use of a new technique. *Sleep* 15(4):312–318, 1992.

43. Wechsler L, Stakes J, Shahani B, Busis N: Periodic leg movements of sleep (nocturnal myoclonus): An electrophysiological study. *Ann Neurol* 19:168–173, 1986.

44. Smith R: Relationship of periodic movements in sleep (nocturnal myoclonus) and the Babinski sign. *Sleep* 8:239–243, 1985.

45. Smith R: Confirmation of Babinski-like response in periodic movements in sleep (nocturnal myoclonus). *Biol Psychiatry* 22:1271–1273, 1987.

46. Wechsler L, Stakes J, Shahani B, Busis N: Nocturnal myoclonus, restless legs syndrome, and abnormal electrophysiological findings. *Ann Neurol* 21:515, 1987.

47. Lugaresi E, Coccagna G, Mantovani M, Lebrun R: Some periodic phenomena arising during drowsiness and sleep in man. *Electroencephalogr Clin Neurophysiol* 32:701–705, 1972.

48. Ali N, Davies R, Fleetham J, Stradling J: Periodic movements of the legs during sleep associated with rises in systemic blood pressure. *Sleep* 14(2):163–165, 1991.

49. Montplaisir J, Godbout R: Restless legs syndrome and periodic movements during sleep, in Kryger M, Roth T, Dement W (eds): *Principles and Practice of Sleep Medicine.* Philadelphia: WB Saunders, 1994, pp 402–409.

50. Staedt J, Stoppe G, Kogler A, et al: Nocturnal myoclonus syndrome (periodic movements in sleep) related to central dopamine D2-receptor alteration. *Eur Arch Psychiatry Clin Neurosci* 245:8–10, 1995.

51. Ekbom K: Restless legs. *Acta Med Scand Suppl* 158:1–123, 1945.

52. Roehrs T, Zorick F, Sicklesteel J, et al: Age-related sleep-wake disorders at a sleep disorder center. *J Am Geriatr Soc* 31:364–370, 1983.

53. Trenkwalder C, Bucher S, Oertel W, et al: Bereitschaftspotential in idiopathic and symptomatic restless legs syndrome. *Electroencephalogr Clin Neurophysiol* 89:95–103, 1993.

54. Montplaisir J, Godbout R, Boghen D, et al: Familial restless legs with periodic movements in sleep: Electrophysiologic, biochemical, and pharmacologic study. *Neurology* 35:130–134, 1985.

55. Jones K, Castleden C: A double-blind comparison of quinine sulphate and placebo in muscle cramps. *Age Ageing* 12:155–158, 1983.

56. Sidorov J: Quinine sulfate for leg cramps: Does it work? *J Am Geriatr Soc* 41:498–500, 1993.

57. Jacobsen J, Rosenberg R, Huttenlocher P, Spire J-P: Familial nocturnal cramping. *Sleep* 9(1):54–60, 1986.

58. Brown T, Fleishman S: Caffeine consumption and periodic limb movements of sleep. *Sleep Res* 24:208, 1995.

59. Hening W, Walters A, Kavey N, et al: Dyskinesias while awake and periodic movements in sleep in restless legs syndrome: Treatment with opiods. *Neurology* 36:1363–1366, 1986.

60. Kavey N, Whyte J, Gidro-Frank S, et al: Treatment of restless legs syndrome and periodic movements in sleep with propoxyphene (abstr.). *Sleep Res* 16:367, 1987.

61. Mitler M, Browman C, Menn S, et al: Nocturnal myoclonus: Treatment efficacy of clonazepam and temazepam. *Sleep* 9:385–392, 1986.

62. Ehrenberg B, Eisensehr I, Walters A: Influence of valproate on sleep and periodic limb movements disorder. *Sleep Res* 24:227, 1995.

62a.Mellick GA, Mellick LB: Successful treatment of restless leg syndrome with gabapentin. *Sleep Res* 24:290, 1995.

63. Schenck C, Bundlie S, Ettinger M, Mahowald M: Chronic behavioral disorders of human REM sleep: A new category of parasomnia. *Sleep* 9:293–308, 1986.

64. Diagnostic Classification Steering Committee: *The International Classification of Sleep Disorders.* Lawrence, KS: Allen Press, 1990.

65. Webster H, Frideman L, Jones B: Modification of paradoxical sleep following transections of the reticular formation at the pontomedullary junction. *Sleep* 9:1–23, 1986.

66. Hendricks J, Morrison A, Mann G: Different behaviors during paradoxical sleep without atonia depend on pontine lesion site. *Brain Res* 239:81–105, 1982.

67. Gross M, Goodenough D, Tobin M, et al: Sleep disturbances and hallucinations in the acute alcoholic psychoses. *J Nerv Ment Dis* 142:493–514, 1966.

68. Greenberg R, Pearlman C: Delirium tremens and dreaming. *Am J Psychiatry* 124:37–46, 1967.

69. Guilleminault C, Raynal D, Takahaski S, et al: Evaluation of short-term and long-term treatment of the narcolepsy syndrome with clomipramine hydrochloride. *Acta Neurol Scand* 54:71–87, 1976.

70. Akindele M, Evans J, Oswald I: Mono-amine oxidase inhibitors, sleep and mood. *Electroencephalogr Clin Neurophysiol* 29:47–56, 1970.

71. Schenck C, Mahowald M, Kim S, et al: Prominent eye movements during NREM sleep and REM sleep behavior disorder associated with fluoxetine treatment of depression and obsessive-compulsive disorder. *Sleep* 15:226–235, 1992.

72. Mahowald M, Schenck C: REM sleep behavior disorder, in Kryger M, Roth T, Dement W (eds): *Principles and Practices of Sleep Medicine.* Philadelphia: WB Saunders, 1994, pp 574–588.

73. Schenck C, Bundlie S, Mahowald M: Delayed Emergence of Parkinson's disease In 38% Of 29 older males initially diagnosed with idiopathic rapid eye movement sleep behavior disorder. *Neurology* 46:388–393, 1996.

74. Tison F, Wenning G, Quinn N, Smith S: REM sleep behaviour disorder as the presenting symptom of multiple system atrophy. *J Neurol Neurosurg Psychiatry* 58:379–385, 1995.

75. Uhde T: The anxiety disorders, in Kryger M, Roth T, Dement W (eds): *Principles and Practice of Sleep Medicine.* Philadelphia: WB Saunders, 1994, pp 871–898.

76. Culebras A, Moore J: Magnetic resonance findings in REM sleep behavior disorder. *Neurology* 39:1519–1523, 1989.

77. Shimizu T, Inami Y, Sugita Y, et al: REM sleep without muscle atonia (stage 1-REM) and its relation to delirious behavior during sleep in patients with degenerative diseases involving the brain stem. *Jpn J Psychiatry Neurol* 44(4):681–692, 1990.

78. Schenck C, Mahowald M: Motor dyscontrol in narcolepsy: Rapid-eye-movement (REM) sleep without atonia and REM sleep behavior disorder. *Ann Neurol* 32:3–10, 1992.

79. Broughton R, Tolentino M, Krelina M: Excessive fragmentary myoclonus in NREM sleep: A report of 38 cases. *Electroencephalogr Clin Neurophysiol* 61:123–309, 1985.

80. Lugaresi E, Cirignotta F: Hypnogenic paroxysmal dystonia: Epileptic seizure or a new syndrome? *Sleep* 4(2):129–138, 1981.

81. Tinuper P, Cerullo A, Cirignotta F, et al: Nocturnal paroxysmal dystonia with short-lasting attacks: Three cases with evidence for an epileptic frontal lobe origin of seizures. *Epilepsia* 31:549–556, 1990.

82. Lugaresi E, Cirignotta F, Montagna P: Nocturnal paroxysmal dystonia. *J Neurol Neurosurg Psychiatry* 49:375–380, 1986.

83. Sforza E, Montagna P, Rinaldi R, et al: Paroxysmal periodic motor attacks during sleep: Clinical and polygraphic features. *Electroencephalogr Clin Neurophysiol* 86:161–166, 1993.

84. Terzano M, Parrino L, Spaggiari M: The cyclic alternating pattern sequences in the dynamic organization of sleep. *Electroencephalogr Clin Neurophysiol* 69:437–447, 1988.

85. Thorpy M, Glovinsky P: Parasomnias. *Psychiatr Clin North Am* 10(4):623–639, 1987.

86. Regestein Q, Hartmann E, Reich P: A head movement disorder occurring in dreaming sleep. *J Nerv Ment Disease* 16:432–435, 1977.

87. Gagnon P, Koninck JD: Repetitive head movements during REM sleep. *Biol Psychiatry* 20:176–178, 1985.

88. Klackenberg G: Rhythmic movements in infancy and early childhood. *Acta Pediatr Scand* 224(suppl):74, 1971.

89. Drake J, ME: Jactatio nocturna after head injury. *Neurology* 36:867–867, 1986.

90. Tuxhorn I, Hoppe M: Parasomnia with rhythmic movements manifesting as nocturnal tongue biting. *Neuropediatrics* 24:167–168, 1993.

91. Satoh T, Harada Y: Electrophysiological study on tooth-grinding during sleep. *Electroencephalogr Clin Neurophysiol* 35:267–274, 1973.

92. Wieselmann G, Permann R, Körner E, et al: Distribution of muscle activity during seep in bruxism. *Eur Neurol* 25(suppl 2): 111–116, 1986.

93. Tachibana N, Yamanaka K, Kaji R, et al: Sleep bruxism as a manifestation of subclinical rapid eye movement sleep behavior disorder. *Sleep* 17(6):555–558, 1994.

94. Ware J, Rugh J: Destructive bruxism: Sleep stage relationship. *Sleep* 11(2):172–181, 1988.

95. Sjöholm T, Polo O, Alihanka J: Sleep movements in teethgrinders. *J Craniomandib Disord Facial Oral Pain* 6:184–191, 1992.

96. Hartmann E: Bruxism, in Kryer M, Roth T, Dement W (eds): *Principles of Practice of Sleep Medicine,* 2d ed. Philadelphia: WB Saunders, 1994, pp 598–601.

97. Glaros A, Rao S: Bruxism: A critical review. *Psychol Bull* 84:767–781, 1977.

98. Hartmann E: Alcohol and bruxism. *N Engl J Med* 301:334, 1979.

99. Ellison J, Stanziani P: SSRI-associated nocturnal bruxism in four patients. *J Clin Psychiatry* 54:432–434, 1993.

100. Kamen S: Tardive dyskinesia, a significant syndrome for geriatric dentistry. *Oral Surg Oral Med Oral Pathol* 39:52, 1975.

101. Pohto P: Experimental aggression and bruxism in rats. *Acta Odontol Scand* 37:117–126, 1979.

102. Magee K: Bruxism related to L-dopa therapy. *J Am Med Assoc* 214:147, 1970.

103. Arkin A (ed): *Sleep-Talking: Psychology and Psychophysiology.* Hillsdale, NJ: Lawrence Erlbaum Associates, 1981.

104. MacNeilage L: Activity of the Speech Apparatus during Sleep and Its Relation to Dream Reports, doctoral dissertation, Columbia University, 1971.

105. Jacobson A, Kales A: Somnambulism: All-night EEG and related studies, in *Sleep and Altered States of Consciousness,* Baltimore: Williams & Wilkins, 1967, pp 424–455.

106. Kavey N, Whyte J, Resor SR, Gidro-Frank S: Somnambulism in adults. *Neurology* 40:749–752, 1990.

107. Broughton R: Sleep disorders: Disorders of arousal? *Science* 159:1070, 1968.

108. Cirignotta F, Zucconi M, Mondini S, et al: Enuresis, sleepwalking, and nightmares: An epidemiological survey in the Republic of San Marino, in Guilleminault C, Lugaresi E (eds): *Sleep/Wake Disorders: Natural History, Epidemiology, and Long-Term Evolution.* New York: Raven Press, 1983, pp 237–241.

109. Kales A, Soldatos C, Caldwell A, et al: Somnambulism. *Arch Gen Psychiatry* 37.1406–1410, 1980.

110. Blatt I, Peled R, Gadoth N, Lavie P: The value of sleep recording in evaluating somnambulism in young adults. *Electroencephalogr Clin Neurophysiol* 78:407–412, 1991.

111. Bliwise D: What is sundowning? *J Am Geriatr Soc* 42:1009–1011, 1994.

112. Kales J, Kales A, Soldatos C, et al: Night terrors. *Arch Gen Psychiatry* 37:1413–1417, 1980.

113. Rogozea R, Florea-Ciocoiu V: Orienting reaction in patients with night terrors. *Biol Psychiatry* 20:894–905, 1985.

114. Llorente M, Currier MB, Norman S, Mellman T: Night terrors in adults: Phenomenology and relationship to psychopathology. *J Clin Psychiatry* 53:392–394, 1992.

115. Schenck C, Hurwitz T, Bundlie S, Mahowald M: Sleep-related eating disorders: Polysomnographic correlates of a heterogeneous syndrome distinct from daytime eating disorders. *Sleep* 14:419–431, 1991.

116. Winkelman J, Dorsey C, Cunningham S, Lukas S: Nocturnal binge eating: Sleep disorder or eating disorder? *Sleep Res* 22:291, 1993.

117. Spaggiari M, Granella F, Parrino L, et al: Nocturnal eating syndrome in adults. *Sleep* 17(4):339–344, 1994.

118. Huapaya L: Somnambulsim and bedtime medication. *Am J Psychiatry* 133:1207, 1976.

119. Huapaya L: Seven cases of somnambulsim induced by drugs. *Am J Psychiatry* 36:985, 1979.

120. Dagino N, Loeb C, Massazza G, Sacco G: Hypnic physiological myoclonus in man: An EEG-EMG study in normals and neurological patients. *Eur Neurol* 2:47–58, 1969.

121. Rosenberg C: Elimination of a rhythmic movement disorder with hypnosis—a case report. *Sleep* 18(7):608–609, 1995.

122. Keefauver SP, Guilleminault C: Parasomnias: Sleep terrors and sleepwalking, in Kryger M, Roth T, Dement W (eds): *Principles and Practice of Sleep Medicine,* 2d ed. Philadelphia: WB Saunders, 1994, pp 567–573.

123. Fisher C, Kahn E, Edwards A, Davis D: A psychophysiological study of nightmares and night terrors. *Psychoanal Contemp Sci* 3:317–398, 1974.

124. Reid W: Treatment of somnambulism in military trainees. *Am J Psychiatry* 29:101–105, 1975.

125. Schenck C, Hurwitz T, O'Connor K, Mahowald M: Additional categories of sleep-related eating disorders and the current status of treatment. *Sleep* 16(5):457–466, 1993.

126. Lees A, Blackburn N, Campbell V: The nightime problems of Parkinson's disease. *Clin Neuropharmacol* 11:512–519, 1988.

127. Mouret J: Differences in sleep in patients with Parkinson's disease. *Electroencephalogr Clin Neurophysiol* 38:653–657, 1975.

128. Kales A, Ansel R, Markham C, et al: Sleep in patients with Parkinson's disease and normal subjects prior to and following L-dopa administration. *Clin Pharmacol Ther* 12:397–406, 1971.

129. Bergonzi P, Chiurulla C, Cianchetti C, et al: Clinical pharmacology as an approach to the study of biochemical sleep mechanisms: The action of L-dopa. *Confin Neurol* 36:5–22, 1974.

130. Bergonzi P, Chiurulla C, Gambi D, et al: L-dopa plus dopadecarboxylase inhibitor: Sleep organization in Parkinson's syndrome before and after treatment. *Acta Neurol Belg* 75(1):5–10, 1975.

131. Wilson W, Nashold B, Green R: Studies of the cortical and subcortical electrical activity during sleep of patients with dyskinesias, in *Third Symposium on Parkinson's Disease*. Edinburgh, Scotland: Livingstone Pub. Co., 1969, pp 160–164.

132. Traczynska-Kubin D, Atef E, Petre-Quadens O: Le sommeil dans la maladie de Parkinson. *Acta Neurol Belg* 69:727–733, 1969.

133. Puca F, Bricolo A, Rurella G: Effect of L-dopa or amantadine therapy on sleep spindles in parkinsonism. *Electroencephalogr Clin Neurophysiol* 35:327–330, 1973.

134. Friedman A: Sleep pattern in Parkinson's disease. *Acta Med Pol* 21:193–199, 1980.

135. Rabey J, Vardi J, Glaubman H, Streifler M: EEG Sleep: Study in parkinsonian patients under bromocryptine treatment. *Eur Neurol* 17:345–350, 1978.

136. Schneider E, Ziegler B, Maxion H, et al: *Sleep in Parkinsonian Patients under L-dopa: Results of a Long-Term Follow-Up Study*. Presented at the 3rd European Congress on Sleep Research, Montpellier, 1976. Basel, Switzerland: Karger, 1976, pp 447–450.

137. Gillin J, Post R, Wyatt R, et al: REM inhibitory effect of L-Dopa infusion during human sleep. *Electroencephalogr Clin Neurophysiol* 35:181–186, 1973.

138. Lavie P, Bental E, Goshen H, Sharf B: REM ocular activity in parkinsonian patients chronically treated with L-dopa. *J Neural Transm* 47:61–67, 1980.

139. Lavie P, Wajsbort J, Youdim M: Deprenyl does not cause insomnia in parkinsonian patients. *Commun Psychopharmacol* 4:303–307, 1980.

140. Lesser R, Fahn S, Sniker S, et al: Analysis of the clinical problems in parkinsonism and the complications of long-term L-dopa therapy. *Neurology* 29:1253–1260, 1979.

141. Moskovitz C, Moses H, Klawans H: L-dopa-induced psychosis: A kindling phenomenon. *Am J Psychiatry* 135(6):669–675, 1978.

142. Sharf B, Moskovitz C, Lupton M, et al: Dream phenomena induced by chronic L-dopa therapy. *J Neural Transm* 43:143–151, 1978.

143. Nausieda P, Weiner W, Kaplan L: Sleep disruption in the course of chronic L-dopa therapy: An early feature of the L-dopa psychosis. *Clin Neuropharmacol* 5:183–194, 1982.

144. Nausieda P, Tanner C, Klawans H: Serotonergically active agents in L-dopa-induced psychiatric toxicity reactions, in Fahn S, Calne DB, Shoulson I (eds): Advances in Neurology, Vol. 37:*Experimental Therapeutics of Movement Disorders*. New York: Raven Press, 1983, pp 23–32.

145. Nausieda P, Glantz R, Weber S, et al: Psychiatric complications of L-dopa therapy of Parkinson' disease, in Hassler, RG, Christ QF (eds): Advances in Neurology, Vol. 40 *Parkinson-Specific Motor and Mental Disorders*, New York, Raven Press, 1984, pp 271–277.

146. Comella C, Tanner C, Ristanovic R: Polysomnographic sleep measures in Parkinson's disease patients with treatment-induced hallucinations. *Ann Neurol* 34:710–714, 1993.

147. Tassinari C, Broughton R, Roger J, Gastaut H: A polygraphic study of the evolution of abnormal movements during sleep. *Electroencephalogr Clin Neurophysiol* 17:716–723, 1964.

148. Askenasy J: Sleep patterns in extrapyramidal disorders. *Int J Neurol* 15:62–76, 1981.

149. Mano T, Shiozawa Z, Sobue I: Extrapyramidal involuntary movements during sleep, in Broughton R (ed): *Neurosciences*. Amsterdam: Elsevier Biomedical Press, 1982, pp 431–442.

150. Fish D, Sawyers D, Allen P, et al: The effect of sleep on the dyskinetic movements of Parkinson's disease, Gilles de la Tourette's syndrome, Huntington's disease, and torsion dystonia. *Arch Neurol* 48:210–214, 1991.

151. Silber M, Ahlskog J: REM sleep behavior disorder in parkinsonian syndromes (abstr.). *Sleep Res* 21:313, 1992.

152. Salva M, Guilleminault C: Olivopontocerebellar degeneration, abnormal sleep and REM sleep without atonia. *Neurology* 36:576–577, 1986.

153. Askenasy J, Weitzman E, Yahr M: Are periodic movements in sleep a basal ganglia dysfunction? *J Neural Transm* 70:337–347, 1987.

154. Askenasy J, Yahr M: Parkinsonian tremor loses its alternating aspect during non-REM sleep and is inhibited by REM sleep. *J Neurol Neurosurg Psychiatry* 53:749–753, 1990.

155. Askenasy J: Sleep in Parkinson's disease. *Acta Neurol Scand* 87:167–170, 1993.

156. Askenasy J, Yahr M: Reversal of sleep disturbance in Parkinson's disease by antiparkinsonian therapy: A preliminary study. *Neurology* 35:527–532, 1985.

157. Irbe D, Rye D, Bliwise D: Sinemet in advanced Parkinson's disease (PD): Effects on sleep-related movement and tremor. *Sleep Res* 23:368, 1994.

158. Nausieda P: Sleep in Parkinson's disease, in Thorpy M (ed): *Handbook of Sleep Disorders*. New York: Marcel Dekker, 1990, pp 719–733.

159. Marsden C, Parkes J, Quinn N: Fluctuations of disability in Parkinson's disease—clinical aspects, in Marsden C, Fahn S (eds): *Movement Disorders*. London: Butterworth Scientific, 1982, pp 96–122.

160. Factor S, McAlarney T, Sanchez-Ramos J, Weiner W: Sleep disorders and sleep effect in Parkinson's disease. *Mov Disord* 5(4):280–285, 1990.

161. van Hilten J, Weggeman M, Velde Evd, et al: Sleep, excessive daytime sleepiness and fatigue in Parkinson's disease. *J Neural Transm* 5:235–244, 1993.

162. Aldrich M: Parkinsonism, in Kryger M, Roth, T, Dement WC (eds): *Principles and Practice of Sleep Medicine*. Philadelphia: WB Saunders, 1994, pp 783–789.

163. Schwab R, Zieper I: Effects of mood, motivation, stress and alertness on the performance in Parkinson's disease. *Psychiatr Neurol Basel* 150:345–357, 1965.

164. Ploski H, Levita E, Riklan M: Impairment of voluntary movement in Parkinson's disease in relation to activation level, autonomic malfunction, and personality rigidity. *Psychosom Med* 28:70–77, 1966.

165. Horne JA: Human sleep, sleep loss and behavior: Implications for the prefrontal cortex and psychiatric disorder. *Br J Psychiatry* 162:413–419, 1993.

166. Harrison Y, Horne JA: Sleep loss affects frontal lobe function, as shown in complex "real world" tasks. *Sleep Res* 25:467, 1996.

167. Karni A, Tanne D, Rubenstein B, et al: Dependence on REM sleep of overnight improvement of a perceptual skill. *Science* 265:679–682, 1994.

168. Cummings J, Huber S: Visuospatial abnormalities in Parkinson's disease, in Huber S, Cummings J (eds): *Parkinson's Disease: Neurobehavioral Aspects*. New York: Oxford University Press, 1992, pp 59–73.

169. Carskadon M, Dement W: Daytime sleepiness: Quantification of a behavioral state. *Neurosci Biobehav Rev* 11:307–317, 1987.

170. Roth T, Roehrs T, Carskadon M, Dement W: Daytime sleepiness and alertness, in Kryger M, Roth T, Dement W (eds): *Principles*

and Practice of Sleep Medicine. Philadelphia: WB Saunders, 1994, pp 40–49.

171. Brown TH, Zador AM: Hippocampus, in Shepherd GM (ed): *The Synaptic Organization of the Brain, 3d ed. Oxford, England: Oxford University Press, 1990, pp 346–388.*

172. Zarcone V, Benson K, Berger P: Abnormal rapid eye movement latencies in schizophrenia. *Arch Gen Psychiatry* 44:45–48, 1987.

173. Steur E: Increase of Parkinson disability after fluoxetine medication. *Neurology* 43:211–213, 1993.

174. Richelson E: Pharmacology of antidepressants—characteristics of the ideal drug. *Mayo Clin Proc* 69:1069–1081, 1994.

175. Lees A: A sustained release formulation of L-dopa (Madopar HBS) in the treatment of nocturnal and early morning disabilities in Parkinson's disease. *Eur Neurol* 27(suppl 1):126–134, 1987.

176. Kerchove MVd, Jacquy J, Gonce M, Deyn PD: Sustained-release L-dopa in Parkinsonian patients with nocturnal disabilities. *Acta Neurol Belg* 93:32–39, 1993.

177. Gaillard J: Benzodiazepines and GABA-ergic transmission, in Kryger M, Roth T, Dement W (eds): *Principles and Practice of Sleep Medicine.* Philadelphia: WB Saunders, 1994, pp 349–354.

178. Bonnet M, Arand D: The use of triazolam in older patients with periodic leg movements, fragmented sleep, and daytime sleepiness. *J Gerontol* 45(4):M139–144, 1990.

179. Ware J, Brown F, Moorad PJ Jr, Wallace ER: Nocturnal myoclonus and tricyclic antidepressants. *Sleep Res* 13:72, 1984.

180. Morgan J, Brown T, Iv EW: Monoamine oxidase inhibitors and sleep movements. *Am J Psychiatry* 151(5):782–783, 1994.

181. Delwaide P, Pepin J, Noordhout AM: Short-latency autogenic inhibition in patients with parkinsonian ridigity. *Ann Neurol* 30:83–89, 1991.

182. Delwaide P, Pepin J, Noordhout Md: The audiospinal reaction in parkinsonian patients reflects functional changes in reticular nuclei. *Ann Neurol* 33:63–69, 1993.

183. Lang A, Johnson K: Akathisia in idiopathic Parkinson's disease. *Neurology* 37:477–481, 1987.

184. Linazasoro G, Masso JM, Suarez J: Nocturnal akathisia in Parkinson's disease: Treatment with clozapine. *Mov Disord* 8(2):171–174, 1993.

185. Fischer P, Naske R: Akathisia-like motor restlessness in major depression responding to serotonin-reuptake inhibition. *J Clin Psychopharmacol* 12(4):295–296, 1992.

186. Vazquez A, Jimenez-Jimenez F, Garcia-Ruiz P, Garcia-Urra D: 'Panik attacks' in Parkinson's disease. A long-term complication of L-dopatherapy. *Acta Neurol Scand* 87:14–18, 1993.

187. Bliwise D, Watts R, Watts N, et al: Disruptive nocturnal behavior in Parkinson's disease and Alzheimer's disease. *J Geriatr Psychiatry Neurol* 8:107–110, 1995.

188. Lauterbach E: Sleep benefit and sleep deprivation in subgroups of depressed patients with Parkinson's disease. *Am J Psychiatry* 151(5):782–783, 1994.

189. Friedman J, Lannon M: Clozapine in the treatment of psychosis in Parkinson's disease. *Neurology* 39:1219–1221, 1989.

190. Wolters E, Hurwitz T, Mak E, et al: Clozapine in the treament of parkinsonian patients with dopaminomimetic psychosis. *Neurology* 40:832–834, 1990.

191. Meco G, Alessandria A, Bonifati V, Giustini P: Risperidone for hallucinations in L-dopa-treated Parkinson's disease patients. *Lancet* 343(8909):1370–1371, 1994.

192. Tavares AR Jr: Risperidone in Parkinson's disease. *J Neurol Neurosurg Psychiatry* 58(4):521, 1995.

193. Touyz S, Beumont P, Saayman G, Zabow T: A psychophysiological investigation of the short-term effects of clozapine upon sleep parameters of normal young adults. *Biol Psychiatry* 12(6):801–822, 1977.

194. Touyz S, Saayman G, Zabow T: A psychophysiological investigation of the long-term effects of clozapine upon sleep patterns of normal young adults. *Psychopharmacology* 56:69–73, 1978.

195. Blum A, Girke W: Marked increase in REM sleep produced by a new antipsychotic compound. *Clin Electroencephalogr* 4(2):80–84, 1973.

196. Blum A: Triad of hyperthermia, increased REM sleep, and cataplexy during clozapine treatment? *J Clin Psychiatry* 51(6):259–260, 1990.

197. Zoldan J, Friedberg G, Goldberg-Stern H, Melamed E: Ondansetron for hallucinosis in advanced Parkinson's disease. *Lancet* 341:562–563, 1993.

198. Hardie R, Efthimiou J, Stern G: Respiration and sleep in Parkinson's disease (letter). *J Neurol Neurosurg Psychiatry* 49:1326, 1986.

199. Apps M, Sheaff P, Ingram D, et al: Respiration and sleep in parkinson's disease. *J Neurol Neurosurg Psychiatry* 48:1240–1245, 1985.

200. Bliwise D, Watts R, Watts N, Rye D: Nocturnal behavior disruption in Parkinson's disease and Alzheimer's disease (abstr.). *Sleep Res* 23:352, 1994.

201. Vincken W, Gauthier S, Dollfuss R, et al: Involvment of upper-airway muscles in extrapyramidal disorders. *N Engl J Med* 311:438–442, 1984.

202. Hovestadt A, Bogaard J, Meerwaldt J, et al: Pulmonary function in Parkinson's disease. *J Neurol Neurosurg Psychiatry* 52:329–333, 1989.

203. Rosen J, Feinsilver S, Friedman J: Increased CO_2 responsiveness in Parkinson's disease: Evidence for a role of dopamine in respiratory control. *Am Rev Respir Dis* 131:A297, 1985.

204. Feinsilver S, Friedman J, Rosen J: Respiration and sleep in Parkinson's disease. *J Neurol Neurosurg Psychiatry* 49:964, 1986.

205. Guilleminault C, Tilkian A, Lehrman K, et al: Sleep apnea syndrome: States of sleep and autonomic dysfunction. *J Neurol Neurosurg Psychiatry* 40:718–725, 1977.

206. Guilleminault C, Briskin J, Greenfield M, Silvestri R: The impact of autonomic nervous system dysfunction on breathing during sleep. *Sleep* 4(3):263–278, 1981.

207. McNicholas W, Rutherford R, Grossman R, et al: Abnormal respiratory pattern generation during sleep in patients with autonomic dysfunction. *Am Rev Respir Dis* 128:429–433, 1983.

208. Bergonzi P, Gigli G, Laudisio A, et al: Sleep and human cerebellar pathology. *Int J Neurosci* 15:159–163, 1981.

209. Chokroverty S, Sachdeo R, Masdeu J: Autonomic dysfunction and sleep apnea in olivopontocerebellar degeneration. *Arch Neurol* 41:926–931, 1984.

210. Salazar-Grueso E, Rosenberg R, Roos R: Sleep apnea in olivopontocerebellar degeneration: Treatment with trazodone. *Ann Neurol* 23:399–401, 1988.

211. Miller E, Nieburg H: Amphetamines: Valuable adjunct in treatment of Parkinsonism. *N Y State J Med* 73:2657–2661, 1973.

212. Cantello R, Aguggia M, Gilli M, et al: Major depression in Parkinson's disease and the mood response to intravenous methylphenidate: Possible role of the 'hedonic' dopamine synapse. *J Neurol Neurosurg Psychiatry* 52:724–731, 1989.

213. Hietanen M: Selegiline and cognitive function in Parkinson's disease. *Acta Neurol Scand* 84:407–410, 1991.

214. Portin R, Rinne U: The effect of deprenyl (selegiline) on cognition and emotion in parkinsonian patients undergoing long-term L-dopa treatment. *Acta Neurol Scand Suppl* 95:135–144, 1983.

215. Nickel B, Borbe H, Szelenyi I: Effect of selegiline and desmethylselegiline on cortical electric activity in rats. *J Neural Transm Suppl* 32:139–144, 1990.

216. Hublin C, Partinen M, Heinonen E, et al: Selegiline in the treatment of narcolepsy. *Neurology* 44:2095–2101, 1994.

217. Reinish L, MacFarlane J, Sandor P, Shapiro C: REM changes in narcolepsy with selegiline. *Sleep* 18(5):362–367, 1995.

218. Mayer G, Meier K, Hephata K: Selegeline hydrochloride treatment in narcolepsy: A double-blind placebo-controlled study. *Clin Neuropharmacol* 18(4):306–319, 1995.

219. Wiegand M, Moller A, Lauer C-J, et al: Nocturnal sleep in Huntington's disease. *J Neurol* 238:203–208, 1991.

220. Starr A: A disorder of rapid eye movements in Huntington's chorea. *Brain* 90(3):545–564, 1967.

221. Emser W, Brenner M, Stober T, Schimrigk K: Changes in nocturnal sleep in Huntington's and Parkinson's disease. *J Neurol* 235:177–179, 1988.

222. Aldrich M, Foster N, White R, et al: Sleep abnormalities in progressive supranuclear palsy. *Ann Neurol* 25:577–581, 1989.

223. Gross R, Spehlmann R, Daniels J: Sleep disturbances in progressive supranuclear palsy. *Electroencephalogr Clin Neurophysiol* 45:16–25, 1978.

224. Jankel W, Allen R, Niedermeyer E, Kalsher M: Polysomnographic findings in dystonia musculorum deformans. *Sleep* 6(3):281–285, 1983.

225. Segawa M, Hosaka A, Miyagawa F, et al: Hereditary progressive dystonia with marked diurnal fluctuation in Eldridge R, Fahn S (eds): Advances in Neurology, Vol. 14, *Dystonia*, New York: Raven Press, 1976, pp 215–233.

226. Montagna P, Imbriaco A, Zucconi M, et al: Hemifacial spasm in sleep. *Neurology* 36:270–273, 1986.

227. Fish D, Sawyers D, Smith S, et al: Motor inhibition from the brainstem is normal in torsion dystonia during REM sleep. *J Neurol Neurosurg Psychiatry* 54(2):140–144, 1991.

228. Forgach L, Eisen A, Fleetham J, Calne D: Studies on dystonic torticollis during sleep. *Neurology* 36(suppl 1):120, 1986.

229. Emser W, Hoffmann K, Stolz T, et al: Sleep disorders in diseases of the basal ganglia, in *Interdisciplinary Topics in Gerontology.* Basel, Switzerland: Karger, 1987, pp 144–157.

230. Sunohara N, Mano Y, Ando K, Satoyoshi E: Idiopathic dystonia—parkinsonism with marked diurnal fluctuation of symptoms. *Ann Neurol* 17:39–45, 1985.

231. Calleja J, Carpizo R, Berciano J, et al: Serial waking-sleep EEGs and evolution of somatosensory potentials in Creutzfeldt-Jakob disease. *Electroencephalogr Clin Neurophysiol* 60:504–508, 1985.

232. Silvestri R, Domenico PD, Rosa AD, et al: The effect of nocturnal physiological sleep on various movement disorders. *Mov Disord* 5(1):8–14, 1990.

233. Jankovic J, Rohaidy H: Motor, behavioral and pharmacologic findings in Tourette's syndrome. *Can J Neurol Sci* 14:541–546, 1987.

234. Sandyk R, Bamford C: Sleep disorders in Tourette's syndrome. *Intern J Neurosci* 37:59–65, 1987.

235. Mendelson W, Caine E, Goyer P, et al: Sleep in Gilles de la Tourette's syndrome. *Biol Psychiatry* 15(2):339–343, 1980.

236. Glaze D, Frost J, Jankovic J: Sleep in Gilles de la Tourette's syndrome: Disorder of arousal. *Neurology* 33:586–592, 1983.

237. Silvestri R, Domenico PD, Gugliotta M, et al: Gilles de la Tourette's syndrome: Arousal and sleep polygraphic findings: A case report. *Acta Neurol (Napoli)* 9(4):263–272, 1987.

238. Hashimoto T, Endo S, Fukuda K, et al: Increased body movements during sleep in Gilles de la Tourette's syndrome. *Brain Dev* 3:31–35, 1981.

239. Drake M, Hietter S, Bogner J, Andrews J: Cassette EEG sleep recordings in Gilles de la Tourette's syndrome. *Clin Electroencephalogr* 23(3):142–146, 1992.

240. Chokroverty S, Barron K: Palatal myoclonus and rhythmic ocular movements: A polygraphic study. *Neurology* 19:975–982, 1969.

241. Kayed K, Sjaastad O, Magnussen I, Marvik R: Palatal myoclonus during sleep. *Sleep* 6(2):130–136, 1983.

242. Yokota T, Atsumi Y, Uchiyama M, et al: Electroencephalographic activity related to palatal myoclonus in REM sleep. *J Neurol* 237:290–294, 1990.

243. Jellinger K: Pathology of Parkinson's disease. Changes other than the nigrostriatal pathway. *Mol Chem Neuropathol* 14:153–197, 1991.

244. Cipolli C, Bolzani R, Massetani R, Murri L: Age-related modifications in sleep of Parkinson patients, in Smirne S, Franceschi M, Ferini-Strambi L (eds): *Sleep and Ageing.* Milan: Masson, 1989, pp 93–96.

245. Kostic V, Susie V, Covickovic-Sternic N, et al: Reduced rapid eye movement sleep latency in patients with Parkinson's disease. *J Neurol* 236:421–423, 1989.

246. Kostic V, Susic V, Przedborski S, Sternic N: Sleep EEG in depressed and nondepressed patients with Parkinson's disease. *J Neuropsychiatry Clin Neurosci* 3:176–179, 1991.

247. Starkstein S, Preiosi T, Forrester W, Robinson R: Specificity of affective and autonomic symptoms of depression in Parkinson's disease. *J Neurol Neurosurg Psychiatry* 53:869–873, 1990.

248. Starkstein S, Preziosi T, Robinson R: Sleep disorders, pain, and depression in Parkinson's disease. *Eur Neurol* 31:352–355, 1991.

249. Menza M, Rosen R: Sleep in Parkinson's disease: The role of depression and anxiety. *Psychosomatics* 36:262–266, 1995.

250. McCance-Katz E, Marek K, Price L: Serotonergic dysfunction in depression associated with Parkinson's disease. *Neurology* 42:1813–1814, 1992.

251. Goetz C, Wilson R, Tanner C, Garron D: Relationships among pain, depression and sleep alterations in Parkinson's disease, in Yahr M, Bergmann K (eds): Advances in Neurology, Vol. 45, *Parkinson's Disease*, New York: Raven Press, 1986, pp 345–347.

252. Jouvet M: Biogenic amines and the states of sleep: Pharmacological and neurophysiological studies suggest a relationship between brain serotonin and sleep. *Science* 163:32–41, 1969.

253. Wauquier A, Clincke G, van den Broek W, de Prins E. Active and permissive roles of dopamine in sleep-wakefulness regulation, in Wauquier A, Gaillard JM, Monti JM, Radulovacki M (eds): *Sleep: Neurotransmitters and Neuromodulators.* New York: Raven Press, 1985, pp 107–120.

254. Nicholson A, Pascoe P: Dopaminergic transmission and the sleep-wakefulness continuum in man. *Neuropharmacology* 29:411–417, 1990.

255. Cianchetti C: Dopamine agonists and sleep in man, in Wauqier A, Gaillard J, Monti J, Radulovacki M (eds): *Sleep: Neurotransmitters and Neuromodulators.* New York: Raven Press, 1989, pp 121–133.

256. German D, Manaye K, Smith W, et al: Midbrain dopaminergic cell loss in Parkinson's disease: Computer visualization. *Ann Neurol* 26:507–514, 1989.

257. Gibb W, Lees A: Anatomy, pigmentation, ventral and dorsal subpopulations of the substantia nigra, and differential cell death in Parkinson's disease. *J Neurol Neurosurg Psychiatry* 54:388–396, 1991.

258. King C, Jewett R: The effects of α-methyltyrosine on sleep and brain norepinephrine in cats. *J Pharmacol Exp Ther* 177(1):188–194, 1971.

259. Hartmann E, Chung R, Draskoczy P, Schildkraut J: Effects of 6-hydroxydopamine on sleep in the rat. *Nature* 233:425–427, 1971.

260. Nishino S, Sampathkumaran R, Tafti M, et al: Is presynaptic activation of dopaminergic transmission important for the EEG arousal effect of stimulants? *Sleep Res* 24:310, 1995.

261. Trampus M, Ferri N, Monopoli A, Ongini E: The dopamine D1 receptor is involved in the regulation of REM sleep in the rat. *Eur J Pharmacol* 194:189–194, 1991.

262. Trampus M, Ferri N, Adami M, Ongini E: The dopamine D1 receptor agonists, A68930 and SKF 38393, induce arousal and suppress REM sleep in the rat. *Eur J Pharmacol* 235:83–87, 1993.

263. Ongini E, Bonizzoni E, Ferri N, et al: Differential effects of dopamine D_1 and D_2 receptor antagonist antipsychotics on sleep-wake patterns in the rat. *J Pharmacol Exp Ther* 266:726–731, 1993.

264. Gunne L-M, Lidvall H, Widen L: Preliminary clinical trial with L-dopa in narcolepsy. *Psychopharmacologia* 19:204–206, 1971.

265. Boivin D, Montplaisir J: The effects of L-dopa on excessive daytime sleepiness in narcolepsy. *Neurology* 41:1267–1269, 1991.

266. Di Chiara G, Porceddu M, Vargiu L, et al: Evidence for dopamine receptors mediating sedation in the mouse brain. *Nature* 264:564–566, 1976.

267. Mignot E, Reid M, Tafti M, et al: Local administration of dopaminergic drugs into the ventral tegmental area modulates cataplexy in narcoleptic canines (abstr.). *Sleep Res* 24:298, 1995.

268. Bagetta G, DeSarro G, Priolo E, Nistico G: Ventral tegmental area: Site through which dopamine D_2-receptor agonists evoke behavioral and electrocortical sleep in rats. *Br J Pharmacol* 95:860–866, 1988.

269. Nicholson A, Bradley C, Pascoe P: Medications: Effect on sleep and wakefulness, in Kryger M, Roth T, Dement W (eds): *Principles and Practice of Sleep Medicine*. Philadelphia: WB Saunders, 1994, pp 364–372.

270. Bjorklund A, Lindvall O: Dopamine-containing systems in the CNS, in Bjorklund A, Hokfelt T (eds): *Handbook of Chemical Neuroanatomy*. Amsterdam: Elsevier, 1984, pp 55–122.

271. Trulson M, Preussler D: Dopamine-containing ventral temental area neurons in freely moving cats: Activity during the sleep-walking cycle and effects of stress. *Exp Neurol* 83:367–377, 1984.

272. Miller J, Farber J, Gatz P, et al: Activity of mesencephalic dopamine and non-dopamine neurons across stages of sleep and waking in the rat. *Brain Res* 273:133–141, 1983.

273. Steinfels G, Heym J, Strecker R, Jacobs B: Behavioral correlates of dopaminergic unit activity in freely moving cats. *Brain Res* 258:217–228, 1983.

274. Grace A, Bunney B: Nigral dopamine neurons. Intracellular recording and identification with L-dopa injection and histofluorescence. *Science* 210:654–656, 1980.

275. Myslobodsky M, Mintz M, Ben-Mayor V, Radwan H: Unilateral dopamine deficit and lateral EEG asymmetry: Sleep abnormalities in hemi-Parkinson's patients. *Electroencephalogr Clin Neurophysiol* 54:227–231, 1982.

276. Jones B, Bobillier P, Pin C, Jouvet M: The effect of lesions of catecholamine-containing neurons upon monoamine content of the brain and EEG and behavioral waking in the cat. *Brain Res* 58:157–177, 1973.

277. Lai Y, Shalita T, Wu J-P et al: Altered sleep-wake pattern produced by neurotoxic lesions of the ventral portion of the mesopontine reticular formation. *Sleep Res* 24:10, 1995.

278. Montaron M, Bouyer J, Rougeul A, Buser P: Ventral mesencephalic tegmentum (VMT) controls electrocortical beta rhythms and associated attentive behavior in the cat. *Behav Brain Res* 6:129–145, 1982.

279. Galy D, Simon H, Lemoal M: Behavioral effects of lesions in the A10 dopaminergic area of the rat. *Brain Res* 124:83–97, 1977.

280. Tassin J, Stinus L, Simon H, et al: Relationship between the locomotor hyperactivity induced by A10 lesions and the destruction of the frontocortical dopaminergic innervation in the rat. *Brain Res* 141:267–281, 1978.

281. Pungor K, Papp M, Kekesi K, Juhasz G: A novel effect of MPTP: The selective suppression of paradoxical sleep in cats. *Brain Res* 525:310–314, 1990.

282. Ciliax BJ, Heilman C, Demchyshyn LL, et al: The dopamine transporter: Immunochemical characterization and localization in brain. *J Neurosci* 15:1714–1723, 1995.

283. Levey AI, Hersch SM, Rye DB, et al: Localization of D1 and D2 dopamine receptors in brain with subtype-specific antibodies. *Proc Natl Acad Sci U S A* 90:8861–8865, 1993.

284. Maeda T, Kitahama K, Geffard M: Dopaminergic innervation of rat locus ceruleus: A light and electron microscopic immunohistochemical study. *Microsc Res Tech* 29:211–218, 1994.

285. Matzuk M, Saper C: Preservation of hypothalamic dopaminergic neurons in Parkinson's disease. *Ann Neurol* 18:552–555, 1985.

286. Scatton B, Dennis T, L'Heureux R, et al: Degeneration of noradrenergic and serotonergic but not dopaminergic neurones in the lumbar spinal cord of parkinsonian patients. *Brain Res* 380:181–185, 1986.

287. McGeer E, McGeer P: Some characteristics of brain tyrosine hydroxylase, in Mandel A (eds): *New Concepts in Neurotransmitter Regulation*. New York: Plenum Press, 1973, pp 53–68.

288. Zwicker A, Calil H: The effects of REM sleep deprivation on striatal dopamine receptor sites. *Pharmacol Biochem Behav* 24:809–812, 1986.

289. Kilduff T, Bowersox S, Faull K, et al: Modulation of the activity of the striatal dopaminergic system during the hibernation cycle. *Sleep Res* 16:63, 1987.

290. Comella C, Bohmer J, Stebbins G: The frequency and factors associated with sleep benefit in Parkinson's disease. *Sleep Res* 24:386, 1995.

291. Gancher S, Nutt J: Diurnal responsiveness to apomorphine. *Neurology* 37:1250–1253, 1987.

292. Paulus W, Jellinger K: The neuropathologic basis of different clinical subgroups of Parkinson's disease. *J Neuropathol Exp Neurol* 50(6):743–755, 1991.

293. Jellinger K: The pedunculopontine nucleus in Parkinson's disease, progressive supranuclear palsy and Alzheimer's disease. *J Neurol Neurosurg Psychiatry* 51:540–543, 1988.

294. Hirsch E, Graybiel A, Duyckaerts C, Jovoy-Agid F: Neuronal loss in Parkinson's disease and in progressive supranucleur palsy. *Proc Natl Acad Sci U S A* 84:5976–5980, 1987.

295. Gai W, Halliday G, Blumbergs P, et al: Substance P-containing neurons in the mesopontine tegmentum are severely affected in Parkinson's disease. *Brain* 114:2253–2267, 1991.

296. Zweig R, Whitehouse P, Casanova M, et al: Loss of pedunculopontine neurons in progressive supranuclear palsy. *Ann Neurol* 22:18–25, 1987.

297. Zweig R, Hedreen J, Jankel W, et al: Pathology in brainstem regions of individuals with primary dystonia. *Neurology* 38:702–706, 1988.

298. Zweig R, Ross C, Hedreen J, et al: Locus coeruleus involvement in Huntington's disease. *Arch Neurol* 49(2):152–156, 1992.

299. Saper C: Diffuse cortical projection systems: Anatomical organization and role in cortical function, in *Handbook of Physiology: The Nervous System*. Bethesda, MD: American Physiological Society, 1987, sect V, pp 169–210.

300. Szymusiak R: State of the art review: Magnocellular nuclei of the basal forebrain: Substrates of sleep and arousal regulation. *Sleep* 18(6):478–500, 1995.

301. Ugedo L, Grenhoff J, Svensson T: Ritanserin, a 5-HT_2 receptor antagonist, activates midbrain dopamine neurons by blocking serotonergic inhibition. *Psychopharmacology* 98:45–50, 1989.

302. Koyama Y, Kayama Y: Mutual interactions among cholinergic noradrenergic and serotonergic neurons studied by ionophoresis of these transmitters in rat brainstem nuclei. *Neuroscience* 55(4):1117–1126, 1993.

303. Blaha C, Winn P: Modulation of dopamine efflux in the striatum following cholinergic stimulation of the substantia nigra in intact and pedunculopontine tegmental nucleus-lesioned rats. *J Neurosci* 13(3):1035–1044, 1993.

304. Corvaja N, Doucet G, Bolam J: Ultrastructure and synaptic targets of the *raphe*-nigral projection in the rat. *Neuroscience* 55(2):417–427, 1993.

305. Tokuna H, Morizumi T, Kudo M, Nakamura Y: A morphological evidence for monosynaptic projections from the nucleus tegmenti pedunculopontinus pars compacta (TPC) to nigrostriatal projection neurons. *Neurosci Lett* 85:1–4, 1988.

306. Clarke P, Hommer D, Pert A, Skirboll L: Innervation of substantia nigra neurons by cholinergic afferents from pedunculopontine nucleus in the rat: Neuroanatomical and electrophysiological evidence. *J Neurosci* 23(3):1011–1019, 1987.

307. Villablanca J, Olmstead C: The striatum: A fine tuner of the brain. *Acta Neurobiol Exp* 42:227–299, 1982.

308. Oniani T, Keshelava-Gogiohadze M: Effect of low-frequency electrical stimulation of the caudate nucleus on cortical electrical activity and the waking-sleep cycle. *Fiziol Zh SSSR* 62:29–37, 1976.

309. Heath R, Hodes R: Induction of sleep by stimulation of the caudate nucleus in macaqus rhesus and man. *Trans Am Neurol Assoc* 77:351–379, 1952.

310. Siegel J, Lineberry C: Caudate-capsular-induced modulation of single-unit activity in mesencephalic reticular formation. *Exp Neurol* 22:444–463, 1968.

311. Siegel J, Wang R: Electroencephalographic, behavioral, and single-unit effects produced by stimulation of forebrain inhibitory structure in cats. *Exp Neurol* 42:28–50, 1974.

312. Corsi-Cabrera M, Grinberg-Zylberbaum J, Arditti L: Caudate nucleus lesion selectively increases paradoxical sleep episodes in the rat. *Physiol Behav* 14:7–11, 1975.

313. Hall R, Keane P. Dopaminergic and cholinergic interactions in the caudate nucleus in relation to the induction of sleep in the cat (abstr.), in *Proceedings of the British Physiological Society*, 1975, pp 247P–248P.

314. Hauri P, Hawkins D: Human sleep after leucotomy. *Arch Gen Psychiatry* 26:469–473, 1972.

315. Hosowaka K, Sawada J, Ohara J, Matsada K: Follow-up studies on the sleep EEG after prefrontal lobotomy. *Psychiatr Neurol Japonica* 22:233–243, 1968.

316. Ith T, Hsu W, Holden J, Gannon P: Digital computer sleep prints in lobotomized and nonlobotomized schizoprenics. *Biol Psychiatry* 2:141–152, 1970.

317. Villablanca J, Marcus R: Effects of caudate nuclei removal in cats. Comparison with effects of frontal cortex ablation. *UCLA Forum Med Sci* 18:273–311, 1975.

318. Bricolo A: Insomnia after bilateral sterotactic thalamotomy in man. *J Neurol Neurosurg Psychiatry* 30:154–158, 1967.

319. McGinty D, Sterman M, Iwamura Y: Activity and atonia in the decerebrate cat. *Sleep Study Abstr* :309, 1970.

320. Albin R, Young A, Penney J: The functional anatomy of basal ganglia disorders. *Trends Neurosci* 12:366–375, 1989.

321. Crossman A: Neural mechanisms in disorders of movement. *Comp Biochem Physiol* 93A:141–149, 1989.

322. Steriade M, McCormick D, Sejnowski T: Thalamocortical oscillations in the sleeping and aroused brain. *Science* 262:679–684, 1993.

323. Hazrati L-N, Parent A: Projection from the external pallidum to the reticular thalamic nucleus in the squirrel monkey. *Brain* 550:142–146, 1994.

324. Paré D, Hazrati L-N, Parent A, Steriade M: Substantia nigra pars reticulata projects to the reticular thalamic nucleus of the cat: A morphological and electrophysiological study. *Brain Res* 2:141–152, 1990.

325. Jones BE, Cuello AC: Afferents to the basal forebrain cholinergic cell areas from pontomesencephalic-catecholamine, serotonin, and acetylcholine-neurons. *Neuroscience* 31:37–61, 1989.

326. Steriade M: Basic mechanisms of sleep generation. *Neurology* 42(suppl 6):9–18, 1992.

327. Steriade M, McCarley R: *Brainstem Control of Wakefulness and Sleep*. New York: Plenum Press, 1990, pp 205–223.

328. Jones B: Paradoxical sleep and its chemical and structural substrates in the brain. *Neuroscience* 40:637–656, 1991.

329. Nakamura Y, Tokuno H, Moriizumi T, et al: Monosynaptic nigral inputs to the pedunculopontine tegmental nucleus neurons which send their axons to the medial reticular formation in the medulla oblongata: An electron microscopic study in the cat. *Neurosci Lett* 103:145–150, 1989.

330. von Krosigk M, Smith Y, Bolam J, Smith A: Synaptic organization of gabaergic inputs from the striatum and the globus pallidus onto neurons in the sustantia nigra and retrorubral field which project to the medullary reticular formation. *Neuroscience* **50:531–549, 1992.**

331. Rye D, Saper C, Lee H, Wainer B: Pedunculopontine tegmental nucleus of the rat: Cytoarchitecture, cytochemistry, and some extrapyramidal connections of the mesopontine tegmentum. *J Comp Neurol* 259:483–528, 1987.

332. Harnois C, Filion M: Pallidofugal projections to thalamus and midbrain: A quantitative antidromic activation study in monkeys and cats. *Exp Brain Res* 47:277–285, 1982.

333. Hazrati L-N, Parent A: Contralateral pallidothalamic and pallidotegmental projections in primates: An anterograde and retrograde labeling study. *Brain Res* 567:212–223, 1991.

334. Crutcher M, Turner R, Perez J, Rye D: Relationship of the primate pedunculopontine nucleus (PPN) to tegmental connections with the internal pallidum (GPi). *Soc Neurosci Abstr* 20:334, 1994.

335. Parent A: Extrinsic connections of the basal ganglia. *Trends Neurosci* 13:254–258, 1990.

336. Rye D, Turner R, Vitek J, et al: Anatomical investigations of the pallidotegmental pathway in monkey and man, in Ohye H, Kimura M, McKenzie J (eds): *Basal Ganglia V. Proceedings of the Fifth Triennial Meeting of the International Basal Ganglia Society*. New York: Plenum Press, 1996, pp 59–75.

337. Sakai K: Some anatomical and physiological properties of pontomesencephalic tegmental neurons with special reference to the PGO waves and postural atonia during paradoxical sleep in the cat, in McGinty D, Drucker-Colin R, Morrison A, Parmeggiani P (eds): *Brain Mechanisms of Sleep*. New York: Raven Press, 1980, pp 111–138.

338. Magoun H, Rhines R: An inhibitory mechanism in the bulbar reticular formation. *J Neurophysiol* 9:165–171, 1946.

339. Lai Y, Siegel J: Medullary regions mediating atonia. *J Neurosci* 8(12):4790–4796, 1988.

340. Toyahma M, Sakai K, Salvert D, et al: Spinal projections from the lower brain stem in the cat as demonstrated by the horseradish peroxidase technique. I. Origins of the reticulospinal tracts and their funicular trajectories. *Brain Res* 173:383–403, 1979.

341. Rye D, Lee H, Saper C, Wainer B: Medullary and spinal efferents of the pedunculopontine tegmental nucleus and adjacent mesopontine tegmentum in the rat. *J Comp Neurol* 269:315–341, 1988.

342. Chase M, Morales F: The control of motoneurons during sleep, in Kryger M, Roth T, Dement W (eds): *Principles and Practice of Sleep Medicine*. Philadelphia: WB Saunders, 1994, pp 163–175.

343. Sakai K: Anatomical and physiological basis of paradoxical sleep, in McGinty D, Drucker-Colin R, Morrison A, Parmeggiani P (eds): *Brain Mechanisms of Sleep*. New York: Raven Press, 1985, pp 111–138.

344. Holmes C, Webster H, Zikman S, Jones B: Quisqualic acid lesions of the ventromedial and medullary reticular formation: Effects upon sleep-wakefulness states. *Soc Neurosci Abstr* 14:308, 1988.

345. Nakashima K, Shimoyama R, Yokoyama Y, Takahashi K: Auditory effects on the electrically elicited blink reflex in patients with Parkinson's disease. *Electroencephalogr Clin Neurophysiol* 89:108–112, 1993.

346. Penders C, Delwaide P: Blink reflex studies in patients with parkinsonism before and during therapy. *J Neurol Neurosurg Psychiatry* 34:674–678, 1971.

347. Kimura J: Disorder of interneurons in parkinsonism: The orbicularis oculi reflex to paired stimuli. *Brain* 96:87–96, 1973.

348. Datta S, Dossi RC, Pare D, et al: Substantia nigra reticulata neurons during sleep-waking states: Relation with ponto-geniculo-occipital waves. *Brain Res* 566:344–347, 1991.

349. Jones B, Webster H: Neurotaxic lesions of the dorsolateral pontomesencephalic tegmentum-cholinergic cell area in the cat. I. Effects upon the cholinergic innervation of the brain. *Brain Res* 451:13–32, 1988.

350. Shouse M, Siegel J: Pontine regulation of REM sleep components in cats: Integrity of the pedunculopontine tegmentum (PPT) is important for phasic events but unnecessary for atonia during REM sleep. *Brain Res* 571:50–63, 1992.

351. DeLong M: Activity of pallidal neurons in the monkey during movement and sleep (abstr.). *Physiologist* 207, 1969.

352. Wyzinski P, McCarley R, Hobson J: Discharge properties of pontine reticulospinal neurons during the sleep-waking cycle. *J Neurophysiol* 41:821–834, 1978.

353. Gassel M, Marchiafava P, Pompeiano O: Activity of the red nucleus during deep desynchronied sleep in unrestrained cats. *Arch Ital Biol* 103:369–396, 1965.

354. Evarts E: Temporal patterns of discharge of pyramidal tract neurons during sleep and waking in the monkey. *J Neurophysiol* 27:152–171, 1963.

355. Whitlock D, Arduini A, Moruzi G: Microelectrode analysis of pyramidal system during transition from sleep to wakefulness. *Boll Soc Ital Biol Sper* 28:414–429, 1952.

356. Iwama K, Kawamoto T: Responsiveness of cat motor cortex to electrical stimulation in sleep and wakefulness. *Progress in Brain Research*, 21:54–63, 1966, pp 54–63.

357. Baron M, Vitek J, Turner R, et al: Lesions in the sensorimotor region of the internal segment of the globus pallidus (GPi) in parkinsonian patients are effective in alleviating the cardinal signs of Parkinson's disease. *Soc Neurosci Abstr* 19:1584, 1993.

358. Vitek J, Kaneoke Y, Turner R, et al: Neuronal activity in the internal (GPi) and external (GPe) segments of the globus pallidus (GP) of parkinsonian patients is similar to that in the MPTP-treated primate model of parkinsonism. *Soc Neurosci Abstr* 19:1584, 1993.

359. Trulson M, Preussler D, Howell G: Activity of substantia nigra units across the sleep-waking cycle in freely moving cats. *Neurosci Lett* 26:183–188, 1981.

360. Kostowski W, Gracalone E, Garattini S, Valzelli L: Electrical stimulation of midbrain raphe: Biochemical, behavioral and bioelectrical effects. *Eur J Pharmacol* 7:170–175, 1969.

361. McGinty D, Harper R: Dorsal raphe neurons: Depression of firing during sleep in cats. *Brain Res* 101:569–575, 1976.

362. Trulson M, Jacobs B: Raphe unit activity in freely moving cats: Correlation with level of behavioral arousal. *Brain Res* 163:135–150, 1979.

363. Polc P, Monnier M: An activating mechanism in the ponto-bulbar raphe system of the rabbit. *Brain Res* 22:47–61, 1970.

364. Sheu Y-S, Nelson J, Bloom F: Discharge patterns of cat raphe neurons during sleep and waking. *Brain Res* 73:263–276, 1974.

365. Jacobs B, Azmitia E: Structure and function of the brain serotonin system. *Physiol Rev* 72:165–229, 1992.

366. Aston-Jones G, Bloom F: Activity of norepinephrine-containing locus coeruleus neurons in behaving rats anticipates fluctuations in the sleep-waking cycle. *J Neurosci* 1:876–886, 1981.

367. Jacobs B: Single unit activity of locus coeruleus neurons in behaving animals. *Prog Neurobiol* 27:183–194, 1986.

368. Aston-Jones G, Rajkowski J, Kubiak P, Alexinsky T: Locus coeruleus neurons in the monkey are selectively activated by attended stimuli in a vigilance task. *J Neurosci* 14:4467–4480, 1994.

369. Webster H, Jones B: Neurotoxic lesions of the dorsolateral pontomesencephalic tegmentum-cholinergic cell area in the cat. II. Effects upon sleep-waking states. *Brain Res* 458:285–302, 1988.

370. Steriade M, Datta S, Pare D, et al: Neuronal activities in brainstem cholinergic nuclei related to tonic activation processes in thalamocortical systems. *J Neurosci* 10(8):2541–2559, 1990.

371. Steriade M, Paré D, Datta S, et al: Different cellular types in mesopontine cholinergic nuclei related to ponto-geniculo-occipital waves. *J Neurosci* 10(8):2560–2579, 1990.

Chapter 52

PSYCHOGENIC MOVEMENT DISORDERS

NESTOR GÁLVEZ-JIMÉNEZ and ANTHONY E. LANG

HISTORY
PSYCHIATRIC DEFINITIONS
EPIDEMIOLOGY
CATEGORIES OF DIAGNOSTIC CERTAINTY
CLUES TO THE DIAGNOSIS
PSYCHOGENIC HYPERKINETIC MOVEMENT
   DISORDERS
     Psychogenic Dystonia
     Psychogenic Tremor
     Psychogenic Myoclonus
     Psychogenic Chorea/Ballism
     Psychogenic Tics
PSYCHOGENIC PARKINSONISM
PSYCHOGENIC GAIT DISORDERS (INCLUDING
   PSYCHOGENIC ATAXIA)
APPROACH TO THERAPY OF PSYCHOGENIC
   MOVEMENT DISORDERS

In 1922 Sir Henry Head wrote: ". . . Hysteria is sometimes said to imitate organic affections; but this is a highly misleading statement. The mimicry can only deceive an observer ignorant of the signs of hysteria or content with perfunctory examination."[1] Although in many cases of psychogenic movement disorders (PMDs) the nature of the problem is quite obvious from the first patient encounter, in the majority the diagnosis requires careful analysis of the history and the phenomenology of the abnormal movements and occasionally prolonged periods of observation and assessment. In general, abnormal movements and postures resulting from primary psychiatric disease are among the most difficult diagnostic problems in neurology, even for the most experienced neurologist. In this chapter we will review the varied manifestations of PMDs and provide guidelines for the diagnosis and approach to therapy of these patients.

History

In the 1880s Charcot was fascinated by "hysteria," directing much attention to its definition, analysis, treatment, and research.[2] In one of his Tuesday lessons at the Salpêtrière he presented a young woman who developed a contracture and deformity of her right foot 5 days after a fall. In his teachings, such a contracture should have been corrected as soon as it appeared. In this particular case he decided to watch the progression of the disorder over 4 days without interfering. He taught that in such instances the treatment involved inducing a second attack to make the "fixed" contracture completely disappear. He used "hysterogenic points" to provoke such a transient attack as a form of therapy in the treatment of static hysteric signs. From the patient description it appears that Charcot was dealing with a case of what we would now term "psychogenic dystonia."

According to Charcot, posttraumatic contractures were more frequently seen in hysterics. He concluded that hysteria was entirely in the mind. Charcot commented on how important it was for these symptoms to be treated as soon as they appeared.[2] Charcot proposed that hysteria was not restricted to women but was also common in males, especially in workingmen,[3] children,[4] and effeminate men.[5] Freud[3] also reported Charcot's observation that many conditions previously ascribed to alcoholic or lead poisoning were, in fact, hysterical.

Charcot's approach to hysteria was critized by many (among others, Paul Broca,[6] Sigmund Freud[7] and, later, Gowers[8]), especially in regards to the therapeutic use of suggestion and hypnosis.[9] Freud in his writings on hypnosis and suggestion, said that ". . . if the supporters of the suggestion theory are right, all the observations made at the Salpêtrière are worthless," because there were many who believed (especially in Germany) that the power of suggestion was the result of ". . . a combination of credulity on the part of the observers and of simulation on the part of the subjects of the experiments."[7] Charcot had the patients repeat their crises in front of physicians and medical students.[4] Furthermore, Charcot's experiments on hypnosis were performed by his chiefs of clinic, interns, and other assistants, but they were never personally checked, with the result that inadequacies and failures of this form of therapy were not known to him.[4] Because the majority of his hysterics were housed together with the epileptics (". . . the old wards of the chronic patients[7]"), it was well known that many of the postures or attacks demonstrated by hysterics were nothing more than colorful imitations of real epileptic seizures further reinforced by public demonstrations in his Tuesday clinics in front of not only his pupils but also society people, actors, writers, magistrates, and journalists.[4] Since then, the clinical manifestations and pathophysiological mechanisms underlying hysteria have been a matter of controversy.

Gowers[10] wrote that "there are few organic diseases of the brain that the great mimetic neurosis may not simulate. Palsy and spasm, coma . . . almost every symptom of positive disease finds its counter part in the repertoire of . . . the nervous system." He insisted that ". . . given symptoms of hysteria, we must never infer that this is the primary disease until we have searched for, and excluded, the symptoms of organic disease."[10] He described "psychogenic laryngeal spasms" and "psychogenic pharyngeal spasms" in his writings on epilepsy and hysteria[8] and used hypnosis to determine whether these spasms could be altered during sleep, attempting to distinguish attacks resulting from hysteria from those resulting from real organic disease (although we now recognize that true organic dystonia can disappear during sleep or with hypnosis). Gowers believed that hysteria could occur in both sexes,[11] observing that ". . . hysteroid attacks are not very rare in lads and young men including transient paralysis, or contractures, of a limb, precisely similar to those met with in the female sex."[8]

In his address to the London Hospital Medical Society, Sir Henry Head[1] described a variety of PMDs. He described hysterical tremor as a positive repetitive movement of a high "voluntary" type, varying in rapidity, and ceasing with distraction: ". . . a soldier with a severe tremor of the right hand and arm was able to play the banjo perfectly and I used this musical aptitude for effecting his cure." He also described abnormal focal postures in a limb or a single joint: ". . . any attempt to break down a spasm of this kind, to open the closed hand, or to straighten the flexed knee, meets with intense resistance," and in describing what he felt was "psychogenic torticollis" he stated that ". . . resistance may be experienced not only in pushing the head towards the normal shoulder, but also in moving it farther in the direction of the affected side."[1] In the same address he referred to "psychogenic ataxia," which differs fundamentally from "ataxy of organic origin."[1] On attempting to touch the nose with the index finger, there was past-pointing ". . . to the same side of the head," but if the head was pushed in the direction of the past-pointed finger so as to make contact with it, the affected limb would deviate even further away from the head.

In general, many of the observations of these earlier writers have been corroborated with time as experience with specific PMDs has accumulated. However, older and even more modern medical literature contains many examples of organic movement disorders mistakenly attributed to primary psychological factors. Tourette's syndrome is possibly the best example of a disorder once thought to have a psychological origin but which is now accepted to be the result of an inherited disturbance of the central nervous system. The same applies to the wide range of idiopathic dystonias, all of which, at one time or another, have been considered psychogenic. Reasons for this include the unusual nature of the movements, their appearance only on certain actions but not others using the same muscles, their relief by means of certain peculiar "sensory tricks," the common worsening of the movements in response to mental or social stress and, until very recently, the failure to find any underlying anatomic, physiological, or biochemical abnormalities. These factors "supported" the common belief that such patients had an underlying psychiatric disturbance, which then encouraged the development of psychopathological hypotheses to explain the significance of the abnormal movements. Examples of these included the "turning away" from responsibilities or avoidance of conflict in the patient with dystonic head turning or the phallic symbolism of a pen extruding ink and causing writer's cramp.

However, in recent years several studies of patients with focal dystonias, such as torticollis[12] and writer's cramp,[13,14] have failed to demonstrate evidence for abnormal premorbid personalities or an association with underlying causative psychopathology. Where abnormalities are found (e.g., depression, poor body image, and self-esteem), it is more likely that they are a result of the dystonia, rather than the cause.

Psychiatric Definitions

It is helpful to begin a review of PMDs with a brief discussion of the current terminology recommended by the American Psychiatric Association's Diagnostic and Statistical Manual of Mental Disorders, Fourth Edition (DSM-IV)[15] related to psychiatric disturbances that can be seen in such patients.

Somatoform disorders have as a feature the occurrence of symptoms suggesting a systemic medical condition, but these symptoms do not fit or cannot be fully explained by the presence of a known medical disorder, the exposure to a substance or drug, or by another psychiatric condition. These symptoms must cause significant distress or impairment in social, occupational, or other areas of functioning. Somatoform disorders include somatization disorders, factitious disorders, malingering, and conversion disorders. *Somatization disorders* (Table 52-1) were formerly referred to as hysteria or Briquet's syndrome. Somatization disorders begin before age 30 and consist of recurrent and multiple clinically significant somatic complaints that result in medical intervention or social or occupational impairment. The differential diagnosis of these disorders must include major depressive, anxiety and adjustment disorders.

Somatization disorders must be differentiated from *factitious disorders*, including Münchausen's syndrome (Table 52-2) and *malingering* (Table 52-3), where the symptoms are intentionally produced or feigned. The difference between these two is that in the former there is a motivation to assume a sick role to obtain medical evaluation and treatment, whereas in the latter there are external incentives such as financial gain or compensation, avoidance of duty, evasion of criminal prosecution, or obtaining drugs.

Conversion disorders (Table 52-4) are characterized by the presence of symptoms or signs affecting voluntary motor or sensory function suggesting a neurological deficit ("pseudoneurological") associated with psychological conflicts or other stressors resulting in significant alterations in social or occupational functioning. These symptoms are not intentionally produced or feigned, as in factitious disorders or malingering. Some patients with a *histrionic personality disorder* add to the clinical presentation a pattern of excessive emotionality and attention-seeking behavior (Table 52-5). Histrionic personality disorder occurs more frequently in women.[15,16]

Epidemiology

It has been reported that at Charcot's Tuesday clinic, 7 percent (244 patients of 3168) of the total population seen during

---

TABLE 52-1 Diagnostic Criteria for Somatization Disorder (DSM-IV)

1—History of many physical complaints beginning before age 30 years and occurring over a period of many years, resulting in medical treatment or significant impairment in social, occupational, or other areas of functioning.
2—The following criteria must have been met, with the symptoms occurring any time during the course of the disturbance:
    A—four pain symptoms in at least four different sites.
    B—two gastrointestinal symptoms other than pain.
    C—one sexual symptom other than pain.
    D—one pseudoneurological symptom, suggesting a neurological condition not limited to pain.

SOURCE: *From the American Psychiatric Association.*[15] *Used with permission.*

TABLE 52-2 Diagnostic Criteria for Factitous Disorder (DSM-IV)

1—Intentional production or feigning of physical or psychological symptoms or signs (Münchausen syndrome).
2—The motivation for the behavior is to assume the sick role.
3—External incentives for the behavior are absent (economic gain, avoidance of legal responsibilities, or improving physical well-being).

SOURCE: *From the American Psychiatric Association.[15] Used with permission.*

one academic year were diagnosed as having hysteria.[4,5,17] This figure is probably influenced by ascertainment bias, because Charcot's interest in hysteria was well-known at the time. The extent of Charcot's overdiagnosis or false-positive labeling of patients as hysterical is also uncertain. More recently, in Marsden's experience, "hysterical symptoms," defined as complaints that were not fully explained by organic or functional neurological disease, accounted for approximately 1 percent of all neurological diagnoses.[18] Others have found that psychogenic disorders account for up to 9 percent of admissions to a neurological unit.[19] In one series of 405 such patients requiring admission to hospital, Lempert et al. found that the most common underlying psychiatric disorder was depression (38 percent), followed by "anxiety and compulsion" (13 percent) and hysterical personality disorders (9 percent).[19] The nature of the primary psychiatric abnormality did not predict the type of presenting neurological symptoms, although paroxysmal vertigo was seen more often in patients with anxiety and compulsion. In Marsden's experience, depression was present in 18 percent of the 34 "hysterical" patients admitted to hospital over a 5-year period, whereas 20 percent had Briquet's syndrome and 6 percent had anxiety.[18] Therefore, it appears that the three most common psychiatric disturbances seen in patients presenting with psychogenic neurological disorders are, in order of frequency, depression (56 percent), followed by hysterical (somatization) personality disorders (29 percent) and anxiety disorders (19 percent).

Ford et al.,[20] from the Movement Disorders Unit at Columbia-Presbyterian Medical Center (CPMC), found that the majority of patients with PMDs had no underlying organic neurological disorder. However, ". . . there are individuals who manifest psychogenic symptomatology that repre-

TABLE 52-3 Features Suggestive of Malingering (DSM-IV)

1—Intentional production of false or grossly exaggerated physical or psychological symptoms, motivated by external incentives (i.e., avoiding work, obtaining financial compensation).
2—Malingering may represent adaptive behavior.
3—Malingering should be suspected when there is a medicolegal issue, that is, a person has been referred by his or her attorney.
4—Marked discrepancy between a person's claimed stress and disability and the objective findings.
5—Lack of cooperation during the diagnostic evaluation and in complying with the prescribed treatment.
6—Presence of antisocial personality disorder.

SOURCE: *Modified from the American Psychiatric Association.[15]*

TABLE 52-4 Diagnostic Criteria for Conversion Disorder (DSM-IV)

1—One or more symptoms or deficits affecting voluntary motor or sensory functions that suggest a neurological or other general medical condition.
2—Psychological factors judged to be associated with the symptom or deficit because the onset of symptoms is preceded by conflicts or other stressors.
3—The symptom is not intentionally produced or feigned.
4—The symptom cannot be explained by a general medical condition after a thorough medical and laboratory evaluation, or as a direct effect of a substance, or a culturally sanctioned behavior or experience.
5—The symptom causes significant distress or impairment in social, occupational, or other important areas of functioning or warrants medical evaluation.
6—The symptom is not limited to pain or sexual dysfunction, does not occur exclusively during the course of somatization disorder, and is not better accounted for by another mental disorder.

SOURCE: *From the American Psychiatric Association[15]. Used with permission.*

sents an exaggeration or elaboration of a neurological condition."[20] In this series of 24 patients with PMDs, the profile of a typical patient consisted of a young person (mean age 36 years, range 11–60 years), most often female (79 percent), of average or above average intelligence (96 percent combined), with a mean duration of symptoms of 5 years (range < 1 month–23 years) being unable to work and on disability (70 percent of patients). The principal psychiatric diagnoses were conversion disorder (75 percent), followed by somatization (12.5 percent), factitious disorder (8 percent), and malingering (4 percent). Dysthymia, as a secondary psychiatric diagnosis, was present in 67 percent of patients. The rest included a variety of different psychiatric conditions, such as major depression, adjustment disorder, organic mood or organic delusional disorders, obsessive-compulsive disorder, panic attacks, bipolar disorder, and others.

Another recent report from the same institution,[21] which houses a dystonia research center, described experience with

TABLE 52-5 Criteria for Histrionic Personality Disorder (DSM-IV)

1—Constantly seeks or demands reassurance, approval, or praise.
2—Is inappropriately sexually seductive in appearance or behavior.
3—Overly concerned with physical attractiveness.
4—Expresses emotion with inappropriate exaggeration, for example, embraces casual acquaintances with excessive ardor, sobbing on minor sentimental occasions, or has temper tantrums.
5—Is uncomfortable in situations in which he or she is not the center of attention.
6—Displays rapidly shifting and shallow expression of emotions.
7—Is self-centered, actions being directed toward obtaining immediate satisfaction; has no tolerance for the frustration of delayed gratification.
8—Has a style of speech that is exceedingly impressionistic and lacking in detail.

SOURCE: *From the American Psychiatric Association.[15] Used with permission.*

131 patients diagnosed as having PMDs. Many patients had more than one movement disorder subtype. Eighty-two (53 percent) had psychogenic dystonia, 21 (13 percent) psychogenic tremor, 14 (9 percent) psychogenic gait disturbances, 11 (7 percent) psychogenic myoclonus, 4 (2 percent) blepharospasm and facial movements, 3 (1.9 percent) parkinsonism, 2 (1.3 percent) tics, and stiff-person syndrome was seen in one case (0.6 percent). Nine percent of their cases (14) were categorized as having paroxysmal dyskinesias/shaking and undifferentiated movements. In our experience (AEL), with a total of 107 patients with PMD disorders seen at The Toronto Hospital (TTH) over a 10-year period (1983–1993), tremor (31) was the most common type of PMD, followed by patients with mixed or bizarre movements (30), psychogenic dystonia (18), psychogenic myoclonus (18), and psychogenic parkinsonism (10).

Table 52-6 combines the data on a total of 259 PMDs from CPMC and TTH. These data give a rough guide to the relative frequencies of psychogenic movements; however, it is important to recognize that there are intrinsic biases in the reporting and pattern of referrals in both practices and that the approach to classification was somewhat different (all subtypes versus predominant subtype). The combination of the New York and Toronto experience suggests that psychogenic dystonia is the most common PMD (39 percent), followed by psychogenic tremor (20 percent), psychogenic myoclonus (11 percent), and other bizarre/mixed or difficult to classify movement disorders (17 percent). Recently, Factor et al.[22] found that 28 of 842 (3.3 percent) consecutive patients seen at the Albany Medical College Movement Disorders Center had PMDs. The most common PMDs were psychogenic tremor, followed by dystonia, myoclonus, and parkinsonism more in keeping with our experience at The Toronto Hospital. On the other hand, in a review from Baylor College of Medicine Movement Disorders Center, psychogenic myoclonus predominated (8.5 percent of all patients with myoclonus and 20.2 percent of all PMDs).[23] Unfortunately, no further data were given for the frequencies of other nonorganic movements disorders.

TABLE 52-6 Combined Data on Psychogenic Movement Disorders Seen at CPMC and TTH

PMD	CPMC (%)*	TTH (%)**	Total (%)***
Dystonia	82 (53)	18 (17)	100 (39)
Tremor	21 (13)	31 (29)	52 (20)
Gait	14 (9)	0****	14 (5)
Myoclonus	11 (7)	18 (17)	29 (11)
Blepharospasm/facial movements	4 (2)	0	4 (1.5)
Parkinsonism	3 (1.9)	10 (9)	13 (5)
Tics	2 (1.3)	0	2 (0.7)
Stiff-person syndrome	1 (0.6)	0	1 (0.3)
Other mixed/bizzare symptoms	14 (9)	30 (28)	44 (17)
Total number	152	107	259

*Listed all types of PMD. **Listed only the predominant PMD. ***Totals represent types of PMD. Some patients have more than one pattern of PMD.[86]
****No pure gait disturbances included.

Categories of Diagnostic Certainty

The level of diagnostic certainty that the physician has for a psychogenic cause of a movement disorder varies greatly, depending on the clinical features of the movement disorder and the accompanying symptoms and signs. The four degrees of certainty for the diagnosis of psychogenic dystonia, developed by Fahn and Williams,[21] are now commonly applied to all forms of PMDs. These degrees of certainty are divided into documented, clinically established, probable, and possible PMDs. In *documented* PMDs the movements must be persistently relieved by psychotherapy, suggestion, or administration of placebos, or the patient is witnessed as being free of symptoms when left alone unobserved. *Clinically established* PMDs are inconsistent over time or are incongruent with the classical definitions of movement disorders. For example, in the case of dystonia the patient cannot move the limb on request and resists passive movements but easily grooms himself or herself in daily life. Along with these incongruities the patient must show additional features that suggest psychogenicity, such as other neurological signs that are definitely psychogenic (e.g., false weakness or false sensory findings or self-inflicted injuries, multiple somatizations, and an obvious psychiatric condition). Caution needs to be exercised in the case of self-inflicted injuries, because these can occasionally be symptoms of an organic movement disorder such as Tourette's syndrome or neuroacanthocytosis. *Probable* PMDs applies to those patients that fall into the following categories: (1) The movement disorder is inconsistent or incongruent with classical definitions, but there are no other features suggesting psychogenicity. (2) The movement disorder is consistent and congruent with organic disease, but accompanying neurological signs are definitely psychogenic, such as false weakness or sensory findings. (3) The movement disorder is consistent with a classical condition, but multiple somatizations are present. In the case of the second and third categories, it is important to consider the diagnostic alternative of an organic movement disorder accompanied by coincidental or associated psychiatric disturbances (see below). Finally, the diagnosis of a PMD is *possible* when an obvious emotional disturbance is present in a patient with a movement disorder that is otherwise consistent with a known organic disease.

Clues to the Diagnosis

There are a number of important historical and clinical features that can give a clue to the psychogenic nature of a movement disorder (Table 52-7).[21,24,25] Many of these are generally applicable to all patients, and others relate to a specific type of abnormal movement (e.g., tremor, dystonia). These clues may be evident on taking the patient's history, on clinical examination, or on assessment of response to therapeutic interventions. The general clues are listed in Table 52-7 whereas the more specific clues are considered in the sections dealing with specific disorders. Taken individually, most of these "clues" are no more than that; more substantive evidence is generally required before a diagnosis of a psycho-

TABLE 52-7 General Clues Suggesting That a Movement Disorder May Be Psychogenic

Historical
  1—Abrupt onset.
  2—Static course.
  3—Spontaneous remissions (inconsistency over time).
  4—Obvious psychiatric disturbance.
  5—Multiple somatizations.
  6—Employed in a health profession.
  7—Pending litigation or compensation.
  8—Presence of secondary gain.
Clinical
  1—Inconsistent character of the movement (amplitude, frequency, distribution, selective disability).
  2—Paroxysmal movement disorder.
  3—Movements increase with attention or decrease with distraction.
  4—Ability to trigger or relieve the abnormal movements with unusual or nonphysiological interventions (e.g., trigger points on the body, tuning fork).
  5—False weakness.
  6—False sensory complaints.
  7—Self-inflicted injuries.
  8—Deliberate slowness of movements.
  9—Functional disability out of proportion to exam findings.
Therapeutic responses
  1—Unresponsiveness to appropriate medications.
  2—Response to placebos.
  3—Remission with psychotherapy.

SOURCE: *Adapted from Fahn and Williams,*[21] *Barclay and Lang,*[24] *and Koller.*[25]

genic disorder can be confirmed. Examples of organic disorders demonstrating the point in question readily come to mind for many of the points listed in Table 52-7. For example, hemiballismus and other movement disorders induced by stroke or exogenous insult may begin abruptly and, in some of these, the course may be quite static. Although uncommon, spontaneous remissions may occur in a number of organic disorders, including idiopathic dystonias (especially cervical dystonia) and Tourette's syndrome. Selective disabilities are a typical feature of organic action-specific movement disorders, such as task-specific dystonias or primary writing tremor. Some functional disability out of proportion to clinical features documented on examination is a related point that can have similar organic exceptions. The converse, selective or surprising ability to perform certain tasks contrary to what might have been predicted from the severity of the abnormal movements or postures or the degree of disability experienced with most other activities, is very suggestive of a psychogenic etiology. Once again, however, this observation also may apply to patients with organic disorders, and it is remarkable how some individuals successfully overcome their disability to perform tasks requiring considerable skill and dexterity. Although PMDs are often exclusively paroxysmal or have some paroxysmal component, there are a large number of idiopathic and symptomatic forms of organic paroxysmal dyskinesias that are commonly misdiagnosed as psychogenic. The ability or inability to exert voluntary control over a particular abnormal movement cannot be used

as basis for the diagnosis of a psychogenic cause. Most but not all patients with PMDs deny any ability to suppress their movements volitionally. Patients with organic movement disorders vary in their ability to voluntarily control their movements. It is widely recognized that tics can be suppressed for prolonged periods. In addition, parkinsonian rest tremor, tardive dyskinesias, L-dopa-induced dyskinesias, some other choreas and certain dystonic movements may be voluntarily suppressed for many minutes at a time.[26]

The use of suggestion in attempting to induce or alter movements is helpful in the diagnosis of PMDs. However, unless the examiner is able to suppress the movements for extremely long periods (out of keeping with any past experience of the patient) or to induce movements that were not evident previously and that fulfill criteria for a psychogenic disorder in their own right, it is unwise to overemphasize the patient's response to suggestion. Suggestion is often combined with *placebo challenge* testing. The use of placebos in these circumstances is somewhat controversial. This is particularly the case, because most authorities do not inform the patient in advance of the possible "inactive" nature of the therapy, because this clearly reduces the likelihood of a response. Patients are generally told that they are going to receive a drug that has the potential to markedly improve or ameliorate their symptoms. Sometimes, patients are told that they will receive a drug that can worsen their symptoms (useful when the movements are exclusively paroxysmal), followed by another ("an antidote") that will have the opposite effect. Usually, these challenges are given intravenously. An alternative (that we have not used) is a small alcohol swab or gauze patch soaked in a very mild chemical irritant that causes a slight tingling or burning sensation on the skin. One of the major concerns or criticisms of the use of placebo is that the patient may respond to being told (or, especially, if they learn "by accident" in some other way) of the nature of the placebo test with the conviction that they have been tricked by the medical profession.[27] The resulting resentment is very counterproductive to the therapeutic relationship necessary for ongoing management of these patients. However, when the nature and results of placebo testing are shared with the patient in a supportive milieu as part of the overall treatment program, this can be an extremely effective tool with both diagnostic and therapeutic effects.

Little has been written on the use of placebos in PMDs, possibly because there is no "gold standard" for the confirmation of diagnosis with which to compare the results of this testing, as in the case of EEG and epilepsy. Recently, Lancman et al.[28] reported that in patients with psychogenic seizures, an "induction test" had a sensitivity of 77.4 percent and a specificity of 100 percent, with a positive predictive value of 100 percent. The negative predictive value was 48.7 percent. They used a "patch" placed on the skin, and the patients were told that the medication would be absorbed into the circulation and reach the brain in 30 seconds. They were also told not to control the seizures and that removal of the patch would stop the resulting seizure when one developed. Similar approaches[29,30] usually using intravenous injections of saline, are considered safe and effective,[28] although Walczak et al.[31] found that in a minority of patients, placebo injections produced atypical events or epileptic seizures that could lead to an incorrect diagnosis. In general, we reserve the use of placebo saline injections for patients in whom there remains diagnostic uncertainty after a full clinical assessment. This would include patients with a history of paroxysmal events that could not be triggered by simpler means, such as the application of a tuning fork to the forehead or sternum, combined with the suggestion that vibration often triggers such attacks in other patients. The use of pressure points in a somewhat similar fashion is effective in some patients. Attacks are sometimes precipitated by asking the patient to look up quickly. In others, applying pressure to the top of the head when the head is held steady for evaluation of eye movements is an effective precipitant.

The results of these triggering or relieving maneuvers, including placebo challenges, should be incorporated into the presentation of the diagnosis to the patient. This approach is discussed further toward the end of the chapter.

As with placebo challenges, little has been written on the use of sodium amytal testing in patients with PMDs. It is critical to remember that amytal may have a nonspecific but pronounced ameliorative effect on a variety of organic movement disorders. Alternatively, PMDs, especially when longstanding, may change little in response to this agent. When the diagnosis is confirmed by other means, amytal testing may provide useful insights into the psychodynamic factors causing the problem. However, caution must be exercised not to overinterpret information volunteered during this testing, especially when the diagnosis of a PMD is not supported or established by other evidence. Recently, symptom persistence during a sodium amytal infusion test[32] was reported as being useful in differentiating organic spasmodic dysphonia from psychogenic vocal cord dystonia, in which improvement in speech symptoms was commonly evident. Family history, neurological and psychiatric evaluations, electrical stimulation of the superior laryngeal nerve, and standard speech testing did not help in distinguishing these two conditions.

Throughout these assessments, as mentioned earlier, it is important to remember that patients with organic neurological disorders can have hysterical or psychogenic dysfunction as well. Weir Mitchell is quoted by Gowers[8] as noting that ". . . the symptoms of many organic diseases of the nervous system are pictures painted on an hysterical background." Gowers,[8] in his work on epilepsy and hysteria, noted that ". . . hysteria, it must be remembered, is common not only as an isolated, but also as a conjoined, morbid state and that hysteria can be the consequence of organic disease. Striking symptoms of hysteria are often seen, for instance, in cases of tumors of the brain." Just as pseudoseizures often occur on a background of true epilepsy, PMDs may occur in patients with underlying organic movement disorders. For example, Ranawaya et al. reported six such cases.[33] The new movement disorders were considered psychogenic because of historical, clinical, and behavioral features and responses to placebo and suggestion. Importantly, the PMD was typically the source of greater concern and disability than the preexisting organic condition. In the series of psychogenic dystonia studied by Fahn and Williams,[21] one patient developed "psychogenic worsening" of organic idiopathic familial dystonia because of his inability to compete with other students and teasing by his friends. "Pseudo-tics" have been reported in patients with Tourette's syndrome.[34] The clinician should be cautious in attributing all symptoms to "hysteria" alone, because up to 30 percent of patients thought to have a psychogenic disorder are eventually found to have a disease that could account for their symptoms.[25] It is also important to remember the potential for an initial presentation with psychiatric alterations to be followed only later by abnormal movement disorders in a variety of diseases, including Wilson's disease, Huntington's disease, dentatorubropallidoluysian atrophy (DRPLA), Tourette's syndrome, and neuroacanthocythosis.

The differential diagnosis of PMDs encompasses the whole field of movement disorders; therefore, the neurologist should be alert to these diagnostic possibilities in any patient who fulfills some of the characteristics mentioned above.

Psychogenic Hyperkinetic Movement Disorders

PSYCHOGENIC DYSTONIA

Dystonia refers to a syndrome dominated by sustained muscle contractions, frequently causing twisting and repetitive movements resulting in abnormal or dystonic postures.[35] Dystonias can be classified as primary or idiopathic where no cause can be found after exhaustive neurological evaluation and secondary or symptomatic where a cause is evident. Dystonia can also be classified according to age of onset (childhood, adolescence, and adult) or according to distribution (focal, segmental, multifocal, generalized, or hemidystonia).

Earlier we mentioned that certain symptoms and signs may occur in organic movement disorders, which can encourage the misdiagnosis of a psychogenic cause. This error probably occurs more often in the case of dystonia, especially the idiopathic dystonias, than in other hyperkinesias. Although a full discussion of dystonia and dystonic syndromes[24,36] is beyond the scope of this chapter (see Chaps. 30, 31, and 33). Table 52-8 outlines some of the features of dystonia that encourage this confusion by those unfamiliar with the disorder.

There are certain other clinical features of organic dystonias that can be extremely useful in raising the consideration of a psychogenic diagnosis. Idiopathic dystonia rarely begins in the lower limb in adult life. When this is a manifestation of a secondary dystonia, other neurological features (e.g., parkinsonism) or laboratory abnormalities (e.g., computed tomography (CT) or magnetic resonance imaging (MRI)) regularly accompany the dystonia. The onset of organic dystonia is almost always gradual or slow. A notable but rare exception to these two rules is an autosomal-dominant disorder known as "rapid-onset dystonia-parkinsonism."[37] Dystonia after peripheral injury can also have an abrupt onset, beginning in the lower limb. However, the role of psychiatric factors in these cases remains a major source of controversy (see below). Idiopathic dystonia typically begins with action-induced movements (see Table 52-8), and only after a prolonged period (sometimes never) progresses to dystonia at

TABLE 52-8 Clinical Features of Organic Dystonias That Sometimes Encourage a Misdiagnosis of a PMD

1—The movements in dystonic syndromes can be quite varied, including prolonged spasms, sinuous writhing, brief myoclonic jerks, slow rhythmical movements, and faster tremors.

2—Dystonia can remit in up to 20 percent of patients, especially in those with cervical dystonia (spasmodic torticollis).

3—Patients with ITD have no other neurological deficits and normal ancillary investigations.

4—Dystonia can be task-specific (i.e., writer's cramp) or may be purely action-induced (e.g., foot dystonia when walking forwards but not backwards or oromandibular dystonia only when attempting to speak or, alternatively, only upon eating).

5—Occasional patients experience dystonia at rest with improvement on action ("paradoxical dystonia").

6—Dystonia can be relieved by "sensory tricks" (geste antagoniste). The best known of these tricks occurs in patients with cervical dystonia, in whom light touch or pressure very often will correct the abnormal head position. Many other examples are seen in a variety of dystonias.

7—Organic dystonia can be relieved by relaxation and hypnosis and is typically worsened by emotional stress.

8—Dystonia can be paroxysmal (e.g., paroxysmal kinesigenic choreoathetosis, paroxysmal nonkinesigenic choreoathetosis) or can show diurnal variation, as seen most prominently in L-dopa-responsive dystonia.

ITD, idiopathic torsion dystonia
SOURCE: *Adapted from Weiner et al.,[36] Herz et al.,[87] and Marsden and Harrison.[88]*

rest Secondary dystonia may present with rest dystonia; however, this is typically accompanied by another neurological dysfunction or abnormalities on investigation. Here again, dystonia after peripheral injury is an exception that we will consider in greater detail below. Despite the extremely disfiguring postures, pain, other than muscle ache, is surprisingly uncommon in patients with dystonia. An important exception here is cervical dystonia, in which pain can be the principal source of disability. Finally, although primary sporadic forms of paroxysmal nonkinesigenic dystonia do occur, psychogenic dystonia is a more common cause of this presentation. In a review of 25 patients with nonkinesigenic paroxysmal dystonia, 7 were found to have a definable symptomatic central nervous system cause, 7 were diagnosed as having primary sporadic paroxysmal dystonia, and 11 (44 percent) had PMD.[38]

Before the seminal study of Fahn and Williams,[21] very few cases of true psychogenic dystonia had appeared in the literature. A critical review of most reports claiming a psychogenic origin in individual cases suggests that an organic source was, in fact, more likely. Indeed, because many patients with idiopathic torsion dystonia (ITD) had been misdiagnosed as hysterical and received years of unnecessary psychotherapy, it was generally emphasized by authorities in the field that psychogenic dystonia did not exist.[21] However, rare well-documented cases of psychogenic dystonia were occasionally reported.[39] Possibly the best known of these was a case of Münchausen syndrome, simulating ITD reported by Batshaw et al.[40] This woman's symptoms began at age 29 with dystonia in the right foot, accompanied by left-sided torticollis. Her symptoms progressed to generalized dystonia over a 7-year period despite aggressive medical therapy.

The organic basis of her symptoms was questioned, and a diagnosis of psychogenic dystonia was considered. Because of the bizarre and relentless progression of her disease despite aggressive psychotherapy, she underwent many consultations at centers with expertise in movement disorders and many psychiatric evaluations and admissions to inpatient psychiatric units, all without benefit. She subsequently underwent bilateral thalamotomies in hopes of improving her limb dystonia. The thalamotomies were "complicated" by the onset of dysarthria, progressing to aphonia 2 months after surgery. She had episodes of periodic breathing and acute opisthotonic posturing, lasting up to 6 hours. During one of these episodes she had a "seizure" and had a respiratory arrest after intravenous diazepam requiring subsequent tracheostomy. Trismus developed, and she had to be fed by nasogastric and, later, gastrotomy tube feedings. She lost 30 lbs. despite these procedures. It was not until nursing home placement became a consideration that one day the patient awoke with normal speech, volume, and articulation. She was transferred to a psychiatric unit, where she appeared delusional, hallucinatory, and with features of a histrionic personality disorder. During behavioral modification therapy she sat up, began to use her arms normally, and walked. Her psychotic symptoms disappeared, and medications were discontinued. By the time of discharge, all symptoms of dystonia had resolved, except for a 20-degree contracture of the right Achilles tendon that had resulted from the volitional maintenance of an equino posture. Later, the patient admitted to have feigned all of her symptoms. It was also learned that she had previously feigned a number of disorders in order to gain sympathy and attention from her family and friends. This history had not been evident earlier because the patient had kept her family apart from her physicians. During subsequent psychiatric evaluations it was found that she was bisexual, with difficulty maintaining long-term relationships, and had difficulty communicating her needs. She had been abandoned by her father early in her life and had been diagnosed with a number of other medical disorders, including lymphoma and multiple sclerosis, for which she claimed to have received therapy.

In 1988, Fahn and Williams[21] clearly defined the features of psychogenic dystonia, reviewing 39 patients, 21 of whom fulfilled their criteria for documented or clinically established psychogenic dystonia. The mean age of onset in these 21 patients was 26 years (with ages ranging from 8 to 56 years). All patients but two were female (10.5:1). The duration of symptoms before a correct diagnosis of psychogenic dystonia varied between less than 1 month and 15 years. The most common clue suggesting psychogenic dystonia was the incongruity or inconsistency of the dystonic movements, which were present in 85 percent (18). Other clues included false weakness (14), onset of dystonia at rest (11), pain (9), multiple somatizations (8), bizarre nature of the movements (7), sudden weakness (6), nonanatomic sensory changes (5), "seizures" (5), excessive slowness of movements (5), tenderness to light touch (4), and startle-induced "elaborate" movements (2). All patients except two had more than one such clue to the diagnosis. Fahn and Williams emphasized the presence of pain or tenderness in 62 percent (13/21), onset at rest in 11 of the 15 patients who had continual, instead of paroxysmal, psychogenic dystonia, and onset in a lower limb, mostly the foot in 66 percent (14). In this series, before the author's diagnosis of psychogenic dystonia all but two patients had a diagnosis of an organic movement disorder (12) or a combination of psychogenic and organic dystonia (7). None had been diagnosed as pure psychogenic dystonia.

Recently, Lang[41] reported his 10-year experience with 18 patients diagnosed as having clinically definite psychogenic dystonia, excluding cases with isolated paroxysmal movements. The clinical characteristics of the dystonia were inconsistent or incongruous with established forms of organic dystonia. The female to male ratio was 2.6:1. The mean age of onset was 35 years (range, 17–59). The onset of dystonia was abrupt in one-half of cases and progressed rapidly to fixed dystonic postures in six. In 4 patients the dystonia progressed over a period of weeks up to 5 years. A known precipitant for the dystonic symptoms was evident in 14 cases, with trauma being the most common (a motor vehicle accident in five and a local injury in six, including one patient with hand surgery, a fall, a poorly described work injury, and a fractured patella with later surgery). The dystonia began in a leg in seven, and the upper extremity was initially affected in four. Four had generalized dystonia from the onset, and three had dystonia of the neck and shoulder. The dystonia was present at rest from the onset in 12 patients, and 7 of them had persistent unchanging dystonia without spontaneous or action-induced changes in posturing. A total of 5 patients had periods in which they were free of dystonia; 11 had dystonia at least part of the time brought out or aggravated by action, with only 1 experiencing dystonia exclusively at these times (i.e., pure action-induced dystonia). Some 10 patients had paroxysmal symptoms superimposed on the persistent dystonia. The final distribution of dystonia at the time of diagnosis was segmental in 28 percent (5), focal in 22 percent (4), generalized in 44 percent (8), and 1 (6 percent) had hemidystonia. Pain was present in 88 percent of patients (16) and was a prominent feature in 14 of the 18 patients. One of these had well-established reflex sympathetic dystrophy (RSD). A total of 10 patients had accompanying other PMDs, including 3 with multiple forms (5 tremor, 2 myoclonus, and 6 miscellaneous). Other psychogenic neurological features included give-way weakness in 61 percent (11/18), excessive slowness in 28 percent (5/18), marked resistance to passive movements in 17 percent (3), and nonanatomic neurological changes in 44 percent (8/18). The primary psychiatric diagnosis most often was a conversion disorder or a somatoform disorder, and none had known factitious or malingering disorders.

Table 52-9 summarizes and combines the data from these two large series. As can be seen, psychogenic dystonia affects mostly young women, with abrupt "onset-at-rest" dystonia involving the lower limb, most often a foot, accompanied by excessive pain and tenderness with nonanatomic sensory dysfunction, give-way weakness or paralysis, excessive slowness of movement and multiple somatizations. The dystonia will most often become generalized, followed in frequency by segmental or focal distribution. Rarely, symptoms will begin as hemidystonia or progress to hemidystonia.

TABLE 52-9 Clinical Features of Psychogenic Dystonia

	Fahn and Williams[21]	Lang[41]	Totals/Means
No. of patients	21	18	39
Mean age of onset	23 y	35 y	29 y
Female to male ratio	10.5:1	2.6:1	5:1
Duration between onset and diagnosis	<1m–15y	2m–30y	<1m–30y
Onset-at-rest dystonia	11/14 (78%)	12/18 (66%)	23/39 (59%)
Pain/tenderness	13/21 (62%)	16/18 (88%)	29/39 (74%)
Distribution of dystonia at onset			
Upper limb	0	4 (22%)	4 (10%)
Neck/shoulder	4 (19%)	3 (17%)	7 (18%)
Trunk	1 (5%)	0	1 (2%)
Lower limb	14 (67%)	7 (39%)	21 (54%)
Hemidystonia	2 (9%)	0	2 (5%)
Generalized	0	4 (22%)	4 (10%)
Final distribution			
Focal	6 (28%)	4 (22%)	10 (26%)
Segmental	5 (24%)	5 (28%)	10 (26%)
Hemidystonia	0	1 (6%)	1 (3%)
Generalized	10 (48%)	8 (44%)	18 (46%)
Other psychogenic neurological findings			
Give-way weakness/paralysis	20/21 (95%)	11/18 (61%)	31/39 (79%)
Excessive slowness	5/21 (24%)	5/18 (28%)	10/39 (26%)
Marked resistance to passive movements	0	3 (17%)	3/39 (7.6%)
Nonanatomic sensory changes	5/21 (24%)	8/18 (44%)	13/39 (33%)
Multiple somatizations	8/21 (38%)	8/18 (14%)	16/39 (41%)

SOURCE: *From Fahn and Williams[21] and Lang.[41] Used with permission.*

DYSTONIA +/− REFLEX SYMPATHETIC DYSTROPHY AFTER PERIPHERAL INJURY

In recent years there have been a number of reports describing a variety of movement disorders, most notably, dystonia, after peripheral injury. When dystonia predominates it may occur in isolation, but more often it occurs in association with other movement disorders (particularly tremor), severe pain ("causalgia") and, sometimes, full-blown RSD. A variety of case series of patients with typical idiopathic dystonia have mentioned the potential role of preceding local trauma in anywhere from 5[42,43] to 16.4 percent.[44] However, in the only available case-control study, Fletcher and colleagues failed to show an association between idiopathic dystonia and a history of previous injury.[45] Importantly, when one reviews the descriptions of movement disorders after peripheral trauma, it is clear that the majority of patients have a clinical syndrome quite distinct from "classical" movement disorder syndromes such as ITD. Bhatia et al.[46] outlined a number of clinical characteristics that distinguished "causalgia-dystonia" from primary torsion dystonia (Table 52-10). Importantly, many of the clinical characteristics of this form of dystonia are similar to those seen in patients with well-defined psychogenic dystonia (see above). This, then, represents one of the most problematic and controversial areas in movement disorders.

There is extensive early literature on the role of trauma in a large number of neurological diseases.[47] With respect to modern movement disorder literature, Marsden et al. described five female patients developing dystonic posturing variably combined with tremor and myoclonus associated with RSD.[48] This syndrome followed minor injury to the limb in three of five patients. Schott in 1986, described a series of 10 patients, with 6 demonstrating features of dystonia.[49,50] In 1988, Jankovic and Van der Linden described 23 patients with movement disorders after peripheral injury.[51] Of the 23 patients studied, 10 had RSD. Of 23, 15 had dystonia as the primary movement disorder, with 4 demonstrating additional tremor. In contrast to other studies of such patients,

those authors believed that the movement disorders seen in their cases were "clinically similar to those typically seen in patients with ITD or ET [essential tremor]" Also, in contrast to other studies, they found that fully 65 percent had evidence of "predisposing factors," such as a family history of a movement disorder or previous neuroleptic use. Although Jankovic and Van der Linden believed that their patients represented examples or organic disorders, they admitted that "psychiatric disease may have contributed." In 1990, Schwartzman and Kerrigan described 43 of 200 RSD patients who demonstrated a movement disorder.[52] All 43 had dystonia, 10 of whom showed only "subtle features." Of the 43 patients, 31 also had tremor. The features of dystonia were similar to those outlined in Table 52-7. In addition to the dystonia, all patients demonstrated "spasms," as well as difficulty initiating movement. Most demonstrated increased tone and reflexes. As in other reports, minor injuries were causative in most cases. No predisposing factors were mentioned in this report. Sympathetic blocks were said to improve the symptoms temporarily in 90 percent of patients. In 1993, Bhatia et al. coined the term "causalgia-dystonia syndrome," describing 18 patients who developed fixed dystonic postures, usually after minor injury.[46] In contrast to the report of Schwartzman and Kerrigan, they found that sympathetic blockade, sympathectomies, and a variety of medications were entirely unhelpful. These authors admitted the potential for psychogenic factors to have played an important role in the development of this problem, recognizing that the absence of overt psychopathology is not uncommon in isolated conversion reactions, contrary to the opinion of Schwartzman and Kerrigan.[53]

A number of peripheral and suprasegmental mechanisms have been proposed to explain the development of movement disorders after peripheral injury.[54] Importantly, none of these have been proven to account for the clinical features demonstrated in patients experiencing such problems. It is also important to recognize that many patients with movement disorders after peripheral injury demonstrate features that are common accompaniments of psychogenic movement disorders.[55] With respect to RSD/causalgia-related dystonia, their similarities to psychogenic dystonia include the frequency and types of precipitant, the lack of overt evidence of nerve injury, the frequency and nature of associated pain, the presence of weakness that usually has features of "giveway" weakness, the pronounced deliberate slowness in initiating movements, the onset of dystonia at rest with fixed dystonic posturing, the abrupt onset and rapid spread to other body parts, the presence of other movements, including tremor and "spasms," and the presence of additional complaints such as "dysphasia" and swallowing difficulties.[52]

In addressing the role of psychological factors, we carried out a pilot study in our unit in which seven unselected patients presenting with RSD and a movement disorder were admitted to the Pain Service (J Wbjcieszek, A Mailis, and AE Lang, unpublished observations). After extensive investigation, which included placebo treatments and placebo-controlled sympathetic blocks, the final diagnosis of the movement disorder was organic in three patients and psychogenic in four. The organic movement disorders were all considered "atypical" for classical syndromes, such as ITD or ET. All

TABLE 52-10 Differences between "Causalgia-Dystonia" and Primary Torsion Dystonia

Causalgia-Dystonia	Idiopathic Dystonia
Clear preponderance of women	No preponderance of women
No family history	Positive family history not uncommon
Painful (causalgia)	Usually painless
Vasomotor, sudomotor and trophic changes	Such changes not seen
Fixed spasm	Mobile spasms
Contractures common and early	Contractures uncommon and late
No geste antagoniste	Geste frequent
No improvement with sleep	Sleep often improves
Poor response to botulinum toxin and other therapy	Often responds to botulinum toxin, others
Onset in leg in adult	Adult leg onset very rare
Rapid spread	Slow progression

SOURCE: Adapted from Bhatia et al.[46]

three of these patients had a well-defined physiological source of pain or had a predisposition to develop a movement disorder (e.g., a family and personal history of tremor, laboratory evidence for multiple sclerosis). In the four patients who had a PMD, there was no identifiable source of pain, and the final pain diagnosis was a chronic pain syndrome in one, pain avoidance behavior in 1, and a somatoform disorder in 2.

The controversy surrounding this syndrome is not limited to the movement disorders aspect. Similar controversy flourishes in the field of RSD, in which some authors have argued that patients who lack clear evidence of nerve injury constitute a "pseudoneuropathy of psychogenic origin."[56] Our experience with a large number of patients thought to have posttraumatic dystonia indicates that a significant proportion have very clear evidence of an important psychogenic component, and in many the problem is entirely psychogenic in origin. We would argue that an unquestioning acceptance of all cases of dystonia after injury as organic "peripheral trauma-induced dystonia," explaining them with a variety of peripheral and secondary suprasegmental pathophysiological mechanisms of unproven relevance, legitimizes and intellectualizes the problem without sufficient justification. With respect to the acceptance of the diagnosis of RSD without nerve injury, Ochoa stated: "It is dangerous to diagnose RSD, because that term carries the illusion of pathophysiology and the illusion of efficacious treatment. These unfortunate patients are the pariahs of our incompetent health system. While they do carry a genuine health disorder, they have been cursed by diagnostic adjudication of a disease of medical understanding."[56] We would argue that a similar statement could be made of many patients who have been diagnosed as having "posttraumatic dystonia."

PSYCHOGENIC TREMOR

Tremor is defined as an involuntary, rhythmic, sinusoidal movement resulting in part from regular rhythmical contractions of reciprocally innervated muscles.[35,57] Psychogenic tremor accounted for 20 percent of a total of 259 psychogenic movement disorders in the combined New York and Toronto series presented in Table 52-6.

There has been much written about this subject. For example, Charcot described proximal tremors (involving the shoulder or hip) as almost unique to hysterical disorders, referring to them (unfortunately) as "rhythmical chorea." Another variant was "hammering chorea," in which the patient alternately flexed and extended the elbow as though using a hammer. We now recognized that both of these forms of tremor, although uncommon, may also be seen in organic neurological disease (e.g., the wing-beating tremor sometimes seen in Wilson's disease). Of the two, a rhythmic hammering movement is more characteristic of psychogenic tremor.

Gowers[10] described the presence of hysterical tremor in patients with hysterical paralysis. He stated that ". . . when the paralysis is incomplete, movement is slow, and is attended by characteristic irregular . . . coarser tremor than simple tremor." This is accompanied by interference of voluntary movements by the ". . . undue contractions in the opponents of the muscles that should effect the movement."

Kinnier Wilson,[58] referring to hysterical tremors said that ". . . they present no separate or contrasting features when set alongside those of so-called 'organic' type." He disagreed with Gowers, who firmly believed that hysterical tremor could be differentiated from organic tremor based on its variability, the influence of physical and emotional stimuli, and dependence on the attention paid to it because ". . . numerous organic tremors can be affected by a whole series of factors, exhibit marked fluctuations and fluidity, are highly irregular, shift their incidence and are aggravated when the subject is under observation." He considered both hysterical and organic tremors, "escape phenomena of infracortical level" and, therefore, they were part of an individual's "physiologic" repertoire. This would explain why ". . . hysterical subjects exhibiting such movements do not complain of fatigue, or at least appear to be less conscious of it than does a normal subject who executes them intentionally." In the person who intentionally produces a tremor, fatigue sets in easily because the "artifactual" tremor forms no part of their habitual function.

More recently, Fahn reported two cases of psychogenic tremor[59] and, subsequently, Koller et al.[60] described 24 patients with clinically established or documented psychogenic tremor. In this latter series the female to male ratio was 1.7:1. The mean age was 43.4 years, with a range of 15–78 years. The onset of tremor was abrupt in 87.5 percent of cases, and the duration of tremor ranged from 1 month to 10 years. The majority of patients showed no change in their tremors over time (45 percent), whereas 25 percent experienced improvement to complete resolution, 4 percent worsened, and 16 percent had a fluctuating course. A total of 91 percent of the patients had other features suggestive of a functional disorder, such as nonphysiological weakness, atypical gait disturbances, and nonanatomical sensory changes. The psychiatric diagnosis, in order of frequency, was a conversion reaction, depression, an anxiety disorder, and malingering. The tremors were characterized as having rest, postural, and kinetic components. The postural component was the most prominent, followed by rest and action tremors (i.e., postural rest > action). Twelve percent of patients had an associated head tremor. With distraction all patients showed a reduction in the amplitude of tremor, as well as variability in tremor frequency.

Our subsequent experience with psychogenic tremor continues to support these earlier observations. All of the general historical and clinical features of PMD apply. Possibly more than in most forms of PMD the abrupt onset and the early (sometimes immediate) attainment of maximal severity are very useful clues, because these features are rarely, if ever, seen in organic tremors. As with other PMDs, abrupt onset often follows a known precipitant (e.g., minor trauma). Psychogenic tremors are often present equally at rest, at postural maintenance, and during action, whereas organic tremors uncommonly persist in all states, and when they do, the tremor tends to increase in amplitude from one to another (i.e., rest < posture < intention). We would agree with Wilson's criticism of overemphasis on tremor variability, given the pronounced variation seen in organic tremors. On the other hand, complete suppression with distraction is not seen in organic tremors. More often, the opposite is seen; the tremor increases with patient concentration on mental or physical tasks. Suppression with distraction is an especially useful sign when a movement disorder is continuous or constant, as are most examples of psychogenic tremor. Another extremely useful clinical sign is the entrainment of the tremor to a new frequency or pattern. When the patient is asked to beat out a slow rhythmical or complex irregular pattern with the uninvolved limb (or the opposite limb to that being observed in cases of bilateral psychogenic tremor), the tremor will often change frequency or character to match the imposed contralateral movement. Rarely, organic mirror movements might be confused with this phenomenon, although they would not normally suppress the underlying tremor. Occasionally, forcefully restraining a tremulous limb will result in a tremor developing in a previously unaffected limb. Psychogenic tremor may affect a single limb or multiple limbs and axial structures. The arms are most often involved, followed by the head and then the legs. Psychogenic tremor may be continuous or intermittent; in the upper limbs it is often continuous, but it rarely, if ever, follows this course in the legs, typically occurring intermittently or paroxysmally, often precipitated by attention, movement, or some other activity.

The combination of general clues to psychogenicity with the specific features listed above permit the experienced clinician sufficient diagnostic certainty to categorize most typical patients as "clinically established" psychogenic tremor. In long-standing, well-established patients it is remarkable how persistent and seemingly invariable the tremor is and, like Wilson, one cannot help remarking on the lack of an expected fatiguing component. However, careful, sometimes prolonged or repeated assessments will demonstrate clinical inconsistencies or incongruities with organic tremors. These criteria must be reliably demonstrated and must be convincingly evident before one accepts a psychogenic diagnosis.

PSYCHOGENIC MYOCLONUS

Myoclonus is defined as brief, shock-like muscle contractions (positive myoclonus) or sudden lapses in tone (negative myoclonus), as exemplified by asterixis. Psychogenic myoclonus represented 11 percent of all PMDs seen in the combined New York and Toronto data, although in Jankovic's series, it was the most common form of PMD, accounting for 8.5 percent of all patients with myoclonus and 20.2 percent of all PMDs.

The only reported series of psychogenic myoclonus is that of Monday and Jankovic,[23] who described 18 patients seen over a 10-year period. The female to male ratio was 2.6:1, with a mean age of 42.5 years (range, 22–75 years). None had a family history of myoclonus. Eighty-three percent of patients (15/18) had a precipitating event, and the abnormal involuntary movement began suddenly in 61 percent of patients (11) with gradual onset over several days in 38 percent. Eighty-three percent of patients (15) experienced exacerbations of the myoclonus with stress, and 77 percent (14) had definite worsening of myoclonus during periods of anxiety. The most common distribution of myoclonus was segmental in 10 (55 percent), followed by generalized in 39 percent and focal in 5 percent of patients. The myoclonus was present at

rest in all patients and was exacerbated by movement in 77 percent (14). Light and noise worsened myoclonus in one and four patients, respectively.

Other neurological findings included tremor (postural, 3; kinetic, 2; rest 1), focal (posttraumatic) dystonia in 1, and gait abnormalities in 6. In most patients, these neurological findings were believed to be also of psychogenic origin. Neurological evaluation showed no abnormalities, except for these movement disorders. All patients had normal EEG tests, and other neurological investigations were unrevealing.

Overt psychiatric disturbances were present in 55 percent of patients before the onset of myoclonus, and 61 percent had a demonstrable psychiatric pathology, as shown by psychiatric interview or neuropsychological testing. The most common diagnoses were depression in four, anxiety disorder and panic attacks in two, and personality disorders in two. Eighty-eight percent of patients had a variety of different predisposing factors. Six had trauma before onset of myoclonus: 3 had "on-the-job" related injuries, one slipped in a shopping mall and two patients were involved in motor vehicle accidents. Only one had filed a worker's compensation suit.

Follow-up was available in 12/18 patients (67 percent). Fifty-eight percent reported improvement of the myoclonus over time, whereas 25 percent thought that the myoclonus was much worse after evaluation. The authors emphasized that spontaneous resolution of the myoclonus can be regarded as a strong indication of psychogenicity, provided that reversible causes of myoclonus are ruled out, such as infections, metabolic encephalopathies, or neurodegenerative disorders and provided there is no family history of myoclonus. Reduction of myoclonus with distraction was found to be a very helpful finding in establishing the diagnosis. However, because psychogenic myoclonus is often intermittent or discontinuous, this sign is probably less useful than in cases of more persistent psychogenic movements (e.g., psychogenic tremor).

Electrophysiological testing may be very helpful in problematic cases. The temporal pattern of muscle activation in various forms of pathological myoclonus is stereotypical and depends on the location of the generator or the origin of myoclonus (e.g., cortex, brain stem, spinal cord). Myoclonic jerks originating in the cortex (electromyogram (EMG) burst of 10–50 ms[61]) and brain stem (EMG burst >100 ms[61]) and induced by sensory input (i.e., reflex myoclonus) usually have a short latency (~60–70 ms[62]) between stimulus and a resulting jerk that is typically just long enough for the sensory input to reach the site of origin and for a return volley to travel down rapidly conducting descending pathways (e.g., the corticospinal tract) to the anterior horn cells and, from there, to the muscle. Less commonly, electrophysiological testing demonstrates evidence of much slower, presumably polysynaptic propagation of the response, as in propriospinal myoclonus. Electrophysiological studies, using EMG surface electrodes in patients with psychogenic myoclonus, may show variable and inconsistent muscle activation patterns and more importantly the stimulus-induced responses tend to habituate, as seen in the normal startle response.[63] More useful is the timing of responses (in stimulus-sensitive forms), when the latency from stimulus to jerk is much longer than that seen in pathological forms of myoclonus and typically falls within the range of voluntary reaction time (~100–120 ms; P Ashby, personal communication). Recently, Terada et al.[64] reported an assessment of the readiness potential or Bereitschaftspotential (BP) in patients with psychogenic myoclonus. The BP is a negative shift in the EEG that occurs 1.5 seconds before a voluntary movement takes place.[65] Terada et al. hypothesized that an involuntary movement (such as that seen in pathological forms of myoclonus) would lack a preceding BP.[64] They found that BPs preceded the jerks in patients with psychogenic myoclonus and concluded that this feature was consistent with the movements being generated through voluntary mechanisms. Although BPs can rarely be associated with involuntary movements because of neuroacanthocytosis[66] and mirror movements,[67,68] the presence of a BP can be extremely useful in identifying a movement as psychogenic.

This same type of electrophysiological assessment is very helpful in cases in which sound is the inducing stimulus (i.e., psychogenic startle). The normal startle response might be considered a form of physiological myoclonus which occurs in an exaggerated fashion in a familial disorder known as hyperekplexia, or startle disease. Electrophysiological study[69-71] of a startle response demonstrates progression of muscle contraction, first involving closure of the eyes (onset latency of 30–40 ms), followed by facial grimacing and forward flexion of the head (55–85 ms), flexion of the elbows (85–100 ms), abduction of the shoulders, pronation of the forearms and clenching of the fists. Onset latency of the muscle activity in hamstrings and quadriceps is about 100–125 ms and for the tibialis anterior 130–140 ms. Some patients only manifest closure of the eyes. The rostrocaudal progression of the muscle contraction follows a pattern similar to that seen in reticular reflex myoclonus or reflex myoclonus of brain stem origin.[63] The normal physiological behavior of the startle response includes sensitization (resulting in increased amplitude and/or shorter latency of a response), which is masked by the habituation resulting from several repetitive stimuli. In startle disease patients have an exaggerated response and lack of habituation. Many patients with psychogenic myoclonus demonstrate an exaggerated response to startle. Typically, this startle response habituates over several trials, as expected in normal physiological startle. Simple visual analysis of the muscle contractions may show moment-to-moment variability (i.e., inconsistency) in the latency from stimulus to response and in the pattern of muscle activation, and these inconsistencies can be confirmed by multichannel EMG assessment.

Brief mention should be made of three related disorders first described approximately 100 years ago in different populations. Latah, Jumping Frenchmen of Maine, and Myriachit all variably demonstrate excessive startle, echolalia, echopraxia, and automatic obedience.[72] Considerable debate exists about the true origins of these disorders. Careful clinical and modern electrophysiological assessments of these uncommon conditions are lacking. Some authors believe that they are organically mediated neuropsychiatric disorders akin to Tourette's syndrome.[73] In fact Gilles de la Tourette himself thought of these disorders as part of the "syndrome of tic convulsive."[74,75] Others argue that they represent forms of "culturally mediated behavior"[72,73,75,76] and, as such, they might be considered types of PMD in the broadest sense (Kinnier Wilson called them "collective psychoneurosis"[75]). Having reviewed videotapes of Latah patients from Indonesia and cases from Louisiana with a disorder related to Jumping Frenchmen of Maine ("Ragin' Cajuns"), the authors favor the latter opinion. However, further study of these unusual conditions is clearly required.

PSYCHOGENIC CHOREA/BALLISM

As mentioned in the section on psychogenic tremors, earlier medical writing used the term chorea to described bizarre movement disorders that would not be consistent with the current definition of chorea. Terms such as "rhythmical chorea," "hammering chorea," and "dancing chorea" were popularized by Charcot for very spectacular movements seen in hysterical patients. True chorea, as defined as random fleeting movements that flow from one part of the body to another in an unpredictable fashion, is exceedingly rare in PMD patients. We have seen only one patient who could be considered as having psychogenic chorea. Importantly, unlike most cases of organic chorea, his movements were purely paroxysmal. There was a very clear psychiatric history, and the patient lacked other features of organic paroxysmal dyskinesias. Given the exceedingly rare occurrence of psychogenic chorea, we would recommend exercising caution in making this diagnosis, even by clinicians with considerable experience in the field of movement disorders.

PSYCHOGENIC TICS

Little has been written about psychogenic tics. Psychogenic tics accounted for only 2 of 152 PMDs in the CPMC series (see above). At our center, over a 10-year period (1983–1993), no cases of psychogenic tics were seen.

Recently, Kurlan et al.[34] reported a young woman with long-standing Tourette's syndrome and obsessive-compulsive disorder (OCD) who developed complex movements such as slumping in a chair or to the floor or bed, along with tonic-clonic-like movements suggestive of pseudoseizures. No alteration of consciousness or incontinence were noted. These episodes were referred to by the patient as "bad spells," and her physicians believed they represented poorly controlled tics. However, multiple adjustments of her anti-tic medications failed to improve the movements. After careful analysis it became clear that these "bad spells" were psychogenic in nature. The patient received psychotherapy and was found to fulfill criteria for a borderline personality disorder. There were clear secondary "gains," such as the need for financial support from her parents and avoidance of social, educational, and domestic responsibilities.

What is not clear from the description of this case is whether the patient had any premonitory feelings or symptoms of an urge to perform her usual tics or the newly developed movements and, if in trying to control the movements she had a buildup of tension with a subsequent worsening. The absence of this urge may have helped differentiate these "tics" from true tics. In our experience, a very high proportion of tic patients experience a subjective urge to perform the tics (at one time or another). The performance of the tic is commonly appreciated as a partially volitional capitulation to this urge. In some of our tic patients who have had other concomitant movement disorders (e.g., dystonia, tardive dyskinesia), a similar subjective feeling has never been present, and the patient has always been able to distinguish between their tics and these other movements. In addition, none of our PMD patients have admitted to the "voluntary" performance of the movement (see below for a possible exception), and we are aware of only one patient in the literature with psychogenic tremor associated with posttraumatic stress disorder[77] who admitted to the purposeful performance of the movement. Thus, patients' responses to this line of questioning may be very helpful in defining bizarre or unusual movements, such as forms of tics or psychogenic movements.

Although Kurlan et al. chose to term the movements "psychogenic tics" based on the diagnostic confusion that had existed in their patient, it could be argued that the movements would be better classified as "pseudoseizures" or a mixed form of bizarre psychogenic movements, given their paroxysmal nature and the complexity of the movements that did not conform to those usually seen in the Tourette's syndrome.

Recently, we consulted about a 52-year-old man who, over a 2-week period after sustaining a minor injury to his lower back, developed paroxysmal episodes of flexion of the shoulders and extension with twisting of the neck. These movements were associated with an inner urge and a preceding feeling of tightness in the neck that forced him to contract the shoulders and neck. The urges gradually disappeared, but the movements continued to occur spontaneously in paroxysms with periods of remission. At this time the movements were described as "having a mind of their own" (in contrast to the purposeful or volitional performance of the same movements earlier in the course of his symptoms). There was a pronounced reduction in the frequency and severity of the movements after the patient's disability support was approved. He had been exposed to phentermine hydrochloride for appetite suppression but had only taken it intermittently for a total of 90 days over a 12-month period and had stopped taking the medication two months before the trauma and onset of the movements. He had no family history of neurological or psychiatric disorders and denied any tic-like symptomatology or OCB at any time earlier in life. During the examination he demonstrated intermittent, abrupt, brief contraction of the trapezius muscle with "pulling" of the shoulders backwards, followed by extension of the neck and contraction of the platysma muscle. At times he had alternating contraction of the sternocleidomastoid muscles, giving a brief rotatory component to the neck movement. During the examination he sometimes stated that he needed to move his neck because of a "buildup" feeling in his neck. As in most cases of both tics and PMDs, distraction completely suppressed the movements. In contrast to tics, but like many psychogenic movements, the neck movements "entrained" with synkinetic and alternating finger-counting movements of his hands.

Although this may be an unusual case of trauma-induced adult-onset tics with the additional theoretic predisposition from prior stimulant use, some of the clinical features outlined above encourage a diagnosis of psychogenic tics. Without further support one could only classify such a case as "probable" or "possible."

Psychogenic Parkinsonism

Walters et al.[78] described a case of psychogenic parkinsonism in a 64-year-old man with onset of symptoms in his lower limbs, later accompanied by stuttering, halting speech and tremor over a 3-year period. His gait was slow and shuffling but atypical for parkinsonism. The patient would slide one foot "glued" to the floor a long distance and then would slide the other foot in the same manner to a point "equally" distant from the first foot. Finger tapping, alternating movements, and foot tapping were slowed. His speech was also very uncharacteristic of Parkinson's disease. Tremor in his hands was equally prominent at rest, at postural maintenance, and at action. The rest of the neurological examination was normal. The patient's symptoms did not respond to L-dopa therapy but resolved spontaneously 1 year after discontinuing L-dopa.

More recently, 14 cases of psychogenic parkinsonism have been described from three university Movement Disorders Centers.[79] Thirteen had pure psychogenic parkinsonism, and one had psychogenic parkinsonism superimposed on milder features of true parkinsonism. There was a 1:1 male to female ratio. The average age of the patients was 47 years, with a range of 21–63 years. The mean duration of symptoms before diagnosis was 5 years, with a range between 4 months and 13 years. In 71 percent (10) the symptoms of parkinsonism began suddenly after a minor work-related injury or motor vehicle accident, except in one case who had sustained a serious head injury 9 years earlier that had been complicated by a subdural hematoma. Parkinsonian symptoms were bilateral in 57 percent of patients and unilateral in the remainder, typically involving the dominant side. Reduced facial expression, probably related to depression in most, was present in 6 of the 14 patients. Tremor was present in 85 percent. An isolated postural and action tremor was seen in only one case. More often, the tremor had characteristic features of a psychogenic tremor, as outlined earlier. It was typically present at rest and persisted in postures and with action, lacking the characteristic dampening of true parkinsonian rest tremor, which occurs on adopting a new posture or with movement. In all cases the tremor dampened or disappeared with distraction. This is the opposite of what is usually seen in patients with true rest tremor of Parkinson's disease, in which the performance of mental exercises typically accentuates or brings out the tremor. The entrainment of the tremor to the frequency of other repetitive movements performed in another limb (typical of psychogenic tremor) contrasts with what may be seen with true parkinsonian tremor, in which it is the tremor that entrains the rate and rhythm of an attempted repetitive task (e.g., finger tapping). "Bradykinesia" was seen in all cases, but the marked degree of slowness seen in most was atypical for true parkinsonian bradykinesia. Movements were often performed painstakingly slowly. However, the fatigue with decremental amplitude and arrest in ongoing movement so common in organic bradykinesia was lacking. Rigidity was present in 42 percent of cases; this often had features of voluntary resistance or difficulty relaxing. Several patients complained of associated pain in the limb that contributed to this increased resistance to passive movements. The increased tone usually diminished during the performance of synkinetic movements of an opposite limb in contrast to the normal accentuation of true parkinsonian rigidity (i.e., "activated rigidity"). No true cogwheeling was appreciated. Abnormal gait and postural instability were present in 85 percent of patients. Arm swing was diminished or absent on the affected side. However, the arm might have been held stiffly extended and adducted at the side (even while running) or flexed across the chest, rather than in the typical flexed posture with reduced swing characteristic of true Parkinson's disease. The gait also demonstrated a variety of other bizarre or atypical features, including a component of antalgia when pain was associated. Minimal force applied to the pull test often resulted in very exaggerated or extreme responses; however, no patient fell. The nature of this response often confirmed the psychogenicity of other features. For example, the distraction might have suppressed tremor. In one patient whose dominant arm was slow and stiff and held tightly at the side while she was walking and running, both arms flailed upward equally rapidly in her extreme response to minimal posterior trunk displacements.

The 15 patients with psychogenic parkinsonism reported to date have demonstrated a combination of features (i.e., tremor, rigidity, bradykinesia, postural disturbances, and gait instability) that justifies their classification as a form of parkinsonism. However, all of these features were somewhat atypical for Parkinson's disease and other akinetic-rigid syndromes. As with all PMDs, the recognition of the clinical incongruities with known disease required considerable experience in the assessment and management of the "organic" counterparts (i.e., parkinsonian disorders). Other important clues to the psychogenicity of the movement disorder (see Table 52-7) were present in all patients. Abrupt onset, inconsistencies in the character of the movements, alterations of the movements with attention or distraction, and associated false neurological signs were characteristically present in all patients in different combinations. Disability from psychogenic parkinsonism was often considerable. Patients were either on full disability pensions or had been forced to take early retirement. Despite the recognition of a psychogenic cause in all 15 (documented in nine, additional mild organic parkinsonism in one, and clinically established in six), outcome varied considerably. In some patients, the symptoms and signs resolved completely, either spontaneously or with psychiatric therapy, and in others, symptoms and resulting disability persisted unabated.

Psychogenic Gait Disorders (Including Psychogenic Ataxia)

The French school headed by Charcot devoted some time to these disorders[80] (Table 52-11). In Woolsey's experience, the

TABLE 52-11 French School Classification of Hysterical Gait Disorders at the Turn of the Twentieth Century

Charcot and Tourette	Roussy and Lhermitte
Astasia-abasia	Astasia-abasia
Paralytic	Pseudotabetic
Ataxic	Pseudopolyneuritic
Choreiform	Tightrope walker
Trepidant	Robot
	Habit limping
	Choreic
	Knock-kneed
	As on a sticky surface
	As through water

SOURCE: Adapted from Keone[80] (after Southard, Roussy and Lhermitte).

nature of the gait disturbance seen in hysteria related to the type of motor disability the patient imagined himself/herself to have.[17] For example, in the most common hysterical gait disorder observed by Woolsey a supposed paretic limb was dragged behind with the foot rotated outward contacting the floor on the medial aspect of the heel and the base of the great toe. Alternatively, when the patient believed himself to be unsteady or "ataxic," the gait would zig-zag from side to side with frequent lurches from one support to another, ". . . making it in the nick of time to the next" but without falls or injuries.

Psychogenic gait disorders accounted for 9 percent of all PMDs reported from Fahn's series. At the Los Angeles County/University of Southern California Medical Center, of all patients admitted to a neurological service with "functional neurological disorders" over a 10-year period, 26 percent (60/228) of patients had hysterical gait disorders.[80] Hysterical gait disorders accounted for 1.5 percent (68/4470) of neurological admissions to the Munich University Clinic, over a 3-year period.[81]

Keane[80] reported his experience with 60 patients with hysterical gait disorders seen over a 10-year period. There were 37 women and 23 males (1.6:1) with a mean age of 36.3 (19–80 years). He found that 43 percent (26/60) of patients had associated hysterical eye findings, including 13 with visual field cuts, 6 with decreased visual acuity, 4 with eye movement limitation, and 3 with monocular diplopia. Other "false" neurological signs were present in 71 percent (43/60) of patients; motor abnormalities were the most common (hemiparesis in 12, quadriparesis in 7, paraparesis in 4, and triparesis in 1). Other findings included voice abnormalities, tremor, contractures, and abnormal finger-to-nose testing, in which three patients had either finger-to-eye or finger-to-cheek alterations. The most common gait abnormalities (some patients had more than one type of gait disturbance) included ataxia (38 percent), hemiparesis (20 percent), paraparesis (16 percent), and trembling gait (14 percent). Other unusual patterns seen included dystonic, myoclonic, stiff-legged, and slapping gaits and one case of camptocormia (from the Greek, for "bent tree trunk"). Camptocormia as a feature of "hysteria" has been emphasized previously, for example, by Eames,[82] whose patient developed a hysterical gait after head trauma resulting in her walking around the hospital bent over with her palms down and almost touching the floor. It is important to recognize that camptocormia may also occur in organic dystonia or parkinsonian disorders, and we have seen one case of a unilateral basal ganglia infarct in which the onset of camptocormia was abrupt.

Other associated features in Keane's series, which were present in 23 of 60 patients, included a scissoring gait, a knee giving-way with quick recovery, posturing of an "arm-above-head" while walking, and ataxic (tandem) gaits that blended into trembling, although "tremblers" usually had additional arm or truncal tremors while lying in bed. Six patients in the ataxic group had a history of intentional overdose with phenytoin which had been prescribed for pseudoseizures.

In another series of psychogenic gait disturbances,[81] 37 patients seen at the Munich University Clinic over 9 years (1980–1989), were videoanalyzed (22 prospectively and 15 retrospectively) for the purposes of establishing diagnostic criteria and to determined whether a diagnosis of psychogenic gait disturbance was possible on phenomenological grounds alone. In this series, the most salient features seen included (1) hesitation (16.2 percent), (2) excessive slowness of movements (35 percent), (3) fluctuations in gait impairment with "uneconomic" postures and wasting of muscle energy (51 percent), (4) a "walking on ice" gait pattern (30 percent), and (5) a "psychogenic Romberg" test (32 percent). The authors concluded that if one or more of these six features were present, a diagnosis of a psychogenic gait disturbance could be made on phenomenological grounds alone with greater than 90 percent certainty (97 percent of patients had one or more of these six characteristics).

Other features included sudden knee buckling in 27 percent; however more than 80 percent of patients did not fall despite this feature. Eleven percent of patients had astasia, and vertical shaking tremor was present in 8 percent of cases. A suffering or strained facial expression was seen in 19 patients, associated in all with moaning, mannered posturing of hands, and grasping of the leg along with hyperventilation.

These 37 patients had a total of 116 associated hysterical findings. The most common abnormalities included other motor disturbances in 53 (45 percent) which often added to the gait disorder. These included hemiparesis (23 percent), quadriparesis (13 percent), scissoring (9 percent), knee giveway with recovery (9 percent), assuming a tandem gait (9 percent), dragging a leg (7.5 percent), paraparesis (7.5 percent) and flailing of the arms (5 percent). Other associated hysterical findings included eye movement abnormalities (22 percent), bizarre tremors (12 percent), pseudoataxia (8 percent) and voice abnormalities (7 percent).

In Keane's experience the most common initial diagnostic error was in not insisting that the patient attempt to walk.[80] Wilson's disease and Huntington's disease were the most frequent neurological disorders in which a misdiagnosis of a hysterical gait was made. In his experience, a few minutes of observation are sufficient to determine that the pattern of gait disturbance is psychogenic in origin, provided that spontaneous gait, tandem, heel, and toe walking are examined. This is in keeping with the finding of Lempert et al.[81] that the diagnosis of a hysterical gait disorder can reliably be made on phenomenological grounds when unusual postures and gait patterns, striking slowness of locomotion, momentary fluctuations, and a psychogenic Romberg test are seen. Other clues helpful in diagnosis are incongruities in the neurological examination (e.g., normal reflexes in a chronically paralyzed leg), give-way weakness, and elimination of symptoms with suggestion or placebo. We agree with Lempert et al.[81] and their word of caution that the presence of muscle atrophy or joint contractures does not necessarily argue against a psychogenic disorder; these conditions can represent secondary changes from lack of use or prolonged maintenance of a tonic posture.

Approach to Therapy of Psychogenic Movement Disorders

The first step in the evaluation and management of a suspected PMD is to confirm the diagnosis. A careful history is critical to this process. It has been noted that the correct clinical diagnosis in medicine can be predicted by careful history in up to 74 percent of patients and that the accuracy of diagnostic prediction increases to as high as 95 percent when the findings of the physical examination are added to the history.[83] The neurologist must pay close attention to family history in an attempt to uncover a possible underlying cause or predisposition to a movement disorder, recognizing both the variable penetrance and, particularly, the variable expressivity of many hereditary diseases that cause movement disorders. With respect to the examination, attention should be placed on a careful analysis of the phenomenology of the movement disorder in question, following the guidelines presented in Table 52-7, looking very carefully for clues to the psychogenic nature of the abnormal movements. Because the differential diagnosis of PMDs encompasses a large number of disease states, the neurologist making the diagnosis should have experience in the investigation and management of all types of movement disorders. The combination of expertise in the field of movement disorders and the application of the historical and clinical clues outlined in previous sections allows a classification of "documented" or "clinically established" PMD in most cases. This is frequently *not* a diagnosis of exclusion, and when these principles are rigorously applied, many unnecessary investigations can be avoided.

In our experience, the most difficult diagnostic problems arise in two situations: (1) when there is a clear evidence of a psychogenic movement disorder but an underlying organic component cannot be excluded and (2) when the movement disorder is an unchanging tonic ("dystonic") contraction of a muscle, usually precipitated by a seemingly inconsequential injury. In most examples of the former, it is the psychogenic movements that are the predominant complaint and the chief source of disability and concern.[33] We suggest dealing with these cases in a manner similar to that used with other PMDs, keeping in mind the potential contribution (sometimes progressively so) of the underlying organic condition. This point was recently emphasized by Mai,[84] who stated that "the diagnosis of conversion disorders and neurological disorders are not mutually exclusive; they may occur in the same patient either concurrently or consecutively and are particularly common in chronic relapsing diseases such as multiple sclerosis and epilepsy." In the second situation, the nature of tonic muscle contraction ("dystonia" or "spasm") occurring after injury represents a major source of controversy in the field of movement disorders. Although some authorities accept all of these cases as examples of organic dystonia after peripheral trauma, we have seen several patients diagnosed as such who later proved to have a psychogenic cause, and we have been impressed by the high incidence of some, albeit incomplete, supportive evidence for psychogenicity in a high proportion of the remainder of these cases. At this time we can only state that when movement disorder experts cannot agree on the nature of this difficult disorder, it would be unwise for a physician with little experience in the field to make a definitive diagnosis without extended periods of assessment and evaluation, which must include placebo-controlled trials or therapeutic interventions.

In many patients with PMDs, the underlying psychopathology is not overt, even after an extended psychiatric assessment. It is not uncommon for such patients to have received "psychiatric clearance," with the final opinion expressed that there is no underlying psychiatric problem and, therefore, an organic cause of the movement disorder must be present. This is comparable to a time when psychiatrists found evidence for psychopathology in patients with organic dystonia and blamed these "disturbances" for the movement disorder, whereas we would now either disregard this evidence or recognize it as a consequence, rather than a cause, of the motor dysfunction. In the final analysis the diagnosis of a PMD cannot be made or refuted by a psychiatrist. The diagnosis can only be made by a neurologist, preferably one with experience in the field of movement disorders. As Ford et al.[20] pointed out, there are three basic errors in dealing with such patients that can lead to devastating consequences: (1) The patient may be misdiagnosed as having a psychogenic disorder when, in fact, it is organic. (2) A truly psychogenic disorder can be misdiagnosed as organic. (3) The clinician fails to provide the appropriate care and therapy for these patients.

When it is clear that the patient has a PMD, empathy and understanding on the part of the physician are of paramount importance. The diagnosis should be presented carefully, avoiding conveyance of uncertainty. We agree with Ford et al.[20] that the use of a neurobiological explanation for the patient's symptoms helps in establishing trust, acceptance, and understanding of their diagnosis and will help in the recovery of the symptoms. The nature of the movement disorder should be confirmed (i.e., the patient is told he or she has a form of dystonia, tremor, myoclonus, etc.) but that the problem is not a result of severe or permanent structural brain disease. In some cases it may be necessary to hospitalize the patient for investigations and observation before further discussion of the nature of the disorder is undertaken. This largely depends on the duration of the disorder and the extent of the resulting disability. The more chronic or severe the problem, the more likely the need for inpatient assessment. The nature of the suspected psychopathology may also influence the decision to hospitalize. For example, when the patient is very strongly suspected of malingering it may not be appropriate to admit him or her to the hospital, unless it

is with the specific purpose of attempting to observe the patient surreptitiously. (This is now often performed out of hospital by insurance agency detectives). Patients with a long-standing somatoform disorder may not benefit from acute hospitalization for a PMD, and such an approach may only further serve to encourage such behavior, especially when multiple investigations are undertaken. It is important to obtain a psychiatric consultation both to develop and assist in a long-term treatment program. The importance of working closely with a psychiatrist interested in the care and management of such patients cannot be overemphasized. Depending on the circumstances, one may have to introduce the need for psychiatric consultation by stating that it is strictly for the purposes of evaluating and assisting the patient in his or her strategy for coping with the disability caused by the abnormal movements. This approach is often necessary in patients with long-standing symptoms who have had multiple investigations, have been given a diagnosis of an organic movement disorder, and have undergone extensive therapeutic trials. In others, it may be possible to introduce the concept of a psychological cause, even before obtaining psychiatric consultation. In both circumstances we eventually emphasized a neurobiological explanation for the movement disorder, stressing the notion that many underlying stressors or conflicts can result in central nervous system dysfunction and unequivocal disability in the same fashion as stress can contribute to such better known (to the public) conditions as hypertension, peptic ulcer disease, coronary artery disease, irritable bowel syndrome, and neurodermatitis. This should be done in a nonjudgmental fashion, reassuring the patient that it is not believed that he or she is "crazy" or that he or she is purposefully feigning or causing the movements to occur.

The patient should be reassured and counseled to the effect that there is a high likelihood of improvement. Further management approaches depend largely on the nature and severity of the underlying psychopathology. Treatment may require the variable combination of physiotherapy, psychotherapy, suggestion, psychopharmacology and, at times, even coercion and placebo treatments. Some patients with acute short-lived symptoms may only require reassurance, support, and active follow-up. Further discussion of the management of the causative psychiatric disorders is beyond the scope of this text.

The outcome of PMDs also depends greatly on the underlying psychiatric basis. Somatoform disorders may respond to therapy. A recent study showed that patients with a conversion disorder who are admitted to the hospital when they were young (<40 years) and who had recent onset of symptoms (usually, a few days before admission to the hospital) generally have a good prognosis.[85] The strongest predictive factor was found to be the condition of the patient on discharge. When the symptoms improved while the patient was in the hospital, a good outcome was observed in up to 96 percent of patients. In this study only two patients mistakenly diagnosed as having a conversion disorder were later found to have developed organic neurological disease (left middle cerebral artery territory infarct and multiple sclerosis, respectively). The authors concluded that neurological disease will emerge only rarely in patients with conversion disorders and, although neuroimaging is helpful in difficult cases, it can also be a source of confusion by ". . . showing harmless anatomical variants." They found that apraxia, focal dystonia, and the combination of organic deficits with a conversion disorder are areas of most frequent diagnostic error and confusion. Finally, it was emphasized that recovery of a conversion disorder is rare when improvement does not occur during the initial hospital evaluation.

As expected, factitious disorders and malingering respond poorly. When litigation or compensation issues are pending, it is important to resolve them as quickly as possible. However, the response to this approach is often disappointing or unpredictable. Malingerers may either keep up the act in order to justify the settlement or will have a striking improvement once a settlement has been reached. In our experience, although somatoform disorders also rarely improve in response to a financial settlement, spontaneous or therapeutically induced remissions are much less likely to occur while economic issues remain unresolved.

Despite the reassurance given to patients suffering from PMDs it should be emphasized that the prognosis must be guarded. Some patients will remain refractory to all treatment. However, a systematic approach involving a team composed of a neurologist, psychiatrist, nurses, physiotherapists, and others may be rewarded with striking successes, even in long-lasting, extremely disabled cases. In the experience of Ford et al.,[20] age, gender, intelligence, chronicity of illness, and PMD symptomatology had no influence on outcome. In PMD patients with either a conversion or a somatoform disorder, the response to treatment was considered "successful" in all, (except in three patients with either malingering or a fictitious disorder), and they concluded that ". . . patients with many years of established psychogenic symptomatology were able to make full recoveries."[20] Although it is important to keep an open mind to the possibility of an incorrect diagnosis, a protracted course, pronounced disability, or resistance to therapy should never be used as criteria against a diagnosis of a PMD when all other historical and clinical criteria have been satisfied.

References

1. Head HH: The diagnosis of hysteria. *Br Med J* 1:827–829, 1992.
2. Charcot J-M: Hystero-epilepsy: A young woman with a convulsive attack in the auditorium, in Goetz CG (ed): *Charcot The Clinician: The Tuesday Lessons*. New York: Raven Press, 1987, pp 102–122.
3. Freud S: Charcot, in Sutherland JD (ed): *Collected Papers*. London: The Hogarth Press, 1957, vol 1, pp 9–23.
4. Guillain G: *J. M. Charcot, 1825–1893: His Life—His Work*. New York: Paul B. Hoeber, 1959.
5. Havens LL: Charcot and hysteria. *J Nerv Ment Dis* 141:505–516, 1966.
6. Schiller F: *Paul Broca—Founder of French Anthropology, Explorer of the Brain*. New York: Oxford University Press, 1992.
7. Freud S: Hypnotism and suggestion (1888), in Strachey J (ed): *Collected Papers*. London: Hogarth Press, 1957, pp 11–24.
8. Gowers WR: *Epilepsy and Other Chronic Convulsive Diseases: Their Causes, Symptoms & Treatment*. New York: Dover Publications, 1964.
9. Lecrubier Y: Images in psychiatry—Jean-Martin Charcot, 1825–1893. *Am J Psychiatry* 152(1):121, 1995.
10. Gowers WR: *A Manual of Diseases of the Nervous System*. Philadelphia: Blakiston, 1888, p 1022.
11. Walshe F: Diagnosis of hysteria. *Br Med J* 2:1451–1454, 1965.
12. Cockburn JJ: Spasmodic torticollis: A psychogenic condition? *J Psychosom Res* 15:471–477, 1971.
13. Harrington RC, Wieck A, Marks IM, Marsden CD: Writer's cramp: Not associated with anxiety. *Mov Disord* 3:195–200, 1988.
14. Grafman J, Cohen LG, Hallett M: Is focal hand dystonia associated with psychopathology? *Mov Disord* 6:29–35, 1991.
15. American Psychiatric Association: *Diagnostic and Statistical Manual of Mental Disorders, (DSM-IV)*, 4th ed. Washington, DC, American Psychiatric Association, 1994.
16. Thompson DJ, Goldberg D: Hysterical personality disorder. *Br J Psychiatry* 150:241–245, 1987.
17. Woolsey RM. Hysteria: 1875 to 1975. *Dis Nerv Syst* 37:379–386, 1976.
18. Marsden CD: Hysteria—a neurologist's view. *Psychol Med* 16:277–288, 1986.
19. Lempert T, Dieterich M, Huppert D, Brandt T: Psychogenic disorders in neurology: Frequency and clinical spectrum. *Acta Neurol Scand* 82:335–340, 1990.
20. Ford B, Williams DT, Fahn S: Treatment of psychogenic movement disorders, in Kurlan R (ed): *Treatment of Movement Disorders*. Philadelphia: JB Lippincott, 1995, pp 475–485.
21. Fahn S, Williams PJ: Psychogenic dystonia. *Adv Neurol* 50:431–455, 1988.
22. Factor SA, Podshalny GD, Molho ES. Psychogenic movement disorders: Frequency, clinical profile and characteristics. *J Neurol Neurosurg Psychiatry* 59:401–412, 1995.
23. Monday K, Jankovic J: Psychogenic myoclonus. *Neurology* 43:349–3521, 993.
24. Barclay CL, Lang AE: Other secondary dystonias, in Tsui J, Calne DB (eds): *Handbook of Dystonia*. New York: Marcel Dekker, 1995 pp 267–305.
25. Koller W: Movement disorders: Which ones are real? in *Malingering and Conversion Reactions*. Washington, DC: American Academy of Neurology Annual Meeting, pp 3–25, 1994.
26. Koller WC, Biary NM: Volitional control of involuntary movements. *Mov Disord* 4:153–156, 1989.
27. Bok S: The ethics of giving placebos. *Sci Am* 231:17–23, 1974.
28. Lancman ME, Asconape JJ, Craven WJ, et al: Predictive value of induction of psychogenic seizures by suggestion. *Ann Neurol* 35:359–361, 1994.
29. Levy RS, Jankovic J: Placebo-induced conversion reaction: A neurobehavioural and EEG study of hysterical aphasia, seizure, and coma. *J Abnorm Psychol* 92:243–249, 1983.
30. Friedman WE, Rothner AD, Luders H, et al: Psychogenic seizures in children and adolescents: Outcome after diagnosis by ictal video and electroencephalographic recording. *Pediatrics* 85:480–484, 1990.
31. Walczak TS, Williams DT, Berten W: Utility and reliability of placebo infusion in the evaluation of patients with seizures. *Neurology* 44:394–399, 1994.
32. Ludlow CL, Martinez P, Braun AR, et al: Differential diagnosis between psychogenic and neurogenic dysphonias. *Neurology* 45:A393, 1995.
33. Ranawaya R, Riley D, Lang AE: Psychogenic dyskinesias in patients with organic movement disorders. *Mov Disord* 5:127–133, 1990.
34. Kurlan R, Deeley C, Comon PG: Psychogenic movement disorder (pseudo-tics) in a patient with Tourette's syndrome. *J Neuropsychiatry Clin Neurosci* 4:347–348, 1992.
35. Weiner WJ, Lang AE: *Movement Disorders—A Comprehensive Survey*. Mt Kisco, New York: Futura Publishing, 1989.

36. Weiner WJ, Lang AE: Idiopathic torsion dystonia, in Weiner WJ, Lang AE (eds): *Movement Disorders: A Comprehensive Survey*. Mt Kisco, NY: Futura Publishing, 1989, pp 1–725.

37. Dobyns WB, Ozelius LJ, Kramer PL, et al: Rapid-onset dystonia-parkinsonism. *Neurology* 43:2596–2602, 1993.

38. Bressman SB, Fahn S, Burke RE: Paroxysmal non-kinesigenic dystonia. *Adv Neurol* 50:403–413, 1988.

39. Lesser RP, Fahn S: Dystonia: A disorder often misdiagnosed as a conversion reaction. *Am J Psychiatry* 153:349–352, 1978.

40. Batshaw ML, Wachtel RC, Deckel AW, et al: Munchausen's syndrome simulating torsion dystonia. *N Engl J Med* 312:1437–1439, 1985.

41. Lang AE: Psychogenic dystonia: A review of 18 cases. *Can J Neurol Sci* 22:136–143, 1995.

42. Sheehy MP, Marsden CD: Writer's cramp—A focal dystonia. *Brain* 461:480, 1982.

43. Sheehy MP, Marsden CD: Trauma and pain in spasmodic torticollis. *Lancet* 1:777–778, 1980.

44. Fletcher NA, Harding AE, Marsden CD: The relationship between trauma and idiopathic torsion dystonia. *J Neurol Neurosurg Psychiatry* 54:713–717, 1991.

45. Fletcher NA, Harding AE, Marsden CD: A case-control study of idiopathic torsion dystonia. *Mov Disord* 6:304–309, 1991.

46. Bhatia KP, Bhatt MH, Marsden CD: The causalgia-dystonia syndrome. *Brain* 116:843–851, 1993.

47. Koller WC, Wong GF, Lang A: Posttraumatic movement disorders: A review. *Mov Disord* 4:20–36, 1989.

48. Marsden CD, Obeso JA, Traub MM, et al: Muscle spasms associated with Sudeck's atrophy after injury. *BMJ* 288:173–176, 1984.

49. Schott JD: Induction of involuntary movements by peripheral trauma: An analogy with causalgia. *Lancet* 2:712–715, 1986.

50. Schott GD: The relationship of peripheral trauma and pain to dystonia. *J Neurol Neurosurg Psychiatry* 48:698–701, 1985.

51. Jankovic J, Van der Linden C: Dystonia and tremor induced by peripheral trauma: Predisposing factors. *J Neurol Neurosurg Psychiatry* 51:1512–1519, 1988.

52. Schwartzman RJ, Kerrigan J: The movement disorder of reflex sympathetic dystrophy. *Neurology* 40:57–61, 1990.

53. Schwartzman RJ: Movement disorder of RSD (letter). *Neurology* 40:1477–1478, 1990.

54. Jankovic J: Post-traumatic movement disorders: Central and peripheral mechanisms. *Neurology* 44:2006–2014, 1994.

55. Lang A, Fahn S: Movement disorder of RSD (letter). *Neurology* 40:1476–1477, 1990.

56. Ochoa J: Reflex sympathetic dystrophy—fact or fiction, in *Malingering and Conversion Reactions*. Course #22. Washington, DC: American Academy of Neurology Annual Meeting, 1994, 222-41–222-56.

57. Elble RJ, Koller WC: The definition and classification of tremor, in *Tremor*. Baltimore: The Johns Hopkins University Press, 1990, pp 1–9.

58. Wilson SAK: The approach to the study of hysteria. *J Neurol Psychopathol* 11:193–206, 1931.

59. Fahn S: Atypical tremors, rare tremors and unclassified tremors, in Findley LJ, Capildeo R (eds): *Movement Disorders*. London: The MacMillan Press, 1984, pp 431–443.

60. Koller W, Lang AE, Vetere-Overfield B, et al: Psychogenic tremors. *Neurology* 39:1094–1099, 1989.

61. Obeso JA, Artieda J, Martinez-Lage JM: The physiology of myoclonus in man, in Quinn NP, Jenner PG (eds): *Disorders of Movement: Clinical, Pharmacological and Physiological Aspects*. London: Academic Press, 1989, pp 437–444.

62. Hallett M, Chadwick D, Marsden CD: Cortical reflex myoclonus. *Neurology* 29:1107–1125, 1979.

63. Thompson PD, Colebatch JG, Brown P, et al: Voluntary stimulus-sensitive jerks and jumps mimicking myoclonus or pathological startle syndromes. *Mov Disord* 7:257–262, 1992.

64. Terada K, Ikeda A, Van Ness PC, et al: Presence of bereitschafts-potential preceding psychogenic myoclonus: Clinical application of jerk-locked back averaging. *J Neurol Neurosurg Psychiatry* 58:745–747, 1995.

65. Rothwell J: Cerebral cortex, in *Control of Human Voluntary Movement*. London: Chapman & Hall, 1994, pp 293–386.

66. Shibasaki H, Sakai T, Nishimura H, et al: Involuntary movements in chorea-acanthocytosis:a comparison with Huntington's chorea. *Ann Neurol* 12:311–314, 1982.

67. Shibasaki H, Nagae K: Mirror movement: Application of movement-related cortical potentials. *Ann Neurol* 15:299–302, 1984.

68. Cohen LG, Meer J, Tarkka I, et al: Congenital mirror movements: Abnormal organization of motor pathways in two patients. *Brain* 114:381–403, 1991.

69. Hallett MD: *The Pathophysiology of Tics, Startle Reactions, and Other Complex Involuntary Movements*. Course #243. Seattle American Academy of Neurology, 1995, pp 77–92.

70. Matsumoto J, Hallett M: Startle syndromes, in Marsden CD, Fahn S (eds): *Movement Disorders 3*. Boston: Butterworth-Heinemann, 1994, pp 418–433.

71. Matsumoto J, Fuhr P, Nigro M, Hallett M: Physiological abnormalities in hereditary hyperekplexia. *Ann Neurol* 32:41–50, 1992.

72. Chapel JL: Latah, Myriachit, and jumpers Revisited. *NY State J Med* 70:2201–2204, 1970.

73. Andermann F, Andermann E: Excessive startle syndromes: Startle disease, jumping and startle epilepsy. *Adv Neurol* 43:321–338, 1986.

74. Stevens H: Jumping Frenchmen of Maine. *Arch Neurol* 12:311–314, 1965.

75. Kunkle EC: The Jumpers of Maine: A reappraisal. *Arch Intern Med* 119:355–358, 1967.

76. Saint-Hilaire MH, Saint-Hilaire JM, Granger L: Jumping Frenchmen of Maine. *Neurology* 36:1269–1271, 1986.

77. Walters AS, Hening WA: Noise-induced psychogenic tremor associated with post-traumatic stress disorder. *Mov Disord* 7:333–338, 1992.

78. Walters AS, Boudwin J, Wright D, Jones K: Three hysterical movement disorders. *Psychol Rep* 62:979–985, 1988.

79. Lang AE, Koller WC, Fahn S: Psychogenic parkinsonism. *Arch Neurol* 52:802–810, 1995.

80. Keane JR: Hysterical gait disorders: 60 cases. *Neurology* 39:586–589, 1989.

81. Lempert T, Brandt T, Dieterich M, Huppert D: How to identify psychogenic disorders of stance and gait. *J Neurol* 238:140–146, 1991.

82. Eames P: Hysteria following brain injury. *J Neurol Neurosurg Psychiatry* 55:1046–1053, 1992.

83. Bordage G: Where are the history and the physical? *Can Med Assoc J* 152:1595–1598, 1995.

84. Mai FM: "Hysteria" in clinical neurology. *Can J Neurol Sci* 22:101–110, 1995.

85. Couprie W, Wijdicks EFM, Rooijmans HGM, vanGijn J: Outcome in conversion disorder: A follow up study. *J Neurol Neurosurg Psychiatry* 58:750–752, 1995.

86. Williams DT, Ford B, Fahn S: Phenomenology and psychopathology related to psychogenic movement disorders, in Weiner WJ, Lang AE (eds): *Behavioural Neurology in Movement Disorders*. New York: Raven Press, 1994, pp 231–257.

87. Herz E: Dystonia. II: Clinical classification. *Arch Neurol Psychiat (Chicago)* 51:319–355, 1944.

88. Marsden CD, Harrison MJG: Idiopathic torsion dystonia (dystonia musculorum deformans): A review of forty-two patients. *Brain* 97:793–810, 1974.

Chapter 53

SYSTEMIC ILLNESSES THAT CAUSE MOVEMENT DISORDERS

AMY COLCHER and HOWARD I. HURTIG

ENDOCRINE DISORDERS
    Hyperthyroidism
    Hypothyroidism
    Diabetes
    Hypoparathyroidism
METABOLIC/NUTRITIONAL DISORDERS
    Tetrahydrobiopterin (BH$_4$) Deficiency
    Malabsorption Syndromes
    Hepatic Failure
    Kwashiorkor
    Alcoholism
    Kernicterus
    Homocystinuria
HEMATOLOGIC DISORDERS
    Polycythemia
    Mastocytosis
INFECTION
    Sydenham's Chorea
    Lyme Disease
    Human Immunodeficiency Virus-Type 1 (HIV-1)
    Encephalitis
    Whipple's Disease
    Hemolytic Uremic Syndrome (HUS)
    Sarcoidosis
AUTOIMMUNE DISORDERS
    Autoimmune Disease
    Sjogren's Syndrome
    Systemic Lupus Erythematosis
    Antiphospholipid Antibody Syndrome
PREGNANCY
NEOPLASMS

Movement disorders often complicate systemic illnesses. They occur in conjunction with metabolic encephalopathy, infection, neoplasms, and disorders of the endocrine, immune, and hematologic systems. Movement disorders associated with systemic illness run the gamut from an exaggerated physiological tremor to hemiballismus and also include the akinetic-rigid syndromes. In some cases, the movement disorder is what causes the patient to consult a physician. The underlying disorder may or may not be known at the time the movement disorder becomes obvious. In some cases the pathophysiology of the systemic disorder causing the movement disorder is known. In some cases there is a structural lesion in the brain responsible for the neurological problem. In other cases, there is no clear explanation for the movement disorder in the context of the systemic disease.

Endocrine Disorders

HYPERTHYROIDISM

Endocrine abnormalities are commonly recognized causes of hyperkinetic movement disorders. Hyperthyroidism is associated with an exaggerated physiological tremor. Up to 97 percent of patients with hyperthyroidism will exhibit a tremor,[1] the oscillatory frequency of which is the same as a physiological tremor (8–12 Hz), but the amplitude is greater. The hands are predominantly affected, although the feet, tongue, and eyelids can be affected as well. The pathophysiology is thought to be mediated by changes in peripheral beta-adrenergic receptor tone. This theory is supported by the fact that beta blockers, including propranolol, will dampen the tremor. It is unclear as to whether there is a central generator for tremor; positron emission tomography (PET) studies of patients with essential tremor reveal abnormal bilateral cerebellar, red nuclear, and thalamic activation.[2] When thyrotoxicosis is the etiology of the tremor, the tremor is reversible by returning thyroid function to normal.

Chorea is a rare complication of hyperthyroidism, occurring in less than 2 percent of patients with thyrotoxicosis.[1] The pathophysiology is not well understood, but the chorea is reversible with treatment of the hyperthyroidism.[1,3–5] Baba et al. described a young woman with unilateral chorea and thyrotoxicosis with normal computed tomography (CT), magnetic resonance imaging (MRI), and single-photon emission computed tomography (SPECT) scans.[3] Autopsy studies of patients with hyperthyroid chorea reveal no pathological lesion within the basal ganglia.[6] Measurements of dopamine metabolites in the cerebrospinal fluid (CSF) in patients with and without hyperthyroidism reveal lower levels of homovanillic acid (HVA) in patients with hyperthyroidism than in normals.[6] Decreased HVA levels suggest an alteration in dopamine metabolism in hyperthyroid individuals.[6] Thyroid abnormalities may alter the sensitivity of dopaminergic receptors.[1,6] An alteration in basal ganglia metabolism or function, such as heightened sensitivity of dopamine receptors in the basal ganglia of hyperthyroid individuals, is one postulated mechanism for the chorea.[6] It is possible that there may need to be preexisting damage to the basal ganglia to predispose a hyperthyroid individual to develop chorea. Fishbeck described a patient who had an anoxic event before the development of hyperthyroidism and later developed chorea.[7] The initial insult may have made the basal ganglia more susceptible to the altered receptor sensitivity induced by the change in thyroid function.[6] The chorea of hyperthyroidism is responsive to dopamine receptor-blocking agents such as haloperidol.

HYPOTHYROIDISM

Myxedema is associated with cerebellar dysfunction in a percentage of patients,[1] most of whom complain of unsteadiness,[8] difficulty walking, and incoordination. Examination of patients with these complaints reveals a truncal ataxia, although appendicular ataxia is also seen. Rare patients will exhibit dysarthria. A 3-Hz body oscillation has been described.[8] Dysfunction of the cerebellum or cerebellar connections is a postulated mechanism for the ataxia seen with myxedema. Autopsy of patients with myxedema and alcoholism reveals degeneration of the cerebellar cortex and glycogen-containing inclusions within cerebellar cortical neurons.[1] It is not clear that the pathology is related purely to the thyroid disorder. The ataxia improves as the patient becomes euthyroid.

DIABETES

Hyper- and hypoglycemia have both been reported as uncommon causes of choreoathetosis.[9,10] SPECT studies done on a patient with hemichorea/hemiballism secondary to hyperglycemia reveal increased blood flow in the contralateral striatum and thalamus.[11] Haan's description of an 80-year-old woman who had paroxysmal choreoathetosis when her blood sugar was both high and low raises interesting questions about pathogenesis. A possible theory is that a prolonged blood glucose level resets the osmoreceptors in the brain and that any rapid change from that level is poorly tolerated.[12]

Hyperglycemia without ketosis is a recognized cause of chorea. The chorea associated with blood sugar abnormalities may resolve with correction of the blood sugar; it may be slow, taking months to resolve[13]; or it may be permanent.[14] The patients described with chorea associated with abnormal blood sugar have, for the most part, been elderly. A multifactorial etiology may play a role here in that some preexisting structural damage, such as lacunar infarction or hemorrhage, may be necessary to make the striatum more susceptible to the effects of hyperglycemia,[15] or an ischemic episode in small arterioles occurring at the time of the hyperglycemia may contribute.

HYPOPARATHYROIDISM

Hypoparathyroidism results in hypocalcemia, hypophosphatemia, and hypomagnesemia. Metabolic derangements, primarily hypocalcemia, are responsible for the frequently encountered neurological complications such as tetany, neuromuscular irritability, and seizures. Pseudohypoparathyroidism is a hereditary parathyroid resistance syndrome caused by a defect in the parathyroid hormone (PTH) receptor. Pseudohypoparathyroidism produces the same metabolic abnormalities in association with pathognomonic phenotypic changes such as short metacarpal bones, short stature, round face, mental retardation, dental abnormalities, and obesity. Inheritance is X-linked or autosomal-dominant. Most patients have a defect of the PTH receptor-adenylate cyclase system.[16] Calcifications of the basal ganglia are seen in the majority of patients with primary hypoparathyroidism.[17] Calcification, described as early as 1855, is not limited to the basal ganglia. It can be present in the cerebral hemispheres and in the dentate nucleus of the cerebellum.[16] Basal ganglia calcification does not correlate with the presence of movement disorders.[18] Chorea is a described complication of both hypoparathyroidism[19] and pseudohypoparathyroidism.[18]

Paroxysmal dystonias are seen in some metabolic disorders, including hypoparathyroidism and hyperthyroidism. Hypoparathyroidism with basal ganglia calcification has been associated with paroxysmal dystonic choreoathetosis.[20] This has been described infrequently but seems to represent basal ganglia dysfunction secondary to disordered calcium metabolism.[21] The movement disorder responds to treatment of the underlying disorder with calciferol. The structural alterations in the basal ganglia from the calcification do not seem to be responsible for the dystonic syndrome, as the calcifications do not resolve with treatment of the hypoparathyroidism.

Parkinsonism can occur in the setting of hypoparathyroidism[22] and pseudohypoparathyroidism (4–12 percent of patients) with or without basal ganglia calcifications.[23] It has been reported to occur at ages ranging from 20 to 73. The pathogenesis of parkinsonism in these patients initially was presumed to result in some way from calcification in the basal ganglia, although cases without basal ganglia calcification have been reported. Evans and Donley hypothesize that parkinsonism may be related to a defective G protein,[23] intermediaries in neurotransmission, or hormonal neuromodulation. An alteration in G protein function could impair neurotransmission in the striatum and produce parkinsonism. Untreated hypoparathyroidism often results in basal ganglia calcification, but it is rare that it is associated with parkinsonism. When the two occur together, it is usually in the setting of symptomatic hypocalcemia. In this setting the parkinsonism is slowly progressive, as in idiopathic PD, and is responsive to L-dopa therapy. Cases have been described without symptomatic hypocalcemia in which the parkinsonism was responsive to vitamin D, calcium, and magnesium replacement.[22]

Metabolic/Nutritional Disorders

TETRAHYDROBIOPTERIN (BH₄) DEFICIENCY

Tetrahydrobiopterin (BH$_4$) is a cofactor necessary for the enzymatic synthesis of biogenic amines. Deficiency states lead to defective production of serotonin and catecholamines in addition to hyperphenylalaninemia. Symptoms occur in infancy and include developmental delay, seizures, hypotonia, and dystonia. Three patients have been reported with tremor and orofacial dyskinesias as presenting symptoms. In the case described by Factor et al. an episodic high-amplitude coarse flapping tremor initially appeared at 3 months of age and recurred twice before 6 months.[24] Each episode lasted several hours and improved with sedation. The tremor was present both at rest and with action. The child was also found to be hypotonic. Treatment with L-dopa led to cessation of the movements. Improvement was seen within 24 hours, and further development was normal when followed up at 18 months. The significant improvement with L-dopa implies that the pathogenesis of movement disorders associated with BH$_4$ deficiency relates to insufficient dopamine synthesis.

MALABSORPTION SYNDROMES

Any disease that causes fat malabsorption or steatorrhea has the potential to cause tocopherol (vitamin E) deficiency. Deficiency of tocopherol must be present for years before neurological sequelae are evident. The associated syndrome of spinocerebellar ataxia and peripheral neuropathy may resemble vitamin B_{12} deficiency. Patients are dysarthric with oculomotor abnormalities, ataxia, and position and vibratory sense loss. Pathologically, there is a loss of myelinated nerve fibers in the posterior columns and CNS. Ataxia has been reported in patients with cystic fibrosis, chronic cholestasis, small bowel resection, blind loop syndromes, and intestinal lymphangiectasia, in addition to other malabsorption syndromes.[25]

HEPATIC FAILURE

Hepatic failure is a well-known cause of tremor, asterixis, and other involuntary movements. Asterixis is seen in the setting of an underlying encephalopathy and can be associated with metabolic derangements secondary to failure of various organ systems. It is encountered in hepatic encephalopathy, uremia, hypercarbia, alcohol withdrawal, cardiac failure, sepsis and, sometimes, as a result of the treatment used for these disorders, such as hemodialysis.[26] The mechanism of pathogenesis is unknown. Asterixis can be caused by a variety of focal lesions in the thalamus (especially the ventrolateral portion), midbrain, parietal cortex, and medial frontal cortex,[26] but in cases of encephalopathy no structural lesion is evident on imaging studies. In most cases EEGs reveal diffuse, rather than focal, brain disturbance.[27] MRI scans can show increased signal on T_1-weighted images of the caudate. Generalized myoclonus, ataxia, and chorea can be seen in the setting of hepatic or renal failure.[27]

KWASHIORKOR

Kwashiorkor is a nutritional deficiency of protein and calories that can produce movement disorders. Kwashiorkor can produce a combination of myoclonus, rigidity, and bradykinesia.[28] Tremors are also apparent in children when they are treated for malnutrition.[28,29]

ALCOHOLISM

A tremor can be prominent among alcoholics when they are not actively drinking or withdrawing from alcohol. The alcoholic tremor is postural, usually mild, and it causes little, if any, functional limitation. It is often of a higher frequency than essential tremor (ET), the majority of ET patients having a tremor frequency of less than 7 Hz,[30] although patterns similar to those seen with essential tremor are described. Postural tremor with a frequency of 6–11 Hz can be seen. The tremor of chronic alcoholism has two components. There is a 4- to 7-Hz peak and a 9.4- to 9.6-Hz peak. Increasing the speed of movement of the arm decreases the low-frequency peak without changing the high-frequency peak. Increasing effort increases the amplitude of the low-frequency peak.[31] The tremor of chronic alcoholism is usually asymmetric and can persist for years during complete abstinence. Treatment with beta-blockers is usually effective.

A second type of tremor that is seen in alcoholics is a 3-Hz tremor of the legs. The tremor is slow and rhythmic, involves flexion and extension of the muscles of the hip

girdle, and can affect the gait. It does not disappear with cessation of alcohol consumption.[32]

Transient parkinsonism has been described in intoxicated patients or within days of the last drink.[33,34] Symptoms include bradykinesia, shuffling gait, stooped posture, cogwheel rigidity, and rest tremor. The condition is self-limited and usually resolves within a few weeks.[32] Alcohol causes decreased dopamine release; which may explain the parkinsonism.[35]

Alcoholic cerebellar degeneration is a well-known complication of alcohol abuse. It is postulated as nutritional in origin. PET scans of ataxic patients reveal hypometabolism in the superior vermis.[36] MRI reveals atrophy of the cerebellar vermis and, when severe, of the cerebellar hemispheres. Pathologically, there is degeneration of the anterior superior aspect of the cerebellar vermis and, when severe, atrophy of the cerebellar hemispheres. There is a striking loss of Purkinje cells, as well as other neurons.

KERNICTERUS

Prolonged untreated hyperbilirubinemia in the perinatal period damages nuclei of the basal ganglia, especially the globus pallidus and subthalamic nucleus. The cerebellum and the auditory and vestibular pathways are also involved. Children may show signs of damage early with high-tone hearing loss, dysarthria, and athetosis. Usually, symptomatic children will have delayed motor development and show signs of dystonia, choreoathetosis, tremor, and rigidity by the time they are 10 years old.[37] Other children may be asymptomatic, and dystonia can occur up to 20 years after the initial insult.[38] In children who die early in the course of the disease, pathological findings reveal yellow staining of the subthalamic nucleus, Ammon's horn, globus pallidus, dentate nucleus, and inferior olives. In children who live longer these areas reveal cell loss, demyelination, and gliosis.[37]

HOMOCYSTINURIA

Many metabolic disorders of childhood have dystonia as a prominent symptom. These will not all be discussed here but are listed in Table 53-1 (see also Chap. 33). Homocystinuria is not commonly associated with dystonia, but the combination has been described. A deficiency of cystathione synthetase leads to a buildup of homocysteine and methionine. Patients

TABLE 53-1 Metabolic Disorders of Childhood That Cause Dystonia

Hexosaminidase A and B deficiency
GM_1 and GM_2 gangliosidosis
Phenylketonuria
Triosephosphate isomerase deficiency
Tetrahydrobiopterin deficiency
Metachromatic leukodystrophy
Glutaric acidemia
Methylmalonic acidemia
Wilson's disease
Lesch-Nyhan syndrome
Ceroid lipofuscinosis

generally are mentally retarded; have lens dislocations, sei-zures, and bony abnormalities; and are predisposed to strokes. In a report of two sisters, symptoms began at ages 3 and 4 with dysarthria in one and foot inversion in the other.[39] Dystonia progressed over the next few years, until it was generalized and both girls had become severely disabled. MRI studies revealed bilateral low-intensity lesions in the basal ganglia on T_2-weighted imaging. Other patients with dystonia had later onset of dystonic symptoms, starting in their teenage years.[38] Other patients described had typical features of homocystinuria that the two sisters did not. As homocystinuria is associated with thromboembolic events, it is possible that the dystonia is secondary to basal ganglia infarcts.[38] Other researchers postulate that a neurochemical derangement, that is, a defect in sulfur amino acid metabolism, is responsible.[39]

Hematologic Disorders

POLYCYTHEMIA

Polycythemia vera usually has its onset in middle age. There is an increase in all myeloid elements, although the increase in hemoglobin concentration is the primary hematologic manifestation of this disease. Neurological symptoms are primarily related to increased blood volume and viscosity. These include headache, dizziness, visual changes, and syncope.[40] Chorea occurs in less than 1 percent of patients with polycythemia vera, and it is more common in females than males.[6] It is usually bilaterally symmetrical and can be short-lived, lasting only weeks, or it can be persistent. Two-thirds of patients who have chorea in the setting of polycythemia do not know that they have polycythemia when the chorea is initially evaluated, although the associated symptoms of a ruddy complexion and splenomegaly are often seen.

The pathophysiology of polycythemic chorea is unclear. Some patients have a history of rheumatic fever in childhood, which may in some way predispose them to the development of chorea later on. Hyperviscosity resulting from the polycythemia can lead to small infarctions or hemorrhage in the basal ganglia, especially the caudate and putamen. Neuropathological specimens support this, although demyelination in the interior globus pallidus has also been reported.[6] Treatment of the polycythemia is not always correlated with amelioration of the chorea. A presynaptic catecholamine-depleting drug like reserpine or tetrabenazine is the treatment of choice, although dopamine receptor-blocking agents (neuroleptics) may be required in resistant cases.

MASTOCYTOSIS

Mastocytosis is a hematologic disorder in which mast cells proliferate and deposit themselves in various tissues in the body. Most often, their distribution is limited to cutaneous structures. CNS dysfunction has been reported with systemic mastocytosis but usually takes the form of headache, seizures, and encephalopathy. One case of chorea has been described in association with this disorder in a 13-year-old girl.[41] The chorea resolved spontaneously within 5 days and did not recur. According to one theory of pathogenesis, mast cells release various substances (histamine, prostaglandins, and other peptide mediators) that induce alterations in the basal ganglia neurotransmission. This may be responsible for the chorea.

Infection

SYDENHAM'S CHOREA

Sydenham's chorea (SC), a sequela of infection with group A streptococcus, is the most celebrated example of a movement disorder resulting from an infection. Chorea occurs 1–6 months after the initial febrile illness, which most often presents with pharyngitis. The onset is usually insidious, progressing over weeks to months. Women are more often affected than men. The movements are usually bilateral but they can be unilateral, and the face is usually involved. Dysarthria and hypotonia are frequently seen. Behavioral changes include psychosis, irritability, confusion, and obsessive-compulsive disorder.[42] These symptoms usually begin several days to weeks before the onset of the chorea. The behavioral, as well as the motoric symptoms, can wax and wane during the course of the syndrome.[42] Antineuronal antibodies are present in the majority of children affected. The initial bout of chorea is self-limiting, but recurrences are well-documented, independent of the natural history of rheumatic fever, which is, for the most part, a monophasic illness. Recurrences usually occur within 2 years of the initial chorea.[43] SC is known to recur during pregnancy in women who have had rheumatic fever as a child[43] and in patients who later take medications such as oral contraceptives and phenytoin.[43]

Few PET studies have been done on patients with SC. Weindl et al., using two patients, found increased striatal regional cerebral glucose consumption in both patients.[44] This study was done without age-matched controls.

Circulating antibodies to brain and cardiolipin have been described in association with SC. Streptococcal proteins can induce antibodies that will cross-react with human brain.[45] Others have reported finding immunoglobulin G (IGG) antibodies that cross-react with nuclear protein of caudate and subthalamus.[46] This may begin to explain the pathophysiology of SC. Figueroa et al. found that 80 percent of patients with acute rheumatic fever had anticardiolipin antibodies during an acute attack.[47] There was no difference in the percentage of patients with antibodies when comparing those with SC (76 percent) and those without chorea (83 percent). All patients with cardiac valvular abnormalities had antibodies. The neuropathology in patients with SC is not specific. There are reports of a broad spectrum of abnormalities, including hemorrhage, inflammation, and vasculopathy.[6]

SC is self-limited in most cases. Therefore, treatment with dopamine blockers, which may have permanent tardive sequelae, should be avoided unless the chorea is incapacitating. Presynaptic dopamine-depleting agents (reserpine and tetrabenazine) can be used. There is no treatment that has been proven to shorten the course of the chorea. (See also Chap. 38.)

LYME DISEASE

Lyme disease, which in the last decade has become the great imitator, can produce chorea along with a myriad of other neurological abnormalities.[48] The disease is transmitted through the bite of the deer tick *Ixodes damani*. The causative organism is a spirochete, *Borrelia burgdorferi*. The initial manifestation is usually an expanding red rash, erythema chronicum migrans. As the rash expands, the center clears creating the appearance of a target. The rash occurs most commonly 1–3 weeks after the tick bite. At the time of the rash, constitutional symptoms, headache, fever, arthralgias, and myalgias may occur. Secondary Lyme disease causes myocarditis, cranial neuritis, and myositis. Stage 3 or chronic Lyme disease occurs months after the initial onset and may persist for years. Clinical findings associated with this stage are arthritis, myositis, peripheral neuropathies, chronic meningitis, and acrodermatitis chronica atrophicans. Cranial nerve palsies are common, including facial diplegia. Patients with meningitis will have positive CSF antibody to *B. burgdorferi*.[49] Serological testing for Lyme disease (enzyme-linked immunosorbent assay [ELISA]) and indirect fluorescent antibody staining) should be positive in most cases of disseminated Lyme infection.[50] False-positive tests do occur in patients with other infections (syphilis), autoimmune disorders (SLE), and some malignancies.[49] A Western blot analysis should be done to confirm the diagnosis before therapy is initiated. MRI findings in patients with focal CNS findings reveal white matter changes representing leukoencephalitis, which can improve with antibiotic therapy.[51] Movement disorders have been reported in the setting of Lyme disease.[18] Chorea and synkinesis are associated with encephalitis.[48] Cerebellar ataxia also has been described.[51] These symptoms usually improve with treatment of the underlying infection and/or with steroids.

HUMAN IMMUNODEFICIENCY VIRUS-TYPE 1 (HIV-1)

A tremor at rest resembling a parkinsonian tremor is seen in the HIV-1 associated cognitive/motor complex. The rest tremor and slowness of movement parallel the slowness in thought processing associated with HIV-1 dementia. Pathological studies reveal white matter pallor, reactive gliosis, and microglial nodules. The caudate, putamen, and pons are involved early and cortical structures later.[52]

HIV can cause movement disorders, as can the opportunistic infections associated with it. Toxoplasmosis, the most common opportunistic infection causing neurological symptoms in HIV-positive patients, has been associated with akathisia, chorea, athetosis, and hemiballism, especially when the lesions are in the basal ganglia.[53] When ring-enhancing lesions are seen on CT or MRI, empiric antitoxoplasmosis therapy is indicated. When treatment causes resolution of the lesions on imaging studies but the movement disorder persists, treatment with dopamine-depleting or dopamine-blocking agents may become necessary. In general, patients without HIV who have cerebral toxoplasmosis do not have movement disorders associated with it.[53] There may be an interaction between the two infections, making HIV-positive patients more susceptible to developing a movement disorder when they are coinfected with toxoplasmosis.

Cerebral toxoplasmosis has also been associated with dystonia. Nath and others described a man with HIV and toxoplasmosis who presented with dystonic posturing of the left arm.[53] An enhancing lesion was seen on CT scan in the right globus pallidus and right thalamus. In this patient, the dystonia was not improved by treatment of the toxoplasmosis.

Cerebral toxoplasmosis in combination with HIV infection is also a rare cause of parkinsonism. A woman with enhancing lesions in the anterior limb of both internal capsules was found to have decreased facial expression, cogwheel rigidity, monotone speech, and drooling.[53] Toxoplasmosis was found in these lesions. Neither antitoxoplasmosis therapy nor L-dopa/carbidopa combinations improved her condition. Bradykinesia, rigidity, facial masking and grimacing, and gait instability were described in a young girl with HIV and progressive multifocal leukoencephalopathy (PML).[54] MRI lesions involved the basal ganglia and deep white matter, centrum semiovale, and corona radiata and enhanced slightly with the administration of gadolinium. Brain biopsy in this case revealed demyelination, Alzheimer type 1 astrocytes, and intranuclear eosinophilic inclusions within oligodendroglial cells. The biopsy, CSF, and white blood cells were positive for the JC virus, a papovavirus, when tested by polymerase chain reaction (PCR).

ENCEPHALITIS

Mycoplasma is a microorganism that accounts for a large number of cases of pneumonia each year. Uncommon complications of infection with this organism include myopathy and encephalitis. Beskind and Keim described a boy with encephalitis who presented with acute choreoathetosis, dysarthria, and fever who was found to have serological evidence of *Mycoplasma pneumoniae* infection.[55] Choreoathetosis and hemiballismus is rarely associated with encephalitis of viral etiology. This may be a direct result of the infection or a postinfectious phenomenon.[56] The movements may be difficult to control necessitating the use of dopamine-depleting agents (reserpine).

WHIPPLE'S DISEASE

Whipple's disease (WD) is an infectious disease of the small intestine causing malabsorption, lymphadenopathy, arthritis, and neurological symptoms. Gastrointestinal (GI) manifestations usually bring the patient to medical attention. These include diarrhea, steatorrhea, abdominal pain, and weight loss. WD and its symptoms respond to antibiotics when therapy is initiated early in the course of the illness. The pathology in the small intestine reveals periodic acid-Schiff (PAS)-positive macrophages and gram-positive bacilli. Neurological complications of WD occur in 10 percent of patients,[57] including encephalopathy, myoclonus, seizures, tremor, and ophthalmoplegia. A dystonic syndrome characterized by involuntary bruxism[58] and abnormalities of extraocular movement has been designated as oculomasticatory myorhythmia (OMM).[59] Myorhythmia is a repetitive, regular 2- to 4-Hz involuntary movement affecting the face (lips, chin, jaw) and neck. Myorhythmia in WD occurs in conjunction with cognitive deterioration and opthalmoparesis. Neurological symptoms occur late in the disease and generally indicate a poor prognosis. OMM can improve with antibiotic therapy. Neurological sequelae can occur even after successful treatment of GI symptoms with antibiotics. This may be because of poor CNS penetration of some antibiotics. Penicillin, trimethoprim-sulfamethoxazole, and streptomycin should be used. There is a high incidence of CNS relapse, so antibiotic therapy should be continued for a prolonged course of many months.[25] Patients have been reported with neurological symptoms and no GI complaints.[60] In patients with OMM WD should be suspected with or without GI symptoms.

Pathological studies of patients with WD affecting the nervous system have revealed nodules and granulomas throughout the brain. Locations include the cortex, basal ganglia, cerebellum, and hypothalamus. Cases of WD with myorhythmia are rare, and consistent clinicopathological correlation has not been done.

HEMOLYTIC UREMIC SYNDROME (HUS)

HUS is a postinfectious illness causing acute renal failure in children and adults. Hemolytic anemia, thrombocytopenic purpura, and oliguric renal failure are the major components of the illness, which mimics thrombocytopenic thrombotic purpura. CNS involvement in HUS is uncommon and can cause seizures, encephalopathy, and stroke. Pathological studies in these patients reveal multiple small infarctions secondary to the ischemic effect of small arteriolar thrombi. Dystonia has been described in association with seizures in HUS.[61]

SARCOIDOSIS

Sarcoidosis is a systemic granulomatous disease without known etiology. Granulomas form in various organ systems, resulting in a varied clinical picture. CNS involvement is rare. Most patients with neurological symptoms have evidence of sarcoidosis in other organ systems, that is, hilar adenopathy, hypercalcemia, or anergy. As in polycythemia, neurological symptoms can be the reason the patient seeks medical attention. Sarcoid most often causes a meningitis, primarily at the base of the brain, affecting cranial nerves, hypothalamus, and the pituitary.[62] Facial nerve palsies and optic neuritis are the most common cranial neuropathies. Movement disorders can take the form of chorea and hemiballismus when granulomas infiltrate the basal ganglia.[62] Myelopathy and myopathy can also occur.

Neurosarcoid can produce akinetic-rigid syndromes or parkinsonism. Schlegel reported a case of cerebral sarcoidosis that presented with vertical-gaze palsy, bradykinesia, and rest tremor.[63] The patient had had systemic sarcoidosis for 11 years before these symptoms became apparent. The parkinsonism and gaze palsy resolved with the use of corticosteroids and antiparkinson medications. Treatment of neurosarcoidosis usually requires the temporary use of corticosteroids. The response of the movement disorder to this treatment is variable.

One concept of pathogenesis is that basilar meningitis leads to obstructive hydrocephalus, which compresses the tectal region of the brain stem and nuclei in the basal ganglia, causing upgaze palsy and parkinsonism, respectively. This is a rare complication of neurosarcoidosis. Other reports of sarcoidosis causing parkinsonism have noted granulomatous infiltration of the basal ganglia.[62]

Autoimmune Disorders

AUTOIMMUNE DISEASE

Autoimmune diseases have also been reported to cause dystonic syndromes. Craniocervical dystonia (Meige's syndrome) was described in a patient with rheumatoid arthritis and Sjogren's syndrome (SS). Other combinations of autoimmune disease and cranial dystonia have been described.[64] Patients with myasthenia gravis have been reported to have coexistent dystonic syndromes.[65] Autoimmune thyroid disease also has an unusually high association with dystonia.[66] For two patients who had blepharospasm described by Jankovic and Patten, one with SLE and one with myasthenia, both patients responded to immunosuppressive therapy.[67] The mechanism underlying blepharospasm and other dystonic disorders in the setting of autoimmune disease is unclear.

Sjogren's Syndrome

Sjogren's syndrome is an immune-mediated disorder in which salivary and lacrimal glands are destroyed, resulting in mucosal and conjunctival dryness (the sicca syndrome). Xerostomia, xerophthalmia, and conjunctivitis are the principal manifestations. Other organs can be involved including kidney, lungs, and blood vessels. Sjogren's syndrome is often associated with other autoimmune diseases. The most common neurological manifestations are mononeuritis multiplex, peripheral neuropathy, and myositis. CNS dysfunction has been reported and can be either focal or diffuse. Some patients have anti-Ro(SS-A) antibodies that are directed against a 60-kd peptide and may be implicated in the production of a small vessel angiitis.[68] Cerebellar degeneration has been described in associations with Sjogren's syndrome. In one reported case of Sjogren's syndrome, antineuronal antibodies were found.[69] These antibodies stained cytoplasmic elements in the cerebellum and hippocampus primarily. The antibodies found in this patient were not anti-Yo or anti-Hu antibodies, although they were similarly immunoreactive. The patient described improved after immunosuppression with corticosteroids. Parkinsonism has also been described in association with Sjogren's syndrome.[70] MRI in this patient showed increased signal on T_2-weighted images in the pons and basal ganglia. The parkinsonism did not respond to treatment with L-dopa but did respond to immunosuppression with corticosteroids.

Systemic Lupus Erythematosis (SLE)

SLE is an autoimmune disease that affects multiple organ systems, including both the CNS and peripheral nervous system. Chorea is by far the most common movement disorder associated with SLE.[5] Involuntary movements account for 2 percent of all neurologic symptoms in SLE and frequently precede the diagnosis of lupus. The patients who develop chorea are usually young and female. Chorea may be intermittent or persistent and is usually unilateral, although it can be generalized. The pathology is inconsistent, although widespread microinfarcts are the classic pathological hallmark of CNS SLE. There is no consistent change in the basal ganglia. PET scans do not reveal any change in striatal glucose metabolism that could be responsible for the chorea. Antiphospholipid antibodies are seen in 45–70 percent of patients with SLE, but they can occur without other findings of lupus in primary antiphospholipid antibody syndrome[71] (see below). The lupus anticoagulant is any antiphospholipid antibody that prolongs the phospholipid dependent coagulation steps when there is not a coagulation factor deficiency. The antiphospholipid antibody reacts with the platelet membrane and leads to recurrent thrombotic events. Blepharospasm and torticollis have been described in the setting of SLE.[72] The clinicopathological correlation is not known, but vasculitis involving the brain stem and diencephalon is one postulated mechanism.[67] As in SC, another postulated mechanism is the cross-reactivity of antibodies with neurons.[72]

ANTIPHOSPHOLIPID ANTIBODY SYNDROME

Antiphospholipid antibody syndrome is a condition in which antibodies that bind to the negatively charged phospholipids in the membrane of endothelial cells somehow cause recurrent arterial and venous thrombotic and embolic events. The syndrome is clinically expressed by thrombocytopenia, spontaneous abortion, thromboembolism, and chorea.[71] In SLE, imaging studies of the brain do not reveal infarcts in the basal ganglia in patients with chorea, despite the frequency of infarction in this patient population as a whole. In some cases, an embolic source is identified, such as a cardiac valvular vegetation, and an infarct can be demonstrated on brain imaging studies. Kirk and Harding reported a patient with antiphospholipid antibody and chorea who had an infarct in the head of the caudate.[73] Recent PET studies in patients with antiphospholipid antibody syndrome, using 18F-fluorodeoxyglucose, revealed contralateral striatal hypermetabolism.[74] Scans were done when the patient had chorea and, later, when the chorea had resolved. The hypermetabolism was present regardless of the presence of chorea. Chorea can occur in association with anticardiolipin antibodies with or without the associated thromboembolic events.

Pregnancy

This heading does not imply that pregnancy is a systemic illness; rather, it is a systemic change from a woman's usual state that makes a woman susceptible to particular illnesses. Chorea gravidarum (CG) is a rare example of a movement disorder that occurs during pregnancy. The term does not specify etiology and is clinically indistinguishable from any other kind of chorea. CG occurs most frequently in young women during first pregnancies. One-half of the cases will start in the first trimester and one-third in the second trimester.[75] The majority of women with CG have previously had chorea as a result of SC before pregnancy. The chorea sponta-

neously remits in about a one-third of patients. In the rest, the chorea will last until the child is born. In about one-fifth of patients, the chorea will recur with subsequent pregnancies. SLE, which can also be worsened by pregnancy, can be responsible for CG in some cases.

Neoplasms

Cerebellar dysfunction is seen in systemic illness, most commonly in the form of pancerebellar degeneration, one of the paraneoplastic syndromes. This syndrome can occur with any malignancy, but it is most often associated with small cell lung cancer, ovarian cancer, and Hodgkin's lymphoma. The paraneoplastic cerebellar syndrome frequently precedes the diagnosis of cancer.

The ataxia in this syndrome usually has a subacute onset, progressing from truncal and gait ataxia to dysarthria, nystagmus, and limb ataxia over a few months. Frequently, the neurological deficit stabilizes, but the patient may remain significantly impaired. Treatment of the underlying malignancy is rarely helpful.

Pathologically, there is cerebellar atrophy with almost total loss of Purkinje cells in the cerebellum. There is thinning of the molecular layer with gliosis and mild thinning of the granular layer. The deep cerebellar nuclei are spared. Other areas of the CNS may be affected, including the corticospinal tracts, dorsal columns, and spinocerebellar tracts, which show varying degrees of degeneration. Patchy demyelination is seen in the brain stem, spinal cord, and dorsal root ganglia.[76]

In some patients antibodies associated with the underlying malignancy cross-react with Purkinje cells and result in their destruction.[77,78] These antibodies bind to membrane-bound and free ribosomes within the Purkinje cell.[79] A putative protein kinase c substrate protein has been detected in some patients with paraneoplastic cerebellar degeneration.[80] Anti-Yo antibodies are present in the serum and CSF of some patients.[81] The onset of this syndrome is similar to that in patients without antibody, in that the syndrome is subacute, progressing over a few weeks. These patients typically have ataxia of the trunk and limbs, dysarthric speech, and nystagmus.[81] Common malignancies associated with the anti-Yo antibody are, in order of frequency, ovarian, breast, endometrial, and adenocarcinoma with unknown primary. In the majority of patients the neurological symptoms preceded the diagnosis of cancer. Neuropathological findings in these patients reveal critical atrophy of the cerebellum with reduction in the number of Purkinje cells, as in antibody-negative cases.

Treatment of underlying malignancy rarely will improve ataxia. Plasmapheresis to remove the anti-Yo antibody does not usually improve ataxia.[81] Corticosteroids and immunosuppression have not been beneficial. It is not clear how the anti-Yo antibody causes cerebellar disease.

Hodgkin's disease is also associated with a cerebellar degeneration.[82] In most of these patients, the cerebellar syndrome begins after the diagnosis of lymphoma. The onset of the ataxia is sudden or subacute. Gait instability is the most common complaint, followed by limb ataxia and truncal ataxia. Nystagmus and dysarthria are frequently present in this syndrome, especially downbeat nystagmus. Some of these patients have anti-Purkinje cell antibodies.[82] This adds support to an autoimmune mechanism, as there are similar antigens in both Purkinje cells and T lymphocytes.[82] The patients with Hodgkin's disease have had more variable responses to treatment of their malignancies. Some patients will stabilize, some will recover, and some will recover and then remit.

References

1. Swanson JW, Kelly JJ, McConahey WM: Neurologic aspects of thyroid dysfunction. *Mayo Clin Proc* 56:504–512, 1981.
2. Wills AJ, Jenkins IH, Thompson PD, et al: A positron emission tomography study of cerebral activation associated with essential and writing tremor. *Arch Neurol* 52(3):299–305, 1995.
3. Baba M, Terada A, Hishida R, et al: Persistant hemichorea associated with thyrotoxicosis. *Intern Med* 31(9):1144–1146, 1992.
4. Lucantoni C, Grottoli S, Moretti A: Chorea due to hyperthyroidism in old age: A case report. *Acta Neurologica* 16(3):129–133, 1994.
5. Pozzan GB, Battistella PA, Rigon F, et al: Hyperthyroid-induced chorea in an adolescent girl. *Brain Dev* 14(2):126–127, 1992.
6. Weiner WJ, Lang AE: *Movement Disorders: A Comprehensive Survey*. Mt Kisco: Futura Publishing, 1989.
7. Fishbeck KH, Layzer RB: Paroxysmal choreoathetosis associated with thyrotoxicosis. *Ann Neurol* 6:453–454, 1979.
8. Harayama H, Ohno T, Miyatake T: Quantitative analysis of stance in ataxic myxoedema. *J Neurol Neurosurg Psychiatry* 46:579–581, 1983.
9. Rector WG, Herlong HF, Moses H: Nonketotic hyperglycemia appearing as choreoathetosis or ballism. *Arch Intern Med* 142:154–155, 1982.
10. Newman RP, Kinkel WR: Paroxysmal choreoathetosis due to hypoglycemia. *Arch Neurol* 41:341–342, 1984.
11. Nabatame H, Nakamura K, Matsuda M, et al: Hemichorea in hyperglycemia associated with increased blood flow in the contralateral striatum and thalamus. *Intern Med* 33(8):472–475, 1994.
12. Haan J, Kremer HPH, Padberg GWAM: Paroxysmal choreoathetosis as presenting symptom of diabetes mellitus. *J Neurol Neurosurg Psychiatry* 52:133, 1989.
13. Linazasoro G, Urtasun M, Poza JJ, et al: Generalized chorea induced by nonketotic hyperglycemia (letter). *Mov Disord* 8(1):119–120, 1993.
14. Hefter H, Mayer P, Benecke R: Persistant chorea after recurrent hypoglycemia: A case report. *Eur Neurol* 33(3):244–247, 1993.
15. Lin JJ, Chang MK: Hemiballism-hemichorea and non-ketotic hyperglycemia. *J Neurol Neurosurg Psychiatry* 57(6):748–750, 1994.
16. O'Doherty DS, Canary JJ: Neurologic aspects of endocrine disturbances, in Joynt RJ (ed): *Clinical Neurology*. Philadelphia: JB Lippincott, 1990, vol. 4.
17. Sachs C, Sjoberg HE, Erison K: Basal ganglia calcifications on CT: Relation to hypoparathyroidism. *Neurology* 32:779–782, 1982.
18. Kaminski HJ, Ruff RL: Neurologic complications of endocrine disease. *Neurol Clin* 7(3):489–508, 1989.
19. Salti I, Faris A, Tannir N: Rapid correction by 1-alpha-hydroxy-cholecalciferol of hemichorea in surgical hypoparathyroidism. *J Neurol Neurosurg Psychiatry* 45:89, 1982.
20. Barabas G, Tucker SM: Idiopathic hypoparathyroidism and paroxysmal dystonic choreoathetosis. *Ann Neurol* 24:585, 1988.
21. Yamamoto K, Kawazawa S: Basal ganglion calcification in paroxysmal dystonic choreoathetosis. *Ann Neurol* 22(4):556, 1987.

22. Tambyah PA, Ong BKC, Lee KO: Reversible parkinsonism and asymptomatic hypocalcemia with basal ganglia calcification from hypoparathyroidism 26 years after thyroid surgery. *Am J Med* 94:444, 1993.
23. Evans BK, Donley DK: Pseudohypoparathyroidism, parkinsonism syndrome, with no basal ganglia calcification. *J Neurol Neurosurg Psychiatry* 51:709–713, 1988.
24. Factor SA, Coni RJ, Cowger M, Rosenblum EL: Paroxysmal tremor and orofacial dyskinesias secondary to a biopterin synthesis defect. *Neurology* 41(6):930–932, 1991.
25. Albers JW, Nostrant TT, Riggs JE: Neurologic manifestations of gastrointestinal disease. *Neurol Clin* 7(3):525–548, 1989.
26. Young RR, Shahani BT: Asterixis: one type of negative myoclonus, in Fahn S, Marsden CD, Van Woert M (eds.): *Adv Neurol* 43:137–156, 1986.
27. Rothstein JD, Herlong HF: Neurologic manifestations of hepatic disease. *Neurol Clin* 7(3):563–578, 1989.
28. Swaiman KF: Disorders of the basal ganglia, in Swaiman KF (ed.): *Pediatric Neurology: Principles and Practice*. St. Louis, CV Mosby, 1989, chap 53, pp 819–837.
29. Thame M, Gray R, Forrester T: Parkinsonian-like tremors in the recovery phase of kwashiorkor. *West Ind Med J* 43(3):102–103, 1994.
30. Koller WC, Busenbark K, Gray C, et al: Classification of essential tremor: *Clin Neuropharmacol* 15(2):81–87, 1992.
31. Aisen ML, Adelstein BD, Romero J, et al: Peripheral mechanical loading and the mechanism of the tremor of chronic alcoholism. *Arch Neurol* 49(7):740–742, 1992.
32. Neiman J, Lang AE, Fornazzari L, Carlen PL: Movement disorders in alcoholism: A review. *Neurology* 40:741–746, 1990.
33. Shandling M, Carlen PL, Lang AE: Parkinsonism in alcohol withdrawal: A follow up study. *Mov Disord* 5:36, 1990.
34. Carlen PL, Lee MA, Jacob MA, Livshits O: Parkinsonism provoked by alcoholism. *Ann Neurol* 9:84, 1981.
35. Brust ACM: *Neurological Aspects of Substance Abuse*. Stoneham, England: Butterworth-Heinemann, 1993, p 201.
36. Gilman S, Adams K, Koeppe RA, et al: Cerebellar and frontal hypometabolism in alcoholic cerebellar degeneration studied with positron emission tomography. *Ann Neurol* 28(6):775–785, 1990.
37. Swaiman KF, Jacobson RI: Developmental abnormalities of the central nervous system, in Joynt RJ (ed): *Clinical Neurology*. Philadelphia: JB Lippincott, 1988, chap 55.
38. Calne DB, Lang AE: Secondary dystonia. *Adv Neurol* 50:9–33, 1988.
39. Berardelli A, Thompson PD, Zaccagnini M, Giardini O, D'Eufemia PD, Massoud R, Manfredi M: Two sisters with generalized dystonia associated with homocystinuria. *Mov Disord* 6(2):163–165, 1991.
40. Massey EW, Riggs JE: Neurologic manifestations of hematologic disease. *Neurol Clin* 7(3):549–561, 1989.
41. Iriarte LM, Mateu J, Cruz G, Escudero J: Chorea: A new manifestation of mastocytosis. *J Neurol Neurosurg Psychiatry* 51:1457–1458, 1988.
42. Swedo SE, Leonard HL, Schapiro MB, et al: Sydenham's chorea: Physical and psychological symptoms of St. Vitus dance. *Pediatrics* 91(4):706–713, 1993.
43. Riley DE, Lang AE: Movement disorders, in Bradley WG, Daroff RB, Fenichel GM, Marsden CD (eds): *Neurology in Clinical Practice*. Stoneham, England: Butterworth-Heinemann, 1991, vol 2, chap 76, p 1584.
44. Weindl A, Kuwert T, Leenders KL, et al: Increases in striatal glucose consumption in Sydenham's chorea. *Mov Disord* 8(4):437–444, 1993.
45. Bronze MS, Dale JB: Epitopes of streptococcal M proteins that evoke antibodies that cross react with human brain. *J Immunol* 151(5):2820–2828, 1993.

46. Husby G, van De Rijn L, Zabriskie JB: Antibodies reaction with cytoplasm of subthalamic and caudate nuclei neurons in chorea and acute rheumatic chorea. *J Exp Med* 144:1094–1110, 1976.

47. Figueroa F, Berrios X, Gutierrez M, et al: Anticardiolipin antibodies in acute rheumatic fever. *J Rheumatol* 19(8):1175–1180, 1992.

48. Reik L, Steere AC, Bartenhagen NH, et al: Neurologic abnormalities of Lyme disease. *Medicine* 58(4):281–294, 1979.

49. Pachner AR: Early disseminated Lyme disease: Lyme meningitis. *Am J Med* 98(4A):30S–37S, 1995.

50. Magnarelli LA: Current status of laboratory diagnosis for Lyme disease. *Am J Med* 98(4A):10S–12S, 1995.

51. Garcia-Monco JC, Benach JL: Lyme neuroborreliosis. *Ann Neurol* 37:691–702, 1995.

52. Kieburtz K, Schiffer RB: Neurologic manifestations of human immunodeficiency virus infections. *Neurol Clin* 7(3):447–468, 1989.

53. Nath A, Hobson DE, Russell A: Movement disorders with cerebral toxoplasmosis and AIDS. *Mov Disord* 8(1):107–112, 1993.

54. Singer C, Berger JR, Bowen BC et al: Akinetic-rigid syndrome in a 13-year-old girl with HIV-related progressive multifocal leukoencephalopathy: *Mov Disord* 8(1):113–116, 1993.

55. Beskind DL, Keim SM: Choreoathetotic movement disorder in a boy with Mycoplasma pneumoniae encephalitis. *Ann Emerg Med* 23(6):1375–1378, 1994.

56. Thiele EA, Sutton ME, Siffert JO, et al: Severe choreoathetosis associated with presumed encephalitis: A series of five cases. *Ann Neurol* 36(3):541, 1994.

57. Weiner SR, Utsinger P: Whipple disease. *Arthritis Rheum* 15:157–167, 1986.

58. Tison F, Louvet-Giendaj C, Henry P, et al: Permanent bruxism as a manifestation of the oculofacial syndrome related to systemic Whipple's disease. *Mov Disord* 7(1):82–85, 1992.

59. Hausser-Hauw C, Roulett E, Robert R, Marteau R: Oculo-facio-skeletal myorhythmia as a cerebral complication of systemic Whipple's disease. *Mov Disord* 3(2):179–184, 1988.

60. Adams M, Rhyner PA, Day J: Whipple's disease confined to the central nervous system. *Ann Neurol* 21:104–108, 1987.

61. Whiting S, Farrell K, McCormic AQ, Carter JEJ: Retinal and neurologic involvement in the hemolytic uremic syndrome (HUS). *Neurology* 35(suppl 1):248, 1985.

62. Delaney P: Neurologic manifestations in sarcoidosis: Review of the literature, with a report of 23 cases. *Ann Intern Med* 87:336–345, 1977.

63. Schlegel U, Clarenbach P, Cordt A, Steudel A: Cerebral sarcoidosis presenting as supranuclear gaze palsy with hypokinetic rigid syndrome. *Mov Disord* 4(3):274–277, 1989.

64. Jankovic J, Ford J: Blepharospasm and orofacial-cervical dystonia: Clinical and pharmacologic findings in 100 patients, *Ann Neurol* 13:402–411, 1983.

65. Jankovic J: Etiology and differential diagnosis of blepharospasm and oromandibular dystonia. *Adv Neurol* 49:103–116, 1988.

66. Nutt JG, Carter J, DeGarmo, Hammerstad JP: Meige syndrome and thyroid dysfunction. *Neurology* 34(suppl 1):222, 1984.

67. Jankovic J, Patten BM: Blepharospasm and autoimmune diseases. *Mov Disord* 2(3):159–163, 1987.

68. Alexander EL, Razenbach MR, Kumar AJ, et al: Anti-Ro(SS-A) autoantibodies in central nervous system disease associated with Sjogren's syndrome (CNS-SS): Clinical, neuroimaging, and angiographic correlates. *Neurology* 44(5):899–908, 1994.

69. Terao Y, Sakai K, Kato S, et al: Antineuronal antibody in Sjogren's syndrome masquerading as paraneoplastic cerebellar degeneration. *Lancet* 343(8900):790, 1994.

70. Nishimura H, Tachibana H, Makiura N, et al: Corticosteroid-responsive parkinsonism associated with primary Sjogren's syndrome. *Clin Neurol Neurosurg* 96(4):327–331, 1994.

71. Coull BM, Levine SR, Brey RL: The role of antiphospholipid antibodies in stroke. *Neurol Clin* 10(1):125–143

72. Rajagopalan N, Humphrey PRD, Bucknall RC: Torticollis and blepharospasm in systemic lupus erythematosus. *Mov Disord* 4(4):345–348, 1989.

73. Kirk A, Harding SR: Cardioembolic caudate infarction as a cause of himichorea in lupus anticoagulant syndrome. *Can J Neurol Sci* 20(2):162–164, 1993.

74. Furie R, Ishikawa T, Dhawan V, Eudelberg D: Alternating hemichorea in primary antiphospholipid antibody syndrome: Evidence for contralateral striatal hypermetabolism. *Neurology* 44(11):2197–2199, 1994.

75. Donaldson JO: *Neurology of Pregnancy*, 2d ed. London: WB Saunders, 1989.

76. Posner JB: Paraneoplastic syndromes. *Neurol Clin* 9(4):919–936, 1991.

77. Hetzel DJ, Stanhope CR, O'Neill BP, Lennon VA: Gynecologic cancer in patients with subacute cerebellar degeneration predicted by anti-Purkinje cell antibodies and limited in metastatic volume. *Mayo Clin Proc* 65(12):1558–1563, 1990.

78. Furneaux HM, Rosenblum MK, Dalmau J, et al: Selective expression of Purkinje-cell antigens in tumor tissue from patients with paraneoplastic cerebellar degeneration. *N Engl J Med* 322(26):1844–1851, 1990.

79. Hida C, Tsukamoto T, Awano H, Yamamoto T: Ultrastructural localization of anti-Purkinje cell antibody-binding sites in paraneoplastic cerebellar degeneration. *Arch Neurol* 51(6):555–558, 1994.

80. Gandy SE, Grebb JA, Rosen N, et al: General assay for phosphoproteins in cerebrospinal fluid: A candidate marker for paraneoplastic cerebellar degeneration. *Ann Neurol* 28(6):829–833, 1990.

81. Peterson K, Rosenblum MK, Kotanides H, Posner JB: Paraneoplastic cerebellar degeneration. I. A clinical analysis of 55 anti-Yo antibody-positive patients. *Neurology* 42:1931–1937, 1992.

82. Hammack J, Kotanides H, Rosenblum MK, Posner JB: Paraneoplastic cerebellar degeneration. II. Clinical and immunologic findings in 21 patients with Hodgkin's disease. *Neurology* 42:1938–1943, 1992.

Appendix _____

Patient Support Organizations

Parkinson's Disease

ARGENTINA
Grupo Autoyauda Parkinson Argentina
Fundacion Alfredo Thomson
La Riojoa 951
1221 Buenos Aires

AUSTRALIA
National Australian Parkinson's Association, Inc.
P.O. Box 363
Newtown, NSW 2042

Parkinson's Syndrome Society of N.S.W. Inc.
Level 3, Room 316
Community Health Services Building
Cm George Street & Marsden Street,
Paramatta, NSW 2150

Parkinson's Disease Association (Victoria), Inc.
Suite 1, 82 Stud Road
Dandenong, Victoria 3175

Parkinson's Association of Western Australia
Neurological Loteries House
320 Rokeby Road,
Subiaco, Western Australia 6008

Parkinson's Association of A.C.T.
South Office
P.O. Box 717
Mawson, A.C.T. 2607

The Parkinson's Society of the Gold Coast
P.O. Box 6096
Gold Coast Mail Centre,
Bundall, QLD 4217

Parkinson's Disease Association of Tasmania, Inc.
82–86 Hampden Road
Battery Point, Hobart Tasmania 7000

Parkinson's Syndrome Society of South Australia, Inc.
37 Woodville Road
Woodville, South Australia 5011

Parkinson's Syndrome Society of QLD, Inc.
Yungaba
120 Main Street
Kangaroo Point 4169
Queensland

AUSTRIA
Austrian Parkinson Patients Association
Marzstrasse 49
A-1150 Vienna

BELGIUM
Association Parkinson Belge
Avenue Jan Stobbaertslaan 43
B-1030 Brussels

BRAZIL
Associação Brasil Parkinson
Rua Visconde de Indaiaruba, 279
05083 São Paulo

CANADA
The Parkinson Foundation of Canada
390 Bay Street
Toronto, Ontario M5H-242
Tel. (416) 366-0099

Parkinson's Society of Ottawa-Carleton
Ottawa Civic Hospital
1053 Carling Avenue
Ottawa, Ontario K1Y 4E9

The Parkinson's Society of Southern Alberta
600 Sloane Square
5920-IA Street, S.W.
Calgary, Alberta T2H OG3
Tel. (416) 258-2595

Victoria Chapter/British Columbia Parkinson's Disease
  Association
1740 Richmond Avenue,
Victoria, British Columbia V8R 4P8
Tel. (604) 370-2211

CHILE
Liga Contra el Mal del Parkinson
Moneda 973, Oficina 335
Santiago
Tel. (56) 2-399036

COLOMBIA
Asociación Colombiana de la Enfermedad de Parkinson
Calle 106 #31-45
Santefe de Bogota

DENMARK
Dansk Parkinsoonforening
Hornemansgade 36 St.
2100 Copenhagen 0

ESTONIA
Estonian Parkinson's Society
Sole 15-1
Tallinn EE0006

EUROPE
European Parkinson's Disease Association
c/o Parkinson Patienten Verenigung
Postbus 46
3980 CA Bunnik
Netherlands

FINLAND
Finnish Parkinson's Association
Pitkamsenk, 4Λ
20250 Turku
Tel. (358) 291-391-233

FRANCE
France Parkinson
37 bis, rue la Fontaine
75016 Paris
Tel. (33) 45.20.22.20

Association des Groupements de Parkinsoniens
3, Ch. du Grand Fosse
44600 Saint-Nazaire

GERMANY
Deutsche Parkinson Vereiningung
Moselstrasse 31
4040 Neuss

HONG KONG
The Parkinson's Disease Society of Hong Kong
703 East Town Building
41 Lockhart Rd.
Wanchai

ICELAND
Parkinsonsamtokin a Islandi
Grandavegi 47
107 Reykjavik

INDIA
P. K. Kanodia
Lion's Club, Dist. 322 E.
Lai Bazar, P. O.
Bettiah, Bihar

IRELAND
Parkinson's Association of Ireland
Carmichael House
N. Brunswick Street
Dublin 7

ISRAEL
Parkinson Disease Association
P.O. Box 635
Kiriat Bialik, 27100

ITALY
Associazione Italiana Parkinsoniani
Via Zuretti 35
20125 Milan

Associazione Azione Parkinson
Via Sesto Celere 6
00152 Rome

Unione Parkinsoniani
Via Aurelio Saffi, 43
43100 Parma

JAMAICA
Parkinson's Society of Jamaica
7 Glendon Circle Hope Pastures
Kingston 6

JAPAN
Japan Parkinson's Association
Satoshi Fujii
979-227 Misawa
Hino-Shi, Tokyo 191

LUXEMBOURG
Association Luxembourgeoise de la
    Maladie de Parkinson
42, rue de Solei
7250 Walferbange

MEXICO
Numa Usi
Paseo de la Soladad-86
La Herradura 53020

NETHERLANDS
Parkinson Patienten Verenigung
Postbus 46
3980 CA Bunnik

NEW ZEALAND
The Parkinsonism Society of New Zealand, Inc.
Wellington Division
P.O. Box 7061
Wellington South

NORWAY
Norway Parkinsonforbund
Schweigaardsgt 34
BYGG F, OPPG 1
0191 Oslo

SOUTH AFRICA
Suid-Afrikaanse Vereenigung Vir Parkinsoniste
P.O. Box 1446
Lonehill
Bryanston 2062
Transvaal

SPAIN
Parkinson España
Cl de la Torre 14
08006 Barcelona

SWEDEN
Neurologiskt Handikappade
Riksforbund
Kingsgatan 32
1135 Stockholm

Svenska Parkinsonforbundet
Karlagatan 23
416 61 Goteborg

SWITZERLAND
Association Suisse de la Maladie de Parkinson
Case Postale
8128 Hinteregg
Tel. (41) 01-40169

TAIWAN
Taiwan Parkinsonian Association
P.O. Box 67-512
Taipei

UNITED KINGDOM
Parkinson Disease Society
22 Upper Woburn Place
London WG1H 0RA
Tel. (44) 171-383-3513
Fax (44) 171-383-5754

UNITED STATES
American Parkinson Disease Association (APDA)
1250 Hylan Blvd.
Staten Island, NY 10305
Tel. (718) 981-8001, (800) 223-2732

National Parkinson Foundation (NPF)
1501 NW Ninth Avenue
Bob Hope Road
Miami, FL 33136
Tel. (305) 547-6666, (800) 327-4545

Parkinson's Disease Foundation (PDF)
650 West 168th Street
New York, NY 10032
Tel. (212) 923-4700, (800) 457-6676

United Parkinson Foundation (UPF)
833 West Washington Boulevard
Chicago, IL 60607
Tel. (312) 733-1893

Huntington's Disease

Support Groups

AUSTRALIA
Australian Huntington's Disease Association
Robyn Kapp
P.O. Box 247 Lindcombe Hospital
Lindcombe 2141, NSW
Tel. (61) 26468394

AUSTRIA
Oestereiche Huntington Hilfe
Christian Stockinger
Hasnerstrasse 88/23, Vienna 1160
Tel. (43) 14929153

BELGIUM
Huntington Liga
Marcel Gulickx
Krijkelberg 1, B 3360 Leuven
Belgium
Tel. (32) 16-452759

CANADA
Huntington Society of Canada (HSC)
Ralph Walker
Box 1296
Cambridge, Ontario N1R 7G6
Tel. (519) 622-1002

Huntington Society of Quebec
4841 Rivard Street
Montreal, Quebec H2J 2N7
Tel. (514) 842-5740
Fax (514) 842-5961

CZECH REPUBLIC
Spolecnost Pro Pomoc Pri
Hintingtonove Chorobe
Jana Zidovská
Doln' Brezany 153, 25241 Doln' Brezany
Prague-West
Tel. (42) 24715291
Fax (42) 2294905

DENMARK
Landsforeningen Mod
Huntington's Chorea
Jytte Broholm
Rosenvaenget 14, 4270 Hong
Tel. (53) 553-003

FRANCE
Association Huntington de France
Micheline Destreil
14, Route de Gometz
91 Bures sur Yvette
Tel. (33) 69.86.90.47
Fax (33) 69.86.90.50

GERMANY
Deutsche Huntington Hilfe
Georg Hirschler
Postfacg 281251
447241 Duisberg

IRELAND
Huntington's Disease Association of Ireland
Bernadette Moran
Carmichael House
N. Brunswick St.,
Dublin 7
Tel. (353) 721303
Tel. (353) 735737

ISRAEL
Israeli Huntington Families Group
Nira Dangoor
19237 Kibbutz Ein Hashojet
Tel. (092) 48-95-372
Fax (092) 48-94-882

ITALY
Associazione Italiana Corea di Huntington
Gabriella Conte Marotta
c/o Instituto Neurological, C. Besta
Via Celoria 11, Milano 20133
Tel. (39) 394448

NETHERLANDS
Vereniging Van Huntington
Gerrit Dommerholt
Callunahof 8
7217 St. Harfsen
Tel. (31) 331595
Fax (31) 35-00-050

NEW ZEALAND
Huntington's Disease Association
Judith Baker
P.O. Box 25-088, Christchurch
Tel. (64) 366516

Wellington Huntington's Disease Association, Inc.
Marjorie Heads
Social Work Dept.
Wellington Hospital
7902 Wellington South
Tel. (64) 3855850

NORTHERN IRELAND
Huntington's Disease Association of Northern Ireland
Dept. of Medical Genetics
Belfast BT9 7AB
Tel. (44) 2653826

NORWAY
Landsforeningen for Huntington's Sykdom
Sigrun Rosenlund
Postbox 114, Kjelsas
N 0411 Oslo
Tel. (47) 2223506

SCOTLAND
Scottish Huntington's Disease Association
Ron Livingston
Thistle House, 61 Main Road
Ederslie, Jonstone PA5 9BA
Tel. (44) 522245

SOUTH AFRICA
Huntington's Society of South Africa
Juan Schrönen
P.O. Box 44501
Claremonte, Cape Town
Tel. (27) 17996413

SPAIN
Asociación de Corea de Huntington Española
Asuncion Martinez-Descals
Servicio Neurologia
Fundacion Jimenez Diaz
Avda Reyes Catolicos 2
Madrid 28040
Tel. (34) 449008
Fax (34) 494764

SWEDEN
Huntington Foreningen I Sverige
Mia Lundstrom
c/o NHR Postbox 3284
Kungsgatan 32
10365 Stockholm
Tel. (46) 8140320

SWITZERLAND
Schweizerische Huntington Vereinigung
Heide Moser
Welti, Beunderweg 1
Tel. (41) 8881383

UNITED KINGDOM
Huntington's Disease Association
Prue Willday
108 Battersea High St.
London SW 11 3HP
Tel. (44) 171-223-7000

UNITED STATES
Huntington's Disease Society of America (HDSA)
140 W. 22nd Street
New York, NY 10011
Tel. (212) 242-1968
Fax (212) 243-2443

Organizations

Foundation for the Care and Cure of Huntington's
   Disease, Inc. (FCCHD)
Liz Mueller
8 Jennifer Drive
Homdel, NJ 07733
Tel. (908) 739-5621

Hereditary Disease Foundation
1427 7th Street, #2,
Santa Monica, CA 90401
Tel. (213) 458-4183
http://ourworld.compuserve.com/homepages/
   hereditary_disease_foundation/

International Huntington Association (IHA)
Gerrit Dommerholt
Callunahof 8
7217 St. Harfsen
Netherlands
Tel. (31) 57331595
Fax (31) 573500050

Dystonia

BELGIUM
Belgische Zelphulgroep Voor Dystonie Patiënten
Christine Wauters
Blokmakerstraat 6
9120 Haasdonk
Tel. (32) 37755125

BRAZIL
Associação Brasileira dos Portadores de Distonias
Helen de Barros
Al Gabriel Monteiro da Silva 1834
São Paolo-SP Cep: 01442-001
Tel. (55) 8521051
Fax (55) 2825995

CROATIA
Hrvatske Grupa Za Istrazivanje Distonije
Prof. Maja Relja
Dept. of Neurology
University of Zagreb
Kispaticeva 12
41000 Zagreb
Tel. (385) 012335595

DENMARK
Dansk Dystoniforening
Kaj Nauning
Lodsgârden B 5, 2791 Dragor
Tel. (45) 32536624

EUROPE
European Dystonia Federation
Alan Leng
The Dystonia Society
Weddel House
13-14 West Smithfield
London EC1A 9JJ
England
Tel. (44) 171-329-0797
Fax (44) 171-329-0689

FRANCE
La Ligue Française contre la Dystonie
Jean-Pierre Bleton
Hospital Sainte Anne
Centre Raymond Garcin
1, rue Cabanis
75014 Paris
Tel. (33) 14.56.585.05

GERMANY
Deutsche Dystonie Ges. e. V.
Didi Jackson
Bockhorst 45A
22589 Hamburg
Tel. (49) 408702133
Fax (49) 4075602

IRELAND
The Dystonia Society of Ireland
Maria Hickey
33 Larkfield Grove-Harold Cross
Dublin 6W
Tel. (353) 1353964387

ITALY
Italiana per la Ricerca sulla Distonia Associazione
Laura Latini
Vicolo Sant'Agata 21
24129 Bergamo
Tel. (39) 35241561
Fax (39) 35526736

JAPAN
Dystonia Support Group of Japan
Masako Kaji
2-19-7 Sencho
Ohtsu City, Shiga 520
Tel. (81) 775330297

NETHERLANDS
Nederlandse Verening van Dystonie Patienten
Josie Timmermans
Sportlaan 17
5242 CN Rosmalen
Tel. (31) 419215645

NORWAY
Norsk Dystoniforening
Tore Wirgenes
P.O. Box 1545 Glombo
1677 Kråkeroy
Tel. (47) 35020538
Fax (47) 35013960

SLOVENIA
Drusto Misicno Obolelik Slovenije
Lnhartova I/3
61000 Ljubljana

SOUTH AFRICA
South African Parkinsonian and Dystonia Association
Maureen Langford
P.O. Box 1446
Lonehill 2062
Tel. (27) 7924982
Fax (27) 4933929

SPAIN
Asociación de Lucha contra la Distonia en España
Felisa Justo Alonso
Santa Isabel 15 1° B Centro
28012 Madrid, Spain
Tel. (34) 15276161
     (34) 17598866
Fax (34) 18076200

SWEDEN
Svensk Dystonia Förening
Gunilla Norén
Gavelvägen 6
S-743 30 Storvreta
Tel. (46) 18314820

SWITZERLAND
SDG Schweizerische Dystonie Gesellschaft
Dr. Brigitte Gygli
Tramstr. 39
CH-4132 Muttenz
(41) 614616993

UNITED KINGDOM
The Dystonia Society
Weddel House
13-14 West Smithfield
London EC1A9JJ
Tel. (44) 171-329-0797
Fax (44) 171-329-0689

UNITED STATES
Dystonia Medical Research Foundation
One East Wacker Dr. #2900
Chicago, IL 60601-2001
Tel. (312) 755-0198, (800) 361-8061 in Canada
Fax (312) 803-0138

Blepharospasm

AUSTRALIA
Blepharospasm Support Group
David McGee
Royal Victorian Eye & Ear Hospital
32 Gilsborne Street
East Melbourne, Victoria 3002
Tel. (61) 36637203
Fax (61) 36659666

FRANCE
Association des Malades Atteints de Blepharospasme
Dr. Henri Bigorre
Sault Premilhat, 03410 Domerat
Tel. (33) 70.29.20.37

UNITED STATES
Benign Essential Blepharospasm Research Foundation, Inc.
P.O. Box 12468
Beaumont, TX 77726-2468
Tel. (409) 832-0788
Fax (409) 832-0890

Spasmodic Torticollis

AUSTRALIA
Australian Spasmodic Torticollis Association
P.O. Box 195
Epping, N.S.W. 2121
Tel. (61) 26859020
Fax (61) 26859023

GERMANY
Bundesverband Torticollis e.V.
Eckernkamp 39
59007 Hamm
Tel. (49) 23892935
Fax (49) 2389536289

UNITED STATES
National Spasmodic Torticollis Association
P.O. Box 873
Royal Oak, MI 48068
Tel. (800) HURTFUL (487-8385), (313) 647-2280,
    or (414) 797-9912
Fax (414) 797-9861

Tardive Dyskinesia

Tardive Dyskinesia/Tardive Dystonia National
    Association
4244 University Way NE
P.O. Box 45732
Seattle, WA 98145-0732
Tel. (206) 522-3166

Tourette's Syndrome

AUSTRALIA
Tourette Syndrome Association of Australia
P.O. Box 1173
Maroubra, 2035 NSW
Tel. (61) 23112745

BELGIUM
Gilles de la Tourette Vlaamse Vereniging
P.O. Box 1173
Jozef Nauwelaertstraat 7
B2110 Wijnegem
Tel. (32) 33536791

CANADA
Tourette Syndrome Foundation of Canada
3675 Keele Street Suite 203
Downsview, Ontario M3J 1M6
Tel. (416) 636-2800

DENMARK
Dansk Tourette Forening
Prestehusene 31
DK 2820
Tel. (45) 43965709

FRANCE
Aftoc Tourette
24, rue Leon Gambetta
F 59790 Ronchin
Tel. (33) 20.85.96.42

GERMANY
Tourette-Gesellschaft Deutschland
Kinder-u. Jugendpsychiatrische Klinik
Zentralinstitut für Seelische Gesundheit
Postfach 12 21 20
68072 Mannheim

ICELAND
Tourette Samtokin a Islandi
Postholf 3128
IS 123 Reykjavik
Tel. (35) 45888581

ISRAEL
Tourette Syndrome Association of Israel
P.O. Box 4079
Ramat Gan 52140

NETHERLANDS
Tourette Syndrome Association of the Netherlands
P.O. Box 925
3160 AC, Rhood
Tel. (31) 189013043

NEW ZEALAND
Tourette Syndrome Association of New Zealand
146 Weymouth Road
Manurowa, South Auckland

NORWAY
Norsk Tourett Forening
Munkerudesen 33, Oslo 1165
Tel. (47) 2285043

SOUTH AFRICA
Southern Africa Tourette Syndrome Institute
228 Oak Avenue
Ferndale 2194
Tel. (27) 118866353

SPAIN
Asociacion Española para Tics y Tourette
Gran Via de les Corts Catalanes
562 pral. 2a, 08011 Barcelona
Tel. (34) 3515550

SWEDEN
The Swedish Tourette Association
Soerkroken 2
S-440, 74 Hjaetleby
Tel. (46) 304678130

UNITED KINGDOM
Tourette Syndrome Association of Great Britain
27 Monkton Street
Ryde, Isle of Wight PO33 2BY
Tel. (44) 83568866

UNITED STATES
Tourette Syndrome Association, Inc.
42-40 Bell Boulevard
Bayside, NY 11361
Tel. (800) 237-0717, (718) 224-2999

Ataxia

CANADA
Canadian Association of Friedreich's Ataxia
Claude St John
5620, rue C. A. Jobin
Montreal, Quebec H1P 1H8
Tel. (514) 321-8684

IRELAND
Friedreich's Ataxia Society of Ireland
Clare Creedon
San Martin
Mart Lane, Foxrock
Dublin 18
Tel (353) 17894788

UNITED KINGDOM
Friedreich's Ataxia Group
Shirley Dalby
Copse Edge
Thursley Rd, Elstead
Godalming, Surrey GU8 6DJ
Tel. (44) 125-270-2864
Fax (44) 125-270-3715

UNITED STATES
National Ataxia Foundation
750 Twelve Oaks Center
15500 Wayzata Blvd
Wayzata, MN 55391
Tel. (612) 473-9289
http://www.ataxia.org/)

AT Medical Research Foundation
5241 Round Meadow Rd
Hidden Hills, CA 91302
Tel. (818) 704-8146

Myoclonus

UNITED STATES
Moving Forward
2934 Glenmore Avenue
Kettering, OH 45409
Tel. (513) 293-0409

Myoclonus Research Foundation
200 Old Palisade Road Suite 17D
Fort Lee, NJ 07024
Tel. (201) 585-0770
Fax (201) 585-8114

Myoclonus Families United
1564 E. 24th Street
Brooklyn, NY 11234
Tel. (718) 252-2133

Progressive Supranuclear Palsy

UNITED KINGDOM
Progressive Supranuclear Palsy Europe Association
22 Upper Woburn Place
London WC1H 0RA
Tel. (44) 171-383-3513

UNITED STATES
The Society for Progressive Supranuclear Palsy, Inc.
Johns Hopkins Outpatient Center, Suite 5065
601 North Caroline Street
Baltimore, MD 21287
Tel. (800) 457-4777, (410) 955-2954
Fax (407) 732-6750

Restless Legs Syndrome

UNITED STATES
Restless Legs Syndrome Foundation
1904 Banbury Road
Raleigh, NC 27608
Tel. (919) 571-1599, (919) 781-4428
Fax (919) 571-9057

Tremor

UNITED KINGDOM
International Tremor Foundation
Karen Walsh
Disablement Services Centre
Harold Wood Hospital
Romford RM3 OBE, Essex
Tel. (44) 170-837-8050
Fox (44) 170-837-8032

UNITED STATES
International Tremor Foundation
833 West Washington Boulevard
Chicago, IL 60607
Tel. (312) 733-1893

Educational Organizations for Physicians

The Movement Disorder Society
Secretariat
Central Headquarters Office
Clarastrasse 57
CH-4005, Basel
Switzerland
Tel. (41) 61-691-51-11
Fax (41) 61-691-81-89

WE MOVE (Worldwide Education and Awareness for
 Movement Disorders)
Mount Sinai Neurology
One Gustave L. Levy Place, Box 1052
New York, NY 10029
Tel. (800) 437-MOV2, (212) 241-8567

INDEX

The letter *f* or *t* following a page number indicates that either a figure or a table is being referenced.

A

Abductor spasmodic dysphonia, 398
Acanthocytes, 337
Acetazolamide
  essential tremor treatment with, 378
  myoclonus treatment with, 549
Acetylcholine
  basal ganglia function, 104–107
  Parkinson's disease, 157
Acetylcholine receptors, molecular diversity of, 105, 105*t*
Achromatic neurons, 614
Acidophilic granules, Parkinson's disease, 265
Acquired dystonia, neuroimaging, 31
Action dystonia, 5, 430
Action myoclonus, 7, 542, 549
Action tremor, 541, 589
Activated oxygen species, 168
Acute akathisia, 10
Acute chorea. *See* Sydenham's chorea
ADHD. *See* Attention deficit hyperactivity disorder
Age
  essential tremor, 367, 369
  Huntington's disease, 492, 492*f*
  idiopathic torsion dystonia, 419, 421*t*
  mitochondrial abnormalities and, 53
  Parkinson's disease, 139, 140*t*, 188–189, 268–269
  progressive supranuclear palsy, 287
Aging. *See also* Elderly
  hypokinetic disorders and, 674*t*
  mitochondrial theory, 53
  movement disorders and, 673–682
  Parkinson's disease progression, 36
AIDS, parkinsonism associated with, 311
Akathisia, 10
  in childhood, 669
  drug-related, 191
  nocturnal, 697
  tardive akathisia, 10, 519, 523
Akinesia
  in the elderly, 673
  facial, 187
  multiple-system atrophy, 299
  Parkinson's disease, 88, 90–91, 186, 186*t*, 258, 259
  pharyngeal, 187
  supplementary motor area lesions and, 77
Alcohol
  essential tremor treatment with, 376
  tremor induced by, 389
Alcoholism, 389, 735
Alien limb, 9

Alpha-ketoglutarate dehydrogenase complex, Parkinson's
    disease and, 167
Alpha-methyldopa, parkinsonism induced by, 328
Alpha motor system, 591, 591–593, 594
Alprazolam, essential tremor treatment with, 378
Aluminum, Parkinson's disease and, 170
Alzheimer's disease, 54, 681–682
  clinical signs, 618*t*
  dementia, 23, 24, 187, 190
  Lewy body dementia distinguished from, 25
  magnetic resonance imaging, 283t
  myoclonus and, 546
  neuropathology, 125, 128
  OXPHOS defects and, 54, 61, 62
  with parkinsonism, 11
  Parkinson's disease symptoms and, 61
Amantadine, 289
  cerebellar disorder treatment, 581
  cyanide-induced parkinsonism, 319
  idiopathic Parkinson's disease, 211–212
  Parkinson's disease, 209–210
Ambulation, 649–650, 650t, 651*t*. *See also* Gait disorder.
Amiodarone, tremor induced by, 328, 391, 413
AMPA, 107
AMPA receptors, 108–109
Amphetamines, postencephalitic parkinsonism, 310
Amputees, phantom dyskinesia, 10
Amyotrophic chorea. *See* Neuroacanthocytosis
Anterior cingulate circuit, of the brain, 16, 16*f*
Anticholinergic drugs
  carbon monoxide-induced parkinsonism, 318
  cyanide-induced parkinsonism, 319
  dystonia, 444–445
  in Parkinson's disease, 209, 209*t*, 212
  postencephalitic parkinsonism, 310
  progressive supranuclear palsy, 289
Anticonvulsants
  dystonia, 445
  stiff-person syndrome, 646
  tremor induced by, 390–391
Antidepressants
  progressive supranuclear palsy, 289
  tremor induced by, 390
Antidopaminergic drugs, dystonia treatment with, 444
Antioxidants, Parkinson's disease and, 211
Antiphospholipid antibody syndrome, 528, 739
Antipsychotic drugs
  in Huntington's disease, 497
  parkinsonism induced by, 325–327, 326t
  tardive dyskinesia induced by, 7, 10, 327, 328,
    519–524

Antiserotonergic drugs, progressive supranuclear palsy, 289

Anxiety, movement disorders and, 20, 258–259

Apathy, movement disorders and, 19

Aphasia, 22, 25

Apomorphine, 207–208

Applause sign, progressive supranuclear palsy and, 284

Apraxia, 23, 432f

Archicerebellum, anatomy, 73, 578, 596

Aromatic amino acid decarboxylase, 203

Arotinolol, essential tremor treatment with, 377

Arteriosclerotic parkinsonism, 273–274

Ascending reticular activating system, behavioral state control and, 702, 703f

Associative circuits, 78

Asterixis, 7, 557–558, 558f, 735

Asynergia, 580

Ataxia, 56f, 590
 Brun's ataxia, 590
 causes, 668t
 cerebellar origin, 580
 in childhood, 667–668, 668t
 mitochondrial mutations and, 62–65, 65f
 myoclonic, 549
 optic, ataxia, 654
 psychogenic, 728
 sensory, 590
 vestibular function, distorted, 652

Ataxia telangiectasia, 463–464
 differential diagnosis, 456t
 dystonia in, 463

Ataxic dysarthria, 581

Atenolol, essential tremor treatment with, 377

Athetosis, 8, 527

ATP, 165, 167

ATP synthase, 51, 52f

Attention deficit, gait disorder, 657

Attention deficit hyperactivity (ADHD), 570, 573–574

Atypical parkinsonism, 126, 298

Auditory blink reflex, progressive supranuclear palsy, 286

Auditory startle reflex, progressive supranuclear palsy, 286

Autism, cerebellar abnormalities in, 578

Autoimmunity
 dystonia, 434–435
 movement disorders secondary to, 738–739
 in stiff-person syndrome, 645

Autonomic dysfunction
 L-dopa and, 221
 multiple-system atrophy and, 299–300
 in Parkinson's disease, 188

Axial myoclonus, 548

B

Baclofen
 dystonia, 445, 445t, 452
 stiff-person syndrome, 646

Balance disorders
 ambulation components, 649–650, 650t
 anatomic correlates, 650t
 attention impairment and, 657–658
 cautious gait, 658
 clinical features, 650, 651t, 652–653
 dementia and, 657
 fear of falling, 658
 force production and scaling, 654–656
 orientation, 653–654
 synergies, 656–657
 vestibular function, 652

Balance synergies, 656

Balance tasks, 649

Ballism, 7
 conditions associated with, 532–583, 533t
 psychogenic, 726
 types, 7–8

Ballistic movements, 527, 580

Ballooned neurons, 272, 614

Basal ganglia, 73, 88f, 90f, 92f, 100f, 102f
 acetylcholine and, 104–107
 anatomy, 77–80, 78f, 87, 153
 behavioral state control and, 702–703, 704f, 705
 calcification, 12t, 734
  dystonia and, 462
  parkinsonism and, 348
 dopamine and, 80, 87, 100–104, 103t
 dopamine receptors, 156
 dystonia and, 436, 457, 458
 "focusing" hypothesis, 89
 functional segregation of pathways, 80, 88–89
 glutamate and, 99, 107–111, 110t
 lesions, 22
 memory and, 22
 movement, role in, 31–32
 movement disorders and, 87–94, 239–244, 239f–241f, 243f
 MRI, 12t
 neuropathology, 126
 obsessive-compulsive disorder and, 20
 oxidative phosphorylation dysfunction and, 51, 54
 Parkinson's disease and, 153
 progressive supranuclear palsy and and, 285
 "scaling" hypothesis, 89

Bassen-Kornzweig syndrome, 337

BDNF, 118–119, 120
 fetal grafts and, 230–231
 Parkinson's disease and, 174

Benign familial chorea, 41, 666

Benign hereditary chorea, 41, 529–530

Benign Parkinson's disease, 272

Benserazide, 203

Benzodiazepines
 dystonia, 445, 445t
 essential tremor, 378
 stiff person syndrome, 646

Benzotropine, 105

Bereitschaftspotential, 75–76, 91, 561

Beta-adrenergic blockers, essential tremor treatment with, 376–377
Beta-blockers
  essential tremor treatment with, 376, 377
  tremor induced by, 391
Beta-carbolines, as neurotoxin, 172
Bethanechol, parkinsonism induced by, 328
Beverages, tremor induced by, 389–390
Biballism, 7, 527
Bililrubin encephalopathy, 666
Binswanger's disease, 346
Binuclear cluster, 164
Biopsy, 4t. *See also* Testing
Biperiden, 105
Biphasic dyskinesia, 214
Bladder symptoms, Parkinson's disease, 188
Blepharospasm, 431, 434–437
  botulinum treatment of, 447–448
  encephalitis lethargica, 307
  dystonia in, 431, 432f, 434, 437
  progressive supranuclear palsy, 286, 290
  sleep in, 699
  suppression of spasm, 5
Blinking
  Parkinson's disease, 187
  progressive supranuclear palsy, 290
Blink reflexes, dystonia and, 436, 436f
Body rocking, 690
Bones, Wilson's disease, 627
Botulinum toxin treatment
  blepahrospasm, 447–448
  dystonia, 445t, 445–447, 446t, 447t, 523
    cervical dystonia, 449–450, 449t
    laryngeal dystonia, 449
    limb dystonia, 450
  essential tremor, 379
  hemifacial spasm, 450
  oromandibular dystonia, 448–449
  primary writing tremor, 399
  progressive supranuclear palsy, 289
  spasmodic dysphonia, 449
  stiff person syndrome, 647
  tardive dyskinesia, 523
  tics, 451
  tremor, 450–451
  writers' cramp, 450
Bowel problems, in Parkinson's disease, 188
Bradykinesia, 10
  DDPAC, 331
  in the elderly, 673
  in Parkinson's disease, 91
  in postencephalitic parkinsonism, 309
  progressive supranuclear palsy and, 284–285
Bradyphrenia
  in Parkinson's disease, 187
  in postencephalitic parkinsonism, 308
Brain
  acetylcholine and, 104–107
  anterior cingulate circuit, 16, 16f
  aphasia, 22

basal ganglia. *See* Basal ganglia
cerebellum. *See* Cerebellum
cognitive behavior, 21
cortical motor areas, 73–77
corticobasal degeneration. *See* Corticobasal degeneration, 614
depression and, 17
dopamine and, 100–104, 103t
dorsolateral prefrontal circuit, 15, 16f
dystonia and, 455, 457–459, 459t
echolalia, 22
executive function, 21
frontal subcortical circuits, 15–16, 16f
glutamate and, 99, 107–111
gross neuropathologic examination, 125–132
Huntington's disease, 503–511
lateral orbitofrontal circuit, 15–16, 16f
memory, 22
microscopic examination, 126–127
mitochondrial DNA mutations and, 54
movement, role in, 31–32
neuroimaging. *See* Neuroimaging
obsessive-compulsive disorder and, 20
psychosis, 18, 19
sexual disturbances, 20, 21
sleep disorders, 20–21
thalamus. *See* Thalamus
tics, 562
tumors, 348
Brain-derived neurotrophic factor. *See* BDNF
Brain lesions, symptomatic dystonia related to, 455, 457–459, 459t
Brain stem, Huntington's disease, 511
Brainstem lesions, 457, 656
Briquet's syndrome, 716, 717
British antilewisite, Wilson's disease therapy, 630
Brodmann's area 4, 6, 73, 75, 76
Bromocriptine
  dystonia, 445t
  neuroleptic malignant syndrome, 349
  pharmacology, 206, 206t
Brun's ataxia, 590
Bruxism, 690, 691
Burning, in Parkinson's disease, 188
Buspirone, tardive dyskinesia treatment with, 523

C

Cabergoline, pharmacology, 208
Caffeine, tremor induced by, 389
CAG repeat, movement disorders, 481–487, 491
Calcium channel blockers
  essential tremor treatment with, 379
  parkinsonism induced by, 328
Calcium homeostasis, mitochondrial functions, 168
Calcium metabolism, parkinsonism and, 348
Calpines, 167
CAPIT. *See* Core Assessment Protocol for Intracerebral Transplantation.

Carbamazepine
  dystonia treatment with, 445*t*
  myoclonus treatment with, 549
  tics induced by, 566
  tremor induced by, 391
Carbidopa, 203
  carbon monoxide-induced parkinsonism, 318
  cyanide-induced parkinsonism, 319
  dystonia treatment with, 445*t*
  with L-dopa, 204
  myoclonus treatment with, 549
Carbon disulfide
  mechanism of toxicity, 318–319
  parkinsonism induced by, 318–319
  tremors induced by, 393
Carbonic anhydrase inhibitors, essential tremor treatment
    with, 378
Carbon monoxide-induced parkinsonism, 317–318
Carbon tetrachloride, tremors induced by, 393
Catapres, 573
Catatonia, neuroleptic malignant syndrome, 348
Catechol-*O*-methyltransferase. *See* COMT
Caudal cingulate motor area, 74, 74*f*
Cautious gait, 658
CBD. *See* Corticobasal degeneration
CCK-8. *See* Cholecystokinin-8
Cerebellar ataxia, mitochondrial mutations and, 62–63, 64
Cerebellar cortex, anatomy, 73, 578, 595, 597, 599–600
Cerebellar disorders, 579, 608
  cerebellar syndromes, 600–601, 601*t*
  clinical signs, 579–581, 587–591
  differential diagnosis, 582*t*
  gait disorders, 655
  mechanism of dysfunction, 603–604
  multiple-system atrophy, 300
  neuroimaging, 582*t*, 605*f*–607*f*
  pathophysiology, 587, 591–594
  treatment, 581, 582*t*
  Wilson's disease, 625
Cerebellar mutism, 581
Cerebellar syndromes, 600–602, 601*t*
Cerebellar tremor, 388–389, 410
Cerebellum
  anatomy, 578–579, 578*t*, 579*t*, 595–600, 596*f*–599*f*
  disorders. *See* Cerebellar disorders.
  functions, 577–578, 594–595
  Huntington's disease, 510–511
  learning and, 604–607, 605*f*, 606
Cerebral cortex
  Huntington's disease, 509–510
  progressive supranuclear palsy and, 283–284
Cerebral palsy, 668
Cerebral toxoplasmosis, 737
Ceroid lipofuscinosis, 457*t*, 465
Ceruletide, tardive dyskinesia treatment with, 523
Ceruloplasmin, 623–624, 628
Ceruloplasmin deficiency, 624
Cervical dystonia, 432–433
  botulinum treatment, 449–450, 449*t*
  surgical treatment, 451

Cervical lipomas, 56*f*
Check, 580–581
Cherry-red-spot myoclonus syndrome, 545
Childhood movement disorders, 661
  akathisia, 669
  ataxia, 667–668, 668*t*
  chorea, 665–667, 665*t*
  classification, 662*t*, 663–667, 663*t*-667*t*
  dystonia, 419–426, 664–665, 665*t*, 735*t*
  idiopathic torsion dystonia, 419–424, 420*t*, 421*t*, 426*t*
  juvenile Parkinson's disease, 272–273, 667
  myoclonus, 667
  parkinsonism, 11
  paroxysmal movement disorder, 668–669
  postpump chorea, 531–532
  psychiatric problems associated with, 669–670
  spasticity, 667–668
  tics, 663, 663*t*
  tremor, 663–664, 664*t*
Chlordiazepoxide, dystonia treatment with, 445*t*
Chlordecone, tremors induced by, 392–393
Chlorpromazine
  tardive dystonia induced by, 467
  tremor induced by, 390
Cholecystokinin-8 (CCK-8), Parkinson's disease and, 157
Choline acetyltransferase, Parkinson's disease, 157
Cholinergic drugs, progressive supranuclear palsy, 289
Cholinesterase inhibitors, tremors induced by, 328, 393
Chorea, 78, 527, 532*t*, 533*t*, 534, 655
  antiphospholipid antibody syndrome, 528
  benign hereditary chorea, 41, 529–530
  causes, 7, 7t
  childhood, 665–667, 665*t*
  chorea gravidarum, 528, 739
  dentatorubropallidoluysian atrophy, 530
  differential diagnosis, 666*t*
    from myoclonus, 541
    from tics, 565
  drug-induced, 532, 532*t*
  etiology, 532t-533t
  hemiballismus, 530
  hemichorea, 530, 734
  Huntington's disease. *See* Huntington's disease
  hyperglycemia and, 734
  hyperthyroidism and, 531, 733
  immune-mediated mechanism, 528
  mastocytosis and, 736
  metabolic disorders and, 531
  multiple sclerosis and, 531
  neuroacanthocytosis, 529
  neuroimaging, 41–43
  painful legs and moving toes, 534
  paroxysmal dyskinesia and, 532, 534
  polycythemia vera and, 531, 736
  postpump chorea and, 531
  psychogenic chorea, 726
  senile chorea, 530
  Sydenham's chorea, 42, 527–528, 665, 736
  systemic lupus erythematosus, 528
  tardive chorea, 7

vascular chorea, 530
Wilson's disease, 625
Chorea gravidarum, 528, 739
Chorea minor. *See* Sydenham's chorea
Choreoacanthocytosis. *See* Neuroacanthocytosis
Choreoathetosis, 527
Choreoathetotic dyskinesia, difference from tardive
    dyskinesia, 10
Choreoballism, 7
Chronic motor tics, 572
Chronic progressive external ophthalmoplegia, 63, 72
Chronic sensorimotor neuropathy, 395
Chronic tic disorder, 9
Cigarette, Parkinson's disease and, 171–172
Ciliary neurotrophic factor. *See* CNTF
Cingulate motor areas, anatomy, 77
Cinnarizine
    parkinsonism induced by, 328
    tremor induced by, 391
Clonazepam
    cerebellar disorder treatment, 581
    dystonia treatment with, 445, 445t
    essential tremor treatment with, 378
    myoclonus treatment with, 549
    stiff person syndrome, 646
    tremor treatment with, 412
Clonic tics, 9, 561
Clonidine, essential tremor treatment with, 378
Clozapine, 191–192, 215, 215t
    dystonia treatment with, 444
    essential tremor treatment with, 379
    Huntington's disease, 497
    parkinsonism induced by, 325
CNTF, 120
Cock walk, manganese-induced parkinsonism, 317
Coenzyme Q10, 66, 498
Coffee, tremor induced by, 389
Cognitive dysfunction, 612
    differential diagnosis, 616–617, 618t
    gait disorder, 657
    in Huntington's disease, 493
    L-dopa related, 191–192
    movement disorders and, 21–23
    multiple-system atrophy, 301
    in Parkinson's disease, 21, 22, 187, 191–192, 226
Cognitive functions, control by cerebellum, 577–578
Cogwheeling
    in the elderly, 675
    Parkinson's disease, 185, 189
Complex I, 51, 52, 158
    chemical structure, 164, 165
    inhibition by pesticides, 171
    MPP+, 163, 164
    neuroleptic medications, 61
    Parkinson's disease and, 165–166, 171, 174
Complex II, 51, 52, 164
Complex III, 51, 52, 164
Complex IV, 51, 52
Complex motor tics, 9, 569
Complex vocal tics, 9, 569

Compulsions
    movement disorders and, 19
Computed tomography
    cerebellar disorders, 582t
    corticobasal degeneration, 613
    DDPAC, 332
    familial L-dopa-resonsive parkinsonian-pyramidal
        syndrome, 340
    Hallervorden-Spatz disease, 333
    hemiparkinsonism-hemiatrophy syndrome, 335
    Huntington's disease, 495
    multiple-system atrophy, 301
    neuroacanthocytosis, 338
    pallidal degeneration, 340
    Parkinson's disease, 189
    progressive supranuclear palsy, 281–282
    Wilson's disease, 628
    x-linked dystonia-parkinsonism syndrome, 337
COMT, 154, 155
COMT inhibitors, 201, 205, 206t
Constipation
    in multiple-system atrophy, 300, 300t
    in Parkinson's disease, 188
Convergence of information, in basal ganglia, 88–89
Conversion disorders, 716, 717t
Copper, metabolism, 624
Copper chelation therapy, Wilson's disease, 630
Copper toxicity
    dystonia and, 467
Copper-zinc superoxide dismutase, 169
Copropraxia, 9
Core Assessment Protocol for Intracerebral
        Transplantation (CAPIT), 226
Corollary discharge, 75
Corpus striatum, Parkinson's disease and, 267
Cortical atrophy, Huntington's disease, 509
Cortical-basal ganglionic degeneration. *See also*
        Corticobasal degeneration
    magnetic resonance imaging, 283t
    myoclonus and, 546
    persistent asymmetry, 191
    tremor, 189–190
Cortical dysfunction, encephalitis lethargica, 307
Cortical Lewy body, dementia, 23, 24–25
Cortical motor areas, anatomy, 73–77
Cortical motor fields, 73, 74, 74f, 75
Cortical myoclonus, 6–7, 543–544, 547, 549, 552
Cortical reflex myoclonus, 552, 553, 554
Cortical-subcortical dementia, 23
Cortical tremor, 389, 413
Corticobasal degeneration, 11, 611, 618
    alien limb, 9
    clinical features, 611–613, 612t, 618t
    differential diagnosis, from multiple-system atrophy, 304
    disordered praxis, 23
    dystonia in, 461
    neuroimaging, 12t, 39, 39t, 613–614, 613f, 614f
    neuropathology, 126, 130–131, 614–616, 614f–616f
    visuospatial disturbance, 23
Corticospinal system, anatomy, 74–75

CPEO plus, 63
Cranial dystonia, encephalitis lethargica, 308
C-reflex, myoclonus, 557, 558
Creutzfeldt-Jakob disease
    apraxia, 23
    clinical signs, 618t
    dementia, 190, 191
    myoclonus and, 547
    neuropathology, 129f
    parkinsonism associated with, 311
    progression, 190–191
    sleep in, 699
    speech disorders, 22
Crossed cerebellar diaschisis, 603–604
Cyanide-induced parkinsonism, 319
Cyclobenzaprine, dystonia treatment with, 445t
Cyclosporine-A, tremor induced by, 391
CYP2D6 alleles, Parkinson's disease and, 148, 173

D

D1 receptors, 156, 201, 202, 202t
D2 receptors, 156, 201, 202, 202t
D3 receptors, 202t
D4 receptors, 202t
D5 receptors, 202t
Dantrolene, neuroleptic malignant syndrome, 349
DDPAC. See Disinhibition-dementia-parkinsonism-
        amyotrophy complex
DDT, tremors induced by, 393
Debrisoquine, Parkinson's disease and, 147–148, 173
Declarative memory, 22
Decomposition of movement, 580, 591, 593
Deep brain stimulation, movement disorder therapy, 251–
        252, 380
Dementia
    Alzheimer's disease, 23, 24, 187, 190
    in Creutzfeldt-Jakob disease, 190, 191
    cortical-subcortical, 23
    defined, 23
    dementia pugilistica, 346
    differential diagnosis, 190–191
    in the elderly, 679
    gait disorder, 657
    Huntington's disease, 23–24
    with Lewy bodies. See Diffuse Lewy body disease, Lewy
        body dementia
    movement disorders and, 23–25, 24t
    multiple-system atrophy, 25
    olivopontocerebellar atrophy, 25
    Parkinson's disease, 23, 24–25, 187, 190
    progressive myoclonic encephalopathy with, 545, 546
    progressive supranuclear palsy, 24, 190
        kindred evaluations, 352–353
    subcortical, 23
    Wilson's disease, 625
Dementia pugilistica, 346
Dentatorubropallidoluysian atrophy, 41, 42, 456t, 463, 486,
        494, 530, 545

Deprenyl, 210, 259
Depression
    Huntington's disease, 17, 497
    movement disorders and, 16–18, 17t
    Parkinson's disease, 16, 17, 187, 257
    progressive supranuclear palsy, 353
    Wilson's disease, 17–18, 625
Desipramine, progressive supranuclear palsy, 289
Dextromethorphan, Huntington's disease, 498
Diabetes mellitus
    movement disorders secondary to, 734
    MTTL1*MELAS3243G mutation, 63
    stiff person syndrome and, 640, 642
Diaschisis, 603
Diazepam
    dystonia treatment with, 445t
    essential tremor treatment with, 378
    parkinsonism induced by, 328
    stiff person syndrome treatment with, 646
Diencephalon, Huntington's disease, 508–509
Diffuse Lewy body disease, 32–33, 61, 335–336
    clinical features, 619t
    neurobehavioral changes, 336
    neuropathology, 128–129, 335
Dilapidation in cognition, defined, 23
Dimercaprol, Wilson's disease therapy, 631
Dioxin, tremors induced by, 393
Diphasic dyskinesia, L-dopa related, 204
Diphenhydramine, dystonia treatment with, 444–445, 445t
Disinhibition-dementia-parkinsonism-amyotrophy complex
        (DDPAC), 331–332
Disordered praxis, 23
DNA, oxidative damage, 170–171
Domperidone, with L-dopa, 204
Dopamine
    basal ganglia and, 87, 100–104, 103t
    behavioral state control and, 701–702
    free radical formation, 170
    free radicals derived from, 170
    metabolism, 153–155, 154f
    Parkinson's disease, 153
    role of, 80
Dopamine agonists
    clinical pharmacology, 206–207, 206t
    experimental, 207–208
    Hallervorden-Spatz disease, 333
    idiopathic Parkinson's disease, 213
    side effects, 207
Dopamine receptor-blocking drugs, tremor induced by,
        390
Dopamine receptors
    function, 154
    molecular diversity, 101–104, 103t
    Parkinson's disease, 158
    pharmacology, 101, 201–202, 202f, 202t
    subtypes, 103t
Dopaminergic drugs
    dystonia treatment with, 443–444
    Parkinson's disease treatment with, 212
    progressive supranuclear palsy treatment with, 288–289

Dopaminergic system
  idiopathic torsion dystonia and, 41
  Parkinson's disease and, 34
Dopamine storage and transport inhibitors, parkinsonism
      induced by, 327–328
Dopamine system, Parkinson's disease, 37
Dopa-responsive dystonia (DRD), 5, 41, 270, 425–426, 426t,
      443, 444
Dorsal premotor area (PMd), 76
Dorsolateral prefrontal circuit, of the brain, 15, 16f
Dorsolateral prefrontal syndrome, 15
Downgaze palsy
  multiple-system atrophy, 300
  progressive supranuclear palsy, 286, 290
Downgaze paresis, 187, 189
DRD gene, 426
Dreaming, Parkinson's disease, 258–259, 260
Drooling
  Parkinson's disease, 187
  postencephalitic parkinsonism, 310
  Wilson's disease, 625
Drug-induced parkinsonism, 328, 328t, 679
  amiodarone, 329
  calcium channel blockers, 328
  cholinergic drugs, 328
  diazepam, 328
  dopamine storage and transport inhibitors, 327–328
  lithium, 328
  neuroleptics, 325–327, 326t
Dysarthria, 589, 602–603
  ataxic, 581
  Huntington's disease, 493
  multiple-system atrophy, 300
  pathophysiology, 578
  progressive supranuclear palsy, 286
  Wilson's disease, 625
Dysarthric speech, 22
Dysautonomia, progressive supranuclear palsy, 286
Dysdiadochokinesia, 589, 589f, 591, 592
Dysdiadochokinesis, 580
Dyskinesia
  childhood, 663
  differential diagnosis, 565
  drug-induced, 92–93
  interdose choreic, 214
  L-dopa-related, 191, 204–205, 214
  management, 214
  multiple-system atrophy, 299
  Parkinson's disease, 191, 204–205
  paroxysmal, 8, 532, 534
  tardive dyskinesia. See Tardive dyskinesia
Dysmetria, 580, 587, 588f, 591, 592, 600, 603, 608
Dysphagia
  dystonia, 434
  in Huntington's disease, 493
  Parkinson's disease, 187
  progressive supranuclear palsy, 286, 290
Dysphonia
  abductor spasmodic dysphonia, 398
  adductor spasmodic dysphonia, 398

whispering dysphonia, 625
Dysrhythmokinesis, 580
Dysynergia, 7, 580
Dystonia, 4–5, 655
  acquired dystonia, 31
  action dystonia, 31
  autoimmunity and, 434–435
  blepharospasm, 431, 432f, 434, 437
  brain and, 445, 457–459, 459t
  basal ganglion and, 436, 457, 458, 462
  causes, 5, 459
  cerebral toxoplasmosis, 737
  cervical dystonia, 432–433, 449–451, 449t
  in childhood, 419–426, 664–665, 665t, 735t
  classification, 665t
  cranial dystonia, 308
  differential diagnosis, 456t–457t, 541t, 665t
  diurnal pattern, 5
  dopa-resistant. See Dopa-resistant dystonia
  dopa-responsive, 5, 41, 270
  dysphagia in, 434
  in the elderly, 674
  familial paroxysmal dystonial, 8
  foot, 465f, 469f
  following stroke, 680–681
  genetics, 423–425, 434
  hemidystonia, 5, 457
  Huntington's disease, 492
  idiopathic torsion dystonia. See Idiopathic torsion
      dystonia
  laryngeal dystonia, 432, 437, 449
  limb dystonia, 433, 450, 497
  mitochondrial mutation and, 58–59
  movements of, 5
  multifocal dystonia, 5
  multiple-system atrophy, 461
  myoclonic dystonia, 5, 541, 543, 545
  neuroimaging, 31, 39–41, 435, 458
  nocturnal paroxysmal dystonia, 8, 690
  oculofaciocervical dystonia, 460
  off-period, 191
  oromandibular dystonia, 431–432, 434, 435, 437, 448–449
  OXPHOS defects, 58
  paroxysmal dystonia, 8, 445, 734
  pathophysiology, 93, 242–243
  postural tremor, 372
  progressive supranuclear palsy, kindred evaluations,
      353, 359
  psychogenic, 5, 437, 468, 720–724, 721t-723t
  pseudodystonia, 468–469
  rapid-onset dystonia-parkinsonism, 429
  relation to activity, 5
  segmental dystonia, 5
  spasmodic dysphonia, 432, 436, 436f
  stroke-induced dystonia, 680–681
  surgical treatment
    pallidotomy, 238
    stereotaxic surgery, 246–247, 248–250
    thalamotomy, 238
  symptomatic, 5, 455

Dystonia, symptomatic (*Cont.*)
    ataxia telangiectasia, 463–464
    calcification of basal ganglia, 462
    ceroid lipofuscinosis, 465
    chemical agent-induced, 467–468, 468t
    corticobasal degeneration, 461
    dentatorubropallidoluysian atrophy, 463
    focal brain lesions and, 455, 457–459
    fumarase deficiency, 466–467
    gangliosidosis, 464–465
    glutaric aciduria, 466
    Hallervorden-Spatz disease, 462
    Hartnup disease, 467
    homocystinuria, 467
    Huntington's disease, 461
    intraneuronal inclusion disease, 463
    Leigh's syndrome, 466
    Lesch-Nyhan syndrome, 467
    Machado-Joseph disease, 463
    metachromatic leukodystrophy, 465
    methylmalonic aciduria, 466
    mitochondrial encephalomyopathies, 465–466
    neuroacanthocytosis, 461
    Niemann-Pick disease, 465
    of organic origin, 468–469
    pallidal atrophy, 462–463
    Parkinson's disease, 460
    peripheral injury and, 459–460
    Pilizaeus-Merzbacher disease, 465
    progressive supranuclear palsy, 460–461
    psychogenic, 468, 720–724
    Rett syndrome, 463
    Seitelberger's disease, 462
    trauma-induced, 467
    Wilson's disease, 351
    Wolfram's syndrome, 464
    xeroderma pigmentosum, 464
  tardive dystonia, 467
  torsion dystonia, 425t
  treatment, 443, 444t, 452
    botulinum toxin, 445t, 445–447, 446t, 447t, 448–450, 523
    pharmacological, 443–445, 445t
    suppression of spasm, 5
    surgical, 451–452
  tremor of, 421–422, 450–451, 461, 462f
  types, 5
  Wilson's disease, 461, 462f, 625
  writer's cramp, 433
Dystonia at rest, 5
Dystonia musculorum deformans, 419, 423
Dystonic tics, 9, 565, 571
Dystonic tremor, 5, 389, 412–413, 431
DYT1 gene, 424–425, 429

E

Early morning dystonia, L-dopa, 191, 204–205
Echolalia, 9, 22

Echopraxia, 9
Economo's encephalitis, 161, 307
Ekbom's syndrome, 9
Edema, in Parkinson's disease, 188
Efaroxan, progressive supranuclear palsy, 289
EGF, 120–121
Elderly
  Alzheimer's disease. *See* Alzheimer's disease
  balance, 676
  bradykinesia, 673
  cautious gait, 658
  dementia in, 679
  essential tremor in, 679–680
  gait abnormality, 658, 676, 677t
  gait apraxia, 676, 677t
  hyperkinesia, 675
  muscle tone in, 673–675, 674t
  ophthalmoplegia, 676–677
  parkinsonism, 677t, 678–679, 681
  posture, 675–676, 677t
  reflexes, 674, 674t, 675t, 677–678
  senile chorea, 530
  senile gait, 675
  senile tremor, 6
  spontaneous orofacial dyskinesia, 681
  station, 675
  stroke. *See* Stroke
  treatment for, 682
  visual disorders, 651t, 653
Electroconvulsive therapy
  neuroleptic malignant syndrome, 349
  progressive supranuclear palsy, 290
  tardive dyskinesia treatment with, 523
Electroencephalogram (EEG)
  corticobasal degeneration, 613
  myoclonus, 551, 552, 555–556, 556f, 558
Electromyogram (EMG)
  asterixis, 558f
  cerebellar disorders, 591
  corticobasal degeneration, 613
  dystonia, 5
  hemifacial spasm, 10
  multiple-system atrophy, 302
  myoclonus, 542, 542f, 543f, 551, 552, 554–555, 554f, 555f, 558
  orthostatic tremor, 412
  stiff-person syndrome, 641, 641f
Electrophysiological tests, 4t
En bloc gait, 652
Encephalitis, movement disorders secondary to, 161, 747
Encephalitis lethargica, 307–308, 310
Encephalopathy, myoclonic, 545–548
Endocrine disorders, movement disorders secondary to, 733–734
End-of-dose dyskinesia, 191
Enhanced physiological tremor, 6
Entacapone, 205
Epidermal growth factor. *See* EGF
Epilepsia partialis continua, 547
Epilepsia partialis continua, 7

Epilepsy
  myoclonus, 6–7, 552–553
  progressive myoclonic encephalopathy with, 545, 546
  stiff person syndrome and, 642
Epileptic myoclonus, 6–7, 552–553
Erythrocytes, neuroacanthocytosis, 529
Essential myoclonus, 544–545, 553
Essential palatal tremor, 548, 553
Essential tremor, 6, 365–380, 407–409, 588. *See also* Tremor
  alcoholism, 735
  assessment, 374–375
  associated conditions, 371–373
  benign, 664
  classification, 368
  clinical manifestations, 368–371
  clinical variants, 370–371
  defined, 387
  in the elderly, 679–680
  epidemiology, 365–367, 366*t*
  familial, 365
  genetics, 367–368
  handwriting, 368, 373, 375
  history, 365
  orthostatic tremor different from, 393*t*
  Parkinson's disease, 189
  pathophysiology, 243 244, 373–374, 407–409, 408*f*
  progression, 369
  stereotaxic surgery for, 238, 247, 248–250
  treatment, 375–380
Estrogens, chorea following use, 528
Exaggerated startle, 553
Excitotoxicity, Huntington's disease, 511
Executive function
  defined, 21
  dementia, 23
  movement disorders and, 21–22
  progressive supranuclear palsy and, 284
External pallidum, anatomy, 79, 87
Extracellular superoxide dismutase, 169
Extraocular movement disturbances, 580
Extrapyramidal myoclonus, 551
Eye blinking, in Parkinson's disease, 187
Eyelid movement, progressive supranuclear palsy, 286
Eye movement abnormalities, 612, 653
  in Huntington's disease, 493
  progressive supranuclear palsy, kindred evaluations, 359
  Wilson's disease, 627

F

Facial akinesia, in Parkinson's disease, 187
Facial myoclonus, 548
Factitious disorders, 716, 717t
Fahr's disease, 63, 64*f*, 348, 456t
Familial amyotrophic chorea. *See* Neuroacanthocytosis
Familial L-dopa-resonsive parkinsonian-pyramidal
      syndrome, 340–341
Familial Lewy body dementia, 272

Familial parkinsonism, 144t–147, 270–272, 271*t*
  with apathy and central hypoventilation, 270–271
  ballooned neurons, 272
  dopa-responsive dystonia, 270
  genetics, 143–145, 144*t*, 145*t*, 173
  kindred evaluations, 351, 352, 360
  L-dopa-responsive parkinsonian-pyramidal syndrome,
      340–341
  Lewy body negative parkinsonism, 271–272
  Lewy body parkinsonism, 271
  mitochondrial inheritance and, 147
  neurofibrillary tangle, 272
  susceptibility genes
Familial paroxysmal dystonia, 8
Familial progressive supranuclear palsy, 288t
  kindred evaluations, 351, 352–353, 353t–357t, 359–360
Familial tremor, 588
Fastigial nucleus, 595
Fear of falling gait, 658
Feet, deformed, in Parkinson's disease, 188
Ferritin, Parkinson's disease, 269
Festinating gait, Parkinson's disease, 186
Fetal nigral transplantation, 36–37, 221–232
  clinical issues
    clinical evaluation, 226 227
    immunosuppression, 225–226
    infectious disease issues, 225
    L-dopa use, 227
    patient selection, 225
  future directions, 230–232, 231*f*
  neuroanatomic issues, 229–230
  outcomes, 227–229, 227*t*
  preclinical issues, 222
    donor age, 222–223
    site of implant, 223–224, 224*f*
    tissue acquisition, 222
    tissue distribution, 224–225
    tissue storage, 223, 223*f*
    volume of tissue, 24
FGF-1, 120
FGF-2, 120
Fibroblast growth factors, 120
Flocculonodular lesions, 655
Flocculonodular lobe, 578, 596, 598–599
Flocculonodular syndrome, 599
Flocculus, 602, 603
Flunarizine
  essential tremor treatment with, 379
  parkinsonism induced by, 328
  tremor induced by, 391
Fluoxetine
  Huntington's disease, 497
  parkinsonism induced by, 328
  progressive supranuclear palsy, 289
Fluphenazine, tic treatment, 573
Flycatcher tongue, 7–8
Focal dystonia. *See* Idiopathic adult-onset focal dystonia
Focal myoclonus, 547, 549
"Focusing" hypothesis, for basal ganglial function, 89
Foods, tremor induced by, 389–390

Force production, 651t, 654
Fragmentary nocturnal myoclonus, Parkinson's disease, 697
Fragmentary NREM myoclonus, 690, 691
Free radicals, 158, 168–170
Free-radical scavengers, 158, 210, 498
Freezing, 657
    L-dopa and, 221
    Parkinson's disease, 186–187, 191
    progressive supranuclear palsy and, 284
Frontal lesions, 656
Frontal subcortical circuits, of the brain, 15–16, 16f
Fumarase deficiency, 466–467
Fungal infection, parkinsonism associated with, 311

G

GABA. *See* Gamma-aminobutyric acid
Gait apraxia, in the elderly, 675
Gait disorder, 590, 649, 658
    ambulation components, 649–650, 650t
    attention impairment and, 657–658
    cautious gait, 658
    cerebellar origin, 579
    clinical features, 650, 651t, 652–653
    corticobasal degeneration, 611, 612
    dementia and, 657
    dopa-resonsive dystonia, 426
    in the elderly, 675, 677t
    fear of falling, 658
    force production and scaling, 654–656
    Hallervorden-Spatz disease, 333
    manganese-induced parkinsonism, 317
    normal pressure hydrocephalus, 347
    orientation, 653–654
    Parkinson's disease, 186–187, 189
    progressive supranuclear palsy, 279
    psychogenic, 728–729, 728t
    synergies, 656–657
    vestibular function, distorted, 652
    Wilson's disease, 625
Gallyas silver stain, 126
Gamma-aminobutyric acid (GABA)
    dystonia treatment with, 445, 445t
    essential tremor treatment with, 379
    Parkinson's disease and, 157
Gamma motor neurons, 593
Gamma motor system, 591, 593–594
Gangliosidosis, 456t, 464–465
GDNF, 117–118
    fetal grafts and, 230, 231
    Parkinson's disease and, 174
Gender
    Parkinson's disease, 139, 140t
    progressive supranuclear palsy, 287
Generalized dystonia, 5
Genetics
    adult-onset dystonia, 434
    dentatorubropallidoluysian atrophy (DRPLA), 486
    dopamine receptors, 201

essential tremor, 367, 369
Hallervorden-Spatz disease, 332
Huntington's disease, 503
    CAG repeat, 481–484, 481f–483f, 485–487, 491–492
    familial studies, 477–478, 478f
    genetic mapping, 478–480, 479f
    genetic markers, 480
    HD defect, 480–481, 481f, 484–485
    HD gene, 479, 484, 491
    huntingtin protein, 484–485, 491, 512–514
    idiopathic adult-onset focal dystonia, 434
    idiopathic torsion dystonia, 423–425
    Kennedy's disease, 485
    kindred evaluations, 351–353, 353t-359t, 359–360
    Machado-Joseph disease, 485–486
    mitochondrial DNA, 51–61, 165, 170, 173
    mutations, 61–62
    neuroacanthocytosis, 337
    Parkinson's disease, 143–148, 144t, 145t, 147t
        familial PD, 143–147, 144t, 145t, 173
        mitochondrial inheritance, 147
        predisposition, 172–173
        susceptibility gene, 147–148
        twin studies, 146–147, 147t
    postencephalitic parkinsonism, 309
    progressive supranuclear palsy, 360
    Rett syndrome, 341
    spinal bulbar muscular atrophy, 485
    spinocerebellar ataxia type, 1, 485
    susceptibility genes, 147–148
    Tourette's syndrome, 572, 573
    Wilson's disease, 623
    x-linked dystonia-parkinsonism syndrome, 336
Genetic testing, 12
    Huntington's disease, 486–487, 496, 666
    for myoclonic epilepsy and ragged-red fiber disease, 57
    OXPHOS diseases, 66
Giant SEPs, myoclonus, 552, 552f, 556
Glabellar reflex, 187, 677
Glial cell line-derived neurotrophic factor. *See* GDNF
Glial cytoplasmic inclusion (GCI), 302–303
Globus pallidus
    anatomy, 153
    biochemistry of, 99–100, 100f
    Huntington's disease, 507–508, *508*
    Parkinson's disease and, 33–34
Glucose, cerebral utilization in PD, 158
Glutamate, 153
    basal ganglia function and, 99, 107–111
    toxicity, 173
Glutamate antagonists, Parkinson's disease, 209–210
Glutamate receptors, 108f, 109f, 110t, 173
Glutamic acid decarboxylase, Parkinson's disease and, 157
Glutamine, Parkinson's disease and, 110–111
Glutamate toxicity, 173–174
Glutaric aciduria, 457t, 466
Glutathione
    free radical scavenging, 158
    molecular structure, 169, 169f
    in Parkinson's disease, 169–170, 169f

Glutathione peroxidase, 158
GM1 gangliosidosis, 456t, 464
GM2 gangliosidosis, 456t, 464–465
Golgi cell, 600
Granule cell, 600
Grumose degeneration, progressive supranuclear palsy and, 283
Guam parkinsonism-dementia complex. *See* Parkinson-dementia/ALS complex of Guam
GYKI52466, 109

H

Haber-Weiss reaction, 168f, 170
Hallervorden-Spatz disease, 332–333
    in childhood, 665
    dementia, 25
    differential diagnosis, 189, 456t
    dystonia in, 462
    genetics, 332
    neuroimaging, 333–334
    neuropathology, 126, 332–333
Hallucinations
    ʟ-dopa, 191, 259
    Parkinson's disease, 191, 259–260
Haloperidol, 521, 528, 573
Hands, deformed, in Parkinson's disease, 188
Harmaline, tremor and, 391
Hartnup disease, 457t, 467
HD gene, 479–484, 491
Head, rotated or tilted postures, 579
Head banging, 690
Head injury, tremor associated with, 397
Head rolling, 669
Heavy metals, tremors induced by, 392
Hematoma, parkinsonism induced by, 348
Hemiballism, 7, 527, 530
    basal ganglia and, 92
    diabetes and, 734
    following stroke, 680
    pathophysiology, 244
    sleep in, 700
    stereotaxic surgery for, 248–250
Hemichorea, 530, 734
Hemidystonia, 5, 457
Hemifacial spasm, 10
    botulinum treatment of, 450
    differential diagnosis, 541
    sleep in, 699
Hemiparkinsonism, depression and, 17
Hemiparkinsonism-hemiatrophy (HPHA), 191, 334–335
Hemiplegia, 668
Hemolytic uremic syndrome, movement disorders secondary to, 738
Herbicides, tremors induced by, 392–393
Hereditary essential myoclonus, 544, 545
Hereditary motor sensory neuropathy, type I, 394
Herpex simplex virus, Parkinson's disease and, 161

Hippocampus, progressive supranuclear palsy and and, 284
Histrionic personality disorder, 716, 717t
HIV-1, movement disorders secondary to, 737
Hodgkin's disease, movement disorders secondary to, 739–740
Hoehn and Yahr staging scale, 192
Holmes, Gordon, 588f
Homocystinuria, 457t, 467, 735–736
Homovanillic acid, 154, 155, 733
Huntingtin protein, 484–485, 491, 512–514, 513f
    mutant, 513–514
    transcription, 512–513
Huntington's disease, 3, 54, 491–492
    anxiety and, 20
    brain and, 503–511
    apathy and, 19
    basal ganglia and, 92
    in childhood, 666
    clinical features, 492–494, 492f
    cognitive disturbance, 21
    dementia, 23–24
    depression and, 17, 497
    diagnosis, 494–496
    differential diagnosis, 456t
    dorsolateral prefrontal syndrome, 15
    dysarthria, 493
    dystonia in, 461, 492
    epidemiology, 477, 491
    executive function, 21
    genetics, 477–487, 503
        CAG repeat, 481–484, 481f–483f, 485–487, 491–492
        familial studies, 477–478, 478f
        genetic mapping, 478–480, 479
        genetic markers, 480
        HD defect, 480–481, 481f, 484–485
        HD gene, 479, 484, 491
        huntingtin protein, 484–485, 491, 512–514
    genetic testing, 486–487, 496, 666
    history, 477
    lateral orbitofrontal circuit, 16
    mania and, 18
    memory impairment and, 22
    neurobehavioral changes, 16, 19, 493, 494
    myoclonus and, 546
    neuroimaging, 12t, 41–43, 495–496
    neuropathology, 126, 503–511
    obsessive-compulsive disorder and, 20
    OXPHOS dysfunction and, 54
    pathophysiology, 511–512, 512f
    personality changes, 16, 19, 494, 497
    progressive functional decline, 494, 495t
    psychosis, 18, 19
    sexual disturbance and, 21, 494
    sleep in, 699
    speech disorders, 22
    suicide and, 17, 493
    support organizations, 497t
    treatment, 496–498
    visuospatial dysfunction, 23

Hydrocephalic parkinsonism, 190
8-hydroxydeoxyguanosine, in mitochondrial DNA, 170–171, 171*f*
Hydroxyl radicals, 168
5-hydroxytryptamine (5-HT), Parkinson's disease psychosis and, 260
5-hydroxytryptophan (5-HTP)
  cerebellar disorder treatment with, 591
  myoclonus treatment with, 547, 549
Hyperekplexia, 10, 548, 565, 667
Hyperglycemia, chorea and, 734
Hyperkinesia, defined, 3
  in the elderly, 675
Hyperkinetic movement disorders, 655
  basal ganglia and, 92–93
  in the elderly, 675
  hyperthyrodism and, 733
  pathophysiology, 239–244, 239*f*–241*f*, 243
  types, 3–10
Hypermetria, 580, 587
Hypersexuality, movement disorders and, 21
Hypersomnia, 20
Hyperthyroidism, chorea and, 531
Hypobetalipoproteinemia, 337
Hypokinesia
  defined, 3
  in the elderly, 673
Hypokinetic movement disorders, 10–11
  aging and, 674*t*
  basal ganglia and, 90–92
  pathophysiology, 239–244, 239*f*–241*f*, 243*f*
Hypomania, movement disorders and, 18, 18*t*
Hypometria, 580, 587
Hypoparathyroidism
  movement disorders and, 734
  parkinsonism and, 348
Hyposexuality, movement disorders and, 21
Hypotension, Parkinson's disease, 188, 192
Hypothalamus, Huntington's disease, 509
Hypothyroidism, movement disorders secondary to, 733–734
Hypotonia, 300, 581, 589–590
Hypoxanthine-guanine phosphoribosyltransferase (HGPRT), 467
Hysteria, 715, 716

I

Idazoxan, progressive supranuclear palsy, 289
Ideational apraxia, defined, 23
Ideomotor apraxia, defined, 23
Idiopathic adult-onset focal dystonia, 5, 429
  blepharospasm, 431, 432*f*, 434–437
  cervical dystonia, 432–433
  clinical features, 429–434, 430t, 431*t*
  differential diagnosis, 436–438
  epidemiology, 429
  etiology, 434–435
  genetics, 434

laryngeal dystonia, 432, 437, 449
limb dystonia, 433, 450, 457
oromandibular dystonia, 431–432, 434, 435, 437, 448–449
pathophysiology, 435–436, 436*f*
spasmodic dysphonia, 432, 436, 436*f*, 449, 452
writer's cramp, 433, 445
Idiopathic calcification of the basal ganglia, 25
  behavioral changes in, 16, 18
  dementia, 25
  psychosis and, 18
Idiopathic dystonia, neuroimaging, 31
Idiopathic parkinsonism, 11
  clinical signs, 351
  dystonia associated with, 5
  exclusion criteria, 11*t*
  kindred evaluations, 351, 352, 360
  neuroimaging, 12*t*
  psychosis and, 18
Idiopathic Parkinson's disease
  Lewy bodies, 127
  neuroimaging, 31
  neuropathology, 127–128
  neuroprotective drugs for, 210–215
  OXPHOS defects, 61
Idiopathic torsion dystonia, 3, 5, 368, 419
  adult onset. *See* Idiopathic adult-onset focal dystonia
  age and, 419, 421*t*
  childhood onset
    bochemistry, 422–423
    clinical features, 419–422, 420*t*, 421*t*, 430*t*
    dopa-resonsive dystonia as variant, 425–426, 426*t*
    epidemiology, 422
    evaluation, 425
    genetics, 423–425
    pathology, 422
  neuroimaging, 12*t*, 39–41
Immunohistochemistry, movement disorders and, 126, 128
Immunosuppression
  fetal nigral transplantation and, 225–226
  stiff person syndrome treatment with, 647
  tremor induced by, 391
Impotence, multiple-system atrophy, 299
Incertohypothalamic system, 155
Incidental Lewy body disease, 171
Infantile neuroaxonal dystrophy (INAD), dystonia in, 462
Infantile neuropathic Gauchers disease, 545
Infectious diseases, 307–311, 311*f*
  fetal nigral transplantation screening, 225
  movement disorders secondary to, 736
  postencephalitic parkinsonism 18–21
Influenza virus, Parkinson's disease and, 161
Initiation of movement, 88
Insecticides, tremors induced by, 392–393
Insomnia, 695–697. *See also* Sleep
  Huntington's disease, 494
  movement disorders and, 20, 21
Insulin, 121
Insulin-dependent diabetes mellitus
  MTTL1*MELAS3243G mutation, 63
  stiff person syndrome and, 640, 642

Intentional tremor, 387
Intention tremor, 6, 410, 581, 589
    stereotaxic surgery for, 238, 247, 248–250
Internal pallidum, anatomy, 79
Interneurons, Huntington's disease, 505
Interpositus nucleus, 595
Interstitial nucleus of Cajal, 653–654
Intraneuronal inclusion disease
    differential diagnosis, 456*t*
    dystonia in, 463
Intravenous immunoglobulin, stiff person syndrome
        treatment with, 647
Iron
    accumulation in Hallervorden-Spatz disease, 332–333
    Parkinson's disease and, 170, 269–270
Iron-sulfur clusters, 164–165
Iron-transferrin complex, 170
Isoniazid, cerebellar disorder treatment, 581
Isotributyline, tremor induced by, 390

J

Jactatio capitis nocturna, 690
Jumping Frenchmen of Maine, 10, 565
Juvenile Parkinson's disease, 272–273, 667

K

Kayser-Fleischer ring, 626–627, 626*f*
Kearns-Sayre syndrome, 63, 72
Kelley-Seegmiller syndrome, 467
Kennedy's disease, genetics, 485
Kepone, tremors induced by, 392–393
Kernicterus, 666, 735
Kindred evaluations, 351–353, 353*t*, 359–360
Kinesia paradoxica, Parkinson's disease, 187, 191
Kinetic tremor, 189, 368, 387, 581, 589, 591
Kufs' disease, 457, 545
Kwashkiorkor, movement disorders secondary to, 735
Kyphosis, in Parkinson's disease, 188

L

L-AAAD, 153
Laboratory tests, 4*t*
Lafora's disease, 545
Lamotrigine, Huntington's disease, 498
Lance-Adams syndrome, 7
Language disorders, movement disorders and, 22
Large neutral amino acid (LNAA) transport system, 203
Laryngeal dystonia, 432, 437, 449
Laryngeal nerve section, 452
Lateral orbitofrontal circuit, of the brain, 15–16, 16*f*
Lateral premotor areas, anatomy, 76
Lateral zone, 601*t*, 602

Lazabemide, 209
L-dopa, 153, 155
    carbon disulfide-induced parkinsonism, 319
    carbon monoxide-induced parkinsonism, 318
    cyanide-induced parkinsonism, 319
    DDPAC, 332
    depression, effect on, 257
    diffuse Lewy body disease, 336
    dopamine and, 257
    dystonia treatment with, 445*t*
    essential tremor treatment with, 378
    familial L-dopa-resonsive parkinsonian-pyramidal
        syndrome, 340–341
    freezing and, 221
    Hallervorden-Spatz disease, 333
    hemiparkinsonism-hemiatrophy syndrome, 335
    history, 201
    idiopathic parkinsonism, 351, 352, 360
    manganese-induced parkinsonism, 317
    mechanisms of action, 203, 203*f*–204*f*
    methanol-induced parkinsonism, 319
    multiple-system atrophy, 299
    neuroacanthocytosis, 338
    Parkinson's disease, 101
        after fetal graft, 227, 228
        bromocriptine with, 206
        drug-resistant periods, 191–192, 204
        idiopathic, 212–213
        late failure, 191–192, 204, 212, 213, 228
    pharmacology, 203
    postencephalitic parkinsonism, 310
    progressive supranuclear palsy, 351, 352–353, 353*t*-357*t*,
        359–360
    response oscillations, 213–214
    side effects, 191–192, 204, 221
        drug-resistant periods, 191
        dyskinesia, 191
        dystonia, 467
        motor fluctuations, 191
        psychiatric, 191–192, 259–260
    slow-release preparations, 205, 212
    tics induced by, 566
    x-linked dystonia-parkinsonism syndrome, 337
Lead, tremors induced by, 392
Learning, cerebellum, 604
Leber's hereditary optic neuropathy, 58–59, 58*f*, 59*f*, 466
Leigh's disease, 466
    differential diagnosis, 457*t*
    mitochondrial mutations and, 59, 60
Lesch-Nyhan syndrome, 457*t*, 467
Levine-Critchley syndrome. *See* Neuroacanthocytosis
Lewy bodies
    diffuse Lewy body disease. *See* Diffuse Lewy body
        disease
    idiopathic Parkinson's disease, 127
    incidental, 137
    Parkinson's disease, 127, 159, 263–265, 264*f*, 264*t*, 265*f*,
        265*t*
Lewy body dementia, 19, 23, 24–25, 127–129, 128*f*, 272
Lidocaine, dystonia treatment with, 445

Limb dystonia, 433
  botulinum toxin treatment, 450
  thalamic lesions, 457
Limbic circuit, 78
Limbic striatum, anatomy, 77
Lipofuscinosis, 457t, 465, 545
Lisuride hydrogen maleate, pharmacology, 206–207, 206t
Lithium
  dystonia treatment with, 445t
  parkinsonism induced by, 328
  tremor induced by, 390, 413
Liver transplantation, Wilson's disease, 631
Locomotion, 649. *See also* Gait disorder
Locomotor synergies, 656
Locus ceruleus, norepinephrine, 156
Long-latency reflexes, abnormalities of, 91
Lorazepam, dystonia treatment with, 445, 445t
Lower body parkinsonism, 345
Lubag, 336–337
Lyme disease, movement disorders secondary to, 736–737

M

Machado-Joseph disease, 21
  differential diagnosis, 189, 456t
  dystonia in, 463
  genetics, 485–486
Madopar CR, 205
Magnetic gait, 190
Magnetic resonance imaging (MRI)
  Alzheimer's disease, 283t
  cerebellar disorders, 582t
  corticobasal degeneration, 283t, 613
  DDPAC, 332
  dystonia, 458
  familial L-dopa-resonsive parkinsonian-pyramidal
    syndrome, 340
  Hallervorden-Spatz disease, 333
  hemiparkinsonism-hemiatrophy syndrome, 335
  Huntington's disease, 495
  movement disorders and, 31, 283t
  multiple-system atrophy, 301, 301f
  pallidal degeneration, 340
  Parkinson's disease, 189
  progressive supranuclear palsy, 281–282, 283t
  Rett syndrome, 342
  stiff person syndrome, 641
  stroke-associated tremor, 396
  Sydenham's chorea, 528
  tardive dyskinesia, 521
  Tourette's syndrome, 562
  Wilson's disease, 628
Malabsorption syndromes, movement disorders and, 734–735
Malingering, 716, 717t
Manganese intoxication
  dystonia and, 467
  mechanism of toxicity, 317

Parkinson's disease and, 161
  tremors induced by, 317, 392
Manganese superoxide dismutase, 169
Mania, movement disorders and, 18t, 18–19
MAO inhibitors
  idiopathic Parkinson's disease, 213
  Parkinson's disease, 208–209
  tremor induced by, 390
Mastocytosis, movement disorders secondary to, 736
Medium spiny neurons
  Huntington's disease, 504–505, 504f–506f
  physiology, 78, 80, 99, 503
Meige's syndrome, 435
Melanocyte-stimulating hormone [MSH]-release inhibiting
    factor. *See* MIF
MELAS, 63
Memory, movement disorders and, 22
Menkes' disease, 623
Mephenesin, essential tremor treatment with, 379
Mercury, tremors induced by, 392
Metabotropic receptors, 109–110
Metachromatic leukodystrophy, 457t, 465
Metaclopramide, tremor induced by, 390
Metal intoxication, Parkinson's disease and, 161
Metamphetamine, free radical formation, 170
Methanol-induced parkinsonism, 319
Methazolamide, essential tremor treatment with, 378
Methylbromide, tremors induced by, 393
Methyl ethyl ketone, tremors induced by, 393
Methylmalonic aciduria, 457t, 466
Methylphenidate, ADHD treatment with, 573
Metoclopramide, parkinsonism induced by, 325
Metoprolol, essential tremor treatment with, 376, 377
Midbrain tremor, 391, 392t, 410–411
MIF, 161
Milacemide, myoclonus treatment with, 549
Minipolymyoclonus, 553
Mirror movements, 668
Mitochondria
  calcium homeostasis, 168
  calpines, 167
  free radicals in, 171
  function, 165
  MPP+ and, 162–163, 163f, 163t, 316
  NaK ATPase, 167
  in Parkinson's disease, 158, 165–168, 165t, 166f, 167f,
    174, 174f, 270
  respiratory failure, 167–168
  structure and function, 164–165, 164f, 164t
Mitochondrial DNA (mtDNA), 51, 57f, 165, 167f
  abnormalities, age-related, 53
  gene arrangement, 52f
  genetics, 51–52
  mutations, 51, 53–55
  neurodegenerative diseases
    ataxia, 62–63, 64
    chronic progressive external ophthalmoplegia, 63–65
    Kearns-Sayre syndrome, 63–65
    Leber's hereditary optic neuropathy, 58–59, 58f, 59f
    Leigh's diseased, 59–61, 60

myoclonic epilepsy and ragged-red fiber disease, 55–58, 56f, 57
oxidative stress, 170
Parkinson's disease, 61–62, 166, 173
structure, 51
Mitochondrial encephalomyopathy, 465–466
Mitochondrial encephalomyopathy, lactic acidosis, and stroke-like episodes. *See* MELAS
Mitochondrial inheritance, Parkinson's disease, 147
Mitochondrial myopathy, 65f
Mitochondrial theory of aging, 53
Molecular genetics, 12t
Monoamine oxidase, 154, 155
Parkinson's disease and, 148, 173
Monoballism, 7
Motor blocks, gait disorder, 186–187
Motor circuits
anatomy, 239–240
movement disorders and, 87, 239–241
neurochemistry, 99–100, 100f
acetylcholine, 104–107
dopamine, 100–104, 103t
glutamate, 99, 107–111
Motor cortex, anatomy, 75–76
Motor fluctuations, Parkinson's disease, 191, 205
Motor functions, basal ganglia and, 88
Motor grasping, progressive supranuclear palsy and, 284
Motor learning, 577
Motor perseveration, progressive supranuclear palsy and, 284
Motor potential, 76
Motor system
alpha system, 591, 591–593, 594
descending and reentrant pathways, 73, 74f
gamma system, 591, 593–594
parallel organization, 73
Motor tics, 9, 561, 562t
in childhood, 663
differential diagnosis, 571
Motor tremor, 589
Mount Reback syndrome, 667
Movement
control by cerebellum, 577
decomposition of, 580, 591, 593
normal developmental steps, 661–663
Movement disorders
aging. *See* Aging; Elderly
basal ganglia. *See* Basal ganglia
brain. *See* Brain
childhood. *See* Childhood movement disorders
classification of, 662t
genetics. *See* Genetics
hyperkinetic. *See* Hyperkinetic movement disorders
hypokinetic. *See* Hypokinetic movement disorders
microscopic examination of the brain, 126–127
neurobehavioral aspects. *See* Neurobehavioral changes
neuroimaging. *See* Neuroimaging
neuropathology. *See* Neuropathology
psychogenic. *See* Psychogenic movement disorders
of sleep. *See* Sleep, movement disorders specific to sleep

surgery. *See* Surgery
systemic illnesses associated with, 733–740
Movement execution, basal ganglia and, 88
MPP+, 61, 210, 316
action in mitochondria, 162–163, 163, 163t, 270
mitochondria and, 162–163, 163f, 163t, 316
MPPP, 315
MPTP, 61, 153
mechanism of toxicity, 316
metabolism, 158, 162–163, 163f
parkinsonism induced by, 162–164, 163t, 210, 270, 315–316, 316t
MT12S*ADPD956–965ins mutation, 62
MT16S*AD3196A mutation, 62
MTATP6*NARP8993C mutation, 63, 65
MTATP6*NARP8993G mutation, 63, 65
MTATP6*NRP8993C mutation, 59
MTATP6*NRP8993G mutation, 59–60
MTDN1*ADPD3397G mutation, 62
MTND4*LHON11778G mutation, 59
MTND6*LDYT14459A mutation, 58–59
MTTK*MERRF8344G mutation, 55–57, 60, 63, 65
MTTK*MERRF8356C mutation, 55, 57
MTTL1*MELAS3243G mutation, 60, 63, 65
MTTL1*MELAS3271C mutation, 60
MTTQ*ADPD4336G mutation, 62
Multifocal action myoclonus, 549
Multifocal dystonia, 5
Multiple sclerosis, chorea and, 531
Multiple-system atrophy, 11, 297–304
autonomic failure in, 299
cardinal features of, 298f
cerebeller atrophy in, 302f
chorea and, 531
clinical features, 299, 618t
dementia, 25
diagnosis, 298–302, 298, 302
differential diagnosis, 189, 303–304
from progressive supranuclear palsy, 281
from symptomatic dystonias, 456t
dysarthria in, 300
dystonia in, 461
history, 298
management and symptomatic treatment of, 300t
neurobehavioral changes, 301
neuroimaging, 12t, 37–38, 283t, 301–302, 301f, 302
neuropathology, 131–132, 302–303, 303f, 304f
nosology, 297–298
postural instability, 190
pyramidal signs in, 300
Muscarinic receptors, 105–107, 105t, 106f
Muscle cramps, in Parkinson's disease, 188, 258
Muscle tone abnormalities, 581
Musculoskeletal deformities, Parkinson's disease, 188
Mutations
ataxia, 62–65, 65t
chronic progressive external ophthalmoplegia, 63–65
Kearns-Sayre syndrome, 63–65
Leber's hereditary optic neuropathy, 58–59, 58f, 59
Leigh's disease, 59–61, 60f

Mutations (*Cont.*)
    myoclonic epilepsy and ragged-red fiber disease, 55–58,
        56, 57f
    Parkinson's disease, 61–62
Mutism
    cerebellar, 581
    supplementary motor area lesions and, 77
Mycoplasma infection, movement disorder secondary to,
        311, 737
Mycotoxins, tremor and, 391
Myerson's sign, in Parkinson's disease, 187
Myoclonic epilepsy, 544
Myoclonic ataxia, 549
Myoclonic dystonia, 5, 541, 543*f*, 545
Myoclonic encephalopathy
    progressive, 545–546
    static, 547–548
Myoclonic epilepsy and ragged-red fiber disease (MERRF),
        55, 545
    mitochondrial mutations and, 55–58, 56*f*, 57*f*
Myoclonus, 6–7, 56*f*, 612
    in Alzheimer's disease, 546
    in childhood, 667
    classification, 541, 542*t*, 551–554, 552*t*
    clinical signs, 542–543
    cortical reflex myaclonus, 552, 553, 554
    differential diagnosis, 541–542, 667*t*
    electromyogram, 542, 542*f*, 543*f*, 551, 552, 554–555, 554*f*,
        555*f*, 558
    epileptic myoclonus, 6–7, 552–553
    etiology, 544–548
    evaluation, 554–557
    multiple-system atrophy, 300
    in myoclonic epilepsy and ragged-red fiber disease, 55
    negative myoclonus, 7, 542–543, 557–558
    neuroimaging, SEP, 556–557, 557*f*, 558, 558*f*
    nocturnal myoclonus. *See* Nocturnal myoclonus
    nonepileptic myoclonus, 552, 553–554
    palatal myoclonus, 7, 411–412, 548, 549, 553, 700
    pathophysiology, 543–544, 551
    physiologic myoclonus, 554
    posthypoxic myoclonus, 547
    progressive supranuclear palsy, 360
    psychogenic myoclonus, 554, 725–726
    reflex myoclonus, 542
    reticular reflex myoclonus, 544, 548, 552, 553
    rhythmic myoclonus, 543
    segmental myoclonus, 7
    stiff person syndrome and, 642
    subcortical myoclonus, 544, 552
    transcranial magnetic stimulation, 557
    treatment, 548–549
    types, 7
Myxedema, movement disorders secondary to, 733–734

N

Nadolol, essential tremor treatment with, 377
Negative myoclonus, 7, 542–543, 557–558

Neocerebellum, anatomy, 73, 578
Neostriatum, anatomy, 77
Nerve growth factor, 117, 118, 231
Neural transplantation
    fetal nigral transplantation, 36–37, 221–232
        clinical evaluation, 226–227
        donor age, 222–223
        future directions, 230–232, 231*f*
        immunosuppression, 225–226
        infectious disease issues, 225
        L-dopa use, 227
        neuroanatomic issues, 229–230
        outcomes, 227–229, 227*t*
        patient selection, 225
        site of implant, 223–224, 224*f*
        tissue acquisition, 222
        tissue distribution, 224–225
        tissue storage, 223, 223*f*
        volume of tissue, 224
    striatal implants, 290
Neuroacanthocytosis, 41–42, 337–338, 494, 529, 565
    in childhood, 667
    differential diagnosis, 456*t*
    dystonia in, 461
Neuroaxonal dystrophy, 462
Neurobehavioral changes, 15–26
    in childhood, 669–670
    cognitive disturbances, 21–23
    DDPAC, 332
    depression. *See* Depression
    dementia, 23–25
    diffuse Lewy body disease, 336
    familial L-dopa-resonsive parkinsonian-pyramidal
        syndrome, 340
    frontal subcortical circuits, 15–16, 16*f*
    in Huntington's disease, 16, 19, 493, 494
    manganese-induced parkinsonism, 317
    multiple-system atrophy, 301
    neuroacanthocytosis, 338
    obsessive-compulsive disorder. *See* Obsessive-
        compulsive disorder
    Parkinson's disease, 16, 17, 187, 257, anxiety, 20, 258–259
    personality traits, 18, 258
    psychosis, 18, 259–261, 260*t*, 261*t*
    sleep disorders, 20–21, 258–259, 692–699, 701
    pallidal degeneration, 339
    progressive supranuclear palsy, 19, 279, 280*t*
        kindred evaluations, 353
    psychosis. *See* Psychosis
    Rett syndrome, 341
    suicide, 17, 493
    Wilson's disease, 19, 625
    x-linked dystonia-parkinsonism syndrome, 337
Neurobehavioral disturbance, L-dopa related, 191–192
Neurocysticercosis, parkinsonism associated with, 311
Neurofibrillary tangles
    corticobasal degeneration, 615
    Parkinson's disease, 272
    postencephalitic parkinsonism, 309
    progressive supranuclear palsy, 282

Neuroimaging, 4t, 12, 12*t*, 31, 31–43, 43. *See* also Magnetic resonance imaging, Position emission tomography, Single-photon emission computed tomography
  basal ganglia, role in movement, 31–32
  cerebellar disorders, 582*t*, 605*f*, 607*f*
  chorea, 41–43
  corticobasal degeneration, 12*t*, 39, 39*t*, 613–614, *613f*
  DDPAC, 332
  dystonia, 31, 39–41, 435, 458
  familial L-dopa-resonsive parkinsonian-pyramidal syndrome, 340
  Hallervorden-Spatz disease, 333–334
  hemiparkinsonism-hemiatrophy syndrome, 335
  Huntington's disease, 41–43, 495, 12*t*, 496
  idiopathic Parkinson's disease, 31
  multiple-system atrophy, 12*t*, 37–38, 39*t*, 301–302, *301f*, 302
  neuroacanthocytosis, 338, 529
  olivopontocerebeller atrophy, 37–38, 39*t*
  pallidal degeneration, 340
  Parkinson's disease, 32–37, 39*t*, 90, 189, 226–227, 226*f*, 263, 283*t*
  progressive supranuclear palsy, 38–39, 39*t*, 281–282, 283*t*
  Rett syndrome, 342
  stiff-person syndrome, 641, 641*f*
  striatal degeneration, 37–38, 39*t*, 311
  tardive dyskinesia, 521, 524
  Tourette's syndrome, 31, 562–563
  Wilson's disease, 12*t*, 628
  x-linked dystonia-parkinsonism syndrome, 337
Neuroleptic drugs
  acute dystonic reactions, 5
  choosing, 521–522
  dystonia treatment with, 444
  essential tremor treatment with, 379
  Huntington's disease, 496
  side effects, 61, 467
  tardive dyskinesia, 7, 10, 327, 328, 519–524
  tics induced by, 565–566
  tic treatment, 573
Neuroleptic-induced parkinsonism, 325–327, 326*t*
Neuroleptic malignant syndrome, 348–349
Neuromelanin, 158, 170, 268–269
Neuronal storage diseases, 545
Neurons
  ballooned, 272, 614
  basal ganglial, 78–79, 88
  functional segregation of pathways, 80, 88–89
  Huntington's disease, 503–506
  medium spiny neurons, 78, 80, 99, 503–505, 504*f*, 505*f*
  nitric oxide, 169
  progressive supranuclear palsy and, 283
Neuropathology
  Alzheimer's disease, 125, 129
  brain, striatal degeneration, 131–132
  diffuse Lewy body disease, 127–129, 335
  familial L-dopa-resonsive parkinsonian-pyramidal syndrome, 340
  gross neuropathologic examination, 125–132

Hallervorden-Spatz disease, 126, 332–333
  Huntington's disease, 126, 503–511
    brain stem, 511
    cerebellum, 510–511
    cerebral cortex, 509–510, 510*f*
    diencephalon, 508–509
    globus pallidus, 507–508, 508*f*
    striatum, 503–509, 504*f*–506*f*
    substantia nigra, 508, *508f*
  multiple-system atrophy, 131–132, 302–303, 303*f*, 304*f*
  neuroacanthocytosis, 338
  olivopontocerebellar atrophy, 126, 131–132
  pallidal degeneration, 339
  Parkinson's disease, 241–242
    acidophilic granules, 265
    corpus striatum, 267
    Lewy body, 127, 159, 263–265, *265*, 264t, *265*, 265t
    mitochondria, 165–168, 165t, 166*f*, 167*f*, 174, 174*f*, 270
    neurofibrillary tangles, 272
    pale body, 265–266
    spheroid bodies, 266
    substantia nigra, 127, 127*f*, 266–267
  Pick's disease, 131
  postencephalitic parkinsonism, 309–310
  progressive supranuclear palsy, 282–285
  Rett syndrome, 341
  x-linked dystonia-parkinsonism syndrome, 336
Neuropathy
  essential tremor and, 373
  hereditary motor sensory neuropathy, 394
  Leber's hereditary optic neuropathy, 58, 466
  tremor associated with, 312, 394–395, 395*t*
Neuropeptides, Parkinson's disease and, 157
Neuropsychiatric disturbances, movement disorders and, 16–21
Neurotoxins
  Parkinson's disease and, 172
  tremor induced by, 391–393
Neurotransmitters, 153, 154*f*, 155–157, 159
Neurotrophic factors, 117, 121, 174
Neurotrophins, 118–120
Nicardipine, essential tremor treatment with, 379
Nicotine
  Parkinson's disease and, 171
  tremor induced by, 390
Nictitating membrane response, 604
Niemann-Pick disease, 456*t*, 465
Nifedipine
  essential tremor treatment with, 379
  tremor induced by, 391
Night terrors, 691
Nigrostriatal system, progressive supranuclear palsy and, 284–285
Nitric oxide, as free radical, 168–169
NMDA, 107
NMDA glutamate antagonists, 209–210
NMDA receptors, 107–108, 173
Nocturnal akathisia, 697
Nocturnal eating, 691

Nocturnal myoclonus, 9, 554, 668–669
  insomnia and, 21
  Parkinson's disease, 258
  stiff person syndrome and, 642
  treatment, 549
Nocturnal paroxysmal dystonia, 690
Nonepileptic myoclonus, 552, 553–554
Noninsulin-dependent diabetes mellitus (NIDDM),
    MTTL1*MELAS3243G mutation, 63
Nonmotor phenomena, Parkinson's disease, 92
Nonviral infections, parkinsonism associated with, 311
Noradrenergic agents, progressive supranuclear palsy, 289
Norepinephrine, Parkinson's disease and, 156–157
Normal pressure hydrocephalus, 190, 347
Nucleus reticularis of the thalamus, anatomy, 79
Numbness, in Parkinson's disease, 188
Nystagmus, 580, 592, 602–603

O

Obsessive-compulsive disorder
  in Huntington's disease, 494
  movement disorders and, 19–20, 20t
  in postencephalitic parkinsonism, 20
  in Tourette's syndrome, 570
  treatment, 574
Oculofaciocervical dystonia, 460
Oculogyric crisis, encephalitis lethargica, 308
Oculomotor circuit, 77
Oculomotor dysfunction, 602
  multiple-system atrophy, 300
  Parkinson's disease, 187
  progressive supranuclear palsy, 285–286, 285t, 290
  Wilson's disease, 626–627
Off-period dyskinesia, 191
Off-period dystonia, 191, 204, 214
Olfactory function, Parkinson's disease, 187
Ondansetron, 215, 215t
OPCA. See Sporadic olivopontocerebellar atrophy
Optic ataxia, 654
Oral-buccal-lingual dyskinesia, 7
Oral contraceptives, chorea following use, 528
Orientation, disordering of, 651t, 653–654
Orofacial dyskinesia, in the elderly, 681
Oromandibular dystonia, 431–432, 434, 435, 437
  botulinum treatment, 448–449
Orthostatic hypotension
  multiple-system atrophy, 299, 300t
  Parkinson's disease, 188, 192
Orthostatic tremor, 6, 393, 393t, 412
Oscillatory myoclonus, 547
Osteoporosis, Wilson's disease, 627
Overflow dystonia, 5, 430
Oxidative phosphorylation (OXPHOS), 51. See also
    OXPHOS diseases
  age-related abnormalities in, 53
  biochemistry and genetics, 51–52, 52f
  movement disorders and, 54–55

Oxidative stress
  defined, 168
  glutathione, 169–170, 170f
  Parkinson's disease, 168–171, 210, 269–270
  superoxide dismutase, 169, 174, 174f
Oxotremorine, tremor and, 391
OXPHOS. See Oxidative phosphorylation
OXPHOS diseases, 51
  ataxia, 62–63, 64
  chronic progressive external ophthalmoplegia, 63–65
  diagnosis, 65–66
  Kearns-Sayre syndrome, 63–65
  Leber's hereditary optic neuropathy, 58–59, 58f, 59
  Leigh's disease, 59–61, 60f
  myoclonic epilepsy and ragged-red fiber disease, 55–58,
    56f, 57
  Parkinson's disease. See Parkinson's disease
  therapy, 66
Oxygen, activated species, 168, 168f

P

Pain
  idiopathic torsion dystonia, 421
  Parkinson's disease, 188
Painful arms and moving fingers, 834
Painful legs and moving toes, 8, 534
Painless legs and moving toes, 534
Palatal myoclonus, 7, 411–412, 548, 549, 553, 700
Palatal tremor, 393–394, 394t, 511–512, 553
Pale body, Parkinson's disease, 264f, 265–266
Paleocerebellum, anatomy, 73, 578, 596
Palilalia, 9, 22, 187, 284
Pallidal atrophy
  dystonia, 462–463
  Huntington's disease, 507
Pallidal degeneration, 338–340
Pallidoluysian atrophy, 462
Pallidoluysionigral atrophy, 463
Pallidotomy, 33, 237, 238, 246, 249–250
Panic attacks
  L-dopa related, 258
  Parkinson's disease, 192, 258
Paraballism, 527
Paraflocculus, 602
Parasitic infection, parkinsonism associated with, 311
Parasomnia, 21, 698
Parathyroid hormone, movement disorders and, 734
Paravermal syndrome, 601–602, 601t
Paresthesias, in Parkinson's disease, 188
Parietal Pick's disease, 617
Parkinsonian tremor, 6
Parkinsonism, 11, 18
  with Alzheimer's disease, 11
  arteriosclerotic parkinsonism, 273–274
  atypical, 126, 298
  in children, 11
  central nervous system manifestations of, 331–332

clinical signs, 655
with Creutzfeldt-Jakob disease, 311
defined, 183
differential diagnosis, 189, 618t
diffuse Lewy body disease, 32–33, 61, 128–129, 335–336
disinhibition-dementia-parkinsonism amyotrophy
   complex, 331–332
drug-induced, 325–328, 326t, 328t, 679
   amiodarone, 329
   calcium channel blockers, 328
   cholinergic drugs, 328
   diazepam, 328
   dopamine storage and transport inhibitors, 327–328
   lithium, 328
   neuroleptics, 325–327, 326t
dystonia associated with, 5
in the elderly, 678–679, 677t, 681
etiology, 311–312, 319
   basal ganglial calcification, 348
   hematoma, 348
   lesions, structural, 347–348
   trauma, 346–347
   tumors, 348
familial. See Familial parkinsonism
following stroke, 681
genetics, 309, 336
Hallervorden-Spatz disease, 25, 126, 189, 332–333
head trauma, 397
hemiparkinsonism-hemiatrophy syndrome, 191, 334–335
herodofamilial syndromes, 351–360
in Huntington's disease, 492–493
hydrocephalic, 190
hydrocephalus, induced, 347
hypoparathyroidism and, 348, 734
idiopathic. See Idiopathic parkinsonism
infectious and postinfectious encephalitis, 307, 308t,
   310–311, 311f–312
   AIDS, 311
   Creutzfeldt-Jakob disease, 311
   encephalitis lethargica, 308–308, 310
   fungal infection, 311
   mycoplasma, 311
   nonviral, 311
   parasitic infection, 311
   postencephalitic parkinsonism, 307, 308–310
   syphilis, 311
kindred evaluations
   idiopathic parkinsonism, 351, 352, 360
   progressive supranuclear palsy, 351, 352–353,
      353t–357t, 359–360
lower-body parkinsonism, 345
lubag, 336–337
neuroacanthocytosis, 41–42, 337–338
neuroimaging, 335, 337
neuroleptic malignant syndrome, 348–349
neuropathology, 309–310, 334
pallidal, pallidonigral, and pallidoluysionigral
   degenerations, 338–340
postencephalitic, 17–21, 308–310
psychogenic, 727–728

Rett syndrome, 10, 341–342
toxin-induced, 309–310, 315, 319, 336
   carbon disulfide, 318–319, 320t
   carbon monoxide, 317–318
   cyanide, 319
   manganese, 317
   methanol, 3219
   MPTP, 162–164, 163t, 163f, 210, 270, 315–316, 316t
trauma-induced, 346–347
vascular, 189, 345–346
linked dystonia-parkinsonism syndrome, 336–337
Parkinsonism-dementia/ALS complex of Guam, 331
dementia, 25
etiology, 309–310
personality changes, 19
sleep disorders, 20
Parkinsonism-hyperpyrexia syndrome, 348–349
Parkinson-plus syndromes, 189, 298, 612, 617
Parkinson's disease, 11, 61, 90, 90, 137–138
arteriosclerotic, 273
basal ganglia and, 88, 153
benign, 272
in childhood. See Juvenile Parkinson's disease
clinical manifestations of, 183–197
clinical rating scales, 192, 193t–197t
clinical signs, 88, 90–91, 137–138, 137t–142t, 258, 259
   absent or atypical tremor, 189–190
   akinesia, 186, 186t
   apraxia, 23
   atypical features, 188, 189t
   autonomic dysfunction, 188
   bradykinesia, 91
   cardinal manifestations, 185t
   cognitive dysfunction, 21, 22, 187, 191–192, 226
   dementia, 23, 24–25, 187, 190–191
   dermatologic problems, 188
   dorsolateral prefrontal syndrome, 15
   dyskinesia, 191, 204–205
   dysphagia, 187
   dystonia, 460
   essential tremor, 372
   facial and oropharyngeal dysfunction, 187
   gender and, 139, 140t
   hallucinations, 191, 259–260
   hypersexuality, 21
   kyphosis, 188
   mania, 18
   motor fluctuations, 191
   ocular dysfunction, 187
   onset, 184
   orthostatic hypotension, 192
   pain and sensory symptoms, 188
   persistent asymmetry, 191
   postural instability, 186–187, 190
   rest tremor, 396
   rigidity, 185–186
   secondary manifestations, 185t, 187
   speech disorders, 22
   tremor, 91–92, 183, 184–185, 387
   visuospatial dysfunction, 23

Parkinson's disease (*Cont.*)
  cognitive disturbance, 21, 22, 187
    assessment, 226
    drug-related, 191–192
  depression in, 16, 17, 187, 258
  defined, 137, 183
  differential diagnosis, 188, 263, 456*t*
    from corticobasal degeneration, 612, 617, 618*t*
    from multiple-system atrophy, 304
    from progressive supranuclear palsy, 279
    from symptomatic dystonias, 456*t*
  dopamine, 153, 155–156, 156*t*
  environmental factors and neurotoxins in 171–172
  epidemiology, 138–143
    age and, 139, 140*t*
    race and, 139, 140*t*
    risk factors, 141–143, 141*t*–143*t*
  etiology, 161–174, 183, 268
    aging, 139, 140*t*, 188–189, 268
    aluminum and, 170
    cohort theory, 307
    excessive free radical production, 158
    glutamine and, 110–111
    iron, 170, 269–270
    mitochondrial function, 270
    MPTP, 270
    neuromelanin, 158, 170, 268–269
    nitric oxide, 168
    oxidative stress, 210, 269–270
  executive function, 21, 22
  familial. *See* Familial parkinsonism
  freezing and, 186–187, 191
  genetics, 143–148, 144*t*, 1415*t*, 147*t*
    familial, 143–147, 144*t*, 145*t*, 173
    mitochondrial inheritance, 147
    mutations, 61–62
    susceptibility gene, 147–148
    twin studies, 146, 147, 147*t*
  idiopathic. *See* Idiopathic Parkinson's disease
  incidence and prevalence of, 138*t*, 139*t*, 140*t*
  juvenile, 272–273, 667
  L-dopa therapy, biochemistry, 101
  Lewy bodies, 137, 159
  Lewy body dementia, 272
  mortality, 140–141, 141*t*
  musculoskeletal deformities, 188
  neurobehavioral abnormalities
    anxiety, 20, 258–259
    depression, 16, 17, 187, 257
    personality traits, 18, 258
    psychosis, 18, 259–261, 260*t*, 261*t*
    sleep disorders, 20–21, 258–259, 692–699, 701
    neurochemistry of, 153–159, 154*f*, 155*t*, 156*t*
  neuroimaging, 32–37, 39*t*, 263
    cerebral activation, 33–34
    detection of preclinical disease, 34–36
    etiology, aging, 36
    fetal graft function, 36–37
    MRI, 189, 283*t*
    PET, 32–37, 90, 226–227, 226*f*
    postsynaptic striated dopamine system, 37
    presynaptic dopaminergic system, 34
    resting metabolism, 33
    tremor, 36
  neuropathology, 241–242
    acidophilic granules, 265
    corpus striatum, 267
    Lewy body, 127, 159, 263–265, 264, 264*t*, 265, 265*t*
    mitochondria, 158, 165–168, 166*f*, 167*f*, 174, 174*f*, 270
    pale body, 265–266
    substantia nigra, 127, 127*f*, 266–267
    spheroid bodies, 266
  neuropharmacology, 159
    acetylcholine, 157
    cerebral glucose utilization, 158
    dopamine, 155–156, 156*t*
    free radical scavengers, 158
    gamma-aminobutyric acid, 157
    mitochondrial function, 158
    neuropeptides, 157
    norepinephrine, 156–157
    serotonin, 157
  nigral neuronal death in, 174*f*
  obsessive-compulsive disorder and, 20
  pathophysiology, 241–242, 409–410
  personality and, 19, 258
  pharmacological treatment, 201–215
    advanced IPD, 213–215
    amantadine, 209–210, 211–212
    anticholinergics, 209, 209*t*, 212
    antipsychotic drugs, 325
    apomorphine, 207–208
    behavioral disturbance due to, 191–192
    bromocriptine, 206, 206*t*
    cabergoline, 208
    COMT-inhibitors, 205, 206*t*
    de novo patients, 211–213
    dopamine agonists, 206–208, 213
    dopaminergic agents, 212–213
    glutamate antagonists, 209–210
    history, 201
    L-dopa, 203–205, 204*f*, 204*t*, 212
    lisuride, 206–207, 206*t*
    MAO-B inhibitors, 208–209
    neuroprotective, 201, 210–211
    nondopaminergic agents, 209, 211–212
    parkinsonism resulting from, 325
    pergolide, 207
    pramipexole, 208
    psychosis, 260–261
    ropinirole, 208
    selegiline, 208–209, 213
    symptomatic, 201–210
  presytmptomatic, 267–268
  progression, 221, 268
  reflexes in, 677
  risk of, 141, 141*t*
  sleep in, 692–699, 693*f*–697*f*, 699*f*, 701
  smoking and, 171–172
  suicide and, 17

surgical treatment, 237–238
deep brain stimulation, 251–252
fetal nigral transplantation, 36–37, 221–232
history, 237–238
pallidotomy, 33, 237, 238, 246, 249 250
stereotaxic surgery, 244–246, 248–250
thalamotomy, 237, 238, 246, 250
treatment-related manifestations, 191
twin studies, 146–147, 147t
young-onset patient, 189
Paroxysmal dyskinesias, 8, 532, 534
Paroxysmal dystonia, 8, 445, 734
Paroxysmal dystonic choreoathetosis, 532, 669
Paroxysmal kinesigenic choreoathetosis, 8, 532, 669
Paroxysmal movement disorders, in childhood, 668–669
Paroxysmal nocturnal dystonia, 8
Pars reticulata, anatomy, 79
Pavor nocturnus, 691
Peak-dose dyskinesia, 191
Pedunculopontine nucleus
anatomy, 79–80, 87
progressive supranuclear palsy and and, 285
Pelizaeus-Merzbacher disease, 465
Pemoline, ADHD treatment with, 573
Penicillamine, Wilson's disease therapy, 630
Penile erection, spontaneous, 299
Pergolide, dystonia treatment with, 445t
Pergolide mesylate, pharmacology, 205t, 207
Periodic leg movements during sleep, 9, 668, 697
Perioxynitrite, 169
Peripheral denervation, 450–451
Peripheral myoclonus, 553
Peripheral neuropathy, tremor associated with, 312, 394–395, 395t
Periventricular system, 155
Personality alterations, movement disorders and, 19
Pesticides, tremors induced by, 392–393
PET. *See* Positron emission tomography
Phantom dyskinesia, 10
Phantom tics, 561
Pharyngeal akinesia, Parkinson's disease, 187
Phenelzine, Huntington's disease, 497
Phenobarbital, essential tremor treatment with, 377–378
Phenol, dystonia treatment with, 445
Phenoxybenzamine, essential tremor treatment with, 378
Phenyethylmalonamide, essential tremor treatment with, 377
Phenytoin, tremor induced by, 391
Physiological myoclonus, 544
Physiological tremor, 6, 387–388
hyperthyroidism and, 733
pathophysiology, 405, 405f
Pick's disease, 332
clinical features, 618t
differential diagnosis, 615, 616–617, 618t
neuropathology, 131
parietal, 617
Pill-rolling tremor
Parkinson's disease, 184, 409
postencephalitic parkinsonism, 308

Pimozide
Sydenham's chorea treatment with, 528
tic treatment with, 573
Pindolol
essential tremor treatment with, 377
tremor induced by, 391
Piperazine derivatives, parkinsonism induced by, 328
Piracetam, myoclonus treatment with, 549
Polycythemia vera, 531, 736
Polyminimyoclonus, 546
Pontocerebellum, anatomy, 73, 578
Positron emission tomography (PET), 12t, 31
cerebellar disorders, 582t
corticobasal degeneration, 613–614
cyanide intoxication, 319
dystonia, 39–41
familial L-dopa-resonsive parkinsonian-pyramidal
syndrome, 340
focal dystonia, 435
Huntington's disease, 41–43, 43f, 495–496
movement studies with, 31–32
multiple-system atrophy, 37–38, 301
neuroacanthocytosis, 338, 529
orthostatic tremor, 412
palatal tremor, 411
Parkinson's disease, 32–37, 90, 226 227, 226
progressive supranuclear palsy, 38–39, 281
regional cerebral glucose utilization, 158
Rett syndrome, 342
stroke-associated tremor, 396
Sydenham's chorea, 528
Tourette's syndrome, 562
x-linked dystonia-parkinsonism syndrome, 337
Postencephalitic parkinsonism, 307, 308–310
apathy, 19
behavioral changes, 18
obsessive-compulsive disorder, 20
pathology, 309–310
pathophysiology, 309
sexual disturbance, 21
sleep disorders, 20
treatment, 310
Posthypoxic myoclonus, 547
Postpump chorea, 531–532
Postsynaptic striatal dopamine system, Parkinson's
disease, 37
Posttraumatic parkinsonism, 346–347
Posttraumatic tremor, 397
Postural hypotension, multiple-system atrophy, 299, 300t
Postural instability, 11
DDPAC, 331
differential diagnosis, 190
in the elderly, 677t
L-dopa and, 221
multiple-system atrophy, 299
Parkinson's disease, 186–187, 190
olivo pontoce rebellar atrophy, 190
postencephalitic parkinsonism, 309
progressive supranuclear palsy, 284, 290
Postural reflexes, in the elderly, 675

Postural tremor, 368, 387, 588
  differential diagnosis, from myoclonus, 541
  dystonia and, 372
  progressive supranuclear palsy, kindred evaluations,
    359–360
Posture
  control by cerebellum, 577
  in the elderly, 675, 677t
Potassium, inhibition of intestinal copper absorption with,
    629
Pramipexole, pharmacology, 208
Praxis, movement disorders and, 23
Prednisone, stiff person syndrome treatment with, 647
Pregnancy, chorea gravidarum, 528, 739
Premotor areas, 73
Presynaptic dopaminergic system, Parkinson's disease
    and, 34
Primary antiphospholipid antibody syndrome, 528
Primary dystonia, 5
Primary motor cortex, 73, 74, 74f, 75
Primary tic disorder, 565
Primary writing tremor, 398–399, 412
Primidone
  dystonia treatment with, 445t
  essential tremor treatment with, 377, 380
  myoclonus treatment with, 549
Procainamide, tremor induced by, 391
Procedural memory, 22
Prochlorperazine, parkinsonism induced by, 325
Progressive autonomic failure, neuroimaging and, 37–38, 39t
Progressive myoclonic ataxia, 546
Progressive myoclonic encephalopathy, 545–546
Progressive myoclonic epilepsy syndrome, causes, 7
Progressive supranuclear palsy, 11, 129f, 130f, 279
  atypical features, 279–280, 281t
  blepharospasm and, 286, 290
  clinical signs, 279, 285–286, 285t, 290, 351, 618t
  cognitive disturbance, 22
  dementia, 24, 190
  depression in, 353
  diagnosis, 280–282, 281t–283t
  differential diagnosis, 189
    from corticobasal degeneration, 612, 615, 616–617, 618t
    from multiple-system atrophy, 304
    from symptomatic dystonias, 456t
  dystonia, 460–461
  epidemiology, 287–288
  familial, 288, 288t
    freezing and, 284
    kindred evaluations, 351, 352–353, 353t–357t, 359–360
  genetics, 360
  history, 280
  kindred evaluations, 351, 352–353, 353t–357t, 359–360
  myoclonus and, 360
  neurobehavioral changes, 19, 279, 280t, 353
  neuroimaging, 12t, 31, 38–39, 39t, 283t
  neuropathology, 125, 126, 129–130, 129f, 130f, 282–285
    basal ganglia, 285
    cerebral cortex, 283–284
    lesion description, 282–283
  nigrostriatal system, 284–285
  obsessive-compulsive disorder and, 20
  patient resources, 290, 290t
  physical therapy, 290
    electroconvulsive therapy, 290
    striatal implants, 290
  postural instability, 190
  sleep in, 286, 699
  treatment
    botulinum toxin, 289
    electroconvulsive therapy, 290
    gaze and lid paresis, 290
    pharmacotherapy, 288–289, 289t
Progressive Supranuclear Palsy Association, 290
Propranolol
  cerebellar disorder treatment, 581
  essential tremor treatment with, 376, 380
Propriospinal myoclonus, 548, 553
Proton magnetic resonance spectroscopy, Huntington's
    disease, 496
Pseudoathetosis, 8
Pseudodystonia, 468–469, 469t
Pseudohypoparathyroidism, movement disorders and, 734
Psychiatric side effects, L-dopa, 191–192, 205
Psychogenic movement disorders, 715
  ataxia, 728
  chorea, 726
  diagnosis, 718–720, 719t
  dystonia, 5, 437, 468, 720–724, 721t–723t
  epidemiology, 716–718, 717t, 718t
  gait disorders, 728–729
  history, 715–716
  myoclonus, 554, 725–726
  parkinsonism, 727–728
  psychiatric definitions, 716
  tics, 726–727
  treatment, 729–731
  tremor, 6, 395, 395t, 724–725
Psychosis
  in Huntington's disease, 16, 19, 494, 497
  L-dopa-related, 191, 214–215
  movement disorders and, 18t, 18–19
  Parkinson's disease, 18, 258–261, 260t, 261t
  Wilson's disease, 625
"Punch drunk" syndrome, 397
Purine metabolism, Lesch-Nyhan syndrome, 467
Purkinje cells, 303f, 599, 604
Putamen
  anatomy, 78–79, 87
  function, 99
Putamen lesions, dystonia and, 457
Pyramidal myoclonus, 551
Pyramidal tract neurons, 75
Pyridostigmine, parkinsonism induced by, 328

R

Rabbit syndrome, 390
Race, Parkinson's disease, 139, 140t

Radioimmunoassays, neuropeptide studies, 157
Ramsay-Hunt syndrome, 7, 542f
Rapid eye movement behavior disorder, 689–690, 697–698
Rapid-onset dystonia-parkinsonism, 429
Readiness potential, 75–76, 91
Rebound, 580–581
Reflexes, 612
   in the elderly, 674, 674t, 675t, 677–678
   multiple-system atrophy, 300
   myoclonus, 557
   Parkinson's disease, 187
   progressive supranuclear palsy, 296
Reflex gaze, progressive supranuclear palsy, 286
Reflex myoclonus, 542
Reflex sympathetic dystrophy, 397
Reiterative speech disorders, movement disorders and, 22
Remacemide, Huntington's disease, 498
Reserpine, 257
   parkinsonism induced by, 327
   tremor induced by, 390
Respiratory abnormalities, progressive supranuclear palsy,
     kindred evaluations, 360
Respiratory dyskinesia, 8
Restless leg syndrome, 9, 21, 697
Rest tremor, 6, 387, 395–396, 396t, 588
   in the elderly, 678, 680
   Parkinson's disease, 185, 189
   progressive supranuclear palsy and, 289
Reticular reflex myoclonus, 544, 548, 552, 553
Rett syndrome, 10, 341–342
   differential diagnosis, 456t
   dystonia in, 463
Rheumatic chorea. See Sydenham's chorea
Rhythmic myoclonus, 543
Rigidity
   DDPAC, 331
   in the elderly, 674
   multiple-system atrophy, 299
   neuroleptic malignant syndrome, 348
   Parkinson's disease, 91, 185–186, 189
   postencephalitic parkinsonism, 308, 309
   progressive supranuclear palsy and, 284
Risus sardonicus, 625
Ritanserin, essential tremor treatment with, 379
Rocking, 669
Romberg sign, 653, 729
Ropinirole, pharmacology, 208
Rostral (CMAr) motor area, 74, 74f
Rotenone, 171
Roussy-Levy syndrome, 373, 394
Rubral tremor, pathophysiology, 410–411

S

St. Vitus' dance. See Sydenham's chorea
Salsolinol, as neurotoxin, 172
Sandhoff's disease, 545
Sandifer's syndrome, 665
Sarcoidosis, movement disorders secondary to, 738

Scaling abnormalities, 651t, 654–655
"Scaling" hypothesis, for basal ganglial function, 89
Schizophrenia
   cerebellar abnormalities in, 568
   movement disorders and, 18, 19
Schwab and England Capacity for Daily Living Scale, 192
Scoliosis, in Parkinson's disease, 188
Scopolamine, 289
Seborrhea, Parkinson's disease, 188
Secondary dystonia. See Dystonia, symptomatic
Secondary myoclonus, 544
Secondary tic disorder, 565
Segmental dystonia, 5
Segmental myoclonus, 7
Segregation of information, in basal ganglia, 88–89
Seitelberger's disease, 462
Seizures
   myoclonus, 6–7
   progressive supranuclear palsy, 360
   Wilson's disease, 625
Selegiline, 210
   anxiety, 20
   idiopathic Parkinson's disease, 213
   side effects, 259
Senile chorea, 530
Senile gait, 675
Senile tremor, 6
Sensory ataxia, 590
Sensory tics, 561, 562t, 569–570, 581
SEP, myoclonus, 556–557, 557f, 558
Sequential movements, suplementary motor area and, 77
Serotonin, Parkinson's disease and, 157
Sexual disturbances
   Huntington's disease, 494
   movement disorders and, 20, 21
   multiple-system atrophy, 299, 300t
Parkinson's disease, 188
   Wilson's disease, 625
Shaky leg syndrome, 393
Shy-Drager syndrome, 11, 282t
   dementia, 25
   differential diagnosis, 189
   dystonia in, 461
   familial, 297
   history, 297
   neuroimaging, 12t, 283t
   neuropathology, 131–132
   postural instability, 190
Sialidosis, 545
Simple motor tics, 569
Simple vocal tics, 9, 569
Simultaneous movements, basal ganglia and, 88
Sinemet CR, 205
Single-photon emission computed tomography (SPECT),
     31
   corticobasal degeneration, 613
   multiple-system atrophy, 301
   progressive supranuclear palsy, 282
   Rett syndrome, 342
Singlet oxygen, 168

Sjögren's syndrome, movement disorders secondary to, 738
Skeletomotor circuit, anatomy, 77, 78–80, 78
Sleep
    dreaming, 258–259, 260
    problems in, 687–691
    insomnia. *See* Insomnia
    somnolence. *See* Somnolence
    in waking movement disorders, 20–21
        ascending reticular activating system and, 702, 703t
        basal ganglia and, 702–703
        blepharospasm, 699, 700
        Creutzfeldt-Jakob disease, 700
        dopamine and, 701–702
        hemiballismus, 700
        hemifacial spasm, 700
        Huntington's disease, 494, 699
        olivopontecerebellar atrophy, 700
        palatal myoclonus, 700
        Parkinson's disease, 20–21, 258–259, 692–699, 701
        progressive supranuclear palsy, 286, 699
        Rett syndrome, 341
        torsion dystonia, 699–700
        Tourette's syndrome, 700
        treatment, 700
Sleep apnea, 698
Sleeptalking, 690–691, 692
Sleepwalking, 691, 692
Smell. *See* Olfactory function
Smoking, Parkinson's disease and, 171–172
Snout reflex, 187, 677
Society for Progressive Supranuclear Palsy (SPSP), 290
Solvents, tremors induced by, 393
Soman, tremors induced by, 393
Somatization, 716, 717t
Somatosensory disorders, 651t, 652–653
Somatosensory evoked potential, 613
Somatostatin, Parkinson's disease and, 157
Somnambulism, 691
Somniloquy, 690–691
Somnolence. *See also* Sleep
    encephalitis lethargica, 307
    Huntington's disease, 494
    movement disorders and, 20, 259
    Parkinson's disease, 698–699
Spasm, stiff person syndrome, 640, 644
Spasmodic dysphonia, 432, 436, 436f
    botulinum treatment, 449
    surgical treatment, 452
Spasmodic torticollis, 5
Spasticity, 655–656, 667–668
SPECT. *See* Single-photon emission computed tomography
Speech, 22, 612; *See also* Dysarthria
    multiple-system atrophy, 300
    Parkinson's disease, 187
    Wilson's disease, 625
Spheroid bodies, Parkinson's disease, 266
Spinal bulbar muscular atrophy, genetics, 485
Spinal myoclonus, 7, 544, 548, 549, 553
Spinocerebellar ataxia, 65

Spinocerebellar ataxia type 1, genetics, 485
Spinocerebellum, 596
Spontaneous myoclonus, 543
Spontaneous orofacial dyskinesia, in the elderly, 681
Sporadic olivopontocerebellar degeneration (OPCA), 11, 131–132, 303f
    dementia, 25
    differential diagnosis, 189
    dystonia in, 461
    familial, 297
    neuroimaging, 37–38, 39t, 283t, 301f, 302f
    myoclonus and, 547–548
    neuropathology, 126, 131–132
    postural instability, 190
    sleep in, 699
    visuospatial dysfunction, 23
Stance, abnormalities of, 579
Startle disease, 10
Startle epilepsy, 10, 554
Startle syndrome, 667
Static myoclonic encephalopathies, 547
Static tremor, 410, 581, 588
Station, in the elderly, 675
Steele-Richardson-Olszewski syndrome, 38
Stereotaxic surgery, 237–239
    for dystonia, 246–247, 248–250
    history, 237–248
    for Parkinson's disease, 237–238, 244–246, 248–240
    technique, 248–250
    thalamotomy, 237, 238, 246, 250, 379–380, 396, 409, 451
    for tremor, 238, 247–248, 248–250
Stereotypy, 10, 669
Steroids, stiff person syndrome, 647
Stiff-person syndrome, 10, 639–642, 641f, 643t, 645–647
Stimulants, tremor induced by, 390
Striatal dopamine system, Parkinson's disease, 37
Striatal implants, progressive supranuclear palsy, 290
Striatonigral degeneration, 11, 132f, 189
    dementia, 25
    dystonia in, 461
    familial, 297–298
    history, 297
    neuroimaging, 311, 37–38, 39t
    neuropathology, 131–132
    postural instability, 190
    visuospatial dysfunction, 23
Striatopallidal pathways, 202f
Striatum
    anatomy, 78, 87, 103f, 153
    dopamine and, 80
    Huntington's disease, 503–506, 504f–506f
Striosomes, 506
Stroke
    and hemiballism, 680
    movement disorders and, 680–681
    and orofacial dyskinesia, 681
    and parkinsonism, 691
Stroke-associated tremor, 396–397, 412
Subacute necrotizing encephalopathy, mitochondrial mutations and, 59

Subacute sclerosing panencephalitis, 551–552
Subcortical dementia, 23
Subcortical lesions, 653–654
Subcortical myoclonus, 544, 552
Substantia nigra
    aluminum and, 170
    anatomy, 77, 266, 266f
    cell death in, 171, 174, 174f
    degeneration, 614, 615f
    dopamine toxicity, 170
    fetal nigral transplantation, 221–232
    Huntington's disease, 508, 508f
    idiopathic Parkinson's disease, 127, 127f
    iron accumulation and, 170, 269
    Lewy bodies, 264, 264f
    Parkinson's disease, 266–267, 268–269
    pars compacta, 80, 87
    pars reticulata, 87–89, 93–94, 99, 153
    superoxide dismutase, 169, 174, 174f
Subthalamic nucleus
    anatomy, 77, 79, 87
    progressive supranuclear palsy and and, 285
Suicide
    Huntington's disease and, 493
    Parkinson's disease and, 17
Sunflower cataract, 626
Superoxide dismutase, 169, 174, 174f
Supplementary motor area, 74, 74f, 76–77
Surgery
    deep brain stimulation, 251–252, 380
    fetal nigral transplantation, 36–37, 221–232
    history, 237–238
    liver transplantation, 631
    pallidotomy, 33, 237, 238, 246, 249–250
    stereotaxic, 237–250
    striatal implants, 290
    thalamotomy, 237, 238, 246, 250, 379–380, 396, 409, 451
Susceptibility genes
    Parkinson's disease, 147–148
    peripheral denervation, 451–452
Sydenham's chorea, 42, 527–528, 665, 736
Symptomatic dystonia. See Dystonia, symptomatic
Symptomatic palatal tremor, 393–394, 394t
Symptomatic palatal tremor, 548, 553
Syphilis, parkinsonism associated with, 311
Systemic illnesses, 733–740
Systemic lupus erythematosus, 42, 528, 738–739

T

Tardive akathisia, 10, 467, 519, 523
Tacrine, 289
Tardive chorea, 7
Tardive dyskinesia, 7, 327, 328, 524
    defined, 519
    difference from choreoathetotic dyskinesia, 10
    in the elderly, 681
    epidemiology, 519–520
    movements of, 10

neuroimaging, 521, 524
    pathophysiology, 520–521
    preventions, 521–522
    symptoms, 519
    treatment, 521t, 522–523
Tardive dystonia, 8, 437
Tardive tics, 566
Tardive tremor, 390, 519
Tau protein
    corticobasal degeneration, 615
    postencephalitic parkinsonism, 309
    progressive supranuclear palsy and, 283
Tay-Sachs disease, 545
Tension tremor, 588
Terminal tremor, 387, 388
Testing. See Biopsy
Tetrabenazine
    dystonia treatment with, 444, 445t
    myoclonus treatment with, 549
    parkinsonism induced by, 328
    tremor induced by, 390
Tetrahydriosoquinolines, 172, 172f
Tetrahydrobiopterin deficiency, 734
Tetranuclear cluster, 164
Tetrathiomolybdate, inhibition of intestinal copper
        absorption with, 629–630
Thalamic degeneration, dementia, 25
Thalamic stimulation, essential tremor, 380
Thalamotomy, 237, 238, 246, 250, 379–380, 396, 409, 451.
        See also Stereotoxic thalamotomy
Thalamus, Huntington's disease, 508–509
Theophylline
    essential tremor treatment with, 379
    tremor induced by, 390
Thioridazine, tremor induced by, 390
Thymoxamine, essential tremor treatment with, 378
Thyroid disorders, movement disorders secondary to, 531,
        733–734
Thyrotoxicosis, hyperthyrodism and, 733
Tics, 9–10, 451, 561, 569
    in childhood, 663, 633t
    chronic motor tics, 522
    classification of, 561, 561t
    clinical signs, 561, 562t
    clonic tics, 9, 561
    complex motor and vocal tics, 9, 569
    differential diagnosis, 6, 541, 564–565, 571–572
    drug-induced, 565–566
    dystonic tics, 9, 565, 571
    etiology of, 565–566, 566t
    features, 9–10
    motor tics, 5, 561, 562t, 571, 663
    neuroleptic-induced tics, 565
    obsessive-compulsive disorder and, 20
    pathophysiology, 562–564
    phantom tics, 561
    primary tic disorder, 565
    psychogenic tics, 726–727
    psychogenic, 726–727
    secondary tic disorder, 569

Tics (*Cont.*)
   sensory tics, 561, 562*t*, 569–570, 581
   tardive tics, 566
   treatment, 566, 573
   vocal tics, 9, 561, 562*t*
Timolol, essential tremor treatment with, 377
Tingling, in Parkinson's disease, 188
Titubation, 579, 589
Tobacco, tremor induced by, 390
Tocopherol, 523, 546, 734–735
Tolcapone, 205
Toluene, tremor induced by, 393
Torsion dystonia, 699, 425*t. See also* Idiopathic torsion
    dystonia
Torticollis, in childhood, 664
Tourette's syndrome (TS), 9, 562, 569, 572, 572*t*
   behavioral changes in, 18, 19
   in childhood, 663
   clinical features, 569–570, 570*t*
   differential diagnosis, 541, 542, 571–572
   epidemiology, 570–571
   etiology, 562
   genetics, 572–573
   neurobiology, 573
   neuroimaging, 31, 562–563
   obsessive-compulsive disorder and, 20, 570
   pathophysiology, 562–564
   progression, 570
   sleep in, 700
   treatment, 451, 573–574, 573*t*, 663
Toxoplasmosis, movement disorders secondary to, 737
Transcranial magnetic stimulation, myoclonus, 557
Transforming growth factor, 117, 118, 120–121
Transient tic disorder, 9
Transplantation. *See* Neural transplantation
Tranylcypromine, Huntington's disease, 497
Trauma
   dystonia and, 459–460, 467
   tremor associated with, 397
Trauma-induced parkinsonism, 346–347
Trazodone
   essential tremor, 378–379
   progressive supranuclear palsy, 289
Tremor, 6, 387, 405, 588–589, 612
   action tremor, 541, 589
   tremor, 388–389, 410, 581
   botulinum toxin treatment, 379, 399, 450–451
   alcoholism, 735
   in CBGD, 189–190
   cerebellar tremor, 388–389, 410, 581
   cortical tremor, 389, 413
   in childhood, 663–664, 664*t*
   defined, 368, 450
   differential diagnosis, 189–190
   drug-induced, 391–393, 413
   dystonia, 450–451
   dystonic tremor, 5, 389, 412–413, 431
   in the elderly, 678
   essential palatal tremor, 548, 533
   essential tremor. *See* Essential tremor

etiology, 387, 389–403, 407
familiar tremor, 588
foods and beverages and, 389–390
intention tremor. *See* Intention tremor
kinetic tremor, 189, 248, 387, 581, 589, 591
midbrain tremor, 391, 392*t*, 410–411
multiple-system atrophy, 299
neuroimaging studies, 36
neurotoxins, 391–393
orthostatic tremor, 6, 393, 393*t*, 412
palatal tremor, 393–394, 394*t*, 511–512, 553
parkinsonian tremor, 409–410
Parkinson's disease, 91–92, 184, 387
   absent or atypical, 183, 189–190
pathophysiology, 242, 244
peripheral neuropathy and, 312, 394–395, 395*t*
PET, 396, 411, 412
physiological tremor, 6, 398–399, 405, 405*f*, 733
pill-rolling tremor, 184, 308, 409
posttraumatic tremor, 397
primary writing tremor, 398–399, 412
primary torsion dystonia, 421–422
psychogenic, 724–725
rubral (midbrain), 410–411
rest tremor. *See* Rest tremor
senile tremor, 6
static tremor, 410, 581, 588
stereotaxic surgery for, 238, 247, 248–250
stroke, 396–397, 412
symptomatic palatal tremor, 393–394, 394*t*, 548, 553
tardive tremor, 390, 519
tension tremor, 588
terminal tremor, 387, 388
uncommon forms, 387–399
Vocal tremor, 397–398, 398*f*
Wilson's disease, 625
Wing-beating tremor, 6, 625
Tricarboxylic acid, alpha-ketoglutarate dehydrogenase
    complex, 167
Tricarboxylic acid cycle, MPP +, 163, 163t, 164, 164*f, 165*
Tricyclic antidepressants, tremor induced by, 390
Trientine, Wilson's disease therapy, 631
Trihexyphenidyl, 105, 444–445
Triplet oxygen, 168
Trophic factor. *See* Neurotrophic factor
Tryptophan, essential tremor treatment with, 378
Tuberohypophysial system, 155
Tumors, parkinsonism induced by, 348
Twin studies, Parkinson's disease, 146–147, 147*t*
Tyrosine hydroxylase (TH, TOH), 153, 232, 267

U

Ubiquinone, Huntington's disease, 498
Ubiquitin, immunohistochemistry, 126, 128
Unified Parkinson's Disease Rating Scale (UPDRS), 192,
    193*t*–197*t*, 494
Unverritch-Lundborg's disease, 546
Upgaze limitation, in Parkinson's disease, 187

Urinary dysfunction
    Parkinson's disease, 188
    multiple-system atrophy, 299–300, 300*t*

V

Valproate, myoclonus treatment with, 549
Valproic acid
    stiff-person syndrome, 646
    tremor induced by, 390–391
Vascular chorea, 530
Vascular parkinsonism, 189, 345–346
Ventral (PMv) premotor areas, 74, 74*f*, 76
Ventral striatum, anatomy, 77
Verapamil, essential tremor treatment with, 379
Vermal syndrome, 601, 601*t*
Vermal zone, 597
Vertical gaze palsy, 187, 675
Vestibular disorders, 650, 651*t*, 652–653
Vestibulocerebellum, 570
Vestibulo-ocular reflex, progressive supranuclear palsy, 286
Vim thalamotomy, 409
Visual disorders, 651*t*, 653
Visual grasping, progressive supranuclear palsy and, 284
Visuospatial function, movement disorders and, 22–23
Vitamin E, 498, 546, 581
Vocal tics, 9, 561, 562*t*
Vocal tremor, 397–398, 398*f*
Voluntary gaze, progressive supranuclear palsy, 285–286, 286*t*
Voluntary movements, supplementary motor area and, 77
Von Economo's encephalitis, 161, 307
Vop thalamotomy, 409

W

Walking, 649–650, 650*t*, 651*t*. *See also* Gait disorder
Whipple's disease, 20, 737–738

Whispering dysphonia, 625
Wilson's disease, 623, 632
    anxiety, 20
    clinical features, 624–627, 626*f*
    dementia, 25
    depression, 17–18
    diagnosis, 627–629
    differential diagnosis, 189, 456*t*
    dysarthria in, 625
    dystonia, 351, 461, 462*f*
    epidemiology, 623
    genetics, 623
    hypersexuality, 21
    neurobehavioral changes in, 19, 625
    neuroimaging, 12*t*
    pathophysiology, 623–624
    treatment, 629–632
"Wing beating" tremor, 6, 625
Wisconsin Card Sort Test (WCST), 15, 21
Writer's cramp, 433, 450

X

Xeroderma pigmentosum, 464
X-linked dystonia-parkinsonism, 336–337

Y

Yohimbine, progressive supranuclear palsy, 289

Z

Zinc, inhibition of intestinal copper absorption with, 629–630

ISBN 0-07-035203-8

9 780070 352032

WATTS MOVE & DISORDER